QUICK LOOK DRUG BOOK

2010

Leonard L. Lance, RPh, BSPharm
Senior Editor
Pharmacist
Lexi-Comp, Inc.
Hudson, Ohio

Charles F. Lacy, RPh, MS, PharmD, FCSHP
Editor
Vice President for Executive Affairs
Professor, Pharmacy Practice
Professor, Business Leadership
University of Southern Nevada
Las Vegas, Nevada

Morton P. Goldman, RPh, PharmD, BCPS, FCCP
Associate Editor
Director of Pharmacotherapy Services
Department of Pharmacy
Cleveland Clinic Foundation
Cleveland, Ohio

Lora L. Armstrong, RPh, PharmD, BCPS
Associate Editor
Vice President, Clinical Affai
Pharmacy & Therapeutics Formul
Clinical Program Oversig
CaremarkRx
Northbrook, Illinois

Wolters Kluwer Health | Lippincott Williams & Wilkins

Philadelphia • Baltimore • New York • London
Buenos Aires • Hong Kong • Sydney • Tokyo

QUICK LOOK DRUG BOOK

2010

Leonard L. Lance, RPh, BSPharm
Senior Editor
Pharmacist
Lexi-Comp, Inc.
Hudson, Ohio

Charles F. Lacy, RPh, MS, PharmD, FCSHP
Editor
Vice President for Executive Affairs
Professor, Pharmacy Practice
Professor, Business Leadership
University of Southern Nevada
Las Vegas, Nevada

Morton P. Goldman, RPh, PharmD, BCPS, FCCP
Associate Editor
Director of Pharmacotherapy Services
Department of Pharmacy
Cleveland Clinic Foundation
Cleveland, Ohio

Lora L. Armstrong, RPh, PharmD, BCPS
Associate Editor
Vice President, Clinical Affairs
Pharmacy & Therapeutics Formulary Process
Clinical Program Oversight
CaremarkRx
Northbrook, Illinois

NOTICE

This data is intended to serve the user as a handy reference and not as a complete drug information resource. It does not include information on every therapeutic agent available. The publication covers over 1700 commonly used drugs and is specifically designed to present important aspects of drug data in a more concise format than is typically found in medical literature or product material supplied by manufacturers.

The nature of drug information is that it is constantly evolving because of ongoing research and clinical experience and is often subject to interpretation. While great care has been taken to ensure the accuracy of the information and recommendations presented, the reader is advised that the authors, editors, reviewers, contributors, and publishers cannot be responsible for the continued currency of the information or for any errors, omissions, or the application of this information, or for any consequences arising therefrom. Therefore, the author(s) and/or the publisher shall have no liability to any person or entity with regard to claims, loss, or damage caused, or alleged to be caused, directly or indirectly, by the use of information contained herein. Because of the dynamic nature of drug information, readers are advised that decisions regarding drug therapy must be based on the independent judgment of the clinician, changing information about a drug (eg, as reflected in the literature and manufacturer's most current product information), and changing medical practices. Therefore, this data is designed to be used in conjunction with other necessary information and is not designed to be solely relied upon by any user. The user of this data hereby and forever releases the authors and publishers of this data from any and all liability of any kind that might arise out of the use of this data. The editors are not responsible for any inaccuracy of quotation or for any false or misleading implication that may arise due to the text or formulas as used or due to the quotation of revisions no longer official.

Certain of the authors, editors, and contributors have written this book in their private capacities. No official support or endorsement by any federal or state agency or pharmaceutical company is intended or inferred.

The publishers have made every effort to trace any third party copyright holders, if any, for borrowed material. If they have inadvertently overlooked any, they will be pleased to make the necessary arrangements at the first opportunity.

This manual was produced using Lexi-Comp's Information Management System™ (LIMS) — a complete publishing service of Lexi-Comp Inc.

LEXI-COMP

1100 Terex Road
Hudson, Ohio 44236
(330) 650-6506

TABLE OF CONTENTS

Visit thePoint http://thepoint.lww.com/QL2010 for exclusive access to:

- Apothecary/Metric Conversions
- Pounds/Kilograms Conversion
- Temperature Conversion
- Pharmaceutical Manufacturers and Distributors
- Multivitamin Products

Refer to the inside front cover of this book for your online access code.

ABOUT THE AUTHORS

Leonard L. Lance, RPh, BSPharm

Leonard L. (Bud) Lance has been directly involved in the pharmaceutical industry since receiving his bachelor's degree in pharmacy from Ohio Northern University in 1970. Upon graduation from ONU, Mr Lance spent four years as a navy pharmacist in various military assignments and was instrumental in the development and operation of the first whole hospital I.V. admixture program in a military (Portsmouth Naval Hospital) facility.

After completing his military service, he entered the retail pharmacy field and has managed both an independent and a home I.V. franchise pharmacy operation. Since the late 1970s, Mr Lance has focused much of his interest on using computers to improve pharmacy service. The independent pharmacy he worked for was one of the first retail pharmacies in the State of Ohio to computerize (1977).

His love for computers and pharmacy led him to Lexi-Comp, Inc. in 1988. He was the first pharmacist at Lexi-Comp and helped develop Lexi-Comp's first drug database in 1989 and was involved in the editing and publishing of Lexi-Comp's first *Drug Information Handbook* in 1990.

As a result of his strong publishing interest, he presently serves in the capacity of pharmacy editor and technical advisor as well as pharmacy (information) database coordinator for Lexi-Comp. Mr Lance provides technical support to Lexi-Comp's reference publications. Mr Lance also assists over 300 major hospitals in producing their own formulary (pharmacy) publications through Lexi-Comp's custom publishing service. Mr Lance is also Manager of the Dosage Forms database in the Medical Sciences Division at Lexi-Comp.

Mr Lance is past president (1984) of the Summit Pharmaceutical Association (SPA). He is a member of the Ohio Pharmacists Association (OPA), the American Pharmaceutical Association (APhA), and the American Society of Health-System Pharmacists (ASHP).

Charles F. Lacy, RPh, MS, PharmD, FCSHP

Dr Lacy is the co-founder and the current Vice President of Executive Affairs at the University of Southern Nevada. In this capacity, Dr Lacy fosters, develops, and maintains new opportunities for the university in the areas of business partnerships, foundational development, external programs development and outreach project design and coordination. Dr Lacy is Professor of Pharmacy Practice in the Nevada College of Pharmacy and Guest Professor in the MBA program and the College of Nursing.

Prior to his promotion to Executive Affairs, Dr Lacy was Vice President for Information Technologies at the University and the Facilitative Officer for Clinical Programs where he managed the clinical curriculum, clinical faculty activities, student experiential programs, pharmacy residency programs, and the college continuing education programs.

Additionally, he spent 20 years at Cedars-Sinai Medical Center, where he was the Department of Pharmacy's Clinical Coordinator. With over 20 years of clinical experience at one of the nation's largest teaching hospitals, he developed a reputation as an acknowledged expert in drug information, pharmacotherapy, and critical care drug interventions.

Dr Lacy received his doctorate from the University of Southern California School of Pharmacy. Presently, Dr Lacy holds teaching affiliations with the Nevada College of Pharmacy, the University of Southern Nevada, Showa University in Tokyo Japan, the University of Alberta at Edmonton School of Pharmacy and Health Sciences, and the Hokkaido College of Pharmacy in Sapporo Japan. He also received his master's degree from Phillips Graduate Institute in Psychology with an emphasis in Marriage and Family Therapy.

Dr Lacy is an active member of numerous professional associations including the American Society of Health-System Pharmacists (ASHP), the American College of Clinical Pharmacy (ACCP), the American Association of Colleges of Pharmacy (AACP), the American Society of Consultant Pharmacists (ASCP), the American Association of Colleges of Pharmacy (AACP), American Pharmaceutical Association (APhA), the Federation of International Pharmacy (FIP), the Japanese Pharmaceutical Association (JPA), the Nevada Pharmacy Alliance (NPA), and the California Society of Hospital Pharmacists (CSHP), through which he has chaired many committees and subcommittees. He is also an active member of the California Association of Marriage and Family Therapists (CAMFT), American Association of Marriage and Family Therapists (AAMFT), the North American Congress of Clinical Toxicology (NACCT) and the European Congress of Clinical Toxicology (ECCT).

Morton P. Goldman, RPh, PharmD, BCPS, FCCP

Dr Goldman received his bachelor's degree in pharmacy from the University of Pittsburgh, College of Pharmacy and his Doctor of Pharmacy degree from the University of Cincinnati, Division of Graduate Studies and Research. He completed his concurrent 2-year hospital pharmacy residency at the VA Medical Center in Cincinnati. Dr Goldman is presently the Director of Pharmacotherapy Services for the Department of Pharmacy at the Cleveland Clinic Foundation (CCF) after having spent over 4 years at CCF as an Infectious Disease pharmacist and 10 years as Clinical Manager/Assistant Director. He holds faculty appointments from The University of Toledo and Ohio Northern University, Colleges of Pharmacy and Case Western Reserve University, College of Medicine and is the Pharmacology Curriculum Director Coordinator for the Cleveland Clinic Lerner College of Medicine. Dr Goldman is a Board-Certified Pharmacotherapy Specialist (BCPS) with added qualifications in infectious diseases.

In his capacity as Director of Pharmacotherapy Services at CCF, Dr Goldman remains actively involved in patient care and clinical research with the Department of Infectious Disease, as well as the continuing education of the medical and pharmacy staff. He is an editor of CCF's *Guidelines for Antibiotic Use* and participates in their annual Antimicrobial Review retreat. He is a member of the Pharmacy and Therapeutics Committee and many of its subcommittees. Dr Goldman has authored numerous journal articles and lectures locally and nationally on infectious diseases topics and current drug therapies. He is currently coauthor of the *Infectious Diseases Handbook* produced by Lexi-Comp, Inc and provides technical support to Lexi-Comp's Clinical Reference Library™ publications.

Dr Goldman is an active member of the Ohio College of Clinical Pharmacy, the Society of Infectious Disease Pharmacists, the American College of Clinical Pharmacy (and is a Fellow of the College), and the American Society of Health-Systems Pharmacists.

Lora L. Armstrong, RPh, PharmD, BCPS

Dr Armstrong received her bachelor's degree in pharmacy from Ferris State University and her Doctor of Pharmacy degree from Midwestern University. Dr Armstrong is a Board-Certified Pharmacotherapy Specialist (BCPS).

In her current position, Dr Armstrong serves as Vice President of Clinical Affairs with responsibility for the National Pharmacy & Therapeutics Committee process, Clinical Program Oversight process, and Pharmaceutical Pipeline Services at CVS Caremark. Prior to joining Caremark, Inc, Dr Armstrong served as the Director of Drug Information Services at the University of Chicago Hospitals. She obtained experience in a variety of clinical settings including critical care, hematology, oncology, infectious diseases, and clinical pharmacokinetics. Dr Armstrong played an active role in the education and training of medical, pharmacy, and nursing staff. She coordinated the Drug Information Center, the medical center's Adverse Drug Reaction Monitoring Program, and the continuing Education Program for pharmacists. She also maintained the hospital's strict formulary program and was the editor of the University of Chicago Hospitals' *Formulary of Accepted Drugs* and the drug information center's monthly newsletter *Topics in Drug Therapy*.

Dr Armstrong is an active member of the Academy of Managed Care Pharmacy (AMCP), the American Society of Health-Systems Pharmacists (ASHP), the American Pharmaceutical Association (APhA), the American College of Clinical Pharmacy (ACCP), and the Pharmacy & Therapeutics Society (P & T Society). Dr Armstrong wrote the chapter entitled "Drugs and Hormones Used in Endocrinology" in the 4th edition of the textbook *Endocrinology*. She is an Adjunct Clinical Instructor of Pharmacy Practice at Midwestern University. Dr Armstrong currently serves on the Drug Information Advisory Board for the American Pharmaceutical Association Scientific Review Panel for Evaluations of Drug Interactions (EDI).

EDITORIAL ADVISORY PANEL

Erin Fabian, PharmD, RPh
Pharmacotherapy Specialist
Lexi-Comp, Inc
Hudson, Ohio

Margaret A. Fitzgerald, MS, APRN, BC, NP-C, FAANP
President
Fitzgerald Health Education Associates, Inc.
North Andover, Massachusetts
Family Nurse Practitioner
Greater Lawrence Family Health Center
Lawrence, Massachusetts

Lawrence A. Frazee, PharmD
Pharmacotherapy Specialist in Internal Medicine
Akron General Medical Center
Akron, Ohio

Matthew A. Fuller, PharmD, BCPS, BCPP, FASHP
Clinical Pharmacy Specialist, Psychiatry
Cleveland Department of Veterans Affairs Medical Center
Brecksville, Ohio
Associate Clinical Professor of Psychiatry
Clinical Instructor of Psychology
Case Western Reserve University
Cleveland, Ohio
Adjunct Associate Professor of Clinical Pharmacy
University of Toledo
Toledo, Ohio

Meredith D. Girard, MD, FACP
Medical Staff
Department of Internal Medicine
Summa Health Systems
Akron, Ohio
Assistant Professor Internal Medicine
Northeast Ohio Universities College of Medicine (NEOUCOM)
Rootstown, Ohio

Morton P. Goldman, RPh, PharmD, BCPS, FCCP
Director of Pharmacotherapy Services
The Cleveland Clinic Foundation
Cleveland, Ohio

Julie A. Golembiewski, PharmD
Clinical Associate Professor
Colleges of Pharmacy and Medicine
Clinical Pharmacist, Anesthesia/Pain
University of Illinois
Chicago, Illinois

Jeffrey P. Gonzales, PharmD, BCPS
Critical Care Clinical Pharmacy Specialist
University of Maryland Medical Center
Baltimore, Maryland

Roland Grad, MDCM, MSc, CCFP, FCFP
Department of Family Medicine
McGill University
Montreal, Quebec, Canada

Larry D. Gray, PhD, ABMM
Director of Clinical Microbiology
TriHealth
Bethesda and Good Samaritan Hospitals
Cincinnati, Ohio

Tracy Hagemann, PharmD
Associate Professor
College of Pharmacy
The University of Oklahoma
Oklahoma City, Oklahoma

Martin D. Higbee, PharmD
Associate Professor
Department of Pharmacy Practice and Science
The University of Arizona
Tucson, Arizona

Jane Hurlburt Hodding, PharmD
Executive Director, Inpatient Pharmacy Services and Clinical Nutrition Services
Long Beach Memorial Medical Center
and Miller Children's Hospital
Long Beach, California

Mark T. Holdsworth, PharmD, BCOP
Associate Professor of Pharmacy & Pediatrics
Pharmacy Practice Area Head
College of Pharmacy
The University of New Mexico
Albuquerque, New Mexico

Collin A. Hovinga, PharmD
Assistant Professor of Pharmacy and Pediatrics
College of Pharmacy
University of Tennessee Health Science Center
Memphis, Tennessee

Darrell T. Hulisz, PharmD
Department of Family Medicine
Case Western Reserve University
Cleveland, Ohio

Michael A. Kahn, DDS
Professor and Chairman
Department of Oral and Maxillofacial Pathology
Tufts University School of Dental Medicine
Boston, Massachusetts

Polly E. Kintzel, PharmD, BCPS, BCOP
Clinical Pharmacy Specialist-Oncology
Spectrum Health
Grand Rapids, Michigan

Daren Knoell, PharmD
Associate Professor of Pharmacy Practice and Internal Medicine
Davis Heart and Lung Research Institute
The Ohio State University
Columbus, Ohio

Sandra Knowles, RPh, BScPhm
Drug Safety Pharmacist
Sunnybrook and Women's College HSC
Toronto, Ontario

Jill M. Kolesar, PharmD, FCCP, BCPS
Associate Professor
School of Pharmacy
Associate Professor
University of Wisconsin Paul P. Carbone
Comprehensive Cancer Center
University of Wisconsin
Madison, Wisconsin

Todd P. Semla, MS, PharmD, BCPS, FCCP, AGSF
Clinical Pharmacy Specialist
Department of Veterans Affairs
Pharmacy Benefits Management Services
Associate Professor, Clinical
Department of Medicine and Psychiatry and Behavioral Health
Feinberg School of Medicine
Northwestern University
Chicago, Illinois

Joe Snoke, RPh, BCPS
Manager
Core Pharmacology Group
Lexi-Comp, Inc
Hudson, Ohio

Dominic A. Solimando, Jr, MA, FAPhA, FASHP, BCOP
Oncology Pharmacist
President, Oncology Pharmacy Services, Inc
Arlington, Virginia

Joni Lombardi Stahura, BS, PharmD, RPh
Pharmacotherapy Specialist
Lexi-Comp, Inc
Hudson, Ohio

Dan Streetman, PharmD, RPh
Pharmacotherapy Specialist
Lexi-Comp, Inc
Hudson, Ohio

Darcie-Ann Streetman, PharmD, RPh
Pharmacotherapy Specialist
Lexi-Comp, Inc
Hudson, Ohio

Carol K. Taketomo, PharmD
Director of Pharmacy and Nutrition Services
Children's Hospital Los Angeles
Los Angeles, California

Mary Temple, PharmD
Pediatric Clinical Research Specialist
Hillcrest Hospital
Mayfield Heights, Ohio

Elizabeth A. Tomsik, PharmD, BCPS
Manager
Adverse Drug Reactions Group
Lexi-Comp, Inc
Hudson, Ohio

Dana Travis, RPh
Pharmacotherapy Specialist
Lexi-Comp, Inc
Hudson, Ohio

Jennifer Trofe, PharmD
Clinical Transplant Pharmacist
Hospital of The University of Pennsylvania
Philadelphia, Pennsylvania

Beatrice B. Turkoski, RN, PhD
Associate Professor, Graduate Faculty, Pharmacology for Advanced Practice Nurses
College of Nursing
Kent State University
Kent, Ohio

Amy Van Orman, PharmD
Pharmacotherapy Specialist
Lexi-Comp, Inc
Hudson, Ohio

Christine Weinstein, BS, RPh
Pharmacotherapy Specialist
Lexi-Comp, Inc
Hudson, Ohio

David M. Weinstein, PhD, RPh
Manager
Metabolism, Interactions, and Genomics Group
Lexi-Comp, Inc
Hudson, Ohio

Anne Marie Whelan, PharmD
College of Pharmacy
Dalhouise University
Halifax, Nova Scotia

Nathan Wirick, PharmD
Infectious Disease and Antibiotic Management Clinical Specialist
Hillcrest Hospital
Cleveland, Ohio

Richard L. Wynn, BSPharm, PhD
Professor of Pharmacology
Baltimore College of Dental Surgery
Dental School
University of Maryland Baltimore
Baltimore, Maryland

PREFACE

Working with clinical pharmacists, hospital pharmacy and therapeutics committees, and hospital drug information centers, the editors of this handbook have directly assisted in the development and production of hospital-specific formulary documentation for several hundred major U.S. and International medical institutions. The resultant documentation provides relevant detail concerning use of medications within the hospital and other clinical settings. Current information on medications has been extracted from pertinent sources, reviewed, coalesced, and cross-referenced by the editors to create this *Quick Look Drug Book*.

Designed to meet the unique needs of medical transcription, this handbook gives the user quick access to data on over 1700 medications with cross-referencing to 6469 U.S. and Canadian brand or trade names. Selection of the included medications was based on the analysis of those medications offered in a wide range of hospital formularies. The concise standardized format for data used in this handbook was developed to ensure a consistent presentation of information for all medications.

All generic drug names and synonyms appear in lower case, whereas brand or trade names appear in upper/lower case with the proper trademark information. These three items appear as individual entries in the alphabetical listing of drugs and, thus, there is no requirement for an alphabetical index of drugs names.

Chemotherapy regimens along with an index are provided in the section directly following the alphabetical listing of drugs. The mailing and web site addresses for pharmaceutical manufacturers and drug distributors can be accessed online using the code located on the inside front cover of this book.

The Indication/Therapeutic Category Index is an expedient mechanism for locating the medication of choice along with its classification. This index will help the user, with knowledge of the disease state, to identify medications which are most commonly used in treatment. All disease states are cross-referenced to a varying number of medications with the most frequently used medication(s) noted.

— L.L. Lance

USE OF THE HANDBOOK

The *Quick Look Drug Book* is organized into a drug information section, an appendix, and an indication/ therapeutic category index.

The drug information section of the handbook, wherein all drugs are listed alphabetically, details information pertinent to each drug. Extensive cross-referencing is provided by brand name and synonyms.

Drug information is presented in a consistent format and for quick reference will provide the following:

Generic Name	U.S. Adopted Name (USAN) or International Nonproprietary Name (INN) If a drug product is only available in Canada, a ***(Canada only)*** will be attached to that product and will appear with every occurrence of that drug throughout the book
Pronunciation Guide	Subjective aid for pronouncing drug names
Sound-Alike/Look-Alike Issues	Lists drugs with similar sounding names or names that look alike
Synonyms	Official names and some slang
Tall-Man	"Tall-Man" lettering revisions recommended by the FDA
U.S./Canadian Brand Names	Common trade names used in the United States and Canada
Therapeutic Category	Lexi-Comp's own system of logical medication classification
Controlled Substance	Drug Enforcement Agency (DEA) classification for federally scheduled controlled substances
Use	Information pertaining to appropriate use of the drug
Usual Dosage	The amount of the drug to be typically given or taken during therapy
Product Availability	Provides availability information on products that have been approved by the FDA, but not yet available for use. Estimates for when a product may be available are included, when this information is known. May also provide any unique or critical drug availability issues (eg, drug shortage of a critical drug).
Dosage Forms	Information with regard to form, strength, and availability of the drug

Appendix

The appendix offers a compilation of tables, guidelines, and conversion information that can often be helpful when considering patient care.

Indication/Therapeutic Category Index

This index provides a listing of accepted drugs for various disease states thus focusing attention on selection of medications most frequently prescribed in relation to a clinical diagnosis. Diseases may have other nonofficial drugs for their treatment and this indication/therapeutic category index should not be used by itself to determine the appropriateness of a particular therapy. The listed indications may encompass varying degrees of severity and, since certain medications may not be appropriate for a given degree of severity, it should not be assumed that the agents listed for specific indications are interchangeable. Also included as a valuable reference is each medication's therapeutic category.

FDA NAME DIFFERENTIATION PROJECT: THE USE OF TALL-MAN LETTERS

Confusion between similar drug names is an important cause of medication errors. For years, The Institute For Safe Medication Practices (ISMP), has urged generic manufacturers to use a combination of large and small letters as well as bolding (ie, chlorpro**MAZINE** and chlorpro**PAMIDE**) to help distinguish drugs with look-alike names, especially when they share similar strengths. Recently the FDA's Division of Generic Drugs began to issue recommendation letters to manufacturers suggesting this novel way to label their products to help reduce this drug name confusion. Although this project has had marginal success, the method has successfully eliminated problems with products such as diphenhydr**AMINE** and dimenhy**DRINATE**. Hospitals should also follow suit by making similar changes in their own labels, preprinted order forms, computer screens and printouts, and drug storage location labels.

In the *Quick Look Drug Book*, the "Tall-Man" lettering revisions for the drugs suggested by the FDA or recommended by ISMP will be listed in a field called **Tall-Man**.

The following is a list of generic product names and recommended revisions.

Drug Product	Recommended Revision
acetazolamide	aceta**ZOLAMIDE**
acetohexamide	aceto**HEXAMIDE**
alprazolam	**ALPRAZ**olam
amiloride	a**MIL**oride
amlodipine	am**LODIP**ine
azacitidine	aza**CITID**ine
azathioprine	aza**THIO**prine
bupropion	bu**PROP**ion
buspirone	bus**PIR**one
carbamazepine	car**BAM**azepine
carboplatin	**CARBO**platin
cefazolin	ce**FAZ**olin
ceftriaxone	cef**TRIAX**one
chlordiazepoxide	chlordiaze**POXIDE**
chlorpromazine	chlorpro**MAZINE**
chlorpropamide	chlorpro**PAMIDE**
cisplatin	**CIS**platin
clomiphene	clomi**PHENE**
clomipramine	clomi**PRAMINE**
clonazepam	clonaze**PAM**
clonidine	clo**NID**ine
cycloserine	cyclo**SERINE**
cyclosporine	cyclo**SPORINE**
dactinomycin	**DACTIN**omycin
daptomycin	**DAPTO**mycin
daunorubicin	**DAUNO**rubicin
dimenhydrinate	dimenhy**DRINATE**
diphenhydramine	diphenhydr**AMINE**
dobutamine	**DOBUT**amine
dopamine	**DOP**amine
doxorubicin	**DOXO**rubicin
duloxetine	**DUL**oxetine
ephedrine	e**PHED**rine
epinephrine	**EPINEPH**rine
fentanyl	fenta**NYL**

Drug Product	Recommended Revision
fluoxetine	**FLU**oxetine
glipizide	glipi**ZIDE**
glyburide	gly**BURIDE**
guaifenesin	guai**FEN**esin
guanfacine	guan**FACINE**
hydralazine	hydr**ALAZINE**
hydrocodone	**HYDRO**codone
hydromorphone	**HYDRO**morphone
hydroxyzine	hydr**OXY**zine
idarubicin	**IDA**rubicin
infliximab	in**FLIX**imab
lamivudine	lami**VUD**ine
lamotrigine	lamo**TRI**gine
lorazepam	**LOR**azepam
medroxyprogesterone	medroxy**PROGESTER**one
metformin	met**FORMIN**
methylprednisolone	methyl**PREDNIS**olone
methyltestosterone	methyl**TESTOSTER**one
metronidazole	metro**NIDAZOLE**
nicardipine	ni**CAR**dipine
nifedipine	**NIFE**dipine
nimodipine	ni**MOD**ipine
olanzapine	**OLANZ**apine
oxcarbazepine	**OX**carbazepine
oxycodone	oxy**CODONE**
paroxetine	**PAR**oxetine
pentobarbital	**PENT**obarbital
phenobarbital	**PHEN**obarbital
prednisolone	predniso**LONE**
prednisone	predni**SONE**
quetiapine	**QUE**tiapine
quinidine	qui**NID**ine
quinine	qui**NINE**
rituximab	ri**TUX**imab
sitagliptin	sita**GLIP**tin
sufentanil	**SUF**entanil
sulfadiazine	sulf**ADIAZINE**
sulfisoxazole	sulfi**SOXAZOLE**
sumatriptan	**SUMA**triptan
tiagabine	tia**GAB**ine
tizanidine	ti**ZAN**idine
tolazamide	**TOLAZ**amide
tolbutamide	**TOLBUT**amide
tramadol	tra**MAD**ol
trazodone	tra**ZOD**one
valacyclovir	val**ACY**clovir
valganciclovir	val**GANCI**clovir

FDA NAME DIFFERENTIATION PROJECT: THE USE OF TALL-MAN LETTERS

Drug Product	Recommended Revision
vinblastine	vin**BLAS**tine
vincristine	vin**CRIS**tine

Institute for Safe Medication Practices. "New Tall-Man Lettering Will Reduce Mix-Ups Due to Generic Drug Name Confusion," *ISMP Medication Safety Alert*, September 19, 2001. Available at: http://www.ismp.org.

Institute for Safe Medication Practices. "Prescription Mapping, Can Improve Efficiency While Minimizing Errors With Look-Alike Products," *ISMP Medication Safety Alert*, October 6, 1999. Available at: http://www.ismp.org.

Institute for Safe Medication Practices. "Use of Tall Man Letters Is Gaining Wide Acceptance," *ISMP Medication Safety Alert*, July 31, 2008. Available at: http://www.ismp.org.

U.S. Pharmacopeia, "USP Quality Review: Use Caution-Avoid Confusion," March 2001, No. 76. Available at: http://www.usp.org.

PREVENTING PRESCRIBING ERRORS

Prescribing errors account for the majority of reported medication errors and have prompted healthcare professionals to focus on the development of steps to make the prescribing process safer. Prescription legibility has been attributed to a portion of these errors and legislation has been enacted in several states to address prescription legibility. However, eliminating handwritten prescriptions and ordering medications through the use of technology [eg, computerized prescriber order entry (CPOE)] has been the primary recommendation. Whether a prescription is electronic, typed, or hand-printed, additional safe practices should be considered for implementation to maximize the safety of the prescribing process. Listed below are suggestions for safer prescribing:

- Ensure correct patient by using at least 2 patient identifiers on the prescription (eg, full name, birth date, or address). Review prescription with the patient or patient's caregiver.
- If pediatric patient, document patient's birth date or age and most recent weight. If geriatric patient, document patient's birth date or age.
- Prevent drug name confusion:
  - Use TALLman lettering (eg, buPROPion, busPIRone, predniSONE, prednisoLONE). For more information see: http://www.fda.gov/Drugs/DrugSafety/MedicationErrors/ucm164587.htm
  - Avoid abbreviated drug names (eg, MSO_4, $MgSO_4$, MS, HCT, 6MP, MTX), as they may be misinterpreted and cause error.
  - Avoid investigational names for drugs with FDA approval (eg, FK-506, CBDCA)
  - Avoid chemical names such as 6-mercaptopurine or 6-thioguanine, as sixfold overdoses have been given when these were not recognized as chemical names. The proper names of these drugs are mercaptopurine or thioguanine.
  - Use care when prescribing drugs that look or sound similar (eg, look- alike, sound-alike drugs). Common examples include: Celebrex® vs Celexa®, hydroxyzine vs hydralazine, Zyprexa® vs Zyrtec®.
- Avoid dangerous, error-prone abbreviations (eg, regardless of letter-case: U, IU, QD, QOD, µg, cc, @). Do not use apothecary system or symbols. Additionally, text messaging abbreviations (eg, "2Day") should never be used.
  - For more information see: http://www.ismp.org/Tools/errorproneabbreviations.pdf
- Always use a leading zero for numbers less than 1 (0.5 mg is correct and .5 mg is **incorrect**) and never use a trailing zero for whole numbers (2 mg is correct and 2.0 mg is **incorrect**)
- Always use a space between a number and its units as it is easier to read. There should be no periods after the abbreviations mg or mL (10 mg is correct and 10mg is **incorrect**)
- For doses that are greater than 1,000 dosing units, use properly placed commas to prevent 10-fold errors (100,000 units is correct and 100000 units is **incorrect**)
- Do not prescribe drug dosage by the type of container in which the drug is available (eg, do not prescribe "1 amp", "2 vials", etc).
- Do not write vague or ambiguous orders which have the potential for misinterpretation by other healthcare providers. Examples of vague orders to avoid: "resume pre-op medications," "give drug per protocol," or "continue home medications."
- Review each prescription with patient (or patient's caregiver) including the medication name, indication, and directions for use.
- Take extra precautions when prescribing *high alert drugs* (drugs that can cause significant patient harm when prescribed in error). Common examples of these drugs include: Anticoagulants, chemotherapy, insulins, opiates, and sedatives.
  - For more information see: http://www.ismp.org/Tools/highalertmedications.pdf

To Err is Human: Building a Safer Health System, Kohn LT, Corrigan JM, and Donaldson MS, eds, Washington, D.C.: National Academy Press, 2000.

A Complete Outpatient Prescription[1]

A complete outpatient prescription can prevent the prescriber, the pharmacist, and/or the patient from making a mistake and can eliminate the need for further clarification. The complete outpatient prescription should contain:

- Patient's full name
- Medication indication
- Allergies
- Prescriber name and telephone or pager number
- For pediatric patients: Their birth date or age and current weight
- For geriatric patients: Their birth date or age
- Drug name, dosage form and strength
- For pediatric patients: Intended daily weight-based dose so that calculations can be checked by the pharmacist (ie, mg/kg/day or units/kg/day)
- Number or amount to be dispensed
- Complete instructions for the patient or caregiver, including the purpose of the medication, directions for use (including dose), dosing frequency, route of administration, duration of therapy, and number of refills.
- Dose should be expressed in convenient units of measure.
- When there are recognized contraindications for a prescribed drug, the prescriber should indicate knowledge of this fact to the pharmacist (ie, when prescribing a potassium salt for a patient receiving an ACE inhibitor, the prescriber should write "K serum leveling being monitored").

Upon dispensing of the final product, the pharmacist should ensure that the patient or caregiver can effectively demonstrate the appropriate administration technique. An appropriate measuring device should be provided or recommended. Household teaspoons and tablespoons should not be used to measure liquid medications due to their variability and inaccuracies in measurement; oral medication syringes are recommended.

For additional information see: http://www.ppag.org/attachments/files/111/Guidelines_Peds.pdf

[1]Levine SR, Cohen MR, Blanchard NR, et al, "Guidelines for Preventing Medication Errors in Pediatrics," *J Pediatr Pharmacol Ther*, 2001, 6:426-42.

ALPHABETICAL LISTING OF DRUGS

A_1-PI *see* alpha$_1$-proteinase inhibitor *on page 50*
α_1-PI *see* alpha$_1$-proteinase inhibitor *on page 50*
A200® Lice [US-OTC] *see* permethrin *on page 769*
A-200® Lice Treatment Kit [US-OTC] *see* pyrethrins and piperonyl butoxide *on page 839*
A-200® Maximum Strength [US-OTC] *see* pyrethrins and piperonyl butoxide *on page 839*
A and D® Original [US-OTC] *see* vitamin A and vitamin D *on page 1017*

abacavir (a BAK a veer)

Synonyms abacavir sulfate; ABC
U.S./Canadian Brand Names Ziagen® [US/Can]
Therapeutic Category Antiretroviral Agent, Nucleoside Reverse Transcriptase Inhibitor (NRTI)
Use Treatment of HIV infections in combination with other antiretroviral agents
Usual Dosage Oral:
Children: 3 months to 16 years: 8 mg/kg body weight twice daily (maximum: 300 mg twice daily) in combination with other antiretroviral agents
Adults: 300 mg twice daily or 600 mg once daily in combination with other antiretroviral agents
Dosage Forms
Solution, oral:
Ziagen®: 20 mg/mL
Tablet:
Ziagen®: 300 mg

abacavir and lamivudine (a BAK a veer & la MI vyoo deen)

Synonyms abacavir sulfate and lamivudine; lamivudine and abacavir
U.S./Canadian Brand Names Epzicom® [US]; Kivexa™ [Can]
Therapeutic Category Antiretroviral Agent, Nucleoside Reverse Transcriptase Inhibitor (NRTI)
Use Treatment of HIV infections in combination with other antiretroviral agents
Usual Dosage Oral: Adults: HIV: One tablet (abacavir 600 mg and lamivudine 300 mg) once daily
Dosage Forms
Tablet:
Epzicom®: Abacavir 600 mg and lamivudine 300 mg

abacavir, lamivudine, and zidovudine
(a BAK a veer, la MI vyoo deen, & zye DOE vyoo deen)

Synonyms 3TC, abacavir, and zidovudine; azidothymidine, abacavir, and lamivudine; AZT, abacavir, and lamivudine; compound S, abacavir, and lamivudine; lamivudine, abacavir, and zidovudine; ZDV, abacavir, and lamivudine; zidovudine, abacavir, and lamivudine
U.S./Canadian Brand Names Trizivir® [US/Can]
Therapeutic Category Antiretroviral Agent, Nucleoside Reverse Transcriptase Inhibitor (NRTI)
Use Treatment of HIV infection (either alone or in combination with other antiretroviral agents) in patients whose regimen would otherwise contain the components of Trizivir®
Usual Dosage Oral: Adolescents ≥40 kg and Adults: 1 tablet twice daily
Dosage Forms
Tablet:
Trizivir®: Abacavir 300 mg, lamivudine 150 mg, and zidovudine 300 mg

abacavir sulfate *see* abacavir *on page 16*
abacavir sulfate and lamivudine *see* abacavir and lamivudine *on page 16*
abarelix *(Discontinued)*

abatacept (ab a TA sept)

Sound-Alike/Look-Alike Issues
Orencia® may be confused with Oracea™
Synonyms CTLA-4Ig
U.S./Canadian Brand Names Orencia® [US/Can]
Therapeutic Category Antirheumatic, Disease Modifying

Use

Treatment of moderately- to severely-active adult rheumatoid arthritis (RA); may be used as monotherapy or in combination with other DMARDs

Treatment of moderately- to severely-active juvenile idiopathic arthritis (JIA); may be used as monotherapy or in combination with methotrexate

Note: Abatacept should **not** be used in combination with anakinra or TNF-blocking agents

Usual Dosage I.V.:

Children 6-17 years: JIA:

<75 kg: 10 mg/kg, repeat dose at 2 and 4 weeks after initial infusion, and every 4 weeks thereafter

≥75 kg: Refer to adult dosing; maximum dose: 1000 mg

Adults: RA: Dosing is according to body weight: Repeat dose at 2 weeks and 4 weeks after initial dose, and every 4 weeks thereafter:

<60 kg: 500 mg

60-100 kg: 750 mg

>100 kg: 1000 mg

Dosage Forms

Injection, powder for reconstitution [preservative free]:

Orencia®: 250 mg

Abbokinase® *(Discontinued)* *see* urokinase *on page 999*

abbott-43818 *see* leuprolide *on page 575*

ABC *see* abacavir *on page 16*

ABCD *see* amphotericin B cholesteryl sulfate complex *on page 73*

abciximab (ab SIK si mab)

Synonyms 7E3; C7E3

U.S./Canadian Brand Names ReoPro® [US/Can]

Therapeutic Category Platelet Aggregation Inhibitor

Use Prevention of cardiac ischemic complications in patients undergoing percutaneous coronary intervention (PCI); prevention of cardiac ischemic complications in patients with unstable angina not responding to conventional therapy when PCI is scheduled within 24 hours

Note: Intended for use with aspirin and heparin, at a minimum.

Usual Dosage

Percutaneous coronary intervention (PCI): I.V.: 0.25 mg/kg bolus administered 10-60 minutes prior to start of PCI followed by an infusion of 0.125 mcg/kg/minute (maximum: 10 mcg/minute) for 12 hours

Patients with unstable angina not responding to conventional medical therapy with planned PCI within 24 hours: 0.25 mg/kg bolus followed by an 18- to 24-hour infusion of 10 mcg/minute, concluding 1 hour after PCI.

Dosage Forms

Injection, solution:

ReoPro®: 2 mg/mL (5 mL)

Abelcet® [US/Can] *see* amphotericin B lipid complex *on page 74*

Abenol® [Can] *see* acetaminophen *on page 19*

ABI-007 *see* paclitaxel (protein bound) *on page 743*

Abilify® [US] *see* aripiprazole *on page 97*

Abilify Discmelt® [US] *see* aripiprazole *on page 97*

ABLC *see* amphotericin B lipid complex *on page 74*

abobotulinumtoxinA (aye bo BOT yoo lin num TOKS in aye)

Synonyms botulinum toxin type A

U.S./Canadian Brand Names Dysport™ [US]

Therapeutic Category Neuromuscular Blocker Agent, Toxin

Use Treatment of cervical dystonia to reduce the severity of abnormal head position and neck pain in both toxin-naive and previously treated patients; temporary improvement in the appearance of moderate-to-severe glabellar lines associated with procerus and corrugator muscle activity in adults <65 years of age

Product Availability Dysport™: FDA approved April 2009; availability anticipated in late 2009

A/B Otic [US] *see* antipyrine and benzocaine *on page 85*

Abraxane® [US] *see* paclitaxel (protein bound) *on page 743*

Abraxane® For Injectable Suspension [Can] *see* paclitaxel *on page 742*
Abreva® [US-OTC] *see* docosanol *on page 326*
absorbable cotton *see* cellulose, oxidized regenerated *on page 201*
absorbable gelatin sponge *see* gelatin (absorbable) *on page 457*
Absorbine® Antifungal *(Discontinued)* *see* tolnaftate *on page 968*
Absorbine® Jock Itch *(Discontinued)* *see* tolnaftate *on page 968*
ABT-335 *see* fenofibric acid *on page 409*
ABX-EGF *see* panitumumab *on page 748*
AC 2993 *see* exenatide *on page 401*
ACAM2000™ [US] *see* smallpox vaccine *on page 906*

acamprosate (a kam PROE sate)

Synonyms acamprosate calcium; calcium acetylhomotaurinate

U.S./Canadian Brand Names Campral® [US/Can]

Therapeutic Category GABA Agonist/Glutamate Antagonist

Use Maintenance of alcohol abstinence

Usual Dosage Oral: Adults: Alcohol abstinence: 666 mg 3 times/day (a lower dose may be effective in some patients)

Dosage Forms

Tablet, enteric coated, delayed release:
Campral®: 333 mg

acamprosate calcium *see* acamprosate *on page 18*
Acanya™ [US] *see* clindamycin and benzoyl peroxide *on page 240*

acarbose (AY car bose)

Sound-Alike/Look-Alike Issues
Precose® may be confused with PreCare®

U.S./Canadian Brand Names Glucobay™ [Can]; Precose® [US]

Therapeutic Category Antidiabetic Agent, Oral

Use Adjunct to diet and exercise to lower blood glucose in patients with type 2 diabetes mellitus (noninsulin-dependent, NIDDM)

Usual Dosage Oral:

Adults: Dosage must be individualized on the basis of effectiveness and tolerance while not exceeding the maximum recommended dose

Initial dose: 25 mg 3 times/day with the first bite of each main meal; to reduce GI effects, some patients may benefit from initiating at 25 mg once daily with gradual titration to 25 mg 3 times/day as tolerated

Maintenance dose: Should be adjusted at 4- to 8-week intervals based on 1-hour postprandial glucose levels and tolerance until maintenance dose is reached. Dosage may be increased from 25 mg 3 times/day to 50 mg 3 times/day. Some patients may benefit from increasing the dose to 100 mg 3 times/day.

Maintenance dose ranges: 50-100 mg 3 times/day.

Maximum dose:
≤60 kg: 50 mg 3 times/day
>60 kg: 100 mg 3 times/day

Patients receiving sulfonylureas or insulin: Acarbose given in combination with a sulfonylurea or insulin will cause a further lowering of blood glucose and may increase the hypoglycemic potential of the sulfonylurea or insulin. If hypoglycemia occurs, appropriate adjustments in the dosage of these agents should be made.

Dosage Forms

Tablet: 25 mg, 50 mg, 100 mg
Precose®: 25 mg, 50 mg, 100 mg

A-Caro-25 [US] *see* beta-carotene *on page 136*
Accolate® [US/Can] *see* zafirlukast *on page 1026*
AccuHist® Pediatric *(Discontinued)* *see* brompheniramine and pseudoephedrine *on page 150*
AccuNeb® [US] *see* albuterol *on page 41*
Accupril® [US/Can] *see* quinapril *on page 844*
Accuretic® [US/Can] *see* quinapril and hydrochlorothiazide *on page 845*

Accutane® [Can] *see* isotretinoin *on page 551*
Accutane® ***(Discontinued)*** *see* isotretinoin *on page 551*
Accuzyme® ***(Discontinued)*** *see* papain and urea *on page 749*
Accuzyme® SE ***(Discontinued)*** *see* papain and urea *on page 749*
ACE *see* captopril *on page 178*

acebutolol (a se BYOO toe lole)

Sound-Alike/Look-Alike Issues
Sectral® may be confused with Factrel®, Seconal®, Septra®
Synonyms acebutolol hydrochloride
U.S./Canadian Brand Names Apo-Acebutolol® [Can]; Gen-Acebutolol [Can]; Monitan® [Can]; Novo-Acebutolol [Can]; Nu-Acebutolol [Can]; Rhotral [Can]; Rhoxal-acebutolol [Can]; Sandoz-Acebutolol [Can]; Sectral® [US/Can]
Therapeutic Category Antiarrhythmic Agent, Class II; Beta-Adrenergic Blocker
Use Treatment of hypertension; management of ventricular arrhythmias
Usual Dosage Oral: Adults:
Hypertension: 400-800 mg/day (larger doses may be divided); maximum: 1200 mg/day; usual dose range (JNC 7): 200-800 mg/day in 2 divided doses
Ventricular arrhythmias: Initial: 400 mg/day in divided doses; maintenance: 600-1200 mg/day in divided doses; maximum: 1200 mg/day
Dosage Forms
Capsule, as hydrochloride: 200 mg, 400 mg
Sectral®: 200 mg, 400 mg

acebutolol hydrochloride *see* acebutolol *on page 19*
Aceon® [US] *see* perindopril erbumine *on page 768*
Acephen™ [US-OTC] *see* acetaminophen *on page 19*
Acerola [US-OTC] *see* ascorbic acid *on page 100*
Acetadote® [US] *see* acetylcysteine *on page 31*
Aceta-Gesic [US-OTC] *see* acetaminophen and phenyltoloxamine *on page 23*

acetaminophen (a seet a MIN oh fen)

Sound-Alike/Look-Alike Issues
Acephen® may be confused with AcipHex®
FeverAll® may be confused with Fiberall®
Tylenol® may be confused with atenolol, timolol, Tuinal®, Tylox®
Synonyms APAP; n-acetyl-p-aminophenol; paracetamol
U.S./Canadian Brand Names Abenol® [Can]; Acephen™ [US-OTC]; APAP 500 [US-OTC]; Apo-Acetaminophen® [Can]; Aspirin Free Anacin® Extra Strength [US-OTC]; Atasol® [Can]; Cetafen® Extra [US-OTC]; Cetafen® [US-OTC]; Excedrin® Tension Headache [US-OTC]; FeverAll® [US-OTC]; Genapap™ Children [US-OTC]; Genapap™ Extra Strength [US-OTC]; Genebs Extra Strength [US-OTC]; Infantaire [US-OTC]; Little Fevers™ [US-OTC]; Mapap Children's [US-OTC]; Mapap Extra Strength [US-OTC]; Mapap Infants [US-OTC]; Mapap Jr. Strength [US-OTC]; Mapap [US-OTC]; Nortemp Children's [US-OTC]; Novo-Gesic [Can]; Pain Eze [US-OTC]; Pediatrix [Can]; Silapap Children's [US-OTC]; Silapap Infants [US-OTC]; Tempra® [Can]; Tycolene Maximum Strength [US-OTC]; Tylenol® Jr. Meltaways [US-OTC]; Tylenol® 8 Hour [US-OTC]; Tylenol® Arthritis Pain Extended Relief [US-OTC]; Tylenol® Children's Meltaways [US-OTC]; Tylenol® Children's with Flavor Creator [US-OTC]; Tylenol® Children's [US-OTC]; Tylenol® Extra Strength [US-OTC]; Tylenol® Infants Concentrated [US-OTC]; Tylenol® [US-OTC/Can]; Valorin Extra [US-OTC]; Valorin [US-OTC]
Therapeutic Category Analgesic, Nonnarcotic; Antipyretic
Use Treatment of mild-to-moderate pain and fever (antipyretic/analgesic); does not have antirheumatic or antiinflammatory effects
Usual Dosage Oral, rectal:
Children <12 years: 10-15 mg/kg/dose every 4-6 hours as needed; do **not** exceed 5 doses (2.6 g) in 24 hours; alternatively, the following age-based doses may be used:
0-3 months: 40 mg
4-11 months: 80 mg
1-2 years: 120 mg
2-3 years: 160 mg

4-5 years: 240 mg
6-8 years: 320 mg
9-10 years: 400 mg
11 years: 480 mg
Note: Higher rectal doses have been studied for use in preoperative pain control in children. However, specific guidelines are not available and dosing may be product dependent. The safety and efficacy of alternating acetaminophen and ibuprofen dosing has not been established.

Adults: 325-650 mg every 4-6 hours or 1000 mg 3-4 times/day; do **not** exceed 4 g/day

Dosage Forms

Caplet, oral: 500 mg
Cetafen® Extra [OTC], Genebs Extra Strength [OTC], Mapap Extra Strength [OTC], Tylenol® Extra Strength [OTC]: 500 mg
Pain Eze [OTC]: 650 mg
Tylenol® [OTC]: 325 mg

Caplet, extended release, oral:
Tylenol® 8 Hour [OTC], Tylenol® Arthritis Pain Extended Relief [OTC]: 650 mg

Captab, oral: 500 mg

Elixir, oral:
Mapap Children's [OTC]: 160 mg/5 mL (118 mL, 480 mL)

Gelcap, oral:
Tylenol® Extra Strength [OTC]: 500 mg

Geltab, oral:
Excedrin® Tension Headache [OTC], Tylenol® Extra Strength [OTC]: 500 mg

Liquid, oral:
APAP 500 [OTC]: 500 mg/5 mL
Silapap Children's [OTC]: 160 mg/5 mL
Tylenol® Extra Strength [OTC]: 500 mg/15 mL

Solution, oral: 160 mg/5 mL

Solution, oral [drops]: 80 mg/0.8 mL
Infantaire [OTC], Silapap Infant's [OTC]: 80 mg/0.8mL
Little Fevers™ [OTC]: 80 mg/1 mL

Suppository, rectal: 120 mg (12s, 50s, 100s); 325 mg (12s); 650 mg (12s, 50s, 100s)
Acephen™ [OTC]: 120 mg (12s, 50s, 100s); 325 mg (6s, 12s, 50s, 100s); 650 mg (12s, 50s, 100s, 500s)
FeverALL® [OTC]: 120 mg (6s, 12s, 50s); 325 mg (6s, 12s, 50s); 650 mg (12s, 50s, 500s); 80 mg (6s, 50s)
Mapap [OTC]: 125 mg (12s)

Suspension, oral: 160 mg/5 mL
Mapap Children's [OTC], Nortemp Children's [OTC], Tylenol® Children's Suspension [OTC]: 160 mg/5 mL

Suspension, oral [drops]:
Mapap Infant's [OTC], Tylenol® Infant's Concentrated [OTC]: 80 mg/0.8 mL

Tablet, oral: 325 mg, 500 mg
Aspirin Free Anacin® Extra Strength [OTC], Genapap™ Extra Strength [OTC], Genebs Extra Strength [OTC], Valorin Extra® [OTC]: 500 mg
Cetafen® [OTC], Mapap [OTC], Tylenol® [OTC], Valorin® [OTC]: 325 mg

Tablet, chewable, oral: 80 mg
Mapap Children's [OTC]: 80 mg
Mapap Junior Strength [OTC]: 160 mg

Tablet, orally disintegrating, oral: 80 mg, 160 mg, 325 mg, 500 mg
Tylenol® Children's Meltaways [OTC]: 80 mg
Tylenol® Jr. Meltaways [OTC]: 160 mg

acetaminophen and butalbital *see* butalbital and acetaminophen *on page* 162
acetaminophen and chlorpheniramine *see* chlorpheniramine and acetaminophen *on page* 214

acetaminophen and codeine (a seet a MIN oh fen & KOE deen)

Sound-Alike/Look-Alike Issues
Capital® may be confused with Capitrol®
Tylenol® may be confused with atenolol, timolol, Tuinal®, Tylox®

T3 is an error-prone abbreviation (mistaken as liothyronine)

Synonyms codeine and acetaminophen

U.S./Canadian Brand Names Capital® and Codeine [US]; ratio-Emtec [Can]; ratio-Lenoltec [Can]; Triatec-30 [Can]; Triatec-8 Strong [Can]; Triatec-8 [Can]; Tylenol® Elixir with Codeine [Can]; Tylenol® No. 1 Forte [Can]; Tylenol® No. 1 [Can]; Tylenol® No. 2 with Codeine [Can]; Tylenol® No. 3 with Codeine [Can]; Tylenol® No. 4 with Codeine [Can]; Tylenol® with Codeine No. 3 [US]; Tylenol® with Codeine No. 4 [US]

Therapeutic Category Analgesic, Narcotic

Controlled Substance C-III; C-V

Use Relief of mild-to-moderate pain

Usual Dosage Doses should be adjusted according to severity of pain and response of the patient. Adult doses ≥60 mg codeine fail to give commensurate relief of pain but merely prolong analgesia and are associated with an appreciably increased incidence of side effects. Oral:

Children: Analgesic:

Codeine: 0.5-1 mg codeine/kg/dose every 4-6 hours

Acetaminophen: 10-15 mg/kg/dose every 4 hours up to a maximum of 2.6 g/24 hours for children <12 years; **alternatively, the following can be used:**

3-6 years: 5 mL 3-4 times/day as needed of elixir

7-12 years: 10 mL 3-4 times/day as needed of elixir

>12 years: 15 mL every 4 hours as needed of elixir

Adults:

Antitussive: Based on codeine (15-30 mg/dose) every 4-6 hours (maximum: 360 mg/24 hours based on codeine component)

Analgesic: Based on codeine (30-60 mg/dose) every 4-6 hours (maximum: 4000 mg/24 hours based on acetaminophen component)

1-2 tablets every 4 hours to a maximum of 12 tablets/24 hours

Dosage Forms [CAN] = Canadian brand name

Caplet:

ratio-Lenoltec No. 1 [CAN], Tylenol No. 1 [CAN]: Acetaminophen 300 mg, codeine 8 mg, and caffeine 15 mg [not available in the U.S.]

Tylenol No. 1 Forte [CAN]: Acetaminophen 500 mg, codeine 8 mg, and caffeine 15 mg [not available in the U.S.]

Solution, oral [C-V]: Acetaminophen 120 mg and codeine 12 mg per 5 mL

Tylenol Elixir with Codeine [CAN]: Acetaminophen 160 mg and codeine 8 mg per 5 mL [not available in the U.S.]

Suspension, oral [C-V]: Acetaminophen 120 mg and codeine 12 mg per 5 mL

Capital® and Codeine [C-V]: Acetaminophen 120 mg and codeine 12 mg per 5 mL

Tablet [C-III]: Acetaminophen 300 mg and codeine 15 mg; acetaminophen 300 mg and codeine 30 mg; acetaminophen 300 mg and codeine 60 mg

ratio-Emtec [CAN], Triatec-30 [CAN]: Acetaminophen 300 mg and codeine 30 mg [not available in the U.S.]

ratio-Lenoltec No. 1 [CAN]: Acetaminophen 300 mg, codeine 8 mg, and caffeine 15 mg [not available in the U.S.]

ratio-Lenoltec No. 2 [CAN], Tylenol No. 2 with Codeine [CAN]: Acetaminophen 300 mg, codeine 15 mg, and caffeine 15 mg [not available in the U.S.]

ratio-Lenoltec No. 3 [CAN], Tylenol No. 3 with Codeine [CAN]: Acetaminophen 300 mg, codeine 30 mg, and caffeine 15 mg [not available in the U.S.]

ratio-Lenoltec No. 4 [CAN], Tylenol No. 4 with Codeine [CAN]: Acetaminophen 300 mg and codeine 60 mg [not available in the U.S.]

Triatec-8 [CAN]: Acetaminophen 325 mg, codeine 8 mg, and caffeine 30 mg [not available in the U.S.]

Triatec-8 Strong [CAN]: Acetaminophen 500 mg, codeine 8 mg, and caffeine 30 mg [not available in the U.S.]

Tylenol® with Codeine No. 3: Acetaminophen 300 mg and codeine 30 mg

Tylenol® with Codeine No. 4: Acetaminophen 300 mg and codeine 60 mg

acetaminophen and diphenhydramine (a seet a MIN oh fen & dye fen HYE dra meen)

Sound-Alike/Look-Alike Issues

Excedrin® may be confused with Dexatrim®, Dexedrine®

Percogesic® may be confused with paregoric, Percodan®

Tylenol® may be confused with atenolol, timolol, Tuinal®, Tylox®

Synonyms diphenhydramine and acetaminophen

U.S./Canadian Brand Names Excedrin PM® [US-OTC]; Goody's PM® [US-OTC]; Legatrin PM® [US-OTC]; Mapap PM [US-OTC]; Percogesic® Extra Strength [US-OTC]; Tylenol® PM [US-OTC]; Tylenol® Severe Allergy [US-OTC]

Therapeutic Category Analgesic, Nonnarcotic

Use Aid in the relief of insomnia accompanied by minor pain

Usual Dosage Oral: Adults: 50 mg of diphenhydramine HCl (76 mg diphenhydramine citrate) at bedtime or as directed by physician; do not exceed recommended dosage; not for use in children <12 years of age

Dosage Forms

Caplet, oral: Acetaminophen 500 mg and diphenhydramine 25 mg
Excedrin PM® [OTC]: Acetaminophen 500 mg and diphenhydramine 38 mg
Legatrin PM® [OTC]: Acetaminophen 500 mg and diphenhydramine 50 mg
Mapap PM [OTC], Tylenol® PM [OTC]: Acetaminophen 500 mg and diphenhydramine 25 mg
Percogesic® Extra Strength [OTC]: Acetaminophen 500 mg and diphenhydramine 12.5 mg
Tylenol® Severe Allergy [OTC]: Acetaminophen 500 mg and diphenhydramine 12.5 mg

Gelcap, rapid release, oral:
Tylenol® PM [OTC]: Acetaminophen 500 mg and diphenhydramine 25 mg

Geltab, oral: Acetaminophen 500 mg and diphenhydramine 25 mg
Excedrin® PM [OTC]: Acetaminophen 500 mg and diphenhydramine 38 mg
Tylenol® PM [OTC]: Acetaminophen 500 mg and diphenhydramine 25 mg

Liquid, oral:
Tylenol® PM [OTC]: Acetaminophen 500 mg and diphenhydramine 25 mg per 15 mL

Powder for solution, oral:
Goody's PM® [OTC]: Acetaminophen 500 mg and diphenhydramine 38 mg

Tablet, oral: Acetaminophen 500 mg and diphenhydramine 25 mg
Excedrin® PM [OTC]: Acetaminophen 500 mg and diphenhydramine 38 mg

acetaminophen and hydrocodone *see* hydrocodone and acetaminophen *on page 501*

acetaminophen and oxycodone *see* oxycodone and acetaminophen *on page 738*

acetaminophen and pamabrom (a seet a MIN oh fen & PAM a brom)

Synonyms pamabrom and acetaminophen

U.S./Canadian Brand Names Cramp Tabs [US-OTC]; Midol® Teen Formula [US-OTC]; Tylenol® Women's Menstrual Relief [US-OTC]

Therapeutic Category Analgesic, Miscellaneous; Diuretic, Combination

Use Temporary relief of symptoms associated with premenstrual and menstrual symptoms (eg, cramps, bloating, water-weight gain, headache, backache, muscle aches)

Usual Dosage Oral: Children ≥12 years and Adults: Acetaminophen 650-1000 mg and pamabrom 50 mg every 4-6 hours as needed (maximum: 8 caplets/tablets/24 hours)

Dosage Forms

Caplet:
Midol® Teen Formula: Acetaminophen 500 mg and pamabrom 25 mg
Tylenol® Women's Menstrual Relief: Acetaminophen 500 mg and pamabrom 25 mg

Tablet:
Cramp Tabs: Acetaminophen 325 mg and pamabrom 25 mg

acetaminophen and pentazocine *see* pentazocine and acetaminophen *on page 765*

acetaminophen and phenylephrine (a seet a MIN oh fen & fen il EF rin)

Synonyms phenylephrine hydrochloride and acetaminophen

U.S./Canadian Brand Names Alka-Seltzer Plus® Sinus Formula [US-OTC]; Cetafen Cold® [US-OTC]; Contac® Cold + Flu Maximum Strength Non-Drowsy [US-OTC]; Excedrin® Sinus Headache [US-OTC]; Mapap® Sinus Congestion and Pain Daytime [US-OTC]; Sinus Pain & Pressure [US-OTC]; Sinutab® Sinus [US-OTC]; Sudafed PE® Sinus Headache [US-OTC]; Tylenol® Sinus Congestion & Pain Daytime [US-OTC]; Vicks® DayQuil® Sinus [US-OTC]

Therapeutic Category Analgesic, Miscellaneous; Decongestant

Use Temporary relief of sinus/nasal congestion and pressure, headache, and minor aches and pains

Usual Dosage Oral: Children ≥12 years and Adults: General dosing guidelines, refer to specific product labeling: Sinus pain/pressure: Acetaminophen 325 mg and phenylephrine 5 mg/caplet: Take 2 caplets every 4 hours as needed; maximum: 12 caplets/24 hours

Dosage Forms

Caplet, oral:

Contac® Cold + Flu Maximum Strength Non Drowsy [OTC]: Acetaminophen 500 mg and phenylephrine 5 mg

Excedrin® Sinus Headache [OTC], Mapap® Sinus Congestion and Pain Daytime [OTC], Sinutab® Sinus [OTC], Sudafed PE® Sinus Headache [OTC]: Acetaminophen 325 mg and phenylephrine 5 mg

Tylenol® Sinus Congestion & Pain Daytime [OTC]: Acetaminophen 325 mg and phenylephrine 5 mg [Cool Burst™ flavor]

Capsule, liquicap, oral:

Vicks® DayQuil® Sinus [OTC]: Acetaminophen 325 mg and phenylephrine 5 mg

Gelcap, oral:

Tylenol® Sinus Congestion & Pain Daytime [OTC]: Acetaminophen 325 mg and phenylephrine 5 mg

Gelcap, rapid release, oral:

Tylenol® Sinus Congestion & Pain Daytime [OTC]: Acetaminophen 325 mg and phenylephrine 5 mg

Tablet for solution, oral [effervescent]:

Alka-Seltzer Plus® Sinus Formula [OTC]: Acetaminophen 250 mg and phenylephrine 5 mg

Tablet, oral:

Cetafen Cold® [OTC], Sinus Pain & Pressure [OTC]: Acetaminophen 500 mg and phenylephrine 5 mg

acetaminophen and phenyltoloxamine (a seet a MIN oh fen & fen il to LOKS a meen)

Sound-Alike/Look-Alike Issues

Percogesic® may be confused with paregoric, Percodan®

Synonyms phenyltoloxamine citrate and acetaminophen

U.S./Canadian Brand Names Aceta-Gesic [US-OTC]; Alpain [US]; BeFlex [US]; Dologesic® [US]; Flextra-650 [US]; Flextra-DS [US]; Genesec™ [US-OTC]; Lagesic™ [US]; Percogesic® [US-OTC]; Phenagesic [US-OTC]; Phenylgesic [US-OTC]; RhinoFlex™ [US]; RhinoFlex™-650 [US]; Staflex [US]; Zgesic [US]

Therapeutic Category Analgesic, Nonnarcotic

Use Relief of mild-to-moderate pain

Usual Dosage Oral:

Analgesic: Based on acetaminophen component:

Children: 10-15 mg/kg/dose every 4-6 hours as needed (maximum: 5 doses/24 hours)

Adults: 325-650 mg every 4-6 hours as needed (maximum: 4 g/day)

Product-specific labeling:

Dologesic®:

Children <12 years: 1 caplet/capsule **or** 5 mL every 4 hours

Children ≥12 years and Adults: 1-2 caplets/capsules **or** 15-30 mL every 4 hours (maximum: 8 caplets/24 hours **or** 120 mL/24 hours)

Flextra 650:

Children 6 to <12 years: 1/2 tablet every 6 hours (maximum: 2 tablets/day)

Children ≥12 years and Adults: 1/2-1 tablet every 6 hours (maximum: 4 tablets/day)

Flextra-DS, RhinoFlex™, RhinoFlex 650:

Children 6 to <12 years: 1/2 tablet every 4 hours (maximum: 2.5 tablets/day)

Children ≥12 years and Adults: 1/2-1 tablet every 4 hours (maximum: 5 tablets/day)

Lagesic™:

Children 6-12 years: 1/2 caplet every 12 hours (maximum: 2 caplets/24 hours)

Children ≥12 years and Adults: 1-2 caplets every 8-12 hours (maximum: 6 caplets/24 hours)

Percogesic®:

Children 6-12 years: 1 tablet every 4 hours (maximum: 4 tablets/24 hours)

Adults: 1-2 tablets every 4 hours (maximum: 8 tablets/24 hours)

Zgesic: Children >12 years and Adults: 1-2 tablets every 8-12 hours (maximum: 6 tablets/24 hours)

Dosage Forms

Caplet:

Alpain: Acetaminophen 500 mg and phenyltoloxamine 60 mg

BeFlex, Staflex: Acetaminophen 500 mg and phenyltoloxamine 55 mg

Dologesic®: Acetaminophen 500 mg and phenyltoloxamine 30 mg

Caplet, extended release [scored]:

Lagesic™: Acetaminophen 600 mg and phenyltoloxamine 66 mg

Capsule:

Dologesic®: Acetaminophen 500 mg and phenyltoloxamine 30 mg

Liquid:
Dologesic®: Acetaminophen 500 mg and phenyltoloxamine 30 mg per 15 mg
Tablet: Acetaminophen 325 mg and phenyltoloxamine 30 mg
Aceta-Gesic [OTC], Genasec™ [OTC], Percogesic® [OTC], Phenagesic [OTC], Phenylgesic [OTC]: Acetaminophen 325 mg and phenyltoloxamine 30 mg
Flextra-650: Acetaminophen 650 mg and phenyltoloxamine 60 mg
Flextra-DS, RhinoFlex™: Acetaminophen 500 mg and phenyltoloxamine 50 mg
RhinoFlex™-650: Acetaminophen 650 mg and phenyltoloxamine 50 mg
Tablet, prolonged release, oral:
Zgesic: Acetaminophen 600 mg and phenyltoloxamine 66 mg

acetaminophen and propoxyphene *see* propoxyphene and acetaminophen *on page 828*

acetaminophen and pseudoephedrine (a seet a MIN oh fen & soo doe e FED rin)

Sound-Alike/Look-Alike Issues
Ornex® may be confused with Orexin®, Orinase®
Sudafed® may be confused with Sufenta®
Tylenol® may be confused with atenolol, timolol, Tuinal®, Tylox®

Synonyms pseudoephedrine and acetaminophen; pseudoephedrine hydrochloride and acetaminophen

U.S./Canadian Brand Names Contac® Cold and Sore Throat, Non Drowsy, Extra Strength [Can]; Dristan® N.D. [Can]; Dristan® N.D., Extra Strength [Can]; Ornex® Maximum Strength [US-OTC]; Ornex® [US-OTC]; Sinutab® Non Drowsy [Can]; Sudafed® Head Cold and Sinus Extra Strength [Can]; Tylenol® Decongestant [Can]; Tylenol® Sinus [Can]

Therapeutic Category Decongestant/Analgesic

Use Temporary relief of nasal congestion, and minor aches and pains associated with colds, flu, sinusitis, or allergies

Usual Dosage Oral:
Children 6-11 years (Ornex®): One caplet every 4-6 hours as needed (maximum: 4 caplets/day)
Children ≥12 years and Adults (Ornex®, Ornex® Maximum Strength): Two caplets every 4-6 hours as needed (maximum: 8 caplets/day)

Dosage Forms
Caplet:
Ornex® [OTC]: Acetaminophen 325 mg and pseudoephedrine 30 mg
Ornex® Maximum Strength [OTC]: Acetaminophen 500 mg and pseudoephedrine 30 mg

acetaminophen and tramadol (a seet a MIN oh fen & TRA ma dole)

Sound-Alike/Look-Alike Issues
Ultracet® may be confused with Ultane®, Ultram®

Synonyms APAP and tramadol; tramadol hydrochloride and acetaminophen

U.S./Canadian Brand Names Tramacet [Can]; Ultracet® [US]

Therapeutic Category Analgesic, Miscellaneous; Analgesic, Nonnarcotic

Use Short-term (≤5 days) management of acute pain

Usual Dosage Oral: Adults: Acute pain: Two tablets every 4-6 hours as needed for pain relief (maximum: 8 tablets/day); treatment should not exceed 5 days

Dosage Forms
Tablet: Acetaminophen 325 mg and tramadol 37.5 mg
Ultracet®: Acetaminophen 325 mg and tramadol 37.5 mg

acetaminophen, aspirin, and caffeine (a seet a MIN oh fen, AS pir in, & KAF een)

Sound-Alike/Look-Alike Issues
Excedrin® may be confused with Dexatrim®, Dexedrine®

Synonyms aspirin, acetaminophen, and caffeine; aspirin, caffeine, and acetaminophen; caffeine, acetaminophen, and aspirin; caffeine, aspirin, and acetaminophen

U.S./Canadian Brand Names Anacin® Advanced Headache Formula [US-OTC]; Excedrin® Extra Strength [US-OTC]; Excedrin® Migraine [US-OTC]; Fem-Prin® [US-OTC]; Genaced™ [US-OTC]; Goody's® Extra Strength Headache Powder [US-OTC]; Goody's® Extra Strength Pain Relief [US-OTC]; Pain-Off [US-OTC]; Vanquish® Extra Strength Pain Reliever [US-OTC]

Therapeutic Category Analgesic, Nonnarcotic

Use Relief of mild-to-moderate pain; mild-to-moderate pain associated with migraine headache

Usual Dosage Oral: Adults:

Analgesic:

Based on **acetaminophen** component:

Mild-to-moderate pain: 325-650 mg every 4-6 hours as needed; do **not** exceed 4 g/day

Mild-to-moderate pain associated with migraine headache: 500 mg/dose (in combination with 500 mg aspirin and 130 mg caffeine) every 6 hours while symptoms persist; do not use for longer than 48 hours

Based on **aspirin** component:

Mild-to-moderate pain: 325-650 mg every 4-6 hours as needed; do **not** exceed 4 g/day

Mild-to-moderate pain associated with migraine headache: 500 mg/dose (in combination with 500 mg acetaminophen and 130 mg caffeine) every 6 hours while symptoms persist; do not use for longer than 48 hours

Product labeling:

Excedrin® Extra Strength, Excedrin® Migraine: Children >12 years and Adults: 2 doses every 6 hours (maximum: 8 doses/24 hours)

Note: When used for migraine, do not use for longer than 48 hours

Goody's® Extra Strength Headache Powder: Children >12 years and Adults: 1 powder, placed on tongue or dissolved in water, every 4-6 hours (maximum: 4 powders/24 hours)

Goody's® Extra Strength Pain Relief Tablets: Children >12 years and Adults: 2 tablets every 4-6 hours (maximum: 8 tablets/24 hours)

Vanquish® Extra Strength Pain Reliever: Children >12 years and Adults: 2 tablets every 4 hours (maximum: 12 tablets/24 hours)

Dosage Forms

Caplet: Acetaminophen 250 mg, aspirin 250 mg, and caffeine 65 mg; acetaminophen 194 mg, aspirin 227 mg, and caffeine 33 mg

Excedrin® Extra Strength [OTC], Excedrin® Migraine [OTC]: Acetaminophen 250 mg, aspirin 250 mg, and caffeine 65 mg

Vanquish® Extra Strength Pain Reliever [OTC]: Acetaminophen 194 mg, aspirin 227 mg, and caffeine 33 mg

Geltab: Acetaminophen 250 mg, aspirin 250 mg, and caffeine 65 mg

Excedrin® Extra Strength [OTC], Excedrin® Migraine [OTC]: Acetaminophen 250 mg, aspirin 250 mg, and caffeine 65 mg

Powder: Acetaminophen 260 mg, aspirin 520 mg, and caffeine 32.5 mg

Goody's® Extra Strength Headache Powder [OTC]: Acetaminophen 260 mg, aspirin 520 mg, and caffeine 32.5 mg

Tablet:

Anacin® Advanced Headache Formula [OTC], Excedrin® Extra Strength [OTC], Excedrin® Migraine [OTC], Genaced™ [OTC], Pain-Off [OTC]: Acetaminophen 250 mg, aspirin 250 mg, and caffeine 65 mg

Fem-Prin® [OTC]: Acetaminophen 194.4 mg, aspirin 226.8 mg, and caffeine 32.4 mg

Goody's® Extra Strength Pain Relief [OTC]: Acetaminophen 130 mg, aspirin 260 mg, and caffeine 16.25 mg

acetaminophen, butalbital, and caffeine *see* butalbital, acetaminophen, and caffeine *on page* *161*

acetaminophen, caffeine, and dihydrocodeine

(a seet a MIN oh fen, KAF een, & dye hye droe KOE deen)

Sound-Alike/Look-Alike Issues

Panlor® DC may be confused with Pamelor®

Synonyms caffeine, dihydrocodeine, and acetaminophen; dihydrocodeine bitartrate, acetaminophen, and caffeine

U.S./Canadian Brand Names Panlor® DC [US]; Panlor® SS [US]; Trezix® [US]; ZerLor™ [US]

Therapeutic Category Analgesic Combination (Opioid)

Controlled Substance C-III

Use Relief of moderate- to moderately-severe pain

Usual Dosage Oral: Adults: Relief of pain:

Panlor® DC, Trezix®: 2 capsules every 4 hours as needed; adjust dose based on severity of pain (maximum dose: 10 capsules/24 hours)

Panlor® SS, ZerLor™: 1 tablet every 4 hours as needed; adjust dose based on severity of pain (maximum dose: 5 tablets/24 hours)

Dosage Forms
Capsule:
Panlor® DC, Trezix®: Acetaminophen 356.4 mg, caffeine 30 mg, and dihydrocodeine 16 mg
Tablet:
Panlor® SS, ZerLor™: Acetaminophen 712.8 mg, caffeine 60 mg, and dihydrocodeine 32 mg

acetaminophen, caffeine, codeine, and butalbital *see* butalbital, acetaminophen, caffeine, and codeine *on page 162*

acetaminophen, chlorpheniramine, and pseudoephedrine
(a seet a MIN oh fen, klor fen IR a meen, & soo doe e FED rin)

Synonyms acetaminophen, chlorpheniramine maleate, and pseudoephedrine hydrochloride; acetaminophen, pseudoephedrine, and chlorpheniramine; chlorpheniramine, acetaminophen, and pseudoephedrine; chlorpheniramine, pseudoephedrine, and acetaminophen; pseudoephedrine, acetaminophen, and chlorpheniramine; pseudoephedrine, chlorpheniramine, and acetaminophen

U.S./Canadian Brand Names Drinex [US-OTC]; Relief-SF® [US]

Therapeutic Category Antihistamine/Decongestant/Analgesic

Use Temporary relief of cold, allergy, or sinus symptoms

Usual Dosage Oral: Children ≥12 years and Adults: Product labeling:
Drinex: 1 tablet 3-4 times/day (maximum: 4 tablets/24 hours); do not take for >7 days
Relief-SF®: 1-2 caplets every 6 hours (maximum: 8 caplets/24 hours)

Dosage Forms
Caplet: Acetaminophen 325 mg, chlorpheniramine 2 mg, and pseudoephedrine 30 mg
Relief-SF®: Acetaminophen 500 mg, chlorpheniramine 2 mg, and pseudoephedrine 30 mg
Tablet:
Drinex [OTC]: Acetaminophen 650 mg, chlorpheniramine 4 mg, and pseudoephedrine 60 mg

acetaminophen, chlorpheniramine maleate, and pseudoephedrine hydrochloride *see* acetaminophen, chlorpheniramine, and pseudoephedrine *on page 26*

acetaminophen, codeine, and doxylamine *(Canada only)*
(a seet a MIN oh fen, KOE deen, & dox IL a meen)

Synonyms codeine, doxylamine, and acetaminophen; doxylamine succinate, codeine phosphate, and acetaminophen

U.S./Canadian Brand Names Mersyndol® With Codeine [Can]

Therapeutic Category Analgesic, Opioid; Antihistamine

Controlled Substance CDSA-1

Use Relief of headache, cold symptoms, neuralgia, and muscular aches/pain

Usual Dosage Oral: Children >12 years and Adults: 1-2 tablets every 4 hours as needed; total dose should not exceed 12 tablets in a 24-hour period

Dosage Forms [CAN] = Canadian brand name
Tablet:
Mersyndol® With Codeine [CAN]: Acetaminophen 325 mg, codeine 8 mg, and doxylamine 5 mg [not available in the U.S.]

acetaminophen, dextromethorphan, and doxylamine
(a seet a MIN oh fen, deks troe meth OR fan, & dox IL a meen)

Synonyms dextromethorphan hydrobromide, acetaminophen, and doxylamine succinate; doxylamine, acetaminophen, and dextromethorphan

U.S./Canadian Brand Names All-Nite [US-OTC]; Tylenol® Cough & Sore Throat Nighttime [US-OTC]; Vicks® NyQuil® Cold & Flu Multi-Symptom [US-OTC]

Therapeutic Category Analgesic, Miscellaneous; Antitussive; Histamine H_1 Antagonist; Histamine H_1 Antagonist, First Generation

Use Temporary relief of common cold and flu symptoms (eg, minor aches and pain, fever, cough, runny nose, sneezing, sore throat)

Usual Dosage Oral: Children ≥12 years and Adults: Relief of cold and flu symptoms: Two capsules/caplets **or** 30 mL every 6 hours (maximum: 8 capsules **or** 240 mL/24 hours)

Dosage Forms
Caplet:
Vicks® NyQuil® Cold & Flu Multi-Symptom [OTC]: Acetaminophen 325 mg dextromethorphan 15 mg, and doxylamine 6.25 mg

Capsule, liquicap:

Vicks® NyQuil® Cold & Flu Multi-Symptom [OTC]: Acetaminophen 325 mg, dextromethorphan 15 mg, and doxylamine 6.25 mg

Liquid:

All-Nite [OTC]: Acetaminophen 500 mg, dextromethorphan 15 mg, and doxylamine 6.25 mg per 15 mL

Tylenol® Cough & Sore Throat Nighttime [OTC]: Acetaminophen 500 mg, dextromethorphan 15 mg, and doxylamine 6.25 mg per 15 mL

Vicks® NyQuil® Cold & Flu Multi-Symptom [OTC]: Acetaminophen 500 mg, dextromethorphan hydrobromide 15 mg, and doxylamine succinate 6.25 mg per 15 mL

acetaminophen, dextromethorphan, and phenylephrine

(a seet a MIN oh fen, deks troe meth OR fan, & fen il EF rin)

Synonyms dextromethorphan hydrobromide, acetaminophen, and phenylephrine hydrochloride; phenylephrine, acetaminophen, and dextromethorphan; phenylephrine, dextromethorphan, and acetaminophen

U.S./Canadian Brand Names Alka-Seltzer Plus® Day Cold [US-OTC]; Comtrex® Maximum Strength, Non-Drowsy Cold & Cough Relief [US-OTC]; Mapap® Multi-Symptom Cold [US-OTC]; Theraflu® Daytime Severe Cold & Cough [US-OTC]; Theraflu® Warming Relief Daytime Severe Cold & Cough [US-OTC]; Tylenol® Cold Head Congestion Daytime [US-OTC]; Tylenol® Cold Multi-Symptom Daytime [US-OTC]; Vicks® DayQuil® Cold/Flu Multi-Symptom Relief [US-OTC]

Therapeutic Category Analgesic, Miscellaneous; Antitussive; Decongestant

Use Temporary relief of common cold and flu symptoms (eg, pain, fever, cough, congestion)

Usual Dosage Product labeling: Oral:

Alka-Seltzer Plus® Day Cold: Children ≥12 years and Adults: 2 capsules or 20 mL every 4 hours (maximum: 6 doses/24 hours)

Tylenol® Cold Head Congestion Daytime: Children ≥12 years and Adults: 2 caplets every 4 hours (maximum: 6 doses/24 hours)

Tylenol® Cold Multi-Symptom Daytime: Children ≥12 years and Adults: 2 caplets/gelcaps or 30 mL every 4 hours (maximum: 6 doses/24 hours)

Vicks® DayQuil® Cold/Flu Multi-Symptom Relief LiquiCaps: Children ≥12 years and Adults: 2 capsules every 4 hours (maximum: 6 doses/24 hours)

Vicks® DayQuil® Cold/Flu Multi-Symptom Relief Liquid:

Children 6-11 years: 15 mL every 4 hours, up to 5 doses/day (maximum: 75 mL/24 hours)

Children ≥12 years and Adults: 30 mL every 4 hours (maximum: 6 doses/24 hours)

Dosage Forms

Caplet:

Comtrex® Maximum Strength, Non-Drowsy Cold & Cough Relief [OTC], Mapap® Multi-Symptom Cold [OTC], Theraflu® Daytime Severe Cold & Cough [OTC], Tylenol® Cold Head Congestion Daytime [OTC], Tylenol® Cold Multi-Symptom Daytime [OTC]: Acetaminophen 325 mg, dextromethorphan 10 mg, and phenylephrine 5 mg

Capsule, liquid gel:

Alka-Seltzer Plus® Day Cold [OTC]: Acetaminophen 325 mg, dextromethorphan 10 mg, and phenylephrine 5 mg

Capsule, liquicap:

Vicks® DayQuil® Cold/Flu Multi-Symptom Relief [OTC]: Acetaminophen 325 mg, dextromethorphan 10 mg, and phenylephrine 5 mg

Gelcap:

Tylenol® Cold Multi-Symptom Daytime [OTC]: Acetaminophen 325 mg, dextromethorphan 10 mg, and phenylephrine 5 mg

Liquid:

Alka-Seltzer Plus® Day Cold [OTC]: Acetaminophen 162.5 mg, dextromethorphan 5 mg, and phenylephrine 2.5 mg per 5 mL

Tylenol® Cold Multi-Symptom Daytime [OTC], Vicks® DayQuil® Cold/Flu Multi-Symptom Relief [OTC]: Acetaminophen 325 mg, dextromethorphan 10 mg, and phenylephrine 5 mg per 15 mL

Powder for solution:

Theraflu® Daytime Severe Cold & Cough [OTC]: Acetaminophen 650 mg, dextromethorphan 20 mg, and phenylephrine 10 mg/packet (6s)

Syrup:

Theraflu® Warming Relief Daytime Severe Cold & Cough [OTC]: Acetaminophen 325 mg, dextromethorphan 10 mg, and phenylephrine 5 mg per 15 mL

acetaminophen, dextromethorphan, and pseudoephedrine *(Discontinued)*

acetaminophen, dextromethorphan, doxylamine, and pseudoephedrine

(a seet a MIN oh fen, deks troe meth OR fan, dox IL a meen & soo doe e FED rin)

Synonyms dextromethorphan hydrobromide, acetaminophen, doxylamine succinate, and pseudoephedrine hydrochloride; doxylamine, acetaminophen, dextromethorphan, and pseudoephedrine; pseudoephedrine, dextromethorphan, doxylamine, and acetaminophen

U.S./Canadian Brand Names All-Nite Cold [US-OTC]; Vicks® NyQuil® D Cold & Flu Multi-Symptom [US-OTC]

Therapeutic Category Analgesic, Miscellaneous; Antitussive; Decongestant; Histamine H_1 Antagonist; Histamine H_1 Antagonist, First Generation

Use Temporary relief of common cold and flu symptoms (eg, minor aches and pain, fever, cough, congestion, runny nose, sneezing, sore throat)

Usual Dosage Oral: Children ≥12 years and Adults: Relief of cold and flu symptoms: 30 mL every 6 hours (maximum: 120 mL/24 hours)

Dosage Forms

Liquid:

All-Nite Multi-Symptom Cold/Flu [OTC]: Acetaminophen 500 mg, dextromethorphan hydrobromide 15 mg, doxylamine succinate 6.25 mg and pseudoephedrine hydrochloride 30 mg per 15 mL

Vicks® NyQuil® D Cold & Flu Multi-Symptom [OTC]: Acetaminophen 500 mg, dextromethorphan hydrobromide 15 mg, doxylamine succinate 6.25 mg and pseudoephedrine hydrochloride 30 mg per 15 mL

acetaminophen, dichloralphenazone, and isometheptene *see* acetaminophen, isometheptene, and dichloralphenazone *on page* 29

acetaminophen, diphenhydramine, and phenylephrine

(a seet a MIN oh fen, dye fen HYE dra meen, & fen il EF rin)

Synonyms acetaminophen, phenylephrine, and diphenhydramine; diphenhydramine, phenylephrine hydrochloride, and acetaminophen; phenylephrine hydrochloride, acetaminophen, and diphenhydramine

U.S./Canadian Brand Names Benadryl® Allergy and Cold [US-OTC]; Benadryl® Allergy and Sinus Headache [US-OTC]; Benadry® Maximum Strength Severe Allergy and Sinus Headache [US-OTC]; Cold Control PE [US-OTC]; Sudafed PE® Nighttime Cold [US-OTC]; Sudafed PE® Severe Cold [US-OTC]; Tylenol® Allergy Multi-Symptom Nighttime [US-OTC]; Tylenol® Children's Plus Cold and Allergy [US-OTC]

Therapeutic Category Analgesic, Miscellaneous; Decongestant; Histamine H_1 Antagonist

Use Temporary relief of symptoms of hay fever and the common cold, including sinus/nasal congestion and pain/pressure, headache, sneezing, runny nose, itchy/watery eyes, sore throat, cough, and minor aches and pains

Usual Dosage Oral: General dosing guidelines; refer to specific product labeling:

Hay fever/cold symptoms:

Children 6-11 years (Benadryl® Allergy and Cold, Benadryl® Allergy and Sinus Headache, Sudafed PE® Severe Cold): One caplet every 4 hours as needed; maximum: 5 caplets/24 hours

Children 6-11 years; 48-95 lbs (Tylenol® Children's Plus Cold and Allergy): 10 mL every 4 hours as needed; maximum: 5 doses/24 hours

Children ≥12 years and Adults (Benadryl® Allergy and Cold, Benadryl® Allergy and Sinus Headache, Sudafed PE® Nighttime Cold, Sudafed PE® Severe Cold, Tylenol® Allergy Multi-Symptom Nighttime): Two caplets every 4 hours as needed; maximum: 12 caplets/24 hours

Dosage Forms

Caplet:

Benadryl® Allergy and Cold [OTC], Benadryl® Allergy and Sinus Headache [OTC], Sudafed PE® Severe Cold [OTC]: Acetaminophen 325 mg, diphenhydramine 12.5 mg, and phenylephrine 5 mg

Benadry® Maximum Strength Severe Allergy and Sinus Headache [OTC], Sudafed PE® Nighttime Cold [OTC], Tylenol® Allergy Multi-Symptom Nighttime [OTC]: Acetaminophen 325 mg, diphenhydramine 25 mg, and phenylephrine 5 mg

Cold Control PE [OTC]: Acetaminophen 650 mg, diphenhydramine 25 mg, and phenylephrine 10 mg

Liquid:

Tylenol® Children's Plus Cold and Allergy [OTC]: Acetaminophen 160 mg, diphenhydramine 12.5 mg, and phenylephrine 2.5 mg per 5 mL

Powder for solution, oral:

Theraflu® Nighttime Severe Cold & Cough [OTC], Theraflu® Sugar-Free Nighttime Severe Cold & Cough [OTC]: Acetaminophen 650 mg, diphenhydramine 25 mg, and phenylephrine 10 mg per packet (6s)

Syrup, oral:

Theraflu® Warming Relief Flu & Sore Throat [OTC], Theraflu® Warming Relief Nighttime Severe Cold & Cough [OTC]: Acetaminophen 325 mg, diphenhydramine 12.5 mg, and phenylephrine 5 mg per 15 mL (245.5 mL)

acetaminophen, isometheptene, and dichloralphenazone

(a seet a MIN oh fen, eye soe me THEP teen, & dye KLOR al FEN a zone)

Sound-Alike/Look-Alike Issues

Midrin® may be confused with Mydfrin®

Synonyms acetaminophen, dichloralphenazone, and isometheptene; dichloralphenazone, acetaminophen, and isometheptene; dichloralphenazone, isometheptene, and acetaminophen; isometheptene, acetaminophen, and dichloralphenazone; isometheptene, dichloralphenazone, and acetaminophen

U.S./Canadian Brand Names Epidrin [US]; Midrin® [US]; Migratine [US]

Therapeutic Category Analgesic, Nonnarcotic

Controlled Substance C-IV

Use Relief of migraine and tension headache

Usual Dosage Oral: Adults:

Migraine headache: 2 capsules to start, followed by 1 capsule every hour until relief is obtained (maximum: 5 capsules/12 hours)

Tension headache: 1-2 capsules every 4 hours (maximum: 8 capsules/24 hours)

Dosage Forms

Capsule:

Epidrin, Midrin®, Migratine: Acetaminophen 325 mg, isometheptene 65 mg, and dichloralphenazone 100 mg

acetaminophen, phenylephrine, and diphenhydramine *see* acetaminophen, diphenhydramine, and phenylephrine *on page* 28

acetaminophen, pseudoephedrine, and chlorpheniramine *see* acetaminophen, chlorpheniramine, and pseudoephedrine *on page* 26

Acetasol® HC [US] *see* acetic acid, propylene glycol diacetate, and hydrocortisone *on page* 30

acetazolamide (a set a ZOLE a mide)

Sound-Alike/Look-Alike Issues

acetaZOLAMIDE may be confused with acetoHEXAMIDE

Diamox® Sequels® may be confused with Diabinese®, Dobutrex®, Trimox®

Tall-Man aceta**ZOLAMIDE**

U.S./Canadian Brand Names Apo-Acetazolamide® [Can]; Diamox® Sequels® [US]; Diamox® [Can]

Therapeutic Category Anticonvulsant; Carbonic Anhydrase Inhibitor

Use Treatment of glaucoma (chronic simple open-angle, secondary glaucoma, preoperatively in acute angle-closure); drug-induced edema or edema due to congestive heart failure (adjunctive therapy); centrencephalic epilepsies (immediate release dosage form); prevention or amelioration of symptoms associated with acute mountain sickness

Usual Dosage Note: I.M. administration is not recommended because of pain secondary to the alkaline pH

Children:

Glaucoma:

Oral: 8-30 mg/kg/day or 300-900 mg/m^2/day divided every 8 hours

I.V.: 20-40 mg/kg/24 hours divided every 6 hours, not to exceed 1 g/day

Edema: Oral, I.V.: 5 mg/kg or 150 mg/m^2 once every day

Epilepsy: Oral: 8-30 mg/kg/day in 1-4 divided doses, not to exceed 1 g/day; extended release capsule is not recommended for treatment of epilepsy

Adults:

Glaucoma:

Chronic simple (open-angle): Oral: 250 mg 1-4 times/day or 500 mg extended release capsule twice daily

Secondary, acute (closed-angle): I.V.: 250-500 mg, may repeat in 2-4 hours to a maximum of 1 g/day

Edema: Oral, I.V.: 250-375 mg once daily

Epilepsy: Oral: 8-30 mg/kg/day in 1-4 divided doses; **extended release capsule is not recommended for treatment of epilepsy**

Mountain sickness: Oral: 250 mg every 8-12 hours (or 500 mg extended release capsules every 12-24 hours)

Therapy should begin 24-48 hours before and continue during ascent and for at least 48 hours after arrival at the high altitude

Note: In situations of rapid ascent (such as rescue or military operations), 1000 mg/day is recommended.

Dosage Forms

Capsule, extended release: 500 mg

Diamox® Sequels®: 500 mg

Injection, powder for reconstitution: 500 mg

Tablet: 125 mg, 250 mg

acetic acid (a SEE tik AS id)

Sound-Alike/Look-Alike Issues

VoSol® may be confused with Vexol®

Synonyms ethanoic acid

Therapeutic Category Antibacterial, Otic; Antibacterial, Topical

Use Irrigation of the bladder; treatment of superficial bacterial infections of the external auditory canal

Usual Dosage

Irrigation (**Note:** Dosage of an irrigating solution depends on the capacity or surface area of the structure being irrigated):

For continuous irrigation of the urinary bladder with 0.25% acetic acid irrigation, the rate of administration will approximate the rate of urine flow; usually 500-1500 mL/24 hours

For periodic irrigation of an indwelling urinary catheter to maintain patency, about 50 mL of 0.25% acetic acid irrigation is required

Otic: Insert saturated wick; keep moist 24 hours; remove wick and instill 5 drops 3-4 times/day

Dosage Forms

Solution for irrigation: 0.25% (250 mL, 500 mL, 1000 mL)

Solution, otic: 2% (15 mL)

acetic acid, hydrocortisone, and propylene glycol diacetate *see* acetic acid, propylene glycol diacetate, and hydrocortisone *on page 30*

acetic acid, propylene glycol diacetate, and hydrocortisone

(a SEE tik AS id, PRO pa leen GLY kole dye AS e tate, & hye droe KOR ti sone)

Sound-Alike/Look-Alike Issues

VoSol® may be confused with Vexol®

Synonyms acetic acid, hydrocortisone, and propylene glycol diacetate; hydrocortisone, acetic acid, and propylene glycol diacetate; propylene glycol diacetate, acetic acid, and hydrocortisone

U.S./Canadian Brand Names Acetasol® HC [US]; VoSol® HC [US]

Therapeutic Category Antibiotic/Corticosteroid, Otic

Use Treatment of superficial infections of the external auditory canal caused by organisms susceptible to the action of the antimicrobial, complicated by swelling

Usual Dosage Otic: Children ≥3 years and Adults: Instill 3-5 drops in ear(s) every 4-6 hours

Dosage Forms

Solution, otic [drops]:

Acetasol® HC, VoSol® HC: Acetic acid 2%, propylene glycol diacetate 3%, and hydrocortisone 1% (10 mL)

acetohydroxamic acid (a SEE toe hye droks am ik AS id)

Sound-Alike/Look-Alike Issues

Lithostat® may be confused with Lithobid®

Synonyms AHA

U.S./Canadian Brand Names Lithostat® [US/Can]

Therapeutic Category Urinary Tract Product

Use Adjunctive therapy in chronic urea-splitting urinary infection

Usual Dosage Oral:

Children: Initial: 10 mg/kg/day

Adults: 250 mg 3-4 times/day for a total daily dose of 10-15 mg/kg/day

Dosage Forms

Tablet:

Lithostat®: 250 mg

Acetoxyl® [Can] *see* benzoyl peroxide *on page 132*

acetoxymethylprogesterone *see* medroxyprogesterone *on page 620*

acetylcholine (a se teel KOE leen)

Sound-Alike/Look-Alike Issues

acetylcholine may be confused with acetylcysteine

Synonyms acetylcholine chloride

U.S./Canadian Brand Names Miochol®-E [US/Can]

Therapeutic Category Cholinergic Agent

Use Produces complete miosis in cataract surgery, keratoplasty, iridectomy, and other anterior segment surgery where rapid miosis is required

Usual Dosage Intraocular: Adults: 0.5-2 mL of 1% injection (5-20 mg) instilled into anterior chamber before or after securing one or more sutures

Dosage Forms

Powder for intraocular solution:

Miochol®-E: 1:100 [20 mg; packaged with diluent (2 mL)]

acetylcholine chloride *see* acetylcholine *on page 31*

acetylcysteine (a se teel SIS teen)

Sound-Alike/Look-Alike Issues

acetylcysteine may be confused with acetylcholine
Mucomyst® may be confused with Mucinex®

Synonyms *N*-acetyl-L-cysteine; *N*-acetylcysteine; acetylcysteine sodium; mercapturic acid; NAC

U.S./Canadian Brand Names Acetadote® [US]; Acetylcysteine Solution [Can]; Mucomyst® [Can]; Parvolex® [Can]

Therapeutic Category Mucolytic Agent

Use Antidote for acute acetaminophen (APAP) poisoning; repeated supratherapeutic ingestion (RSTI) of APAP; adjunctive mucolytic therapy in patients with abnormal or viscid mucous secretions in acute and chronic bronchopulmonary diseases; pulmonary complications of surgery and cystic fibrosis; diagnostic bronchial studies

Usual Dosage

Acetaminophen poisoning: **Note:** Only the 72-hour oral and 21-hour I.V. regimens are FDA-approved. Ideally, in patients with an acute APAP ingestion, treatment should begin within 8 hours of ingestion. In patients who present following RSTI and treatment is deemed appropriate, acetylcysteine should be initiated immediately.

Children and Adults:

Oral: **Note:** Consultation with a poison control center or clinical toxicologist is highly recommended when considering the discontinuation of oral acetylcysteine prior to the conclusion of a full 18-dose course of therapy.

72-hour regimen: Consists of 18 doses; total dose delivered: 1330 mg/kg

Loading dose: 140 mg/kg

Maintenance dose: 70 mg/kg every 4 hours; repeat dose if emesis occurs within 1 hour of administration

I.V. (Acetadote®):

21-hour regimen: Consists of 3 doses; total dose delivered: 300 mg/kg

Loading dose: 150 mg/kg infused over 60 minutes

Second dose: 50 mg/kg infused over 4 hours

Third dose: 100 mg/kg infused over 16 hours

Adjuvant therapy in respiratory conditions: **Note:** Patients should receive an aerosolized bronchodilator 10-15 minutes prior to acetylcysteine.

Inhalation, nebulization (face mask, mouth piece, tracheostomy): Acetylcysteine 10% and 20% solution (dilute 20% solution with sodium chloride or sterile water for inhalation); 10% solution may be used undiluted

Infants: 1-2 mL of 20% solution or 2-4 mL of 10% solution until nebulized given 3-4 times/day

Children and Adults: 3-5 mL of 20% solution or 6-10 mL of 10% solution until nebulized given 3-4 times/day; dosing range: 1-10 mL of 20% solution or 2-20 mL of 10% solution every 2-6 hours

Inhalation, nebulization (tent, croupette): Children and Adults: Dose must be individualized; may require up to 300 mL solution/treatment

Direct instillation: Adults:

Into tracheostomy: 1-2 mL of 10% to 20% solution every 1-4 hours

Through percutaneous intratracheal catheter: 1-2 mL of 20% or 2-4 mL of 10% solution every 1-4 hours via syringe attached to catheter

Diagnostic bronchogram: Nebulization or intratracheal: Adults: 1-2 mL of 20% solution or 2-4 mL of 10% solution administered 2-3 times prior to procedure

Dosage Forms

Injection, solution:

Acetadote®: 20% (30 mL) [200 mg/mL]

Solution, inhalation/oral: 10% [100 mg/mL]; 20% [200 mg/mL]

acetylcysteine, methylcobalamin, and methylfolate *see* methylfolate, methylcobalamin, and acetylcysteine *on page* 644

acetylcysteine, methylfolate, and methylcobalamin *see* methylfolate, methylcobalamin, and acetylcysteine *on page* 644

acetylcysteine sodium *see* acetylcysteine *on page* 31

Acetylcysteine Solution [Can] *see* acetylcysteine *on page* 31

acetylsalicylic acid *see* aspirin *on page* 103

Aches-N-Pain® *(Discontinued)* *see* ibuprofen *on page* 515

achromycin *see* tetracycline *on page* 950

aciclovir *see* acyclovir *on page* 33

Acid Gone [US-OTC] *see* aluminum hydroxide and magnesium carbonate *on page* 55

Acid Gone Extra Strength [US-OTC] *see* aluminum hydroxide and magnesium carbonate *on page* 55

Acid Reducer [Can] *see* ranitidine *on page* 852

Acid Reducer Maximum Strength Non Prescription [Can] *see* ranitidine *on page* 852

acidulated phosphate fluoride *see* fluoride *on page* 430

Aci-jel® *(Discontinued)* *see* acetic acid *on page* 30

Acilac [Can] *see* lactulose *on page* 565

AcipHex® [US/Can] *see* rabeprazole *on page* 847

acitretin (a si TRE tin)

Sound-Alike/Look-Alike Issues

Soriatane® may be confused with Loxitane®

U.S./Canadian Brand Names Soriatane® CK Convenience Kit™ [US]; Soriatane® [Can]

Therapeutic Category Retinoid-like Compound

Use Treatment of severe psoriasis

Usual Dosage Oral: Adults: Individualization of dosage is required to achieve maximum therapeutic response while minimizing side effects

Initial therapy: Therapy should be initiated at 25-50 mg/day, given as a single dose with the main meal

Maintenance doses of 25-50 mg/day may be given after initial response to treatment; the maintenance dose should be based on clinical efficacy and tolerability

Dosage Forms

Capsule:

Soriatane® CK Convenience Kit™: 10 mg, 25 mg

Aclaro PD™ [US] *see* hydroquinone *on page* 508

Aclasta® [Can] *see* zoledronic acid *on page* 1032

Aclovate® [US] *see* alclometasone *on page* 42

Acne Clear Maximum Strength [US-OTC] *see* benzoyl peroxide *on page* 132

acrivastine and pseudoephedrine (AK ri vas teen & soo doe e FED rin)

Synonyms pseudoephedrine hydrochloride and acrivastine

U.S./Canadian Brand Names Semprex®-D [US]

Therapeutic Category Antihistamine/Decongestant Combination

Use Temporary relief of nasal congestion, decongest sinus openings, running nose, itching of nose or throat, and itchy, watery eyes due to hay fever or other upper respiratory allergies

Usual Dosage Oral: Adults: 1 capsule 3-4 times/day

Dosage Forms

Capsule:

Semprex®-D: Acrivastine 8 mg and pseudoephedrine 60 mg

ACT® [US-OTC] *see* fluoride *on page 430*

ACT-D *see* dactinomycin *on page 273*

Actagen® Syrup *(Discontinued)* *see* triprolidine and pseudoephedrine *on page 989*

Actagen® Tablet *(Discontinued)* *see* triprolidine and pseudoephedrine *on page 989*

Act-A-Med® *(Discontinued)* *see* triprolidine and pseudoephedrine *on page 989*

ACTH *see* corticotropin *on page 258*

ActHIB® [US/Can] *see* *Haemophilus* B conjugate vaccine *on page 483*

Acthrel® [US] *see* corticorelin *on page 258*

Acticin® [US] *see* permethrin *on page 769*

Actidose-Aqua® [US-OTC] *see* charcoal *on page 206*

Actidose® with Sorbitol [US-OTC] *see* charcoal *on page 206*

Actifed® [Can] *see* triprolidine and pseudoephedrine *on page 989*

Actifed® Allergy Tablet (Night) *(Discontinued)*

Actifed® Cold & Allergy [US-OTC] *[reformulation]* *see* chlorpheniramine and phenylephrine *on page 214*

Actifed® Cold and Allergy *(Discontinued)* *see* triprolidine and pseudoephedrine *on page 989*

Actigall® [US] *see* ursodiol *on page 1000*

Actimmune® [US/Can] *see* interferon gamma-1b *on page 536*

actinomycin *see* dactinomycin *on page 273*

actinomycin D *see* dactinomycin *on page 273*

actinomycin CI *see* dactinomycin *on page 273*

Actiq® [US/Can] *see* fentanyl *on page 410*

Activase® [US] *see* alteplase *on page 53*

Activase® rt-PA [Can] *see* alteplase *on page 53*

activated carbon *see* charcoal *on page 206*

activated charcoal *see* charcoal *on page 206*

activated dimethicone *see* simethicone *on page 901*

activated ergosterol *see* ergocalciferol *on page 364*

activated methylpolysiloxane *see* simethicone *on page 901*

activated protein C, human, recombinant *see* drotrecogin alfa *on page 340*

Activella® [US] *see* estradiol and norethindrone *on page 376*

Actonel® [US/Can] *see* risedronate *on page 869*

Actonel® and Calcium [US] *see* risedronate and calcium *on page 870*

Actoplus Met® [US] *see* pioglitazone and metformin *on page 786*

Actoplus Met® XR [US] *see* pioglitazone and metformin *on page 786*

Actos® [US/Can] *see* pioglitazone *on page 785*

ACT® Plus [US-OTC] *see* fluoride *on page 430*

ACT® x2™ [US-OTC] *see* fluoride *on page 430*

Acular® [US/Can] *see* ketorolac *on page 558*

Acular LS® [US/Can] *see* ketorolac *on page 558*

Acular® PF [US] *see* ketorolac *on page 558*

ACV *see* acyclovir *on page 33*

acycloguanosine *see* acyclovir *on page 33*

acyclovir (ay SYE kloe veer)

Sound-Alike/Look-Alike Issues

acyclovir may be confused with ganciclovir, Retrovir®, valacyclovir

Zovirax® may be confused with Valtrex®, Zithromax®, Zostrix®, Zyloprim®, Zyvox®

Synonyms aciclovir; ACV; acycloguanosine

U.S./Canadian Brand Names Apo-Acyclovir® [Can]; Gen-Acyclovir [Can]; Novo-Acyclovir [Can]; Nu-Acyclovir [Can]; ratio-Acyclovir [Can]; Zovirax® [US/Can]

Therapeutic Category Antiviral Agent

Use Treatment of genital herpes simplex virus (HSV), herpes labialis (cold sores), herpes zoster (shingles), HSV encephalitis, neonatal HSV, mucocutaneous HSV in immunocompromised patients, varicella-zoster (chickenpox)

Usual Dosage Note: Obese patients should be dosed using ideal body weight

Genital HSV:

I.V.: Children ≥12 years and Adults (immunocompetent): Initial episode, severe: 5 mg/kg/dose every 8 hours for 5-7 days

Oral: Adults:

Initial episode: 200 mg every 4 hours while awake (5 times/day) for 10 days (per manufacturer's labeling); 400 mg 3 times/day for 5-10 days has also been reported

Recurrence: 200 mg every 4 hours while awake (5 times/day) for 5 days (per manufacturer's labeling; begin at earliest signs of disease); 400 mg 3 times/day for 5 days has also been reported

Chronic suppression: 400 mg twice daily or 200 mg 3-5 times/day, for up to 12 months followed by re-evaluation (per manufacturer's labeling); 400-1200 mg/day in 2-3 divided doses has also been reported

Topical: Adults (immunocompromised): Ointment: Initial episode: 1/2" ribbon of ointment for a 4" square surface area every 3 hours (6 times/day) for 7 days

Herpes labialis (cold sores): Topical: Children ≥12 years and Adults: Cream: Apply 5 times/day for 4 days

Herpes zoster (shingles):

Oral: Adults (immunocompetent): 800 mg every 4 hours (5 times/day) for 7-10 days

I.V.:

Children <12 years (immunocompromised): 20 mg/kg/dose every 8 hours for 7 days

Children ≥12 years and Adults (immunocompromised): 10 mg/kg/dose or 500 mg/m^2/dose every 8 hours for 7 days

HSV encephalitis: I.V.:

Children 3 months to 12 years: 20 mg/kg/dose every 8 hours for 10 days (per manufacturer's labeling); dosing for 14-21 days also reported

Children ≥12 years and Adults: 10 mg/kg/dose every 8 hours for 10 days (per manufacturer's labeling); 10-15 mg/kg/dose every 8 hours for 14-21 days also reported

Mucocutaneous HSV:

I.V.:

Children <12 years (immunocompromised): 10 mg/kg/dose every 8 hours for 7 days

Children ≥12 years and Adults (immunocompromised): 5 mg/kg/dose every 8 hours for 7 days (per manufacturer's labeling); dosing for up to 14 days also reported

Topical: Ointment: Adults (nonlife-threatening, immunocompromised): 1/2" ribbon of ointment for a 4" square surface area every 3 hours (6 times/day) for 7 days

Neonatal HSV: I.V.: Neonate: Birth to 3 months: 10 mg/kg/dose every 8 hours for 10 days (manufacturer's labeling); 15 mg/kg/dose or 20 mg/kg/dose every 8 hours for 14-21 days has also been reported

Varicella-zoster (chickenpox): Begin treatment within the first 24 hours of rash onset:

Oral: **Note:** The AIDS*info* guidelines recommended duration of therapy is 7-10 days or until no new lesions for 48 hours (for patients with mild varicella and no or moderate immune suppression).

Children ≥2 years and ≤40 kg (immunocompetent): 20 mg/kg/dose (up to 800 mg/dose) 4 times/day for 5 days

Children >40 kg and Adults (immunocompetent): 800 mg/dose 4 times a day for 5 days

I.V.:

Manufacturer's labeling (immunocompromised):

Children <12 years: 20 mg/kg/dose every 8 hours for 7 days

Children ≥12 years and Adults: 10 mg/kg/dose every 8 hours for 7 days

AIDSinfo guidelines (immunocompromised):

Children <1 year: 10 mg/kg/dose every 8 hours for 7-10 days or until no new lesions for 48 hours

Children ≥1 year: 10 mg/kg/dose or 500 mg/m^2/dose every 8 hours for 7-10 days or until no new lesions for 48 hours

Adolescents and Adults: 10-15 mg/kg/dose every 8 hours for 7-10 days

Dosage Forms

Capsule: 200 mg
Zovirax®: 200 mg
Cream, topical:
Zovirax®: 5% (2 g, 5 g)
Injection, powder for reconstitution: 500 mg, 1000 mg
Injection, solution [preservative free]: 50 mg/mL (10 mL, 20 mL)
Ointment, topical:
Zovirax®: 5% (15 g)
Suspension, oral: 200 mg/5 mL
Zovirax®: 200 mg/5 mL
Tablet: 400 mg, 800 mg
Zovirax®: 400 mg, 800 mg

ACZ885 *see* canakinumab *on page 176*

Aczone® [US] *see* dapsone *on page 276*

AD32 *see* valrubicin *on page 1003*

Adacel® [US/Can] *see* diphtheria, tetanus toxoids, and acellular pertussis vaccine *on page 321*

Adagen® [US/Can] *see* pegademase (bovine) *on page 754*

Adalat® XL® [Can] *see* nifedipine *on page 697*

Adalat® CC [US] *see* nifedipine *on page 697*

Adalat® ***(Discontinued)*** *see* nifedipine *on page 697*

adalimumab (a da LIM yoo mab)

Sound-Alike/Look-Alike Issues

Humira® may be confused with Humulin®, Humalog®
Humira® Pen may be confused with HumaPen® Memoir®

Synonyms antitumor necrosis factor apha (human); D2E7; human antitumor necrosis factor alpha

U.S./Canadian Brand Names Humira® [US/Can]

Therapeutic Category Antirheumatic, Disease Modifying; Monoclonal Antibody

Use

Treatment of active rheumatoid arthritis (moderate-to-severe) and active psoriatic arthritis; may be used alone or in combination with disease-modifying antirheumatic drugs (DMARDs); treatment of ankylosing spondylitis

Treatment of moderately- to severely-active Crohn disease in patients with inadequate response to conventional treatment, or patients who have lost response to or are intolerant of infliximab

Treatment of moderate-to-severe plaque psoriasis

Treatment of moderately- to severely-active juvenile idiopathic arthritis

Usual Dosage SubQ:

Children ≥4 years: Juvenile idiopathic arthritis:
15 kg to <30 kg: 20 mg every other week
≥30 kg: 40 mg every other week

Adults:
Rheumatoid arthritis: 40 mg every other week; may be administered with other DMARDs; patients not taking methotrexate may increase dose to 40 mg every week
Ankylosing spondylitis, psoriatic arthritis: 40 mg every other week
Crohn disease: Initial: 160 mg given as 4 injections on day 1 or over 2 days, then 80 mg 2 weeks later (day 15); maintenance: 40 mg every other week beginning day 29
Plaque psoriasis: Initial: 80 mg as a single dose; maintenance: 40 mg every other week beginning 1 week after initial dose

Dosage Forms

Injection, solution [pediatric; preservative free]:
Humira®: 20 mg/0.4 mL (0.4 mL)
Injection, solution [preservative free]:
Humira®: 40 mg/0.8 mL (0.8 mL)

adamantanamine hydrochloride *see* amantadine *on page 57*

adapalene (a DAP a leen)

U.S./Canadian Brand Names Differin® XP [Can]; Differin® [US/Can]

Therapeutic Category Acne Products

Use Treatment of acne vulgaris

Usual Dosage Topical: Children >12 years and Adults: Apply once daily at bedtime; therapeutic results should be noticed after 8-12 weeks of treatment

Dosage Forms

Cream, topical:

Differin®: 0.1% (15 g, 45 g)

Gel, topical:

Differin®: 0.1% (15 g, 45 g); 0.3% (45 g)

adapalene and benzoyl peroxide (a DAP a leen & BEN zoe il peer OKS ide)

Synonyms benzoyl peroxide and adapalene

U.S./Canadian Brand Names Epiduo™ [US]

Therapeutic Category Acne Products; Topical Skin Product; Topical Skin Product, Acne

Use Topical treatment of acne vulgaris

Usual Dosage Topical: Children ≥12 years and Adults: Apply once daily to affected areas after skin has been cleaned and dried

Dosage Forms

Gel, topical:

Epiduo™: Adapalene 0.1% and benzoyl peroxide 2.5% (45 g)

Adcirca™ [US] *see* tadalafil *on page* 936
ADD 234037 *see* lacosamide *on page* 563
Addaprin [US-OTC] *see* ibuprofen *on page* 515
Adderall® [US] *see* dextroamphetamine and amphetamine *on page* 293
Adderall XR® [US/Can] *see* dextroamphetamine and amphetamine *on page* 293

adefovir (a DEF o veer)

Synonyms adefovir dipivoxil; bis-POM PMEA

U.S./Canadian Brand Names Hepsera™ [US/Can]

Therapeutic Category Antiretroviral Agent, Nonnucleoside Reverse Transcriptase Inhibitor (NNRTI)

Use Treatment of chronic hepatitis B with evidence of active viral replication (based on persistent elevation of ALT/AST or histologic evidence), including patients with lamivudine-resistant hepatitis B

Usual Dosage Oral: Children ≥12 years and Adults: 10 mg once daily. **Note:** Usual treatment duration is at least 1 year and varies with HBeAg status, consult current guidelines and literature.

Dosage Forms

Tablet:

Hepsera®: 10 mg

adefovir dipivoxil *see* adefovir *on page* 36
ADEKs® [US-OTC] *see* vitamins (multiple/pediatric) *on page* 1020
Adenocard® [US/Can] *see* adenosine *on page* 36
Adenoscan® [US/Can] *see* adenosine *on page* 36

adenosine (a DEN oh seen)

Synonyms 9-beta-d-ribofuranosyladenine

U.S./Canadian Brand Names Adenocard® [US/Can]; Adenoscan® [US/Can]; Adenosine Injection, USP [Can]

Therapeutic Category Antiarrhythmic Agent, Class IV; Diagnostic Agent

Use

Adenocard®: Treatment of paroxysmal supraventricular tachycardia (PSVT) including that associated with accessory bypass tracts (Wolff-Parkinson-White syndrome); when clinically advisable, appropriate vagal maneuvers should be attempted prior to adenosine administration; **not effective for conversion of atrial fibrillation, atrial flutter, or ventricular tachycardia**

Adenoscan®: Pharmacologic stress agent used in myocardial perfusion thallium-201 scintigraphy

Usual Dosage

Adenocard®: **Rapid I.V. push (over 1-2 seconds) via peripheral line:**

Infants and Children:

Paroxysmal supraventricular tachycardia: Manufacturer's recommendation:

<50 kg: Initial: 0.05-0.1 mg/kg (maximum initial dose: 6 mg). If conversion of PSVT does not occur within 1-2 minutes, may increase dose by 0.05-0.1 mg/kg. May repeat until sinus rhythm is established or to a maximum single dose of 0.3 mg/kg or 12 mg. Follow each dose with normal saline flush.

≥50 kg: Refer to Adult dosing

Pediatric advanced life support: Treatment of SVT: I.V., I.O.: Initial: 0.1 mg/kg (maximum initial dose: 6 mg); if not effective within 1-2 minutes, administer 0.2 mg/kg; may repeat 0.2 mg/kg if needed (maximum single dose: 12 mg). Follow each dose with normal saline flush.

Adults:

Paroxysmal supraventricular tachycardia: Initial: 6 mg; if not effective within 1-2 minutes, 12 mg may be given; may repeat 12 mg bolus if needed (maximum single dose: 12 mg). Follow each dose with normal saline flush.

Recommended dosage adjustment for adenosine when administered via central line or with concurrent carbamazepine or dipyridamole: Initial dose: 3 mg

Adenoscan®: Pharmacologic stress testing: Continuous I.V. infusion via peripheral line: 140 mcg/kg/minute for 6 minutes using syringe or columetric infusion pump; total dose: 0.84 mg/kg. Thallium-201 is injected at midpoint (3 minutes) of infusion.

Dosage Forms

Injection, solution [preservative free]: 3 mg/mL (2 mL, 4 mL)

Adenocard®: 3 mg/mL (2 mL, 4 mL)

Adenoscan®: 3 mg/mL (20 mL, 30 mL)

Adenosine Injection, USP [Can] *see* adenosine *on page 36*

Adept® [US] *see* icodextrin *on page 517*

ADH *see* vasopressin *on page 1008*

Adipex-P® [US] *see* phentermine *on page 773*

ADL-2698 *see* alvimopan *on page 57*

Adlone® Injection *(Discontinued)* *see* methylprednisolone *on page 647*

Adoxa® [US] *see* doxycycline *on page 336*

Adrenalin® [US/Can] *see* epinephrine *on page 358*

adrenaline *see* epinephrine *on page 358*

adrenocorticotropic hormone *see* corticotropin *on page 258*

AdreView™ [US] *see* iobenguane I 123 *on page 537*

adria *see* doxorubicin *on page 335*

Adriamycin® [US/Can] *see* doxorubicin *on page 335*

Adrucil® [US] *see* fluorouracil *on page 431*

adsorbent charcoal *see* charcoal *on page 206*

Adsorbocarpine® Ophthalmic *(Discontinued)* *see* pilocarpine *on page 783*

Adsorbonac® *(Discontinued)* *see* sodium chloride *on page 908*

Adsorbotear® Ophthalmic Solution *(Discontinued)* *see* artificial tears *on page 100*

Advagraf™ [Can] *see* tacrolimus *on page 935*

Advair® [Can] *see* fluticasone and salmeterol *on page 436*

Advair Diskus® [US/Can] *see* fluticasone and salmeterol *on page 436*

Advair® HFA [US] *see* fluticasone and salmeterol *on page 436*

Advanced Formula Oxy® Sensitive Gel *(Discontinued)* *see* benzoyl peroxide *on page 132*

Advanced NatalCare® *(Discontinued)* *see* vitamins (multiple/prenatal) *on page 1020*

Advanced-RF NatalCare® *(Discontinued)* *see* vitamins (multiple/prenatal) *on page 1020*

Advantage-S® [US-OTC] *see* nonoxynol 9 *on page 703*

Advate [US] *see* antihemophilic factor (recombinant) *on page 82*

Advicor® [US/Can] *see* niacin and lovastatin *on page 694*

Advil® [US-OTC/Can] *see* ibuprofen *on page 515*

Advil® Allergy Sinus [US] *see* ibuprofen, pseudoephedrine, and chlorpheniramine *on page 517*

Advil® Children's [US-OTC] *see* ibuprofen *on page 515*

Advil® Cold and Sinus Plus [Can] *see* ibuprofen, pseudoephedrine, and chlorpheniramine *on page 517*

Advil® Cold, Children's *(Discontinued)* *see* pseudoephedrine and ibuprofen *on page 835*

Advil® Cold & Sinus [US-OTC/Can] *see* pseudoephedrine and ibuprofen *on page 835*

Advil® Infants' [US-OTC] *see* ibuprofen *on page 515*

Advil® Junior *(Discontinued)* *see* ibuprofen *on page 515*

Advil® Migraine [US-OTC] *see* ibuprofen *on page 515*

Advil® Multi-Symptom Cold [US] *see* ibuprofen, pseudoephedrine, and chlorpheniramine *on page 517*

Aerius® [Can] *see* desloratadine *on page 284*

Aeroaid® *(Discontinued)*

AeroBid® [US] *see* flunisolide *on page 427*

AeroBid®-M [US] *see* flunisolide *on page 427*

Aerodine® *(Discontinued)* *see* povidone-iodine *on page 807*

aerohist plus™ [US] *see* chlorpheniramine, phenylephrine, and methscopolamine *on page 218*

aeroKid™ [US] *see* chlorpheniramine, phenylephrine, and methscopolamine *on page 218*

Afeditab® CR [US] *see* nifedipine *on page 697*

Afinitor® [US] *see* everolimus *on page 400*

Afluria® [US] *see* influenza virus vaccine *on page 528*

A-Free Prenatal [US] *see* vitamins (multiple/prenatal) *on page 1020*

Afrin® Children's Nose Drops *(Discontinued)* *see* oxymetazoline *on page 740*

Afrin® Extra Moisturizing [US-OTC] *see* oxymetazoline *on page 740*

Afrinol® *(Discontinued)* *see* pseudoephedrine *on page 833*

Afrin® Original [US-OTC] *see* oxymetazoline *on page 740*

Afrin® Saline Mist *(Discontinued)* *see* sodium chloride *on page 908*

Afrin® Severe Congestion [US-OTC] *see* oxymetazoline *on page 740*

Afrin® Sinus [US-OTC] *see* oxymetazoline *on page 740*

Aftate® Antifungal *(Discontinued)* *see* tolnaftate *on page 968*

agalsidase alfa *(Canada only)* (aye GAL si days AL fa)

Sound-Alike/Look-Alike Issues
agalsidase alfa may be confused with agalsidase beta, alglucerase, alglucosidase alfa

Synonyms agalsidase alpha; alpha-galactosidase-A (gene-activated)

U.S./Canadian Brand Names Replagal™ [Can]

Therapeutic Category Enzyme

Use Replacement therapy for Fabry disease

Usual Dosage Note: Premedication with oral antihistamines and corticosteroids may alleviate infusion-related reactions associated with agalsidase alfa.
I.V.: Children and Adults: Fabry disease: 0.2 mg/kg every 2 weeks

Dosage Forms [CAN] = Canadian brand name
Injection, solution [preservative free]:
Replagal™ [CAN]: 1 mg/1mL (3.5 mL) [not available in the U.S.]

agalsidase alpha *see* agalsidase alfa *(Canada only) on page 38*

agalsidase beta (aye GAL si days BAY ta)

Sound-Alike/Look-Alike Issues
agalsidase beta may be confused with agalsidase alfa, alglucerase, alglucosidase alfa

Synonyms alpha-galactosidase-A (recombinant); r-h α-GAL

U.S./Canadian Brand Names Fabrazyme® [US/Can]

Therapeutic Category Enzyme

Use Replacement therapy for Fabry disease

Usual Dosage I.V.: Children ≥8 years and Adults: 1 mg/kg every 2 weeks

Dosage Forms
Injection, powder for reconstitution:
Fabrazyme®: 5 mg, 35 mg

Agenerase® ***(Discontinued)***
Aggrastat® [US/Can] *see* tirofiban *on page 964*
Aggrenox® [US/Can] *see* aspirin and dipyridamole *on page 105*
AGN 1135 *see* rasagiline *on page 853*
$AgNO_3$ *see* silver nitrate *on page 901*
Agrylin® [US/Can] *see* anagrelide *on page 78*
AHA *see* acetohydroxamic acid *on page 30*
AH-Chew® [US] *see* chlorpheniramine, phenylephrine, and methscopolamine *on page 218*
AH-Chew™ Ultra [US] *see* chlorpheniramine, phenylephrine, and methscopolamine *on page 218*
AHF (human) *see* antihemophilic factor (human) *on page 81*
AHF (human) *see* antihemophilic factor/von Willebrand factor complex (human) *on page 83*
AHF (recombinant) *see* antihemophilic factor (recombinant) *on page 82*
Ahist™ [US] *see* chlorpheniramine *on page 213*
AICC *see* antiinhibitor coagulant complex *on page 85*
Airet® ***(Discontinued)*** *see* albuterol *on page 41*
Airomir [Can] *see* albuterol *on page 41*
AKBeta® ***(Discontinued)*** *see* levobunolol *on page 578*
Ak-Chlor® Ophthalmic ***(Discontinued)*** *see* chloramphenicol *on page 208*
AK-Con™ [US] *see* naphazoline *on page 680*
AK-Dilate® [US] *see* phenylephrine *on page 774*
AK-Fluor® [US] *see* fluorescein *on page 429*
Ak-Homatropine® Ophthalmic ***(Discontinued)*** *see* homatropine *on page 495*
Akineton® ***(Discontinued)***
AK-Nefrin ***(Discontinued)*** *see* phenylephrine *on page 774*
Akne-Mycin® [US] *see* erythromycin *on page 368*
AK-Pentolate™ [US] *see* cyclopentolate *on page 265*
AK-Poly-Bac™ [US] *see* bacitracin and polymyxin B *on page 119*
AK-Pred® [US] *see* prednisolone (ophthalmic) *on page 813*
AK-Spore® H.C. Ophthalmic ***(Discontinued)*** *see* bacitracin, neomycin, polymyxin B, and hydrocortisone *on page 120*
AK-Spore® H.C. Otic ***(Discontinued)*** *see* neomycin, polymyxin B, and hydrocortisone *on page 688*
AK-Spore® Ophthalmic Ointment ***(Discontinued)*** *see* bacitracin, neomycin, and polymyxin B *on page 119*
AK-Taine® ***(Discontinued)*** *see* proparacaine *on page 826*
Akten™ [US] *see* lidocaine *on page 584*
AKTob® [US] *see* tobramycin *on page 965*
AK-Tracin® ***(Discontinued)*** *see* bacitracin *on page 118*
AK-Trol® Ophthalmic Ointment ***(Discontinued)*** *see* neomycin, polymyxin B, and dexamethasone *on page 687*
AK-Trol® Ophthalmic Suspension ***(Discontinued)*** *see* neomycin, polymyxin B, and dexamethasone *on page 687*
Akurza ***(Discontinued)*** *see* salicylic acid *on page 884*
Akwa Tears® [US-OTC] *see* artificial tears *on page 100*
Alamag [US-OTC] *see* aluminum hydroxide and magnesium hydroxide *on page 55*
Alamag Plus [US-OTC] *see* aluminum hydroxide, magnesium hydroxide, and simethicone *on page 56*
Alamast® [US/Can] *see* pemirolast *on page 759*
Alavert® Allergy 24 Hour [US-OTC] *see* loratadine *on page 599*
Alavert™ Allergy and Sinus [US-OTC] *see* loratadine and pseudoephedrine *on page 599*
Alavert® Children's Allergy [US-OTC] *see* loratadine *on page 599*
Alaway™ [US-OTC] *see* ketotifen *on page 559*
Alazide® ***(Discontinued)*** *see* hydrochlorothiazide and spironolactone *on page 500*
Albalon-A® Ophthalmic ***(Discontinued)***
Albalon® ***(Discontinued)*** *see* naphazoline *on page 680*

albendazole (al BEN da zole)

Sound-Alike/Look-Alike Issues
Albenza® may be confused with Aplenzin™, Relenza®

U.S./Canadian Brand Names Albenza® [US]

Therapeutic Category Anthelmintic

Use Treatment of parenchymal neurocysticercosis caused by *Taenia solium* and cystic hydatid disease of the liver, lung, and peritoneum caused by *Echinococcus granulosus*

Usual Dosage Oral: Children and Adults:
Neurocysticercosis:
<60 kg: 15 mg/kg/day in 2 divided doses (maximum: 800 mg/day) for 8-30 days
≥60 kg: 800 mg/day in 2 divided doses for 8-30 days
Note: Give concurrent anticonvulsant and steroid therapy during first week.
Hydatid:
<60 kg: 15 mg/kg/day in 2 divided doses (maximum: 800 mg/day)
≥60 kg: 800 mg/day in 2 divided doses
Note: Administer dose for three 28-day cycles with a 14-day drug-free interval in between. The manufacturer recommends a total of 3 cycles.

Dosage Forms
Tablet:
Albenza®: 200 mg

Albenza® [US] *see* albendazole *on page 40*
Albert® Glyburide [Can] *see* glyburide *on page 467*
Albert® Pentoxifylline [Can] *see* pentoxifylline *on page 766*
Albumarc® [US] *see* albumin *on page 40*

albumin (al BYOO min)

Sound-Alike/Look-Alike Issues
Albutein® may be confused with albuterol
Buminate® may be confused with bumetanide

Synonyms albumin (human); normal human serum albumin; normal serum albumin (human); salt-poor albumin; SPA

U.S./Canadian Brand Names Albumarc® [US]; Albuminar® [US]; AlbuRx™ [US]; Albutein® [US]; Buminate® [US]; Flexbumin [US]; Plasbumin® [US]; Plasbumin®-25 [Can]; Plasbumin®-5 [Can]

Therapeutic Category Blood Product Derivative

Use Plasma volume expansion and maintenance of cardiac output in the treatment of certain types of shock or impending shock; may be useful for burn patients, ARDS, and cardiopulmonary bypass; other uses considered by some investigators (but not proven) are retroperitoneal surgery, peritonitis, and ascites; unless the condition responsible for hypoproteinemia can be corrected, albumin can provide only symptomatic relief or supportive treatment

Usual Dosage I.V.:
5% should be used in hypovolemic patients or intravascularly-depleted patients
25% should be used in patients in whom fluid and sodium intake must be minimized
Dose depends on condition of patient:
Children: Hypovolemia: 0.5-1 g/kg/dose (10-20 mL/kg/dose of albumin 5%); maximum dose: 6 g/kg/day
Adults: Usual dose: 25 g; initial dose may be repeated in 15-30 minutes if response is inadequate; no more than 250 g should be administered within 48 hours
Hypoproteinemia: 0.5-1 g/kg/dose; repeat every 1-2 days as calculated to replace ongoing losses
Hypovolemia: 5% albumin: 0.5-1 g/kg/dose; repeat as needed. **Note:** May be considered after inadequate response to crystalloid therapy and when nonprotein colloids are contraindicated. The volume administered and the speed of infusion should be adapted to individual response.

Dosage Forms
Injection, solution [preservative free; human]: 5% (250 mL, 500 mL); 25% (50 mL, 100 mL)
Albuminar®: 5% (50 mL, 250 mL, 500 mL) [50 mg/mL]; 25% (20 mL, 50 mL, 100 mL) [250 mg/mL]
AlbuRx™: 5% (250 mL, 500 mL) [50 mg/mL]; 25% (50 mL, 100 mL) [250 mg/mL]
Albutein®: 5% (250 mL, 500 mL) [50 mg/mL]
Buminate®: 5% (250 mL, 500 mL) [50 mg/mL]; 25% (20 mL, 50 mL, 100 mL) [250 mg/mL]
Flexbumin: 25% (50 mL, 100 mL) [250 mg/mL]
Human Albumin Grifols®: 25% (50 mL, 100 mL) [250 mg/mL]
Plasbumin®: 5% (50 mL, 250 mL) [50 mg/mL]; 25% (20 mL, 50 mL, 100 mL) [250 mg/mL]

Albuminar® [US] *see* albumin *on page 40*
albumin-bound paclitaxel *see* paclitaxel (protein bound) *on page 743*
albumin (human) *see* albumin *on page 40*
albumin-stabilized nanoparticle paclitaxel *see* paclitaxel (protein bound) *on page 743*
Albumisol® ***(Discontinued)*** *see* albumin *on page 40*
Albunex® ***(Discontinued)*** *see* albumin *on page 40*
AlbuRx™ [US] *see* albumin *on page 40*
Albutein® [US] *see* albumin *on page 40*

albuterol (al BYOO ter ole)

Sound-Alike/Look-Alike Issues
albuterol may be confused with Albutein®, atenolol
Proventil® may be confused with Bentyl®, Prilosec® Prinivil®
salbutamol may be confused with salmeterol
Ventolin® may be confused with phentolamine, Benylin®, Vantin®
Volmax® may be confused with Flomax®

Synonyms albuterol sulfate; salbutamol; salbutamol sulphate

U.S./Canadian Brand Names AccuNeb® [US]; Airomir [Can]; Alti-Salbutamol [Can]; Apo-Salvent® CFC Free [Can]; Apo-Salvent® Respirator Solution [Can]; Apo-Salvent® Sterules [Can]; Apo-Salvent® [Can]; Gen-Salbutamol [Can]; PMS-Salbutamol [Can]; ProAir® HFA [US]; Proventil® HFA [US]; ratio-Inspra-Sal [Can]; ratio-Salbutamol [Can]; Rhoxal-salbutamol [Can]; Salbu-2 [Can]; Salbu-4 [Can]; Ventolin® Diskus [Can]; Ventolin® HFA [US/Can]; Ventolin® I.V. Infusion [Can]; Ventolin® [Can]; Ventrodisk [Can]; VoSpire ER® [US]

Therapeutic Category Adrenergic Agonist Agent

Use Bronchodilator in reversible airway obstruction due to asthma or COPD; prevention of exercise-induced bronchospasm

Usual Dosage

Oral:
Children: Bronchospasm:
2-6 years: 0.1-0.2 mg/kg/dose 3 times/day; maximum dose not to exceed 12 mg/day (divided doses)
6-12 years: 2 mg/dose 3-4 times/day; maximum dose not to exceed 24 mg/day (divided doses)
Extended release: 4 mg every 12 hours; maximum dose not to exceed 24 mg/day (divided doses)
Children >12 years and Adults: Bronchospasm (treatment): 2-4 mg/dose 3-4 times/day; maximum dose not to exceed 32 mg/day (divided doses)
Extended release: 8 mg every 12 hours; maximum dose not to exceed 32 mg/day (divided doses). A 4 mg dose every 12 hours may be sufficient in some patients, such as adults of low body weight.

Metered-dose inhaler (90 mcg/puff):
Children ≤4 years:
Quick relief: 1-2 puffs every 4-6 hours as needed
Exacerbation of asthma (acute, severe): 4-8 puffs every 20 minutes for 3 doses, then every 1-4 hours as needed
Exercise-induced bronchospasm (prevention): 1-2 puffs 5 minutes prior to exercise
Children 5-11 years:
Bronchospasm, quick relief: 2 puffs every 4-6 hours as needed
Exacerbation of asthma (acute, severe): 4-8 puffs every 20 minutes for 3 doses, then every 1-4 hours as needed
Exercise-induced bronchospasm (prevention): 2 puffs 5-30 minutes prior to exercise
Children ≥12 years and Adults:
Bronchospasm, quick relief: 2 puffs every 4-6 hours as needed
Exacerbation of asthma (acute, severe): 4-8 puffs every 20 minutes for up to 4 hours, then every 1-4 hours as needed
Exercise-induced bronchospasm (prevention): 2 puffs 5-30 minutes prior to exercise

Solution for nebulization:
Children 2-12 years (AccuNeb®): Bronchospasm: 0.63-1.25 mg every 4-6 hours as needed
Children ≤4 years:
Quick relief: 0.63-2.5 mg every 4-6 hours as needed
Exacerbation of asthma (acute, severe): 0.15 mg/kg (minimum: 2.5 mg) every 20 minutes for 3 doses, then 0.15-0.3 mg/kg (maximum: 10 mg) every 1-4 hours as needed **or** 0.5 mg/kg/hour by continuous nebulization

Children 5-11 years:
Quick relief: 1.25-5 mg every 4-8 hours as needed
Exacerbation of asthma (acute, severe): 0.15 mg/kg (minimum: 2.5 mg) every 20 minutes for 3 doses, then 0.15-0.3 mg/kg (maximum: 10 mg) every 1-4 hours as needed **or** 0.5 mg/kg/hour by continuous nebulization
Children ≥12 years and Adults:
Bronchospasm: 2.5 mg every 4-8 hours as needed
Quick relief: 1.25-5 mg every 4-8 hours as needed
Exacerbation of asthma (acute, severe): 2.5-5 mg every 20 minutes for 3 doses then 2.5-10 mg every 1-4 hours as needed, **or** 10-15 mg/hour by continuous nebulization

I.V. continuous infusion: Adults (Ventolin® I.V. solution [not available in U.S.]): Severe bronchospasm and status asthmaticus: Initial: 5 mcg/minute; may increase up to 10-20 mcg/minute at 15- to 30-minute intervals if needed

Dosage Forms [CAN] = Canadian brand name
Aerosol, for oral inhalation:
ProAir® HFA: 90 mcg/metered inhalation (8.5 g)
Proventil® HFA: 90 mcg/metered inhalation (6.7 g)
Ventolin® HFA: 90 mcg/metered inhalation (8 g, 18 g)
Injection, solution, as sulphate:
Ventolin® I.V. [CAN]: 1 mg/1mL (5 mL) [not available in U.S.]
Solution for nebulization [preservative free]: 0.021% (3 mL); 0.042% (3 mL); 0.083% (3 mL); 0.5% (0.5 mL, 20 mL)
AccuNeb®: 0.021% (3 mL); 0.042% (3 mL)
Syrup, oral: 2 mg/5 mL
Tablet, oral: 2 mg, 4 mg
Tablet, extended release, oral: 4 mg, 8 mg
VoSpire ER®: 4 mg, 8 mg

albuterol and ipratropium *see* ipratropium and albuterol *on page 545*
albuterol sulfate *see* albuterol *on page 41*
Alcaine® [US/Can] *see* proparacaine *on page 826*
Alcalak [US-OTC] *see* calcium carbonate *on page 170*

alclometasone (al kloe MET a sone)

Sound-Alike/Look-Alike Issues
Aclovate® may be confused with Accolate®
Synonyms alclometasone dipropionate
U.S./Canadian Brand Names Aclovate® [US]
Therapeutic Category Corticosteroid, Topical
Use Treatment of inflammation of corticosteroid-responsive dermatosis (low to medium potency topical corticosteroid)
Usual Dosage Note: Therapy should be discontinued when control is achieved; if no improvement is seen within 2 weeks, reassessment of diagnosis may be necessary.
Topical:
Children ≥1 year: Apply thin film to affected area 2-3 times/day; do not use for >3 weeks
Adults: Apply a thin film to the affected area 2-3 times/day
Dosage Forms
Cream: 0.05% (15 g, 45 g, 60 g)
Aclovate®: 0.05% (15 g, 60 g)
Ointment: 0.05% (15 g, 45 g, 60 g)
Aclovate®: 0.05% (15 g, 45 g, 60 g)

alclometasone dipropionate *see* alclometasone *on page 42*
alcohol, absolute *see* alcohol (ethyl) *on page 42*
alcohol, dehydrated *see* alcohol (ethyl) *on page 42*

alcohol (ethyl) (AL koe hol, ETH il)

Sound-Alike/Look-Alike Issues
ethanol may be confused with Ethyol®, Ethamolin®
Synonyms alcohol, absolute; alcohol, dehydrated; ethanol; ethyl alcohol; EtOH

U.S./Canadian Brand Names Biobase-G™ [Can]; Biobase™ [Can]; EpiClenz™ [US-OTC]; Gel-Stat™ [US-OTC]; GelRite [US-OTC]; Isagel® [US-OTC]; Lavacol® [US-OTC]; Prevacare® [US-OTC]; Protection Plus® [US-OTC]; Purell® 2 in 1 [US-OTC]; Purell® with Aloe [US-OTC]; Purell® [US-OTC]

Therapeutic Category Intravenous Nutritional Therapy; Pharmaceutical Aid

Use Topical antiinfective; pharmaceutical aid; therapeutic neurolysis (nerve or ganglion block); replenishment of fluid and carbohydrate calories

Usual Dosage

Antiseptic: Children and Adults: Liquid denatured alcohol: Topical: Apply 1-3 times/day as needed

Therapeutic neurolysis (nerve or ganglion block): Adults: Dehydrated alcohol injection 98%: Intraneural: Dosage variable depending upon the site of injection (eg, trigeminal neuralgia: 0.05-0.5 mL as a single injection per interspace vs subarachnoid injection: 0.5-1 mL as a single injection per interspace); single doses >1.5 mL are seldom required

Replenishment of fluid and carbohydrate calories: Adults: Dehydrated alcohol infusion: Alcohol 5% and dextrose 5%: 1-2 L/day by slow infusion

Dosage Forms

Foam, topical:

Epi-Clenz™ [OTC]: 62% (240 mL, 480 mL)

Gel, topical:

Epi-Clenz™ [OTC]: 70% (45 mL, 120 mL, 480 mL)
GelRite [OTC]: 67% (120 mL, 480 mL, 800 mL)
Gel-Stat™ [OTC]: 62% (120 mL, 480 mL)
Isagel® [OTC]: 60% (59 mL, 118 mL, 621 mL, 800 mL)
Prevacare® [OTC]: 60% (120 mL, 240 mL, 960 mL, 1200 mL, 1500 mL)
Protection Plus® [OTC]: 62% (800 mL)
Purell® [OTC]: 62% (15 mL, 30 mL, 59 mL, 120 mL, 236 mL, 250 mL, 360 mL, 500 mL, 800 mL, 1000 mL, 2000 mL)
Purell® Moisture Therapy [OTC]: 62% (75 mL)
Purell® with Aloe [OTC]: 62% (15 mL, 59 mL, 236 mL, 360 mL, 800 mL, 1000 mL, 2000 mL)

Injection, solution [dehydrated]: 98% (1 mL, 5 mL)

Liquid, topical [denatured]: 70% (3840 mL)

Lavacol® [OTC]: 70% (473 mL)

Lotion, topical:

Purell® 2 in 1 [OTC]: 62% (60 mL, 360 mL, 1000 mL)

Towlettes, topical:

Isagel® [OTC]: 60% (50s, 300s)
Purell® [OTC]: 62% (35s, 175s)

Alcomicin® [Can] *see* gentamicin *on page 461*
Alconefrin® Nasal Solution *(Discontinued)* *see* phenylephrine *on page 774*
Alcortin™ [US] *see* iodoquinol and hydrocortisone *on page 539*
Aldactazide® [US] *see* hydrochlorothiazide and spironolactone *on page 500*
Aldactazide 25® [Can] *see* hydrochlorothiazide and spironolactone *on page 500*
Aldactazide 50® [Can] *see* hydrochlorothiazide and spironolactone *on page 500*
Aldactone® [US/Can] *see* spironolactone *on page 920*
Aldara® [US/Can] *see* imiquimod *on page 522*

aldesleukin (al des LOO kin)

Sound-Alike/Look-Alike Issues

aldesleukin may be confused with oprelvekin
Proleukin® may be confused with oprelvekin

Synonyms epidermal thymocyte activating factor; IL-2; interleukin-2; lymphocyte mitogenic factor; NSC-373364; T-cell growth factor; TCGF; thymocyte stimulating factor

U.S./Canadian Brand Names Proleukin® [US/Can]

Therapeutic Category Biological Response Modulator

Use Treatment of metastatic renal cell cancer, metastatic melanoma

Usual Dosage Refer to individual protocols. I.V.:

Renal cell carcinoma: 600,000 int. units/kg every 8 hours for a maximum of 14 doses; repeat after 9 days for a total of 28 doses per course. Retreat if needed 7 weeks after previous course.

Melanoma: Single-agent use: 600,000 int. units/kg every 8 hours for a maximum of 14 doses; repeat after 9 days for a total of 28 doses per course. Retreat if needed 7 weeks after previous course.

Dosage Forms

Injection, powder for reconstitution:

Proleukin®: 22 x 10^6 int. units

Aldex™ [US] *see* guaifenesin and phenylephrine *on page* 475
Aldex® AN [US] *see* doxylamine *on page* 338
Aldex® CT [US] *see* diphenhydramine and phenylephrine *on page* 317
Aldex®D [US] *see* phenylephrine and pyrilamine *on page* 776
Aldex® DM [US] *see* phenylephrine, pyrilamine, and dextromethorphan *on page* 778
Aldomet® *(Discontinued)* *see* methyldopa *on page* 643
Aldoril® D50 *(Discontinued)* *see* methyldopa and hydrochlorothiazide *on page* 643
Aldoril® *(Discontinued)* *see* methyldopa and hydrochlorothiazide *on page* 643
Aldroxicon I [US-OTC] *see* aluminum hydroxide, magnesium hydroxide, and simethicone *on page* 56
Aldroxicon II [US-OTC] *see* aluminum hydroxide, magnesium hydroxide, and simethicone *on page* 56
Aldurazyme® [US/Can] *see* laronidase *on page* 573

alefacept (a LE fa sept)

Synonyms B 9273; BG 9273; human LFA-3/IgG(1) fusion protein; LFA-3/IgG(1) fusion protein, human

U.S./Canadian Brand Names Amevive® [US/Can]

Therapeutic Category Monoclonal Antibody

Use Treatment of moderate-to-severe chronic plaque psoriasis in adults who are candidates for systemic therapy or phototherapy

Usual Dosage Adults:

I.M.: 15 mg once weekly; usual duration of treatment: 12 weeks

A second course of treatment may be initiated at least 12 weeks after completion of the initial course of treatment, provided $CD4^+$ T-lymphocyte counts are within the normal range.

Note: $CD4^+$ T-lymphocyte counts should be monitored before initiation of treatment and every 2 weeks during therapy. Dosing should be withheld if $CD4^+$ counts are <250 cells/µL, and dosing should be permanently discontinued if $CD4^+$ lymphocyte counts remain at <250 cells/µL for longer than 1 month.

Dosage Forms

Injection, powder for reconstitution [I.M. administration]:

Amevive®: 15 mg

alemtuzumab (ay lem TU zoo mab)

Synonyms C1H; campath-1H; humanized IgG1 anti-CD52 monoclonal antibody; NSC-715969

U.S./Canadian Brand Names Campath® [US]; MabCampath® [Can]

Therapeutic Category Antineoplastic Agent, Monoclonal Antibody

Use Treatment of B-cell chronic lymphocytic leukemia (B-CLL)

Usual Dosage Note: Dose escalation is required; usually accomplished in 3-7 days. Single doses >30 mg or cumulative doses >90 mg/week increase the incidence of pancytopenia. Pretreatment (with acetaminophen and diphenhydramine) is recommended prior to the first dose, with dose escalations, and as clinically indicated; I.V. hydrocortisone may be used for severe infusion-related reactions.

I.V. infusion: Adults: B-cell CLL: Initial: 3 mg/day beginning on day 1; if tolerated (infusion reaction ≤grade 2), increase to 10 mg/day; if tolerated (infusion reaction ≤grade 2), increase to maintenance of 30 mg/dose 3 times/week on alternate days for a total duration of therapy of up to 12 weeks

Dosage Forms

Injection, solution [preservative free]:

Campath®: 30 mg/mL (1 mL)

alendronate (a LEN droe nate)

Sound-Alike/Look-Alike Issues

alendronate may be confused with risedronate

Fosamax® may be confused with Flomax®, Fosamax Plus D™, fosinopril, Zithromax®

Synonyms alendronate sodium; alendronic acid monosodium salt trihydrate; MK-217

U.S./Canadian Brand Names Apo-Alendronate® [Can]; CO Alendronate [Can]; Dom-Alendronate [Can]; Fosamax® [US/Can]; Gen-Alendronate [Can]; Novo-Alendronate [Can]; PHL-Alendronate [Can]; PHL-Alendronate-FC [Can]; PMS-Alendronate [Can]; PMS-Alendronate-FC [Can]; ratio-Alendronate [Can]; Riva-Alendronate [Can]; Sandoz Alendronate [Can]

Therapeutic Category Bisphosphonate Derivative

Use Treatment and prevention of osteoporosis in postmenopausal females; treatment of osteoporosis in males; Paget disease of the bone in patients who are symptomatic, at risk for future complications, or with alkaline phosphatase ≥2 times the upper limit of normal; treatment of glucocorticoid-induced osteoporosis in males and females with low bone mineral density who are receiving a daily dosage ≥7.5 mg of prednisone (or equivalent)

Usual Dosage Oral: Adults: **Note:** Patients treated with glucocorticoids and those with Paget disease should receive adequate amounts of calcium and vitamin D.

Osteoporosis in postmenopausal females:

Prophylaxis: 5 mg once daily **or** 35 mg once weekly

Treatment: 10 mg once daily **or** 70 mg once weekly

Osteoporosis in males: 10 mg once daily **or** 70 mg once weekly

Osteoporosis secondary to glucocorticoids in males and females: Treatment: 5 mg once daily; a dose of 10 mg once daily should be used in postmenopausal females who are not receiving estrogen.

Paget disease of bone in males and females: 40 mg once daily for 6 months

Retreatment: Relapses during the 12 months following therapy occurred in 9% of patients who responded to treatment. Specific retreatment data are not available. Following a 6-month post-treatment evaluation period, retreatment with alendronate may be considered in patients who have relapsed based on increases in serum alkaline phosphatase, which should be measured periodically. Retreatment may also be considered in those who failed to normalize their serum alkaline phosphatase.

Dosage Forms

Solution, oral:

Fosamax®: 70 mg/75 mL

Tablet: 5 mg, 10 mg, 35 mg, 40 mg, 70 mg

Fosamax®: 5 mg, 10 mg, 35 mg, 40 mg, 70 mg

alendronate and cholecalciferol (a LEN droe nate & kole e kal SI fer ole)

Sound-Alike/Look-Alike Issues

Fosamax Plus D™ may be confused with Fosamax®

Synonyms alendronate sodium and cholecalciferol; cholecalciferol and alendronate; vitamin D_3 and alendronate

U.S./Canadian Brand Names Fosamax Plus D™ [US]; Fosavance [Can]

Therapeutic Category Bisphosphonate Derivative; Vitamin D Analog

Use Treatment of osteoporosis in postmenopausal females; increase bone mass in males with osteoporosis

Usual Dosage Oral: Adults: One tablet (alendronate 70 mg/cholecalciferol 2800 int. units **or** alendronate 70 mg/cholecalciferol 5600 int. units) once weekly. Appropriate dose in most osteoporotic women or men: Alendronate 70 mg/cholecalciferol 5600 int. units once weekly.

Dosage Forms

Tablet:

Fosamax Plus D™ 70/2800: Alendronate 70 mg and cholecalciferol 2800 int. units

Fosamax Plus D™ 70/5600: Alendronate 70 mg and cholecalciferol 5600 int. units

alendronate sodium *see* alendronate *on page* 44
alendronate sodium and cholecalciferol *see* alendronate and cholecalciferol *on page* 45
alendronic acid monosodium salt trihydrate *see* alendronate *on page* 44
Alenic Alka *(Discontinued)* *see* aluminum hydroxide and magnesium carbonate *on page* 55
Alenic Alka Tablet [US-OTC] *see* aluminum hydroxide and magnesium trisilicate *on page* 56
Aler-Cap [US-OTC] *see* diphenhydramine *on page* 315
Aler-Dryl [US-OTC] *see* diphenhydramine *on page* 315
Aler-Tab [US-OTC] *see* diphenhydramine *on page* 315
Alertec® [Can] *see* modafinil *on page* 664
Alesse® [US/Can] *see* ethinyl estradiol and levonorgestrel *on page* 387
Aleve® [US-OTC] *see* naproxen *on page* 681
Aleve®-D Sinus & Cold [US-OTC] *see* naproxen and pseudoephedrine *on page* 682
Aleve®-D Sinus & Headache [US-OTC] *see* naproxen and pseudoephedrine *on page* 682
Aleve® Cold & Sinus *(Discontinued)* *see* naproxen and pseudoephedrine *on page* 682
Alfenta® [US/Can] *see* alfentanil *on page* 46

alfentanil (al FEN ta nil)

Sound-Alike/Look-Alike Issues

alfentanil may be confused with Anafranil®, fentanyl, remifentanil, sufentanil

Alfenta® may be confused with Sufenta®

Synonyms alfentanil hydrochloride

U.S./Canadian Brand Names Alfentanil Injection, USP [Can]; Alfenta® [US/Can]

Therapeutic Category Analgesic, Narcotic; General Anesthetic

Controlled Substance C-II

Use Analgesic adjunct for the induction and maintenance of general anesthesia; analgesic component for monitored anesthesia care (MAC)

Usual Dosage Doses should be titrated to appropriate effects; wide range of doses is dependent upon desired degree of analgesia/anesthesia. Adults: Dose should be based on ideal body weight.

Dosage Forms

Injection, solution [preservative free]: 500 mcg/mL (2 mL, 5 mL)

Alfenta®: 500 mcg/mL (2 mL, 5 mL, 10 mL, 20 mL)

alfentanil hydrochloride *see* alfentanil *on page 46*

Alfentanil Injection, USP [Can] *see* alfentanil *on page 46*

Alferon® N [US/Can] *see* interferon alfa-n3 *on page 535*

alfuzosin (al FYOO zoe sin)

Synonyms alfuzosin hydrochloride

U.S./Canadian Brand Names Apo-Alfuzosin [Can]; Sandoz-Alfuzosin [Can]; Uroxatral® [US]; Xatral [Can]

Therapeutic Category Alpha-Adrenergic Blocking Agent

Use Treatment of the functional symptoms of benign prostatic hyperplasia (BPH)

Usual Dosage Oral: Adults: 10 mg once daily

Dosage Forms

Tablet, extended release:

Uroxatral®: 10 mg

alfuzosin hydrochloride *see* alfuzosin *on page 46*

alglucerase (al GLOO ser ase)

Sound-Alike/Look-Alike Issues

alglucerase may be confused with agalsidase alfa, agalsidase beta, alglucosidase alfa

Ceredase® may be confused with Cerezyme®

Synonyms glucocerebrosidase

U.S./Canadian Brand Names Ceredase® [US]

Therapeutic Category Enzyme

Use Replacement therapy for Gaucher disease (type 1)

Usual Dosage I.V.: Children and Adults: Initial: 30-60 units/kg every 2 weeks; dosing is individualized based on disease severity; average dose: 60 units/kg every 2 weeks. Range: 2.5 units/kg 3 times/week to 60 units/kg once weekly to every 4 weeks. Once patient response is well established, dose may be reduced every 3-6 months to determine maintenance therapy.

Dosage Forms

Injection, solution [preservative free]:

Ceredase®: 80 units/mL (5 mL)

alglucosidase *see* alglucosidase alfa *on page 46*

alglucosidase alfa (al gloo KOSE i dase AL fa)

Sound-Alike/Look-Alike Issues

alglucosidase alfa may be confused with agalsidase alfa, agalsidase beta, alglucerase

Synonyms alglucosidase; GAA; rhGAA

U.S./Canadian Brand Names Myozyme® [US]

Therapeutic Category Enzyme

Use Replacement therapy for Pompe disease (infantile onset)

Usual Dosage I.V.: Children 1 month to 3.5 years (at first infusion): 20 mg/kg over ~4 hours every 2 weeks

Product Availability Myozyme®: January 2009: Critical shortage in international markets, including the U.S.; recommended guidelines for drug distribution can be found at http://www.myozyme.com/pdf/MTAP_Supply_Update_January%202009.pdf

Dosage Forms

Injection, powder for reconstitution [preservative free]:

Myozyme®: 50 mg

Aliclen™ [US] *see* salicylic acid *on page 884*

Alimta® [US/Can] *see* pemetrexed *on page 758*

Alinia® [US] *see* nitazoxanide *on page 698*

aliskiren (a lis KYE ren)

Synonyms aliskiren hemifumarate; SPP100

U.S./Canadian Brand Names Rasilez® [Can]; Tekturna® [US]

Therapeutic Category Renin Inhibitor

Use Treatment of hypertension, alone or in combination with other antihypertensive agents

Usual Dosage Oral: Adults: Initial: 150 mg once daily; may increase to 300 mg once daily (maximum: 300 mg/day). **Note:** Prior to initiation, correct hypovolemia and/or closely monitor volume status in patients on concurrent diuretics during treatment initiation.

Dosage Forms

Tablet:

Tekturna®: 150 mg, 300 mg

aliskiren and hydrochlorothiazide (a lis KYE ren & hye droe klor oh THYE a zide)

Synonyms aliskiren hemifumarate and hydrochlorothiazide; hydrochlorothiazide and aliskiren

U.S./Canadian Brand Names Tekturna HCT® [US]

Therapeutic Category Antihypertensive Agent, Combination; Diuretic, Thiazide; Renin Inhibitor

Use Treatment of hypertension (not recommended for initial treatment)

Usual Dosage Oral: Adults: One tablet daily; dosage must be individualized (see below). May be substituted for previously titrated dosages of the individual components. Titrate at 2- to 4-week intervals as necessary.

Patients not controlled with single-agent therapy: Initiate by adding the lowest available dose of the alternative component (aliskiren 150 mg or hydrochlorothiazide 12.5 mg); titrate to effect (maximum daily aliskiren dose: 300 mg; maximum daily hydrochlorothiazide dose: 25 mg)

Dosage Forms

Tablet:

Tekturna HCT®: 150/12.5: Aliskiren 150 mg and hydrochlorothiazide 12.5 mg; 150/25: Aliskiren 150 mg and hydrochlorothiazide 25 mg; 300/12.5: Aliskiren 300 mg and hydrochlorothiazide 12.5 mg; 300/25: Aliskiren 300 mg and hydrochlorothiazide 25 mg

aliskiren hemifumarate *see* aliskiren *on page 47*

aliskiren hemifumarate and hydrochlorothiazide *see* aliskiren and hydrochlorothiazide *on page 47*

alitretinoin (a li TRET i noyn)

Sound-Alike/Look-Alike Issues

Panretin® may be confused with pancreatin

U.S./Canadian Brand Names Panretin® [US/Can]

Therapeutic Category Antineoplastic Agent; Retinoic Acid Derivative

Use **Orphan drug:** Topical treatment of cutaneous lesions in AIDS-related Kaposi sarcoma

Usual Dosage Topical: Apply gel twice daily to cutaneous lesions

Dosage Forms

Gel:

Panretin®: 0.1% (60 g)

Alka-Mints® [US-OTC] *see* calcium carbonate *on page 170*

Alka-Seltzer Plus® Day Cold [US-OTC] *see* acetaminophen, dextromethorphan, and phenylephrine *on page 27*

Alka-Seltzer Plus® Sinus Formula [US-OTC] *see* acetaminophen and phenylephrine *on page 22*

Alka-Seltzer® P.M. [US-OTC] *see* aspirin and diphenhydramine *on page 105*

Alkeran® [US/Can] *see* melphalan *on page* 622
Allanderm-T™ ***(Discontinued)*** *see* trypsin, balsam Peru, and castor oil *on page* 993
AllanEnzyme ***(Discontinued)*** *see* papain and urea *on page* 749
Allanfil 405 ***(Discontinued)*** *see* chlorophyllin, papain, and urea *on page* 211
Allanfil Spray ***(Discontinued)*** *see* chlorophyllin, papain, and urea *on page* 211
AllanFol RX ***(Discontinued)*** *see* folic acid, cyanocobalamin, and pyridoxine *on page* 440
AllanHist PDX [US] *see* brompheniramine, pseudoephedrine, and dextromethorphan *on page* 152
AllanTan Pediatric ***(Discontinued)*** *see* chlorpheniramine and phenylephrine *on page* 214
AllanVan-DM [US] *see* phenylephrine, pyrilamine, and dextromethorphan *on page* 778
AllanVan-S ***(Discontinued)*** *see* phenylephrine and pyrilamine *on page* 776
Allbee® C-800 [US-OTC] *see* vitamin B complex combinations *on page* 1017
Allbee® C-800 + Iron [US-OTC] *see* vitamin B complex combinations *on page* 1017
Allbee® with C [US-OTC] *see* vitamin B complex combinations *on page* 1017
Allegra® [US/Can] *see* fexofenadine *on page* 416
Allegra® 60 mg Capsule ***(Discontinued)*** *see* fexofenadine *on page* 416
Allegra-D® [Can] *see* fexofenadine and pseudoephedrine *on page* 417
Allegra-D® 12 Hour [US] *see* fexofenadine and pseudoephedrine *on page* 417
Allegra-D® 24 Hour [US] *see* fexofenadine and pseudoephedrine *on page* 417
Allegra® ODT [US] *see* fexofenadine *on page* 416
Aller-Chlor® [US-OTC] *see* chlorpheniramine *on page* 213
Allercon® Tablet ***(Discontinued)*** *see* triprolidine and pseudoephedrine *on page* 989
Allerdryl® [Can] *see* diphenhydramine *on page* 315
AllerDur™ ***(Discontinued)*** *see* dexchlorpheniramine and pseudoephedrine *on page* 290
Allerest® 12 Hour Nasal Solution ***(Discontinued)*** *see* oxymetazoline *on page* 740
Allerest® Eye Drops ***(Discontinued)*** *see* naphazoline *on page* 680
Allerest® Maximum Strength Allergy and Hay Fever [US-OTC] *see* chlorpheniramine and pseudoephedrine *on page* 215
Allerfrim [US-OTC] *see* triprolidine and pseudoephedrine *on page* 989
Allerfrin® Syrup ***(Discontinued)*** *see* triprolidine and pseudoephedrine *on page* 989
Allerfrin® Tablet ***(Discontinued)*** *see* triprolidine and pseudoephedrine *on page* 989
Allerfrin® with Codeine ***(Discontinued)*** *see* triprolidine, pseudoephedrine, and codeine *(Canada only) on page* 990
Allergen® [US] *see* antipyrine and benzocaine *on page* 85
AllerMax® [US-OTC] *see* diphenhydramine *on page* 315
Allernix [Can] *see* diphenhydramine *on page* 315
AllerTan™ ***(Discontinued)*** *see* chlorpheniramine, pyrilamine, and phenylephrine *on page* 221
AlleRx™-D [US] *see* pseudoephedrine and methscopolamine *on page* 835
AlleRx™ Dose Pack ***(Discontinued)*** *see* chlorpheniramine, pseudoephedrine, and methscopolamine *on page* 221
AlleRx™ Suspension ***(Discontinued)*** *see* chlorpheniramine and phenylephrine *on page* 214
Allfen [US-OTC] *see* guaifenesin *on page* 473
Allfen DM [US-OTC] *see* guaifenesin and dextromethorphan *on page* 474
Allfen ***(reformulation) (Discontinued)***
Alli™ [US-OTC] *see* orlistat *on page* 729
All-Nite [US-OTC] *see* acetaminophen, dextromethorphan, and doxylamine *on page* 26
All-Nite Cold [US-OTC] *see* acetaminophen, dextromethorphan, doxylamine, and pseudoephedrine *on page* 28
Alloprin® [Can] *see* allopurinol *on page* 48

allopurinol (al oh PURE i nole)

Sound-Alike/Look-Alike Issues

allopurinol may be confused with Apresoline
Zyloprim® may be confused with Xylo-Pfan®, ZORprin®, Zovirax®

Synonyms allopurinol sodium

U.S./Canadian Brand Names Alloprin® [Can]; Aloprim™ [US]; Apo-Allopurinol® [Can]; Novo-Purol [Can]; Zyloprim® [US/Can]

Therapeutic Category Xanthine Oxidase Inhibitor

Use

Oral: Prevention of attack of gouty arthritis and nephropathy; treatment of secondary hyperuricemia which may occur during treatment of tumors or leukemia; prevention of recurrent calcium oxalate calculi

I.V.: Treatment of elevated serum and urinary uric acid levels when oral therapy is not tolerated in patients with leukemia, lymphoma, and solid tumor malignancies who are receiving cancer chemotherapy

Usual Dosage

Oral: Doses >300 mg should be given in divided doses.

Children ≤10 years: Secondary hyperuricemia associated with chemotherapy: 10 mg/kg/day in 2-3 divided doses **or** 200-300 mg/m^2/day in 2-4 divided doses, maximum: 800 mg/24 hours

Alternative (manufacturer labeling): <6 years: 150 mg/day in 3 divided doses; 6-10 years: 300 mg/day in 2-3 divided doses

Children >10 years and Adults:

Secondary hyperuricemia associated with chemotherapy: 600-800 mg/day in 2-3 divided doses for prevention of acute uric acid nephropathy for 2-3 days starting 1-2 days before chemotherapy

Gout: Mild: 200-300 mg/day; Severe: 400-600 mg/day; to reduce the possibility of acute gouty attacks, initiate dose at 100 mg/day and increase weekly to recommended dosage. Maximum daily dose: 800 mg/day.

Recurrent calcium oxalate stones: 200-300 mg/day in single or divided doses

I.V.: Hyperuricemia secondary to chemotherapy: Intravenous daily dose can be given as a single infusion or in equally divided doses at 6-, 8-, or 12-hour intervals. A fluid intake sufficient to yield a daily urinary output of at least 2 L in adults and the maintenance of a neutral or, preferably, slightly alkaline urine are desirable.

Children ≤10 years: Starting dose: 200 mg/m^2/day

Children >10 years and Adults: 200-400 mg/m^2/day (maximum: 600 mg/day)

Dosage Forms

Injection, powder for reconstitution: 500 mg (base)

Aloprim®: 500 mg (base)

Tablet: 100 mg, 300 mg

Zyloprim®: 100 mg, 300 mg

allopurinol sodium *see* allopurinol *on page 48*

all-*trans*-retinoic acid *see* tretinoin (systemic) *on page 980*

Almacone® [US-OTC] *see* aluminum hydroxide, magnesium hydroxide, and simethicone *on page 56*

Almacone Double Strength® [US-OTC] *see* aluminum hydroxide, magnesium hydroxide, and simethicone *on page 56*

almotriptan (al moh TRIP tan)

Sound-Alike/Look-Alike Issues

Axert® may be confused with Antivert®

Synonyms almotriptan malate

U.S./Canadian Brand Names Axert® [US/Can]

Therapeutic Category Serotonin 5-HT_{1D} Receptor Agonist

Use Acute treatment of migraine with or without aura in adults (with a history of migraine) and adolescents (with a history of migraine lasting ≥4 hours when left untreated)

Usual Dosage Oral: Children ≥12 years and Adults: Migraine: Initial: 6.25-12.5 mg in a single dose; if the headache returns, repeat the dose after 2 hours (maximum daily dose: 25 mg)

Note: The safety of treating more than 4 migraines/month has not been established.

Dosage Forms

Tablet:

Axert®: 6.25 mg, 12.5 mg

almotriptan malate *see* almotriptan *on page 49*

Alocril® [US/Can] *see* nedocromil (ophthalmic) *on page 685*

Alodox™ [US] *see* doxycycline *on page 336*

Aloe Vesta® Antifungal [US-OTC] *see* miconazole *on page 654*

Alomide® [US/Can] *see* lodoxamide *on page 596*

Alophen® [US-OTC] *see* bisacodyl *on page 142*

Aloprim™ [US] *see* allopurinol *on page 48*
Alor® 5/500 ***(Discontinued)***
Alora® [US] *see* estradiol *on page 373*

alosetron (a LOE se tron)

Sound-Alike/Look-Alike Issues
Lotronex® may be confused with Lovenox®, Protonix®

U.S./Canadian Brand Names Lotronex® [US]

Therapeutic Category 5-HT_3 Receptor Antagonist

Use Treatment of women with severe diarrhea-predominant irritable bowel syndrome (IBS) who have failed to respond to conventional therapy

Usual Dosage Oral: Adults: Female: Initial: 0.5 mg twice daily for 4 weeks, with or without food; if tolerated, but response is inadequate, may be increased after 4 weeks to 1 mg twice daily. If response is inadequate after 4 weeks of 1 mg twice-daily dosing, discontinue treatment.

Note: Discontinue immediately if constipation or signs/symptoms of ischemic colitis occur. Do not reinitiate in patients who develop ischemic colitis.

Dosage Forms
Tablet:
Lotronex®: 0.5 mg, 1 mg

Aloxi® [US] *see* palonosetron *on page 744*
Alpain [US] *see* acetaminophen and phenyltoloxamine *on page 23*
$alpha_1$-antitrypsin *see* $alpha_1$-proteinase inhibitor *on page 50*
$alpha_1$-PI *see* $alpha_1$-proteinase inhibitor *on page 50*
$alpha_1$-proteinase inhibitor, human *see* $alpha_1$-proteinase inhibitor *on page 50*

$alpha_1$-proteinase inhibitor (al fa won PRO tee in ase in HI bi tor)

Synonyms A_1-PI; $alpha_1$-antitrypsin; $alpha_1$-PI; $alpha_1$-proteinase inhibitor, human; α_1-PI

U.S./Canadian Brand Names Aralast NP [US]; Aralast [US]; Prolastin® [US/Can]; Zemaira® [US]

Therapeutic Category Antitrypsin Deficiency Agent

Use Replacement therapy in congenital $alpha_1$-antitrypsin deficiency with clinical emphysema

Usual Dosage I.V.: Adults: 60 mg/kg once weekly

Dosage Forms
Injection, powder for reconstitution [preservative free]:
Aralast, Aralast NP, Prolastin®: 500 mg, 1000 mg
Zemaira®: 1000 mg

alpha-galactosidase (AL fa ga lak TOE si days)

Sound-Alike/Look-Alike Issues
beano® may be confused with B&O (belladonna and opium)

Synonyms *Aspergillus niger*

U.S./Canadian Brand Names beano® [US-OTC]

Therapeutic Category Enzyme

Use Prevention of flatulence and bloating attributed to a variety of grains, cereals, nuts, and vegetables containing the sugars raffinose, stachyose, and/or verbascose

Usual Dosage Oral: Children ≥12 years and Adults:
Drops: Take 5 drops per serving of problem food; adjust according to number of problem foods per meal; usual dose/meal: 10-15 drops
Tablet: One tablet per serving of problem food; adjust according to number of problem foods per meal; usual dose/meal: 2-3 tablets

Dosage Forms
Liquid, oral [drops]:
beano®: 150 galactosidase units/5 drops
Tablet, oral:
beano®: 150 galactosidase units/tablet

alpha-galactosidase-A (gene-activated) *see* agalsidase alfa *(Canada only) on page 38*
alpha-galactosidase-A (recombinant) *see* agalsidase beta *on page 38*
1α-hydroxyergocalciferol *see* doxercalciferol *on page 334*

Alphagan® [Can] *see* brimonidine *on page 147*
Alphagan® *(Discontinued)* *see* brimonidine *on page 147*
Alphagan® P [US] *see* brimonidine *on page 147*
α-2-interferon *see* interferon alfa-2b *on page 534*
Alphamul® *(Discontinued)* *see* castor oil *on page 190*
Alphanate® *[new formulation]* [US] *see* antihemophilic factor/von Willebrand factor complex (human) *on page 83*
AlphaNine® SD [US] *see* factor IX *on page 403*
Alphaquin HP® [US] *see* hydroquinone *on page 508*
Alph-E [US-OTC] *see* vitamin E *on page 1018*
Alph-E-Mixed [US-OTC] *see* vitamin E *on page 1018*

alprazolam (al PRAY zoe lam)

Sound-Alike/Look-Alike Issues
ALPRAZolam may be confused with alprostadil, LORazepam, triazolam
Xanax® may be confused with Lanoxin®, Tenex®, Tylox®, Xopenex®, Zantac®, Zyrtec®

Tall-Man **ALPRAZ**olam

U.S./Canadian Brand Names Alprazolam Intensol® [US]; Alti-Alprazolam [Can]; Apo-Alpraz® TS [Can]; Apo-Alpraz® [Can]; Gen-Alprazolam [Can]; Niravam™ [US]; Novo-Alprazol [Can]; Nu-Alprax [Can]; Xanax TS™ [Can]; Xanax XR® [US]; Xanax® [US/Can]

Therapeutic Category Benzodiazepine

Controlled Substance C-IV

Use Treatment of anxiety disorder (GAD); panic disorder, with or without agoraphobia; anxiety associated with depression

Usual Dosage Oral: **Note:** Treatment >4 months should be reevaluated to determine the patient's continued need for the drug

Adults:

Anxiety: Immediate release: Effective doses are 0.5-4 mg/day in divided doses; the manufacturer recommends starting at 0.25-0.5 mg 3 times/day; titrate dose upward; usual maximum: 4 mg/day. Patients requiring doses >4 mg/day should be increased cautiously. Periodic reassessment and consideration of dosage reduction is recommended.

Anxiety associated with depression: Immediate release: Average dose required: 2.5-3 mg/day in divided doses

Panic disorder:

Immediate release: Initial: 0.5 mg 3 times/day; dose may be increased every 3-4 days in increments ≤1 mg/day. Mean effective dosage: 5-6 mg/day; many patients obtain relief at 2 mg/day, as much as 10 mg/day may be required

Extended release: 0.5-1 mg once daily; may increase dose every 3-4 days in increments ≤1 mg/day (range: 3-6 mg/day)

Switching from immediate release to extended release: Patients may be switched to extended release tablets by taking the total daily dose of the immediate release tablets and giving it once daily using the extended release preparation.

Preoperative sedation: 0.5 mg in evening at bedtime and 0.5 mg 1 hour before procedure

Dose reduction: Abrupt discontinuation should be avoided. Daily dose may be decreased by 0.5 mg every 3 days, however, some patients may require a slower reduction. If withdrawal symptoms occur, resume previous dose and discontinue on a less rapid schedule.

Dosage Forms

Solution, oral [concentrate]:
Alprazolam Intensol®: 1 mg/mL

Tablet: 0.25 mg, 0.5 mg, 1 mg, 2 mg
Xanax®: 0.25 mg, 0.5 mg, 1 mg, 2 mg

Tablet, extended release: 0.5 mg, 1 mg, 2 mg, 3 mg
Xanax XR®: 0.5 mg, 1 mg, 2 mg, 3 mg

Tablet, orally disintegrating [scored]: 0.25 mg, 0.5 mg, 1 mg, 2 mg
Niravam™: 0.25 mg, 0.5 mg, 1 mg, 2 mg

Alprazolam Intensol® [US] *see* alprazolam *on page 51*

alprostadil (al PROS ta dill)

Sound-Alike/Look-Alike Issues
alprostadil may be confused with alPRAZolam

Synonyms PGE_1; prostaglandin E_1

U.S./Canadian Brand Names Caverject Impulse® [US]; Caverject® [US/Can]; Edex® [US]; Muse® Pellet [Can]; Muse® [US]; Prostin VR Pediatric® [US]; Prostin® VR [Can]

Therapeutic Category Prostaglandin

Use

Prostin VR Pediatric®: Temporary maintenance of patency of ductus arteriosus in neonates with ductal-dependent congenital heart disease until surgery can be performed. These defects include cyanotic (eg, pulmonary atresia, pulmonary stenosis, tricuspid atresia, Fallot tetralogy, transposition of the great vessels) and acyanotic (eg, interruption of aortic arch, coarctation of aorta, hypoplastic left ventricle) heart disease.

Caverject®: Treatment of erectile dysfunction of vasculogenic, psychogenic, or neurogenic etiology; adjunct in the diagnosis of erectile dysfunction

Edex®, Muse®: Treatment of erectile dysfunction of vasculogenic, psychogenic, or neurogenic etiology

Usual Dosage

Patent ductus arteriosus (Prostin VR Pediatric®):

I.V. continuous infusion into a large vein, or alternatively through an umbilical artery catheter placed at the ductal opening: 0.05-0.1 mcg/kg/minute with therapeutic response, rate is reduced to lowest effective dosage; with unsatisfactory response, rate is increased gradually; maintenance: 0.01-0.4 mcg/kg/minute

PGE_1 is usually given at an infusion rate of 0.1 mcg/kg/minute, but it is often possible to reduce the dosage to 1/2 or even 1/10 without losing the therapeutic effect. The mixing schedule is as follows. Infusion rates deliver 0.1 mcg/kg/minute. **Note:** 500 mcg equals 1 ampul.

For a concentration of 2 mcg/mL, add 500 mcg to 250 mL; infuse at 0.05 mL/kg/minute (72 mL/kg/24 hours)

For a concentration of 5 mcg/mL, add 500 mcg to 100 mL; infuse at 0.02 mL/kg/minute (28.8 mL/kg/24 hours)

For a concentration of 10 mcg/mL, add 500 mcg to 50 mL; infuse at 0.01 mL/kg/minute (14.4 mL/kg/24 hours)

For a concentration of 20 mcg/mL, add 500 mcg to 25 mL; infuse at 0.005 mL/kg/minute (7.2 mL/kg/24 hours)

Therapeutic response is indicated by increased pH in those with acidosis or by an increase in oxygenation (PO_2) usually evident within 30 minutes

Erectile dysfunction:

Caverject®, Edex®: Intracavernous: Individualize dose by careful titration; doses >40 mcg (Edex®) or >60 mcg (Caverject®) are not recommended: Initial dose must be titrated in physicians office. Patient must stay in the physician's office until complete detumescence occurs; if there is no response, then the next higher dose may be given within 1 hour; if there is still no response, a 1-day interval before giving the next dose is recommended; increasing the dose or concentration in the treatment of impotence results in increasing pain and discomfort

Vasculogenic, psychogenic, or mixed etiology: Initiate dosage titration at 2.5 mcg, increasing by 2.5 mcg to a dose of 5 mcg and then in increments of 5-10 mcg depending on the erectile response until the dose produces an erection suitable for intercourse, not lasting >1 hour; if there is absolutely no response to initial 2.5 mcg dose, the second dose may be increased to 7.5 mcg, followed by increments of 5-10 mcg

Neurogenic etiology (eg, spinal cord injury): Initiate dosage titration at 1.25 mcg, increasing to a dose of 2.5 mcg and then 5 mcg; increase further in increments 5 mcg until the dose is reached that produces an erection suitable for intercourse, not lasting >1 hour

Maintenance: Once appropriate dose has been determined, patient may self-administer injections at a frequency of no more than 3 times/week with at least 24 hours between doses

Muse® Pellet: Intraurethral:

Initial: 125-250 mcg

Maintenance: Administer as needed to achieve an erection; duration of action is about 30-60 minutes; use only two systems per 24-hour period

Dosage Forms

Injection, powder for reconstitution:

Caverject®: 20 mcg, 40 mcg

Caverject Impulse®: 10 mcg, 20 mcg

Edex®: 10 mcg, 20 mcg, 40 mcg

Injection, solution: 500 mcg/mL (1 mL)
Prostin VR Pediatric®: 500 mcg/mL (1 mL)
Pellet, urethral:
Muse®: 250 mcg (6s), 500 mcg (6s), 1000 mcg (6s)

Alrex® [US/Can] *see* loteprednol *on page 601*
AL-Rr® Oral ***(Discontinued)*** *see* chlorpheniramine *on page 213*
Altabax™ [US] *see* retapamulin *on page 860*
Altace® [US/Can] *see* ramipril *on page 850*
Altace® HCT [Can] *see* ramipril and hydrochlorothiazide *(Canada only) on page 851*
Altace® Plus Felodipine [Can] *see* ramipril and felodipine *(Canada only) on page 850*
Altachlore [US-OTC] *see* sodium chloride *on page 908*
Altafrin [US] *see* phenylephrine *on page 774*
Altamist [US-OTC] *see* sodium chloride *on page 908*
Altaryl [US-OTC] *see* diphenhydramine *on page 315*

alteplase (AL te plase)

Sound-Alike/Look-Alike Issues
alteplase may be confused with Altace®

"tPA" abbreviation should not be used when writing orders for this medication; has been misread as TNKase (tenecteplase)

Synonyms alteplase, recombinant; alteplase, tissue plasminogen activator, recombinant; tPA

U.S./Canadian Brand Names Activase® rt-PA [Can]; Activase® [US]; Cathflo® Activase® [US/Can]

Therapeutic Category Fibrinolytic Agent

Use Management of ST-elevation myocardial infarction (STEMI) for the lysis of thrombi in coronary arteries; management of acute ischemic stroke (AIS); management of acute pulmonary embolism

Recommended criteria for treatment:

STEMI: Chest pain ≥20 minutes duration, onset of chest pain within 12 hours of treatment (or within prior 12-24 hours in patients with continuing ischemic symptoms), and ST-segment elevation >0.1 mV in at least two contiguous precordial leads or two adjacent limb leads on ECG or new or presumably new left bundle branch block (LBBB)

AIS: Onset of stroke symptoms within 3 hours of treatment

Acute pulmonary embolism: Age ≤75 years: Documented massive pulmonary embolism by pulmonary angiography or echocardiography or high probability lung scan with clinical shock

Cathflo® Activase®: Restoration of central venous catheter function

Usual Dosage

I.V. (Activase®):

ST-elevation myocardial infarction (STEMI): Front loading dose (weight-based):

Patients >67 kg: Total dose: 100 mg over 1.5 hours; infuse 15 mg over 1-2 minutes. Infuse 50 mg over 30 minutes. Infuse remaining 35 mg of alteplase over the next hour. See **"Note."**

Patients ≤67 kg: Infuse 15 mg I.V. bolus over 1-2 minutes, then infuse 0.75 mg/kg (not to exceed 50 mg) over next 30 minutes, followed by 0.5 mg/kg over next 60 minutes (not to exceed 35 mg). See **"Note."**

Note: All patients should receive 162-325 mg of chewable nonenteric coated aspirin as soon as possible and then daily. Administer concurrently with heparin 60 units/kg bolus (maximum: 4000 units) followed by continuous infusion of 12 units/kg/hour (maximum: 1000 units/hour) and adjust to aPTT target of 50-70 seconds (or 1.5-2 times the upper limit of control).

Acute pulmonary embolism: 100 mg over 2 hours.

Acute ischemic stroke: Doses should be given within the first 3 hours of the onset of symptoms; **Note:** Initiation of anticoagulants (eg, heparin) or antiplatelet agents (eg, aspirin) within 24 hours after starting alteplase is not recommended; however, initiation of aspirin between 24-48 hours after stroke onset is recommended.

Recommended total dose: 0.9 mg/kg (maximum total dose: 90 mg)

Patients ≤100 kg: Load with 0.09 mg/kg (10% of 0.9 mg/kg dose) as an I.V. bolus over 1 minute, followed by 0.81 mg/kg (90% of 0.9 mg/kg dose) as a continuous infusion over 60 minutes.

Patients >100 kg: Load with 9 mg (10% of 90 mg) as an I.V. bolus over 1 minute, followed by 81 mg (90% of 90 mg) as a continuous infusion over 60 minutes.

Intracatheter: Central venous catheter clearance (Cathflo® Activase® 1 mg/mL):

Patients <30 kg: 110% of the internal lumen volume of the catheter, not to exceed 2 mg/2 mL; retain in catheter for 0.5-2 hours; may instill a second dose if catheter remains occluded

Patients ≥30 kg: 2 mg (2 mL); retain in catheter for 0.5-2 hours; may instill a second dose if catheter remains occluded

Dosage Forms

Injection, powder for reconstitution, recombinant:

Activase®: 50 mg [29 million int. units]; 100 mg [58 million int. units]

Cathflo® Activase®: 2 mg

alteplase, recombinant *see* alteplase *on page* *53*

alteplase, tissue plasminogen activator, recombinant *see* alteplase *on page* *53*

ALternaGel® [US-OTC] *see* aluminum hydroxide *on page* *55*

Alti-Alprazolam [Can] *see* alprazolam *on page* *51*

Alti-Amiodarone [Can] *see* amiodarone *on page* *64*

Alti-Amoxi-Clav [Can] *see* amoxicillin and clavulanate potassium *on page* *71*

Alti-Azathioprine [Can] *see* azathioprine *on page* *115*

Alti-Captopril [Can] *see* captopril *on page* *178*

Alti-Clindamycin [Can] *see* clindamycin *on page* *239*

Alti-Clobazam [Can] *see* clobazam *(Canada only) on page* *241*

Alti-Clonazepam [Can] *see* clonazepam *on page* *245*

Alti-Desipramine [Can] *see* desipramine *on page* *284*

Alti-Divalproex [Can] *see* valproic acid and derivatives *on page* *1002*

Alti-Doxazosin [Can] *see* doxazosin *on page* *333*

Alti-Flunisolide [Can] *see* flunisolide *on page* *427*

Alti-Flurbiprofen [Can] *see* flurbiprofen *on page* *435*

Alti-Fluvoxamine [Can] *see* fluvoxamine *on page* *439*

Alti-Ipratropium [Can] *see* ipratropium *on page* *544*

Alti-Minocycline [Can] *see* minocycline *on page* *659*

Alti-MPA [Can] *see* medroxyprogesterone *on page* *620*

Alti-Nadolol [Can] *see* nadolol *on page* *675*

Alti-Nortriptyline [Can] *see* nortriptyline *on page* *706*

Alti-Salbutamol [Can] *see* albuterol *on page* *41*

Alti-Sulfasalazine [Can] *see* sulfasalazine *on page* *930*

Alti-Terazosin [Can] *see* terazosin *on page* *945*

Alti-Ticlopidine [Can] *see* ticlopidine *on page* *960*

Alti-Timolol [Can] *see* timolol *on page* *961*

Altocor™ *(Discontinued)* *see* lovastatin *on page* *602*

Altoprev® [US] *see* lovastatin *on page* *602*

altretamine (al TRET a meen)

Synonyms hexamethylmelamine; HEXM; HMM; HXM; NSC-13875

U.S./Canadian Brand Names Hexalen® [US/Can]

Therapeutic Category Antineoplastic Agent

Use Palliative treatment of persistent or recurrent ovarian cancer

Usual Dosage Refer to individual protocols. Oral: Adults: Ovarian cancer: 260 mg/m^2/day in 4 divided doses for 14 or 21 days of a 28-day cycle

Dosage Forms

Gelcap:

Hexalen®: 50 mg

Alu-Cap® *(Discontinued)* *see* aluminum hydroxide *on page* *55*

Aludrox® *(Discontinued)* *see* aluminum hydroxide and magnesium hydroxide *on page* *55*

aluminum chloride hexahydrate (a LOO mi num KLOR ide heks a HYE drate)

Sound-Alike/Look-Alike Issues

Drysol™ may be confused with Drisdol®

U.S./Canadian Brand Names Certain Dri® [US-OTC]; Drysol™ [US]; Hypercare™ [US]; Xerac AC™ [US]

Therapeutic Category Topical Skin Product

Use Astringent in the management of hyperhidrosis

Usual Dosage Topical: Adults: Apply once daily at bedtime; once excessive sweating has stopped, may decrease to once or twice weekly, or as needed. Wash treated area in the morning.

Dosage Forms

Solution, topical:

Certain Dri® [OTC]: 12% (36 mL)

Drysol™, Hypercare™: 20% (35 mL, 37.5 mL, 60 mL)

Xerac AC™: 6.25% (35 mL, 60 mL)

aluminum hydroxide (a LOO mi num hye DROKS ide)

U.S./Canadian Brand Names ALternaGel® [US-OTC]; Amphojel® [Can]; Basaljel® [Can]; Dermagran® [US-OTC]

Therapeutic Category Antacid

Use Treatment of hyperacidity; hyperphosphatemia; temporary protection of minor cuts, scrapes, and burns

Usual Dosage

Oral:

Hyperphosphatemia:

Children: 50-150 mg/kg/24 hours in divided doses every 4-6 hours, titrate dosage to maintain serum phosphorus within normal range

Adults: Initial: 300-600 mg 3 times/day with meals

Antacid: Adults: 600-1200 mg between meals and at bedtime

Topical: Apply to affected area as needed; reapply at least every 12 hours

Dosage Forms

Ointment:

Dermagran® [OTC]: 0.275% (120 g)

Suspension, oral: 320 mg/5 mL

ALternaGel® [OTC]: 600 mg/5 mL

aluminum hydroxide and magnesium carbonate

(a LOO mi num hye DROKS ide & mag NEE zhum KAR bun nate)

Synonyms magnesium carbonate and aluminum hydroxide

U.S./Canadian Brand Names Acid Gone Extra Strength [US-OTC]; Acid Gone [US-OTC]; Gaviscon® Extra Strength [US-OTC]; Gaviscon® Liquid [US-OTC]; Genaton™ [US-OTC]

Therapeutic Category Antacid

Use Temporary relief of symptoms associated with gastric acidity

Usual Dosage Oral: Adults:

Liquid:

Gaviscon® Regular Strength: 15-30 mL 4 times/day after meals and at bedtime

Gaviscon® Extra Strength: 15-30 mL 4 times/day after meals

Tablet (Gaviscon® Extra Strength): Chew 2-4 tablets 4 times/day

Dosage Forms

Liquid: Aluminum hydroxide 31.7 mg and magnesium carbonate 119.3 mg per 5 mL; aluminum hydroxide 84.6 mg and magnesium carbonate 79.1 mg per 5 mL

Acid Gone [OTC], Gaviscon® [OTC], Genaton™ [OTC]: Aluminum hydroxide 31.7 mg and magnesium carbonate 119.3 mg per 5 mL

Gaviscon® Extra Strength [OTC]: Aluminum hydroxide 84.6 mg and magnesium carbonate 79.1 mg per 5 mL

Tablet, chewable: Aluminum hydroxide 160 mg and magnesium carbonate 105 mg

Acid Gone Extra Strength [OTC], Gaviscon® Extra Strength [OTC]: Aluminum hydroxide 160 mg and magnesium carbonate 105 mg

aluminum hydroxide and magnesium hydroxide

(a LOO mi num hye DROKS ide & mag NEE zhum hye DROK side)

Sound-Alike/Look-Alike Issues

Maalox® may be confused with Maox®, Monodox®

Synonyms magnesium hydroxide and aluminum hydroxide

U.S./Canadian Brand Names Alamag [US-OTC]; Diovol® Ex [Can]; Diovol® [Can]; Gelusil® Extra Strength [Can]; Mylanta™ [Can]; Rulox [US-OTC]

Therapeutic Category Antacid

Use Antacid, hyperphosphatemia in renal failure

Usual Dosage Oral: 5-10 mL 4-6 times/day, between meals and at bedtime; may be used every hour for severe symptoms

Dosage Forms

Suspension: Aluminum hydroxide 225 mg and magnesium hydroxide 200 mg per 5 mL

Alamag [OTC], Rulox [OTC]: Aluminum hydroxide 225 mg and magnesium hydroxide 200 mg per 5 mL

Tablet, chewable:

Alamag [OTC]: Aluminum hydroxide 300 mg and magnesium hydroxide 150 mg

aluminum hydroxide and magnesium trisilicate

(a LOO mi num hye DROKS ide & mag NEE zhum trye SIL i kate)

Synonyms magnesium trisilicate and aluminum hydroxide

U.S./Canadian Brand Names Alenic Alka Tablet [US-OTC]; Gaviscon® Tablet [US-OTC]; Genaton Tablet [US-OTC]

Therapeutic Category Antacid

Use Temporary relief of hyperacidity

Usual Dosage Oral: Adults: Chew 2-4 tablets 4 times/day or as directed by healthcare provider

Dosage Forms

Tablet, chewable: Aluminum hydroxide 80 mg and magnesium trisilicate 20 mg

Alenic Alka [OTC], Gaviscon® [OTC], Genaton [OTC]: Aluminum hydroxide 80 mg and magnesium trisilicate 20 mg

aluminum hydroxide, magnesium hydroxide, and simethicone

(a LOO mi num hye DROKS ide, mag NEE zhum hye DROKS ide, & sye METH i kone)

Sound-Alike/Look-Alike Issues

Maalox® may be confused with Maox®, Monodox®

Mylanta® may be confused with Mynatal®

Synonyms magnesium hydroxide, aluminum hydroxide, and simethicone; simethicone, aluminum hydroxide, and magnesium hydroxide

U.S./Canadian Brand Names Alamag Plus [US-OTC]; Aldroxicon I [US-OTC]; Aldroxicon II [US-OTC]; Almacone Double Strength® [US-OTC]; Almacone® [US-OTC]; Diovol Plus® [Can]; Gelusil® [US-OTC/Can]; Maalox® Max [US-OTC]; Maalox® [US-OTC]; Mi-Acid Maximum Strength [US-OTC]; Mi-Acid [US-OTC]; Mintox Extra Strength [US-OTC]; Mintox Plus [US-OTC]; Mylanta® Double Strength [Can]; Mylanta® Extra Strength [Can]; Mylanta® Liquid [US-OTC]; Mylanta® Maximum Strength Liquid [US-OTC]; Mylanta® Regular Strength [Can]

Therapeutic Category Antacid; Antiflatulent

Use Temporary relief of hyperacidity associated with gas; may also be used for indications associated with other antacids

Usual Dosage Oral: Adults: 10-20 mL or 2-4 tablets 4-6 times/day between meals and at bedtime; may be used every hour for severe symptoms

Dosage Forms

Liquid: Aluminum hydroxide 200 mg, magnesium hydroxide 200 mg, and simethicone 20 mg per 5 mL; aluminum hydroxide 400 mg, magnesium hydroxide 400 mg, and simethicone 40 mg per 5 mL

Aldroxicon I [OTC], Almacone® [OTC], Maalox® [OTC], Mi-Acid [OTC], Mylanta® [OTC]: Aluminum hydroxide 200 mg, magnesium hydroxide 200 mg, and simethicone 20 mg per 5 mL

Aldroxicon II [OTC], Almacone Double Strength [OTC], Maalox® Max® [OTC], Mi-Acid Maximum Strength [OTC], Mylanta® Maximum Strength [OTC]: Aluminum hydroxide 400 mg, magnesium hydroxide 400 mg, and simethicone 40 mg per 5 mL

Mintox Extra Strength [OTC]: Aluminum hydroxide 500 mg, magnesium hydroxide 450 mg, and simethicone 40 mg per 5 mL

Suspension:

Alamag Plus [OTC]: Aluminum hydroxide 225 mg, magnesium hydroxide 200 mg, and simethicone 25 mg per 5 mL

Tablet, chewable: Aluminum hydroxide 200 mg, magnesium hydroxide 200 mg, and simethicone 25 mg

Alamag Plus [OTC], Gelusil® [OTC], Mintox Plus [OTC]: Aluminum hydroxide 200 mg, magnesium hydroxide 200 mg, and simethicone 25 mg

Almacone® [OTC]: Aluminum hydroxide 200 mg, magnesium hydroxide 200 mg, and simethicone 20 mg

aluminum sucrose sulfate, basic *see* sucralfate *on page 925*

aluminum sulfate and calcium acetate (a LOO mi num SUL fate & KAL see um AS e tate)

Synonyms calcium acetate and aluminum sulfate

U.S./Canadian Brand Names Domeboro® [US-OTC]; Gordon Boro-Packs [US-OTC]; Pedi-Boro® [US-OTC]

Therapeutic Category Topical Skin Product

Use Astringent wet dressing for relief of inflammatory conditions of the skin; reduce weeping that may occur in dermatitis

Usual Dosage Topical: Soak affected area in the solution 2-4 times/day for 15-30 minutes or apply wet dressing soaked in the solution for more extended periods; rewet dressing with solution 2-4 times/day every 15-30 minutes

Dosage Forms

Powder, for topical solution:

Domeboro® [OTC]: Aluminum sulfate 1191 mg and calcium acetate 839 mg per packet (12s, 100s)

Gordon Boro-Packs: Aluminum sulfate 49% and calcium acetate 51% per packet (100s)

Pedi-Boro® [OTC]: Aluminum sulfate 1191 mg and calcium acetate 839 mg per packet (12s, 100s)

Alupent® ***(Discontinued)*** *see* metaproterenol *on page 632*

Alupent® Inhalation Solution ***(Discontinued)*** *see* metaproterenol *on page 632*

Alu-Tab® ***(Discontinued)*** *see* aluminum hydroxide *on page 55*

Alvesco® [US/Can] *see* ciclesonide *on page 226*

alvimopan (al vi MOE pan)

Sound-Alike/Look-Alike Issues

alvimopan may be confused with almotriptan

Synonyms ADL-2698; LY246736

U.S./Canadian Brand Names Entereg® [US]

Therapeutic Category Gastrointestinal Agent, Miscellaneous; Opioid Antagonist, Peripherally-Acting

Use Accelerate the time to upper and lower GI recovery following partial large or small bowel resection surgery with primary anastomosis

Usual Dosage **Note:** For hospital use only. Oral: Adults:

Initial: 12 mg administered 30 minutes to 5 hours prior to surgery

Maintenance: 12 mg twice daily beginning the day after surgery for a maximum of 7 days or until discharged from hospital (maximum total treatment doses: 15 doses)

Dosage Forms

Capsule:

Entereg®: 12 mg

amantadine (a MAN ta deen)

Sound-Alike/Look-Alike Issues

amantadine may be confused with ranitidine, rimantadine

Symmetrel® may be confused with Synthroid®

Synonyms adamantanamine hydrochloride; amantadine hydrochloride

U.S./Canadian Brand Names Endantadine® [Can]; PMS-Amantadine [Can]; Symmetrel® [US/Can]

Therapeutic Category Anti-Parkinson Agent (Dopamine Agonist); Antiviral Agent

Use Prophylaxis and treatment of influenza A viral infection (per manufacturer labeling; also refer to current ACIP guidelines for recommendations during current flu season); treatment of parkinsonism; treatment of drug-induced extrapyramidal symptoms

Note: In certain circumstances, the ACIP recommends use of amantadine in combination with oseltamivir for the treatment or prophylaxis of influenza A infection when resistance to oseltamivir is suspected.

Usual Dosage Oral:

Children: Influenza A treatment/prophylaxis: **Note:** Due to issues of resistance, amantadine is no longer recommended for the treatment or prophylaxis of influenza A. Please refer to the current ACIP recommendations. The following is based on the manufacturer's labeling and past ACIP dosing recommendations:

Influenza A treatment:

1-9 years: 5 mg/kg/day in 2 divided doses (manufacturers range: 4.4-8.8 mg/kg/day); maximum dose: 150 mg/day

≥10 years and <40 kg: 5 mg/kg/day in 2 divided doses; maximum dose: 150 mg/day

≥10 years and ≥40 kg: 100 mg twice daily

Note: Initiate within 24-48 hours after onset of symptoms; continue for 24-48 hours after symptom resolution (duration of therapy is generally 3-5 days)

Influenza A prophylaxis: Refer to "Influenza A treatment" dosing. **Note:** Continue prophylaxis throughout the peak influenza activity in the community or throughout the entire influenza season in patients who cannot be vaccinated. Development of immunity following vaccination takes ~2 weeks; amantadine therapy should be considered for high-risk patients from the time of vaccination until immunity has developed. For children <9 years receiving influenza vaccine for the first time, amantadine prophylaxis should continue for 6 weeks (4 weeks after the first dose and 2 weeks after the second dose).

Adults:

Drug-induced extrapyramidal symptoms: 100 mg twice daily; may increase to 300 mg/day in divided doses, if needed

Parkinson disease: Usual dose: 100 mg twice daily as monotherapy; may increase to 400 mg/day in divided doses, if needed, with close monitoring. **Note:** Patients with a serious concomitant illness or those receiving high doses of other anti-Parkinson drugs should be started at 100 mg/day; may increase to 100 mg twice daily, if needed, after one to several weeks.

Influenza A treatment/prophylaxis: **Note:** Due to issues of resistance, amantadine is no longer recommended for the treatment or prophylaxis of influenza A. Please refer to the current ACIP recommendations. The following is based on the manufacturer's labeling:

Influenza A treatment: 200 mg once daily **or** 100 mg twice daily (may be preferred to reduce CNS effects); **Note:** Initiate within 24-48 hours after onset of symptoms; continue for 24-48 hours after symptom resolution (duration of therapy is generally 3-5 days).

Influenza A prophylaxis: 200 mg once daily **or** 100 mg twice daily (may be preferred to reduce CNS effects). **Note:** Continue prophylaxis throughout the peak influenza activity in the community or throughout the entire influenza season in patients who cannot be vaccinated. Development of immunity following vaccination takes ~2 weeks; amantadine therapy should be considered for high-risk patients from the time of vaccination until immunity has developed.

Dosage Forms

Capsule: 100 mg

Capsule, softgel: 100 mg

Solution, oral: 50 mg/5 mL

Syrup, oral: 50 mg/5 mL

Tablet: 100 mg

Symmetrel®: 100 mg

amantadine hydrochloride *see* amantadine *on page* 57

Amaphen® ***(Discontinued)***

Amaryl® [US/Can] *see* glimepiride *on page* 464

Amatine® [Can] *see* midodrine *on page* 657

ambenonium (am be NOE nee um)

Synonyms ambenonium chloride

U.S./Canadian Brand Names Mytelase® [US/Can]

Therapeutic Category Cholinergic Agent

Use Treatment of myasthenia gravis

Usual Dosage Oral: Adults: 5-25 mg 3-4 times/day

Dosage Forms

Caplet [scored]:

Mytelase®: 10 mg

ambenonium chloride *see* ambenonium *on page* 58

Ambi 10® ***(Discontinued)*** *see* benzoyl peroxide *on page* 132

Ambien® [US] *see* zolpidem *on page 1033*
Ambien CR® [US] *see* zolpidem *on page 1033*
Ambifed-G [US] *see* guaifenesin and pseudoephedrine *on page 477*
Ambifed-G DM [US] *see* guaifenesin, pseudoephedrine, and dextromethorphan *on page 479*
Ambi® Skin Tone *(Discontinued)* *see* hydroquinone *on page 508*
AmBisome® [US/Can] *see* amphotericin B liposomal *on page 75*

ambrisentan (am bri SEN tan)

Synonyms BSF208075

U.S./Canadian Brand Names Letairis™ [US]; Volibris™ [Can]

Therapeutic Category Endothelin Antagonist

Use Treatment of pulmonary artery hypertension (PAH) World Health Organization (WHO) Group I in patients with WHO Class II or III symptoms to improve exercise capacity and decrease the rate of clinical deterioration

Usual Dosage Oral: Adults: Initial: 5 mg once daily; if tolerated, may increase to maximum 10 mg once daily

Modifications based on transaminase elevation:

If any elevation, regardless of degree, is accompanied by clinical symptoms of hepatic injury (unusual fatigue, nausea, vomiting, abdominal pain, fever, or jaundice) or a serum bilirubin >2 times ULN, treatment should be stopped and not reintroduced.

AST/ALT >3 but ≤5 times ULN: Confirm with additional test; if confirmed, reduce dose or interrupt treatment. Monitor transaminase levels at least every 2 weeks until levels are <3 times ULN. Reinitiate treatment as appropriate with return to pretreatment values and with more frequent checks of transaminase levels.

AST/ALT >5 but ≤8 times ULN: Confirm with additional test; if confirmed, stop treatment. Monitor transaminase levels until they are <3 times ULN. May reintroduce treatment, as appropriate, at starting dose, following return to pretreatment values. More frequent checks of transaminase levels are required after resuming therapy.

AST/ALT >8 times ULN: Stop treatment and do not reintroduce.

Dosage Forms

Tablet:

Letairis®: 5 mg, 10 mg

amcinonide (am SIN oh nide)

U.S./Canadian Brand Names Amcort® [Can]; Cyclocort® [Can]; ratio-Amcinonide [Can]; Taro-Amcinonide [Can]

Therapeutic Category Corticosteroid, Topical

Use Relief of the inflammatory and pruritic manifestations of corticosteroid-responsive dermatoses (high potency corticosteroid)

Usual Dosage Topical: Adults: Apply in a thin film 2-3 times/day. Therapy should be discontinued when control is achieved; if no improvement is seen, reassessment of diagnosis may be necessary.

Dosage Forms

Cream: 0.1% (15 g, 30 g, 60 g)
Lotion: 0.1% (60 mL)
Ointment: 0.1% (30 g, 60 g)

Amcort® [Can] *see* amcinonide *on page 59*
Amcort® Injection *(Discontinued)*
AMD3100 *see* plerixafor *on page 789*
Amdry-C [US] *see* chlorpheniramine, pseudoephedrine, and methscopolamine *on page 221*
Amdry-D *(Discontinued)* *see* pseudoephedrine and methscopolamine *on page 835*
Amerge® [US/Can] *see* naratriptan *on page 682*
Americaine® Anesthetic Lubricant *(Discontinued)* *see* benzocaine *on page 129*
Americaine® Hemorrhoidal [US-OTC] *see* benzocaine *on page 129*
A-Methapred® [US] *see* methylprednisolone *on page 647*
A-methapred *see* methylprednisolone *on page 647*
amethocaine hydrochloride *see* tetracaine *on page 950*
amethopterin *see* methotrexate *on page 639*

Ametop™ [Can] *see* tetracaine *on page 950*
Amevive® [US/Can] *see* alefacept *on page 44*
amfepramone *see* diethylpropion *on page 306*
AMG 073 *see* cinacalcet *on page 229*
AMG 531 *see* romiplostim *on page 876*
Amibid DM *(Discontinued)* *see* guaifenesin and dextromethorphan *on page 474*
Amibid LA *(Discontinued)* *see* guaifenesin *on page 473*
Amicar® [US] *see* aminocaproic acid *on page 63*
Amidal *(Discontinued)* *see* guaifenesin and phenylephrine *on page 475*
Amidate® [US/Can] *see* etomidate *on page 398*
Amidrine *(Discontinued)* *see* acetaminophen, isometheptene, and dichloralphenazone *on page 29*

amifostine (am i FOS teen)

Sound-Alike/Look-Alike Issues

Ethyol® may be confused with ethanol

Synonyms ethiofos; gammaphos; WR-2721; YM-08310

U.S./Canadian Brand Names Ethyol® [US/Can]

Therapeutic Category Antidote

Use Reduce the incidence of moderate-to-severe xerostomia in patients undergoing postoperative radiation treatment for head and neck cancer, where the radiation port includes a substantial portion of the parotid glands; reduce the cumulative renal toxicity associated with repeated administration of cisplatin

Usual Dosage Note: Antiemetic medication, including dexamethasone 20 mg I.V. and a serotonin 5-HT_3 receptor antagonist, is recommended prior to and in conjunction with amifostine.

Adults:

Cisplatin-induced renal toxicity, reduction: I.V.: 910 mg/m^2 over 15 minutes once daily 30 minutes prior to cisplatin

For 910 mg/m^2 doses, the manufacturer suggests the following blood pressure-based adjustment schedule:

The infusion of amifostine should be interrupted if the systolic blood pressure decreases significantly from baseline, as defined below:

- Decrease of 20 mm Hg if baseline systolic blood pressure <100
- Decrease of 25 mm Hg if baseline systolic blood pressure 100-119
- Decrease of 30 mm Hg if baseline systolic blood pressure 120-139
- Decrease of 40 mm Hg if baseline systolic blood pressure 140-179
- Decrease of 50 mm Hg if baseline systolic blood pressure ≥180

If blood pressure returns to normal within 5 minutes (assisted by fluid administration and postural management) and the patient is asymptomatic, the infusion may be restarted so that the full dose of amifostine may be administered. If the full dose of amifostine cannot be administered, the dose of amifostine for subsequent cycles should be 740 mg/m^2.

Xerostomia from head and neck cancer, reduction: I.V.: 200 mg/m^2 over 3 minutes once daily 15-30 minutes prior to radiation therapy

Dosage Forms

Injection, powder for reconstitution: 500 mg

Ethyol®: 500 mg

Amigesic® [Can] *see* salsalate *on page 888*
Amigesic® *(Discontinued)* *see* salsalate *on page 888*

amikacin (am i KAY sin)

Sound-Alike/Look-Alike Issues

amikacin may be confused with Amicar®, anakinra

Amikin® may be confused with Amicar®

Synonyms amikacin sulfate

U.S./Canadian Brand Names Amikacin Sulfate Injection, USP [Can]; Amikin® [Can]

Therapeutic Category Aminoglycoside (Antibiotic)

Use Treatment of serious infections (bone infections, respiratory tract infections, endocarditis, and septicemia) due to organisms resistant to gentamicin and tobramycin, including *Pseudomonas*, *Proteus*, *Serratia*, and other gram-negative bacilli; documented infection of mycobacterial organisms susceptible to amikacin

Usual Dosage Note: Individualization is critical because of the low therapeutic index

Use of ideal body weight (IBW) for determining the mg/kg/dose appears to be more accurate than dosing on the basis of total body weight (TBW)

In morbid obesity, dosage requirement may best be estimated using a dosing weight of IBW + 0.4 (TBW - IBW)

Initial and periodic peak-and-trough plasma drug levels should be determined, particularly in critically-ill patients with serious infections or in disease states known to significantly alter aminoglycoside pharmacokinetics (eg, cystic fibrosis, burns, or major surgery)

Usual dosage range:

Infants and Children: I.M., I.V.: 5-7.5 mg/kg/dose every 8 hours

Adults: I.M., I.V.: 5-7.5 mg/kg/dose every 8 hours

Note: Some clinicians suggest a daily dose of 15-20 mg/kg for all patients with normal renal function. This dose is at least as efficacious with similar, if not less, toxicity than conventional dosing.

Indication-specific dosing:

Adults:

Hospital-acquired pneumonia (HAP): I.V.: 20 mg/kg/day with antipseudomonal beta-lactam or carbapenem (American Thoracic Society/ATS guidelines)

Meningitis *(Pseudomonas aeruginosa)*: I.V.: 5 mg/kg every 8 hours (administered with another bacteriocidal drug)

Mycobacterium fortuitum, M. chelonae, or M. abscessus: I.V.: 10-15 mg/kg daily for at least 2 weeks with high dose cefoxitin

Dosage Forms

Injection, solution: 50 mg/mL (2 mL); 250 mg/mL (2 mL, 4 mL)

amikacin sulfate *see* amikacin *on page 60*

Amikacin Sulfate Injection, USP [Can] *see* amikacin *on page 60*

Amikin® [Can] *see* amikacin *on page 60*

amiloride (a MIL oh ride)

Sound-Alike/Look-Alike Issues

aMILoride may be confused with amiodarone, amLODIPine, amrinone

Synonyms amiloride hydrochloride

Tall-Man a**MIL**oride

U.S./Canadian Brand Names Apo-Amiloride® [Can]

Therapeutic Category Diuretic, Potassium Sparing

Use Counteracts potassium loss induced by other diuretics in the treatment of hypertension or edematous conditions including CHF, hepatic cirrhosis, and hypoaldosteronism; usually used in conjunction with more potent diuretics such as thiazides or loop diuretics

Usual Dosage Oral: Adults: 5-10 mg/day (up to 20 mg)

Hypertension (JNC 7): 5-10 mg/day in 1-2 divided doses

Dosage Forms

Tablet: 5 mg

amiloride and hydrochlorothiazide (a MIL oh ride & hye droe klor oh THYE a zide)

Synonyms hydrochlorothiazide and amiloride

U.S./Canadian Brand Names Apo-Amilzide® [Can]; Gen-Amilazide [Can]; Moduret [Can]; Novamilor [Can]; Nu-Amilzide [Can]

Therapeutic Category Diuretic, Combination

Use Potassium-sparing diuretic; antihypertensive

Usual Dosage Oral: Adults: Start with 1 tablet/day, then may be increased to 2 tablets/day if needed; usually given in a single dose

Dosage Forms

Tablet: 5/50: Amiloride 5 mg and hydrochlorothiazide 50 mg

amiloride hydrochloride *see* amiloride *on page 61*

2-amino-6-mercaptopurine *see* thioguanine *on page 955*

2-amino-6-methoxypurine arabinoside *see* nelarabine *on page 685*

2-amino-6-trifluoromethoxy-benzothiazole *see* riluzole *on page 868*

amino acid injection (a MEE noe AS id in JEK shun)

Sound-Alike/Look-Alike Issues

TrophAmine® may be confused with tromethamine

U.S./Canadian Brand Names Aminosyn® II [US]; Aminosyn® [US/Can]; Aminosyn®-HBC [US]; Aminosyn®-PF [US/Can]; Aminosyn®-RF [US/Can]; BranchAmin® [US]; Clinisol® [US]; FreAmine® HBC® [US]; FreAmine® III [US]; FreAmine® [US]; HepatAmine® [US]; Hepatasol® [US]; NephrAmine® [US]; Premasol™ [US]; Primene® [Can]; Prosol [US]; Renamin® [US]; Travasol® [US]; TrophAmine® [US]

Therapeutic Category Intravenous Nutritional Therapy

Use As part of parenteral nutrition to prevent nitrogen loss or treat negative nitrogen balance when alimentary tract cannot be used (eg, GI absorption is impaired, bowel rest is needed). Specialty amino acid formulas may be considered only in certain instances.

Usual Dosage Intravenous as a component of parenteral nutrition: Protein as amino acids:

Children:

- Term: Initial: 2.5 g/kg/day; Goal: 3 g/kg/day
- Extremely (<1000 g) and very (<1500 g) low-birth-weight (stable): Initial: 1-1.5 g/kg/day; Goal: 3.5-3.85 g/kg/day to promote utero growth rates
- Sepsis, hypoxia: Initial: 1 g/kg/day; goal: 3-3.85 g/kg/day

Adults:

- Maintenance: 0.8-1 g/kg/day
- Normal/mild stress level: 1-1.2 g/kg/day
- Moderate stress level: 1.2-1.5 g/kg/day
- Severe stress level: 1.5-2 g/kg/day
- Burn patients (severe): Increase protein until significant wound healing achieved
- Solid organ transplant: Perioperative: 1.5-2 g/kg/day
- Renal failure:
  - Acute (severely malnourished or hypercatabolic): 1.5-1.8 g/kg/day
  - Chronic, with dialysis: 1.2-1.3 g/kg/day
  - Chronic, without dialysis: 0.6-0.8 g/kg/day
  - Continuous hemofiltration: ≥1 g/kg/day
- Hepatic failure:
  - Acute management when other treatments have failed:
    - With encephalopathy: 0.6-1 g/kg/day
    - Without encephalopathy: 1-1.5 g/kg/day
  - Chronic encephalopathy: Use branch chain amino acid enriched diets only if unresponsive to pharmacotherapy
- Pregnant women in second or third trimester: Add an additional 10-14 g/day

Dosage Forms Excipient information presented when available (limited, particularly for generics); consult specific product labeling. Peripheral parenteral nutrition and total parenteral nutrition are usually compounded from optimal combinations of macronutrients (water, protein, dextrose, and lipids) and micronutrients (electrolytes, trace elements, and vitamins) to meet the specific nutritional requirements of a patient. Individual hospitals may have designated standard TPN formulas. There are a few commercially-available amino acids with electrolytes solutions; however, these products may not meet an individual's specific nutritional requirements. Consult with nutrition support service to determine adequate formula based upon patient specifics.

Injection, solution [branched chain]:

Aminosyn®-HBC: 7%
BranchAmin®: 4%
FreAmine® HBC: 6.9%

Injection, solution [crystalline]:

Aminosyn®: 3.5%, 5%, 7%, 8.5%, 10%
Aminosyn® II: 7%, 8.5%, 10%, 15%
Clinisol®: 15%
FreAmine® III: 8.5%, 10%
PremaSol™: 6%, 10%
Prosol: 20%
Travasol®: 10%

Injection, solution [hepatic]:

Aminosyn®-HF, HepatAmine®, Hepatasol®: 8%

Injection, solution [pediatric]:
Aminosyn®-PF: 7%, 10%
TrophAmine®: 6%, 10%
Injection, solution [renal]:
Aminosyn®-RF: 5.2%
NephrAmine®: 5.4%
Renamin®: 6.5%

aminobenzylpenicillin *see* ampicillin *on page* 76

aminocaproic acid (a mee noe ka PROE ik AS id)

Sound-Alike/Look-Alike Issues
Amicar® may be confused with amikacin, Amikin®, Omacor®

Synonyms EACA; epsilon aminocaproic acid

U.S./Canadian Brand Names Amicar® [US]

Therapeutic Category Hemostatic Agent

Use To enhance hemostasis when fibrinolysis contributes to bleeding (causes may include cardiac surgery, hematologic disorders, neoplastic disorders, abruption placentae, hepatic cirrhosis, and urinary fibrinolysis)

Usual Dosage Oral, I.V.: Adults: Acute bleeding syndrome: Loading dose: 4-5 g during the first hour, followed by 1 g/hour (or 1.25 g/hour using oral solution) for 8 hours or until bleeding controlled (maximum daily dose: 30 g)

Dosage Forms
Injection, solution: 250 mg/mL (20 mL)
Solution, oral: 1.25 g/5 mL (480 mL)
Syrup:
Amicar®: 1.25 g/5 mL
Tablet [scored]: 500 mg
Amicar®: 500 mg, 1000 mg

aminoglutethimide ***(Discontinued)***

aminolevulinic acid (a MEE noh lev yoo lin ik AS id)

Sound-Alike/Look-Alike Issues
Sound-alike/look-alike issues:
Aminolevulinic acid may be confused with methyl aminolevulinate

Synonyms aminolevulinic acid hydrochloride

U.S./Canadian Brand Names Levulan® Kerastick® [US]; Levulan® [Can]

Therapeutic Category Photosensitizing Agent, Topical; Porphyrin Agent, Topical

Use Treatment of minimally to moderately thick actinic keratoses (grade 1 or 2) of the face or scalp; to be used in conjunction with blue light illumination

Usual Dosage Topical: Adults: Apply to actinic keratoses (**not** perilesional skin) followed 14-18 hours later by blue light illumination. Application/treatment may be repeated at a treatment site after 8 weeks.

Dosage Forms
Powder for topical solution:
Levulan® Kerastick®: 20% (1s, 6s)

aminolevulinic acid hydrochloride *see* aminolevulinic acid *on page* 63

aminophylline (am in OFF i lin)

Sound-Alike/Look-Alike Issues
aminophylline may be confused with amitriptyline, ampicillin

Synonyms theophylline ethylenediamine

U.S./Canadian Brand Names Phyllocontin® [Can]; Phyllocontin®-350 [Can]

Therapeutic Category Theophylline Derivative

Use Bronchodilator in reversible airway obstruction due to asthma or COPD; increase diaphragmatic contractility

Usual Dosage
Treatment of acute bronchospasm: I.V.:
Loading dose (in patients not currently receiving aminophylline or theophylline): 6 mg/kg (based on aminophylline) administered I.V. over 20-30 minutes; administration rate should not exceed 25 mg/minute (aminophylline)
Approximate I.V. maintenance dosages are based upon **continuous infusions**; bolus dosing (often used in children <6 months of age) may be determined by multiplying the hourly infusion rate by 24 hours and dividing by the desired number of doses/day
6 weeks to 6 months: 0.5 mg/kg/hour
6 months to 1 year: 0.6-0.7 mg/kg/hour
1-9 years: 1 mg/kg/hour
9-16 years and smokers: 0.8 mg/kg/hour
Adults, nonsmoking: 0.5 mg/kg/hour
Older patients and patients with cor pulmonale: 0.3 mg/kg/hour
Patients with congestive heart failure: 0.1-0.2 mg/kg/hour
Dosage should be adjusted according to serum level measurements during the first 12- to 24-hour period.
Bronchodilator: Oral: Children ≥45 kg and Adults: Initial: 380 mg/day (equivalent to theophylline 300 mg/day) in divided doses every 6-8 hours; may increase dose after 3 days; maximum dose: 928 mg/day (equivalent to theophylline 800 mg/day)

Dosage Forms
Injection, solution: 25 mg/mL (10 mL, 20 mL)
Injection, solution, [preservative free]: 25 mg/mL (10 mL, 20 mL)
Tablet: 100 mg

aminosalicylate sodium *see* aminosalicylic acid *on page* 64

aminosalicylic acid (a mee noe sal i SIL ik AS id)

Synonyms 4-aminosalicylic acid; aminosalicylate sodium; para-aminosalicylate sodium; PAS; sodium PAS
U.S./Canadian Brand Names Paser® [US]
Therapeutic Category Nonsteroidal Antiinflammatory Drug (NSAID)
Use Adjunctive treatment of tuberculosis used in combination with other antitubercular agents
Usual Dosage Oral: Tuberculosis:
Children: 200-300 mg/kg/day in 3-4 equally divided doses
Adults: 150 mg/kg/day in 2-3 equally divided doses

Dosage Forms
Granules, delayed release:
Paser®: 4 g/packet

4-aminosalicylic acid *see* aminosalicylic acid *on page* 64
5-aminosalicylic acid *see* mesalamine *on page* 631
Aminosyn® [US/Can] *see* amino acid injection *on page* 62
Aminosyn® II [US] *see* amino acid injection *on page* 62
Aminosyn®-HBC [US] *see* amino acid injection *on page* 62
Aminosyn®-PF [US/Can] *see* amino acid injection *on page* 62
Aminosyn®-RF [US/Can] *see* amino acid injection *on page* 62
Aminoxin [US-OTC] *see* pyridoxine *on page* 840

amiodarone (a MEE oh da rone)

Sound-Alike/Look-Alike Issues
amiodarone may be confused with aMILoride, amrinone
Cordarone® may be confused with Cardura®, Cordran®
Synonyms amiodarone hydrochloride
U.S./Canadian Brand Names Alti-Amiodarone [Can]; Amiodarone Hydrochloride for Injection® [Can]; Apo-Amiodarone® [Can]; Cordarone® [US/Can]; Dom-Amiodarone [Can]; Gen-Amiodarone [Can]; Novo-Amiodarone [Can]; Pacerone® [US]; PHL-Amiodarone [Can]; PMS-Amiodarone [Can]; PRO-Amiodarone [Can]; ratio-Amiodarone I.V. [Can]; ratio-Amiodarone [Can]; Riva-Amiodarone [Can]; Sandoz-Amiodarone [Can]
Therapeutic Category Antiarrhythmic Agent, Class III

Use Management of life-threatening recurrent ventricular fibrillation (VF) or hemodynamically-unstable ventricular tachycardia (VT) refractory to other antiarrhythmic agents or in patients intolerant of other agents used for these conditions

Usual Dosage Note: Lower loading and maintenance doses are preferable in women and all patients with low body weight.

Oral: Adults: Ventricular arrhythmias: 800-1600 mg/day in 1-2 doses for 1-3 weeks, then when adequate arrhythmia control is achieved, decrease to 600-800 mg/day in 1-2 doses for 1 month; maintenance: 400 mg/day. Lower doses are recommended for supraventricular arrhythmias.

I.V.:

Children:

Pulseless VF or VT (PALS dosing): 5 mg/kg (maximum: 300 mg/dose) rapid I.V. bolus or I.O.; repeat up to a maximum daily dose of 15 mg/kg. (**Note:** Maximum recommended daily dose in adolescents is 2.2 g).

Perfusing tachycardias (PALS dosing): Loading dose: 5 mg/kg (maximum: 300 mg/dose) I.V. over 20-60 minutes or I.O.; may repeat up to maximum dose of 15 mg/kg/day. (**Note:** Maximum recommended daily dose in adolescents is 2.2 g).

Adults: Ventricular arrhythmias:

Breakthrough VF or VT: 150 mg supplemental doses in 100 mL D_5W over 10 minutes

Pulseless VF or VT: I.V. push: Initial: 300 mg in 20-30 mL NS or D_5W; if VF or VT recurs, supplemental dose of 150 mg followed by infusion of 1 mg/minute for 6 hours, then 0.5 mg/minute (maximum daily dose: 2.1 g)

I.V. to oral therapy conversion: Use the following as a guide:

<1 week I.V. infusion: 800-1600 mg/day

1- to 3-week I.V. infusion: 600-800 mg/day

>3-week I.V. infusion: 400 mg/day

Recommendations for conversion to intravenous amiodarone after oral administration: During long-term amiodarone therapy (ie, ≥4 months), the mean plasma-elimination half-life of the active metabolite of amiodarone is 61 days. Replacement therapy may not be necessary in such patients if oral therapy is discontinued for a period <2 weeks, since any changes in serum amiodarone concentrations during this period may **not** be clinically significant.

Dosage Forms

Injection, solution: 50 mg/mL (3 mL, 9 mL, 18 mL)

Tablet [scored]: 200 mg, 400 mg

Cordarone®: 200 mg

Pacerone®: 100 mg [not scored], 200 mg, 400 mg

amiodarone hydrochloride *see* amiodarone *on page 64*

Amiodarone Hydrochloride for Injection® [Can] *see* amiodarone *on page 64*

Ami-Tex LA *(Discontinued)* *see* guaifenesin and phenylephrine *on page 475*

Amitiza® [US] *see* lubiprostone *on page 603*

Amitone® *(Discontinued)* *see* calcium carbonate *on page 170*

amitriptyline (a mee TRIP ti leen)

Sound-Alike/Look-Alike Issues

amitriptyline may be confused with aminophylline, imipramine, nortriptyline

Elavil® may be confused with Aldoril®, Eldepryl®, enalapril, Equanil®, Mellaril®, Oruvail®, Plavix®

Synonyms amitriptyline hydrochloride

U.S./Canadian Brand Names Apo-Amitriptyline® [Can]; Levate® [Can]; Novo-Triptyn [Can]; PMS-Amitriptyline [Can]

Therapeutic Category Antidepressant, Tricyclic (Tertiary Amine)

Use Relief of symptoms of depression

Usual Dosage Oral:

Adolescents: Depressive disorders: Initial: 25-50 mg/day; may administer in divided doses; increase gradually to 100 mg/day in divided doses

Adults: Depression: 50-150 mg/day single dose at bedtime or in divided doses; dose may be gradually increased up to 300 mg/day

Dosage Forms

Tablet: 10 mg, 25 mg, 50 mg, 75 mg, 100 mg, 150 mg

amitriptyline and chlordiazepoxide (a mee TRIP ti leen & klor dye az e POKS ide)

Synonyms chlordiazepoxide and amitriptyline hydrochloride

U.S./Canadian Brand Names Limbitrol® [US/Can]

Therapeutic Category Antidepressant, Tricyclic (Tertiary Amine)

Controlled Substance C-IV

Use Treatment of moderate-to-severe anxiety and/or agitation and depression

Usual Dosage Initial: 3-4 tablets in divided doses; this may be increased to 6 tablets/day as required; some patients respond to smaller doses and can be maintained on 2 tablets

Dosage Forms

Tablet: 12.5/5: Amitriptyline 12.5 mg and chlordiazepoxide 5 mg; 25/10: Amitriptyline 25 mg and chlordiazepoxide 10 mg

Limbitrol®: 12.5/5: Amitriptyline 12.5 mg and chlordiazepoxide 5 mg

amitriptyline and perphenazine (a mee TRIP ti leen & per FEN a zeen)

Synonyms perphenazine and amitriptyline hydrochloride

U.S./Canadian Brand Names Etrafon® [Can]

Therapeutic Category Antidepressant/Phenothiazine

Use Treatment of patients with moderate-to-severe anxiety and depression

Usual Dosage Oral: 1 tablet 2-4 times/day

Dosage Forms

Tablet: 2-10: Amitriptyline 10 mg and perphenazine 2 mg; 2-25: Amitriptyline 25 mg and perphenazine 2 mg; 4-10: Amitriptyline 10 mg and perphenazine 4 mg; 4-25: Amitriptyline 25 mg and perphenazine 4 mg; 4-50: Amitriptyline 50 mg and perphenazine 4 mg

amitriptyline hydrochloride *see* amitriptyline *on page 65*

AMJ 9701 *see* palifermin *on page 743*

AmLactin® [US-OTC] *see* lactic acid and ammonium hydroxide *on page 564*

amlexanox (am LEKS an oks)

U.S./Canadian Brand Names Aphthasol® [US]

Therapeutic Category Antiinflammatory Agent, Locally Applied

Use Treatment of aphthous ulcers (ie, canker sores)

Usual Dosage Topical: Administer ~1/4 inch (0.5 cm) directly on ulcers 4 times/day following oral hygiene, after meals, and at bedtime

Dosage Forms

Paste, oral:

Aphthasol®: 5% (3 g)

amlodipine (am LOE di peen)

Sound-Alike/Look-Alike Issues

amLODIPine may be confused with aMILoride

Norvasc® may be confused with Navane®, Norvir®, Vascor®

Synonyms amlodipine besylate

Tall-Man am**LODIP**ine

U.S./Canadian Brand Names CO Amlodipine [Can]; GD-Amlodipine [Can]; Gen-Amlodipine [Can]; Norvasc® [US/Can]; Novo-Amlodipine [Can]; PHL-Amlodipine [Can]; PMS-Amlodipine [Can]; ratio-Amlodipine [Can]; ZYM-Amlodipine [Can]

Therapeutic Category Calcium Channel Blocker

Use Treatment of hypertension; treatment of symptomatic chronic stable angina, vasospastic (Prinzmetal) angina (confirmed or suspected); prevention of hospitalization due to angina with documented CAD (limited to patients without heart failure or ejection fraction <40%)

Usual Dosage Oral:

Children 6-17 years: Hypertension: 2.5-5 mg once daily

Adults:

Hypertension: Initial dose: 5 mg once daily; maximum dose: 10 mg once daily. In general, titrate in 2.5 mg increments over 7-14 days. Usual dosage range (JNC 7): 2.5-10 mg once daily.

Angina: Usual dose: 5-10 mg; lower dose suggested in elderly or hepatic impairment; most patients require 10 mg for adequate effect

Dosage Forms

Tablet: 2.5 mg, 5 mg, 10 mg

Norvasc®: 2.5 mg, 5 mg, 10 mg

amlodipine and atorvastatin (am LOW di peen & a TORE va sta tin)

Synonyms atorvastatin calcium and amlodipine besylate

U.S./Canadian Brand Names Caduet® [US/Can]

Therapeutic Category Antilipemic Agent, HMG-CoA Reductase Inhibitor; Calcium Channel Blocker

Use For use when treatment with both amlodipine and atorvastatin is appropriate:

Amlodipine: Treatment of hypertension; treatment of symptomatic chronic stable angina, vasospastic (Prinzmetal) angina (confirmed or suspected); prevention of hospitalization due to angina with documented CAD (limited to patients without heart failure or ejection fraction <40%)

Atorvastatin: Treatment of dyslipidemias or primary prevention of cardiovascular disease (atherosclerotic) as detailed here:

Primary prevention of cardiovascular disease (high-risk for CVD): To reduce the risk of MI or stroke in patients without evidence of heart disease who have multiple CVD risk factors or type 2 diabetes. Treatment reduces the risk for angina or revascularization procedures in patients with multiple risk factors.

Treatment of dyslipidemias: To reduce elevations in total cholesterol, LDL-C, apolipoprotein B, and triglycerides in patients with elevations of one or more components, and/or to increase HDL-C as present in heterozygous hypercholesterolemia (Fredrickson type IIa hyperlipidemias); treatment of primary dysbetalipoproteinemia (Fredrickson type III), elevated serum TG levels (Fredrickson type IV), and homozygous familial hypercholesterolemia

Treatment of heterozygous familial hypercholesterolemia (HeFH) in adolescent patients (10-17 years of age, females >1 year postmenarche) having LDL-C ≥190 mg/dL or LDL-C ≥160 mg/dL with positive family history of premature cardiovascular disease (CVD) or with two or more CVD risk factors.

Usual Dosage Oral:

Amlodipine:

Children >10 years: Hypertension: 2.5-5 mg once daily. **Note:** Use in ages >10 years because of atorvastatin content.

Adults:

Hypertension: Initial dose: 5 mg once daily; maximum dose: 10 mg once daily; in general, titrate in 2.5 mg increments over 7-14 days. Usual dosage range (JNC 7): 2.5-10 mg once daily

Angina: Usual dose: 5-10 mg; most patients require 10 mg for adequate effect

Atorvastatin:

Children 10-17 years (females >1 year postmenarche): HeFH: 10 mg once daily (maximum: 20 mg/day)

Adults:

Hyperlipidemias: Initial: 10-20 mg once daily; patients requiring >45% reduction in LDL-C may be started at 40 mg once daily; range: 10-80 mg once daily

Primary prevention of CVD: 10 mg once daily

Dosage Forms

Tablet:

Caduet®:

2.5/10: Amlodipine 2.5 mg and atorvastatin 10 mg; 2.5/20: Amlodipine 2.5 mg and atorvastatin 20 mg; 2.5/40: Amlodipine 2.5 mg and atorvastatin 40 mg

5/10: Amlodipine 5 mg and atorvastatin 10 mg; 5/20: Amlodipine 5 mg and atorvastatin 20 mg; 5/40: Amlodipine 5 mg and atorvastatin 40 mg; 5/80: Amlodipine 5 mg and atorvastatin 80 mg

10/10: Amlodipine 10 mg and atorvastatin 10 mg; 10/20: Amlodipine 10 mg and atorvastatin 20 mg; 10/40: Amlodipine 10 mg and atorvastatin 40 mg; 10/80: Amlodipine 10 mg and atorvastatin 80 mg

amlodipine and benazepril (am LOE di peen & ben AY ze pril)

Synonyms benazepril hydrochloride and amlodipine besylate

U.S./Canadian Brand Names Lotrel® [US]

Therapeutic Category Antihypertensive Agent, Combination

Use Treatment of hypertension

Usual Dosage Oral: Adults: 2.5-10 mg (amlodipine) and 10-40 mg (benazepril) once daily; maximum: Amlodipine: 10 mg/day; benazepril: 40 mg/day

Dosage Forms

Capsule: 2.5/10: Amlodipine 2.5 mg and benazepril 10 mg; 5/10: Amlodipine 5 mg and benazepril 10 mg; 5/20: Amlodipine 5 mg and benazepril 20 mg; 10/20: Amlodipine 10 mg and benazepril 20 mg

Lotrel®: 2.5/10: Amlodipine 2.5 and benazepril 10 mg; 5/10: Amlodipine 5 mg and benazepril 10 mg; 5/20: Amlodipine 5 mg and benazepril 20 mg; 5/40: Amlodipine 5 mg and benazepril 40 mg; 10/20: Amlodipine 10 mg and benazepril 20 mg; 10/40: Amlodipine 10 mg and benazepril 40 mg

amlodipine and olmesartan (am LOE di peen & olme SAR tan)

Synonyms amlodipine besylate and olmesartan medoxomil; olmesartan and amlodipine

U.S./Canadian Brand Names Azor™ [US]

Therapeutic Category Angiotensin II Receptor Blocker Combination; Antihypertensive Agent, Combination; Calcium Channel Blocker

Use Treatment of hypertension, including initial treatment in patients who will require multiple antihypertensives for adequate control

Usual Dosage Oral: Dose is individualized; combination product may be substituted for individual components in patients currently maintained on both agents separately or in patients not adequately controlled with monotherapy (using one of the agents or an agent the within same antihypertensive class). May also be used as initial therapy in patients who are likely to need >1 antihypertensive to control blood pressure.

Adults: Hypertension:

Initial therapy (antihypertensive naive): Amlodipine 5 mg/olmesartan 20 mg once daily; dose may be increased after 1-2 weeks of therapy. Maximum recommended dose: Amlodipine 10 mg/day; olmesartan 40 mg/day.

Add-on/replacement therapy: Amlodipine 5-10 mg and olmesartan 20-40 mg once daily depending upon previous doses, current control, and goals of therapy; dose may be titrated after 2 weeks of therapy. Maximum recommended doses: Amlodipine 10 mg/day; olmesartan 40 mg/day.

Dosage Forms

Tablet:

Azor™: 5/20: Amlodipine besylate 5 mg and olmesartan medoxomil 20 mg; 5/40: Amlodipine besylate 5 mg and olmesartan medoxomil 40 mg; 10/20: Amlodipine besylate 10 mg and olmesartan medoxomil 20 mg; 10/40: Amlodipine besylate 10 mg and olmesartan medoxomil 40 mg

amlodipine and valsartan (am LOE di peen & val SAR tan)

Synonyms amlodipine besylate and valsartan; valsartan and amlodipine

U.S./Canadian Brand Names Exforge® [US]

Therapeutic Category Angiotensin II Receptor Blocker Combination; Antihypertensive Agent, Combination; Calcium Channel Blocker

Use Treatment of hypertension

Usual Dosage Oral: Dose is individualized; combination product may be used as initial therapy or substituted for individual components in patients currently maintained on both agents separately or in patients not adequately controlled with monotherapy (using one of the agents or an agent within same antihypertensive class).

Adults: Hypertension:

Initial therapy: Amlodipine 5 mg and valsartan 160 mg once daily, dose may be titrated after 1-2 weeks of therapy. Maximum recommended doses: Amlodipine 10 mg/day; valsartan 320 mg/day

Add-on/replacement therapy: Amlodipine 5-10 mg and valsartan 160-320 mg once daily; dose may be titrated after 3-4 weeks of therapy. Maximum recommended doses: Amlodipine 10 mg/day; valsartan 320 mg/day

Dosage Forms

Tablet:

Exforge®: 5/160: Amlodipine 5 mg and valsartan 160 mg; 5/320 mg: Amlodipine 5 mg and valsartan 320 mg; 10/160: Amlodipine 10 mg and valsartan 160 mg; 10/320: Amlodipine 10 mg and valsartan 320 mg

amlodipine besylate *see* amlodipine *on page* 66

amlodipine besylate and olmesartan medoxomil *see* amlodipine and olmesartan *on page* 68

amlodipine besylate and valsartan *see* amlodipine and valsartan *on page* 68

amlodipine besylate, valsartan, and hydrochlorothiazide *see* amlodipine, valsartan, and hydrochlorothiazide *on page* 69

amlodipine, valsartan, and hydrochlorothiazide

(am LOE di peen, val SAR tan, & hye droe klor oh THYE a zide)

Synonyms amlodipine besylate, valsartan, and hydrochlorothiazide; hydrochlorothiazide, amlodipine, and valsartan; valsartan, hydrochlorothiazide, and amlodipine

U.S./Canadian Brand Names Exforge HCT® [US]

Therapeutic Category Angiotensin II Receptor Blocker; Calcium Channel Blocker; Diuretic, Thiazide

Use Treatment of hypertension (not for initial therapy)

Usual Dosage Oral: **Note:** Not for initial therapy. Dose is individualized; combination product may be substituted for individual components in patients currently maintained on all three agents separately or in patients not adequately controlled with any two of the following antihypertensive classes: calcium channel blockers, angiotensin II receptor blockers, and diuretics.

Adults: Hypertension: Add-on/switch/replacement therapy: Amlodipine 5-10 mg and Valsartan 160-320 mg and hydrochlorothiazide 12.5-25 mg once daily; dose may be titrated after 2 weeks of therapy. Maximum recommended daily dose: Amlodipine 10 mg/valsartan 320 mg/hydrochlorothiazide 25 mg

Dosage Forms

Tablet, oral:

Exforge HCT®: Amlodipine 5 mg, valsartan 160 mg, and hydrochlorothiazide 12.5 mg; Amlodipine 5 mg, valsartan 160 mg, and hydrochlorothiazide 25 mg; Amlodipine 10 mg, valsartan 160 mg, and hydrochlorothiazide 12.5 mg; Amlodipine 10 mg, valsartan 160 mg, and hydrochlorothiazide 25 mg; Amlodipine 10 mg, valsartan 320 mg, and hydrochlorothiazide 25 mg

Ammens® Medicated Deodorant [US-OTC] *see* zinc oxide *on page* *1030*

ammonapse *see* sodium phenylbutyrate *on page* *912*

ammonia spirit (aromatic) (a MOE nee ah SPEAR it, air oh MAT ik)

Synonyms smelling salts

Therapeutic Category Respiratory Stimulant

Use Respiratory and circulatory stimulant; treatment of fainting

Usual Dosage Used as "smelling salts" to treat or prevent fainting

Dosage Forms

Solution, for inhalation: 1.7% to 2.1% (0.33 mL, 60 mL)

ammonium chloride (a MOE nee um KLOR ide)

Therapeutic Category Electrolyte Supplement, Oral

Use Treatment of hypochloremic states or metabolic alkalosis

Usual Dosage Metabolic alkalosis: The following equations represent different methods of correction utilizing either the serum HCO_3^-, the serum chloride, or the base excess

Dosing of mEq NH_4 Cl via the chloride-deficit method (hypochloremia):

Dose of mEq NH_4Cl = [0.2 L/kg x body weight (kg)] x [103 - observed serum chloride]; administer 50% of dose over 12 hours, then reevaluate

Note: 0.2 L/kg is the estimated chloride volume of distribution and 103 is the average normal serum chloride concentration (mEq/L)

Dosing of mEq NH_4 Cl via the bicarbonate-excess method (refractory hypochloremic metabolic alkalosis):

Dose of NH_4Cl = [0.5 L/kg x body weight (kg)] x (observed serum HCO_3^- - 24); administer 50% of dose over 12 hours, then reevaluate

Note: 0.5 L/kg is the estimated bicarbonate volume of distribution and 24 is the average normal serum bicarbonate concentration (mEq/L)

These equations will yield different requirements of ammonium chloride

Dosage Forms

Injection, solution: Ammonium 5 mEq/mL and chloride 5 mEq/mL (20 mL)

ammonium hydroxide and lactic acid *see* lactic acid and ammonium hydroxide *on page* *564*

ammonium lactate *see* lactic acid and ammonium hydroxide *on page* *564*

Ammonul® [US] *see* sodium phenylacetate and sodium benzoate *on page* *912*

AMN107 *see* nilotinib *on page* *697*

Amnesteem™ [US] *see* isotretinoin *on page* *551*

amobarbital (am oh BAR bi tal)

Synonyms amobarbital sodium; amylobarbitone

U.S./Canadian Brand Names Amytal® [US/Can]

Therapeutic Category Barbiturate

Controlled Substance C-II

Use Hypnotic in short-term treatment of insomnia; reduce anxiety and provide sedation preoperatively

Usual Dosage I.M., I.V.:

Children 6-12 years: Sedative: Manufacturer's dosing range: 65-500 mg

Adults:

Hypnotic: 65-200 mg at bedtime (maximum single dose: 1000 mg)

Sedative: 30-50 mg 2-3 times/day (maximum single dose: 1000 mg)

Dosage Forms

Injection, powder for reconstitution:

Amytal®: 500 mg

amobarbital sodium *see* amobarbital *on page 70*

Amoclan [US] *see* amoxicillin and clavulanate potassium *on page 71*

AMO Vitrax® *(Discontinued)* *see* hyaluronate and derivatives *on page 496*

amoxapine (a MOKS a peen)

Sound-Alike/Look-Alike Issues

amoxapine may be confused with amoxicillin, Amoxil®

Asendin may be confused with aspirin

Therapeutic Category Antidepressant, Tricyclic (Secondary Amine)

Use Treatment of depression, psychotic depression, depression accompanied by anxiety or agitation

Usual Dosage Once symptoms are controlled, decrease gradually to lowest effective dose. Maintenance dose is usually given at bedtime to reduce daytime sedation. Oral:

Adolescents: Initial: 25-50 mg/day; increase gradually to 100 mg/day; may administer as divided doses or as a single dose at bedtime

Adults: Initial: 25 mg 2-3 times/day, if tolerated, dosage may be increased to 100 mg 2-3 times/day; may be given in a single bedtime dose when dosage <300 mg/day

Maximum daily dose:

Inpatient: 600 mg

Outpatient: 400 mg

Dosage Forms

Tablet: 25 mg, 50 mg, 100 mg, 150 mg

amoxicillin (a moks i SIL in)

Sound-Alike/Look-Alike Issues

amoxicillin may be confused with amoxapine, Amoxil®, Atarax®

Amoxil® may be confused with amoxapine, amoxicillin

Synonyms *p*-hydroxyampicillin; amoxicillin trihydrate; amoxycillin

U.S./Canadian Brand Names Amoxil® [US]; Apo-Amoxi® [Can]; Gen-Amoxicillin [Can]; Lin-Amox [Can]; Moxatag™ [US]; Novamoxin® [Can]; Nu-Amoxi [Can]; PHL-Amoxicillin [Can]; PMS-Amoxicillin [Can]

Therapeutic Category Penicillin

Use Treatment of otitis media, sinusitis, and infections caused by susceptible organisms involving the upper and lower respiratory tract, skin, and urinary tract; prophylaxis of infective endocarditis in patients undergoing surgical or dental procedures; as part of a multidrug regimen for *H. pylori* eradication

Usual Dosage

Usual dosage range:

Children ≤3 months: Oral: 20-30 mg/kg/day divided every 12 hours

Children >3 months and <40 kg: Oral: 20-50 mg/kg/day in divided doses every 8-12 hours

Children ≥12 years: Oral: Extended-release tablet: 775 mg once daily

Adults: Oral: 250-500 mg every 8 hours or 500-875 mg twice daily

Extended-release tablet: 775 mg once daily

Indication-specific dosing:

Children >3 months and <40 kg: Oral:

Acute otitis media: 80-90 mg/kg/day divided every 12 hours

Anthrax exposure (CDC guidelines): Note: Postexposure prophylaxis only with documented susceptible organisms: 80 mg/kg/day in divided doses every 8 hours (maximum: 500 mg/dose)

Community-acquired pneumonia:

4 months to <5 years: 80-100 mg/kg/day divided every 8 hours

5-15 years: 100 mg/kg/day divided every 8 hours; **Note:** Treatment with a macrolide or doxycycline (if age >8 years) is preferred due to higher prevalence of atypical pathogens in this age group

Ear, nose, throat, genitourinary tract, or skin/skin structure infections:

Mild-to-moderate: 25 mg/kg/day in divided doses every 12 hours **or** 20 mg/kg/day in divided doses every 8 hours

Severe: 45 mg/kg/day in divided doses every 12 hours **or** 40 mg/kg/day in divided doses every 8 hours

Tonsillitis and/or pharyngitis: Children ≥12 years: Extended-release tablet: 775 mg once daily

Lower respiratory tract infections: 45 mg/kg/day in divided doses every 12 hours **or** 40 mg/kg/day in divided doses every 8 hours

Lyme disease: 25-50 mg/kg/day divided every 8 hours (maximum: 500 mg)

Prophylaxis against infective endocarditis: 50 mg/kg 1 hour before procedure. **Note:** American Heart Association (AHA) guidelines now recommend prophylaxis only in patients undergoing invasive procedures and in whom underlying cardiac conditions may predispose to a higher risk of adverse outcomes should infection occur. As of April 2007, routine prophylaxis for GI/GU procedures is no longer recommended by the AHA.

Adults: Oral:

Anthrax exposure (CDC guidelines): Note: Postexposure prophylaxis in pregnant or nursing women only with documented susceptible organisms: 500 mg every 8 hours

Ear, nose, throat, genitourinary tract, or skin/skin structure infections:

Mild-to-moderate: 500 mg every 12 hours **or** 250 mg every 8 hours

Severe: 875 mg every 12 hours **or** 500 mg every 8 hours

Tonsillitis and/or pharyngitis: Extended-release tablet: 775 mg once daily

***Helicobacter pylori* eradication:** 1000 mg twice daily; requires combination therapy with at least one other antibiotic and an acid-suppressing agent (proton pump inhibitor or H_2 blocker)

Lower respiratory tract infections: 875 mg every 12 hours **or** 500 mg every 8 hours

Lyme disease: 500 mg every 6-8 hours (depending on size of patient) for 21-30 days

Prophylaxis against infective endocarditis: 2 g 30-60 minutes before procedure. **Note:** American Heart Association (AHA) guidelines now recommend prophylaxis only in patients undergoing invasive procedures and in whom underlying cardiac conditions may predispose to a higher risk of adverse outcomes should infection occur. As of April 2007, routine prophylaxis for GI/GU procedures is no longer recommended by the AHA.

Prophylaxis in total joint replacement patients undergoing dental procedures which produce bacteremia: 2 g 1 hour prior to procedure

Product Availability Moxatag™: FDA approved January 2009; availability anticipated in March 2009

Moxatag™ is an extended-release tablet of amoxicillin intended for once-daily administration.

Dosage Forms

Capsule: 250 mg, 500 mg

Powder for suspension, oral: 125 mg/5 mL, 200 mg/5 mL, 250 mg/5 mL, 400 mg/5 mL

Tablet: 500 mg, 875 mg

Tablet, chewable: 125 mg, 200 mg, 250 mg, 400 mg

Tablet, extended release:

Moxatag™: 775 mg

amoxicillin and clavulanate potassium

(a moks i SIL in & klav yoo LAN ate poe TASS ee um)

Sound-Alike/Look-Alike Issues

Augmentin® may be confused with Azulfidine®

Synonyms amoxicillin and clavulanic acid; clavulanic acid and amoxicillin

U.S./Canadian Brand Names Alti-Amoxi-Clav [Can]; Amoclan [US]; Apo-Amoxi-Clav® [Can]; Augmentin ES-600® [US]; Augmentin XR® [US]; Augmentin® [US/Can]; Clavulin® [Can]; Novo-Clavamoxin [Can]; ratio-Aclavulanate [Can]

Therapeutic Category Penicillin

Use Treatment of otitis media, sinusitis, and infections caused by susceptible organisms involving the lower respiratory tract, skin and skin structure, and urinary tract; spectrum same as amoxicillin with additional coverage of beta-lactamase producing *B. catarrhalis*, *H. influenzae*, *N. gonorrhoeae*, and *S. aureus* (not MRSA). The expanded coverage of this combination makes it a useful alternative when amoxicillin resistance is present and patients cannot tolerate alternative treatments.

Usual Dosage Note: Dose is based on the amoxicillin component

Usual dosage range:

Infants <3 months: Oral: 30 mg/kg/day divided every 12 hours using the 125 mg/5 mL suspension

Children ≥3 months and <40 kg: Oral: 20-90 mg/kg/day divided every 8-12 hours

Children >40 kg and Adults: Oral: 250-500 mg every 8 hours or 875 mg every 12 hours

Indication-specific dosing:

Children ≥3 months and <40 kg: Oral:

Lower respiratory tract infections, severe infections, sinusitis: 45 mg/kg/day divided every 12 hours **or** 40 mg/kg/day divided every 8 hours

Mild-to-moderate infections: 25 mg/kg/day divided every 12 hours or 20 mg/kg/day divided every 8 hours

Otitis media (Augmentin ES-600®): 90 mg/kg/day divided every 12 hours for 10 days in children with severe illness and when coverage for β-lactamase-positive *H. influenzae* and *M. catarrhalis* is needed.

Children ≥16 years and Adults: Oral:

Acute bacterial sinusitis: Extended release tablet: Two 1000 mg tablets every 12 hours for 10 days

Bite wounds (animal/human): 875 mg every 12 hours **or** 500 mg every 8 hours

Chronic obstructive pulmonary disease: 875 mg every 12 hours **or** 500 mg every 8 hours

Diabetic foot: Extended release tablet: Two 1000 mg tablets every 12 hours for 7-14 days

Diverticulitis, perirectal abscess: Extended release tablet: Two 1000 mg tablets every 12 hours for 7-10 days

Erysipelas: 875 mg every 12 hours **or** 500 mg every 8 hours

Febrile neutropenia: 875 mg every 12 hours

Pneumonia:

Aspiration: 875 mg every 12 hours

Community-acquired: Extended release tablet: Two 1000 mg tablets every 12 hours for 7-10 days

Pyelonephritis (acute, uncomplicated): 875 mg every 12 hours **or** 500 mg every 8 hours

Skin abscess: 875 mg every 12 hours

Dosage Forms

Powder for oral suspension: 200: Amoxicillin 200 mg and clavulanate potassium 28.5 mg per 5 mL; 400: Amoxicillin 400 mg and clavulanate potassium 57 mg per 5 mL; 600: Amoxicillin 600 mg and clavulanate potassium 42.9 mg per 5 mL

Amoclan:

200: Amoxicillin 200 mg and clavulanate potassium 28.5 mg per 5 mL

400: Amoxicillin 400 mg and clavulanate potassium 57 mg per 5 mL

600: Amoxicillin 600 mg and clavulanate potassium 42.9 mg per 5 mL

Augmentin®:

125: Amoxicillin 125 mg and clavulanate potassium 31.25 mg per 5 mL

250: Amoxicillin 250 mg and clavulanate potassium 62.5 mg per 5 mL

Augmentin ES-600®: Amoxicillin 600 mg and clavulanate potassium 42.9 mg per 5 mL

Tablet: 500: Amoxicillin 500 mg and clavulanate potassium 125 mg; 875: Amoxicillin 875 mg and clavulanate potassium 125 mg

Augmentin®:

250: Amoxicillin 250 mg and clavulanate potassium 125 mg

500: Amoxicillin 500 mg and clavulanate potassium 125 mg

875: Amoxicillin 875 mg and clavulanate potassium 125 mg

Tablet, chewable: 200: Amoxicillin 200 mg and clavulanate potassium 28.5 mg; 400: Amoxicillin 400 mg and clavulanate potassium 57 mg

Tablet, extended release:

Augmentin XR®: 1000: Amoxicillin 1000 mg and clavulanate acid 62.5 mg

amoxicillin and clavulanic acid *see* amoxicillin and clavulanate potassium *on page 71*

amoxicillin, clarithromycin, and lansoprazole *see* lansoprazole, amoxicillin, and clarithromycin *on page 571*

amoxicillin trihydrate *see* amoxicillin *on page 70*

Amoxil® [US] *see* amoxicillin *on page 70*

amoxycillin *see* amoxicillin *on page 70*

Amphadase™ [US] *see* hyaluronidase *on page 497*

amphetamine and dextroamphetamine *see* dextroamphetamine and amphetamine *on page 293*

Amphocin® *(Discontinued)* *see* amphotericin B (conventional) *on page 73*

Amphojel® [Can] *see* aluminum hydroxide *on page* 55
Amphojel® ***(Discontinued)*** *see* aluminum hydroxide *on page* 55
Amphotec® [US/Can] *see* amphotericin B cholesteryl sulfate complex *on page* 73
Amphotec® [Can] *see* amphotericin B lipid complex *on page* 74

amphotericin B cholesteryl sulfate complex

(am foe TER i sin bee kole LES te ril SUL fate KOM plecks)

Synonyms ABCD; amphotericin B colloidal dispersion

U.S./Canadian Brand Names Amphotec® [US/Can]

Therapeutic Category Antifungal Agent

Use Treatment of invasive aspergillosis in patients who have failed amphotericin B deoxycholate treatment, or who have renal impairment or experience unacceptable toxicity which precludes treatment with amphotericin B deoxycholate in effective doses.

Usual Dosage I.V.: Children and Adults:

Premedication: For patients who experience chills, fever, hypotension, nausea, or other nonanaphylactic infusion-related immediate reactions, premedicate with the following drugs 30-60 minutes prior to drug administration: A nonsteroidal (eg, ibuprofen, choline magnesium trisalicylate) with or without diphenhydramine **or** acetaminophen with diphenhydramine **or** hydrocortisone 50-100 mg. If the patient experiences rigors during the infusion, meperidine may be administered.

Range: 3-4 mg/kg/day (infusion of 1 mg/kg/hour); maximum: 7.5 mg/kg/day

A regimen of 6 mg/kg/day has been used for treatment of life-threatening invasive mold infections in immunocompromised patients; maximum: 7.5 mg/kg/day

Initially infuse at 1 mg/kg/hour. Rate of infusion may be increased with subsequent doses to 3 mg/kg/hour as patient tolerance allows. Treatment should continue as patient tolerance allows, until complete resolution of microbiologic and clinical evidence of fungal disease.

Dosage Forms

Injection, powder for reconstitution:

Amphotec®: 50 mg, 100 mg

amphotericin B colloidal dispersion *see* amphotericin B cholesteryl sulfate complex *on page* 73

amphotericin B (conventional) (am foe TER i sin bee con VEN sha nal)

Synonyms amphotericin B desoxycholate

U.S./Canadian Brand Names Fungizone® [Can]

Therapeutic Category Antifungal Agent

Use Treatment of severe systemic and central nervous system infections caused by susceptible fungi such as *Candida* species, *Histoplasma capsulatum*, *Cryptococcus neoformans*, *Aspergillus* species, *Blastomyces dermatitidis*, *Torulopsis glabrata*, and *Coccidioides immitis*; fungal peritonitis; irrigant for bladder fungal infections; used in fungal infection in patients with bone marrow transplantation, amebic meningoencephalitis, ocular aspergillosis (intraocular injection), candidal cystitis (bladder irrigation), chemoprophylaxis (low-dose I.V.), immunocompromised patients at risk of aspergillosis (intranasal/ nebulized), refractory meningitis (intrathecal), coccidioidal arthritis (intraarticular/I.M.).

Low-dose amphotericin B has been administered after bone marrow transplantation to reduce the risk of invasive fungal disease.

Usual Dosage Premedication: For patients who experience infusion-related immediate reactions, premedicate with the following drugs 30-60 minutes prior to drug administration: NSAID (with or without diphenhydramine) **or** acetaminophen with diphenhydramine **or** hydrocortisone 50-100 mg. If the patient experiences rigors during the infusion, meperidine may be administered.

Usual dosage ranges:

Infants and Children:

Test dose: I.V.: 0.1 mg/kg/dose to a maximum of 1 mg; infuse over 30-60 minutes. Many clinicians believe a test dose is unnecessary.

Maintenance dose: 0.25-1 mg/kg/day given once daily; infuse over 2-6 hours. Once therapy has been established, amphotericin B can be administered on an every-other-day basis at 1-1.5 mg/kg/dose; cumulative dose: 1.5-2 g over 6-10 weeks.

Duration of therapy: Varies with nature of infection, usual duration is 4-12 weeks or cumulative dose of 1-4 g

Adults:

Test dose: 1 mg infused over 20-30 minutes. Many clinicians believe a test dose is unnecessary.

Maintenance dose: Usual: 0.05-1.5 mg/kg/day; 1-1.5 mg/kg over 4-6 hours every other day may be given once therapy is established; aspergillosis, rhinocerebral mucormycosis, often require 1-1.5 mg/kg/day; do not exceed 1.5 mg/kg/day

Indication-specific dosing:

Children: **Meningitis, coccidioidal or cryptococcal:** I.T.: 25-100 mcg every 48-72 hours; increase to 500 mcg as tolerated

Adults:

Aspergillosis, disseminated: I.V.: 0.6-0.7 mg/kg/day for 3-6 months

Bone marrow transplantation (prophylaxis): I.V.: Low-dose amphotericin B 0.1-0.25 mg/kg/day has been administered after bone marrow transplantation to reduce the risk of invasive fungal disease.

Candidemia (neutropenic or nonneutropenic): I.V.: 0.5-1 mg/kg/day until 14 days after last positive blood culture and resolution of signs and symptoms

Candidiasis, chronic, disseminated: I.V.: 0.5-0.7 mg/kg/day for 3-6 months and resolution of radiologic lesions

Dematiaceous fungi: I.V.: 0.7 mg/kg/day in combination with an azole

Endocarditis: I.V.: 0.6-1 mg/kg/day (with or without flucytosine) for 6 weeks after valve replacement; **Note:** If isolates susceptible and/or clearance demonstrated, guidelines recommend step-down to fluconazole; also for long-term suppression therapy if valve replacement is not possible

Endophthalmitis, fungal: I.V.: 0.7-1 mg/kg/day (with or without flucytosine) for at least 4-6 weeks

Esophageal: I.V.: 0.3-0.7 mg/kg/day for 14-21 days after clinical improvement

Histoplasmosis: Chronic, severe pulmonary or disseminated: I.V.: 0.5-1 mg/kg/day for 7 days, then 0.8 mg/kg every other day (or 3 times/week) until total dose of 10-15 mg/kg; may continue itraconazole as suppressive therapy (lifelong for immunocompromised patients)

Meningitis:

Candidal: I.V.: 0.7-1 mg/kg/day (with or without flucytosine) for at least 4 weeks; **Note:** Liposomal amphotericin favored by IDSA guidelines based on decreased risk of nephrotoxicity and potentially better CNS penetration

Cryptococcal or Coccidioides: I.T.: Initial: 25-300 mcg every 48-72 hours; increase to 500 mcg to 1 mg as tolerated; maximum total dose: 15 mg has been suggested

Histoplasma: I.V.: 0.5-1 mg/kg/day for 7 days, then 0.8 mg/kg every other day (or 3 times/week) for 3 months total duration; follow with fluconazole suppressive therapy for up to 12 months

Meningoencephalitis, cryptococcal: I.V.:

HIV positive: 0.7-1 mg/kg/day (plus flucytosine 100 mg/kg/day) for 2 weeks, then change to oral fluconazole for at least 10 weeks; alternatively, amphotericin and flucytosine may be continued uninterrupted for 6-10 weeks

HIV negative: 0.5-0.7 mg/kg/day (plus flucytosine) for 2 weeks

Oropharyngeal candidiasis: I.V.: 0.3 mg/kg/day for 7-14 days

Osteoarticular candidiasis: I.V.: 0.5-1 mg/kg/day for several weeks, followed by fluconazole for 6-12 months (osteomyelitis) or 6 weeks (septic arthritis)

Penicillium marneffei: I.V.: 0.6 mg/kg/day for 2 weeks

Pneumonia: Cryptococcal (mild-to-moderate): I.V.:

HIV positive: 0.5-1 mg/kg/day

HIV negative: 0.5-0.7 mg/kg/day (plus flucytosine) for 2 weeks

Sporotrichosis: Pulmonary, meningeal, osteoarticular, or disseminated: I.V.: Total dose of 1-2 g, then change to oral itraconazole or fluconazole for suppressive therapy

Urinary tract candidiasis:

Fungus balls: I.V.: 0.5-0.7 mg/kg/day with or without flucytosine 25 mg/kg 4 times daily

Pyelonephritis: I.V.: 0.5-0.7 mg/kg/day with or without flucytosine 25 mg/kg 4 times daily for 2 weeks

Symptomatic cystitis: I.V.: 0.3-0.6 mg/kg/day for 1-7 days

Bladder irrigation: Irrigate with 50 mcg/mL solution instilled periodically or continuously for 5-10 days or until cultures are clear for fluconazole-resistant *Candida*

Dosage Forms

Injection, powder for reconstitution: 50 mg

amphotericin B desoxycholate *see* amphotericin B (conventional) *on page* 73

amphotericin B lipid complex (am foe TER i sin bee LIP id KOM pleks)

Synonyms ABLC

U.S./Canadian Brand Names Abelcet® [US/Can]; Amphotec® [Can]

Therapeutic Category Antifungal Agent

Use Treatment of aspergillosis or any type of progressive fungal infection in patients who are refractory to or intolerant of conventional amphotericin B therapy

Usual Dosage I.V.: Children and Adults:

Premedication: For patients who experience infusion-related immediate reactions, premedicate with the following drugs 30-60 minutes prior to drug administration: A nonsteroidal antiinflammatory agent ± diphenhydramine **or** acetaminophen with diphenhydramine **or** hydrocortisone 50-100 mg. If the patient experiences rigors during the infusion, meperidine may be administered.

Range: 2.5-5 mg/kg/day as a single infusion

Dosage Forms

Injection, suspension [preservative free]:

Abelcet®: 5 mg/mL (20 mL)

amphotericin B liposomal (am foe TER i sin bee lye po SO mal)

Synonyms L-AmB

U.S./Canadian Brand Names AmBisome® [US/Can]

Therapeutic Category Antifungal Agent, Systemic

Use Empirical therapy for presumed fungal infection in febrile, neutropenic patients; treatment of patients with *Aspergillus* species, *Candida* species, and/or *Cryptococcus* species infections refractory to amphotericin B desoxycholate (conventional amphotericin), or in patients where renal impairment or unacceptable toxicity precludes the use of amphotericin B desoxycholate; treatment of cryptococcal meningitis in HIV-infected patients; treatment of visceral leishmaniasis

Usual Dosage

Usual dosage range:

Children ≥1 month: I.V.: 3-6 mg/kg/day

Adults: I.V.: 3-6 mg/kg/day; **Note:** Higher doses (15 mg/kg/day) have been used clinically

Note: Premedication: For patients who experience nonanaphylactic infusion-related immediate reactions, premedicate with the following drugs 30-60 minutes prior to drug administration: A nonsteroidal antiinflammatory agent ± diphenhydramine; **or** acetaminophen with diphenhydramine; **or** hydrocortisone 50-100 mg. If the patient experiences rigors during the infusion, meperidine may be administered.

Indication-specific dosing:

Children ≥1 month: I.V.:

Cryptococcal meningitis (HIV-positive): 6 mg/kg/day

Empiric therapy: 3 mg/kg/day

Systemic fungal infections *(Aspergillus, Candida, Cryptococcus, Histoplasmosis):* 3-5 mg/kg/day

General invasive Candidal disease: 3-5 mg/kg/day

Candidal meningitis: 5 mg/kg/day

Visceral leishmaniasis:

Immunocompetent: 3 mg/kg/day on days 1-5, and 3 mg/kg/day on days 14 and 21; a repeat course may be given in patients who do not achieve parasitic clearance

Note: Alternate regimen of 10 mg/kg/day for 2 days has been reportedly effective.

Immunocompromised: 4 mg/kg/day on days 1-5, and 4 mg/kg/day on days 10, 17, 24, 31, and 38

Adults: I.V.:

Cryptococcal meningitis (HIV-positive): 6 mg/kg/day

Empiric therapy: 3 mg/kg/day

Fungal sinusitis: Limited data in immunocompromised patients have shown efficacy with 3-10 mg/kg/day. **Note:** An azole antifungal is recommended if causative organism is *Aspergillus* spp or *Pseudallescheria boydii* (*Scedosporium* sp).

Systemic fungal infections *(Aspergillus, Candida, Cryptococcus, Histoplasmosis):* 3-5 mg/kg/day

Visceral leishmaniasis:

Immunocompetent: 3 mg/kg/day on days 1-5, and 3 mg/kg/day on days 14 and 21; a repeat course may be given in patients who do not achieve parasitic clearance

Note: Alternate regimen of 2 mg/kg/day for 5 days has been reportedly effective.

Immunocompromised: 4 mg/kg/day on days 1-5, and 4 mg/kg/day on days 10, 17, 24, 31, and 38

Dosage Forms

Injection, powder for reconstitution:

AmBisome®: 50 mg

ampicillin (am pi SIL in)

Sound-Alike/Look-Alike Issues
ampicillin may be confused with aminophylline

Synonyms aminobenzylpenicillin; ampicillin sodium; ampicillin trihydrate

U.S./Canadian Brand Names Apo-Ampi® [Can]; Novo-Ampicillin [Can]; Nu-Ampi [Can]

Therapeutic Category Penicillin

Use Treatment of susceptible bacterial infections (nonbeta-lactamase-producing organisms); treatment or prophylaxis of infective endocarditis; susceptible bacterial infections caused by streptococci, pneumococci, nonpenicillinase-producing staphylococci, *Listeria*, meningococci; some strains of *H. influenzae*, *Salmonella*, *Shigella*, *E. coli*, *Enterobacter*, and *Klebsiella*

Usual Dosage

Usual dosage range:

Infants and Children:

Oral: 50-100 mg/kg/day in doses divided every 6 hours (maximum: 2-4 g/day)

I.M., I.V.: 100-400 mg/kg/day in divided doses every 6 hours (maximum: 12 g/day)

Adults: Oral, I.M., I.V.: 250-500 mg every 6 hours

Indication-specific dosing:

Infants and Children:

Prophylaxis against Infective endocarditis:

Dental, oral, or respiratory tract procedures: I.M., I.V.: 50 mg/kg within 30-60 minutes prior to procedure in patients not allergic to penicillin and unable to take oral amoxicillin. Intramuscular injections should be avoided in patients who are receiving anticoagulant therapy. In these circumstances, orally administered regimens should be given whenever possible. Intravenously administered antibiotics should be used for patients who are unable to tolerate or absorb oral medications.

Note: American Heart Association (AHA) guidelines now recommend prophylaxis only in patients undergoing invasive procedures and in whom underlying cardiac conditions may predispose to a higher risk of adverse outcomes should infection occur.

Genitourinary and gastrointestinal tract procedures: I.M., I.V.:

High-risk patients: 50 mg/kg (maximum: 2 g) within 30 minutes prior to procedure, followed by ampicillin 25 mg/kg (or amoxicillin 25 mg/kg orally) 6 hours later; must be used in combination with gentamicin. **Note:** As of April 2007, routine prophylaxis for GI/GU procedures is no longer recommended by the AHA.

Moderate-risk patients: 50 mg/kg within 30 minutes prior to procedure

Mild-to-moderate infections:

Oral: 50-100 mg/kg/day in doses divided every 6 hours (maximum: 2-4 g/day)

I.M., I.V.: 100-150 mg/kg/day in divided doses every 6 hours (maximum: 2-4 g/day)

Severe infections, meningitis: I.M., I.V.: 200-400 mg/kg/day in divided doses every 6 hours (maximum: 6-12 g/day)

Adults:

Actinomycosis: I.V.: 50 mg/kg/day for 4-6 weeks then oral amoxicillin

Cholangitis (acute): I.V.: 2 g every 4 hours with gentamicin

Diverticulitis: I.M., I.V.: 2 g every 6 hours with metronidazole

Endocarditis:

Infective: I.V.: 12 g/day via continuous infusion or divided every 4 hours

Prophylaxis: Dental, oral, or respiratory tract: I.M., I.V.: 2 g within 30-60 minutes prior to procedure in patients not allergic to penicillin and unable to take oral amoxicillin. Intramuscular injections should be avoided in patients who are receiving anticoagulant therapy. In these circumstances, orally administered regimens should be given whenever possible. Intravenously administered antibiotics should be used for patients who are unable to tolerate or absorb oral medications.

Note: American Heart Association (AHA) guidelines now recommend prophylaxis only in patients undergoing invasive procedures and in whom underlying cardiac conditions may predispose to a higher risk of adverse outcomes should infection occur.

Prophylaxis in total joint replacement patient: I.M., I.V.: 2 g 1 hour prior to the procedure

Genitourinary and gastrointestinal tract procedures:

High-risk patients: I.M., I.V.: 2 g within 30 minutes prior to procedure, followed by ampicillin 1 g (or amoxicillin 1g orally) 6 hours later; must be used in combination with gentamicin. **Note:** As of April 2007, routine prophylaxis for GI/GU procedures is no longer recommended by the AHA.

Moderate-risk patients: I.M., I.V.: 2 g within 30 minutes prior to procedure

Group B strep prophylaxis (intrapartum): I.V.: 2 g initial dose, then 1 g every 4 hours until delivery

***Listeria* infections:** I.V.: 2 g every 4 hours (consider addition of aminoglycoside)

Sepsis/meningitis: I.M., I.V.: 150-250 mg/kg/day divided every 3-4 hours (range: 6-12 g/day)

Urinary tract infections (enterococcus suspected): I.V.: 1-2 g every 6 hours with gentamicin

Dosage Forms

Capsule: 250 mg, 500 mg

Injection, powder for reconstitution: 125 mg, 250 mg, 500 mg, 1 g, 2 g, 10 g

Powder for oral suspension: 125 mg/5 mL, 250 mg/5 mL

ampicillin and sulbactam (am pi SIL in & SUL bak tam)

Synonyms sulbactam and ampicillin

U.S./Canadian Brand Names Unasyn® [US/Can]

Therapeutic Category Penicillin

Use Treatment of susceptible bacterial infections involved with skin and skin structure, intraabdominal infections, gynecological infections; spectrum is that of ampicillin plus organisms producing beta-lactamases such as *S. aureus*, *H. influenzae*, *E. coli*, *Klebsiella*, *Acinetobacter*, *Enterobacter*, and anaerobes

Usual Dosage Note: Unasyn® (ampicillin/sulbactam) is a combination product. Dosage recommendations for Unasyn® are based on the ampicillin component.

Usual dosage range:

Children ≥1 year: I.V.: 100-400 mg ampicillin/kg/day divided every 6 hours (maximum: 8 g ampicillin/day, 12 g Unasyn®). **Note:** The American Academy of Pediatrics recommends a dose of up to 300 mg/kg/day for severe infection in infants >1 month of age.

Adults: I.M., I.V.: 1-2 g ampicillin (1.5-3 g Unasyn®) every 6 hours (maximum: 8 g ampicillin/day, 12 g Unasyn®)

Indication-specific dosing:

Children: ≥1 year:

Epiglottitis: I.V.: 100-200 mg ampicillin/kg/day divided in 4 doses

Mild-to-moderate infections: I.V.: 100-200 mg ampicillin/kg/day (150-300 mg Unasyn®) divided every 6 hours (maximum: 8 g ampicillin/day, 12 g Unasyn®)

Peritonsillar and retropharyngeal abscess: I.V.: 50 mg ampicillin/kg/dose every 6 hours

Severe infections: I.V.: 200-400 mg ampicillin/kg/day divided every 6 hours (maximum: 8 g ampicillin/day, 12 g Unasyn®)

Adults: Doses expressed as ampicillin/sulbactam combination:

Amnionitis, cholangitis, diverticulitis, endometritis, endophthalmitis, epididymitis/orchitis, liver abscess, osteomyelitis (diabetic foot), peritonitis: I.V.: 3 g every 6 hours

Endocarditis: I.V.: 3 g every 6 hours with gentamicin or vancomycin for 4-6 weeks

Orbital cellulitis: I.V.: 1.5 g every 6 hours

Parapharyngeal space infections: I.V.: 3 g every 6 hours

***Pasteurella multocida* (human, canine/feline bites):** I.V.: 1.5-3 g every 6 hours

Pelvic inflammatory disease: I.V.: 3 g every 6 hours with doxycycline

Peritonitis (CAPD): Intraperitoneal:

Anuric, intermittent: 3 g every 12 hours

Anuric, continuous: Loading dose: 1.5 g; maintenance dose: 150 mg

Pneumonia:

Aspiration, community-acquired: I.V.: 1.5-3 g every 6 hours

Hospital-acquired: I.V.: 3 g every 6 hours

Urinary tract infections, pyelonephritis: I.V.: 3 g every 6 hours for 14 days

Dosage Forms

Injection, powder for reconstitution: 1.5 g [ampicillin 1 g and sulbactam 0.5 g]; 3 g [ampicillin 2 g and sulbactam 1 g]; 15 g [ampicillin 10 g and sulbactam 5 g]

Unasyn®: 1.5 g [ampicillin 1 g and sulbactam 0.5 g]; 3 g [ampicillin 2 g and sulbactam 1 g]; 15 g [ampicillin 10 g and sulbactam 5 g]; 15 g [ampicillin 10 g and sulbactam 5 g

ampicillin sodium *see* ampicillin *on page 76*

ampicillin trihydrate *see* ampicillin *on page 76*

amprenavir *(Discontinued)*

AMPT *see* metyrosine *on page 653*

amrinone lactate *see* inamrinone *on page 525*

Amrix® [US] *see* cyclobenzaprine *on page 264*

Amvisc® *(Discontinued)* *see* hyaluronate and derivatives *on page 496*

Amvisc® Plus *(Discontinued)* *see* hyaluronate and derivatives *on page 496*

amyl nitrite (AM il NYE trite)

Synonyms isoamyl nitrite

Therapeutic Category Vasodilator

Use Coronary vasodilator in angina pectoris; adjunct in treatment of cyanide poisoning; produce changes in the intensity of heart murmurs

Usual Dosage Nasal inhalation:

Cyanide poisoning: Children and Adults: Inhale the vapor from a 0.3 mL crushed ampul every minute for 15-30 seconds until I.V. sodium nitrite infusion is available

Angina: Adults: 1-6 inhalations from 1 crushed ampul; may repeat in 3-5 minutes

Dosage Forms

Vapor for inhalation [crushable covered glass capsules]: Amyl nitrite USP (0.3 mL)

amyl nitrite, sodium nitrite, and sodium thiosulfate *see* sodium nitrite, sodium thiosulfate, and amyl nitrite *on page 911*

amylobarbitone *see* amobarbital *on page 70*

Amytal® [US/Can] *see* amobarbital *on page 70*

AN100226 *see* natalizumab *on page 683*

Anabolin® *(Discontinued)* *see* nandrolone *(Canada only) on page 680*

Anacin® Advanced Headache Formula [US-OTC] *see* acetaminophen, aspirin, and caffeine *on page 24*

Anacin® PM Aspirin Free *(Discontinued)* *see* acetaminophen and diphenhydramine *on page 21*

Anadrol®-50 [US] *see* oxymetholone *on page 740*

Anafranil® [US/Can] *see* clomipramine *on page 244*

anagrelide (an AG gre lide)

Sound-Alike/Look-Alike Issues

anagrelide may be confused with anastrozole

Synonyms anagrelide hydrochloride; BL4162A; NSC-724577

U.S./Canadian Brand Names Agrylin® [US/Can]; Dom-Anagrelide [Can]; Gen-Anagrelide [Can]; PHL-Anagrelide [Can]; PMS-Anagrelide [Can]; Sandoz-Anagrelide [Can]

Therapeutic Category Platelet Reducing Agent

Use Treatment of thrombocythemia associated with myeloproliferative disorders (eg, chronic myelogenous leukemia, essential thrombocythemia, polycythemia vera, myeloid metaplasia with myelofibrosis, or other myeloproliferative disorder)

Usual Dosage Note: Maintain for ≥1 week, then adjust to the lowest effective dose to reduce and maintain platelet count <600,000/μL ideally to the normal range; the dose must not be increased by >0.5 mg/day in any 1 week; maximum dose: 10 mg/day or 2.5 mg/dose

Oral: Thrombocythemia:

Children: Initial: 0.5 mg/day (range: 0.5 mg 1-4 times/day)

Adults: 0.5 mg 4 times/day or 1 mg twice daily (most patients will experience adequate response at dose ranges of 1.5-3 mg/day)

Dosage Forms

Capsule: 0.5 mg, 1 mg

Agrylin®: 0.5 mg

anagrelide hydrochloride *see* anagrelide *on page 78*

anakinra (an a KIN ra)

Sound-Alike/Look-Alike Issues

anakinra may be confused with amikacin

Synonyms IL-1Ra; interleukin-1 receptor antagonist

U.S./Canadian Brand Names Kineret® [US/Can]

Therapeutic Category Antirheumatic, Disease Modifying

Use Treatment of moderately- to severely-active rheumatoid arthritis in adult patients who have failed one or more disease-modifying antirheumatic drugs (DMARDs); may be used alone or in combination with DMARDs (other than tumor necrosis factor-blocking agents)

Usual Dosage SubQ: Adults: Rheumatoid arthritis: 100 mg once daily (administer at approximately the same time each day)

Dosage Forms

Injection, solution [preservative free]:

Kineret®: 100 mg/0.67 mL (0.67 mL)

Ana-Kit® [US] *see* epinephrine and chlorpheniramine *on page 360*

Analpram-HC® [US] *see* pramoxine and hydrocortisone *on page 810*

AnaMantle HC® Cream [US] *see* lidocaine and hydrocortisone *on page 587*

AnaMantle HC® Forte [US] *see* lidocaine and hydrocortisone *on page 587*

AnaMantle HC® Gel [US] *see* lidocaine and hydrocortisone *on page 587*

Anamine® Syrup *(Discontinued)* *see* chlorpheniramine and pseudoephedrine *on page 215*

Anandron® [Can] *see* nilutamide *on page 697*

Anaplex® DM [US] *see* brompheniramine, pseudoephedrine, and dextromethorphan *on page 152*

Anaplex® DMX *(Discontinued)* *see* brompheniramine, pseudoephedrine, and dextromethorphan *on page 152*

Anaplex® Liquid *(Discontinued)* *see* chlorpheniramine and pseudoephedrine *on page 215*

Anaprox® [US/Can] *see* naproxen *on page 681*

Anaprox® DS [US/Can] *see* naproxen *on page 681*

Anaspaz® [US] *see* hyoscyamine *on page 512*

anastrozole (an AS troe zole)

Sound-Alike/Look-Alike Issues

anastrozole may be confused with anagrelide, letrozole

Arimidex® may be confused with Aromasin®

Synonyms ICI-D1033; NSC-719344; ZD1033

U.S./Canadian Brand Names Arimidex® [US/Can]

Therapeutic Category Antineoplastic Agent

Use Treatment of locally-advanced or metastatic breast cancer (hormone receptor-positive or unknown) in postmenopausal women; treatment of advanced breast cancer in postmenopausal women with disease progression following tamoxifen therapy; adjuvant treatment of early hormone receptor-positive breast cancer in postmenopausal women

Usual Dosage Oral: Adults: Breast cancer: 1 mg once daily

Dosage Forms

Tablet:

Arimidex®: 1 mg

Anatrast [US] *see* barium *on page 122*

Anbesol® [US-OTC] *see* benzocaine *on page 129*

Anbesol® Baby [US-OTC/Can] *see* benzocaine *on page 129*

Anbesol® Cold Sore Therapy [US-OTC] *see* benzocaine *on page 129*

Anbesol® Jr. [US-OTC] *see* benzocaine *on page 129*

Anbesol® Maximum Strength [US-OTC] *see* benzocaine *on page 129*

Ancobon® [US/Can] *see* flucytosine *on page 425*

Andehist DM NR [US] *see* brompheniramine, pseudoephedrine, and dextromethorphan *on page 152*

Andehist DM NR Drops *(Discontinued)*

Andehist NR Drops *(Discontinued)*

Andehist NR Syrup *(Discontinued)* *see* brompheniramine and pseudoephedrine *on page 150*

Andriol® [Can] *see* testosterone *on page 947*

Androcur® [Can] *see* cyproterone *(Canada only) on page 268*

Androcur® Depot [Can] *see* cyproterone *(Canada only) on page 268*

Androderm® [US/Can] *see* testosterone *on page 947*

AndroGel® [US/Can] *see* testosterone *on page 947*

Android® [US] *see* methyltestosterone *on page 648*

Andro-L.A.® Injection *(Discontinued)* *see* testosterone *on page 947*

Androlone®-D *(Discontinued)* *see* nandrolone *(Canada only) on page 680*

Androlone® *(Discontinued)* *see* nandrolone *(Canada only) on page 680*

Andropository [Can] *see* testosterone *on page 947*

Andropository® Injection *(Discontinued)* *see* testosterone *on page 947*

Androvite® [US-OTC] *see* vitamins (multiple/oral) *on page 1019*
Androxy™ [US] *see* fluoxymesterone *on page 433*
Anectine® [US] *see* succinylcholine *on page 924*
Anestacon® [US] *see* lidocaine *on page 584*
Anestafoam™ [US-OTC] *see* lidocaine *on page 584*
aneurine hydrochloride *see* thiamine *on page 954*
Anexate® [Can] *see* flumazenil *on page 426*
Angeliq® [US/Can] *see* drospirenone and estradiol *on page 340*
Angiofluor™ [US] *see* fluorescein *on page 429*
Angiofluor™ Lite [US] *see* fluorescein *on page 429*
Angiomax® [US/Can] *see* bivalirudin *on page 144*
anhydrous glucose *see* dextrose *on page 298*

anidulafungin (ay nid yoo la FUN jin)

Synonyms LY303366

U.S./Canadian Brand Names Eraxis™ [US/Can]

Therapeutic Category Antifungal Agent, Parenteral; Echinocandin

Use Treatment of candidemia and other forms of *Candida* infections (including those of intraabdominal, peritoneal, and esophageal locus)

Usual Dosage I.V.: Adults:

Candidemia, intraabdominal or peritoneal candidiasis: 200 mg loading dose on day 1, followed by 100 mg daily for at least 14 days after last positive culture

Esophageal candidiasis: 100 mg loading dose on day 1, followed by 50 mg daily for at least 14 days and for at least 7 days after symptom resolution

Dosage Forms

Injection, powder for reconstitution [preservative free]:

Eraxis™: 50 mg, 100 mg

Anodynos-DHC® ***(Discontinued)*** *see* hydrocodone and acetaminophen *on page 501*
Anolor 300 [US] *see* butalbital, acetaminophen, and caffeine *on page 161*
Anoquan® ***(Discontinued)***
Ansaid® [Can] *see* flurbiprofen *on page 435*
Ansaid® ***(Discontinued)*** *see* flurbiprofen *on page 435*
ansamycin *see* rifabutin *on page 866*
Antabuse® [US] *see* disulfiram *on page 325*
antagon *see* ganirelix *on page 455*
Antara® [US] *see* fenofibrate *on page 408*
Antazoline-V® Ophthalmic ***(Discontinued)***
Anthra-Derm® ***(Discontinued)*** *see* anthralin *on page 80*
Anthraforte® [Can] *see* anthralin *on page 80*

anthralin (AN thra lin)

Synonyms dithranol

U.S./Canadian Brand Names Anthraforte® [Can]; Anthranol® [Can]; Anthrascalp® [Can]; Dritho-Scalp® [US]; Micanol® [Can]; Psoriatec™ [US]

Therapeutic Category Keratolytic Agent

Use Treatment of psoriasis (quiescent or chronic psoriasis)

Usual Dosage Topical: Adults: Generally, apply once a day or as directed. The irritant potential of anthralin is directly related to the strength being used and each patient's individual tolerance. Always commence treatment using a short, daily contact time (5-10 minutes) for at least 1 week using the lowest strength possible. Contact time may be gradually increased (to 20-30 minutes) as tolerated.

Skin application: Apply sparingly only to psoriatic lesions and rub gently and carefully into the skin until absorbed. Avoid applying an excessive quantity which may cause unnecessary soiling and staining of the clothing or bed linen.

Scalp application: Comb hair to remove scalar debris, wet hair and, after suitably parting, rub cream well into the lesions, taking care to prevent the cream from spreading onto the forehead.

Remove by washing or showering; optimal period of contact will vary according to the strength used and the patient's response to treatment. Continue treatment until the skin is entirely clear (ie, when there is nothing to feel with the fingers and the texture is normal).

Dosage Forms

Cream:

Dritho-Scalp®: 0.5% (50 g)

Psoriatec™: 1% (50 g)

Anthranol® [Can] *see* anthralin *on page 80*

Anthrascalp® [Can] *see* anthralin *on page 80*

anthrax vaccine, adsorbed (AN thraks vak SEEN ad SORBED)

Synonyms AVA

U.S./Canadian Brand Names BioThrax® [US]

Therapeutic Category Vaccine

Use Immunization against *Bacillus anthracis* in persons at high risk for exposure.

The Advisory Committee on Immunization Practices (ACIP) recommends routine vaccination for the following:

- Persons who work directly with the organism in the laboratory
- Persons who may come in contact with animal products which come from anthrax endemic areas and may be contaminated with *Bacillus anthracis* spores, such as veterinarians who travel to other countries or persons who work with imported animal hides/furs from areas where standards are insufficient to prevent anthrax spores.
- Military personnel deployed to areas with high risk of exposure

Routine immunization for the general population is not recommended.

Usual Dosage I.M.: Adults:

Primary immunization: Five injections of 0.5 mL each given at 0- and 4 weeks, then 6-, 12-, and 18 months

Subsequent booster injections: 0.5 mL at 1-year intervals are recommended for immunity to be maintained in persons who remain at risk

Dosage Forms

Injection, suspension:

BioThrax®: *Bacillus anthracis* proteins (5 mL)

anti-4 alpha integrin *see* natalizumab *on page 683*

131 I anti-B1 antibody *see* tositumomab and iodine I 131 tositumomab *on page 971*

131 I-anti-B1 monoclonal antibody *see* tositumomab and iodine I 131 tositumomab *on page 971*

Antiben® *(Discontinued)* *see* antipyrine and benzocaine *on page 85*

anti-CD11a *see* efalizumab *on page 348*

anti-CD20 monoclonal antibody *see* rituximab *on page 872*

anti-CD20-murine monoclonal antibody I-131 *see* tositumomab and iodine I 131 tositumomab *on page 971*

antidigoxin fab fragments, ovine *see* digoxin immune Fab *on page 308*

antidiuretic hormone *see* vasopressin *on page 1008*

antihemophilic factor (human) (an tee hee moe FIL ik FAK tor HYU man)

Synonyms AHF (human); factor VIII (human)

U.S./Canadian Brand Names Hemofil M [US/Can]; Koāte®-DVI [US]; Monarc-M™ [US]; Monoclate-P® [US]

Therapeutic Category Blood Product Derivative

Use Prevention and treatment of hemorrhagic episodes in patients with hemophilia A (classic hemophilia); perioperative management of hemophilia A; can be of significant therapeutic value in patients with acquired factor VIII inhibitors not exceeding 10 Bethesda units/mL

Usual Dosage I.V.: Children and Adults: Individualize dosage based on coagulation studies performed prior to treatment and at regular intervals during treatment. In general, administration of factor VIII 1 int. unit/kg will increase circulating factor VIII levels by ~2 int. units/dL. (General guidelines presented; consult individual product labeling for specific dosing recommendations.)

Dosage based on desired factor VIII increase (%):
To calculate dosage needed based on desired factor VIII increase (%):
Body weight (kg) x 0.5 int. units/kg x desired factor VIII increase (%) = int. units factor VIII required
For example:
50 kg x 0.5 int. units/kg x 30 (% increase) = 750 int. units factor VIII
Dosage based on expected factor VIII increase (%):
It is also possible to calculate the **expected** % factor VIII increase:
(# int. units administered x 2%/int. units/kg) divided by body weight (kg) = expected % factor VIII increase
For example:
(1400 int. units x 2%/int. units/kg) divided by 70 kg = 40%
General guidelines:
Minor hemorrhage: 10-20 int. units/kg as a single dose to achieve FVIII plasma level ~20% to 40% of normal. Mild superficial or early hemorrhages may respond to a single dose; may repeat dose every 12-24 hours for 1-3 days until bleeding is resolved or healing achieved.
Moderate hemorrhage/minor surgery: 15-25 int. units/kg to achieve FVIII plasma level 30% to 50% of normal. If needed, may continue with a maintenance dose of 10-15 int. units/kg every 8-12 hours.
Major to life-threatening hemorrhage: Initial dose 40-50 int. units/kg, followed by a maintenance dose of 20-25 int. units/kg every 8-12 hours until threat is resolved, to achieve FVIII plasma level 80% to 100% of normal.
Major surgery: 50 int. units/kg given preoperatively to raise factor VIII level to 100% before surgery begins. May repeat as necessary after 6-12 hours initially and for a total of 10-14 days until healing is complete. Intensity of therapy may depend on type of surgery and postoperative regimen.
Bleeding prophylaxis: May be administered on a regular basis for bleeding prophylaxis. Doses of 24-40 int. units/kg 3 times/week have been reported in patients with severe hemophilia to prevent joint bleeding.
If bleeding is not controlled with adequate dose, test for presence of inhibitor. It may not be possible or practical to control bleeding if inhibitor titers are >10 Bethesda units/mL.

Dosage Forms
Injection, powder for reconstitution:
Hemofil M: Vial labeled with international units
Koāte®-DVI: ~250 int. units, ~500 int. units, ~1000 int. units
Monarc-M™: Vial labeled with international units
Monoclate-P®: ~250 int. units, ~500 int. units, ~1000 int. units, ~1500 int. units

antihemophilic factor (recombinant) (an tee hee moe FIL ik FAK tor ree KOM be nant)

Synonyms AHF (recombinant); factor VIII (recombinant); rAHF

U.S./Canadian Brand Names Advate [US]; Helixate® FS [US/Can]; Kogenate® FS [US/Can]; Kogenate® [Can]; Recombinate [US/Can]; ReFacto® [Can]; Xyntha™ [US]

Therapeutic Category Blood Product Derivative

Use Prevention and treatment of hemorrhagic episodes in patients with hemophilia A (classic hemophilia); can be of significant therapeutic value in patients with acquired factor VIII inhibitors ≤10 Bethesda units/mL

Usual Dosage I.V.:
Hemophilia: Children and Adults: Individualize dosage based on coagulation studies performed prior to treatment and at regular intervals during treatment. In general, administration of factor VIII 1 int. unit/kg will increase circulating factor VIII levels by ~2 int. units/dL. (General guidelines presented; consult individual product labeling for specific dosing recommendations).
Joint bleeding prophylaxis (Kogenate® FS): Children: 25 int. units/kg every other day

Dosage based on desired factor VIII increase (%):
To calculate dosage needed based on desired factor VIII increase (%):
[Body weight (kg) x desired factor VIII increase (%)] divided by 2%/int. units/kg = int. units factor VIII required
For example:
50 kg x 30 (% increase) divided by 2%/int. units/kg = 750 int. units factor VIII
Dosage based on expected factor VIII increase (%):
It is also possible to calculate the **expected** % factor VIII increase:
(# int. units administered x 2%/int. units/kg) divided by body weight (kg) = expected % factor VIII increase
For example:
(1400 int. units x 2%/int. units/kg) divided by 70 kg = 40%

General guidelines:

Minor hemorrhage: 10-20 int. units/kg as a single dose to achieve FVIII plasma level ~20% to 40% of normal. Mild superficial or early hemorrhages may respond to a single dose; may repeat dose every 12-24 hours for 1-3 days until bleeding is resolved or healing achieved.

Moderate hemorrhage/minor surgery: 15-30 int. units/kg to achieve FVIII plasma level 30% to 60% of normal. May repeat 1 dose at 12-24 hours if needed. Some products suggest continuing for ≥3 days until pain and disability are resolved.

Major to life-threatening hemorrhage: Initial dose 40-50 int. units/kg followed by a maintenance dose of 20-25 int. units/kg every 8-24 hours until threat is resolved, to achieve FVIII plasma level 60% to 100% of normal.

Major surgery: 50 int. units/kg given preoperatively to raise factor VIII level to 100% before surgery begins. May repeat as necessary after 6-12 hours initially and for a total of 10-14 days until healing is complete. Intensity of therapy may depend on type of surgery and postoperative regimen.

Bleeding prophylaxis: May be administered on a regular basis for bleeding prophylaxis. Doses of 24-40 int. units/kg 3 times/week have been reported in patients with severe hemophilia to prevent joint bleeding.

If bleeding is not controlled with adequate dose, test for presence of inhibitor. It may not be possible or practical to control bleeding if inhibitor titers >10 Bethesda units/mL.

Product Availability Xyntha™: FDA approved February 2008; availability anticipated in September 2008

Wyeth is replacing ReFacto® with Xyntha™.

Dosage Forms

Injection, powder for reconstitution, recombinant [preservative free]:

Advate: 250 int. units, 500 int. units, 1000 int. units, 1500 int. units, 3000 int. units

Helixate® FS, Recombinate: 250 int. units, 500 int. units, 1000 int. units

Kogenate® FS: 250 int. units, 500 int. units, 1000 int. units, 2000 int. units, 3000 int. units

Xyntha™: 250 int. units, 500 int. units, 1000 int. units, 2000 int. units

antihemophilic factor/von Willebrand factor complex (human)

(an tee hee moe FIL ik FAK tor von WILL le brand FAK tor KOM plex HYU man)

Synonyms AHF (human); factor VIII (human); FVIII/vWF; vWF:RCof

U.S./Canadian Brand Names Alphanate® *[new formulation]* [US]; Humate-P® [US/Can]

Therapeutic Category Antihemophilic Agent; Blood Product Derivative

Use

Prevention and treatment of hemorrhagic episodes in patients with hemophilia A (classical hemophilia) (Alphanate®, Humate-P®) or acquired factor VIII deficiency (Alphanate®)

Prophylaxis with surgical and/or invasive procedures in patients with von Willebrand disease (vWD) when desmopressin is either ineffective or contraindicated (Alphanate®)

Treatment of spontaneous or trauma-induced bleeding, as well as prevention of excessive bleeding during and after surgery, in patients with vWD (mild, moderate, or severe) where use of desmopressin is known or suspected to be inadequate (Humate-P®)

Usual Dosage

Hemophilia A: General guidelines (consult specific product labeling): Children and Adults: I.V.:

Individualize dosage based on coagulation studies performed prior to treatment and at regular intervals during treatment; in general, administration of factor VIII 1 int. unit/kg will increase circulating factor VIII levels by ~2 int. units/dL.

Minor hemorrhage: Loading dose: FVIII:C 15 int. units/kg to achieve FVIII:C plasma level ~30% of normal. If second infusion is needed, half the loading dose may be given once or twice daily for 1-2 days.

Moderate hemorrhage: Loading dose: FVIII:C 25 int. units/kg to achieve FVIII:C plasma level ~50% of normal; Maintenance: FVIII:C 15 int. units/kg every 8-12 hours for 1-2 days in order to maintain FVIII:C plasma levels at 30% of normal. Repeat the same dose once or twice daily for up to 7 days or until adequate wound healing.

Life-threatening hemorrhage/major surgery: Loading dose: FVIII:C 40-50 int. units/kg; Maintenance: FVIII:C 20-25 int. units/kg every 8 hours to maintain FVIII:C plasma levels at 80% to 100% of normal for 7 days. Continue same dose once or twice daily for another 7 days in order to maintain FVIII:C levels at 30% to 50% of normal.

von Willebrand disease (vWD): Treatment (Humate-P®): Children and Adults: I.V.: Individualize dosage based on coagulation studies performed prior to treatment and at regular intervals during treatment; in general, administration of factor VIII 1 int. unit/kg would be expected to raise circulating vWF:RCof ~5 int. units/dL

Type 1, mild (if desmopressin is not appropriate): Major hemorrhage:
Loading dose: vWF:RCof 40-60 int. units/kg
Maintenance dose: vWF:RCof 40-50 int. units/kg every 8-12 hours for 3 days, keeping vWF:RCof nadir >50%; follow with 40-50 int. units/kg daily for up to 7 days
Type 1, moderate or severe:
Minor hemorrhage: vWF:RCof 40-50 int. units/kg for 1-2 doses
Major hemorrhage:
Loading dose: vWF:RCof 50-75 int. units/kg
Maintenance dose: vWF:RCof 40-60 int. units/kg every 8-12 hours for 3 days to keep the vWF:RCof nadir >50%, then 40-60 int. units/kg daily for a total of up to 7 days
Types 2 and 3:
Minor hemorrhage: vWF:RCof 40-50 int. units/kg for 1-2 doses
Major hemorrhage:
Loading dose: vWF:RCof 60-80 int. units/kg
Maintenance dose: vWF:RCof 40-60 int. units/kg every 8-12 hours for 3 days, keeping the vWF:RCof nadir >50%; follow with 40-60 int. units/kg daily for a total of up to 7 days

von Willebrand disease (vWD): Surgery/procedure prophylaxis (except patients with type 3 undergoing major surgery) (Alphanate®):
Children: I.V.:
Preoperative dose: vWF:RCof 75 int. units/kg 1 hour prior to surgery
Maintenance dose: vWF:RCof 50-75 int. units/kg every 8-12 hours as clinically needed. May reduce dose after third postoperative day; continue treatment until healing is complete.
Adults: I.V.:
Preoperative dose: vWF:RCof 60 int. units/kg 1 hour prior to surgery
Maintenance dose: vWF:RCof 40-60 int. units/kg every 8-12 hours as clinically needed. May reduce dose after third postoperative day; continue treatment until healing is complete. For minor procedures, maintain vWF of 40% to 50% during postoperative days 1-3; for major procedures maintain vWF of 40% to 50% for ≥3-7 days.

von Willebrand disease (vWD): Surgery/procedure prevention of bleeding (Humate-P®): Children and Adults: I.V.:
Emergency surgery: Administer vWF:RCof 50-60 int units/kg; monitor trough coagulation factor levels for subsequent doses
Surgical management (nonemergency):
Loading dose calculation based on baseline target vWF:RCo: (Target peak vWF:RCof - Baseline vWF: RCof) x weight (in kg) / IVR = int. units vWF:RCof required. Administer loading dose 1-2 hours prior to surgery. **Note:** If IVR not available, assume 2 int. units/dL per int. units/kg of vWF:RCof product administered.
Target concentrations for vWF:RCof following loading dose:
Major surgery: 100 int. units/dL
Minor surgery: 50-60 int. units/dL
Maintenance dose: Initial: 1/2 loading dose followed by dosing determined by target tough concentrations, generally every 8-12 hours. Patients with shorter half-lives may require dosing every 6 hours.
Target maintenance trough vWF:RCof concentrations:
Major surgery: >50 int. units/dL for up to 3 days, followed by >30 int. units/dL for a minimum total treatment of 72 hours
Minor surgery: ≥30 int. units/dL for a minimum duration of 48 hours
Oral surgery: ≥30 int. units/dL for a minimum duration of 8-12 hours

Dosage Forms

Injection, powder for reconstitution [human derived]:
Alphanate®:
250 int. units [Factor VIII and vWF:RCof ratio varies by lot]
500 int. units [Factor VIII and vWF:RCof ratio varies by lot]
1000 int. units [Factor VIII and vWF:RCof ratio varies by lot]
1500 int. units [Factor VIII and vWF:RCof ratio varies by lot]
Humate-P®:
FVIII 250 int. units and vWF:RCof 600 int. units
FVIII 500 int. units and vWF:RCof 1200 int. units
FVIII 1000 int. units and vWF:RCof 2400 int. units

Anti-Hist [US-OTC] *see* diphenhydramine *on page* 315

Antihist-1® ***(Discontinued)*** *see* clemastine *on page* 237

antiinhibitor coagulant complex (an TEE in HI bi tor coe AG yoo lant KOM pleks)

Synonyms AICC; coagulant complex inhibitor

U.S./Canadian Brand Names Feiba VH Immuno [Can]; Feiba VH [US]

Therapeutic Category Hemophilic Agent

Use Hemophilia A & B patients with inhibitors who are to undergo surgery or those who are bleeding

Usual Dosage I.V.: Children and Adults:

General dosing guidelines: 50-100 units/kg (maximum: 200 units/kg)

Joint hemorrhage: 50 units/kg every 12 hours; may increase to 100 units/kg; continue until signs of clinical improvement occur

Mucous membrane bleeding: 50 units/kg every 6 hours; may increase to 100 units/kg (maximum: 2 administrations/day or 200 units/kg/day)

Soft tissue hemorrhage: 100 units/kg every 12 hours (maximum: 200 units/kg/day)

Other severe hemorrhage: 100 units/kg every 12 hours; may be used every 6 hours if needed; continue until clinical improvement

Dosage Forms

Injection, powder for reconstitution:

Feiba VH: Each bottle is labeled with Immuno units of factor VIII [heparin free; contains sodium 8 mg/mL]

Antilirium® ***(Discontinued)*** *see* physostigmine *on page 782*

Antiminth® ***(Discontinued)*** *see* pyrantel pamoate *on page 838*

Antiphlogistine Rub A-535 No Odour [Can] *see* trolamine *on page 991*

antipyrine and benzocaine (an tee PYE reen & BEN zoe kane)

Synonyms benzocaine and antipyrine

U.S./Canadian Brand Names A/B Otic [US]; Allergen® [US]; Auralgan® [Can]; Aurodex [US]

Therapeutic Category Otic Agent, Analgesic; Otic Agent, Ceruminolytic

Use Temporary relief of pain and reduction of swelling associated with acute congestive and serous otitis media, swimmer's ear, otitis externa; facilitates ear wax removal

Usual Dosage Otic: Children and Adults:

Otitis media: Fill ear canal with solution; moisten cotton pledget with solution, place in external ear, repeat every 1-2 hours until pain and congestion are relieved

Ear wax removal: Instill drops 3-4 times/day for 2-3 days

Dosage Forms

Solution, otic [drops]: Antipyrine 5.4% and benzocaine 1.4% (10 mL)

A/B Otic, Allergen®, Aurodex: Antipyrine 5.4% and benzocaine 1.4% (15 mL)

Antispas® Injection ***(Discontinued)*** *see* dicyclomine *on page 305*

antithrombin III *see* antithrombin III *on page 85*

antithrombin III (an tee THROM bin)

Synonyms antithrombin III; AT; AT-III; heparin cofactor I

U.S./Canadian Brand Names ATryn® [US]; Thrombate III® [US/Can]

Therapeutic Category Blood Product Derivative

Use Treatment of hereditary antithrombin (AT or AT-III) deficiency in connection with surgical procedures, obstetrical procedures, or thromboembolism

Usual Dosage I.V.: Adults:

Initial loading dose: Dosing is individualized based on pretherapy antithrombin (AT) levels. The initial dose should raise AT levels to 120% and may be calculated based on the following formula:

[(desired AT level % - baseline AT level %) x body weight (kg)] **divided** by 1.4 = int. units of antithrombin required

For example, if a 70 kg adult patient had a baseline AT level of 57%, the initial dose would be [(120% - 57%) x 70] divided by 1.4 = 3150 int. units

Maintenance dose: In general, subsequent dosing should be targeted to keep levels between 80% to 120% which may be achieved by administering 60% of the initial loading dose every 24 hours. Adjustments may be made by adjusting dose or interval. Maintain level within normal range for 2-8 days depending on type of procedure.

Product Availability
ATryn®: FDA approved February 2009; anticipated availability is currently undetermined
ATryn® is the first recombinant antithrombin product approved in the U.S.

Dosage Forms
Injection, powder for reconstitution [preservative free]:
ATryn®: ~1750 int. units [exact potency labeled on each vial]
Thrombate III®: 500 int. units, 1000 int. units

antithymocyte globulin (equine) (an te THY moe site GLOB yu lin, E kwine)

Sound-Alike/Look-Alike Issues
Atgam® may be confused with Ativan®

Synonyms antithymocyte immunoglobulin; ATG; horse antihuman thymocyte gamma globulin; lymphocyte immune globulin

U.S./Canadian Brand Names Atgam® [US/Can]

Therapeutic Category Immunosuppressant Agent

Use Prevention and treatment of acute renal allograft rejection; treatment of moderate-to-severe aplastic anemia in patients not considered suitable candidates for bone marrow transplantation

Usual Dosage An intradermal skin test is recommended prior to administration of the initial dose of ATG; use 0.1 mL of a 1:1000 dilution of ATG in normal saline. A positive skin reaction consists of a wheal ≥10 mm in diameter. If a positive skin test occurs, the first infusion should be administered in a controlled environment with intensive life support immediately available. A systemic reaction precludes further administration of the drug. The absence of a reaction does **not** preclude the possibility of an immediate sensitivity reaction.

Premedication with diphenhydramine, hydrocortisone, and acetaminophen is recommended prior to first dose.

Children: I.V.:
Aplastic anemia protocol: 10-20 mg/kg/day for 8-14 days; then administer every other day for 7 more doses; additional doses may be given every other day for 21 total doses in 28 days
Renal allograft: 5-25 mg/kg/day

Adults: I.V.:
Aplastic anemia protocol: 10-20 mg/kg/day for 8-14 days, then administer every other day for 7 more doses, for a total of 21 doses in 28 days
Renal allograft:
Rejection prophylaxis: 15 mg/kg/day for 14 days, then give every other day for 7 more doses for a total of 21 doses in 28 days; the initial dose should be administered within 24 hours before or after transplantation
Rejection treatment: 10-15 mg/kg/day for 14 days, then administer every other day for 7 more doses for a total of 21 doses in 28 days

Dosage Forms
Injection, solution:
Atgam®: 50 mg/mL (5 mL)

antithymocyte globulin (rabbit) (an te THY moe site GLOB yu lin RAB bit)

Synonyms rATG

U.S./Canadian Brand Names Thymoglobulin® [US]

Therapeutic Category Immunosuppressant Agent

Use Treatment of acute rejection of renal transplant; used in conjunction with concomitant immunosuppression

Usual Dosage I.V.: Children and Adults: Treatment of acute rejection: 1.5 mg/kg/day for 7-14 days

Dosage Forms
Injection, powder for reconstitution:
Thymoglobulin®: 25 mg

antithymocyte immunoglobulin *see* antithymocyte globulin (equine) *on page* *86*
antitumor necrosis factor apha (human) *see* adalimumab *on page* *35*
Anti-Tuss® Expectorant *(Discontinued)* *see* guaifenesin *on page* *473*
anti-VEGF monoclonal antibody *see* bevacizumab *on page* *140*
anti-VEGF rhuMAb *see* bevacizumab *on page* *140*
antivenin (crotalidae) polyvalent *see* crotalidae polyvalent immune FAB (ovine) *on page* *262*

antivenin *(Latrodectus mactans)* (an tee VEN in lak tro DUK tus MAK tans)

Synonyms *Latrodectus mactans* antivenin; black widow spider species antivenin

Therapeutic Category Antivenin

Use Treatment of patients with symptoms of black widow spider bites

Usual Dosage

Skin test: Intradermal: Children and Adults: 0.02 mL of a 1:10 dilution in NS (also use a control solution of NS); evaluate in 10 minutes. Positive reaction is urticarial wheal surrounded by zone of erythema

Conjunctival test: Ophthalmic:

Children: Instill 1 drop of a 1:100 dilution into the conjunctival sac

Adults: Instill 1 drop of a 1:10 dilution into the conjunctival sac

Note: Itching of the eye and/or reddening of conjunctiva indicates a positive reaction, usually occurring within 10 minutes.

Desensitization: Children and Adults: **Note:** In separate vials or syringes, prepare 1:10 and 1:100 dilutions of antivenin in NS.

SubQ: Inject 0.1, 0.2, and 0.5 mL of the 1:100 dilution at 15- to 30-minute intervals. Proceed with the next dose only if no reaction has occurred following the previous. Repeat procedure using the 1:10 dilution and then undiluted antivenin.

If a reaction occurs, apply tourniquet proximal to the injection site and administer epinephrine 1:1000. Wait at least 30 minutes, then administer another antivenin injection at the last dose which did not evoke a reaction.

If no reaction has occurred following 0.5 mL of undiluted antivenin, continue the dose at 15-minute intervals until entire dose has been administered.

Treatment of symptoms due to black widow spider bite: Administer only following the skin test or conjunctival test:

Children <12 years: I.V.: 2.5 mL

Children >12 years and Adults: I.M., I.V.: 2.5 mL

Dosage Forms

Injection, powder for reconstitution:

6000 antivenin units

antivenin *(Micrurus fulvius)* (an tee VEN in mye KRU rus FUL vee us)

Synonyms *Micrurus fulvius* antivenin; North American coral snake antivenin

Therapeutic Category Antivenin

Use Neutralization of venoms of Eastern coral snake and Texas coral snake

Usual Dosage I.V.: Children and Adults: 3-5 vials by slow injection (dependent on severity of signs/ symptoms; some patients may need more than 10 vials)

Note: Each vial of antivenom neutralizes ~2 mg of venom.

Antivert® [US] *see* meclizine *on page 619*

Antizol® [US] *see* fomepizole *on page 442*

Antrizine® *(Discontinued)* *see* meclizine *on page 619*

Anturane® *(Discontinued)*

Anucort-HC® [US] *see* hydrocortisone (rectal) *on page 503*

Anu-Med [US-OTC] *see* phenylephrine *on page 774*

Anusol-HC® [US] *see* hydrocortisone (rectal) *on page 503*

Anusol® HC-1 [US-OTC] *see* hydrocortisone (rectal) *on page 503*

Anusol® Ointment [US-OTC] *see* pramoxine *on page 809*

Anuzinc [Can] *see* zinc sulfate *on page 1031*

Anxanil® Oral *(Discontinued)* *see* hydroxyzine *on page 511*

Anzemet® [US/Can] *see* dolasetron *on page 328*

Apacet® *(Discontinued)* *see* acetaminophen *on page 19*

APAP *see* acetaminophen *on page 19*

APAP 500 [US-OTC] *see* acetaminophen *on page 19*

APAP and tramadol *see* acetaminophen and tramadol *on page 24*

Apaphen® *(Discontinued)* *see* acetaminophen and phenyltoloxamine *on page 23*

Apatate® [US-OTC] *see* vitamin B complex combinations *on page 1017*

ApexiCon™ [US] *see* diflorasone *on page 307*

ApexiCon™ E [US] *see* diflorasone *on page 307*

apomorphine (a poe MOR feen)

Synonyms apomorphine hydrochloride; apomorphine hydrochloride hemihydrate

U.S./Canadian Brand Names Apokyn® [US]

Therapeutic Category Anti-Parkinson Agent (Dopamine Agonist)

Use Treatment of hypomobility, "off" episodes with Parkinson disease

Usual Dosage SubQ: Adults: Begin antiemetic therapy 3 days prior to initiation and continue for 2 months before reassessing need.

Parkinson disease, "off" episode: Initial test dose 2 mg, **medical supervision required; see "Note"**. Subsequent dosing is based on both tolerance and response to initial test dose.

If patient tolerates test dose and responds: Starting dose: 2 mg as needed; may increase dose in 1 mg increments every few days; maximum dose: 6 mg

If patient tolerates but does not respond to 2 mg test dose: Second test dose: 4 mg

If patient tolerates and responds to 4 mg test dose: Starting dose: 3 mg, as needed for "off" episodes; may increase dose in 1 mg increments every few days; maximum dose 6 mg

If patient does not tolerate 4 mg test dose: Third test dose: 3 mg

If patient tolerates 3 mg test dose: Starting dose: 2 mg as needed for "off" episodes; may increase dose in 1 mg increments to a maximum of 3 mg

If therapy is interrupted for >1 week, restart at 2 mg and gradually titrate dose.

Note: Medical supervision is required for all test doses with standing and supine blood pressure monitoring predose and 20-, 40-, and 60 minutes postdose. If subsequent test doses are required, wait >2 hours before another test dose is given; next test dose should be timed with another "off" episode. If a single dose is ineffective for a particular "off" episode, then a second dose should not be given. The average dosing frequency was 3 times/day in the development program with limited experience in dosing >5 times/day and with total daily doses >20 mg. Apomorphine is intended to treat the "off" episodes associated with levodopa therapy of Parkinson disease and has not been studied in levodopa-naive Parkinson patients.

Dosage Forms

Injection, solution:

Apokyn®: 10 mg/mL (2 mL, 3 mL)

apomorphine hydrochloride *see* apomorphine *on page* *91*
apomorphine hydrochloride hemihydrate *see* apomorphine *on page* *91*
Apo-Nabumetone® [Can] *see* nabumetone *on page* *675*
Apo-Nadol® [Can] *see* nadolol *on page* *675*
Apo-Napro-Na® [Can] *see* naproxen *on page* *681*
Apo-Napro-Na DS® [Can] *see* naproxen *on page* *681*
Apo-Naproxen® [Can] *see* naproxen *on page* *681*
Apo-Naproxen EC® [Can] *see* naproxen *on page* *681*
Apo-Naproxen SR® [Can] *see* naproxen *on page* *681*
Apo-Nifed® [Can] *see* nifedipine *on page* *697*
Apo-Nifed PA® [Can] *see* nifedipine *on page* *697*
Apo-Nitrazepam® [Can] *see* nitrazepam *(Canada only) on page* *699*
Apo-Nitrofurantoin® [Can] *see* nitrofurantoin *on page* *700*
Apo-Nizatidine® [Can] *see* nizatidine *on page* *702*
Apo-Norflox® [Can] *see* norfloxacin *on page* *705*
Apo-Nortriptyline® [Can] *see* nortriptyline *on page* *706*
Apo-Oflox® [Can] *see* ofloxacin *on page* *718*
Apo-Ofloxacin® [Can] *see* ofloxacin *on page* *718*
Apo-Omeprazole® [Can] *see* omeprazole *on page* *723*
Apo-Ondansetron® [Can] *see* ondansetron *on page* *726*
Apo-Orciprenaline® [Can] *see* metaproterenol *on page* *632*
Apo-Oxaprozin® [Can] *see* oxaprozin *on page* *734*
Apo-Oxazepam® [Can] *see* oxazepam *on page* *734*
Apo-Oxybutynin® [Can] *see* oxybutynin *on page* *736*
Apo-Paclitaxel® [Can] *see* paclitaxel *on page* *742*
Apo-Pantoprazole® [Can] *see* pantoprazole *on page* *748*
Apo-Paroxetine® [Can] *see* paroxetine *on page* *752*
Apo-Pentoxifylline SR® [Can] *see* pentoxifylline *on page* *766*
Apo-Pen VK® [Can] *see* penicillin V potassium *on page* *763*
Apo-Perindopril® [Can] *see* perindopril erbumine *on page* *768*
Apo-Perphenazine® [Can] *see* perphenazine *on page* *769*
Apo-Pimozide® [Can] *see* pimozide *on page* *784*
Apo-Pindol® [Can] *see* pindolol *on page* *785*
Apo-Pioglitazone [Can] *see* pioglitazone *on page* *785*
Apo-Piroxicam® [Can] *see* piroxicam *on page* *788*
Apo-Pramipexole [Can] *see* pramipexole *on page* *808*
Apo-Pravastatin® [Can] *see* pravastatin *on page* *811*
Apo-Prazo® [Can] *see* prazosin *on page* *812*
Apo-Prednisone® [Can] *see* prednisone *on page* *814*
Apo-Primidone® [Can] *see* primidone *on page* *818*
Apo-Procainamide® [Can] *see* procainamide *on page* *819*

Apo-Prochlorperazine® [Can] *see* prochlorperazine *on page 820*
Apo-Propafenone® [Can] *see* propafenone *on page 825*
Apo-Propranolol® [Can] *see* propranolol *on page 828*
Apo-Quetiapine® [Can] *see* quetiapine *on page 844*
Apo-Quinidine® [Can] *see* quinidine *on page 845*
Apo-Quinine® [Can] *see* quinine *on page 846*
Apo-Raloxifene [Can] *see* raloxifene *on page 849*
Apo-Ramipril® [Can] *see* ramipril *on page 850*
Apo-Ranitidine® [Can] *see* ranitidine *on page 852*
Apo-Risperidone® [Can] *see* risperidone *on page 870*
Apo-Salvent® [Can] *see* albuterol *on page 41*
Apo-Salvent® CFC Free [Can] *see* albuterol *on page 41*
Apo-Salvent® Respirator Solution [Can] *see* albuterol *on page 41*
Apo-Salvent® Sterules [Can] *see* albuterol *on page 41*
Apo-Selegiline® [Can] *see* selegiline *on page 895*
Apo-Sertraline® [Can] *see* sertraline *on page 898*
Apo-Simvastatin® [Can] *see* simvastatin *on page 902*
Apo-Sotalol® [Can] *see* sotalol *on page 919*
Apo-Sulfatrim® [Can] *see* sulfamethoxazole and trimethoprim *on page 929*
Apo-Sulfatrim® DS [Can] *see* sulfamethoxazole and trimethoprim *on page 929*
Apo-Sulfatrim® Pediatric [Can] *see* sulfamethoxazole and trimethoprim *on page 929*
Apo-Sulin® [Can] *see* sulindac *on page 932*
Apo-Sumatriptan® [Can] *see* sumatriptan *on page 932*
Apo-Tamox® [Can] *see* tamoxifen *on page 937*
Apo-Temazepam® [Can] *see* temazepam *on page 942*
Apo-Terazosin® [Can] *see* terazosin *on page 945*
Apo-Tetra® [Can] *see* tetracycline *on page 950*
Apo-Theo LA® [Can] *see* theophylline *on page 953*
Apo-Tiaprofenic® [Can] *see* tiaprofenic acid *(Canada only) on page 959*
Apo-Ticlopidine® [Can] *see* ticlopidine *on page 960*
Apo-Timol® [Can] *see* timolol *on page 961*
Apo-Timop® [Can] *see* timolol *on page 961*
Apo-Tizanidine® [Can] *see* tizanidine *on page 964*
Apo-Tolbutamide® [Can] *see* tolbutamide *on page 967*
Apo-Topiramate® [Can] *see* topiramate *on page 969*
Apo-Trazodone® [Can] *see* trazodone *on page 979*
Apo-Trazodone D® [Can] *see* trazodone *on page 979*
Apo-Triazide® [Can] *see* hydrochlorothiazide and triamterene *on page 500*
Apo-Triazo® [Can] *see* triazolam *on page 984*
Apo-Trifluoperazine® [Can] *see* trifluoperazine *on page 986*
Apo-Trihex® [Can] *see* trihexyphenidyl *on page 986*
Apo-Trimebutine® [Can] *see* trimebutine *(Canada only) on page 987*
Apo-Trimethoprim® [Can] *see* trimethoprim *on page 988*
Apo-Trimip® [Can] *see* trimipramine *on page 988*
Apo-Valacyclovir® [Can] *see* valacyclovir *on page 1001*
Apo-Valproic® [Can] *see* valproic acid and derivatives *on page 1002*
Apo-Verap® [Can] *see* verapamil *on page 1010*
Apo-Verap® SR [Can] *see* verapamil *on page 1010*
Apo-Warfarin® [Can] *see* warfarin *on page 1022*
Apo-Zidovudine® [Can] *see* zidovudine *on page 1028*
Apo-Zopiclone® [Can] *see* zopiclone *(Canada only) on page 1034*
APPG *see* penicillin G procaine *on page 762*

apraclonidine (a pra KLOE ni deen)

Sound-Alike/Look-Alike Issues

Iopidine® may be confused with indapamide, iodine, Lodine®

Synonyms aplonidine; apraclonidine hydrochloride; p-aminoclonidine

U.S./Canadian Brand Names Iopidine® [US/Can]

Therapeutic Category $Alpha_2$ Agonist, Ophthalmic

Use Prevention and treatment of postsurgical intraocular pressure (IOP) elevation; short-term, adjunctive therapy in patients who require additional reduction of IOP

Usual Dosage Ophthalmic: Adults:

0.5%: Instill 1-2 drops in the affected eye(s) 3 times/day

1%: Instill 1 drop in operative eye 1 hour prior to anterior segment laser surgery, second drop in eye immediately upon completion of procedure

Dosage Forms

Solution, ophthalmic:

Iopidine®: 0.5% (5 mL, 10 mL); 1% (0.1 mL)

apraclonidine hydrochloride *see* apraclonidine *on page 94*

Apra *(Discontinued)* *see* acetaminophen *on page 19*

aprepitant (ap RE pi tant)

Sound-Alike/Look-Alike Issues

aprepitant may be confused with fosaprepitant

Emend® (aprepitant) oral capsule formulation may be confused with Emend® for injection (fosaprepitant).

Synonyms L 754030; MK 869

U.S./Canadian Brand Names Emend® [US/Can]

Therapeutic Category Antiemetic

Use Prevention of acute and delayed nausea and vomiting associated with moderately- and highly-emetogenic chemotherapy (in combination with other antiemetics); prevention of postoperative nausea and vomiting (PONV)

Usual Dosage Oral: Adults:

Prevention of chemotherapy-induced nausea/vomiting: 125 mg on day 1, followed by 80 mg on days 2 and 3 (in combination with a corticosteroid and 5-HT_3 antagonist antiemetic regimen)

Prevention of PONV: 40 mg within 3 hours prior to induction

Dosage Forms

Capsule:

Emend®: 40 mg, 80 mg, 125 mg

Combination package:

Emend®:

Capsule: 80 mg (2s)

Capsule: 125 mg (1s)

aprepitant injection *see* fosaprepitant *on page 445*

Apresazide *(Discontinued)* *see* hydralazine and hydrochlorothiazide *on page 499*

Apresoline® [Can] *see* hydralazine *on page 498*

Apresoline® *(Discontinued)* *see* hydralazine *on page 498*

Apri® [US] *see* ethinyl estradiol and desogestrel *on page 383*

Apriso™ [US] *see* mesalamine *on page 631*

Aprodine [US-OTC] *see* triprolidine and pseudoephedrine *on page 989*

aprotinin (a proe TYE nin)

U.S./Canadian Brand Names Trasylol® [US/Can]

Therapeutic Category Hemostatic Agent

Use Prevention of perioperative blood loss in patients who are at increased risk for blood loss and blood transfusions in association with cardiopulmonary bypass in coronary artery bypass graft surgery

Usual Dosage Adults: Test dose: **All** patients should receive a 1 mL (1.4 mg) I.V. test dose at least 10 minutes prior to the loading dose to assess the potential for allergic reactions.

Notes:

The loading dose should be given after induction of anesthesia but prior to sternotomy. In patients with previous exposure to aprotinin, administer loading dose just prior to cannulation. A constant infusion is continued until surgery is complete.

To avoid physical incompatibility with heparin when adding to pump-prime solution, each agent should be added during recirculation to assure adequate dilution.

Regimen A (standard dose):

2 million KIU (280 mg; 200 mL) loading dose I.V. over 20-30 minutes
2 million KIU (280 mg; 200 mL) into pump prime volume
500,000 KIU/hour (70 mg/hour; 50 mL/hour) I.V. during operation

Regimen B (low dose):

1 million KIU (140 mg; 100 mL) loading dose I.V. over 20-30 minutes
1 million KIU (140 mg; 100 mL) into pump prime volume
250,000 KIU/hour (35 mg/hour; 25 mL/hour) I.V. during operation

Dosage Forms

Injection, solution:

Trasylol®: 1.4 mg/mL [10,000 KIU/mL] (100 mL, 200 mL)

Aptivus® [US/Can] *see* tipranavir *on page 963*
Aqua-Ban® Maximum Strength [US-OTC] *see* pamabrom *on page 745*
Aquacare® [US-OTC] *see* urea *on page 998*
Aquachloral® Supprettes® *(Discontinued)* *see* chloral hydrate *on page 208*
Aquacort® [Can] *see* hydrocortisone (topical) *on page 505*
AquADEKs™ [US-OTC] *see* vitamins (multiple/pediatric) *on page 1020*
AquaLase™ [US] *see* balanced salt solution *on page 121*
AquaMEPHYTON® [Can] *see* phytonadione *on page 782*
AquaMEPHYTON® *(Discontinued)* *see* phytonadione *on page 782*
Aquanil™ HC [US-OTC] *see* hydrocortisone (topical) *on page 505*
Aquaphilic® With Carbamide [US-OTC] *see* urea *on page 998*
Aquaphyllin® *(Discontinued)* *see* theophylline *on page 953*
Aquasol A® [US] *see* vitamin A *on page 1016*
Aquasol E® [US-OTC] *see* vitamin E *on page 1018*
Aquatab® C *(Discontinued)* *see* guaifenesin, pseudoephedrine, and dextromethorphan *on page 479*
Aquatab® D *(Discontinued)* *see* guaifenesin and pseudoephedrine *on page 477*
Aquatab® DM *(Discontinued)* *see* guaifenesin and dextromethorphan *on page 474*
AquaTar® *(Discontinued)* *see* coal tar *on page 250*
aquavan *see* fospropofol *on page 447*
Aquavit-E [US-OTC] *see* vitamin E *on page 1018*
aqueous procaine penicillin G *see* penicillin G procaine *on page 762*
Aquoral™ [US] *see* saliva substitute *on page 887*
ara-C *see* cytarabine *on page 270*
arabinosylcytosine *see* cytarabine *on page 270*
Aralast [US] *see* alpha$_1$-proteinase inhibitor *on page 50*
Aralast NP [US] *see* alpha$_1$-proteinase inhibitor *on page 50*
Aralen® [US/Can] *see* chloroquine *on page 212*
Aranelle™ [US] *see* ethinyl estradiol and norethindrone *on page 390*
Aranesp® [US/Can] *see* darbepoetin alfa *on page 277*
Arava® [US/Can] *see* leflunomide *on page 574*
Arcalyst™ [US] *see* rilonacept *on page 868*
Arduan® *(Discontinued)*
Aredia® [US/Can] *see* pamidronate *on page 745*

arformoterol (ar for MOE ter ol)

Synonyms (R,R)-formoterol L-tartrate; arformoterol tartrate

U.S./Canadian Brand Names Brovana® [US]

Therapeutic Category Beta$_2$-Adrenergic Agonist

Use Long-term maintenance treatment of bronchoconstriction in chronic obstructive pulmonary disease (COPD), including chronic bronchitis and emphysema

Usual Dosage Nebulization: Adults: COPD: 15 mcg twice daily; maximum: 30 mcg/day

Dosage Forms

Solution for nebulization:

Brovana®: 15 mcg/2 mL (30s, 60s)

arformoterol tartrate *see* arformoterol *on page* 95

argatroban (ar GA troh ban)

Sound-Alike/Look-Alike Issues

argatroban may be confused with Aggrastat®, Orgaran®

Therapeutic Category Anticoagulant, Thrombin Inhibitor

Use Prophylaxis or treatment of thrombosis in patients with heparin-induced thrombocytopenia (HIT); adjunct to percutaneous coronary intervention (PCI) in patients who have or are at risk of thrombosis associated with HIT

Usual Dosage I.V.:

Children: **Heparin-induced thrombocytopenia** (dosing based on limited data from critically-ill patients):

Initial dose: 0.75 mcg/kg/minute

Maintenance dose: Patient may not be at steady-state but measure aPTT after 2 hours; adjust dose until the steady-state aPTT is 1.5-3.0 times the initial baseline value, not exceeding 100 seconds; dosage may be adjusted in increments of 0.1-0.25 mcg/kg/minute. **Note:** Frequent dosage adjustments may be required to maintain desired anticoagulant activity.

Adults:

Heparin-induced thrombocytopenia:

Initial dose: 2 mcg/kg/minute

Maintenance dose: Patient may not be at steady-state but measure aPTT after 2 hours; adjust dose until the steady-state aPTT is 1.5-3.0 times the initial baseline value, not exceeding 100 seconds; dosage should not exceed 10 mcg/kg/minute

Note: Critically-ill patients with normal hepatic function became excessively anticoagulated with FDA-approved or lower starting doses of argatroban. Doses between 0.15-1.3 mcg/kg/minute were required to maintain aPTTs in the target range. In a prospective observational study of critically-ill patients with MODS and suspected or proven HIT, an initial infusion dose of 0.2 mcg/kg/minute was found to be sufficient and safe in this population. Consider reducing starting dose to 0.2 mcg/kg/minute in critically-ill patients with multiple organ dysfunction (MODS) defined as a minimum number of two organ failures. Another report of a cardiac patient with anasarca secondary to acute renal failure had a reduction in argatroban clearance similar to patients with hepatic dysfunction. Reduced clearance may have been due to reduced liver perfusion. The American College of Chest Physicians has recommended an initial infusion rate of 0.5-1.2 mcg/kg/minute for patients with heart failure, MODS, severe anasarca, or postcardiac surgery.

Conversion to oral anticoagulant: Because there may be a combined effect on the INR when argatroban is combined with warfarin, loading doses of warfarin should not be used. Warfarin therapy should be started at the expected daily dose.

Patients receiving ≤2 mcg/kg/minute of argatroban: Argatroban therapy can be stopped when the combined INR on warfarin and argatroban is >4; repeat INR measurement in 4-6 hours; if INR is below therapeutic level, argatroban therapy may be restarted. Repeat procedure daily until desired INR on warfarin alone is obtained.

Patients receiving >2 mcg/kg/minute of argatroban: In order to predict the INR on warfarin alone, reduce dose of argatroban to 2 mcg/kg/minute; measure INR for argatroban and warfarin 4-6 hours after dose reduction; argatroban therapy can be stopped when the combined INR on warfarin and argatroban is >4. Repeat INR measurement in 4-6 hours; if INR is below therapeutic level, argatroban therapy may be restarted. Repeat procedure daily until desired INR on warfarin alone is obtained.

Note: The American College of Chest Physicians recommends monitoring chromogenic factor X assay when transitioning from argatroban to warfarin. Factor X levels <45% have been associated with INR values >2 after the effects of argatroban have been eliminated.

Percutaneous coronary intervention (PCI):

Initial: Begin infusion of 25 mcg/kg/minute and administer bolus dose of 350 mcg/kg (over 3-5 minutes). ACT should be checked 5-10 minutes after bolus infusion; proceed with procedure if ACT >300 seconds. Following initial bolus:

ACT <300 seconds: Give an additional 150 mcg/kg bolus, and increase infusion rate to 30 mcg/kg/minute (recheck ACT in 5-10 minutes)

ACT >450 seconds: Decrease infusion rate to 15 mcg/kg/minute (recheck ACT in 5-10 minutes)

Once a therapeutic ACT (300-450 seconds) is achieved, infusion should be continued at this dose for the duration of the procedure.

If dissection, impending abrupt closure, thrombus formation during PCI, or inability to achieve ACT >300 seconds: An additional bolus of 150 mcg/kg, followed by an increase in infusion rate to 40 mcg/kg/minute may be administered.

Note: Post-PCI anticoagulation, if required, may be achieved by continuing infusion at a reduced dose of 2-10 mcg/kg/minute, with close monitoring of aPTT.

Dosage Forms

Injection, solution:

100 mg/mL (2.5 mL)

arginine (AR ji neen)

Synonyms arginine hydrochloride

U.S./Canadian Brand Names R-Gene® 10 [US]

Therapeutic Category Diagnostic Agent

Use Pituitary function test (growth hormone)

Usual Dosage I.V.: Pituitary function test:

Children: 500 mg/kg/dose administered over 30 minutes

Adults: 30 g (300 mL) administered over 30 minutes

Dosage Forms

Injection, solution:

R-Gene® 10: 10% (300 mL) [100 mg/mL = 950 mOsm/L]

arginine hydrochloride *see* arginine *on page* 97

8-arginine vasopressin *see* vasopressin *on page* 1008

Aricept® [US/Can] *see* donepezil *on page* 330

Donazepil

Aricept® ODT [US] *see* donepezil *on page* 330

Aricept® RDT [Can] *see* donepezil *on page* 330

Arimidex® [US/Can] *see* anastrozole *on page* 79

aripiprazole (ay ri PIP ray zole)

Sound-Alike/Look-Alike Issues

aripiprazole may be confused with rabeprazole

Synonyms BMS-337039; OPC-14597

U.S./Canadian Brand Names Abilify Discmelt® [US]; Abilify® [US]

Therapeutic Category Antipsychotic Agent, Quinolone

Use

Oral: Acute and maintenance treatment of schizophrenia; stabilization, maintenance, and adjunctive therapy (to lithium or valproate) of bipolar disorder (with acute manic or mixed episodes); adjunctive treatment of major depressive disorder

Injection: Agitation associated with schizophrenia or bipolar mania

Usual Dosage Note: Oral solution may be substituted for the oral tablet on a mg-per-mg basis, up to 25 mg. Patients receiving 30 mg tablets should be given 25 mg oral solution. Orally disintegrating tablets (Abilify Discmelt®) are bioequivalent to the immediate release tablets (Abilify®).

Children ≥10 years: Oral: Bipolar I disorder (acute manic or mixed episodes): Initial: 2 mg daily for 2 days, followed by 5 mg daily for 2 days with a further increase to target dose of 10 mg daily as monotherapy or adjunctive therapy; subsequent dose increases may be made in 5 mg increments, up to a maximum of 30 mg/day

Adolescents ≥13 years: Oral: Schizophrenia: Initial: 2 mg daily for 2 days, followed by 5 mg daily for 2 days with a further increase to target dose of 10 mg daily; subsequent dose increases may be made in 5 mg increments up to a maximum of 30 mg/day (30 mg/day not shown to be more efficacious than 10 mg/day)

Adults:

Acute agitation (schizophrenia/bipolar mania): I.M.: 9.75 mg as a single dose (range: 5.25-15 mg); repeated doses may be given at ≥2-hour intervals to a maximum of 30 mg/day. **Note:** If ongoing therapy with aripiprazole is necessary, transition to oral therapy as soon as possible.

Bipolar disorder (acute manic or mixed episodes): Oral:
Stabilization: Initial: 15 mg once daily as monotherapy or adjunctive to lithium or valproic acid. May increase to 30 mg once daily if clinically indicated; safety of doses >30 mg/day has not been evaluated.
Maintenance: Continue stabilization dose for up to 6 weeks; efficacy of continued treatment >6 weeks has not been established
Depression (adjunctive with antidepressants): Oral: Initial: 2-5 mg/day (range: 2-15 mg/day); dose adjustments of up to 5 mg/day may be made in intervals of ≥1 week. **Note:** Dosing based on patients already receiving antidepressant therapy.
Schizophrenia: Oral: 10-15 mg once daily; may be increased to a maximum of 30 mg once daily (efficacy at dosages above 10-15 mg has not been shown to be increased). Dosage titration should not be more frequent than every 2 weeks.

Dosage Forms
Injection, solution:
Abilify®: 7.5 mg/mL (1.3 mL)
Solution, oral:
Abilify®: 1 mg/mL
Tablet:
Abilify®: 2 mg, 5 mg, 10 mg, 15 mg, 20 mg, 30 mg
Tablet, orally disintegrating:
Abilify Discmelt®: 10 mg, 15 mg

Aristocort® A [US] *see* triamcinolone (topical) *on page 983*
Aristospan® [US/Can] *see* triamcinolone (systemic) *on page 982*
Arixtra® [US/Can] *see* fondaparinux *on page 442*
Arm-a-Med® Isoproterenol *(Discontinued)* *see* isoproterenol *on page 549*
Arm-a-Med® Metaproterenol *(Discontinued)*

armodafinil (ar moe DAF i nil)

Synonyms R-modafinil
U.S./Canadian Brand Names Nuvigil™ [US]
Therapeutic Category Stimulant
Controlled Substance C-IV
Use Improve wakefulness in patients with excessive daytime sleepiness associated with narcolepsy and shift work sleep disorder (SWSD); adjunctive therapy for obstructive sleep apnea/hypopnea syndrome (OSAHS)
Usual Dosage Oral: Adults:
Narcolepsy: 150-250 mg once daily in the morning
Obstructive sleep apnea/hypopnea syndrome (OSAHS): 150-250 mg once daily in the morning; 250 mg was not shown to have any increased benefit over 150 mg
Shift work sleep disorder (SWSD): 150 mg given once daily ~1 hour prior to work shift
Dosage Forms
Tablet:
Nuvigil™: 50 mg, 150 mg, 250 mg

Armour® Thyroid [US] *see* thyroid, desiccated *on page 957*
Aromasin® [US/Can] *see* exemestane *on page 400*
Arranon® [US] *see* nelarabine *on page 685*
Arrestin® *(Discontinued)* *see* trimethobenzamide *on page 987*

arsenic trioxide (AR se nik tri OKS id)

Synonyms As_2O_3; NSC-706363
U.S./Canadian Brand Names Trisenox® [US]
Therapeutic Category Antineoplastic Agent, Miscellaneous
Use Induction of remission and consolidation in patients with relapsed or refractory acute promyelocytic leukemia (APL) which is specifically characterized by t(15;17) translocation or PML/RAR-alpha gene expression
Usual Dosage I.V.: Children ≥5 years and Adults: APL:
Induction: 0.15 mg/kg/day; administer daily until bone marrow remission; maximum induction: 60 doses

Consolidation: 0.15 mg/kg/day starting 3-6 weeks after completion of induction therapy; maximum consolidation: 25 doses over 5 weeks

Dosage Forms

Injection, solution [preservative free]:

Trisenox®: 1 mg/mL (10 mL)

Artane® ***(Discontinued)*** *see* trihexyphenidyl *on page 986*

artemether and benflumetol *see* artemether and lumefantrine *on page 99*

artemether and lumefantrine (ar TEM e ther & loo me FAN treen)

Synonyms artemether and benflumetol; benflumetol and artemether; lumefantrine and artemether

U.S./Canadian Brand Names Coartem® [US]

Therapeutic Category Antimalarial Agent

Use Treatment of acute, uncomplicated malaria infections due to *Plasmodium falciparum*

Usual Dosage Oral: Three-day schedule for the treatment of uncomplicated malaria:

Children 2 months to <16 years:

- 5 to <15 kg: One tablet at hour 0 and hour 8 on the first day, then 1 tablet twice daily on day 2 and day 3 (total of 6 tablets per treatment course)
- 15 to <25 kg: Two tablets at hour 0 and hour 8 on the first day, then 2 tablets twice daily on day 2 and day 3 (total of 12 tablets per treatment course)
- 25 to <35 kg: Three tablets at hour 0 and hour 8 on the first day, then 3 tablets twice daily on day 2 and day 3 (total of 18 tablets per treatment course)
- ≥35 kg: Four tablets at hour 0 and hour 8 on the first day, then 4 tablets twice daily on day 2 and day 3 (total of 24 tablets per treatment course)

Children ≥16 years and Adults:

- 25 to <35 kg: Three tablets at hour 0 and hour 8 on the first day, then 3 tablets twice daily on day 2 and day 3 (total of 18 tablets per treatment course)
- ≥35 kg: Four tablets at hour 0 and hour 8 on the first day, then 4 tablets twice daily on day 2 and day 3 (total of 24 tablets per treatment course)

Dosage Forms

Tablet:

Coartem®: Artemether 20 mg and lumefantrine 120 mg

Artha-G® ***(Discontinued)*** *see* salsalate *on page 888*

ArthriCare® for Women Extra Moisturizing ***(Discontinued)*** *see* capsaicin *on page 178*

ArthriCare® for Women Multi-Action ***(Discontinued)*** *see* capsaicin *on page 178*

ArthriCare® for Women Silky Dry ***(Discontinued)*** *see* capsaicin *on page 178*

ArthriCare® for Women Ultra Strength ***(Discontinued)*** *see* capsaicin *on page 178*

Arthropan® ***(Discontinued)***

Arthrotec® [US/Can] *see* diclofenac and misoprostol *on page 304*

articaine and epinephrine (AR ti kane & ep i NEF rin)

Synonyms epinephrine and articaine hydrochloride

U.S./Canadian Brand Names Astracaine® with epinephrine 1:200,000 [Can]; Astracaine® with epinephrine forte 1:100,000 [Can]; Septanest® N [Can]; Septanest® SP [Can]; Septocaine® with epinephrine 1:100,000 [US]; Septocaine® with epinephrine 1:200,000 [US]; Ultracaine® DS Forte [Can]; Ultracaine® DS [Can]; Zorcaine™ [US/Can]

Therapeutic Category Local Anesthetic

Use Local, infiltrative, or conductive anesthesia in both simple and complex dental and periodontal procedures

Usual Dosage Summary of recommended volumes and concentrations for various types of anesthetic procedures; dosages (administered by submucosal injection and/or nerve block) apply to normal healthy adults:

Infiltration: Injection volume of 4% solution: 0.5-2.5 mL; total dose: 20-100 mg

Nerve block: Injection volume of 4% solution: 0.5-3.4 mL; total dose: 20-136 mg

Oral surgery: Injection volume of 4% solution: 1-5.1 mL; total dose: 40-204 mg

Note: These dosages are guides only; other dosages may be used; however, do not exceed maximum recommended dose

Dosage Forms [CAN] = Canadian brand name

Injection, solution [for dental use]:

Astracaine® with epinephrine 1:200,000 [CAN]: Articaine 4% and epinephrine 1:200,000 (1.8 mL) [not available in the U.S.]

Astracaine® Forte with epinephrine forte 1:100,000 [CAN]: Articaine 4% and epinephrine 1:100,000 (1.8 mL) [not available in the U.S.]

Septanest® N [CAN]: Articaine 4% and epinephrine 1:200,000 (1.7 mL) [not available in the U.S.]

Septanest® SP [CAN]: Articaine 4% and epinephrine 1:100,000 (1.7 mL) [not available in the U.S.]

Septocaine® with epinephrine 1:100,000: Articaine 4% and epinephrine 1:100,000 (1.7 mL)

Septocaine® with epinephrine 1:200,000: Articaine 4% and epinephrine 1:200,000 (1.7 mL)

Ultracaine® DS [CAN]: Articaine 4% and epinephrine 1:200,000 (1.7 mL) [not available in the U.S.]

Ultracaine® DS Forte [CAN]: Articaine 4% and epinephrine 1:100,000 (1.7 mL) [not available in the U.S.]

Zorcaine™: Articaine 4% and epinephrine 1:100,000 (1.7 mL) [contains sodium metabisulfite]

artificial saliva *see* saliva substitute *on page* 887

artificial tears (ar ti FISH il tears)

Sound-Alike/Look-Alike Issues

Isopto® Tears may be confused with Isoptin®

Murocel® may be confused with Murocoll-2®

Synonyms hydroxyethylcellulose; polyvinyl alcohol

U.S./Canadian Brand Names Akwa Tears® [US-OTC]; Bion® Tears [US-OTC]; HypoTears PF [US-OTC]; HypoTears [US-OTC]; Liquifilm® Tears [US-OTC]; Moisture® Eyes PM [US-OTC]; Moisture® Eyes [US-OTC]; Murine® Tears [US-OTC]; Murocel® [US-OTC]; Nature's Tears® [US-OTC]; Nu-Tears® II [US-OTC]; Nu-Tears® [US-OTC]; Puralube® Tears [US-OTC]; Refresh Plus® [US-OTC]; Refresh Tears® [US-OTC]; Refresh® [US-OTC]; Soothe® [US-OTC]; Systane® Free [US-OTC]; Systane® [US-OTC]; Teardrops® [Can]; Teargen® II [US-OTC]; Teargen® [US-OTC]; Tearisol® [US-OTC]; Tears Again® [US-OTC]; Tears Naturale® Free [US-OTC]; Tears Naturale® II [US-OTC]; Tears Naturale® [US-OTC]; Tears Plus® [US-OTC]; Tears Renewed® [US-OTC]; Ultra Tears® [US-OTC]; Viva-Drops® [US-OTC]

Therapeutic Category Ophthalmic Agent, Miscellaneous

Use Ophthalmic lubricant; for relief of dry eyes and eye irritation

Usual Dosage Ophthalmic: Children and Adults: Use as needed to relieve symptoms, 1-2 drops into eye(s) 3-4 times/day

Dosage Forms

Solution, ophthalmic: 15 mL and 30 mL dropper bottles

Artiss™ [US] *see* fibrin sealant kit *on page* 417

As_2O_3 *see* arsenic trioxide *on page* 98

ASA *see* aspirin *on page* 103

5-ASA *see* mesalamine *on page* 631

ASA and diphenhydramine *see* aspirin and diphenhydramine *on page* 105

Asacol® [US/Can] *see* mesalamine *on page* 631

Asacol® 800 [Can] *see* mesalamine *on page* 631

Asacol® HD [US] *see* mesalamine *on page* 631

A.S.A.® *(Discontinued)* *see* aspirin *on page* 103

Asaphen [Can] *see* aspirin *on page* 103

Asaphen E.C. [Can] *see* aspirin *on page* 103

Asco-Caps [US-OTC] *see* ascorbic acid *on page* 100

Ascocid® [US-OTC] *see* ascorbic acid *on page* 100

Ascomp® with Codeine [US] *see* butalbital, aspirin, caffeine, and codeine *on page* 163

Ascor L 500® [US] *see* ascorbic acid *on page* 100

Ascor L NC® [US] *see* ascorbic acid *on page* 100

ascorbic acid (a SKOR bik AS id)

Synonyms vitamin C

U.S./Canadian Brand Names Acerola [US-OTC]; Asco-Caps [US-OTC]; Asco-Tabs [US-OTC]; Ascocid® [US-OTC]; Ascor L 500® [US]; Ascor L NC® [US]; C-Gel [US-OTC]; C-Gram [US-OTC]; C-Time [US-OTC]; Cecon® [US-OTC]; Cemill [US-OTC]; Cenolate® [US]; Chew-C [US-OTC]; Dull-C® [US-OTC]; Mild-C® [US-OTC]; One Gram C [US-OTC]; Proflavanol C™ [Can]; Revitalose C-1000® [Can]; Time-C [US-OTC]; Time-C-Bio [US-OTC]; Vicks® Vitamin C [US-OTC]; Vita-C® [US-OTC]

Therapeutic Category Vitamin, Water Soluble

Use Prevention and treatment of scurvy; acidify the urine

Usual Dosage Oral, I.M., I.V., SubQ:

Recommended adequate intake (AI):
- 0-6 months: 40 mg
- 6-12 months: 50 mg

Recommended daily allowance (RDA):
- 1-3 years: 15 mg; upper limit of intake should not exceed 400 mg/day
- 4-8 years: 25 mg; upper limit of intake should not exceed 650 mg/day
- 9-13 years: 45 mg; upper limit of intake should not exceed 1200 mg/day
- 14-18 years: Upper limit of intake should not exceed 1800 mg/day
  - Male: 75 mg
  - Female: 65 mg
- Adults: Upper limit of intake should not exceed 2000 mg/day
  - Male: 90 mg
  - Female: 75 mg
- Pregnant female:
  - ≤18 years: 80 mg; upper limit of intake should not exceed 1800 mg/day
  - 19-50 years: 85 mg; upper limit of intake should not exceed 2000 mg/day
- Lactating female:
  - ≤18 years: 115 mg; upper limit of intake should not exceed 1800 mg/day
  - 19-50 years: 120 mg; upper limit of intake should not exceed 2000 mg/day
- Adult smoker: Add an additional 35 mg/day

Children:
- Scurvy: 100-300 mg/day in divided doses for at least 2 weeks
- Urinary acidification: 500 mg every 6-8 hours
- Dietary supplement: 35-100 mg/day

Adults:
- Scurvy: 100-250 mg 1-2 times/day for at least 2 weeks
- Urinary acidification: 4-12 g/day in 3-4 divided doses
- Prevention and treatment of colds: 1-3 g/day
- Dietary supplement: 50-200 mg/day

Dosage Forms

Caplet: 1000 mg

Caplet, timed release: 500 mg, 1000 mg

Capsule:
- Mild-C® [OTC]: 500 mg

Capsule, softgel:
- C-Gel [OTC]: 1000 mg

Capsule, sustained release:
- C-Time [OTC]: 500 mg

Capsule, timed release: 500 mg
- Asco-Caps [OTC]: 500 mg, 1000 mg
- Time-C® [OTC]: 500 mg

Crystals for solution, oral: 4 g/teaspoonful
- Mild-C® [OTC]: 3600 mg/teaspoonful
- Vita-C® [OTC]: 4 g/teaspoonful

Injection, solution: 500 mg/mL (50 mL)
- Cenolate®: 500 mg/mL (1 mL, 2 mL)

Injection, solution [preservative free]:
- Ascor L 500®: 500 mg/mL (50 mL)
- Ascor L NC®: 500 mg/mL (50 mL)

Liquid, oral: 500 mg/5 mL

Lozenge:
- Vicks® Vitamin C [OTC]: 25 mg

Powder, for solution, oral:
Ascocid® [OTC}: 4000 mg/5 mL; 4300 mg/5 mL; 5000 mg/5 mL
Dull-C® [OTC]: 4 g/teaspoonful
Solution, oral:
Cecon® [OTC]: 90 mg/mL
Tablet: 100 mg, 250 mg, 500 mg, 1000 mg
Asco-Tabs [OTC]: 1000 mg
Ascocid® [OTC]: 500 mg
C-Gram [OTC]: 1000 mg
One Gram C [OTC]: 1000 mg
Tablet, chewable: 250 mg, 500 mg
Acerola [OTC]: 500 mg
Chew-C [OTC]: 500 mg
Mild-C® [OCT]: 250 mg
Tablet, timed release: 500 mg, 1000 mg
Cemill [OTC]: 500 mg, 1000 mg
Mild-C® [OTC]: 1000 mg
Time-C-Bio [OTC]: 500 mg

ascorbic acid and ferrous sulfate *see* ferrous sulfate and ascorbic acid *on page 415*

Ascorbicap® *(Discontinued)* *see* ascorbic acid *on page 100*

Asco-Tabs [US-OTC] *see* ascorbic acid *on page 100*

Ascriptin® [US-OTC] *see* aspirin *on page 103*

Ascriptin® Maximum Strength [US-OTC] *see* aspirin *on page 103*

asenapine (a SEN a peen)

Sound-Alike/Look-Alike Issues
asenapine may be confused with Inapsine®

U.S./Canadian Brand Names Saphris® [US]

Therapeutic Category Antimanic Agent; Antipsychotic Agent, Atypical

Use Acute treatment of schizophrenia; treatment of acute mania or mixed episodes associated with bipolar I disorder

Product Availability
Saphris®: FDA approved August 2009; availability expected by end of 2009; consult prescribing information for additional information

Asendin® *(Discontinued)* *see* amoxapine *on page 70*

Asmalix® *(Discontinued)* *see* theophylline *on page 953*

Asmanex® Twisthaler® [US] *see* mometasone *on page 665*

asparaginase (a SPEAR a ji nase)

Sound-Alike/Look-Alike Issues
asparaginase may be confused with pegaspargase
Elspar® may be confused with Elaprase™, Oncaspar®

Synonyms *E. coli* asparaginase; *Erwinia* asparaginase; L-asparaginase; NSC-106977 (*Erwinia*); NSC-109229 (*E. coli*)

U.S./Canadian Brand Names Elspar® [US]; Kidrolase® [Can]

Therapeutic Category Antineoplastic Agent

Use Treatment of acute lymphocytic leukemia (ALL)

Usual Dosage Refer to individual protocols. **Note:** Dose, frequency, number of doses, and start date may vary by protocol and treatment phase.
Children:
I.V.:
6000 units/m^2/dose 3 times/week for ~6-9 doses **or**
1000 units/kg/day for 10 days
I.M.: 6000 units/m^2/dose 3 times/week **or** 6000 units/m^2/dose every ~3 days for ~6-9 doses
Adults:
I.V.:
6000 units/m^2/dose 3 times/week for ~6-9 doses **or**
1000 units/kg/day for 10 days
Single agent therapy (rare): 200 units/kg/day for 28 days

I.M.: 6000 units/m^2/dose 3 times/week for ~6-9 doses **or** 6000 units/m^2/dose every ~3 days for ~6-9 doses

Test dose: A test dose is often recommended prior to the first dose of asparaginase, or prior to restarting therapy after a hiatus of several days. Most commonly, 0.1 mL of a 20 units/mL (2 units) asparaginase dilution is injected intradermally, and the patient observed for at least 1 hour. False-negative rates of up to 80% to test doses of 2-50 units are reported.

Some practitioners recommend an asparaginase desensitization regimen for patients who react to a test dose, or are being retreated following a break in therapy. Doses are doubled and given every 10 minutes until the total daily dose for that day has been administered. One schedule begins with a total of 1 unit given I.V. and doubles the dose every 10 minutes until the total amount given is the planned dose for that day. For example, if a patient was to receive a total dose of 4000 units, he/she would receive injections 1 through 12 during the desensitization.

Dosage Forms

Injection, powder for reconstitution:

Elspar®: 10,000 int. units

aspart insulin *see* insulin aspart *on page 530*

A-Spas® ***(Discontinued)*** *see* hyoscyamine *on page 512*

Aspercin [US-OTC] *see* aspirin *on page 103*

Aspercreme® [US-OTC] *see* trolamine *on page 991*

Aspergillus niger *see* alpha-galactosidase *on page 50*

Aspergum® [US-OTC] *see* aspirin *on page 103*

aspirin (AS pir in)

Sound-Alike/Look-Alike Issues

aspirin may be confused with Afrin®, Asendin®
Ascriptin® may be confused with Aricept®
Ecotrin® may be confused with Akineton®, Edecrin®, Epogen®
Halfprin® may be confused with Halfan®, Haltran®
ZORprin® may be confused with Zyloprim®

Synonyms acetylsalicylic acid; ASA

U.S./Canadian Brand Names Asaphen E.C. [Can]; Asaphen [Can]; Ascriptin® Maximum Strength [US-OTC]; Ascriptin® [US-OTC]; Aspercin [US-OTC]; Aspergum® [US-OTC]; Aspirtab [US-OTC]; Bayer® Aspirin Extra Strength [US-OTC]; Bayer® Aspirin Regimen Adult Low Dose [US-OTC]; Bayer® Aspirin Regimen Children's [US-OTC]; Bayer® Aspirin Regimen Regular Strength [US-OTC]; Bayer® Genuine Aspirin [US-OTC]; Bayer® Plus Extra Strength [US-OTC]; Bayer® with Heart Advantage [US-OTC]; Bayer® Women's Aspirin Plus Calcium [US-OTC]; Buffasal [US-OTC]; Bufferin® Extra Strength [US-OTC]; Bufferin® [US-OTC]; Buffinol [US-OTC]; Easprin® [US]; Ecotrin® Low Strength [US-OTC]; Ecotrin® Maximum Strength [US-OTC]; Ecotrin® [US-OTC]; Entrophen® [Can]; Genacote™ [US-OTC]; Halfprin® [US-OTC]; Novasen [Can]; St. Joseph® Adult Aspirin [US-OTC]; ZORprin® [US]

Therapeutic Category Analgesic, Nonnarcotic; Antiplatelet Agent; Antipyretic; Nonsteroidal Antiinflammatory Drug (NSAID)

Use Treatment of mild-to-moderate pain, inflammation, and fever; prevention and treatment of myocardial infarction (MI), acute ischemic stroke, and transient ischemic episodes; management of rheumatoid arthritis, rheumatic fever, osteoarthritis, and gout (high dose); adjunctive therapy in revascularization procedures (coronary artery bypass graft [CABG], percutaneous transluminal coronary angioplasty [PTCA], carotid endarterectomy), stent implantation

Usual Dosage

Children:

Analgesic and antipyretic: Oral, rectal: 10-15 mg/kg/dose every 4-6 hours, up to a total of 4 g/day

Antiinflammatory: Oral: Initial: 60-90 mg/kg/day in divided doses; usual maintenance: 80-100 mg/kg/day divided every 6-8 hours; monitor serum concentrations

Antiplatelet effects: Adequate pediatric studies have not been performed; pediatric dosage is derived from adult studies and clinical experience and is not well established; suggested doses have ranged from 3-5 mg/kg/day to 5-10 mg/kg/day given as a single daily dose. Doses are rounded to a convenient amount (eg, 1/2 of 81 mg tablet).

Mechanical prosthetic heart valves: 6-20 mg/kg/day given as a single daily dose (used in combination with an oral anticoagulant in children who have systemic embolism despite adequate oral anticoagulation therapy (INR 2.5-3.5) and used in combination with low-dose anticoagulation (INR 2-3) and dipyridamole when full-dose oral anticoagulation is contraindicated)

Blalock-Taussig shunts: 1-5 mg/kg/day given as a single daily dose

Kawasaki disease: Oral: 80-100 mg/kg/day divided every 6 hours; monitor serum concentrations; after fever resolves: 3-5 mg/kg/day once daily; in patients without coronary artery abnormalities, give lower dose for at least 6-8 weeks or until ESR and platelet count are normal; in patients with coronary artery abnormalities, low-dose aspirin should be continued indefinitely

Antirheumatic: Oral: 60-100 mg/kg/day in divided doses every 4 hours

Adults:

Acute ischemic stroke: Oral: 150-325 mg once daily, initiated within 48 hours (in patients who are not candidates for alteplase and not receiving systemic anticoagulation)

Analgesic and antipyretic:

Oral: 325-650 mg every 4-6 hours up to 4 g/day

Rectal: 300-600 mg every 4-6 hours up to 4 g/day

Antiinflammatory: Oral: Initial: 2.4-3.6 g/day in divided doses; usual maintenance: 3.6-5.4 g/day; monitor serum concentrations

Atrial fibrillation (in patients not candidates for warfarin or at low risk of ischemic stroke): Oral: 75-325 mg once daily

Bioprosthetic aortic valve: Oral: 50-100 mg once daily; usual dose: 81 mg once daily

Bioprosthetic mitral valve (following 3 months of anticoagulation): Oral: 50-100 mg once daily; usual dose: 81 mg once daily

CABG: Oral: 75-100 mg once daily (usual dose: 81 mg) initiated 6 hours following surgery; if bleeding prevents administration at 6 hours after CABG, initiate as soon as possible

CABG (internal mammary bypass graft): Oral: 75-162 mg once daily

Carotid artery stenting: Oral: 81-325 mg once daily beginning at least 24 hours (preferably 4 days) prior to procedure with concomitant clopidogrel

Carotid endarterectomy: Oral: 50-100 mg once daily preoperatively and daily thereafter; usual dose: 81 mg once daily

Infrainguinal arterial reconstruction/bypass: Oral: 75-100 mg once daily (begin preoperatively); usual dose: 81 mg once daily

Mechanical heart valve (with additional risk factors for thromboembolism): Oral: 50-100 mg once daily (in addition to warfarin); usual dose: 81 mg once daily

Mitral annular calcification (with documented stroke, TIA, or systemic embolism): Oral: 50-100 mg once daily; usual dose: 81 mg once daily

Mitral valve prolapse (with documented stroke or TIA): Oral: 50-100 mg once daily; usual dose: 81 mg once daily

Myocardial infarction (primary prevention): Oral: 75-162 mg once daily **or** 75-100 mg (usual dose: 81 mg) once daily

Non-ST-segment elevation myocardial infarction (NSTEMI): Oral: Initial: 162-325 mg; Maintenance: 75-100 mg once daily indefinitely; usual maintenance dose: 81 mg once daily

PCI: Oral: Initial: 75-325 mg (300-325 mg in aspirin naive patients) starting at least 2 hours (preferably 24 hours) before procedure; post procedure: 162-325 mg once daily (dose and duration varies with type of stent implanted); **Note:** Dose may be reduced to 75-162 mg once daily after appropriate duration based on stent-type is complete

Pericarditis associated with myocardial infarction: Oral: 162-325 mg once daily; doses as high as 650 mg every 4-6 hours may be required

Peripheral arterial disease: Oral: 75-100 mg once daily; usual dose: 81 mg once daily

Prosthetic valve thromboprophylaxis in pregnancy: Oral:75-100 mg once daily; usual dose: 81 mg once daily

ST-segment elevation myocardial infarction (STEMI): Oral: Initial: 162-325 mg given on presentation (patient should chew nonenteric-coated aspirin especially if not taking before presentation); for patients unable to take oral, may use rectal suppository (300 mg). Maintenance (secondary prevention): 75-162 mg once daily indefinitely

Stroke (cardioembolic, anticoagulation contraindicated): Oral: 75-325 mg once daily

Stroke/TIA (noncardioembolic, secondary prevention): Oral: 50-325 mg once daily **or** 50-100 mg once daily; usual dose: 81 mg once daily

Dosage Forms

Caplet: 81 mg, 325 mg, 500 mg

Bayer® Aspirin Extra Strength [OTC], Bayer® Plus Extra Strength [OTC]: 500 mg

Bayer® Aspirin Regimen Regular Strength [OTC], Bayer® Genuine Aspirin [OTC]: 325 mg

Bayer® with Heart Advantage [OTC], Bayer® Women's Aspirin Plus Calcium [OTC]: 81 mg

Caplet, buffered: 500 mg

Ascriptin® Maximum Strength [OTC]: 500 mg

Gum:
Aspergum® [OTC]: 227 mg
Suppository, rectal: 300 mg, 600 mg
Tablet: 325 mg
Aspercin [OTC], Aspirtab [OTC], Bayer® Genuine Aspirin [OTC]: 325 mg
Tablet, buffered: 325 mg
Ascriptin® [OTC], Bufferin® [OTC], Buffasal [OTC], Buffinol [OTC]: 325 mg
Bufferin® Extra Strength [OTC]: 500 mg
Tablet, chewable: 81 mg
Bayer® Aspirin Regimen Children's [OTC], St. Joseph® Adult Aspirin [OTC]: 81 mg
Tablet, controlled release: 800 mg
ZORprin®: 800 mg
Tablet, delayed release, enteric coated:
Easprin®: 975 mg
Tablet, enteric coated: 81 mg, 325 mg, 500 mg, 650 mg
Bayer® Aspirin Regimen Adult Low Dose [OTC], Ecotrin® Low Strength [OTC], St. Joseph Adult Aspirin [OTC]: 81 mg
Ecotrin® [OTC], Genacote™ [OTC]: 325 mg
Ecotrin® Maximum Strength [OTC]: 500 mg
Halfprin® [OTC]: 81 mg, 162 mg

aspirin, acetaminophen, and caffeine *see* acetaminophen, aspirin, and caffeine *on page 24*
aspirin and carisoprodol *see* carisoprodol and aspirin *on page 187*

aspirin and diphenhydramine (AS pir in & dye fen HYE dra meen)

Synonyms ASA and diphenhydramine; aspirin and diphenhydramine citrate; diphenhydramine and ASA; diphenhydramine and aspirin; diphenhydramine citrate and aspirin

U.S./Canadian Brand Names Alka-Seltzer® P.M. [US-OTC]; Bayer® PM [US-OTC]

Therapeutic Category Analgesic, Miscellaneous

Use Aid in the relief of insomnia accompanied by minor pain or headache

Usual Dosage Oral: Children ≥12 years and Adults: Pain-associated insomnia: Two tablets (650 mg aspirin/76 mg diphenhydramine citrate) **or** 2 caplets (1000 mg aspirin/76 mg diphenhydramine citrate) at bedtime or as directed by physician; do not exceed recommended dosage; not for use in children <12 years of age

Dosage Forms
Caplet:
Bayer® PM [OTC]: Aspirin 500 mg and diphenhydramine 38.3 mg
Tablet, effervescent:
Alka-Seltzer® P.M. [OTC]: Aspirin 325 mg and diphenhydramine 38 mg

aspirin and diphenhydramine citrate *see* aspirin and diphenhydramine *on page 105*

aspirin and dipyridamole (AS pir in & dye peer ID a mole)

Sound-Alike/Look-Alike Issues
Aggrenox® may be confused with Aggrastat®

Synonyms aspirin and extended-release dipyridamole; dipyridamole and aspirin

U.S./Canadian Brand Names Aggrenox® [US/Can]

Therapeutic Category Antiplatelet Agent

Use Reduction in the risk of stroke in patients who have had transient ischemia of the brain or ischemic stroke due to thrombosis

Usual Dosage Oral: Adults: 1 capsule (dipyridamole 200 mg, aspirin 25 mg) twice daily
Alternative regimen for patients with intolerable headache: 1 capsule at bedtime and low-dose aspirin in the morning. Return to usual dose (1 capsule twice daily) as soon as tolerance to headache develops (usually within a week).

Dosage Forms
Capsule:
Aggrenox®: Aspirin 25 mg (immediate release) and dipyridamole 200 mg (extended release)

aspirin and extended-release dipyridamole *see* aspirin and dipyridamole *on page 105*
aspirin and meprobamate *see* meprobamate and aspirin *on page 629*
aspirin and oxycodone *see* oxycodone and aspirin *on page 739*

aspirin, caffeine, and acetaminophen *see* acetaminophen, aspirin, and caffeine *on page 24*
aspirin, caffeine, and butalbital *see* butalbital, aspirin, and caffeine *on page 162*
aspirin, caffeine, and orphenadrine *see* orphenadrine, aspirin, and caffeine *on page 730*
aspirin, caffeine, codeine, and butalbital *see* butalbital, aspirin, caffeine, and codeine *on page 163*
aspirin, carisoprodol, and codeine *see* carisoprodol, aspirin, and codeine *on page 187*
Aspirin Free Anacin® *(Discontinued)* *see* acetaminophen *on page 19*
Aspirin Free Anacin® Extra Strength [US-OTC] *see* acetaminophen *on page 19*
aspirin, orphenadrine, and caffeine *see* orphenadrine, aspirin, and caffeine *on page 730*
Aspirtab [US-OTC] *see* aspirin *on page 103*
Astelin® [US/Can] *see* azelastine *on page 115*
Astepro™ [US] *see* azelastine *on page 115*
AsthmaHaler® Mist *(Discontinued)* *see* epinephrine *on page 358*
AsthmaNefrin® *(Discontinued)* *see* epinephrine *on page 358*
Astracaine® with epinephrine 1:200,000 [Can] *see* articaine and epinephrine *on page 99*
Astracaine® with epinephrine forte 1:100,000 [Can] *see* articaine and epinephrine *on page 99*
Astramorph/PF™ [US] *see* morphine sulfate *on page 667*
AT *see* antithrombin III *on page 85*
AT-III *see* antithrombin III *on page 85*
Atacand® [US/Can] *see* candesartan *on page 176*
Atacand HCT® [US] *see* candesartan and hydrochlorothiazide *on page 177*
Atacand® Plus [Can] *see* candesartan and hydrochlorothiazide *on page 177*
Atapryl® *(Discontinued)*
Atarax® [Can] *see* hydroxyzine *on page 511*
Atarax® *(Discontinued)* *see* hydroxyzine *on page 511*
Atasol® [Can] *see* acetaminophen *on page 19*

atazanavir (at a za NA veer)

Synonyms atazanavir sulfate; BMS-232632

U.S./Canadian Brand Names Reyataz® [US/Can]

Therapeutic Category Antiretroviral Agent, Protease Inhibitor

Use Treatment of HIV-1 infections in combination with at least two other antiretroviral agents

Note: In patients with prior virologic failure, coadministration with ritonavir is recommended.

Usual Dosage Oral:

Children 6-15 years:

Antiretroviral-naive patients:

15-24 kg: Atazanavir 150 mg once daily **plus** ritonavir 80 mg once daily
25-31 kg: Atazanavir 200 mg once daily **plus** ritonavir 100 mg once daily
32-38 kg: Atazanavir 250 mg once daily **plus** ritonavir 100 mg once daily
≥39 kg: Atazanavir 300 mg once daily **plus** 100 mg ritonavir once daily. **Note:** Treatment-naive patients ≥39 kg and ≥13 years of age who are unable to tolerate ritonavir, refer to adult dosing.

or

15-19 kg: Atazanavir 8.5 mg/kg/dose once daily (rounded to available capsule strengths) **plus** ritonavir 4 mg/kg once daily
≥20 kg: Atazanavir 7 mg/kg/dose once daily (round to available capsule strengths) (maximum: 300 mg/day) **plus** ritonavir 4 mg/kg once daily (maximum: 100 mg/day)

Antiretroviral-experienced patients: **Note:** Atazanavir without ritonavir is not recommended in antiretroviral-experienced patients with prior virologic failure:

25-31 kg: Atazanavir 200 mg once daily **plus** ritonavir 100 mg once daily
32-38 kg: Atazanavir 250 mg once daily **plus** ritonavir 100 mg once daily
≥39 kg: Atazanavir 300 mg once daily **plus** 100 mg ritonavir once daily

Adolescents ≥16 years and Adults:

Antiretroviral-naive patients: Atazanavir 300 mg once daily **plus** ritonavir 100 mg once daily **or** 400 mg once daily in patients unable to tolerate ritonavir.

Antiretroviral-experienced patients: Atazanavir 300 mg once daily **plus** ritonavir 100 mg once daily. **Note:** Atazanavir without ritonavir is not recommended in antiretroviral-experienced patients with prior virologic failure.

Dosage Forms

Capsule:

Reyataz®: 100 mg, 150 mg, 200 mg, 300 mg

atazanavir sulfate *see* atazanavir *on page 106*

atenolol (a TEN oh lole)

Sound-Alike/Look-Alike Issues

atenolol may be confused with albuterol, Altenol®, timolol, Tylenol®

Tenormin® may be confused with Imuran®, Norpramin®, thiamine, Trovan®

U.S./Canadian Brand Names Apo-Atenol® [Can]; Gen-Atenolol [Can]; Novo-Atenol [Can]; Nu-Atenol [Can]; PMS-Atenolol [Can]; RAN™-Atenolol [Can]; Rhoxal-atenolol [Can]; Riva-Atenolol [Can]; Sandoz-Atenolol [Can]; Tenolin [Can]; Tenormin® [US/Can]

Therapeutic Category Beta-Adrenergic Blocker

Use Treatment of hypertension, alone or in combination with other agents; management of angina pectoris; secondary prevention postmyocardial infarction

Usual Dosage

Oral:

Children: Hypertension: 0.5-1 mg/kg/dose given daily; range of 0.5-1.5 mg/kg/day; maximum dose: 2 mg/kg/day up to 100 mg/day

Adults:

Hypertension: 25-50 mg once daily, may increase to 100 mg/day. Doses >100 mg are unlikely to produce any further benefit.

Angina pectoris: 50 mg once daily, may increase to 100 mg/day. Some patients may require 200 mg/day.

Postmyocardial infarction: Follow I.V. dose with 100 mg/day or 50 mg twice daily for 6-9 days postmyocardial infarction.

I.V.:

Hypertension: Dosages of 1.25-5 mg every 6-12 hours have been used in short-term management of patients unable to take oral enteral beta-blockers

Postmyocardial infarction: Early treatment: 5 mg slow I.V. over 5 minutes; may repeat in 10 minutes. If both doses are tolerated, may start oral atenolol 50 mg every 12 hours or 100 mg/day for 6-9 days postmyocardial infarction.

Dosage Forms

Tablet: 25 mg, 50 mg, 100 mg

Tenormin®: 25 mg, 50 mg, 100 mg

atenolol and chlorthalidone (a TEN oh lole & klor THAL i done)

Synonyms chlorthalidone and atenolol

U.S./Canadian Brand Names Apo-Atenidone® [Can]; Novo-Atenolthalidone [Can]; Tenoretic® [US/Can]

Therapeutic Category Antihypertensive Agent, Combination

Use Treatment of hypertension with a cardioselective beta-blocker and a diuretic

Usual Dosage Oral: Adults: Initial (based on atenolol component): 50 mg once daily, then individualize dose until optimal dose is achieved

Dosage Forms

Tablet:

50: Atenolol 50 mg and chlorthalidone 25 mg

100: Atenolol 100 mg and chlorthalidone 25 mg

Tenoretic®:

50: Atenolol 50 mg and chlorthalidone 25 mg

100: Atenolol 100 mg and chlorthalidone 25 mg

ATG *see* antithymocyte globulin (equine) *on page 86*

Atgam® [US/Can] *see* antithymocyte globulin (equine) *on page 86*

Ativan® [US/Can] *see* lorazepam *on page 599*

ATNAA [US] *see* atropine and pralidoxime *on page 112*

Atolone® Oral *(Discontinued)*

atomoxetine (AT oh mox e teen)

Sound-Alike/Look-Alike Issues
atomoxetine may be confused with atorvastatin

Synonyms atomoxetine hydrochloride; LY139603; methylphenoxy-benzene propanamine; tomoxetine

U.S./Canadian Brand Names Strattera® [US/Can]

Therapeutic Category Norepinephrine Reuptake Inhibitor, Selective

Use Treatment of attention-deficit/hyperactivity disorder (ADHD)

Usual Dosage Oral: **Note:** Atomoxetine may be discontinued without the need for tapering dose. ADHD:

Children ≥6 years and ≤70 kg: Initial: 0.5 mg/kg/day, increase after minimum of 3 days to ~1.2 mg/kg/day; may administer as either a single daily dose or 2 evenly divided doses in morning and late afternoon/ early evening. Maximum daily dose: 1.4 mg/kg or 100 mg, whichever is less.

Children ≥6 years and >70 kg and Adults: Initial: 40 mg/day, increased after minimum of 3 days to ~80 mg/day; may administer as either a single daily dose or two evenly divided doses in morning and late afternoon/early evening. May increase to 100 mg/day in 2-4 additional weeks to achieve optimal response.

Dosage Forms

Capsule:

Strattera®: 10 mg, 18 mg, 25 mg, 40 mg, 60 mg, 80 mg, 100 mg

atomoxetine hydrochloride *see* atomoxetine *on page 108*

atorvastatin (a TORE va sta tin)

Sound-Alike/Look-Alike Issues
Lipitor® may be confused with Levatol®

Synonyms atorvastatin calcium

U.S./Canadian Brand Names Lipitor® [US/Can]

Therapeutic Category HMG-CoA Reductase Inhibitor

Use Treatment of dyslipidemias or primary prevention of cardiovascular disease (atherosclerotic) as detailed below:

Primary prevention of cardiovascular disease (high-risk for CVD): To reduce the risk of MI or stroke in patients without evidence of heart disease who have multiple CVD risk factors or type 2 diabetes. Treatment reduces the risk for angina or revascularization procedures in patients with multiple risk factors.

Secondary prevention of cardiovascular disease: To reduce the risk of MI, stroke, revascularization procedures, and angina in patients with evidence of coronary heart disease. To reduce the risk of hospitalization for heart failure.

Treatment of dyslipidemias: To reduce elevations in total cholesterol (C), LDL-C, apolipoprotein B, and triglycerides in patients with elevations of one or more components, and/or to increase low HDL-C as present in Fredrickson type IIa, IIb, III, and IV hyperlipidemias, heterozygous familial and nonfamilial hypercholesterolemia, and homozygous familial hypercholesterolemia

Treatment of heterozygous familial hypercholesterolemia (HeFH) in adolescent patients (10-17 years of age, females >1 year postmenarche) having LDL-C ≥190 mg/dL or LDL-C ≥160 mg/dL with positive family history of premature cardiovascular disease (CVD) or with two or more CVD risk factors.

Usual Dosage Oral: **Note:** Doses should be individualized according to the baseline LDL-cholesterol levels, the recommended goal of therapy, and patient response; adjustments should be made at intervals of 2-4 weeks

Children 10-17 years (females >1 year postmenarche): Heterozygous familial hypercholesterolemia (HeFH): 10 mg once daily (maximum: 20 mg/day)

Adults:

Hypercholesterolemia (heterozygous familial and nonfamilial) and mixed hyperlipidemia (Fredrickson types IIa and IIb): Initial: 10-20 mg once daily; patients requiring >45% reduction in LDL-C may be started at 40 mg once daily; range: 10-80 mg once daily

Homozygous familial hypercholesterolemia: 10-80 mg once daily

Dosage Forms

Tablet:

Lipitor®: 10 mg, 20 mg, 40 mg, 80 mg

atorvastatin calcium *see* atorvastatin *on page 108*

atorvastatin calcium and amlodipine besylate *see* amlodipine and atorvastatin *on page 67*

atovaquone (a TOE va kwone)

U.S./Canadian Brand Names Mepron® [US/Can]

Therapeutic Category Antiprotozoal

Use Acute oral treatment of mild-to-moderate *Pneumocystis jirovecii* pneumonia (PCP) in patients who are intolerant to co-trimoxazole; prophylaxis of PCP in patients who are intolerant to co-trimoxazole

Usual Dosage Oral: Adolescents 13-16 years and Adults:

Prevention of PCP: 1500 mg once daily with food

Treatment of mild-to-moderate PCP: 750 mg twice daily with food for 21 days

Dosage Forms

Suspension, oral:

Mepron®: 750 mg/5 mL

atovaquone and proguanil (a TOE va kwone & pro GWA nil)

Synonyms atovaquone and proguanil hydrochloride; proguanil and atovaquone; proguanil hydrochloride and atovaquone

U.S./Canadian Brand Names Malarone® Pediatric [Can]; Malarone® [US/Can]

Therapeutic Category Antimalarial Agent

Use Prevention or treatment of acute, uncomplicated *P. falciparum* malaria

Usual Dosage Oral:

Children (dosage based on body weight):

Prevention of malaria: Start 1-2 days prior to entering a malaria-endemic area, continue throughout the stay and for 7 days after returning. Take as a single dose, once daily.

11-20 kg: Atovaquone/proguanil 62.5 mg/25 mg
21-30 kg: Atovaquone/proguanil 125 mg/50 mg
31-40 kg: Atovaquone/proguanil 187.5 mg/75 mg
>40 kg: Atovaquone/proguanil 250 mg/100 mg

Treatment of acute malaria: Take as a single dose, once daily for 3 consecutive days.

5-8 kg: Atovaquone/proguanil 125 mg/50 mg
9-10 kg: Atovaquone/proguanil 187.5 mg/75 mg
11-20 kg: Atovaquone/proguanil 250 mg/100 mg
21-30 kg: Atovaquone/proguanil 500 mg/200 mg
31-40 kg: Atovaquone/proguanil 750 mg/300 mg
>40 kg: Atovaquone/proguanil 1 g/400 mg

Adults:

Prevention of malaria: Atovaquone/proguanil 250 mg/100 mg once daily; start 1-2 days prior to entering a malaria-endemic area, continue throughout the stay and for 7 days after returning

Treatment of acute malaria: Atovaquone/proguanil 1 g/400 mg as a single dose, once daily for 3 consecutive days

Dosage Forms

Tablet:

Malarone®: Atovaquone 250 mg and proguanil 100 mg

Tablet [pediatric]:

Malarone®: Atovaquone 62.5 mg and proguanil 25 mg

atovaquone and proguanil hydrochloride *see* atovaquone and proguanil *on page 109*

Atozine® Oral *(Discontinued)* *see* hydroxyzine *on page 511*

ATRA *see* tretinoin (systemic) *on page 980*

atracurium (a tra KYOO ree um)

Synonyms atracurium besylate

U.S./Canadian Brand Names Atracurium Besylate Injection [Can]

Therapeutic Category Skeletal Muscle Relaxant

Use Adjunct to general anesthesia to facilitate endotracheal intubation and to relax skeletal muscles during surgery; to facilitate mechanical ventilation in ICU patients; does not relieve pain or produce sedation

Usual Dosage I.V. (not to be used I.M.): Dose to effect; doses must be individualized due to interpatient variability; use ideal body weight for obese patients

Children 1 month to 2 years: Initial: 0.3-0.4 mg/kg followed by maintenance doses as needed to maintain neuromuscular blockade

Children >2 years to Adults: 0.4-0.5 mg/kg, then 0.08-0.1 mg/kg 20-45 minutes after initial dose to maintain neuromuscular block, followed by repeat doses of 0.08-0.1 mg/kg at 15- to 25-minute intervals
Initial dose after succinylcholine for intubation (balanced anesthesia): Adults: 0.2-0.4 mg/kg
Pretreatment/priming: 10% of intubating dose given 3-5 minutes before initial dose

Continuous infusion:
Surgery: Initial: 9-10 mcg/kg/minute at initial signs of recovery from bolus dose; block usually maintained by a rate of 5-9 mcg/kg/minute under balanced anesthesia
ICU: Block usually maintained by rate of 11-13 mcg/kg/minute (rates for pediatric patients may be higher)

Dosage Forms

Injection: 10 mg/mL (10 mL)
Injection [preservative free]: 10 mg/mL (5 mL)

atracurium besylate *see* atracurium *on page 109*
Atracurium Besylate Injection [Can] *see* atracurium *on page 109*
Atralin™ [US] *see* tretinoin (topical) *on page 981*
Atriance™ [Can] *see* nelarabine *on page 685*
Atripla® [US/Can] *see* efavirenz, emtricitabine, and tenofovir *on page 349*
Atropair® ***(Discontinued)*** *see* atropine *on page 110*
AtroPen® [US] *see* atropine *on page 110*

atropine (A troe peen)

Synonyms atropine sulfate

U.S./Canadian Brand Names AtroPen® [US]; Atropine-Care® [US]; Dioptic's Atropine Solution [Can]; Isopto® Atropine [US/Can]; Sal-Tropine™ [US]

Therapeutic Category Anticholinergic Agent

Use

Injection: Preoperative medication to inhibit salivation and secretions; treatment of symptomatic sinus bradycardia, AV block (nodal level); antidote for acetylcholinesterase inhibitor poisoning (carbamate insecticides, nerve agents, organophosphate insecticides); adjuvant use with anticholinesterases (eg, edrophonium, neostigmine) to decrease their side effects during reversal of neuromuscular blockade
Ophthalmic: Produce mydriasis and cycloplegia for examination of the retina and optic disc and accurate measurement of refractive errors; uveitis
Oral: Inhibit salivation and secretions

Usual Dosage

Neonates, Infants, and Children: Doses <0.1 mg have been associated with paradoxical bradycardia.
Inhibit salivation and secretions (preanesthesia): Oral, I.M., I.V., SubQ:
<5 kg: 0.02 mg/kg/dose 30-60 minutes preop then every 4-6 hours as needed. Use of a minimum dosage of 0.1 mg in neonates <5 kg will result in dosages >0.02 mg/kg. There is no documented minimum dosage in this age group.
>5 kg: 0.01-0.02 mg/kg/dose to a maximum 0.4 mg/dose 30-60 minutes preop; minimum dose: 0.1 mg
Alternate dosing:
3-7 kg (7-16 lb): 0.1 mg
8-11 kg (17-24 lb): 0.15 mg
11-18 kg (24-40 lb): 0.2 mg
18-29 kg (40-65 lb): 0.3 mg
>30 kg (>65 lb): 0.4 mg
Bradycardia: I.V., intratracheal: 0.02 mg/kg, minimum dose 0.1 mg, maximum single dose: 0.5 mg in children and 1 mg in adolescents; may repeat in 5-minute intervals to a maximum total dose of 1 mg in children or 2 mg in adolescents. (**Note:** For intratracheal administration, the dosage must be diluted with normal saline to a total volume of 1-5 mL). When treating bradycardia in neonates, reserve use for those patients unresponsive to improved oxygenation and epinephrine.
Infants and Children: Nerve agent toxicity management: See **Note** under adult dosing.
Prehospital ("in the field"): I.M.:
Birth to <2 years: Mild-to-moderate symptoms: 0.05 mg/kg; severe symptoms: 0.1 mg/kg
2-10 years: Mild-to-moderate symptoms: 1 mg; severe symptoms: 2 mg
>10 years: Mild-to-moderate symptoms: 2 mg; severe symptoms: 4 mg
Hospital/emergency department: I.M.:
Birth to <2 years: Mild-to-moderate symptoms: 0.05 mg/kg I.M. **or** 0.02 mg/kg I.V.; severe symptoms: 0.1 mg/kg I.M. **or** 0.02 mg/kg I.V.

2-10 years: Mild-to-moderate symptoms: 1 mg; severe symptoms: 2 mg
>10 years: Mild-to-moderate symptoms: 2 mg; severe symptoms: 4 mg

Note: Pralidoxime is a component of the management of nerve agent toxicity; consult pralidoxime for specific route and dose. For prehospital ("in the field") management, repeat atropine I.M. (children: 0.05-0.1 mg/kg) at 5-10 minute intervals until secretions have diminished and breathing is comfortable or airway resistance has returned to near normal. For hospital management, repeat atropine I.M. (infants 1 mg; all others: 2 mg) at 5-10 minute intervals until secretions have diminished and breathing is comfortable or airway resistance has returned to near normal.

Children: Organophosphate or carbamate poisoning:

I.V.: 0.03-0.05 mg/kg every 10-20 minutes until atropine effect, then every 1-4 hours for at least 24 hours

I.M. (AtroPen®): Mild symptoms: Administer dose listed below as soon as exposure is known or suspected. If severe symptoms develop after first dose, 2 additional doses should be repeated in 10 minutes; do not administer more than 3 doses. Severe symptoms: Immediately administer 3 doses as follows:

<6.8 kg (15 lb): Use of **AtroPen® formulation not recommended;** administer atropine 0.05 mg/kg
6.8-18 kg (15-40 lb): 0.5 mg/dose
18-41 kg (40-90 lb): 1 mg/dose
>41 kg (>90 lb): 2 mg/dose

Adults (doses <0.5 mg have been associated with paradoxical bradycardia):

Asystole or pulseless electrical activity:

I.V.: 1 mg; repeat in 3-5 minutes if asystole persists; total dose of 0.04 mg/kg.

Intratracheal: Administer 2-2.5 times the recommended I.V. dose; dilute in 10 mL NS or distilled water. **Note:** Absorption is greater with distilled water, but causes more adverse effects on PaO_2.

Inhibit salivation and secretions (preanesthesia):

I.M., I.V., SubQ: 0.4-0.6 mg 30-60 minutes preop and repeat every 4-6 hours as needed

Oral: 0.4 mg; may repeat in 4 hours if necessary; 0.4 mg initial dose may be exceeded in certain cases and may repeat in 4 hours if necessary

Bradycardia: I.V.: 0.5-1 mg every 5 minutes, not to exceed a total of 3 mg or 0.04 mg/kg; may give intratracheally in 10 mL NS (intratracheal dose should be 2-2.5 times the I.V. dose)

Neuromuscular blockade reversal: I.V.: 25-30 mcg/kg 30-60 seconds before neostigmine or 7-10 mcg/kg 30-60 seconds before edrophonium

Organophosphate or carbamate poisoning: **Note:** The dose of atropine required varies considerably with the severity of poisoning. Total amount of atropine used in carbamate poisoning is usually less. Severely poisoned patients may exhibit significant tolerance to atropine; ≥2 times the suggested doses may be needed. Titrate to pulmonary status (decreased bronchial secretions). Once patient is stable for a period of time, the dose/dosing frequency may be decreased. If atropinization occurs after 1-2 mg of atropine then reevaluate working diagnosis.

I.V.: Initial: 1-5 mg; doses should be doubled every 5 minutes until signs of muscarinic excess abate (clearing of bronchial secretions, bronchospasm, and adequate oxygenation). Overly aggressive dosing may cause anticholinergic toxicity (eg, delirium, hyperthermia, and muscle twitching).

I.V. Infusion: 0.5-1 mg/hour or 10% to 20% of loading dose/hour

I.M. (AtroPen®): Mild symptoms: Administer 2 mg as soon as exposure is known or suspected. If severe symptoms develop after first dose, 2 additional doses should be repeated in 10 minutes; do not administer more than 3 doses. Severe symptoms: Immediately administer three 2 mg doses.

Nerve agent toxicity management: I.M.: See **Note**. Prehospital ("in the field") or hospital/emergency department: Mild-to-moderate symptoms: 2-4 mg; severe symptoms: 6 mg

Note: Pralidoxime is a component of the management of nerve agent toxicity; consult Pralidoxime for specific route and dose. For prehospital ("in the field") management, repeat atropine I.M. (2 mg) at 5-10 minute intervals until secretions have diminished and breathing is comfortable or airway resistance has returned to near normal. For hospital management, repeat atropine I.M. (2 mg) at 5-10 minute intervals until secretions have diminished and breathing is comfortable or airway resistance has returned to near normal.

Mydriasis, cycloplegia (preprocedure): Ophthalmic (1% solution): Instill 1-2 drops 1 hour before procedure.

Uveitis: Ophthalmic:

1% solution: Instill 1-2 drops 4 times/day

Ointment: Apply a small amount in the conjunctival sac up to 3 times/day; compress the lacrimal sac by digital pressure for 1-3 minutes after instillation

Dosage Forms

Injection, solution: 0.05 mg/mL (5 mL); 0.1 mg/mL (5 mL, 10 mL); 0.4 mg/0.5 mL (0.5 mL); 0.4 mg/mL (0.5 mL, 1 mL, 20 mL); 1 mg/mL (1 mL)

AtroPen®: 0.25 mg/0.3 mL (0.3 mL); 0.5 mg/0.7 mL (0.7 mL); 1 mg/0.7 mL (0.7 mL); 2 mg/0.7 mL (0.7 mL) [prefilled autoinjector]

Ointment, ophthalmic: 1% (3.5 g)

Solution, ophthalmic: 1% (2 mL, 5 mL, 15 mL)

Atropine-Care®: 1% (2 mL) [contains benzalkonium chloride]

Isopto® Atropine: 1% (5 mL, 15 mL) [contains benzalkonium chloride]

Tablet:

Sal-Tropine™: 0.4 mg

atropine and difenoxin *see* difenoxin and atropine *on page 307*

atropine and diphenoxylate *see* diphenoxylate and atropine *on page 318*

atropine and pralidoxime (A troe peen & pra li DOKS eem)

Synonyms atropine and pralidoxime chloride; Mark 1™; NAAK; nerve agent antidote kit; pralidoxime and atropine

U.S./Canadian Brand Names ATNAA [US]; Duodote™ [US]

Therapeutic Category Anticholinergic Agent; Antidote

Use

ATNAA: Treatment of poisoning by susceptible organophosphorous nerve agents having acetylcholinesterase-inhibiting activity for self- or buddy-administration by military personnel

Duodote™: Treatment of poisoning by organophosphorous nerve agents (eg, tabun, sarin, soman) or organophosphorous insecticide for use by trained emergency medical services personnel

Usual Dosage I.M.: Adults: Organophosphorous poisoning: **Note:** If suspected, antidotal therapy should be given immediately as soon as symptoms appear (critical to administer immediately in case of soman exposure). Definitive medical care should be sought after any injection given. One injection only may be given as self-aid. If repeat injections needed, administration must be done by another trained individual. Emergency medical personnel who have self-administered a dose must determine capacity to continue to provide care.

ATNAA:

Mild symptoms (some or all mild symptoms): Self-Aid or Buddy-Aid: 1 injection (wait 10-15 minutes for effect); if patient is able to ambulate, and knows who and where they are, then no more injections are needed. If symptoms still present: Buddy-Aid: May repeat 1-2 more injections

Severe symptoms (if most or all): Buddy-Aid: If no self-aid given, 3 injections in rapid succession; if 1 self-aid injection given, 2 injections in rapid succession

Maximum cumulative dose: 3 injections

Symptoms provided by manufacturer in ATNAA product labeling to guide therapy:

Mild symptoms: Breathing difficulties, chest tightness, coughing, difficulty in seeing, drooling, headache, localized sweating and muscular twitching, miosis, nausea (with or without vomiting), runny nose, stomach cramps, tachycardia (followed by bradycardia), wheezing

Severe symptoms: Bradycardia, confused/strange behavior, convulsions, increased wheezing and breathing difficulties, involuntary urination/defecation, miosis (severe), muscular twitching/generalized weakness (severe), red/teary eyes, respiratory failure, unconsciousness, vomiting

Duodote™:

Mild symptoms (≥2 mild symptoms): 1 injection (wait 10-15 minutes for effect); if after 10-15 minutes no severe symptoms emerge, no further injections are indicated; if any severe symptoms emerge at any point following initial injection, repeat dose by giving 2 additional injections in rapid succession. Transport to medical care facility.

Severe symptoms (≥1 severe symptom): 3 injections in rapid succession. Transport to medical care facility.

Maximum cumulative dose: 3 injections unless medical care support (eg, hospital, respiratory support) is available

Symptoms provided by manufacturer in Duodote™ product labeling to guide therapy:

Mild symptoms: Airway secretions increased, blurred vision, bradycardia, breathing difficulties, chest tightness, drooling miosis, nausea, vomiting, runny nose, salivation, stomach cramps (acute onset), tachycardia, teary eyes, tremors/muscular twitching, wheezing/coughing

Severe symptoms: Breathing difficulties (severe), confused/strange behavior, convulsions, copious secretions from lung or airway, involuntary urination/defecation, muscular twitching/generalized weakness (severe)

Dosage Forms

Injection, solution:

ATNAA, Duodote™: Atropine 2.1 mg/0.7 mL and pralidoxime chloride 600 mg/2 mL [contains benzyl alcohol; prefilled auto-injector]

atropine and pralidoxime chloride *see* atropine and pralidoxime *on page* 112

Atropine-Care® [US] *see* atropine *on page* 110

atropine, hyoscyamine, scopolamine, and phenobarbital *see* hyoscyamine, atropine, scopolamine, and phenobarbital *on page* 513

atropine soluble tablet *(Discontinued)*

atropine sulfate *see* atropine *on page* 110

atropine sulfate and edrophonium chloride *see* edrophonium and atropine *on page* 348

Atropisol® *(Discontinued)* *see* atropine *on page* 110

Atrovent® [US/Can] *see* ipratropium *on page* 544

Atrovent® HFA [US/Can] *see* ipratropium *on page* 544

ATryn® [US] *see* antithrombin III *on page* 85

Attenuvax® [US] *see* measles virus vaccine (live) *on page* 616

Atuss® HD *(Discontinued)*

Atuss® HX *(Discontinued)*

Augmentin® [US/Can] *see* amoxicillin and clavulanate potassium *on page* 71

Augmentin ES-600® [US] *see* amoxicillin and clavulanate potassium *on page* 71

Augmentin XR® [US] *see* amoxicillin and clavulanate potassium *on page* 71

Auralgan® [Can] *see* antipyrine and benzocaine *on page* 85

auranofin (au RANE oh fin)

Sound-Alike/Look-Alike Issues

Ridaura® may be confused with Cardura®

U.S./Canadian Brand Names Ridaura® [US/Can]

Therapeutic Category Gold Compound

Use Management of active stage of classic or definite rheumatoid arthritis in patients who do not respond to or tolerate other agents; psoriatic arthritis; adjunctive or alternative therapy for pemphigus

Usual Dosage Oral:

Children: Initial: 0.1 mg/kg/day divided daily; usual maintenance: 0.15 mg/kg/day in 1-2 divided doses; maximum: 0.2 mg/kg/day in 1-2 divided doses

Adults: 6 mg/day in 1-2 divided doses; after 3 months may be increased to 9 mg/day in 3 divided doses; if still no response after 3 months at 9 mg/day, discontinue drug

Dosage Forms

Capsule:

Ridaura®: 3 mg

Auraphene® B [US-OTC] *see* carbamide peroxide *on page* 181

Auro® [US-OTC] *see* carbamide peroxide *on page* 181

Aurodex [US] *see* antipyrine and benzocaine *on page* 85

Autoplex® T *(Discontinued)* *see* antiinhibitor coagulant complex *on page* 85

AVA *see* anthrax vaccine, adsorbed *on page* 81

Avagard™ [US-OTC] *see* chlorhexidine gluconate *on page* 210

Avage™ [US] *see* tazarotene *on page* 939

avakine *see* infliximab *on page* 527

Avalide® [US/Can] *see* irbesartan and hydrochlorothiazide *on page* 545

Avandamet® [US/Can] *see* rosiglitazone and metformin *on page* 879

Avandaryl® [US] *see* rosiglitazone and glimepiride *on page* 879

Avandia® [US/Can] *see* rosiglitazone *on page* 878

Avapro® [US/Can] *see* irbesartan *on page* 545

Avapro® HCT *see* irbesartan and hydrochlorothiazide *on page* 545

AVAR™ *(Discontinued)* *see* sulfur and sulfacetamide *on page* 931

AVAR™-e [US] *see* sulfur and sulfacetamide *on page* 931

AVAR™-e Green *(Discontinued)* *see* sulfur and sulfacetamide *on page* 931

Avastin® [US/Can] *see* bevacizumab *on page 140*
Avaxim® [Can] *see* hepatitis A vaccine *on page 489*
Avaxim®-Pediatric [Can] *see* hepatitis A vaccine *on page 489*
Avelox® [US/Can] *see* moxifloxacin *on page 670*
Avelox® I.V. [US/Can] *see* moxifloxacin *on page 670*
Aventyl® [Can] *see* nortriptyline *on page 706*
Aventyl® HCl *(Discontinued)* *see* nortriptyline *on page 706*
Aviane™ [US/Can] *see* ethinyl estradiol and levonorgestrel *on page 387*
avian influenza virus vaccine *see* influenza virus vaccine (H5N1) *on page 529*
Avinza® [US] *see* morphine sulfate *on page 667*
Avita® [US] *see* tretinoin (topical) *on page 981*
Avitene® [US] *see* collagen hemostat *on page 255*
Avitene® Flour [US] *see* collagen hemostat *on page 255*
Avitene® Ultrafoam [US] *see* collagen hemostat *on page 255*
Avitene® UltraWrap™ [US] *see* collagen hemostat *on page 255*
Avlosulfon® *(Discontinued)* *see* dapsone *on page 276*
Avodart® [US/Can] *see* dutasteride *on page 343*
Avonex® [US/Can] *see* interferon beta-1a *on page 535*
Axert® [US/Can] *see* almotriptan *on page 49*
Axid® [US/Can] *see* nizatidine *on page 702*
Axid® AR [US-OTC] *see* nizatidine *on page 702*
AY-25650 *see* triptorelin *on page 990*
Aygestin® [US] *see* norethindrone *on page 704*
Ayr® Allergy Sinus [US-OTC] *see* sodium chloride *on page 908*
Ayr® Baby Saline [US-OTC] *see* sodium chloride *on page 908*
Ayr® Saline [US-OTC] *see* sodium chloride *on page 908*
Ayr® Saline No-Drip [US-OTC] *see* sodium chloride *on page 908*
5-aza-2'-deoxycytidine *see* decitabine *on page 279*
5-azaC *see* decitabine *on page 279*

azacitidine (ay za SYE ti deen)

Sound-Alike/Look-Alike Issues
azaCITIDine may be confused with azaTHIOprine

Synonyms 5-azacytidine; 5-AZC; AZA-CR; azacytidine; ladakamycin; NSC-102816

Tall-Man aza**CITID**ine

U.S./Canadian Brand Names Vidaza® [US]

Therapeutic Category Antineoplastic Agent, Antimetabolite (Pyrimidine)

Use Treatment of myelodysplastic syndrome (MDS)

Usual Dosage I.V., SubQ: Adults: MDS: 75 mg/m^2/day for 7 days repeated every 4 weeks. Dose may be increased to 100 mg/m^2/day if no benefit is observed after 2 cycles and no toxicity other than nausea and vomiting have occurred. Treatment is recommended for at least 4 cycles; treatment may be continued as long as patient continues to benefit.

Dosage Forms

Injection, powder for suspension:
Vidaza®: 100 mg

AZA-CR *see* azacitidine *on page 114*
Azactam® [US/Can] *see* aztreonam *on page 118*
azacytidine *see* azacitidine *on page 114*
5-azacytidine *see* azacitidine *on page 114*
azaepothilone B *see* ixabepilone *on page 554*
Azasan® [US] *see* azathioprine *on page 115*
AzaSite® [US] *see* azithromycin *on page 116*

azathioprine (ay za THYE oh preen)

Sound-Alike/Look-Alike Issues

azaTHIOprine may be confused with azaCITIDine, azatadine, azidothymidine, azithromycin, Azulfidine®

Imuran® may be confused with Elmiron®, Enduron®, Imdur®, Inderal®, Tenormin®

Synonyms azathioprine sodium

Tall-Man aza**THIO**prine

U.S./Canadian Brand Names Alti-Azathioprine [Can]; Apo-Azathioprine® [Can]; Azasan® [US]; Gen-Azathioprine [Can]; Imuran® [US/Can]; Novo-Azathioprine [Can]

Therapeutic Category Immunosuppressant Agent

Use Adjunctive therapy in prevention of rejection of kidney transplants; management of active rheumatoid arthritis (RA)

Usual Dosage Note: Patients with intermediate TPMT activity may be at risk for increased myelosuppression; those with low or absent TPMT activity receiving conventional azathioprine doses are at risk for developing severe, life-threatening myelotoxicity. Dosage reductions are recommended for patients with reduced TPMT activity.

I.V. dose is equivalent to oral dose (dosing should be transitioned from I.V. to oral as soon as tolerated):

Adults:

Renal transplantation (treatment usually started the day of transplant, however, has been initiated [rarely] 1-3 days prior to transplant): Oral, I.V.: Initial: 3-5 mg/kg/day usually given as a single daily dose, then 1-3 mg/kg/day maintenance

Rheumatoid arthritis: Oral:

Initial: 1 mg/kg/day given once daily or divided twice daily for 6-8 weeks; increase by 0.5 mg/kg every 4 weeks until response or up to 2.5 mg/kg/day; an adequate trial should be a minimum of 12 weeks

Maintenance dose: Reduce dose by 0.5 mg/kg every 4 weeks until lowest effective dose is reached; optimum duration of therapy not specified; may be discontinued abruptly

Dosage Forms

Injection, powder for reconstitution: 100 mg

Tablet [scored]: 50 mg

Azasan®: 75 mg, 100 mg

Imuran®: 50 mg

azathioprine sodium *see* azathioprine *on page* 115

5-AZC *see* azacitidine *on page* 114

Azdone® ***(Discontinued)***

azelaic acid (a zeh LAY ik AS id)

U.S./Canadian Brand Names Azelex® [US]; Finacea® [US/Can]

Therapeutic Category Topical Skin Product

Use Topical treatment of inflammatory papules and pustules of mild-to-moderate rosacea; mild-to-moderate inflammatory acne vulgaris

Finacea®: Not FDA-approved for the treatment of acne

Usual Dosage Topical:

Adolescents ≥12 years and Adults: Acne vulgaris: Cream 20%: After skin is thoroughly washed and patted dry, gently but thoroughly massage a thin film of azelaic acid cream into the affected areas twice daily, in the morning and evening. The duration of use can vary and depends on the severity of the acne. In the majority of patients with inflammatory lesions, improvement of the condition occurs within 4 weeks.

Adults: Rosacea: Gel 15%: Massage gently into affected areas of the face twice daily; use beyond 12 weeks has not been studied

Dosage Forms

Cream:

Azelex®: 20% (30 g, 50 g)

Gel:

Finacea®, Finacea® Plus™: 15% (50 g)

azelastine (a ZEL as teen)

Sound-Alike/Look-Alike Issues

Astelin® may be confused with Astepro™

Optivar® may be confused with Optiray®, Optive™

Synonyms azelastine hydrochloride

U.S./Canadian Brand Names Astelin® [US/Can]; Astepro™ [US]; Optivar® [US]

Therapeutic Category Antihistamine; Antihistamine, Ophthalmic

Use

Nasal spray: Treatment of the symptoms of seasonal allergic rhinitis such as rhinorrhea, sneezing, and nasal pruritus; treatment of the symptoms of vasomotor rhinitis

Ophthalmic: Treatment of itching of the eye associated with seasonal allergic conjunctivitis

Usual Dosage

Children 5-11 years: Seasonal allergic rhinitis: Intranasal: 1 spray each nostril twice daily

Children ≥3 years and Adults: Itching eyes due to seasonal allergic conjunctivitis: Ophthalmic: Instill 1 drop into affected eye(s) twice daily

Children ≥12 years and Adults:

Seasonal allergic rhinitis: Intranasal: 1-2 sprays each nostril twice daily

Vasomotor rhinitis: Intranasal: 2 sprays each nostril twice daily.

Dosage Forms

Solution, intranasal [spray]:

Astelin®, Astepro™: 1 mg/mL [137 mcg/spray] (30 mL)

Solution, ophthalmic:

Optivar®: 0.05% (6 mL)

azelastine hydrochloride *see* azelastine *on page 115*

Azelex® [US] *see* azelaic acid *on page 115*

azidothymidine *see* zidovudine *on page 1028*

azidothymidine, abacavir, and lamivudine *see* abacavir, lamivudine, and zidovudine *on page 16*

Azilect® [US] *see* rasagiline *on page 853*

azithromycin (az ith roe MYE sin)

Sound-Alike/Look-Alike Issues

azithromycin may be confused with azathioprine, erythromycin

Zithromax® may be confused with Fosamax®, Zinacef®, Zovirax®

Synonyms azithromycin dihydrate; azithromycin hydrogen citrate; azithromycin monohydrate; Zithromax® TRI-PAK™; Zithromax® Z-PAK®

U.S./Canadian Brand Names Apo-Azithromycin® [Can]; AzaSite® [US]; CO Azithromycin [Can]; Dom-Azithromycin [Can]; GEN-Azithromycin [Can]; Novo-Azithromycin [Can]; PHL-Azithromycin [Can]; PMS-Azithromycin [Can]; PRO-Azithromycin [Can]; ratio-Azithromycin [Can]; Riva-Azithromycin [Can]; Sandoz-Azithromycin [Can]; Zithromax® [US/Can]; Zmax® [US]

Therapeutic Category Macrolide (Antibiotic)

Use

Oral, I.V.: Treatment of acute otitis media due to *H. influenzae*, *M. catarrhalis*, or *S. pneumoniae*; pharyngitis/tonsillitis due to *S. pyogenes*; treatment of mild-to-moderate upper and lower respiratory tract infections, infections of the skin and skin structure, community-acquired pneumonia, pelvic inflammatory disease (PID), sexually-transmitted diseases (urethritis/cervicitis), pharyngitis/tonsillitis (alternative to first-line therapy), and genital ulcer disease (chancroid) due to susceptible strains of *Chlamydophila pneumoniae*, *C. trachomatis*, *M. catarrhalis*, *H. influenzae*, *S. aureus*, *S. pneumoniae*, *Mycoplasma pneumoniae*, and *C. psittaci*; acute bacterial exacerbations of chronic obstructive pulmonary disease (COPD) due to *H. influenzae*, *M. catarrhalis,* or *S. pneumoniae*; acute bacterial sinusitis

Ophthalmic: Bacterial conjunctivitis

Usual Dosage Note: Extended release suspension (Zmax®) is not interchangeable with immediate release formulations. Use should be limited to approved indications. All doses are expressed as immediate release azithromycin unless otherwise specified.

Usual dosage range:

Children ≥6 months: Oral: 5-12 mg/kg given once daily (maximum: 500 mg/day) **or** 30 mg/kg as a single dose (maximum: 1500 mg)

Extended release suspension (Zmax®): 60 mg/kg as a single dose; **Note:** Extended release suspension (Zmax®): Dose in mL is equal to the weight in lbs for patients <75 lbs (34 kg). Pediatric patients ≥75 lbs should receive the adult dose.

Children ≥1 year and Adults: Ophthalmic: Instill 1 drop into affected eye(s) twice daily (8-12 hours apart) for 2 days, then 1 drop once daily for 5 days

Adolescents ≥16 years and Adults:
Oral: 250-600 mg once daily **or** 1-2 g as a single dose
Extended release suspension (Zmax®): 2 g as a single dose
I.V.: 250-500 mg once daily

Indication-specific dosing:

Children: Oral:

Bacterial sinusitis: 10 mg/kg once daily for 3 days (maximum: 500 mg/day)

Community-acquired pneumonia: 10 mg/kg on day 1 (maximum: 500 mg/day) followed by 5 mg/kg/day once daily on days 2-5 (maximum: 250 mg/day)
Extended release suspension (Zmax®):
<75 lbs (34 kg): 60 mg/kg as a single dose; dose in mL is equal to the weight in lbs for patients <75 lbs (34 kg)
≥75 lbs (34 kg): Refer to adult dose

Otitis media:
1-day regimen: 30 mg/kg as a single dose (maximum: 1500 mg)
3-day regimen: 10 mg/kg once daily for 3 days (maximum: 500 mg/day)
5-day regimen: 10 mg/kg on day 1 (maximum: 500 mg/day) followed by 5 mg/kg/day once daily on days 2-5 (maximum: 250 mg/day)

Pharyngitis, tonsillitis: Children ≥2 years: 12 mg/kg/day once daily for 5 days (maximum: 500 mg/day)

Pertussis (CDC guidelines):
Children <6 months: 10 mg/kg/day for 5 days
Children ≥6 months: 10 mg/kg on day 1 (maximum: 500 mg/day) followed by 5 mg/kg/day once daily on days 2-5 (maximum: 250 mg/day)

Children ≥1 year and Adults: Ophthalmic:

Bacterial conjunctivitis: Instill 1 drop into affected eye(s) twice daily (8-12 hours apart) for 2 days, then 1 drop once daily for 5 days

Adolescents ≥16 years and Adults:

Bacterial sinusitis: Oral: 500 mg/day for a total of 3 days
Extended release suspension (Zmax®): 2 g as a single dose

Chancroid due to *H. ducreyi*: Oral: 1 g as a single dose

Community-acquired pneumonia:
Oral: Extended release suspension (Zmax®): 2 g as a single dose
I.V.: 500 mg as a single dose for at least 2 days, follow I.V. therapy by the oral route with a single daily dose of 500 mg to complete a 7- to 10-day course of therapy.

Mild-to-moderate respiratory tract, skin, and soft tissue infections: Oral: 500 mg in a single loading dose on day 1 followed by 250 mg/day as a single dose on days 2-5
Alternative regimen: Bacterial exacerbation of COPD: 500 mg/day for a total of 3 days

Pelvic inflammatory disease (PID): I.V.: 500 mg as a single dose for 1-2 days, follow I.V. therapy by the oral route with a single daily dose of 250 mg to complete a 7-day course of therapy

Pertussis (CDC guidelines): Oral: 500 mg on day 1 followed by 250 mg/day on days 2-5 (maximum: 500 mg/day)

Urethritis/cervicitis: Oral:
Due to C. trachomatis: 1 g as a single dose
Due to N. gonorrhoeae: 2 g as a single dose

Dosage Forms

Injection, powder for reconstitution: 500 mg, 2.5 g
Zithromax®: 500 mg

Microspheres for oral suspension, extended release:
Zmax®: 2 g/bottle (60 mL)

Powder for oral suspension: 100 mg/5 mL (15 mL); 200 mg/5 mL (15 mL, 22.5 mL, 30 mL); 1 g/packet (3s)
Zithromax®: 100 mg/5 mL, 200 mg/5 mL, 1 g/packet (3s, 10s)

Solution, ophthalmic:
AzaSite®: 1% (2.5 mL)

Tablet: 250 mg, 500 mg, 600 mg
Zithromax®: 250 mg, 500 mg, 600 mg
Zithromax® TRI-PAK™ [unit-dose pack]: 500 mg (3s)
Zithromax® Z-PAK® [unit-dose pack]: 250 mg (6s)

azithromycin dihydrate *see* azithromycin *on page 116*
azithromycin hydrogen citrate *see* azithromycin *on page 116*

azithromycin monohydrate *see* azithromycin *on page 116*
Azmacort® [US] *see* triamcinolone (inhalation, oral) *on page 982*
AZO-Gesic® [US-OTC] *see* phenazopyridine *on page 770*
Azopt® [US/Can] *see* brinzolamide *on page 147*
Azor™ [US] *see* amlodipine and olmesartan *on page 68*
AZO-Standard® [US-OTC] *see* phenazopyridine *on page 770*
AZO-Standard® Maximum Strength [US-OTC] *see* phenazopyridine *on page 770*
AZT™ [Can] *see* zidovudine *on page 1028*
AZT, abacavir, and lamivudine *see* abacavir, lamivudine, and zidovudine *on page 16*
azthreonam *see* aztreonam *on page 118*

aztreonam (AZ tree oh nam)

Sound-Alike/Look-Alike Issues
aztreonam may be confused with azidothymidine
Synonyms azthreonam
U.S./Canadian Brand Names Azactam® [US/Can]
Therapeutic Category Antibiotic, Miscellaneous
Use Treatment of patients with urinary tract infections, lower respiratory tract infections, septicemia, skin/skin structure infections, intraabdominal infections, and gynecological infections caused by susceptible gram-negative bacilli
Usual Dosage
Children >1 month:
Mild-to-moderate infections: I.M., I.V.: 30 mg/kg every 8 hours
Moderate-to-severe infections: I.M., I.V.: 30 mg/kg every 6-8 hours; maximum: 120 mg/kg/day (8 g/day)
Cystic fibrosis: I.V.: 50 mg/kg/dose every 6-8 hours (ie, up to 200 mg/kg/day); maximum: 8 g/day
Adults:
Urinary tract infection: I.M., I.V.: 500 mg to 1 g every 8-12 hours
Moderately-severe systemic infections: 1 g I.V. or I.M. or 2 g I.V. every 8-12 hours
Severe systemic or life-threatening infections (especially caused by *Pseudomonas aeruginosa*): I.V.: 2 g every 6-8 hours; maximum: 8 g/day
Meningitis (gram-negative): I.V.: 2 g every 6-8 hours
Dosage Forms
Infusion premixed iso-osmotic solution:
Azactam®: 1 g (50 mL); 2 g (50 mL)
Injection, powder for reconstitution:
Azactam®: 1 g, 2 g

Azulfidine® [US] *see* sulfasalazine *on page 930*
Azulfidine® EN-tabs® [US] *see* sulfasalazine *on page 930*
B-D™ Glucose [US-OTC] *see* dextrose *on page 298*
B2036-PEG *see* pegvisomant *on page 758*
B 9273 *see* alefacept *on page 44*
BabyBIG® [US] *see* botulism immune globulin (intravenous-human) *on page 146*
BAC *see* benzalkonium chloride *on page 129*
Bacid® [US-OTC/Can] *see* Lactobacillus *on page 564*
Baciguent® [US-OTC/Can] *see* bacitracin *on page 118*
BaciiM® [US] *see* bacitracin *on page 118*
Baciject® [Can] *see* bacitracin *on page 118*
bacillus calmette-Guérin (BCG) live *see* BCG vaccine *on page 124*
Baci-Rx [US] *see* bacitracin *on page 118*

bacitracin (bas i TRAY sin)

Sound-Alike/Look-Alike Issues
bacitracin may be confused with Bactrim®, Bactroban®
U.S./Canadian Brand Names Baci-Rx [US]; Baciguent® [US-OTC/Can]; BaciiM® [US]; Baciject® [Can]
Therapeutic Category Antibiotic, Miscellaneous; Antibiotic, Ophthalmic; Antibiotic, Topical

Use Treatment of susceptible bacterial infections mainly; has activity against gram-positive bacilli; due to toxicity risks, systemic and irrigant uses of bacitracin should be limited to situations where less toxic alternatives would not be effective

Usual Dosage **Do not administer I.V.:**

Infants: I.M.:

≤2.5 kg: 900 units/kg/day in 2-3 divided doses

>2.5 kg: 1000 units/kg/day in 2-3 divided doses

Children: I.M.: 800-1200 units/kg/day divided every 8 hours

Adults: Oral: Antibiotic-associated colitis: 25,000 units 4 times/day for 7-10 days

Children and Adults:

Topical: Apply 1-5 times/day

Ophthalmic, ointment: Instill 1/4" to 1/2" ribbon every 3-4 hours into conjunctival sac for acute infections, or 2-3 times/day for mild-to-moderate infections for 7-10 days

Irrigation, solution: 50-100 units/mL in normal saline, lactated Ringer's, or sterile water for irrigation; soak sponges in solution for topical compresses 1-5 times/day or as needed during surgical procedures

Dosage Forms

Injection, powder for reconstitution: 50,000 units

BaciiM®: 50,000 units

Ointment, ophthalmic: 500 units/g (3.5 g)

Ointment, topical: 500 units/g (0.9 g, 15 g, 30 g, 120 g, 454 g)

Baciguent® [OTC]: 500 units/g (15 g, 30 g)

Powder, for prescription compounding [micronized]:

Baci-Rx: 5 million units

bacitracin and polymyxin B (bas i TRAY sin & pol i MIKS in bee)

Sound-Alike/Look-Alike Issues

Betadine® may be confused with Betagan®, betaine

Synonyms polymyxin B and bacitracin

U.S./Canadian Brand Names AK-Poly-Bac™ [US]; LID-Pack® [Can]; Optimyxin® [Can]; Polysporin® [US-OTC]

Therapeutic Category Antibiotic, Ophthalmic; Antibiotic, Topical

Use Treatment of superficial infections caused by susceptible organisms

Usual Dosage Children and Adults:

Ophthalmic ointment: Instill 1/2" ribbon in the affected eye(s) every 3-4 hours for acute infections or 2-3 times/day for mild-to-moderate infections for 7-10 days

Topical ointment/powder: Apply to affected area 1-4 times/day; may cover with sterile bandage if needed

Dosage Forms

Ointment, ophthalmic: Bacitracin 500 units and polymyxin B 10,000 units per g (3.5 g)

AK-Poly-Bac™: Bacitracin 500 units and polymyxin 10,000 units per g (3.5 g)

Ointment, topical: Bacitracin 500 units and polymyxin B 10,000 units per g in white petrolatum (15 g, 30 g)

Polysporin®: Bacitracin 500 units and polymyxin B 10,000 units per g (0.9 g, 15 g, 30 g)

Powder, topical:

Polysporin®: Bacitracin 500 units and polymyxin B 10,000 units per g (10 g)

bacitracin, neomycin, and polymyxin B

(bas i TRAY sin, nee oh MYE sin, & pol i MIKS in bee)

Synonyms neomycin, bacitracin, and polymyxin B; polymyxin B, bacitracin, and neomycin; triple antibiotic

U.S./Canadian Brand Names Neosporin® Neo To Go® [US-OTC]; Neosporin® Topical [US-OTC]

Therapeutic Category Antibiotic, Ophthalmic; Antibiotic, Topical

Use Helps prevent infection in minor cuts, scrapes, and burns; short-term treatment of superficial external ocular infections caused by susceptible organisms

Usual Dosage Children and Adults:

Ophthalmic: Ointment: Instill 1/2" into the conjunctival sac every 3-4 hours for 7-10 days for acute infections

Topical: Apply 1-3 times/day to infected area; may cover with sterile bandage as needed

Dosage Forms

Ointment, ophthalmic: Bacitracin 400 units, neomycin 3.5 mg, and polymyxin B 10,000 units per g (3.5 g)

Ointment, topical: Bacitracin 400 units, neomycin 3.5 mg, and polymyxin B 5000 units per g (0.9 g, 15 g, 30 g, 454 g)

Neosporin® [OTC]: Bacitracin 400 units, neomycin 3.5 mg, and polymyxin B 5000 units per g (15 g, 30 g)

Neosporin® Neo To Go® [OTC]: Bacitracin 400 units, neomycin 3.5 mg, and polymyxin B 5000 units per g (0.9 g)

bacitracin, neomycin, polymyxin B, and hydrocortisone

(bas i TRAY sin, nee oh MYE sin, pol i MIKS in bee, & hye droe KOR ti sone)

Synonyms hydrocortisone, bacitracin, neomycin, and polymyxin B; neomycin, bacitracin, polymyxin B, and hydrocortisone; polymyxin B, bacitracin, neomycin, and hydrocortisone

U.S./Canadian Brand Names Cortisporin® Ointment [US]; Cortisporin® Topical Ointment [Can]

Therapeutic Category Antibiotic/Corticosteroid, Ophthalmic; Antibiotic/Corticosteroid, Topical

Use Prevention and treatment of susceptible inflammatory conditions where bacterial infection (or risk of infection) is present

Usual Dosage Children and Adults:

Ophthalmic: Ointment: Instill 1/2 inch ribbon to inside of lower lid every 3-4 hours until improvement occurs

Topical: Apply sparingly 2-4 times/day. Therapy should be discontinued when control is achieved; if no improvement is seen, reassessment of diagnosis may be necessary.

Dosage Forms

Ointment, ophthalmic: Bacitracin 400 units, neomycin sulfate 3.5 mg, polymyxin B 10,000 units, and hydrocortisone 10 mg per g (3.5 g)

Ointment, topical:

Cortisporin®: Bacitracin 400 units, neomycin 3.5 mg, polymyxin B 5000 units, and hydrocortisone 10 mg per g (15 g)

bacitracin, neomycin, polymyxin B, and pramoxine

(bas i TRAY sin, nee oh MYE sin, pol i MIKS in bee, & pra MOKS een)

Synonyms neomycin, bacitracin, polymyxin B, and pramoxine; polymyxin B, neomycin, bacitracin, and pramoxine; pramoxine, neomycin, bacitracin, and polymyxin B

U.S./Canadian Brand Names Neosporin® + Pain Relief Ointment [US-OTC]; Tri Biozene [US-OTC]

Therapeutic Category Antibiotic, Topical

Use Prevention and treatment of susceptible superficial topical infections and provide temporary relief of pain or discomfort

Usual Dosage Children ≥2 years and Adults: Apply 1-3 times/day to infected areas; cover with sterile bandage if needed

Dosage Forms

Ointment, topical: Bacitracin 500 units, neomycin 3.5 mg, polymyxin B 10,000 units, and pramoxine 10 mg (15 g, 30 g)

Neosporin® + Pain Relief Ointment [OTC]: Bacitracin 500 units, neomycin 3.5 mg, polymyxin B 10,000 units, and pramoxine 10 mg (15 g, 30 g)

Tri Biozene [OTC]: Bacitracin 500 units, neomycin 3.5 mg, polymyxin B 10,000 units, and pramoxine 10 mg (15 g)

baclofen (BAK loe fen)

Sound-Alike/Look-Alike Issues

baclofen may be confused with Bactroban®

Lioresal® may be confused with lisinopril, Lotensin®

U.S./Canadian Brand Names Apo-Baclofen® [Can]; Gen-Baclofen [Can]; Lioresal® [US/Can]; Liotec [Can]; Nu-Baclo [Can]; PMS-Baclofen [Can]

Therapeutic Category Skeletal Muscle Relaxant

Use Treatment of reversible spasticity associated with multiple sclerosis or spinal cord lesions

Orphan drug: Intrathecal: Treatment of intractable spasticity caused by spinal cord injury, multiple sclerosis, and other spinal disease (spinal ischemia or tumor, transverse myelitis, cervical spondylosis, degenerative myelopathy)

Usual Dosage

Oral (avoid abrupt withdrawal of drug): Adults: 5 mg 3 times/day, may increase 5 mg/dose every 3 days to a maximum of 80 mg/day

Intrathecal: Children and Adults:

Test dose: 50-100 mcg, doses >50 mcg should be given in 25 mcg increments, separated by 24 hours. A screening dose of 25 mcg may be considered in very small patients. Patients not responding to screening dose of 100 mcg should not be considered for chronic infusion/implanted pump.

Maintenance: After positive response to test dose, a maintenance intrathecal infusion can be administered via an implanted intrathecal pump. Initial dose via pump: Infusion at a 24-hour rate dosed at twice the test dose. Avoid abrupt discontinuation.

Dosage Forms

Injection, solution, intrathecal [preservative free]:

Lioresal®: 50 mcg/mL (1 mL); 500 mcg/mL (20 mL); 2000 mcg/mL (5 mL, 20 mL)

Tablet: 10 mg, 20 mg

BactoShield® CHG [US-OTC] *see* chlorhexidine gluconate *on page* *210*

BactoShield® *(Discontinued)* *see* chlorhexidine gluconate *on page* *210*

Bactrim™ [US] *see* sulfamethoxazole and trimethoprim *on page* *929*

Bactrim™ DS [US] *see* sulfamethoxazole and trimethoprim *on page* *929*

Bactrim™ I.V. Infusion *(Discontinued)* *see* sulfamethoxazole and trimethoprim *on page* *929*

Bactroban® [US/Can] *see* mupirocin *on page* *672*

Bactroban Cream® [US] *see* mupirocin *on page* *672*

Bactroban Nasal® [US] *see* mupirocin *on page* *672*

baking soda *see* sodium bicarbonate *on page* *907*

BAL *see* dimercaprol *on page* *313*

BAL5788 *see* ceftobiprole *(Canada only) on page* *198*

BAL9141 *see* ceftobiprole *(Canada only) on page* *198*

Balacet 325™ [US] *see* propoxyphene and acetaminophen *on page* *828*

balanced salt solution (BAL anced salt soe LOO shun)

U.S./Canadian Brand Names AquaLase™ [US]; BSS Plus® [US/Can]; BSS® [US/Can]; Eye-Stream® [Can]; Navstel® [US]

Therapeutic Category Ophthalmic Agent, Miscellaneous

Use

Irrigation solution for ophthalmic surgery:

AquaLase™, BSS®: Intraocular or extraocular irrigating solution

BSS Plus®, Navstel®: Intraocular irrigating solution

Irrigation solution for eyes, ears, nose, or throat

Usual Dosage Irrigation: Adults: Based on standard for each surgical procedure

Dosage Forms

Solution, irrigation [preservative free]: Sodium chloride 0.64%, potassium chloride 0.075%, calcium chloride 0.048%, magnesium chloride 0.03%, sodium acetate 0.39%, sodium citrate 0.17% (500 mL)

Solution, ophthalmic [irrigation; preservative free]: Sodium chloride 0.64%, potassium chloride 0.075%, calcium chloride 0.048%, magnesium chloride 0.03%, sodium acetate 0.39%, sodium citrate 0.17% (18 mL, 500 mL)

AquaLase™: Sodium chloride 0.64%, potassium chloride 0.075%, calcium chloride 0.048%, magnesium chloride 0.03%, sodium acetate 0.39%, sodium citrate 0.17% (90 mL)

BSS®: Sodium chloride 0.64%, potassium chloride 0.075%, calcium chloride 0.048%, magnesium chloride 0.03%, sodium acetate 0.39%, sodium citrate 0.17% (15 mL, 30 mL, 250 mL, 500 mL)

BSS Plus®: Sodium chloride 0.71%, potassium chloride 0.038%, calcium chloride 0.015%, magnesium chloride 0.02%, sodium phosphate 0.042%, sodium bicarbonate 0.21%, dextrose 0.092%, glutathione 0.018% (250 mL, 500 mL)

Navstel®: Sodium chloride 0.71%, potassium chloride 0.038%, calcium chloride 0.015%, magnesium chloride 0.02%, sodium phosphate 0.042%, sodium bicarbonate 0.21%, dextrose 0.092%, glutathione 0.018%, hypromellose 0.125% to 0.173% (250 mL, 500 mL)

Baldex® *(Discontinued)*

BAL in Oil® [US] *see* dimercaprol *on page* *313*

Balmex® [US-OTC] *see* zinc oxide *on page* *1030*

Balminil Decongestant [Can] *see* pseudoephedrine *on page* *833*

Balminil DM D [Can] *see* pseudoephedrine and dextromethorphan *on page* *834*

Balminil DM + Decongestant + Expectorant [Can] *see* guaifenesin, pseudoephedrine, and dextromethorphan *on page* *479*

Balminil DM E [Can] *see* guaifenesin and dextromethorphan *on page 474*
Balminil Expectorant [Can] *see* guaifenesin *on page 473*
Balnetar® [US-OTC/Can] *see* coal tar *on page 250*

balsalazide (bal SAL a zide)

Sound-Alike/Look-Alike Issues
Colazal® may be confused with Clozaril®

Synonyms balsalazide disodium

U.S./Canadian Brand Names Colazal® [US]

Therapeutic Category 5-Aminosalicylic Acid Derivative; Antiinflammatory Agent

Use Treatment of mild-to-moderate active ulcerative colitis

Usual Dosage Oral:
Children 5-17 years: 750 mg 3 times/day for up to 8 weeks **or** 2.25 g (three 750 mg capsules) 3 times/day for 8 weeks
Adults: 2.25 g (three 750 mg capsules) 3 times/day for 8-12 weeks

Dosage Forms
Capsule: 750 mg
Colazal®: 750 mg

balsalazide disodium *see* balsalazide *on page 122*
balsam Peru, castor oil, and trypsin *see* trypsin, balsam Peru, and castor oil *on page 993*
Baltussin [US] *see* dihydrocodeine, chlorpheniramine, and phenylephrine *on page 309*
Balziva™ [US] *see* ethinyl estradiol and norethindrone *on page 390*
Band-Aid® Hurt-Free™ Antiseptic Wash [US-OTC] *see* lidocaine *on page 584*
Banophen™ [US-OTC] *see* diphenhydramine *on page 315*
Banophen™ Anti-Itch [US-OTC] *see* diphenhydramine *on page 315*
Banophen® Decongestant Capsule *(Discontinued)*
Banzel™ [US] *see* rufinamide *on page 882*
Baraclude® [US/Can] *see* entecavir *on page 356*
Barbidonna® *(Discontinued)* *see* hyoscyamine, atropine, scopolamine, and phenobarbital *on page 513*
Barbita® *(Discontinued)* *see* phenobarbital *on page 771*
Barc™ Liquid *(Discontinued)*
Baricon™ [US] *see* barium *on page 122*
Baridium® [US-OTC] *see* phenazopyridine *on page 770*

barium (BA ree um)

Synonyms barium sulfate

U.S./Canadian Brand Names Anatrast [US]; Bar-Test [US]; Baricon™ [US]; Baro-Cat® [US]; Barobag® [US]; Barosperse® [US]; CheeTah® [US]; E-Z-Cat® Dry [US]; E-Z-Cat® [US]; E-Z-Disk™ [US]; Enhancer [US]; Entero Vu™ [US]; Entrobar® [US]; EntroEase® [US]; Esopho-Cat® [US]; HD 200® Plus [US]; Intropaste [US]; Liqui-Coat HD® [US]; Liquid Barosperse® [US]; Medebar® Plus [US]; Prepcat [US]; Readi-Cat® 2 [US]; Readi-Cat® [US]; Tomocat® 1000 [US]; Tomocat® [US]; Tonojug [US]; Tonopaque [US]; Varibar® Honey [US]; Varibar® Nectar [US]; Varibar® Pudding [US]; Varibar® Thin Honey [US]; Varibar® Thin Liquid [US]; VoLumen™ [US]

Therapeutic Category Radiopaque Agents

Use Diagnostic aid for computed tomography or x-ray examinations of the GI tract

Dosage Forms
Cream, oral:
Esopho-Cat®: 3% w/w
Paste, oral:
Varibar® Pudding: 40% w/v
Powder for suspension, oral:
Baricon™, Enhancer, HD 200® Plus: 98% w/w
E-Z-Cat® Dry: 2% w/w
Tonopaque: 95% w/w
Varibar® Thin Liquid: 40% w/v

Powder for suspension, oral/rectal:
Barosperse®, Tonojug: 95% w/w
Powder for suspension, rectal:
Barobag®: 97% w/w
Suspension, oral:
Entero Vu™: 24% w/v
EntroEase®: 13% w/v
E-Z-Cat®: 4.9% w/v
Liqui-Coat HD®: 210% w/v
Readi-Cat® 2: 2.1% w/v
Varibar® Honey, Varibar® Nectar, Varibar® Thin Honey: 40% w/v
VoLumen™: 0.1% w/v
Suspension, oral/rectal:
Baro-Cat®, Prepcat: 1.5% w/v
CheeTah®: 2.2% w/w
Liquid Barosperse®: 60% w/v
Readi-Cat®: 1.3% w/v
Readi-Cat® 2: 2.1% w/v
Tomocat®, Tomocat® 1000: 5% w/v
Suspension, paste:
Anatrast: 100% w/v
Intropaste: 70% w/v
Suspension, rectal:
Entrobar®: 50% w/v
Medebar® Plus: 100% w/v
Tablet, oral, as sulfate:
Bar-Test, E-Z-Disk™: 648 mg

barium sulfate *see* barium *on page* *122*
Barobag® [US] *see* barium *on page* *122*
Baro-Cat® [US] *see* barium *on page* *122*
Barosperse® [US] *see* barium *on page* *122*
Bar-Test [US] *see* barium *on page* *122*
Basaljel® [Can] *see* aluminum hydroxide *on page* *55*
base ointment *see* zinc oxide *on page* *1030*

basiliximab (ba si LIK si mab)

U.S./Canadian Brand Names Simulect® [US/Can]

Therapeutic Category Immunosuppressant Agent

Use Prophylaxis of acute organ rejection in renal transplantation

Usual Dosage **Note:** Patients previously administered basiliximab should only be reexposed to a subsequent course of therapy with extreme caution.

I.V.:

Children <35 kg: Renal transplantation: 10 mg within 2 hours prior to transplant surgery, followed by a second 10 mg dose 4 days after transplantation; the second dose should be withheld if complications occur (including severe hypersensitivity reactions or graft loss)

Children ≥35 kg and Adults: Renal transplantation: 20 mg within 2 hours prior to transplant surgery, followed by a second 20 mg dose 4 days after transplantation; the second dose should be withheld if complications occur (including severe hypersensitivity reactions or graft loss)

Dosage Forms

Injection, powder for reconstitution [preservative free]:
Simulect®: 10 mg, 20 mg

Bausch & Lomb® Computer Eye Drops [US-OTC] *see* glycerin *on page* *468*
BAY 43-9006 *see* sorafenib *on page* *918*
BAY 59-7939 *see* rivaroxaban *(Canada only) on page* *873*
Bayer® Aspirin Extra Strength [US-OTC] *see* aspirin *on page* *103*
Bayer® Aspirin Regimen Adult Low Dose [US-OTC] *see* aspirin *on page* *103*
Bayer® Aspirin Regimen Children's [US-OTC] *see* aspirin *on page* *103*
Bayer® Aspirin Regimen Regular Strength [US-OTC] *see* aspirin *on page* *103*

Bayer® Genuine Aspirin [US-OTC] *see* aspirin *on page 103*
Bayer® Plus Extra Strength [US-OTC] *see* aspirin *on page 103*
Bayer® PM [US-OTC] *see* aspirin and diphenhydramine *on page 105*
Bayer® with Heart Advantage [US-OTC] *see* aspirin *on page 103*
Bayer® Women's Aspirin Plus Calcium [US-OTC] *see* aspirin *on page 103*
BayGam® [Can] *see* immune globulin (intramuscular) *on page 522*
BayGam® ***(Discontinued)*** *see* immune globulin (intramuscular) *on page 522*
BayHepB® ***(Discontinued)*** *see* hepatitis B immune globulin (human) *on page 489*
BayRab® ***(Discontinued)*** *see* rabies immune globulin (human) *on page 848*
BayRho-D® Full Dose ***(Discontinued)*** *see* Rh_o(D) immune globulin *on page 862*
BayRho-D® Mini Dose ***(Discontinued)*** *see* Rh_o(D) immune globulin *on page 862*
BayTet™ ***(Discontinued)*** *see* tetanus immune globulin (human) *on page 948*
Baza® Antifungal [US-OTC] *see* miconazole *on page 654*
Baza® Clear [US-OTC] *see* vitamin A and vitamin D *on page 1017*
β,β-dimethylcysteine *see* penicillamine *on page 759*
B-Caro-T™ [US] *see* beta-carotene *on page 136*
BCG, live *see* BCG vaccine *on page 124*

BCG vaccine (bee see jee vak SEEN)

Synonyms bacillus calmette-Guérin (BCG) live; BCG vaccine U.S.P. *(percutaneous use product)*; BCG, live

U.S./Canadian Brand Names ImmuCyst® [Can]; Oncotice™ [Can]; Pacis™ [Can]; TheraCys® [US]; TICE® BCG [US]

Therapeutic Category Biological Response Modulator

Use Immunization against tuberculosis and immunotherapy for cancer; treatment and prophylaxis of carcinoma *in situ* of the bladder; prophylaxis of primary or recurrent superficial papillary tumors following transurethral resection

Usual Dosage

Immunization against tuberculosis: Percutaneous: **Note:** Initial lesion usually appears after 10-14 days consisting of small, red papule at injection site and reaches maximum diameter of 3 mm in 4-6 weeks.

Children <1 month: 0.2-0.3 mL (half-strength dilution). Administer tuberculin test (5 TU) after 2-3 months; repeat vaccination after 1 year of age for negative tuberculin test if indications persist.

Children >1 month and Adults: 0.2-0.3 mL (full-strength dilution); conduct postvaccinal tuberculin test (5 TU of PPD) in 2-3 months; if test is negative, repeat vaccination.

Immunotherapy for bladder cancer: Intravesicular Adults:

TheraCys®: One dose instilled into bladder (for 2 hours) once weekly for 6 weeks followed by one treatment at 3, 6, 12, 18, and 24 months after initial treatment

TICE® BCG: One dose instilled into the bladder (for 2 hours) once weekly for 6 weeks followed by once monthly for 6-12 months

Dosage Forms

Injection, powder for reconstitution, intravesical [preservative free]:
TheraCys®: 81 mg
TICE® BCG: 50 mg

Injection, powder for reconstitution, percutaneous [preservative free]:
BCG Vaccine: 50 mg

BCG vaccine U.S.P. ***(percutaneous use product)*** *see* BCG vaccine *on page 124*
BCNU *see* carmustine *on page 187*
B complex combinations *see* vitamin B complex combinations *on page 1017*
beano® [US-OTC] *see* alpha-galactosidase *on page 50*
Bebulin® VH [US] *see* factor IX complex (human) *on page 404*

becaplermin (be KAP ler min)

Sound-Alike/Look-Alike Issues
Regranex® may be confused with Granulex®, Repronex®

Synonyms recombinant human platelet-derived growth factor B; rPDGF-BB

U.S./Canadian Brand Names Regranex® [US/Can]

Therapeutic Category Topical Skin Product

Use Adjunctive treatment of diabetic neuropathic ulcers occurring on the lower limbs and feet that extend into subcutaneous tissue (or beyond) and have adequate blood supply

Usual Dosage Topical: Adults: Diabetic ulcers: Apply appropriate amount of gel once daily with a cotton swab or similar tool, as a coating over the ulcer. The amount of becaplermin to be applied will vary depending on the size of the ulcer area.

Note: If the ulcer does not decrease in size by ~30% after 10 weeks of treatment or complete healing has not occurred in 20 weeks, continued treatment with becaplermin gel should be reassessed.

To calculate the length of gel applied to the ulcer, measure the greatest length of the ulcer by the greatest width of the ulcer. Tube size and unit of measure will determine the formula used in the calculation. Recalculate amount of gel needed every 1-2 weeks, depending on the rate of change in ulcer area.

Centimeters:

15 g tube: [ulcer length (cm) x width (cm)] divided by 4 = length of gel (cm)

2 g tube: [ulcer length (cm) x width (cm)] divided by 2 = length of gel (cm)

Inches:

15 g tube: [length (in) x width (in)] x 0.6 = length of gel (in)

2 g tube: [length (in) x width (in)] x 1.3 = length of gel (in)

Dosage Forms

Gel, topical:

Regranex®: 0.01% (2 g, 15 g)

beclomethasone (be kloe METH a sone)

Sound-Alike/Look-Alike Issues

Vanceril® may be confused with Vancenase®

Synonyms beclomethasone dipropionate

U.S./Canadian Brand Names Apo-Beclomethasone® [Can]; Beconase® AQ [US]; Gen-Beclo [Can]; Nu-Beclomethasone [Can]; Propaderm® [Can]; QVAR® [US/Can]; Rivanase AQ [Can]; Vanceril® AEM [Can]

Therapeutic Category Adrenal Corticosteroid

Use

Oral inhalation: Maintenance and prophylactic treatment of asthma; includes those who require corticosteroids and those who may benefit from a dose reduction/elimination of systemically-administered corticosteroids. Not for relief of acute bronchospasm.

Nasal aerosol: Symptomatic treatment of seasonal or perennial rhinitis; prevent recurrence of nasal polyps following surgery.

Usual Dosage Nasal inhalation and oral inhalation dosage forms are not to be used interchangeably

Inhalation, nasal: Rhinitis, nasal polyps (Beconase® AQ): Children ≥6 years and Adults: 1-2 inhalations each nostril twice daily; total dose 168-336 mcg/day

Inhalation, oral: Asthma (doses should be titrated to the lowest effective dose once asthma is controlled) (QVAR®):

Children 5-11 years: Initial: 40 mcg twice daily; maximum dose: 80 mcg twice daily

Children ≥12 years and Adults:

Patients previously on bronchodilators only: Initial dose 40-80 mcg twice daily; maximum dose: 320 mcg twice day

Patients previously on inhaled corticosteroids: Initial dose 40-160 mcg twice daily; maximum dose: 320 mcg twice daily

NIH Asthma Guidelines: HFA formulation (eg, QVAR®): Administer in divided doses:

Children 5-11 years:

"Low" dose: 80-160 mcg/day

"Medium" dose: >160-320 mcg/day

"High" dose: >320 mcg/day

Children ≥12 years and Adults:

"Low" dose: 80-240 mcg/day

"Medium" dose: >240-480 mcg/day

"High" dose: >480 mcg/day

Dosage Forms

Aerosol for oral inhalation:

QVAR®: 40 mcg/inhalation (7.3 g); 80 mcg/inhalation (7.3 g)

Suspension, intranasal, aqueous [spray]:

Beconase® AQ: 42 mcg/inhalation (25 g)

beclomethasone dipropionate *see* beclomethasone *on page* 125

Beclovent® *(Discontinued)* *see* beclomethasone *on page* 125
Beconase® AQ [US] *see* beclomethasone *on page* 125
Beconase® *(Discontinued)* *see* beclomethasone *on page* 125
Becotin® Pulvules® *(Discontinued)*
Beepen-VK® *(Discontinued)* *see* penicillin V potassium *on page* 763
BeFlex [US] *see* acetaminophen and phenyltoloxamine *on page* 23
behenyl alcohol *see* docosanol *on page* 326
Belix® Oral *(Discontinued)* *see* diphenhydramine *on page* 315
belladonna alkaloids with phenobarbital *see* hyoscyamine, atropine, scopolamine, and phenobarbital *on page* 513

belladonna and opium (bel a DON a & OH pee um)

Sound-Alike/Look-Alike Issues
B&O may be confused with beano®

Synonyms opium and belladonna

Therapeutic Category Analgesic, Narcotic

Controlled Substance C-II

Use Relief of moderate-to-severe pain associated with ureteral spasms not responsive to nonopioid analgesics and to space intervals between injections of opiates

Usual Dosage Rectal: Children >12 years and Adults: 1 suppository 1-2 times/day, up to 4 doses/day

Dosage Forms
Suppository: Belladonna extract 16.2 mg and opium 30 mg; belladonna extract 16.2 mg and opium 60 mg

belladonna, phenobarbital, and ergotamine *(Discontinued)*
Bellamine S *(Discontinued)*
Bellatal® *(Discontinued)* *see* hyoscyamine, atropine, scopolamine, and phenobarbital *on page* 513
Bellergal-S® *(Discontinued)*
Bel-Tabs *(Discontinued)*
Benadryl® [Can] *see* diphenhydramine *on page* 315
Benadryl® Allergy [US-OTC] *see* diphenhydramine *on page* 315
Benadryl® Allergy and Cold [US-OTC] *see* acetaminophen, diphenhydramine, and phenylephrine *on page* 28
Benadryl® Allergy and Sinus Headache [US-OTC] *see* acetaminophen, diphenhydramine, and phenylephrine *on page* 28
Benadryl® Allergy Quick Dissolve [US-OTC] *see* diphenhydramine *on page* 315
Benadryl® Children's Allergy [US-OTC] *see* diphenhydramine *on page* 315
Benadryl® Children's Allergy Fastmelt® [US-OTC] *see* diphenhydramine *on page* 315
Benadryl® Children's Allergy Perfect Measure™ [US] *see* diphenhydramine *on page* 315
Benadryl® Children's Allergy Quick Dissolve *(Discontinued)* *see* diphenhydramine *on page* 315
Benadryl® Children's Dye-Free Allergy [US-OTC] *see* diphenhydramine *on page* 315
Benadryl® Dye-Free Allergy [US-OTC] *see* diphenhydramine *on page* 315
Benadryl® Itch Relief Extra Strength [US-OTC] *see* diphenhydramine *on page* 315
Benadryl® Itch Stopping [US-OTC] *see* diphenhydramine *on page* 315
Benadryl® Itch Stopping Extra Strength [US-OTC] *see* diphenhydramine *on page* 315
Benadry® Maximum Strength Severe Allergy and Sinus Headache [US-OTC] *see* acetaminophen, diphenhydramine, and phenylephrine *on page* 28
Ben-Allergin-50® Injection *(Discontinued)* *see* diphenhydramine *on page* 315
Ben-Aqua® *(Discontinued)* *see* benzoyl peroxide *on page* 132

benazepril (ben AY ze pril)

Sound-Alike/Look-Alike Issues
benazepril may be confused with Benadryl®
Lotensin® may be confused with Lioresal®, lovastatin

Synonyms benazepril hydrochloride

U.S./Canadian Brand Names Apo-Benazepril® [Can]; Lotensin® [US/Can]

Therapeutic Category Angiotensin-Converting Enzyme (ACE) Inhibitor

Use Treatment of hypertension, either alone or in combination with other antihypertensive agents

Usual Dosage Oral: Hypertension:

Children ≥6 years: Initial: 0.2 mg/kg/day (up to 10 mg/day) as monotherapy; dosing range: 0.1-0.6 mg/kg/day (maximum dose: 40 mg/day)

Adults: Initial: 10 mg/day in patients not receiving a diuretic; 20-80 mg/day as a single dose or 2 divided doses; the need for twice-daily dosing should be assessed by monitoring peak (2-6 hours after dosing) and trough responses.

Note: Patients taking diuretics should have them discontinued 2-3 days prior to starting benazepril. If they cannot be discontinued, then initial dose should be 5 mg; restart after blood pressure is stabilized if needed.

Dosage Forms

Tablet: 5 mg, 10 mg, 20 mg, 40 mg

Lotensin®: 5 mg, 10 mg, 20 mg, 40 mg

benazepril and hydrochlorothiazide (ben AY ze pril & hye droe klor oh THYE a zide)

Synonyms hydrochlorothiazide and benazepril

U.S./Canadian Brand Names Lotensin® HCT [US]

Therapeutic Category Antihypertensive Agent, Combination

Use Treatment of hypertension

Usual Dosage Oral: Dose is individualized (range: benazepril: 5-20 mg; hydrochlorothiazide: 6.25-25 mg/day)

Dosage Forms

Tablet:

Generics:

5/6.25: Benazepril 5 mg and hydrochlorothiazide 6.25 mg
10/12.5: Benazepril 10 mg and hydrochlorothiazide 12.5 mg
20/12.5: Benazepril 20 mg and hydrochlorothiazide 12.5 mg
20/25: Benazepril 20 mg and hydrochlorothiazide 25 mg

Brands:

Lotensin® HCT 5/6.25: Benazepril 5 mg and hydrochlorothiazide 6.25 mg
Lotensin® HCT 10/12.5: Benazepril 10 mg and hydrochlorothiazide 12.5 mg
Lotensin® HCT 20/12.5: Benazepril 20 mg and hydrochlorothiazide 12.5 mg
Lotensin® HCT 20/25: Benazepril 20 mg and hydrochlorothiazide 25 mg

benazepril hydrochloride *see* benazepril *on page* 126

benazepril hydrochloride and amlodipine besylate *see* amlodipine and benazepril *on page* 67

bendamustine (ben da MUS teen)

Sound-Alike/Look-Alike Issues

bendamustine may be confused with carmustine

Synonyms bendamustine hydrochloride; cytostasan; SDX-105

U.S./Canadian Brand Names Treanda® [US]

Therapeutic Category Antineoplastic Agent, Alkylating Agent

Use Treatment of chronic lymphocytic leukemia (CLL); treatment of progressed indolent B-cell non-Hodgkin lymphoma (NHL)

Usual Dosage I.V.: Adults:

CLL: 100 mg/m^2 on days 1 and 2 of a 28-day treatment cycle (for up to 6 cycles)
NHL: 120 mg/m^2 on days 1 and 2 of a 21-day treatment cycle (for up to 8 cycles)

Dosage Forms

Injection, powder for reconstitution:

Treanda®: 100 mg

bendamustine hydrochloride *see* bendamustine *on page* 127

bendroflumethiazide and nadolol *see* nadolol and bendroflumethiazide *on page* 676

BeneFix® [US/Can] *see* factor IX *on page* 403

Benemid® ***(Discontinued)*** *see* probenecid *on page* 818

benflumetol and artemether *see* artemether and lumefantrine *on page* 99

Benicar® [US] *see* olmesartan *on page* 721
Benicar HCT® [US] *see* olmesartan and hydrochlorothiazide *on page* 721
Benoquin® ***(Discontinued)*** *see* monobenzone *on page* 666
Benoxyl® [Can] *see* benzoyl peroxide *on page* 132

benserazide and levodopa *(Canada only)* (ben SER a zide & lee voe DOE pa)

Synonyms levodopa and benserazide
U.S./Canadian Brand Names Prolopa® [Can]
Therapeutic Category Anti-Parkinson Agent (Dopamine Agonist)
Use Treatment of Parkinson disease (except drug-induced parkinsonism)
Usual Dosage Oral: Adults: **Note:** Dosage expressed as levodopa/benserazide:

Initial: 100/25 mg 1-2 times/day, increase every 3-4 days until therapeutic effect; optimal dosage: 400/100 mg to 800/200 mg/day divided into 4-6 doses

Note: 200/50 mg used only when maintenance therapy is reached and not to exceed levodopa 1000-1200 mg/benserazide 250-300 mg per day

Patients previously on levodopa: Allow 12 hours or more to lapse between last dose of levodopa; start at 15% of previous levodopa dosage

Note: Dosages should be introduced gradually, individualized, and continued for 3-6 weeks before assessing benefit. Decrease dosage in patients with dystonia.

Dosage Forms [CAN] = Canadian brand name

Capsule:

Prolopa® [CAN]: 50-12.5: Levodopa 50 mg and benserazide 12.5 mg [not available in the U.S.]; 100-25: Levodopa 100 mg and benserazide 25 mg [not available in the U.S.]; 200-50: Levodopa 200 mg and benserazide 50 mg [not available in the U.S.]

Ben-Tann ***(Discontinued)*** *see* diphenhydramine *on page* 315

bentoquatam (BEN toe kwa tam)

Synonyms quaternium-18 bentonite
U.S./Canadian Brand Names IvyBlock® [US-OTC]
Therapeutic Category Protectant, Topical
Use Skin protectant for the prevention of allergic contact dermatitis to poison oak, ivy, and sumac
Usual Dosage Topical: Children >6 years and Adults: Apply to skin 15 minutes prior to potential exposure to poison ivy, poison oak, or poison sumac, and reapply every 4 hours

Dosage Forms

Lotion:

IvyBlock® [OTC]: 5% (120 mL)

Bentyl® [US] *see* dicyclomine *on page* 305
Bentyl® Injection ***(Discontinued)*** *see* dicyclomine *on page* 305
Bentylol® [Can] *see* dicyclomine *on page* 305
Benuryl™ [Can] *see* probenecid *on page* 818
Benylin® 3.3 mg-D-E [Can] *see* guaifenesin, pseudoephedrine, and codeine *on page* 479
Benylin® D for Infants [Can] *see* pseudoephedrine *on page* 833
Benylin® Adult ***(Discontinued)*** *see* dextromethorphan *on page* 295
Benylin® Cough Syrup ***(Discontinued)*** *see* diphenhydramine *on page* 315
Benylin® DM-D [Can] *see* pseudoephedrine and dextromethorphan *on page* 834
Benylin® DM-D-E [Can] *see* guaifenesin, pseudoephedrine, and dextromethorphan *on page* 479
Benylin® DM ***(Discontinued)*** *see* dextromethorphan *on page* 295
Benylin® DM-E [Can] *see* guaifenesin and dextromethorphan *on page* 474
Benylin® E Extra Strength [Can] *see* guaifenesin *on page* 473
Benylin® Expectorant ***(Discontinued)*** *see* guaifenesin and dextromethorphan *on page* 474
Benylin® Pediatric ***(Discontinued)*** *see* dextromethorphan *on page* 295
Benzac® AC [US/Can] *see* benzoyl peroxide *on page* 132
Benzac® AC Gel ***(Discontinued)*** *see* benzoyl peroxide *on page* 132
BenzaClin® [US/Can] *see* clindamycin and benzoyl peroxide *on page* 240
Benzac® W ***(Discontinued)*** *see* benzoyl peroxide *on page* 132

Benzac W® Gel [Can] *see* benzoyl peroxide *on page 132*
Benzac W® Wash [Can] *see* benzoyl peroxide *on page 132*
5 Benzagel® [US] *see* benzoyl peroxide *on page 132*
10 Benzagel® [US] *see* benzoyl peroxide *on page 132*
Benzagel® Wash *(Discontinued)* *see* benzoyl peroxide *on page 132*

benzalkonium chloride (benz al KOE nee um KLOR ide)

Synonyms BAC

U.S./Canadian Brand Names HandClens® [US-OTC]; Pedi-Pro® [US]; Pronto® Plus Lice Egg Remover Kit [US-OTC]; Zephiran® [US-OTC]

Therapeutic Category Antibacterial, Topical

Use Antiseptic of skin, mucous membranes, and wounds; surface antiseptic; germicidal preservative

Usual Dosage Topical:

Children ≥2 years and Adults: Pronto® Plus Lice Egg Remover Kit (benzalkonium chloride 0.1% solution): Apply topically to clean affected area after shampooing with a lice killing shampoo

Adults: Zephiran® (benzalkonium chloride solution 1:750): Antiseptic on skin, mucous membranes, or wounds (the following is a guide for appropriate concentrations, depending on intended use and application site):

- Bladder and urethral irrigation: Aqueous solution 1:5000 to 1:20,000
- Bladder retention lavage: Aqueous solution 1:20,000 to 1:40,000
- Breast and nipple hygiene: Aqueous solution 1:1000 to 1:2000
- Denuded skin and mucous membranes: Aqueous solution 1:5000 to 1:10,000
- Eye irrigation: Aqueous solution 1:5000 to 1:10,000
- Irrigation of deep, infected wounds: Aqueous solution 1:3000 to 1:20,000
- Oozing and open infections: Aqueous solution 1:2000 to 1:5000
- Postepisiotomy care: Aqueous solution 1:5000 to 1:10,000
- Preoperative preparation of skin (unbroken): Aqueous solution 1:750
- Preservation of ophthalmic solutions: Aqueous solution 1:5000 to 1:7500
- Surgeons' hands and arms soaks: Aqueous solution 1:750
- Vaginal douche and irrigation: Aqueous solution 1:2000 to 1:5000
- Wet dressings by irrigation or open dressing (do not use in occlusive dressings): Aqueous solution ≤1:5000

Dosage Forms

Lotion, topical [foam]:
HandClens® [OTC]: 0.13% (50 mL, 240 mL, 1800 mL)

Lotion, topical [spray]:
HandClens® [OTC]: 0.13% (15 mL)

Powder, topical:
Pedi-Pro®: 1% (60 g)

Solution, topical:
Pronto® Plus Lice Egg Remover Kit [OTC]: 0.1% (60 mL)
Zephiran® [OTC]: 1:750 (240 mL, 3840 mL)

Benzamycin® [US] *see* erythromycin and benzoyl peroxide *on page 370*
Benzamycin® Pak [US] *see* erythromycin and benzoyl peroxide *on page 370*
BenzaShave® [US] *see* benzoyl peroxide *on page 132*
benzathine benzylpenicillin *see* penicillin G benzathine *on page 760*
benzathine penicillin G *see* penicillin G benzathine *on page 760*
Benzedrex® [US-OTC] *see* propylhexedrine *on page 830*
benzene hexachloride *see* lindane *on page 590*
benzhexol hydrochloride *see* trihexyphenidyl *on page 986*
Benziq™ [US] *see* benzoyl peroxide *on page 132*
Benziq™ LS [US] *see* benzoyl peroxide *on page 132*
benzmethyzin *see* procarbazine *on page 820*

benzocaine (BEN zoe kane)

Sound-Alike/Look-Alike Issues
Orabase®-B may be confused with Orinase®

Synonyms ethyl aminobenzoate

U.S./Canadian Brand Names Americaine® Hemorrhoidal [US-OTC]; Anbesol® Baby [US-OTC/Can]; Anbesol® Cold Sore Therapy [US-OTC]; Anbesol® Jr. [US-OTC]; Anbesol® Maximum Strength [US-OTC]; Anbesol® [US-OTC]; Benzodent® [US-OTC]; Bi-Zets [US]; Boil-Ease® Pain Relieving [US]; Cepacol® Sore Throat [US-OTC]; Chiggerex® Plus [US]; Chiggerex® [US-OTC]; Chiggertox® [US-OTC]; Cylex® [US-OTC]; Dent's Extra Strength Toothache [US-OTC]; Dentapaine [US-OTC]; Dermoplast® Antibacterial [US-OTC]; Dermoplast® Pain Relieving [US-OTC]; Detane® [US-OTC]; Foille® [US-OTC]; HDA® Toothache [US-OTC]; Hurricaine® [US-OTC]; Ivy-Rid® [US-OTC]; Kank-A® Soft Brush™ [US-OTC]; Lanacane® Maximum Strength [US-OTC]; Lanacane® [US-OTC]; Little Teethers® [US-OTC]; Mycinettes® [US-OTC]; Orabase® with Benzocaine [US-OTC]; Orajel PM® Maximum Strength [US-OTC]; Orajel® Baby Daytime and Nighttime [US-OTC]; Orajel® Baby Teething Nighttime [US-OTC]; Orajel® Baby Teething [US-OTC]; Orajel® Denture Plus [US-OTC]; Orajel® Maximum Strength [US-OTC]; Orajel® Medicated Toothache [US-OTC]; Orajel® Mouth Sore [US-OTC]; Orajel® Multi-Action Cold Sore [US-OTC]; Orajel® Ultra Mouth Sore [US-OTC]; Outgro® [US-OTC]; Red Cross™ Canker Sore [US-OTC]; Rid-A-Pain Dental [US-OTC]; Sepasoothe® [US]; Skeeter Stik [US-OTC]; Sting-Kill [US-OTC]; Tanac® [US-OTC]; Thorets [US-OTC]; Trocaine® [US-OTC]; Zilactin Baby® [Can]; Zilactin Toothache and Gum Pain® [US-OTC]; Zilactin®-B [US-OTC/Can]

Therapeutic Category Local Anesthetic

Use Temporary relief of pain associated with pruritic dermatosis, pruritus, minor burns, acute congestive, bee stings, and insect bites; mouth and gum irritations (toothache, minor sore throat pain, canker sores, dentures, orthodontia, teething, mucositis, stomatitis); sunburn; hemorrhoids; anesthetic lubricant for passage of catheters and endoscopic tubes

Usual Dosage Note: These are general dosing guidelines; refer to specific product labeling for dosing instructions.

Children ≥4 months: Topical (oral): Teething pain: 7.5% to 10%: Apply to affected gum area up to 4 times daily

Children ≥2 years and Adults:

Topical:

Bee stings, insect bites, minor burns, sunburn: 5% to 20%: Apply to affected area 3-4 times a day as needed. In cases of bee stings, remove stinger before treatment.

Lubricant for passage of catheters and instruments: 20%: Apply evenly to exterior of instrument prior to use.

Topical (oral): Mouth and gum irritation: 10% to 20%: Apply thin layer to affected area up to 4 times daily

Children ≥5 years and Adults: Oral: Sore throat: Allow 1 lozenge (10-15 mg) to dissolve slowly in mouth; may repeat every 2 hours as needed

Children ≥12 years and Adults: Rectal: Hemorrhoids: 5% to 20%: Apply externally to affected area up to 6 times daily

Dosage Forms

Aerosol, oral spray:

Hurricaine® [OTC]: 20% (60 mL)

Aerosol, topical spray:

Dermoplast® Antibacterial [OTC]: 20% (83 mL)

Dermoplast® Pain Relieving [OTC]: 20% (60 mL, 83 mL)

Foille® [OTC]: 5% (92 g)

Ivy-Rid® [OTC]: 2% (83 mL)

Lanacane® Maximum Strength [OTC]: 20% (120 mL)

Combination package:

Orajel® Baby Daytime and Nighttime [OTC]:

Gel, oral [Daytime Regular Formula]: 7.5% (5.3 g)

Gel, oral [Nighttime Formula]: 10% (5.3 g)

Cream, oral:

Benzodent® [OTC]: 20% (7.5 g, 30 g)

Orajel PM® Maximum Strength [OTC]: 20% (5.3 g, 7 g)

Cream, topical:

Lanacane® [OTC]: 6% (30 g, 60 g)

Lanacane® Maximum Strength [OTC]: 20% (30 g)

Gel, oral:

Anbesol® [OTC], Zilactin®-B [OTC]: 10% (7.5 g)

Anbesol® Baby [OTC]: 7.5% (7.5 g)

Anbesol® Jr. [OTC]: 10% (7 g)

Anbesol® Maximum Strength [OTC]: 20% (7.5 g, 10 g)

Dentapaine [OTC]: 20% (11 g)

HDA® Toothache [OTC]: 6.5% (15 mL)

Hurricaine® [OTC]: 20% (5 g, 30 g)
Kank-A® Soft Brush™ [OTC]: 20% (2 mL)
Little Teethers® [OTC]: 7.5% (9.4 g)
Orabase® with Benzocaine [OTC]: 20% (7 g)
Orajel® [OTC]: 10% (5.3 g, 7 g, 9.4 g)
Orajel® Baby Teething [OTC]: 7.5% (9.4 g, 11.9 g)
Orajel® Baby Teething Nighttime [OTC]: 10% (5.3 g)
Orajel® Denture Plus [OTC]: 15% (9 g)
Orajel® Maximum Strength [OTC]: 20% (5.3 g, 7 g, 9.4 g, 11.9 g)
Orajel® Mouth Sore [OTC]: 20% (5.3 g, 9.4 g, 11.9 g)
Orajel® Multi-Action Cold Sore [OTC]: 20% (9.4 g)
Orajel® Ultra Mouth Sore [OTC]: 15% (9.4 g)

Gel, topical:
Detane® [OTC]: 7.5% (15 g)

Liquid, oral:
Anbesol® [OTC], Tanac® [OTC]: 10%
Anbesol® Maximum Strength [OTC], Hurricaine® [OTC], Orajel® Maximum Strength [OTC]: 20%
Orajel® Baby Teething [OTC]: 7.5%

Liquid, oral [drops]:
Rid-A-Pain Dental [OTC]: 6.3%

Liquid, topical:
Chiggertox® [OTC]: 2% (30 mL)
Outgro® [OTC]: 20% (9 mL)
Skeeter Stik [OTC]: 5% (14 mL)

Lozenge: 6 mg (18s), 15 mg (10s)
Bi-Zets: 15 mg (10s)
Cepacol® Sore Throat [OTC]: 15 mg (16s, 18s)
Cylex® [OTC], Mycinettes® [OTC]: 15 mg (12s)
Sepasoothe®: 10 mg (6s, 24s, 100s, 250s, 500s)
Thorets [OTC]: 18 mg (300s)
Trocaine® [OTC]: 10 mg (50s, 300s)

Ointment, oral:
Anbesol® Cold Sore Therapy [OTC]: 20% (7.1 g)
Red Cross™ Canker Sore [OTC]: 20% (7.5 g)

Ointment, rectal:
Americaine® Hemorrhoidal [OTC]: 20% (30 g)

Ointment, topical:
Boil-Ease® Pain Relieving: 20% (30 g)
Chiggerex® Plus: 6% (50 g)
Foille® [OTC]: 5% (3.5 g, 14 g, 28 g)

Pads, topical:
Sting-Kill [OTC]: 20% (8s)

Paste, oral:
Orabase® with Benzocaine [OTC]: 20% (6 g)

Swabs, oral:
Hurricaine® [OTC]: 20% (6s, 100s)
Orajel® Baby Teething [OTC]: 7.5% (12s)
Orajel® Mouth Sore [OTC], Orajel® Medicated Toothache [OTC]: 20% (8s, 12s)
Zilactin Toothache and Gum Pain® [OTC]: 20% (8s)

Swabs, topical:
Boil-Ease® Pain Relieving: 20% (12s)
Sting-Kill [OTC]: 20% (5s)

Wax, oral:
Dent's Extra Strength Toothache Gum [OTC]: 20% (1 g)

benzocaine and antipyrine *see* antipyrine and benzocaine *on page 85*

benzocaine, butamben, and tetracaine (BEN zoe kane, byoo TAM ben, & TET ra kane)

Synonyms benzocaine, butamben, and tetracaine hydrochloride; benzocaine, butyl aminobenzoate, and tetracaine; butamben, tetracaine, and benzocaine; tetracaine, benzocaine, and butamben

U.S./Canadian Brand Names Cetacaine® [US]; Exactacain™ [US]

Therapeutic Category Local Anesthetic

Use Topical anesthetic to control pain in surgical or endoscopic procedures; anesthetic for accessible mucous membranes except for the eyes

Usual Dosage Topical anesthetic: **Note:** Decrease dose in the acutely-ill patient: Adults:
Cetacaine®:
Aerosol: Apply for ≤1 second; use of sprays >2 seconds is contraindicated
Gel: Apply ~1/2 inch (13 mm) x 3/16 inch (5 mm); application of >1 inch (26 cm) x 3/16 inch (5 mm) is contraindicated
Liquid: Apply 6-7 drops (0.2 mL); application of >12-14 drops (0.4 mL) is contraindicated
Exactacain™: 3 metered sprays (use of >6 metered sprays is contraindicated)

Dosage Forms
Aerosol, topical [spray]:
Cetacaine®: Benzocaine 14%, butamben 2%, and tetracaine 2% (56 g)
Exactacain™: Benzocaine 14%, butamben 2%, and tetracaine 2% (60 g)
Gel, topical:
Cetacaine®: Benzocaine 14%, butamben 2%, and tetracaine 2% (29 g)
Liquid, topical:
Cetacaine®: Benzocaine 14%, butamben 2%, and tetracaine 2% (56 g)

benzocaine, butamben, and tetracaine hydrochloride *see* benzocaine, butamben, and tetracaine *on page 131*

benzocaine, butyl aminobenzoate, and tetracaine *see* benzocaine, butamben, and tetracaine *on page 131*

Benzocol® *(Discontinued)* *see* benzocaine *on page 129*

Benzodent® [US-OTC] *see* benzocaine *on page 129*

benzoic acid, hyoscyamine, methenamine, methylene blue, and phenyl salicylate *see* methenamine, phenyl salicylate, methylene blue, benzoic acid, and hyoscyamine *on page 637*

benzoic acid, methenamine, methylene blue, phenyl salicylate, and hyoscyamine *see* methenamine, phenyl salicylate, methylene blue, benzoic acid, and hyoscyamine *on page 637*

benzoin (BEN zoin)

Synonyms gum benjamin

U.S./Canadian Brand Names Benz-Protect Swabs™ [US-OTC]; Sprayzoin™ [US-OTC]

Therapeutic Category Pharmaceutical Aid; Protectant, Topical

Use Protective application for irritations of the skin; sometimes used in boiling water as steam inhalants for its expectorant and soothing action

Usual Dosage Apply 1-2 times/day

Dosage Forms
Tincture: Benzoin USP [OTC] (60 mL); Benzoin Compound USP [OTC] (30 mL, 60 mL, 120 mL, 480 mL)
Tincture [swab]:
Benz-Protect Swabs™ [OTC]: Benzoin Compound USP (50s)
Tincture [spray]: Benzoin USP [OTC] (120 mL)
Sprayzoin™ [OTC]: Benzoin Compound USP (120 mL)

benzonatate (ben ZOE na tate)

Synonyms Tessalon Perles

U.S./Canadian Brand Names Tessalon® [US/Can]

Therapeutic Category Antitussive

Use Symptomatic relief of nonproductive cough

Usual Dosage Oral: Children >10 years and Adults: 100 mg 3 times/day or every 4 hours up to 600 mg/day

Dosage Forms
Capsule, softgel: 100 mg, 200 mg
Tessalon®: 100 mg, 200 mg

benzoyl peroxide (BEN zoe il peer OKS ide)

Sound-Alike/Look-Alike Issues
benzoyl peroxide may be confused with benzyl alcohol
Benoxyl® may be confused with Brevoxyl®, Peroxyl®
Benzac® may be confused with Benza®

Brevoxyl® may be confused with Benoxyl®
Fostex® may be confused with pHisoHex®

U.S./Canadian Brand Names 10 Benzagel® [US]; 5 Benzagel® [US]; Acetoxyl® [Can]; Acne Clear Maximum Strength [US-OTC]; Benoxyl® [Can]; Benzac W® Wash [Can]; Benzac W® Gel [Can]; Benzac® AC [US/Can]; BenzaShave® [US]; Benziq™ LS [US]; Benziq™ [US]; Brevoxyl® [US]; Brevoxyl®-4 [US]; Brevoxyl®-8 [US]; Clearskin [US-OTC]; Clinac BPO [US]; Desquam-X® [US/Can]; Inova™ [US]; NeoBenz® Micro Wash [US]; Neutrogena® Body Clear® [US-OTC]; Neutrogena® Clear Pore™ [US-OTC]; Neutrogena® Oil-Free Acne Wash [US-OTC]; Neutrogena® On The Spot® Acne Treatment [US-OTC]; Oxyderm™ [Can]; Palmer's® Skin Success Invisible Acne [US-OTC]; PanOxyl® Aqua Gel [US]; PanOxyl® Bar [US-OTC]; PanOxyl® [Can]; Solugel® [Can]; Triaz® [US]; Zapzyt® [US-OTC]; Zoderm® Hydrating Wash™ [US]; Zoderm® Redi-Pads™ [US]; Zoderm® [US]

Therapeutic Category Acne Products

Use Adjunctive treatment of mild-to-moderate acne vulgaris and acne rosacea

Usual Dosage Children and Adults:

Cleansers: Wash once or twice daily; control amount of drying or peeling by modifying dose frequency or concentration

Topical: Apply sparingly once daily; gradually increase to 2-3 times/day if needed. If excessive dryness or peeling occurs, reduce dose frequency or concentration; if excessive stinging or burning occurs, remove with mild soap and water; resume use the next day.

Dosage Forms

Bar, topical [wash]:
PanOxyl® Bar [OTC]: 5% (113 g); 10% (113 g)
Zapzyt® [OTC]: 10% (113 g)

Cream, topical:
BenzaShave®: 5% (120 g); 10% (120 g)
Clearskin [OTC]: 10% (28 g)
Neutrogena® On The Spot® Acne Treatment [OTC]: 2.5% (22.5 g)
Zoderm®: 4.5% (125 mL); 6.5% (125 mL); 8.5% (125 mL)

Cream, topical [cleanser, mask]:
Neutrogena® Clear Pore™ [OTC]: 3.5% (125mL)

Gel, topical: 5% (45 g, 60 g); 10% (42.5 g, 45 g, 60 g, 90 g)
5 Benzagel®: 5% (45 g)
10 Benzagel®: 10% (45 g)
Acne Clear Maximum Strength [OTC]: 10% (42.5 g)
Brevoxyl®-4: 4% (42.5 g)
Brevoxyl®-8: 8% (42.5 g)
Clearplex: 5% (45 g); 10% (45 g)
Clinic BPO: 7% (45 g)
Desquam-X®: 10% (42.5 g, 90 g)
Neutrogena® Oil-Free Acne Wash [OTC]: 2% (177 mL)
Zapzyt® [OTC]: 10% (30 g)
Zoderm®: 4.5% (125 mL); 6.5% (125 mL); 8.5% (125 mL)

Gel, topical [alcohol-based]: 5% (60 g); 10% (60 g)
Triaz®: 3% (170 g, 340 g); 6% (170 g, 340 g); 9% (170 g, 340 g)

Gel, topical [wash]: 5% (150 g, 240 g); 10% (150 g, 240 g)

Gel, topical [water-based]: 2.5% (60 g; 5% (60 g, 90 g); 10% (60 g, 90 g)
Benzac® AC: 5% (60 g); 10% (60 g)
Benziq™: 5.25% (50 g)
Benziq™ LS: 2.75% (50 g)
PanOxyl® Aqua Gel: 10% (42.5 g)

Liquid, topical:
Desquam-X®: 5% (150 mL)

Liquid, topical [body wash]: 5.75% (473 mL)
Neutrogena® Body Clear® [OTC]: 2% (250 mL)

Liquid, topical [wash]: 2.5% (240 mL); 5% (120 mL, 150 mL, 240 mL); 10% (150 mL, 240 mL)
Zoderm® Hydrating Wash™: 5.75% (473 mL)

Liquid, topical [wash/water-based]:
Benzac® AC: 10% (240 mL)
Benziq™: 5.25% (175 g)

Lotion, topical: 5% (30 mL); 10% (30 mL)
Palmer's® Skin Success Invisible Acne [OTC]: 10% (30 mL)

Lotion, topical [wash]: 4% (170 g); 5% (227 g); 8% (170 g); 10% (227 g)
NeoBenz® Micro Wash: 7% (180 g)
Pacnex™: 7% (454 g)
Pad, topical:
Inova™: 4% (30s); 8% (30s)
Triaz®: 3% (30s, 60s); 6% (30s, 60s); 9% (30s)
ZoDerm®: 4.5% (30s); 6.5% (30s); 8.5% (30s)
Soap, topical [cleanser/emulsion-based]:
ZoDerm®: 4.5% (400 mL); 6.5% (400 mL); 8.5% (400 mL)

benzoyl peroxide and adapalene *see* adapalene and benzoyl peroxide *on page* 36
benzoyl peroxide and clindamycin *see* clindamycin and benzoyl peroxide *on page* 240
benzoyl peroxide and erythromycin *see* erythromycin and benzoyl peroxide *on page* 370

benzoyl peroxide and hydrocortisone (BEN zoe il peer OKS ide & hye droe KOR ti sone)

Synonyms hydrocortisone and benzoyl peroxide
U.S./Canadian Brand Names Vanoxide-HC® [US/Can]
Therapeutic Category Acne Products
Use Treatment of acne vulgaris and oily skin
Usual Dosage Topical: Adolescents and Adults: Shake well; apply thin film 1-3 times/day, gently massage into skin
Dosage Forms
Lotion:
Vanoxide-HC®: Benzoyl peroxide 5% and hydrocortisone 0.5% (25 mL)

benzphetamine (benz FET a meen)

Synonyms benzphetamine hydrochloride
U.S./Canadian Brand Names Didrex® [US/Can]
Therapeutic Category Anorexiant
Controlled Substance C-III
Use Short-term (few weeks) adjunct in exogenous obesity
Usual Dosage Oral: Children ≥12 years and Adults: Dose should be individualized based on patient response: Initial: 25-50 mg once daily; titrate to 25-50 mg 1-3 times/day; once-daily dosing should be administered midmorning or midafternoon; maximum dose: 50 mg 3 times/day
Dosage Forms
Tablet: 50 mg
Didrex®: 50 mg

benzphetamine hydrochloride *see* benzphetamine *on page* 134
Benz-Protect Swabs™ [US-OTC] *see* benzoin *on page* 132

benztropine (BENZ troe peen)

Sound-Alike/Look-Alike Issues
benztropine may be confused with bromocriptine
Synonyms benztropine mesylate
U.S./Canadian Brand Names Apo-Benztropine® [Can]; Cogentin® [US]
Therapeutic Category Anti-Parkinson Agent; Anticholinergic Agent
Use Adjunctive treatment of Parkinson disease; treatment of drug-induced extrapyramidal symptoms (except tardive dyskinesia)
Usual Dosage Use in children ≤3 years of age should be reserved for life-threatening emergencies
Drug-induced extrapyramidal symptom: Oral, I.M., I.V.:
Children >3 years: 0.02-0.05 mg/kg/dose 1-2 times/day
Adults: 1-4 mg/dose 1-2 times/day
Acute dystonia: Adults: I.M., I.V.: 1-2 mg
Parkinsonism: Adults: Oral: 0.5-6 mg/day in 1-2 divided doses; if one dose is greater, administer at bedtime; titrate dose in 0.5 mg increments at 5- to 6-day intervals
Dosage Forms
Injection, solution:
Cogentin®: 1 mg/mL (2 mL)
Tablet: 0.5 mg, 1 mg, 2 mg

benztropine mesylate *see* benztropine *on page 134*

benzydamine *(Canada only)* (ben ZID a meen)

Synonyms benzydamine hydrochloride

U.S./Canadian Brand Names Apo-Benzydamine® [Can]; Dom-Benzydamine [Can]; Novo-Benzydamine [Can]; PMS-Benzydamine [Can]; ratio-Benzydamine [Can]; Sun-Benz® [Can]; Tantum® [Can]

Therapeutic Category Analgesic, Topical

Use Symptomatic treatment of pain associated with acute pharyngitis; treatment of pain associated with radiation-induced oropharyngeal mucositis

Usual Dosage Oral rinse: Adults:

Acute pharyngitis: Gargle with 15 mL of undiluted solution every 1½-3 hours until symptoms resolve. Patient should expel solution from mouth following use; solution should not be swallowed.

Mucositis: 15 mL of undiluted solution as a gargle or rinse 3-4 times/day; contact should be maintained for at least 30 seconds, followed by expulsion from the mouth. Clinical studies maintained contact for ~2 minutes, up to 8 times/day. Patient should not swallow the liquid. Begin treatment 1 day prior to initiation of radiation therapy and continue daily during treatment. Continue oral rinse treatments after the completion of radiation therapy until desired result/healing is achieved.

Dosage Forms

Oral rinse: 0.15% (100 mL, 250 mL) [not available in the U.S.]

benzydamine hydrochloride *see* benzydamine *(Canada only) on page 135*

benzyl alcohol (BEN zill AL koe hol)

Sound-Alike/Look-Alike Issues

benzyl alcohol may be confused with benzoyl peroxide

Therapeutic Category Antiparasitic Agent, Topical; Pediculocide

Use Treatment of head lice infestation

Usual Dosage Topical: Children ≥6 months and Adults: Apply appropriate volume for hair length to dry hair and completely saturate the scalp; leave on for 10 minutes; rinse thoroughly with water; repeat in 7 days

Hair length 0-2 inches: 4-6 ounces
Hair length 2-4 inches: 6-8 ounces
Hair length 4-8 inches: 8-12 ounces
Hair length 8-16 inches: 12-24 ounces
Hair length 16-22 inches: 24-32 ounces
Hair length >22 inches: 32-48 ounces

Dosage Forms

Lotion, topical:

Ulesfia™: 5% (240 mL)

benzylpenicillin benzathine *see* penicillin G benzathine *on page 760*
benzylpenicillin potassium *see* penicillin G (parenteral/aqueous) *on page 761*
benzylpenicillin sodium *see* penicillin G (parenteral/aqueous) *on page 761*
benzylpenicilloyl-polylysine *(Discontinued)*

beractant (ber AKT ant)

Sound-Alike/Look-Alike Issues

Survanta® may be confused with Sufenta®

Synonyms bovine lung surfactant; natural lung surfactant

U.S./Canadian Brand Names Survanta® [US/Can]

Therapeutic Category Lung Surfactant

Use Prevention and treatment of respiratory distress syndrome (RDS) in premature infants

Prophylactic therapy: Body weight <1250 g in infants at risk for developing, or with evidence of, surfactant deficiency (administer within 15 minutes of birth)

Rescue therapy: Treatment of infants with RDS confirmed by x-ray and requiring mechanical ventilation (administer as soon as possible - within 8 hours of age)

Usual Dosage

Prophylactic treatment: Administer 100 mg phospholipids (4 mL/kg) intratracheal as soon as possible; as many as 4 doses may be administered during the first 48 hours of life, no more frequently than 6 hours apart. The need for additional doses is determined by evidence of continuing respiratory distress; if the

infant is still intubated and requiring at least 30% inspired oxygen to maintain a PaO_2 ≤80 torr.
Rescue treatment: Administer 100 mg phospholipids (4 mL/kg) as soon as the diagnosis of RDS is made; may repeat if needed, no more frequently than every 6 hours to a maximum of 4 doses

Dosage Forms

Suspension, intratracheal [preservative free; bovine derived]:
Survanta®: 25 mg/mL

Berocca® ***(Discontinued)***

Berocca® Plus ***(Discontinued)***

Berotec® [Can] *see* fenoterol *(Canada only) on page 410*

Berubigen® ***(Discontinued)*** *see* cyanocobalamin *on page 263*

besifloxacin (be si FLOX a sin)

Synonyms besifloxacin hydrochloride; BOL-303224-A; SS734

U.S./Canadian Brand Names Besivance™ [US]

Therapeutic Category Antibiotic, Ophthalmic; Antibiotic, Quinolone

Use Treatment of bacterial conjunctivitis

Usual Dosage Ophthalmic: Children ≥1 year and Adults: Bacterial conjunctivitis: Instill 1 drop into affected eye(s) 3 times/day (4-12 hours apart) for 7 days

Dosage Forms

Suspension, ophthalmic:
Besivance™: 0.6% (5 mL) [contains benzalkonium chloride]

besifloxacin hydrochloride *see* besifloxacin *on page 136*

Besivance™ [US] *see* besifloxacin *on page 136*

Betacaine® [Can] *see* lidocaine *on page 584*

beta-carotene (BAY ta KARE oh teen)

U.S./Canadian Brand Names A-Caro-25 [US]; B-Caro-T™ [US]; Lumitene™ [US]

Therapeutic Category Vitamin, Fat Soluble

Usual Dosage Oral:
Children <14 years: 30-150 mg/day
Adults: 30-300 mg/day

Dosage Forms

Capsule, softgel: 10,000 int. units (6 mg); 25,000 int. units (15 mg)
A-Caro-25: 25,000 int. units (15 mg)
B-Caro-T™: 25,000 int. units (15 mg)

Capsule:
Lumitene™: 50,000 int. units (30 mg)

Tablet: 10,000 int. units

Betachron® ***(Discontinued)*** *see* propranolol *on page 828*

Betaderm [Can] *see* betamethasone (topical) *on page 138*

Betadine® [US/Can] *see* povidone-iodine *on page 807*

Betadine® First Aid Antibiotics + Moisturizer ***(Discontinued)*** *see* bacitracin and polymyxin B *on page 119*

9-beta-d-ribofuranosyladenine *see* adenosine *on page 36*

Betagan® [US/Can] *see* levobunolol *on page 578*

Beta-HC® [US] *see* hydrocortisone (topical) *on page 505*

betahistine *(Canada only)* (bay ta HISS teen)

Synonyms betahistine dihydrochloride

U.S./Canadian Brand Names Novo-Betahistine [Can]; Serc® [Can]

Therapeutic Category Antihistamine

Use Treatment of Ménière disease (to decrease episodes of vertigo)

Usual Dosage Oral: Adults: 8-16 mg 3 times/day; administration with meals is recommended

Dosage Forms [CAN] = Canadian brand name

Tablet:
Serc® [CAN]: 16 mg, 24 mg [not available in the U.S.]

betahistine dihydrochloride *see* betahistine *(Canada only) on page 136*

betaine (BAY ta een)

Sound-Alike/Look-Alike Issues

betaine may be confused with Betadine®

Cystadane® may be confused with cysteamine, cysteine

Synonyms betaine anhydrous

U.S./Canadian Brand Names Cystadane® [US/Can]

Therapeutic Category Homocystinuria Agent

Use Treatment of homocystinuria (eg, deficiencies or defects in cystathionine beta-synthase [CBS], 5,10-methylene tetrahydrofolate reductase [MTHFR], and cobalamin cofactor metabolism [CBL])

Usual Dosage Oral:

Children <3 years: Initial dose: 100 mg/kg/day given once daily or in 2 divided doses; increase weekly by 50 mg/kg increments, as needed

Children ≥3 years and Adults: Usual dose: 6 g/day administered in divided doses of 3 g twice daily; dosages of up to 20 g/day have been necessary to control homocysteine levels in some patients

Note: Dosage in all patients can be gradually increased until plasma total homocysteine is undetectable or present only in small amounts. One study in six patients with CBS deficiency, ranging from 6-17 years of age, showed minimal benefit from exceeding a twice daily dosing schedule and a 150 mg/kg/day dosage.

Dosage Forms

Powder for oral solution, anhydrous:

Cystadane®: 1 g/scoop

betaine anhydrous *see* betaine *on page 137*

Betaject™ [Can] *see* betamethasone (systemic) *on page 138*

Betalin® S *(Discontinued)* *see* thiamine *on page 954*

Betaloc® [Can] *see* metoprolol *on page 650*

Betaloc® Durules® [Can] *see* metoprolol *on page 650*

BetaMed [US-OTC] *see* pyrithione zinc *on page 842*

betamethasone and clotrimazole (bay ta METH a sone & kloe TRIM a zole)

Sound-Alike/Look-Alike Issues

clotrimazole may be confused with co-trimoxazole

Lotrisone® may be confused with Lotrimin®

Synonyms clotrimazole and betamethasone

U.S./Canadian Brand Names Lotriderm® [Can]; Lotrisone® [US]

Therapeutic Category Antifungal/Corticosteroid

Use Topical treatment of various dermal fungal infections (including tinea pedis, cruris, and corpora in patients ≥17 years of age)

Usual Dosage Topical: Children ≥17 years and Adults:

Allergic or inflammatory diseases: Apply to affected area twice daily, morning and evening

Tinea corporis, tinea cruris: Massage into affected area twice daily, morning and evening; do not use for longer than 2 weeks; reevaluate after 1 week if no clinical improvement; do not exceed 45 g cream/week or 45 mL lotion/week

Tinea pedis: Massage into affected area twice daily, morning and evening; do not use for longer than 4 weeks; reevaluate after 2 weeks if no clinical improvement; do not exceed 45 g cream/week or 45 mL lotion/week

Dosage Forms

Cream: Betamethasone 0.05% and clotrimazole 1% (15 g, 45 g)

Lotrisone®: Betamethasone 0.05% and clotrimazole 1% (15 g, 45 g)

Lotion: Betamethasone 0.05% and clotrimazole 1% (30 mL)

Lotrisone®: Betamethasone 0.05% and clotrimazole 1% (30 mL)

betamethasone dipropionate *see* betamethasone (topical) *on page 138*

betamethasone dipropionate and calcipotriene hydrate *see* calcipotriene and betamethasone *on page 167*

betamethasone dipropionate, augmented *see* betamethasone (topical) *on page 138*

betamethasone sodium phosphate *see* betamethasone (systemic) *on page 138*

betamethasone (systemic) (bay ta METH a sone sis TEM ik)

Synonyms betamethasone sodium phosphate

U.S./Canadian Brand Names Betaject™ [Can]; Celestone® Soluspan® [US/Can]; Celestone® [US]

Therapeutic Category Adrenal Corticosteroid

Use Antiinflammatory; immunosuppressant agent; corticosteroid replacement

Usual Dosage Base dosage on severity of disease and patient response

Children: Use lowest dose listed as initial dose for adrenocortical insufficiency (physiologic replacement)

I.M.: 0.0175-0.125 mg base/kg/day divided every 6-12 hours **or** 0.5-7.5 mg base/m^2/day divided every 6-12 hours

Oral: 0.0175-0.25 mg/kg/day divided every 6-8 hours **or** 0.5-7.5 mg/m^2/day divided every 6-8 hours

Adolescents and Adults:

Oral: 2.4-4.8 mg/day in 2-4 doses; range: 0.6-7.2 mg/day

I.M.: Betamethasone sodium phosphate and betamethasone acetate: 0.6-9 mg/day (generally, 1/3 to 1/2 of oral dose) divided every 12-24 hours

Adults:

Intrabursal, intraarticular, intradermal: 0.25-2 mL

Intralesional: Rheumatoid arthritis/osteoarthritis:

Very large joints: 1-2 mL

Large joints: 1 mL

Medium joints: 0.5-1 mL

Small joints: 0.25-0.5 mL

Dosage Forms

Injection, suspension:

Celestone® Soluspan®: Betamethasone sodium phosphate 3 mg and betamethasone acetate 3 mg per 1 mL (5 mL) [6 mg/mL]

Solution:

Celestone®: 0.6 mg/5 mL

betamethasone (topical) (bay ta METH a sone TOP i kal)

Sound-Alike/Look-Alike Issues

Luxiq® may be confused with Lasix®

Synonyms betamethasone dipropionate; betamethasone dipropionate, augmented; betamethasone valerate; flubenisolone

U.S./Canadian Brand Names Beta-Val® [US]; Betaderm [Can]; Betnesol® [Can]; Betnovate® [Can]; Diprolene® AF [US]; Diprolene® Glycol [Can]; Diprolene® [US]; Diprosone® [Can]; Ectosone [Can]; Luxiq® [US]; Maxivate® [US]; Prevex® B [Can]; Taro-Sone® [Can]; Topilene® [Can]; Topisone® [Can]; Valisone® Scalp Lotion [Can]

Therapeutic Category Corticosteroid, Topical

Use Inflammatory dermatoses such as seborrheic or atopic dermatitis, neurodermatitis, anogenital pruritus, psoriasis, inflammatory phase of xerosis

Usual Dosage Topical:

≥13 years: Use minimal amount for shortest period of time to avoid HPA axis suppression

Gel, augmented formulation: Apply once or twice daily; rub in gently. **Note:** Do not exceed 2 weeks of treatment or 50 g/week.

Lotion: Apply a few drops twice daily

Augmented formulation: Apply a few drops once or twice daily; rub in gently. **Note:** Do not exceed 2 weeks of treatment or 50 mL/week.

Cream/ointment: Apply one or twice daily.

Augmented formulation: Apply once or twice daily. **Note:** Do not exceed 2 weeks of treatment or 45 g/week.

Adults:

Foam: Apply to the scalp twice daily, once in the morning and once at night

Gel, augmented formulation: Apply once or twice daily; rub in gently. **Note:** Do not exceed 2 weeks of treatment or 50 g/week.

Lotion: Apply a few drops twice daily

Augmented formulation: Apply a few drops once or twice daily; runb in gently. **Note:** Do not exceed 2 weeks of treatment or 50 mL/week.

Cream/ointment: Apply once or twice daily

Augmented formulation: Apply once or twice daily. **Note:** Do not exceed 2 weeks of treatment or 45 g/week.

Dosage Forms

Aerosol, topical [foam]:
Luxiq®: 0.12% (50 g, 100 g, 150 g)
Cream, topical: 0.05% (15 g, 45 g; 50 g [augmented])
Beta-Val®: 0.1% (15 g, 45 g)
Diprolene® AF: 0.05% (15 g, 50 g)
Gel, topical: 0.05% (15 g, 50 g)
Lotion, topical: 0.05% (30 mL, 60 mL); 0.1% (60 mL)
Beta-Val®: 0.1% (60 mL)
Diprolene®: 0.05% (30 mL, 60 mL)
Ointment, topical: 0.05% (15 g, 45 g), 0.1% (15 g, 45 g)
Diprolene®: 0.05% (15 g, 50 g)

betamethasone valerate *see* betamethasone (topical) *on page 138*
Betapace® [US] *see* sotalol *on page 919*
Betapace AF® [US/Can] *see* sotalol *on page 919*
Beta Sal® [US-OTC] *see* salicylic acid *on page 884*
Betasept® [US-OTC] *see* chlorhexidine gluconate *on page 210*
Betaseron® [US/Can] *see* interferon beta-1b *on page 536*
Betatar® Gel [US-OTC] *see* coal tar *on page 250*
Beta-Val® [US] *see* betamethasone (topical) *on page 138*
Betaxin® [Can] *see* thiamine *on page 954*

betaxolol (be TAKS oh lol)

Sound-Alike/Look-Alike Issues
betaxolol may be confused with bethanechol, labetalol
Betoptic® S may be confused with Betagan®, Timoptic®

Synonyms betaxolol hydrochloride

U.S./Canadian Brand Names Betoptic® S [US/Can]; Kerlone® [US]; Sandoz-Betaxolol [Can]

Therapeutic Category Beta-Adrenergic Blocker

Use
Ophthalmic: Treatment of chronic open-angle glaucoma or ocular hypertension
Oral: Management of hypertension

Usual Dosage
Children and Adults: Ophthalmic suspension (Betoptic® S): Instill 1 drop into affected eye(s) twice daily.
Adults:
Ophthalmic solution: Instill 1-2 drops into affected eye(s) twice daily.
Oral: 5-10 mg/day; may increase dose to 20 mg/day after 7-14 days if desired response is not achieved.

Dosage Forms
Solution, ophthalmic: 0.5% (5 mL, 10 mL, 15 mL)
Suspension, ophthalmic:
Betoptic® S: 0.25% (10 mL, 15 mL)
Tablet: 10 mg, 20 mg
Kerlone®: 10 mg, 20 mg

betaxolol hydrochloride *see* betaxolol *on page 139*

bethanechol (be THAN e kole)

Sound-Alike/Look-Alike Issues
bethanechol may be confused with betaxolol

Synonyms bethanechol chloride

U.S./Canadian Brand Names Duvoid® [Can]; PMS-Bethanechol [Can]; Urecholine® [US]

Therapeutic Category Cholinergic Agent

Use Treatment of acute postoperative and postpartum nonobstructive (functional) urinary retention; treatment of neurogenic atony of the urinary bladder with retention

Usual Dosage Oral: Adults: Urinary retention, neurogenic bladder: Initial: 10-50 mg 3-4 times/day (some patients may require dosages of 50-100 mg 4 times/day). To determine effective dose, may initiate at a dose of 5-10 mg, with additional doses of 5-10 mg hourly until an effective cumulative dose is reached. Cholinergic effects at higher oral dosages may be cumulative.

Dosage Forms [CAN] = Canadian brand name
Tablet: 5 mg, 10 mg, 25 mg, 50 mg
Duvoid® [CAN]: 10 mg, 25 mg, 50 mg [not available in U.S.]
Urecholine®: 5 mg, 10 mg, 25 mg, 50 mg

bethanechol chloride *see* bethanechol *on page* *139*
Betimol® [US] *see* timolol *on page* *961*
Betnesol® [Can] *see* betamethasone (topical) *on page* *138*
Betnovate® [Can] *see* betamethasone (topical) *on page* *138*
Betoptic® S [US/Can] *see* betaxolol *on page* *139*

bevacizumab (be vuh SIZ uh mab)

Sound-Alike/Look-Alike Issues
bevacizumab may be confused with cetuximab
Synonyms anti-VEGF monoclonal antibody; anti-VEGF rhuMAb; rhuMAb-VEGF
U.S./Canadian Brand Names Avastin® [US/Can]
Therapeutic Category Antineoplastic Agent, Monoclonal Antibody; Vaccine, Recombinant
Use Treatment of metastatic colorectal cancer; treatment of advanced nonsquamous, nonsmall cell lung cancer; treatment of metastatic HER-2 negative breast cancer (who have not received chemotherapy for metastatic disease); treatment of progressive glioblastoma (not an approved use in Canada); treatment of metastatic renal cell cancer (not an approved use in Canada)
Usual Dosage I.V.: Adults: Details concerning dosing in combination regimens should also be consulted.
Breast cancer: 10 mg/kg every 2 weeks (in combination with paclitaxel)
Colorectal cancer: 5 or 10 mg/kg every 2 weeks (in combination with fluorouracil-based chemotherapy)
Canadian labeling: 5 mg/kg every 2 weeks (in combination with fluorouracil-based chemotherapy)
Lung cancer, nonsquamous cell nonsmall cell: 15 mg/kg every 3 weeks (in combination with carboplatin and paclitaxel)
Dosage Forms
Injection, solution [preservative free]:
Avastin®: 25 mg/mL (4 mL, 16 mL)

bexarotene (beks AIR oh teen)

U.S./Canadian Brand Names Targretin® [US/Can]
Therapeutic Category Retinoic Acid Derivative; Vitamin A Derivative; Vitamin, Fat Soluble
Use
Oral: Treatment of cutaneous manifestations of cutaneous T-cell lymphoma in patients who are refractory to at least one prior systemic therapy
Topical: Treatment of cutaneous lesions in patients with refractory cutaneous T-cell lymphoma (stage 1A and 1B) or who have not tolerated other therapies
Usual Dosage Adults:
Oral: 300-400 mg/m^2/day taken as a single daily dose.
Topical: Apply once every other day for first week, then increase on a weekly basis to once daily, 2 times/day, 3 times/day, and finally 4 times/day, according to tolerance
Dosage Forms
Capsule:
Targretin®: 75 mg
Gel:
Targretin®: 1% (60 g)

Bextra® ***(Discontinued)***
Bexxar® [US] *see* tositumomab and iodine I 131 tositumomab *on page* *971*

bezafibrate *(Canada only)* (be za FYE brate)

U.S./Canadian Brand Names Bezalip® [Can]; PMS-Bezafibrate [Can]
Therapeutic Category Antihyperlipidemic Agent, Miscellaneous
Use Adjunct to diet and other therapeutic measures for treatment of type IIa and IIb mixed hyperlipidemia, to regulate lipid and apoprotein levels (reduce serum TG, LDL-cholesterol, and apolipoprotein B, increase HDL-cholesterol and apolipoprotein A); treatment of adult patients with high to very high triglyceride levels (Fredrickson classification type IV and V hyperlipidemias) who are at high risk of sequelae and complications from their dyslipidemia

Usual Dosage Oral: Adults:

Immediate release: 200 mg 2-3 times/day; may reduce to 200 mg twice daily in patients with good response

Sustained release: 400 mg once daily

Dosage Forms [CAN] = Canadian brand name

Tablet, immediate release: 200 mg [not available in the U.S.]

PMA-Bezafibrate [CAN]: 200 mg [not available in the U.S.]

Tablet, sustained release:

Bezalip® [CAN]: 400 mg [not available in the U.S.]

Bezalip® [Can] *see* bezafibrate *(Canada only) on page 140*

BG 9273 *see* alefacept *on page 44*

Biavax® II *(Discontinued)*

Biaxin® [US/Can] *see* clarithromycin *on page 236*

Biaxin® XL [US/Can] *see* clarithromycin *on page 236*

bicalutamide (bye ka LOO ta mide)

Sound-Alike/Look-Alike Issues

Casodex® may be confused with Kapidex™

Synonyms CDX; ICI-176334

U.S./Canadian Brand Names Casodex® [US/Can]; CO Bicalutamide [Can]; Gen-Bicalutamide [Can]; Novo-Bicalutamide [Can]; PHL-Bicalutamide [Can]; PMS-Bicalutamide [Can]; Pro-Bicalutamide [Can]; ratio-Bicalutamide [Can]; Sandoz-Bicalutamide [Can]

Therapeutic Category Androgen

Use Treatment of metastatic prostate cancer (in combination with an LHRH agonist)

Usual Dosage Oral: Adults: Metastatic prostate cancer: 50 mg once daily (in combination with an LHRH analogue)

Dosage Forms

Tablet: 50 mg

Casodex®: 50 mg

Bicillin® L-A [US/Can] *see* penicillin G benzathine *on page 760*

Bicillin® C-R [US] *see* penicillin G benzathine and penicillin G procaine *on page 761*

Bicillin® C-R 900/300 [US] *see* penicillin G benzathine and penicillin G procaine *on page 761*

BiCNU® [US/Can] *see* carmustine *on page 187*

BiDil® [US] *see* isosorbide dinitrate and hydralazine *on page 550*

BIG-IV *see* botulism immune globulin (intravenous-human) *on page 146*

Biltricide® [US/Can] *see* praziquantel *on page 811*

bimatoprost (bi MAT oh prost)

U.S./Canadian Brand Names Latisse™ [US]; Lumigan® [US/Can]

Therapeutic Category Ophthalmic Agent, Miscellaneous

Use Reduction of intraocular pressure (IOP) in patients with open-angle glaucoma or ocular hypertension; hypotrichosis treatment of the eyelashes

Usual Dosage Adults:

Ophthalmic: Open-angle glaucoma or ocular hypertension: Instill 1 drop into affected eye(s) once daily in the evening; do not exceed once-daily dosing (may decrease IOP-lowering effect). If used with other topical ophthalmic agents, separate administration by at least 5 minutes.

Ophthalmic, topical: Hypotrichosis of the eyelashes: Place one drop on applicator and apply evenly along the skin of the upper eyelid at base of eyelashes once daily at bedtime; repeat procedure for second eye (use a clean applicator)

Dosage Forms

Solution, ophthalmic:

Latisse™: 0.03% (3 mL)

Lumigan®: 0.03% (2.5 mL, 5 mL, 7.5 mL)

Biobase™ [Can] *see* alcohol (ethyl) *on page 42*

Biobase-G™ [Can] *see* alcohol (ethyl) *on page 42*

Bio-Carbamazepine [Can] *see* carbamazepine *on page 180*

Bioclate® *(Discontinued)* *see* antihemophilic factor (recombinant) *on page 82*
Biodine® *(Discontinued)* *see* povidone-iodine *on page 807*
Biolon™ *(Discontinued)* *see* hyaluronate and derivatives *on page 496*
Bionect® [US] *see* hyaluronate and derivatives *on page 496*
Bioniche Promethazine [Can] *see* promethazine *on page 823*
Bion® Tears [US-OTC] *see* artificial tears *on page 100*
Bio-Oxazepam [Can] *see* oxazepam *on page 734*
Biopatch® *(Discontinued)* *see* chlorhexidine gluconate *on page 210*
BioQuin® Durules™ [Can] *see* quinidine *on page 845*
Bio-Statin® [US] *see* nystatin *on page 715*
BioThrax® [US] *see* anthrax vaccine, adsorbed *on page 81*
Biozyme-C® *(Discontinued)* *see* collagenase *on page 255*
biperiden *(Discontinued)*
Biphentin® [Can] *see* methylphenidate *on page 645*
bird flu vaccine *see* influenza virus vaccine (H5N1) *on page 529*
Bisac-Evac™ [US-OTC] *see* bisacodyl *on page 142*

bisacodyl (bis a KOE dil)

Sound-Alike/Look-Alike Issues
Doxidan® may be confused with doxepin

U.S./Canadian Brand Names Alophen® [US-OTC]; Apo-Bisacodyl® [Can]; Bisac-Evac™ [US-OTC]; Biscolax™ [US-OTC]; Carter's Little Pills® [Can]; Correctol® Tablets [US-OTC]; Dacodyl™ [US-OTC]; Doxidan® [US-OTC]; Dulcolax® [US-OTC/Can]; ex-lax® Ultra [US-OTC]; Fematrol [US-OTC]; Femilax™ [US-OTC]; Fleet® Bisacodyl [US-OTC]; Fleet® Stimulant Laxative [US-OTC]; Gentlax® [Can]; Veracolate [US-OTC]

Therapeutic Category Laxative

Use Treatment of constipation; colonic evacuation prior to procedures or examination

Usual Dosage
Children:
Oral: >6 years: 5-10 mg (0.3 mg/kg) at bedtime or before breakfast
Rectal suppository:
<2 years: 5 mg as a single dose
>2 years: 10 mg
Adults:
Oral: 5-15 mg as single dose (up to 30 mg when complete evacuation of bowel is required)
Rectal suppository: 10 mg as single dose

Dosage Forms
Solution, rectal [enema]:
Fleet® Bisacodyl [OTC]: 10 mg/30 mL (37 mL)
Suppository, rectal: 10 mg
Bisac-Evac™ [OTC], Biscolax™ [OTC], Dulcolax® [OTC]: 10 mg
Tablet [enteric coated]: 5 mg
Alophen® [OTC], Bisac-Evac™ [OTC], Correctol® [OTC], Dacodyl™ [OTC], Dulcolax® [OTC], ex-lax® Ultra [OTC], Fematrol [OTC], Femilax™ [OTC], Veracolate [OTC]: 5 mg
Tablet, delayed release: 5 mg
Doxidan® [OTC], Fleet® Stimulant Laxative [OTC]: 5 mg

Bisacodyl Uniserts® *(Discontinued)* *see* bisacodyl *on page 142*
bis-chloronitrosourea *see* carmustine *on page 187*
Biscolax™ [US-OTC] *see* bisacodyl *on page 142*
Bismatrol [US-OTC] *see* bismuth *on page 142*
Bismatrol Maximum Strength [US-OTC] *see* bismuth *on page 142*

bismuth (BIZ muth)

Sound-Alike/Look-Alike Issues
Kaopectate® may be confused with Kayexalate®

Synonyms bismuth subsalicylate; pink bismuth

U.S./Canadian Brand Names Bismatrol Maximum Strength [US-OTC]; Bismatrol [US-OTC]; Diotame® [US-OTC]; Kao-Tin [US-OTC]; Kaopectate® Extra Strength [US-OTC]; Kaopectate® [US-OTC]; Maalox® Total Stomach Relief® [US-OTC]; Peptic Relief [US-OTC]; Pepto Relief [US-OTC]; Pepto-Bismol® Maximum Strength [US-OTC]; Pepto-Bismol® [US-OTC]

Therapeutic Category Antidiarrheal

Use Subsalicylate formulation: Symptomatic treatment of mild, nonspecific diarrhea; control of traveler's diarrhea (enterotoxigenic *Escherichia coli*); as part of a multidrug regimen for *H. pylori* eradication to reduce the risk of duodenal ulcer recurrence

Usual Dosage Oral:

Treatment of nonspecific diarrhea, control/relieve traveler's diarrhea: Subsalicylate (doses based on 262 mg/15 mL liquid or 262 mg tablets):

Children: Up to 8 doses/24 hours:

3-6 years: 1/3 tablet or 5 mL every 30 minutes to 1 hour as needed

6-9 years: 2/3 tablet or 10 mL every 30 minutes to 1 hour as needed

9-12 years: 1 tablet or 15 mL every 30 minutes to 1 hour as needed

Children >12 years and Adults: 2 tablets or 30 mL every 30 minutes to 1 hour as needed up to 8 doses/ 24 hours

Helicobacter pylori eradication: Subsalicylate: Adults: 524 mg 4 times/day with meals and at bedtime; requires combination therapy

Dosage Forms

Caplet:

Kaopectate® [OTC]: 262 mg

Pepto-Bismol® [OTC]: 262 mg

Liquid: 262 mg/15 mL

Bismatrol [OTC], Diotame® [OTC], Kaopectate® [OTC], Kao-Tin [OTC], Peptic Relief [OTC], Pepto-Bismol® [OTC]: 262 mg/15 mL

Bismatrol Maximum Strength [OTC], Kaopectate® Extra Strength [OTC], Maalox® Total Stomach Relief® [OTC], Pepto-Bismol® Maximum Strength [OTC]: 525 mg/15 mL

Suspension: 262 mg/15 mL

Tablet, chewable: 262 mg

Bismatrol [OTC], Diotame® [OTC], Peptic Relief [OTC], Pepto Relief [OTC], Pepto-Bismol® [OTC]: 262 mg

bismuth, metronidazole, and tetracycline

(BIZ muth, me troe NI da zole, & tet ra SYE kleen)

Synonyms bismuth subcitrate potassium, tetracycline, and metronidazole; bismuth subsalicylate, tetracycline, and metronidazole; metronidazole, bismuth subcitrate potassium, and tetracycline; metronidazole, bismuth subsalicylate, and tetracycline; tetracycline, metronidazole, and bismuth subcitrate potassium; tetracycline, metronidazole, and bismuth subsalicylate

U.S./Canadian Brand Names Helidac® [US]; Pylera™ [US]

Therapeutic Category Antidiarrheal

Use As part of a multidrug regimen for *H. pylori* eradication to reduce the risk of duodenal ulcer recurrence in combination with an H_2 agonist (Helidac®) or omeprazole (Pylera™)

Usual Dosage Oral: Adults:

Helidac®: Two bismuth subsalicylate 262.4 mg tablets, 1 metronidazole 250 mg tablet, and 1 tetracycline 500 mg capsule 4 times/day at meals and bedtime, plus an H_2 antagonist (at the appropriate dose) for 14 days; follow with 8 oz of water; the H_2 antagonist should be continued for a total of 28 days

Pylera™: Three capsules 4 times/day after meals and at bedtime, plus omeprazole 20 mg twice daily for 10 days; follow each dose with 8 oz of water (each capsule contains bismuth subcitrate potassium 140 mg, metronidazole 125 mg, and tetracycline 125 mg)

Dosage Forms

Capsule:

Pylera™: Bismuth subcitrate potassium 140 mg, metronidazole 125 mg, and tetracycline hydrochloride 125 mg

Combination package:

Helidac® [each package contains 14 blister cards (2-week supply); each card contains the following]:

Capsule: Tetracycline: 500 mg (4)

Tablet, chewable: Bismuth subsalicylate]: 262.4 mg (8)

Tablet: Metronidazole: 250 mg (4)

bismuth subcitrate potassium, tetracycline, and metronidazole *see* bismuth, metronidazole, and tetracycline *on page 143*

bismuth subsalicylate *see* bismuth *on page 142*

bismuth subsalicylate, tetracycline, and metronidazole *see* bismuth, metronidazole, and tetracycline *on page 143*

bisoprolol (bis OH proe lol)

Sound-Alike/Look-Alike Issues
Zebeta® may be confused with DiaBeta®, Zetia®

Synonyms bisoprolol fumarate

U.S./Canadian Brand Names Apo-Bisoprolol® [Can]; Monocor® [Can]; Novo-Bisoprolol [Can]; PMS-Bisoprolol [Can]; PRO-Bisoprolol [Can]; Sandoz-Bisoprolol [Can]; Zebeta® [US/Can]; ZYM-Bisoprolol [Can]

Therapeutic Category Beta-Adrenergic Blocker

Use Treatment of hypertension, alone or in combination with other agents

Usual Dosage Oral: Adults: 2.5-5 mg once daily, may be increased to 10 mg, and then up to 20 mg once daily, if necessary
Hypertension (JNC 7): 2.5-10 mg once daily

Dosage Forms
Tablet: 5 mg, 10 mg
Zebeta®: 5 mg, 10 mg

bisoprolol and hydrochlorothiazide (bis OH proe lol & hye droe klor oh THYE a zide)

Sound-Alike/Look-Alike Issues
Ziac® may be confused with Tiazac®, Zerit®

Synonyms hydrochlorothiazide and bisoprolol

U.S./Canadian Brand Names Ziac® [US/Can]

Therapeutic Category Antihypertensive Agent, Combination

Use Treatment of hypertension

Usual Dosage Oral: Adults: Hypertension: Dose is individualized, given once daily

Dosage Forms
Tablet, oral: 2.5/6.25: Bisoprolol 2.5 mg and hydrochlorothiazide 6.25 mg; 5/6.25: Bisoprolol 5 mg and hydrochlorothiazide 6.25 mg; 10/6.25: Bisoprolol 10 mg and hydrochlorothiazide 6.25 mg
Ziac®: 2.5/6.25: Bisoprolol 2.5 mg and hydrochlorothiazide 6.25 mg; 5/6.25: Bisoprolol 5 mg and hydrochlorothiazide 6.25 mg; 10/6.25: Bisoprolol 10 mg and hydrochlorothiazide 6.25 mg

bisoprolol fumarate *see* bisoprolol *on page 144*

bis-POM PMEA *see* adefovir *on page 36*

bistropamide *see* tropicamide *on page 992*

bivalirudin (bye VAL i roo din)

Synonyms hirulog

U.S./Canadian Brand Names Angiomax® [US/Can]

Therapeutic Category Anticoagulant (Other)

Use Anticoagulant used in conjunction with aspirin for patients with unstable angina undergoing percutaneous transluminal coronary angioplasty (PTCA) or percutaneous coronary intervention (PCI) with provisional glycoprotein IIb/IIIa inhibitor; anticoagulant used in patients undergoing PCI with (or at risk of) heparin-induced thrombocytopenia (HIT) / thrombosis syndrome (HITTS)

Usual Dosage I.V.: Adults: Anticoagulant in patients undergoing PTCA/PCI or PCI with HITS/HITTS (treatment should be started just prior to procedure): Initial: Bolus: 0.75 mg/kg, followed by continuous infusion: 1.75 mg/kg/hour for the duration of procedure and up to 4 hours post-procedure if needed; determine ACT 5 minutes after bolus dose; may administer additional bolus of 0.3 mg/kg if necessary.
A glycoprotein IIb/IIIa inhibitor may be administered concomitantly during the procedure.
If needed, infusion may be continued beyond initial 4 hours at 0.2 mg/kg/hour for up to 20 hours.

Dosage Forms
Injection, powder for reconstitution:
Angiomax®: 250 mg

Bi-Zets [US] *see* benzocaine *on page 129*

BL4162A *see* anagrelide *on page 78*
Black-Draught™ Tablets [US-OTC] *see* senna *on page 896*
black widow spider species antivenin *see* antivenin *(Latrodectus mactans) on page 87*
BlemErase® Lotion *(Discontinued)* *see* benzoyl peroxide *on page 132*
Blenoxane® [Can] *see* bleomycin *on page 145*
Blenoxane® *(Discontinued)* *see* bleomycin *on page 145*
bleo *see* bleomycin *on page 145*

bleomycin (blee oh MYE sin)

Sound-Alike/Look-Alike Issues
bleomycin may be confused with Cleocin®

Synonyms bleo; bleomycin sulfate; BLM; NSC-125066

U.S./Canadian Brand Names Blenoxane® [Can]; Bleomycin Injection, USP [Can]

Therapeutic Category Antineoplastic Agent

Use Treatment of squamous cell carcinomas, melanomas, sarcomas, testicular carcinoma, Hodgkin lymphoma, and non-Hodgkin lymphoma; sclerosing agent for malignant pleural effusion

Usual Dosage Maximum cumulative lifetime dose: 400 units; refer to individual protocols; 1 unit = 1 mg
May be administered I.M., I.V., SubQ, or intracavitary
Children and Adults:
Test dose for lymphoma patients: I.M., I.V., SubQ: Because of the possibility of an anaphylactoid reaction, administer 1-2 units of bleomycin before the first 1-2 doses; monitor vital signs every 15 minutes; wait a minimum of 1 hour before administering remainder of dose; if no acute reaction occurs, then the regular dosage schedule may be followed. **Note:** Test doses may produce false-negative results.
Single-agent therapy:
I.M./I.V./SubQ: Squamous cell carcinoma, lymphoma, testicular carcinoma: 0.25-0.5 units/kg (10-20 units/m^2) 1-2 times/week
CIV: 15 units/m^2 over 24 hours daily for 4 days
Pleural sclerosing: Intrapleural: 60 units as a single instillation (some recommend limiting the dose in the elderly to 40 units/m^2; usual maximum: 60 units). Dose may be repeated at intervals of several days if fluid continues to accumulate (mix in 50-100 mL of NS); may add lidocaine 100-200 mg to reduce local discomfort.

Dosage Forms
Injection, powder for reconstitution: 15 units, 30 units

Bleomycin Injection, USP [Can] *see* bleomycin *on page 145*
bleomycin sulfate *see* bleomycin *on page 145*
Bleph®-10 [US] *see* sulfacetamide *on page 927*
Blephamide® [US/Can] *see* sulfacetamide and prednisolone *on page 927*
Blis-To-Sol® [US-OTC] *see* tolnaftate *on page 968*
BLM *see* bleomycin *on page 145*
BMS-232632 *see* atazanavir *on page 106*
BMS-247550 *see* ixabepilone *on page 554*
BMS-337039 *see* aripiprazole *on page 97*
BMS-354825 *see* dasatinib *on page 278*
BMS-477118 *see* saxagliptin *on page 892*
Boil-Ease® Pain Relieving [US] *see* benzocaine *on page 129*
BOL-303224-A *see* besifloxacin *on page 136*
Bonamine™ [Can] *see* meclizine *on page 619*
Bondronat® [Can] *see* ibandronate *on page 514*
Bonefos® [Can] *see* clodronate *(Canada only) on page 243*
Bonine® [US-OTC/Can] *see* meclizine *on page 619*
Boniva® [US] *see* ibandronate *on page 514*
Bontril® [Can] *see* phendimetrazine *on page 770*
Bontril® PDM [US] *see* phendimetrazine *on page 770*
Bontril® Slow Release [US] *see* phendimetrazine *on page 770*
Boostrix® [US] *see* diphtheria, tetanus toxoids, and acellular pertussis vaccine *on page 321*

bortezomib (bore TEZ oh mib)

Synonyms LDP-341; MLN341; NSC-681239; PS-341

U.S./Canadian Brand Names Velcade® [US/Can]

Therapeutic Category Proteasome Inhibitor

Use Treatment of multiple myeloma; treatment of relapsed or refractory mantle cell lymphoma

Usual Dosage Details concerning dosing in combination regimens should also be consulted. I.V.: Adults:

Multiple myeloma (first-line therapy; in combination with melphalan and prednisone): 1.3 mg/m^2 days 1, 4, 8, 11, 22, 25, 29, and 32 of a 42-day treatment cycle for 4 cycles, followed by 1.3 mg/m^2 days 1, 8, 22, and 29 of a 42-day treatment cycle for 5 cycles.

Relapsed multiple myeloma and mantle cell lymphoma: 1.3 mg/m^2 twice weekly for 2 weeks on days 1, 4, 8, and 11 of a 21-day treatment cycle. Consecutive doses should be separated by at least 72 hours. Therapy extending beyond 8 cycles may be given once weekly for 4 weeks (days 1, 8, 15, and 22), followed by a 13-day rest (days 23 through 35).

Dosage Forms

Injection, powder for reconstitution [preservative free]:

Velcade®: 3.5 mg

bosentan (boe SEN tan)

Sound-Alike/Look-Alike Issues

Tracleer® may be confused with TriCor©

U.S./Canadian Brand Names Tracleer® [US/Can]

Therapeutic Category Endothelin Antagonist

Use Treatment of pulmonary artery hypertension (PAH) (WHO Group I) in patients with World Health Organization (WHO) Class II, III, or IV symptoms to improve exercise capacity and decrease the rate of clinical deterioration

Usual Dosage Oral: Adolescents >12 years and ≥40 kg and Adults: Initial: 62.5 mg twice daily for 4 weeks; increase to maintenance dose of 125 mg twice daily; patients <40 kg should be maintained at 62.5 mg twice daily. Doses >125 mg twice daily do not appear to confer additional clinical benefit but may increase risk of liver toxicity.

Note: When discontinuing treatment, consider a reduction in dosage to 62.5 mg twice daily for 3-7 days (to avoid clinical deterioration).

Dosage Forms

Tablet:

Tracleer®: 62.5 mg, 125 mg

B&O Supprettes® ***(Discontinued)*** *see* belladonna and opium *on page* 126
Botox® [US/Can] *see* onabotulinumtoxinA *on page* 725
Botox® Cosmetic [US/Can] *see* onabotulinumtoxinA *on page* 725
botulinum toxin type A *see* abobotulinumtoxinA *on page* 17
botulinum toxin type A *see* onabotulinumtoxinA *on page* 725
botulinum toxin type B *see* rimabotulinumtoxinB *on page* 868

botulism immune globulin (intravenous-human)

(BOT yoo lism i MYUN GLOB you lin, in tra VEE nus, YU man)

Sound-Alike/Look-Alike Issues

BabyBIG® may be confused with HBIG

Synonyms BIG-IV

U.S./Canadian Brand Names BabyBIG® [US]

Therapeutic Category Immune Globulin

Use Treatment of infant botulism caused by toxin type A or B

Usual Dosage I.V.: Children <1 year: Infant botulism: 1 mL/kg (50 mg/kg) as a single dose; infuse at 0.5 mL/kg/hour (25 mg/kg/hour) for the first 15 minutes; if well tolerated, may increase to 1 mL/kg/hour (50 mg/kg/hour)

Dosage Forms

Injection, powder for reconstitution [preservative free]:

BabyBIG® [OTC]: ~100 mg

Boudreaux's® Butt Paste [US-OTC] *see* zinc oxide *on page* 1030
bovine lung surfactant *see* beractant *on page* 135

BPM PE [US] *see* brompheniramine and phenylephrine *on page 150*
BranchAmin® [US] *see* amino acid injection *on page 62*
Bravelle® [US/Can] *see* urofollitropin *on page 999*
Breathe Free® [US-OTC] *see* sodium chloride *on page 908*
Breezee® Mist Antifungal *(Discontinued)* *see* miconazole *on page 654*
Breonesin® *(Discontinued)* *see* guaifenesin *on page 473*
Brethaire® *(Discontinued)* *see* terbutaline *on page 945*
brethine *see* terbutaline *on page 945*
Brevibloc® [US/Can] *see* esmolol *on page 371*
Brevicon® [US] *see* ethinyl estradiol and norethindrone *on page 390*
Brevicon® 0.5/35 [Can] *see* ethinyl estradiol and norethindrone *on page 390*
Brevicon® 1/35 [Can] *see* ethinyl estradiol and norethindrone *on page 390*
Brevital® [Can] *see* methohexital *on page 638*
Brevital® Sodium [US] *see* methohexital *on page 638*
Brevoxyl® [US] *see* benzoyl peroxide *on page 132*
Brevoxyl®-4 [US] *see* benzoyl peroxide *on page 132*
Brevoxyl®-8 [US] *see* benzoyl peroxide *on page 132*
Brevoxyl® Acne Wash Kit *(Discontinued)* *see* benzoyl peroxide *on page 132*
breze™ *(Discontinued)* *see* benzoyl peroxide *on page 132*
Bricanyl® [Can] *see* terbutaline *on page 945*
Bricanyl® *(Discontinued)* *see* terbutaline *on page 945*

brimonidine (bri MOE ni deen)

Sound-Alike/Look-Alike Issues
brimonidine may be confused with bromocriptine

Synonyms brimonidine tartrate

U.S./Canadian Brand Names Alphagan® P [US]; Alphagan® [Can]; Apo-Brimonidine P [Can]; Apo-Brimonidine® [Can]; PMS-Brimonidine Tartrate [Can]; ratio-Brimonidine [Can]; Sandoz-Brimonidine [Can]

Therapeutic Category $Alpha_2$ Agonist, Ophthalmic

Use Lowering of intraocular pressure (IOP) in patients with open-angle glaucoma or ocular hypertension

Usual Dosage Ophthalmic: Children ≥2 years of age and Adults: Glaucoma: Instill 1 drop in affected eye(s) 3 times/day (approximately every 8 hours)

Dosage Forms
Solution, ophthalmic: 0.2% (5 mL, 10 mL, 15 mL)
Alphagan® P: 0.1% (5 mL, 10 mL, 15 mL); 0.15% (5 mL, 10 mL, 15 mL)

brimonidine and timolol (bri MOE ni deen & TIM oh lol)

Synonyms brimonidine tartrate and timolol maleate; timolol and brimonidine

U.S./Canadian Brand Names Combigan™ [US/Can]

Therapeutic Category $Alpha_2$ Agonist, Ophthalmic; Beta Blocker, Nonselective; Ophthalmic Agent, Antiglaucoma

Use Reduction of intraocular pressure (IOP) in patients with glaucoma or ocular hypertension

Usual Dosage Ophthalmic: Children ≥2 years and Adults: Instill 1 drop into affected eye(s) twice daily
Note: In the Canadian labeling, use in children (at any age) is not recommended

Dosage Forms [CAN] = Canadian availability
Solution, ophthalmic [drops]:
Combigan™: Brimonidine 0.2% and timolol 0.5% (5 mL,10 mL)
Combigan® [CAN]: Brimonidine 0.2% and timolol 0.5% (2.5 mL, 5 mL,10 mL)

brimonidine tartrate *see* brimonidine *on page 147*
brimonidine tartrate and timolol maleate *see* brimonidine and timolol *on page 147*

brinzolamide (brin ZOH la mide)

U.S./Canadian Brand Names Azopt® [US/Can]

Therapeutic Category Carbonic Anhydrase Inhibitor

Use Lowers intraocular pressure in patients with ocular hypertension or open-angle glaucoma

Usual Dosage Ophthalmic: Adults: Instill 1 drop in affected eye(s) 3 times/day

Dosage Forms

Suspension, ophthalmic:

Azopt®: 1% (10 mL, 15 mL)

Brioschi® [US-OTC] *see* sodium bicarbonate *on page* 907

British anti-lewisite *see* dimercaprol *on page* 313

BRL 43694 *see* granisetron *on page* 471

Bromaline® [US-OTC] *see* brompheniramine and pseudoephedrine *on page* 150

Bromaline® DM [US-OTC] *see* brompheniramine, pseudoephedrine, and dextromethorphan *on page* 152

Bromarest® *(Discontinued)* *see* brompheniramine *on page* 149

Bromatane DX [US] *see* brompheniramine, pseudoephedrine, and dextromethorphan *on page* 152

Bromaxefed RF *(Discontinued)* *see* brompheniramine and pseudoephedrine *on page* 150

bromazepam *(Canada only)* (broe MA ze pam)

U.S./Canadian Brand Names Apo-Bromazepam® [Can]; Gen-Bromazepam [Can]; Lectopam® [Can]; Novo-Bromazepam [Can]; Nu-Bromazepam [Can]; Pro Doc Limitee Bromazepam [Can]

Therapeutic Category Benzodiazepine; Sedative

Use Short-term, symptomatic treatment of anxiety

Usual Dosage Oral: Adults: Initial: 6-18 mg/day in equally divided doses; initial course of treatment should not last longer than 1 week; optimal dosage range: 6-30 mg/day

Dosage Forms [CAN] = Canadian brand name

Tablet: 1.5 mg, 3 mg, 6 mg [not available in the U.S.]

Apo-Bromazepam® [CAN], Gen-Bromazepam [CAN], Lectopam® [CAN], Novo-Bromazepam [CAN], Nu-Bromazepam [CAN]: 1.5 mg, 3 mg, 6 mg [not available in the U.S.]

Brombay® *(Discontinued)* *see* brompheniramine *on page* 149

Brometane DX *(Discontinued)* *see* brompheniramine, pseudoephedrine, and dextromethorphan *on page* 152

Bromfed® [US] *see* brompheniramine and phenylephrine *on page* 150

Bromfed® DM [US] *see* brompheniramine, pseudoephedrine, and dextromethorphan *on page* 152

Bromfed®-PD [US] *see* brompheniramine and phenylephrine *on page* 150

bromfenac (BROME fen ak)

Synonyms bromfenac sodium

U.S./Canadian Brand Names Xibrom™ [US]

Therapeutic Category Analgesic, Nonnarcotic; Nonsteroidal Antiinflammatory Drug (NSAID), Ophthalmic

Use Treatment of postoperative inflammation and reduction in ocular pain following cataract removal

Usual Dosage Ophthalmic: Adults: Instill 1 drop into affected eye(s) twice daily beginning 24 hours after surgery and continuing for 2 weeks postoperatively

Dosage Forms

Solution, ophthalmic:

Xibrom™: 0.09% (2.5 mL, 5 mL)

bromfenac sodium *see* bromfenac *on page* 148

Bromfenex® *(Discontinued)* *see* brompheniramine and pseudoephedrine *on page* 150

Bromfenex® PD *(Discontinued)* *see* brompheniramine and pseudoephedrine *on page* 150

Bromhist DM [US] *see* brompheniramine, pseudoephedrine, and dextromethorphan *on page* 152

Bromhist-NR [US] *see* brompheniramine and pseudoephedrine *on page* 150

Bromhist PDX *(Discontinued)* *see* brompheniramine, pseudoephedrine, and dextromethorphan *on page* 152

Bromhist Pediatric [US] *see* brompheniramine and pseudoephedrine *on page* 150

bromocriptine (broe moe KRIP teen)

Sound-Alike/Look-Alike Issues

bromocriptine may be confused with benztropine, brimonidine

Parlodel® may be confused with pindolol, Provera®

Synonyms bromocriptine mesylate

U.S./Canadian Brand Names Apo-Bromocriptine® [Can]; Cycloset® [US]; Parlodel® SnapTabs® [US]; Parlodel® [US/Can]; PMS-Bromocriptine [Can]

Therapeutic Category Anti-Parkinson Agent (Dopamine Agonist); Ergot Alkaloid and Derivative

Use Treatment of hyperprolactinemia associated with amenorrhea with or without galactorrhea, infertility, or hypogonadism; treatment of prolactin-secreting adenomas; treatment of acromegaly; treatment of Parkinson disease

Usual Dosage Oral:

Children: Hyperprolactinemia:

- 11-15 years (based on limited information): Initial: 1.25-2.5 mg daily; dosage may be increased as tolerated to achieve a therapeutic response (range: 2.5-10 mg daily).
- ≥16 years: Refer to adult dosing

Adults:

- Parkinsonism: 1.25 mg twice daily, increased by 2.5 mg/day in 2- to 4-week intervals (usual dose range is 30-90 mg/day in 3 divided doses; maximum: 100 mg/day), though elderly patients can usually be managed on lower doses
- Acromegaly: Initial: 1.25-2.5 mg daily increasing by 1.25-2.5 mg daily as necessary every 3-7 days; usual dose: 20-30 mg/day (maximum: 100 mg/day)
- Hyperprolactinemia: Initial: 1.25-2.5 mg/day; may be increased by 2.5 mg/day as tolerated every 2-7 days until optimal response (range: 2.5-15 mg/day)

Product Availability

Cycloset®: FDA approved May 2009; availability anticipated in the third quarter of 2009

Cycloset® has been approved for the treatment of type 2 diabetes.

Dosage Forms

Capsule: 5 mg

Parlodel®: 5 mg

Tablet: 2.5 mg

Parlodel® SnapTabs®: 2.5 mg

bromocriptine mesylate *see* bromocriptine *on page 148*

Bromphen® *(Discontinued)* *see* brompheniramine *on page 149*

Bromphenex™ DM [US] *see* brompheniramine, pseudoephedrine, and dextromethorphan *on page 152*

brompheniramine (brome fen IR a meen)

Synonyms brompheniramine maleate; brompheniramine tannate

U.S./Canadian Brand Names Lodrane® 24 [US]; LoHist-12 [US]; TanaCof-XR [US]; VaZol™ [US]

Therapeutic Category Antihistamine

Use Symptomatic relief of perennial and seasonal allergic rhinitis, vasomotor rhinitis, and other respiratory allergies

Usual Dosage Oral: Allergic rhinitis, allergic symptoms, vasomotor rhinitis:

Children:

- <2 years (VaZol™): 0.5 mg/kg/day in divided doses 4 times/day
- 2-6 years:
  - TanaCof-XR: 1.25 mL every 12 hours (maximum: 2.5 mL/day)
  - VaZol™: 2.5 mL 4 times/day
- 6-12 years:
  - Lodrane® 24: One capsule once daily
  - LoHist-12: One tablet every 12 hours (maximum: 2 tablets/day)
  - TanaCof-XR: 2.5 mL every 12 hours (maximum: 5 mL/day)
  - VaZol™: 5 mL 4 times/day
- >12 years (Lodrane® 24, LoHist-12, TanaCof-XR, VaZol™): Refer to adult dosing

Adults:

- Lodrane® 24: 1-2 capsules once daily
- LoHist-12: 1-2 tablets every 12 hours (maximum: 4 tablets/day)
- TanaCof-XR: 5 mL every 12 hours (maximum: 10 mL/day)
- VaZol™: 10 mL 4 times/day

Dosage Forms

Capsule, extended release:

Lodrane® 24: 12 mg

Liquid, as maleate:
VaZol™: 2 mg/5 mL
Suspension, as tannate: 12 mg/5 mL
TanaCof-XR: 8 mg/5 mL
Tablet, chewable: 12 mg
Tablet, extended release [scored]:
LoHist-12: 6 mg
Tablet, timed release: 6 mg

brompheniramine and phenylephrine (brome fen IR a meen & fen il EF rin)

Sound-Alike/Look-Alike Issues
Bromfed® may be confused with Bromphen®

Synonyms brompheniramine maleate and phenylephrine hydrochloride; brompheniramine tannate and phenylephrine tannate; phenylephrine and brompheniramine

U.S./Canadian Brand Names BPM PE [US]; Bromfed® [US]; Bromfed®-PD [US]; Brotapp PE [US-OTC]; C-Tan D Plus [US]; C-Tan D [US]; Dimaphen Cold & Allergy [US-OTC]; Dimetapp® Children's Cold & Allergy [US-OTC]

Therapeutic Category Alpha/Beta Agonist; Histamine H_1 Antagonist; Histamine H_1 Antagonist, First Generation

Use Temporary relief of upper respiratory conditions such as nasal congestion, runny nose, itchy/watery eyes, and sneezing due to the common cold, hay fever, or upper respiratory allergies

Usual Dosage Antihistamine/decongestant: Oral:
Children:
2-6 years: B-Vex D: 2.5 mL every 12 hours (maximum: 5 mL/24 hours)
6-11 years:
B-Vex D, C-Tann D, C-Tann D Plus: 5 mL every 12 hours (maximum: 10 mL/24 hours)
BPM PE: 2.5 mL every 6 hours as needed (maximum: 15 mL/24 hours)
Bromfed®-PD: One capsule every 12 hours
Dimaphen Cold & Allergy: 10 mL every 4-6 hours as needed (maximum: 60 mL/24 hours)
Dimetapp® chewable tablet: Two tablets every 4 hours as needed (maximum: 12 tablets/24 hours)
Dimetapp® syrup: 10 mL every 4 hours as needed (maximum: 60 mL/24 hours)
Children ≥12 years and Adults:
B-Vex, C-Tann D, C-Tann D Plus: 5-10 mL every 12 hours (maximum: 20 mL/24 hours)
BPM PE: 5 mL every 6 hours as needed (maximum: 30 mL/24 hours)
Bromfed®: One capsule every 12 hours
Bromfed®-PD: 1-2 capsules every 12 hours
Dimaphen Cold & Allergy: 20 mL every 4-6 hours as needed (maximum: 120 mL/24 hours)
Dimetapp® syrup: 20 mL every 4 hours as needed (maximum: 120 mL/24 hours)

Dosage Forms
Capsule, extended release: Brompheniramine 6 mg and phenylephrine 7.5 mg; Brompheniramine 12 mg and phenylephrine 15 mg
Bromfed®: Brompheniramine 12 mg and phenylephrine 15 mg
Bromfed®-PD: Brompheniramine 6 mg and phenylephrine 7.5 mg
Elixir, oral:
Dimaphen Cold & Allergy [OTC]: Brompheniramine 1 mg and phenylephrine 2. 5 mg per 5 mL
Liquid, oral:
BPM PE: Brompheniramine 4 mg and phenylephrine 7.5 mg per 5 mL
Brotapp PE [OTC]: Brompheniramine 1 mg and phenylephrine 2. 5 mg per 5 mL
Suspension, oral: Brompheniramine 12 mg and phenylephrine 20 mg per 5 mL
C-Tan D: Brompheniramine 4 mg and phenylephrine 5 mg per 5 mL
C-Tan D Plus: Brompheniramine 5 mg and phenylephrine 5 mg per 5 mL
Syrup:
Dimetapp® Children's Cold & Allergy [OTC]: Brompheniramine 1 mg and phenylephrine 2.5 mg per 5 mL
Tablet, chewable:
Dimetapp® Children's Cold & Allergy [OTC]: Brompheniramine 1 mg and phenylephrine 2.5 mg

brompheniramine and pseudoephedrine (brome fen IR a meen & soo doe e FED rin)

Synonyms brompheniramine maleate and pseudoephedrine hydrochloride; brompheniramine maleate and pseudoephedrine sulfate; pseudoephedrine and brompheniramine

U.S./Canadian Brand Names Bromaline® [US-OTC]; Bromhist Pediatric [US]; Bromhist-NR [US]; Brotapp [US]; Dimaphen [US-OTC]; Histex® SR [US]; Lodrane® 12D [US]; Lodrane® 24D [US]; Lodrane® D [US]; LoHist 12D [US]; LoHist LQ [US]; LoHist PD [US]; Respahist® [US]; Sildec Syrup [US]; Touro® Allergy [US]

Therapeutic Category Antihistamine/Decongestant Combination

Use Temporary relief of symptoms of seasonal and perennial allergic rhinitis, and vasomotor rhinitis, including nasal obstruction

Usual Dosage Oral:

Capsule, long acting:
- Based on 60 mg pseudoephedrine:
  - Children 6-12 years: 1 capsule every 12 hours
  - Children ≥12 years and Adults: 1-2 capsules every 12 hours
- Based on 120 mg pseudoephedrine: Children ≥12 years and Adults: 1 capsule every 12 hours

Liquid:
- Based on brompheniramine 1 mg/pseudoephedrine 15 mg per 1 mL: Children:
  - 1-3 months: 0.25 mL 4 times/day
  - 3-6 months: 0.5 mL 4 times/day
  - 6-12 months: 0.75 mL 4 times/day
  - 12-24 months: 1 mL 4 times/day
- Based on brompheniramine 1 mg/pseudoephedrine 15 mg per 5 mL: Children:
  - 6-11 months (6-8 kg): 2.5 mL every 6-8 hours (maximum: 4 doses/24 hours)
  - 12-23 months (8-10 kg): 3.75 mL every 6-8 hours (maximum: 4 doses/24 hours)
  - 2-6 years: 5 mL every 6-8 hours (maximum: 4 doses/24 hours)
  - 6-12 years: 10 mL every 6-8 hours (maximum: 4 doses/24 hours)
  - >12 years and Adults: 20 mL every 4 hours (maximum: 4 doses/24 hours)
- Based on brompheniramine 4 mg/pseudoephedrine 30 mg:
  - Children 2-6 years: 2.5 mL 3 times/day
  - Children >6 years and Adults: 5 mL 3 times/day
- Brompheniramine 4 mg/pseudoephedrine 45 mg per 5 mL:
  - Children 2-6 years: 2.5 mL 4 times/day
  - Children >6 years and Adults: 5 mL 4 times/day

Tablet, extended release: Based on pseudoephedrine 45 mg:
- Children 6-12 years: 1 tablet every 12 hours
- Children ≥12 years and Adults: 1-2 tablets every 12 hours

Dosage Forms

Caplet, extended release:
Histex® SR: Brompheniramine 10 mg and pseudoephedrine 120 mg

Capsule, extended release:
Lodrane® 24D: Brompheniramine 12 mg and pseudoephedrine 90 mg

Capsule, sustained release:
Respahist®: Brompheniramine 6 mg and pseudoephedrine 60 mg

Elixir:
Dimaphen [OTC]: Brompheniramine 1 mg and pseudoephedrine 15 mg per 5 mL

Liquid: Brompheniramine 4 mg and pseudoephedrine 60 mg per 5 mL (480 mL)
Brotapp: Brompheniramine 1 mg and pseudoephedrine 15 mg per 5 mL
LoHist LQ: Brompheniramine 4 mg and pseudoephedrine 60 mg per 5 mL

Liquid, oral [drops]:
Bromhist NR, LoHist LQ: Brompheniramine 1 mg and pseudoephedrine 12.5 mg per 1 mL
Bromhist Pediatric: Brompheniramine 1 mg and pseudoephedrine 15 mg per 1 mL

Solution:
Bromaline® [OTC]: Brompheniramine 1 mg and pseudoephedrine 15 mg per 5 mL

Suspension:
Lodrane® D: Brompheniramine 8 mg and pseudoephedrine 90 mg per 5 mL

Syrup:
Sildec: Brompheniramine 4 mg and pseudoephedrine 45 mg per 5 mL

Tablet, extended release:
Lodrane® 12D, LoHist 12D: Brompheniramine 6 mg and pseudoephedrine 45 mg

Tablet, prolonged release:
Touro® Allergy: Brompheniramine 6 mg and pseudoephedrine 45 mg

Tablet, sustained release: Brompheniramine 6 mg and pseudoephedrine 45 mg

brompheniramine maleate *see* brompheniramine *on page 149*

brompheniramine maleate and phenylephrine hydrochloride *see* brompheniramine and phenylephrine *on page 150*

brompheniramine maleate and pseudoephedrine hydrochloride *see* brompheniramine and pseudoephedrine *on page 150*

brompheniramine maleate and pseudoephedrine sulfate *see* brompheniramine and pseudoephedrine *on page 150*

brompheniramine, pseudoephedrine, and dextromethorphan

(brome fen IR a meen, soo doe e FED rin, & deks troe meth OR fan)

Synonyms dextromethorphan hydrobromide, brompheniramine maleate, and pseudoephedrine hydrochloride; pseudoephedrine tannate, dextromethorphan tannate, and brompheniramine tannate

U.S./Canadian Brand Names AllanHist PDX [US]; Anaplex® DM [US]; Andehist DM NR [US]; Bromaline® DM [US-OTC]; Bromatane DX [US]; Bromfed® DM [US]; Bromhist DM [US]; Bromphenex™ DM [US]; Bromplex DX [US]; Brotapp-DM [US]; Carbofed DM [US]; EndaCof-DM [US]; EndaCof-PD [US]; Histacol™ BD [US]; Myphetane DX [US]; PediaHist DM [US]

Therapeutic Category Antihistamine; Cough Preparation; Decongestant

Use Relief of cough and upper respiratory symptoms (including nasal congestion) associated with allergy or the common cold

Usual Dosage

Children:

1-3 months (EndaCof-PD): 0.25 mL 4 times/day
3-6 months (EndaCof-PD): 0.5 mL 4 times/day
6-12 months (EndaCof-PD): 0.75 mL 4 times/day
12-24 months (EndaCof-PD): 1 mL 4 times/day
2-6 years (Anaplex® DM, EndaCof-DM): 1.25 mL every 4-6 hours (maximum: 4 doses/24 hours)
6-12 years:
Anaplex® DM, EndaCof-DM: 2.5 mL every 4-6 hours (maximum: 4 doses/24 hours)
Bromaline® DM: 10 mL every 4-6 hours (maximum: 4 doses/24 hours)

Children ≥12 years and Adults:
Anaplex® DM: 5 mL every 4-6 hours (maximum: 4 doses/24 hours)
Bromaline® DM: 20 mL every 4-6 hours (maximum: 4 doses/24 hours)

Dosage Forms

Elixir, oral:

Bromaline® DM [OTC]: Brompheniramine 1 mg, pseudoephedrine 15 mg, and dextromethorphan 5 mg per 5 mL

Liquid, oral:

Bromphenex™ DM [OTC], Bromplex DM: Brompheniramine 4 mg, pseudoephedrine 60 mg, and dextromethorphan 30 mg per 5 mL

Brotapp-DM: Brompheniramine 1 mg, pseudoephedrine 15 mg, and dextromethorphan 5 mg per 5 mL

Solution, oral [drops]:

AllanHist PDX, EndaCof-PD, Histacol™ BD: Brompheniramine 1 mg, pseudoephedrine 12.5 mg, and dextromethorphan 3 mg per 1 mL

Bromhist DM, PediaHist DM: Brompheniramine 1 mg, pseudoephedrine 15 mg, and dextromethorphan 4 mg per 1 mL

Suspension, oral: Brompheniramine 8 mg, pseudoephedrine 90 mg, and dextromethorphan 60 mg per 5 mL

Syrup, oral:

Anaplex® DM, EndaCof-DM: Brompheniramine 4 mg, pseudoephedrine 60 mg, and dextromethorphan 30 mg per 5 mL

Andehist DM NR, Carbofed DM: Brompheniramine 4 mg, pseudoephedrine 45 mg, and dextromethorphan 15 mg per 5 mL

Bromatane DX, Bromfed® DM, Myphetane DX: Brompheniramine 2 mg, pseudoephedrine 30 mg, and dextromethorphan 10 mg per 5 mL

brompheniramine tannate *see* brompheniramine *on page 149*

brompheniramine tannate and phenylephrine tannate *see* brompheniramine and phenylephrine *on page 150*

Brompheril® ***(Discontinued)*** *see* dexbrompheniramine and pseudoephedrine *on page 289*

Bromplex DX [US] *see* brompheniramine, pseudoephedrine, and dextromethorphan *on page 152*

Bronchial® ***(Discontinued)***

Bronchial Mist® ***(Discontinued)*** *see* epinephrine *on page 358*

Broncho Saline® *(Discontinued)* *see* sodium chloride *on page 908*
Bronitin® Mist *(Discontinued)* *see* epinephrine *on page 358*
Brontex® *(Discontinued)* *see* guaifenesin and codeine *on page 473*
Brotane® *(Discontinued)* *see* brompheniramine *on page 149*
Brotapp [US] *see* brompheniramine and pseudoephedrine *on page 150*
Brotapp-DM [US] *see* brompheniramine, pseudoephedrine, and dextromethorphan *on page 152*
Brotapp PE [US-OTC] *see* brompheniramine and phenylephrine *on page 150*
Brovana® [US] *see* arformoterol *on page 95*
BroveX™ CT *(Discontinued)* *see* brompheniramine *on page 149*
BroveX™ *(Discontinued)* *see* brompheniramine *on page 149*
Brovex SR *(Discontinued)* *see* brompheniramine and pseudoephedrine *on page 150*
BSF208075 *see* ambrisentan *on page 59*
BSS® [US/Can] *see* balanced salt solution *on page 121*
BSS Plus® [US/Can] *see* balanced salt solution *on page 121*
B-Tuss™ [US] *see* phenylephrine, hydrocodone, and chlorpheniramine *on page 778*
BTX-A *see* onabotulinumtoxinA *on page 725*
B-type natriuretic peptide (human) *see* nesiritide *on page 690*
Bubbli-Pred™ [US] *see* prednisolone (systemic) *on page 813*
Budeprion XL® [US] *see* bupropion *on page 158*
Budeprion SR® [US] *see* bupropion *on page 158*

budesonide (byoo DES oh nide)

U.S./Canadian Brand Names Entocort® EC [US]; Entocort® [Can]; Gen-Budesonide AQ [Can]; Pulmicort Flexhaler™ [US]; Pulmicort Respules® [US]; Pulmicort® [Can]; Rhinocort® Aqua® [US/Can]; Rhinocort® Turbuhaler® [Can]

Therapeutic Category Adrenal Corticosteroid

Use

Intranasal: Management of symptoms of seasonal or perennial rhinitis
Canadian labeling: Additional use (not in U.S. labeling): Prevention and treatment of nasal polyps
Nebulization: Maintenance and prophylactic treatment of asthma
Oral capsule: Treatment of active Crohn disease (mild-to-moderate) involving the ileum and/or ascending colon; maintenance of remission (for up to 3 months) of Crohn disease (mild-to-moderate) involving the ileum and/or ascending colon
Oral inhalation: Maintenance and prophylactic treatment of asthma; includes patients who require oral corticosteroids and those who may benefit from systemic dose reduction/elimination

Usual Dosage

Nasal inhalation:

U.S. labeling (Rhinocort® Aqua®): Rhinitis: Children ≥6 years and Adults: 64 mcg/day as a single 32 mcg spray in each nostril. Some patients who do not achieve adequate control may benefit from increased dosage. A reduced dosage may be effective after initial control is achieved.
Maximum dose: Children <12 years: 128 mcg/day; Adults: 256 mcg/day

Canadian labeling:
Rhinocort® Aqua®: Children ≥6 years and Adults:
Nasal polyps: 256 mcg/day administered as a single 64 mcg spray in each nostril twice daily
Rhinitis: Initial: 256 mcg/day administered as two 64 mcg sprays in each nostril once daily or a single 64 mcg spray in each nostril twice daily; Maintenance: Individualize, lowest effective dose
Maximum dose: 256 mcg/day
Rhinocort® Turbuhaler®: Children ≥6 years and Adults:
Nasal polyps: 100 mcg into each nostril twice daily (maximum: 400 mcg/day)
Rhinitis: Initial: 200 mcg into each nostril once daily; Maintenance: Individualize, lowest effective dose (maximum: 400 mcg/day)

Nebulization: Children 12 months to 8 years: Asthma: Pulmicort Respules®: Titrate to lowest effective dose once patient is stable; start at 0.25 mg/day or use as follows:
Previous therapy of bronchodilators alone: 0.5 mg/day administered as a single dose or divided twice daily (maximum daily dose: 0.5 mg)
Previous therapy of inhaled corticosteroids: 0.5 mg/day administered as a single dose or divided twice daily (maximum daily dose: 1 mg)

Previous therapy of oral corticosteroids: 1 mg/day administered as a single dose or divided twice daily (maximum daily dose: 1 mg)

NIH Asthma Guidelines:

Children 0-4 years:

"Low" dose: 0.25-0.5 mg/day

"Medium" dose: >0.5-1 mg/day

"High" dose: >1 mg/day

Children 5-11 years:

"Low" dose: 0.5 mg/day

"Medium" dose: 1 mg/day

"High" dose: 2 mg/day

Oral inhalation: Asthma:

Children ≥6 years:

Pulmicort Flexhaler™: Initial: 180 mcg twice daily (some patients may be initiated at 360 mcg twice daily); maximum: 360 mcg twice daily

NIH Asthma Guidelines (administer in divided doses twice daily):

Children 5-11 years:

"Low" dose: 180-400 mcg/day

"Medium" dose: >400-800 mcg/day

"High" dose: >800 mcg/day

Children ≥12 years: Refer to adult dosing.

Pulmicort® Turbuhaler®: [CAN, not available in the U.S.]: Initial (during periods of severe asthma or when switching from oral corticosteroid therapy): 200-400 mcg daily in 2 divided doses; Maintenance: Individualized, lowest effective dose.

Adults:

Pulmicort Flexhaler™: Initial: 360 mcg twice daily (selected patients may be initiated at 180 mcg twice daily); maximum 720 mcg twice daily

NIH Asthma Guidelines (administer in divided doses twice daily):

"Low" dose: 180-600 mcg/day

"Medium" dose: >600-1200 mcg/day

"High" dose: >1200 mcg/day

Pulmicort® Turbuhaler® [CAN, not available in the U.S.]: Initial (during periods of severe asthma or when switching from oral corticosteroid therapy): 400-2400 mcg daily in 2-4 divided doses; Maintenance: 200-400 mcg twice daily (higher doses may be needed for short periods of time). **Note:** Patients taking 400 mcg/day may take as a single daily dose

Oral: Crohn disease (active): Adults: 9 mg once daily in the morning for up to 8 weeks; recurring episodes may be treated with a repeat 8-week course of treatment

Note: Patients receiving CYP3A4 inhibitors should be monitored closely for signs and symptoms of hypercorticism; dosage reduction may be required. If switching from oral prednisolone, prednisolone dosage should be tapered while budesonide (Entocort® EC) treatment is initiated.

Maintenance of remission: Following treatment of active disease (control of symptoms with CDAI <150), treatment may be continued at a dosage of 6 mg once daily for up to 3 months. If symptom control is maintained for 3 months, tapering of the dosage to complete cessation is recommended. Continued dosing beyond 3 months has not been demonstrated to result in substantial benefit.

Dosage Forms [CAN] = Canadian brand name

Capsule, enteric coated:

Entocort® EC: 3 mg

Powder for nasal inhalation:

Rhinocort® Turbuhaler® [CAN]: 100 mcg/inhalation [not available in the U.S.]

Powder for oral inhalation:

Pulmicort Flexhaler™: 90 mcg/inhalation (165 mg)

Pulmicort Flexhaler™: 180 mcg/inhalation (225 mg)

Pulmicort Turbuhaler® [CAN]: 100 mcg/inhalation, 200 mcg/inhalation, 400 mcg/inhalation [not available in the U.S.]

Suspension, intranasal [spray]:

Rhinocort® Aqua®: 32 mcg/inhalation (8.6 g)

Rhinocort® Aqua® [CAN]: 64 mcg/inhalation [not available in the U.S.]

Suspension for nebulization:

Pulmicort Respules®: 0.25 mg/2 mL; 0.5 mg/2 mL; 1 mg/2 mL

budesonide and eformoterol *see* budesonide and formoterol *on page* 155

budesonide and formoterol (byoo DES oh nide & for MOH te rol)

Synonyms budesonide and eformoterol; eformoterol and budesonide; formoterol and budesonide; formoterol fumarate dihydrate and budesonide

U.S./Canadian Brand Names Symbicort® [US/Can]

Therapeutic Category $Beta_2$-Adrenergic Agonist Agent; Corticosteroid, Inhalant (Oral)

Use Treatment of asthma in patients ≥12 years of age where combination therapy is indicated; maintenance treatment of airflow obstruction associated with chronic obstructive pulmonary disease (COPD; including chronic bronchitis and emphysema)

Usual Dosage Oral inhalation:

Asthma:

Children 5-11 years (NIH Guidelines): Symbicort® 80/4.5: Two inhalations twice daily. Do not exceed 4 inhalations per day.

Children ≥12 years and Adults:

U.S. labeling: Symbicort® 80/4.5, Symbicort® 160/4.5: Two inhalations twice daily. Patients currently receiving a low-to-medium dose inhaled corticosteroid may be started on the lower strength combination; those receiving a medium-to-high dose inhaled corticosteroid may be started on the higher strength combination. Consider the higher dose combination for patients not adequately controlled on the lower combination following 1-2 weeks of therapy. Do not use more than 2 inhalations twice daily of either strength.

Canadian labeling:

Symbicort® 100 Turbuhaler® [CAN; not available in U.S.], Symbicort® 200 Turbuhaler® [CAN; not available in U.S.]:

Initial: 1-2 inhalations twice daily until symptom control, then titrate to lowest effective dosage to maintain control

Maintenance: 1-2 inhalations once or twice daily (maximum: 8 inhalations/day as temporary treatment in periods of worsening asthma)

Symbicort® Maintenance and Reliever Therapy (Symbicort® SMART): **Note:** Not approved in the U.S.:

Maintenance: Symbicort® 100 Turbuhaler® [CAN] **or** Symbicort® 200 Turbuhaler® [CAN]: 1-2 inhalations twice daily **or** 2 inhalations once daily

Reliever therapy: Symbicort® 100 Turbuhaler [CAN] **or** Symbicort® 200 Turbuhaler® [CAN.]: One additional inhalation as needed, may repeat if no relief for up to 6 inhalations total (maximum: 8 inhalations/day)

COPD: Adults: Symbicort® 160/4.5: Two inhalations twice daily (maximum: 4 inhalations/day)

Dosage Forms [CAN] = Canadian product

Aerosol for oral inhalation:

Symbicort® 80/4.5: Budesonide 80 mcg and formoterol fumarate dihydrate 4.5 mcg per actuation (6.9 g) [60 metered inhalations]; budesonide 80 mcg and formoterol fumarate dihydrate 4.5 mcg per actuation (10.2 g) [120 metered inhalations]

Symbicort® 160/4.5: Budesonide 160 mcg and formoterol fumarate dihydrate 4.5 mcg per actuation (6 g) [60 metered inhalations]; budesonide 160 mcg and formoterol fumarate dihydrate 4.5 mcg per actuation (10.2 g) [120 metered inhalations]

Powder for oral inhalation:

Symbicort® 100 Turbuhaler® [CAN]: Budesonide 100 mcg and formoterol dihydrate 6 mcg per inhalation (available in 60 or 120 metered doses) [delivers ~80 mcg budesonide and 4.5 mcg formoterol per inhalation; contains lactose] [not available in the U.S]

Symbicort® 200 Turbuhaler® [CAN]: Budesonide 200 mcg and formoterol dihydrate 6 mcg per inhalation (available in 60 or 120 metered doses) [delivers ~160 mcg budesonide and 4.5 mcg formoterol per inhalation; contains lactose] [not available in the U.S]

Buffasal [US-OTC] *see* aspirin *on page 103*

Bufferin® [US-OTC] *see* aspirin *on page 103*

Bufferin® Extra Strength [US-OTC] *see* aspirin *on page 103*

Buffinol [US-OTC] *see* aspirin *on page 103*

Bulk-K [US-OTC] *see* psyllium *on page 837*

bumetanide (byoo MET a nide)

Sound-Alike/Look-Alike Issues

bumetanide may be confused with Buminate®

Bumex® may be confused with Brevibloc®, Buprenex®, Permax®

U.S./Canadian Brand Names Bumex® [Can]; Burinex® [Can]

Therapeutic Category Diuretic, Loop

Use Management of edema secondary to heart failure or hepatic or renal disease including nephrotic syndrome; may be used alone or in combination with antihypertensives in the treatment of hypertension; can be used in furosemide-allergic patients

Usual Dosage

Oral, I.M., I.V.:

Neonates: 0.01-0.05 mg/kg/dose every 24-48 hours

Infants and Children: 0.015-0.1 mg/kg/dose every 6-24 hours (maximum dose: 10 mg/day)

Adults:

Edema:

Oral: 0.5-2 mg/dose (maximum dose: 10 mg/day) 1-2 times/day

I.M., I.V.: 0.5-1 mg/dose; may repeat in 2-3 hours for up to 2 doses if needed (maximum dose: 10 mg/day)

Continuous I.V. infusion: Initial: 1 mg I.V. load then 0.5-2 mg/hour

Hypertension: Oral: 0.5 mg daily (maximum dose: 5 mg/day); usual dosage range (JNC 7): 0.5-2 mg/day in 2 divided doses

Dosage Forms

Injection, solution: 0.25 mg/mL (2 mL, 4 mL, 10 mL)

Tablet: 0.5 mg, 1 mg, 2 mg

Bumex® [Can] *see* bumetanide *on page* 155

Bumex® ***(Discontinued)*** *see* bumetanide *on page* 155

Bumex® Injection ***(Discontinued)*** *see* bumetanide *on page* 155

Buminate® [US] *see* albumin *on page* 40

Bupap [US] *see* butalbital and acetaminophen *on page* 162

Buphenyl® [US] *see* sodium phenylbutyrate *on page* 912

bupivacaine (byoo PIV a kane)

Sound-Alike/Look-Alike Issues

bupivacaine may be confused with mepivacaine, ropivacaine

Marcaine® may be confused with Narcan®

Synonyms bupivacaine hydrochloride

U.S./Canadian Brand Names Marcaine® Spinal [US]; Marcaine® [US/Can]; Sensorcaine® [US/Can]; Sensorcaine®-MPF Spinal [US]; Sensorcaine®-MPF [US]

Therapeutic Category Local Anesthetic

Use Peripheral nerve block; infiltration; sympathetic block; spinal, caudal or epidural block; retrobulbar block

Usual Dosage Dose varies with procedure, depth of anesthesia, vascularity of tissues, duration of anesthesia, and condition of patient. Do not use solutions containing preservatives for caudal or epidural block.

Children >12 years and Adults:

Local anesthesia: Infiltration: 0.25% infiltrated locally; maximum: 175 mg

Caudal block (preservative free): 15-30 mL of 0.25% or 0.5%

Epidural block (other than caudal block; preservative free): Administer in 3-5 mL increments, allowing sufficient time to detect toxic manifestations of inadvertent I.V. or I.T. administration: 10-20 mL of 0.25% or 0.5%

Surgical procedures requiring a high degree of muscle relaxation and prolonged effects **only**: 10-20 mL of 0.75% (**Note:** Not to be used in obstetrical cases)

Peripheral nerve block: 5 mL of 0.25% or 0.5%; maximum: 400 mg/day

Sympathetic nerve block: 20-50 mL of 0.25%

Retrobulbar anesthesia: 2-4 mL of 0.75%

Adults: Spinal anesthesia: Preservative free solution of 0.75% bupivacaine in 8.25% dextrose:

Lower extremity and perineal procedures: 1 mL

Lower abdominal procedures: 1.6 mL

Normal vaginal delivery: 0.8 mL (higher doses may be required in some patients)

Cesarean section: 1-1.4 mL

Dosage Forms

Injection, solution [preservative free]: 0.25% (10 mL, 20 mL, 30 mL, 50 mL); 0.5% (10 mL, 20 mL, 30 mL); 0.75% (10 mL, 20 mL, 30 mL)

Marcaine®: 0.25% (10 mL, 30 mL, 50 mL); 0.5% (10 mL, 30 mL); 0.75% (10 mL, 30 mL)
Sensorcaine®-MPF: 0.25% (10 mL, 30 mL); 0.5% (10 mL, 30 mL); 0.75% (10 mL, 30 mL)
Injection, solution, premixed in D8.25 [preservative free]: 0.75% (2 mL)
Marcaine® Spinal: 0.75% (2 mL)
Sensorcaine®-MPF Spinal: 0.75% (2 mL)
Injection, solution: 0.25% (50 mL); 0.5% (50 mL)
Marcaine®: 0.5% (50 mL)
Sensorcaine®: 0.25% (50 mL); 0.5% (50 mL)

bupivacaine and epinephrine (byoo PIV a kane & ep i NEF rin)

Synonyms epinephrine bitartrate and bupivacaine hydrochloride

U.S./Canadian Brand Names Marcaine® with Epinephrine [US]; Sensorcaine® with Epinephrine [US/Can]; Sensorcaine®-MPF with Epinephrine [US]; Vivacaine™ [US]

Therapeutic Category Local Anesthetic

Use Local anesthetic (injectable) for peripheral nerve block, infiltration, sympathetic block, caudal or epidural block, retrobulbar block

Usual Dosage Dose varies with procedure, depth of anesthesia, vascularity of tissues, duration of anesthesia, and condition of patient. Do not use solutions containing preservatives for caudal or epidural block.

Children >12 years and Adults:

Caudal block (preservative free): 15-30 mL of 0.25% or 0.5%

Epidural block (other than caudal block, preservative free): 10-20 mL of 0.25% or 0.5%. Administer in 3-5 mL increments, allowing sufficient time to detect toxic manifestations of inadvertent I.V. or I.T. administration.

Surgical procedures requiring a high degree of muscle relaxation and prolonged effects only: 10-20 mL of 0.75% (**Note:** Not to be used in obstetrical cases)

Local anesthesia: Infiltration: 0.25% infiltrated locally (maximum: 175 mg of bupivacaine)

Peripheral nerve block: 5 mL of 0.25 or 0.5% (maximum: 400 mg/day of bupivacaine)

Retrobulbar anesthesia: 2-4 mL of 0.75%

Sympathetic nerve block: 20-50 mL of 0.25%

Infiltration and nerve block in maxillary and mandibular area: 9 mg (1.8 mL) of bupivacaine as a 0.5% solution with epinephrine 1:200,000 per injection site. A second dose may be administered if necessary to produce adequate anesthesia after allowing up to 10 minutes for onset. Up to a maximum of 90 mg of bupivacaine hydrochloride per dental appointment. The effective anesthetic dose varies with procedure, intensity of anesthesia needed, duration of anesthesia required, and physical condition of the patient; always use the lowest effective dose along with careful aspiration.

Dosage Forms

Injection, solution [preservative free]: Bupivacaine 0.25% and epinephrine 1:200,000 (10 mL, 30 mL); bupivacaine 0.5% and epinephrine 1:200,000 (10 mL, 30 mL)

Marcaine® with Epinephrine: Bupivacaine 0.25% and epinephrine 1:200,000 (10 mL, 30 mL); bupivacaine 0.5% and epinephrine 1:200,000 (3 mL, 10 mL, 30 mL)

Sensorcaine® MPF with Epinephrine: Bupivacaine 0.25% and epinephrine 1:200,000 (10 mL, 30 mL); bupivacaine 0.5% and epinephrine 1:200,000 (10 mL, 30 mL); bupivacaine 0.75% and epinephrine 1:200,000 (30 mL)

Injection, solution: Bupivacaine 0.25% and epinephrine 1:200,000 (50 mL); bupivacaine 0.5% and epinephrine 1:200,000 (50 mL)

Marcaine® with Epinephrine, Sensorcaine® with Epinephrine: Bupivacaine 0.25% and epinephrine 1:200,000 (50 mL); bupivacaine 0.5% and epinephrine 1:200,000 (50 mL)

Injection, solution [for dental use]:

Marcaine® with Epinephrine, Vivacaine™: Bupivacaine 0.5% and epinephrine 1:200,000 (1.8 mL)

bupivacaine hydrochloride *see* bupivacaine *on page* 156
Buprenex® [US/Can] *see* buprenorphine *on page* 157

buprenorphine (byoo pre NOR feen)

Sound-Alike/Look-Alike Issues

Buprenex® may be confused with Brevibloc®, Bumex®

Synonyms buprenorphine hydrochloride

U.S./Canadian Brand Names Buprenex® [US/Can]; Subutex® [US/Can]

Therapeutic Category Analgesic, Narcotic

Controlled Substance Injection: C-V/C-III; Tablet: C-III

Use

Injection: Management of moderate-to-severe pain

Tablet: Treatment of opioid dependence

Usual Dosage Long-term use is not recommended

Note: These are guidelines and do not represent the maximum doses that may be required in all patients. Doses should be titrated to pain relief/prevention. In high-risk patients (eg, elderly, debilitated, presence of respiratory disease) and/or concurrent CNS depressant use, reduce dose by one-half. Buprenorphine has an analgesic ceiling.

Acute pain (moderate-to-severe):

Children 2-12 years: I.M., slow I.V.: 2-6 mcg/kg every 4-6 hours

Children ≥13 years and Adults:

I.M.: Initial: Opiate-naive: 0.3 mg every 6-8 hours as needed; initial dose (up to 0.3 mg) may be repeated once in 30-60 minutes after the initial dose if needed; usual dosage range: 0.15-0.6 mg every 4-8 hours as needed

Slow I.V.: Initial: Opiate-naive: 0.3 mg every 6-8 hours as needed; initial dose (up to 0.3 mg) may be repeated once in 30-60 minutes after the initial dose if needed

Sublingual: Children ≥16 years and Adults: Opioid dependence:

Induction: Range: 12-16 mg/day (doses during an induction study used 8 mg on day 1, followed by 16 mg on day 2; induction continued over 3-4 days). Treatment should begin at least 4 hours after last use of heroin or short-acting opioid, preferably when first signs of withdrawal appear. Titrating dose to clinical effectiveness should be done as rapidly as possible to prevent undue withdrawal symptoms and patient drop-out during the induction period.

Maintenance: Target dose: 16 mg/day; range: 4-24 mg/day; patients should be switched to the buprenorphine/naloxone combination product for maintenance and unsupervised therapy

Dosage Forms

Injection, solution: 0.3 mg/mL (1 mL)

Buprenex®: 0.3 mg/mL (1 mL)

Tablet, sublingual:

Subutex®: 2 mg, 8 mg

buprenorphine and naloxone (byoo pre NOR feen & nal OKS one)

Synonyms buprenorphine hydrochloride and naloxone hydrochloride dihydrate; naloxone and buprenorphine; naloxone hydrochloride dihydrate and buprenorphine hydrochloride

U.S./Canadian Brand Names Suboxone® [US]

Therapeutic Category Analgesic, Narcotic

Controlled Substance C-III

Use Treatment of opioid dependence

Usual Dosage Sublingual: Children ≥16 years and Adults: Opioid dependence: **Note:** This combination product is not recommended for use during the induction period; initial treatment should begin using buprenorphine oral tablets. Patients should be switched to the combination product for maintenance and unsupervised therapy.

Maintenance: Target dose (based on buprenorphine content): 16 mg/day; range: 4-24 mg/day

Dosage Forms

Tablet, sublingual:

Suboxone®: Buprenorphine 2 mg and naloxone 0.5 mg; buprenorphine 8 mg and naloxone 2 mg

buprenorphine hydrochloride *see* buprenorphine *on page 157*

buprenorphine hydrochloride and naloxone hydrochloride dihydrate *see* buprenorphine and naloxone *on page 158*

Buproban™ [US] *see* bupropion *on page 158*

bupropion (byoo PROE pee on)

Sound-Alike/Look-Alike Issues

buPROPion may be confused with busPIRone

Aplenzin® may be confused with Albenza®, Relenza®

Wellbutrin SR® may be confused with Wellbutrin XL®

Wellbutrin XL® may be confused with Wellbutrin SR®

Zyban® may be confused with Zagam®, Diovan®

Tall-Man bu**PROP**ion

U.S./Canadian Brand Names Aplenzin® [US]; Budeprion SR® [US]; Budeprion XL® [US]; Buproban™ [US]; Novo-Bupropion SR [Can]; PMS-Bupropion SR [Can]; ratio-Bupropion SR [Can]; SANDOZ-Bupropion SR [Can]; Wellbutrin SR® [US]; Wellbutrin XL® [US/Can]; Wellbutrin® [US/Can]; Zyban® [US/Can]

Therapeutic Category Antidepressant, Aminoketone

Use Treatment of major depressive disorder, including seasonal affective disorder (SAD); adjunct in smoking cessation

Usual Dosage Oral: Adults:

Depression:

Immediate release hydrochloride salt: 100 mg 3 times/day; begin at 100 mg twice daily; may increase to a maximum dose of 450 mg/day

Sustained release hydrochloride salt: Initial: 150 mg/day in the morning; may increase to 150 mg twice daily by day 4 if tolerated; target dose: 300 mg/day given as 150 mg twice daily; maximum dose: 400 mg/day given as 200 mg twice daily

Extended release:

Hydrochloride salt: Initial: 150 mg/day in the morning; may increase as early as day 4 of dosing to 300 mg/day; maximum dose: 450 mg/day

Hydrobromide salt (Aplenzin®): Target dose: 348 mg/day in the morning. Patients not previously on bupropion: Initial: 174 mg/day in the morning; may increase as early as day 4 of dosing to 348 mg/day; maximum dose: 522 mg/day. **Note:** 174 mg strength currently not available; 348 mg tablet cannot be split.

Switching from hydrochloride salt formulation (eg, Wellbutrin® immediate release, SR®, XL®) to hydrobromide salt formulation (Aplenzin®): **Note:** Patients being treated twice daily with bupropion hydrochloride would be switched to the equivalent once daily dose of bupropion hydrobromide.

Bupropion hydrochloride 150 mg is equivalent to bupropion hydrobromide 174 mg

Bupropion hydrochloride 300 mg is equivalent to bupropion hydrobromide 348 mg

Bupropion hydrochloride 450 mg is equivalent to bupropion hydrobromide 522 mg

SAD (Wellbutrin XL®): Initial: 150 mg/day in the morning; if tolerated, may increase after 1 week to 300 mg/day

Note: Prophylactic treatment should be reserved for those patients with frequent depressive episodes and/or significant impairment. Initiate treatment in the Autumn prior to symptom onset, and discontinue in early Spring with dose tapering to 150 mg/day for 2 weeks

Smoking cessation (Zyban®): Initiate with 150 mg once daily for 3 days; increase to 150 mg twice daily; treatment should continue for 7-12 weeks

Note: Therapy should begin at least 1 week before target quit date. Target quit dates are generally in the second week of treatment. If patient successfully quits smoking after 7-12 weeks, may consider ongoing maintenance therapy based on individual patient risk/benefit. Efficacy of maintenance therapy (300 mg/day) has been demonstrated for up to 6 months. Conversely, if significant progress has not been made by the seventh week of therapy, success is unlikely and treatment discontinuation should be considered.

Dosage Forms

Tablet: 75 mg, 100 mg [generic for Wellbutrin®]

Wellbutrin®: 75 mg, 100 mg

Tablet, extended release: 100 mg [generic for Wellbutrin SR®], 150 mg [generic for Wellbutrin SR®], 150 mg [generic for Wellbutrin XL®], 150 mg [generic for Zyban®], 200 mg [generic for Wellbutrin SR®], 300 mg [generic for Wellbutrin XL®]

Aplenzin®: 174 mg, 348 mg, 522 mg

Budeprion SR®: 100 mg, 150 mg [generic for Wellbutrin SR®]

Budeprion XL®: 150 mg, 300 mg [generic for Wellbutrin XL®]

Buproban®: 150 mg [generic for Zyban®]

Wellbutrin XL®: 150 mg, 300 mg

Tablet, sustained release: 100 mg [generic for Wellbutrin SR®], 150 mg [generic for Wellbutrin SR®], 150 mg [generic for Zyban®], 200 mg [generic for Wellbutrin SR®]

Wellbutrin SR®: 100 mg, 150 mg, 200 mg

Zyban®: 150 mg

Burinex® [Can] *see* bumetanide *on page 155*

BurnaMycin [US-OTC] *see* lidocaine *on page 584*

Burn Jel® [US-OTC] *see* lidocaine *on page 584*

Burn-O-Jel [US-OTC] *see* lidocaine *on page 584*

Buscopan® [Can] *see* scopolamine derivatives *on page 892*

buserelin acetate *(Canada only)* (BYOO se rel in AS e tate)

Sound-Alike/Look-Alike Issues
Suprefact® may be confused with Suprane®

U.S./Canadian Brand Names Suprefact® Depot [Can]; Suprefact® [Can]

Therapeutic Category Luteinizing Hormone-Releasing Hormone Analog

Use Palliative treatment in patients with hormone-dependent advanced prostate cancer (stage D); treatment of endometriosis in women who do not require surgical intervention as first-line therapy (length of therapy is usually 6 months, but no longer than 9 months)

Usual Dosage Adults:
Prostate cancer: **Note:** Administration of an antiandrogen agent beginning 7 days prior to initiation of buserelin therapy and continuing for ~5 weeks with buserelin therapy is recommended in patients with prostate cancer.
SubQ:
Suprefact®: Initial: 500 mcg every 8 hours for 7 days. Maintenance: 200 mcg once daily
Suprefact® Depot
2-month: 6.3 mg implant injected into lateral abdominal wall every 8 weeks
3-month: 9.45 mg injected into lateral abdominal wall every 12 weeks
Intranasal (Suprefact®): Maintenance: 400 mcg (200 mcg into each nostril) 3 times/day
Endometriosis: Intranasal (Suprefact®): 400 mcg (200 mcg into each nostril) 3 times/day for 6-9 months

Dosage Forms [CAN] = Canadian brand name
Injection, solution:
Suprefact® [CAN]: 1 mg/mL (5.5 mL, 10 mL) [not available in U.S.]
Solution, intranasal:
Suprefact® [CAN]: 1mg/1mL (10 mL) [not available in U.S.]
Implant, subcutaneous:
Suprefact® [CAN] Depot: 6.3 mg, 9.45 mg [not available in U.S.]

BuSpar® [US/Can] *see* buspirone *on page* *160*
Buspirex [Can] *see* buspirone *on page* *160*

buspirone (byoo SPYE rone)

Sound-Alike/Look-Alike Issues
busPIRone may be confused with buPROPion

Synonyms buspirone hydrochloride

Tall-Man bus**PIR**one

U.S./Canadian Brand Names Apo-Buspirone® [Can]; BuSpar® [US/Can]; Buspirex [Can]; Bustab® [Can]; CO Buspirone [Can]; Dom-Buspirone [Can]; Gen-Buspirone [Can]; Lin-Buspirone [Can]; Novo-Buspirone [Can]; Nu-Buspirone [Can]; PMS-Buspirone [Can]; ratio-Buspirone [Can]; Riva-Buspirone [Can]

Therapeutic Category Antianxiety Agent

Use Management of generalized anxiety disorder (GAD)

Usual Dosage Oral: Generalized anxiety disorder:
Children ≥6 years and Adolescents: Initial: 5 mg daily; increase in increments of 5 mg/day at weekly intervals as needed, to a maximum dose of 60 mg/day divided into 2-3 doses
Adults: 15 mg/day (7.5 mg twice daily); may increase in increments of 5 mg/day every 2-3 days to a maximum of 60 mg/day; target dose for most people is 20-30 mg/day (10-15 mg twice daily)

Dosage Forms
Tablet: 5 mg, 7.5 mg, 10 mg, 15 mg, 30 mg
BuSpar®: 5 mg, 10 mg, 15 mg

buspirone hydrochloride *see* buspirone *on page* *160*
Bustab® [Can] *see* buspirone *on page* *160*

busulfan (byoo SUL fan)

Sound-Alike/Look-Alike Issues
busulfan may be confused with Butalan®
Myleran® may be confused with Alkeran®, Leukeran®, melphalan, Mylicon®

Synonyms NSC-750

U.S./Canadian Brand Names Busulfex® [US/Can]; Myleran® [US/Can]

Therapeutic Category Antineoplastic Agent

Use

Oral: Chronic myelogenous leukemia (CML); conditioning regimens for bone marrow transplantation

I.V.: Combination therapy with cyclophosphamide as a conditioning regimen prior to allogeneic hematopoietic progenitor cell transplantation for chronic myelogenous leukemia

Usual Dosage Note: Premedicate with prophylactic anticonvulsant therapy (eg, phenytoin) prior to high-dose busulfan treatment.

Children:

CML, remission induction: Oral: 0.06-0.12 mg/kg/day **or** 1.8-4.6 mg/m^2/day; titrate dosage to maintain leukocyte count above 40,000/mm^3; reduce dosage by 50% if the leukocyte count reaches 30,000-40,000/mm^3; discontinue drug if counts fall to ≤20,000/mm^3

BMT marrow-ablative conditioning regimen:

Oral: 1 mg/kg/dose (ideal body weight) every 6 hours for 16 doses

I.V.:

≤12 kg: 1.1 mg/kg/dose (ideal body weight) every 6 hours for 16 doses

>12 kg: 0.8 mg/kg/dose (ideal body weight) every 6 hours for 16 doses

Adjust dose to desired AUC [1125 μmol(min)] using the following formula:

Adjusted dose (mg) = Actual dose (mg) x [target AUC μmol(min) / actual AUC μmol(min)]

Adults:

CML, remission induction: Oral: 60 mcg/kg/day or 1.8 mg/m^2/day; usual range: 4-8 mg/day (may be as high as 12 mg/day); Maintenance doses: 1-4 mg/day to 2 mg/week to maintain WBC 10,000-20,000 cells/mm^3

BMT marrow-ablative conditioning regimen:

Oral: 1 mg/kg/dose (ideal body weight) every 6 hours for 16 doses

I.V.: 0.8 mg/kg (ideal body weight or actual body weight, whichever is lower); for obese or severely-obese patients adjusted ideal body weight is recommended) every 6 hours for 4 days (a total of 16 doses)

Dosage Forms

Injection, solution:

Busulfex®: 6 mg/mL (10 mL)

Tablet:

Myleran®: 2 mg

Busulfex® [US/Can] *see* busulfan *on page 160*

butabarbital (byoo ta BAR bi tal)

Sound-Alike/Look-Alike Issues

butabarbital may be confused with butalbital

U.S./Canadian Brand Names Butisol Sodium® [US]

Therapeutic Category Barbiturate

Controlled Substance C-III

Use Sedative; hypnotic

Usual Dosage Oral:

Children: Preoperative sedation: 2-6 mg/kg/dose (maximum: 100 mg)

Adults:

Sedative: 15-30 mg 3-4 times/day

Hypnotic: 50-100 mg at bedtime. When used for insomnia, treatment should be limited since barbiturates lose effectiveness for sleep induction and maintenance after 2 weeks.

Preop: 50-100 mg 1-1$^1/_2$ hours before surgery

Dosage Forms

Elixir:

Butisol Sodium®: 30 mg/5 mL

Tablet:

Butisol Sodium®: 30 mg, 50 mg

Butalan® ***(Discontinued)***

butalbital, acetaminophen, and caffeine

(byoo TAL bi tal, a seet a MIN oh fen, & KAF een)

Sound-Alike/Look-Alike Issues

Fioricet® may be confused with Fiorinal®, Lorcet®

Repan® may be confused with Riopan®

Synonyms acetaminophen, butalbital, and caffeine

U.S./Canadian Brand Names Anolor 300 [US]; Dolgic® Plus [US]; Esgic-Plus™ [US]; Esgic® [US]; Fioricet® [US]; Medigesic® [US]; Repan® [US]; Zebutal™ [US]

Therapeutic Category Barbiturate/Analgesic

Use Relief of the symptomatic complex of tension or muscle contraction headache

Usual Dosage Oral: Adults: 1-2 tablets or capsules (or 15-30 mL solution) every 4 hours; not to exceed 6 tablets or capsules (or 180 mL solution) daily

Dosage Forms

Capsule, oral:

Alagesic, Anolor 300, Esgic®, Margesic: Butalbital 50 mg, acetaminophen 325 mg, and caffeine 40 mg

Esgic-Plus™, Zebutal®: Butalbital 50 mg, acetaminophen 500 mg, and caffeine 40 mg

Liquid, oral:

Alagesic LQ: Butalbital 50 mg, acetaminophen 325 mg, and caffeine 40 mg per 15 mL

Tablet, oral: Butalbital 50 mg, acetaminophen 325 mg, and caffeine 40 mg; butalbital 50 mg, acetaminophen 500 mg, and caffeine 40 mg

Dolgic® Plus: Butalbital 50 mg, acetaminophen 750 mg, and caffeine 40 mg

Esgic®, Fioricet®, Repan®: Butalbital 50 mg, acetaminophen 325 mg, and caffeine 40 mg

Esgic-Plus™: Butalbital 50 mg, acetaminophen 500 mg, and caffeine 40 mg

butalbital, acetaminophen, caffeine, and codeine

(byoo TAL bi tal, a seet a MIN oh fen, KAF een, & KOE deen)

Sound-Alike/Look-Alike Issues

Fioricet® may be confused with Fiorinal®, Florinef®, Lorcet®, Percocet®

Phrenilin® may be confused with Phenergan®, Trinalin®

Synonyms acetaminophen, caffeine, codeine, and butalbital; caffeine, acetaminophen, butalbital, and codeine; codeine, acetaminophen, butalbital, and caffeine

U.S./Canadian Brand Names Fioricet® with Codeine [US]

Therapeutic Category Analgesic Combination (Opioid); Barbiturate

Controlled Substance C-III

Use Relief of symptoms of complex tension (muscle contraction) headache

Usual Dosage Oral: Adults: 1-2 capsules every 4 hours. Total daily dosage should not exceed 6 capsules.

Dosage Forms

Capsule: Butalbital 50 mg, acetaminophen 325 mg, caffeine 40 mg, and codeine 30 mg

Fioricet® with Codeine: Butalbital 50 mg, acetaminophen 325 mg, caffeine 40 mg, and codeine 30 mg

butalbital and acetaminophen (byoo TAL bi tal & a seet a MIN oh fen)

Synonyms acetaminophen and butalbital

U.S./Canadian Brand Names Bupap [US]; Cephadyn [US]; Phrenilin® Forte [US]; Phrenilin® [US]; Promacet [US]; Sedapap® [US]

Therapeutic Category Analgesic, Miscellaneous; Barbiturate

Use Relief of the symptomatic complex of tension or muscle contraction headache

Usual Dosage Oral: Adults: One tablet/capsule every 4 hours as needed (maximum dose: 6 tablets/day)

Phrenilin®: 1-2 tablets every 4 hours as needed (maximum: 6 tablets in 24 hours)

Dosage Forms

Tablet:

Phrenilin®: Butalbital 50 mg and acetaminophen 325 mg

Bupap, Cephadyn, Promacet, Sedapap®: Butalbital 50 mg and acetaminophen 650 mg

Capsule:

Phrenilin® Forte: Butalbital 50 mg and acetaminophen 650 mg

butalbital, aspirin, and caffeine (byoo TAL bi tal, AS pir in, & KAF een)

Sound-Alike/Look-Alike Issues

Fiorinal® may be confused with Fioricet®, Florical®, Florinef®

Synonyms aspirin, caffeine, and butalbital; butalbital compound

U.S./Canadian Brand Names Fiorinal® [US/Can]

Therapeutic Category Barbiturate/Analgesic

Controlled Substance C-III

Use Relief of the symptomatic complex of tension or muscle contraction headache

Usual Dosage Oral: Adults: 1-2 tablets or capsules every 4 hours; not to exceed 6 tablets or capsules/day

Dosage Forms

Capsule: Butalbital 50 mg, aspirin 325 mg, and caffeine 40 mg
Fiorinal®: Butalbital 50 mg, aspirin 325 mg, and caffeine 40 mg

Tablet: Butalbital 50 mg, aspirin 325 mg, and caffeine 40 mg

butalbital, aspirin, caffeine, and codeine

(byoo TAL bi tal, AS pir in, KAF een, & KOE deen)

Sound-Alike/Look-Alike Issues
Fiorinal® may be confused with Fioricet®, Florical®, Florinef®

Synonyms aspirin, caffeine, codeine, and butalbital; butalbital compound and codeine; codeine and butalbital compound; codeine, butalbital, aspirin, and caffeine

U.S./Canadian Brand Names Ascomp® with Codeine [US]; Fiorinal® with Codeine [US]; Fiorinal®-C 1/2 [Can]; Fiorinal®-C 1/4 [Can]; Tecnal C 1/2 [Can]; Tecnal C 1/4 [Can]

Therapeutic Category Analgesic, Narcotic; Barbiturate

Controlled Substance C-III

Use Relief of symptoms of complex tension (muscle contraction) headache

Usual Dosage Oral: Adults: 1-2 capsules every 4 hours as needed (maximum: 6 capsules/day)

Dosage Forms

Capsule: Butalbital 50 mg, aspirin 325 mg, caffeine 40 mg, and codeine 30 mg
Ascomp® with Codeine, Fiorinal® with Codeine: Butalbital 50 mg, aspirin 325 mg, caffeine 40 mg, and codeine 30 mg

butalbital compound *see* butalbital, aspirin, and caffeine *on page 162*

butalbital compound and codeine *see* butalbital, aspirin, caffeine, and codeine *on page 163*

butamben, tetracaine, and benzocaine *see* benzocaine, butamben, and tetracaine *on page 131*

butenafine (byoo TEN a feen)

Sound-Alike/Look-Alike Issues
Lotrimin® may be confused with Lotrisone®, Otrivin®

Synonyms butenafine hydrochloride

U.S./Canadian Brand Names Lotrimin® Ultra™ [US-OTC]; Mentax® [US]

Therapeutic Category Antifungal Agent

Use Topical treatment of tinea pedis (athlete's foot), tinea cruris (jock itch), tinea corporis (ringworm), and tinea versicolor

Usual Dosage Topical: Children >12 years and Adults:
Tinea corporis, tinea cruris (Lotrimin® Ultra™): Apply once daily for 2 weeks to affected area and surrounding skin
Tinea versicolor (Mentax®): Apply once daily for 2 weeks to affected area and surrounding skin
Tinea pedis (Lotrimin® Ultra™): Apply to affected skin between and around the toes, twice daily for 1 week, or once daily for 4 weeks

Dosage Forms

Cream:
Lotrimin® Ultra™ [OTC]: 1% (12 g, 24 g)
Mentax®: 1% (15 g, 30 g)

butenafine hydrochloride *see* butenafine *on page 163*

Buticaps® ***(Discontinued)***

Butisol Sodium® [US] *see* butabarbital *on page 161*

butoconazole (byoo toe KOE na zole)

Synonyms butoconazole nitrate

U.S./Canadian Brand Names Femstat® One [Can]; Gynazole-1® [US/Can]

Therapeutic Category Antifungal Agent

Use Local treatment of vulvovaginal candidiasis

Usual Dosage Adults: Female: Gynazole-1®: Insert 1 applicatorful (~5 g) intravaginally as a single dose; treatment may need to be extended for up to 6 days in pregnant women (use in pregnancy during 2nd or 3rd trimester only)

Dosage Forms
Cream, vaginal:
Gynazole-1®: 2% (5 g)

butoconazole nitrate *see* butoconazole *on page* 163

butorphanol (byoo TOR fa nole)

Sound-Alike/Look-Alike Issues
Stadol® may be confused with Haldol®, sotalol
Synonyms butorphanol tartrate
U.S./Canadian Brand Names Apo-Butorphanol® [Can]; PMS-Butorphanol [Can]
Therapeutic Category Analgesic, Narcotic
Controlled Substance C-IV
Use
Parenteral: Management of moderate-to-severe pain; preoperative medication; supplement to balanced anesthesia; management of pain during labor
Nasal spray: Management of moderate-to-severe pain, including migraine headache pain
Usual Dosage Note: These are guidelines and do not represent the maximum doses that may be required in all patients. Doses should be titrated to pain relief/prevention. Butorphanol has an analgesic ceiling.
Adults:
Parenteral:
Acute pain (moderate-to-severe):
I.M.: Initial: 2 mg, may repeat every 3-4 hours as needed; usual range: 1-4 mg every 3-4 hours as needed
I.V.: Initial: 1 mg, may repeat every 3-4 hours as needed; usual range: 0.5-2 mg every 3-4 hours as needed
Preoperative medication: I.M.: 2 mg 60-90 minutes before surgery
Supplement to balanced anesthesia: I.V.: 2 mg shortly before induction and/or an incremental dose of 0.5-1 mg (up to 0.06 mg/kg), depending on previously administered sedative, analgesic, and hypnotic medications
Pain during labor (fetus >37 weeks gestation and no signs of fetal distress):
I.M., I.V.: 1-2 mg; may repeat in 4 hours
Note: Alternative analgesia should be used for pain associated with delivery or if delivery is anticipated within 4 hours
Nasal spray:
Moderate-to-severe pain (including migraine headache pain): Initial: 1 spray (~1 mg per spray) in 1 nostril; if adequate pain relief is not achieved within 60-90 minutes, an additional 1 spray in 1 nostril may be given; may repeat initial dose sequence in 3-4 hours after the last dose as needed
Alternatively, an initial dose of 2 mg (1 spray in each nostril) may be used in patients who will be able to remain recumbent (in the event drowsiness or dizziness occurs); additional 2 mg doses should not be given for 3-4 hours
Note: In some clinical trials, an initial dose of 2 mg (as 2 doses 1 hour apart or 2 mg initially - 1 spray in each nostril) has been used, followed by 1 mg in 1 hour; side effects were greater at these dosages
Dosage Forms
Injection, solution [preservative free]: 1 mg/mL (1 mL); 2 mg/mL (1 mL, 2 mL)
Injection, solution [with preservative]: 2 mg/mL (10 mL)
Solution, intranasal [spray]: 10 mg/mL (2.5 mL)

butorphanol tartrate *see* butorphanol *on page* 164
B-Vex D *(Discontinued)* *see* brompheniramine and phenylephrine *on page* 150
B-Vex *(Discontinued)* *see* brompheniramine *on page* 149
B vitamin combinations *see* vitamin B complex combinations *on page* 1017
BW-430C *see* lamotrigine *on page* 567
BW524W91 *see* emtricitabine *on page* 352
Byclomine® Injection *(Discontinued)* *see* dicyclomine *on page* 305
Bydramine® Cough Syrup *(Discontinued)* *see* diphenhydramine *on page* 315
Byetta® [US] *see* exenatide *on page* 401
Bystolic™ [US] *see* nebivolol *on page* 684
C1 esterase inhibitor *see* C1 inhibitor (human) *on page* 165
C1H *see* alemtuzumab *on page* 44

C1-INH *see* C1 inhibitor (human) *on page 165*
C1-inhibitor *see* C1 inhibitor (human) *on page 165*
C1INHRP *see* C1 inhibitor (human) *on page 165*
C2B8 monoclonal antibody *see* rituximab *on page 872*
C7E3 *see* abciximab *on page 17*
C8-CCK *see* sincalide *on page 903*
311C90 *see* zolmitriptan *on page 1033*
C225 *see* cetuximab *on page 205*

C1 inhibitor (human) (cee won in HIB i ter HYU man)

Synonyms C1 esterase inhibitor; C1-INH; C1-inhibitor; C1INHRP; human C1 inhibitor

U.S./Canadian Brand Names Cinryze™ [US]

Therapeutic Category Blood Product Derivative

Use Routine prophylaxis against angioedema attacks in patients with hereditary angioedema (HAE) or inherited C1 inhibitor deficiency

Usual Dosage I.V.: Adolescents and Adults: Routine prophylaxis against HAE attacks: 1000 units every 3-4 days

Dosage Forms

Injection, powder for reconstitution:
Cinryze™: 500 units [contains sucrose 21 mg/mL]

cabergoline (ca BER goe leen)

U.S./Canadian Brand Names CO Cabergoline [Can]; Dostinex® [Can]

Therapeutic Category Ergot-like Derivative

Use Treatment of hyperprolactinemic disorders, either idiopathic or due to pituitary adenomas

Usual Dosage Oral: Initial dose: 0.25 mg twice weekly; the dose may be increased by 0.25 mg twice weekly up to a maximum of 1 mg twice weekly according to the patient's serum prolactin level. Dosage increases should not occur more rapidly than every 4 weeks. Once a normal serum prolactin level is maintained for 6 months, the dose may be discontinued and prolactin levels monitored to determine if cabergoline is still required. The durability of efficacy beyond 24 months of therapy has not been established.

Dosage Forms

Tablet: 0.5 mg

Ca-DTPA *see* diethylene triamine penta-acetic acid *on page 306*
Caduet® [US/Can] *see* amlodipine and atorvastatin *on page 67*
CaEDTA *see* edetate CALCIUM disodium *on page 346*
Caelyx® [Can] *see* doxorubicin (liposomal) *on page 336*
Cafatine-PB® *(Discontinued)* *see* ergotamine *on page 366*
Cafcit® [US] *see* caffeine *on page 165*
CAFdA *see* clofarabine *on page 243*
Cafergor® [Can] *see* ergotamine and caffeine *on page 366*
Cafergot® [US] *see* ergotamine and caffeine *on page 366*
Cafetrate® *(Discontinued)* *see* ergotamine *on page 366*

caffeine (KAF een)

Synonyms caffeine and sodium benzoate; caffeine citrate; sodium benzoate and caffeine

U.S./Canadian Brand Names Cafcit® [US]; Enerjets [US-OTC]; No Doz® Maximum Strength [US-OTC]; Vivarin® [US-OTC]

Therapeutic Category Stimulant

Use

Caffeine citrate: Treatment of idiopathic apnea of prematurity
Caffeine and sodium benzoate: Treatment of acute respiratory depression (not a preferred agent)
Caffeine [OTC labeling]: Restore mental alertness or wakefulness when experiencing fatigue

Usual Dosage Note: Caffeine citrate should not be interchanged with the caffeine sodium benzoate formulation.

Caffeine citrate: Neonates: Apnea of prematurity: Oral, I.V.:

Loading dose: 10-20 mg/kg as caffeine citrate (5-10 mg/kg as caffeine base). If theophylline has been administered to the patient within the previous 3 days, a full or modified loading dose (50% to 75% of a loading dose) may be given.

Maintenance dose: 5 mg/kg/day as caffeine citrate (2.5 mg/kg/day as caffeine base) once daily starting 24 hours after the loading dose. Maintenance dose is adjusted based on patient's response and serum caffeine concentrations.

Caffeine and sodium benzoate:

Children: Stimulant: I.M., I.V., SubQ: 8 mg/kg every 4 hours as needed

Children ≥12 years and Adults: OTC labeling (stimulant): Oral: 100-200 mg every 3-4 hours as needed

Adults:

Electroconvulsive therapy: I.V.: 300-2000 mg

Respiratory depression: I.M., I.V.: 250 mg as a single dose; may repeat as needed. Maximum single dose should be limited to 500 mg; maximum amount in any 24-hour period should generally be limited to 2500 mg.

Dosage Forms

Caplet:

No Doz® Maximum Strength [OTC], Vivarin® [OTC]: 200 mg

Injection, solution [preservative free]: 20 mg/mL (3 mL)

Cafcit®: 20 mg/mL (3 mL)

Lozenge:

Enerjets® [OTC]: 75 mg

Solution, oral [preservative free]: 20 mg/mL (3 mL)

Cafcit®: 20 mg/mL

Tablet: 200 mg

Vivarin® [OTC]: 200 mg

caffeine, acetaminophen, and aspirin *see* acetaminophen, aspirin, and caffeine *on page* 24

caffeine, acetaminophen, butalbital, and codeine *see* butalbital, acetaminophen, caffeine, and codeine *on page* 162

caffeine and ergotamine *see* ergotamine and caffeine *on page* 366

caffeine and sodium benzoate *see* caffeine *on page* 165

caffeine, aspirin, and acetaminophen *see* acetaminophen, aspirin, and caffeine *on page* 24

caffeine citrate *see* caffeine *on page* 165

caffeine, dihydrocodeine, and acetaminophen *see* acetaminophen, caffeine, and dihydrocodeine *on page* 25

caffeine, orphenadrine, and aspirin *see* orphenadrine, aspirin, and caffeine *on page* 730

Cal-C-Caps [US-OTC] *see* calcium citrate *on page* 172

Caladryl® Clear [US-OTC] *see* pramoxine *on page* 809

CalaMycin® Cool and Clear [US-OTC] *see* pramoxine *on page* 809

Calan® [US/Can] *see* verapamil *on page* 1010

Calan® SR [US] *see* verapamil *on page* 1010

Calcarb 600 [US-OTC] *see* calcium carbonate *on page* 170

Cal-Cee [US-OTC] *see* calcium citrate *on page* 172

Calci-Chew® [US-OTC] *see* calcium carbonate *on page* 170

Calciday-667® *(Discontinued)* *see* calcium carbonate *on page* 170

Calciferol™ Injection *(Discontinued)* *see* ergocalciferol *on page* 364

CalciFolic-D™ [US] *see* vitamins (multiple/oral) *on page* 1019

Calcijex® [US/Can] *see* calcitriol *on page* 168

Calcimar® [Can] *see* calcitonin *on page* 167

Calcimar® *(Discontinued)* *see* calcitonin *on page* 167

Calci-Mix® [US-OTC] *see* calcium carbonate *on page* 170

Calcionate [US-OTC] *see* calcium glubionate *on page* 173

calcipotriene (kal si POE try een)

U.S./Canadian Brand Names Dovonex® [US/Can]

Therapeutic Category Antipsoriatic Agent

Use Treatment of plaque psoriasis; chronic, moderate-to-severe psoriasis of the scalp

Usual Dosage Topical: Adults:

Cream: Apply a thin film to the affected skin twice daily and rub in gently and completely, for up to 8 weeks

Solution: Apply to the affected scalp twice daily and rub in gently and completely, for up to 8 weeks

Dosage Forms

Cream:

Dovonex® [OTC]: 0.005% (60 g, 120 g)

Solution, topical: 0.005% (60 mL)

Dovonex® [OTC]: 0.005% (60 mL)

calcipotriene and betamethasone (kal si POE try een & bay ta METH a sone)

Synonyms betamethasone dipropionate and calcipotriene hydrate; calcipotriol and betamethasone dipropionate

U.S./Canadian Brand Names Dovobet® [Can]; Taclonex Scalp® [US]; Taclonex® [US]

Therapeutic Category Corticosteroid, Topical; Vitamin D Analog

Use Treatment of psoriasis vulgaris

Usual Dosage Topical: Adults: Psoriasis vulgaris:

Cream/ointment: Apply to affected area once daily for up to 4 weeks (maximum recommended dose: 100 g/week). Application to >30% of body surface area is not recommended.

Suspension: Apply to affected area of the scalp once daily for 2 weeks or until clear; may continue for up to 8 weeks (maximum recommended dose: 100 g/week)

Dosage Forms [CAN] = Canadian brand name

Cream, topical:

Dovobet® [CAN]: Calcipotriol 50 mcg and betamethasone 0.5 mg per gram (3 g, 30 g, 60 g, 100 g, 120 g) [not available in the U.S.]

Ointment, topical:

Taclonex®: Calcipotriene 0.005% and betamethasone 0.064% (60 g, 100 g)

Suspension, topical:

Taclonex Scalp®: Calcipotriene 0.005% and betamethasone 0.064% (15 g, 30 g, 60 g, 2 x 60 g)

calcipotriol and betamethasone dipropionate *see* calcipotriene and betamethasone *on page 167*

Calcite-500 [Can] *see* calcium carbonate *on page 170*

calcitonin (kal si TOE nin)

Sound-Alike/Look-Alike Issues

calcitonin may be confused with calcitriol

Miacalcin® may be confused with Micatin®

Synonyms calcitonin (salmon)

U.S./Canadian Brand Names Apo-Calcitonin® [Can]; Calcimar® [Can]; Caltine® [Can]; Fortical® [US]; Miacalcin® NS [Can]; Miacalcin® [US]; Pro-Calcitonin [Can]

Therapeutic Category Polypeptide Hormone

Use Calcitonin (salmon): Treatment of Paget disease of bone (osteitis deformans); adjunctive therapy for hypercalcemia; treatment of osteoporosis in women >5 years postmenopause

Usual Dosage Adults:

Paget disease (Miacalcin®): I.M., SubQ: Initial: 100 units/day; maintenance: 50 units/day or 50-100 units every 1-3 days

Hypercalcemia (Miacalcin®): I.M., SubQ: Initial: 4 units/kg every 12 hours; may increase up to 8 units/kg every 12 hours to a maximum of every 6 hours

Postmenopausal osteoporosis:

I.M., SubQ: Miacalcin®: 100 units/every other day

Intranasal: Fortical®, Miacalcin®: 200 units (1 spray) in one nostril daily

Dosage Forms

Injection, solution [calcitonin-salmon]:

Miacalcin®: 200 int. units/mL (2 mL)

Solution, intranasal [spray, calcitonin-salmon]: 2200 int. units/mL (3.7 mL)

Fortical®: 200 int. units/0.09 mL (3.7 mL)

Miacalcin®: 200 int. units/0.09 mL (3.7 mL)

calcitonin (salmon) *see* calcitonin *on page 167*

Cal-Citrate-225 [US] *see* calcium citrate *on page 172*

calcitriol (kal si TRYE ole)

Sound-Alike/Look-Alike Issues

calcitriol may be confused with calcifediol, Calciferol®, calcitonin, calcium carbonate, captopril, colestipol, paricalcitol, ropinirole

Synonyms 1,25 dihydroxycholecalciferol

U.S./Canadian Brand Names Calcijex® [US/Can]; Rocaltrol® [US/Can]; Vectical™ [US]

Therapeutic Category Vitamin D Analog

Use

Oral, injection: Management of hypocalcemia in patients on chronic renal dialysis; management of secondary hyperparathyroidism in patients with chronic kidney disease (CKD); management of hypocalcemia in hypoparathyroidism and pseudohypoparathyroidism

Topical: Management of mild-to-moderate plaque psoriasis

Usual Dosage

Hypocalcemia in patients on chronic renal dialysis (manufacturer labeling): *Adults:*

Oral: 0.25 mcg/day or every other day (may require 0.5-1 mcg/day); increases should be made at 4- to 8-week intervals

I.V.: Initial: 1-2 mcg 3 times/week (0.02 mcg/kg) approximately every other day. Adjust dose at 2-4 week intervals; dosing range: 0.5-4 mcg 3 times/week

Hypocalcemia in hypoparathyroidism/pseudohypoparathyroidism (manufacturers labeling): Oral (evaluate dosage at 2- to 4-week intervals):

Children 1-5 years: 0.25-0.75 mcg once daily

Children ≥6 years and Adults: Initial: 0.25 mcg/day, range: 0.5-2 mcg once daily

Secondary hyperparathyroidism associated with moderate-to-severe CKD in patients not on dialysis (manufacturer labeling): Oral:

Children <3 years: Initial dose: 0.01-0.015 mcg/kg/day

Children ≥3 years and Adults: 0.25 mcg/day; may increase to 0.5 mcg/day

K/DOQI guidelines for vitamin D therapy in CKD:

Children:

CKD stage 2, 3: Oral:

<10 kg: 0.05 mcg every other day

10-20 kg: 0.1-0.15 mcg/day

>20 kg: 0.25 mcg/day

Note: Treatment should only be started with serum 25(OH) D >30 ng/mL, serum iPTH >70 pg/mL, serum calcium <10 mg/dL and serum phosphorus less than or equal to the age appropriate level.

CKD stage 4: Oral:

<10 kg: 0.05 mcg every other day

10-20 kg: 0.1-0.15 mcg/day

>20 kg: 0.25 mcg/day

Note: Treatment should only be started with serum 25(OH) D >30 ng/mL, serum iPTH >110 pg/mL, serum calcium <10 mg/dL and serum phosphorus less than or equal to the age appropriate level.

CKD stage 5: Oral, I.V.: **Note:** The following initial doses are based on plasma PTH and serum calcium levels for patients with serum phosphorus <5.5 mg/dL in adolescents or <6.5 in infants and children, and Ca-P product <55 in adolescents or <65 in infants and children <12 years. Adjust dose based on serum phosphate, calcium and PTH levels. Administer dose with each dialysis session (3 times/week). Intermittent I.V./oral administration is more effective than daily oral dosing.

Plasma PTH 300-500 pg/mL and serum Ca <10 mg/dL: 0.0075 mcg/kg (maximum: 0.25 mcg/day)

Plasma PTH >500-1000 pg/mL and serum Ca <10 mg/dL: 0.015 mcg/kg (maximum: 0.5 mcg/day)

Plasma PTH >1000 pg/mL and serum Ca <10.5 mg/dL: 0.025 mcg/kg (maximum: 1 mcg/day)

Adults:

CKD stage 3: Oral: 0.25 mcg/day. Treatment should only be started with serum 25(OH) D >30 ng/mL, serum iPTH >70 pg/mL, serum calcium <9.5 mg/dL and serum phosphorus <4.6 mg/dL

CKD stage 4: Oral: 0.25 mcg/day. Treatment should only be started with serum 25(OH) D >30 ng/mL, serum iPTH >110 pg/mL, serum calcium <9.5 mg/dL and serum phosphorus <4.6 mg/dL

CKD stage 5:

Peritoneal dialysis: Oral: Initial: 0.5-1 mcg 2-3 times/week or 0.25 mcg/day

Hemodialysis: **Note:** The following initial doses are based on plasma PTH and serum calcium levels for patients with serum phosphorus <5.5 mg/dL and Ca-P product <55. Adjust dose based on serum phosphate, calcium, and PTH levels. Intermittent I.V. administration may be more effective than daily oral dosing.

Plasma PTH 300-600 pg/mL and serum Ca <9.5 mg/dL: Oral, I.V.: 0.5-1.5 mcg

Plasma PTH 600-1000 pg/mL and serum Ca <9.5 mg/dL:
Oral: 1-4 mcg
I.V: 1-3 mcg
Plasma PTH >1000 pg/mL and serum Ca <10 mg/dL:
Oral: 3-7 mcg
I.V.: 3-5 mcg
Psoriasis: Adults: Topical: Apply twice daily to affected areas (maximum: 200 g/week)

Dosage Forms
Capsule: 0.25 mcg, 0.5 mcg
Rocaltrol®: 0.25 mcg, 0.5 mcg
Injection, solution: 1 mcg/mL (1 mL)
Calcijex®: 1 mcg/mL (1 mL)
Ointment, topical:
Vectical™: 3 mcg/g (100 g)
Solution, oral: 1 mcg/mL
Rocaltrol®: 1 mcg/mL

calcium acetate (KAL see um AS e tate)

Sound-Alike/Look-Alike Issues
PhosLo® may be confused with Phos-Flur®, ProSom™

U.S./Canadian Brand Names PhosLo® [US/Can]

Therapeutic Category Electrolyte Supplement, Oral

Use Control of hyperphosphatemia in end-stage renal failure; does not promote aluminum absorption

Usual Dosage
Dietary Reference Intake:
0-6 months: 210 mg/day
7-12 months: 270 mg/day
1-3 years: 500 mg/day
4-8 years: 800 mg/day
Adults, Male/Female:
9-18 years: 1300 mg/day
19-50 years: 1000 mg/day
≥51 years: 1200 mg/day
Female: Pregnancy/lactating: Same as for Adults, Male/Female
Oral: Adults, on dialysis: Initial: 1334 mg with each meal, can be increased gradually to bring the serum phosphate value to <6 mg/dL as long as hypercalcemia does not develop (usual dose: 2001-2868 mg calcium acetate with each meal); do not give additional calcium supplements

Dosage Forms
Gelcap: 667 mg
PhosLo®: 667 mg

calcium acetate and aluminum sulfate *see* aluminum sulfate and calcium acetate *on page 57*
calcium acetylhomotaurinate *see* acamprosate *on page 18*
calcium and risedronate *see* risedronate and calcium *on page 870*

calcium and vitamin D (KAL see um & VYE ta min dee)

Synonyms vitamin D and calcium carbonate

U.S./Canadian Brand Names Cal-CYUM [US-OTC]; Caltrate® 600+ Soy™ [US-OTC]; Caltrate® 600+D [US-OTC]; Caltrate® ColonHealth™ [US-OTC]; Chew-Cal [US-OTC]; Liqua-Cal [US-OTC]; Os-Cal® 500+D [US-OTC]; Oysco 500+D [US-OTC]; Oysco D [US-OTC]; Oyst-Cal-D 500 [US-OTC]; Oyst-Cal-D [US-OTC]

Therapeutic Category Calcium Salt; Electrolyte Supplement, Oral; Vitamin, Fat Soluble

Use Dietary supplement, antacid

Usual Dosage Oral: Adults: Refer to individual monographs for dietary reference intake.

Dosage Forms
Capsule, softgel: Calcium 500 mg and vitamin D 500 int. units; calcium 600 mg and vitamin D 100 int. units; calcium 600 mg and vitamin D 200 int. units
Liqua-Cal: Calcium 600 mg and vitamin D 200 int. units

Tablet: Calcium 250 mg and vitamin D 125 int. units; calcium 500 mg and vitamin D 125 int. units; calcium 500 mg and vitamin D 200 int. units; calcium 600 mg and vitamin D 125 int. units; calcium 600 mg and vitamin D 200 int. units

Caltrate® 600+D: Calcium 600 mg and vitamin D 200 int. units
Caltrate® 600+ Soy™: Calcium 600 mg and vitamin D 200 int. units
Caltrate® ColonHealth™: Calcium 600 mg and vitamin D 200 int. units
Oysco D: Calcium 250 mg and vitamin D 125 int. units
Oysco 500+D: Calcium 500 mg and vitamin D 200 int. units
Oyst-Cal-D: Calcium 250 mg and vitamin D 125 int. units
Oyst-Cal-D 500: Calcium 500 mg and vitamin D 200 int. units

Tablet, chewable: Calcium 500 mg and vitamin D 100 int. units; calcium 600 mg and vitamin D 400 int. units

Os-Cal® 500+D: Calcium 500 mg and vitamin D 400 int. units

Wafer, chewable:

Cal-CYUM: Calcium 519 mg and vitamin D 150 int. units (50s)
Chew-Cal: Calcium 333 mg and vitamin D 40 int. units (100s, 250s)

calcium carbonate (KAL see um KAR bun ate)

Sound-Alike/Look-Alike Issues

calcium carbonate may be confused with calcitriol
Florical® may be confused with Fiorinal®
Mylanta® may be confused with Mynatal®
Nephro-Calci® may be confused with Nephrocaps®
Os-Cal® may be confused with Asacol®

Synonyms oscal

U.S./Canadian Brand Names Alcalak [US-OTC]; Alka-Mints® [US-OTC]; Apo-Cal® [Can]; Cal-Gest [US-OTC]; Cal-Mint [US-OTC]; Calcarb 600 [US-OTC]; Calci-Chew® [US-OTC]; Calci-Mix® [US-OTC]; Calcite-500 [Can]; Caltrate® 600 [US-OTC]; Caltrate® Select [Can]; Caltrate® [Can]; Children's Pepto [US-OTC]; Chooz® [US-OTC]; Florical® [US-OTC]; Maalox® Regular Chewable [US-OTC]; Mylanta® Children's [US-OTC]; Nephro-Calci® [US-OTC]; Nutralox® [US-OTC]; Os-Cal® [Can]; Oysco 500 [US-OTC]; Oyst-Cal 500 [US-OTC]; Rolaids® Softchews [US-OTC]; Titralac™ [US-OTC]; Tums® E-X [US-OTC]; Tums® Extra Strength Sugar Free [US-OTC]; Tums® Smoothies™ [US-OTC]; Tums® Ultra [US-OTC]; Tums® [US-OTC]

Therapeutic Category Antacid; Electrolyte Supplement, Oral

Use As an antacid; treatment and prevention of calcium deficiency or hyperphosphatemia (eg, osteoporosis, osteomalacia, mild/moderate renal insufficiency, hypoparathyroidism, postmenopausal osteoporosis, rickets); has been used to bind phosphate

Usual Dosage Oral (dosage is in terms of elemental calcium):

Dietary Reference Intake:

0-6 months: 210 mg/day
7-12 months: 270 mg/day
1-3 years: 500 mg/day
4-8 years: 800 mg/day
Adults, Male/Female:
9-18 years: 1300 mg/day
19-50 years: 1000 mg/day
≥51 years: 1200 mg/day
Female: Pregnancy/Lactating: Same as for Adults, Male/Female

Hypocalcemia (dose depends on clinical condition and serum calcium level): Dose expressed in mg of **elemental calcium**

Neonates: 50-150 mg/kg/day in 4-6 divided doses; not to exceed 1 g/day
Children: 45-65 mg/kg/day in 4 divided doses
Adults: 1-2 g or more/day in 3-4 divided doses

Antacid:

Children 2-5 years (24-47 lb): Elemental calcium 161 mg as needed; maximum 483 mg per 24 hours
Children 6-11 years (48-95 lb): Elemental calcium 322 mg as needed; maximum: 966 mg per 24 hours
Adults: Dosage based on acid-neutralizing capacity of specific product; generally, 1-2 tablets or 5-10 mL every 2 hours; maximum: 7000 mg calcium carbonate per 24 hours; specific product labeling should be consulted

Dietary supplementation: Adults: 500 mg to 2 g divided 2-4 times/day

Osteoporosis: Adults >51 years: 1200 mg/day

Dosage Forms

Capsule: 364 mg, 1250 mg
Calci-Mix® [OTC]: 1250 mg
Florical® [OTC]: 364 mg
Gum, chewing: 250 mg (30s)
Chooz® [OTC]: 500 mg (12s)
Powder: 4000 mg/teaspoonful
Suspension, oral: 1250 mg/5 mL
Tablet: 1250 mg, 1500 mg
Calcarb 600 [OTC], Caltrate® 600 [OTC], Nephro-Calci® [OTC]: 1500 mg
Florical® [OTC]: 364 mg
Oysco 500 [OTC], Oyst-Cal 500 [OTC]: 1250 mg
Tablet, chewable: 500 mg, 650 mg, 750 mg
Alcalak [OTC], Nutralox® [OTC], Titralac™ [OTC]: 420 mg
Alka-Mints® [OTC]: 850 mg
Cal-Gest [OTC], Tums® [OTC]: 500 mg
Calci-Chew® [OTC]: 1250 mg
Cal-Mint [OTC]: 650 mg
Children's Pepto [OTC], Mylanta® Children's [OTC]: 400 mg
Maalox® Regular [OTC]: 600 mg
Tums® E-X [OTC], Tums® Extra Strength Sugar Free [OTC], Tums® Smoothies™ [OTC]: 750 mg
Tums® Ultra [OTC]: 1000 mg
Tablet, softchew: 1177 mg
Rolaids® [OTC]: 1177 mg

calcium carbonate and etidronate disodium *see* etidronate and calcium *(Canada only) on page 396*

calcium carbonate and magnesium hydroxide

(KAL see um KAR bun ate & mag NEE zhum hye DRÓKS ide)

Sound-Alike/Look-Alike Issues

Mylanta® may be confused with Mynatal®

Synonyms magnesium hydroxide and calcium carbonate

U.S./Canadian Brand Names Mi-Acid™ Double Strength [US-OTC]; Mylanta® Gelcaps® [US-OTC]; Mylanta® Supreme [US-OTC]; Mylanta® Ultra [US-OTC]; Rolaids® Extra Strength [US-OTC]; Rolaids® [US-OTC]

Therapeutic Category Antacid

Use Hyperacidity

Usual Dosage Oral: Adults: 2-4 tablets between meals, at bedtime, or as directed by healthcare provider

Dosage Forms

Gelcap:
Mylanta® Gelcaps® [OTC]: Calcium carbonate 550 mg and magnesium hydroxide 125 mg
Liquid:
Mylanta® Supreme [OTC]: Calcium carbonate 400 mg and magnesium hydroxide 135 mg per 5 mL
Tablet, chewable: Calcium carbonate 550 mg and magnesium hydroxide 110 mg; calcium carbonate 675 mg and magnesium hydroxide 135 mg; calcium carbonate 700 mg and magnesium hydroxide 300 mg
Mi-Acid™ Double Strength [OTC], Mylanta® Ultra [OTC]: Calcium carbonate 700 mg and magnesium hydroxide 300 mg
Rolaids® [OTC]: Calcium carbonate 550 mg and magnesium hydroxide 110 mg
Rolaids® Extra Strength [OTC]: Calcium carbonate 675 mg and magnesium hydroxide 135 mg

calcium carbonate and simethicone (KAL see um KAR bun ate & sye METH i kone)

Synonyms simethicone and calcium carbonate

U.S./Canadian Brand Names Gas Ban™ [US-OTC]; Titralac® Plus [US-OTC]

Therapeutic Category Antacid; Antiflatulent

Use Relief of acid indigestion, heartburn

Usual Dosage Oral (OTC labeling): Adults: Two tablets every 2-3 hours as needed (maximum: 19 tablets/ 24 hours)

Dosage Forms

Tablet, chewable:

Gas Ban™ [OTC]: Calcium carbonate 300 mg and simethicone 40 mg

Titralac® Plus [OTC]: Calcium carbonate 420 mg and simethicone 21 mg

calcium carbonate, magnesium hydroxide, and famotidine *see* famotidine, calcium carbonate, and magnesium hydroxide *on page 406*

calcium chloride (KAL see um KLOR ide)

Therapeutic Category Electrolyte Supplement, Oral

Use Treatment of acute symptomatic hypocalcemia; cardiac disturbances of hyperkalemia or hypocalcemia; emergent treatment of hypocalcemic tetany; treatment of severe hypermagnesemia

Usual Dosage **Note:** One gram of calcium chloride is equal to 270 mg of elemental calcium.

Dosages are expressed in terms of the calcium chloride salt based on a solution concentration of 100 mg/mL (10%) containing 1.4 mEq (27.3 mg)/mL elemental calcium.

Acute, symptomatic ionized hypocalcemia, hyperkalemia, or magnesium toxicity: **Note:** Routine use in cardiac arrest is not recommended due to the lack of improved survival: I.V.:

Neonates: 20 mg/kg; may repeat as necessary

Infants and Children: 20 mg/kg; may repeat as necessary

Adults: 500-1000 mg, may repeat as necessary

Hypocalcemia secondary to citrated blood transfusion: I.V.: **Note:** Routine administration of calcium, in the absence of signs/symptoms of hypocalcemia, is generally not recommended. A number of recommendations have been published seeking to address potential hypocalcemia during massive transfusion of citrated blood; however, many practitioners recommend replacement only as guided by clinical evidence of hypocalcemia and/or serial monitoring of ionized calcium. In adults, clinically-significant hypocalcemia usually dose not occur until >5 units of packed red blood cells have been administered.

Neonates, Infants, and Children: Give 32 mg (0.45 mEq elemental calcium) for each 100 mL citrated blood infused

Adults: 200-500 mg per 500 mL of citrated blood (infused into another vein)

Hypocalcemic tetany: I.V.:

Neonates: 40-60 mg/kg/dose repeated every 6-8 hours

Infants and Children: 10 mg/kg over 5-10 minutes; may repeat after 6-8 hours or follow with an infusion with a maximum dose of 200 mg/kg/day; alternatively, higher doses of 35-50 mg/kg/dose repeated every 6-8 hours have been used

Adults: 1000 mg over 10-30 minutes; may repeat after 6 hours

Dosage Forms

Injection, solution [preservative free]: 10% (10 mL)

Injection, solution: [with preservative]: 10% (10 mL)

calcium citrate (KAL see um SIT rate)

Sound-Alike/Look-Alike Issues

Citracal® may be confused with Citrucel®

U.S./Canadian Brand Names Cal-C-Caps [US-OTC]; Cal-Cee [US-OTC]; Cal-Citrate-225 [US]; Osteocit® [Can]

Therapeutic Category Electrolyte Supplement, Oral

Use Antacid; treatment and prevention of calcium deficiency or hyperphosphatemia (eg, osteoporosis, osteomalacia, mild/moderate renal insufficiency, hypoparathyroidism, postmenopausal osteoporosis, rickets)

Usual Dosage Oral: Dosage is in terms of elemental calcium

Dietary Reference Intake:

0-6 months: 210 mg/day

7-12 months: 270 mg/day

1-3 years: 500 mg/day

4-8 years: 800 mg/day

Adults, Male/Female:

- 9-18 years: 1300 mg/day
- 19-50 years: 1000 mg/day
- ≥51 years: 1200 mg/day

Female: Pregnancy/Lactating: Same as for Adults, Male/Female

Dietary supplement: Usual dose: 500-2000 mg divided 2-4 times/day

Dosage Forms

Capsule:

Cal-C-Caps [OTC]: Elemental calcium 180 mg

Cal-Citrate-225: Elemental calcium 225 mg

Granules: Elemental calcium 760 mg/teaspoonful

Tablet: Elemental calcium 200 mg, 250 mg

Cal-Cee [OTC]: Elemental calcium 250 mg

calcium disodium edetate *see* edetate CALCIUM disodium *on page 346*

Calcium Disodium Versenate® [US] *see* edetate CALCIUM disodium *on page 346*

calcium glubionate (KAL see um gloo BYE oh nate)

Sound-Alike/Look-Alike Issues

calcium glubionate may be confused with calcium gluconate

U.S./Canadian Brand Names Calcionate [US-OTC]

Therapeutic Category Electrolyte Supplement, Oral

Use Dietary supplement

Usual Dosage Dosage is in terms of **elemental** calcium

Dietary Reference Intake:

0-6 months: 210 mg/day

7-12 months: 270 mg/day

1-3 years: 500 mg/day

4-8 years: 800 mg/day

Adults, Male/Female:

9-18 years: 1300 mg/day

19-50 years: 1000 mg/day

≥51 years: 1200 mg/day

Female: Pregnancy/Lactating: Same as for Adults, Male/Female

Dietary supplement: Oral:

Infants <12 months: 1 teaspoonful 5 times a day; may mix with juice or formula

Children <4 years: 2 teaspoonsful 3 times a day

Children ≥4 years and Adults: 1 tablespoonful 3 times a day

Pregnant or lactating women: 1 tablespoonful 4 times a day

Dosage Forms

Syrup:

Calcionate: 1.8 g/5 mL

calcium gluconate (KAL see um GLOO koe nate)

Sound-Alike/Look-Alike Issues

calcium gluconate may be confused with calcium glubionate

U.S./Canadian Brand Names Cal-G [US-OTC]; Cal-GLU™ [US]

Therapeutic Category Electrolyte Supplement, Oral

Use Treatment and prevention of hypocalcemia; treatment of tetany, cardiac disturbances of hyperkalemia, cardiac resuscitation when epinephrine fails to improve myocardial contractions, hypocalcemia; calcium supplementation; hydrofluoric acid (HF) burns

Usual Dosage

Adequate Intake (as elemental calcium):

0-6 months: 210 mg/day

7-12 months: 270 mg/day

1-3 years: 500 mg/day

4-8 years: 800 mg/day

9-18 years: 1300 mg/day

Adults, Male/Female:

19-50 years: 1000 mg/day

≥51 years: 1200 mg/day

Female: Pregnancy/Lactating: Same as for Adults, Male/Female

Dosage note: Calcium chloride has 3 times more elemental calcium than calcium gluconate. Calcium chloride is 27% elemental calcium; calcium gluconate is 9% elemental calcium. One gram of calcium chloride is equal to 270 mg of elemental calcium; 1 gram of calcium gluconate is equal to 90 mg of elemental calcium. The following dosages are expressed in terms of the calcium gluconate salt based on a solution concentration of 100 mg/mL (10%) containing 0.465 mEq (9.3 mg)/mL elemental calcium:

Hypocalcemia: I.V.:

Neonates: 200-800 mg/kg/day as a continuous infusion or in 4 divided doses (maximum: 1 g/dose)

Infants and Children: 200-500 mg/kg/day as a continuous infusion or in 4 divided doses (maximum: 2-3 g/dose)

Adults: 2-15 g/24 hours as a continuous infusion or in divided doses

Hypocalcemia: Oral:

Children: 200-500 mg/kg/day divided every 6 hours

Adults: 500 mg to 2 g 2-4 times/day

Hypocalcemia secondary to citrated blood infusion: I.V.: **Note:** Routine administration of calcium, in the absence of signs/symptoms of hypocalcemia, is generally not recommended. A number of recommendations have been published seeking to address potential hypocalcemia during massive transfusion of citrated blood; however, many practitioners recommend replacement only as guided by clinical evidence of hypocalcemia and/or serial monitoring of ionized calcium.

Neonates, Infants, and Children: Give 98 mg (0.45 mEq **elemental** calcium) for each 100 mL citrated blood infused

Adults: 500 mg to 1 g per 500 mL of citrated blood (infused into another vein). Single doses up to 2 g have also been recommended.

Hypocalcemic tetany: I.V.:

Neonates, Infants, and Children: 100-200 mg/kg/dose over 5-10 minutes; may repeat every 6-8 hours **or** follow with an infusion of 500 mg/kg/day

Adults: 1-3 g may be administered until therapeutic response occurs

Magnesium intoxication, cardiac arrest in the presence of hyperkalemia or hypocalcemia: I.V.:

Infants and Children: 60-100 mg/kg/dose (maximum: 3 g/dose)

Adults: 500-800 mg/dose (maximum: 3 g/dose)

Maintenance electrolyte requirements for total parenteral nutrition: I.V.: Daily requirements: Adults: 1.7-3.4 g/1000 kcal/24 hours

Dosage Forms

Capsule, oral:

Cal-G: 700 mg

Capsule, oral [preservative free]:

Cal-GLU™: 515 mg

Injection, solution [preservative free]: 10% (10 mL, 50 mL, 100 mL, 200 mL) [100 mg/mL]

Powder: 347 mg/tablespoonful

Tablet: 500 mg, 650 mg, 975 mg

calcium lactate (KAL see um LAK tate)

Therapeutic Category Electrolyte Supplement, Oral

Use Adjunct in prevention of postmenopausal osteoporosis; treatment and prevention of calcium depletion

Usual Dosage Oral (in terms of calcium lactate):

Dietary Reference Intake (in terms of elemental calcium):

0-6 months: 210 mg/day

7-12 months: 270 mg/day

1-3 years: 500 mg/day

4-8 years: 800 mg/day

9-18 years: 1300 mg/day

Adults, Male/Female:

19-50 years: 1000 mg/day

≥51 years: 1200 mg/day

Female: Pregnancy/Lactating: Same as Adults, Male/Female

Dosage Forms

Tablet: 650 mg

calcium leucovorin *see* leucovorin calcium *on page* 575

calcium levoleucovorin *see* LEVOleucovorin *on page* 581

calcium pantothenate *see* pantothenic acid *on page* 749

calcium phosphate (tribasic) (KAL see um FOS fate tri BAY sik)

Synonyms tricalcium phosphate

U.S./Canadian Brand Names Posture® [US-OTC]

Therapeutic Category Electrolyte Supplement, Oral

Use Dietary supplement

Usual Dosage Oral:

Adequate Intake (as elemental calcium):

0-6 months: 210 mg/day
7-12 months: 270 mg/day
1-3 years: 500 mg/day
4-8 years: 800 mg/day
9-18 years: 1300 mg/day
Adults, Male/Female:
19-50 years: 1000 mg/day
≥51 years: 1200 mg/day
Female: Pregnancy/Lactating: Same as for Adults, Male/Female

Dietary supplement: Adults: 2 tablets daily

Dosage Forms

Caplet:

Posture® [OTC]: Calcium 600 mg and phosphorus 280 mg

Cal-CYUM [US-OTC] *see* calcium and vitamin D *on page 169*

Caldecort® [US-OTC] *see* hydrocortisone (topical) *on page 505*

Caldolor™ [US] *see* ibuprofen *on page 515*

calfactant (kaf AKT ant)

U.S./Canadian Brand Names Infasurf® [US]

Therapeutic Category Lung Surfactant

Use Prevention of respiratory distress syndrome (RDS) in premature infants at high risk for RDS and for the treatment ("rescue") of premature infants who develop RDS

Prophylaxis: Therapy at birth with calfactant is indicated for premature infants <29 weeks of gestational age at significant risk for RDS. Should be administered as soon as possible, preferably within 30 minutes after birth.

Treatment: For infants ≤72 hours of age with RDS (confirmed by clinical and radiologic findings) and requiring endotracheal intubation.

Usual Dosage Intratracheal administration **only**: Each dose is 3 mL/kg body weight at birth; should be administered every 12 hours for a total of up to 3 doses

Dosage Forms

Suspension, intratracheal [preservative free]:

Infasurf®: 35 mg/mL

Cal-G [US-OTC] *see* calcium gluconate *on page 173*

Cal-Gest [US-OTC] *see* calcium carbonate *on page 170*

Cal-GLU™ [US] *see* calcium gluconate *on page 173*

Callergy Clear [US-OTC] *see* pramoxine *on page 809*

Calm-X® Oral *(Discontinued)* *see* dimenhydrinate *on page 312*

Cal-Mint [US-OTC] *see* calcium carbonate *on page 170*

Calmylin with Codeine [Can] *see* guaifenesin, pseudoephedrine, and codeine *on page 479*

Calna [US-OTC] *see* vitamins (multiple/prenatal) *on page 1020*

Cal-Nate™ *(Discontinued)* *see* vitamins (multiple/prenatal) *on page 1020*

CaloMist™ [US] *see* cyanocobalamin *on page 263*

Calphron® *(Discontinued)* *see* calcium acetate *on page 169*

Cal-Plus® *(Discontinued)* *see* calcium carbonate *on page 170*

Caltine® [Can] *see* calcitonin *on page 167*

Caltrate® [Can] *see* calcium carbonate *on page 170*

Caltrate® 600 [US-OTC] *see* calcium carbonate *on page 170*

Caltrate® 600+D [US-OTC] *see* calcium and vitamin D *on page 169*

Caltrate® 600+ Soy™ [US-OTC] *see* calcium and vitamin D *on page 169*

Caltrate® ColonHealth™ [US-OTC] *see* calcium and vitamin D *on page 169*
Caltrate® Jr. ***(Discontinued)*** *see* calcium carbonate *on page 170*
Caltrate® Select [Can] *see* calcium carbonate *on page 170*
Camila™ [US] *see* norethindrone *on page 704*
Campath® [US] *see* alemtuzumab *on page 44*
campath-1H *see* alemtuzumab *on page 44*
Campho-Phenique® [US-OTC] *see* camphor and phenol *on page 176*

camphor and phenol (KAM for & FEE nole)

Synonyms phenol and camphor

U.S./Canadian Brand Names Campho-Phenique® [US-OTC]

Therapeutic Category Topical Skin Product

Use Relief of pain and itching associated with minor burns, sunburn, minor cuts, insect bites, minor skin irritation; temporary relief of pain from cold sores

Usual Dosage Topical: Adults: Relief of pain/itching: Apply 1-3 times/day

Dosage Forms

Gel, topical:

Campho-Phenique® [OTC]: Camphor 10.8% and phenol 4.7% (7 g, 14 g)

Liquid, topical: Camphor 10.8% and phenol 4.7% (45 mL)

Campho-Phenique® [OTC]: Camphor 10.8% and phenol 4.7% (22.5 mL, 45 mL)

Campral® [US/Can] *see* acamprosate *on page 18*
Camptosar® [US/Can] *see* irinotecan *on page 546*
camptothecin-11 *see* irinotecan *on page 546*

canakinumab (can a KIN ue mab)

Synonyms ACZ885

U.S./Canadian Brand Names Ilaris® [US]

Therapeutic Category Interleukin-1 Beta Inhibitor; Interleukin-1 Inhibitor; Monoclonal Antibody

Use Treatment of cryopyrin-associated periodic syndromes (CAPS), including familial cold autoinflammatory syndrome (FCAS) and Muckle-Wells syndrome (MWS)

Product Availability Ilaris®: FDA approved June 2009; availability currently undetermined; consult prescribing information for additional information

Canasa® [US] *see* mesalamine *on page 631*
Cancidas® [US/Can] *see* caspofungin *on page 189*

candesartan (kan de SAR tan)

Sound-Alike/Look-Alike Issues

Atacand® may be confused with antacid

Synonyms candesartan cilexetil

U.S./Canadian Brand Names Atacand® [US/Can]

Therapeutic Category Angiotensin II Receptor Antagonist

Use Alone or in combination with other antihypertensive agents in treating essential hypertension; treatment of heart failure (NYHA class II-IV)

Usual Dosage Oral: Adults:

Hypertension: Usual dose is 4-32 mg once daily; dosage must be individualized. Blood pressure response is dose-related over the range of 2-32 mg. The usual recommended starting dose of 16 mg once daily when it is used as monotherapy in patients who are not volume depleted. It can be administered once or twice daily with total daily doses ranging from 8-32 mg. Larger doses do not appear to have a greater effect and there is relatively little experience with such doses.

Congestive heart failure: Initial: 4 mg once daily; double the dose at 2-week intervals, as tolerated; target dose: 32 mg

Note: In selected cases, concurrent therapy with an ACE inhibitor may provide additional benefit.

Dosage Forms

Tablet:

Atacand®: 4 mg, 8 mg, 16 mg, 32 mg

candesartan and hydrochlorothiazide (kan de SAR tan & hye droe klor oh THYE a zide)

Synonyms candesartan cilexetil and hydrochlorothiazide

U.S./Canadian Brand Names Atacand HCT® [US]; Atacand® Plus [Can]

Therapeutic Category Antihypertensive Agent, Combination

Use Treatment of hypertension; combination product should not be used for initial therapy

Usual Dosage Oral: Adults: Replacement therapy: Combination product can be substituted for individual agents; maximum therapeutic effect would be expected within 4 weeks

Usual dosage range:

Candesartan: 16-32 mg/day, given once daily or twice daily in divided doses

Hydrochlorothiazide: 12.5-25 mg once daily

Dosage Forms

Tablet:

Atacand HCT®: 16/12.5: Candesartan 16 mg and hydrochlorothiazide 12.5 mg; 32/12.5: Candesartan 32 mg and hydrochlorothiazide 12.5 mg; 32/25: Candesartan 32 mg and hydrochlorothiazide 25 mg

candesartan cilexetil *see* candesartan *on page 176*

candesartan cilexetil and hydrochlorothiazide *see* candesartan and hydrochlorothiazide *on page 177*

Candida albicans (Monilia) (KAN dee da AL bi kans mo NIL ya)

Synonyms *Monilia* skin test

U.S./Canadian Brand Names Candin® [US]

Therapeutic Category Diagnostic Agent

Use Screen for detection of nonresponsiveness to antigens in immunocompromised individuals

Usual Dosage Intradermal: 0.1 mL, examine reaction site in 24-48 hours; induration of ≥5 mm in diameter is a positive reaction

Dosage Forms

Injection, solution:

Candin®: 0.1 mL/dose (1 mL)

Candin® [US] *see Candida albicans (Monilia) on page 177*

Candistatin® [Can] *see* nystatin *on page 715*

Canesten® Topical [Can] *see* clotrimazole *on page 248*

Canesten® Vaginal [Can] *see* clotrimazole *on page 248*

Cankaid® [US-OTC] *see* carbamide peroxide *on page 181*

cannabidiol and tetrahydrocannabinol *see* tetrahydrocannabinol and cannabidiol *(Canada only) on page 951*

Cantil® [US/Can] *see* mepenzolate *on page 626*

Capastat® Sulfate [US] *see* capreomycin *on page 178*

capecitabine (ka pe SITE a been)

Sound-Alike/Look-Alike Issues

Xeloda® may be confused with Xenical®

Synonyms NSC-712807

U.S./Canadian Brand Names Xeloda® [US/Can]

Therapeutic Category Antineoplastic Agent, Antimetabolite

Use Treatment of metastatic colorectal cancer; adjuvant therapy of Dukes C colon cancer; treatment of metastatic breast cancer

Usual Dosage Oral: Adults: **Note:** Details concerning dosing in combination regimens should also be consulted. Capecitabine toxicities, particularly hand-foot syndrome, may be higher in North American populations (for the treatment of colorectal cancer); therapy initiation at doses of 1000 mg/m^2 twice daily (for 2 weeks every 21 days) may be considered

Metastatic breast cancer, metastatic colorectal cancer: 1250 mg/m^2 twice daily (morning and evening) for 2 weeks, every 21 days

Adjuvant therapy of Dukes C colon cancer: Recommended for a total of 24 weeks (8 cycles of 2 weeks of drug administration and 1 week rest period.

Dosage Forms
Tablet:
Xeloda®: 150 mg, 500 mg

Capex® [US/Can] *see* fluocinolone *on page* *428*
Caphosol® [US] *see* saliva substitute *on page* *887*
Capital® and Codeine [US] *see* acetaminophen and codeine *on page* *20*
Capitrol® ***(Discontinued)***
Capoten® [Can] *see* captopril *on page* *178*
Capoten® ***(Discontinued)*** *see* captopril *on page* *178*
Capozide® [US/Can] *see* captopril and hydrochlorothiazide *on page* *179*

capreomycin (kap ree oh MYE sin)

Sound-Alike/Look-Alike Issues
Capastat® may be confused with Cepastat®

Synonyms capreomycin sulfate

U.S./Canadian Brand Names Capastat® Sulfate [US]

Therapeutic Category Antibiotic, Miscellaneous

Use Treatment of tuberculosis in conjunction with at least one other antituberculosis agent

Usual Dosage I.M., I.V.: Adults: 1 g/day (maximum: 20 mg/kg/day) for 60-120 days, followed by 1 g 2-3 times/week **or** 15 mg/kg/day (maximum: 1 g/dose) for 2-4 months, followed by 15 mg/kg (maximum: 1 g/dose) 2-3 times/week

Dosage Forms
Injection, powder for reconstitution:
Capastat® Sulfate: 1 g

capreomycin sulfate *see* capreomycin *on page* *178*

capsaicin (kap SAY sin)

Sound-Alike/Look-Alike Issues
Zostrix® may be confused with Zestril®, Zovirax®

U.S./Canadian Brand Names Capzasin-HP® [US-OTC]; Capzasin-P® [US-OTC]; DiabetAid Pain and Tingling Relief [US-OTC]; Zostrix® Neuropathy [US-OTC]; Zostrix® [US-OTC/Can]; Zostrix®-HP [US-OTC/Can]

Therapeutic Category Analgesic, Topical

Use Topical treatment of pain associated with postherpetic neuralgia, rheumatoid arthritis, osteoarthritis, diabetic neuropathy; postsurgical pain

Usual Dosage Topical: Children >10 years and Adults: Apply to affected area at least 3-4 times/day; application frequency less than 3-4 times/day prevents the total depletion, inhibition of synthesis, and transport of substance P resulting in decreased clinical efficacy and increased local discomfort

Dosage Forms
Cream, topical: 0.025% (60 g); 0.075% (60 g)
Capzasin-P® [OTC]: 0.025% (45 g)
Capzasin-HP® [OTC]: 0.075% (45 g)
Zostrix® [OTC]: 0.025% (60 g)
Zostrix®-HP [OTC]: 0.075% (60 g)
Zostrix® Neuropathy [OTC]: 0.25% (60 g)
Lotion, topical:
DiabetAid Pain and Tingling Relief: 0.025% (120 mL)
Patch, topical:
Salonpas® Hot [OTC]: 0.025% (1s)

captopril (KAP toe pril)

Sound-Alike/Look-Alike Issues
captopril may be confused with calcitriol, Capitrol®, carvedilol

Synonyms ACE

U.S./Canadian Brand Names Alti-Captopril [Can]; Apo-Capto® [Can]; Capoten® [Can]; Gen-Captopril [Can]; Novo-Captopril [Can]; Nu-Capto [Can]; PMS-Captopril [Can]

Therapeutic Category Angiotensin-Converting Enzyme (ACE) Inhibitor

Use Management of hypertension; treatment of heart failure, left ventricular dysfunction after myocardial infarction, diabetic nephropathy

Usual Dosage Note: Titrate dose according to patient's response; use lowest effective dose. Oral:

Infants: Initial: 0.15-0.3 mg/kg/dose; titrate dose upward to maximum of 6 mg/kg/day in 1-4 divided doses; usual required dose: 2.5-6 mg/kg/day

Children: Initial: 0.5 mg/kg/dose; titrate upward to maximum of 6 mg/kg/day in 2-4 divided doses

Older Children: Initial: 6.25-12.5 mg/dose every 12-24 hours; titrate upward to maximum of 6 mg/kg/day

Adolescents: Initial: 12.5-25 mg/dose given every 8-12 hours; increase by 25 mg/dose to maximum of 450 mg/day

Adults:

Acute hypertension (urgency/emergency): 12.5-25 mg, may repeat as needed (may be given sublingually, but no therapeutic advantage demonstrated)

Heart failure:

Initial dose: 6.25-12.5 mg 3 times/day in conjunction with cardiac glycoside and diuretic therapy; initial dose depends upon patient's fluid/electrolyte status

Target dose: 50 mg 3 times/day

Hypertension:

Initial dose: 12.5-25 mg 2-3 times/day; may increase by 12.5-25 mg/dose at 1- to 2-week intervals up to 50 mg 3 times/day; maximum dose: 150 mg 3 times/day; add diuretic before further dosage increases

Usual dose range (JNC 7): 25-100 mg/day in 2 divided doses

LV dysfunction after MI: Initial dose: 6.25 mg followed by 12.5 mg 3 times/day; then increase to 25 mg 3 times/day during next several days and then gradually increase over next several weeks to target dose of 50 mg 3 times/day (Some dose schedules are more aggressive to achieve an increased goal dose within the first few days of initiation.)

Diabetic nephropathy: 25 mg 3 times/day; other antihypertensives often given concurrently

Dosage Forms

Tablet, oral: 12.5 mg, 25 mg, 50 mg, 100 mg

captopril and hydrochlorothiazide (KAP toe pril & hye droe klor oh THYE a zide)

Synonyms hydrochlorothiazide and captopril

U.S./Canadian Brand Names Capozide® [US/Can]

Therapeutic Category Antihypertensive Agent, Combination

Use Management of hypertension

Usual Dosage Oral: Adults: Hypertension, CHF: May be substituted for previously titrated dosages of the individual components; alternatively, may initiate as follows:

Initial: Single tablet (captopril 25 mg/hydrochlorothiazide 15 mg) taken once daily; daily dose of captopril should not exceed 150 mg; daily dose of hydrochlorothiazide should not exceed 50 mg

Dosage Forms

Tablet:

Generics:

25/15: Captopril 25 mg and hydrochlorothiazide 15 mg
25/25: Captopril 25 mg and hydrochlorothiazide 25 mg
50/15: Captopril 50 mg and hydrochlorothiazide 15 mg
50/25: Captopril 50 mg and hydrochlorothiazide 25 mg

Brands:

Capozide®:

25/15: Captopril 25 mg and hydrochlorothiazide 15 mg
25/25: Captopril 25 mg and hydrochlorothiazide 25 mg
50/15: Captopril 50 mg and hydrochlorothiazide 15 mg
50/25: Captopril 50 mg and hydrochlorothiazide 25 mg

Capzasin-HP® [US-OTC] *see* capsaicin *on page* 178

Capzasin-P® [US-OTC] *see* capsaicin *on page* 178

Carac® [US] *see* fluorouracil *on page* 431

Carafate® [US] *see* sucralfate *on page* 925

Carapres® [Can] *see* clonidine *on page* 245

carbachol (KAR ba kole)

Sound-Alike/Look-Alike Issues

Isopto® Carbachol may be confused with Isopto® Carpine

Synonyms carbacholine; carbamylcholine chloride

U.S./Canadian Brand Names Isopto® Carbachol [US/Can]; Miostat® [US/Can]

Therapeutic Category Cholinergic Agent

Use Lowers intraocular pressure in the treatment of glaucoma; cause miosis during surgery

Usual Dosage Adults:

Ophthalmic: Instill 1-2 drops up to 3 times/day

Intraocular: 0.5 mL instilled into anterior chamber before or after securing sutures

Dosage Forms

Solution, intraocular:

Miostat® [OTC]: 0.01% (1.5 mL)

Solution, ophthalmic:

Isopto® Carbachol [OTC]: 1.5% (15 mL); 3% (15 mL)

carbacholine *see* carbachol *on page 180*

carbamazepine (kar ba MAZ e peen)

Sound-Alike/Look-Alike Issues

carBAMazepine may be confused with OXcarbazepine

Carbatrol® may be confused with Cartrol®

Epitol® may be confused with Epinal®

Tegretol®, Tegretol®-XR may be confused with Mebaral®, Tegrin®, Toprol-XL®, Toradol®, Trental®

Synonyms CBZ; SPD417

Tall-Man car**BAM**azepine

U.S./Canadian Brand Names Apo-Carbamazepine® [Can]; Bio-Carbamazepine [Can]; Carbamazepine [Can]; Carbatrol® [US]; Dom-Carbamazepine [Can]; Epitol® [US]; Equetro® [US]; Gen-Carbamazepine CR [Can]; Mapezine® [Can]; Novo-Carbamaz [Can]; Nu-Carbamazepine [Can]; PHL-Carbamazepine [Can]; PMS-Carbamazepine [Can]; Sandoz-Carbamazepine [Can]; Taro-Carbamazepine Chewable [Can]; Tegretol® [US/Can]; Tegretol®-XR [US]

Therapeutic Category Anticonvulsant

Use

Carbatrol®, Tegretol®, Tegretol®-XR: Partial seizures with complex symptomatology (psychomotor, temporal lobe), generalized tonic-clonic seizures (grand mal), mixed seizure patterns, trigeminal neuralgia

Equetro®: Acute manic and mixed episodes associated with bipolar 1 disorder

Usual Dosage Dosage must be adjusted according to patient's response and serum concentrations. Administer tablets (chewable or conventional) in 2-3 divided doses daily and suspension in 4 divided doses daily. Oral:

Epilepsy:

Children:

<6 years: Initial: 10-20 mg/kg/day divided twice or 3 times daily as tablets or 4 times/day as suspension; increase dose every week until optimal response and therapeutic levels are achieved

Maintenance dose: Divide into 3-4 doses daily (tablets or suspension); maximum recommended dose: 35 mg/kg/day

6-12 years: Initial: 200 mg/day in 2 divided doses (tablets or extended release tablets) or 4 divided doses (oral suspension); increase by up to 100 mg/day at weekly intervals using a twice daily regimen of extended release tablets or 3-4 times daily regimen of other formulations until optimal response and therapeutic levels are achieved

Maintenance: Usual: 400-800 mg/day; maximum recommended dose: 1000 mg/day

Note: Children <12 years who receive ≥400 mg/day of carbamazepine may be converted to extended release capsules (Carbatrol®) using the same total daily dosage divided twice daily

Children >12 years and Adults: Initial: 400 mg/day in 2 divided doses (tablets or extended release tablets) or 4 divided doses (oral suspension); increase by up to 200 mg/day at weekly intervals using a twice daily regimen of extended release tablets or capsules, or a 3-4 times/day regimen of other formulations until optimal response and therapeutic levels are achieved; usual dose: 800-1200 mg/day

Maximum recommended doses:

Children 12-15 years: 1000 mg/day

Children >15 years: 1200 mg/day

Adults: 1600 mg/day; however, some patients have required up to 1.6-2.4 g/day

Trigeminal or glossopharyngeal neuralgia: Adults: Initial: 200 mg/day in 2 divided doses (tablets, extended release tablets, or extended release capsules) or 4 divided doses (oral suspension) with food, gradually increasing in increments of 200 mg/day as needed

Maintenance: Usual: 400-800 mg daily in 2 divided doses (tablets, extended release tablets, or extended release capsules) or 4 divided doses (oral suspension); maximum dose: 1200 mg/day

Bipolar disorder: Adults: Initial: 400 mg/day in 2 divided doses (tablets, extended release tablets, or extended release capsules) or 4 divided doses (oral suspension), may adjust by 200 mg/day increments; maximum dose: 1600 mg/day.

Note: Equetro® is the only formulation specifically approved by the FDA for the management of bipolar disorder.

Dosage Forms

Capsule, extended release:

Carbatrol®, Equetro®: 100 mg, 200 mg, 300 mg

Suspension, oral: 100 mg/5 mL

Tegretol®: 100 mg/5 mL

Tablet: 200 mg

Epitol®, Tegretol®: 200 mg

Tablet, chewable: 100 mg

Tegretol®: 100 mg

Tablet, extended release:

Tegretol®-XR: 100 mg, 200 mg, 400 mg

Carbamazepine [Can] *see* carbamazepine *on page 180*

carbamide *see* urea *on page 998*

carbamide peroxide (KAR ba mide per OKS ide)

Synonyms urea peroxide

U.S./Canadian Brand Names Auraphene® B [US-OTC]; Auro® [US-OTC]; Cankaid® [US-OTC]; Debrox® [US-OTC]; E•R•O [US-OTC]; Gly-Oxide® [US-OTC]; Murine® Ear Wax Removal System [US-OTC]; Orajel® Perioseptic® Spot Treatment [US-OTC]; Otix® [US-OTC]

Therapeutic Category Antiinfective Agent, Oral; Otic Agent, Ceruminolytic

Use Relief of minor inflammation of gums, oral mucosal surfaces, and lips including canker sores and dental irritation; emulsify and disperse ear wax

Usual Dosage Children and Adults:

Oral: Inflammation/dental irritation: Solution (should not be used for >7 days): Oral preparation should not be used in children <2 years of age; apply several drops undiluted on affected area 4 times/day after meals and at bedtime; expectorate after 2-3 minutes **or** place 10 drops onto tongue, mix with saliva, swish for several minutes, expectorate

Otic:

Children <12 years: Tilt head sideways and individualize the dose according to patient size; 3 drops (range: 1-5 drops) twice daily for up to 4 days, tip of applicator should not enter ear canal; keep drops in ear for several minutes by keeping head tilted and placing cotton in ear

Children ≥12 years and Adults: Tilt head sideways and instill 5-10 drops twice daily up to 4 days, tip of applicator should not enter ear canal; keep drops in ear for several minutes by keeping head tilted and placing cotton in ear

Dosage Forms

Liquid, oral: 10% (60 mL)

Cankaid® [OTC]: 10% (22 mL)

Gly-Oxide® [OTC]: 10% (15 mL, 60 mL)

Solution, otic [drops]: 6.5% (15 mL)

Auraphene® B [OTC]: 6.5% (15 mL)

Auro® [OTC]: 6.5% (22.2 mL)

Debrox® [OTC]: 6.5% (15 mL, 30 mL)

E•R•O [OTC], Murine® Ear Wax Removal System [OTC], Otix® [OTC]: 6.5% (15 mL)

carbamylcholine chloride *see* carbachol *on page 180*

Carbaphen 12® [US] *see* carbetapentane, phenylephrine, and chlorpheniramine *on page 183*

Carbaphen 12 Ped® [US] *see* carbetapentane, phenylephrine, and chlorpheniramine *on page 183*

Carbastat® ***(Discontinued)*** *see* carbachol *on page 180*

Carbatrol® [US] *see* carbamazepine *on page 180*

Carbaxefed DM RF *(Discontinued)*
Carbaxefed RF *(Discontinued)*
carbenicillin *(Discontinued)*

carbetapentane and chlorpheniramine (kar bay ta PEN tane & klor fen IR a meen)

Synonyms carbetapentane tannate and chlorpheniramine tannate; chlorpheniramine and carbetapentane

U.S./Canadian Brand Names C-Tanna 12 [US]; Tannic-12 S [US]; Tussi-12 S™ [US]; Tussi-12® [US]; Tussizone-12 RF™ [US]; Tustan 12S™ [US]

Therapeutic Category Antihistamine/Antitussive

Use Symptomatic relief of cough associated with upper respiratory tract conditions, such as the common cold, bronchitis, bronchial asthma

Usual Dosage Oral:

Children: Based on carbetapentane 30 mg and chlorpheniramine 4 mg per 5 mL suspension:

2-6 years: 2.5-5 mL every 12 hours

>6 years: 5-10 mL every 12 hours

Adults: Based on carbetapentane 60 mg and chlorpheniramine 5 mg per tablet: 1-2 tablets every 12 hours

Dosage Forms

Suspension:

C-Tanna 12, Tannic-12 S, Tussi-12 S™, Tustan 12S™: Carbetapentane 30 mg and chlorpheniramine 4 mg per 5 mL

Tablet:

Tussi-12®, Tussizone-12 RF™: Carbetapentane 60 mg and chlorpheniramine 5 mg

carbetapentane and phenylephrine (kar bay ta PEN tane & fen il EF rin)

Synonyms phenylephrine tannate and carbetapentane tannate

Therapeutic Category Antitussive; Antitussive/Decongestant; Sympathomimetic

Use Symptomatic relief of upper respiratory tract conditions such as the common cold, bronchial asthma, and bronchitis (acute and chronic)

Usual Dosage Oral: Suspension: Based on carbetapentane 30 mg/phenylephrine 25 mg per 5 mL:

Children:

2-6 years: 2.5 mL every 12 hours, not to exceed 5 mL/24 hours

6-12 years: 5 mL every 12 hours, not to exceed 10 mL/24 hours

Children >12 years and Adults: 5-10 mL every 12 hours, not to exceed 20 mL/24 hours

carbetapentane and pseudoephedrine (kar bay ta PEN tane & soo doe e FED rin)

Synonyms carbetapentane tannate and pseudoephedrine tannate; pseudoephedrine and carbetapentane

U.S./Canadian Brand Names Pseudacarb™ [US]

Therapeutic Category Antitussive/Decongestant

Use Relief of cough and congestion due to the common cold, influenza, sinusitis, or bronchitis

Usual Dosage Oral: Relief of cough and congestion:

Children:

2-6 years: 1/2 tablet or 2.5 mL suspension every 12 hours (maximum: 4 doses/24 hours)

6-12 years: 1 tablet or 5 mL suspension every 12 hours (maximum: 4 doses/24 hours)

Children >12 years and Adults: 2 tablets or 10 mL suspension every 12 hours (maximum: 4 doses/24 hours)

Dosage Forms

Suspension: Carbetapentane 25 mg and pseudoephedrine 75 mg per 5 mL

Tablet, chewable:

Pseudacarb™: Carbetapentane 25 mg and pseudoephedrine 75 mg

carbetapentane, ephedrine, phenylephrine, and chlorpheniramine *see* chlorpheniramine, ephedrine, phenylephrine, and carbetapentane *on page* 216

carbetapentane, guaifenesin, and phenylephrine

(kar bay ta PEN tane, gwye FEN e sin, & fen il EF rin)

Synonyms guaifenesin, carbetapentane citrate, and phenylephrine hydrochloride; phenylephrine hydrochloride, carbetapentane citrate, and guaifenesin

U.S./Canadian Brand Names Carbetaplex [US]; Extendryl® GCP [US]; Gentex LQ [US]; Phencarb GG [US]

Therapeutic Category Antitussive; Expectorant; Expectorant/Decongestant/Antitussive; Sympathomimetic

Use Relief of nonproductive cough accompanying respiratory tract congestion associated with the common cold, influenza, sinusitis, and bronchitis

Usual Dosage Oral:

Children 2-6 years: Gentex LQ: 2.5 mL every 4-6 hours
Children 6-12 years: Gentex LQ: 5 mL every 4-6 hours
Children ≥12 years and Adults: Gentex LQ: 5-10 mL every 4-6 hours

Dosage Forms

Liquid:

Carbetaplex: Carbetapentane 20 mg, guaifenesin 100 mg, and phenylephrine 15 mg per 5 mL
Gentex LQ: Carbetapentane 20 mg, guaifenesin 100 mg, and phenylephrine 10 mg per 5 mL
Phencarb GG: Carbetapentane 20 mg, guaifenesin 100 mg, and phenylephrine 10 mg per 5 mL

Solution, oral:

Extendryl® GCP: Carbetapentane 15 mg, guaifenesin 100 mg, and phenylephrine 5 mg per 5 mL

carbetapentane, phenylephrine, and chlorpheniramine

(kar bay ta PEN tane, fen il EF rin, & klor fen IR a meen)

Synonyms chlorpheniramine, carbetapentane, and phenylephrine; phenylephrine, chlorpheniramine, and carbetapentane

U.S./Canadian Brand Names Carbaphen 12 Ped® [US]; Carbaphen 12® [US]

Therapeutic Category Antihistamine/Decongestant/Antitussive; Antitussive; Sympathomimetic

Use Symptomatic relief of cough, nasal congestion, and discharge associated with the common cold, bronchial asthma, acute and chronic bronchitis, and other respiratory tract conditions

Usual Dosage Oral: Relief of cough, congestion:

Children 2-6 years (Carbaphen 12 Ped®): 1-2 mL every 12 hours
Children 6-12 years (Carbaphen 12 Ped®): 2-4 mL every 12 hours
Children >12 years and Adults (Carbaphen 12®): 5-10 mL every 12 hours

Dosage Forms

Suspension:

Carbaphen 12®: Carbetapentane 60 mg, phenylephrine 20 mg, and chlorpheniramine 8 mg per 5 mL
Carbaphen 12 Ped®: Carbetapentane 15 mg, phenylephrine 2.5 mg, and chlorpheniramine 2 mg per 1 mL

carbetapentane, phenylephrine, and pyrilamine

(kar bay ta PEN tane, fen il EF rin, & peer Il a meen)

Synonyms phenylephrine tannate, carbetapentane tannate, and pyrilamine tannate; pyrilamine, phenylephrine, and carbetapentane

U.S./Canadian Brand Names C-Tanna 12D [US]; Tussi-12® D [US]; Tussi-12® DS [US]

Therapeutic Category Antihistamine; Antihistamine/Decongestant/Antitussive; Antitussive; Decongestant

Use Symptomatic relief of cough associated with respiratory tract conditions such as the common cold, bronchial asthma, acute and chronic bronchitis

Usual Dosage Oral: Relief of cough:

Children:
2-6 years (Tussi-12® DS): 2.5-5 mL every 12 hours
6-11 years:
Tussi-12® D: 1/2 to 1 tablet every 12 hours
Tussi-12® DS: 5-10 mL every 12 hours
Children ≥12 years and Adults (Tussi-12® D): 1-2 tablets every 12 hours

Dosage Forms

Suspension:

C-Tanna 12D: Carbetapentane 30 mg, pyrilamine 30 mg, and phenylephrine 5 mg per 5 mL
Tussi-12® DS: Carbetapentane 30 mg, pyrilamine 30 mg, and phenylephrine 5 mg per 5 mL

Tablet:

C-Tanna 12D, Tussi-12® D: Carbetapentane 60 mg, pyrilamine 40 mg, and phenylephrine 10 mg

carbetapentane tannate and chlorpheniramine tannate *see* carbetapentane and chlorpheniramine *on page 182*

carbetapentane tannate and pseudoephedrine tannate *see* carbetapentane and pseudoephedrine *on page 182*

Carbetaplex [US] *see* carbetapentane, guaifenesin, and phenylephrine *on page 182*

carbidopa (kar bi DOE pa)

U.S./Canadian Brand Names Lodosyn® [US]

Therapeutic Category Anti-Parkinson Agent (Dopamine Agonist)

Use Given with levodopa in the treatment of parkinsonism to enable a lower dosage of levodopa to be used and a more rapid response to be obtained and to decrease side effects; for details of administration and dosage, see Levodopa; has no effect without levodopa

Usual Dosage Oral: Adults: 70-100 mg/day; maximum daily dose: 200 mg

Dosage Forms

Tablet:

Lodosyn®: 25 mg

carbidopa and levodopa (kar bi DOE pa & lee voe DOE pa)

Sound-Alike/Look-Alike Issues

Sinemet® may be confused with Serevent®

Synonyms levodopa and carbidopa

U.S./Canadian Brand Names Apo-Levocarb® CR [Can]; Apo-Levocarb® [Can]; Endo®-Levodopa/Carbidopa [Can]; Novo-Levocarbidopa [Can]; Nu-Levocarb [Can]; Parcopa™ [US]; Pro-Levocarb [US]; Sinemet® CR [US/Can]; Sinemet® [US/Can]

Therapeutic Category Anti-Parkinson Agent (Dopamine Agonist)

Use Idiopathic Parkinson disease; postencephalitic parkinsonism; symptomatic parkinsonism

Usual Dosage Oral: Adults: Parkinson disease:

Immediate release tablet:

Initial: Carbidopa 25 mg/levodopa 100 mg 3 times/day

Dosage adjustment: Alternate tablet strengths may be substituted according to individual carbidopa/levodopa requirements. Increase by 1 tablet every other day as necessary, except when using the carbidopa 25 mg/levodopa 250 mg tablets where increases should be made using 1/2-1 tablet every 1-2 days. Use of more than 1 dosage strength or dosing 4 times/day may be required (maximum: 8 tablets of any strength/day or 200 mg of carbidopa and 2000 mg of levodopa)

Sustained release tablet:

Initial: Carbidopa 50 mg/levodopa 200 mg 2 times/day, at intervals not <6 hours

Dosage adjustment: May adjust every 3 days; intervals should be between 4-8 hours during the waking day (maximum: 8 tablets/day)

Dosage Forms

Tablet: 10/100: Carbidopa 10 mg and levodopa 100 mg; 25/100: Carbidopa 25 mg and levodopa 100 mg; 25/250: Carbidopa 25 mg and levodopa 250 mg

Sinemet®:

10/100: Carbidopa 10 mg and levodopa 100 mg

25/100: Carbidopa 25 mg and levodopa 100 mg

25/250: Carbidopa 25 mg and levodopa 250 mg

Tablet, extended release: 25/100: Carbidopa 25 mg and levodopa 100 mg; 50/200: Carbidopa 50 mg and levodopa 200 mg

Tablet, orally disintegrating: 10/100: Carbidopa 10 mg and levodopa 100 mg; 25/100: Carbidopa 25 mg and levodopa 100 mg; 25/250: Carbidopa 25 mg and levodopa 250 mg

Parcopa™:

10/100: Carbidopa 10 mg and levodopa 100 mg [contains phenylalanine 3.4 mg/tablet; mint flavor]

25/100: Carbidopa 25 mg and levodopa 100 mg [contains phenylalanine 3.4 mg/tablet; mint flavor]

25/250: Carbidopa 25 mg and levodopa 250 mg [contains phenylalanine 8.4 mg/tablet; mint flavor]

Tablet, sustained release: 25/100: Carbidopa 25 mg and levodopa 100 mg; 50/200: Carbidopa 50 mg and levodopa 200 mg

Sinemet® CR:

25/100: Carbidopa 25 mg and levodopa 100 mg

50/200: Carbidopa 50 mg and levodopa 200 mg

carbidopa, entacapone, and levodopa *see* levodopa, carbidopa, and entacapone *on page 579*

carbidopa, levodopa, and entacapone *see* levodopa, carbidopa, and entacapone *on page 579*

Carbihist *(Discontinued)* *see* carbinoxamine *on page 185*

carbinoxamine (kar bi NOKS a meen)

Synonyms carbinoxamine maleate

U.S./Canadian Brand Names Palgic® [US]

Therapeutic Category Antihistamine

Use Seasonal and perennial allergic rhinitis; vasomotor rhinitis; urticaria; decrease severity of other allergic reactions

Usual Dosage Oral (Palgic®):

Children:

>3-6 years: 2-5 mg 3-4 times/day

>6 years: 4-6 mg 3-4 times/day

Adults: 4-8 mg 3-4 times/day

Dosage Forms

Solution:

Palgic®: 4 mg/5 mL

Tablet [scored]:

Palgic®: 4 mg

carbinoxamine and pseudoephedrine *(Discontinued)*

carbinoxamine maleate *see* carbinoxamine *on page 185*

Carbinoxamine PD *(Discontinued)* *see* carbinoxamine *on page 185*

carbinoxamine, pseudoephedrine, and dextromethorphan *(Discontinued)*

Carbiset® Tablet *(Discontinued)*

Carbiset-TR® Tablet *(Discontinued)*

Carbocaine® [US/Can] *see* mepivacaine *on page 628*

Carbocaine® 2% with Neo-Cobefrin® [US] *see* mepivacaine and levonordefrin *on page 628*

Carbodec® Syrup *(Discontinued)*

Carbodec® Tablet *(Discontinued)*

Carbodec® TR Tablet *(Discontinued)*

Carbofed DM [US] *see* brompheniramine, pseudoephedrine, and dextromethorphan *on page 152*

carbolic acid *see* phenol *on page 772*

Carbolith™ [Can] *see* lithium *on page 594*

carboplatin (KAR boe pla tin)

Sound-Alike/Look-Alike Issues

CARBOplatin may be confused with CISplatin, oxaliplatin

Paraplatin® may be confused with Platinol®

Synonyms CBDCA; NSC-241240

Tall-Man CARBOplatin

U.S./Canadian Brand Names Paraplatin-AQ [Can]

Therapeutic Category Antineoplastic Agent

Use Treatment of ovarian cancer

Usual Dosage Details concerning dosing in combination regimens should also be consulted. **Note:** Doses for adults are usually determined by the AUC using the Calvert formula.

IVPB, I.V. infusion: Adults:

Ovarian cancer: 300-360 mg/m^2 every 4 weeks

In adults, dosing is commonly calculated using the Calvert formula:

Total dose (mg) = Target AUC x (GFR+ 25)

Usual target AUCs:

Previously untreated patients: 6-8

Previously treated patients: 4-6

Dosage Forms

Injection, powder for reconstitution: 50 mg, 150 mg, 450 mg

Injection, solution: 10 mg/mL (5 mL, 15 mL, 45 mL, 60 mL)

Injection, solution [preservative free] 10 mg/mL (5 mL, 15 mL, 45 mL)

carboprost *see* carboprost tromethamine *on page 186*

carboprost tromethamine (KAR boe prost tro METH a meen)

Synonyms carboprost; prostaglandin F_2

U.S./Canadian Brand Names Hemabate® [US/Can]

Therapeutic Category Prostaglandin

Use Termination of pregnancy; treatment of refractory postpartum uterine bleeding

Usual Dosage I.M.: Adults:

Abortion: Initial: 250 mcg, then 250 mcg at 1.5- to 3.5-hour intervals, depending on uterine response; a 500 mcg dose may be given if uterine response is not adequate after several 250 mcg doses; do not exceed 12 mg total dose or continuous administration for >2 days

Refractory postpartum uterine bleeding: Initial: 250 mcg; if needed, may repeat at 15- to 90-minute intervals; maximum total dose: 2 mg (8 doses)

Dosage Forms

Injection, solution:

Hemabate®: Carboprost 250 mcg and tromethamine 83 mcg per mL (1 mL)

carbose D *see* carboxymethylcellulose *on page 186*

Carboxine *(Discontinued)* *see* carbinoxamine *on page 185*

Carboxine-PSE *(Discontinued)*

carboxymethylcellulose (kar boks ee meth il SEL yoo lose)

Sound-Alike/Look-Alike Issues

Optive™ may be confused with Optivar®

Synonyms carbose D; carboxymethylcellulose sodium

U.S./Canadian Brand Names Celluvisc™ [Can]; Optive™ [US-OTC]; Refresh Liquigel® [US-OTC]; Refresh Plus® [US-OTC/Can]; Refresh Tears® [US-OTC/Can]; Tears Again® Gel Drops™ [US-OTC]; Tears Again® Night and Day™ [US-OTC]; Theratears® [US]

Therapeutic Category Ophthalmic Agent, Miscellaneous

Use Artificial tear substitute

Usual Dosage Ophthalmic: Adults: Instill 1-2 drops into eye(s) 3-4 times/day

Dosage Forms

Gel, ophthalmic:

Tears Again® Night and Day™ [OTC]: 1.5% (3.5 g)

Solution ophthalmic [drops]:

Optive™ [OTC]: 0.5% (15 mL, 30 mL)
Refresh Liquigel® [OTC]: 1% (15 mL)
Refresh Tears® [OTC]: 0.5% (15 mL)
Tears Again® Gel Drops™ [OTC]: 0.7% (15 mL)
Theratears®: 0.25% (15 mL)

Solution ophthalmic [drops; preservative free]:

Refresh Plus®: 0.5% (0.4 mL)
Theratears®: 0.25% (0.6 mL)

carboxymethylcellulose sodium *see* carboxymethylcellulose *on page 186*
Cardene® [US] *see* nicardipine *on page 695*
Cardene® I.V. [US] *see* nicardipine *on page 695*
Cardene® SR [US] *see* nicardipine *on page 695*
Cardio-Green® *(Discontinued)* *see* indocyanine green *on page 526*
Cardioquin® *(Discontinued)* *see* quinidine *on page 845*
Cardizem® [US] *see* diltiazem *on page 311*
Cardizem® CD [US/Can] *see* diltiazem *on page 311*
Cardizem® Injection *(Discontinued)* *see* diltiazem *on page 311*
Cardizem® LA [US] *see* diltiazem *on page 311*
Cardizem® SR *(Discontinued)* *see* diltiazem *on page 311*
Cardura® [US] *see* doxazosin *on page 333*
Cardura-1™ [Can] *see* doxazosin *on page 333*
Cardura-2™ [Can] *see* doxazosin *on page 333*
Cardura-4™ [Can] *see* doxazosin *on page 333*
Cardura® XL [US] *see* doxazosin *on page 333*

CareNatal™ DHA *(Discontinued)* *see* vitamins (multiple/prenatal) *on page 1020*
Carimune™ *(Discontinued)* *see* immune globulin (intravenous) *on page 523*
Carimune® NF [US] *see* immune globulin (intravenous) *on page 523*
carisoprodate *see* carisoprodol *on page 187*

carisoprodol (kar eye soe PROE dole)

Synonyms carisoprodate; isobamate
U.S./Canadian Brand Names Soma® [US/Can]
Therapeutic Category Skeletal Muscle Relaxant
Use Short-term (2-3 weeks) relief of skeletal muscle pain
Usual Dosage Note: Carisoprodol should only be used for short periods (2-3 weeks) due to lack of evidence of effectiveness with prolonged use.
Oral: Children ≥16 years and Adults: 250-350 mg 3 times/day and at bedtime
Dosage Forms
Tablet: 350 mg
Soma®: 250 mg, 350 mg

carisoprodol and aspirin (kar eye soe PROE dole & AS pir in)

Synonyms aspirin and carisoprodol
U.S./Canadian Brand Names Soma® Compound [US]
Therapeutic Category Skeletal Muscle Relaxant
Use Relief of discomfort associated with acute, painful skeletal muscle conditions
Usual Dosage Oral: Children ≥16 years and Adults: Acute skeletal muscle pain: 1-2 tablets 4 times/day for 2-3 weeks (maximum: 8 tablets/24 hours)
Dosage Forms
Tablet: Carisoprodol 200 mg and aspirin 325 mg
Soma® Compound: Carisoprodol 200 mg and aspirin 325 mg

carisoprodol, aspirin, and codeine (kar eye soe PROE dole, AS pir in, and KOE deen)

Synonyms aspirin, carisoprodol, and codeine; codeine, aspirin, and carisoprodol
Therapeutic Category Skeletal Muscle Relaxant
Controlled Substance C-III
Use Skeletal muscle relaxant
Usual Dosage Oral: Adults: 1 or 2 tablets 4 times/day (maximum: 8 tablets/day); treatment should be temporary (2-3 weeks)
Dosage Forms
Tablet: Carisoprodol 200 mg, aspirin 325 mg, and codeine 16 mg

Carmol® 10 [US-OTC] *see* urea *on page 998*
Carmol® 20 [US-OTC] *see* urea *on page 998*
Carmol® 40 [US] *see* urea *on page 998*
Carmol® Deep Cleaning [US] *see* urea *on page 998*
Carmol-HC® [US] *see* urea and hydrocortisone *on page 999*
Carmol® Scalp Treatment [US] *see* sulfacetamide *on page 927*

carmustine (kar MUS teen)

Sound-Alike/Look-Alike Issues
carmustine may be confused with bendamustine, lomustine
Synonyms BCNU; bis-chloronitrosourea; carmustinum; NSC-409962; WR-139021
U.S./Canadian Brand Names BiCNU® [US/Can]; Gliadel Wafer® [Can]; Gliadel® [US]
Therapeutic Category Antineoplastic Agent
Use
Injection: Treatment of brain tumors (glioblastoma, brainstem glioma, medulloblastoma, astrocytoma, ependymoma, and metastatic brain tumors), multiple myeloma, Hodgkin disease (relapsed or refractory), non-Hodgkin lymphomas (relapsed or refractory),
Wafer (implant): Adjunct to surgery in patients with recurrent glioblastoma multiforme; adjunct to surgery and radiation in patients with high-grade malignant glioma

Usual Dosage I.V. (refer to individual protocols): Adults:

Usual dosage (per manufacturer labeling): 150-200 mg/m² every 6 weeks **or** 75-100 mg/m²/day for 2 days every 6 weeks

Primary brain cancer:

150-200 mg/m² every 6-8 weeks as a single dose **or**

75-120 mg/m² days 1 and 2 every 6-8 weeks **or**

20-65 mg/m² every 4-6 weeks **or**

0.5-1 mg/kg every 4-6 weeks **or**

40-80 mg/m²/day for 3 days every 6-8 weeks

Autologous BMT:

Combination therapy: Up to 300-900 mg/m²

Single-agent therapy: Up to 1200 mg/m² (fatal necrosis is associated with doses >2 g/m²)

Implantation (wafer): Recurrent glioblastoma multiforme, malignant glioma: Up to 8 wafers may be placed in the resection cavity (total dose 62.6 mg); should the size and shape not accommodate 8 wafers, the maximum number of wafers allowed should be placed

Dosage Forms

Implant:

Gliadel®: 7.7 mg (8s)

Injection, powder for reconstitution:

BiCNU®: 100 mg

carmustinum *see* carmustine *on page* 187
Carnation Instant Breakfast® [US-OTC] *see* nutritional formula, enteral/oral *on page* 715
Carnitine-300 [US-OTC] *see* levocarnitine *on page* 578
Carnitor® [US/Can] *see* levocarnitine *on page* 578
Carnitor® SF [US] *see* levocarnitine *on page* 578
Carrington Antifungal [US-OTC] *see* miconazole *on page* 654
Carrington® Oral Wound Rinse [US] *see* maltodextrin *on page* 612

carteolol (KAR tee oh lole)

Sound-Alike/Look-Alike Issues

carteolol may be confused with carvedilol

Synonyms carteolol hydrochloride

U.S./Canadian Brand Names Ocupress® Ophthalmic [Can]

Therapeutic Category Beta-Adrenergic Blocker

Use Treatment of chronic open-angle glaucoma and intraocular hypertension

Usual Dosage Ophthalmic: Adults: Instill 1 drop in affected eye(s) twice daily.

Dosage Forms

Solution, ophthalmic, as hydrochloride: 1% (5 mL, 10 mL, 15 mL)

carteolol hydrochloride *see* carteolol *on page* 188
Carter's Little Pills® [Can] *see* bisacodyl *on page* 142
Carter's Little Pills® *(Discontinued)* *see* bisacodyl *on page* 142
Cartia XT® [US] *see* diltiazem *on page* 311

carvedilol (KAR ve dil ole)

Sound-Alike/Look-Alike Issues

carvedilol may be confused with atenolol, captopril, carbidopa, carteolol

Coreg® may be confused with Corgard®, Cortef®, Cozaar®

U.S./Canadian Brand Names Apo-Carvedilol® [Can]; Coreg CR® [US]; Coreg® [US/Can]; Dom-Carvedilol [Can]; Novo-Carvedilol [Can]; PHL-Carvedilol [Can]; PMS-Carvedilol [Can]; RAN™-Carvedilol [Can]; ratio-Carvedilol [Can]

Therapeutic Category Beta-Adrenergic Blocker

Use Mild-to-severe heart failure of ischemic or cardiomyopathic origin (usually in addition to standard therapy); left ventricular dysfunction following myocardial infarction (MI) (clinically stable with LVEF ≤40%); management of hypertension

Usual Dosage Oral: Adults: Reduce dosage if heart rate drops to <55 beats/minute.

Hypertension:

Immediate release: 6.25 mg twice daily; if tolerated, dose should be maintained for 1-2 weeks, then increased to 12.5 mg twice daily. If necessary, dosage may be increased to a maximum of 25 mg twice daily after 1-2 weeks.

Extended release: Initial: 20 mg once daily, if tolerated, dose should be maintained for 1-2 weeks then increased to 40 mg once daily if necessary; maximum dose: 80 mg once daily

Heart failure:

Immediate release: 3.125 mg twice daily for 2 weeks; if this dose is tolerated, may increase to 6.25 mg twice daily. Double the dose every 2 weeks to the highest dose tolerated by patient. (Prior to initiating therapy, other heart failure medications should be stabilized and fluid retention minimized.)

Maximum recommended dose:

Mild-to-moderate heart failure:

<85 kg: 25 mg twice daily

>85 kg: 50 mg twice daily

Severe heart failure: 25 mg twice daily

Extended release: Initial: 10 mg once daily for 2 weeks; if the dose is tolerated, increase dose to 20 mg, 40 mg, and 80 mg over successive intervals of at least 2 weeks. Maintain on lower dose if higher dose is not tolerated.

Left ventricular dysfunction following MI: **Note**: Should be initiated only after patient is hemodynamically stable and fluid retention has been minimized.

Immediate release: Initial 3.125-6.25 mg twice daily; increase dosage incrementally (ie, from 6.25-12.5 mg twice daily) at intervals of 3-10 days, based on tolerance, to a target dose of 25 mg twice daily.

Extended release: Initial: 10-20 mg once daily; increase dosage incrementally at intervals of 3-10 days, based on tolerance, to a target dose of 80 mg once daily.

Conversion from immediate release to extended release (Coreg CR®):

Current dose immediate release tablets 3.125 mg twice daily: Convert to extended release capsules 10 mg once daily

Current dose immediate release tablets 6.25 mg twice daily: Convert to extended release capsules 20 mg once daily

Current dose immediate release tablets 12.5 mg twice daily: Convert to extended release capsules 40 mg once daily

Current dose immediate release tablets 25 mg twice daily: Convert to extended release capsules 80 mg once daily

Dosage Forms

Capsule, extended release:

Coreg CR®: 10 mg, 20 mg, 40 mg, 80 mg

Tablet: 3.125 mg, 6.25 mg, 12.5 mg, 25 mg

Coreg®: 3.125 mg, 6.25 mg, 12.5 mg, 25 mg

Casodex® [US/Can] *see* bicalutamide *on page* 141

caspofungin (kas poe FUN jin)

Synonyms caspofungin acetate

U.S./Canadian Brand Names Cancidas® [US/Can]

Therapeutic Category Antifungal Agent, Systemic

Use Treatment of invasive *Aspergillus* infections in patients who are refractory or intolerant of other therapy; treatment of candidemia and other *Candida* infections (intraabdominal abscesses, esophageal, peritonitis, pleural space); empirical treatment for presumed fungal infections in febrile neutropenic patient

Usual Dosage I.V.:

Children: 3 months to 17 years: Initial dose: 70 mg/m^2 on day 1, subsequent dosing: 50 mg/m^2 once daily, if clinical response inadequate, may increase to 70 mg/m^2 once daily if tolerated, but increased efficacy not demonstrated (maximum dose: 70 mg/day)

Adults: **Note:** Duration of caspofungin treatment should be determined by patient status and clinical response. Empiric therapy should be given until neutropenia resolves. In patients with positive cultures, treatment should continue until 14 days after last positive culture. In neutropenic patients, treatment should be given at least 7 days after both signs and symptoms of infection **and** neutropenia resolve.

Aspergillosis, invasive: Initial dose: 70 mg on day 1; subsequent dosing: 50 mg/day. If clinical response inadequate, may increase up to 70 mg/day if tolerated, but increased efficacy not demonstrated. **Note:** Duration of therapy should be a minimum of 6-12 weeks or throughout period of immunosuppression.

Candidiasis: Initial dose: 70 mg on day 1; subsequent dosing: 50 mg/day

Esophageal: 50 mg/day; **Note:** The majority of patients studied for this indication also had oropharyngeal involvement.

Empiric therapy: Initial dose: 70 mg on day 1; subsequent dosing: 50 mg/day; if clinical response inadequate, may increase up to 70 mg/day if tolerated, but increased efficacy not demonstrated

Dosage Forms

Injection, powder for reconstitution:

Cancidas®: 50 mg, 70 mg

caspofungin acetate *see* caspofungin *on page 189*
Castellani Paint Modified [US-OTC] *see* phenol *on page 772*

castor oil (KAS tor oyl)

Synonyms oleum ricini

Therapeutic Category Laxative

Use Preparation for rectal or bowel examination or surgery; rarely used to relieve constipation; also applied to skin as emollient and protectant

Usual Dosage Oral: Oil:

Children 2-11 years: 5-15 mL as a single dose

Children ≥12 years and Adults: 15-60 mL as a single dose

Dosage Forms

Oil, oral: 100%

castor oil, trypsin, and balsam Peru *see* trypsin, balsam Peru, and castor oil *on page 993*
Cataflam® [US/Can] *see* diclofenac *on page 303*
Catapres® [US] *see* clonidine *on page 245*
Catapres-TTS® [US] *see* clonidine *on page 245*
catechins *see* sinecatechins *on page 903*
Cathflo® Activase® [US/Can] *see* alteplase *on page 53*
Caverject® [US/Can] *see* alprostadil *on page 51*
Caverject Impulse® [US] *see* alprostadil *on page 51*
CaviRinse™ [US] *see* fluoride *on page 430*
CB-1348 *see* chlorambucil *on page 208*
CBDCA *see* carboplatin *on page 185*
CBZ *see* carbamazepine *on page 180*
CC-5013 *see* lenalidomide *on page 574*
CCI-779 *see* temsirolimus *on page 943*
CCNU *see* lomustine *on page 596*
C-Crystals® *(Discontinued)* *see* ascorbic acid *on page 100*
2-CdA *see* cladribine *on page 235*
CDDP *see* cisplatin *on page 233*
CDP870 *see* certolizumab pegol *on page 203*
CDX *see* bicalutamide *on page 141*
CE *see* estrogens (conjugated/equine) *on page 378*
Cebid® *(Discontinued)* *see* ascorbic acid *on page 100*
Ceclor® [Can] *see* cefaclor *on page 191*
Ceclor® *(Discontinued)* *see* cefaclor *on page 191*
Cecon® [US-OTC] *see* ascorbic acid *on page 100*
Cedax® [US] *see* ceftibuten *on page 197*
Cedocard®-SR [Can] *see* isosorbide dinitrate *on page 550*
CEE *see* estrogens (conjugated/equine) *on page 378*
CeeNU® [US/Can] *see* lomustine *on page 596*
Ceepryn® *(Discontinued)* *see* cetylpyridinium *on page 205*

cefaclor (SEF a klor)

Sound-Alike/Look-Alike Issues

cefaclor may be confused with cephalexin

U.S./Canadian Brand Names Apo-Cefaclor® [Can]; Ceclor® [Can]; Novo-Cefaclor [Can]; Nu-Cefaclor [Can]; PMS-Cefaclor [Can]; Raniclor™ [US]

Therapeutic Category Cephalosporin (Second Generation)

Use Treatment of susceptible bacterial infections including otitis media, lower respiratory tract infections, acute exacerbations of chronic bronchitis, pharyngitis and tonsillitis, urinary tract infections, skin and skin structure infections

Usual Dosage

Usual dosage range:

Children >1 month: Oral: 20-40 mg/kg/day divided every 8-12 hours (maximum dose: 1 g/day)
Adults: Oral: 250-500 mg every 8 hours

Indication-specific dosing:

Children: Oral:

Otitis media: 40 mg/kg/day divided every 12 hours
Pharyngitis: 20 mg/kg/day divided every 12 hours

Dosage Forms

Capsule: 250 mg, 500 mg
Powder for oral suspension: 125 mg/5 mL, 250 mg/5 mL, 375 mg/5 mL
Tablet, chewable:
Raniclor™: 250 mg, 375 mg
Tablet, extended release: 500 mg

cefadroxil (sef a DROKS il)

Synonyms cefadroxil monohydrate

U.S./Canadian Brand Names Apo-Cefadroxil® [Can]; Novo-Cefadroxil [Can]; Pro-Cefadroxil [Can]

Therapeutic Category Cephalosporin (First Generation)

Use Treatment of susceptible bacterial infections, including those caused by group A beta-hemolytic *Streptococcus*

Usual Dosage

Usual dosage range: Oral:

Children: 30 mg/kg/day divided twice daily up to a maximum of 2 g/day
Adults: 1-2 g/day in 2 divided doses

Indication-specific dosing: Orofacial infections: Adults: 250-500 mg every 8 hours

Dosage Forms Note: Strength is expressed as base

Capsule: 500 mg
Powder for oral suspension: 250 mg/5 mL, 500 mg/5 mL
Tablet: 1 g

cefadroxil monohydrate *see* cefadroxil *on page* *191*

Cefanex® ***(Discontinued)*** *see* cephalexin *on page* *202*

cefazolin (sef A zoe lin)

Sound-Alike/Look-Alike Issues

ceFAZolin may be confused with cefprozil, cefTRIAXone, cephalexin, cephalothin
Kefzol® may be confused with Cefzil®

Synonyms cefazolin sodium

Tall-Man ce**FAZ**olin

Therapeutic Category Cephalosporin (First Generation)

Use Treatment of respiratory tract, skin, genital, urinary tract, biliary tract, bone and joint infections, and septicemia due to susceptible gram-positive cocci (except enterococcus); some gram-negative bacilli including *E. coli*, *Proteus*, and *Klebsiella* may be susceptible; surgical prophylaxis

Usual Dosage

Usual dosage range: I.M., I.V.:

Children >1 month: 25-100 mg/kg/day divided every 6-8 hours; maximum: 6 g/day
Adults: 250 mg to 1.5 g every 6-12 (usually 8) hours, depending on severity of infection; maximum dose: 12 g/day

Indication-specific dosing:

I.M., I.V.: Adults:

Moderate-to-severe infections: 500 mg to 1 g every 6-8 hours

Mild infection with gram-positive cocci: 250-500 mg every 8 hours

Perioperative prophylaxis: 1-2 g within 60 minutes prior to surgery (may repeat in 2-5 hours intraoperatively); followed by 500 mg to 1 g every 6-8 hours for 24 hours postoperatively

Cardiothoracic surgery: 1 g within 60 minutes prior to incision, followed by 1 g at sternotomy and 1 g after cardiopulmonary bypass; may continue 1 g every 6 hours for 24-72 hours postoperatively

Total joint replacement: 1 g 1 hour prior to the procedure

Pneumococcal pneumonia: 500 mg every 12 hours

Severe infection: 1-1.5 g every 6 hours

UTI (uncomplicated): 1 g every 12 hours

Dosage Forms

Infusion [iso-osmotic dextrose solution]: 1 g (50 mL)

Injection, powder for reconstitution: 500 mg, 1 g, 10 g, 20 g

cefazolin sodium *see* cefazolin *on page 191*

cefdinir (SEF di ner)

Synonyms CFDN

U.S./Canadian Brand Names Omnicef® [US/Can]

Therapeutic Category Cephalosporin (Third Generation)

Use Treatment of community-acquired pneumonia, acute exacerbations of chronic bronchitis, acute bacterial otitis media, acute maxillary sinusitis, pharyngitis/tonsillitis, and uncomplicated skin and skin structure infections.

Usual Dosage

Usual dosage range:

Children 6 months to 12 years: Oral: 7 mg/kg/dose twice daily or 14 mg/kg/dose once daily (maximum: 600 mg/day)

Adolescents and Adults: Oral: 300 mg twice daily or 600 mg once daily

Indication-specific dosing:

Children 6 months to 12 years: Oral:

Acute bacterial otitis media, pharyngitis/tonsillitis: 7 mg/kg/dose twice daily for 5-10 days **or** 14 mg/kg/dose once daily for 10 days (maximum: 600 mg/day)

Acute maxillary sinusitis: 7 mg/kg/dose twice daily **or** 14 mg/kg/dose once daily for 10 days (maximum: 600 mg/day)

Uncomplicated skin and skin structure infections: 7 mg/kg/dose twice daily for 10 days (maximum: 600 mg/day)

Adolescents and Adults:

Acute exacerbations of chronic bronchitis, pharyngitis/tonsillitis: 300 mg twice daily for 5-10 days **or** 600 mg once daily for 10 days

Acute maxillary sinusitis: 300 mg twice daily **or** 600 mg once daily for 10 days

Community-acquired pneumonia, uncomplicated skin and skin structure infections: 300 mg twice daily for 10 days

Dosage Forms

Capsule: 300 mg

Omnicef®: 300 mg

Powder for oral suspension: 125 mg/5 mL; 250 mg/5 mL

Omnicef®: 125 mg/5 mL (60 mL, 100 mL), 250 mg/5 mL (60 mL, 100 mL)

cefditoren (sef de TOR en)

Synonyms cefditoren pivoxil

U.S./Canadian Brand Names Spectracef® [US]

Therapeutic Category Antibiotic, Cephalosporin

Use Treatment of acute bacterial exacerbation of chronic bronchitis or community-acquired pneumonia (due to susceptible organisms including *Haemophilus influenzae*, *Haemophilus parainfluenzae*, *Streptococcus pneumoniae*-penicillin susceptible only, *Moraxella catarrhalis*); pharyngitis or tonsillitis (*Streptococcus pyogenes*); and uncomplicated skin and skin-structure infections (*Staphylococcus aureus* - not MRSA, *Streptococcus pyogenes*)

Usual Dosage

Usual dosage range:

Children ≥12 years and Adults: Oral: 200-400 mg twice daily

Indication-specific dosing:

Children ≥12 years and Adults: Oral:

Acute bacterial exacerbation of chronic bronchitis: 400 mg twice daily for 10 days

Community-acquired pneumonia: 400 mg twice daily for 14 days

Pharyngitis, tonsillitis, uncomplicated skin and skin structure infections: 200 mg twice daily for 10 days

Dosage Forms

Tablet:

Spectracef®: 200 mg, 400 mg

cefditoren pivoxil *see* cefditoren *on page 192*

cefepime (SEF e pim)

Synonyms cefepime hydrochloride

U.S./Canadian Brand Names Maxipime® [US/Can]

Therapeutic Category Cephalosporin (Fourth Generation)

Use Treatment of uncomplicated and complicated urinary tract infections, including pyelonephritis caused by typical urinary tract pathogens; monotherapy for febrile neutropenia; uncomplicated skin and skin structure infections caused by *Streptococcus pyogenes*; moderate-to-severe pneumonia caused by pneumococcus, *Pseudomonas aeruginosa*, and other gram-negative organisms; complicated intra-abdominal infections (in combination with metronidazole). Also active against methicillin-susceptible staphylococci, *Enterobacter* sp, and many other gram-negative bacilli.

Children 2 months to 16 years: Empiric therapy of febrile neutropenia patients, uncomplicated skin/soft tissue infections, pneumonia, and uncomplicated/complicated urinary tract infections.

Usual Dosage

Usual dosage range:

Children: I.M., I.V.: 50 mg/kg every 8-12 hours (maximum not to exceed adult dosing)

Adults: I.V.: 1-2 g every 8-12 hours; I.M.: 500-1000 mg every 12 hours

Indication-specific dosing:

Children ≥2 months to 16 years (<40 kg):

Febrile neutropenia: I.V.: 50 mg/kg every 8 hours for 7 days or until neutropenia resolves

Skin and skin structure infections (uncomplicated) and pneumonia: I.V.: 50 mg/kg every 12 hours for 10 days

Urinary tract infections, complicated and uncomplicated: I.M., I.V.: 50 mg/kg every 12 hours for 7-10 days; **Note:** I.M. may be considered for mild-to-moderate infection only

Adults:

Febrile neutropenia, monotherapy: I.V: 2 g every 8 hours for 7 days or until the neutropenia resolves

Intraabdominal infections, complicated: I.V.: 2 g every 12 hours for 7-10 days with metronidazole

Pneumonia: I.V.:

Nosocomial (HAP/VAP): 1-2 g every 8-12 hours; **Note:** Duration of therapy may vary considerably (7-21 days); usually longer courses are required if *Pseudomonas*. In absence of *Pseudomonas*, and if appropriate empiric treatment used and patient responsive, it may be clinically appropriate to reduce duration of therapy to 7-10 days.

Community-acquired (including pseudomonal): 1-2 g every 12 hours for 10 days

Skin and skin structure, uncomplicated: I.V.: 2 g every 12 hours for 10 days

Urinary tract infections, complicated and uncomplicated:

Mild-to-moderate: I.M., I.V.: 500-1000 mg every 12 hours for 7-10 days

Severe: I.V.: 2 g every 12 hours for 10 days

Dosage Forms

Infusion, premixed iso-osomotic dextrose solution: 1 g (50 mL); 2 g (100 mL)

Injection, powder for reconstitution: 500 mg, 1 g, 2 g

Maxipime®: 500 mg, 1 g, 2 g

cefepime hydrochloride *see* cefepime *on page 193*

Cefizox® [US/Can] *see* ceftizoxime *on page 197*

Cefotan® ***(Discontinued)***

cefotaxime (sef oh TAKS eem)

Sound-Alike/Look-Alike Issues
cefotaxime may be confused with cefoxitin, ceftizoxime, cefuroxime

Synonyms cefotaxime sodium

U.S./Canadian Brand Names Claforan® [US/Can]

Therapeutic Category Cephalosporin (Third Generation)

Use Treatment of susceptible infection in respiratory tract, skin and skin structure, bone and joint, urinary tract, gynecologic as well as septicemia, and documented or suspected meningitis. Active against most gram-negative bacilli (not *Pseudomonas*) and gram-positive cocci (not enterococcus). Active against many penicillin-resistant pneumococci.

Usual Dosage

Usual dosage range:
Infants and Children 1 month to 12 years <50 kg: I.M., I.V.: 50-200 mg/kg/day in divided doses every 6-8 hours
Children >12 years and Adults: I.M., I.V.: 1-2 g every 4-12 hours

Indication-specific dosing:
Infants and Children 1 month to 12 years:
Epiglottitis: I.M., I.V.: 150-200 mg/kg/day in 4 divided doses with clindamycin for 7-10 days
Meningitis: I.M., I.V.: 200 mg/kg/day in divided doses every 6 hours
Pneumonia: I.V.: 200 mg/kg/day divided every 8 hours
Sepsis: I.V.: 150 mg/kg/day divided every 8 hours
Typhoid fever: I.M., I.V.: 150-200 mg/kg/day in 3-4 divided doses (maximum: 12 g/day); fluoroquinolone resistant: 80 mg/kg/day in 3-4 divided doses (maximum: 12 g/day)
Children >12 years and Adults:
Arthritis (septic): I.V.: 1 g every 8 hours
Brain abscess, meningitis: I.V.: 2 g every 4-6 hours
Caesarean section: I.M., I.V.: 1 g as soon as the umbilical cord is clamped, then 1 g at 6- and 12-hour intervals
Epiglottitis: I.V.: 2 g every 4-8 hours
Gonorrhea: I.M.: 1 g as a single dose
Disseminated: I.V.: 1 g every 8 hours
Life-threatening infections: I.V.: 2 g every 4 hours
Liver abscess: I.V.: 1-2 g every 6 hours
Lyme disease:
Cardiac manifestations: I.V.: 2 g every 4 hours
CNS manifestations: I.V.: 2 g every 8 hours for 14-28 days
Moderate-to-severe infections: I.M., I.V.: 1-2 g every 8 hours
Orbital cellulitis: I.V.: 2 g every 4 hours
Peritonitis (spontaneous): I.V.: 2 g every 8 hours, unless life-threatening then 2 g every 4 hours
Septicemia: I.V.: 2 g every 6-8 hours
Skin and soft tissue:
Mixed, necrotizing: I.V.: 2 g every 6 hours, with metronidazole or clindamycin
Bite wounds (animal): I.V.: 2 g every 6 hours
Surgical prophylaxis: I.M., I.V.: 1 g 30-90 minutes before surgery
Uncomplicated infections: I.M., I.V.: 1 g every 12 hours

Dosage Forms
Infusion [premixed iso-osmotic solution]:
Claforan®: 1 g (50 mL); 2 g (50 mL)
Injection, powder for reconstitution: 500 mg, 1 g, 2 g, 10 g, 20 g
Claforan®: 500 mg, 1 g, 2 g, 10 g

cefotaxime sodium *see* cefotaxime *on page 194*

cefoxitin (se FOKS i tin)

Sound-Alike/Look-Alike Issues
cefoxitin may be confused with cefotaxime, cefotetan, Cytoxan®

Synonyms cefoxitin sodium

U.S./Canadian Brand Names Apo-Cefoxitin® [Can]

Therapeutic Category Cephalosporin (Second Generation)

Use Less active against staphylococci and streptococci than first generation cephalosporins, but active against anaerobes including *Bacteroides fragilis*; active against gram-negative enteric bacilli including *E. coli*, *Klebsiella*, and *Proteus*; used predominantly for respiratory tract, skin, bone and joint, urinary tract and gynecologic as well as septicemia; surgical prophylaxis; intraabdominal infections and other mixed infections; indicated for bacterial *Eikenella corrodens* infections

Usual Dosage

Usual dosage range:

Infants >3 months and Children: I.M., I.V.: 80-160 mg/kg/day in divided doses every 4-6 hours (maximum dose: 12 g/day)

Adults: I.M., I.V.: 1-2 g every 6-8 hours (maximum dose: 12 g/day)

Note: I.M. injection is painful

Indication-specific dosing:

Infants >3 months and Children:

Mild-to-moderate infection: I.M., I.V.: 80-100 mg/kg/day in divided doses every 4-6 hours

Perioperative prophylaxis: I.V.: 30-40 mg/kg 30-60 minutes prior to surgery followed by 30-40 mg/kg/dose every 6 hours for no more than 24 hours after surgery depending on the procedure

Severe infection: I.M., I.V.: 100-160 mg/kg/day in divided doses every 4-6 hours

Adolescents and Adults:

Perioperative prophylaxis: I.M., I.V.: 1-2 g 30-60 minutes prior to surgery followed by 1-2 g every 6-8 hours for no more than 24 hours after surgery depending on the procedure

Adults:

Amnionitis, endomyometritis: I.M., I.V.: 2 g every 6-8 hours

Aspiration pneumonia, empyema, orbital cellulitis, parapharyngeal space, human bites: I.M., I.V.: 2 g every 8 hours

Liver abscess: I.V.: 1 g every 4 hours

Mycobacterium species, not MTB or MAI: I.V.: 12 g/day with amikacin

Pelvic inflammatory disease:

Inpatients: I.V.: 2 g every 6 hours **plus** doxycycline 100 mg I.V. or 100 mg orally every 12 hours until improved, followed by doxycycline 100 mg orally twice daily to complete 14 days

Outpatients: I.M.: 2 g **plus** probenecid 1 g orally as a single dose, followed by doxycycline 100 mg orally twice daily for 14 days

Dosage Forms

Injection, powder for reconstitution: 1 g, 2 g, 10 g

Powder for prescription compounding: 100 g

cefoxitin sodium *see* cefoxitin *on page 194*

cefpodoxime (sef pode OKS eem)

Sound-Alike/Look-Alike Issues

Vantin® may be confused with Ventolin®

Synonyms cefpodoxime proxetil

U.S./Canadian Brand Names Vantin® [US/Can]

Therapeutic Category Cephalosporin (Second Generation)

Use Treatment of susceptible acute, community-acquired pneumonia caused by *S. pneumoniae* or nonbeta-lactamase producing *H. influenzae*; acute uncomplicated gonorrhea caused by *N. gonorrhoeae*; uncomplicated skin and skin structure infections caused by *S. aureus* or *S. pyogenes*; acute otitis media caused by *S. pneumoniae*, *H. influenzae*, or *M. catarrhalis*; pharyngitis or tonsillitis; and uncomplicated urinary tract infections caused by *E. coli*, *Klebsiella*, and *Proteus*

Usual Dosage

Usual dosage range:

Children 2 months to 12 years: Oral: 10 mg/kg/day divided every 12 hours (maximum dose: 400 mg/day)

Children ≥12 years and Adults: Oral: 100-400 mg every 12 hours

Indication-specific dosing:

Children 2 months to 12 years: Oral:

Acute maxillary sinusitis: 10 mg/kg/day divided every 12 hours for 10 days (maximum: 200 mg/dose)

Acute otitis media: 10 mg/kg/day divided every 12 hours (400 mg/day) for 5 days (maximum: 200 mg/dose)

Pharyngitis/tonsillitis: 10 mg/kg/day in 2 divided doses for 5-10 days (maximum: 100 mg/dose)

Children ≥12 years and Adults: Oral:

Acute community-acquired pneumonia and bacterial exacerbations of chronic bronchitis: 200 mg every 12 hours for 14 days and 10 days, respectively

Acute maxillary sinusitis: 200 mg every 12 hours for 10 days

Pharyngitis/tonsillitis: 100 mg every 12 hours for 5-10 days

Skin and skin structure: 400 mg every 12 hours for 7-14 days

Uncomplicated gonorrhea (male and female) and rectal gonococcal infections (female): 200 mg as a single dose

Uncomplicated urinary tract infection: 100 mg every 12 hours for 7 days

Dosage Forms

Granules for suspension, oral: 50 mg/5 mL (50 mL, 75 mL, 100 mL); 100 mg/5 mL (50 mL, 75 mL, 100 mL)

Tablet: 100 mg, 200 mg

Vantin®: 200 mg

cefpodoxime proxetil *see* cefpodoxime *on page 195*

cefprozil (sef PROE zil)

Sound-Alike/Look-Alike Issues

cefprozil may be confused with ceFAZolin, cefuroxime

Cefzil® may be confused with Cefol®, Ceftin®, Kefzol®

U.S./Canadian Brand Names Apo-Cefprozil® [Can]; Cefzil® [Can]; Ran-Cefprozil [Can]; Sandoz-Cefprozil [Can]

Therapeutic Category Cephalosporin (Second Generation)

Use Treatment of otitis media and infections involving the respiratory tract and skin and skin structure; active against methicillin-sensitive staphylococci, many streptococci, and various gram-negative bacilli including *E. coli*, some *Klebsiella*, *P. mirabilis*, *H. influenzae*, and *Moraxella*.

Usual Dosage

Usual dosage range:

Infants and Children >6 months to 12 years: Oral: 7.5-15 mg/kg/day divided every 12 hours

Children >12 years and Adults: Oral: 250-500 mg every 12 hours or 500 mg every 24 hours

Indication-specific dosing:

Infants and Children >6 months to 12 years: Oral: **Otitis media:** 15 mg/kg every 12 hours for 10 days

Children 2-12 years: Oral:

Pharyngitis/tonsillitis: 7.5-15 mg/kg/day divided every 12 hours for 10 days (administer for >10 days if due to *S. pyogenes*); maximum: 1 g/day

Uncomplicated skin and skin structure infections: 20 mg/kg every 24 hours for 10 days; maximum: 1 g/day

Children >12 years and Adults: Oral:

Pharyngitis/tonsillitis: 500 mg every 24 hours for 10 days

Secondary bacterial infection of acute bronchitis or acute bacterial exacerbation of chronic bronchitis: 500 mg every 12 hours for 10 days

Uncomplicated skin and skin structure infections: 250 mg every 12 hours or 500 mg every 12-24 hours for 10 days

Dosage Forms

Powder for oral suspension: 125 mg/5 mL, 250 mg/5 mL

Tablet: 250 mg, 500 mg

ceftazidime (SEF tay zi deem)

Sound-Alike/Look-Alike Issues

ceftazidime may be confused with ceftizoxime

Ceptaz® may be confused with Septra®

Tazicef® may be confused with Tazidime®

U.S./Canadian Brand Names Fortaz® [US/Can]; Tazicef® [US]

Therapeutic Category Cephalosporin (Third Generation)

Use Treatment of documented susceptible *Pseudomonas aeruginosa* infection and infections due to other susceptible aerobic gram-negative organisms; empiric therapy of a febrile, granulocytopenic patient

Usual Dosage

Usual dosage range:

Infants and Children 1 month to 12 years: I.V.: 30-50 mg/kg/dose every 8 hours (maximum dose: 6 g/day)

Adults: I.M., I.V.: 500 mg to 2 g every 8-12 hours

Indication-specific dosing:

Bacterial arthritis (gram-negative bacilli): I.V.: 1-2 g every 8 hours

Cystic fibrosis: I.V.: 30-50 mg/kg every 8 hours (maximum: 6 g/day)

Melioidosis: I.V.: 40 mg/kg every 8 hours for 10 days, followed by oral therapy with doxycycline or TMP/SMX

Otitis externa: I.V.: 2 g every 8 hours

Peritonitis (CAPD):

Anuric, intermittent: 1000-1500 mg/day

Anuric, continuous (per liter exchange): Loading dose: 250 mg; maintenance dose: 125 mg

Severe infections, including meningitis, complicated pneumonia, endophthalmitis, CNS infection, osteomyelitis, intraabdominal and gynecological, skin and soft tissue: I.V.: 2 g every 8 hours

Dosage Forms

Infusion [premixed iso-osmotic solution, frozen]:

Fortaz®: 1 g (50 mL); 2 g (50 mL)

Injection, powder for reconstitution: 1 g, 2 g, 6 g

Fortaz®: 500 mg, 1 g, 2 g, 6 g

Tazicef®: 1 g, 2 g, 6 g

ceftibuten (sef TYE byoo ten)

Sound-Alike/Look-Alike Issues

Cedax® may be confused with Cidex®

U.S./Canadian Brand Names Cedax® [US]

Therapeutic Category Cephalosporin (Third Generation)

Use Treatment of acute exacerbations of chronic bronchitis, acute bacterial otitis media, and pharyngitis/tonsillitis

Usual Dosage

Usual dosage range:

Children 6 months to <12 years: Oral: 9 mg/kg/day for 10 days (maximum dose: 400 mg/day)

Children ≥12 years and Adults: Oral: 400 mg once daily for 10 days

Dosage Forms

Capsule:

Cedax®: 400 mg

Powder for oral suspension:

Cedax®: 90 mg/5 mL

Ceftin® [US/Can] *see* cefuroxime *on page 199*

Ceftin® Tablet 125 mg *(Discontinued)* *see* cefuroxime *on page 199*

ceftizoxime (sef ti ZOKS eem)

Sound-Alike/Look-Alike Issues

ceftizoxime may be confused with cefotaxime, ceftazidime, cefuroxime

Synonyms ceftizoxime sodium

U.S./Canadian Brand Names Cefizox® [US/Can]

Therapeutic Category Cephalosporin (Third Generation)

Use Treatment of susceptible bacterial infections, mainly respiratory tract, skin and skin structure, bone and joint, urinary tract and gynecologic, as well as septicemia; active against many gram-negative bacilli (not *Pseudomonas*), some gram-positive cocci (not *Enterococcus*), and some anaerobes

Usual Dosage

Usual dosage range:

Children ≥6 months: I.M., I.V.: 150-200 mg/kg/day divided every 6-8 hours (maximum: 12 g/24 hours)

Adults: I.M., I.V.: 1-4 g every 8-12 hours

Indication-specific dosing:

Adults:

Gonococcal:

Disseminated infection: I.M., I.V.: 1 g every 8 hours

Uncomplicated: I.M.: 1 g as single dose

Life-threatening infections: I.V.: 2 g every 4 hours or 4 g every 8 hours

Dosage Forms

Infusion [premixed iso-osmotic solution]:

Cefizox®: 1 g (50 mL); 2 g (50 mL)

ceftizoxime sodium *see* ceftizoxime *on page* 197

ceftobiprole *(Canada only)* (sef toe BYE prole)

Synonyms BAL5788; BAL9141; ceftobiprole medocaril

U.S./Canadian Brand Names Zeftera™ [Can]

Therapeutic Category Antibiotic, Cephalosporin

Use Treatment of complicated skin and skin structure infections, including diabetic foot infections without concurrent osteomyelitis, caused by *Enterobacter cloacae, Escherichia coli, Klebsiella pneumoniae, Proteus mirabilis, Staphylococcus aureus* (including methicillin-resistant *Staphylococcus aureus* [MRSA]) and *Streptococcus pyogenes*

Usual Dosage I.V.: Adults:

Usual dosage range: 500 mg every 8-12 hours

Indication specific dosing:

Complicated skin and skin structure infections (not including diabetic foot infections):

Gram positive: 500 mg every 12 hours for 7-14 days

Gram negative or mixed infection: 500 mg every 8 hours for 7-14 days

Complicated skin and skin structure infections including diabetic foot infections (nonlimb-threatening and without concurrent osteomyelitis): Gram positive, gram negative, and mixed infection: 500 mg every 8 hours for 7-14 days

Dosage Forms [CAN] = Canadian product

Injection, powder for reconstitution:

Zeftera™ [CAN]: 500 mg [not available in U.S.]

ceftobiprole medocaril *see* ceftobiprole *(Canada only) on page* 198

ceftriaxone (sef trye AKS one)

Sound-Alike/Look-Alike Issues

Rocephin® may be confused with Roferon®

Synonyms ceftriaxone sodium

Tall-Man cef**TRIAX**one

U.S./Canadian Brand Names Rocephin® [US/Can]

Therapeutic Category Cephalosporin (Third Generation)

Use Treatment of lower respiratory tract infections, acute bacterial otitis media, skin and skin structure infections, bone and joint infections, intraabdominal and urinary tract infections, pelvic inflammatory disease (PID), uncomplicated gonorrhea, bacterial septicemia, and meningitis; used in surgical prophylaxis

Usual Dosage

Usual dosage range:

Infants and Children: I.M., I.V.: 50-100 mg/kg/day in 1-2 divided doses (maximum: 4 g/day [meningitis]; 2 g/day [nonmeningeal infections])

Adults: I.M., I.V.: 1-2 g every 12-24 hours

Indication-specific dosing:

Infants and Children:

Gonococcal infections:

Prophylaxis (due to maternal gonococcal infection): I.M., I.V.: 25-50 mg/kg as a single dose (maximum: 125 mg)

Uncomplicated: I.M.: 125 mg in a single dose

Infective endocarditis: I.M., I.V.:

Native valve: 100 mg/kg once daily for 2-4 weeks; **Note:** If using 2-week regimen, concurrent gentamicin is recommended

Prosthetic valve: 100 mg/kg once daily for 6 weeks (with or without 2 weeks of gentamicin [dependent on penicillin MIC]); **Note:** For HACEK organisms, duration of therapy is 4 weeks

Enterococcus faecalis (resistant to penicillin, aminoglycoside, and vancomycin), native or prosthetic valve: 100 mg/kg once daily for ≥8 weeks administered concurrently with ampicillin

Prophylaxis: 50 mg/kg 30-60 minutes before procedure; maximum dose: 1 g. Intramuscular injections should be avoided in patients who are receiving anticoagulant therapy. In these circumstances, orally administered regimens should be given whenever possible. Intravenously administered antibiotics should be used for patients who are unable to tolerate or absorb oral medications.

Note: American Heart Association (AHA) guidelines now recommend prophylaxis only in patients undergoing invasive procedures and in whom underlying cardiac conditions may predispose to a higher risk of adverse outcomes should infection occur. As of April 2007, routine prophylaxis for GI/ GU procedures is no longer recommended by the AHA.

Mild-to-moderate infections: I.M., I.V.: 50-75 mg/kg/day in 1-2 divided doses every 12-24 hours (maximum: 2 g/day); continue until at least 2 days after signs and symptoms of infection have resolved

Meningitis:

Gonococcal, complicated:

<45 kg: I.V.: 50 mg/kg/day given every 12 hours (maximum: 2 g/day); usual duration of treatment is 10-14 days

>45 kg: I.V.: 1-2 g every 12 hours; usual duration of treatment is 10-14 days

Uncomplicated: I.M., I.V.: Loading dose of 100 mg/kg (maximum: 4 g), followed by 100 mg/kg/day divided every 12-24 hours (maximum: 4 g/day); usual duration of treatment is 7-14 days

Otitis media: *Acute:* I.M.: 50 mg/kg in a single dose (maximum: 1 g)

Pneumonia: I.V.: 50-75 mg/kg once daily

Serious infections: I.V.: 80-100 mg/kg/day in 1-2 divided doses (maximum: 4 g/day)

Skin/skin structure infections: I.M., I.V.: 50-75 mg/kg/day in 1-2 divided doses (maximum: 2 g/day)

Adults:

Gonococcal infections: *Uncomplicated:* I.M.: 125-250 mg in a single dose

Infective endocarditis: I.M., I.V.:

Native valve: 2 g once daily for 2-4 weeks; **Note:** If using 2-week regimen, concurrent gentamicin is recommended

Prosthetic valve: I.M., I.V.: 2 g once daily for 6 weeks (with or without 2 weeks of gentamicin [dependent on penicillin MIC]); **Note:** For HACEK organisms, duration of therapy is 4 weeks

Enterococcus faecalis (resistant to penicillin, aminoglycoside, and vancomycin), native or prosthetic valve: 2 g twice daily for ≥8 weeks administered concurrently with ampicillin

Prophylaxis: I.M., I.V.: 1 g 30-60 minutes before procedure. Intramuscular injections should be avoided in patients who are receiving anticoagulant therapy. In these circumstances, orally administered regimens should be given whenever possible. Intravenously administered antibiotics should be used for patients who are unable to tolerate or absorb oral medications.

Note: American Heart Association (AHA) guidelines now recommend prophylaxis only in patients undergoing invasive procedures and in whom underlying cardiac conditions may predispose to a higher risk of adverse outcomes should infection occur. As of April 2007, routine prophylaxis for GI/ GU procedures is no longer recommended by the AHA.

Meningitis: I.V.: 2 g every 12 hours for 7-14 days (longer courses may be necessary for selected organisms)

Pelvic inflammatory disease: I.M.: 250 mg in a single dose

Pneumonia, community-acquired: I.V.: 1 g once daily, usually in combination with a macrolide; consider 2 g/day for patients at risk for more severe infection and/or resistant organisms (ICU status, age >65 years, disseminated infection)

Pyelonephritis (acute, uncomplicated): Females: I.V.: 1-2 g once daily. Many physicians administer a single parenteral dose before initiating oral therapy.

STD prophylaxis in sexual assault victims: I.M.: 125 mg as a single dose

Surgical prophylaxis: I.V.: 1 g 30 minutes to 2 hours before surgery

Dosage Forms

Infusion [premixed in dextrose]: 1 g (50 mL); 2 g (50 mL)

Injection, powder for reconstitution: 250 mg, 500 mg, 1 g, 2 g, 10 g

Rocephin®: 500 mg, 1 g

ceftriaxone sodium *see* ceftriaxone *on page 198*

cefuroxime (se fyoor OKS eem)

Sound-Alike/Look-Alike Issues

cefuroxime may be confused with cefotaxime, cefprozil, ceftizoxime, deferoxamine

Ceftin® may be confused with Cefzil®, Cipro®

Zinacef® may be confused with Zithromax®

Synonyms cefuroxime axetil; cefuroxime sodium

U.S./Canadian Brand Names Apo-Cefuroxime® [Can]; Ceftin® [US/Can]; Cefuroxime For Injection [Can]; Pro-Cefuroxime [Can]; ratio-Cefuroxime [Can]; Zinacef® [US/Can]

Therapeutic Category Cephalosporin (Second Generation)

Use Treatment of infections caused by staphylococci, group B streptococci, *H. influenzae* (type A and B), *E. coli*, *Enterobacter*, *Salmonella*, and *Klebsiella*; treatment of susceptible infections of the upper and lower respiratory tract, otitis media, urinary tract, uncomplicated skin and soft tissue, bone and joint, sepsis, uncomplicated gonorrhea, and early Lyme disease; surgical prophylaxis

Usual Dosage Note: Cefuroxime axetil film-coated tablets and oral suspension are not bioequivalent and are not substitutable on a mg/mg basis

Usual dosage range:

Children 3 months to 12 years:

Oral: 20-30 mg/kg/day in 2 divided doses

I.M., I.V.: 75-150 mg/kg/day divided every 8 hours (maximum dose: 6 g/day)

Children ≥13 years and Adults:

Oral: 250-500 mg twice daily

I.M., I.V.: 750 mg to 1.5 g every 6-8 hours or 100-150 mg/kg/day in divided doses every 6-8 hours (maximum: 6 g/day)

Indication-specific dosing:

Children ≥3 months to 12 years:

Acute bacterial maxillary sinusitis, acute otitis media, and impetigo:

Oral: Suspension: 30 mg/kg/day in 2 divided doses for 10 days (maximum dose: 1 g/day); tablet: 250 mg twice daily for 10 days

I.M., I.V.: 75-150 mg/kg/day divided every 8 hours (maximum dose: 6 g/day)

Epiglottitis: Oral: 150 mg/kg/day in 3 divided doses for 7-10 days

Pharyngitis/tonsillitis:

Oral: Suspension: 20 mg/kg/day (maximum: 500 mg/day) in 2 divided doses for 10 days; tablet: 125 mg every 12 hours for 10 days

I.M., I.V.: 75-150 mg/kg day divided every 8 hours (maximum: 6 g/day)

Children ≥13 years and Adults (all oral doses listed are for tablet formulation):

Bronchitis (acute and exacerbations of chronic bronchitis):

Oral: 250-500 mg every 12 hours for 10 days

I.V.: 500-750 mg every 8 hours (complete therapy with oral dosing)

Cellulitis, orbital: I.V.: 1.5 g every 8 hours

Gonorrhea:

Disseminated: I.M., I.V.: 750 mg every 8 hours

Uncomplicated:

Oral: 1 g as a single dose

I.M.: 1.5 g as single dose (administer in 2 different sites with probenecid)

Lyme disease (early): Oral: 500 mg twice daily for 20 days

Pharyngitis/tonsillitis and sinusitis: Oral: 250 mg twice daily for 10 days

Pneumonia (uncomplicated): I.V.: 750 mg every 8 hours

Severe or complicated infections: I.M., I.V.: 1.5 g every 8 hours (up to 1.5 g every 6 hours in life-threatening infections)

Skin/skin structure infection (uncomplicated):

Oral: 250-500 mg every 12 hours for 10 days

I.M., I.V.: 750 mg every 8 hours

Surgical prophylaxis:

I.V.: 1.5 g 30 minutes to 1 hour prior to procedure (if procedure is prolonged can give 750 mg every 8 hours I.M.)

Open heart: I.V.: 1.5 g every 12 hours to a total of 6 g

Urinary tract infection (uncomplicated):

Oral: 125-250 mg every 12 hours for 7-10 days

I.M., I.V.: 750 mg every 8 hours

Dosage Forms Note: Strength expressed as base

Infusion [premixed]: 750 mg (50 mL); 1.5 g (50 mL)

Zinacef®: 750 mg (50 mL); 1.5 g (50 mL)

Injection, powder for reconstitution: 750 mg, 1.5 g, 7.5 g, 75 g, 225 g

Zinacef®: 750 mg, 1.5 g, 7.5 g

Powder for suspension, oral: 125 mg/5 mL, 250 mg/5 mL

Ceftin®: 125 mg/5 mL, 250 mg/5 mL

Tablet: 250 mg, 500 mg

Ceftin®: 250 mg, 500 mg

cefuroxime axetil *see* cefuroxime *on page 199*
Cefuroxime For Injection [Can] *see* cefuroxime *on page 199*
cefuroxime sodium *see* cefuroxime *on page 199*
Cefzil® [Can] *see* cefprozil *on page 196*
Celebrex® [US/Can] *see* celecoxib *on page 201*

celecoxib (se le KOKS ib)

Sound-Alike/Look-Alike Issues
Celebrex® may be confused with Celexa®, cerebra, Cerebyx®, Clarinex®

U.S./Canadian Brand Names Celebrex® [US/Can]; GD-Celecoxib [Can]

Therapeutic Category Nonsteroidal Antiinflammatory Drug (NSAID), COX-2 Selective

Use Relief of the signs and symptoms of osteoarthritis, ankylosing spondylitis, juvenile rheumatoid arthritis (JRA), and rheumatoid arthritis; management of acute pain; treatment of primary dysmenorrhea; to reduce the number of intestinal polyps in familial adenomatous polyposis (FAP)

Canadian note: Celecoxib is only indicated for relief of symptoms of rheumatoid arthritis, osteoarthritis, and relief of acute pain in adults

Usual Dosage Note: Use the lowest effective dose for the shortest duration of time, consistent with individual patient goals. Oral:

Children ≥2 years: JRA
- ≥10 kg to ≤25 kg: 50 mg twice daily
- >25 kg: 100 mg twice daily

Adults:
- Acute pain or primary dysmenorrhea: Initial dose: 400 mg, followed by an additional 200 mg if needed on day 1; maintenance dose: 200 mg twice daily as needed
- Ankylosing spondylitis: 200 mg/day as a single dose or in divided doses twice daily; if no effect after 6 weeks, may increase to 400 mg/day. If no response following 6 weeks of treatment with 400 mg/day, consider discontinuation and alternative treatment.
- Familial adenomatous polyposis: 400 mg twice daily
- Osteoarthritis: 200 mg/day as a single dose or in divided dose twice daily
- Rheumatoid arthritis: 100-200 mg twice daily

Dosage Forms
Capsule:
Celebrex®: 50 mg, 100 mg, 200 mg, 400 mg

Celestone® [US] *see* betamethasone (systemic) *on page 138*
Celestone® Soluspan® [US/Can] *see* betamethasone (systemic) *on page 138*
Celexa® [US/Can] *see* citalopram *on page 234*
CellCept® [US/Can] *see* mycophenolate *on page 673*
Cellugel® [US] *see* hydroxypropyl methylcellulose *on page 510*

cellulose, oxidized regenerated (SEL yoo lose, OKS i dyzed re JEN er aye ted)

Sound-Alike/Look-Alike Issues
Surgicel® may be confused with Serentil®

Synonyms absorbable cotton; oxidized regenerated cellulose

U.S./Canadian Brand Names Surgicel® Fibrillar [US]; Surgicel® NuKnit [US]; Surgicel® [US]

Therapeutic Category Hemostatic Agent

Use Hemostatic; temporary packing for the control of capillary, venous, or small arterial hemorrhage

Usual Dosage Minimal amounts of the fabric strip are laid on the bleeding site or held firmly against the tissues until hemostasis occurs; remove excess material

Dosage Forms
Fabric, fibrous:
Surgicel® Fibrillar:
- 1" x 2" (10s)
- 2" x 4" (10s)
- 4" x 4" (10s)

Fabric, knitted:
Surgicel® NuKnit:
1" x 1" (24s)
1" x 3½" (10s)
3" x 4" (24s)
6" x 9" (10s)
Fabric, sheer weave:
Surgicel®:
½" x 2" (24s)
2" x 3" (24s)
2" x 14" (24s)
4" x 8" (24s)

Celluvisc™ [Can] *see* carboxymethylcellulose *on page 186*
Celontin® [US/Can] *see* methsuximide *on page 642*
Celsentri™ [Can] *see* maraviroc *on page 614*
Cemill [US-OTC] *see* ascorbic acid *on page 100*
Cena-K® *(Discontinued)* *see* potassium chloride *on page 803*
Cenestin® [US/Can] *see* estrogens (conjugated A/synthetic) *on page 378*
Cenolate® [US] *see* ascorbic acid *on page 100*
Centamin [US-OTC] *see* vitamins (multiple/oral) *on page 1019*
Centany™ *(Discontinued)* *see* mupirocin *on page 672*
Centrum® [US-OTC] *see* vitamins (multiple/oral) *on page 1019*
Centrum Cardio® [US-OTC] *see* vitamins (multiple/oral) *on page 1019*
Centrum Kids® Complete Dora the Explorer™ [US-OTC] *see* vitamins (multiple/pediatric) *on page 1020*
Centrum Kids® Complete Rugrats™ [US-OTC] *see* vitamins (multiple/pediatric) *on page 1020*
Centrum Kids® Complete SpongeBob SquarePants™ [US-OTC] *see* vitamins (multiple/pediatric) *on page 1020*
Centrum Performance® [US-OTC] *see* vitamins (multiple/oral) *on page 1019*
Centrum® Silver® [US-OTC] *see* vitamins (multiple/oral) *on page 1019*
Centrum® Silver® Ultra Men's [US-OTC] *see* vitamins (multiple/oral) *on page 1019*
Centrum® Silver® Ultra Women's [US-OTC] *see* vitamins (multiple/oral) *on page 1019*
Centrum® Ultra Men's [US-OTC] *see* vitamins (multiple/oral) *on page 1019*
Centrum® Ultra Women's [US-OTC] *see* vitamins (multiple/oral) *on page 1019*
Cepacol® Antibacterial Mouthwash Gold [US-OTC] *see* cetylpyridinium *on page 205*
Cepacol® Sore Throat [US-OTC] *see* benzocaine *on page 129*
Cephadyn [US] *see* butalbital and acetaminophen *on page 162*

cephalexin (sef a LEKS in)

Sound-Alike/Look-Alike Issues
cephalexin may be confused with cefaclor, cefazolin, cephalothin, ciprofloxacin

Synonyms cephalexin monohydrate

U.S./Canadian Brand Names Apo-Cephalex® [Can]; Keflex® [US]; Keftab® [Can]; Novo-Lexin [Can]; Nu-Cephalex [Can]

Therapeutic Category Cephalosporin (First Generation)

Use Treatment of susceptible bacterial infections including respiratory tract infections, otitis media, skin and skin structure infections, bone infections, and genitourinary tract infections, including acute prostatitis; alternative therapy for acute infective endocarditis prophylaxis

Usual Dosage
Usual dosage range:
Children >1 year: Oral: 25-100 mg/kg/day every 6-8 hours (maximum: 4 g/day)
Adults: Oral: 250-1000 mg every 6 hours; maximum: 4 g/day
Indication-specific dosing:
Children >1 year: Oral:
Furunculosis: 25-50 mg/kg/day in 4 divided doses
Impetigo: 25 mg/kg/day in 4 divided doses
Otitis media: 75-100 mg/kg/day in 4 divided doses

Prophylaxis against infective endocarditis (dental, oral, or respiratory tract procedures): 50 mg/kg 30-60 minutes prior to procedure (maximum: 2 g). **Note:** American Heart Association (AHA) guidelines now recommend prophylaxis only in patients undergoing invasive procedures and in whom underlying cardiac conditions may predispose to a higher risk of adverse outcomes should infection occur.

Severe infections: 50-100 mg/kg/day in divided doses every 6-8 hours

Skin abscess: 50 mg/kg/day in 4 divided doses (maximum: 4 g)

Streptococcal pharyngitis, skin and skin structure infections: 25-50 mg/kg/day divided every 12 hours

Children >15 years and Adults: Oral:

Cellulitis and mastitis: 500 mg every 6 hours

Furunculosis/skin abscess: 250 mg 4 times/day

Prophylaxis against infective endocarditis (dental, oral, or respiratory tract procedures): 2 g 30-60 minutes prior to procedure. **Note:** American Heart Association (AHA) guidelines now recommend prophylaxis only in patients undergoing invasive procedures and in whom underlying cardiac conditions may predispose to a higher risk of adverse outcomes should infection occur.

Prophylaxis in total joint replacement patients undergoing dental procedures which produce bacteremia: 2 g 1 hour prior to procedure

Streptococcal pharyngitis, skin and skin structure infections: 500 mg every 12 hours

Uncomplicated cystitis: 500 mg every 12 hours for 7-14 days

Dosage Forms

Capsule: 250 mg, 500 mg

Keflex®: 250 mg, 500 mg, 750 mg

Powder for oral suspension: 125 mg/5 mL, 250 mg/5 mL

Keflex®: 125 mg/5 mL, 250 mg/5 mL

Tablet: 250 mg, 500 mg

cephalexin monohydrate *see* cephalexin *on page 202*

cephalothin ***(Discontinued)***

Cephulac® ***(Discontinued)*** *see* lactulose *on page 565*

Ceprotin [US] *see* protein C concentrate (human) *on page 831*

Ceptaz® ***(Discontinued)*** *see* ceftazidime *on page 196*

Cerebyx® [US/Can] *see* fosphenytoin *on page 446*

Ceredase® [US] *see* alglucerase *on page 46*

Cerefolin® NAC [US] *see* methylfolate, methylcobalamin, and acetylcysteine *on page 644*

Cerezyme® [US/Can] *see* imiglucerase *on page 520*

Ceron [US] *see* chlorpheniramine and phenylephrine *on page 214*

Ceron-DM [US] *see* chlorpheniramine, phenylephrine, and dextromethorphan *on page 217*

Cerovel™ [US] *see* urea *on page 998*

Certain Dri® [US-OTC] *see* aluminum chloride hexahydrate *on page 54*

certolizumab pegol (cer to LIZ u mab PEG ol)

Synonyms CDP870

U.S./Canadian Brand Names Cimzia® [US]

Therapeutic Category Gastrointestinal Agent, Miscellaneous; Tumor Necrosis Factor (TNF) Blocking Agent

Use Treatment of moderately- to severely-active Crohn disease in patients who have inadequate response to conventional therapy; moderately- to severely-active rheumatoid arthritis (as monotherapy or in combination with nonbiological disease-modifying antirheumatic drugs [DMARDS])

Usual Dosage **Note:** Each 400 mg dose should be administered as 2 injections of 200 mg each

SubQ: Adults:

Crohn disease: Initial: 400 mg, repeat dose 2 and 4 weeks after initial dose; Maintenance: 400 mg every 4 weeks

Rheumatoid arthritis: Initial: 400 mg, repeat dose 2 and 4 weeks after initial dose; Maintenance: 200 mg every other week. May consider maintenance dose of 400 mg every 4 weeks.

Dosage Forms

Injection, powder for reconstitution [preservative free]:

Cimzia®: 200 mg [contains sucrose 100 mg]

Injection, solution [preservative-free]:

Cimzia®: 200 mg/mL (1 mL)

Certuss-D® [US] *see* guaifenesin, dextromethorphan, and phenylephrine *on page 478*
Cerubidine® [US/Can] *see* daunorubicin hydrochloride *on page 278*
Cerumenex® *(Discontinued)*
Cervidil® [US/Can] *see* dinoprostone *on page 314*
C.E.S.® [Can] *see* estrogens (conjugated/equine) *on page 378*
C.E.S. *see* estrogens (conjugated/equine) *on page 378*
Cesia™ [US] *see* ethinyl estradiol and desogestrel *on page 383*
Cetacaine® [US] *see* benzocaine, butamben, and tetracaine *on page 131*
Cetacort® [US] *see* hydrocortisone (topical) *on page 505*
Cetafen® [US-OTC] *see* acetaminophen *on page 19*
Cetafen Cold® [US-OTC] *see* acetaminophen and phenylephrine *on page 22*
Cetafen® Extra [US-OTC] *see* acetaminophen *on page 19*
Cetamide™ [Can] *see* sulfacetamide *on page 927*
Cetapred® Ophthalmic *(Discontinued)* *see* sulfacetamide and prednisolone *on page 927*

cetirizine (se TI ra zeen)

Sound-Alike/Look-Alike Issues
Zyrtec® may be confused with Serax®, Xanax®, Zantac®, Zerit®, Zyprexa®

Synonyms cetirizine hydrochloride; P-071; UCB-P071

U.S./Canadian Brand Names Apo-Cetirizine® [Can]; PMS-Cetirizine [Can]; Reactine™ [Can]; Zyrtec® Allergy [US-OTC]; Zyrtec® Children's Allergy [US-OTC]; Zyrtec® Children's Hives Relief [US-OTC]

Therapeutic Category Antihistamine

Use Perennial and seasonal allergic rhinitis and other allergic symptoms including urticaria; chronic idiopathic urticaria

Usual Dosage Oral:
Children:
6-12 months: Chronic urticaria, perennial allergic rhinitis: 2.5 mg once daily
12 months to <2 years: Chronic urticaria, perennial allergic rhinitis: 2.5 mg once daily; may increase to 2.5 mg every 12 hours if needed
2-5 years: Chronic urticaria, perennial or seasonal allergic rhinitis: Initial: 2.5 mg once daily; may be increased to 2.5 mg every 12 hours **or** 5 mg once daily
Children ≥6 years and Adults: Chronic urticaria, perennial or seasonal allergic rhinitis: 5-10 mg once daily, depending upon symptom severity

Dosage Forms
Syrup, oral: 5 mg/5 mL
Zyrtec® Children's Allergy [OTC], Zyrtec® Children's Hives Relief [OTC]: 5 mg/5 mL
Tablet, oral: 5 mg, 10 mg
All Day Allergy, Zyrtec® Allergy [OTC]: 10 mg
Tablet, chewable, oral:
Zyrtec® Children's Allergy [OTC]: 5 mg, 10 mg

cetirizine and pseudoephedrine (se TI ra zeen & soo doe e FED rin)

Sound-Alike/Look-Alike Issues
Zyrtec® may be confused with Serax®, Xanax®, Zantac®, Zyprexa®

Synonyms cetirizine hydrochloride and pseudoephedrine hydrochloride; pseudoephedrine hydrochloride and cetirizine hydrochloride

U.S./Canadian Brand Names Reactine® Allergy and Sinus [Can]; Zytrec-D® Allergy & Congestion [US-OTC]

Therapeutic Category Antihistamine/Decongestant Combination

Use Treatment of symptoms of seasonal or perennial allergic rhinitis

Usual Dosage Oral: Children ≥12 years and Adults: Seasonal/perennial allergic rhinitis: 1 tablet twice daily (maximum: 2 tablets/day)

Dosage Forms
Tablet, extended release: Cetirizine hydrochloride 5 mg and pseudoephedrine hydrochloride 120 mg
Zyrtec-D® Allergy & Congestion [OTC]: Cetirizine 5 mg and pseudoephedrine 120 mg

cetirizine hydrochloride *see* cetirizine *on page 204*

cetirizine hydrochloride and pseudoephedrine hydrochloride *see* cetirizine and pseudoephedrine *on page* 204

Cetraxal® [US] *see* ciprofloxacin *on page* 229

cetrorelix (set roe REL iks)

Synonyms cetrorelix acetate

U.S./Canadian Brand Names Cetrotide® [US/Can]

Therapeutic Category Antigonadotropic Agent

Use Inhibits premature luteinizing hormone (LH) surges in women undergoing controlled ovarian stimulation

Usual Dosage SubQ: Adults: Female: Used in conjunction with controlled ovarian stimulation therapy using gonadotropins (FSH, HMG):

Single-dose regimen: 3 mg given when serum estradiol levels show appropriate stimulation response, usually stimulation day 7 (range days 5-9). If hCG is not administered within 4 days, continue cetrorelix at 0.25 mg/day until hCG is administered.

Multiple-dose regimen: 0.25 mg morning or evening of stimulation day 5, or morning of stimulation day 6; continue until hCG is administered.

Dosage Forms

Injection, powder for reconstitution:

Cetrotide®: 0.25 mg, 3 mg

cetrorelix acetate *see* cetrorelix *on page* 205

Cetrotide® [US/Can] *see* cetrorelix *on page* 205

cetuximab (se TUK see mab)

Sound-Alike/Look-Alike Issues

cetuximab may be confused with bevacizumab

Synonyms C225; IMC-C225; NSC-714692

U.S./Canadian Brand Names Erbitux® [US/Can]

Therapeutic Category Antineoplastic Agent, Monoclonal Antibody; Epidermal Growth Factor Receptor (EGFR) Inhibitor

Use Treatment of metastatic colorectal cancer; treatment of squamous cell cancer of the head and neck

Note: Subset analyses (retrospective) in metastatic colorectal cancer trials have not shown a benefit with EGFR inhibitor treatment in patients whose tumors have codon 12 or 13 *KRAS* mutations; use is not recommended in these patients.

Usual Dosage I.V.: Adults: **Note:** Premedicate with an H_1 antagonist (eg, diphenhydramine) I.V. 30-60 minutes prior to the first dose; premedication for subsequent doses is based on clinical judgement.

Colorectal cancer:

Initial loading dose: 400 mg/m^2 infused over 120 minutes

Maintenance dose: 250 mg/m^2 infused over 60 minutes weekly

Head and neck cancer:

Initial loading dose: 400 mg/m^2 infused over 120 minutes

Maintenance dose: 250 mg/m^2 infused over 60 minutes weekly

Note: If given in combination with radiation therapy, administer loading dose 1 week prior to initiation of radiation course. Weekly maintenance dose should be completed 1 hour prior to radiation for the duration of radiation therapy (6-7 weeks).

Dosage Forms

Injection, solution [preservative free]:

Erbitux®: 2 mg/mL (50 mL, 100 mL)

cetyl alcohol, glycerin, lanolin, mineral oil, and petrolatum *see* lanolin, cetyl alcohol, glycerin, petrolatum, and mineral oil *on page* 570

cetylpyridinium (SEE til peer i DI nee um)

Synonyms cetylpyridinium chloride; CPC

U.S./Canadian Brand Names Cepacol® Antibacterial Mouthwash Gold [US-OTC]; DiabetAid Gingivitis Mouth Rinse [US-OTC]

Therapeutic Category Local Anesthetic

Use Antiseptic to aid in the prevention and reduction of plaque and gingivitis, and to freshen breath

Usual Dosage Oral (OTC labeling): Children ≥6 years and Adults: Rinse or gargle to freshen mouth; may be used before or after brushing

Dosage Forms

Liquid, oral [mouthwash/gargle]:

Cepacol® Antibacterial Mouthwash Gold [OTC]: 0.05%

DiabetAid Gingivitis Mouth Rinse [OTC]: 0.1%

cetylpyridinium chloride *see* cetylpyridinium *on page* *205*

Cevalin® ***(Discontinued)*** *see* ascorbic acid *on page* *100*

cevimeline (se vi ME leen)

Sound-Alike/Look-Alike Issues

cevimeline may be confused with Savella™

Evoxac® may be confused with Eurax®

Synonyms cevimeline hydrochloride

U.S./Canadian Brand Names Evoxac® [US/Can]

Therapeutic Category Cholinergic Agent

Use Treatment of symptoms of dry mouth in patients with Sjögren syndrome

Usual Dosage Oral: Adults: 30 mg 3 times/day

Dosage Forms

Capsule:

Evoxac®: 30 mg

cevimeline hydrochloride *see* cevimeline *on page* *206*

CFDN *see* cefdinir *on page* *192*

CG *see* chorionic gonadotropin (human) *on page* *225*

CG5503 *see* tapentadol *on page* *938*

C-Gel [US-OTC] *see* ascorbic acid *on page* *100*

CGP 33101 *see* rufinamide *on page* *882*

CGP-42446 *see* zoledronic acid *on page* *1032*

CGP-57148B *see* imatinib *on page* *519*

C-Gram [US-OTC] *see* ascorbic acid *on page* *100*

CGS-20267 *see* letrozole *on page* *575*

Champix® [Can] *see* varenicline *on page* *1006*

Chantix® [US] *see* varenicline *on page* *1006*

Charcadole® [Can] *see* charcoal *on page* *206*

Charcadole®, Aqueous [Can] *see* charcoal *on page* *206*

Charcadole® TFS [Can] *see* charcoal *on page* *206*

Char-Caps [US-OTC] *see* charcoal *on page* *206*

CharcoAid® ***(Discontinued)*** *see* charcoal *on page* *206*

CharcoAid® G [US-OTC] *see* charcoal *on page* *206*

charcoal (CHAR kole)

Sound-Alike/Look-Alike Issues

Actidose® may be confused with Actos®

Synonyms activated carbon; activated charcoal; adsorbent charcoal; liquid antidote; medicinal carbon; medicinal charcoal

U.S./Canadian Brand Names Actidose-Aqua® [US-OTC]; Actidose® with Sorbitol [US-OTC]; Char-Caps [US-OTC]; Charcadole® TFS [Can]; Charcadole® [Can]; Charcadole®, Aqueous [Can]; CharcoAid® G [US-OTC]; Charcoal Plus® DS [US-OTC]; CharcoCaps® [US-OTC]; EZ-Char™ [US-OTC]; Kerr Insta-Char® [US-OTC]; Requa® Activated Charcoal [US-OTC]

Therapeutic Category Antidote

Use Emergency treatment in poisoning by drugs and chemicals; aids the elimination of certain drugs and improves decontamination of excessive ingestions of sustained-release products or in the presence of bezoars; repetitive doses have proven useful to enhance the elimination of certain drugs (eg, carbamazepine, dapsone, phenobarbital, quinine, or theophylline); repetitive doses for gastric dialysis in uremia to adsorb various waste products; dietary supplement (digestive aid)

Usual Dosage Oral:

Acute poisoning: **Note:** ~10 g of activated charcoal for each 1 g of toxin is considered adequate; this may require multiple doses. If sorbitol is also used, sorbitol dose should not exceed 1.5 g/kg. When using multiple doses of charcoal, sorbitol should be given with every other dose (not to exceed 2 doses/day).

Children:

<1 year: 0.5-1 g/kg (10-25 g) as a single dose; if multiple doses are needed, give as 0.25 g/kg/hour or equivalent (eg, 0.5 g/kg every 2 hours)

1-12 years: 0.5-1 g/kg (25-50 g) as a single dose; if multiple doses are needed, give as 0.25 g/kg/hour or equivalent (eg, 0.5 g/kg every 2 hours)

Children >12 years and Adults: 25-100 g as a single dose; if multiple doses are needed, additional doses may be given as 12.5 g/hour or equivalent (eg, 25 g every 2 hours)

Dietary supplement: Adults: 500-520 mg after meals; may repeat in 2 hours if needed (maximum: 10 g/day)

Dosage Forms

Capsule:

Char-Caps [OTC], CharcoCaps® [OTC]: 260 mg

Pellets, for suspension:

EZ-Char™ [OTC]: 25 g

Powder for suspension: 30 g, 240 g

CharcoAid® G [OTC]: 15 g

Suspension:

Actidose-Aqua® [OTC]: 15 g, 25 g, 50 g

Kerr Insta-Char® [OTC]: 25 g, 50 g

Suspension [with sorbitol]:

Actidose® with Sorbitol [OTC], Kerr Insta-Char® [OTC]: 25 g, 50 g

Tablet:

Requa® Activated Charcoal [OTC]: 250 mg

Tablet, enteric coated:

Charcoal Plus® DS [OTC]: 250 mg

Charcoal Plus® DS [US-OTC] *see* charcoal *on page 206*

CharcoCaps® [US-OTC] *see* charcoal *on page 206*

Chealamide® ***(Discontinued)*** *see* edetate disodium *on page 347*

CheeTah® [US] *see* barium *on page 122*

Chemet® [US/Can] *see* succimer *on page 924*

Cheracol® D [US-OTC] *see* guaifenesin and dextromethorphan *on page 474*

Cheracol® Plus [US-OTC] *see* guaifenesin and dextromethorphan *on page 474*

Cheracol® Spray [US-OTC] *see* phenol *on page 772*

Cheracol® Syrup [US] *see* guaifenesin and codeine *on page 473*

Chew-C [US-OTC] *see* ascorbic acid *on page 100*

Chew-Cal [US-OTC] *see* calcium and vitamin D *on page 169*

CHG *see* chlorhexidine gluconate *on page 210*

Chibroxin® ***(Discontinued)*** *see* norfloxacin *on page 705*

chickenpox vaccine *see* varicella virus vaccine *on page 1007*

Chiggerex® [US-OTC] *see* benzocaine *on page 129*

Chiggerex® Plus [US] *see* benzocaine *on page 129*

Chiggertox® [US-OTC] *see* benzocaine *on page 129*

Children's Advil® Cold [Can] *see* pseudoephedrine and ibuprofen *on page 835*

Children's Dimetapp® Elixir Cold & Allergy ***(Discontinued)*** *see* brompheniramine and pseudoephedrine *on page 150*

Children's Hold® ***(Discontinued)*** *see* dextromethorphan *on page 295*

Children's Kaopectate® ***(Discontinued)***

Children's Motion Sickness Liquid [Can] *see* dimenhydrinate *on page 312*

Children's Pepto [US-OTC] *see* calcium carbonate *on page 170*

children's vitamins *see* vitamins (multiple/pediatric) *on page 1020*

ChiRhoStim® [US] *see* secretin *on page 894*

Chirocaine® ***(Discontinued)***

Chlo-Amine® Oral ***(Discontinued)*** *see* chlorpheniramine *on page 213*

chloditan *see* mitotane *on page* 662
chlodithane *see* mitotane *on page* 662
Chlorafed® Liquid *(Discontinued)* *see* chlorpheniramine and pseudoephedrine *on page* 215
chloral *see* chloral hydrate *on page* 208

chloral hydrate (KLOR al HYE drate)

Synonyms chloral; hydrated chloral; trichloroacetaldehyde monohydrate

U.S./Canadian Brand Names PMS-Chloral Hydrate [Can]; Somnote® [US]

Therapeutic Category Hypnotic, Nonbarbiturate

Controlled Substance C-IV

Use Short-term sedative and hypnotic (<2 weeks); sedative/hypnotic for diagnostic procedures; sedative prior to EEG evaluations

Usual Dosage

Children:

Sedation or anxiety: Oral, rectal: 5-15 mg/kg/dose every 8 hours (maximum: 500 mg/dose)

Prior to EEG: Oral, rectal: 20-25 mg/kg/dose, 30-60 minutes prior to EEG; may repeat in 30 minutes to maximum of 100 mg/kg or 2 g total

Hypnotic: Oral, rectal: 20-40 mg/kg/dose up to a maximum of 50 mg/kg/24 hours or 1 g/dose or 2 g/24 hours

Conscious sedation: Oral: 50-75 mg/kg/dose 30-60 minutes prior to procedure; may repeat 30 minutes after initial dose if needed, to a total maximum dose of 120 mg/kg or 1 g total

Adults: Oral, rectal:

Sedation, anxiety: 250 mg 3 times/day

Hypnotic: 500-1000 mg at bedtime or 30 minutes prior to procedure, not to exceed 2 g/24 hours

Discontinuation: Withdraw gradually over 2 weeks if patient has been maintained on high doses for prolonged period of time. Do not stop drug abruptly; sudden withdrawal may result in delirium.

Dosage Forms

Capsule:

Somnote®: 500 mg

Suppository, rectal: 500 mg

Syrup: 500 mg/5 mL

chlorambucil (klor AM byoo sil)

Sound-Alike/Look-Alike Issues

chlorambucil may be confused with Chloromycetin®

Leukeran® may be confused with Alkeran®, leucovorin, Leukine®, Myleran®

Synonyms CB-1348; chlorambucilum; chloraminophene; chlorbutinum; NSC-3088; WR-139013

U.S./Canadian Brand Names Leukeran® [US/Can]

Therapeutic Category Antineoplastic Agent

Use Management of chronic lymphocytic leukemia (CLL), Hodgkin lymphoma, non-Hodgkin lymphoma (NHL)

Usual Dosage Oral (refer to individual protocols): Adults:

CLL, NHL: 0.1 mg/kg/day for 3-6 weeks **or** 0.4 mg/kg (increased by 0.1 mg/kg/dose until response/toxicity observed) biweekly **or** 0.4 mg/kg (increased by 0.1 mg/kg/dose until response/toxicity observed) monthly **or** 0.03-0.1 mg/kg/day continuously

Hodgkin lymphoma: 0.2 mg/kg/day for 3-6 weeks **or** 0.4 mg/kg (increased by 0.1 mg/kg/dose until response/toxicity observed) biweekly **or** 0.4 mg/kg (increased by 0.1 mg/kg/dose until response/toxicity observed) monthly **or** 0.03-0.1 mg/kg/day continuously

Dosage Forms

Tablet:

Leukeran®: 2 mg

chlorambucilum *see* chlorambucil *on page* 208
chloraminophene *see* chlorambucil *on page* 208

chloramphenicol (klor am FEN i kole)

Sound-Alike/Look-Alike Issues

Chloromycetin® may be confused with chlorambucil, Chlor-Trimeton®

U.S./Canadian Brand Names Chloromycetin® Succinate [Can]; Chloromycetin® [Can]; Diochloram® [Can]; Pentamycetin® [Can]

Therapeutic Category Antibiotic, Miscellaneous; Antibiotic, Ophthalmic; Antibiotic, Otic

Use Treatment of serious infections due to organisms resistant to other less toxic antibiotics or when its penetrability into the site of infection is clinically superior to other antibiotics to which the organism is sensitive; useful in infections caused by *Bacteroides*, *H. influenzae*, *Neisseria meningitidis*, *Salmonella*, and *Rickettsia*; active against many vancomycin-resistant enterococci

Usual Dosage

Neonates: Initial loading dose: I.V. (I.M. administration is not recommended): 20 mg/kg (the first maintenance dose should be given 12 hours after the loading dose)

Maintenance dose: Postnatal age:

≤7 days: 25 mg/kg/day once every 24 hours

>7 days, ≤2000 g: 25 mg/kg/day once every 24 hours

>7 days, >2000 g: 50 mg/kg/day divided every 12 hours

Children: Usual dosing range: I.V.: 50-100 mg/kg/day in divided doses every 6 hours; maximum daily dose: 4 g/day

Meningitis: I.V.: Infants >30 days and Children: 75-100 mg/kg/day divided every 6 hours

Adults: 50-100 mg/kg/day in divided doses every 6 hours; maximum daily dose: 4 g/day

Dosage Forms

Injection, powder for reconstitution: 1 g

ChloraPrep® [US-OTC] *see* chlorhexidine gluconate *on page 210*

ChloraPrep® Frepp® [US-OTC] *see* chlorhexidine gluconate *on page 210*

ChloraPrep® Sepp® [US-OTC] *see* chlorhexidine gluconate *on page 210*

Chlorascrub™ [US-OTC] *see* chlorhexidine gluconate *on page 210*

Chlorascrub™ Maxi [US-OTC] *see* chlorhexidine gluconate *on page 210*

Chloraseptic® Gargle [US-OTC] *see* phenol *on page 772*

Chloraseptic® Mouth Pain [US-OTC] *see* phenol *on page 772*

Chloraseptic® Pocket Pump [US-OTC] *see* phenol *on page 772*

Chloraseptic® Spray [US-OTC] *see* phenol *on page 772*

Chloraseptic® Spray for Kids [US-OTC] *see* phenol *on page 772*

Chlorate® Oral *(Discontinued)* *see* chlorpheniramine *on page 213*

chlorbutinum *see* chlorambucil *on page 208*

Chlordex GP [US] *see* dextromethorphan, chlorpheniramine, phenylephrine, and guaifenesin *on page 297*

chlordiazepoxide (klor dye az e POKS ide)

Sound-Alike/Look-Alike Issues

chlordiazePOXIDE may be confused with chlorproMAZINE

Librium® may be confused with Librax®

Synonyms methaminodiazepoxide hydrochloride

Tall-Man chlordiaze**POXIDE**

U.S./Canadian Brand Names Apo-Chlordiazepoxide® [Can]; Librium® [US]

Therapeutic Category Benzodiazepine

Controlled Substance C-IV

Use Management of anxiety disorder or for the short-term relief of symptoms of anxiety; withdrawal symptoms of acute alcoholism; preoperative apprehension and anxiety

Usual Dosage

Children >6 years: Anxiety: Oral, I.M.: 0.5 mg/kg/24 hours divided every 6-8 hours

Adults:

Anxiety:

Oral: 15-100 mg divided 3-4 times/day

I.M., I.V.: Initial: 50-100 mg followed by 25-50 mg 3-4 times/day as needed

Preoperative anxiety: I.M.: 50-100 mg prior to surgery

Ethanol withdrawal symptoms: Oral, I.V.: 50-100 mg to start, dose may be repeated in 2-4 hours as necessary to a maximum of 300 mg/24 hours

Note: Up to 300 mg may be given I.M. or I.V. during a 6-hour period, but not more than this in any 24-hour period.

Dosage Forms

Capsule, oral: 5 mg, 10 mg, 25 mg

Librium®: 10 mg

chlordiazepoxide and amitriptyline hydrochloride *see* amitriptyline and chlordiazepoxide *on page 66*

chlordiazepoxide and clidinium *see* clidinium and chlordiazepoxide *on page 238*

chlorethazine *see* mechlorethamine *on page 618*

chlorethazine mustard *see* mechlorethamine *on page 618*

Chlorex-A [US] *see* chlorpheniramine, phenylephrine, and phenyltoloxamine *on page 219*

Chlorex-A 12 ***(Discontinued)*** *see* chlorpheniramine, pyrilamine, and phenylephrine *on page 221*

chlorhexidine gluconate (klor HEKS i deen GLOO koe nate)

Sound-Alike/Look-Alike Issues

Peridex® may be confused with Precedex™

Synonyms CHG

U.S./Canadian Brand Names Avagard™ [US-OTC]; BactoShield® CHG [US-OTC]; Betasept® [US-OTC]; ChloraPrep® Frepp® [US-OTC]; ChloraPrep® Sepp® [US-OTC]; ChloraPrep® [US-OTC]; Chlorascrub™ Maxi [US-OTC]; Chlorascrub™ [US-OTC]; Dyna-Hex® [US-OTC]; Hibiclens® [US-OTC]; Hibidil® 1:2000 [Can]; Hibistat® [US-OTC]; Operand® Chlorhexidine Gluconate [US-OTC]; ORO-Clense [Can]; Peridex® Oral Rinse [Can]; Peridex® [US]; PerioChip® [US]; PerioGard® [US]

Therapeutic Category Antibiotic, Oral Rinse; Antibiotic, Topical

Use Skin cleanser for line placement, skin wounds, preoperative skin preparation; germicidal hand rinse; antibacterial dental rinse. Chlorhexidine is active against gram-positive and gram-negative organisms, facultative anaerobes, aerobes, and yeast.

Orphan drug: Peridex®: Oral mucositis with cytoreductive therapy when used for patients undergoing bone marrow transplant

Usual Dosage Adults:

Oral rinse (Peridex®, PerioGard®):

Floss and brush teeth, completely rinse toothpaste from mouth and swish 15 mL (one capful) undiluted oral rinse around in mouth for 30 seconds, then expectorate. Caution patient not to swallow the medicine and instruct not to eat for 2-3 hours after treatment. (Cap on bottle measures 15 mL.)

Treatment of gingivitis: Oral prophylaxis: Swish for 30 seconds with 15 mL chlorhexidine, then expectorate; repeat twice daily (morning and evening). Patient should have a reevaluation followed by a dental prophylaxis every 6 months.

Periodontal chip: One chip is inserted into a periodontal pocket with a probing pocket depth ≥5 mm. Up to 8 chips may be inserted in a single visit. Treatment is recommended every 3 months in pockets with a remaining depth ≥5 mm. If dislodgment occurs 7 days or more after placement, the subject is considered to have had the full course of treatment. If dislodgment occurs within 48 hours, a new chip should be inserted. The chip biodegrades completely and does not need to be removed. Patients should avoid dental floss at the site of PerioChip® insertion for 10 days after placement because flossing might dislodge the chip.

Insertion of periodontal chip: Pocket should be isolated and surrounding area dried prior to chip insertion. The chip should be grasped using forceps with the rounded edges away from the forceps. The chip should be inserted into the periodontal pocket to its maximum depth. It may be maneuvered into position using the tips of the forceps or a flat instrument.

Cleanser:

Surgical scrub: Scrub 3 minutes and rinse thoroughly, wash for an additional 3 minutes

Hand sanitizer (Avagard™): Dispense 1 pumpful in palm of one hand; dip fingertips of opposite hand into solution and work it under nails. Spread remainder evenly over hand and just above elbow, covering all surfaces. Repeat on other hand. Dispense another pumpful in each hand and reapply to each hand up to the wrist. Allow to dry before gloving.

Hand wash: Wash for 15 seconds and rinse

Hand rinse: Rub 15 seconds and rinse

Dosage Forms

Chip, for periodontal pocket insertion:

PerioChip®: 2.5 mg

Liquid, topical [surgical scrub]:

BactoShield® CHG [OTC]: 2% (120 mL, 480 mL, 750 mL, 960 mL, 3840 mL); 4% (120 mL, 480 mL, 960 mL, 3840 mL)

Betasept® [OTC]: 4% 120 mL, 240 mL, 480 mL, 960 mL, 3840 mL)

ChloraPrep® [OTC]: 2% (0.67 mL, 1.5 mL, 3 mL, 10.5 mL, 26 mL)
Dyna-Hex® [OTC]: 2% (120 mL, 480 mL, 960 mL, 3840 mL); 4% (120 mL, 480 mL, 960 mL, 3840 mL)
Hibiclens® [OTC]: 4% (15 mL, 120 mL, 240 mL, 480 mL, 960 mL, 3840 mL)
Operand® Chlorhexidine Gluconate [OTC]: 2% (120 mL); 4% (120 mL, 240 mL, 480 mL, 960 mL, 3840 mL)

Liquid, oral [rinse]: 0.12%
Peridex®, PerioGard®: 0.12%

Lotion, topical [surgical scrub]:
Avagard™ [OTC]: 1% (500 mL)

Sponge/Brush, topical:
BactoShield® CHG [OTC]: 4%

Sponge, topical [surgical scrub]:
ChloraPrep® [OTC] 3 mL: 2% (25s)
ChloraPrep® [OTC] 10.5 mL: 2% (25s)
ChloraPrep® [OTC] 26 mL: 2% (25s)
ChloraPrep® Frepp® [OTC] 1.5 mL: 2% (20s)
ChloraPrep® Sepp® [OTC] 0.67 mL: 2% (200s)

Swab, topical [prep pad]:
Chlorascrub™ [OTC]: 3.15% (100s)

Swabstick, topical [surgical scrub]:
ChloraPrep® [OTC] 1.75 mL: 2% (48s)
ChloraPrep® [OTC] 5.25 mL: 2% (40s)
Chlorascrub™ [OTC] 1.6 mL: 3.15% (50s)
Chlorascrub™ Maxi [OTC] 5.1 mL: 3.15% (30s)

Wipe, topical [towlette]:
Hibistat® [OTC]: 0.5% (50s)

chlormeprazine *see* prochlorperazine *on page 820*

Chlor-Mes [US] *see* chlorpheniramine, phenylephrine, and methscopolamine *on page 218*

Chlor-Mes-D [US] *see* chlorpheniramine, phenylephrine, and methscopolamine *on page 218*

2-chlorodeoxyadenosine *see* cladribine *on page 235*

chloroethane *see* ethyl chloride *on page 396*

Chloromag® [US] *see* magnesium chloride *on page 606*

Chloromycetin® [Can] *see* chloramphenicol *on page 208*

Chloromycetin® Succinate [Can] *see* chloramphenicol *on page 208*

chlorophyll (KLOR oh fil)

Synonyms chlorophyllin

U.S./Canadian Brand Names Nullo® [US-OTC]

Therapeutic Category Gastrointestinal Agent, Miscellaneous

Use Control fecal odors in colostomy or ileostomy

Usual Dosage

Oral: Children >12 years and Adults: 100-200 mg/day in divided doses; may increase to 300 mg/day if odor is not controlled (maximum: 300 mg/day)

Ostomy: Tablet: May also place 1-2 tablets in empty pouch each time it is reused or changed.

Dosage Forms

Caplet:
Nullo® [OTC]: Chlorophyllin copper complex 100 mg

chlorophyllin *see* chlorophyll *on page 211*

chlorophyllin copper complex sodium, papain, and urea *see* chlorophyllin, papain, and urea *on page 211*

chlorophyllin, papain, and urea (KLOR oh fil in, pa PAY in, & yoor EE a)

Sound-Alike/Look-Alike Issues

Ziox™ may be confused with Zyvox®

Synonyms chlorophyllin copper complex sodium, papain, and urea; papain, urea, and chlorophyllin; urea, chlorophyllin, and papain

U.S./Canadian Brand Names Ziox 405™ [US]; Ziox™ [US]

Therapeutic Category Enzyme, Topical Debridement

Use Treatment of acute and chronic lesions, such as venous, diabetic, and decubitus ulcers, burns, postoperative wounds, pilonidal cyst wounds, carbuncles, and miscellaneous traumatic or infected wounds

Usual Dosage Topical: Adults: Apply with each dressing change; daily or twice daily dressing changes are preferred, but some products may be applied every 2-3 days. Cover with dressing following application.

Foam: Apply a single even layer

Ointment: Apply 1/8" thickness over the wound with clean applicator.

Spray: Completely cover the wound site so that the wound is not visible.

Dosage Forms

Ointment:

Ziox™: Chlorophyllin copper complex sodium 0.5%, papain ≥521,700 USP units/g, and urea 10% (30 g)

Ziox 405™: Chlorophyllin copper complex sodium 0.5%, papain ≥521,700 USP units/g, and urea 10% (3.5 g, 30 g)

chloroprocaine (klor oh PROE kane)

Sound-Alike/Look-Alike Issues

Nesacaine® may be confused with Neptazane®

Synonyms chloroprocaine hydrochloride

U.S./Canadian Brand Names Nesacaine® [US]; Nesacaine®-CE [Can]; Nesacaine®-MPF [US]

Therapeutic Category Local Anesthetic

Use Infiltration anesthesia, peripheral nerve block, epidural anesthesia

Usual Dosage Dosage varies with anesthetic procedure, the area to be anesthetized, the vascularity of the tissues, depth of anesthesia required, degree of muscle relaxation required, and duration of anesthesia; range.

Children >3 years (normally developed): Maximum dose (without epinephrine): 11 mg/kg; for infiltration, concentrations of 0.5% to 1% are recommended; for nerve block, concentrations of 1% to 1.5% are recommended

Adults:

Maximum single dose (without epinephrine): 11 mg/kg; maximum dose: 800 mg

Maximum single dose (with epinephrine): 14 mg/kg; maximum dose: 1000 mg

Infiltration and peripheral nerve block:

Mandibular: 2%: 2-3 mL; total dose 40-60 mg

Infraorbital: 2%: 0.5-1 mL; total dose 10-20 mg

Brachial plexus: 2%; 30-40 mL; total dose 600-800 mg

Digital (without epinephrine): 1%; 3-4 mL; total dose: 30-40 mg

Pudendal: 2%; 10 mL each side; total dose: 400 mg

Paracervical: 1%; 3 mL per each of four sites

Caudal block: Preservative-free: 2% or 3%: 15-25 mL; may repeat at 40-60 minute intervals

Lumbar epidural block: Preservative-free: 2% or 3%: 2-2.5 mL per segment; usual total volume: 15-25 mL; may repeat with doses that are 2-6 mL less than initial dose every 40-50 minutes.

Dosage Forms

Injection, solution: 1% (30 mL); 2% (30 mL)

Nesacaine®: 1% (30 mL); 2% (30 mL)

Injection, solution [preservative free]: 2% (20 mL); 3% (20 mL)

Nesacaine®-MPF: 2% (20 mL); 3% (20 mL)

chloroprocaine hydrochloride *see* chloroprocaine *on page* 212

Chloroptic® Ophthalmic Solution *(Discontinued)* *see* chloramphenicol *on page* 208

Chloroptic® SOP *(Discontinued)* *see* chloramphenicol *on page* 208

chloroquine (KLOR oh kwin)

Synonyms chloroquine phosphate

U.S./Canadian Brand Names Aralen® [US/Can]; Novo-Chloroquine [Can]

Therapeutic Category Aminoquinoline (Antimalarial)

Use Suppression or chemoprophylaxis of malaria; treatment of uncomplicated or mild-to-moderate malaria; extraintestinal amebiasis

Usual Dosage Oral:

Suppression or prophylaxis of malaria:

Children: Administer 5 mg base/kg/week on the same day each week (not to exceed 300 mg base/dose); begin 1-2 weeks prior to exposure; continue for 4-6 weeks after leaving endemic area; if suppressive therapy is not begun prior to exposure, double the initial loading dose to 10 mg base/kg and administer in 2 divided doses 6 hours apart, followed by the usual dosage regimen

Adults: 500 mg/week (300 mg base) on the same day each week; begin 1-2 weeks prior to exposure; continue for 4-6 weeks after leaving endemic area; if suppressive therapy is not begun prior to exposure, double the initial loading dose to 1 g (600 mg base) and administer in 2 divided doses 6 hours apart, followed by the usual dosage regimen

Acute attack:

Children: 10 mg/kg (base) on day 1, followed by 5 mg/kg (base) 6 hours later, and 5 mg/kg (base) on days 2 and 3

Adults: 1 g (600 mg base) on day 1, followed by 500 mg (300 mg base) 6 hours later, followed by 500 mg (300 mg base) on days 2 and 3

Extraintestinal amebiasis:

Children: 10 mg/kg (base) once daily for 2-3 weeks (up to 300 mg base/day)

Adults: 1 g/day (600 mg base) for 2 days followed by 500 mg/day (300 mg base) for at least 2-3 weeks

Dosage Forms

Tablet: 250 mg, 500 mg

Aralen®: 500 mg

chloroquine phosphate *see* chloroquine *on page 212*

chlorothiazide (klor oh THYE a zide)

U.S./Canadian Brand Names Diuril® [US/Can]; Sodium Diuril® [US]

Therapeutic Category Diuretic, Thiazide

Use Management of mild-to-moderate hypertension; adjunctive treatment of edema

Usual Dosage Note: The manufacturer states that I.V. and oral dosing are equivalent. Some clinicians may use lower I.V. doses; however, because of chlorothiazide's poor oral absorption. I.V. dosing in infants and children has not been well established.

Infants >6 months and Children: Oral: 10-20 mg/kg/day in 1-2 divided doses (maximum dose: 375 mg/day in children <2 years or 1 g/day in children 2-12 years)

Adults:

Hypertension: Oral: 500-2000 mg/day divided in 1-2 doses (manufacturer labeling); doses of 125-500 mg/day have also been recommended (JNC 7)

Edema: Oral, I.V.: 500-1000 mg once or twice daily; intermittent treatment (eg, therapy on alternative days) may be appropriate for some patients

ACC/AHA 2009 Heart Failure guidelines:

Oral: 250-500 mg once or twice daily (maximum daily dose: 1000 mg)

I.V.: 500-1000 mg once or twice daily plus a loop diuretic

Dosage Forms

Injection, powder for reconstitution:

Sodium Diuril®: 500 mg

Suspension, oral:

Diuril®: 250 mg/5 mL

Tablet: 250 mg, 500 mg

Chlorphed® *(Discontinued)* *see* brompheniramine *on page 149*

Chlorphed®-LA Nasal Solution *(Discontinued)* *see* oxymetazoline *on page 740*

Chlorphen [US-OTC] *see* chlorpheniramine *on page 213*

chlorpheniramine (klor fen IR a meen)

Sound-Alike/Look-Alike Issues

Chlor-Trimeton® may be confused with Chloromycetin®

Synonyms chlorpheniramine maleate; CTM

U.S./Canadian Brand Names Ahist™ [US]; Aller-Chlor® [US-OTC]; Chlor-Trimeton® Allergy [US-OTC]; Chlor-Tripolon® [Can]; Chlorphen [US-OTC]; CPM-12 [US]; Diabetic Tussin® Allergy Relief [US-OTC]; Ed Chlorped [US]; Ed-Chlor-Tan [US]; Novo-Pheniram [Can]; P-Tann [US]; PediaTan™ [US]; Teldrin® HBP [US-OTC]

Therapeutic Category Antihistamine

Use Perennial and seasonal allergic rhinitis and other allergic symptoms including urticaria

Usual Dosage Oral:

Children: 0.35 mg/kg/day in divided doses every 4-6 hours

2-6 years: 1 mg every 4-6 hours, not to exceed 6 mg in 24 hours

6-12 years: 2 mg every 4-6 hours, not to exceed 12 mg/day or sustained release 8 mg at bedtime

Children >12 years and Adults: 4 mg every 4-6 hours, not to exceed 24 mg/day or sustained release 8-12 mg every 8-12 hours, not to exceed 24 mg/day

Dosage Forms

Capsule, extended release, oral: 8 mg, 12 mg

CPM-12: 12 mg

Suspension, oral:

PediaTan™, P-Tann: 8 mg/5 mL

Suspension, oral [drops]:

Ed Chlorped: 2 mg/mL

Syrup:

Aller-Chlor® [OTC], Diabetic Tussin® Allergy Relief [OTC]: 2 mg/5 mL

Tablet: 4 mg

Aller-Chlor® [OTC], Chlor-Trimeton® Allergy [OTC], Chlorphen [OTC], Teldrin® HBP [OTC]: 4 mg

Tablet, extended release, oral:

Chlor-Trimeton® Allergy [OTC]: 12 mg

Ed-Chlor-Tan: 8 mg

Tablet, long acting [scored]:

Ahist™: 12 mg

chlorpheniramine, acetaminophen, and pseudoephedrine *see* acetaminophen, chlorpheniramine, and pseudoephedrine *on page* 26

chlorpheniramine and acetaminophen (klor fen IR a meen & a seet a MIN oh fen)

Synonyms acetaminophen and chlorpheniramine

U.S./Canadian Brand Names Coricidin HBP® Cold and Flu [US-OTC]

Therapeutic Category Antihistamine/Analgesic

Use Symptomatic relief of congestion, headache, aches and pains of colds and flu

Usual Dosage Oral: Adults: 2 tablets every 4 hours

Dosage Forms

Tablet:

Coricidin HBP® Cold and Flu [OTC]: Chlorpheniramine 2 mg and acetaminophen 325 mg

chlorpheniramine and carbetapentane *see* carbetapentane and chlorpheniramine *on page* 182

chlorpheniramine and dextromethorphan *see* dextromethorphan and chlorpheniramine *on page* 296

chlorpheniramine and phenylephrine (klor fen IR a meen & fen il EF rin)

Sound-Alike/Look-Alike Issues

Rynatan® may be confused with Rynatuss®

Synonyms chlorpheniramine maleate and phenylephrine hydrochloride; chlorpheniramine tannate and phenylephrine tannate; phenylephrine and chlorpheniramine

U.S./Canadian Brand Names Actifed® Cold & Allergy [US-OTC] *[reformulation]*; C-Phen [US]; Ceron [US]; Dallergy Drops [US]; Dallergy®-JR [US]; Dec-Chlorphen [US]; Ed A-Hist™ [US]; Ed ChlorPed D [US]; NoHist [US]; PD-Hist-D [US]; PediaTan™ D [US]; Phenabid® [US]; R-Tanna Pediatric [US]; R-Tanna [US]; Rescon-Jr® [US]; Rinate™ Pediatric [US]; Rondec® [US]; Rynatan® Pediatric [US]; Rynatan® [US]; Sudafed PE® Sinus & Allergy [US-OTC]; Tannate Pediatric [US]; Triaminic® Cold and Allergy [US-OTC]

Therapeutic Category Antihistamine/Decongestant Combination

Use Temporary relief of upper respiratory conditions such as nasal congestion, runny nose, and sneezing due to the common cold, hay fever, or allergic or vasomotor rhinitis

Usual Dosage Oral: Antihistamine/decongestant:

Children:

6-12 months: Rondec® drops: 0.75 mL 4 times/day

1-2 years: Rondec® drops: 1 mL 4 times/day

2-6 years:

Dallergy®-JR suspension: 2.5 mL every 12 hours

Rondec® syrup: 1.25 mL every 4-6 hours; maximum: 7.5 mL/24 hours

Rynatan® suspension: 2.5 -5 mL every 12 hours

6-12 years:
  Dallergy®-JR: One capsule every 12 hours; maximum: 2 capsules/24 hours
  Dallergy®-JR suspension: 5 mL every 12 hours
  Ed A-Hist™: One-half caplet every 12 hours
  Rondec® syrup: 2.5 mL every 4-6 hours; maximum: 15 mL/24 hours
  Rynatan® suspension: 5-10 mL every 12 hours
≥12 years: Refer to adult dosing.

Adults:
  Dallergy®-JR: Two capsules every 12 hours; maximum: 4 capsules/24 hours
  Dallergy®-JR suspension: 10 mL every 12 hours
  Ed A-Hist™: One caplet every 12 hours
  R-Tanna: 1-2 tablets every 12 hours
  Rondec® syrup: 5 mL every 4-6 hours; maximum: 30 mL/24 hours
  Rynatan® tablet: 1-2 tablets every 12 hours

Dosage Forms

Caplet, prolonged release:
Ed A-Hist™, NoHist: Chlorpheniramine 8 mg and phenylephrine 20 mg

Capsule, extended release:
Dallergy®-JR: Chlorpheniramine 4 mg and phenylephrine 20 mg

Liquid:
Ed A-Hist™: Chlorpheniramine 4 mg and phenylephrine 10 mg per 5 mL
Triaminic® Cold and Allergy [OTC]: Chlorpheniramine 1 mg and phenylephrine 2.5 mg per 5 mL

Liquid, oral [drops]:
Dallergy: Chlorpheniramine 1 mg and phenylephrine 2 mg per 1 mL

Solution, oral [drops]:
Ceron, C-Phen, Dec-Chlorphen, PD-Hist-D: Chlorpheniramine 1 mg and phenylephrine 3.5 mg per 1 mL

Suspension, oral: Chlorpheniramine 4 mg and phenylephrine 20 mg per 5 mL
Dallergy®-JR: Chlorpheniramine 4 mg and phenylephrine 20 mg per 5 mL
PediaTan™ D: Chlorpheniramine 8 mg and phenylephrine 10 mg per 5 mL
R-Tanna Pediatric, Rinate™ Pediatric, Rynatan® Pediatric, Tannate Pediatric: Chlorpheniramine 4.5 mg and phenylephrine 5 mg per 5 mL

Suspension, oral [drops]:
Ed ChlorPed D: Chlorpheniramine 2 mg and phenylephrine 6 mg per 1 mL

Syrup:
Ceron, C-Phen, Dec-Chlorphen, PD-Hist-D, Rondec®: Chlorpheniramine 4 mg and phenylephrine 12.5 mg per 5 mL

Tablet:
Actifed® Cold & Allergy [OTC], Sudafed PE® Sinus & Allergy [OTC]: Chlorpheniramine 4 mg and phenylephrine 10 mg
R-Tanna, Rynatan®: Chlorpheniramine 9 mg and phenylephrine 25 mg

Tablet, chewable:
Rynatan®: Chlorpheniramine 4.5 mg and phenylephrine 5 mg

Tablet, sustained release:
Rescon-Jr®: Chlorpheniramine 4 mg and phenylephrine 20 mg

Tablet, timed release:
Phenabid®: Chlorpheniramine 8 mg and phenylephrine 20 mg

chlorpheniramine and pseudoephedrine (klor fen IR a meen & soo doe e FED rin)

Sound-Alike/Look-Alike Issues
Allerest® may be confused with Sinarest®
Chlor-Trimeton® may be confused with Chloromycetin®
Sudafed® may be confused with Sufenta®

Synonyms chlorpheniramine maleate and pseudoephedrine hydrochloride; chlorpheniramine tannate and pseudoephedrine tannate; pseudoephedrine and chlorpheniramine

U.S./Canadian Brand Names Allerest® Maximum Strength Allergy and Hay Fever [US-OTC]; Dicel™ [US]; Duratuss® DA [US]; LoHist-D [US]; Suclor™ [US]; Sudafed® Sinus & Allergy [US-OTC]; SudaHist® [US]; Sudal® 12 [US]; Triaminic® Cold & Allergy [Can]

Therapeutic Category Antihistamine/Decongestant Combination

Use Relief of nasal congestion associated with the common cold, hay fever, and other allergies, sinusitis, eustachian tube blockage, and vasomotor and allergic rhinitis

Usual Dosage General dosing guidelines; consult specific product labeling. Rhinitis/decongestant: Oral:

Children:

2-6 years:

Chlorpheniramine maleate 1 mg and pseudoephedrine hydrochloride 15 mg every 4-6 hours

Chlorpheniramine tannate 4.5 mg and pseudoephedrine tannate 75 mg: 2.5-5 mL every 12 hours (maximum: 10 mL/24 hours)

6-12 years: Chlorpheniramine maleate 2 mg and pseudoephedrine hydrochloride 30 mg every 4-6 hours (immediate release products)

Children ≥12 years and Adults:

Chlorpheniramine maleate 4 mg and pseudoephedrine hydrochloride 60 mg every 4-6 hours (immediate release products)

Chlorpheniramine tannate 4.5 mg and pseudoephedrine tannate 75 mg: 10-20 mL every 12 hours (maximum: 40 mL/24 hours)

Dosage Forms

Capsule, extended release: Chlorpheniramine 8 mg and pseudoephedrine 120 mg; chlorpheniramine 12 mg and pseudoephedrine 100 mg

Duratuss® DA: Chlorpheniramine 12 mg and pseudoephedrine 100 mg

Suclor™: Chlorpheniramine 8 mg and pseudoephedrine 120 mg

Capsule, sustained release: Chlorpheniramine 8 mg and pseudoephedrine 120 mg

Liquid:

LoHist-D: Chlorpheniramine 2 mg and pseudoephedrine 30 mg per 5 mL

Suspension:

Dicel™: Chlorpheniramine 5 mg and pseudoephedrine 75 mg per 5 mL

Syrup: Chlorpheniramine 2 mg and pseudoephedrine 30 mg per 5 mL

Tablet: Chlorpheniramine 4 mg and pseudoephedrine 60 mg

Allerest® Maximum Strength Allergy and Hay Fever [OTC]: Chlorpheniramine 2 mg and pseudoephedrine 30 mg

Sudafed® Sinus & Allergy [OTC]: Chlorpheniramine 4 mg and pseudoephedrine 60 mg

Tablet, chewable:

Sudal® 12: Chlorpheniramine 4 mg and pseudoephedrine 30 mg

Tablet, sustained release:

SudaHist®: Chlorpheniramine 12 mg and pseudoephedrine 120 mg

chlorpheniramine, carbetapentane, and phenylephrine *see* carbetapentane, phenylephrine, and chlorpheniramine *on page 183*

chlorpheniramine, dextromethorphan, phenylephrine, and guaifenesin *see* dextromethorphan, chlorpheniramine, phenylephrine, and guaifenesin *on page 297*

chlorpheniramine, dihydrocodeine, and pseudoephedrine *see* pseudoephedrine, dihydrocodeine, and chlorpheniramine *on page 836*

chlorpheniramine, ephedrine, phenylephrine, and carbetapentane

(klor fen IR a meen, e FED rin, fen il EF rin, & kar bay ta PEN tane)

Sound-Alike/Look-Alike Issues

Rynatuss® may be confused with Rynatan®

Synonyms carbetapentane, ephedrine, phenylephrine, and chlorpheniramine; ephedrine, chlorpheniramine, phenylephrine, and carbetapentane; phenylephrine, ephedrine, chlorpheniramine, and carbetapentane

U.S./Canadian Brand Names Quad Tann® [US]; Rynatuss® [US]; Tetra Tannate Pediatric [US]

Therapeutic Category Antihistamine/Decongestant/Antitussive

Use Symptomatic relief of cough with a decongestant and an antihistamine

Usual Dosage Oral:

Children:

<2 years: Titrate dose individually

2-6 years: 2.5-5 mL every 12 hours

>6 years: 5-10 mL every 12 hours

Adults: 1-2 tablets every 12 hours

Dosage Forms

Suspension:

Tetra Tannate Pediatric: Chlorpheniramine 4 mg, ephedrine 5 mg, phenylephrine 5 mg, and carbetapentane 30 mg per 5 mL

Tablet:

Rynatuss®: Chlorpheniramine 5 mg, ephedrine 10 mg, phenylephrine 10 mg, and carbetapentane 50 mg

Tablet, long acting:

Quad Tann®: Chlorpheniramine 5 mg, ephedrine 10 mg, phenylephrine 10 mg, and carbetapentane 60 mg

chlorpheniramine, hydrocodone, and phenylephrine *see* phenylephrine, hydrocodone, and chlorpheniramine *on page 778*

chlorpheniramine maleate *see* chlorpheniramine *on page 213*

chlorpheniramine maleate and dextromethorphan hydrobromide *see* dextromethorphan and chlorpheniramine *on page 296*

chlorpheniramine maleate and hydrocodone bitartrate *see* hydrocodone and chlorpheniramine *on page 502*

chlorpheniramine maleate and phenylephrine hydrochloride *see* chlorpheniramine and phenylephrine *on page 214*

chlorpheniramine maleate and pseudoephedrine hydrochloride *see* chlorpheniramine and pseudoephedrine *on page 215*

chlorpheniramine maleate, dihydrocodeine bitartrate, and phenylephrine hydrochloride *see* dihydrocodeine, chlorpheniramine, and phenylephrine *on page 309*

chlorpheniramine maleate, ibuprofen, and pseudoephedrine *see* ibuprofen, pseudoephedrine, and chlorpheniramine *on page 517*

chlorpheniramine maleate, phenylephrine hydrochloride, and guaifenesin *see* chlorpheniramine, phenylephrine, and guaifenesin *on page 218*

chlorpheniramine maleate, pseudoephedrine hydrochloride, and dextromethorphan hydrobromide *see* chlorpheniramine, pseudoephedrine, and dextromethorphan *on page 220*

chlorpheniramine, phenylephrine, and dextromethorphan

(klor fen IR a meen, fen il EF rin, & deks troe meth OR fan)

Synonyms dextromethorphan, chlorpheniramine, and phenylephrine; phenylephrine, chlorpheniramine, and dextromethorphan

U.S./Canadian Brand Names C-Phen DM [US]; Ceron-DM [US]; Corfen DM [US]; De-Chlor DM [US]; De-Chlor DR [US]; Dex PC [US]; Ed A-Hist DM [US]; Father John's® Plus [US-OTC]; Mintuss DR [US]; Neo DM [US]; Norel DM™ [US]; PD-Cof [US]; PE-Hist DM [US]; Phenabid DM® [US]; Poly Tussin DM [US]; Robitussin® Cough and Cold Nighttime [US-OTC]; Robitussin® Pediatric Cough and Cold Nighttime [US-OTC]; Rondec®-DM [US]; Statuss™ DM [US]; Trital DM [US]; Tussplex™ DM [US]

Therapeutic Category Antihistamine/Decongestant/Antitussive

Use Temporary relief of cough and upper respiratory symptoms associated with allergies or the common cold

Usual Dosage Oral: Relief of cough and cold symptoms:

Children:

- 6-12 months (Rondec®-DM drops): 0.75 mL 4 times/day
- 1-2 years (Rondec®-DM drops): 1 mL 4 times/day
- 2-6 years (Rondec®-DM syrup): 1.25 mL every 4-6 hours (maximum: 7.5 mL/24 hours)
- 6-12 years (Rondec®-DM syrup): 2.5 mL every 4-6 hours (maximum: 15 mL/24 hours)

Children ≥12 years and Adults (Rondec®-DM syrup): 5 mL every 4-6 hours (maximum: 30 mL/24 hours)

Dosage Forms

Liquid:

Corfen DM, Norel DM™, Trital DM: Chlorpheniramine 4 mg, phenylephrine 10 mg, and dextromethorphan 15 mg per 5 mL

De-Chlor DM: Chlorpheniramine 2 mg, phenylephrine 10 mg, and dextromethorphan 15 mg per 5 mL

De-Chlor DR: Chlorpheniramine 2 mg, phenylephrine 6 mg, and dextromethorphan 15 mg per 5 mL

Father John's® Plus [OTC]: Chlorpheniramine 2 mg, phenylephrine 5 mg, and dextromethorphan 5 mg per 15 mL

Liquid, oral [drops]:

C-Phen DM, PD-Cof, Rondec® DM: Chlorpheniramine 1 mg, phenylephrine 3.5 mg, and dextromethorphan 3 mg per 1 mL

Neo DM: Chlorpheniramine 0.75 mg, phenylephrine 1.75 mg, and dextromethorphan 2.75 mg per 1 mL ▶

Syrup:

Ceron-DM, C-Phen DM, PD-Cof, Rondec®-DM: Chlorpheniramine 4 mg, phenylephrine 12.5 mg, and dextromethorphan 15 mg per 5 mL

Dex PC, Mintuss DR: Chlorpheniramine 2 mg, phenylephrine 6 mg, and dextromethorphan 15 mg per 5 mL

Ed A-Hist DM: Chlorpheniramine 4 mg, phenylephrine 10 mg, and dextromethorphan 15 mg per 5 mL

PE-Hist DM, Poly Tussin DM, Tussplex™ DM: Chlorpheniramine 2 mg, phenylephrine 5 mg, and dextromethorphan 15 mg per 5 mL

Robitussin® Cough and Cold Nighttime [OTC], Robitussin® Pediatric Cough and Cold Nighttime [OTC]: Chlorpheniramine 1 mg, phenylephrine 2.5 mg, and dextromethorphan 5 mg per 5 mL

Statuss™ DM: Chlorpheniramine 2 mg, phenylephrine 10 mg, and dextromethorphan 15 mg per 5 mL

Tablet, timed release:

Phenabid DM®: Chlorpheniramine 8 mg, phenylephrine 20 mg, and dextromethorphan 30 mg

chlorpheniramine, phenylephrine, and guaifenesin

(klor fen IR a meen, fen il EF rin, & gwye FEN e sin)

Synonyms chlorpheniramine maleate, phenylephrine hydrochloride, and guaifenesin; chlorpheniramine tannate, phenylephrine tannate, and guaifenesin; guaifenesin, phenylephrine, and chlorpheniramine; phenylephrine, chlorpheniramine, and guaifenesin

U.S./Canadian Brand Names P Chlor GG [US]

Therapeutic Category Cough and Cold Combination

Use Symptomatic relief of upper respiratory symptoms associated with infections such as the common cold or allergies

Usual Dosage General dosing guidelines; consult specific product labeling. Oral: Antihistamine/decongestant/expectorant:

Children <3 months: 2-3 drops per month of age every 4-6 hours as needed; not to exceed 4 doses/24 hours

Children 3-6 months: 0.3-0.6 mL every 4-6 hours as needed; not to exceed 4 doses/24 hours

Children 6 months to 1 year: 0.6-1 mL every 4-6 hours as needed; not to exceed 4 doses/24 hours

Children 1-2 years: 1-2 mL every 4-6 hours as needed; not to exceed 4 doses/24 hours

Dosage Forms

Liquid:

P Chlor GG [drops]: Chlorpheniramine 1 mg, phenylephrine 2 mg, and guaifenesin 20 mg per 1 mL

chlorpheniramine, phenylephrine, and methscopolamine

(klor fen IR a meen, fen il EF rin, & meth skoe POL a meen)

Synonyms methscopolamine nitrate, chlorpheniramine maleate, and phenylephrine hydrochloride; phenylephrine tannate, chlorpheniramine tannate, and methscopolamine nitrate

U.S./Canadian Brand Names aerohist plus™ [US]; aeroKid™ [US]; AH-Chew® [US]; AH-Chew™ Ultra [US]; Chlor-Mes [US]; Chlor-Mes-D [US]; Dallergy® [US]; Dehistine [US]; Duradyl® [US]; Durahist™ PE [US]; Histatab PH [US]; OMNIhist® II L.A. [US]; Phenylephrine CM [US]; Ralix [US]; Rescon® MX [US]; Rescon® [US]; Triall™ [US]

Therapeutic Category Antihistamine/Decongestant/Anticholinergic

Use Treatment of upper respiratory symptoms such as respiratory congestion, allergic rhinitis, vasomotor rhinitis, sinusitis, and allergic skin reactions of urticaria and angioedema

Usual Dosage

Children 6-11 years: Relief of respiratory symptoms: Oral:

aeroKid™: 2.5-5 mL every 4 hours

AH-Chew® suspension: 2.5-5 mL every 12 hours

Dallergy®, Durahist™ PE, OMNIhist® II L.A., Rescon® MX: One-half caplet/tablet every 12 hours

Duradryl® syrup, Extendryl® syrup: 2.5-5 mL, may repeat up to every 4 hours depending on age and body weight

Children ≥12 years and Adults: Relief of respiratory symptoms: Oral: **Note:** If disturbances in urination occur in patients without renal impairment, medication should be discontinued for 1-2 days and should then be restarted at a lower dose

aeroKid™: 5-10 mL every 3-4 hours

AH-Chew® suspension: 5-10 mL every 12 hours

Dallergy®, Durahist™ PE, Extendryl® SR, OMNIhist® II L.A., Rescon® MX: One capsule/tablet every 12 hours

Duradryl® syrup, Extendryl® syrup: 5-10 mL every 3-4 hours (4 times/day)

Dosage Forms

Caplet, extended release:

aerohist plus™: Chlorpheniramine 8 mg, phenylephrine 20 mg, and methscopolamine 2.5 mg

Chlor-Mes, Dallergy®: Chlorpheniramine 12 mg, phenylephrine 20 mg, and methscopolamine 2.5 mg

Liquid:

Chlor-Mes-D: Chlorpheniramine 2 mg, phenylephrine 10 mg, and methscopolamine 0.625 mg per 5 mL

Suspension:

AH-Chew®: Chlorpheniramine, phenylephrine, and methscopalamine 1.5 mg per 5 mL

Syrup:

aeroKid™: Chlorpheniramine 4 mg, phenylephrine 1 mg, and methscopolamine 1.25 mg per 5 mL

Dallergy®: Chlorpheniramine 2 mg, phenylephrine 8 mg, and methscopolamine 0.75 mg per 5 mL

Dehistine, Duradryl®: Chlorpheniramine 2 mg, phenylephrine 10 mg, and methscopolamine 1.25 mg per 5 mL

Triall™: Chlorpheniramine 2 mg, phenylephrine 8 mg, and methscopolamine 0.75 mg per 5 mL

Tablet [scored]:

Dallergy®: Chlorpheniramine 4 mg, phenylephrine 10 mg, and methscopolamine 1.25 mg

Tablet, chewable:

AH-Chew™ Ultra: Chlorpheniramine 2 mg, phenylephrine 10 mg, and methscopolamine 1.5 mg

Tablet, extended release: Chlorpheniramine 8 mg, phenylephrine 20 mg, and methscopolamine 1.25 mg

Durahist™ PE: Chlorpheniramine 8 mg, phenylephrine 20 mg, and methscopolamine 1.25 mg [scored]

Tablet, long acting [scored]:

OMNIhist® II L.A.: Chlorpheniramine 8 mg, phenylephrine 25 mg, and methscopolamine 2.5 mg

Rescon® MX: Chlorpheniramine 8 mg, phenylephrine 40 mg, and methscopolamine 2.5 mg

Tablet, sustained release:

Histatab PH: Chlorpheniramine 8 mg, phenylephrine 20 mg, and methscopolamine 1.25 mg

Ralix: Chlorpheniramine 8 mg, phenylephrine 40 mg, and methscopolamine 2 mg

Tablet, timed release:

Phenylephrine CM: Chlorpheniramine 8 mg, phenylephrine 40 mg, and methscopolamine 2.5 mg

Tablet, variable release:

Rescon®: Chlorpheniramine 12 mg and phenylephrine 40 mg [sustained release] and methscopolamine 2 mg [immediate release] [MaxRelent release]

chlorpheniramine, phenylephrine, and phenyltoloxamine

(klor fen IR a meen, fen il EF rin, & fen il tole LOKS a meen)

Synonyms phenylephrine, chlorpheniramine, and phenyltoloxamine; phenyltoloxamine, chlorpheniramine, and phenylephrine

U.S./Canadian Brand Names Chlorex-A [US]; Nalex®-A [US]; NoHist-A [US]; Rhinacon A [US]

Therapeutic Category Antihistamine/Decongestant Combination

Use Symptomatic relief of rhinitis and nasal congestion due to colds or allergy

Usual Dosage Oral:

Children:

2-6 years: Nalex®-A liquid: 1.25-2.5 mL every 4-6 hours

6-12 years:

Nalex®-A liquid: 5 mL every 4-6 hours

Nalex®-A tablet: 1/2 tablet 2-3 times/day

Children >12 years and Adults:

Nalex®-A liquid: 10 mL every 4-6 hours

Nalex®-A tablet: 1 tablet 2-3 times/day

Dosage Forms

Liquid: Chlorpheniramine 2.5 mg, phenylephrine 5 mg, and phenyltoloxamine 7.5 mg per 5 mL

Nalex®-A, NoHist-A, Rhinacon A: Chlorpheniramine 2.5 mg, phenylephrine 5 mg, and phenyltoloxamine 7.5 mg per 5 mL

Tablet, extended release:

Rhinacon A: Chlorpheniramine 4 mg, phenylephrine 20 mg, and phenyltoloxamine 40 mg

Tablet, prolonged release:

Nalex®-A: Chlorpheniramine 4 mg, phenylephrine 20 mg, and phenyltoloxamine 40 mg

Tablet, sustained release:

Chlorex-A: Chlorpheniramine 4 mg, phenylephrine 20 mg, and phenyltoloxamine 40 mg

chlorpheniramine, phenylephrine, and pyrilamine *see* chlorpheniramine, pyrilamine, and phenylephrine *on page* 221

chlorpheniramine, phenylephrine, codeine, and potassium iodide

(klor fen IR a meen, fen il EF rin, KOE deen, & poe TASS ee um EYE oh dide)

Synonyms codeine, chlorpheniramine, phenylephrine, and potassium iodide; phenylephrine, chlorpheniramine, codeine, and potassium iodide; potassium iodide, chlorpheniramine, phenylephrine, and codeine

Therapeutic Category Antihistamine/Decongestant/Antitussive

Controlled Substance C-V

Use Symptomatic relief of rhinitis, nasal congestion and cough due to colds or allergy

Usual Dosage Children 6 months to 12 years: 1.25-10 mL every 4-6 hours

chlorpheniramine, pseudoephedrine, and acetaminophen *see* acetaminophen, chlorpheniramine, and pseudoephedrine *on page 26*

chlorpheniramine, pseudoephedrine, and codeine

(klor fen IR a meen, soo doe e FED rin, & KOE deen)

Synonyms codeine, chlorpheniramine, and pseudoephedrine; pseudoephedrine, chlorpheniramine, and codeine

Therapeutic Category Antihistamine/Decongestant/Antitussive

Controlled Substance C-V

Use Temporary relief of cough associated with minor throat or bronchial irritation or nasal congestion due to common cold, allergic rhinitis, or sinusitis

Usual Dosage Oral:

Children:

25-50 lb: 1.25-2.5 mL every 4-6 hours, up to 4 doses in 24-hour period

50-90 lb: 2.5-5 mL every 4-6 hours, up to 4 doses in 24-hour period

Adults: 10 mL every 4-6 hours, up to 4 doses in 24-hour period

chlorpheniramine, pseudoephedrine, and dextromethorphan

(klor fen IR a meen, soo doe e FED rin, & deks troe meth OR fan)

Synonyms chlorpheniramine maleate, pseudoephedrine hydrochloride, and dextromethorphan hydrobromide; chlorpheniramine tannate, pseudoephedrine tannate, and dextromethorphan tannate; dexchlorpheniramine tannate, pseudoephedrine tannate, and dextromethorphan tannate; dextromethorphan, chlorpheniramine, and pseudoephedrine; pseudoephedrine, chlorpheniramine, and dextromethorphan

U.S./Canadian Brand Names Dicel™ DM [US]; DuraTan™ Forte [US]; Kidkare Children's Cough and Cold [US-OTC]; Pedia Relief™ [US-OTC]; Rescon DM [US-OTC]; Tanafed DMX™ [US]; Tannate PD-DM [US]

Therapeutic Category Antihistamine/Decongestant/Antitussive

Use Temporarily relieves nasal congestion, runny nose, cough, and sneezing due to the common cold, hay fever, or allergic rhinitis

Usual Dosage General dosing guidelines; consult specific product labeling. Relief of cold symptoms: Oral:

Children:

2-6 years:

Dexchlorpheniramine tannate 2.5 mg, pseudoephedrine tannate 75 mg, and dextromethorphan tannate 25 mg (Tanafed DMX™): 2.5-5 mL every 12 hours (maximum: 10 mL/24 hours)

Dexchlorpheniramine tannate 3.5 mg, pseudoephedrine tannate 45 mg, and dextromethorphan tannate 30 mg (DuraTan™ Forte): 1.25-2.5 mL every 12 hours (maximum: 5 mL/24 hours)

6-12 years:

Chlorpheniramine maleate 1 mg, pseudoephedrine 15 mg, and dextromethorphan hydrobromide 7.5 mg per 5 mL: 10 mL every 6 hours

Chlorpheniramine maleate 1 mg, pseudoephedrine 15 mg, and dextromethorphan hydrobromide 5 mg per tablet or 5 mL: 2 tablets or 10 mL every 4-6 hours (maximum: 4 doses/24 hours)

Chlorpheniramine maleate 2 mg, pseudoephedrine 30 mg, and dextromethorphan hydrobromide 10 mg per tablet or 5 mL (Rescon DM): 5 mL every 4-6 hours (maximum: 4 doses/24 hours)

Dexchlorpheniramine tannate 2.5 mg, pseudoephedrine tannate 75 mg, and dextromethorphan tannate 25 mg (Tanafed DMX™): 5-10 mL every 12 hours (maximum: 20 mL/24 hours)

Dexchlorpheniramine tannate 3.5 mg, pseudoephedrine tannate 45 mg, and dextromethorphan tannate 30 mg (DuraTan™ Forte): 2.5-5 mL every 12 hours (maximum: 10 mL/24 hours)

>12 years: Refer to adult dosing

Adults:
Chlorpheniramine maleate 1 mg, pseudoephedrine 15 mg, and dextromethorphan hydrobromide 7.5 mg per 5 mL: 20 mL every 6 hours
Chlorpheniramine maleate 2 mg, pseudoephedrine 30 mg, and dextromethorphan hydrobromide 10 mg per tablet or 5 mL (Rescon DM): 10 mL every 4-6 hours (maximum: 4 doses/24 hours)
Dexchlorpheniramine tannate 2.5 mg, pseudoephedrine tannate 75 mg, and dextromethorphan tannate 25 mg (Tanafed DMX™): 10-20 mL every 12 hours (maximum: 40 mL/24 hours)
Dexchlorpheniramine tannate 3.5 mg, pseudoephedrine tannate 45 mg, and dextromethorphan tannate 30 mg (DuraTan™ Forte): 5-15 mL every 12 hours (maximum: 30 mL/24 hours)

Dosage Forms

Liquid: Chlorpheniramine 1 mg, pseudoephedrine 15 mg, and dextromethorphan 5 mg per 5 mL
Kidkare Children's Cough and Cold [OTC], Pedia Relief™ [OTC]: Chlorpheniramine 1 mg, pseudoephedrine 15 mg, and dextromethorphan 5 mg per 5 mL
Rescon DM [OTC]: Chlorpheniramine 2 mg, pseudoephedrine 30 mg, and dextromethorphan 10 mg per 5 mL

Suspension:
Dicel™ DM: Chlorpheniramine 5 mg, pseudoephedrine 75 mg, and dextromethorphan 25 mg per 5 mL
DuraTan™ Forte: Dexchlorpheniramine tannate 3.5 mg, pseudoephedrine tannate 45 mg, and dextromethorphan tannate 30 mg per 5 mL
Tanafed DMX™: Dexchlorpheniramine 2.5 mg, pseudoephedrine 75 mg, and dextromethorphan 25 mg
Tannate PD-DM: Dexchlorpheniramine 3 mg, pseudoephedrine 50 mg, and dextromethorphan 27.5 mg per 5 mL

chlorpheniramine, pseudoephedrine, and methscopolamine

(klor fen IR a meen, soo doe e FED rin, & meth skoe POL a meen)

Synonyms methscopolamine, chlorpheniramine, and pseudoephedrine; methscopolamine, pseudoephedrine, and chlorpheniramine; pseudoephedrine hydrochloride, methscopolamine nitrate, and chlorpheniramine maleate; pseudoephedrine, methscopolamine, and chlorpheniramine

U.S./Canadian Brand Names Amdry-C [US]; Coldamine [US]; Durahist™ [US]

Therapeutic Category Antihistamine/Decongestant/Anticholinergic

Use Relief of symptoms of allergic rhinitis, vasomotor rhinitis, sinusitis, and the common cold

Usual Dosage Oral:
Children 6-11 years (Durahist™): One-half tablet every 12 hours (maximum dose: 1 tablet/24 hours)
Children ≥12 years and Adults (Durahist™): One tablet every 12 hours (maximum dose: 2 tablets/24 hours).

Dosage Forms

Tablet, extended release:
Coldamine: Chlorpheniramine 8 mg, pseudoephedrine 90 mg, and methscopolamine 2.5 mg

Tablet, sustained release: Chlorpheniramine maleate 8 mg, pseudoephedrine hydrochloride 60 mg, and methscopolamine nitrate 1.25 mg; chlorpheniramine maleate 8 mg, pseudoephedrine hydrochloride 90 mg, and methscopolamine nitrate 2.5 mg
Amdry-C: Chlorpheniramine 8 mg, pseudoephedrine 120 mg, and methscopolamine 2.5 mg [scored]

chlorpheniramine, pyrilamine, and phenylephrine

(klor fen IR a meen, pye RIL a meen, & fen il EF rin)

Synonyms chlorpheniramine, phenylephrine, and pyrilamine; phenylephrine, chlorpheniramine, and pyrilamine; pyrilamine, chlorpheniramine, and phenylephrine

U.S./Canadian Brand Names Conal [US]; MyHist-PD [US]; Nalex A 12 [US]; Poly Hist Forte® [US]; Poly Hist PD [US]; Ru-Hist Forte [US]; Triplex™ AD [US]

Therapeutic Category Alpha/Beta Agonist; Histamine H_1 Antagonist; Histamine H_1 Antagonist, First Generation

Use Symptomatic relief of rhinitis and nasal congestion due to colds or allergy

Usual Dosage Oral:
Tablet (Ru-Hist Forte, Poly Hist Forte®):
Children 6-12 years: 1/2 tablet 2-3 times/day
Children >12 years and Adults: 1 tablet 2-3 times/day
Liquid (MyHist-PD, Poly Hist PD):
Children 2-6 years: 2.5 mL every 4-6 hours (maximum: 10 mL/day)
Children 6-12 years: 5 mL every 4-6 hours (maximum: 20 mL/day)
Children >12 years and Adults: 5-10 mL every 4-6 hours (maximum: 40 mL/day)

Liquid (Triplex™ AD):
Children 6-12 years: 5 mL every 4-6 hours (maximum: 20 mL/day)
Children >12 and Adults: 5-10 mL every 4-6 hours (maximum: 40 mL/day)
Suspension (Conal):
Children 2-6 years: 2.5 mL every 12 hours (maximum: 5 mL/day)
Children 6-12 years: 5 mL every 12 hours (maximum: 10 mL/day)
Children >12 years and Adults: 5-10 mL every 12 hours (maximum: 20 mL/day)

Dosage Forms

Liquid, oral:
MyHist-PD, Triplex™ AD: Chlorpheniramine 2 mg, pyrilamine 12.5 mg, and phenylephrine 7.5 mg per 5 mL (473 mL)
Poly Hist PD: Chlorpheniramine 2 mg, pyrilamine 12.5 mg, and phenylephrine 7.5 mg per 5 mL (480 mL)

Suspension, oral:
Conal: Chlorpheniramine 8 mg, pyrilamine 12.5 mg, and phenylephrine 15 mg per 5 mL
Nalex A 12: Chlorpheniramine 2 mg, pyrilamine 12.5 mg, and phenylephrine 5 mg per 5 mL

Tablet, sustained release, oral:
Poly Hist Forte®: Chlorpheniramine 4 mg, pyrilamine 25 mg, and phenylephrine 10 mg

Tablet, time-released, oral: Chlorpheniramine 4 mg, pyrilamine 25 mg, and phenylephrine 10 mg
Ru-Hist Forte: Chlorpheniramine 4 mg, pyrilamine 25 mg, and phenylephrine 10 mg

chlorpheniramine tannate and phenylephrine tannate *see* chlorpheniramine and phenylephrine *on page 214*

chlorpheniramine tannate and pseudoephedrine tannate *see* chlorpheniramine and pseudoephedrine *on page 215*

chlorpheniramine tannate, phenylephrine tannate, and guaifenesin *see* chlorpheniramine, phenylephrine, and guaifenesin *on page 218*

chlorpheniramine tannate, pseudoephedrine tannate, and dextromethorphan tannate *see* chlorpheniramine, pseudoephedrine, and dextromethorphan *on page 220*

Chlor-Pro® Injection *(Discontinued)* *see* chlorpheniramine *on page 213*

chlorpromazine (klor PROE ma zeen)

Sound-Alike/Look-Alike Issues
chlorproMAZINE may be confused with chlordiazePOXIDE, chlorproPAMIDE, clomiPRAMINE, prochlorperazine, promethazine
Thorazine® may be confused with thiamine, thioridazine

Synonyms chlorpromazine hydrochloride; CPZ

Tall-Man chlorpro**MAZINE**

U.S./Canadian Brand Names Largactil® [Can]; Novo-Chlorpromazine [Can]

Therapeutic Category Phenothiazine Derivative

Use Control of mania; treatment of schizophrenia; control of nausea and vomiting; relief of restlessness and apprehension before surgery; acute intermittent porphyria; adjunct in the treatment of tetanus; intractable hiccups; combativeness and/or explosive hyperexcitable behavior in children 1-12 years of age and in short-term treatment of hyperactive children

Usual Dosage
Children ≥6 months:
Schizophrenia/psychoses:
Oral: 0.5-1 mg/kg/dose every 4-6 hours; older children may require 200 mg/day or higher
I.M., I.V.: 0.5-1 mg/kg/dose every 6-8 hours
<5 years (22.7 kg): Maximum: 40 mg/day
5-12 years (22.7-45.5 kg): Maximum: 75 mg/day
Nausea and vomiting:
Oral: 0.5-1 mg/kg/dose every 4-6 hours as needed
I.M., I.V.: 0.5-1 mg/kg/dose every 6-8 hours
<5 years (22.7 kg): Maximum: 40 mg/day
5-12 years (22.7-45.5 kg): Maximum: 75 mg/day
Adults:
Schizophrenia/psychoses:
Oral: Range: 30-800 mg/day in 1-4 divided doses, initiate at lower doses and titrate as needed; usual dose: 200-600 mg/day; some patients may require 1-2 g/day

I.M., I.V.: Initial: 25 mg, may repeat (25-50 mg) in 1-4 hours, gradually increase to a maximum of 400 mg/dose every 4-6 hours until patient is controlled; usual dose: 300-800 mg/day
Intractable hiccups: Oral, I.M.: 25-50 mg 3-4 times/day
Nausea and vomiting:
Oral: 10-25 mg every 4-6 hours
I.M., I.V.: 25-50 mg every 4-6 hours

Dosage Forms
Injection, solution: 25 mg/mL (1 mL, 2 mL)
Tablet: 10 mg, 25 mg, 50 mg, 100 mg, 200 mg

chlorpromazine hydrochloride *see* chlorpromazine *on page 222*

chlorpropamide (klor PROE pa mide)

Sound-Alike/Look-Alike Issues
chlorproPAMIDE may be confused with chlorproMAZINE
Diabinese® may be confused with DiaBeta®, Dialume®, Diamox®

Tall-Man chlorpro**PAMIDE**

U.S./Canadian Brand Names Apo-Chlorpropamide® [Can]; Novo-Propamide [Can]

Therapeutic Category Antidiabetic Agent, Oral

Use Management of blood sugar in type 2 diabetes mellitus (noninsulin-dependent, NIDDM)

Usual Dosage Oral: The dosage of chlorpropamide is variable and should be individualized based upon the patient's response
Initial dose: Adults: 250 mg/day in mild-to-moderate diabetes in middle-aged, stable diabetic
Subsequent dosages may be increased or decreased by 50-125 mg/day at 3- to 5-day intervals
Maintenance dose: 100-250 mg/day; severe diabetics may require 500 mg/day; avoid doses >750 mg/day

Dosage Forms
Tablet: 100 mg, 250 mg

Chlor-Tan A 12 *(Discontinued)* *see* chlorpheniramine, pyrilamine, and phenylephrine *on page 221*

chlorthalidone (klor THAL i done)

U.S./Canadian Brand Names Apo-Chlorthalidone® [Can]; Thalitone® [US]

Therapeutic Category Diuretic, Miscellaneous

Use Management of mild-to-moderate hypertension when used alone or in combination with other agents; treatment of edema associated with heart failure or nephrotic syndrome. Recent studies have found chlorthalidone effective in the treatment of isolated systolic hypertension in the elderly.

Usual Dosage Oral: Adults:
Hypertension: 25-100 mg/day or 100 mg 3 times/week; usual dosage range (JNC 7): 12.5-25 mg/day
Edema: Initial: 50-100 mg/day or 100 mg on alternate days; maximum dose: 200 mg/day
Heart failure-associated edema: 12.5-25 mg once daily; maximum daily dose: 100 mg

Dosage Forms
Tablet: 25 mg, 50 mg, 100 mg
Thalitone®: 15 mg

chlorthalidone and atenolol *see* atenolol and chlorthalidone *on page 107*
chlorthalidone and clonidine *see* clonidine and chlorthalidone *on page 246*
Chlor-Trimeton® Allergy [US-OTC] *see* chlorpheniramine *on page 213*
Chlor-Trimeton® Allergy D *(Discontinued)* *see* chlorpheniramine and pseudoephedrine *on page 215*
Chlor-Trimeton® Syrup *(Discontinued)* *see* chlorpheniramine *on page 213*
Chlor-Tripolon® [Can] *see* chlorpheniramine *on page 213*
Chlor-Tripolon ND® [Can] *see* loratadine and pseudoephedrine *on page 599*

chlorzoxazone (klor ZOKS a zone)

Sound-Alike/Look-Alike Issues
Parafon Forte® may be confused with Fam-Pren Forte

U.S./Canadian Brand Names Parafon Forte® DSC [US]; Parafon Forte® [Can]; Strifon Forte® [Can]

Therapeutic Category Skeletal Muscle Relaxant

Use Symptomatic treatment of muscle spasm and pain associated with acute musculoskeletal conditions

Usual Dosage Oral:
Children: 20 mg/kg/day or 600 mg/m^2/day in 3-4 divided doses
Adults: 250-500 mg 3-4 times/day up to 750 mg 3-4 times/day

Dosage Forms
Caplet: 500 mg
Parafon Forte® DSC: 500 mg
Tablet: 250 mg, 500 mg

cholecalciferol (kole e kal SI fer ole)

Synonyms D_3

U.S./Canadian Brand Names D-3 [US-OTC]; D-Vi-Sol® [Can]; D3-50™ [US-OTC]; D3-5™ [US-OTC]; Delta-D® [US-OTC]; Maximum D3® [US-OTC]; Vitamin D3 [US-OTC]

Therapeutic Category Vitamin D Analog

Use Dietary supplement, treatment of vitamin D deficiency, or prophylaxis of deficiency

Usual Dosage
Oral: Adults: **Dietary Intake Reference: Note:** DIR is currently being reviewed:
18-50 years: 500 int. units/day
51-70 years: 400 int. units/day
Osteoporosis prevention and treatment: Adults ≥50 years: 800-1000 int. units/day

Dosage Forms
Capsule, oral:
D-3 [OTC]: 1000 int. units
D3-5™ [OTC]: 5000 int. units
D3-50™ [OTC]: 50,000 int. units
Maximum D3® [OTC]: 10,000 int. units
Capsule, softgel, oral:
D-3 [OTC]: 2000 int. units
Tablet:
Delta-D® [OTC]: 400 int. units

cholecalciferol and alendronate *see* alendronate and cholecalciferol *on page* 45

cholera and traveler's diarrhea vaccine *see* traveler's diarrhea and cholera vaccine *(Canada only) on page* 978

cholestyramine resin (koe LES teer a meen REZ in)

U.S./Canadian Brand Names Novo-Cholamine Light [Can]; Novo-Cholamine [Can]; PMS-Cholestyramine [Can]; Prevalite® [US]; Questran® Light Sugar Free [Can]; Questran® Light [US]; Questran® [US/Can]

Therapeutic Category Bile Acid Sequestrant

Use Adjunct in the management of primary hypercholesterolemia; pruritus associated with elevated levels of bile acids; diarrhea associated with excess fecal bile acids; binding toxicologic agents; pseudomembraneous colitis

Usual Dosage Oral (dosages are expressed in terms of anhydrous resin):
Children: 240 mg/kg/day in 3 divided doses; need to titrate dose depending on indication
Adults: 4 g 1-2 times/day to a maximum of 24 g/day and 6 doses/day

Dosage Forms
Powder for oral suspension: Cholestyramine resin 4 g/5 g packet (60s); cholestyramine resin 4 g/5 g of powder (210 g); cholestyramine resin 4 g/5.7 g packet (60s); cholestyramine resin 4 g/5.7 g of powder (240 g can); cholestyramine resin 4 g/9 g packet (60s); cholestyramine resin 4 g of resin/9 g of powder (378 g)
Prevalite®: Cholestyramine resin 4 g/5.5 g packet (42s, 60s); cholestyramine resin 4 g/5.5 g of powder
Questran®: Cholestyramine resin 4 g/9 g packet (60s); cholestyramine resin 4 g/9 g of powder
Questran® Light: Cholestyramine resin 4 g/5 g packet (60s); cholestyramine resin 4 g/5 g of powder

choline fenofibrate *see* fenofibric acid *on page* 409

choline magnesium trisalicylate (KOE leen mag NEE zhum trye sa LIS i late)

Synonyms tricosal

Therapeutic Category Analgesic, Nonnarcotic; Nonsteroidal Antiinflammatory Drug (NSAID)

Use Management of osteoarthritis, rheumatoid arthritis, and other arthritis; acute painful shoulder

Usual Dosage Oral (based on total salicylate content):

Children <37 kg: 50 mg/kg/day given in 2 divided doses; 2250 mg/day for heavier children

Adults: 500 mg to 1.5 g 2-3 times/day **or** 3 g at bedtime; usual maintenance dose: 1-4.5 g/day

Dosage Forms

Liquid: 500 mg/5 mL

Tablet: 500 mg, 750 mg, 1000 mg

Cholografin® Meglumine [US] *see* iodipamide meglumine *on page* 538

chondroitin sulfate and sodium hyaluronate *see* sodium chondroitin sulfate and sodium hyaluronate *on page* 910

Chooz® [US-OTC] *see* calcium carbonate *on page* 170

choriogonadotropin alfa *see* chorionic gonadotropin (recombinant) *on page* 225

chorionic gonadotropin (human) (kor ee ON ik goe NAD oh troe pin, HYU man)

Synonyms CG; hCG

U.S./Canadian Brand Names Humegon® [Can]; Novarel® [US]; Pregnyl® [US/Can]; Profasi® HP [Can]

Therapeutic Category Gonadotropin

Use Induces ovulation and pregnancy in anovulatory, infertile females; treatment of hypogonadotropic hypogonadism, prepubertal cryptorchidism; spermatogenesis induction with follitropin alfa

Usual Dosage I.M.:

Children: Various regimens:

Prepubertal cryptorchidism:

4000 units 3 times/week for 3 weeks **or**

5000 units every second day for 4 injections **or**

500 units 3 times/week for 4-6 weeks **or**

15 injections of 500-1000 units given over 6 weeks

Hypogonadotropic hypogonadism: Males:

500-1000 units 3 times/week for 3 weeks, followed by the same dose twice weekly for 3 weeks **or**

4000 units 3 times/week for 6-9 months, then reduce dosage to 2000 units 3 times/week for additional 3 months

Adults:

Induction of ovulation: Females: 5000-10,000 units one day following last dose of menotropins

Spermatogenesis induction associated with hypogonadotropic hypogonadism: Males: Treatment regimens vary (range: 1000-2000 units 2-3 times a week). Administer hCG until serum testosterone levels are normal (may require 2-3 months of therapy), then may add follitropin alfa or menopausal gonadotropin if needed to induce spermatogenesis; continue hCG at the dose required to maintain testosterone levels.

Dosage Forms

Injection, powder for reconstitution: 10,000 units

Novarel®, Pregnyl®: 10,000 units

chorionic gonadotropin (recombinant)

(kor ee ON ik goe NAD oh troe pin ree KOM be nant)

Synonyms choriogonadotropin alfa; r-hCG

U.S./Canadian Brand Names Ovidrel® [US/Can]

Therapeutic Category Gonadotropin; Ovulation Stimulator

Use As part of an assisted reproductive technology (ART) program, induces ovulation in infertile females who have been pretreated with follicle-stimulating hormones (FSH); induces ovulation and pregnancy in infertile females when the cause of infertility is functional

Usual Dosage SubQ: Adults: Female: Assisted reproductive technologies (ART) and ovulation induction: 250 mcg given 1 day following the last dose of follicle-stimulating agent. Use only after adequate follicular development has been determined. Hold treatment when there is an excessive ovarian response.

Dosage Forms

Injection, solution:

Ovidrel®: 257.5 mcg/0.515 mL (0.515 mL)

Choron® *(Discontinued)* *see* chorionic gonadotropin (human) *on page* 225

chromic phosphate P 32 (KROME ik FOS fate pe THUR tee too)

Synonyms P32; phosphorus p32

U.S./Canadian Brand Names Phosphocol® P 32 [US]

Therapeutic Category Radiopharmaceutical

Use Treatment of peritoneal or pleural effusions caused by metastatic disease by intracavitary instillation; may be injected interstitially for the treatment of cancer

Usual Dosage Adults: **Note:** Consult manufacturer potency tables when applicable. All doses should be individualized.

General dosing ranges (based on 70 kg patient):

Intraperitoneal instillation: 370-740 megabecquerels (10-20 millicuries)

Intrapleural instillation: 222-444 megabecquerels (6-12 millicuries)

Interstitial use: ~3.7-18.5 megabecquerels/g of tumor weight (0.1-0.5 millicuries/g)

Dosage Forms

Injection, suspension:

Phosphocol® P 32: 185 MBq (5mCi) per mL

chromium *see* trace metals *on page 974*

Chronovera® [Can] *see* verapamil *on page 1010*

Chronulac® ***(Discontinued)*** *see* lactulose *on page 565*

CI-1008 *see* pregabalin *on page 815*

Cialis® [US/Can] *see* tadalafil *on page 936*

Cibacalcin® ***(Discontinued)*** *see* calcitonin *on page 167*

ciclesonide (sye KLES oh nide)

U.S./Canadian Brand Names Alvesco® [US/Can]; Omnaris™ [US/Can]

Therapeutic Category Corticosteroid, Inhalant (Oral); Corticosteroid, Nasal

Use

Intranasal: Management of seasonal and perennial allergic rhinitis

Oral inhalation: Prophylactic management of bronchial asthma

Usual Dosage

Intranasal (Omnaris™):

Seasonal allergic rhinitis:

U.S. labeling: Children ≥6 years and Adults: 2 sprays (50 mcg/spray) per nostril once daily; maximum: 200 mcg/day

Canadian labeling: Children ≥12 years and Adults: 2 sprays (50 mcg/spray) per nostril once daily; maximum: 200 mcg/day

Perennial allergic rhinitis: Children ≥12 years and Adults: 2 sprays (50 mcg/spray) per nostril once daily; maximum: 200 mcg/day

Oral inhalation (Alvesco®):

Asthma: **Note:** Titrate to the lowest effective dose once asthma stability is achieved:

U.S. labeling: Children ≥12 years and Adults:

Prior therapy with bronchodilators alone: Initial: 80 mcg twice daily (maximum dose: 320 mcg/day)

Prior therapy with inhaled corticosteroids: Initial: 80 mcg twice daily (maximum dose: 640 mcg/day)

Prior therapy with oral corticosteroids: Initial: 320 mcg twice daily (maximum dose: 640 mcg/day)

Canadian labeling: Children ≥12 years and Adults: Initial: 400 mcg once daily; maintenance: 100-800 mcg/day (1-2 puffs once or twice daily)

Conversion from oral to inhaled steroid: Initiation of oral inhalation therapy should begin in patients who have previously been stabilized on oral corticosteroids (OCS). A gradual dose reduction of OCS should begin ~7-10 days after starting inhaled therapy. U.S. labeling recommends reducing prednisone dose no more rapidly than ≤2.5 mg/day on a weekly basis. The Canadian labeling recommends decreasing the daily dose of prednisone by 1 mg (or equivalent of other OCS) every 7 days in closely monitored patients, and every 10 days in patients whom close monitoring is not possible. In the presence of withdrawal symptoms, resume previous OCS dose for 1 week before attempting further dose reductions.

Dosage Forms [CAN] = Canadian brand name

Aerosol for oral inhalation:

Alvesco® [U.S.]: 80 mcg/inhalation (6.1 g) [60 metered actuations]; 160 mcg/inhalation (6.1 g) [60 metered actuations]

Alvesco® [CAN]: 50 mcg/inhalation [30-, 60-, and 120 metered actuations] [not available in the U.S.]; 100 mcg/inhalation [30-, 60-, and 120 metered actuations] [not available in the U.S.]; 200 mcg/inhalation [30-, 60-, and 120 metered actuations] [not available in the U.S.]

Suspension, intranasal [spray]:
Omnaris™: 50 mcg/inhalation (12.5 g) [120 metered actuations]

ciclopirox (sye kloe PEER oks)

Sound-Alike/Look-Alike Issues
Loprox® may be confused with Lonox®

Synonyms ciclopirox olamine

U.S./Canadian Brand Names Loprox® [US/Can]; Penlac® [US/Can]; Stieprox® [Can]

Therapeutic Category Antifungal Agent

Use
Cream/suspension: Treatment of tinea pedis (athlete's foot), tinea cruris (jock itch), tinea corporis (ringworm), cutaneous candidiasis, and tinea versicolor (pityriasis)
Gel: Treatment of tinea pedis (athlete's foot), tinea corporis (ringworm); seborrheic dermatitis of the scalp
Lacquer (solution): Topical treatment of mild-to-moderate onychomycosis of the fingernails and toenails due to *Trichophyton rubrum* (not involving the lunula) and the immediately-adjacent skin
Shampoo: Treatment of seborrheic dermatitis of the scalp

Usual Dosage Topical:
Children >10 years and Adults: Tinea pedis, tinea cruris, tinea corporis, cutaneous candidiasis, and tinea versicolor: Cream/suspension: Apply twice daily, gently massage into affected areas; if no improvement after 4 weeks of treatment, reevaluate the diagnosis.
Children ≥12 years and Adults: Onychomycosis of the fingernails and toenails: Lacquer (solution): Apply to adjacent skin and affected nails daily (as a part of a comprehensive management program for onychomycosis). Remove with alcohol every 7 days.
Children >16 years and Adults:
Tinea pedis, tinea corporis: Gel: Apply twice daily, gently massage into affected areas and surrounding skin; if no improvement after 4 weeks of treatment, reevaluate diagnosis
Seborrheic dermatitis of the scalp:
Gel: Apply twice daily, gently massage into affected areas and surrounding skin; if no improvement after 4 weeks of treatment, reevaluate diagnosis.
Shampoo: Apply ~5 mL (1 teaspoonful) to wet hair; lather, and leave in place ~3 minutes; rinse. May use up to 10 mL for longer hair. Repeat twice weekly for 4 weeks; allow a minimum of 3 days between applications.

Dosage Forms
Cream, topical: 0.77% (15 g, 30 g, 90 g)
Gel, topical: 0.77% (30 g, 45 g, 100 g)
Loprox®: 0.77% (30 g, 45 g, 100 g)
Shampoo, topical:
Loprox®: 1% (120 mL)
Solution, topical [nail lacquer]: 8% (6.6 mL)
Penlac®: 8% (6.6 mL)
Suspension, topical: 0.77% (30 mL, 60 mL)

ciclopirox olamine *see* ciclopirox *on page 227*
cidecin *see* daptomycin *on page 276*

cidofovir (si DOF o veer)

U.S./Canadian Brand Names Vistide® [US]

Therapeutic Category Antiviral Agent

Use Treatment of cytomegalovirus (CMV) retinitis in patients with acquired immunodeficiency syndrome (AIDS). **Note:** Should be administered with probenecid.

Usual Dosage Adults:
Induction: 5 mg/kg I.V. over 1 hour once weekly for 2 consecutive weeks
Maintenance: 5 mg/kg over 1 hour once every other week
Note: Administer with probenecid 2 g orally 3 hours prior to each cidofovir dose and 1 g at 2 hours and 8 hours after completion of the infusion (total: 4 g)
Hydrate with at least 1 L of 0.9% NS I.V. prior to each cidofovir infusion; infuse saline over a 1- to 2-hour period immediately prior to cidofovir infusion. A second liter may be administered over a 1- to 3-hour period at the start of cidofovir infusion or immediately following infusion, if tolerated

Dosage Forms
Injection, solution [preservative free]:
Vistide®: 75 mg/mL (5 mL)

cilazapril and hydrochlorothiazide *(Canada only)*

(sye LAY za pril & hye droe klor oh THYE a zide)

Synonyms cilazapril monohydrate and hydrochlorothiazide; hydrochlorothiazide and cilazapril

U.S./Canadian Brand Names Apo-Cilazapril/Hctz [Can]; Inhibace® Plus [Can]; Novo-Cilazapril/HCTZ [Can]

Therapeutic Category Angiotensin-Converting Enzyme (ACE) Inhibitor

Use Treatment of mild-to-moderate hypertension in patients who have been stabilized on the individual agents given in the same proportions; not indicated for initial treatment of hypertension

Usual Dosage Note: Initiate therapy with combination product only after successful titration of individual agents to adequate blood pressure response.

Oral: Adults: One tablet administered once daily; dose is individualized (range: Cilazapril: 2.5-10 mg; hydrochlorothiazide: 6.25-25 mg/day)

Dosage Forms [CAN] = Canadian brand name

Tablet: 5/12.5: Cilazapril 5 mg and hydrochlorothiazide 12.5 mg [not available in the U.S.]

Inhibace® Plus 5/12.5 [CAN]: Cilazapril 5 mg and hydrochlorothiazide 12.5 mg [not available in the U.S.; contains lactose]

cilazapril *(Canada only)* (sye LAY za pril)

Synonyms cilazapril monohydrate

U.S./Canadian Brand Names Apo-Cilazapril® [Can]; CO Cilazapril [Can]; Gen-Cilazapril [Can]; Inhibace® [Can]; Novo-Cilazapril [Can]; PHL-Cilazapril [Can]; PMS-Cilazapril [Can]

Therapeutic Category Angiotensin-Converting Enzyme (ACE) Inhibitor

Use Management of hypertension; treatment of heart failure

Usual Dosage Oral:

Heart failure: Initial: 0.5 mg once daily; if tolerated, after 5 days increase to 1 mg/day (lowest maintenance dose); may increase to maximum of 2.5 mg once daily

Hypertension: 2.5-5 mg once daily (maximum dose: 10 mg/day)

Dosage Forms [CAN] = Canadian brand name

Tablet:

Inhibace® [CAN], Novo-Cilazapril [CAN]: 1 mg, 2.5 mg, 5 mg [not available in the U.S.]

cilazapril monohydrate *see* cilazapril *(Canada only) on page 228*

cilazapril monohydrate and hydrochlorothiazide *see* cilazapril and hydrochlorothiazide *(Canada only) on page 228*

cilostazol (sil OH sta zol)

Sound-Alike/Look-Alike Issues

Pletal® may be confused with Plendil®

Synonyms OPC-13013

U.S./Canadian Brand Names Pletal® [US/Can]

Therapeutic Category Platelet Aggregation Inhibitor

Use Symptomatic management of peripheral vascular disease, primarily intermittent claudication

Usual Dosage Oral: Adults: 100 mg twice daily

Dosage Forms

Tablet: 50 mg, 100 mg

Pletal®: 50 mg, 100 mg

Ciloxan® [US/Can] *see* ciprofloxacin *on page 229*

cimetidine (sye MET i deen)

Sound-Alike/Look-Alike Issues

cimetidine may be confused with simethicone

U.S./Canadian Brand Names Apo-Cimetidine® [Can]; Gen-Cimetidine [Can]; Novo-Cimetidine [Can]; Nu-Cimet [Can]; PMS-Cimetidine [Can]; Tagamet® HB 200 [US-OTC]; Tagamet® HB [Can]

Therapeutic Category Histamine H_2 Antagonist

Use Short-term treatment of active duodenal ulcers and benign gastric ulcers; long-term prophylaxis of duodenal ulcer; gastric hypersecretory states; gastroesophageal reflux; prevention of upper GI bleeding in critically-ill patients; labeled for OTC use for prevention or relief of heartburn, acid indigestion, or sour stomach

Usual Dosage

Children: Oral, I.M., I.V.: 20-40 mg/kg/day in divided doses every 6 hours

Children ≥12 years and Adults: Oral: Heartburn, acid indigestion, sour stomach (OTC labeling): 200 mg up to twice daily; may take 30 minutes prior to eating foods or beverages expected to cause heartburn or indigestion

Adults:

Short-term treatment of active ulcers:

Oral: 300 mg 4 times/day or 800 mg at bedtime or 400 mg twice daily for up to 8 weeks

Note: Higher doses of 1600 mg at bedtime for 4 weeks may be beneficial for a subpopulation of patients with larger duodenal ulcers (>1 cm defined endoscopically) who are also heavy smokers (≥1 pack/day).

I.M., I.V.: 300 mg every 6 hours or 37.5 mg/hour by continuous infusion; I.V. dosage should be adjusted to maintain an intragastric pH ≥5

Prevention of upper GI bleed in critically-ill patients: 50 mg/hour by continuous infusion; I.V. dosage should be adjusted to maintain an intragastric pH ≥5

Note: Reduce dose by 50% if Cl_{cr} <30 mL/minute; treatment >7 days has not been evaluated.

Duodenal ulcer prophylaxis: Oral: 400 mg at bedtime

Gastric hypersecretory conditions: Oral, I.M., I.V.: 300-600 mg every 6 hours; dosage not to exceed 2.4 g/day

Gastroesophageal reflux disease: Oral: 400 mg 4 times/day or 800 mg twice daily for 12 weeks

Dosage Forms

Note: Strength is expressed as base

Infusion [premixed in NS]: 300 mg (50 mL)

Injection, solution: 150 mg/mL (2 mL, 8 mL)

Solution, oral: 300 mg/5 mL

Tablet: 200 mg [OTC], 300 mg, 400 mg, 800 mg

Tagamet® HB 200 [OTC]: 200 mg

Cimzia® [US] *see* certolizumab pegol *on page* 203

cinacalcet (sin a KAL cet)

Synonyms AMG 073; cinacalcet hydrochloride

U.S./Canadian Brand Names Sensipar® [US/Can]

Therapeutic Category Calcimimetic

Use Treatment of secondary hyperparathyroidism in patients with chronic kidney disease (CKD) on dialysis; treatment of hypercalcemia in patients with parathyroid carcinoma

Note: In Canada, cinacalcet is approved only for the treatment of secondary hyperparathyroidism in patients with chronic kidney disease (CKD) on dialysis

Usual Dosage Oral: Adults: **Do not titrate dose more frequently than every 2-4 weeks.**

Secondary hyperparathyroidism: Initial: 30 mg once daily (maximum daily dose: 180 mg); increase dose incrementally (60 mg, 90 mg, 120 mg, 180 mg once daily) as necessary to maintain iPTH level between 150-300 pg/mL.

Parathyroid carcinoma: Initial: 30 mg twice daily (maximum daily dose: 360 mg daily as 90 mg 4 times/day); increase dose incrementally (60 mg twice daily, 90 mg twice daily, 90 mg 3-4 times/day) as necessary to normalize serum calcium levels.

Dosage Forms

Tablet:

Sensipar®: 30 mg, 60 mg, 90 mg

cinacalcet hydrochloride *see* cinacalcet *on page* 229

Cinryze™ [US] *see* C1 inhibitor (human) *on page* 165

Cipralex® [Can] *see* escitalopram *on page* 370

Cipro® [US/Can] *see* ciprofloxacin *on page* 229

Cipro® XL [Can] *see* ciprofloxacin *on page* 229

Ciprodex® [US/Can] *see* ciprofloxacin and dexamethasone *on page* 232

ciprofloxacin (sip roe FLOKS a sin)

Sound-Alike/Look-Alike Issues

ciprofloxacin may be confused with cephalexin

Ciloxan® may be confused with cinoxacin, Cytoxan®

Cipro® may be confused with Ceftin®

Synonyms ciprofloxacin hydrochloride

U.S./Canadian Brand Names Apo-Ciproflox® [Can]; Cetraxal® [US]; Ciloxan® [US/Can]; Cipro® I.V. [US]; Cipro® XL [Can]; Cipro® XR [US]; Cipro® [US/Can]; CO Ciprofloxacin [Can]; Dom-Ciprofloxacin [Can]; Mint-Ciprofloxacin [Can]; Mylan-Ciprofloxacin [Can]; Novo-Ciprofloxacin [Can]; PHL-Ciprofloxacin [Can]; PMS-Ciprofloxacin [Can]; PRO-Ciprofloxacin [Can]; Proquin® XR [US]; RAN-Ciprofloxacin [Can]; ratio-Ciprofloxacin [Can]; Riva-Ciprofloxacin [Can]; Sandoz-Ciprofloxacin [Can]; Taro-Ciprofloxacin [Can]

Therapeutic Category Antibiotic, Ophthalmic; Quinolone

Use

Children: Complicated urinary tract infections and pyelonephritis due to *E. coli*. **Note:** Although effective, ciprofloxacin is not the drug of first choice in children.

Children and Adults: To reduce incidence or progression of disease following exposure to aerolized *Bacillus anthracis*. Ophthalmologically, for superficial ocular infections (corneal ulcers, conjunctivitis) due to susceptible strains

Adults: Treatment of the following infections when caused by susceptible bacteria: Urinary tract infections; acute uncomplicated cystitis in females; chronic bacterial prostatitis; lower respiratory tract infections (including acute exacerbations of chronic bronchitis); acute sinusitis; skin and skin structure infections; bone and joint infections; complicated intraabdominal infections (in combination with metronidazole); infectious diarrhea; typhoid fever due to *Salmonella typhi* (eradication of chronic typhoid carrier state has not been proven); uncomplicated cervical and urethral gonorrhea (due to *N. gonorrhoeae*); nosocomial pneumonia; empirical therapy for febrile neutropenic patients (in combination with piperacillin)

Note: As of April 2007, the CDC no longer recommends the use of fluoroquinolones for the treatment of gonococcal disease.

Usual Dosage Note: Extended release tablets and immediate release formulations are not interchangeable. Unless otherwise specified, oral dosing reflects the use of immediate release formulations.

Usual dosage range:

Children:

Oral: 20-30 mg/kg/day in 2 divided doses; maximum dose: 1.5 g/day

I.V.: 20-30 mg/kg/day divided every 12 hours; maximum dose: 800 mg/day

Adults:

Oral: 250-750 mg every 12 hours

I.V.: 200-400 mg every 12 hours

Indication-specific dosing:

Children:

Acute otitis externa: Children ≥1 year: Refer to adult dosing

Anthrax:

Inhalational (postexposure prophylaxis):

Oral: 15 mg/kg/dose every 12 hours for 60 days; maximum: 500 mg/dose

I.V.: 10 mg/kg/dose every 12 hours for 60 days; do **not** exceed 400 mg/dose (800 mg/day)

Cutaneous (treatment, CDC guidelines): Oral: 10-15 mg/kg every 12 hours for 60 days (maximum: 1 g/day); amoxicillin 80 mg/kg/day divided every 8 hours is an option for completion of treatment after clinical improvement. **Note:** In the presence of systemic involvement, extensive edema, lesions on head/neck, refer to I.V. dosing for treatment of inhalational/gastrointestinal/oropharyngeal anthrax.

Inhalational/gastrointestinal/oropharyngeal (treatment, CDC guidelines): I.V.: Initial: 10-15 mg/kg every 12 hours for 60 days (maximum: 500 mg/dose); switch to oral therapy when clinically appropriate; refer to adult dosing for notes on combined therapy and duration

Bacterial conjunctivitis: See adult dosing

Corneal ulcer: See adult dosing

Urinary tract infection (complicated) or pyelonephritis:

Oral: 20-30 mg/kg/day in 2 divided doses (every 12 hours) for 10-21 days; maximum: 1.5 g/day

I.V.: 6-10 mg/kg every 8 hours for 10-21 days (maximum: 400 mg/dose)

Adults:

Acute otitis externa: Otic solution: Instill 0.25 mL (contents of 1 single-dose container) into affected ear twice daily for 7 days

Anthrax:

Inhalational (postexposure prophylaxis):

Oral: 500 mg every 12 hours for 60 days

I.V.: 400 mg every 12 hours for 60 days

Cutaneous (treatment, CDC guidelines): Oral: Immediate release formulation: 500 mg every 12 hours for 60 days. **Note:** In the presence of systemic involvement, extensive edema, lesions on head/neck, refer to I.V. dosing for treatment of inhalational/gastrointestinal/oropharyngeal anthrax

Inhalational/gastrointestinal/oropharyngeal (treatment, CDC guidelines): I.V.: 400 mg every 12 hours. **Note:** Initial treatment should include two or more agents predicted to be effective (per CDC recommendations). Continue combined therapy for 60 days.

Bacterial conjunctivitis:

Ophthalmic solution: Instill 1-2 drops in eye(s) every 2 hours while awake for 2 days and 1-2 drops every 4 hours while awake for the next 5 days

Ophthalmic ointment: Apply a 1/2" ribbon into the conjunctival sac 3 times/day for the first 2 days, followed by a 1/2" ribbon applied twice daily for the next 5 days

Bone/joint infections:

Oral: 500-750 mg twice daily for 4-6 weeks

I.V.: Mild-to-moderate: 400 mg every 12 hours for 4-6 weeks; Severe/complicated: 400 mg every 8 hours for 4-6 weeks

Chancroid (CDC guidelines): Oral: 500 mg twice daily for 3 days

Corneal ulcer: Ophthalmic solution: Instill 2 drops into affected eye every 15 minutes for the first 6 hours, then 2 drops into the affected eye every 30 minutes for the remainder of the first day. On day 2, instill 2 drops into the affected eye hourly. On days 3-14, instill 2 drops into affected eye every 4 hours. Treatment may continue after day 14 if re-epithelialization has not occurred.

Febrile neutropenia*: I.V.: 400 mg every 8 hours for 7-14 days

Gonococcal infections:

Urethral/cervical gonococcal infections: Oral: 250-500 mg as a single dose (CDC recommends concomitant doxycycline or azithromycin due to possible coinfection with *Chlamydia*; **Note:** As of April 2007, the CDC no longer recommends the use of fluoroquinolones for the treatment of uncomplicated gonococcal disease.

Disseminated gonococcal infection (CDC guidelines): Oral: 500 mg twice daily to complete 7 days of therapy (initial treatment with ceftriaxone 1 g I.M./I.V. daily for 24-48 hours after improvement begins); **Note:** As of April 2007, the CDC no longer recommends the use of fluoroquinolones for the treatment of more serious gonococcal disease, unless no other options exist and susceptibility can be confirmed via culture.

Infectious diarrhea: Oral:

Salmonella: 500 mg twice daily for 5-7 days

Shigella: 500 mg twice daily for 3 days

Traveler's diarrhea: Mild: 750 mg for one dose; Severe: 500 mg twice daily for 3 days

Vibrio cholerae: 1 g for one dose

Intraabdominal*:

Oral: 500 mg every 12 hours for 7-14 days

I.V.: 400 mg every 12 hours for 7-14 days

Lower respiratory tract, skin/skin structure infections:

Oral: 500-750 mg twice daily for 7-14 days

I.V.: Mild-to-moderate: 400 mg every 12 hours for 7-14 days; Severe/complicated: 400 mg every 8 hours for 7-14 days

Nosocomial pneumonia: I.V.: 400 mg every 8 hours for 10-14 days

Prostatitis (chronic, bacterial): Oral: 500 mg every 12 hours for 28 days

Sinusitis (acute): Oral: 500 mg every 12 hours for 10 days

Typhoid fever: Oral: 500 mg every 12 hours for 10 days

Urinary tract infection:

Acute uncomplicated, cystitis:

Oral:

Immediate release formulation: 250 mg every 12 hours for 3 days

Extended release formulation (Cipro® XR, Proquin® XR): 500 mg every 24 hours for 3 days

I.V.: 200 mg every 12 hours for 7-14 days

Complicated (including pyelonephritis):

Oral:

Immediate release formulation: 500 mg every 12 hours for 7-14 days

Extended release formulation (Cipro® XR): 1000 mg every 24 hours for 7-14 days

I.V.: 400 mg every 12 hours for 7-14 days

*Combination therapy generally recommended.

Dosage Forms

Infusion [premixed in D_5W]: 200 mg (100 mL); 400 mg (200 mL)

Cipro® I.V.: 200 mg (100 mL); 400 mg (200 mL)

Injection, solution [concentrate]: 10 mg/mL (20 mL, 40 mL, 120 mL)
Cipro® I.V.: 10 mg/mL (20 mL)
Microcapsules for suspension, oral:
Cipro®: 250 mg/5 mL, 500 mg/5 mL
Ointment, ophthalmic:
Ciloxan®: 3.33 mg/g (3.5 g) [equivalent to ciprofloxacin base 0.3%]
Solution, ophthalmic: 3.5 mg/mL (2.5 mL, 5mL, 10 mL) [equivalent to ciprofloxacin base 0.3%]
Ciloxan®: 3.5 mg/mL (5 mL) [0.3% base]
Solution, otic: [preservative free]:
Cetraxal®: 0.5 mg/0.25 mL (14s) [equivalent to ciprofloxacin base 0.2%]
Tablet: 100 mg, 250 mg, 500 mg, 750 mg
Cipro®: 250 mg, 500 mg, 750 mg
Tablet, extended release: 500 mg, 1000 mg
Cipro® XR: 500 mg, 1000 mg
Tablet, extended release:
Proquin® XR: 500 mg
Tablet, extended release [dose pack]:
Proquin® XR: 500 mg (3s)

ciprofloxacin and dexamethasone (sip roe FLOKS a sin & deks a METH a sone)

Synonyms ciprofloxacin hydrochloride and dexamethasone; dexamethasone and ciprofloxacin

U.S./Canadian Brand Names Ciprodex® [US/Can]

Therapeutic Category Antibiotic/Corticosteroid, Otic

Use Treatment of acute otitis media in pediatric patients with tympanostomy tubes or acute otitis externa in children and adults

Usual Dosage Otic:
Children: Acute otitis media in patients with tympanostomy tubes or acute otitis externa: Instill 4 drops into affected ear(s) twice daily for 7 days
Adults: Acute otitis externa: Instill 4 drops into affected ear(s) twice daily for 7 days

Dosage Forms
Suspension, otic:
Ciprodex®: Ciprofloxacin 0.3% and dexamethasone 0.1% (7.5 mL)

ciprofloxacin and hydrocortisone (sip roe FLOKS a sin & hye droe KOR ti sone)

Synonyms ciprofloxacin hydrochloride and hydrocortisone; hydrocortisone and ciprofloxacin

U.S./Canadian Brand Names Cipro® HC [US/Can]

Therapeutic Category Antibiotic/Corticosteroid, Otic

Use Treatment of acute otitis externa, sometimes known as "swimmer's ear"

Usual Dosage Otic: Children >1 year of age and Adults: The recommended dosage for all patients is three drops of the suspension in the affected ear twice daily for 7 days; twice-daily dosing schedule is more convenient for patients than that of existing treatments with hydrocortisone, which are typically administered three or four times a day; a twice-daily dosage schedule may be especially helpful for parents and caregivers of young children

Dosage Forms
Suspension, otic:
Cipro® HC: Ciprofloxacin 0.2% and hydrocortisone 1% (10 mL)

ciprofloxacin hydrochloride *see* ciprofloxacin *on page* 229
ciprofloxacin hydrochloride and dexamethasone *see* ciprofloxacin and dexamethasone *on page* 232
ciprofloxacin hydrochloride and hydrocortisone *see* ciprofloxacin and hydrocortisone *on page* 232
Cipro® HC [US/Can] *see* ciprofloxacin and hydrocortisone *on page* 232
Cipro® I.V. [US] *see* ciprofloxacin *on page* 229
Cipro® XR [US] *see* ciprofloxacin *on page* 229

cisapride (SIS a pride)

Sound-Alike/Look-Alike Issues
Propulsid® may be confused with propranolol

U.S./Canadian Brand Names Propulsid® [US]

Therapeutic Category Gastrointestinal Agent, Prokinetic

Use Treatment of nocturnal symptoms of gastroesophageal reflux disease (GERD); has demonstrated effectiveness for gastroparesis, refractory constipation, and nonulcer dyspepsia

Usual Dosage Oral:

Children: 0.15-0.3 mg/kg/dose 3-4 times/day; maximum: 10 mg/dose

Adults: Initial: 10 mg 4 times/day at least 15 minutes before meals and at bedtime; in some patients the dosage will need to be increased to 20 mg to obtain a satisfactory result

cisatracurium (sis a tra KYOO ree um)

Sound-Alike/Look-Alike Issues

Nimbex® may be confused with Revex®

Synonyms cisatracurium besylate

U.S./Canadian Brand Names Nimbex® [US/Can]

Therapeutic Category Skeletal Muscle Relaxant

Use Adjunct to general anesthesia to facilitate endotracheal intubation and to relax skeletal muscles during surgery; to facilitate mechanical ventilation in ICU patients; does not relieve pain or produce sedation

Usual Dosage I.V. (not to be used I.M.):

Operating room administration:

Infants 1-23 months: 0.15 mg/kg over 5-10 seconds during either halothane or opioid anesthesia

Children 2-12 years: Intubating doses: 0.1-0.15 mg/kg over 5-15 seconds during either halothane or opioid anesthesia. (**Note:** When given during stable opioid/nitrous oxide/oxygen anesthesia, 0.1 mg/kg produces maximum neuromuscular block in an average of 2.8 minutes and clinically effective block for 28 minutes.)

Adults: Intubating doses: 0.15-0.2 mg/kg as component of propofol/nitrous oxide/oxygen induction-intubation technique. (**Note:** May produce generally good or excellent conditions for tracheal intubation in 1.5-2 minutes with clinically effective duration of action during propofol anesthesia of 55-61 minutes.); initial dose after succinylcholine for intubation: 0.1 mg/kg; maintenance dose: 0.03 mg/kg 40-60 minutes after initial dose, then at ~20-minute intervals based on clinical criteria

Children ≥2 years and Adults: Continuous infusion: After an initial bolus, a diluted solution can be given by continuous infusion for maintenance of neuromuscular blockade during extended surgery; adjust the rate of administration according to the patient's response as determined by peripheral nerve stimulation. An initial infusion rate of 3 mcg/kg/minute may be required to rapidly counteract the spontaneous recovery of neuromuscular function; thereafter, a rate of 1-2 mcg/kg/minute should be adequate to maintain continuous neuromuscular block in the 89% to 99% range in most pediatric and adult patients. Consider reduction of the infusion rate by 30% to 40% when administering during stable isoflurane, enflurane, sevoflurane, or desflurane anesthesia. Spontaneous recovery from neuromuscular blockade following discontinuation of infusion of cisatracurium may be expected to proceed at a rate comparable to that following single bolus administration.

Intensive care unit administration: Follow the principles for infusion in the operating room. At initial signs of recovery from bolus dose, begin the infusion at a dose of 3 mcg/kg/minute and adjust rates accordingly; dosage ranges of 0.5-10 mcg/kg/minute have been reported. If patient is allowed to recover from neuromuscular blockade, readministration of a bolus dose may be necessary to quickly reestablish neuromuscular block prior to reinstituting the infusion.

Dosage Forms

Injection, solution:

Nimbex®: 2 mg/mL (5 mL, 10 mL); 10 mg/mL (20 mL)

cisatracurium besylate *see* cisatracurium *on page* 233

cisplatin (SIS pla tin)

Sound-Alike/Look-Alike Issues

CISplatin may be confused with CARBOplatin, oxaliplatin

Synonyms CDDP

Tall-Man CISplatin

Therapeutic Category Antineoplastic Agent

Use Treatment of bladder, testicular, and ovarian cancer

Usual Dosage Refer to individual protocols. **VERIFY ANY CISPLATIN DOSE EXCEEDING 100 mg/m^2 PER COURSE.**

Adults:

Advanced bladder cancer: 50-70 mg/m^2 every 3-4 weeks

Malignant pleural mesothelioma in combination with pemetrexed: 75 mg/m^2 on day 1 of each 21-day cycle; see pemetrexed monograph for additional details

Metastatic ovarian cancer: 75-100 mg/m^2 every 3-4 weeks

Intraperitoneal: Cisplatin has been administered intraperitoneal with systemic sodium thiosulfate for ovarian cancer; doses up to 90-270 mg/m^2 have been administered and retained for 4 hours before draining

Testicular cancer: 10-20 mg/m^2/day for 5 days repeated every 3-4 weeks

Dosage Forms

Injection, solution [preservative free]: 1 mg/mL (50 mL, 100 mL, 200 mL)

13-*cis*-retinoic acid *see* isotretinoin *on page 551*

citalopram (sye TAL oh pram)

Sound-Alike/Look-Alike Issues

Celexa® may be confused with Celebrex®, Cerebra®, Cerebyx®, Ranexa™, Zyprexa®

Synonyms citalopram hydrobromide; nitalapram

U.S./Canadian Brand Names Apo-Citalopram® [Can]; Celexa® [US/Can]; Citalopram-ODAN [Can]; CO Citalopram [Can]; CTP 30 [Can]; Dom-Citalopram [Can]; Gen-Citalopram [Can]; IPG-Citalopram [Can]; JAMP-Citalopram [Can]; Mint-Citalopram [Can]; Novo-Citalopram [Can]; PHL-Citalopram [Can]; PMS-Citalopram [Can]; RAN™-Citalopram [Can]; ratio-Citalopram [Can]; Riva-Citalopram [Can]; Sandoz-Citalopram [Can]

Therapeutic Category Antidepressant

Use Treatment of depression

Usual Dosage Oral: Adults: Depression: Initial: 20 mg/day, generally with an increase to 40 mg/day; doses of more than 40 mg are not usually necessary. Should a dose increase be necessary, it should occur in 20 mg increments at intervals of no less than 1 week. Maximum dose: 60 mg/day

Dosage Forms

Solution, oral: 10 mg/5 mL

Tablet: 10 mg, 20 mg, 40 mg

Celexa®: 10 mg

Celexa®: 20 mg, 40 mg [scored]

citalopram hydrobromide *see* citalopram *on page 234*

Citalopram-ODAN [Can] *see* citalopram *on page 234*

Citanest® Plain [Can] *see* prilocaine *on page 817*

Citanest® Plain Dental [US] *see* prilocaine *on page 817*

Citracal® Kosher *(Discontinued)* *see* calcium citrate *on page 172*

Citracal® Prenatal 90+ DHA *(Discontinued)* *see* vitamins (multiple/prenatal) *on page 1020*

Citracal® Prenatal + DHA *(Discontinued)* *see* vitamins (multiple/prenatal) *on page 1020*

CitraNatal™ 90 DHA [US] *see* vitamins (multiple/prenatal) *on page 1020*

CitraNatal™ DHA [US] *see* vitamins (multiple/prenatal) *on page 1020*

CitraNatal™ Rx [US] *see* vitamins (multiple/prenatal) *on page 1020*

citrate of magnesia *see* magnesium citrate *on page 607*

citric acid and D-gluconic acid irrigant *see* citric acid, magnesium carbonate, and glucono-delta-lactone *on page 234*

citric acid and potassium citrate *see* potassium citrate and citric acid *on page 804*

citric acid bladder mixture *see* citric acid, magnesium carbonate, and glucono-delta-lactone *on page 234*

citric acid, magnesium carbonate, and glucono-delta-lactone
(SI trik AS id, mag NEE see um KAR bo nate, and GLOO kon o DEL ta LAK tone)

Sound-Alike/Look-Alike Issues

Renacidin® may be confused with Remicade®

Synonyms citric acid and D-gluconic acid irrigant; citric acid bladder mixture; citric acid, magnesium hydroxycarbonate, D-gluconic acid, magnesium acid citrate, and calcium carbonate; hemiacidrin

U.S./Canadian Brand Names Renacidin® [US]

Therapeutic Category Irrigating Solution

Use Prevention of formation of calcifications of indwelling urinary tract catheters; treatment of renal and bladder calculi of the apatite or struvite type

Usual Dosage Adults:

Dissolution or prevention of calcifications: Irrigation (indwelling urethral catheters): 30-60 mL 2-3 times/day by means of a rubber syringe

Renal calculi: Irrigation: Infuse NS at 60 mL/hour and increase until pain, elevated pressure, or maximum flow rate of 120 mL/hour is reached. Begin flow of solution at maximum rate achieved with NS.

Bladder calculi: 30 mL instilled through urinary catheter; clamp for 30-60 minutes, then release and drain; repeat 4-6 times/day

Dosage Forms

Solution, irrigation:

Renacidin®: Citric acid 6.602 g, magnesium carbonate 3.177 g, glucono-delta-lactone 0.198 g per 100 mL (500 mL)

citric acid, magnesium hydroxycarbonate, D-gluconic acid, magnesium acid citrate, and calcium carbonate *see* citric acid, magnesium carbonate, and glucono-delta-lactone *on page* *234*

citric acid, sodium citrate, and potassium citrate

(SIT rik AS id, SOW dee um SIT rate, & poe TASS ee um SIT rate)

Sound-Alike/Look-Alike Issues

Polycitra® may be confused with Bicitra®

Synonyms potassium citrate, citric acid, and sodium citrate; sodium citrate, citric acid, and potassium citrate

U.S./Canadian Brand Names Cytra-3 [US]; Polycitra® [US]; Polycitra®-LC [US]; Tricitrates [US]

Therapeutic Category Alkalinizing Agent

Use Conditions where long-term maintenance of an alkaline urine is desirable as in control and dissolution of uric acid and cystine calculi of the urinary tract

Usual Dosage Oral:

Children: 5-15 mL diluted in water after meals and at bedtime

Adults: 15-30 mL diluted in water after meals and at bedtime

Dosage Forms

Solution, oral:

Cytra-3, Polycitra®-LC, Tricitrates: Citric acid 334 mg, sodium citrate 500 mg, and potassium citrate 550 mg per 5 mL

Syrup, oral:

Polycitra®: Citric acid 334 mg, sodium citrate 500 mg, and potassium citrate 550 mg per 5 mL

Citroma® [US-OTC] *see* magnesium citrate *on page* *607*

Citro-Mag® [Can] *see* magnesium citrate *on page* *607*

Citrotein® [US-OTC] *see* nutritional formula, enteral/oral *on page* *715*

citrovorum factor *see* leucovorin calcium *on page* *575*

Citrucel® [US-OTC] *see* methylcellulose *on page* *642*

Citrucel® Fiber Shake [US-OTC] *see* methylcellulose *on page* *642*

Citrucel® Fiber Smoothie [US-OTC] *see* methylcellulose *on page* *642*

CL-118,532 *see* triptorelin *on page* *990*

Cl-719 *see* gemfibrozil *on page* *458*

CL-184116 *see* porfimer *on page* *801*

CL-232315 *see* mitoxantrone *on page* *662*

cladribine (KLA dri been)

Sound-Alike/Look-Alike Issues

cladribine may be confused with clevidipine, clofarabine, fludarabine

Leustatin® may be confused with lovastatin

Synonyms 2-CdA; 2-chlorodeoxyadenosine; NSC-105014

U.S./Canadian Brand Names Leustatin® [US/Can]

Therapeutic Category Antineoplastic Agent

Use Treatment of hairy cell leukemia

Usual Dosage I.V. (refer to individual protocols): Adults: Hairy cell leukemia: Continuous infusion: 0.09 mg/kg/day days 1-7; may be repeated every 28-35 days

Dosage Forms

Injection, solution [preservative free]: 1 mg/mL (10 mL)

Leustatin®: 1 mg/mL (10 mL)

Claforan® [US/Can] *see* cefotaxime *on page* 194
Claravis™ [US] *see* isotretinoin *on page* 551
Clarifoam™ EF [US] *see* sulfur and sulfacetamide *on page* 931
Clarinex® [US] *see* desloratadine *on page* 284
Clarinex-D® 12 Hour [US] *see* desloratadine and pseudoephedrine *on page* 284
Clarinex-D® 24 Hour [US] *see* desloratadine and pseudoephedrine *on page* 284
Claripel™ *(Discontinued)* *see* hydroquinone *on page* 508

clarithromycin (kla RITH roe mye sin)

Sound-Alike/Look-Alike Issues
clarithromycin may be confused with Claritin®, clindamycin, erythromycin

U.S./Canadian Brand Names Apo-Clarithromycin [Can]; Biaxin® XL [US/Can]; Biaxin® [US/Can]; Gen-Clarithromycin [Can]; PMS-Clarithromycin [Can]; ratio-Clarithromycin [Can]; Sandoz-Clarithromycin [Can]

Therapeutic Category Macrolide (Antibiotic)

Use

Children:

Acute otitis media (*H. influenzae*, *M. catarrhalis*, or *S. pneumoniae*)

Community-acquired pneumonia due to susceptible *Mycoplasma pneumoniae, S. pneumoniae*, or *Chlamydia pneumoniae* (TWAR)

Pharyngitis/tonsillitis due to susceptible *S. pyogenes*, acute maxillary sinusitis due to susceptible *H. influenzae, S. pneumoniae*, or *Moraxella catarrhalis*, uncomplicated skin/skin structure infections due to susceptible *S. aureus, S. pyogenes,* and mycobacterial infections

Prevention of disseminated mycobacterial infections due to MAC disease in patients with advanced HIV infection

Adults:

Pharyngitis/tonsillitis due to susceptible *S. pyogenes*

Acute maxillary sinusitis and acute exacerbation of chronic bronchitis due to susceptible *H. influenzae*, *H. parainfluenzae*, *M. catarrhalis*, or *S. pneumoniae*

Community-acquired pneumonia due to susceptible *H. influenzae, H. parainfluenzae, Mycoplasma pneumoniae, S. pneumoniae,* or *Chlamydia pneumoniae* (TWAR), *Moraxella catarrhalis*

Uncomplicated skin/skin structure infections due to susceptible *S. aureus*, *S. pyogenes*

Disseminated mycobacterial infections due to *M. avium* or *M. intracellulare*

Prevention of disseminated mycobacterial infections due to *M. avium* complex (MAC) disease (eg, patients with advanced HIV infection)

Duodenal ulcer disease due to *H. pylori* in regimens with other drugs including amoxicillin and lansoprazole or omeprazole, ranitidine bismuth citrate, bismuth subsalicylate, tetracycline, and/or an H_2 antagonist

Usual Dosage

Usual dosage range:

Children ≥6 months: Oral: 7.5 mg/kg every 12 hours (maximum: 500 mg/dose)

Adults: Oral: 250-500 mg every 12 hours **or** 1000 mg (two 500 mg extended release tablets) once daily for 7-14 days

Indication-specific dosing:

Children: Oral:

Community-acquired pneumonia, sinusitis, bronchitis, skin infections: 15 mg/kg/day divided every 12 hours for 10 days

Mycobacterial infection (prevention and treatment): 7.5 mg/kg (up to 500 mg) twice daily. **Note:** Safety of clarithromycin for MAC not studied in children <20 months.

Adults: Oral:

Acute exacerbation of chronic bronchitis:

M. catarrhalis and *S. pneumoniae*: 250 mg every 12 hours for 7-14 days **or** 1000 mg (two 500 mg extended release tablets) once daily for 7 days

H. influenzae: 500 mg every 12 hours for 7-14 days **or** 1000 mg (two 500 mg extended release tablets) once daily for 7 days

H. parainfluenzae: 500 mg every 12 hours for 7 days **or** 1000 mg (two 500 mg extended release tablets) once daily for 7 days

Acute maxillary sinusitis: 500 mg every 12 hours **or** 1000 mg (two 500 mg extended release tablets) once daily for 14 days

Mycobacterial infection (prevention and treatment): 500 mg twice daily (use with other antimycobacterial drugs, eg, ethambutol or rifampin)

Peptic ulcer disease: Eradication of *Helicobacter pylori*: Dual or triple combination regimens with bismuth subsalicylate, amoxicillin, an H_2-receptor antagonist, or proton-pump inhibitor: 500 mg every 8-12 hours for 10-14 days

Pharyngitis, tonsillitis: 250 mg every 12 hours for 10 days

Pneumonia:

C. pneumoniae, *M. pneumoniae*, and *S. pneumoniae*: 250 mg every 12 hours for 7-14 days **or** 1000 mg (two 500 mg extended release tablets) once daily for 7 days

H. influenzae: 250 mg every 12 hours for 7 days **or** 1000 mg (two 500 mg extended release tablets) once daily for 7 days

H. parainfluenzae and *M. catarrhalis*: 1000 mg (two 500 mg extended release tablets) once daily for 7 days

Skin and skin structure infection, uncomplicated: 250 mg every 12 hours for 7-14 days

Dosage Forms

Granules for oral suspension: 125 mg/5 mL (50 mL, 100 mL); 250 mg/5 mL (50 mL, 100 mL)

Biaxin®: 125 mg/5 mL, 250 mg/5 mL

Tablet: 250 mg, 500 mg

Biaxin®: 250 mg, 500 mg

Tablet, extended release: 500 mg

Biaxin® XL: 500 mg

clarithromycin, lansoprazole, and amoxicillin *see* lansoprazole, amoxicillin, and clarithromycin *on page 571*

Claritin® [Can] *see* loratadine *on page 599*

Claritin® 24 Hour Allergy [US-OTC] *see* loratadine *on page 599*

Claritin® Allergic Decongestant [Can] *see* oxymetazoline *on page 740*

Claritin® Children's Allergy [US-OTC] *see* loratadine *on page 599*

Claritin-D® 12 Hour Allergy & Congestion [US-OTC] *see* loratadine and pseudoephedrine *on page 599*

Claritin-D® 24 Hour Allergy & Congestion [US-OTC] *see* loratadine and pseudoephedrine *on page 599*

Claritin® *(Discontinued)* *see* loratadine *on page 599*

Claritin® Extra [Can] *see* loratadine and pseudoephedrine *on page 599*

Claritin™ Eye [US-OTC] *see* ketotifen *on page 559*

Claritin® Hives Relief *(Discontinued)* *see* loratadine *on page 599*

Claritin® Kids [Can] *see* loratadine *on page 599*

Claritin® Liberator [Can] *see* loratadine and pseudoephedrine *on page 599*

Claritin® Liqui-Gels® 24 Hour Allergy [US-OTC] *see* loratadine *on page 599*

Claritin® RediTabs® 24 Hour Allergy [US-OTC] *see* loratadine *on page 599*

Claritin® Reditabs *(Discontinued)* *see* loratadine *on page 599*

Clarus™ [Can] *see* isotretinoin *on page 551*

Clasteon® [Can] *see* clodronate *(Canada only) on page 243*

clavulanic acid and amoxicillin *see* amoxicillin and clavulanate potassium *on page 71*

Clavulin® [Can] *see* amoxicillin and clavulanate potassium *on page 71*

Clear Away® Disc *(Discontinued)* *see* salicylic acid *on page 884*

Clear By Design® Gel *(Discontinued)* *see* benzoyl peroxide *on page 132*

Clear eyes® for Dry Eyes and ACR Relief [US-OTC] *see* naphazoline *on page 680*

Clear eyes® for Dry Eyes and Redness Relief [US-OTC] *see* naphazoline *on page 680*

Clear eyes® Redness Relief [US-OTC] *see* naphazoline *on page 680*

Clear eyes® Seasonal Relief [US-OTC] *see* naphazoline *on page 680*

Clearsil® Maximum Strength *(Discontinued)* *see* benzoyl peroxide *on page 132*

Clearskin [US-OTC] *see* benzoyl peroxide *on page 132*

Clear Tussin® 30 *(Discontinued)* *see* guaifenesin and dextromethorphan *on page 474*

clemastine (KLEM as teen)

Synonyms clemastine fumarate

U.S./Canadian Brand Names Dayhist® Allergy [US-OTC]; Tavist® Allergy [US-OTC]

Therapeutic Category Antihistamine

Use Perennial and seasonal allergic rhinitis and other allergic symptoms including urticaria

Usual Dosage Oral:

Infants and Children <6 years: 0.05 mg/kg/day as **clemastine base** or 0.335-0.67 mg/day clemastine fumarate (0.25-0.5 mg base/day) divided into 2 or 3 doses; maximum daily dosage: 1.34 mg (1 mg base)

Children 6-12 years: 0.67-1.34 mg clemastine fumarate (0.5-1 mg base) twice daily; do not exceed 4.02 mg/day (3 mg/day base)

Children ≥12 years and Adults:

1.34 mg clemastine fumarate (1 mg base) twice daily to 2.68 mg (2 mg base) 3 times/day; do not exceed 8.04 mg/day (6 mg base)

OTC labeling: 1.34 mg clemastine fumarate (1 mg base) twice daily; do not exceed 2 mg base/24 hours

Dosage Forms

Syrup: 0.67 mg/5 mL [0.5 mg base/5 mL; prescription formulation]

Tablet: 1.34 mg [1 mg base; OTC], 2.68 mg [2 mg base; prescription formulation]

Dayhist® Allergy [OTC], Tavist® Allergy [OTC]: 1.34 mg [1 mg base]

clemastine fumarate *see* clemastine *on page 237*
Clenia™ [US] *see* sulfur and sulfacetamide *on page 931*
Cleocin® [US] *see* clindamycin *on page 239*
Cleocin HCl® [US] *see* clindamycin *on page 239*
Cleocin Pediatric® [US] *see* clindamycin *on page 239*
Cleocin Phosphate® [US] *see* clindamycin *on page 239*
Cleocin T® [US] *see* clindamycin *on page 239*
Cleocin® Vaginal Ovule [US] *see* clindamycin *on page 239*

clevidipine (klev ID i peen)

Sound-Alike/Look-Alike Issues

clevidipine may be confused with cladribine, clofarabine, clomiPRAMINE

Cleviprex™ may be confused with Claravis™

Synonyms clevidipine butyrate

U.S./Canadian Brand Names Cleviprex™ [US]

Therapeutic Category Calcium Channel Blocker

Use Management of hypertension when oral treatment is not feasible or not desirable

Usual Dosage I.V.: Adults: Initial: 1-2 mg/hour

Titration: Initial: dose may be doubled at 90-second intervals toward blood pressure goal. As blood pressure approaches goal, dose may be increased by less than double every 5-10 minutes. **Note:** For every 1-2 mg/hour increase in dose, an approximate reduction of 2-4 mm Hg in systolic blood pressure may occur.

Usual maintenance: 4-6 mg/hour; maximum: 21 mg/hour (1000 mL within a 24-hour period). There is limited short-term experience with doses up to 32 mg/hour. Data is limited beyond 72 hours.

Dosage Forms

Injection, emulsion:

Cleviprex™: 0.5 mg/mL (50 mL, 100 mL)

clevidipine butyrate *see* clevidipine *on page 238*
Cleviprex™ [US] *see* clevidipine *on page 238*

clidinium and chlordiazepoxide (kli DI nee um & klor dye az e POKS ide)

Sound-Alike/Look-Alike Issues

Librax® may be confused with Librium®

Synonyms chlordiazepoxide and clidinium

U.S./Canadian Brand Names Apo-Chlorax® [Can]; Librax® *[original formulation]* [US/Can]

Therapeutic Category Anticholinergic Agent

Use Adjunct treatment of peptic ulcer; treatment of irritable bowel syndrome

Usual Dosage Oral: 1-2 capsules 3-4 times/day, before meals or food and at bedtime

Caution: Do not abruptly discontinue after prolonged use; taper dose gradually.

Dosage Forms

Capsule: Clidinium 2.5 mg and chlordiazepoxide 5 mg

Librax® [original formulation]: Clidinium 2.5 mg and chlordiazepoxide 5 mg

Climara® [US/Can] *see* estradiol *on page 373*

ClimaraPro® [US] *see* estradiol and levonorgestrel *on page 376*

Clinac BPO [US] *see* benzoyl peroxide *on page 132*

Clindagel® [US] *see* clindamycin *on page 239*

ClindaMax® [US] *see* clindamycin *on page 239*

clindamycin (klin da MYE sin)

Sound-Alike/Look-Alike Issues

clindamycin may be confused with clarithromycin, Claritin®, vancomycin

Cleocin® may be confused with bleomycin, Clinoril®, Cubicin®, Lincocin®

Synonyms clindamycin hydrochloride; clindamycin palmitate; clindamycin phosphate

U.S./Canadian Brand Names Alti-Clindamycin [Can]; Apo-Clindamycin® [Can]; Cleocin HCl® [US]; Cleocin Pediatric® [US]; Cleocin Phosphate® [US]; Cleocin T® [US]; Cleocin® Vaginal Ovule [US]; Cleocin® [US]; Clindagel® [US]; ClindaMax® [US]; Clindamycin Injection, USP [Can]; ClindaReach™ [US]; Clindasol™ [Can]; Clindesse™ [US]; Dalacin® C [Can]; Dalacin® T [Can]; Dalacin® Vaginal [Can]; Evoclin® [US]; Gen-Clindamycin [Can]; Novo-Clindamycin [Can]; PMS-Clindamycin [Can]; ratio-Clindamycin [Can]; Riva-Clindamycin [Can]; Taro-Clindamycin [Can]

Therapeutic Category Acne Products; Antibiotic, Miscellaneous

Use Treatment of susceptible bacterial infections, mainly those caused by anaerobes, streptococci, pneumococci, and staphylococci; bacterial vaginosis (vaginal cream, vaginal suppository); pelvic inflammatory disease (I.V.); topically in treatment of severe acne; vaginally for *Gardnerella vaginalis*

Usual Dosage

Usual dosage ranges:

Infants and Children:

Oral: 8-20 mg/kg/day as hydrochloride; 8-25 mg/kg/day as palmitate in 3-4 divided doses (minimum dose of palmitate: 37.5 mg 3 times/day)

I.M., I.V.:

<1 month: 15-20 mg/kg/day in 3-4 divided doses

>1 month: 20-40 mg/kg/day in 3-4 divided doses

Adults:

Oral: 150-450 mg/dose every 6-8 hours; maximum dose: 1.8 g/day

I.M., I.V.: 1.2-2.7 g/day in 2-4 divided doses; maximum dose: 4.8 g/day

Indication-specific dosing:

Children:

Anthrax: I.V.: 7.5 mg/kg every 6 hours

Orofacial infections:

Oral: 10-20 mg/kg/day in 3-4 equally divided doses

I.V.: 15-25 mg/kg/day in 3-4 equally divided doses

Children ≥12 years and Adults:

Acne vulgaris: Topical:

Gel, pledget, lotion, solution: Apply a thin film twice daily

Foam (Evoclin®): Apply once daily

Adults:

Amnionitis: I.V.: 450-900 mg every 8 hours

Anthrax: I.V.: 900 mg every 8 hours with ciprofloxacin or doxycycline

Bacterial vaginosis: Intravaginal:

Suppositories: Insert one ovule (100 mg clindamycin) daily into vagina at bedtime for 3 days

Cream:

Cleocin®: One full applicator inserted intravaginally once daily before bedtime for 3 or 7 consecutive days in nonpregnant patients or for 7 consecutive days in pregnant patients

Clindesse™: One full applicator inserted intravaginally as a single dose at anytime during the day in nonpregnant patients

Bite wounds (canine): Oral: 300 mg 4 times/day with a fluoroquinolone

Gangrenous pyomyositis: I.V.: 900 mg every 8 hours with penicillin G

Group B streptococcus (neonatal prophylaxis): I.V.: 900 mg every 8 hours until delivery

Orofacial/parapharyngeal space infections:
Oral: 150-450 mg every 6 hours for 7 days, maximum 1.8 g/day
I.V.: 600-900 mg every 8 hours
Pelvic inflammatory disease: I.V.: 900 mg every 8 hours with gentamicin 2 mg/kg, then 1.5 mg/kg every 8 hours; continue after discharge with doxycycline 100 mg twice daily to complete 14 days of total therapy
Prophylaxis in total joint replacement patients undergoing dental procedures which produce bacteremia:
Oral: 600 mg 1 hour prior to procedure
I.V.: 600 mg 1 hour prior to procedure (for patients unable to take oral medication)
Toxic shock syndrome: I.V.: 900 mg every 8 hours with penicillin G or ceftriaxone

Dosage Forms
Capsule: 75 mg, 150 mg, 300 mg
Cleocin HCl®: 75 mg, 150 mg, 300 mg
Cream, vaginal: 2% (40 g)
Cleocin®: 2% (40 g)
Clindesse™: 2% (5 g)
Foam, topical:
Evoclin®: 1% (50 g, 100 g)
Gel, topical: 1% (30 g, 60 g)
Cleocin T®: 1% (30 g, 60 g)
Clindagel®: 1% (40 mL, 75 mL)
ClindaMax®: 1% (30 g, 60 g)
Granules for oral solution:
Cleocin Pediatric®: 75 mg/5 mL
Infusion [premixed in D_5W]:
Cleocin Phosphate®: 300 mg (50 mL); 600 mg (50 mL); 900 mg (50 mg/mL]
Injection, solution: 150 mg/mL (2 mL, 4 mL, 6 mL, 60 mL)
Cleocin Phosphate®: 150 mg/mL (2 mL, 4 mL, 6 mL, 60 mL)
Lotion: 1% (60 mL)
Cleocin T®, ClindaMax®: 1% (60 mL)
Pledgets, topical: 1% (60s, 69s)
Cleocin T®: 1% (60s)
ClindaReach™: 1% (120s)
Solution, topical: 1% (30 mL, 60 mL)
Cleocin T®: 1% (30 mL, 60 mL)
Suppository, vaginal:
Cleocin® Vaginal Ovule: 100 mg (3s)

clindamycin and benzoyl peroxide (klin da MYE sin & BEN zoe il peer OKS ide)

Synonyms benzoyl peroxide and clindamycin; clindamycin phosphate and benzoyl peroxide
U.S./Canadian Brand Names Acanya™ [US]; BenzaClin® [US/Can]; Clindoxyl® [US]; Duac® CS [US]
Therapeutic Category Topical Skin Product; Topical Skin Product, Acne
Use Topical treatment of acne vulgaris
Usual Dosage Topical: Children ≥12 years and Adults: Apply to affected areas after skin has been cleansed and dried
Acanya™: Acne: Apply pea-sized amount once daily; use >12 weeks has not been studied
BenzaClin®: Acne: Apply twice daily (morning and evening)
Duac® CS: Inflammatory acne: Apply once daily in the evening

Dosage Forms
Gel, topical: Clindamycin 1% and benzoyl peroxide 5% (50 g)
Acanya™: Clindamycin 1% and benzoyl peroxide 2.5% (50 g)
BenzaClin®: Clindamycin 1% and benzoyl peroxide 5% (25 g, 50 g)
Duac® CS: Clindamycin 1% and benzoyl peroxide 5% (45 g)

clindamycin and tretinoin (klin da MYE sin & TRET i noyn)

Synonyms clindamycin phosphate and tretinoin; tretinoin and clindamycin
U.S./Canadian Brand Names Ziana™ [US]
Therapeutic Category Acne Products; Retinoic Acid Derivative; Topical Skin Product; Topical Skin Product, Acne
Use Treatment of acne vulgaris

Usual Dosage Topical: Children ≥12 years and Adults: Apply pea-size amount to entire face once daily at bedtime

Dosage Forms

Gel, topical:

Ziana™: Clindamycin phosphate 1.2% and tretinoin 0.025% (30 g, 60 g)

clindamycin hydrochloride *see* clindamycin *on page 239*

Clindamycin Injection, USP [Can] *see* clindamycin *on page 239*

clindamycin palmitate *see* clindamycin *on page 239*

clindamycin phosphate *see* clindamycin *on page 239*

clindamycin phosphate and benzoyl peroxide *see* clindamycin and benzoyl peroxide *on page 240*

clindamycin phosphate and tretinoin *see* clindamycin and tretinoin *on page 240*

ClindaReach™ [US] *see* clindamycin *on page 239*

Clindasol™ [Can] *see* clindamycin *on page 239*

Clindesse™ [US] *see* clindamycin *on page 239*

Clindets® *(Discontinued)* *see* clindamycin *on page 239*

Clindex® *(Discontinued)* *see* clidinium and chlordiazepoxide *on page 238*

Clindoxyl® [US] *see* clindamycin and benzoyl peroxide *on page 240*

Clinisol® [US] *see* amino acid injection *on page 62*

Clinoril® [US] *see* sulindac *on page 932*

clioquinol and flumethasone *(Canada only)* (klye ok KWIN ole & floo METH a sone)

Synonyms flumethasone and clioquinol; iodochlorhydroxyquin and flumethasone

U.S./Canadian Brand Names Locacorten® Vioform® [Can]

Therapeutic Category Antibiotic, Topical; Corticosteroid, Topical

Use Treatment of corticosteroid-responsive dermatoses complicated by infection with bacterial and/or fungal agents

Usual Dosage Children >2 years and Adults:

Otic solution (drops): Instill 2-3 drops into affected ear(s) 2 times/day; generally limit duration to 10 days

Topical: Apply in a thin layer to affected area 2-3 times/day; generally limit duration to 7 days

Dosage Forms [CAN] = Canadian brand name

Cream, topical:

Locacorten® Vioform® [CAN]: Clioquinol 3% and flumethasone 0.02% (15 g, 50 g) [not available in the U.S.]

Solution, otic:

Locacorten® Vioform® [CAN]: Clioquinol 1% and flumethasone 0.02% (10 mL) [not available in the U.S.]

Clobazam-10 [Can] *see* clobazam *(Canada only) on page 241*

clobazam *(Canada only)* (KLOE ba zam)

U.S./Canadian Brand Names Alti-Clobazam [Can]; Apo-Clobazam® [Can]; Clobazam-10 [Can]; Dom-Clobazam [Can]; Frisium® [Can]; Novo-Clobazam [Can]; PMS-Clobazam [Can]; ratio-Clobazam [Can]

Therapeutic Category Anticonvulsant; Antidepressant

Use Adjunctive treatment of epilepsy

Usual Dosage Oral:

Children:

<2 years: Initial 0.5-1 mg/kg/day

2-16 years: Initial: 5 mg/day; may be increased (no more frequently than every 5 days) to a maximum of 40 mg/day

Adults: Initial: 5-15 mg/day; dosage may be gradually adjusted (based on tolerance and seizure control) to a maximum of 80 mg/day

Note: Daily doses of up to 30 mg may be taken as a single dose at bedtime; higher doses should be divided.

Dosage Forms [CAN] = Canadian brand name

Tablet: 10 mg [not available in the U.S.]

Alti-Clobazam [CAN], Apo-Clobazam® [CAN], Clobazam-10 [CAN], Dom-Clobazam [CAN], Frisium® [CAN], Novo-Clobazam [CAN], PMS-Clobazam [CAN], ration-Clobazam [CAN]: 10 mg [not available in the U.S.]

clobetasol (kloe BAY ta sol)

Synonyms clobetasol propionate

U.S./Canadian Brand Names Clobex® [US/Can]; Cormax® [US]; Dermovate® [Can]; Gen-Clobetasol [Can]; Novo-Clobetasol [Can]; Olux-E™ [US]; Olux® [US]; Olux®/Olux-E™ CP [US]; PMS-Clobetasol [Can]; ratio-Clobetasol [Can]; Taro-Clobetasol [Can]; Temovate E® [US]; Temovate® [US]

Therapeutic Category Corticosteroid, Topical

Use Short-term relief of inflammation of moderate-to-severe corticosteroid-responsive dermatoses (very high potency topical corticosteroid)

Usual Dosage Topical: Discontinue when control achieved; if improvement not seen within 2 weeks, reassessment of diagnosis may be necessary.

Children ≥12 years and Adults:

Steroid-responsive dermatoses:

Cream, emollient cream, gel, ointment: Apply twice daily for up to 2 weeks (maximum dose: 50 g/week)

Foam (Olux-E™): Apply to affected area twice daily for up to 2 weeks (maximum dose: 50 g/week); do not apply to face or intertriginous areas

Steroid-responsive dermatoses: Foam (Olux®), solution: Apply to affected scalp twice daily for up to 2 weeks (maximum dose: 50 g/week or 50 mL/week)

Mild-to-moderate plaque-type psoriasis of nonscalp areas: Foam (Olux®): Apply to affected area twice daily for up to 2 weeks (maximum dose: 50 g/week); do not apply to face or intertriginous areas

Children ≥16 years and Adults: Moderate-to-severe plaque-type psoriasis: Emollient cream, lotion: Apply twice daily for up to 2 weeks, has been used for up to 4 weeks when application is <10% of body surface area; use with caution (maximum dose: 50 g/week)

Children ≥18 years and Adults:

Moderate-to-severe plaque-type psoriasis: Spray: Apply by spraying directly onto affected area twice daily; should be gently rubbed into skin. Should be used for not longer than 4 weeks; treatment beyond 2 weeks should be limited to localized lesions which have not improved sufficiently. Total dose should not exceed 50 g/week or 59 mL/week.

Scalp psoriasis: Shampoo: Apply thin film to dry scalp once daily; leave in place for 15 minutes, then add water, lather; rinse thoroughly

Steroid-responsive dermatoses: Lotion: Apply twice daily for up to 2 weeks (maximum dose: 50 g/week)

Dosage Forms

Aerosol, topical [foam]: 0.05% (50 g, 100 g)

Olux-E™, Olux®: 0.05% (50 g, 100 g)

Combination package, topical:

Olux®/Olux-E™ CP: Aerosol, topical [foam]:

Olux-E™: 0.05% (50 g)

Olux®: 0.05% (50 g)

Cream, topical: 0.05% (15 g, 30 g, 45 g, 60 g, 60s)

Temovate®: 0.05% (30 g, 60 g)

Cream, topical [emulsion-based]: 0.05% (15 g, 30 g, 60 g)

Cream, topical [in emollient base]: 0.05% (15 g, 30 g, 60 g)

Temovate E®: 0.05% (60 g)

Gel, topical: 0.05% (15 g, 30 g, 60 g)

Temovate®: 0.05% (60 g)

Lotion, topical:

Clobex®: 0.05% (30 mL, 59 mL, 118 mL)

Ointment, topical: 0.05% (15 g, 30 g, 45 g, 60 g)

Cormax®: 0.05% (15 g, 45 g)

Temovate®: 0.05% (15 g, 30 g)

Shampoo, topical:

Clobex®: 0.05% (118 mL)

Solution, topical [for scalp application]: 0.05% (25 mL, 50 mL)

Cormax®: 0.05% (25 mL, 50 mL)

Temovate®: 0.05% (50 mL)

Solution, topical [spray]:
Clobex®: 0.05% (59 mL, 125 mL)

clobetasol propionate *see* clobetasol *on page 242*
Clobevate® ***(Discontinued)*** *see* clobetasol *on page 242*
Clobex® [US/Can] *see* clobetasol *on page 242*

clocortolone (kloe KOR toe lone)

Sound-Alike/Look-Alike Issues
Cloderm® may be confused with Clocort®

Synonyms clocortolone pivalate

U.S./Canadian Brand Names Cloderm® [US/Can]

Therapeutic Category Corticosteroid, Topical

Use Inflammation of corticosteroid-responsive dermatoses (intermediate-potency topical corticosteroid)

Usual Dosage Adults: Apply sparingly and gently; rub into affected area from 1-4 times/day. Therapy should be discontinued when control is achieved; if no improvement is seen, reassessment of diagnosis may be necessary.

Dosage Forms
Cream:
Cloderm®: 0.1% (30 g, 45 g, 90 g)

clocortolone pivalate *see* clocortolone *on page 243*
Cloderm® [US/Can] *see* clocortolone *on page 243*

clodronate *(Canada only)* (KLOE droh nate)

Synonyms clodronate disodium

U.S./Canadian Brand Names Bonefos® [Can]; Clasteon® [Can]

Therapeutic Category Bisphosphonate Derivative

Use Management of hypercalcemia of malignancy; management of osteolysis due to bone metastases of malignancy

Usual Dosage Adults:
Clasteon®: Hypercalcemia of malignancy/osteolytic bone metastases:
I.V.:
Single infusion: 1500 mg as a single dose
Multiple infusions: 300 mg/day; should not be prolonged beyond 10 days
Oral: Recommended daily maintenance dose following I.V. therapy: Range: 1600 mg (4 capsules) to 2400 mg (6 capsules) given in a single or 2 divided doses; maximum recommended daily dose: 3200 mg (8 capsules). Should be taken at least 1 hour before or after food since food may decrease clodronate absorption.
Bonefos®:
Hypercalcemia of malignancy:
I.V.: Multiple infusions: 300 mg/day; should not be prolonged beyond 7 days
Oral: Recommended daily maintenance dose following I.V. therapy: Range: 1600 mg (4 capsules) to 2400 mg (6 capsules) given in single or 2 divided doses; maximum recommended daily dose: 3200 mg (8 capsules). Should be taken at least 2 hours before or after food since food may decrease clodronate absorption.
Osteolytic bone metastases:
I.V.: Multiple infusions: 300 mg/day; should not be prolonged beyond 7 days
Oral: Initial: 1600 mg/day; may be increased to a maximum of 3200 mg/day

Dosage Forms [CAN] = Canadian brand name
Injection:
Bonefos® [CAN]: 60 mg/mL (5 mL) [not available in the U.S.]
Clasteon® [CAN]: 30 mg/mL (10 mL) [not available in the U.S.]
Capsule:
Bonefos® [CAN], Clasteon® [CAN]: 400 mg [not available in the U.S.]

clodronate disodium *see* clodronate *(Canada only) on page 243*

clofarabine (klo FARE a been)

Sound-Alike/Look-Alike Issues
clofarabine may be confused with cladribine, clevidipine

Synonyms CAFdA; clofarex; NSC606869

U.S./Canadian Brand Names Clolar® [US]

Therapeutic Category Antineoplastic Agent, Antimetabolite (Purine Antagonist)

Use Treatment of relapsed or refractory acute lymphoblastic leukemia (ALL)

Usual Dosage Consider prophylactic corticosteroids (hydrocortisone 100 mg/m^2 on days 1-3; to prevent signs/symptoms of capillary leak syndrome or SIRS), hydration and allopurinol (to reduce the risk of tumor lysis syndrome/hyperuricemia), and prophylactic antiemetics.

I.V.: Children ≥1 year and Adults ≤21 years: ALL: 52 mg/m^2/day days 1 through 5; repeat every 2-6 weeks; subsequent cycles should begin no sooner than 14 days from day 1 of the previous cycle (subsequent cycles may be administered when ANC ≥750/mm^3)

Dosage Forms

Injection, solution [preservative free]:

Clolar®: 1 mg/mL (20 mL)

clofarex *see* clofarabine *on page 243*

Clolar® [US] *see* clofarabine *on page 243*

Clomid® [US/Can] *see* clomiphene *on page 244*

clomiphene (KLOE mi feen)

Sound-Alike/Look-Alike Issues

clomiPHENE may be confused with clomiPRAMINE, clonidine

Clomid® may be confused with clonidine

Serophene® may be confused with Sarafem®

Synonyms clomiphene citrate

Tall-Man clomi**PHENE**

U.S./Canadian Brand Names Clomid® [US/Can]; Milophene® [Can]; Serophene® [US/Can]

Therapeutic Category Ovulation Stimulator

Use Treatment of ovulatory failure in patients desiring pregnancy

Usual Dosage Oral: Adults: Ovulation induction: Females:

Initial course: 50 mg once daily for 5 days. Begin on or about the fifth day of cycle if progestin-induced bleeding is scheduled or spontaneous uterine bleeding occurs prior to therapy.

Dose adjustment: Subsequent doses may be increased to 100 mg once daily for 5 days only if ovulation does not occur at the initial dose. A low dose or duration of course is recommended in patients where unusual sensitivity to pituitary gonadotropin is suspected (eg, PCOS).

Repeat courses: If needed, the 5-day cycle may be repeated as early as 30 days after the previous one. Exclude the presence of pregnancy.

Maximum dose: 100 mg once daily for 5 days for 6 cycles. Discontinue if ovulation does not occur after 3 courses of treatment; or if 3 ovulatory responses occur but pregnancy is not achieved. Reevaluate if menses does not occur following ovulatory response. Doses larger than 150 mg have been reported, however, pregnancy rates are low.

Dosage Forms

Tablet [scored]: 50 mg

Clomid®, Serophene®: 50 mg

clomiphene citrate *see* clomiphene *on page 244*

clomipramine (kloe MI pra meen)

Sound-Alike/Look-Alike Issues

clomiPRAMINE may be confused with chlorproMAZINE, clevidipine, clomiPHENE, desipramine, Norpramin®

Anafranil® may be confused with alfentanil, enalapril, nafarelin

Synonyms clomipramine hydrochloride

Tall-Man clomi**PRAMINE**

U.S./Canadian Brand Names Anafranil® [US/Can]; Apo-Clomipramine® [Can]; CO Clomipramine [Can]; Gen-Clomipramine [Can]

Therapeutic Category Antidepressant, Tricyclic (Tertiary Amine)

Use Treatment of obsessive-compulsive disorder (OCD)

Usual Dosage Oral: OCD:

Children: ≥10 years:

Initial: 25 mg/day; may gradually increase as tolerated over the first 2 weeks to 3 mg/kg/day or 100 mg/day (whichever is less) in divided doses

Maintenance: May further increase to recommended maximum of 3 mg/kg/day or 200 mg/day (whichever is less); may give as a single daily dose at bedtime once tolerated

Adults:

Initial: 25 mg/day; may gradually increase as tolerated over the first 2 weeks to 100 mg/day in divided doses

Maintenance: May further increase to recommended maximum of 250 mg/day; may give as a single daily dose at bedtime once tolerated

Dosage Forms

Capsule: 25 mg, 50 mg, 75 mg

Anafranil®: 25 mg, 50 mg, 75 mg

clomipramine hydrochloride *see* clomipramine *on page 244*

Clonapam [Can] *see* clonazepam *on page 245*

clonazepam (kloe NA ze pam)

Sound-Alike/Look-Alike Issues

clonazePAM may be confused with clofazimine, cloNIDine, clorazepate, clozapine, LORazepam

Klonopin® may be confused with clofazimine, clonNIDine, clorazepate, clozapine, LORazepam

Tall-Man clonaze**PAM**

U.S./Canadian Brand Names Alti-Clonazepam [Can]; Apo-Clonazepam® [Can]; Clonapam [Can]; CO Clonazepam [Can]; Gen-Clonazepam [Can]; Klonopin® [US/Can]; Novo-Clonazepam [Can]; Nu-Clonazepam [Can]; PMS-Clonazepam [Can]; Pro-Clonazepam [Can]; Rho®-Clonazepam [Can]; Rivotril® [Can]; Sandoz-Clonazepam [Can]

Therapeutic Category Benzodiazepine

Controlled Substance C-IV

Use Alone or as an adjunct in the treatment of petit mal variant (Lennox-Gastaut), akinetic, and myoclonic seizures; petit mal (absence) seizures unresponsive to succimides; panic disorder with or without agoraphobia

Usual Dosage Oral:

Children <10 years or 30 kg: Seizure disorders:

Initial daily dose: 0.01-0.03 mg/kg/day (maximum: 0.05 mg/kg/day) given in 2-3 divided doses; increase by no more than 0.5 mg every third day until seizures are controlled or adverse effects seen

Usual maintenance dose: 0.1-0.2 mg/kg/day divided 3 times/day, not to exceed 0.2 mg/kg/day

Adults:

Burning mouth syndrome (dental use): 0.25-3 mg/day in 2 divided doses, in morning and evening

Seizure disorders:

Initial daily dose not to exceed 1.5 mg given in 3 divided doses; may increase by 0.5-1 mg every third day until seizures are controlled or adverse effects seen (maximum: 20 mg/day)

Usual maintenance dose: 0.05-0.2 mg/kg; do not exceed 20 mg/day

Panic disorder: 0.25 mg twice daily; increase in increments of 0.125-0.25 mg twice daily every 3 days; target dose: 1 mg/day (maximum: 4 mg/day)

Discontinuation of treatment: To discontinue, treatment should be withdrawn gradually. Decrease dose by 0.125 mg twice daily every 3 days until medication is completely withdrawn.

Dosage Forms

Tablet: 0.5 mg, 1 mg, 2 mg

Klonopin®: 0.5 mg, 1 mg, 2 mg

Tablet, orally disintegrating: 0.125 mg, 0.25 mg, 0.5 mg, 1 mg, 2 mg

clonidine (KLON i deen)

Sound-Alike/Look-Alike Issues

cloNIDine may be confused with Clomid®, clomiPHENE, clonazePAM, clozapine, Klonopin®, quiNIDine

Catapres® may be confused with Cataflam®, Cetapred®, Combipres®

Synonyms clonidine hydrochloride

Tall-Man clo**NID**ine

U.S./Canadian Brand Names Apo-Clonidine® [Can]; Carapres® [Can]; Catapres-TTS® [US]; Catapres® [US]; Dixarit® [Can]; DOM-Clonidine [Can]; Duraclon® [US]; Novo-Clonidine [Can]; Nu-Clonidine [Can]

Therapeutic Category Alpha-Adrenergic Agonist

Use Management of mild-to-moderate hypertension; either used alone or in combination with other antihypertensives

Orphan drug: Duraclon®: For continuous epidural administration as adjunctive therapy with intraspinal opiates for treatment of cancer pain in patients tolerant to or unresponsive to intraspinal opiates

Usual Dosage

Children:

Oral:

Hypertension: Children ≥12 years: Initial: 0.2 mg/day in 2 divided doses; increase gradually at 5- to 7-day intervals; usual maintenance dose: 0.2-0.6 mg/day in divided doses; maximum: 2.4 mg/day (rarely required)

Clonidine tolerance test (test of growth hormone release from pituitary): 0.15 mg/m^2 or 4 mcg/kg as single dose

Epidural infusion: Pain management: Reserved for patients with severe intractable pain, unresponsive to other analgesics or epidural or spinal opiates: Initial: 0.5 mcg/kg/hour; adjust with caution, based on clinical effect

Adults:

Oral:

Acute hypertension (urgency): Initial 0.1-0.2 mg; may be followed by additional doses of 0.1 mg every hour, if necessary, to a maximum total dose of 0.6 mg

Hypertension: Initial dose: 0.1 mg twice daily (maximum recommended dose: 2.4 mg/day); usual dose range (JNC 7): 0.1-0.8 mg/day in 2 divided doses

Transdermal: Hypertension: Apply once every 7 days; for initial therapy start with 0.1 mg and increase by 0.1 mg at 1- to 2-week intervals (dosages >0.6 mg do not improve efficacy); usual dose range (JNC 7): 0.1-0.3 mg once weekly

Note: If transitioning from oral to transdermal therapy, overlap oral regimen for 1-2 days; transdermal route takes 2-3 days to achieve therapeutic effects.

Conversion from oral to transdermal:

Day 1: Place Catapres-TTS® 1; administer 100% of oral dose.

Day 2: Administer 50% of oral dose.

Day 3: Administer 25% of oral dose.

Day 4: Patch remains, no further oral supplement necessary.

Epidural infusion: Pain management: Starting dose: 30 mcg/hour; titrate as required for relief of pain or presence of side effects; minimal experience with doses >40 mcg/hour; should be considered an adjunct to intraspinal opiate therapy

Dosage Forms

Injection, solution [epidural; preservative free]:

Duraclon®: 100 mcg/mL (10 mL); 500 mcg/mL (10 mL)

Tablet: 0.1 mg, 0.2 mg, 0.3 mg

Catapres®: 0.1 mg, 0.2 mg, 0.3 mg

Transdermal system, topical [once-weekly patch]:

Catapres-TTS®-1: 0.1 mg/24 hours (4s)

Catapres-TTS®-2: 0.2 mg/24 hours (4s)

Catapres-TTS®-3: 0.3 mg/24 hours (4s)

clonidine and chlorthalidone (KLON i deen & klor THAL i done)

Sound-Alike/Look-Alike Issues

Combipres® may be confused with Catapres®

Synonyms chlorthalidone and clonidine

U.S./Canadian Brand Names Clorpres® [US]

Therapeutic Category Antihypertensive Agent, Combination

Use Management of mild-to-moderate hypertension

Usual Dosage Oral: 1 tablet 1-2 times/day; maximum: 0.6 mg clonidine and 30 mg chlorthalidone

Dosage Forms

Tablet:

Clorpres®: 0.1: Clonidine 0.1 mg and chlorthalidone 15 mg; 0.2: Clonidine 0.2 mg and chlorthalidone 15 mg; 0.3: Clonidine 0.3 mg and chlorthalidone 15 mg

clonidine hydrochloride *see* clonidine *on page 245*

clopidogrel (kloh PID oh grel)

Sound-Alike/Look-Alike Issues

Plavix® may be confused with Elavil®, Paxil®

Synonyms clopidogrel bisulfate

U.S./Canadian Brand Names Plavix® [US/Can]

Therapeutic Category Antiplatelet Agent

Use Reduces rate of atherothrombotic events (myocardial infarction, stroke, vascular deaths) in patients with recent MI or stroke, or established peripheral arterial disease; reduces rate of atherothrombotic events in patients with unstable angina or non-ST-segment elevation acute coronary syndromes (unstable angina and non-ST-segment elevation MI) managed medically or through percutaneous coronary intervention (PCI) (with or without stent) or CABG; reduces rate of death and atherothrombotic events in patients with ST-segment elevation MI (STEMI) managed medically

Usual Dosage Oral: Adults:

Recent MI, recent stroke, or established arterial disease: 75 mg once daily

Acute coronary syndrome (ACS):

Unstable angina, non-ST-segment elevation myocardial infarction (UA/NSTEMI): Initial: 300 mg loading dose, followed by 75 mg once daily (in combination with aspirin 75-325 mg once daily). **Note:** A loading dose of 600 mg given at least 2 hours (or 24 hours in patients unable to take aspirin) prior to PCI followed by 75 mg once daily is recommended

ST-segment elevation myocardial infarction (STEMI): 75 mg once daily (in combination with aspirin 75-162 mg/day). CLARITY used a 300 mg loading dose of clopidogrel (with thrombolysis). The duration of therapy was <28 days (usually until hospital discharge).

The American College of Chest Physicians recommends:

Patients ≤75 years: Initial: 300 mg loading dose, followed by 75 mg once daily for up to 28 days (in combination with aspirin)

Patients >75 years: 75 mg once daily for up to 28 days (with or without thrombolysis)

Note: *Coronary artery stents:* Duration of clopidogrel (in combination with aspirin): According to the ACC/AHA/SCAI guidelines, ideally 12 months following drug-eluting stent (DES) placement in patients not at high risk for bleeding; at a minimum, 1, 3, and 6 months for bare metal (BMS), sirolimus eluting, and paclitaxel eluting stents, respectively, for uninterrupted therapy. For newer drug-eluting stents (eg, everolimus [Xience™], zotarolimus [Endeavor®]), a minimum duration of 3 months is recommended. The 2008 *Chest* guidelines recommend for patients who undergo PCI and receive a BMS (with ongoing ACS) or a DES (with or without ongoing ACS) that clopidogrel be continued for at least 12 months. In patients receiving a BMS without ongoing ACS, clopidogrel may be continued for at least 1 month. In patients receiving a DES, therapy with clopidogrel beyond 12 months may be considered in patients without bleeding or tolerability issues. Premature interruption of therapy may result in stent thrombosis with subsequent fatal and nonfatal myocardial infarction.

Dosage Forms

Tablet:

Plavix®: 75 mg, 300 mg

clopidogrel bisulfate *see* clopidogrel *on page 247*

Clopixol® [Can] *see* zuclopenthixol *(Canada only) on page 1035*

Clopixol-Acuphase® [Can] *see* zuclopenthixol *(Canada only) on page 1035*

Clopixol® Depot [Can] *see* zuclopenthixol *(Canada only) on page 1035*

clorazepate (klor AZ e pate)

Sound-Alike/Look-Alike Issues

clorazepate may be confused with clofibrate, clonazepam

Synonyms clorazepate dipotassium

U.S./Canadian Brand Names Apo-Clorazepate® [Can]; Novo-Clopate [Can]; Tranxene® SD™ [US]; Tranxene® SD™-Half Strength [US]; Tranxene® T-Tab® [US]

Therapeutic Category Anticonvulsant; Benzodiazepine

Controlled Substance C-IV

Use Treatment of generalized anxiety disorder; management of ethanol withdrawal; adjunct anticonvulsant in management of partial seizures

Usual Dosage Oral:
Children 9-12 years: Anticonvulsant: Initial: 3.75-7.5 mg/dose twice daily; increase dose by 3.75 mg at weekly intervals, not to exceed 60 mg/day in 2-3 divided doses
Children >12 years and Adults: Anticonvulsant: Initial: Up to 7.5 mg/dose 2-3 times/day; increase dose by 7.5 mg at weekly intervals, not to exceed 90 mg/day
Adults:
Anxiety:
Regular release tablets (Tranxene® T-Tab®): 7.5-15 mg 2-4 times/day
Sustained release (Tranxene® SD™): 11.25 or 22.5 mg once daily at bedtime
Ethanol withdrawal: Initial: 30 mg, then 15 mg 2-4 times/day on first day; maximum daily dose: 90 mg; gradually decrease dose over subsequent days

Dosage Forms
Tablet: 3.75 mg, 7.5 mg, 15 mg
Tranxene® SD™: 22.5 mg
Tranxene® SD™-Half Strength: 11.25 mg
Tranxene® T-Tab®: 3.75 mg, 7.5 mg, 15 mg

clorazepate dipotassium *see* clorazepate *on page 247*
Clorpactin® WCS-90 [US-OTC] *see* oxychlorosene *on page 737*
Clorpres® [US] *see* clonidine and chlorthalidone *on page 246*
Clotrimaderm [Can] *see* clotrimazole *on page 248*

clotrimazole (kloe TRIM a zole)

Sound-Alike/Look-Alike Issues
clotrimazole may be confused with co-trimoxazole
Lotrimin® may be confused with Lotrisone®, Otrivin®
Mycelex® may be confused with Myoflex®

U.S./Canadian Brand Names Canesten® Topical [Can]; Canesten® Vaginal [Can]; Clotrimaderm [Can]; Cruex® Cream [US-OTC]; Gyne-Lotrimin® 3 [US-OTC]; Gyne-Lotrimin® 7 [US-OTC]; Lotrimin® AF Athlete's Foot Cream [US-OTC]; Lotrimin® AF for Her [US-OTC]; Lotrimin® AF Jock Itch Cream [US-OTC]; Mycelex® [US]; Trivagizole-3® [Can]

Therapeutic Category Antifungal Agent

Use Treatment of susceptible fungal infections, including oropharyngeal candidiasis, dermatophytoses, superficial mycoses, and cutaneous candidiasis, as well as vulvovaginal candidiasis; limited data suggest that clotrimazole troches may be effective for prophylaxis against oropharyngeal candidiasis in neutropenic patients

Usual Dosage
Children >3 years and Adults:
Oral:
Prophylaxis: 10 mg troche dissolved 3 times/day for the duration of chemotherapy or until steroids are reduced to maintenance levels
Treatment: 10 mg troche dissolved slowly 5 times/day for 14 consecutive days
Topical (cream, solution): Apply twice daily; if no improvement occurs after 4 weeks of therapy, reevaluate diagnosis
Children >12 years and Adults:
Vaginal:
Cream:
1%: Insert 1 applicatorful vaginal cream daily (preferably at bedtime) for 7 consecutive days
2%: Insert 1 applicatorful vaginal cream daily (preferably at bedtime) for 3 consecutive days
Tablet: Insert 100 mg/day for 7 days or 500 mg single dose
Topical (cream, solution): Apply to affected area twice daily (morning and evening) for 7 consecutive days

Dosage Forms
Cream, topical: 1% (15 g, 30 g, 45 g)
Cruex® [OTC]: 1% (15 g)
Lotrimin® AF Athlete's Foot [OTC]: 1% (12 g)
Lotrimin® AF Jock Itch [OTC]: 1% (12 g)
Lotrimin® AF for Her [OTC]: 1% (24 g)
Cream, topical/vaginal: 1% (45 g)
Gyne-Lotrimin® 7 [OTC]: 1% (45 g)

Cream, vaginal: 2% (21 g)
Gyne-Lotrimin® 3 [OTC]: 2% (21 g)
Solution, topical: 1% (10 mL, 30 mL)
Troche, oral: 10 mg
Mycelex®: 10 mg

clotrimazole and betamethasone *see* betamethasone and clotrimazole *on page 137*
Cloxacillin [Can] *see* cloxacillin *(Canada only) on page 249*

cloxacillin *(Canada only)* (kloks a SIL in)

Synonyms cloxacillin sodium

U.S./Canadian Brand Names Apo-Cloxi® [Can]; Cloxacillin [Can]; Novo-Cloxin [Can]; Nu-Cloxi [Can]

Therapeutic Category Penicillin

Use Treatment of susceptible bacterial infections, including beta-hemolytic streptococci, pneumococci, and penicillinase-producing staphylococci causing respiratory tract, skin and skin structure, bone and joint, urinary tract infections

Usual Dosage Note: Dose and duration of therapy can vary depending on infecting organism, severity of infection, and clinical response of patient. Treat beta-hemolytic streptococcal infections at least 10 days to prevent the occurrence of rheumatic fever or acute glomerulonephritis. Treat severe staphylococcal infections for at least 14 days; endocarditis and osteomyelitis require an extended duration of therapy

Usual dosage range:
Oral:
Children ≤20 kg: 25-50 mg/kg/day in divided doses every 6 hours
Children >20 kg and Adults: 250-500 mg every 6 hours (manufacturer recommended maximum adult dose: 6 g/day)
I.M., I.V.:
Children ≤20 kg: 25-50 mg/kg/day in divided doses every 6 hours; up to 200 mg/kg/day has been used in some studies for severe infections
Children >20 kg and Adults: 250-500 mg every 6 hours (manufacturer recommended maximum adult dose: 6 g/day)

Dosage Forms
Capsule: 250 mg, 500 mg [not available in the U.S.]
Injection, powder for reconstitution: 50 mg, 500 mg, 1000 mg, 2000 mg [not available in the U.S.]
Powder for suspension, oral: 125 mg/5 mL [not available in the U.S.]

cloxacillin sodium *see* cloxacillin *(Canada only) on page 249*
Cloxapen® ***(Discontinued)*** *see* cloxacillin *(Canada only) on page 249*

clozapine (KLOE za peen)

Sound-Alike/Look-Alike Issues
clozapine may be confused with clofazimine, clonidine, Klonopin®
Clozaril® may be confused with Clinoril®, Colazal®

U.S./Canadian Brand Names Apo-Clozapine® [Can]; Clozaril® [US/Can]; FazaClo® [US]; Gen-Clozapine [Can]; PMS-Clozapine [Can]

Therapeutic Category Antipsychotic Agent, Dibenzodiazepine

Use Treatment-refractory schizophrenia; to reduce risk of recurrent suicidal behavior in schizophrenia or schizoaffective disorder

Usual Dosage Oral: Adults:
Schizophrenia: Initial: 12.5 mg once or twice daily; increased, as tolerated, in increments of 25-50 mg/day to a target dose of 300-450 mg/day after 2-4 weeks, may require doses as high as 600-900 mg/day
Reduce risk of suicidal behavior: Initial: 12.5 mg once or twice daily; increased, as tolerated, in increments of 25-50 mg/day to a target dose of 300-450 mg/day after 2-4 weeks; median dose is ~300 mg/day (range: 12.5-900 mg)

Termination of therapy: If dosing is interrupted for ≥48 hours, therapy must be reinitiated at 12.5-25 mg/day; may be increased more rapidly than with initial titration, unless cardiopulmonary arrest occurred during initial titration.
In the event of planned termination of clozapine, gradual reduction in dose over a 1- to 2-week period is recommended. If conditions warrant abrupt discontinuation (leukopenia), monitor patient for psychosis and cholinergic rebound (headache, nausea, vomiting, diarrhea).
Patients discontinued on clozapine therapy due to WBC <2000/mm^3 or ANC <1000/mm^3 should not be restarted on clozapine.

Dosage Forms

Tablet: 25 mg, 50 mg, 100 mg, 200 mg
Clozaril®: 25 mg [scored], 100 mg [scored]

Tablet, orally disintegrating:
FazaClo®: 12.5 mg, 25 mg, 100 mg

Clozaril® [US/Can] *see* clozapine *on page* *249*
Clysodrast® ***(Discontinued)*** *see* bisacodyl *on page* *142*
CMA-676 *see* gemtuzumab ozogamicin *on page* *459*
CMV-IGIV *see* cytomegalovirus immune globulin (intravenous-human) *on page* *271*
CNJ-016™ [US] *see* vaccinia immune globulin (intravenous) *on page* *1001*
CNTO-148 *see* golimumab *on page* *470*
CNTO 1275 *see* ustekinumab *(Canada only) on page* *1000*
CoActifed® [Can] *see* triprolidine, pseudoephedrine, and codeine *(Canada only) on page* *990*
coagulant complex inhibitor *see* antiinhibitor coagulant complex *on page* *85*
coagulation factor I *see* fibrinogen concentrate (human) *on page* *417*
coagulation factor VIIa *see* factor VIIa (recombinant) *on page* *402*
CO Alendronate [Can] *see* alendronate *on page* *44*

coal tar (KOLE tar)

Synonyms crude coal tar; LCD; pix carbonis

U.S./Canadian Brand Names Balnetar® [US-OTC/Can]; Betatar® Gel [US-OTC]; Cutar® [US-OTC]; Denorex® Original Therapeutic Strength [US-OTC]; DHS™ Tar [US-OTC]; DHS™ Targel [US-OTC]; Doak® Tar [US-OTC]; Estar® [Can]; Exorex® [US]; MG 217® Medicated Tar [US-OTC]; MG 217® [US-OTC]; Neutrogena® T/Gel Extra Strength [US-OTC]; Neutrogena® T/Gel Stubborn Itch Control [US-OTC]; Neutrogena® T/Gel [US-OTC]; Oxipor® VHC [US-OTC]; Reme-T™ [US-OTC]; Scytera™ [US-OTC]; Targel® [Can]; Tera-Gel™ [US-OTC]; Zetar® [US-OTC]

Therapeutic Category Antipsoriatic Agent; Antiseborrheic Agent, Topical

Use Topically for controlling dandruff, seborrheic dermatitis, or psoriasis

Usual Dosage Topical:

Bath: Add appropriate amount to bath water; for adults usually 60-90 mL of a 5% to 20% solution or 15-25 mL of 30% lotion; soak 5-20 minutes, then pat dry; use once daily to 3 days

Shampoo: Rub shampoo onto wet hair and scalp, rinse thoroughly; repeat; leave on 5 minutes; rinse thoroughly; apply twice weekly for the first 2 weeks then once weekly or more often if needed

Soap: Use on affected areas in place of regular soap. Work into a lather using warm water; massage into skin; rinse.

Skin: Apply to the affected area 1-4 times/day; decrease frequency to 2-3 times/week once condition has been controlled

Scalp psoriasis: Tar oil bath or coal tar solution may be painted sparingly to the lesions 3-12 hours before each shampoo

Psoriasis of the body, arms, legs: Apply at bedtime; if thick scales are present, use product with salicylic acid and apply several times during the day

Dosage Forms

Aerosol, topical [foam]:
Scytera™ [OTC]: Coal tar solution 10% (100 g)

Emulsion, topical:
Cutar® [OTC]: Coal tar solution 7.5% (180 mL, 3840 mL)
Exorex®: Coal tar 1% (240 mL)

Gel, shampoo:
DHS™ Targel [OTC]: Coal tar solution 2.9% (240 mL)

Liquid:
Doak® Tar Distillate [OTC]: Coal tar 40% (60 mL)

Lotion, topical:
Doak® Tar [OTC]: Coal tar distillate 5% (240 mL)
Exorex®: Coal tar 1% (240 mL)
MG 217® [OTC]: Coal tar solution 5% (120 mL)
Oxipor® VHC [OTC]: Coal tar solution 25% (60 mL, 120 mL)

Oil, topical:
Balnetar® [OTC]: Coal tar 2.5% (225 mL) [for use in bath]
Doak® Tar [OTC]: Coal tar distillate 2% (240 mL)

Ointment, topical:
MG 217® [OTC]: Coal tar solution 10% (107 g, 430 g)
Shampoo, topical:
Betatar Gel® [OTC]: Coal tar solution 5% (240 mL)
Denorex® Original Therapeutic Strength [OTC]: Coal tar solution 12.5% (120 mL, 240 mL, 360 mL)
DHS™ Tar [OTC]: Coal tar solution 2.9% (120 mL, 240 mL, 480 mL)
Doak® Tar [OTC]: Coal tar distillate 3% (240 mL)
MG 217® Medicated Tar [OTC]: Coal tar solution 15% (120 mL, 240 mL)
Neutrogena® T/Gel [OTC]: Coal tar 0.5% (132 mL, 480 mL)
Neutrogena® T/Gel Extra Strength [OTC]: Coal tar extract 4% (132 mL)
Neutrogena® T/Gel Stubborn Itch Control [OTC]: Coal tar extract 2% (132 mL)
Reme-T™ [OTC]: Coal tar 5% (236 mL)
Tera-Gel™ [OTC]: Solubilized coal tar 0.5% (120 mL, 240 mL)
Zetar® [OTC]: Coal tar 1% (180 mL)

coal tar and salicylic acid (KOLE tar & sal i SIL ik AS id)

Synonyms salicylic acid and coal tar

U.S./Canadian Brand Names Sebcur/T® [Can]; Tarsum® [US-OTC]; X-Seb T® Pearl [US-OTC]; X-Seb T® Plus [US-OTC]

Therapeutic Category Antipsoriatic Agent; Antiseborrheic Agent, Topical

Use Seborrheal dermatitis, dandruff, psoriasis

Usual Dosage Psoriasis: Scalp:

Gel: Apply directly to plaques; may leave in place for up to 1 hour. Apply water and work into a lather; rinse.

Shampoo: Apply to wet hair; massage into scalp; rinse.

Dosage Forms

Gel [shampoo]: Coal tar solution 10% [equivalent to coal tar 2%] and salicylic acid (120 mL, 240 mL)
Tarsum® [OTC]: Coal tar solution 10% [equivalent to coal tar 2%] and salicylic acid (120 mL, 240 mL)
Shampoo, topical: Coal tar solution 10% [equivalent to coal tar 2%] and salicylic acid (120 mL, 240 mL)
X-Seb T® Pearl [OTC], X-Seb T® Plus [OTC]: Coal tar solution 10% [equivalent to coal tar 2%] and salicylic acid (120 mL, 240 mL)

CO Amlodipine [Can] *see* amlodipine *on page* 66
Coartem® [US] *see* artemether and lumefantrine *on page* 99
CO Azithromycin [Can] *see* azithromycin *on page* 116
Cobex® *(Discontinued)* *see* cyanocobalamin *on page* 263
CO Bicalutamide [Can] *see* bicalutamide *on page* 141
CO Buspirone [Can] *see* buspirone *on page* 160
CO Cabergoline [Can] *see* cabergoline *on page* 165

cocaine (koe KANE)

Synonyms cocaine hydrochloride

Therapeutic Category Local Anesthetic

Controlled Substance C-II

Use Topical anesthesia for mucous membranes

Usual Dosage Topical application (ear, nose, throat, bronchoscopy): Dosage depends on the area to be anesthetized, tissue vascularity, technique of anesthesia, and individual patient tolerance; the lowest dose necessary to produce adequate anesthesia should be used; concentrations of 1% to 10% are used (not to exceed 1 mg/kg). Use reduced dosages for children, elderly, or debilitated patients.

Dosage Forms

Powder, for prescription compounding: 1 g, 5 g, 25 g
Solution, topical: 4% (4 mL, 10 mL); 10% (4 mL, 10 mL)

cocaine hydrochloride *see* cocaine *on page* 251
CO Cilazapril [Can] *see* cilazapril *(Canada only) on page* 228
CO Ciprofloxacin [Can] *see* ciprofloxacin *on page* 229
CO Citalopram [Can] *see* citalopram *on page* 234
CO Clomipramine [Can] *see* clomipramine *on page* 244
CO Clonazepam [Can] *see* clonazepam *on page* 245

Codal-DM [US-OTC] *see* phenylephrine, pyrilamine, and dextromethorphan *on page 778*
Codamine® *(Discontinued)*
Codamine® Pediatric *(Discontinued)*
Codehist® DH *(Discontinued)* *see* chlorpheniramine, pseudoephedrine, and codeine *on page 220*

codeine (KOE deen)

Sound-Alike/Look-Alike Issues
codeine may be confused with Cardene®, Cophene®, Cordran®, iodine, Lodine®

Synonyms codeine phosphate; codeine sulfate; methylmorphine

U.S./Canadian Brand Names Codeine Contin® [Can]

Therapeutic Category Analgesic, Narcotic; Antitussive

Controlled Substance C-II

Use Treatment of mild-to-moderate pain; antitussive in lower doses

Usual Dosage Note: These are guidelines and do not represent the maximum doses that may be required in all patients. Doses should be titrated to pain relief/prevention. Doses >1.5 mg/kg body weight are not recommended.

Analgesic:
- Children: Oral, I.M., SubQ: 0.5-1 mg/kg/dose every 4-6 hours as needed; maximum: 60 mg/dose
- Adults:
  - Oral: 30 mg every 4-6 hours as needed; patients with prior opiate exposure may require higher initial doses. Usual range: 15-120 mg every 4-6 hours as needed
  - Oral, controlled release formulation (Codeine Contin®, not available in U.S.): 50-300 mg every 12 hours. **Note:** A patient's codeine requirement should be established using prompt release formulations; conversion to long-acting products may be considered when chronic, continuous treatment is required. Higher dosages should be reserved for use only in opioid-tolerant patients.
  - I.M., SubQ: 30 mg every 4-6 hours as needed; patients with prior opiate exposure may require higher initial doses. Usual range: 15-120 mg every 4-6 hours as needed; more frequent dosing may be needed

Antitussive: Oral (for nonproductive cough):
- Children: 1-1.5 mg/kg/day in divided doses every 4-6 hours as needed: Alternative dose according to age:
  - 2-6 years: 2.5-5 mg every 4-6 hours as needed; maximum: 30 mg/day
  - 6-12 years: 5-10 mg every 4-6 hours as needed; maximum: 60 mg/day
- Adults: 10-20 mg/dose every 4-6 hours as needed; maximum: 120 mg/day

Dosage Forms [CAN] = Canadian brand name

Injection: 15 mg/mL (2 mL); 30 mg/mL (2 mL)
Powder, for prescription compounding: 10 g, 25 g
Tablet: 15 mg, 30 mg, 60 mg
Tablet, controlled release: 50 mg, 100 mg, 150 mg, 200 mg
Codeine Contin® [CAN]: 50 mg, 100 mg, 150 mg, 200 mg [not available in the U.S.]

codeine, acetaminophen, butalbital, and caffeine *see* butalbital, acetaminophen, caffeine, and codeine *on page 162*
codeine and acetaminophen *see* acetaminophen and codeine *on page 20*
codeine and butalbital compound *see* butalbital, aspirin, caffeine, and codeine *on page 163*
codeine and guaifenesin *see* guaifenesin and codeine *on page 473*
codeine and promethazine *see* promethazine and codeine *on page 824*
codeine and pseudoephedrine *see* pseudoephedrine and codeine *on page 834*
codeine, aspirin, and carisoprodol *see* carisoprodol, aspirin, and codeine *on page 187*
codeine, butalbital, aspirin, and caffeine *see* butalbital, aspirin, caffeine, and codeine *on page 163*
codeine, chlorpheniramine, and pseudoephedrine *see* chlorpheniramine, pseudoephedrine, and codeine *on page 220*
codeine, chlorpheniramine, phenylephrine, and potassium iodide *see* chlorpheniramine, phenylephrine, codeine, and potassium iodide *on page 220*
Codeine Contin® [Can] *see* codeine *on page 252*
codeine, doxylamine, and acetaminophen *see* acetaminophen, codeine, and doxylamine *(Canada only) on page 26*
codeine, guaifenesin, and pseudoephedrine *see* guaifenesin, pseudoephedrine, and codeine *on page 479*

codeine, phenylephrine, and promethazine *see* promethazine, phenylephrine, and codeine *on page 825*
codeine phosphate *see* codeine *on page 252*
codeine phosphate and pseudoephedrine hydrochloride *see* pseudoephedrine and codeine *on page 834*
codeine, pseudoephedrine, and triprolidine *see* triprolidine, pseudoephedrine, and codeine *(Canada only) on page 990*
codeine sulfate *see* codeine *on page 252*
codeine, triprolidine, and pseudoephedrine *see* triprolidine, pseudoephedrine, and codeine *(Canada only) on page 990*
Codiclear® DH *(Discontinued)*
codimal® DM [US-OTC] *see* phenylephrine, pyrilamine, and dextromethorphan *on page 778*
Codituss DM [US-OTC] *see* phenylephrine, pyrilamine, and dextromethorphan *on page 778*
cod liver oil *see* vitamin A and vitamin D *on page 1017*
CO Enalapril [Can] *see* enalapril *on page 352*
CO-Etidrocal [Can] *see* etidronate and calcium *(Canada only) on page 396*
CO Famciclovir [Can] *see* famciclovir *on page 404*
CO Fluconazole [Can] *see* fluconazole *on page 424*
CO Fluoxetine [Can] *see* fluoxetine *on page 432*
CO Gabapentin [Can] *see* gabapentin *on page 450*
Cogentin® [US] *see* benztropine *on page 134*
Co-Gesic® *(Discontinued)* *see* hydrocodone and acetaminophen *on page 501*
CO Glimepiride [Can] *see* glimepiride *on page 464*
Cognex® [US] *see* tacrine *on page 935*
CO Ipra-Sal [Can] *see* ipratropium and albuterol *on page 545*
Colace® [US-OTC/Can] *see* docusate *on page 326*
Colace® Adult/Children Suppositories [US-OTC] *see* glycerin *on page 468*
Colace® Infant/Children Suppositories [US-OTC] *see* glycerin *on page 468*
Colax-C® [Can] *see* docusate *on page 326*
Colazal® [US] *see* balsalazide *on page 122*
ColBenemid® *(Discontinued)* *see* colchicine and probenecid *on page 253*

colchicine (KOL chi seen)

Sound-Alike/Look-Alike Issues
colchicine may be confused with Cortrosyn®

Therapeutic Category Antigout Agent

Use Treatment of acute gout flares and familial Mediterranean fever (FMF)

Usual Dosage Oral:
Familial Mediterranean fever (FMF):
Children:
4-6 years: 0.3-1.8 mg/day in 1-2 divided doses
6-12 years: 0.9-1.8 mg/day in 1-2 divided doses
Children >12 years and Adults: 1.2-2.4 mg/day in 1-2 divided doses. Titration: Increase or decrease dose in 0.3 mg increments based on efficacy or adverse effects
Gout: Adults: Flares: Initial: 1.2 mg at the first sign of flare, followed in 1 hour with a single dose of 0.6 mg (maximum: 1.8 mg within 1 hour). **Note:** Current FDA-approved dose for gout flare is substantially lower than what has been historically used clinically. Doses larger than the currently recommended dosage for gout flare have not been proven to be more effective.

Dosage Forms
Tablet: 0.6 mg
Colcrys™: 0.6 mg

colchicine and probenecid (KOL chi seen & proe BEN e sid)

Synonyms probenecid and colchicine

Therapeutic Category Antigout Agent

Use Treatment of chronic gouty arthritis when complicated by frequent, recurrent acute attacks of gout

Usual Dosage Oral: Adults: 1 tablet daily for 1 week, then 1 tablet twice daily thereafter

Dosage Forms

Tablet: Colchicine 0.5 mg and probenecid 0.5 g

Coldamine [US] *see* chlorpheniramine, pseudoephedrine, and methscopolamine *on page 221*

Cold Control PE [US-OTC] *see* acetaminophen, diphenhydramine, and phenylephrine *on page 28*

Coldcough [US] *see* pseudoephedrine, dihydrocodeine, and chlorpheniramine *on page 836*

Coldcough HC ***(Discontinued)***

Coldcough PD [US] *see* dihydrocodeine, chlorpheniramine, and phenylephrine *on page 309*

Coldlac-LA® ***(Discontinued)***

Coldloc® ***(Discontinued)***

Coldmist DM ***(Discontinued)*** *see* guaifenesin, pseudoephedrine, and dextromethorphan *on page 479*

Coldtuss DR ***(Discontinued)*** *see* chlorpheniramine, phenylephrine, and dextromethorphan *on page 217*

colesevelam (koh le SEV a lam)

U.S./Canadian Brand Names WelChol® [US/Can]

Therapeutic Category Antihyperlipidemic Agent, Miscellaneous; Bile Acid Sequestrant

Use Management of elevated LDL in primary hypercholesterolemia (Fredrickson type IIa) when used alone or in combination with an HMG-CoA reductase inhibitor; improve control of type 2 diabetes mellitus (noninsulin-dependent, NIDDM) in conjunction with insulin or oral antidiabetic agents

Usual Dosage Oral: Adults: 3 tablets twice daily with meals or 6 tablets once daily with a meal

Dosage Forms

Tablet:

WelChol®: 625 mg

Colestid® [US/Can] *see* colestipol *on page 254*

colestipol (koe LES ti pole)

Sound-Alike/Look-Alike Issues

colestipol may be confused with calcitriol

Synonyms colestipol hydrochloride

U.S./Canadian Brand Names Colestid® [US/Can]

Therapeutic Category Antihyperlipidemic Agent, Miscellaneous

Use Adjunct in management of primary hypercholesterolemia; regression of arteriolosclerosis; relief of pruritus associated with elevated levels of bile acids; possibly used to decrease plasma half-life of digoxin in toxicity

Usual Dosage Oral: Adults:

Granules: 5-30 g/day given once or in divided doses 2-4 times/day; initial dose: 5 g 1-2 times/day; increase by 5 g at 1- to 2-month intervals

Tablets: 2-16 g/day; initial dose: 2 g 1-2 times/day; increase by 2 g at 1- to 2-month intervals

Dosage Forms

Granules for suspension, oral: 5 g/packet (30s, 90s); 5 g/scoopful (500 g)

Colestid®: 5 g/packet (30s, 90s); 5 g/teaspoon (300 g, 500 g)

Colestid®, flavored: 5 g/packet (60s)

Colestid®, flavored: 5 g/scoopful (450 g)

Tablet: 1 g

Tablet, oral [micronized]:

Colestid®: 1 g

colestipol hydrochloride *see* colestipol *on page 254*

CO Levetiracetam [Can] *see* levetiracetam *on page 577*

CO Lisinopril [Can] *see* lisinopril *on page 593*

colistimethate (koe lis ti METH ate)

Synonyms colistimethate sodium; colistin methanesulfonate; colistin sulfomethate; pentasodium colistin methanesulfonate

U.S./Canadian Brand Names Coly-Mycin® M [US/Can]

Therapeutic Category Antibiotic, Miscellaneous

Use Treatment of infections due to sensitive strains of certain gram-negative bacilli which are resistant to other antibacterials or in patients allergic to other antibacterials

Usual Dosage Note: Doses should be based on ideal body weight in obese patients; dosage expressed in terms of colistin.

I.M., I.V.: Children and Adults: Susceptible infections: 2.5-5 mg/kg/day in 2-4 divided doses

Dosage Forms

Injection, powder for reconstitution, as colistin base: 150 mg

Coly-Mycin® M: 150 mg

colistimethate sodium *see* colistimethate *on page* 254

colistin, hydrocortisone, neomycin, and thonzonium *see* neomycin, colistin, hydrocortisone, and thonzonium *on page* 687

colistin methanesulfonate *see* colistimethate *on page* 254

colistin sulfomethate *see* colistimethate *on page* 254

collagen *see* collagen hemostat *on page* 255

collagen absorbable hemostat *see* collagen hemostat *on page* 255

collagenase (KOL la je nase)

U.S./Canadian Brand Names Santyl® [US]

Therapeutic Category Enzyme

Use Promotes debridement of necrotic tissue in dermal ulcers and severe burns

Orphan drug: Injection: Treatment of Peyronie disease; treatment of Dupuytren disease

Usual Dosage Topical: Apply once daily (or more frequently if the dressing becomes soiled)

Dosage Forms

Ointment:

Santyl®: 250 units/g (15 g, 30 g)

collagen hemostat (KOL la jen HEE moe stat)

Sound-Alike/Look-Alike Issues

Avitene® may be confused with Ativan®

Synonyms collagen; collagen absorbable hemostat; MCH; microfibrillar collagen hemostat

U.S./Canadian Brand Names Avitene® Flour [US]; Avitene® Ultrafoam [US]; Avitene® UltraWrap™ [US]; Avitene® [US]; EndoAvitene® [US]; Helistat® [US]; Helitene® [US]; Instat™ MCH [US]; Instat™ [US]; SyringeAvitene™ [US]

Therapeutic Category Hemostatic Agent

Use Adjunct to hemostasis when control of bleeding by ligature is ineffective or impractical

Usual Dosage Apply dry directly to source of bleeding; remove excess material after ~10-15 minutes

Dosage Forms

Pad:

Instat™: 1 inch x 2 inch (24s); 3 inch x 4 inch (24s)

Powder:

Avitene® Flour [microfibrillar product]: 0.5 g, 1 g, 5 g

Helitene®: 0.5 g, 1 g

Instat™ MCH [microfibrillar product]: 0.5 g, 1 g

SyringeAvitene™ [microfibrillar product, prefilled syringe]: 1 g

Sheet:

Avitene® [microfibrillar product, nonwoven web]: 35 mm x 35 mm (1s); 70 mm x 35 mm (6s, 12s); 70 mm x 70 mm (6s, 12s)

EndoAvitene® [microfibrillar product, preloaded applicator]: 5 mm diameter (6s); 10 mm diameter (6s)

Sponge:

Avitene® Ultrafoam [microfibrillar product]: 2 cm x 6.25 cm x 7 mm (12s); 8 cm x 6.25 cm x 1 cm (6s); 8 cm x 12.5 cm x 1 cm (6s); 8 cm x 12.5 cm x 3 mm (6s)

Avitene® UltraWrap™ [microfibrillar product]: 8 cm x 12.5 cm (6s)

Helistat®: 0.5 inch x 1 inch x 7 mm (18s); 3 inch x 4 inch x 5 inch (10s)

Colocort® [US] *see* hydrocortisone (rectal) *on page* 503

CO Lovastatin [Can] *see* lovastatin *on page* 602

Coly-Mycin® M [US/Can] *see* colistimethate *on page* 254

Coly-Mycin® S [US] *see* neomycin, colistin, hydrocortisone, and thonzonium *on page* 687

Colyte® [US/Can] *see* polyethylene glycol-electrolyte solution *on page* 797
Combantrin™ [Can] *see* pyrantel pamoate *on page* 838
ComBgen™ *(Discontinued)* *see* folic acid, cyanocobalamin, and pyridoxine *on page* 440
Combigan™ [US/Can] *see* brimonidine and timolol *on page* 147
CombiPatch® [US] *see* estradiol and norethindrone *on page* 376
Combipres® *(Discontinued)* *see* clonidine and chlorthalidone *on page* 246
ComBi Rx™ *(Discontinued)* *see* vitamins (multiple/prenatal) *on page* 1020
Combivent® [US] *see* ipratropium and albuterol *on page* 545
Combivent UDV [Can] *see* ipratropium and albuterol *on page* 545
Combivir® [US/Can] *see* zidovudine and lamivudine *on page* 1029
Combunox™ [US] *see* oxycodone and ibuprofen *on page* 739
CO Meloxicam [Can] *see* meloxicam *on page* 622
CO Metformin [Can] *see* metformin *on page* 633
Comfort® Ophthalmic *(Discontinued)* *see* naphazoline *on page* 680
Comfort® Tears Solution *(Discontinued)* *see* artificial tears *on page* 100
Comhist® *(Discontinued)* *see* chlorpheniramine, phenylephrine, and phenyltoloxamine *on page* 219
CO Mirtazapine [Can] *see* mirtazapine *on page* 661
Commit® [US-OTC] *see* nicotine *on page* 695
Compazine® *(Discontinued)* *see* prochlorperazine *on page* 820
Compound 347™ [US] *see* enflurane *on page* 354
compound E *see* cortisone acetate *on page* 259
compound F *see* hydrocortisone (systemic) *on page* 504
compound S *see* zidovudine *on page* 1028
compound S, abacavir, and lamivudine *see* abacavir, lamivudine, and zidovudine *on page* 16
Compound W® [US-OTC] *see* salicylic acid *on page* 884
Compound W® One-Step Wart Remover [US-OTC] *see* salicylic acid *on page* 884
Compound W® One-Step Wart Remover for Feet [US-OTC] *see* salicylic acid *on page* 884
Compound W® One-Step Wart Remover for Kids [US-OTC] *see* salicylic acid *on page* 884
Compoz® Nighttime Sleep Aid [US-OTC] *see* diphenhydramine *on page* 315
Compro™ [US] *see* prochlorperazine *on page* 820
Comtan® [US/Can] *see* entacapone *on page* 356
Comtrex® Maximum Strength, Non-Drowsy Cold & Cough Relief [US-OTC] *see* acetaminophen, dextromethorphan, and phenylephrine *on page* 27
Comtrex® Maximum Strength Sinus and Nasal Decongestant *(Discontinued)* *see* acetaminophen, chlorpheniramine, and pseudoephedrine *on page* 26
Comtrex® Non-Drowsy Cold and Cough Relief *(Discontinued)*
Comvax® [US] *see Haemophilus* B conjugate and hepatitis B vaccine *on page* 482
Conal [US] *see* chlorpheniramine, pyrilamine, and phenylephrine *on page* 221
Conceptrol® [US-OTC] *see* nonoxynol 9 *on page* 703
Concerta® [US/Can] *see* methylphenidate *on page* 645
Condyline™ [Can] *see* podofilox *on page* 795
Condylox® [US] *see* podofilox *on page* 795
Conex® *(Discontinued)*
Congess® Jr *(Discontinued)* *see* guaifenesin and pseudoephedrine *on page* 477
Congess® Sr *(Discontinued)* *see* guaifenesin and pseudoephedrine *on page* 477
Congestac® [US-OTC] *see* guaifenesin and pseudoephedrine *on page* 477

conivaptan (koe NYE vap tan)

Synonyms conivaptan hydrochloride; YM087
U.S./Canadian Brand Names Vaprisol® [US]
Therapeutic Category Vasopressin Antagonist
Use Treatment of euvolemic and hypervolemic hyponatremia in hospitalized patients

Usual Dosage I.V.: Adults: 20 mg infused over 30 minutes as a loading dose, followed by a continuous infusion of 20 mg over 24 hours (0.83 mg/hour); may increase dose to 40 mg over 24 hours (1.7 mg/hour) if serum sodium not rising sufficiently; total duration of therapy not to exceed 4 days. **Note:** If patient requires 40 mg/24 hours and using manufacturer premixed solution, may administer two consecutive 20 mg/100 mL premixed solutions over 24 hours (ie, 20 mg over 12 hours followed by 20 mg over 12 hours).

Dosage Forms

Infusion, premixed in D_5:

Vaprisol®: 20 mg (100 mL)

conivaptan hydrochloride *see* conivaptan *on page* 256

conjugated estrogen *see* estrogens (conjugated/equine) *on page* 378

conjugated estrogen and methyltestosterone *see* estrogens (esterified) and methyltestosterone *on page* 380

CO Norfloxacin [Can] *see* norfloxacin *on page* 705

Conray® [US] *see* iothalamate meglumine *on page* 541

Conray® 30 [US] *see* iothalamate meglumine *on page* 541

Conray® 43 [US] *see* iothalamate meglumine *on page* 541

Conray® 400 [US] *see* iothalamate sodium *on page* 542

Constulose [US] *see* lactulose *on page* 565

Contac® Cold 12 Hour Relief Non Drowsy [Can] *see* pseudoephedrine *on page* 833

Contac® Cold 12 Hour Relief Non Drowsy *(Discontinued)* *see* pseudoephedrine *on page* 833

Contac® Cold and Sore Throat, Non Drowsy, Extra Strength [Can] *see* acetaminophen and pseudoephedrine *on page* 24

Contac® Cold-Chest Congestion, Non Drowsy, Regular Strength [Can] *see* guaifenesin and pseudoephedrine *on page* 477

Contac® Cold *(Discontinued)* *see* pseudoephedrine *on page* 833

Contac® Cold + Flu Maximum Strength Non-Drowsy [US-OTC] *see* acetaminophen and phenylephrine *on page* 22

Contac® Cough Formula Liquid *(Discontinued)* *see* guaifenesin and dextromethorphan *on page* 474

continuous renal replacement therapy *see* electrolyte solution, renal replacement *on page* 350

ControlRx® [US] *see* fluoride *on page* 430

Contuss® *(Discontinued)*

Contuss® XT *(Discontinued)*

CO Pantoprazole [Can] *see* pantoprazole *on page* 748

CO Paroxetine [Can] *see* paroxetine *on page* 752

Copaxone® [US/Can] *see* glatiramer acetate *on page* 464

COPD [US] *see* dyphylline and guaifenesin *on page* 344

Copegus® [US] *see* ribavirin *on page* 864

Cophene-B® *(Discontinued)* *see* brompheniramine *on page* 149

Cophene XP® *(Discontinued)*

CO Pioglitazone [Can] *see* pioglitazone *on page* 785

copolymer-1 *see* glatiramer acetate *on page* 464

copper *see* trace metals *on page* 974

CO Pravastatin [Can] *see* pravastatin *on page* 811

Co-Pyronil® 2 Pulvules® *(Discontinued)* *see* chlorpheniramine and pseudoephedrine *on page* 215

CO Quetiapine [Can] *see* quetiapine *on page* 844

CO Ramipril [Can] *see* ramipril *on page* 850

CO Ranitidine [Can] *see* ranitidine *on page* 852

Cordarone® [US/Can] *see* amiodarone *on page* 64

Cordran® [US/Can] *see* flurandrenolide *on page* 434

Cordran® SP [US] *see* flurandrenolide *on page* 434

Cordron-D NR *(Discontinued)*

Cordron-DM NR *(Discontinued)*

Cordron-HC *(Discontinued)*

Cordron-HC NR ***(Discontinued)***
Coreg® [US/Can] *see* carvedilol *on page* 188
Coreg CR® [US] *see* carvedilol *on page* 188
Corfen DM [US] *see* chlorpheniramine, phenylephrine, and dextromethorphan *on page* 217
Corgard® [US/Can] *see* nadolol *on page* 675
Coricidin HBP® Chest Congestion and Cough [US-OTC] *see* guaifenesin and dextromethorphan *on page* 474
Coricidin HBP® Cold and Flu [US-OTC] *see* chlorpheniramine and acetaminophen *on page* 214
Coricidin® HBP Cough & Cold [US-OTC] *see* dextromethorphan and chlorpheniramine *on page* 296
CO Risperidone [Can] *see* risperidone *on page* 870
Corlopam® [US/Can] *see* fenoldopam *on page* 409
Cormax® [US] *see* clobetasol *on page* 242
Coronex® [Can] *see* isosorbide dinitrate *on page* 550
CO Ropinirole [Can] *see* ropinirole *on page* 877
Correctol® [US-OTC] *see* docusate *on page* 326
Correctol® Tablets [US-OTC] *see* bisacodyl *on page* 142
Cortaid® Intensive Therapy [US-OTC] *see* hydrocortisone (topical) *on page* 505
Cortaid® Maximum Strength [US-OTC] *see* hydrocortisone (topical) *on page* 505
Cortaid® Sensitive Skin [US-OTC] *see* hydrocortisone (topical) *on page* 505
Cortamed® [Can] *see* hydrocortisone (topical) *on page* 505
Cortatrigen® Otic ***(Discontinued)*** *see* neomycin, polymyxin B, and hydrocortisone *on page* 688
Cortef® [US/Can] *see* hydrocortisone (systemic) *on page* 504
Cortenema® [Can] *see* hydrocortisone (rectal) *on page* 503
Corticool® [US-OTC] *see* hydrocortisone (topical) *on page* 505

corticorelin (kor ti koe REL in)

Sound-Alike/Look-Alike Issues
corticorelin may be confused with corticotropin
Acthrel® may be confused with Acthar®

Synonyms corticorelin ovine triflutate; human corticotrophin-releasing hormone, analogue; ovine corticotrophin-releasing hormone

U.S./Canadian Brand Names Acthrel® [US]

Therapeutic Category Diagnostic Agent, ACTH-Dependent Hypercortisolism

Use Diagnostic test used in adrenocorticotropic hormone (ACTH)-dependent Cushing syndrome to differentiate between pituitary and ectopic production of ACTH

Usual Dosage I.V.: Adults: Testing pituitary corticotrophin function: 1 mcg/kg; dosages >100 mcg have been associated with an increase in adverse effects

Note: Venous blood samples should be drawn 15 minutes before and immediately prior to corticorelin administration to determine baseline ACTH and cortisol. At 15-, 30-, and 60 minutes after administration, venous blood samples should be drawn again to determine response. **Basal and peak responses differ depending on AM or PM administration; therefore, any repeat evaluations are recommended to be done at the same time of day as initial testing.**

Dosage Forms
Injection, powder for reconstitution:
Acthrel®: 100 mcg

corticorelin ovine triflutate *see* corticorelin *on page* 258

corticotropin (kor ti koe TROE pin)

Sound-Alike/Look-Alike Issues
corticotropin may be confused with corticorelin

Synonyms ACTH; adrenocorticotropic hormone; corticotropin, repository

U.S./Canadian Brand Names H.P. Acthar® Gel [US]

Therapeutic Category Adrenal Corticosteroid

Use Acute exacerbations of multiple sclerosis; diagnostic aid in adrenocortical insufficiency, severe muscle weakness in myasthenia gravis

Cosyntropin is preferred over corticotropin for diagnostic test of adrenocortical insufficiency (cosyntropin is less allergenic and test is shorter in duration)

Usual Dosage

Children:

Antiinflammatory/immunosuppressant: I.M.: 0.8 units/kg/day or 25 units/m^2/day divided every 12-24 hours

Infantile spasms: Various regimens have been used. Some neurologists recommend low-dose ACTH (5-40 units/day) for short periods (1-6 weeks), while others recommend larger doses of ACTH (40-160 units/day) for long periods of treatment (3-12 months). Well designed comparative dosing studies are needed. Example of low dose regimen:

Initial: I.M.: 20 units/day for 2 weeks, if patient responds, taper and discontinue; if patient does not respond, increase dose to 30 units/day for 4 weeks then taper and discontinue

I.M. usual dose: 20-40 units/day or 5-8 units/kg/day in 1-2 divided doses; range: 5-160 units/day

Oral prednisone (2 mg/kg/day) was as effective as I.M. ACTH gel (20 units/day) in controlling infantile spasms

Adults: Acute exacerbation of multiple sclerosis: I.M.: 80-120 units/day for 2-3 weeks

Repository injection: I.M., SubQ: 40-80 units every 24-72 hours

Dosage Forms

Injection, gelatin:

H.P. Acthar® Gel: 80 units/mL (5 mL)

corticotropin, repository *see* corticotropin *on page 258*

Cortifoam® [US/Can] *see* hydrocortisone (rectal) *on page 503*

Cortimyxin® [Can] *see* neomycin, polymyxin B, and hydrocortisone *on page 688*

cortisol *see* hydrocortisone (systemic) *on page 504*

cortisone acetate (KOR ti sone AS e tate)

Sound-Alike/Look-Alike Issues

cortisone may be confused with Cardizem®, Cortizone®

Synonyms compound E

Therapeutic Category Adrenal Corticosteroid

Use Management of adrenocortical insufficiency

Usual Dosage If possible, administer glucocorticoids before 9 AM to minimize adrenocortical suppression; dosing depends upon the condition being treated and the response of the patient; **Note:** Supplemental doses may be warranted during times of stress in the course of withdrawing therapy

Children:

Antiinflammatory or immunosuppressive: Oral: 2.5-10 mg/kg/day **or** 20-300 mg/m^2/day in divided doses every 6-8 hours

Physiologic replacement: Oral: 0.5-0.75 mg/kg/day **or** 20-25 mg/m^2/day in divided doses every 8 hours

Adults:

Antiinflammatory or immunosuppressive: Oral: 25-300 mg/day in divided doses every 12-24 hours

Physiologic replacement: Oral: 25-35 mg/day

Dosage Forms

Tablet: 25 mg

Cortisporin® Cream [US] *see* neomycin, polymyxin B, and hydrocortisone *on page 688*

Cortisporin® Ointment [US] *see* bacitracin, neomycin, polymyxin B, and hydrocortisone *on page 120*

Cortisporin® Ophthalmic *(Discontinued)* *see* neomycin, polymyxin B, and hydrocortisone *on page 688*

Cortisporin® Otic [US/Can] *see* neomycin, polymyxin B, and hydrocortisone *on page 688*

Cortisporin®-TC [US] *see* neomycin, colistin, hydrocortisone, and thonzonium *on page 687*

Cortisporin® Topical Cream *(Discontinued)* *see* neomycin, polymyxin B, and hydrocortisone *on page 688*

Cortisporin® Topical Ointment [Can] *see* bacitracin, neomycin, polymyxin B, and hydrocortisone *on page 120*

Cortizone®-10 Maximum Strength [US-OTC] *see* hydrocortisone (topical) *on page 505*

Cortizone®-10 Plus Maximum Strength [US-OTC] *see* hydrocortisone (topical) *on page 505*

Cortizone®-10 Quick Shot [US-OTC] *see* hydrocortisone (topical) *on page 505*

Cortone® *(Discontinued)*

Cortrosyn® [US/Can] *see* cosyntropin *on page 260*

Corvert® [US] *see* ibutilide *on page* 517
Corzide® [US] *see* nadolol and bendroflumethiazide *on page* 676
CO Sertraline [Can] *see* sertraline *on page* 898
CO Simvastatin [Can] *see* simvastatin *on page* 902
Cosmegen® [US/Can] *see* dactinomycin *on page* 273
Cosopt® [US/Can] *see* dorzolamide and timolol *on page* 332
CO Sotalol [Can] *see* sotalol *on page* 919
CO Sumatriptan [Can] *see* sumatriptan *on page* 932

cosyntropin (koe sin TROE pin)

Sound-Alike/Look-Alike Issues
Cortrosyn® may be confused with colchicine, Cotazym®

Synonyms synacthen; tetracosactide

U.S./Canadian Brand Names Cortrosyn® [US/Can]

Therapeutic Category Diagnostic Agent

Use Diagnostic test to differentiate primary adrenal from secondary (pituitary) adrenocortical insufficiency

Usual Dosage Adrenocortical insufficiency: I.M., I.V. (over 2 minutes): Peak plasma cortisol concentrations usually occur 45-60 minutes after cosyntropin administration
- Children <2 years: 0.125 mg
- Children >2 years and Adults: 0.25-0.75 mg
- When greater cortisol stimulation is needed, an I.V. infusion may be used:
  - Children >2 years and Adults: 0.25 mg administered at 0.04 mg/hour over 6 hours

Dosage Forms
Injection, powder for reconstitution: 0.25 mg
Cortrosyn®: 0.25 mg

Cotazym® [Can] *see* pancrelipase *on page* 746
Cotazym® *(Discontinued)* *see* pancrelipase *on page* 746
Cotazym-S® *(Discontinued)* *see* pancrelipase *on page* 746
CO Temazepam [Can] *see* temazepam *on page* 942
CO Topiramate [Can] *see* topiramate *on page* 969
co-trimoxazole *see* sulfamethoxazole and trimethoprim *on page* 929
Coughcold HCM *(Discontinued)*
Coughtuss [US] *see* phenylephrine, hydrocodone, and chlorpheniramine *on page* 778
Coumadin® [US/Can] *see* warfarin *on page* 1022
Covan® [Can] *see* triprolidine, pseudoephedrine, and codeine *(Canada only) on page* 990
Covaryx™ [US] *see* estrogens (esterified) and methyltestosterone *on page* 380
Covaryx™ HS [US] *see* estrogens (esterified) and methyltestosterone *on page* 380
CO Venlafaxine XR [Can] *see* venlafaxine *on page* 1009
Covera® [Can] *see* verapamil *on page* 1010
Covera-HS® [US/Can] *see* verapamil *on page* 1010
Coversyl® [Can] *see* perindopril erbumine *on page* 768
Coversyl® Plus [Can] *see* perindopril erbumine and indapamide *(Canada only) on page* 768
co-vidarabine *see* pentostatin *on page* 766
coviracil *see* emtricitabine *on page* 352
Cozaar® [US/Can] *see* losartan *on page* 600
CO Zopiclone [Can] *see* zopiclone *(Canada only) on page* 1034
CP358774 *see* erlotinib *on page* 367
CPC *see* cetylpyridinium *on page* 205
C-Phen [US] *see* chlorpheniramine and phenylephrine *on page* 214
C-Phen DM [US] *see* chlorpheniramine, phenylephrine, and dextromethorphan *on page* 217
CPM *see* cyclophosphamide *on page* 265
CPM-12 [US] *see* chlorpheniramine *on page* 213
CPT-11 *see* irinotecan *on page* 546
CPZ *see* chlorpromazine *on page* 222

Cramp Tabs [US-OTC] *see* acetaminophen and pamabrom *on page* 22
Crantex HC ***(Discontinued)***
Crantex LA [US] *see* guaifenesin and phenylephrine *on page* 475
Creomulsion® Adult Formula [US-OTC] *see* dextromethorphan *on page* 295
Creomulsion® for Children [US-OTC] *see* dextromethorphan *on page* 295
Creon® [US/Can] *see* pancrelipase *on page* 746
Creo-Terpin® [US-OTC] *see* dextromethorphan *on page* 295
Crestor® [US/Can] *see* rosuvastatin *on page* 880
Cresylate® [US] *see* m-cresyl acetate *on page* 615
Crinone® [US/Can] *see* progesterone *on page* 822
Critic-Aid® Clear AF [US-OTC] *see* miconazole *on page* 654
Critic-Aid Skin Care® [US-OTC] *see* zinc oxide *on page* 1030
Criticare HN® [US-OTC] *see* nutritional formula, enteral/oral *on page* 715
Crixivan® [US/Can] *see* indinavir *on page* 525
CroFab™ [US] *see* crotalidae polyvalent immune FAB (ovine) *on page* 262
Crolom® [US] *see* cromolyn sodium *on page* 261
cromoglycic acid *see* cromolyn sodium *on page* 261

cromolyn sodium (KROE moe lin SOW dee um)

Sound-Alike/Look-Alike Issues

Intal® may be confused with Endal®

NasalCrom® may be confused with Nasacort®, Nasalide®

Synonyms cromoglycic acid; disodium cromoglycate; DSCG

U.S./Canadian Brand Names Apo-Cromolyn® [Can]; Crolom® [US]; Gastrocrom® [US]; Intal® [Can]; Nalcrom® [Can]; NasalCrom® [US-OTC]; Nu-Cromolyn [Can]; Opticrom® [Can]; Rhinaris-CS Anti-Allergic Nasal Mist [Can]

Therapeutic Category Mast Cell Stabilizer

Use

Inhalation: May be used as an adjunct in the prophylaxis of allergic disorders, including asthma; prevention of exercise-induced bronchospasm

Nasal: Prevention and treatment of seasonal and perennial allergic rhinitis

Oral: Systemic mastocytosis

Ophthalmic: Treatment of vernal keratoconjunctivitis, vernal conjunctivitis, and vernal keratitis

Usual Dosage

Oral:

Systemic mastocytosis:

Children 2-12 years: 100 mg 4 times/day; not to exceed 40 mg/kg/day; given 1/2 hour prior to meals and at bedtime

Children >12 years and Adults: 200 mg 4 times/day; given 1/2 hour prior to meals and at bedtime; if control of symptoms is not seen within 2-3 weeks, dose may be increased to a maximum 40 mg/kg/day

Inhalation:

For chronic control of asthma, taper frequency to the lowest effective dose (ie, 4 times/day to 3 times/day to twice daily): **Note:** Not effective for immediate relief of symptoms in acute asthmatic attacks; must be used at regular intervals for 2-4 weeks to be effective.

Nebulization solution: Children >2 years and Adults: Initial: 20 mg 4 times/day; usual dose: 20 mg 3-4 times/day

Metered spray:

Children 5-12 years: Initial: 2 inhalations 4 times/day; usual dose: 1-2 inhalations 3-4 times/day

Children ≥12 years and Adults: Initial: 2 inhalations 4 times/day; usual dose: 2-4 inhalations 3-4 times/day

Prevention of allergen- or exercise-induced bronchospasm: Administer 10-15 minutes prior to exercise or allergen exposure but no longer than 1 hour before:

Nebulization solution: Children >2 years and Adults: Single dose of 20 mg

Metered spray: Children >5 years and Adults: Single dose of 2 inhalations

Ophthalmic: Children >4 years and Adults: 1-2 drops in each eye 4-6 times/day

Nasal: Allergic rhinitis (treatment and prophylaxis): Children ≥2 years and Adults: 1 spray into each nostril 3-4 times/day; may be increased to 6 times/day (symptomatic relief may require 2-4 weeks)

Dosage Forms

Solution for nebulization: 20 mg/2 mL (60s, 120s)

Solution, intranasal [spray]:

NasalCrom® [OTC]: 40 mg/mL (13 mL, 26 mL)

Solution, ophthalmic: 4% (10 mL)

Crolom®: 4% (10 mL)

Solution, oral [concentrate]:

Gastrocrom®: 100 mg/5 mL

Crosseal™ [US] *see* fibrin sealant kit *on page* 417

crotalidae polyvalent immune FAB (ovine)

(kroe TAL ih die pol i VAY lent i MYUN fab (oh vine))

Synonyms antivenin (crotalidae) polyvalent; crotaline antivenin, polyvalent; fabAV; North American antisnake-bite serum; snake antivenin

U.S./Canadian Brand Names CroFab™ [US]

Therapeutic Category Antivenin

Use Neutralization of venoms of North American crotalids: Rattlesnakes (*Crotalus*, *Sistrurus*); copperhead and cottonmouth moccasins (*Agkistrodon*)

Usual Dosage I.V.: Children and Adults: **Note:** Clinical trials included patients as young as 11 years of age. Specific pediatric studies have not been conducted. Because the absolute venom dose is expected to be the same in adults and children, adult dosing should be used. Products contain thimerosal, which in high doses has been associated with neurological and renal toxicity. Very young children are most susceptible.

Crotalid envenomation: Minimal or moderate:

Initial dose: 4-6 vials, dependent upon patient response. Treatment should begin within 6 hours of snakebite; monitor for 1 hour following infusion. Repeat with an additional 4-6 vials if control is not achieved with initial dose. Continue to treat with 4- to 6-vial doses until complete arrest of local manifestations, coagulation tests, and systemic signs are normal.

Maintenance dose: Once control is achieved, administer 2 vials every 6 hours for up to 18 hours. Optimal dosing past 18 hours has not been established; however, treatment may be continued if deemed necessary based on the patient's condition.

Dosage Forms

Injection, powder for reconstitution:

CroFab™: Derived from *Crotalus adamanteus*, *C. atrox*, *C. scutulatus*, and *Agkistrodon piscivorus* snake venoms

crotaline antivenin, polyvalent *see* crotalidae polyvalent immune FAB (ovine) *on page* 262

crotamiton (kroe TAM i tonn)

Sound-Alike/Look-Alike Issues

Eurax® may be confused with Efudex®, Eulexin®, Evoxac™, Serax®, Urex®

U.S./Canadian Brand Names Eurax® [US]

Therapeutic Category Scabicides/Pediculicides

Use Treatment of scabies (*Sarcoptes scabiei*) and symptomatic treatment of pruritus

Usual Dosage Topical:

Scabicide: Children and Adults: Wash thoroughly and scrub away loose scales, then towel dry; apply a thin layer and massage drug onto skin of the entire body from the neck to the toes (with special attention to skin folds, creases, and interdigital spaces). Repeat application in 24 hours. Take a cleansing bath 48 hours after the final application. Treatment may be repeated after 7-10 days if live mites are still present.

Pruritus: Massage into affected areas until medication is completely absorbed; repeat as necessary

Dosage Forms

Cream:

Eurax®: 10% (60 g)

Lotion:

Eurax®: 10% (60 mL, 480 mL)

CRRT *see* electrolyte solution, renal replacement *on page* 350

crude coal tar *see* coal tar *on page* 250

Cruex® Cream [US-OTC] *see* clotrimazole *on page* 248

Cryselle® 28 [US] *see* ethinyl estradiol and norgestrel *on page* 394

crystalline penicillin *see* penicillin G (parenteral/aqueous) *on page 761*
Crystamine® *(Discontinued)* *see* cyanocobalamin *on page 263*
Crystapen® [Can] *see* penicillin G (parenteral/aqueous) *on page 761*
Crysti 1000® *(Discontinued)* *see* cyanocobalamin *on page 263*
CS-747 *see* prasugrel *on page 810*
CsA *see* cyclosporine *on page 266*
C-Tan D [US] *see* brompheniramine and phenylephrine *on page 150*
C-Tan D Plus [US] *see* brompheniramine and phenylephrine *on page 150*
C-Tanna 12 [US] *see* carbetapentane and chlorpheniramine *on page 182*
C-Tanna 12D [US] *see* carbetapentane, phenylephrine, and pyrilamine *on page 183*
C-Time [US-OTC] *see* ascorbic acid *on page 100*
CTLA-4Ig *see* abatacept *on page 16*
CTM *see* chlorpheniramine *on page 213*
CTP 30 [Can] *see* citalopram *on page 234*
CTX *see* cyclophosphamide *on page 265*
Cubicin® [US/Can] *see* daptomycin *on page 276*
Culturelle® [US-OTC] *see* Lactobacillus *on page 564*
Cuprimine® [US/Can] *see* penicillamine *on page 759*
Curasore® [US-OTC] *see* pramoxine *on page 809*
Curosurf® [US/Can] *see* poractant alfa *on page 800*
Cutar® [US-OTC] *see* coal tar *on page 250*
Cutivate® [US/Can] *see* fluticasone (topical) *on page 438*
CVT-3146 *see* regadenoson *on page 856*
CyA *see* cyclosporine *on page 266*
cyanide antidote kit *see* sodium nitrite, sodium thiosulfate, and amyl nitrite *on page 911*
Cyanide Antidote Package [US] *see* sodium nitrite, sodium thiosulfate, and amyl nitrite *on page 911*

cyanocobalamin (sye an oh koe BAL a min)

Synonyms vitamin B_{12}

U.S./Canadian Brand Names CaloMist™ [US]; Nascobal® [US]; Twelve Resin-K [US-OTC]

Therapeutic Category Vitamin, Water Soluble

Use Treatment of pernicious anemia; vitamin B_{12} deficiency due to dietary deficiencies or malabsorption diseases, inadequate secretion of intrinsic factor, and inadequate utilization of B_{12} (eg, during neoplastic treatment); increased B_{12} requirements due to pregnancy, thyrotoxicosis, hemorrhage, malignancy, liver or kidney disease

CaloMist™: Maintenance of vitamin B_{12} concentrations after initial correction in patients with B_{12} deficiency without CNS involvement

Usual Dosage

Adequate intake:

Children:

0-6 months: 0.4 mcg/day

7-12 months: 0.5 mcg/day

Recommended intake:

Children:

1-3 years: 0.9 mcg/day

4-8 years: 1.2 mcg/day

9-13 years: 1.8 mcg/day

Children >14 years and Adults: 2.4 mcg/day

Pregnancy: 2.6 mcg/day

Lactation: 2.8 mcg/day

Vitamin B_{12} deficiency:

I.M., deep SubQ:

Children (dosage not well established): 0.2 mcg/kg for 2 days, followed by 1000 mcg/day for 2-7 days, followed by 100 mcg/week for one month; for malabsorptive causes of B_{12} deficiency, monthly maintenance doses of 100 mcg have been recommended **or** as an alternative 100 mcg/day for 10-15 days, then once or twice weekly for several months

Adults: Initial: 30 mcg/day for 5-10 days; maintenance: 100-200 mcg/month

Intranasal: Adults:
Nascobal®: 500 mcg in one nostril once weekly
CaloMist™: Maintenance therapy (following correction of vitamin B_{12} deficiency): 25 mcg in each nostril daily (50 mcg/day). If inadequate response, 25 mcg in each nostril twice daily (100 mcg/day).
Oral: Adults: 250 mcg/day

Pernicious anemia: I.M., deep SubQ (administer concomitantly with folic acid if needed, 1 mg/day for 1 month):
Children: 30-50 mcg/day for 2 or more weeks (to a total dose of 1000-5000 mcg), then follow with 100 mcg/month as maintenance dosage
Adults: 100 mcg/day for 6-7 days; if improvement, administer same dose on alternate days for 7 doses, then every 3-4 days for 2-3 weeks; once hematologic values have returned to normal, maintenance dosage: 100 mcg/month. **Note:** Alternative dosing of 1000 mcg/day for 5 days (followed by 500-1000 mcg/month) has been used.
Hematologic remission (without evidence of nervous system involvement): Adults:
Intranasal (Nascobal®): 500 mcg in one nostril once weekly
Oral: 1000-2000 mcg/day
I.M., SubQ: 100-1000 mcg/month

Schilling test: Adults: I.M.: 1000 mcg

Dosage Forms
Injection, solution: 1000 mcg/mL (1 mL, 10 mL, 30 mL)
Lozenge: 50 mcg, 100 mcg, 250 mcg, 500 mcg
Lozenge, sublingual: 500 mcg
Solution, intranasal [spray]:
CaloMist™: 25 mcg/0.1 mL actuation (10.7 mL)
Nascobal®: 500 mcg/0.1 mL actuation (2.3 mL)
Tablet: 50 mcg, 100 mcg, 250 mcg, 500 mcg, 1000 mcg
Twelve Resin-K (OTC): 1000 mcg
Tablet, timed release: 1000 mcg, 1500 mcg
Tablet, sublingual: 1000 mcg, 2500 mcg, 5000 mcg

cyanocobalamin, folic acid, and pyridoxine *see* folic acid, cyanocobalamin, and pyridoxine *on page 440*

Cyanoject® *(Discontinued)* *see* cyanocobalamin *on page 263*

Cyclen® [Can] *see* ethinyl estradiol and norgestimate *on page 393*

Cyclessa® [US/Can] *see* ethinyl estradiol and desogestrel *on page 383*

cyclobenzaprine (sye kloe BEN za preen)

Sound-Alike/Look-Alike Issues
cyclobenzaprine may be confused with cycloSERINE, cyproheptadine
Flexeril® may be confused with Floxin®

Synonyms cyclobenzaprine hydrochloride

U.S./Canadian Brand Names Amrix® [US]; Apo-Cyclobenzaprine® [Can]; Fexmid® [US]; Flexeril® [US/Can]; Flexitec [Can]; Gen-Cyclobenzaprine [Can]; Novo-Cycloprine [Can]; Nu-Cyclobenzaprine [Can]

Therapeutic Category Skeletal Muscle Relaxant

Use Treatment of muscle spasm associated with acute painful musculoskeletal conditions

Usual Dosage Oral: **Note:** Do not use longer than 2-3 weeks
Capsule, extended release: Adults: Usual: 15 mg once daily; some patients may require up to 30 mg once daily
Tablet, immediate release: Children ≥15 years and Adults: Initial: 5 mg 3 times/day; may increase to 7.5-10 mg 3 times/day if needed

Dosage Forms
Capsule, extended release:
Amrix®: 15 mg, 30 mg
Tablet: 5 mg, 10 mg
Fexmid®: 7.5 mg
Flexeril®: 5 mg, 10 mg

cyclobenzaprine hydrochloride *see* cyclobenzaprine *on page 264*

Cyclocort® [Can] *see* amcinonide *on page 59*

Cyclocort® *(Discontinued)* *see* amcinonide *on page 59*

Cyclogyl® [US/Can] *see* cyclopentolate *on page 265*

Cyclomen® [Can] *see* danazol *on page 275*

Cyclomydril® [US] *see* cyclopentolate and phenylephrine *on page 265*

cyclopentolate (sye kloe PEN toe late)

Synonyms cyclopentolate hydrochloride

U.S./Canadian Brand Names AK-Pentolate™ [US]; Cyclogyl® [US/Can]; Cylate™ [US]; Diopentolate® [Can]

Therapeutic Category Anticholinergic Agent

Use Diagnostic procedures requiring mydriasis and cycloplegia

Usual Dosage Ophthalmic:

Neonates and Infants: **Note:** Cyclopentolate and phenylephrine combination formulation is the preferred agent for use in neonates and infants due to lower cyclopentolate concentration and reduced risk for systemic reactions

Children: Instill 1 drop of 0.5%, 1%, or 2% in eye followed by 1 drop of 0.5% or 1% in 5 minutes, if necessary

Adults: Instill 1 drop of 1% followed by another drop in 5 minutes; 2% solution in heavily pigmented iris

Dosage Forms

Solution, ophthalmic: 1% (2 mL, 15 mL)

AK-Pentolate™, Cylate™: 1% (2 mL, 15 mL)

Cyclogyl®: 0.5% (15 mL); 1% (2 mL, 5 mL, 15 mL); 2% (2 mL, 5 mL, 15 mL)

cyclopentolate and phenylephrine (sye kloe PEN toe late & fen il EF rin)

Synonyms phenylephrine and cyclopentolate

U.S./Canadian Brand Names Cyclomydril® [US]

Therapeutic Category Anticholinergic/Adrenergic Agonist

Use Induce mydriasis greater than that produced with cyclopentolate HCl alone

Usual Dosage Ophthalmic: Neonates, Infants, Children, and Adults: Instill 1 drop into the eye every 5-10 minutes, for up to 3 doses, approximately 40-50 minutes before the examination

Dosage Forms

Solution, ophthalmic:

Cyclomydril®: Cyclopentolate 0.2% and phenylephrine 1% (2 mL, 5 mL)

cyclopentolate hydrochloride *see* cyclopentolate *on page 265*

cyclophosphamide (sye kloe FOS fa mide)

Sound-Alike/Look-Alike Issues

cyclophosphamide may be confused with cycloSPORINE, ifosfamide

Synonyms CPM; CTX; CYT; neosar; NSC-26271

U.S./Canadian Brand Names Cytoxan® [Can]; Procytox® [Can]

Therapeutic Category Antineoplastic Agent

Use

Oncologic: Treatment of Hodgkin and non-Hodgkin lymphoma, Burkitt lymphoma, chronic lymphocytic leukemia (CLL), chronic myelocytic leukemia (CML), acute myelocytic leukemia (AML), acute lymphocytic leukemia (ALL), mycosis fungoides, multiple myeloma, neuroblastoma, retinoblastoma, rhabdomyosarcoma, Ewing sarcoma; breast, testicular, endometrial, ovarian, and lung cancers, and in conditioning regimens for bone marrow transplantation

Nononcologic: Prophylaxis of rejection for kidney, heart, liver, and bone marrow transplants, severe rheumatoid disorders, nephrotic syndrome, Wegener granulomatosis, idiopathic pulmonary hemosideroses, myasthenia gravis, multiple sclerosis, systemic lupus erythematosus, lupus nephritis, autoimmune hemolytic anemia, idiopathic thrombocytic purpura (ITP), macroglobulinemia, and antibody-induced pure red cell aplasia

Usual Dosage Refer to individual protocols

Children:

SLE: I.V.: 500-750 mg/m^2 every month; maximum dose: 1 g/m^2

JRA/vasculitis: I.V.: 10 mg/kg every 2 weeks

Children and Adults:

Oral: 50-100 mg/m^2/day as continuous therapy or 400-1000 mg/m^2 in divided doses over 4-5 days as intermittent therapy

I.V.:

Single doses: 400-1800 mg/m^2 (30-50 mg/kg) per treatment course (1-5 days) which can be repeated at 2-4 week intervals

Continuous daily doses: 60-120 mg/m^2 (1-2.5 mg/kg) per day

Autologous BMT: IVPB: 50 mg/kg/dose x 4 days or 60 mg/kg/dose for 2 days; total dose is usually divided over 2-4 days

Nephrotic syndrome: Oral: 2-3 mg/kg/day every day for up to 12 weeks when corticosteroids are unsuccessful

Dosage Forms

Injection, powder for reconstitution: 500 mg, 1 g, 2 g

Tablet: 25 mg, 50 mg

cycloserine (sye kloe SER een)

Sound-Alike/Look-Alike Issues

cycloSERINE may be confused with cyclobenzaprine, cycloSPORINE

Tall-Man cyclo**SERINE**

U.S./Canadian Brand Names Seromycin® [US]

Therapeutic Category Antibiotic, Miscellaneous

Use Adjunctive treatment in pulmonary or extrapulmonary tuberculosis

Usual Dosage Some neurotoxic effects may be relieved or prevented by concomitant administration of pyridoxine

Tuberculosis: Oral:

Children: 10-20 mg/kg/day in 2 divided doses up to 1000 mg/day for 18-24 months

Adults: Initial: 250 mg every 12 hours for 14 days, then administer 500 mg to 1 g/day in 2 divided doses for 18-24 months (maximum daily dose: 1 g)

Dosage Forms

Capsule:

Seromycin®: 250 mg

Cycloset® [US] *see* bromocriptine *on page 148*

cyclosporin A *see* cyclosporine *on page 266*

cyclosporine (SYE kloe spor een)

Sound-Alike/Look-Alike Issues

cycloSPORINE may be confused with cyclophosphamide, Cyklokapron®, cycloSERINE

cycloSPORINE modified (Neoral®, Gengraf®) may be confused with cycloSPORINE non-modified (Sandimmne®)

Gengraf® may be confused with Prograf®

Neoral® may be confused with Neurontin®, Nizoral®

Sandimmune® may be confused with Sandostatin®

Synonyms CsA; CyA; cyclosporin A

Tall-Man cyclo**SPORINE**

U.S./Canadian Brand Names Apo-Cyclosporine [Can]; Gengraf® [US]; Neoral® [US/Can]; Restasis® [US]; Rhoxal-cyclosporine [Can]; Sandimmune® I.V. [Can]; Sandimmune® [US]; Sandoz-Cyclosporine [Can]

Therapeutic Category Immunosuppressant Agent

Use Prophylaxis of organ rejection in kidney, liver, and heart transplants, has been used with azathioprine and/or corticosteroids; severe, active rheumatoid arthritis (RA) not responsive to methotrexate alone; severe, recalcitrant plaque psoriasis in nonimmunocompromised adults unresponsive to or unable to tolerate other systemic therapy

Ophthalmic emulsion (Restasis®): Increase tear production when suppressed tear production is presumed to be due to keratoconjunctivitis sicca-associated ocular inflammation (in patients not already using topical antiinflammatory drugs or punctal plugs)

Usual Dosage **Neoral®/Genraf® and Sandimmune® are not bioequivalent and cannot be used interchangeably.**

Children: Transplant: Refer to adult dosing; children may require, and are able to tolerate, larger doses than adults.

Adults:

Newly-transplanted patients: Adjunct therapy with corticosteroids is recommended. Initial dose should be given 4-12 hours prior to transplant or may be given postoperatively; adjust initial dose to achieve desired plasma concentration

Oral: Dose is dependent upon type of transplant and formulation:

Cyclosporine (modified):

Renal: 9 ± 3 mg/kg/day, divided twice daily

Liver: 8 ± 4 mg/kg/day, divided twice daily

Heart: 7 ± 3 mg/kg/day, divided twice daily

Cyclosporine (nonmodified): Initial dose: 15 mg/kg/day as a single dose (range 14-18 mg/kg); lower doses of 10-14 mg/kg/day have been used for renal transplants. Continue initial dose daily for 1-2 weeks; taper by 5% per week to a maintenance dose of 5-10 mg/kg/day; some renal transplant patients may be dosed as low as 3 mg/kg/day

Note: When using the nonmodified formulation, cyclosporine levels may increase in liver transplant patients when the T-tube is closed; dose may need decreased

I.V.: Cyclosporine (nonmodified): Manufacturer's labeling: Initial dose: 5-6 mg/kg/day as a single dose (1/3 the oral dose), infused over 2-6 hours; use should be limited to patients unable to take capsules or oral solution; patients should be switched to an oral dosage form as soon as possible

Note: Many transplant centers administer cyclosporine as "divided dose" infusions (in 2-3 doses/day) or as a continuous (24-hour) infusion; dosages range from 3-7.5 mg/kg/day. Specific institutional protocols should be consulted.

Conversion to cyclosporine (modified) from cyclosporine (nonmodified): Start with daily dose previously used and adjust to obtain preconversion cyclosporine trough concentration. Plasma concentrations should be monitored every 4-7 days and dose adjusted as necessary, until desired trough level is obtained. When transferring patients with previously poor absorption of cyclosporine (nonmodified), monitor trough levels at least twice weekly (especially if initial dose exceeds 10 mg/kg/day); high plasma levels are likely to occur.

Rheumatoid arthritis: Oral: Cyclosporine (modified): Initial dose: 2.5 mg/kg/day, divided twice daily; salicylates, NSAIDs, and oral glucocorticoids may be continued; dose may be increased by 0.5-0.75 mg/kg/day if insufficient response is seen after 8 weeks of treatment; additional dosage increases may be made again at 12 weeks (maximum dose: 4 mg/kg/day). Discontinue if no benefit is seen by 16 weeks of therapy.

Note: Increase the frequency of blood pressure monitoring after each alteration in dosage of cyclosporine. Cyclosporine dosage should be decreased by 25% to 50% in patients with no history of hypertension who develop sustained hypertension during therapy and, if hypertension persists, treatment with cyclosporine should be discontinued.

Psoriasis: Oral: Cyclosporine (modified): Initial dose: 2.5 mg/kg/day, divided twice daily; dose may be increased by 0.5 mg/kg/day if insufficient response is seen after 4 weeks of treatment. Additional dosage increases may be made every 2 weeks if needed (maximum dose: 4 mg/kg/day). Discontinue if no benefit is seen by 6 weeks of therapy. Once patients are adequately controlled, the dose should be decreased to the lowest effective dose. Doses lower than 2.5 mg/kg/day may be effective. Treatment longer than 1 year is not recommended.

Note: Increase the frequency of blood pressure monitoring after each alteration in dosage of cyclosporine. Cyclosporine dosage should be decreased by 25% to 50% in patients with no history of hypertension who develop sustained hypertension during therapy and, if hypertension persists, treatment with cyclosporine should be discontinued.

Keratoconjunctivitis sicca: Ophthalmic (Restasis®): Children ≥16 years and Adults: Instill 1 drop in each eye every 12 hours

Dosage Forms

Capsule [modified]:

Gengraf®: 25 mg, 100 mg

Capsule [non-modified]: 25 mg, 100 mg

Capsule, soft gel [modified]: 25 mg, 50 mg, 100 mg

Neoral®: 25 mg, 100 mg

Capsule, soft gel [non-modified]:

Sandimmune®: 25 mg, 100 mg

Emulsion, ophthalmic [preservative free]:

Restasis®: 0.05% (0.4 mL)

Injection, solution [non-modified]: 50 mg/mL (5 mL)

Sandimmune®: 50 mg/mL (5 mL)

Solution, oral [modified]: 100 mg/mL
Gengraf®, Neoral®: 100 mg/mL
Solution, oral [non-modified]: 100 mg/mL
Sandimmune®: 100 mg/mL

Cycofed® Pediatric ***(Discontinued)*** *see* guaifenesin, pseudoephedrine, and codeine *on page* 479
Cyestra-35 [Can] *see* cyproterone and ethinyl estradiol *(Canada only) on page* 268
Cyklokapron® [US/Can] *see* tranexamic acid *on page* 977
Cylate™ [US] *see* cyclopentolate *on page* 265
Cylex® [US-OTC] *see* benzocaine *on page* 129
Cymbalta® [US/Can] *see* duloxetine *on page* 341
Cyomin® ***(Discontinued)*** *see* cyanocobalamin *on page* 263

cyproheptadine (si proe HEP ta deen)

Sound-Alike/Look-Alike Issues
cyproheptadine may be confused with cyclobenzaprine
Periactin may be confused with Perative®, Percodan®, Persantine®

Synonyms cyproheptadine hydrochloride

Therapeutic Category Antihistamine

Use Perennial and seasonal allergic rhinitis and other allergic symptoms including urticaria

Usual Dosage Oral:
Children:
Allergic conditions: 0.25 mg/kg/day or 8 mg/m^2/day in 2-3 divided doses **or**
2-6 years: 2 mg every 8-12 hours (not to exceed 12 mg/day)
7-14 years: 4 mg every 8-12 hours (not to exceed 16 mg/day)
Migraine headaches: 4 mg 2-3 times/day
Children ≥12 years and Adults: Spasticity associated with spinal cord damage: 4 mg at bedtime; increase by a 4 mg dose every 3-4 days; average daily dose: 16 mg in divided doses; not to exceed 36 mg/day
Children >13 years and Adults: Appetite stimulation (anorexia nervosa): 2 mg 4 times/day; may be increased gradually over a 3-week period to 8 mg 4 times/day
Adults:
Allergic conditions: 4-20 mg/day divided every 8 hours (not to exceed 0.5 mg/kg/day)
Cluster headaches: 4 mg 4 times/day
Migraine headaches: 4-8 mg 3 times/day

Dosage Forms
Syrup: 2 mg/5 mL
Tablet: 4 mg

cyproheptadine hydrochloride *see* cyproheptadine *on page* 268
cyproterone acetate *see* cyproterone *(Canada only) on page* 268

cyproterone and ethinyl estradiol *(Canada only)*

(sye PROE ter one & ETH in il es tra DYE ole)

Synonyms ethinyl estradiol and cyproterone acetate

U.S./Canadian Brand Names Cyestra-35 [Can]; Diane-35® [Can]; NOVO-Cyproterone/Ethinyl Estradiol [Can]

Therapeutic Category Acne Products; Estrogen and Androgen Combination

Use Treatment of females with severe acne, unresponsive to other therapies, with associated symptoms of androgenization (including mild hirsutism or seborrhea). **Should not be used solely for contraception;** however, will provide reliable contraception if taken as recommended for approved indications.

Usual Dosage Oral: Adults: Female: Acne: One tablet daily for 21 days, followed by 7 days off; first cycle should begin on the first day of menstrual flow. Discontinue therapy 3-4 cycles after symptoms have resolved.

Dosage Forms CAN = [Canadian brand name]
Tablet:
Diane-35 [CAN]: Cyproterone 2 mg and ethinyl estradiol 0.35 mg (21s) [not available in the U.S.]

cyproterone *(Canada only)* (sye PROE ter one)

Synonyms cyproterone acetate

U.S./Canadian Brand Names Androcur® Depot [Can]; Androcur® [Can]; Apo-Cyproterone® [Can]; Gen-Cyproterone [Can]; Novo-Cyproterone [Can]

Therapeutic Category Antiandrogen; Progestin

Use Palliative treatment of advanced prostate carcinoma

Usual Dosage Adults: Males: Prostatic carcinoma (palliative treatment):

Oral: 200-300 mg/day in 2-3 divided doses; following orchiectomy, reduce dose to 100-200 mg/day; should be taken with meals

I.M. (depot): 300 mg (3 mL) once weekly; reduce dose in orchiectomized patients to 300 mg every 2 weeks

Dosage Forms [CAN] = Canadian brand name:

Injection, solution: 100 mg/mL (3 mL) [not available in the U.S.]

Androcur® Depot [CAN]: 100 mg/mL (3 mL) [not available in the U.S.]

Tablet: 50 mg [not available in the U.S.]

Androcur® [CAN], Apo-Cyproterone® [CAN], Gen-Cyproterone [CAN]: 50 mg [not available in the U.S.]

Cystadane® [US/Can] *see* betaine *on page* 137

Cystagon® [US] *see* cysteamine *on page* 269

cysteamine (sis TEE a meen)

Synonyms cysteamine bitartrate

U.S./Canadian Brand Names Cystagon® [US]

Therapeutic Category Urinary Tract Product

Use Treatment of nephropathic cystinosis

Usual Dosage Oral: Initiate therapy with 1/4 to 1/6 of maintenance dose; titrate slowly upward over 4-6 weeks. **Note:** Dosage may be increased if cystine levels are <1 nmol/1/2 cystine/mg protein, although intolerance and incidence of adverse events may be increased.

Children <12 years: Maintenance: 1.3 g/m^2/day or 60 mg/kg/day divided into 4 doses (maximum dose: 1.95 g/m^2/day or 90 mg/kg/day)

Children >12 years and Adults (>110 lb): 2 g/day in 4 divided doses; maximum dose: 1.95 g/m^2/day or 90 mg/kg/day

Dosage Forms

Capsule:

Cystagon®: 50 mg, 150 mg

cysteamine bitartrate *see* cysteamine *on page* 269

cysteine (SIS te een)

Synonyms cysteine hydrochloride

U.S./Canadian Brand Names Cysteine-500 [US]

Therapeutic Category Nutritional Supplement

Use Supplement to crystalline amino acid solutions, in particular the specialized pediatric formulas (eg, Aminosyn® PF, TrophAmine®) to meet the intravenous amino acid nutritional requirements of infants receiving parenteral nutrition (PN)

Usual Dosage I.V.: Neonates and Infants: Added as a fixed ratio to crystalline amino acid solution: 40 mg cysteine per g of amino acids; dosage will vary with the daily amino acid dosage (eg, 0.5-2.5 g/kg/day amino acids would result in 20-100 mg/kg/day cysteine); individual doses of cysteine of 0.8-1 mmol/kg/day have also been added directly to the daily PN solution; the duration of treatment relates to the need for PN; patients on chronic PN therapy have received cysteine until 6 months of age and in some cases until 2 years of age

Dosage Forms

Capsule:

Cysteine-500: 500 mg

Injection, solution: 50 mg/mL (10 mL, 50 mL)

Cysteine-500 [US] *see* cysteine *on page* 269

cysteine hydrochloride *see* cysteine *on page* 269

Cystistat® [Can] *see* hyaluronate and derivatives *on page* 496

Cysto-Conray® II [US] *see* iothalamate meglumine *on page* 541

Cystografin® [US] *see* diatrizoate meglumine *on page* 300

Cystografin® Dilute [US] *see* diatrizoate meglumine *on page* 300

Cystospaz-M® *(Discontinued)* *see* hyoscyamine *on page 512*

CYT *see* cyclophosphamide *on page 265*

Cytadren® *(Discontinued)*

cytarabine (sye TARE a been)

Sound-Alike/Look-Alike Issues

cytarabine may be confused with Cytadren®, Cytosar®, Cytoxan®, vidarabine
cytarabine (conventional) may be confused with cytarabine liposomal
Cytosar-U may be confused with cytarabine, Cytovene®, Cytoxan®, Neosar®

Synonyms ara-C; arabinosylcytosine; cytarabine (conventional); cytarabine hydrochloride; Cytosar-U; cytosine arabinosine hydrochloride; NSC-63878

U.S./Canadian Brand Names Cytosar® [Can]

Therapeutic Category Antineoplastic Agent

Use Treatment of acute myeloid leukemia (AML), acute lymphocytic leukemia (ALL), chronic myelocytic leukemia (CML; blast phase), and lymphomas; prophylaxis and treatment of meningeal leukemia

Usual Dosage Refer to individual protocols. Children and Adults:

Remission induction:

I.V.: 75-200 mg/m^2/day for 5-10 days; a second course, beginning 2-4 weeks after the initial therapy, may be required in some patients.
or 100 mg/m^2 for 7 days
or 100 mg/m^2/dose every 12 hours for 7 days

I.T.: Usual dose 30 mg/m^2 every 4 days; range: 5-75 mg/m^2 every 2-7 days until CNS findings normalize; or age-based dosing (frequency of administration usually defined by protocol):
<1 year of age: 15-20 mg per dose
1-2 years of age: 16-30 mg per dose
2-3 years of age: 20-50 mg per dose
>3 years of age: 24-75 mg per dose

Remission maintenance:

I.V.: 70-200 mg/m^2/day for 2-5 days at monthly intervals
I.M., SubQ: 1-1.5 mg/kg single dose for maintenance at 1- to 4-week intervals

Dosage Forms

Injection, powder for reconstitution: 100 mg, 500 mg, 1 g, 2 g
Injection, solution: 100 mg/mL (20 mL)
Injection, solution: 20 mg/mL (25 mL)
Injection, solution [preservative free]: 20 mg/mL (5 mL, 50 mL); 100 mg/mL (20 mL)

cytarabine (conventional) *see* cytarabine *on page 270*

cytarabine hydrochloride *see* cytarabine *on page 270*

cytarabine (liposomal) (sye TARE a been lip po SOE mal)

Sound-Alike/Look-Alike Issues

cytarabine may be confused with Cytadren®, Cytosar®, Cytoxan®, vidarabine
cytarabine (liposomal) may be confused with conventional cytarabine
DepoCyt® may be confused with Depoject®

U.S./Canadian Brand Names DepoCyt® [US/Can]

Therapeutic Category Antineoplastic Agent, Antimetabolite (Purine)

Use Treatment of lymphomatous meningitis

Usual Dosage Note: Patients should be started on dexamethasone 4 mg twice daily (oral or I.V.) for 5 days, beginning on the day of cytarabine liposomal injection.

Intrathecal: Adults:

Induction: 50 mg every 14 days for a total of 2 doses (weeks 1 and 3)
Consolidation: 50 mg every 14 days for 3 doses (weeks 5, 7, and 9), followed by an additional dose at week 13
Maintenance: 50 mg every 28 days for 4 doses (weeks 17, 21, 25, and 29)

Dosage Forms

Injection, suspension, intrathecal [preservative free]:
Depocyt®: 10 mg/mL (5 mL)

CytoGam® [US/Can] *see* cytomegalovirus immune globulin (intravenous-human) *on page 271*

cytomegalovirus immune globulin (intravenous-human)

(sye toe meg a low VYE rus i MYUN GLOB yoo lin in tra VEE nus HYU man)

Sound-Alike/Look-Alike Issues

CytoGam® may be confused with Cytoxan®, Gamimune® N

Synonyms CMV-IGIV

U.S./Canadian Brand Names CytoGam® [US/Can]

Therapeutic Category Immune Globulin

Use Prophylaxis of cytomegalovirus (CMV) disease associated with kidney, lung, liver, pancreas, and heart transplants; concomitant use with ganciclovir should be considered in organ transplants (other than kidney) from CMV seropositive donors to CMV seronegative recipients

Usual Dosage I.V.: Adults:

Kidney transplant:

Initial dose (within 72 hours of transplant): 150 mg/kg/dose
2-, 4-, 6-, and 8 weeks after transplant: 100 mg/kg/dose
12 and 16 weeks after transplant: 50 mg/kg/dose

Liver, lung, pancreas, or heart transplant:

Initial dose (within 72 hours of transplant): 150 mg/kg/dose
2-, 4-, 6-, and 8 weeks after transplant: 150 mg/kg/dose
12 and 16 weeks after transplant: 100 mg/kg/dose

Dosage Forms

Injection, solution [preservative free]:

CytoGam®: 50 mg ± 10 mg/mL (50 mL)

Cytomel® [US/Can] *see* liothyronine *on page* *591*
Cytosar® [Can] *see* cytarabine *on page* *270*
Cytosar-U *see* cytarabine *on page* *270*
cytosine arabinosine hydrochloride *see* cytarabine *on page* *270*
cytostasan *see* bendamustine *on page* *127*
Cytotec® [US] *see* misoprostol *on page* *662*
Cytovene® [US/Can] *see* ganciclovir *on page* *454*
Cytoxan® [Can] *see* cyclophosphamide *on page* *265*
Cytoxan® *(Discontinued)* *see* cyclophosphamide *on page* *265*
Cytra-3 [US] *see* citric acid, sodium citrate, and potassium citrate *on page* *235*
Cytra-K [US] *see* potassium citrate and citric acid *on page* *804*
Cytuss HC [US] *see* phenylephrine, hydrocodone, and chlorpheniramine *on page* *778*
Cēpacol® Dual Action Maximum Strength [US-OTC] *see* dyclonine *on page* *343*
Cēpastat® [US-OTC] *see* phenol *on page* *772*
Cēpastat® Extra Strength [US-OTC] *see* phenol *on page* *772*
D2E7 *see* adalimumab *on page* *35*
D-3 [US-OTC] *see* cholecalciferol *on page* *224*
D_3 *see* cholecalciferol *on page* *224*
D3-5™ [US-OTC] *see* cholecalciferol *on page* *224*
D3-50™ [US-OTC] *see* cholecalciferol *on page* *224*
D-3-mercaptovaline *see* penicillamine *on page* *759*
d4T *see* stavudine *on page* *921*
D_5W *see* dextrose *on page* *298*
$D_{10}W$ *see* dextrose *on page* *298*
$D_{25}W$ *see* dextrose *on page* *298*
$D_{30}W$ *see* dextrose *on page* *298*
$D_{40}W$ *see* dextrose *on page* *298*
$D_{50}W$ *see* dextrose *on page* *298*
$D_{60}W$ *see* dextrose *on page* *298*
$D_{70}W$ *see* dextrose *on page* *298*
$DAB_{389}IL$-2 *see* denileukin diftitox *on page* *282*
DAB389 interleukin-2 *see* denileukin diftitox *on page* *282*

dabigatran etexilate *(Canada only)* (da BIG a tran ett EX ill ate)

Synonyms dabigatran etexilate mesilate

U.S./Canadian Brand Names Pradax™ [Can]

Therapeutic Category Anticoagulant, Thrombin Inhibitor

Use Postoperative thromboprophylaxis in patients who have undergone total hip or knee replacement procedures

Usual Dosage Oral: **Note:** Therapy should not be initiated until hemostasis has been established. When transitioning from intravenous anticoagulation therapy, initiate oral dabigatran therapy no sooner than time of next regularly scheduled dose of I.V. anticoagulant. When transitioning from dabigatran to I.V. anticoagulation therapy, allow 24 hours after the last dabigatran dose before initiating I.V. anticoagulation therapy.

Adults: Postoperative thromboprophylaxis:

Knee replacement: Initial: 110 mg given 1-4 hours after completion of surgery and establishment of hemostasis **OR** 220 mg as one dose in postoperative patients in whom therapy is not initiated on day of surgery regardless of reason; maintenance: 220 mg once daily (total duration of therapy: 10 days)

Hip replacement: Initial: 110 mg given 1-4 hours after completion of surgery and establishment of hemostasis **OR** 220 mg as one dose in postoperative patients in whom therapy is not initiated on day of surgery regardless of reason; maintenance: 220 mg once daily (total duration of therapy: 28-35 days)

Dosage Forms [CAN] = Canadian brand name

Capsule:

Pradax™ [CAN]: 75 mg, 110 mg [not available in the U.S.]

dabigatran etexilate mesilate *see* dabigatran etexilate *(Canada only) on page 272*

DABIL2 *see* denileukin diftitox *on page 282*

dacarbazine (da KAR ba zeen)

Sound-Alike/Look-Alike Issues

dacarbazine may be confused with Dicarbosil®, procarbazine

Synonyms DIC; dimethyl triazeno imidazole carboxamide; DTIC; imidazole carboxamide; imidazole carboxamide dimethyltriazene; WR-139007

U.S./Canadian Brand Names DTIC® [Can]

Therapeutic Category Antineoplastic Agent

Use Treatment of malignant melanoma, Hodgkin disease, soft-tissue sarcomas, fibrosarcomas, rhabdomyosarcoma, islet cell carcinoma, medullary carcinoma of the thyroid, and neuroblastoma

Usual Dosage Refer to individual protocols. Some dosage regimens include:

Intraarterial: 50-400 mg/m^2 for 5-10 days

I.V.:

Hodgkin disease, ABVD: 375 mg/m^2 days 1 and 15 every 4 weeks **or** 100 mg/m^2/day for 5 days

Metastatic melanoma (alone or in combination with other agents): 150-250 mg/m^2 days 1-5 every 3-4 weeks

Metastatic melanoma: 850 mg/m^2 every 3 weeks

High dose: Bone marrow/blood cell transplantation: I.V.: 1-3 g/m^2; maximum dose as a single agent: 3.38 g/m^2; generally combined with other high-dose chemotherapeutic drugs

Dosage Forms

Injection, powder for reconstitution: 100 mg, 200 mg

Dacex-DM [US] *see* guaifenesin, dextromethorphan, and phenylephrine *on page 478*

daclizumab (dac KLYE zue mab)

U.S./Canadian Brand Names Zenapax® [US/Can]

Therapeutic Category Immunosuppressant Agent

Use Part of an immunosuppressive regimen (including cyclosporine and corticosteroids) for the prophylaxis of acute organ rejection in patients receiving renal transplant

Usual Dosage Daclizumab is used adjunctively with other immunosuppressants (eg, cyclosporine, corticosteroids, mycophenolate mofetil, and azathioprine): I.V.:

Children: Use same weight-based dose as adults

Adults: Immunoprophylaxis against acute renal allograft rejection: 1 mg/kg infused over 15 minutes within 24 hours before transplantation (day 0), then every 14 days for 4 additional doses

Dosage Forms

Injection, solution [concentrate; preservative free]:

Zenapax®: 5 mg/mL (5 mL)

Dacodyl™ [US-OTC] *see* bisacodyl *on page 142*

Dacogen™ [US] *see* decitabine *on page 279*

DACT *see* dactinomycin *on page 273*

dactinomycin (dak ti noe MYE sin)

Sound-Alike/Look-Alike Issues

DACTINomycin may be confused with DAPTOmycin, DAUNOrubicin

actinomycin may be confused with achromycin

Synonyms ACT-D; actinomycin; actinomycin Cl; actinomycin D; DACT

Tall-Man DACTINomycin

U.S./Canadian Brand Names Cosmegen® [US/Can]

Therapeutic Category Antineoplastic Agent

Use Treatment of Wilms tumor, childhood rhabdomyosarcoma, Ewing sarcoma, metastatic testicular tumors (nonseminomatous), gestational trophoblastic neoplasm; regional perfusion (palliative or adjunctive) of locally recurrent or locoregional solid tumors (sarcomas, carcinomas and adenocarcinomas)

Usual Dosage Details concerning dosing in combination regimens should also be consulted.

Note: Medication orders for dactinomycin are commonly written in MICROgrams (eg, 150 mcg) although many regimens list the dose in MILLIgrams (eg, mg/kg or mg/m²). One-time doses for >1000 mcg, or multiple-day doses for >500 mcg/day are not common. The dose intensity per 2-week cycle for adults and children should not exceed 15 mcg/kg/day for 5 days or 400-600 mcg/m²/day for 5 days. Some practitioners recommend calculation of the dosage for obese or edematous adult patients on the basis of body surface area in an effort to relate dosage to lean body mass.

I.V.:

Children >6 months:

Usual dose: 15 mcg/kg/day for 5 days every 3-6 weeks **or** 400-600 mcg/m²/day for 5 days every 3-6 weeks

Wilms tumor, rhabdomyosarcoma, Ewing sarcoma: 15 mcg/kg/day for 5 days (in various combination regimens and schedules)

Adults:

Usual doses: 15 mcg/kg/day for 5 days every 3-6 weeks **or** 400-600 mcg/m²/day for 5 days every 3-6 weeks **or** 1000 mcg/m² on day 1 **or** 12 mcg/kg/day for 5 days (monotherapy) **or** 500 mcg/dose days 1 and 2 (as part of a combination chemotherapy regimen)

Testicular cancer: 1000 mcg/m² on day 1 (as part of a combination chemotherapy regimen)

Gestational trophoblastic neoplasm: 12 mcg/kg/day for 5 days (monotherapy) **or** 500 mcg/dose days 1 and 2 (as part of a combination chemotherapy regimen)

Wilms tumor, Ewing sarcoma, rhabdomyosarcoma: 15 mcg/kg/day for 5 days (in various combination regimens and schedules)

Regional perfusion: Adults (dosages and techniques may vary by institution; obese patients and patients with prior chemotherapy or radiation therapy may require lower doses): Lower extremity or pelvis: 50 mcg/kg; Upper extremity: 35 mcg/kg

Dosage Forms

Injection, powder for reconstitution:

Cosmegen®: 0.5 mg

Dairyaid® [Can] *see* lactase *on page 563*

Dakin's Solution [US] *see* sodium hypochlorite solution *on page 911*

Dakrina® Ophthalmic Solution *(Discontinued)* *see* artificial tears *on page 100*

Dalacin® C [Can] *see* clindamycin *on page 239*

Dalacin® T [Can] *see* clindamycin *on page 239*

Dalacin® Vaginal [Can] *see* clindamycin *on page 239*

dalfopristin and quinupristin *see* quinupristin and dalfopristin *on page 846*

Dallergy® [US] *see* chlorpheniramine, phenylephrine, and methscopolamine *on page 218*

Dallergy-D® Syrup *(Discontinued)* *see* chlorpheniramine and phenylephrine *on page 214*

Dallergy Drops [US] *see* chlorpheniramine and phenylephrine *on page 214*

Dallergy®-JR [US] *see* chlorpheniramine and phenylephrine *on page* 214
Dalmane® [Can] *see* flurazepam *on page* 435
Dalmane® *(Discontinued)* *see* flurazepam *on page* 435
d-Alpha-Gems™ [US-OTC] *see* vitamin E *on page* 1018
***d*-alpha tocopherol** *see* vitamin E *on page* 1018

dalteparin (dal TE pa rin)

Synonyms dalteparin sodium; NSC-714371

U.S./Canadian Brand Names Fragmin® [US/Can]

Therapeutic Category Anticoagulant (Other)

Use Prevention of deep vein thrombosis which may lead to pulmonary embolism, in patients requiring abdominal surgery who are at risk for thromboembolism complications (eg, patients >40 years of age, obesity, patients with malignancy, history of deep vein thrombosis or pulmonary embolism, and surgical procedures requiring general anesthesia and lasting >30 minutes); prevention of DVT in patients undergoing hip-replacement surgery; patients immobile during an acute illness; acute treatment of unstable angina or non-Q-wave myocardial infarction; prevention of ischemic complications in patients on concurrent aspirin therapy; in patients with cancer, extended treatment (6 months) of acute symptomatic venous thromboembolism (DVT and/or PE) to reduce the recurrence of venous thromboembolism

Usual Dosage SubQ: Adults:

Abdominal surgery:

Low-to-moderate DVT risk: 2500 int. units 1-2 hours prior to surgery, then once daily for 5-10 days postoperatively

High DVT risk: 5000 int. units the evening prior to surgery and then once daily for 5-10 days postoperatively. Alternatively in patients with malignancy: 2500 int. units 1-2 hours prior to surgery, 2500 int. units 12 hours later, then 5000 int. units once daily for 5-10 days postoperatively.

Patients undergoing total hip surgery: **Note:** Three treatment options are currently available. Dose is given for 5-10 days, although up to 14 days of treatment have been tolerated in clinical trials:

Postoperative start:

Initial: 2500 int. units 4-8 hours* after surgery

Maintenance: 5000 int. units once daily; start at least 6 hours after postsurgical dose

Preoperative (starting day of surgery):

Initial: 2500 int. units within 2 hours before surgery

Adjustment: 2500 int. units 4-8 hours* after surgery

Maintenance: 5000 int. units once daily; start at least 6 hours after postsurgical dose

Preoperative (starting evening prior to surgery):

Initial: 5000 int. units 10-14 hours before surgery

Adjustment: 5000 int. units 4-8 hours* after surgery

Maintenance: 5000 int. units once daily, allowing 24 hours between doses.

***Dose may be delayed if hemostasis is not yet achieved.**

Unstable angina or non-Q-wave myocardial infarction: 120 int. units/kg body weight (maximum dose: 10,000 int. units) every 12 hours for 5-8 days with concurrent aspirin therapy. Discontinue dalteparin once patient is clinically stable.

Venous thromboembolism: Cancer patients:

Initial (month 1): 200 int. units/kg (maximum dose: 18,000 int. units) once daily for 30 days

Maintenance (months 2-6): ~150 int. units/kg (maximum dose: 18,000 int. units) once daily. If platelet count between 50,000-100,000/mm^3, reduce dose by 2500 int. units until platelet count recovers to ≥100,000/mm^3. If platelet count <50,000/mm^3, discontinue dalteparin until platelet count recover to >50,000/mm^3.

Immobility during acute illness: 5000 int. units once daily

Dosage Forms

Injection, solution:

Fragmin®: Antifactor Xa 10,000 int. units per 1 mL (9.5 mL); antifactor Xa 25,000 units per 1 mL (3.8 mL)

Injection, solution [preservative free]:

Fragmin®: Antifactor Xa 2500 int. units per 0.2 mL (0.2 mL); antifactor Xa 5000 int. units per 0.2 mL (0.2 mL); antifactor Xa 7500 int. units per 0.3 mL (0.3 mL); antifactor Xa 10,000 int. units per 1 mL (1 mL); antifactor Xa 12,500 int. units per 0.5 mL (0.5 mL); antifactor Xa 15,000 int. units per 0.6 mL (0.6 mL); antifactor Xa 18,000 int. units per 0.72 mL (0.72 mL)

dalteparin sodium *see* dalteparin *on page* 274
Damason-P® *(Discontinued)*

danaparoid *(Canada only)* (da NAP a roid)

Sound-Alike/Look-Alike Issues
Orgaran® may be confused with argatroban

Synonyms danaparoid sodium

U.S./Canadian Brand Names Orgaran® [Can]

Therapeutic Category Anticoagulant (Other)

Use Prevention of postoperative deep vein thrombosis following elective hip replacement surgery

Usual Dosage SubQ: Adults: Prevention of DVT following hip replacement: 750 anti-Xa units twice daily; beginning 1-4 hours before surgery and then not sooner than 2 hours after surgery and every 12 hours until the risk of DVT has diminished. The average duration of therapy is 7-10 days.

Dosage Forms [CAN] = Canadian brand name

Injection, solution:
Orgaran® [CAN]: 750 anti-Xa units/0.6 mL (0.6 mL) [not available in the U.S.]

danaparoid sodium *see* danaparoid *(Canada only) on page 275*

danazol (DA na zole)

Sound-Alike/Look-Alike Issues
danazol may be confused with Dantrium®
Danocrine® may be confused with Dacriose®

U.S./Canadian Brand Names Cyclomen® [Can]

Therapeutic Category Androgen

Use Treatment of endometriosis, fibrocystic breast disease, and hereditary angioedema

Usual Dosage Oral: Adults:

Females: Endometriosis: Initial: 200-400 mg/day in 2 divided doses for mild disease; individualize dosage. Usual maintenance dose: 800 mg/day in 2 divided doses to achieve amenorrhea and rapid response to painful symptoms. Continue therapy uninterrupted for 3-6 months (up to 9 months).

Females: Fibrocystic breast disease: Range: 100-400 mg/day in 2 divided doses

Males/Females: Hereditary angioedema: Initial: 200 mg 2-3 times/day; after favorable response, decrease the dosage by 50% or less at intervals of 1-3 months or longer if the frequency of attacks dictates. If an attack occurs, increase the dosage by up to 200 mg/day.

Dosage Forms

Capsule: 50 mg, 100 mg, 200 mg

Dandrex [US-OTC] *see* selenium sulfide *on page 895*
Danocrine® *(Discontinued)* *see* danazol *on page 275*
Dantrium® [US/Can] *see* dantrolene *on page 275*

dantrolene (DAN troe leen)

Sound-Alike/Look-Alike Issues
Dantrium® may be confused with danazol, Daraprim®

Synonyms dantrolene sodium

U.S./Canadian Brand Names Dantrium® [US/Can]

Therapeutic Category Skeletal Muscle Relaxant

Use Treatment of spasticity associated with upper motor neuron disorders (eg, spinal cord injury, stroke, cerebral palsy, or multiple sclerosis); management of malignant hyperthermia; prevention of malignant hyperthermia in susceptible individuals (preoperative/postoperative administration)

Usual Dosage

Spasticity: Oral:

Children: Initial: 0.5 mg/kg/dose twice daily, increase frequency to 3-4 times/day at 4- to 7-day intervals, then increase dose by 0.5 mg/kg to a maximum of 3 mg/kg/dose 2-4 times/day up to 400 mg/day

Adults: 25 mg/day to start, increase frequency to 2-4 times/day, then increase dose by 25 mg every 4-7 days to a maximum of 100 mg 2-4 times/day or 400 mg/day

Malignant hyperthermia: Children and Adults:

Preoperative prophylaxis:

Oral: 4-8 mg/kg/day in 4 divided doses, begin 1-2 days prior to surgery with last dose 3-4 hours prior to surgery

I.V.: 2.5 mg/kg ~1 1/4 hours prior to anesthesia and infused over 1 hour with additional doses as needed and individualized

Crisis: I.V.: 2.5 mg/kg; may repeat dose up to cumulative dose of 10 mg/kg; if physiologic and metabolic abnormalities reappear, repeat regimen

Postcrisis follow-up: Oral: 4-8 mg/kg/day in 4 divided doses for 1-3 days; I.V. dantrolene may be used when oral therapy is not practical; individualize dosage beginning with 1 mg/kg or more as the clinical situation dictates

Dosage Forms

Capsule: 25 mg, 50 mg, 100 mg

Dantrium®: 25 mg, 50 mg, 100 mg

Injection, powder for reconstitution:

Dantrium®: 20 mg

dantrolene sodium *see* dantrolene *on page* 275

dapcin *see* daptomycin *on page* 276

dapiprazole *(Discontinued)*

dapsone (DAP sone)

Sound-Alike/Look-Alike Issues

dapsone may be confused with Diprosone®

Synonyms diaminodiphenylsulfone

U.S./Canadian Brand Names Aczone® [US]

Therapeutic Category Sulfone

Use Treatment of leprosy and dermatitis herpetiformis (infections caused by *Mycobacterium leprae*); topical treatment of acne vulgaris

Usual Dosage

Oral:

Leprosy:

Children: 1-2 mg/kg/24 hours, up to a maximum of 100 mg/day

Adults: 50-100 mg/day for 3-10 years

Dermatitis herpetiformis: Adults: Start at 50 mg/day, increase to 300 mg/day, or higher to achieve full control, reduce dosage to minimum level as soon as possible

Topical: Acne: Children ≥12 years and Adults: Apply pea-sized amount (approximately) in a thin layer to affected areas twice daily; reevaluate patient if no improvement after 12 weeks of therapy

Dosage Forms

Gel, topical:

Aczone®: 5% (30 g, 60 g)

Tablet: 25 mg, 100 mg

Daptacel® [US] *see* diphtheria, tetanus toxoids, and acellular pertussis vaccine *on page* 321

daptomycin (DAP toe mye sin)

Sound-Alike/Look-Alike Issues

DAPTOmycin may be confused with DACTINomycin

Cubicin® may be confused with Cleocin®

Synonyms cidecin; dapcin; LY146032

Tall-Man DAPTOmycin

U.S./Canadian Brand Names Cubicin® [US/Can]

Therapeutic Category Antibiotic, Cyclic Lipopeptide

Use Treatment of complicated skin and skin structure infections caused by susceptible aerobic gram-positive organisms; *Staphylococcus aureus* bacteremia, including right-sided infective endocarditis caused by MSSA or MRSA

Usual Dosage I.V.: Adults:

Skin and soft tissue: 4 mg/kg once daily for 7-14 days

Bacteremia, right-sided endocarditis caused by MSSA or MRSA: 6 mg/kg once daily for 2-6 weeks

Dosage Forms

Injection, powder for reconstitution:

Cubicin®: 500 mg

Daranide® *(Discontinued)*

Daraprim® [US/Can] *see* pyrimethamine *on page* 841

darbepoetin alfa (dar be POE e tin AL fa)

Sound-Alike/Look-Alike Issues

darbepoetin alfa may be confused with dalteparin, epoetin alfa, epoetin beta

Aranesp® may be confused with Aralast, Aricept®

Synonyms erythropoiesis-stimulating agent (ESA); erythropoiesis-stimulating protein; NSC-729969

U.S./Canadian Brand Names Aranesp® [US/Can]

Therapeutic Category Colony-Stimulating Factor; Growth Factor; Recombinant Human Erythropoietin

Use Treatment of anemia (elevate/maintain red blood cell level and decrease the need for transfusions) associated with chronic renal failure (including patients on dialysis and not on dialysis); treatment of anemia due to concurrent chemotherapy in patients with metastatic cancer (nonmyeloid malignancies)

Note: Darbepoetin is **not** indicated for use in cancer patients under the following conditions:

- receiving hormonal therapy, therapeutic biologic products, or radiation therapy unless also receiving concurrent myelosuppressive chemotherapy
- receiving myelosuppressive therapy when the expected outcome is curative

Usual Dosage Note: Hemoglobin levels should not exceed 12 g/dL and should not rise >1 g/dL per 2-week time period during therapy in any patient. **Anemia associated with CRF:** Individualize dosing to achieve and maintain hemoglobin levels at a target range of 10-12 g/dL. Hemoglobin levels should not exceed 12 g/dL. **Note:** I.V. route is preferred in hemodialysis patients.

Dosage Forms

Injection, solution [preservative free]:

Aranesp®: 25 mcg/0.42 mL (0.42 mL); 40 mcg/ 0.4 mL (0.4 mL); 60 mcg/0.3 mL (0.3 mL); 100 mcg/0.5 mL (0.5 mL); 150 mcg/0.3 mL (0.3 mL); 200 mcg/0.4 mL (0.4 mL); 300 mcg/0.6 mL (0.6 mL); 500 mcg/mL (1 mL) [contains polysorbate 80; prefilled syringe; needle cover contains latex]

Aranesp®: 25 mcg/mL (1 mL); 40 mcg/mL (1 mL); 60 mcg/mL (1 mL); 100 mcg/mL (1 mL); 150 mcg/0.75 mL (0.75 mL); 200 mcg/mL (1 mL); 300 mcg/mL (1 mL) [contains polysorbate 80; single-dose vial]

darifenacin (dar i FEN a sin)

Synonyms darifenacin hydrobromide; UK-88,525

U.S./Canadian Brand Names Enablex® [US/Can]

Therapeutic Category Anticholinergic Agent

Use Management of symptoms of bladder overactivity (urge incontinence, urgency, and frequency)

Usual Dosage Oral: Adults: Initial: 7.5 mg once daily. If response is not adequate after a minimum of 2 weeks, dosage may be increased to 15 mg once daily.

Dosage Forms

Tablet, extended release:

Enablex®: 7.5 mg, 15 mg

darifenacin hydrobromide *see* darifenacin *on page* 277

darunavir (dar OO na veer)

Synonyms darunavir ethanolate; TMC-114

U.S./Canadian Brand Names Prezista® [US/Can]

Therapeutic Category Antiretroviral Agent, Protease Inhibitor

Use Treatment of HIV-1 infections in combination with ritonavir and other antiretroviral agents

Usual Dosage Oral:

Children ≥6 years: **Note:** Do not use once daily dosing in pediatric patients; maximum dose: 600 mg darunavir/100 mg ritonavir twice daily

≥20 kg to <30 kg: 375 mg twice daily with food; coadministration with ritonavir 50 mg twice daily is required

≥30 kg to <40 kg: 450 mg twice daily with food; coadministration with ritonavir 60 mg twice daily is required

≥40 kg: 600 mg twice daily with food; coadministration with ritonavir 100 mg twice daily is required

Adults:

Therapy-naive: 800 mg once daily with food; coadministration with ritonavir 100 mg once daily is required

Therapy-experienced: 600 mg twice daily with food; coadministration with ritonavir 100 mg twice daily is required

Dosage Forms [CAN] = Canadian brand name

Tablet:

Prezista®: 75 mg, 150 mg, 400 mg, 600 mg

Prezista® [CAN]: 300 mg [not available in U.S.], 400 mg, 600 mg

darunavir ethanolate *see* darunavir *on page 277*

Darvocet A500® [US] *see* propoxyphene and acetaminophen *on page 828*

Darvocet-N® 50 [US/Can] *see* propoxyphene and acetaminophen *on page 828*

Darvocet-N® 100 [US/Can] *see* propoxyphene and acetaminophen *on page 828*

Darvon® [US] *see* propoxyphene *on page 827*

Darvon® Compound *(Discontinued)*

Darvon-N® [US/Can] *see* propoxyphene *on page 827*

dasatinib (da SA ti nib)

Synonyms BMS-354825

U.S./Canadian Brand Names Sprycel® [US/Can]

Therapeutic Category Antineoplastic Agent, Tyrosine Kinase Inhibitor

Use Treatment of chronic myelogenous leukemia (CML) in chronic, accelerated or blast (myeloid or lymphoid) phase resistant or intolerant to prior therapy (including imatinib); treatment of Philadelphia chromosome-positive (Ph+) acute lymphoblastic leukemia (ALL) resistant or intolerant to prior therapy

Usual Dosage Oral: Adults:

CML:

Chronic phase: 100 mg once daily. In clinical studies, a dose escalation to 140 mg once daily was allowed in patients not achieving cytogenetic response at recommended initial dosage.

Accelerated or blast phase: 140 mg once daily. In clinical studies, a dose escalation to 180 mg once daily was allowed in patients not achieving cytogenetic response at recommended initial dosage.

Ph+ ALL: 140 mg once daily. In clinical studies, a dose escalation to 180 mg once daily was allowed in patients not achieving cytogenetic response at recommended initial dosage.

Dosage Forms

Tablet, oral:

Sprycel®: 20 mg, 50 mg, 70 mg, 100 mg

daunomycin *see* daunorubicin hydrochloride *on page 278*

daunorubicin citrate (liposomal) (daw noe ROO bi sin SI trate lip po SOE mal)

Sound-Alike/Look-Alike Issues

DAUNOrubicin liposomal may be confused with DACTINomycin, DOXOrubicin, DOXOrubicin liposomal, epirubicin, IDArubicin, valrubicin

Liposomal formulation (DaunoXome®) may be confused with the conventional formulation (Cerubidine®, Rubex®)

Synonyms DAUNOrubicin liposomal; liposomal DAUNOrubicin; NSC-697732

Tall-Man **DAUNO**rubicin citrate (liposomal)

U.S./Canadian Brand Names DaunoXome® [US]

Therapeutic Category Antineoplastic Agent

Use First-line treatment of advanced HIV-associated Kaposi sarcoma (KS)

Usual Dosage I.V. (refer to individual protocols): Adults: HIV-associated KS: 40 mg/m^2 every 2 weeks

Dosage Forms

Injection, solution [preservative free]:

DaunoXome®: 2 mg/mL (25 mL)

daunorubicin hydrochloride (daw noe ROO bi sin hye droe KLOR ide)

Sound-Alike/Look-Alike Issues

DAUNOrubicin may be confused with DACTINomycin, DOXOrubicin, DOXOrubicin liposomal, epirubicin, IDArubicin, valrubicin

Conventional formulation (Cerubidine®, DAUNOrubicin hydrochloride) may be confused with the liposomal formulation (DaunoXome®)

Synonyms daunomycin; NSC-82151; rubidomycin hydrochloride

Tall-Man **DAUNO**rubicin hydrochloride

U.S./Canadian Brand Names Cerubidine® [US/Can]

Therapeutic Category Antineoplastic Agent

Use Treatment of acute lymphocytic leukemia (ALL) and acute myeloid leukemia (AML)

Usual Dosage I.V. (refer to individual protocols):

Children: **Note:** Cumulative dose should not exceed 300 mg/m^2 in children >2 years or 10 mg/kg in children <2 years of age; maximum cumulative doses for younger children are unknown.

Children <2 years or BSA <0.5 m^2: ALL combination therapy: 1 mg/kg/dose per protocol, with frequency dependent on regimen employed

Children ≥2 years and BSA ≥0.5 m^2:

ALL combination therapy: Remission induction: 25 mg/m^2 on day 1 every week for up to 4-6 cycles

AML combination therapy: Induction: I.V. continuous infusion: 30-60 mg/m^2/day on days 1-3 of cycle

Adults: **Note:** Cumulative dose should not exceed 550 mg/m^2 in adults without risk factors for cardiotoxicity and should not exceed 400 mg/m^2 in adults receiving chest irradiation.

Range: 30-60 mg/m^2/day for 3 days, repeat dose in 3-4 weeks

ALL combination therapy: 45 mg/m^2/day for 3 days

AML combination therapy:

Adults <60 years: Induction: 45 mg/m^2/day for 3 days of the first course of induction therapy; subsequent courses: 45 mg/m^2/day for 2 days

Adults ≥60 years: Induction: 30 mg/m^2/day for 3 days of the first course of induction therapy; subsequent courses: 30 mg/m^2/day for 2 days

Dosage Forms

Injection, powder for reconstitution: 20 mg

Cerubidine®: 20 mg

Injection, solution: 5 mg/mL (4 mL, 10 mL)

DAUNOrubicin liposomal *see* daunorubicin citrate (liposomal) *on page 278*

DaunoXome® [US] *see* daunorubicin citrate (liposomal) *on page 278*

1-Day™ [US-OTC] *see* tioconazole *on page 963*

Dayhist® Allergy [US-OTC] *see* clemastine *on page 237*

Daypro® [US/Can] *see* oxaprozin *on page 734*

Dayto Himbin® ***(Discontinued)*** *see* yohimbine *on page 1025*

Daytrana™ [US] *see* methylphenidate *on page 645*

DC 240® Softgel® ***(Discontinued)*** *see* docusate *on page 326*

dCF *see* pentostatin *on page 766*

DDAVP® [US/Can] *see* desmopressin acetate *on page 285*

DDAVP® Melt [Can] *see* desmopressin acetate *on page 285*

ddI *see* didanosine *on page 305*

1-deamino-8-D-arginine vasopressin *see* desmopressin acetate *on page 285*

Debrox® [US-OTC] *see* carbamide peroxide *on page 181*

Decadron® [US] *see* dexamethasone (systemic) *on page 288*

Decadron® Phosphate ***(Discontinued)*** *see* dexamethasone (systemic) *on page 288*

Deca-Durabolin® [Can] *see* nandrolone *(Canada only) on page 680*

Deca-Durabolin® ***(Discontinued)*** *see* nandrolone *(Canada only) on page 680*

Decahist-DM ***(Discontinued)***

Decavac® [US] *see* diphtheria and tetanus toxoid *on page 318*

Dec-Chlorphen [US] *see* chlorpheniramine and phenylephrine *on page 214*

Dec-Chlorphen DM ***(Discontinued)*** *see* chlorpheniramine, phenylephrine, and dextromethorphan *on page 217*

De-Chlor DM [US] *see* chlorpheniramine, phenylephrine, and dextromethorphan *on page 217*

De-Chlor DR [US] *see* chlorpheniramine, phenylephrine, and dextromethorphan *on page 217*

De-Chlor G ***(Discontinued)***

De-Chlor HC [US] *see* phenylephrine, hydrocodone, and chlorpheniramine *on page 778*

decitabine (de SYE ta been)

Synonyms 5-aza-2'-deoxycytidine; 5-azaC; NSC-127716

U.S./Canadian Brand Names Dacogen™ [US]

Therapeutic Category Antineoplastic Agent, Antimetabolite (Pyrimidine)

Use Treatment of myelodysplastic syndrome (MDS)

Usual Dosage I.V.: Adults: MDS: 15 mg/m^2 over 3 hours every 8 hours (45 mg/m^2/day) for 3 days (135 mg/m^2/cycle) every 6 weeks. Treatment is recommended for at least 4 cycles and may continue until the patient no longer continues to benefit.

Dosage Forms

Injection, powder for reconstitution:

Dacogen™: 50 mg

Declomycin® [US/Can] *see* demeclocycline *on page 282*

Deconamine® SR *(Discontinued)* *see* chlorpheniramine and pseudoephedrine *on page 215*

Deconsal® II [US] *see* guaifenesin and phenylephrine *on page 475*

Deconsal® CT [US] *see* phenylephrine and pyrilamine *on page 776*

Deep Sea [US-OTC] *see* sodium chloride *on page 908*

Defen-LA® *(Discontinued)* *see* guaifenesin and pseudoephedrine *on page 477*

deferasirox (de FER a sir ox)

Sound-Alike/Look-Alike Issues

deferasirox may be confused with deferoxamine

Synonyms ICL670

U.S./Canadian Brand Names Exjade® [US/Can]

Therapeutic Category Antidote; Chelating Agent

Use Treatment of chronic iron overload due to blood transfusions (transfusional hemosiderosis)

Usual Dosage Oral: Children ≥2 years and Adults:

Initial: 20 mg/kg daily (calculate dose to nearest whole tablet)

Maintenance: Adjust dose every 3-6 months based on serum ferritin levels; adjust by 5-10 mg/kg/day (calculate dose to nearest whole tablet); titrate. Usual range: 20-30 mg/kg/day; doses up to 40 mg/kg/day may be considered for serum ferritin levels persistently >2500 mcg/L (doses above 40 mg/kg/day are not recommended). In clinical trials, doses were individualized based on iron burden determined by liver iron concentrations (LIC); transfusional iron intake should be considered when individualizing maintenance dose. **Note:** Consider interrupting therapy for serum ferritin <500 mcg/L and dose reduction or interruption for hearing loss or visual disturbances.

Dosage Forms

Tablet, for oral suspension:

Exjade®: 125 mg, 250 mg, 500 mg

deferoxamine (de fer OKS a meen)

Sound-Alike/Look-Alike Issues

deferoxamine may be confused with cefuroxime, deferasirox

Desferal® may be confused with desflurane, Dexferrum®, Disophrol®

Synonyms deferoxamine mesylate; desferrioxamine; NSC-644468

U.S./Canadian Brand Names Desferal® [US/Can]; PMS-Deferoxamine [Can]

Therapeutic Category Antidote

Use Acute iron intoxication or when clinical signs of significant iron toxicity exist; chronic iron overload secondary to multiple transfusions

Usual Dosage

Acute iron toxicity: **Note:** I.V. route is used when severe toxicity is evidenced by systemic symptoms (coma, shock, metabolic acidosis, or severe gastrointestinal bleeding) or potentially severe intoxications (serum iron level >500 mcg/dL). When severe symptoms are not present, the I.M. route may be preferred (per manufacturer); however, the use of deferoxamine in situations where the serum iron concentration is <500 mcg/dL or when severe toxicity is not evident is a subject of some clinical debate.

Children ≥3 years:

I.M.: 90 mg/kg/dose every 8 hours (maximum: 6 g/24 hours)

I.V.: 15 mg/kg/hour (maximum: 6 g/24 hours)

Adults: I.M., I.V.: Initial: 1000 mg, may be followed by 500 mg every 4 hours for up to 2 doses; subsequent doses of 500 mg have been administered every 4-12 hours

Maximum recommended dose: 6 g/day (per manufacturer, however, higher doses have been administered)

Chronic iron overload:

Children ≥3 years:

I.V.: 15 mg/kg/hour (maximum: 12 g/24 hours)

SubQ: 20-40 mg/kg/day over 8-12 hours (maximum: 1000-2000 mg/day)
Adults:
I.M., I.V.: 500-1000 mg/day I.M.; in addition, 2000 mg should be given I.V. with each unit of blood transfused (administer separately from blood); maximum: 1 g/day in absence of transfusions; 6 g/day if patient received transfusions
SubQ: 1-2 g every day or 20-40 mg/kg/day over 8-24 hours

Dosage Forms
Injection, powder for reconstitution: 500 mg, 2 g
Desferal®: 500 mg, 2 g

deferoxamine mesylate *see* deferoxamine *on page 280*
Deficol® *(Discontinued)* *see* bisacodyl *on page 142*
Definity® [US/Can] *see* perflutren lipid microspheres *on page 767*

degarelix (deg a REL ix)

Sound-Alike/Look-Alike Issues
degarelix may be confused with cetrorelix, ganirelix

Synonyms degarelix acetate; FE200486

U.S./Canadian Brand Names Firmagon® [US]

Therapeutic Category Antineoplastic Agent, Gonadotropin-Releasing Hormone Antagonist; Gonadotropin Releasing Hormone Antagonist

Use Treatment of advanced prostate cancer

Usual Dosage SubQ: Adults: Prostate cancer:
Loading dose: 240 mg administered as two 120 mg (3 mL) injections
Maintenance dose: 80 mg every 28 days (beginning 28 days after initial loading dose)

Dosage Forms **Injection, powder for reconstitution:**
Firmagon®: 80 mg, 120 mg

degarelix acetate *see* degarelix *on page 281*
Degest® 2 Ophthalmic *(Discontinued)* *see* naphazoline *on page 680*
Dehistine [US] *see* chlorpheniramine, phenylephrine, and methscopolamine *on page 218*
Dehydral® [Can] *see* methenamine *on page 637*
dehydrobenzperidol *see* droperidol *on page 340*
Delatest® Injection *(Discontinued)* *see* testosterone *on page 947*
Delatestryl® [US/Can] *see* testosterone *on page 947*

delavirdine (de la VIR deen)

Synonyms U-90152S

U.S./Canadian Brand Names Rescriptor® [US/Can]

Therapeutic Category Antiviral Agent

Use Treatment of HIV-1 infection in combination with at least two additional antiretroviral agents

Usual Dosage Oral: Adolescents ≥16 years and Adults: 400 mg 3 times/day

Dosage Forms
Tablet:
Rescriptor®: 100 mg, 200 mg

Delestrogen® [US] *see* estradiol *on page 373*
Delfen® [US-OTC] *see* nonoxynol 9 *on page 703*
Delsym® [US-OTC] *see* dextromethorphan *on page 295*
delta-9-tetrahydro-cannabinol *see* dronabinol *on page 339*
delta-9-tetrahydrocannabinol and cannabinol *see* tetrahydrocannabinol and cannabidiol *(Canada only) on page 951*
delta-9 THC *see* dronabinol *on page 339*
Delta-D® [US-OTC] *see* cholecalciferol *on page 224*
deltacortisone *see* prednisone *on page 814*
deltadehydrocortisone *see* prednisone *on page 814*
deltahydrocortisone *see* prednisolone (systemic) *on page 813*
Del-Vi-A® *(Discontinued)* *see* vitamin A *on page 1016*

Demadex® [US] *see* torsemide *on page* 971

demeclocycline (dem e kloe SYE kleen)

Synonyms demeclocycline hydrochloride; demethylchlortetracycline

U.S./Canadian Brand Names Declomycin® [US/Can]

Therapeutic Category Tetracycline Derivative

Use Treatment of susceptible bacterial infections (acne, gonorrhea, pertussis, and urinary tract infections) caused by both gram-negative and gram-positive organisms

Usual Dosage Oral:

Children ≥8 years: 8-12 mg/kg/day divided every 6-12 hours

Adults: 150 mg 4 times/day or 300 mg twice daily

Dosage Forms

Tablet: 150 mg, 300 mg

Declomycin®: 150 mg, 300 mg

demeclocycline hydrochloride *see* demeclocycline *on page* 282

Demerol® [US/Can] *see* meperidine *on page* 626

4-demethoxydaunorubicin *see* idarubicin *on page* 518

demethylchlortetracycline *see* demeclocycline *on page* 282

Demser® [US/Can] *see* metyrosine *on page* 653

Demulen® 30 [Can] *see* ethinyl estradiol and ethynodiol diacetate *on page* 385

Demulen® *(Discontinued)* *see* ethinyl estradiol and ethynodiol diacetate *on page* 385

Denavir® [US] *see* penciclovir *on page* 759

denileukin diftitox (de ni LOO kin DIF ti toks)

Synonyms DAB389 interleukin-2; DAB_{389}IL-2; DABIL2

U.S./Canadian Brand Names ONTAK® [US]

Therapeutic Category Antineoplastic Agent, Miscellaneous

Use Treatment of persistent or recurrent cutaneous T-cell lymphoma (CTCL) whose malignant cells express the CD25 component of the IL-2 receptor

Usual Dosage Note: Premedicate with an antihistamine and acetaminophen prior to each infusion; corticosteroid premedication (eg, dexamethasone) may reduce the incidence of hypersensitivity and edema. Withhold treatment if serum albumin <3 g/dL.

I.V.: Adults: CTCL: 9 or 18 mcg/kg/day days 1 through 5 every 21 days for 8 cycles

Dosage Forms

Injection, solution [frozen]:

ONTAK®: 150 mcg/mL (2 mL)

Denorex® Daily Protection [US-OTC] *see* pyrithione zinc *on page* 842

Denorex® Original Therapeutic Strength [US-OTC] *see* coal tar *on page* 250

Denta 5000 Plus [US] *see* fluoride *on page* 430

DentaGel [US] *see* fluoride *on page* 430

Dentapaine [US-OTC] *see* benzocaine *on page* 129

Dent's Ear Wax *(Discontinued)* *see* carbamide peroxide *on page* 181

Dent's Extra Strength Toothache [US-OTC] *see* benzocaine *on page* 129

2'-deoxycoformycin *see* pentostatin *on page* 766

deoxycoformycin *see* pentostatin *on page* 766

Depacon® [US] *see* valproic acid and derivatives *on page* 1002

Depade® [US] *see* naltrexone *on page* 679

Depakene® [US/Can] *see* valproic acid and derivatives *on page* 1002

Depakote® [US] *see* valproic acid and derivatives *on page* 1002

Depakote® ER [US] *see* valproic acid and derivatives *on page* 1002

Depakote® Sprinkle [US] *see* valproic acid and derivatives *on page* 1002

depAndro® Injection *(Discontinued)* *see* testosterone *on page* 947

Depen® [US/Can] *see* penicillamine *on page* 759

depGynogen® Injection *(Discontinued)* *see* estradiol *on page* 373

Deplin™ [US] *see* methylfolate *on page* 644

desflurane (DES flure ane)

Sound-Alike/Look-Alike Issues
desflurane may be confused with Desferal®

U.S./Canadian Brand Names Suprane® [US/Can]

Therapeutic Category General Anesthetic

Use Induction and/or maintenance of general anesthesia in adults; maintenance of anesthesia in intubated children; **Note:** Use of desflurane for induction of general anesthesia is not recommended due to its irritant properties and unpleasant odor which causes coughing, breath holding, laryngospasm, oxygen desaturation, increased secretions, hypertension, and tachycardia.

Usual Dosage Note: Concurrent use with benzodiazepines, nitrous oxide, or opioids decreases the desflurane dose.
Children (intubated): Maintenance: Surgical levels of anesthesia range between 5.2% to 10%

Adults: The minimum alveolar concentration (MAC), the concentration at which 50% of patients do not respond to surgical incision, ranges from 6.0% (45 years of age) to 7.3% (25 years of age). The concentration at which amnesia and loss of awareness occur (MAC - awake) is 2.4%. Surgical levels of anesthesia are achieved with concentrations between 2.5% to 8.5%.

Note: Because of the higher vapor pressure of desflurane, its vaporizer is heated in order to deliver a constant concentration

Dosage Forms

Liquid, for inhalation:

Suprane®: 100% (240 mL)

desiccated thyroid *see* thyroid, desiccated *on page 957*

desipramine (des IP ra meen)

Sound-Alike/Look-Alike Issues

desipramine may be confused with clomiPRAMINE, deserpidine, diphenhydrAMINE, disopyramide, imipramine, nortriptyline

Norpramin® may be confused with clomiPRAMINE, imipramine, Norpace®, nortriptyline, Tenormin®

Synonyms desipramine hydrochloride; desmethylimipramine hydrochloride

U.S./Canadian Brand Names Alti-Desipramine [Can]; Apo-Desipramine® [Can]; Norpramin® [US/Can]; Nu-Desipramine [Can]; PMS-Desipramine [Can]

Therapeutic Category Antidepressant, Tricyclic (Secondary Amine)

Use Treatment of depression

Usual Dosage Oral (dose is generally administered at bedtime): Depression:

Adolescents: Initial: 25-50 mg/day; gradually increase to 100 mg/day in single or divided doses (maximum: 150 mg/day)

Adults: Initial: 75 mg/day in divided doses; increase gradually to 150-200 mg/day in divided or single dose (maximum: 300 mg/day)

Dosage Forms

Tablet: 10 mg, 25 mg, 50 mg, 75 mg, 100 mg, 150 mg

Norpramin®: 10 mg, 25 mg, 50 mg, 75 mg, 100 mg, 150 mg

desipramine hydrochloride *see* desipramine *on page 284*

Desitin® [US-OTC] *see* zinc oxide *on page 1030*

Desitin® Creamy [US-OTC] *see* zinc oxide *on page 1030*

desloratadine (des lor AT a deen)

Sound-Alike/Look-Alike Issues

Clarinex® may be confused with Celebrex®

U.S./Canadian Brand Names Aerius® [Can]; Clarinex® [US]

Therapeutic Category Antihistamine, Nonsedating

Use Relief of nasal and non-nasal symptoms of seasonal allergic rhinitis (SAR) and perennial allergic rhinitis (PAR); treatment of chronic idiopathic urticaria (CIU)

Usual Dosage Oral:

Children:

6-11 months: 1 mg once daily

12 months to 5 years: 1.25 mg once daily

6-11 years: 2.5 mg once daily

Children ≥12 years and Adults: 5 mg once daily

Dosage Forms

Syrup:

Clarinex®: 0.5 mg/mL

Tablet:

Clarinex®: 5 mg

Tablet, orally disintegrating:

Clarinex® RediTabs®: 2.5 mg, 5 mg

desloratadine and pseudoephedrine (des lor AT a deen & soo doe e FED rin)

Synonyms pseudoephedrine and desloratadine

U.S./Canadian Brand Names Clarinex-D® 12 Hour [US]; Clarinex-D® 24 Hour [US]

Therapeutic Category Antihistamine/Decongestant Combination, Nonsedating

Use Relief of symptoms of seasonal allergic rhinitis, in children ≥12 years of age and adults

Usual Dosage Oral: Children ≥12 years and Adults:

Clarinex-D® 12 Hour: One tablet twice daily

Clarinex-D® 24 Hour: One tablet daily

Dosage Forms

Tablet, variable release:

Clarinex-D® 12 Hour: Desloratadine 2.5 mg [immediate release] and pseudoephedrine 120 mg [extended release]

Clarinex-D® 24 Hour: Desloratadine 5 mg [immediate release] and pseudoephedrine 240 mg [extended release]

desmethylimipramine hydrochloride *see* desipramine *on page 284*

desmopressin acetate (des moe PRES in AS e tate)

Synonyms 1-deamino-8-D-arginine vasopressin

U.S./Canadian Brand Names Apo-Desmopressin® [Can]; DDAVP® Melt [Can]; DDAVP® [US/Can]; Minirin® [Can]; Nove-Desmopressin [Can]; Octostim® [Can]; PMS-Desmopressin [Can]; Stimate® [US]

Therapeutic Category Vasopressin Analog, Synthetic

Use

Injection: Treatment of diabetes insipidus; maintenance of hemostasis and control of bleeding in hemophilia A with factor VIII coagulant activity levels >5% and mild-to-moderate classic von Willebrand disease (type 1) with factor VIII coagulant activity levels >5%

Nasal solutions (DDAVP® Nasal Spray and DDAVP® Rhinal Tube): Treatment of central diabetes insipidus

Nasal spray (Stimate®): Maintenance of hemostasis and control of bleeding in hemophilia A with factor VIII coagulant activity levels >5% and mild-to-moderate classic von Willebrand disease (type 1) with factor VIII coagulant activity levels >5%

Tablet: Treatment of central diabetes insipidus, temporary polyuria and polydipsia following pituitary surgery or head trauma, primary nocturnal enuresis

Usual Dosage

Children:

Diabetes insipidus:

I.M., I.V., SubQ: Canadian labeling (not in U.S. labeling): ≥3 months: 0.4 mcg (0.1 mL) once daily or 1/10 of the maintenance intranasal dose. Fluid restriction should be observed.

I.V., SubQ: Children <12 years: No definitive dosing available. Adult dosing should **not** be used in this age group; adverse events such as hyponatremia-induced seizures may occur. Dose should be reduced. Some have suggested an initial dosage range of 0.1-1 mcg in 1 or 2 divided doses. Initiate at low dose and increase as necessary. Closely monitor serum sodium levels and urine output; fluid restriction is recommended.

Intranasal (using 100 mcg/mL nasal solution): 3 months to 12 years: Initial: 5 mcg/day (0.05 mL/day) divided 1-2 times/day; range: 5-30 mcg/day (0.05-0.3 mL/day) divided 1-2 times/day; adjust morning and evening doses separately for an adequate diurnal rhythm of water turnover. **Note:** The nasal spray pump can only deliver doses of 10 mcg (0.1 mL) or multiples of 10 mcg (0.1 mL); if doses other than this are needed, the rhinal tube delivery system is preferred. Fluid restriction should be observed.

Oral:

U.S. labeling: ≥4 years: Initial: 0.05 mg twice daily; total daily dose should be increased or decreased as needed to obtain adequate antidiuresis (range: 0.1-1.2 mg divided 2-3 times/day). Fluid restriction should be observed.

Canadian labeling (not in U.S. labeling): ≥5 years: Initial: 0.1 mg 3 times/day; total daily dose should be increased or decreased as needed to obtain adequate antidiuresis (range: 0.3-1.2 mg divided 3 times/day). Divide daily doses so that the evening dose is 2 times higher than the morning or afternoon dose to ensure adequate antidiuresis during the night. Fluid restriction should be observed.

Hemophilia A and von Willebrand disease (type 1): I.V.: ≥3 months: 0.3 mcg/kg by slow infusion; may repeat dose if needed; if used preoperatively, administer 30 minutes before procedure

Children ≥12 years and Adults:

Diabetes insipidus:

I.V., SubQ: 2-4 mcg/day (0.5-1 mL) in 2 divided doses or 1/10 of the maintenance intranasal dose. Fluid restriction should be observed.

Intranasal (using 100 mcg/mL nasal solution): 10-40 mcg/day (0.1-0.4 mL) divided 1-3 times/day; adjust morning and evening doses separately for an adequate diurnal rhythm of water turnover. **Note:** The nasal spray pump can only deliver doses of 10 mcg (0.1 mL) or multiples of 10 mcg (0.1 mL); if doses other than this are needed, the rhinal tube delivery system is preferred. Fluid restriction should be observed.

Oral:

U.S. labeling: Initial: 0.05 mg twice daily; total daily dose should be increased or decreased as needed to obtain adequate antidiuresis (range: 0.1-1.2 mg divided 2-3 times/day). Fluid restriction should be observed.

Canadian labeling (not in U.S. labeling): Initial: 0.1 mg 3 times/day; total daily dose should be increased or decreased as needed to obtain adequate antidiuresis (range: 0.3-1.2 mg divided 3 times/day). Fluid restriction should be observed.

Sublingual formulation: Canadian labeling (not in U.S. labeling): Initial: 60 mcg 3 times/day; total daily dose should be increased or decreased as needed to obtain adequate antidiuresis. Usual maintenance: 60-120 mcg 3 times/day (range: 120-720 mcg divided 2-3 times/day). Fluid restriction should be observed.

Hemophilia A and mild-to-moderate von Willebrand disease (type 1):

I.V.: 0.3 mcg/kg by slow infusion; if used preoperatively, administer 30 minutes before procedure

Canadian labeling (not in U.S. labeling): Maximum I.V. dose: 20 mcg

Intranasal (using high concentration spray [1.5 mg/mL]): <50 kg: 150 mcg (1 spray); >50 kg: 300 mcg (1 spray each nostril); repeat use is determined by the patient's clinical condition and laboratory work; if using preoperatively, administer 2 hours before surgery

Adults: Diabetes insipidus: I.M., I.V., SubQ: Canadian label (not in U.S. labeling): 1-4 mcg (0.25-1 mL) once daily or 1/10 of the maintenance intranasal dose. Fluid restriction should be observed.

Dosage Forms [CAN] = Canadian product

Injection, solution: 4 mcg/mL (1 mL, 10 mL)

DDAVP®: 4 mcg/mL (1 mL, 10 mL)

Solution, intranasal: 100 mcg/mL (2.5 mL)

DDAVP®: 100 mcg/mL (2.5 mL)

Solution, intranasal [spray]: 100 mcg/mL (5 mL)

DDAVP®: 100 mcg/mL (5 mL)

Stimate®: 1.5 mg/mL (2.5 mL)

Tablet, oral: 0.1 mg, 0.2 mg

DDAVP®: 0.1 mg, 0.2 mg

Tablet, sublingual:

DDAVP® Melt (CAN) [not available in U.S.]: 60 mcg, 120 mcg, 240 mcg

Desocort® [Can] *see* desonide *on page* 286

Desogen® [US] *see* ethinyl estradiol and desogestrel *on page* 383

desogestrel and ethinyl estradiol *see* ethinyl estradiol and desogestrel *on page* 383

Desonate™ [US] *see* desonide *on page* 286

desonide (DES oh nide)

U.S./Canadian Brand Names Desocort® [Can]; Desonate™ [US]; DesOwen® [US]; LoKara™ [US]; PMS-Desonide [Can]; Verdeso™ [US]

Therapeutic Category Corticosteroid, Topical

Use Adjunctive therapy for inflammation in acute and chronic corticosteroid responsive dermatosis (low potency corticosteroid); mild-to-moderate atopic dermatitis

Usual Dosage Topical:

Corticosteroid responsive dermatoses: Children and Adults: Therapy should be discontinued when control is achieved. If no improvement is seen within 2 weeks, reassessment of diagnosis may be necessary.

Cream, ointment: Apply 2-4 times/day sparingly

Lotion: Apply 2-3 times/day sparingly

Atopic dermatitis: Children ≥3 months and Adults: Aerosol, gel: Apply 2 times/day sparingly. Therapy should be discontinued when control is achieved. If no improvement is seen within 4 weeks, reassessment of diagnosis may be necessary.

Dosage Forms

Aerosol, topical [foam]:

Verdeso®: 0.05% (50 g, 100 g)

Cream, topical: 0.05% (15 g, 60 g)
DesOwen®: 0.05% (60 g)
Gel, topical [aqueous]:
Desonate™: 0.05% (60 g)
Lotion, topical: 0.05% (60 mL, 120 mL)
LoKara™: 0.05% (60 mL, 120 mL)
Ointment, topical: 0.05% (15 g, 60 g)
DesOwen®: 0.05% (60 g)

DesOwen® [US] *see* desonide *on page 286*

desoximetasone (des oks i MET a sone)

Sound-Alike/Look-Alike Issues
desoximetasone may be confused with dexamethasone
Topicort® may be confused with Topic®

U.S./Canadian Brand Names Taro-Desoximetasone [Can]; Topicort® [US/Can]; Topicort®-LP [US]

Therapeutic Category Corticosteroid, Topical

Use Relieves inflammation and pruritic symptoms of corticosteroid-responsive dermatosis (intermediate- to high-potency topical corticosteroid)

Usual Dosage Desoximetasone is a potent fluorinated topical corticosteroid. Therapy should be discontinued when control is achieved; if no improvement is seen, reassessment of diagnosis may be necessary.

Cream, gel: Children and Adults: Apply a thin film to affected area twice daily
Ointment: Children ≥10 years and Adults: Apply a thin film to affected area twice daily

Dosage Forms
Cream, topical: 0.25% (15 g, 60 g); 0.05% (15 g, 60 g)
Topicort®: 0.25% (15 g, 60 g)
Topicort®-LP: 0.05% (15 g, 60 g)
Gel, topical: 0.05% (15 g, 60 g)
Topicort®: 0.05% (15 g, 60 g)
Ointment, topical: 0.25% (15 g, 60 g)
Topicort®: 0.25% (15 g, 60 g)

desoxyephedrine hydrochloride *see* methamphetamine *on page 636*
Desoxyn® [US/Can] *see* methamphetamine *on page 636*
desoxyphenobarbital *see* primidone *on page 818*
Desquam-X® [US/Can] *see* benzoyl peroxide *on page 132*
Desquam-X® Wash *(Discontinued)* *see* benzoyl peroxide *on page 132*
Desquam-E™ *(Discontinued)* *see* benzoyl peroxide *on page 132*

desvenlafaxine (des ven la FAX een)

Synonyms O-desmethylvenlafaxine; ODV

U.S./Canadian Brand Names Pristiq™ [US]

Therapeutic Category Antidepressant, Serotonin/Norepinephrine Reuptake Inhibitor

Use Treatment of major depressive disorder

Usual Dosage Oral: Adults: Depression: 50 mg once daily; up to 400 mg once daily have been studied; however, the manufacturer states there is no evidence that higher doses confer any additional benefit. A flat dose response curve for efficacy between 50-400 mg/day has been noted as well as an increase in adverse events.
Note: Gradually taper dose (by increasing dosing interval) if discontinuing.

Dosage Forms
Tablet, extended release:
Pristiq™: 50 mg, 100 mg

Desyrel® [Can] *see* trazodone *on page 979*
Desyrel® *(Discontinued)* *see* trazodone *on page 979*
Detane® [US-OTC] *see* benzocaine *on page 129*
detemir insulin *see* insulin detemir *on page 530*
Detrol® [US/Can] *see* tolterodine *on page 969*
Detrol® LA [US/Can] *see* tolterodine *on page 969*

Detuss ***(Discontinued)***
Detussin® Expectorant ***(Discontinued)***
Dex4® [US-OTC] *see* dextrose *on page* *298*
Dexacidin® ***(Discontinued)*** *see* neomycin, polymyxin B, and dexamethasone *on page* *687*
Dexacine™ ***(Discontinued)*** *see* neomycin, polymyxin B, and dexamethasone *on page* *687*
dexamethasone and ciprofloxacin *see* ciprofloxacin and dexamethasone *on page* *232*
dexamethasone and tobramycin *see* tobramycin and dexamethasone *on page* *966*
Dexamethasone Intensol® [US] *see* dexamethasone (systemic) *on page* *288*
dexamethasone, neomycin, and polymyxin B *see* neomycin, polymyxin B, and dexamethasone *on page* *687*

dexamethasone (ophthalmic) (deks a METH a sone op THAL mik)

Sound-Alike/Look-Alike Issues
dexamethasone may be confused with desoximetasone
Maxidex® may be confused with Maxzide®

Synonyms dexamethasone sodium phosphate

U.S./Canadian Brand Names Maxidex® [US/Can]

Therapeutic Category Adrenal Corticosteroid

Use Inflammatory or allergic conjunctivitis

Usual Dosage Ophthalmic: Adults:
Ointment: Apply thin coating into conjunctival sac 3-4 times/day; gradually taper dose to discontinue
Suspension: Instill 2 drops into conjunctival sac every hour during the day and every other hour during the night; gradually reduce dose to every 3-4 hours, then to 3-4 times/day

Dosage Forms
Solution, ophthalmic: 0.1% (5 mL)
Suspension, ophthalmic:
Maxidex®: 0.1% (5 mL)

dexamethasone sodium phosphate *see* dexamethasone (ophthalmic) *on page* *288*
dexamethasone sodium phosphate *see* dexamethasone (systemic) *on page* *288*

dexamethasone (systemic) (deks a METH a sone sis TEM ik)

Sound-Alike/Look-Alike Issues
dexamethasone may be confused with desoximetasone
Decadron® may be confused with Percodan®

Synonyms dexamethasone sodium phosphate

U.S./Canadian Brand Names Apo-Dexamethasone® [Can]; Decadron® [US]; Dexamethasone Intensol® [US]; Dexasone® [Can]; DexPak® TaperPak® [US]; Diodex® [Can]; PMS-Dexamethasone [Can]

Therapeutic Category Adrenal Corticosteroid

Use Systemically and locally for chronic swelling; allergic, hematologic, neoplastic, and autoimmune diseases; may be used in management of cerebral edema, septic shock, as a diagnostic agent, antiemetic

Usual Dosage
Children:
Antiemetic (prior to chemotherapy): I.V. (should be given as sodium phosphate): 5-20 mg given 15-30 minutes before treatment
Antiinflammatory immunosuppressant: Oral, I.M., I.V. (injections should be given as sodium phosphate): 0.08-0.3 mg/kg/day **or** 2.5-10 mg/m^2/day in divided doses every 6-12 hours
Extubation or airway edema: Oral, I.M., I.V. (injections should be given as sodium phosphate): 0.5-2 mg/kg/day in divided doses every 6 hours beginning 24 hours prior to extubation and continuing for 4-6 doses afterwards
Cerebral edema: I.V. (should be given as sodium phosphate): Loading dose: 1-2 mg/kg/dose as a single dose; maintenance: 1-1.5 mg/kg/day (maximum: 16 mg/day) in divided doses every 4-6 hours for 5 days then taper for 5 days, then discontinue
Bacterial meningitis in infants and children >2 months: I.V. (should be given as sodium phosphate): 0.6 mg/kg/day in 4 divided doses every 6 hours for the first 4 days of antibiotic treatment; start dexamethasone at the time of the first dose of antibiotic

Physiologic replacement: Oral, I.M., I.V.: 0.03-0.15 mg/kg/day **or** 0.6-0.75 mg/m^2/day in divided doses every 6-12 hours

Adults:

Antiemetic:

Prophylaxis: Oral, I.V.: 10-20 mg 15-30 minutes before treatment on each treatment day

Continuous infusion regimen: Oral or I.V.: 10 mg every 12 hours on each treatment day

Mildly emetogenic therapy: Oral, I.M., I.V.: 4 mg every 4-6 hours

Delayed nausea/vomiting: Oral: 4-10 mg 1-2 times/day for 2-4 days **or**

8 mg every 12 hours for 2 days; then

4 mg every 12 hours for 2 days **or**

20 mg 1 hour before chemotherapy; then

10 mg 12 hours after chemotherapy; then

8 mg every 12 hours for 4 doses; then

4 mg every 12 hours for 4 doses

Antiinflammatory:

Oral, I.M., I.V. (injections should be given as sodium phosphate): 0.75-9 mg/day in divided doses every 6-12 hours

Intraarticular, intralesional, or soft tissue (as sodium phosphate): 0.4-6 mg/day

Chemotherapy: Oral, I.V.: 40 mg every day for 4 days, repeated every 4 weeks (VAD regimen)

Cerebral edema: I.V. 10 mg stat, 4 mg I.M./I.V. (should be given as sodium phosphate) every 6 hours until response is maximized, then switch to oral regimen, then taper off if appropriate; dosage may be reduced after 24 days and gradually discontinued over 5-7 days

Cushing syndrome, diagnostic: Oral: 1 mg at 11 PM, draw blood at 8 AM; greater accuracy for Cushing syndrome may be achieved by the following:

Dexamethasone 0.5 mg by mouth every 6 hours for 48 hours (with 24-hour urine collection for 17-hydroxycorticosteroid excretion)

Differentiation of Cushing syndrome due to ACTH excess from Cushing due to other causes: Oral: Dexamethasone 2 mg every 6 hours for 48 hours (with 24-hour urine collection for 17-hydroxycorticosteroid excretion)

Multiple sclerosis (acute exacerbation): 30 mg/day for 1 week, followed by 4-12 mg/day for 1 month

Physiological replacement: Oral, I.M., I.V. (should be given as sodium phosphate): 0.03-0.15 mg/kg/day **or** 0.6-0.75 mg/m^2/day in divided doses every 6-12 hours

Treatment of shock:

Addisonian crisis/shock (ie, adrenal insufficiency/responsive to steroid therapy): I.V. (given as sodium phosphate): 4-10 mg as a single dose, which may be repeated if necessary

Unresponsive shock (ie, unresponsive to steroid therapy): I.V. (given as sodium phosphate): 1-6 mg/kg as a single I.V. dose or up to 40 mg initially followed by repeat doses every 2-6 hours while shock persists

Dosage Forms

Elixir: 0.5 mg/5 mL

Injection, solution: 4 mg/mL (1 mL, 5 mL, 10 mL, 25 mL, 30 mL); 10 mg/mL (1 mL, 10 mL)

Injection, solution [preservative free]: 10 mg/mL (1 mL)

Solution, oral: 0.5 mg/5 mL

Solution, oral concentrate:

Dexamethasone Intensol®: 1 mg/mL

Tablet: 0.5 mg, 0.75 mg, 1 mg, 1.5 mg, 2 mg, 4 mg, 6 mg

DexPak® TaperPak®: 1.5 mg

Dexasone® [Can] *see* dexamethasone (systemic) *on page* 288

dexbrompheniramine and pseudoephedrine

(deks brom fen EER a meen & soo doe e FED rin)

Synonyms pseudoephedrine and dexbrompheniramine

U.S./Canadian Brand Names Drixoral® [Can]

Therapeutic Category Antihistamine/Decongestant Combination

Use Relief of symptoms of upper respiratory mucosal congestion in seasonal and perennial nasal allergies, acute rhinitis, rhinosinusitis, and eustachian tube blockage

Usual Dosage Oral: Children >12 years and Adults: 1 timed release tablet every 12 hours, may require 1 tablet every 8 hours

Dosage Forms

Tablet, sustained action: Dexbrompheniramine 6 mg and pseudoephedrine 120 mg

Dexchlor® *(Discontinued)* *see* dexchlorpheniramine *on page 290*

dexchlorpheniramine (deks klor fen EER a meen)

Synonyms dexchlorpheniramine maleate

Therapeutic Category Antihistamine

Use Perennial and seasonal allergic rhinitis and other allergic symptoms including urticaria

Usual Dosage Oral:

Children:

2-5 years: 0.5 mg every 4-6 hours (do not use timed release)

6-11 years: 1 mg every 4-6 hours or 4 mg timed release at bedtime

Adults: 2 mg every 4-6 hours or 4-6 mg timed release at bedtime or every 8-10 hours

Dosage Forms

Syrup: 2 mg/5 mL

dexchlorpheniramine and pseudoephedrine
(deks klor fen EER a meen & soo doe e FED rin)

Synonyms pseudoephedrine tannate and dexchlorpheniramine tannate

U.S./Canadian Brand Names SuTan [US]

Therapeutic Category Alpha/Beta Agonist; Antihistamine

Use Relief of nasal congestion associated with the common cold, hay fever, and other allergies, sinusitis, and vasomotor and allergic rhinitis

Usual Dosage Oral: Rhinitis/decongestant:

Children:

2-6 years: 2.5-5 mL every 12 hours (maximum: 10 mL/24 hours)

6-12 years: 5-7.5 mL every 12 hours (maximum: 15 mL/24 hours)

Children ≥12 years and Adults: 15 mL every 12 hours (maximum: 30 mL/24 hours)

Dosage Forms

Suspension:

SuTan: Dexchlorpheniramine 3 mg and pseudoephedrine 50 mg per 5 mL

dexchlorpheniramine maleate *see* dexchlorpheniramine *on page 290*

dexchlorpheniramine tannate, pseudoephedrine tannate, and dextromethorphan tannate *see* chlorpheniramine, pseudoephedrine, and dextromethorphan *on page 220*

Dexcon-DM *(Discontinued)* *see* guaifenesin, dextromethorphan, and phenylephrine *on page 478*

Dexcon-PE [US] *see* guaifenesin, dextromethorphan, and phenylephrine *on page 478*

Dexedrine® [US/Can] *see* dextroamphetamine *on page 293*

Dexferrum® [US] *see* iron dextran complex *on page 546*

DexFol™ [US] *see* vitamin B complex combinations *on page 1017*

Dexiron™ [Can] *see* iron dextran complex *on page 546*

dexlansoprazole (deks lan SOE pra zole)

Sound-Alike/Look-Alike Issues

dexlansoprazole may be confused with aripiprazole, lansoprazole

Synonyms TAK-390MR

U.S./Canadian Brand Names Kapidex™ [US]

Therapeutic Category Proton Pump Inhibitor; Substituted Benzimidazole

Use Short-term (4 weeks) treatment of heartburn associated with nonerosive GERD; short-term (up to 8 weeks) treatment of all grades of erosive esophagitis; to maintain healing of erosive esophagitis for up to 6 months

Usual Dosage Oral: Adults:

Erosive esophagitis: Short-term treatment: 60 mg once daily for up to 8 weeks; maintenance therapy: 30 mg once daily for up to 6 months

Symptomatic GERD: Short-term treatment: 30 mg once daily for 4 weeks

Dosage Forms

Capsule, delayed release:

Kapidex™: 30 mg, 60 mg

dexmedetomidine (deks MED e toe mi deen)

Sound-Alike/Look-Alike Issues
Precedex® may be confused with Peridex®

Synonyms dexmedetomidine hydrochloride

U.S./Canadian Brand Names Precedex® [US/Can]

Therapeutic Category Alpha-Adrenergic Agonist - Central-Acting ($Alpha_2$-Agonists); Sedative

Use Sedation of initially intubated and mechanically ventilated patients during treatment in an intensive care setting; sedation prior to and/or during surgical or other procedures of nonintubated patients

Usual Dosage Individualized and titrated to desired clinical effect. Manufacturer recommends duration of infusion should not exceed 24 hours; however, randomized clinical trials have demonstrated efficacy and safety comparable to lorazepam and midazolam with longer-term infusions of up to approximately 5 days.
ICU sedation:
Adults: I.V.: Initial: Loading infusion (optional; see **"Note"** below) of 1 mcg/kg over 10 minutes, followed by a maintenance infusion of 0.2-0.7 mcg/kg/hour; adjust rate to desired level of sedation; titration no more frequently than every 30 minutes may reduce the incidence of hypotension
Note: *Loading infusion:* Administration of a loading infusion may increase the risk of hemodynamic compromise. For this indication, the loading dose may be omitted. *Maintenance infusion:* Dosing ranges between 0.2-1.4 mcg/kg/hour have been reported during randomized controlled clinical trials. Although infusion rates as high as 2.5 mcg/kg/hour have been used, it is thought that doses >1.5 mcg/kg/hour do not add to clinical efficacy.
Procedural sedation: Adults: I.V.: Initial: Loading infusion of 1 mcg/kg (or 0.5 mcg/kg for less invasive procedures [eg, ophthalmic]) over 10 minutes, followed by a maintenance infusion of 0.6 mcg/kg/hour, titrate to desired effect; usual range: 0.2-1 mcg/kg/hour
Fiberoptic intubation (awake): I.V. Initial: Loading infusion of 1 mcg/kg over 10 minutes, followed by a maintenance infusion of 0.7 mcg/kg/hour until endotracheal tube is secured.

Dosage Forms
Injection, solution [preservative free]:
Precedex®: 100 mcg/mL (2 mL)

dexmedetomidine hydrochloride *see* dexmedetomidine *on page* 291

dexmethylphenidate (dex meth il FEN i date)

Sound-Alike/Look-Alike Issues
dexmethylphenidate may be confused with methadone

Synonyms dexmethylphenidate hydrochloride

U.S./Canadian Brand Names Focalin® XR [US]; Focalin® [US]

Therapeutic Category Central Nervous System Stimulant, Nonamphetamine

Controlled Substance C-II

Use Treatment of attention-deficit/hyperactivity disorder (ADHD)

Usual Dosage Treatment of ADHD: Oral:
Children ≥6 years: Patients not currently taking methylphenidate:
Tablet: Initial: 2.5 mg twice daily; dosage may be adjusted in increments of 2.5-5 mg at weekly intervals (maximum dose: 20 mg/day); doses should be taken at least 4 hours apart
Capsule: Initial: 5 mg/day; dosage may be adjusted in increments of 5 mg/day at weekly intervals (maximum dose: 20 mg/day)
Adults: Patients not currently taking methylphenidate:
Tablet: Initial: 2.5 mg twice daily; dosage may be adjusted in increments of 2.5-5 mg at weekly intervals (maximum dose: 20 mg/day); doses should be taken at least 4 hours apart
Capsule: Initial: 10 mg/day; dosage may be adjusted in increments of 10 mg/day at weekly intervals (maximum dose: 20 mg/day)

Dosage Forms
Capsule, extended release:
Focalin® XR: 5 mg, 10 mg, 15 mg, 20 mg
Tablet: 2.5 mg, 5 mg, 10 mg
Focalin®: 2.5 mg, 5 mg, 10 mg

dexmethylphenidate hydrochloride *see* dexmethylphenidate *on page* 291

DexPak® TaperPak® [US] *see* dexamethasone (systemic) *on page* 288

dexpanthenol (deks PAN the nole)

Synonyms pantothenyl alcohol

Therapeutic Category Gastrointestinal Agent, Stimulant

Use Prophylactic use to minimize paralytic ileus; treatment of postoperative distention; topical to relieve itching and to aid healing of minor dermatoses

Usual Dosage I.M.: Adults:

Prevention of postoperative ileus: 250-500 mg stat, repeat in 2 hours, followed by doses every 6 hours until danger passes

Paralytic ileus: 500 mg stat, repeat in 2 hours, followed by doses every 6 hours, if needed

Dosage Forms

Injection, solution [preservative free]: 250 mg/mL (2 mL)

Dex PC [US] *see* chlorpheniramine, phenylephrine, and dextromethorphan *on page 217*

dexrazoxane (deks ray ZOKS ane)

Sound-Alike/Look-Alike Issues

Zinecard® may be confused with Gemzar®

Synonyms ICRF-187; NSC-169780

U.S./Canadian Brand Names Totect™ [US]; Zinecard® [US/Can]

Therapeutic Category Cardiovascular Agent, Other

Use

Zinecard®: Reduction of the incidence and severity of cardiomyopathy associated with doxorubicin administration in women with metastatic breast cancer who have received a cumulative doxorubicin dose of 300 mg/m^2 and who would benefit from continuing therapy with doxorubicin. (Not recommended for use with initial doxorubicin therapy.)

Totect™: Treatment of anthracycline-induced extravasation.

Usual Dosage I.V.: Adults:

Prevention of doxorubicin cardiomyopathy: A 10:1 ratio of dexrazoxane:doxorubicin (500 mg/m^2 dexrazoxane: 50 mg/m^2 doxorubicin). **Note:** Cardiac monitoring should continue during dexrazoxane therapy; doxorubicin/dexrazoxane should be discontinued in patients who develop a decline in LVEF or clinical CHF.

Treatment of anthracycline extravasation: 1000 mg/m^2 on days 1 and 2 (maximum dose: 2000 mg), followed by 500 mg/m^2 on day 3 (maximum dose: 1000 mg); begin treatment as soon as possible, within 6 hours of extravasation

Dosage Forms

Injection, powder for reconstitution: 250 mg, 500 mg

Totect™: 500 mg

Zinecard®: 250 mg, 500 mg

dextran (DEKS tran)

Sound-Alike/Look-Alike Issues

dextran may be confused with Dexatrim®, Dexedrine®

Synonyms dextran 40; dextran 70; dextran, high molecular weight; dextran, low molecular weight

U.S./Canadian Brand Names Gentran® [Can]; LMD® [US]

Therapeutic Category Plasma Volume Expander

Use Blood volume expander used in treatment of shock or impending shock when blood or blood products are not available; dextran 40 is also used as a priming fluid in cardiopulmonary bypass and for prophylaxis of venous thrombosis and pulmonary embolism in surgical procedures associated with a high risk of thromboembolic complications

Usual Dosage I.V. (requires an infusion pump): Dose and infusion rate are dependent upon the patient's fluid status and must be individualized:

Volume expansion/shock:

Children (Dextran 40 or 70): Total dose should not exceed 20 mL/kg during first 24 hours

Adults:

Dextran 40: 500-1000 mL at a rate of 20-40 mL/minute (maximum: 20 mL/kg/day for first 24 hours); 10 mL/kg/day thereafter; therapy should not be continued beyond 5 days

Dextran 70: 500-1000 mL at a rate of 20-40 mL/minute (maximum: 20 mL/kg/day for first 24 hours)

Pump prime (Dextran 40): Varies with the volume of the pump oxygenator; generally, the 10% solution is added in a dose of 1-2 g/kg

Prophylaxis of venous thrombosis/pulmonary embolism (Dextran 40): Begin during surgical procedure and give 50-100 g on the day of surgery; an additional 50 g (500 mL) should be administered every 2-3 days during the period of risk (up to 2 weeks postoperatively); usual maximum infusion rate for nonemergency use: 4 mL/minute

Dosage Forms

Infusion [premixed in D_5W; low molecular weight]:
LMD®: 10% Dextran 40 (500 mL)

Infusion [premixed in NS; low molecular weight]:
LMD®: 10% Dextran (500 mL)

dextran 1 ***(Discontinued)***

dextran 40 *see* dextran *on page 292*

dextran 70 *see* dextran *on page 292*

dextran, high molecular weight *see* dextran *on page 292*

dextran, low molecular weight *see* dextran *on page 292*

dextroamphetamine (deks troe am FET a meen)

Sound-Alike/Look-Alike Issues

dextroamphetamine may be confused with dexamethasone
Dexedrine® may be confused with dextran, Excedrin®

Synonyms dextroamphetamine sulfate

U.S./Canadian Brand Names Dexedrine® [US/Can]; DextroStat® [US]; Liquadd™ [US]

Therapeutic Category Amphetamine

Controlled Substance C-II

Use Narcolepsy; attention-deficit/hyperactivity disorder (ADHD)

Usual Dosage Oral:

Children:

Narcolepsy: 6-12 years: Initial: 5 mg/day; may increase at 5 mg increments in weekly intervals until side effects appear (maximum dose: 60 mg/day)

ADHD:

3-5 years: Initial: 2.5 mg/day given every morning; increase by 2.5 mg/day in weekly intervals until optimal response is obtained; usual range: 0.1-0.5 mg/kg/dose every morning with maximum of 40 mg/day

≥6 years: 5 mg once or twice daily; increase in increments of 5 mg/day at weekly intervals until optimal response is obtained; usual range: 0.1-0.5 mg/kg/dose every morning (5-20 mg/day) with maximum of 40 mg/day

Children >12 years and Adults: Narcolepsy: Initial: 10 mg/day, may increase at 10 mg increments in weekly intervals until side effects appear; maximum: 60 mg/day

Dosage Forms

Capsule, extended release: 5 mg, 10 mg, 15 mg

Capsule, sustained release:
Dexedrine® Spansule®: 5 mg, 10 mg, 15 mg

Tablet: 5 mg, 10 mg
DextroStat®: 5 mg, 10 mg

Solution, oral:
Liquadd™: 5 mg/5 mL

dextroamphetamine and amphetamine (deks troe am FET a meen & am FET a meen)

Sound-Alike/Look-Alike Issues

Adderall® may be confused with Inderal®

Synonyms amphetamine and dextroamphetamine

U.S./Canadian Brand Names Adderall XR® [US/Can]; Adderall® [US]

Therapeutic Category Amphetamine

Controlled Substance C-II

Use Attention-deficit/hyperactivity disorder (ADHD); narcolepsy

Usual Dosage Oral: **Note:** Use lowest effective individualized dose; administer first dose as soon as awake

ADHD:

Children: 3-5 years (Adderall®): Initial 2.5 mg/day given every morning; increase daily dose in 2.5 mg increments at weekly intervals until optimal response is obtained (maximum dose: 40 mg/day given in 1-3 divided doses); use intervals of 4-6 hours between additional doses

Children: ≥6 years:

Adderall®: Initial: 5 mg 1-2 times/day; increase daily dose in 5 mg increments at weekly intervals until optimal response is obtained (usual maximum dose: 40 mg/day given in 1-3 divided doses); use intervals of 4-6 hours between additional doses

Adderall XR®: 5-10 mg once daily in the morning; if needed, may increase daily dose in 5-10 mg increments at weekly intervals (maximum dose: 30 mg/day)

Adolescents 13-17 years (Adderall XR®): 10 mg once daily in the morning; may be increased to 20 mg/day after 1 week if symptoms are not controlled; higher doses (up to 60 mg)/day have been evaluated; however, there is not adequate evidence that higher doses afforded additional benefit.

Adults (Adderall XR®): Initial: 20 mg once daily in the morning; higher doses (up to 60 mg once daily) have been evaluated; however, there is not adequate evidence that higher doses afforded additional benefit

Narcolepsy (Adderall®):

Children: 6-12 years: Initial: 5 mg/day; increase daily dose in 5 mg at weekly intervals until optimal response is obtained (maximum dose: 60 mg/day given in 1-3 divided doses with intervals of 4-6 hours between doses)

Children >12 years and Adults: Initial: 10 mg/day; increase daily dose in 10 mg increments at weekly intervals until optimal response is obtained (maximum dose: 60 mg/day given in 1-3 divided doses with intervals of 4-6 hours between doses)

Dosage Forms

Capsule, extended release:

5 mg [dextroamphetamine sulfate 1.25 mg, dextroamphetamine saccharate 1.25 mg, amphetamine aspartate monohydrate 1.25 mg, amphetamine sulfate 1.25 mg]

10 mg [dextroamphetamine sulfate 2.5 mg, dextroamphetamine saccharate 2.5 mg, amphetamine aspartate monohydrate 2.5 mg, amphetamine sulfate 2.5 mg]

15 mg [dextroamphetamine sulfate 3.75 mg, dextroamphetamine saccharate 3.75 mg, amphetamine aspartate monohydrate 3.75 mg, amphetamine sulfate 3.75 mg]

20 mg [dextroamphetamine sulfate 5 mg, dextroamphetamine saccharate 5 mg, amphetamine aspartate monohydrate 5 mg, amphetamine sulfate 5 mg]

25 mg [dextroamphetamine sulfate 6.25 mg, dextroamphetamine saccharate 6.25 mg, amphetamine aspartate monohydrate 6.25 mg, amphetamine sulfate 6.25 mg]

30 mg [dextroamphetamine sulfate 7.5 mg, dextroamphetamine saccharate 7.5 mg, amphetamine aspartate monohydrate 7.5 mg, amphetamine sulfate 7.5 mg]

Adderall XR®:

5 mg [dextroamphetamine 1.25 mg, dextroamphetamine saccharate 1.25 mg, amphetamine aspartate monohydrate 1.25 mg, amphetamine sulfate 1.25 mg]

10 mg [dextroamphetamine sulfate 2.5 mg, dextroamphetamine saccharate 2.5 mg, amphetamine aspartate monohydrate 2.5 mg, amphetamine sulfate 2.5 mg]

15 mg [dextroamphetamine sulfate 3.75 mg, dextroamphetamine saccharate 3.75 mg, amphetamine aspartate monohydrate 3.75 mg, amphetamine sulfate 3.75 mg]

20 mg [dextroamphetamine sulfate 5 mg, dextroamphetamine saccharate 5 mg, amphetamine aspartate monohydrate 5 mg, amphetamine sulfate 5 mg]

25 mg [dextroamphetamine sulfate 6.25 mg, dextroamphetamine saccharate 6.25 mg, amphetamine aspartate monohydrate 6.25 mg, amphetamine sulfate 6.25 mg]

30 mg [dextroamphetamine sulfate 7.5 mg, dextroamphetamine saccharate 7.5 mg, amphetamine aspartate monohydrate 7.5 mg, amphetamine sulfate 7.5 mg]

Tablet: 5 mg, 7.5 mg, 10 mg, 12.5 mg, 15 mg, 20 mg, 30 mg

5 mg [dextroamphetamine sulfate 1.25 mg, dextroamphetamine saccharate 1.25 mg, amphetamine aspartate monohydrate 1.25 mg, amphetamine sulfate 1.25 mg]

7.5 mg [dextroamphetamine sulfate 1.875 mg, dextroamphetamine saccharate 1.875 mg, amphetamine aspartate monohydrate 1.875 mg, amphetamine sulfate 1.875 mg]

10 mg [dextroamphetamine sulfate 2.5 mg, dextroamphetamine saccharate 2.5 mg, amphetamine aspartate monohydrate 2.5 mg, amphetamine sulfate 2.5 mg]

12.5 mg [dextroamphetamine sulfate 3.125 mg, dextroamphetamine saccharate 3.125 mg, amphetamine aspartate monohydrate 3.125 mg, amphetamine sulfate 3.125 mg]

15 mg [dextroamphetamine sulfate 3.75 mg, dextroamphetamine saccharate 3.75 mg, amphetamine aspartate monohydrate 3.75 mg, amphetamine sulfate 3.75 mg]

20 mg [dextroamphetamine sulfate 5 mg, dextroamphetamine saccharate 5 mg, amphetamine aspartate monohydrate 5 mg, amphetamine sulfate 5 mg]
30 mg [dextroamphetamine sulfate 7.5 mg, dextroamphetamine saccharate 7.5 mg, amphetamine aspartate monohydrate 7.5 mg, amphetamine sulfate 7.5 mg]
Adderall®:
5 mg [dextroamphetamine sulfate 1.25 mg, dextroamphetamine saccharate 1.25 mg, amphetamine aspartate monohydrate 1.25 mg, amphetamine sulfate 1.25 mg]
7.5 mg [dextroamphetamine 1.875 mg, dextroamphetamine saccharate 1.875 mg, amphetamine aspartate monohydrate 1.875 mg, amphetamine sulfate 1.875 mg]
10 mg [dextroamphetamine sulfate 2.5 mg, dextroamphetamine saccharate 2.5 mg, amphetamine aspartate monohydrate 2.5 mg, amphetamine sulfate 2.5 mg]
12.5 mg [dextroamphetamine sulfate 3.125 mg, dextroamphetamine saccharate 3.125 mg, amphetamine aspartate monohydrate 3.125 mg, amphetamine sulfate 3.125 mg]
15 mg [dextroamphetamine sulfate 3.75 mg, dextroamphetamine saccharate 3.75 mg, amphetamine aspartate monohydrate 3.75 mg, amphetamine sulfate 3.75 mg]
20 mg [dextroamphetamine sulfate 5 mg, dextroamphetamine saccharate 5 mg, amphetamine aspartate monohydrate 5 mg, amphetamine sulfate 5 mg]
30 mg [dextroamphetamine sulfate 7.5 mg, dextroamphetamine saccharate 7.5 mg, amphetamine aspartate monohydrate 7.5 mg, amphetamine sulfate 7.5 mg]

dextroamphetamine sulfate *see* dextroamphetamine *on page* 293

dextromethorphan (deks troe meth OR fan)

Sound-Alike/Look-Alike Issues
Benylin® may be confused with Benadryl®, Ventolin®
Delsym® may be confused with Delfen®, Desyrel®

U.S./Canadian Brand Names Creo-Terpin® [US-OTC]; Creomulsion® Adult Formula [US-OTC]; Creomulsion® for Children [US-OTC]; Delsym® [US-OTC]; Father John's® [US-OTC]; Hold® DM [US-OTC]; Nycoff [US-OTC]; PediaCare® Children's Long-Acting Cough [US-OTC]; Robafen Cough [US-OTC]; Robitussin® Children's Cough Long Acting [US-OTC]; Robitussin® Cough Long-Acting [US-OTC]; Robitussin® CoughGels™ [US-OTC]; Scot-Tussin® Diabetes [US-OTC]; Silphen DM® [US-OTC]; Triaminic® Children's Cough Long Acting [US-OTC]; Triaminic® Thin Strips® Children's Long Acting Cough [US-OTC]; Trocal® [US-OTC]; Vicks® 44® Cough Relief [US-OTC]; Vicks® DayQuil® Cough [US-OTC]

Therapeutic Category Antitussive

Use Symptomatic relief of coughs caused by the common cold or inhaled irritants

Usual Dosage Oral:
Children:
<4 years: Not for OTC use
4-6 years (syrup): 2.5-7.5 mg every 4-8 hours; extended release is 15 mg twice daily (maximum: 30 mg/24 hours)
6-12 years: 5-10 mg every 4 hours or 15 mg every 6-8 hours; extended release is 30 mg twice daily (maximum: 60 mg/24 hours)
Children >12 years and Adults: 10-20 mg every 4 hours or 30 mg every 6-8 hours; extended release: 60 mg twice daily; maximum: 120 mg/day

Dosage Forms
Capsule, liquid filled, oral:
Robafen Cough [OTC], Robitussin® CoughGels™ [OTC]: 15 mg
Liquid, oral:
Creo-Terpin® [OTC]: 10 mg/15 mL
Scot-Tussin® Diabetes [OTC], Vicks® 44® Cough Relief [OTC]: 10 mg/5 mL
Lozenge, oral:
Hold® DM [OTC]: 5 mg
Trocal® [OTC]: 7.5 mg
Solution, oral:
PediaCare® Children's Long-Acting Cough [OTC]: 7.5 mg/5 mL
Vicks® DayQuil® Cough [OTC]: 15 mg/15 mL
Strips, orally disintegrating:
Triaminic® Thin Strips® Children's Long Acting Cough [OTC]: 7.5 mg
Suspension, extended release, oral:
Delsym® [OTC]: Dextromethorphan polistirex [equivalent to dextromethorphan hydrobromide 30 mg/5 mL]

Syrup, oral:

Creomulsion® Adult Formula [OTC]: 20 mg/15 mL

Creomulsion® for Children [OTC]: 5 mg/5 mL

Father John's® [OTC], Silphen DM® [OTC]: 10 mg/5 mL

Robitussin® Children's Cough Long Acting [OTC], Triaminic® Children's Cough Long Acting [OTC]: 7.5 mg/5 mL

Robitussin® Cough Long-Acting [OTC]: 15 mg/5 mL

Tablet, oral:

Nycoff [OTC]: 15 mg

dextromethorphan and chlorpheniramine (deks troe meth OR fan & klor fen IR a meen)

Synonyms chlorpheniramine and dextromethorphan; chlorpheniramine maleate and dextromethorphan hydrobromide; dextromethorphan hydrobromide and chlorpheniramine maleate

U.S./Canadian Brand Names Coricidin® HBP Cough & Cold [US-OTC]; Dimetapp® Children's Long Acting Cough Plus Cold [US-OTC]; Robitussin® Children's Cough & Cold Long-Acting [US-OTC]; Robitussin® Cough & Cold Long-Acting [US-OTC]; Scot-Tussin® DM Maximum Strength [US-OTC]; Triaminic® Children's Softchews® Cough & Runny Nose [US-OTC]

Therapeutic Category Antitussive; Histamine H_1 Antagonist; Histamine H_1 Antagonist, First Generation

Use Symptomatic relief of runny nose, sneezing, itchy/watery eyes, cough, and other upper respiratory symptoms associated with hay fever, common cold, or upper respiratory allergies

Usual Dosage General dosing guidelines; consult specific product labeling.

Antitussive/antihistamine: Oral:

Children: 6-11 years: Dextromethorphan 15 mg and chlorpheniramine 2 mg every 6 hours as needed (maximum: 60 mg dextromethorphan and 8 mg chlorpheniramine/24 hours)

Children ≥12 years and Adults: Dextromethorphan 30 mg and chlorpheniramine 4 mg every 6 hours as needed (maximum: 120 mg dextromethorphan and 16 mg chlorpheniramine/24 hours)

Dosage Forms

Syrup:

Dimetapp® Children's Long Acting Cough Plus Cold [OTC]: Dextromethorphan 7.5 mg and chlorpheniramine 1 mg per 5 mL (118 mL)

Robitussin® Children's Cough and Cold Long-Acting [OTC]: Dextromethorphan 15 mg and chlorpheniramine 2 mg per 5 mL (118 mL)

Robitussin® Cough and Cold Long-Acting [OTC]: Dextromethorphan 15 mg and chlorpheniramine 2 mg per 5 mL (118 mL)

Scot-Tussin® DM Maximum Strength [OTC]: Dextromethorphan 15 mg and chlorpheniramine 2 mg per 5 mL (118 mL)

Tablet:

Coricidin® HBP Cough and Cold [OTC]: Dextromethorphan 30 mg and chlorpheniramine 4 mg

Tablet, softchew:

Triaminic® Children's Softchews® Cough & Runny Nose [OTC]: Dextromethorphan 5 mg and chlorpheniramine 1 mg

dextromethorphan and guaifenesin *see* guaifenesin and dextromethorphan *on page* 474

dextromethorphan and phenylephrine (deks troe meth OR fan & fen il EF rin)

Synonyms dextromethorphan hydrobromide and phenylephrine hydrochloride; phenylephrine and dextromethorphan

U.S./Canadian Brand Names PediaCare® Children's Multi-Symptom Cold [US-OTC]; Safetussin® CD [US-OTC]; Triaminic Thin Strips® Children's Day Time Cold & Cough [US-OTC]; Triaminic® Day Time Cold & Cough [US-OTC]

Therapeutic Category Antitussive; Decongestant

Use Temporary relief of symptoms of hay fever, the common cold, and upper respiratory allergies including: sinus/nasal congestion, minor bronchial/throat irritation, and cough

Usual Dosage Oral: Relief of nasal/sinus congestion and cough:

Children:

4-6 years:

PediaCare® Children's Multi-Symptom Cold, Triaminic® Day Time Cold & Cough: 5 mL every 4 hours as needed (maximum: 30 mL/24 hours)

Triaminic Thin Strips® Children's Day Time Cold & Cough: Allow 1 strip to dissolve on tongue every 4 hours as needed (maximum: 6 strips/24 hours)

6-12 years:
PediaCare® Children's Multi-Symptom Cold, Triaminic® Day Time Cold & Cough: 10 mL every 4 hours as needed (maximum: 60 mL/24 hours)
Safetussin® CD: 5 mL every 6 hours as needed (maximum: 20 mL/24 hours)
Triaminic Thin Strips® Children's Day Time Cold & Cough: Allow 2 strips to dissolve on tongue every 4 hours as needed (maximum: 12 strips/24 hours)
Children ≥12 years and Adults: Safetussin® CD: 10 mL every 6 hours as needed (maximum: 40 mL/24 hours)

Dosage Forms

Strip, orally disintegrating:
Triaminic Thin Strips® Children's Day Time Cold & Cough [OTC]: Dextromethorphan bromide 5 mg and phenylephrine 2.5 mg (14s, 16s, 48s)

Syrup:
PediaCare® Children's Multi-Symptom Cold [OTC], Triaminic® Day Time Cold & Cough [OTC]: Dextromethorphan 5 mg and phenylephrine 2.5 mg per 5 mL
Safetussin® CD [OTC]: Dextromethorphan 15 mg and phenylephrine 2.5 mg per 5 mL

dextromethorphan and promethazine *see* promethazine and dextromethorphan *on page* 824

dextromethorphan and pseudoephedrine *see* pseudoephedrine and dextromethorphan *on page* 834

dextromethorphan, chlorpheniramine, and phenylephrine *see* chlorpheniramine, phenylephrine, and dextromethorphan *on page* 217

dextromethorphan, chlorpheniramine, and pseudoephedrine *see* chlorpheniramine, pseudoephedrine, and dextromethorphan *on page* 220

dextromethorphan, chlorpheniramine, phenylephrine, and guaifenesin

(deks troe meth OR fan, klor fen IR a meen, fen il EF rin, & gwye FEN e sin)

Synonyms chlorpheniramine, dextromethorphan, phenylephrine, and guaifenesin; guaifenesin, chlorpheniramine, phenylephrine, and dextromethorphan; phenylephrine hydrochloride, chlorpheniramine maleate, dextromethorphan hydrobromide, and guaifenesin

U.S./Canadian Brand Names Chlordex GP [US]; Donatussin [US]; Quartuss™ [US]

Therapeutic Category Antihistamine/Decongestant/Antitussive/Expectorant

Use Symptomatic relief of dry, nonproductive cough and upper respiratory symptoms associated with infections such as the common cold, bronchitis, or sinusitis

Usual Dosage General dosing guidelines; consult specific product labeling.
Antitussive/antihistamine/decongestant/expectorant: Oral (Donatussin):
Children:
2-6 years: 2.5 mL every 6 hours as needed (maximum: 10 mL/24 hours)
6-12 years: 5 mL every 6 hours as needed (maximum: 20 mL/24 hours)
Children ≥12 years and Adults: 10 mL every 6 hours as needed (maximum: 40 mL/24 hours)

Dosage Forms

Syrup:
Chlordex GP: Dextromethorphan 7.5 mg, chlorpheniramine 2 mg, phenylephrine 10 mg, and guaifenesin 100 mg per 5 mL (480 mL)
Donatussin, Quartuss™: Dextromethorphan 15 mg, chlorpheniramine 2 mg, phenylephrine 10 mg, and guaifenesin 100 mg per 5 mL (480 mL)

dextromethorphan, guaifenesin, and pseudoephedrine *see* guaifenesin, pseudoephedrine, and dextromethorphan *on page* 479

dextromethorphan hydrobromide, acetaminophen, and doxylamine succinate *see* acetaminophen, dextromethorphan, and doxylamine *on page* 26

dextromethorphan hydrobromide, acetaminophen, and phenylephrine hydrochloride *see* acetaminophen, dextromethorphan, and phenylephrine *on page* 27

dextromethorphan hydrobromide, acetaminophen, doxylamine succinate, and pseudoephedrine hydrochloride *see* acetaminophen, dextromethorphan, doxylamine, and pseudoephedrine *on page* 28

dextromethorphan hydrobromide and chlorpheniramine maleate *see* dextromethorphan and chlorpheniramine *on page* 296

dextromethorphan hydrobromide and phenylephrine hydrochloride *see* dextromethorphan and phenylephrine *on page* 296

dextromethorphan hydrobromide, brompheniramine maleate, and pseudoephedrine hydrochloride *see* brompheniramine, pseudoephedrine, and dextromethorphan *on page 152*

dextromethorphan tannate, pyrilamine tannate, and phenylephrine tannate *see* phenylephrine, pyrilamine, and dextromethorphan *on page 778*

dextropropoxyphene *see* propoxyphene *on page 827*

dextrose (DEKS trose)

Sound-Alike/Look-Alike Issues

Glutose™ may be confused with Glutofac®

Synonyms anhydrous glucose; $D_{10}W$; $D_{25}W$; $D_{30}W$; $D_{40}W$; $D_{50}W$; D_5W; $D_{60}W$; $D_{70}W$; dextrose monohydrate; glucose; glucose monohydrate; glycosum

U.S./Canadian Brand Names B-D™ Glucose [US-OTC]; Dex4® [US-OTC]; Enfamil® Glucose [US]; GlucoBurst® [US-OTC]; Glutol™ [US-OTC]; Glutose 15™ [US-OTC]; Glutose 45™ [US-OTC]; Insta-Glucose® [US-OTC]; Similac® Glucose [US]

Therapeutic Category Antidote, Hypoglycemia; Intravenous Nutritional Therapy

Use

Oral: Treatment of hypoglycemia

5% and 10% solutions: Peripheral infusion to provide calories and fluid replacement

25% (hypertonic) solution: Treatment of acute symptomatic episodes of hypoglycemia in infants and children to restore depressed blood glucose levels; adjunctive treatment of hyperkalemia when combined with insulin

50% (hypertonic) solution: Treatment of insulin-induced hypoglycemia (hyperinsulinemia or insulin shock) and adjunctive treatment of hyperkalemia in adolescents and adults

≥10% solutions: Infusion after admixture with amino acids for nutritional support

Usual Dosage

Hypoglycemia: Doses may be repeated in severe cases

I.V.:

Infants ≤6 months: 0.25-0.5 g/kg/dose (1-2 mL/kg/dose of 25% solution); maximum: 25 g/dose

Infants >6 months and Children: 0.5-1 g/kg/dose (2-4 mL/kg/dose of 25% solution); maximum: 25 g/dose

Adolescents and Adults: 10-25 g (40-100 mL of 25% solution or 20-50 mL of 50% solution)

Oral: Children >2 years and Adults: 10-20 g as single dose; repeat in 10 minutes if necessary

Treatment of Hyperkalemia: I.V. (in combination with insulin):

Infants and Children: 0.5-1 g/kg (using 25% or 50% solution) combined with regular insulin 1 unit for every 4-5 g dextrose given; infuse over 2 hours (infusions as short as 30 minutes have been recommended); repeat as needed

Adolescents and Adults: 25-50 g dextrose (250-500 mL $D_{10}W$) combined with 10 units regular insulin administered over 30-60 minutes; repeat as needed or as an alternative 25 g dextrose (50 mL $D_{50}W$) combined with 5-10 units regular insulin infused over 5 minutes; repeat as needed

Note: More rapid infusions (<30 minutes) may be associated with hyperglycemia and hyperosmolality and will exacerbate hyperkalemia; avoid use in patients who are already hyperglycemic

Dosage Forms

Gel, oral:

Dex4® [OTC]: 40% (38 g)

GlucoBurst® [OTC]: 40% (375 g)

Glutose 15™ [OTC]: 40% (37.5 g)

Glutose 45™ [OTC]: 40% (112.5 g)

Insta-Glucose® [OTC]: 40% (30 g)

Infusion:

Generics:

2.5% (1000 mL)

5% (25 mL, 50 mL, 100 mL, 150 mL, 250 mL, 500 mL, 1000 mL)

10% (250 mL, 500 mL, 1000 mL)

20% (500 mL)

30% (500 mL)

40% (500 mL)

50% (500 mL, 1000 mL, 2000 mL)

60% (500 mL, 1000 mL)

70% (500 mL, 1000 mL, 2000 mL)

Injection, solution: 10% (5 mL); 25% (10 mL); 50% (50 mL)

Injection, solution: 5% (10 mL)

...al:
...[OTC]: 15 g/60 mL
...ion, oral:
...ifamil® Glucose: 5%
Glutol™ [OTC]: 55%
Similac® Glucose: 5%
Tablet, chewable:
BD™ Glucose [OTC]: 5 g
Dex4® [OTC]: 4 g
GlucoBurst® [OTC]: 5 g

Diastat® AcuDial™ [US] *see* diazepam *on page 301*

Diastat® Rectal Delivery System [Can] *see* diazepam *on page 301*

diatrizoate meglumine (dye a tri ZOE ate MEG loo meen)

U.S./Canadian Brand Names Cystografin® Dilute [US]; Cystografin® [US]

Therapeutic Category Iodinated Contrast Media; Radiological/Contrast Media, Ionic

Use

Solution for instillation: Retrograde cystourethrography; retrograde or ascending pyelography

Solution for injection: Arthrography, cerebral angiography, direct cholangiography, discography, drip infusion pyelography, excretory urography, peripheral arteriography, splenoportography, venography; contrast enhancement of computed tomographic head and body imaging

Usual Dosage Dosing is based upon route of administration, type of examination, age of patient, and product used. Consult specific product information for detailed dosing.

Dosage Forms

Solution, for instillation:

Cystografin®: 30% (100 mL, 300 mL)

Cystografin® Dilute: 18% (300 mL)

diatrizoate meglumine and diatrizoate sodium
(dye a tri ZOE ate MEG loo meen & dye a tri ZOE ate SOW dee um)

Synonyms diatrizoate sodium and diatrizoate meglumine

U.S./Canadian Brand Names Gastrografin® [US]; MD-76®R [US]; MD-Gastroview® [US]

Therapeutic Category Iodinated Contrast Media; Radiological/Contrast Media, Ionic

Use

Oral/rectal: Examination of GI tract; adjunct to contrast enhancement in computed tomography of the torso

Injection: Angiocardiography, aortography, central venography, cerebral angiography, cholangiography, digital arteriography, excretory urography, nephrotomography, peripheral angiography, peripheral arteriography, renal arteriography, renal venography, splenoportography, visceral arteriography; contrast enhancement of computed tomographic imaging

Usual Dosage

Radiographic exam of GI tract segments:

Oral:

Children <5 years: 30 mL, dilute 1:1 (if <10 kg or debilitated, dilute 1:3)

Children 5-10 years: 60 mL, dilute 1:1 (if <10 kg or debilitated, dilute 1:3)

Adults: 30-90 mL

Rectal enema:

Children <5 years: Dilute 1:5 in tap water

Children >5 years: Dilute 90 mL in 500 mL tap water

Adults: Dilute 240 mL in 1000 mL tap water

Tomography: Adults: Oral: 25-77 mL in 1000 mL tap water 15-30 minutes prior to imaging

Dosage Forms

Solution, injection:

MD-76®R: Diatrizoate meglumine 660 mg and diatrizoate sodium 100 mg per 1 mL (50 mL, 100 mL, 200 mL)

Solution, oral/rectal:

Gastrografin®: Diatrizoate meglumine 660 mg and diatrizoate sodium 100 mg per 1 mL

MD-Gastroview®: Diatrizoate meglumine 660 mg and diatrizoate sodium 100 mg per 1 mL

diatrizoate meglumine and iodipamide meglumine
(dye a tri ZOE ate MEG loo meen & eye oh DI pa mide MEG loo meen)

Synonyms iodipamide meglumine and diatrizoate meglumine

U.S./Canadian Brand Names Sinografin® [US]

Therapeutic Category Iodinated Contrast Media; Radiological/Contrast Media, Ionic

Use Hysterosalpingography

Usual Dosage Intrauterine: Adults: Hysterosalpingography: Usual dose: 3-4 mL administered in fractional doses of ~1 mL; may give additional 3-4 mL to visualize tubes; total dosage range: 1.5-10 mL

Dosage Forms

Injection, solution [for intrauterine instillation]:

Sinografin®: Diatrizoate meglumine 524 mg and iodipamide meglumine 268 mg per mL (10 mL)

diatrizoate sodium (dye a tri ZOE ate SOW dee um)

U.S./Canadian Brand Names Hypaque™ Sodium [US]

Therapeutic Category Iodinated Contrast Media; Radiological/Contrast Media, Ionic

Use Radiographic examination of GI tract

Usual Dosage

Oral:

Infants and Children: 20% to 40% solution: 30-75 mL

Adults: 25% to 40% solution: 90-180 mL

Rectal: Enema:

Infants and Children: 10% to 15% solution: 100-500 mL depending on weight of patient

Adults: 15% to 25% solution: 500-1000 mL

Dosage Forms

Powder for solution, oral/rectal:

Hypaque™ Sodium: 100% (250 g)

diatrizoate sodium and diatrizoate meglumine *see* diatrizoate meglumine and diatrizoate sodium *on page 300*

Diatx®Zn [US] *see* vitamins (multiple/oral) *on page 1019*

Diazemuls® [Can] *see* diazepam *on page 301*

Diazemuls® Injection *(Discontinued)* *see* diazepam *on page 301*

diazepam (dye AZ e pam)

Sound-Alike/Look-Alike Issues

diazepam may be confused with diazoxide, diltiazem, Ditropan®, LORazepam

Valium® may be confused with Valcyte™

U.S./Canadian Brand Names Apo-Diazepam® [Can]; Diastat® AcuDial™ [US]; Diastat® Rectal Delivery System [Can]; Diastat® [US/Can]; Diazemuls® [Can]; Diazepam Intensol™ [US]; Novo-Dipam [Can]; Valium® [US/Can]

Therapeutic Category Benzodiazepine

Controlled Substance C-IV

Use Management of anxiety disorders, ethanol withdrawal symptoms; skeletal muscle relaxant; treatment of convulsive disorders; preoperative or preprocedural sedation and amnesia

Rectal gel: Management of selected, refractory epilepsy patients on stable regimens of antiepileptic drugs requiring intermittent use of diazepam to control episodes of increased seizure activity

Usual Dosage Oral absorption is more reliable than I.M.

Children:

Conscious sedation for procedures: Oral: 0.2-0.3 mg/kg (maximum: 10 mg) 45-60 minutes prior to procedure

Muscle spasm associated with tetanus: I.V., I.M.:

Infants >30 days: 1-2 mg/dose every 3-4 hours as needed

Children ≥5 years: 5-10 mg/dose every 3-4 hours as needed

Sedation/muscle relaxant/anxiety:

Oral: 0.12-0.8 mg/kg/day in divided doses every 6-8 hours

I.M., I.V.: 0.04-0.3 mg/kg/dose every 2-4 hours to a maximum of 0.6 mg/kg within an 8-hour period if needed

Status epilepticus:

I.V.: Infants >30 days and Children: 0.1-0.3 mg/kg given over ≤5 mg/minute; may repeat dose after 5-10 minutes; maximum: 10 mg/dose

Rectal gel: 0.5 mg/kg, then 0.25 mg/kg in 10 minutes if needed

Anticonvulsant (acute treatment): Rectal gel:

Children 2-5 years: 0.5 mg/kg

Children 6-11 years: 0.3 mg/kg

Children ≥12 years: 0.2 mg/kg

Note: Dosage should be rounded upward to the next available dose, 2.5, 5, 7.5, 10, 12.5, 15, 17.5, and 20 mg/dose; dose may be repeated in 4-12 hours if needed; do not use for more than 5 episodes per month or more than one episode every 5 days

Adolescents: Conscious sedation for procedures:
Oral: 10 mg
I.V.: 5 mg, may repeat with 1/2 dose if needed
Adults:
Acute ethanol withdrawal: Oral: 10 mg 3-4 times during first 24 hours, then decrease to 5 mg 3-4 times/day as needed
Anticonvulsant (acute treatment): Rectal gel: 0.2 mg/kg
Note: Dosage should be rounded upward to the next available dose, 2.5, 5, 7.5, 10, 12.5, 15, 17.5, and 20 mg/dose; dose may be repeated in 4-12 hours if needed; do not use for more than 5 episodes per month or more than one episode every 5 days.
Anxiety (symptoms/disorders):
Oral: 2-10 mg 2-4 times/day
I.M., I.V.: 2-10 mg, may repeat in 3-4 hours if needed
Muscle spasm: I.V., I.M.: Initial: 5-10 mg; then 5-10 mg in 3-4 hours, if necessary. Larger doses may be required if associated with tetanus.
Sedation in the ICU patient: I.V.: 0.03-0.1 mg/kg every 30 minutes to 6 hours
Skeletal muscle relaxant (adjunct therapy): Oral: 2-10 mg 3-4 times/day
Status epilepticus:
I.V.: 5-10 mg every 5-10 minutes given over ≤5 mg/minute; maximum dose: 30 mg
Rectal gel: Premonitory/out-of-hospital treatment: 10 mg once; may repeat once if necessary
Rapid tranquilization of agitated patient (administer every 30-60 minutes): Oral: 5-10 mg; average total dose for tranquilization: 20-60 mg

Dosage Forms
Gel, rectal [adult rectal tip (6 cm)]:
Diastat® AcuDial™: 20 mg (4 mL)
Gel, rectal [pediatric rectal tip (4.4 cm)]:
Diastat®: 5 mg/mL (0.5 mL)
Gel, rectal [pediatric/adult rectal tip (4.4 cm)]:
Diastat® AcuDial™: 10 mg (2 mL)
Injection, solution: 5 mg/mL (2 mL, 10 mL)
Solution, oral: 5 mg/5 mL
Solution, oral [concentrate]:
Diazepam Intensol™: 5 mg/mL
Tablet: 2 mg, 5 mg, 10 mg
Valium®: 2 mg, 5 mg, 10 mg

Diazepam Intensol™ [US] *see* diazepam *on page* 301

diazoxide (dye az OKS ide)

Sound-Alike/Look-Alike Issues
diazoxide may be confused with diazepam, Dyazide®

U.S./Canadian Brand Names Proglycem® [US/Can]

Therapeutic Category Antihypertensive Agent; Antihypoglycemic Agent

Use Hypoglycemia related to islet cell adenoma, carcinoma, hyperplasia, or adenomatosis; nesidioblastosis; leucine sensitivity; extrapancreatic malignancy

Usual Dosage Oral: Hyperinsulinemic hypoglycemia:
Newborns and Infants: Initial dose: 10 mg/kg/day; dosing range: 8-15 mg/kg/day in divided doses every 8-12 hours
Children and Adults: Initial dose: 3 mg/kg/day; dosing range: 3-8 mg/kg/day in divided doses every 8-12 hours. **Note:** In certain instances, patients with refractory hypoglycemia may require higher doses.

Dosage Forms [CAN] = Canadian brand name
Capsule, oral:
Proglycem® [CAN]: 50 mg [not available in the U.S.]
Suspension, oral:
Proglycem®: 50 mg/mL

Dibent® Injection *(Discontinued)* *see* dicyclomine *on page* 305
Dibenzyline® [US/Can] *see* phenoxybenzamine *on page* 773

dibucaine (DYE byoo kane)

U.S./Canadian Brand Names Nupercainal® [US-OTC]

Therapeutic Category Local Anesthetic

Use Fast, temporary relief of pain and itching due to hemorrhoids, minor burns

Usual Dosage Topical: Children and Adults: Apply gently to the affected areas; no more than 30 g for adults or 7.5 g for children should be used in any 24-hour period

Dosage Forms

Ointment, topical: 1% (30 g)

Nupercainal® [OTC]: 1% (30 g, 60g)

DIC *see* dacarbazine *on page 272*

Dicarbosil® ***(Discontinued)*** *see* calcium carbonate *on page 170*

Dicel™ [US] *see* chlorpheniramine and pseudoephedrine *on page 215*

Dicel™ DM [US] *see* chlorpheniramine, pseudoephedrine, and dextromethorphan *on page 220*

Dicetel® [Can] *see* pinaverium *(Canada only) on page 784*

dichloralphenazone, acetaminophen, and isometheptene *see* acetaminophen, isometheptene, and dichloralphenazone *on page 29*

dichloralphenazone, isometheptene, and acetaminophen *see* acetaminophen, isometheptene, and dichloralphenazone *on page 29*

dichlorodifluoromethane and trichloromonofluoromethane

(dye klor oh dye flor oh METH ane & tri klor oh mon oh flor oh METH ane)

Synonyms trichloromonofluoromethane and dichlorodifluoromethane

U.S./Canadian Brand Names Fluori-Methane® [US]

Therapeutic Category Analgesic, Topical

Use Management of pain associated with injections

Usual Dosage Invert bottle over treatment area approximately 12" away from site of application; open dispenseal spring valve completely, allowing liquid to flow in a stream from the bottle. The rate of spraying is approximately 10 cm/second and should be continued until entire muscle has been covered.

Dosage Forms

Aerosol, topical:

Fluori-Methane®: Dichlorodifluoromethane 15% and trichloromonofluoromethane 85% (103 mL)

dichlorotetrafluoroethane and ethyl chloride *see* ethyl chloride and dichlorotetrafluoroethane *on page 396*

dichlorphenamide ***(Discontinued)***

Dickinson's® Witch Hazel [US-OTC] *see* witch hazel *on page 1023*

Diclectin® [Can] *see* doxylamine and pyridoxine *(Canada only) on page 338*

diclofenac (dye KLOE fen ak)

Sound-Alike/Look-Alike Issues

diclofenac may be confused with Diflucan®, Duphalac®

Cataflam® may be confused with Catapres®

Voltaren® may be confused with traMADol, Ultram®, Verelan®

Synonyms diclofenac epolamine; diclofenac potassium; diclofenac sodium

U.S./Canadian Brand Names Apo-Diclo Rapide® [Can]; Apo-Diclo SR® [Can]; Apo-Diclo® [Can]; Cataflam® [US/Can]; Dom-Diclofenac SR [Can]; Dom-Diclofenac [Can]; Flector® [US]; Novo-Difenac K [Can]; Novo-Difenac [Can]; Novo-Difenac-SR [Can]; Nu-Diclo [Can]; Nu-Diclo-SR [Can]; Pennsaid® [Can]; PMS-Diclofenac SR [Can]; PMS-Diclofenac [Can]; Pro-Diclo-Rapide [Can]; Riva-Diclofenac [Can]; Riva-Diclofenac-K [Can]; Sab-Diclofenac [Can]; Sandoz-Diclofenac [Can]; Solaraze® [US]; Voltaren Ophthalmic® [US]; Voltaren Ophtha® [Can]; Voltaren Rapide® [Can]; Voltaren® Gel [US]; Voltaren® [US/Can]; Voltaren®-XR [US]

Therapeutic Category Analgesic, Nonnarcotic; Nonsteroidal Antiinflammatory Drug (NSAID)

Use

Immediate-release tablet: Ankylosing spondylitis; primary dysmenorrhea; acute and chronic treatment of rheumatoid arthritis, osteoarthritis

Delayed-release tablet: Acute and chronic treatment of rheumatoid arthritis, osteoarthritis, ankylosing spondylitis

Extended-release tablet: Chronic treatment of osteoarthritis, rheumatoid arthritis

Ophthalmic solution: Postoperative inflammation following cataract extraction; temporary relief of pain and photophobia in patients undergoing corneal refractive surgery

Topical gel 1%: Relief of osteoarthritis pain in joints amenable to topical therapy (eg, ankle, elbow, foot, hand, knee, wrist)

Topical gel 3%: Actinic keratosis (AK) in conjunction with sun avoidance
Topical patch: Acute pain due to minor strains, sprains, and contusions

Usual Dosage Adults:

Oral:

Analgesia/primary dysmenorrhea: Starting dose: 50 mg 3 times/day; maximum dose: 150 mg/day

Rheumatoid arthritis: 150-200 mg/day in 2-4 divided doses (100-200 mg/day of sustained release product)

Osteoarthritis: 100-150 mg/day in 2-3 divided doses (100-200 mg/day of sustained release product)

Ankylosing spondylitis: 100-125 mg/day in 4-5 divided doses

Ophthalmic:

Cataract surgery: Instill 1 drop into affected eye 4 times/day beginning 24 hours after cataract surgery and continuing for 2 weeks

Corneal refractive surgery: Instill 1-2 drops into affected eye within the hour prior to surgery, within 15 minutes following surgery, and then continue for 4 times/day, up to 3 days

Topical gel:

Actinic keratoses (Solaraze® Gel): Apply 3% gel to lesion area twice daily for 60-90 days

Osteoarthritis (Voltaren® Gel): **Note:** Maximum total body dose of 1% gel should not exceed 32 g per day

Lower extremities: Apply 4 g of 1% gel to affected area 4 times daily (maximum: 16 g per joint per day)

Upper extremities: Apply 2 g of 1% gel to affected area 4 times daily (maximum: 8 g per joint per day)

Transdermal patch: Acute pain (strains, sprains, contusions): Apply 1 patch twice daily to most painful area of skin

Dosage Forms

Gel:

Solaraze®: 3% (50 g, 100 g)

Voltaren® Gel: 1% (100 g)

Solution, ophthalmic [drops]: 0.1% (2.5 mL, 5 mL)

Voltaren Ophthalmic®: 0.1% (2.5 mL, 5 mL)

Tablet: 50 mg

Cataflam®: 50 mg

Tablet, delayed release, enteric coated: 50 mg, 75 mg

Voltaren®: 75 mg

Tablet, extended release: 100 mg

Voltaren®-XR: 100 mg

Transdermal system, topical:

Flector®: 1.3% (30s) [180 mg]

diclofenac and misoprostol (dye KLOE fen ak & mye soe PROST ole)

Synonyms misoprostol and diclofenac

U.S./Canadian Brand Names Arthrotec® [US/Can]

Therapeutic Category Analgesic, Nonnarcotic; Prostaglandin

Use The diclofenac component is indicated for the treatment of osteoarthritis and rheumatoid arthritis; the misoprostol component is indicated for the prophylaxis of NSAID-induced gastric and duodenal ulceration

Usual Dosage Oral: Adults:

Arthrotec® 50:

Osteoarthritis: 1 tablet 2-3 times/day

Rheumatoid arthritis: 1 tablet 3-4 times/day

For both regimens, if not tolerated by patient, the dose may be reduced to 1 tablet twice daily

Arthrotec® 75:

Patients who cannot tolerate full daily Arthrotec® 50 regimens: 1 tablet twice daily

Note: The use of these tablets may not be as effective at preventing GI ulceration

Dosage Forms

Tablet:

Arthrotec®: Diclofenac 50 mg and misoprostol 200 mcg; diclofenac 75 mg and misoprostol 200 mcg

diclofenac epolamine *see* diclofenac *on page 303*

diclofenac potassium *see* diclofenac *on page 303*

diclofenac sodium *see* diclofenac *on page 303*

dicloxacillin (dye kloks a SIL in)

Synonyms dicloxacillin sodium

U.S./Canadian Brand Names Dycill® [Can]; Pathocil® [Can]

Therapeutic Category Penicillin

Use Treatment of systemic infections such as pneumonia, skin and soft tissue infections, and osteomyelitis caused by penicillinase-producing staphylococci

Usual Dosage

Usual dosage range:

Children <40 kg: Oral: 12.5-100 mg/kg/day divided every 6 hours

Children >40 kg: Oral: 125-250 mg every 6 hours

Adults: Oral: 125-1000 mg every 6 hours

Indication-specific dosing:

Children: Oral:

Furunculosis: 25-50 mg/kg/day divided every 6 hours

Osteomyelitis: 50-100 mg/kg/day in divided doses every 6 hours

Adults: Oral:

Erysipelas, furunculosis, mastitis, otitis externa, septic bursitis, skin abscess: 500 mg every 6 hours

Impetigo: 250 mg every 6 hours

Prosthetic joint (long-term suppression therapy): 250 mg twice daily

***Staphylococcus aureus,* methicillin susceptible infection if no I.V. access:** 500-1000 mg every 6-8 hours

Dosage Forms

Capsule: 250 mg, 500 mg

dicloxacillin sodium *see* dicloxacillin *on page 304*

dicyclomine (dye SYE kloe meen)

Sound-Alike/Look-Alike Issues

dicyclomine may be confused with diphenhydrAMINE, doxycycline, dyclonine

Bentyl® may be confused with Aventyl®, Benadryl®, Bontril®, Cantil®, Proventil®, Trental®

Synonyms dicyclomine hydrochloride; dicycloverine hydrochloride

U.S./Canadian Brand Names Bentylol® [Can]; Bentyl® [US]; Formulex® [Can]; Lomine [Can]; Riva-Dicyclomine [Can]

Therapeutic Category Anticholinergic Agent

Use Treatment of functional bowel/irritable bowel syndrome

Usual Dosage Adults:

Oral: Initiate with 80 mg/day in 4 equally divided doses, then increase up to 160 mg/day. Duration: Safety data not available for duration >2 weeks.

I.M. **(should not be used I.V.)**: 80 mg/day in 4 divided doses (20 mg/dose)

Dosage Forms

Capsule: 10 mg

Bentyl®: 10 mg

Injection, solution: 10 mg/mL (2 mL)

Bentyl®: 10 mg/mL (2 mL)

Syrup:

Bentyl®: 10 mg/5 mL

Tablet: 20 mg

Bentyl®: 20 mg

dicyclomine hydrochloride *see* dicyclomine *on page 305*

dicycloverine hydrochloride *see* dicyclomine *on page 305*

Di-Dak-Sol [US] *see* sodium hypochlorite solution *on page 911*

didanosine (dye DAN oh seen)

Sound-Alike/Look-Alike Issues

Videx® may be confused with Lidex®

Synonyms ddI; dideoxyinosine

U.S./Canadian Brand Names Videx® EC [US/Can]; Videx® [US/Can]

Therapeutic Category Antiviral Agent

Use Treatment of HIV infection; always to be used in combination with at least two other antiretroviral agents

Usual Dosage Treatment of HIV infection: Oral (administer on an empty stomach):
Pediatric powder for oral solution (Videx®):
Infants: 2 weeks to 8 months: 100 mg/m^2 twice daily is recommended by the manufacturer; 50 mg/m^2 may be considered in infants 2 weeks to 4 months (AIDSinfo guidelines)
Infants and Children >8 months: 120 mg/m^2 twice daily is recommended by the manufacturer. **Note:** AIDSinfo guidelines suggest a range of 90-150 mg/m^2 twice daily
Children 3-21 years (AIDS*info* guidelines): Treatment-naive: 240 mg/m^2/dose once daily (maximum: 400 mg/dose)
Adolescents and Adults: Dosing based on patient weight:
<60 kg: 125 mg twice daily (preferred) or 250 mg once daily
≥60 kg: 200 mg twice daily (preferred) or 400 mg once daily
Delayed release capsule (Videx® EC): Children and Adults:
20 kg to <25 kg: 200 mg once daily
25 kg to <60 kg: 250 mg once daily
≥60 kg: 400 mg once daily

When taken with tenofovir: Adults:
<60 kg and Cl_{cr} ≥60 mL/minute: 200 mg once daily
≥60 kg and Cl_{cr} ≥60 mL/minute: 250 mg once daily

Dosage Forms
Capsule, delayed release, enteric coated pellets: 200 mg, 250 mg, 400 mg
Capsule, delayed release, enteric coated beadlets:
Videx® EC: 125 mg, 200 mg, 250 mg, 400 mg
Powder for oral solution, pediatric:
Videx®: 2 g, 4 g

dideoxyinosine *see* didanosine *on page 305*
Didrex® [US/Can] *see* benzphetamine *on page 134*
Didrocal™ [Can] *see* etidronate and calcium *(Canada only) on page 396*
Didronel® [US/Can] *see* etidronate disodium *on page 397*
dietary supplements *see* nutritional formula, enteral/oral *on page 715*

diethylene triamine penta-acetic acid

(dye ETH i leen TRYE a meen PEN ta a SEE tik AS id)

Synonyms Ca-DTPA; diethylenetriamine pentaacetic acid; DTPA; pentetate calcium trisodium; pentetate zinc trisodium; trisodium calcium diethylenetriaminepentaacetate (Ca-DTPA); zinc diethylenetriamine-pentaacetate (Zn-DTPA); Zn-DTPA

Therapeutic Category Antidote

Use Treatment of known or suspected internal contamination with plutonium, americium, or curium

Usual Dosage Internal contamination with plutonium, americium, or curium: Ca-DTPA is the preferred initial agent; sequential administration of Ca-DTPA then Zn-DTPA is recommended. I.V.:
Children <12 years:
Initial: Ca-DTPA: 14 mg/kg/day (maximum dose: 1 g/day)
Maintenance: Zn-DTPA: 14 mg/kg/day (maximum: 1 g/day); length of therapy depends on patient response and degree of contamination. **Note:** An equivalent dose of Ca-DTPA should be used for maintenance therapy only if Zn-DTPA is not available.
Children ≥12 years and Adults:
Initial: Ca-DTPA: 1 g/day
Pregnancy: Zn-DTPA 1 g/day should be used for the initial dose in pregnant women **except** in cases of high internal contamination
Maintenance: Zn-DTPA: 1 g/day; length of therapy depends on patient response and degree of contamination. **Note:** An equivalent dose of Ca-DTPA should be used for maintenance therapy only if Zn-DTPA is not available.

Dosage Forms
Injection, solution:
Ca-DTPA: 200 mg/mL (5 mL)
Zn-DTPA: 200 mg/mL (5 mL)

diethylenetriamine pentaacetic acid *see* diethylene triamine penta-acetic acid *on page 306*

diethylpropion (dye eth il PROE pee on)

Synonyms amfepramone; diethylpropion hydrochloride

U.S./Canadian Brand Names Tenuate® Dospan® [Can]; Tenuate® [Can]

Therapeutic Category Anorexiant

Controlled Substance C-IV

Use Short-term (few weeks) adjunct in the management of exogenous obesity

Usual Dosage Oral: Children >16 years and Adults:

Tablet: 25 mg 3 times/day before meals or food

Tablet, controlled release: 75 mg at midmorning

Dosage Forms

Tablet: 25 mg

Tablet, controlled release: 75 mg

diethylpropion hydrochloride *see* diethylpropion *on page 306*

difenoxin and atropine (dye fen OKS in & A troe peen)

Synonyms atropine and difenoxin

U.S./Canadian Brand Names Motofen® [US]

Therapeutic Category Antidiarrheal

Controlled Substance C-IV

Use Treatment of diarrhea

Usual Dosage Oral: Adults: Initial: 2 tablets (each tablet contains difenoxin hydrochloride 1 mg and atropine sulfate 0.025 mg), then 1 tablet after each loose stool; 1 tablet every 3-4 hours, up to 8 tablets in a 24-hour period; if no improvement after 48 hours, continued administration is not indicated

Dosage Forms

Tablet, oral:

Motofen®: Difenoxin 1 mg and atropine 0.025 mg

Differin® [US/Can] *see* adapalene *on page 35*

Differin® XP [Can] *see* adapalene *on page 35*

Difil-G [US] *see* dyphylline and guaifenesin *on page 344*

Difil®-G Forte [US] *see* dyphylline and guaifenesin *on page 344*

diflorasone (dye FLOR a sone)

Synonyms diflorasone diacetate

U.S./Canadian Brand Names ApexiCon™ E [US]; ApexiCon™ [US]

Therapeutic Category Corticosteroid, Topical

Use Relieves inflammation and pruritic symptoms of corticosteroid-responsive dermatosis (high to very high potency topical corticosteroid)

Usual Dosage Topical: Apply ointment sparingly 1-3 times/day; apply cream sparingly 2-4 times/day. Therapy should be discontinued when control is achieved; if no improvement is seen, reassessment of diagnosis may be necessary.

Dosage Forms

Cream: 0.05% (15 g, 30 g, 60 g)

ApexiCon™ E: 0.05% (30 g, 60 g)

Ointment: 0.05% (15 g, 30 g, 60 g)

ApexiCon™: 0.05% (30 g, 60 g)

diflorasone diacetate *see* diflorasone *on page 307*

Diflucan® [US/Can] *see* fluconazole *on page 424*

diflunisal (dye FLOO ni sal)

Sound-Alike/Look-Alike Issues

Dolobid® may be confused with Slo-Bid®

U.S./Canadian Brand Names Apo-Diflunisal® [Can]; Novo-Diflunisal [Can]; Nu-Diflunisal [Can]

Therapeutic Category Analgesic, Nonnarcotic; Nonsteroidal Antiinflammatory Drug (NSAID)

Use Management of inflammatory disorders usually including rheumatoid arthritis and osteoarthritis; can be used as an analgesic for treatment of mild-to-moderate pain

Usual Dosage Oral: Adults:
Mild-to-moderate pain: Initial: 500-1000 mg followed by 250-500 mg every 8-12 hours; maximum daily dose: 1.5 g
Arthritis: 500-1000 mg/day in 2 divided doses; maximum daily dose: 1.5 g

Dosage Forms
Tablet: 500 mg

difluprednate (dye floo PRED nate)

U.S./Canadian Brand Names Durezol™ [US]

Therapeutic Category Corticosteroid, Ophthalmic

Use Treatment of inflammation and pain following ocular surgery

Usual Dosage Ophthalmic: Adults: Instill 1 drop in conjunctival sac of the affected eye(s) 4 times/day beginning 24 hours after surgery, continue for 2 weeks, then decrease to 2 times/day for 1 week, then taper based on response

Dosage Forms
Emulsion, ophthalmic:
Durezol™: 0.05% (5 mL)

Digibind® [US/Can] *see* digoxin immune Fab *on page 308*
DigiFab™ [US] *see* digoxin immune Fab *on page 308*

digoxin (di JOKS in)

Sound-Alike/Look-Alike Issues
digoxin may be confused with Desoxyn®, doxepin
Lanoxin® may be confused with Lasix®, Levoxyl®, Levsinex®, Lomotil®, Lonox®, Mefoxin®, Xanax®

U.S./Canadian Brand Names Apo-Digoxin® [Can]; Digoxin CSD [Can]; Lanoxicaps® [Can]; Lanoxin® [US/Can]; Novo-Digoxin [Can]; Pediatric Digoxin CSD [Can]

Therapeutic Category Antiarrhythmic Agent, Miscellaneous; Cardiac Glycoside

Use Treatment of congestive heart failure and to slow the ventricular rate in tachyarrhythmias such as atrial fibrillation, atrial flutter, and supraventricular tachycardia (paroxysmal atrial tachycardia); cardiogenic shock

Usual Dosage When changing from oral (tablets or liquid) or I.M. to I.V. therapy, dosage should be reduced by 20% to 25%. Refer to the following:
Adults:
Total digitalizing dose[1]:
Oral: 0.75-1.5 mg
I.V. or I.M.: 0.5-1 mg
Daily maintenance dose[2]:
Oral: 0.125-0.5 mg
I.V. or I.M.: 0.1-0.4 mg

[1]Give one-half of the total digitalizing dose (TDD) in the initial dose, then give one-quarter of the TDD in each of two subsequent doses at 6- to 8-hour intervals. Obtain ECG 6 hours after each dose to assess potential toxicity.
[2]Divided every 12 hours in infants and children <10 years of age. Give once daily to children >10 years of age and adults.

Dosage Forms
Injection: 250 mcg/mL (1 mL, 2 mL)
Lanoxin®: 250 mcg/mL (2 mL)
Injection, pediatric: 100 mcg/mL (1 mL)
Solution, oral: 50 mcg/mL (2.5 mL, 60 mL)
Tablet: 125 mcg, 250 mcg
Lanoxin®: 125 mcg, 250 mcg

Digoxin CSD [Can] *see* digoxin *on page 308*

digoxin immune Fab (di JOKS in i MYUN fab)

Synonyms antidigoxin fab fragments, ovine

U.S./Canadian Brand Names Digibind® [US/Can]; DigiFab™ [US]

Therapeutic Category Antidote

Use Treatment of life-threatening or potentially life-threatening digoxin intoxication, including:

- acute digoxin ingestion (ie, >10 mg in adults or >4 mg in children)
- chronic ingestions leading to steady-state digoxin concentrations >6 ng/mL in adults or >4 ng/mL in children
- manifestations of digoxin toxicity due to overdose (life-threatening ventricular arrhythmias, progressive bradycardia, second- or third-degree heart block not responsive to atropine, serum potassium >5 mEq/L in adults or >6 mEq in children)

Usual Dosage Each vial of Digibind® 38 mg or DigiFab™ 40 mg will bind ~0.5 mg of digoxin or digitoxin.

Estimation of the dose is based on the body burden of digitalis. This may be calculated if the amount ingested is known or the postdistribution serum drug level is known (round dose to the nearest whole vial). Fab dose (in vials) based on number of tablets (0.25 mg) ingested.

Dosage Forms

Injection, powder for reconstitution [ovine derived]:

Digibind®: 38 mg

DigiFab™: 40 mg

dihematoporphyrin ether *see* porfimer *on page 801*

Dihistine® DH *(Discontinued)* *see* chlorpheniramine, pseudoephedrine, and codeine *on page 220*

dihydrocodeine, aspirin, and caffeine (dye hye droe KOE deen, AS pir in, & KAF een)

Sound-Alike/Look-Alike Issues

Synalgos®-DC may be confused with Synagis®

Synonyms dihydrocodeine compound

U.S./Canadian Brand Names Synalgos®-DC [US]

Therapeutic Category Analgesic, Narcotic

Controlled Substance C-III

Use Management of mild-to-moderate pain that requires relaxation

Usual Dosage Oral: Adults: 1-2 capsules every 4-6 hours as needed for pain

Dosage Forms

Capsule:

Synalgos®-DC: Dihydrocodeine 16 mg, aspirin 356.4 mg, and caffeine 30 mg

dihydrocodeine bitartrate, acetaminophen, and caffeine *see* acetaminophen, caffeine, and dihydrocodeine *on page 25*

dihydrocodeine bitartrate, phenylephrine hydrochloride, and chlorpheniramine maleate *see* phenylephrine, hydrocodone, and chlorpheniramine *on page 778*

dihydrocodeine bitartrate, pseudoephedrine hydrochloride, and chlorpheniramine maleate *see* pseudoephedrine, dihydrocodeine, and chlorpheniramine *on page 836*

dihydrocodeine, chlorpheniramine, and phenylephrine

(dye hye droe KOE deen, klor fen IR a meen, & fen il EF rin)

Synonyms chlorpheniramine maleate, dihydrocodeine bitartrate, and phenylephrine hydrochloride; phenylephrine, chlorpheniramine, and dihydrocodeine

U.S./Canadian Brand Names Baltussin [US]; Coldcough PD [US]; Novahistine DH [US]

Therapeutic Category Antihistamine; Antihistamine/Decongestant/Antitussive; Antitussive; Decongestant

Controlled Substance C-III/C-V

Use Symptomatic relief of cough and congestion associated with the upper respiratory tract

Usual Dosage Oral: Cough and congestion:

Children 2-6 years (Novahistine DH): 1.25-2.5 mL every 4-6 hours as needed (maximum: 10 mL/24 hours)

Children 6-12 years:

Baltussin: 2.5 mL every 4-6 hours as needed

Novahistine DH: 2.5-5 mL every 4-6 hours as needed (maximum: 20 mL/24 hours)

Children ≥12 years and Adults:

Baltussin: 5 mL every 4-6 hours as needed

Novahistine DH: 5-10 mL every 4-6 hours as needed (maximum: 40 mL/24 hours)

Dosage Forms

Liquid:

Novahistine DH: Dihydrocodeine 7.5 mg, chlorpheniramine 2 mg and phenylephrine 5 mg per 5 mL

Syrup:

Baltussin: Dihydrocodeine 3 mg, chlorpheniramine 5 mg, and phenylephrine 20 mg per 5 mL

Coldcough PD: Dihydrocodeine 3 mg, chlorpheniramine 2 mg, and phenylephrine 7.5 mg per 5 mL

dihydrocodeine compound *see* dihydrocodeine, aspirin, and caffeine *on page 309*

dihydrocodeine, pseudoephedrine, and guaifenesin

(dye hye droe KOE deen, soo doe e FED rin, & gwye FEN e sin)

Synonyms guaifenesin, dihydrocodeine, and pseudoephedrine; pseudoephedrine hydrochloride, guaifenesin, and dihydrocodeine bitartrate

U.S./Canadian Brand Names DiHydro-GP [US]; Pancof®-EXP [US]

Therapeutic Category Antitussive/Decongestant/Expectorant

Use Temporary relief of cough and congestion associated with upper respiratory tract infections and allergies

Usual Dosage Oral: Cough/congestion (Pancof®-EXP):

Children:

2-6 years: 1.25-2.5 mL every 4-6 hours as needed

6-12 years: 2.5-5 mL every 4-6 hours as needed

Children ≥12 years and Adults: 5-10 mL every 4-6 hours as needed

Dosage Forms

Syrup:

DiHydro-GP, Pancof®-EXP: Dihydrocodeine 7.5 mg, pseudoephedrine 15 mg, and guaifenesin 100 mg per 5 mL

DiHydro-CP [US] *see* pseudoephedrine, dihydrocodeine, and chlorpheniramine *on page 836*

dihydroergotamine (dye hye droe er GOT a meen)

Synonyms DHE; dihydroergotamine mesylate

U.S./Canadian Brand Names D.H.E. 45® [US]; Migranal® [US/Can]

Therapeutic Category Ergot Alkaloid and Derivative

Use Treatment of migraine headache with or without aura; injection also indicated for treatment of cluster headaches

Usual Dosage Adults:

I.M., SubQ: 1 mg at first sign of headache; repeat hourly to a maximum dose of 3 mg total; maximum dose: 6 mg/week

I.V.: 1 mg at first sign of headache; repeat hourly up to a maximum dose of 2 mg total; maximum dose: 6 mg/week

Intranasal: 1 spray (0.5 mg) of nasal spray should be administered into each nostril; if needed, repeat after 15 minutes, up to a total of 4 sprays. **Note:** Do not exceed 3 mg (6 sprays) in a 24-hour period and no more than 8 sprays in a week.

Dosage Forms

Injection, solution: 1 mg/mL (1 mL)

D.H.E. 45®: 1 mg/mL (1 mL)

Solution, intranasal spray:

Migranal®: 4 mg/mL [0.5 mg/spray] (1 mL)

dihydroergotamine mesylate *see* dihydroergotamine *on page 310*
dihydroergotoxine *see* ergoloid mesylates *on page 366*
dihydrogenated ergot alkaloids *see* ergoloid mesylates *on page 366*
DiHydro-GP [US] *see* dihydrocodeine, pseudoephedrine, and guaifenesin *on page 310*
dihydrohydroxycodeinone *see* oxycodone *on page 737*
dihydromorphinone *see* hydromorphone *on page 506*
dihydroxyanthracenedione *see* mitoxantrone *on page 662*
dihydroxyanthracenedione dihydrochloride *see* mitoxantrone *on page 662*
1,25 dihydroxycholecalciferol *see* calcitriol *on page 168*
dihydroxydeoxynorvinkaleukoblastine *see* vinorelbine *on page 1014*
dihydroxypropyl theophylline *see* dyphylline *on page 344*

Dihyrex® Injection *(Discontinued)* *see* diphenhydramine *on page 315*
diiodohydroxyquin *see* iodoquinol *on page 539*
Dilacor XR® [US] *see* diltiazem *on page 311*
Dilantin® [US/Can] *see* phenytoin *on page 780*
Dilatrate®-SR [US] *see* isosorbide dinitrate *on page 550*
Dilaudid® [US/Can] *see* hydromorphone *on page 506*
Dilaudid® Cough Syrup *(Discontinued)* *see* hydromorphone *on page 506*
Dilaudid-HP® [US/Can] *see* hydromorphone *on page 506*
Dilaudid-HP-Plus® [Can] *see* hydromorphone *on page 506*
Dilaudid® Sterile Powder [Can] *see* hydromorphone *on page 506*
Dilaudid-XP® [Can] *see* hydromorphone *on page 506*
Dilex-G [US] *see* dyphylline and guaifenesin *on page 344*
Dilocaine® Injection *(Discontinued)* *see* lidocaine *on page 584*
Dilomine® Injection *(Discontinued)* *see* dicyclomine *on page 305*
Dilor® [Can] *see* dyphylline *on page 344*
Dilor-G® [US] *see* dyphylline and guaifenesin *on page 344*
Dilt-CD [US] *see* diltiazem *on page 311*
Diltia XT® [US] *see* diltiazem *on page 311*

diltiazem (dil TYE a zem)

Sound-Alike/Look-Alike Issues

diltiazem may be confused with Calan®, diazepam, Dilantin®

Cardizem® may be confused with Cardene®, Cardene SR®, Cardizem CD®, Cardizem SR®, cardiem, cortisone

Cartia XT® may be confused with Procardia XL®

Tiazac® may be confused with Tigan®, Tiazac® XC [CAN], Ziac®

Synonyms diltiazem hydrochloride

U.S./Canadian Brand Names Apo-Diltiaz CD® [Can]; Apo-Diltiaz SR® [Can]; Apo-Diltiaz TZ® [Can]; Apo-Diltiaz® Injectable [Can]; Apo-Diltiaz® [Can]; Cardizem® CD [US/Can]; Cardizem® LA [US]; Cardizem® [US]; Cartia XT® [US]; Dilacor XR® [US]; Dilt-CD [US]; Dilt-XR [US]; Diltia XT® [US]; Diltiazem HCl ER® [Can]; Diltiazem Hydrochloride Injection [Can]; Diltzac [US]; Gen-Diltiazem CD [Can]; Gen-Diltiazem SR [Can]; Gen-Diltiazem [Can]; Med-Diltiazem [Can]; Novo-Diltazem [Can]; Novo-Diltazem-CD [Can]; Novo-Diltiazem HCl ER [Can]; Nu-Diltiaz [Can]; Nu-Diltiaz-CD [Can]; ratio-Diltiazem CD [Can]; Sandoz-Diltiazem CD [Can]; Sandoz-Diltiazem T [Can]; Taztia XT® [US]; Tiazac® XC [Can]; Tiazac® [US/Can]

Therapeutic Category Calcium Channel Blocker

Use

Oral: Essential hypertension; chronic stable angina or angina from coronary artery spasm

Injection: Atrial fibrillation or atrial flutter; paroxysmal supraventricular tachycardia (PSVT)

Usual Dosage Adults:

Oral:

Angina:

Capsule, extended release:

Dilacor XR®, Dilt-XR, Diltia XT®: Initial: 120 mg once daily; titrate over 7-14 days; usual dose range: 120-320 mg/day: maximum: 480 mg/day

Cardizem® CD, Cartia XT®, Dilt-CD: Initial: 120-180 mg once daily; titrate over 7-14 days; usual dose range: 120-320 mg/day; maximum: 480 mg/day

Tiazac®, Taztia XT®: Initial: 120-180 mg once daily; titrate over 7-14 days; usual dose range: 120-320 mg/day; maximum: 540 mg/day

Tablet, extended release (Cardizem® LA, Tiazac® XC [CAN; not available in U.S.]): 180 mg once daily; may increase at 7- to 14-day intervals; usual dose range: 120-320 mg/day; maximum: 360 mg/day

Tablet, immediate release (Cardizem®): Usual starting dose: 30 mg 4 times/day; titrate dose gradually at 1- to 2-day intervals; usual dose range: 120-320 mg/day

Hypertension:

Capsule, extended release (once-daily dosing):

Cardizem® CD, Cartia XT®, Dilt-CD: Initial: 180-240 mg once daily; dose adjustment may be made after 14 days; usual dose range (JNC 7): 180-420 mg/day; maximum: 480 mg/day

Dilacor® XR, Diltia XT®, Dilt-XR: Initial: 180-240 mg once daily; dose adjustment may be made after 14 days; usual dose range (JNC 7): 180-420 mg/day; maximum: 540 mg/day

Tiazac®, Taztia XT®: Initial: 120-240 mg once daily; dose adjustment may be made after 14 days; usual dose range (JNC 7): 180-420 mg/day; maximum: 540 mg/day

Capsule, extended release (twice-daily dosing): Initial: 60-120 mg twice daily; dose adjustment may be made after 14 days; usual range: 240-360 mg/day

Note: Diltiazem is available as a generic intended for either once- or twice-daily dosing, depending on the formulation; verify appropriate extended release capsule formulation is administered.

Tablet, extended release (Cardizem® LA, Tiazac® XC [CAN; not available in U.S.]): Initial: 180-240 mg once daily; dose adjustment may be made after 14 days; usual dose range (JNC 7): 120-540 mg/day

I.V.: Atrial fibrillation, atrial flutter, PSVT:

Initial bolus dose: 0.25 mg/kg actual body weight over 2 minutes (average adult dose: 20 mg)

Repeat bolus dose (may be administered after 15 minutes if the response is inadequate.): 0.35 mg/kg actual body weight over 2 minutes (average adult dose: 25 mg)

Continuous infusion (infusions >24 hours or infusion rates >15 mg/hour are not recommended.): Initial infusion rate of 10 mg/hour; rate may be increased in 5 mg/hour increments up to 15 mg/hour as needed; some patients may respond to an initial rate of 5 mg/hour.

If diltiazem injection is administered by continuous infusion for >24 hours, the possibility of decreased diltiazem clearance, prolonged elimination half-life, and increased diltiazem and/or diltiazem metabolite plasma concentrations should be considered.

Conversion from I.V. diltiazem to oral diltiazem:

Oral dose (mg/day) is approximately equal to [rate (mg/hour) x 3 + 3] x 10.

3 mg/hour = 120 mg/day
5 mg/hour = 180 mg/day
7 mg/hour = 240 mg/day
11 mg/hour = 360 mg/day

Dosage Forms

Capsule, extended release [once-daily dosing]: 120 mg, 180 mg, 240 mg, 300 mg, 360 mg, 420 mg

Cardizem® CD, Taztia XT®, Diltzac: 120 mg, 180 mg, 240 mg, 300 mg, 360 mg
Cartia XT®: 120 mg, 180 mg, 240 mg, 300 mg
Dilacor XR®, Dilt-XR, Diltia XT®: 120 mg, 180 mg, 240 mg
Dilt-CD: 120 mg, 180 mg, 240 mg, 300 mg
Tiazac®: 120 mg, 180 mg, 240 mg, 300 mg, 360 mg, 420 mg

Capsule, extended release [twice-daily dosing]: 60 mg, 90 mg, 120 mg

Injection, solution: 5 mg/mL (5 mL, 10 mL, 25 mL)

Injection, powder for reconstitution: 100 mg

Tablet: 30 mg, 60 mg, 90 mg, 120 mg

Cardizem®: 30 mg, 60 mg, 90 mg, 120 mg

Tablet, extended release:

Cardizem® LA: 120 mg, 180 mg, 240 mg, 300 mg, 360 mg, 420 mg
Tiazac® XC [CAN; not available in U.S.]: 120 mg, 180 mg, 240 mg, 300 mg, 360 mg

Diltiazem HCl ER® [Can] *see* diltiazem *on page 311*

diltiazem hydrochloride *see* diltiazem *on page 311*

Diltiazem Hydrochloride Injection [Can] *see* diltiazem *on page 311*

Dilt-XR [US] *see* diltiazem *on page 311*

Diltzac [US] *see* diltiazem *on page 311*

Dimaphen [US-OTC] *see* brompheniramine and pseudoephedrine *on page 150*

Dimaphen Cold & Allergy [US-OTC] *see* brompheniramine and phenylephrine *on page 150*

Dimaphen DM *(Discontinued)* *see* brompheniramine, pseudoephedrine, and dextromethorphan *on page 152*

dimenhydrinate (dye men HYE dri nate)

Sound-Alike/Look-Alike Issues

dimenhyDRINATE may be confused with diphenhydrAMINE

Tall-Man dimenhy**DRINATE**

U.S./Canadian Brand Names Apo-Dimenhydrinate® [Can]; Children's Motion Sickness Liquid [Can]; Dimenhydrinate Injection [Can]; Dinate® [Can]; Dramamine® [US-OTC]; Driminate® [US-OTC]; Gravol® [Can]; Nauseatol [Can]; Novo-Dimenate [Can]; PMS-Dimenhydrinate [Can]; Sandoz-Dimenhydrinate [Can]; TripTone® [US-OTC]

Therapeutic Category Antihistamine

Use Treatment and prevention of nausea, vertigo, and vomiting associated with motion sickness

Usual Dosage

Oral:

Children:

2-5 years: 12.5-25 mg every 6-8 hours, maximum: 75 mg/day

6-12 years: 25-50 mg every 6-8 hours, maximum: 150 mg/day

Adults: 50-100 mg every 4-6 hours, not to exceed 400 mg/day

I.M.:

Children: 1.25 mg/kg **or** 37.5 mg/m^2 4 times/day; maximum: 300 mg/day

Adults: 50 mg every 4 hours; maximum: 100 mg every 4 hours

I.V.: Adults: 50 mg every 4 hours; maximum: 100 mg every 4 hours

Dosage Forms

Injection, solution: 50 mg/mL (1 mL, 10 mL) [contains benzyl alcohol]

Tablet: 50 mg

Driminate® [OTC]: 50 mg [scored]

Tablet, chewable: 50 mg

Dramamine® [OTC]: 50 mg

Dimenhydrinate Injection [Can] *see* dimenhydrinate *on page* 312

dimercaprol (dye mer KAP role)

Synonyms BAL; British anti-lewisite; dithioglycerol

U.S./Canadian Brand Names BAL in Oil® [US]

Therapeutic Category Chelating Agent

Use Antidote to gold, arsenic (except arsine), or acute mercury poisoning (except nonalkyl mercury); adjunct to edetate CALCIUM disodium in lead poisoning

Usual Dosage Note: Premedication with a histamine H_1 antagonist (eg, diphenhydramine) is recommended.

Children and Adults: Deep I.M.:

Mild arsenic or gold poisoning: 2.5 mg/kg every 6 hours for 2 days, then every 12 hours for 1 day, followed by once daily for 10 days

Severe arsenic or gold poisoning: 3 mg/kg every 4 hours for 2 days, then every 6 hours for 1 day, followed every 12 hours for 10 days

Mercury poisoning: 5 mg/kg initially, followed by 2.5 mg/kg 1-2 times/day for 10 days

Lead poisoning: **Note:** For the treatment of high blood lead levels in children, the CDC recommends chelation treatment when blood lead levels are >45 mcg/dL. Combination parenteral therapy is indicated when blood lead levels are ≥70 mcg/dL, or patients are symptomatic. In adults, available guidelines recommend chelation therapy with blood lead levels >50 mcg/dL and significant symptoms; chelation therapy may also be indicated with blood lead levels ≥100 mcg/dL and/or symptoms.

Lead encephalopathy (in conjunction with edetate CALCIUM disodium): Dimercaprol 4 mg/kg (75 mg/m^2) loading dose, followed by dimercaprol 4 mg/kg (75 mg/m^2) every 4 hours for 2-7 days (edetate CALCIUM disodium is **not** administered with the loading dose; begin edetate CALCIUM disodium with the second dose)

Symptomatic lead poisoning or blood lead levels ≥70 mcg/dL (in conjunction with edetate CALCIUM disodium): Dimercaprol 4 mg/kg (75 mg/m^2) loading dose, followed by dimercaprol 3 mg/kg/dose (50 mg/m^2) every 4 hours for 2-7 days (edetate CALCIUM disodium is **not** administered with the loading dose; begin edetate CALCIUM disodium with the second dose)

Dosage Forms

Injection, oil:

BAL in Oil®: 100 mg/mL (3 mL)

Dimetabs® Oral *(Discontinued)* *see* dimenhydrinate *on page* 312

Dimetapp® 12-Hour Non-Drowsy Extentabs® *(Discontinued)* *see* pseudoephedrine *on page* 833

Dimetapp® Children's ND *(Discontinued)* *see* loratadine *on page* 599

Dimetapp® Children's Cold & Allergy [US-OTC] *see* brompheniramine and phenylephrine *on page* 150

Dimetapp® Children's Long Acting Cough Plus Cold [US-OTC] *see* dextromethorphan and chlorpheniramine *on page* 296

Dimetapp® Children's Nighttime Cold & Congestion [US-OTC] *see* diphenhydramine and phenylephrine *on page* 317

Dimetapp® Decongestant Infant *(Discontinued)* *see* pseudoephedrine *on page 833*

Dimetapp® DM Children's Cold and Cough *(Discontinued)* *see* brompheniramine, pseudoephedrine, and dextromethorphan *on page 152*

Dimetapp® Infant Decongestant Plus Cough *(Discontinued)* *see* pseudoephedrine and dextromethorphan *on page 834*

Dimetapp® ND Children's *(Discontinued)* *see* loratadine *on page 599*

Dimetapp® Sinus Caplets *(Discontinued)* *see* pseudoephedrine and ibuprofen *on page 835*

Dimetapp® Toddler's [US-OTC] *see* phenylephrine *on page 774*

dimethyl sulfoxide (dye meth il sul FOKS ide)

Synonyms DMSO

U.S./Canadian Brand Names Dimethyl Sulfoxide Irrigation, USP [Can]; Kemsol® [Can]; Rimso®-50 [US/Can]

Therapeutic Category Urinary Tract Product

Use Symptomatic relief of interstitial cystitis

Usual Dosage Adults: Bladder instillation: Instill 50 mL directly into bladder and allow to remain for 15 minutes; repeat every 2 weeks until symptoms are relieved, then increase intervals between treatments **or** 50 mL directly into bladder for 15-20 minutes every 1-2 weeks for 4-8 treatments

Dosage Forms

Solution, intravesical:

Rimso-50®: 50% [500 mg/mL] (50 mL)

Dimethyl Sulfoxide Irrigation, USP [Can] *see* dimethyl sulfoxide *on page 314*

dimethyl triazeno imidazole carboxamide *see* dacarbazine *on page 272*

Dinate® [Can] *see* dimenhydrinate *on page 312*

Dinate® Injection *(Discontinued)* *see* dimenhydrinate *on page 312*

dinoprostone (dye noe PROST one)

Sound-Alike/Look-Alike Issues

Prepidil® may be confused with Bepridil®

Synonyms PGE_2; prostaglandin E_2

U.S./Canadian Brand Names Cervidil® [US/Can]; Prepidil® [US/Can]; Prostin E_2® [US/Can]

Therapeutic Category Prostaglandin

Use

Gel: Promote cervical ripening in patients at or near term in whom there is a medical or obstetrical indication for the induction of labor

Suppositories: Terminate pregnancy from 12th through 20th week of gestation; evacuate uterus in cases of missed abortion or intrauterine fetal death up to 28 weeks of gestation; manage benign hydatidiform mole (nonmetastatic gestational trophoblastic disease)

Vaginal insert: Initiation and/or continuation of cervical ripening in patients at or near term in whom there is a medical or obstetrical indication for the induction of labor

Usual Dosage Females of reproductive age:

Abortifacient: Vaginal suppository: Insert 20 mg (1 suppository) high in vagina, repeat at 3- to 5-hour intervals until abortion occurs; continued administration for longer than 2 days is not advisable

Cervical ripening:

Endocervical gel: Using catheter supplied with gel, insert 0.5 mg into the cervical canal. May repeat every 6 hours if needed. Maximum cumulative dose: 1.5 mg/24 hours

Vaginal insert: Insert 10 mg transversely into the posterior fornix of the vagina (to be removed at the onset of active labor or after 12 hours)

Dosage Forms

Gel, endocervical:

Prepidil®: 0.5 mg/3 g syringe

Insert, vaginal:

Cervidil®: 10 mg

Suppository, vaginal:

Prostin E_2®: 20 mg

Diocaine® [Can] *see* proparacaine *on page 826*

Diocarpine [Can] *see* pilocarpine *on page 783*

Diochloram® [Can] *see* chloramphenicol *on page 208*
Diocto® [US-OTC] *see* docusate *on page 326*
Diocto C® ***(Discontinued)***
Diocto-K® ***(Discontinued)*** *see* docusate *on page 326*
Diocto-K Plus® ***(Discontinued)*** *see* docusate *on page 326*
dioctyl calcium sulfosuccinate *see* docusate *on page 326*
dioctyl sodium sulfosuccinate *see* docusate *on page 326*
Diodex® [Can] *see* dexamethasone (systemic) *on page 288*
Diodoquin® [Can] *see* iodoquinol *on page 539*
Diogent® [Can] *see* gentamicin *on page 461*
Diomycin® [Can] *see* erythromycin *on page 368*
Dionephrine® [Can] *see* phenylephrine *on page 774*
Diopentolate® [Can] *see* cyclopentolate *on page 265*
Diopred® [Can] *see* prednisolone (systemic) *on page 813*
Dioptic's Atropine Solution [Can] *see* atropine *on page 110*
Dioptimyd® [Can] *see* sulfacetamide and prednisolone *on page 927*
Dioptrol® [Can] *see* neomycin, polymyxin B, and dexamethasone *on page 687*
Diosulf™ [Can] *see* sulfacetamide *on page 927*
Diotame® [US-OTC] *see* bismuth *on page 142*
Diotrope® [Can] *see* tropicamide *on page 992*
Dioval® Injection ***(Discontinued)*** *see* estradiol *on page 373*
Diovan® [US/Can] *see* valsartan *on page 1004*
Diovan HCT® [US/Can] *see* valsartan and hydrochlorothiazide *on page 1004*
Diovol® [Can] *see* aluminum hydroxide and magnesium hydroxide *on page 55*
Diovol® Ex [Can] *see* aluminum hydroxide and magnesium hydroxide *on page 55*
Diovol Plus® [Can] *see* aluminum hydroxide, magnesium hydroxide, and simethicone *on page 56*
Dipentum® [US/Can] *see* olsalazine *on page 722*
Diphen [US-OTC] *see* diphenhydramine *on page 315*
Diphenacen 50® Injection ***(Discontinued)*** *see* diphenhydramine *on page 315*
Diphenatol® ***(Discontinued)*** *see* diphenoxylate and atropine *on page 318*
Diphenhist® [US-OTC] *see* diphenhydramine *on page 315*

diphenhydramine (dye fen HYE dra meen)

Sound-Alike/Look-Alike Issues
diphenhydrAMINE may be confused with desipramine, dicyclomine, dimenhyDRINATE
Benadryl® may be confused with benazepril, Bentyl®, Benylin®, Caladryl®

Synonyms diphenhydramine citrate; diphenhydramine hydrochloride; diphenhydramine tannate

Tall-Man diphenhydr**AMINE**

U.S./Canadian Brand Names Aler-Cap [US-OTC]; Aler-Dryl [US-OTC]; Aler-Tab [US-OTC]; Allerdryl® [Can]; AllerMax® [US-OTC]; Allernix [Can]; Altaryl [US-OTC]; Anti-Hist [US-OTC]; Banophen™ Anti-Itch [US-OTC]; Banophen™ [US-OTC]; Benadryl® Allergy Quick Dissolve [US-OTC]; Benadryl® Allergy [US-OTC]; Benadryl® Children's Allergy Fastmelt® [US-OTC]; Benadryl® Children's Allergy Perfect Measure™ [US]; Benadryl® Children's Allergy [US-OTC]; Benadryl® Children's Dye-Free Allergy [US-OTC]; Benadryl® Dye-Free Allergy [US-OTC]; Benadryl® Itch Relief Extra Strength [US-OTC]; Benadryl® Itch Stopping Extra Strength [US-OTC]; Benadryl® Itch Stopping [US-OTC]; Benadryl® [Can]; Compoz® Nighttime Sleep Aid [US-OTC]; Dermamycin® [US-OTC]; Diphen [US-OTC]; Diphenhist® [US-OTC]; Dytan™ [US]; Genahist™ [US-OTC]; Histaprin [US-OTC]; Hydramine [US-OTC]; Nytol® Extra Strength [Can]; Nytol® Quick Caps [US-OTC]; Nytol® Quick Gels [US-OTC]; Nytol® [Can]; PediaCare® Children's Allergy [US-OTC]; PediaCare® Children's NightTime Cough [US-OTC]; PMS-Diphenhydramine [Can]; Siladryl Allergy [US-OTC]; Silphen Cough [US-OTC]; Simply Sleep™ [US-OTC/Can]; Sleep-ettes D [US-OTC]; Sleep-Tabs [US-OTC]; Sleepinal® [US-OTC]; Sominex® Maximum Strength [US-OTC]; Sominex® [US-OTC]; Theraflu® Thin Strips® Multi Symptom [US-OTC]; Triaminic Thin Strips® Children's Cough and Runny Nose [US-OTC]; Twilite® [US-OTC]; Unisom® SleepGels® Maximum Strength [US-OTC]; Unisom® SleepMelts™ [US-OTC]

Therapeutic Category Antihistamine

Use Symptomatic relief of allergic symptoms caused by histamine release including nasal allergies and allergic dermatosis; adjunct to epinephrine in the treatment of anaphylaxis; nighttime sleep aid; prevention or treatment of motion sickness; antitussive; management of parkinsonian syndrome including drug-induced extrapyramidal symptoms; topically for relief of pain and itching associated with insect bites, minor cuts and burns, or rashes due to poison ivy, poison oak, and poison sumac

Usual Dosage Note: Dosages are expressed as the hydrochloride salt.

Children:

Allergic reactions or motion sickness: Oral, I.M., I.V.: 5 mg/kg/day or 150 mg/m^2/day in divided doses every 6-8 hours, not to exceed 300 mg/day

Alternate dosing by age: Oral:

2 to <6 years: 6.25 mg every 4-6 hours; maximum: 37.5 mg/day

6 to <12 years: 12.5-25 mg every 4-6 hours; maximum: 150 mg/day

≥12 years: 25-50 mg every 4-6 hours; maximum: 300 mg/day

Nighttime sleep aid: Oral: Children ≥12 years: 50 mg at bedtime

Antitussive: Oral:

2 to <6 years: 6.25 mg every 4 hours; maximum 37.5 mg/day

6 to <12 years: 12.5 mg every 4 hours; maximum 75 mg/day

≥12 years: 25 mg every 4 hours; maximum 150 mg/day

Treatment of dystonic reactions: I.M., I.V.: 0.5-1 mg/kg/dose

Relief of pain and itching: Topical: Children ≥2 years: Apply 1% or 2% to affected area up to 3-4 times/day

Adults:

Allergic reactions or motion sickness: Oral: 25-50 mg every 6-8 hours

Antitussive: Oral: 25 mg every 4 hours; maximum 150 mg/24 hours

Nighttime sleep aid: Oral: 50 mg at bedtime

Allergic reactions or motion sickness: I.M., I.V.: 10-50 mg per dose; single doses up to 100 mg may be used if needed; not to exceed 400 mg/day

Dystonic reaction: I.M., I.V.: 50 mg in a single dose; may repeat in 20-30 minutes if necessary

Relief of pain and itching: Topical: Apply 1% or 2% to affected area up to 3-4 times/day

Dosage Forms

Caplet: 25 mg, 50 mg

Aler-Dryl [OTC], AllerMax® [OTC], Compoz® Nighttime Sleep Aid [OTC], Sleep-ettes D [OTC], Sominex® Maximum Strength [OTC], Twilite® [OTC]: 50 mg

Anti-Hist [OTC], Histaprin [OTC], Nytol® Quick Caps [OTC], Simply Sleep™ [OTC]: 25 mg

Capsule: 25 mg, 50 mg

Aler-Cap [OTC], Banophen™ [OTC], Benadryl® Allergy [OTC], Diphen [OTC], Diphenhist® [OTC], Genahist® [OTC]: 25 mg

Sleepinal® [OTC]: 50 mg

Capsule, softgel: 50 mg

Benadryl® Dye-Free Allergy [OTC]: 25 mg

Compoz® Nighttime Sleep Aid [OTC], Nytol® Quick Gels [OTC], Unisom® SleepGels Maximum Strength [OTC]: 50 mg

Captab: 25 mg

Diphenhist® [OTC]: 25 mg

Cream: 2% (30 g)

Banophen™ Anti-Itch [OTC], Diphenhist® [OTC]: 2% (30 g)

Benadryl® Itch Stopping [OTC]: 1% (15 g, 30 g)

Benadryl® Itch Stopping Extra Strength [OTC]: 2% (15 g, 30 g)

Elixir: 12.5 mg/5 mL

Altaryl [OTC], Banophen™ [OTC]: 12.5 mg/5 mL

Gel, topical:

Benadryl® Itch Stopping Extra Strength [OTC]: 2% (120 mL)

Injection, solution: 50 mg/mL (1 mL, 10 mL)

Liquid, oral:

AllerMax® [OTC], Benadryl® Children's Allergy [OTC], Benadryl® Children's Allergy Perfect Measure™, Benadryl® Children's Dye-Free Allergy [OTC], Genahist™ [OTC], Hydramine [OTC], Siladryl Allergy [OTC]: 12.5 mg/5 mL

Liquid, topical [spray]:

Benadryl® Itch Stopping Extra Strength [OTC], Dermamycin® [OTC]: 2% (60 mL)

Liquid, topical [stick]:

Benadryl® Itch Relief Extra Strength [OTC]: 2% (14 mL)

Solution, oral:
Diphenhist® [OTC]: 12.5 mg/5mL
Strips, orally disintegrating:
Benadryl® Allergy Quick Dissolve [OTC]: 25 mg (10s)
Theraflu® Thin Strips® Multi Symptom [OTC]: 25 mg (12s)
Triaminic Thin Strips® Children's Cough and Runny Nose [OTC]: 12. 5 mg (14s)
Syrup:
PediaCare® Children's Allergy [OTC], PediaCare® Children's NightTime Cough [OTC], Silphen Cough [OTC]: 12.5 mg/5 mL
Tablet: 25 mg, 50 mg
Aler-Tab [OTC], Banophen™ [OTC], Benadryl® Allergy [OTC], Genahist™ [OTC], Sominex® [OTC], Sleep-Tabs [OTC]: 25 mg
Tablet, chewable:
Dytan™: 25 mg
Tablet, orally dissolving:
Benadryl® Children's Allergy Fastmelt® [OTC]: 12.5 mg
Unisom® SleepMelts™ [OTC]: 25 mg

diphenhydramine and acetaminophen *see* acetaminophen and diphenhydramine *on page 21*
diphenhydramine and ASA *see* aspirin and diphenhydramine *on page 105*
diphenhydramine and aspirin *see* aspirin and diphenhydramine *on page 105*

diphenhydramine and phenylephrine (dye fen HYE dra meen & fen il EF rin)

Synonyms diphenhydramine hydrochloride and phenylephrine hydrochloride; diphenhydramine tannate and phenylephrine tannate; phenylephrine and diphenhydramine; phenylephrine hydrochloride and diphenhydramine hydrochloride; phenylephrine tannate and diphenhydramine tannate

U.S./Canadian Brand Names Aldex® CT [US]; Dimetapp® Children's Nighttime Cold & Congestion [US-OTC]; Robitussin® Night Time Cough & Cold [US-OTC]

Therapeutic Category Alpha/Beta Agonist; Histamine H_1 Antagonist; Histamine H_1 Antagonist, First Generation

Use Temporary relief of symptoms of allergic rhinitis, sinusitis, and other upper respiratory conditions, including sinus/nasal congestion, sneezing, stuffy/runny nose, itchy/watery eyes, and cough

Usual Dosage Oral:
Aldex® CT:
Children 6-11 years: One-half to 1 tablet every 6 hours
Children ≥12 years and Adults: 1-2 tablets every 6 hours
OTC labeling:
Children 6-11 years (Dimetapp® Children's Nighttime Cold and Congestion): 10 mL every 4 hours as needed, maximum: 6 doses/24 hours
Children ≥12 years and Adults: 20 mL every 4 hours as needed, maximum: 6 doses/24 hours

Dosage Forms
Liquid, oral:
Benadryl-D® Children's Allergy & Sinus [OTC]: Diphenhydramine 12.5 mg and phenylephrine 5 mg per 5 mL (118 mL)
Strip, orally disintegrating:
Triaminic® Children's Thin Strips® Night Time Cold & Cough [OTC]: Diphenhydramine 12.5 mg and phenylephrine 5 mg
Syrup, oral:
Dimetapp® Children's Nighttime Cold and Congestion [OTC]: Diphenhydramine 6.25 mg and phenylephrine 2.5 mg per 5 mL (120 mL)
Robitussin® Night Time Cough & Cold [OTC]: Diphenhydramine 6.25 mg and phenylephrine 2.5 mg per 5 mL (120 mL)
Triaminic® Children's Night Time Cold & Cough [OTC]: Diphenhydramine 6.25 mg and phenylephrine 2.5 mg per 5 mL (118 mL)
Tablet, oral:
Benadryl-D® Allergy & Sinus [OTC]: Diphenhydramine 25 mg and phenylephrine 10 mg
Tablet, chewable, oral:
Aldex® CT: Diphenhydramine 12.5 mg and phenylephrine 5 mg

diphenhydramine and pseudoephedrine *(Discontinued)*
diphenhydramine citrate *see* diphenhydramine *on page 315*
diphenhydramine citrate and aspirin *see* aspirin and diphenhydramine *on page 105*

diphenhydramine hydrochloride *see* diphenhydramine *on page 315*

diphenhydramine hydrochloride and phenylephrine hydrochloride *see* diphenhydramine and phenylephrine *on page 317*

diphenhydramine, phenylephrine hydrochloride, and acetaminophen *see* acetaminophen, diphenhydramine, and phenylephrine *on page 28*

diphenhydramine tannate *see* diphenhydramine *on page 315*

diphenhydramine tannate and phenylephrine tannate *see* diphenhydramine and phenylephrine *on page 317*

diphenoxylate and atropine (dye fen OKS i late & A troe peen)

Sound-Alike/Look-Alike Issues

Lomotil® may be confused with Lamictal®, Lamisil®, lamoTRIgine, Lanoxin®, Lasix®, ludiomil

Lonox® may be confused with Lanoxin®, Loprox®

Synonyms atropine and diphenoxylate

U.S./Canadian Brand Names Lomotil® [US/Can]; Lonox® [US]

Therapeutic Category Antidiarrheal

Controlled Substance C-V

Use Treatment of diarrhea

Usual Dosage Oral:

Children 2-12 years (use with caution in young children due to variable responses): Liquid: Diphenoxylate 0.3-0.4 mg/kg/day in 4 divided doses until control achieved (maximum: 10 mg/day), then reduce dose as needed; some patients may be controlled on doses as low as 25% of the initial daily dose

Adults: Diphenoxylate 5 mg 4 times/day until control achieved (maximum: 20 mg/day), then reduce dose as needed; some patients may be controlled on doses of 5 mg/day

Dosage Forms

Solution, oral: Diphenoxylate 2.5 mg and atropine 0.025 mg per 5 mL

Lomotil®: Diphenoxylate 2.5 mg and atropine 0.025 mg per 5 mL

Tablet: Diphenoxylate 2.5 mg and atropine 0.025 mg

Lomotil®, Lonox®: Diphenoxylate 2.5 mg and atropine 0.025 mg

Diphenylan Sodium® *(Discontinued)* *see* phenytoin *on page 780*

diphenylhydantoin *see* phenytoin *on page 780*

diphtheria and tetanus toxoid (dif THEER ee a & TET a nus TOKS oyds)

Sound-Alike/Look-Alike Issues

diphtheria and Tetanus Toxoids (Td) may be confused with tuberculin purified protein derivative (PPD)

Synonyms DT; Td; tetanus and diphtheria toxoid

U.S./Canadian Brand Names Decavac® [US]; Td Adsorbed [Can]

Therapeutic Category Toxoid

Use

Diphtheria and tetanus toxoids adsorbed for pediatric use (DT): Infants and children through 6 years of age: Active immunization against diphtheria and tetanus when pertussis vaccine is contraindicated

Tetanus and diphtheria toxoids adsorbed for adult use (Td) (Decavac™): Children ≥7 years of age and Adults: Active immunization against diphtheria and tetanus; tetanus prophylaxis in wound management

The Advisory Committee on Immunization Practices (ACIP) recommends routine vaccination for the following:

- Adults and children ≥7 years should receive a booster dose of Td every 10 years; persons <65 years of age may substitute a single Td booster dose with Tdap
- Children 7-10 years, adults, and the elderly (≥65 years) who are wounded in bombings or similar mass casualty events who have penetrating injuries or nonintact skin exposure and who cannot confirm receipt of a tetanus booster within the previous 5 years, may also receive a single dose of Td; children ≥11 years may also received Td if Tdap is unavailable

Usual Dosage I.M.:

Infants and Children ≤6 years (DT): Primary immunization:

6 weeks to 1 year: Three 0.5 mL doses at least 4 weeks apart; administer a reinforcing dose 6-12 months after the third injection

1-6 years: Two 0.5 mL doses at least 4-8 weeks apart; reinforcing dose 6-12 months after second injection; if final dose is given after seventh birthday, use adult preparation

4-6 years (booster immunization): 0.5 mL; not necessary if the fourth dose was given after fourth birthday; routinely administer booster doses at 10-year intervals with the adult preparation

Children ≥7 years and Adults (Td):

Primary immunization: Patients previously not immunized should receive 2 primary doses of 0.5 mL each, given at an interval of 4-8 weeks; third (reinforcing) dose of 0.5 mL 6-12 months later

Booster immunization: 0.5 mL every 10 years; to be given to children 11-12 years of age if at least 5 years have elapsed since last dose of toxoid containing vaccine. Subsequent routine doses are not recommended more often than every 10 years. The ACIP prefers Tdap for use in adolescents 11-18 years; refer to diphtheria, tetanus toxoids, and acellular pertussis vaccine monograph for additional information.

Tetanus prophylaxis in wound management; use of tetanus toxoid (Td) and/or tetanus immune globulin (TIG) depends upon the number of prior tetanus toxoid (TT) doses and type of wound.

Clean, minor wounds:

- Prior number of tetanus toxoid doses is unknown or <3: Td[1] or Tdap
- Prior number of tetanus toxoid doses is ≥3: Td[1] or Tdap only if ≥10 years since last dose
- If only three doses of fluid tetanus toxoid have been received, a fourth dose of toxoid, preferably an adsorbed toxoid, should be given

All other wounds:

- Prior number of tetanus toxoid doses is unknown or <3: Td[1] or Tdap and TIG
- Prior number of tetanus toxoid doses is ≥3: Td[1] or Tdap only if ≥5 years since last dose

[1]Adult tetanus and diphtheria toxoids; use pediatric preparations (DT or DTP) if the patient is <7 years old.

Note: Tdap is preferred in adolescents ≥10 years and adults who have never received Tdap. Td is preferred to TT in adolescents ≥10 years and adults who received Tdap previously or when Tdap is not available. If TT and TIG are both used, tetanus toxoid (adsorbed) rather than tetanus toxoid (fluid) should be used.

Adapted from Centers for Disease Control publications *MMWR*, 1991, 40(RR-10); *MMWR*, 2009, 58 (14):374-5; *MMWR*, 2006, 55(early release);1-34; *MMWR Recomm Rep*, 2006, 55(RR-17):1-37.

Dosage Forms

Injection, suspension [Td, adult]: Diphtheria 2 Lf units and tetanus 2 Lf units per 0.5 mL (5 mL, 7.5 mL); diphtheria 2 Lf units and tetanus 5 Lf units per 0.5 mL (5 mL, 7.5 mL)

Injection, suspension [Td, adult; preservative free]: Diphtheria 2 Lf units and tetanus 2 Lf units per 0.5 mL (0.5 mL); diphtheria 2 Lf units and tetanus 5 Lf units per 0.5 mL (0.5 mL)

Decavac™: Diphtheria 2 Lf units and tetanus 5 Lf units per 0.5 mL (0.5 mL)

Injection, suspension [DT, pediatric; preservative free]: Diphtheria 6.7 Lf units and tetanus 5 Lf units per 0.5 mL (0.5 mL)

diphtheria and tetanus toxoids, acellular pertussis, and poliovirus vaccine

(dif THEER ee a & TET a nus TOKS oyds, ay CEL yoo lar per TUS sis & POE lee oh VYE rus vak SEEN)

Synonyms diphtheria and tetanus toxoids and acellular pertussis adsorbed, and inactivated poliovirus vaccine combined; DTaP-IPV

U.S./Canadian Brand Names Kinrix™ [US]

Therapeutic Category Vaccine, Inactivated

Use Active immunization against diphtheria, tetanus, pertussis, and poliomyelitis, used as the 5th dose in the DTaP series and the 4th dose in the IPV series

The Advisory Committee on Immunization Practices (ACIP) recommends routine vaccination for use as the fifth dose in the DTaP series and the fourth dose in the IPV series in children who received DTaP (Infanrix®) and/or DTaP-Hepatitis B-IPV (Pediarix®) as the first 3 doses and DTaP (Infanrix®) as the fourth dose. Whenever feasible, the same manufacturer should be used to provide the pertussis component; however, vaccination should not be deferred if a specific brand is not known or is not available.

Usual Dosage I.M.: Children 4-6 years: Immunization: 0.5 mL; **Note:** For use as the 5th dose in the DTaP series and the 4th dose in the IPV series

Dosage Forms

Injection, suspension [preservative free]:

Kinrix™: Diphtheria toxoid 25 Lf, tetanus toxoid 10 Lf, acellular pertussis antigens [inactivated pertussis toxin 25 mcg, filamentous hemagglutinin 25 mcg, pertactin 8 mcg], type 1 poliovirus 40 D-antigen units, type 2 poliovirus 8 D-antigen units, and type 3 poliovirus 32 D-antigen units per 0.5 mL (0.5 mL)

diphtheria and tetanus toxoids, acellular pertussis, poliovirus and *Haemophilus* b conjugate vaccine

(dif THEER ee a & TET a nus TOKS oyds ay CEL yoo lar per TUS sis POE lee oh VYE rus & hem OF fi lus in floo EN za bee KON joo gate vak SEEN)

Synonyms *Haemophilus* B conjugate (Hib); *Haemophilus* B polysaccharide; diphtheria toxoid; DTaP-IPV/Hib; pertussis, acellular (adsorbed); tetanus toxoid

U.S./Canadian Brand Names Pentacel® [US]

Therapeutic Category Vaccine, Inactivated

Use Active immunization against diphtheria, tetanus, pertussis, poliomyelitis, and invasive disease caused by *H. influenzae* type b in children 6 weeks through 4 years of age

Advisory Committee on Immunization Practices (ACIP) recommends that Pentacel® (DTaP-IPV/Hib) may be used to provide the recommended DTaP, IPV, and Hib immunization in children <5 years of age. Whenever feasible, the same manufacturer should be used to provide the pertussis component; however, vaccination should not be deferred if a specific brand is not known or is not available. The Hib component in Pentacel® contains a tetanus toxoid conjugate. A Hib vaccine containing the PRP-OMP conjugate (PedvaxHIB®) may provide a more rapid seroconversion following the first dose and may be preferable to use in certain populations (eg, American Indian or Alaska Native children).

Usual Dosage I.M.: Children:

Primary immunization: Children 6 weeks to ≤4 years: 0.5 mL per dose administered at 2, 4, 6 and 15-18 months of age (total of 4 doses). The first dose may be administered as early as 6 weeks of age. Following completion of the 4-dose series, children should receive a dose of DTaP vaccine at 4-6 years of age (Daptacel® recommended due to same pertussis antigen used in both products).

Children previously vaccinated with ≥1 dose of Daptacel® or IPV vaccines: Pentacel® may be used to complete the first 4 doses of the DTaP or IPV series in children scheduled to receive the other components in the vaccine.

Children previously vaccinated with ≥1 dose of *Haemophilus* b conjugate vaccine: Pentacel® may be used to complete the series in children scheduled to receive the other components in the vaccine; however, if different brands of *Haemophilus* b conjugate vaccine are administered to complete the series, 3 primary immunizing doses are needed, followed by a booster dose.

Note: Completion of 3 doses of Pentacel® provides primary immunization against diphtheria, tetanus, *H. influenzae* type B, and poliomyelitis. Completion of the 4-dose series with Pentacel® provides primary immunization against pertussis. It also provides a booster vaccination against diphtheria, tetanus, *H. influenzae* type B, and poliomyelitis.

Dosage Forms

Injection, suspension:

Pentacel®: Diphtheria toxoid 15 Lf, tetanus toxoid 5 Lf, acellular pertussis antigens, poliovirus, and *Haemophilus* b capsular polysaccharide 10 mcg per 0.5 mL (0.5 mL)

diphtheria and tetanus toxoids and acellular pertussis adsorbed, and inactivated poliovirus vaccine combined *see* diphtheria and tetanus toxoids, acellular pertussis, and poliovirus vaccine *on page 319*

diphtheria and tetanus toxoids and acellular pertussis adsorbed, hepatitis B (recombinant) and inactivated poliovirus vaccine combined *see* diphtheria, tetanus toxoids, acellular pertussis, hepatitis B (recombinant), and poliovirus (inactivated) vaccine *on page 320*

diphtheria antitoxin (dif THEER ee a an tee TOKS in)

Therapeutic Category Antitoxin

Use Treatment of diphtheria (neutralizes unbound toxin, available from CDC)

Usual Dosage I.M. or slow I.V. infusion: Dosage varies; range: 20,000-120,000 units

diphtheria CRM$_{197}$ protein *see* pneumococcal conjugate vaccine (7-valent) *on page 793*

diphtheria, tetanus toxoids, acellular pertussis, hepatitis B (recombinant), and poliovirus (inactivated) vaccine

(dif THEER ee a, TET a nus TOKS oyds, ay CEL yoo lar per TUS sis, hep a TYE tis bee ree KOM be nant, & POE lee oh VYE rus vak SEEN)

Synonyms diphtheria and tetanus toxoids and acellular pertussis adsorbed, hepatitis B (recombinant) and inactivated poliovirus vaccine combined; DTap-HepB-IPV

U.S./Canadian Brand Names Pediarix® [US/Can]

Therapeutic Category Vaccine

Use Combination vaccine for the active immunization against diphtheria, tetanus, pertussis, hepatitis B virus (all known subtypes), and poliomyelitis (caused by poliovirus types 1, 2, and 3)

The Advisory Committee on Immunization Practices (ACIP) recommends Pediarix® for the following:

- Primary vaccination for DTaP, Hep B, and IPV in children at 2-, 4-, and 6 months of age.
- To complete the primary vaccination series in children who have received DTaP (Infanrix®) and who are scheduled to received the other components of the vaccine. Whenever feasible, the same manufacturer should be used to provide the pertussis component; however, vaccination should not be deferred if a specific brand is not known or is not available. HepB and IPV from different manufacturers are interchangeable.

Usual Dosage I.M.: Children 6 weeks to <7 years:

Primary immunization: 0.5 mL; repeat in 6-8 week intervals (preferably 8-week intervals) for a total of 3 doses. Vaccination usually begins at 2 months, but may be started as early as 6 weeks of age.

Use in children previously vaccinated with one or more component, and who are also scheduled to receive all vaccine components:

Hepatitis B vaccine: Infants born of HBsAg-negative mothers who received 1 dose of hepatitis B vaccine at birth may be given Pediarix® (safety data limited); use in infants who received more than 1 dose of hepatitis B vaccine has not been studied. Infants who received 1 or more doses of hepatitis B vaccine (recombinant) may be given Pediarix® to complete the hepatitis B series (safety and efficacy not established).

Diphtheria and tetanus toxoids, and acellular pertussis vaccine (DTaP): Infants previously vaccinated with 1 or 2 doses of Infanrix® may use Pediarix® to complete the first 3 doses of the series (safety and efficacy not established); use of Pediarix® to complete DTaP vaccination started with products other than Infanrix® is not recommended.

Inactivated polio vaccine (IPV): Infants previously vaccinated with 1 or 2 doses of IPV may use Pediarix® to complete the first 3 doses of the series (safety and efficacy not established).

Dosage Forms

Injection, suspension [preservative free]:

Pediarix®: Diphtheria toxoid 25 Lf, tetanus toxoid 10 Lf, acellular pertussis antigens per 0.5 mL (0.5 mL)

diphtheria, tetanus toxoids, and acellular pertussis vaccine

(dif THEER ee a & TET a nus TOKS oyds & ay CEL yoo lar per TUS sis vak SEEN)

Sound-Alike/Look-Alike Issues

Adacel® (Tdap) may be confused with Daptacel® (DTap)

Daptacel® (DTap) may be confused with Adacel® (Tdap)

Synonyms DTaP; dTpa; Tdap; tetanus toxoid, reduced diphtheria toxoid, and acellular pertussis, adsorbed

U.S./Canadian Brand Names Adacel® [US/Can]; Boostrix® [US]; Daptacel® [US]; Infanrix® [US]; Tripedia® [US]

Therapeutic Category Toxoid

Use

Daptacel®, Infanrix®, Tripedia® (DTaP): Active immunization against diphtheria, tetanus, and pertussis from age 6 weeks through 6 years of age (prior to seventh birthday)

Adacel®, Boostrix® (Tdap): Active booster immunization against diphtheria, tetanus, and pertussis

The Advisory Committee on Immunization Practices (ACIP) recommends routine vaccination for the following:

Children 6 weeks to <7 years (DTaP): For primary immunization against diphtheria, tetanus and pertussis

Adolescents 11-18 years (Tdap):

- A single dose of Tdap as a booster dose in adolescents who have completed the recommended childhood DTaP vaccination series (preferred age of administration is 11-12 years)
- A single dose of Tdap should be given to replace a single dose of Td if the last dose of Td was ≥5 years earlier; lesser intervals may be used if the benefit outweighs the risk (not for multiple administrations; recommendations are for the replacement of a single dose of Td only)
- Persons wounded in bombings or similar mass casualty events and who cannot confirm receipt of a tetanus booster within the previous 5 years and who have penetrating injuries or nonintact skin exposure should receive a single dose of Tdap

Adults 19-64 years: A single dose of Tdap should be given to replace a single dose of Td if the last dose of Td was ≥10 years earlier (not for multiple administrations; recommendations are for the replacement of a single dose of Td only). A shorter interval (<10 years but at least 2 years since last dose of Td) may be considered in the following situations:

- To protect against pertussis
- To protect against pertussis transmission to infants in adults who anticipate close contact with children <12 months of age; Tdap should be administered at least 2 weeks prior to beginning close contact
- Healthcare providers with direct patient contact
- Persons wounded in bombings or similar mass casualty events and who cannot confirm receipt of a tetanus booster within the previous 5 years and who have penetrating injuries or nonintact skin exposure, should receive a single dose of Tdap

Usual Dosage

Primary immunization: Children 6 weeks to <7 years: I.M.: **Note:** Whenever possible, the same product should be used for all doses. Interruption of recommended schedule does not require starting the series over; a delay between doses should not interfere with final immunity.

Daptacel®, Infanrix®, Tripedia®: 0.5 mL per dose, total of 5 doses administered as follows:

Three doses, usually given at 2-, 4-, and 6 months of age; may be given as early as 6 weeks of age and repeated every 6-8 weeks

Fourth dose: Given at ~15-20 months of age, but at least 6 months after third dose

Fifth dose: Given at 4-6 years of age, prior to starting school or kindergarten; if the fourth dose is given at ≥4 years of age, the fifth dose may be omitted

Booster immunization:

ACIP recommendations:

Adolescents 11-18 years: I.M.: 0.5 mL. A single dose of Tdap should be given instead of Td in adolescents who have completed the recommended childhood DTP/DTaP series and have not received Td or Tdap; preferred age of vaccination with Tdap is 11-12 years. Adolescents who received Td but not Tdap and who have completed the recommended childhood DTP/DTaP series are encouraged to receive Tdap; an interval of at least 5 years between Td and Tdap is recommended, but lesser intervals may be used if the benefit outweighs the risk.

Adults 19-64 years: I.M.: 0.5 mL. A single dose should be given instead of Td in adults if they received their last dose of Td ≥10 years previous. Shorter intervals (as short as 2 years) may used among healthcare providers, adults in contact with infants, or others in settings with increased risk for pertussis, including during pertussis outbreaks. Tdap should only be used to replace a single booster dose of Td.

Manufacturer's labeling:

Children ≥10 and Adults ≤64 years (Boostrix®): I.M.: 0.5 mL as a single dose, administered 5 years after last dose of DTwP or DTaP vaccine.

Children ≥11 years and Adults ≤64 years (Adacel®): I.M.: 0.5 mL as a single dose, administered 5 years after last dose of DTwP or DTaP vaccine.

Wound management: Adacel® (in patients 11-64 years of age) or Boostrix® (in patients 10-64 years of age) may be used as an alternative to Td vaccine when a tetanus toxoid-containing vaccine is needed for wound management, and in whom the pertussis component is also indicated.

Clean, minor wounds:

- Prior number of tetanus toxoid doses is unknown or <3: Td[1] or Tdap
- Prior number of tetanus toxoid doses is ≥3: Td[1] or Tdap only if ≥10 years since last dose
- If only three doses of fluid tetanus toxoid have been received, a fourth dose of toxoid, preferably an adsorbed toxoid, should be given

All other wounds:

- Prior number of tetanus toxoid doses is unknown or <3: Td[1] or Tdap and TIG
- Prior number of tetanus toxoid doses is ≥3: Td[1] or Tdap only if ≥5 years since last dose

[1]Adult tetanus and diphtheria toxoids; use pediatric preparations (DT or DTP) if the patient is <7 years old.

Note: Tdap is preferred in adolescents ≥10 years and adults who have never received Tdap. Td is preferred to TT in adolescents ≥10 years and adults who received Tdap previously or when Tdap is not available. If TT and TIG are both used, tetanus toxoid (adsorbed) rather than tetanus toxoid (fluid) should be used.

Adapted from Centers for Disease Control publications *MMWR*, 1991, 40(RR-10); *MMWR*, 2009, 58 (14):374-5; *MMWR*, 2006, 55(early release);1-34; *MMWR Recomm Rep*, 2006, 55(RR-17):1-37.

Dosage Forms

Injection, suspension [Tdap, booster formulation]:

Adacel®: Diphtheria 2 Lf units, tetanus 5 Lf units, and acellular pertussis antigens per 0.5 mL (0.5 mL)

Boostrix®: Diphtheria 2.5 Lf units, tetanus 5 Lf units, and acellular pertussis antigens per 0.5 mL (0.5 mL)

Injection, suspension [DTaP, active immunization formulation]:

Daptacel®: Diphtheria 15 Lf units, tetanus 5 Lf units, and acellular pertussis antigens per 0.5 mL (0.5 mL)

Infanrix®: Diphtheria 25 Lf units, tetanus 10 Lf units, and acellular pertussis antigens per 0.5 mL (0.5 mL)

Tripedia®: Diphtheria 6.7 Lf units, tetanus 5 Lf units, and acellular pertussis antigens per 0.5 mL (0.5 mL)

Note: Tripedia® vaccine is also used to reconstitute ActHIB® to prepare TriHIBit® vaccine (diphtheria, tetanus toxoids, and acellular pertussis and *Haemophilus influenzae* b conjugate vaccine combination)

diphtheria, tetanus toxoids, and acellular pertussis vaccine and *Haemophilus influenzae* b conjugate vaccine

(dif THEER ee a & TET a nus TOKS oyds, ay CEL yoo lar per TUS sis & hem OF fi lus in floo EN za bee KON joo gate vak SEEN)

Synonyms *Haemophilus influenzae* b conjugate vaccine and diphtheria, tetanus toxoids, and acellular pertussis vaccine; DTaP/Hib

U.S./Canadian Brand Names TriHIBit® [US]

Therapeutic Category Toxoid; Vaccine, Inactivated Bacteria

Use Active immunization of children 15-18 months of age for prevention of diphtheria, tetanus, pertussis, and invasive disease caused by *H. influenzae* type b

The Advisory Committee on Immunization Practices (ACIP) recommends the use of TriHIBit® for the fourth dose of the diphtheria, tetanus, pertussis, and *Haemophilus* vaccine series. Whenever feasible, the same manufacturer should be used to provide the pertussis component; however, vaccination should not be deferred if a specific brand is not known or is not available.

Usual Dosage I.M.: Children 15-18 months: 0.5 mL: **Note:** For use as the fourth dose of the DTaP and Hib series (see individual vaccines). May be used as a booster in children 12-20 months of age as long as 6 months have elapsed since the third dose.

Dosage Forms

Injection, suspension [preservative free]:

TriHIBit®: Diphtheria 6.7 Lf units, tetanus 5 Lf units, acellular pertussis antigens [inactivated pertussis toxin 23.4 mcg, filamentous hemagglutinin 23.4 mcg], and *Haemophilus* b capsular polysaccharide 10 mcg [bound to tetanus toxoid 24 mcg] per 0.5 mL (0.5 mL) [Tripedia® vaccine used to reconstitute ActHIB® forms TriHIBit®]

diphtheria toxoid *see* diphtheria and tetanus toxoids, acellular pertussis, poliovirus and *Haemophilus* b conjugate vaccine *on page 320*

diphtheria toxoid conjugate *see Haemophilus* B conjugate vaccine *on page 483*

dipivalyl epinephrine *see* dipivefrin *on page 323*

dipivefrin (dye PI ve frin)

Synonyms dipivalyl epinephrine; dipivefrin hydrochloride; DPE

U.S./Canadian Brand Names Ophtho-Dipivefrin™ [Can]; PMS-Dipivefrin [Can]; Propine® [Can]

Therapeutic Category Adrenergic Agonist Agent

Use Reduces elevated intraocular pressure in chronic open-angle glaucoma; also used to treat ocular hypertension, low tension, and secondary glaucomas

Usual Dosage Ophthalmic: Adults: Instill 1 drop every 12 hours into the eyes

dipivefrin hydrochloride *see* dipivefrin *on page 323*

Diprivan® [US/Can] *see* propofol *on page 827*

Diprolene® [US] *see* betamethasone (topical) *on page 138*

Diprolene® AF [US] *see* betamethasone (topical) *on page 138*

Diprolene® Glycol [Can] *see* betamethasone (topical) *on page 138*

dipropylacetic acid *see* valproic acid and derivatives *on page 1002*

Diprosone® [Can] *see* betamethasone (topical) *on page 138*

dipyridamole (dye peer ID a mole)

Sound-Alike/Look-Alike Issues

dipyridamole may be confused with disopyramide

Persantine® may be confused with Periactin®, Permitil®

U.S./Canadian Brand Names Apo-Dipyridamole FC® [Can]; Dipyridamole For Injection [Can]; Persantine® [US/Can]

Therapeutic Category Antiplatelet Agent; Vasodilator

Use

Oral: Used with warfarin to decrease thrombosis in patients after artificial heart valve replacement

I.V.: Diagnostic agent in CAD

Usual Dosage

Oral: Children ≥12 years and Adults: Adjunctive therapy for prophylaxis of thromboembolism with cardiac valve replacement: 75-100 mg 4 times/day

I.V.: Adults: Evaluation of coronary artery disease: 0.14 mg/kg/minute for 4 minutes; maximum dose: 60 mg

Following dipyridamole infusion, inject thallium-201 within 5 minutes. **Note:** Aminophylline should be available for urgent/emergent use; dosing of 50-100 mg (range: 50-250 mg) I.V. push over 30-60 seconds.

Dosage Forms

Injection, solution: 5 mg/mL (2 mL, 10 mL)

Tablet: 25 mg, 50 mg, 75 mg

Persantine®: 25 mg, 50 mg, 75 mg

dipyridamole and aspirin *see* aspirin and dipyridamole *on page* 105

Dipyridamole For Injection [Can] *see* dipyridamole *on page* 324

Disalcid® *(Discontinued)* *see* salsalate *on page* 888

disalicylic acid *see* salsalate *on page* 888

DisCoVisc® [US] *see* sodium chondroitin sulfate and sodium hyaluronate *on page* 910

Disobrom® *(Discontinued)* *see* dexbrompheniramine and pseudoephedrine *on page* 289

disodium cromoglycate *see* cromolyn sodium *on page* 261

disodium thiosulfate pentahydrate *see* sodium thiosulfate *on page* 915

***d*-isoephedrine hydrochloride** *see* pseudoephedrine *on page* 833

Disonate® *(Discontinued)* *see* docusate *on page* 326

disopyramide (dye soe PEER a mide)

Sound-Alike/Look-Alike Issues

disopyramide may be confused with desipramine, dipyridamole

Norpace® may be confused with Norpramin®

Synonyms disopyramide phosphate

U.S./Canadian Brand Names Norpace® CR [US]; Norpace® [US/Can]; Rythmodan® [Can]; Rythmodan®-LA [Can]

Therapeutic Category Antiarrhythmic Agent, Class I-A

Use Suppression and prevention of unifocal and multifocal atrial and premature, ventricular premature complexes, coupled ventricular tachycardia; effective in the conversion of atrial fibrillation, atrial flutter, and paroxysmal atrial tachycardia to normal sinus rhythm and prevention of the recurrence of these arrhythmias after conversion by other methods

Usual Dosage Oral:

Children:

<1 year: 10-30 mg/kg/24 hours in 4 divided doses

1-4 years: 10-20 mg/kg/24 hours in 4 divided doses

4-12 years: 10-15 mg/kg/24 hours in 4 divided doses

12-18 years: 6-15 mg/kg/24 hours in 4 divided doses

Adults:

<50 kg: 100 mg every 6 hours or 200 mg every 12 hours (controlled release)

>50 kg: 150 mg every 6 hours or 300 mg every 12 hours (controlled release); if no response, increase to 200 mg every 6 hours. Maximum dose required for patients with severe refractory ventricular tachycardia is 400 mg every 6 hours.

Dosage Forms

Capsule: 100 mg, 150 mg

Norpace®: 100 mg, 150 mg

Capsule, controlled release: 100 mg, 150 mg

Norpace® CR: 100 mg, 150 mg

disopyramide phosphate *see* disopyramide *on page* 324

Disotate® ***(Discontinued)*** *see* edetate disodium *on page* 347

Di-Spaz® Injection ***(Discontinued)*** *see* dicyclomine *on page* 305

Di-Spaz® Oral ***(Discontinued)*** *see* dicyclomine *on page* 305

DisperMox™ ***(Discontinued)*** *see* amoxicillin *on page* 70

disulfiram (dye SUL fi ram)

Sound-Alike/Look-Alike Issues

disulfiram may be confused with Diflucan®

Antabuse® may be confused with Anturane®

U.S./Canadian Brand Names Antabuse® [US]

Therapeutic Category Aldehyde Dehydrogenase Inhibitor Agent

Use Management of chronic alcoholism

Usual Dosage Oral: Adults: Do not administer until the patient has abstained from ethanol for at least 12 hours

Initial: 500 mg/day as a single dose for 1-2 weeks; maximum daily dose is 500 mg

Average maintenance dose: 250 mg/day; range: 125-500 mg; duration of therapy is to continue until the patient is fully recovered socially and a basis for permanent self control has been established; maintenance therapy may be required for months or even years

Dosage Forms

Tablet:

Antabuse®: 250 mg, 500 mg

Dital® ***(Discontinued)*** *see* phendimetrazine *on page* 770

dithioglycerol *see* dimercaprol *on page* 313

dithranol *see* anthralin *on page* 80

Ditropan® [US/Can] *see* oxybutynin *on page* 736

Ditropan XL® [US/Can] *see* oxybutynin *on page* 736

diurex® [US-OTC] *see* pamabrom *on page* 745

diurex® Aquagels® [US-OTC] *see* pamabrom *on page* 745

diurex® Maximum Relief [US-OTC] *see* pamabrom *on page* 745

Diurigen® ***(Discontinued)*** *see* chlorothiazide *on page* 213

Diuril® [US/Can] *see* chlorothiazide *on page* 213

divalproex sodium *see* valproic acid and derivatives *on page* 1002

Divigel® [US] *see* estradiol *on page* 373

Dixarit® [Can] *see* clonidine *on page* 245

Dizac® Injectable Emulsion ***(Discontinued)*** *see* diazepam *on page* 301

Dizmiss® ***(Discontinued)*** *see* meclizine *on page* 619

5071-1DL(6) *see* megestrol *on page* 621

***dl*-alpha tocopherol** *see* vitamin E *on page* 1018

4-DMDR *see* idarubicin *on page* 518

***D*-mannitol** *see* mannitol *on page* 613

D-Med® Injection ***(Discontinued)*** *see* methylprednisolone *on page* 647

DMSA *see* succimer *on page* 924

DMSO *see* dimethyl sulfoxide *on page* 314

Doak® Tar [US-OTC] *see* coal tar *on page* 250

Doan's® Extra Strength [US-OTC] *see* magnesium salicylate *on page* 610

dobutamine (doe BYOO ta meen)

Sound-Alike/Look-Alike Issues

DOBUTamine may be confused with DOPamine

Synonyms dobutamine hydrochloride

Tall-Man DOBUTamine

U.S./Canadian Brand Names Dobutamine Injection, USP [Can]; Dobutrex® [Can]

Therapeutic Category Adrenergic Agonist Agent

Use Short-term management of patients with cardiac decompensation

Usual Dosage Administration requires the use of an infusion pump; I.V. infusion: Children and Adults: 2.5-20 mcg/kg/minute; maximum: 40 mcg/kg/minute, titrate to desired response.

Dosage Forms

Infusion [premixed in dextrose]: 1 mg/mL (250 mL, 500 mL); 2 mg/mL (250 mL); 4 mg/mL (250 mL)

Injection, solution: 12.5 mg/mL (20 mL, 40 mL, 100 mL)

dobutamine hydrochloride *see* dobutamine *on page* 325

Dobutamine Injection, USP [Can] *see* dobutamine *on page* 325

Dobutrex® [Can] *see* dobutamine *on page* 325

docetaxel (doe se TAKS el)

Sound-Alike/Look-Alike Issues

Taxotere® may be confused with Taxol®

Synonyms NSC-628503; RP-6976

U.S./Canadian Brand Names Taxotere® [US/Can]

Therapeutic Category Antineoplastic Agent

Use Treatment of breast cancer; locally-advanced or metastatic nonsmall cell lung cancer (NSCLC); hormone refractory, metastatic prostate cancer; advanced gastric adenocarcinoma; locally-advanced squamous cell head and neck cancer

Usual Dosage I.V. infusion: Adults: Refer to individual protocols: **Note:** Premedicate with corticosteroids, beginning the day before docetaxel administration, (administer for 1-5 days) to reduce the severity of hypersensitivity reactions and pulmonary/peripheral edema

Breast cancer:

Locally-advanced or metastatic: 60-100 mg/m^2 every 3 weeks; patients initially started at 60 mg/m^2 who do not develop toxicity may tolerate higher doses

Operable, node-positive (adjuvant treatment): 75 mg/m^2 every 3 weeks for 6 courses (in combination with doxorubicin and cyclophosphamide)

Nonsmall cell lung cancer: 75 mg/m^2 every 3 weeks (as monotherapy or in combination with cisplatin)

Prostate cancer: 75 mg/m^2 every 3 weeks (in combination with prednisone)

Gastric adenocarcinoma: 75 mg/m^2 every 3 weeks (in combination with cisplatin and fluorouracil)

Head and neck cancer: 75 mg/m^2 every 3 weeks (in combination with cisplatin and fluorouracil) for 3 or 4 cycles, followed by radiation therapy

Dosage Forms

Injection, solution [concentrate]:

Taxotere®: 20 mg/0.5 mL (0.5 mL, 2 mL)

docosanol (doe KOE san ole)

Synonyms *n*-docosanol; behenyl alcohol

U.S./Canadian Brand Names Abreva® [US-OTC]

Therapeutic Category Antiviral Agent, Topical

Use Treatment of herpes simplex of the face or lips

Usual Dosage Topical: Children ≥12 years and Adults: Apply 5 times/day to affected area of face or lips. Start at first sign of cold sore or fever blister and continue until healed.

Dosage Forms

Cream, topical:

Abreva® [OTC]: 10% (2 g)

docusate (DOK yoo sate)

Sound-Alike/Look-Alike Issues

docusate may be confused with Doxinate®

Colace® may be confused with Calan®, Cozaar®

Surfak® may be confused with Surbex®

Synonyms dioctyl calcium sulfosuccinate; dioctyl sodium sulfosuccinate; docusate calcium; docusate potassium; docusate sodium; DOSS; DSS

U.S./Canadian Brand Names Apo-Docusate-Sodium® [Can]; Colace® [US-OTC/Can]; Colax-C® [Can]; Correctol® [US-OTC]; D-S-S® [US-OTC]; Diocto® [US-OTC]; Docu-Soft [US-OTC]; Docusoft-S™ [US-OTC]; DOK™ [US-OTC]; DOS® [US-OTC]; Dulcolax® Stool Softener [US-OTC]; Enemeez® Plus [US-OTC]; Enemeez® [US-OTC]; Fleet® Pedia-Lax™ Liquid Stool Softener [US-OTC]; Fleet® Sof-Lax® [US-OTC]; Genasoft® [US-OTC]; Novo-Docusate Calcium [Can]; Novo-Docusate Sodium [Can]; Phillips'® Stool Softener Laxative [US-OTC]; PMS-Docusate Calcium [Can]; PMS-Docusate Sodium [Can]; Regulex® [Can]; Selax® [Can]; Silace [US-OTC]; Soflax™ [Can]; Surfak® [US-OTC]

Therapeutic Category Stool Softener

Use Stool softener in patients who should avoid straining during defecation and constipation associated with hard, dry stools; prophylaxis for straining (Valsalva) following myocardial infarction. A safe agent to be used in elderly; some evidence that doses <200 mg are ineffective; stool softeners are unnecessary if stool is well hydrated or "mushy" and soft; shown to be ineffective used long-term.

Usual Dosage Docusate salts are interchangeable; the amount of sodium or calcium per dosage unit is clinically insignificant

Infants and Children <3 years: Oral: 10-40 mg/day in 1-4 divided doses

Children: Oral:

- 3-6 years: 20-60 mg/day in 1-4 divided doses
- 6-12 years: 40-150 mg/day in 1-4 divided doses

Adolescents and Adults: Oral: 50-500 mg/day in 1-4 divided doses

Older Children and Adults: Rectal: Add 50-100 mg of docusate liquid to enema fluid (saline or water); administer as retention or flushing enema

Dosage Forms

Capsule, oral: 100 mg, 240 mg, 250 mg
- Colace® [OTC]: 50 mg, 100 mg

Capsule, softgel, oral: 100 mg, 240 mg, 250 mg
- Correctol® [OTC], Docu-Soft [OTC], Docusoft-S™ [OTC], Genasoft® [OTC], Dulcolax® Stool Softener [OTC], Fleet® Sof-Lax® [OTC], Phillips'® Stool Softener Laxative [OTC]: 100 mg
- DOK™ [OTC], DOS® [OTC], D-S-S® [OTC]: 100 mg, 250 mg
- Surfak® [OTC]: 240 mg

Liquid, oral: 150 mg/15 mL
- Colace® [OTC], Diocto® [OTC], Silace [OTC]: 150 mg/15 mL
- Fleet® Pedia-Lax™ Liquid Stool Softener [OTC]: 50 mg/15 mL

Solution, rectal [enema]:
- Enemeez® [OTC], Enemeez® Plus [OTC]: 283 mg/5 mL

Syrup: 20 mg/5 mL, 60 mg/15 mL
- Colace® [OTC], Diocto® [OTC]: 60 mg/15 mL
- Silace [OTC]: 20 mg/5 mL

docusate and senna (DOK yoo sate & SEN na)

Sound-Alike/Look-Alike Issues

Senokot® may be confused with Depakote®

Synonyms senna and docusate; senna-S

U.S./Canadian Brand Names Peri-Colace® [US-OTC]; Senokot-S® [US-OTC]; SenoSol™-SS [US-OTC]

Therapeutic Category Laxative, Stimulant; Stool Softener

Use Short-term treatment of constipation

Usual Dosage Oral: Constipation: OTC ranges:

Children:

- 2-6 years: Initial: 4.3 mg sennosides plus 25 mg docusate (1/2 tablet) once daily (maximum: 1 tablet twice daily)
- 6-12 years: Initial: 8.6 sennosides plus 50 mg docusate (1 tablet) once daily (maximum: 2 tablets twice daily)

Children ≥12 years and Adults: Initial: 2 tablets (17.2 mg sennosides plus 100 mg docusate) once daily (maximum: 4 tablets twice daily)

Dosage Forms

Tablet: Docusate 50 mg and sennosides 8.6 mg
- Peri-Colace® [OTC], Senokot-S® [OTC], SenoSol™-SS: Docusate 50 mg and sennosides 8.6 mg

docusate calcium *see* docusate *on page* 326

docusate potassium *see* docusate *on page* 326

docusate sodium *see* docusate *on page* 326

Docu-Soft [US-OTC] *see* docusate *on page 326*
Docusoft Plus™ ***(Discontinued)***
Docusoft-S™ [US-OTC] *see* docusate *on page 326*

dofetilide (doe FET il ide)

U.S./Canadian Brand Names Tikosyn® [US/Can]

Therapeutic Category Antiarrhythmic Agent, Class III

Use Maintenance of normal sinus rhythm in patients with chronic atrial fibrillation/atrial flutter of longer than 1-week duration who have been converted to normal sinus rhythm; conversion of atrial fibrillation and atrial flutter to normal sinus rhythm

Usual Dosage Oral: Adults: **Note:** QT or QT_c must be determined prior to first dose. If QT_c >440 msec (>500 msec in patients with ventricular conduction abnormalities), dofetilide is contraindicated.

Initial: 500 mcg orally twice daily. Initial dosage must be adjusted in patients with estimated Cl_{cr} <60 mL/minute. Dofetilide may be initiated at lower doses than recommended based on physician discretion.

Modification of dosage in response to initial dose: QT_c interval should be measured 2-3 hours after the initial dose. If the QT_c >15% of baseline, or if the QT_c is >500 msec (550 msec in patients with ventricular conduction abnormalities) dofetilide should be adjusted. If the starting dose is 500 mcg twice daily, then adjust to 250 mcg twice daily. If the starting dose was 250 mcg twice daily, then adjust to 125 mcg twice daily. If the starting dose was 125 mcg twice daily then adjust to 125 mcg every day.

Continued monitoring for doses 2-5: QT_c interval must be determined 2-3 hours after each subsequent dose of dofetilide for in-hospital doses 2-5. If the measured QT_c is >500 msec (550 msec in patients with ventricular conduction abnormalities) at any time, dofetilide should be discontinued.

Chronic therapy (following the 5th dose):

QT or QT_c and creatinine clearance should be evaluated every 3 months. If QT_c >500 msec (>550 msec in patients with ventricular conduction abnormalities), dofetilide should be discontinued.

Dosage Forms

Capsule:

Tikosyn®: 125 mcg, 250 mcg, 500 mcg

Dofus [US-OTC] *see* Lactobacillus *on page 564*
DOK™ [US-OTC] *see* docusate *on page 326*
Doktors® Nasal Solution ***(Discontinued)*** *see* phenylephrine *on page 774*
Dolacet® Forte ***(Discontinued)*** *see* hydrocodone and acetaminophen *on page 501*

dolasetron (dol A se tron)

Sound-Alike/Look-Alike Issues

dolasetron may be confused with granisetron, ondansetron, palonosetron

Anzemet® may be confused with Aldomet® and Avandamet®

Synonyms dolasetron mesylate; MDL 73,147EF

U.S./Canadian Brand Names Anzemet® [US/Can]

Therapeutic Category Selective 5-HT_3 Receptor Antagonist

Use Prevention of nausea and vomiting associated with emetogenic cancer chemotherapy; prevention of postoperative nausea and vomiting; treatment of postoperative nausea and vomiting (injectable form only).

Note: In Canada, the use of dolasetron is contraindicated in children <18 years of age and for the prevention and treatment of postoperative nausea and vomiting in adults. These are not labeled contraindications in the U.S.

Usual Dosage Note: In Canada, the use of dolasetron is contraindicated in children <18 years of age or in the treatment of postoperative nausea and vomiting in adults. These are not labeled contraindications in the U.S.

Prevention of chemotherapy-associated nausea and vomiting (including initial and repeat courses):

Children 2-16 years:

Oral: 1.8 mg/kg within 1 hour before chemotherapy; maximum: 100 mg/dose

I.V.: 1.8 mg/kg ~30 minutes before chemotherapy; maximum: 100 mg/dose

Adults:

Oral:100 mg single dose 1 hour prior to chemotherapy

I.V.: 1.8 mg/kg or 100 mg 30 minutes prior to chemotherapy

Prevention of postoperative nausea and vomiting:
Children 2-16 years:
Oral: 1.2 mg/kg within 2 hours before surgery; maximum: 100 mg/dose
I.V.: 0.35 mg/kg (maximum: 12.5 mg) ~15 minutes before stopping anesthesia
Adults:
Oral: 100 mg within 2 hours before surgery
I.V.: 12.5 mg ~15 minutes before stopping anesthesia
Treatment of postoperative nausea and vomiting: I.V. (only):
Children: 0.35 mg/kg (maximum: 12.5 mg) as soon as needed
Adults: 12.5 mg as soon as needed

Dosage Forms

Injection, solution:

Anzemet®: 20 mg/mL (0.625 mL) [single-use Carpuject® or vial; contains mannitol 38.2 mg/mL]; 20 mg/mL (5 mL) [single-use vial; contains mannitol 38.2 mg/mL]; 20 mg/mL (25 mL) [multidose vial; contains mannitol 29 mg/mL]

Tablet:

Anzemet®: 50 mg, 100 mg

Dom-Mefenamic Acid [Can] *see* mefenamic acid *on page* *621*
Dom-Metformin [Can] *see* metformin *on page* *633*
Dom-Methimazole [Can] *see* methimazole *on page* *637*
Dom-Metoprolol [Can] *see* metoprolol *on page* *650*
DOM-Mirtazapine [Can] *see* mirtazapine *on page* *661*
Dom-Moclobemide [Can] *see* moclobemide *(Canada only) on page* *663*
DOM-Ondansetron [Can] *see* ondansetron *on page* *726*

domperidone *(Canada only)* (dom PE ri done)

Synonyms domperidone maleate

U.S./Canadian Brand Names Apo-Domperidone® [Can]; Dom-Domperidone [Can]; Novo-Domperidone [Can]; Nu-Domperidone [Can]; PHL-Domperidone [Can]; PMS-Domperidone [Can]; RAN™-Domperidone [Can]; ratio-Domperidone [Can]

Therapeutic Category Dopamine Antagonist

Use Symptomatic management of upper GI motility disorders associated with chronic and subacute gastritis and diabetic gastroparesis; prevention of GI symptoms associated with use of dopamine-agonist anti-Parkinson agents

Usual Dosage Oral: Adults:

GI motility disorders: 10 mg 3-4 times/day, 15-30 minutes before meals; severe/resistant cases: 20 mg 3-4 times/day, 15-30 minutes before meals

Nausea/vomiting associated with dopamine-agonist anti-Parkinson agents: 20 mg 3-4 times/day

Dosage Forms [CAN] = Canadian brand name

Tablet: 10 mg [not available in the U.S.]

Alti-Domperidone [CAN], Apo-Domperidone® [CAN], Dom-Domperidone [CAN], Novo-Domperidone [CAN], Nu-Domperidone [CAN], PHL-Domperidone [CAN], PMS-Domperidone [CAN], ratio-Domperidone [CAN]: 10 mg [not available in the U.S.]

domperidone maleate *see* domperidone *(Canada only) on page* *330*
Dom-Piroxicam [Can] *see* piroxicam *on page* *788*
DOM-Pravastatin [Can] *see* pravastatin *on page* *811*
Dom-Propranolol [Can] *see* propranolol *on page* *828*
Dom-Ranitidine [Can] *see* ranitidine *on page* *852*
Dom-Risperidone [Can] *see* risperidone *on page* *870*
Dom-Sertraline [Can] *see* sertraline *on page* *898*
Dom-Simvastatin [Can] *see* simvastatin *on page* *902*
DOM-Sotalol [Can] *see* sotalol *on page* *919*
Dom-Sumatriptan [Can] *see* sumatriptan *on page* *932*
Dom-Temazepam [Can] *see* temazepam *on page* *942*
Dom-Tiaprofenic [Can] *see* tiaprofenic acid *(Canada only) on page* *959*
Dom-Topiramate [Can] *see* topiramate *on page* *969*
Dom-Trazodone [Can] *see* trazodone *on page* *979*
DOM-Ursodiol C [Can] *see* ursodiol *on page* *1000*
Dom-Verapamil SR [Can] *see* verapamil *on page* *1010*
Dom-Zopiclone [Can] *see* zopiclone *(Canada only) on page* *1034*
Donatussin [US] *see* dextromethorphan, chlorpheniramine, phenylephrine, and guaifenesin *on page* *297*
Donatussin DC *(Discontinued)*
Donatussin DM *(Discontinued)* *see* chlorpheniramine, phenylephrine, and dextromethorphan *on page* *217*
Donatussin Drops [US] *see* guaifenesin and phenylephrine *on page* *475*

donepezil (doh NEP e zil)

Sound-Alike/Look-Alike Issues

Aricept® may be confused with AcipHex®, Ascriptin®, and Azilect®

Synonyms E2020

U.S./Canadian Brand Names Aricept® ODT [US]; Aricept® RDT [Can]; Aricept® [US/Can]

Therapeutic Category Acetylcholinesterase Inhibitor; Cholinergic Agent

Use Treatment of mild, moderate, or severe dementia of the Alzheimer type

Usual Dosage Oral: Adults: Dementia of Alzheimer type: Initial: 5 mg/day at bedtime; may increase to 10 mg/day at bedtime after 4-6 weeks

Dosage Forms

Tablet:

Aricept®: 5 mg, 10 mg

Tablet, orally disintegrating:

Aricept® ODT: 5 mg, 10 mg

Donnamar® ***(Discontinued)*** *see* hyoscyamine *on page 512*

Donnapine® ***(Discontinued)*** *see* hyoscyamine, atropine, scopolamine, and phenobarbital *on page 513*

Donnatal® [US] *see* hyoscyamine, atropine, scopolamine, and phenobarbital *on page 513*

Donnatal Extentabs® [US] *see* hyoscyamine, atropine, scopolamine, and phenobarbital *on page 513*

dopamine (DOE pa meen)

Sound-Alike/Look-Alike Issues

DOPamine may be confused with DOBUTamine, Dopram®

Synonyms dopamine hydrochloride

Tall-Man **DOP**amine

Therapeutic Category Adrenergic Agonist Agent

Use Adjunct in the treatment of shock (eg, MI, open heart surgery, renal failure, cardiac decompensation) which persists after adequate fluid volume replacement

Usual Dosage I.V. infusion (administration requires the use of an infusion pump):

Neonates: 1-20 mcg/kg/minute continuous infusion, titrate to desired response.

Children: 1-20 mcg/kg/minute, maximum: 50 mcg/kg/minute continuous infusion, titrate to desired response.

Adults: 1-5 mcg/kg/minute up to 20 mcg/kg/minute, titrate to desired response (maximum: 50 mcg/kg/minute). Infusion may be increased by 1-4 mcg/kg/minute at 10- to 30-minute intervals until optimal response is obtained.

If dosages >20-30 mcg/kg/minute are needed, a more direct-acting pressor may be more beneficial (ie, epinephrine, norepinephrine).

Dosage Forms

Infusion [premixed in D_5W]: 0.8 mg/mL (250 mL, 500 mL); 1.6 mg/mL (250 mL, 500 mL); 3.2 mg/mL (250 mL)

Injection, solution: 40 mg/mL (5 mL, 10 mL); 80 mg/mL (5 mL); 160 mg/mL (5 mL)

dopamine hydrochloride *see* dopamine *on page 331*

Dopram® [US] *see* doxapram *on page 332*

Doral® [US/Can] *see* quazepam *on page 843*

Doribax™ [US] *see* doripenem *on page 331*

doripenem (dore i PEN em)

Synonyms S-4661

U.S./Canadian Brand Names Doribax™ [US]

Therapeutic Category Antibiotic, Carbapenem

Use Treatment of complicated intraabdominal infections and complicated urinary tract infections (including pyelonephritis) due to susceptible gram-positive, gram-negative (including *Pseudomonas aeruginosa*), and anaerobic bacteria

Usual Dosage

Usual dosage: Adults: I.V.: 500 mg every 8 hours

Indication-specific dosing: Adults: I.V.:

Intraabdominal infection (complicated): 500 mg every 8 hours for 5-14 days

Urinary tract infection (complicated) or pyelonephritis: 500 mg every 8 hours for 10-14 days

Dosage Forms

Injection, powder for reconstitution:

Doribax™: 500 mg

Dormarex® 2 Oral ***(Discontinued)*** *see* diphenhydramine *on page 315*

dornase alfa (DOOR nase AL fa)

Synonyms recombinant human deoxyribonuclease; rhDNase

U.S./Canadian Brand Names Pulmozyme® [US/Can]

Therapeutic Category Enzyme

Use Management of cystic fibrosis patients to reduce the frequency of respiratory infections that require parenteral antibiotics in patients with FVC ≥40% of predicted; in conjunction with standard therapies, to improve pulmonary function in patients with cystic fibrosis

Usual Dosage Inhalation:

Children ≥3 months to Adults: 2.5 mg once daily through selected nebulizers; experience in children <5 years is limited

Patients unable to inhale or exhale orally throughout the entire treatment period may use Pari-Baby™ nebulizer. Some patients may benefit from twice daily administration.

Dosage Forms

Solution for nebulization [preservative free]:

Pulmozyme®: 1 mg/mL (2.5 mL)

Doryx® [US] *see* doxycycline *on page 336*

dorzolamide (dor ZOLE a mide)

Synonyms dorzolamide hydrochloride

U.S./Canadian Brand Names Trusopt® [US/Can]

Therapeutic Category Carbonic Anhydrase Inhibitor

Use Treatment of elevated intraocular pressure in patients with ocular hypertension or open-angle glaucoma

Usual Dosage Children and Adults: Reduction of intraocular pressure: Instill 1 drop in the affected eye(s) 3 times/day

Dosage Forms

Solution, ophthalmic: 2% (10 mL)

Trusopt®: 2% (10 mL)

dorzolamide and timolol (dor ZOLE a mide & TYE moe lole)

Synonyms timolol and dorzolamide

U.S./Canadian Brand Names Cosopt® [US/Can]; Preservative-Free Cosopt® [Can]

Therapeutic Category Beta-Adrenergic Blocker; Carbonic Anhydrase Inhibitor

Use Treatment of elevated intraocular pressure in patients with ocular hypertension or open-angle glaucoma

Usual Dosage Ophthalmic: Children ≥2 years and Adults: Instill 1 drop in affected eye(s) twice daily

Dosage Forms

Solution, ophthalmic: Dorzolamide 2% and timolol 0.5% (10 mL)

Cosopt®: Dorzolamide 2% and timolol 0.5% (10 mL)

dorzolamide hydrochloride *see* dorzolamide *on page 332*

DOS® [US-OTC] *see* docusate *on page 326*

DOSS *see* docusate *on page 326*

Dostinex® [Can] *see* cabergoline *on page 165*

Dostinex® *(Discontinued)* *see* cabergoline *on page 165*

Double Tussin DM [US-OTC] *see* guaifenesin and dextromethorphan *on page 474*

Dovobet® [Can] *see* calcipotriene and betamethasone *on page 167*

Dovonex® [US/Can] *see* calcipotriene *on page 166*

doxacurium *(Discontinued)*

doxapram (DOKS a pram)

Sound-Alike/Look-Alike Issues

doxapram may be confused with doxacurium, doxazosin, doxepin, Doxinate®, DOXOrubicin

Dopram® may be confused with DOPamine

Synonyms doxapram hydrochloride

U.S./Canadian Brand Names Dopram® [US]

Therapeutic Category Respiratory Stimulant

Use Respiratory and CNS stimulant for respiratory depression secondary to anesthesia, drug-induced CNS depression; acute hypercapnia secondary to COPD

Usual Dosage

Respiratory depression following anesthesia:

Intermittent injection: Initial: 0.5-1 mg/kg; may repeat at 5-minute intervals (only in patients who demonstrate initial response); maximum total dose: 2 mg/kg

I.V. infusion: Initial: 5 mg/minute until adequate response or adverse effects seen; decrease to 1-3 mg/minute; maximum total dose: 4 mg/kg

Drug-induced CNS depression:

Intermittent injection: Initial: Priming dose of 1-2 mg/kg, repeat after 5 minutes; may repeat at 1-2 hour intervals (until sustained consciousness); maximum: 3 g/day. May repeat in 24 hours if necessary.

I.V. infusion: Initial: Priming dose of 1-2 mg/kg, repeat after 5 minutes. If no response, wait 1-2 hours and repeat. If some stimulation is noted, initiate infusion at 1-3 mg/minute (depending on size of patient/depth of CNS depression); suspend infusion if patient begins to awaken. Infusion should not be continued for >2 hours. May reinstitute infusion as described above, including bolus, after rest interval of 30 minutes to 2 hours; maximum: 3 g/day

Acute hypercapnia secondary to COPD: I.V. infusion: Initial: Initiate infusion at 1-2 mg/minute (depending on size of patient/depth of CNS depression); may increase to maximum rate of 3 mg/minute; infusion should not be continued for >2 hours. Monitor arterial blood gases prior to initiation of infusion and at 30-minute intervals during the infusion (to identify possible development of acidosis/CO_2 retention). Additional infusions are not recommended (per manufacturer).

Dosage Forms

Injection, solution: 20 mg/mL (20 mL)

Dopram®: 20 mg/mL (20 mL)

doxapram hydrochloride *see* doxapram *on page* 332

doxazosin (doks AY zoe sin)

Sound-Alike/Look-Alike Issues

doxazosin may be confused with doxapram, doxepin, DOXOrubicin

Cardura® may be confused with Cardene®, Cordarone®, Cordran®, Coumadin®, K-Dur®, Ridaura®

Synonyms doxazosin mesylate

U.S./Canadian Brand Names Alti-Doxazosin [Can]; Apo-Doxazosin® [Can]; Cardura-1™ [Can]; Cardura-2™ [Can]; Cardura-4™ [Can]; Cardura® XL [US]; Cardura® [US]; Gen-Doxazosin [Can]; Novo-Doxazosin [Can]

Therapeutic Category Alpha-Adrenergic Blocking Agent

Use

Immediate release formulation: Treatment of hypertension as monotherapy or in conjunction with diuretics, ACE inhibitors, beta-blockers, or calcium antagonists

Immediate release and extended release formulations: Treatment of urinary outflow obstruction and/or obstructive and irritative symptoms associated with benign prostatic hyperplasia (BPH)

Usual Dosage Oral: Adults:

Immediate release: 1 mg once daily in morning or evening; may be increased to 2 mg once daily. Thereafter titrate upwards, if needed, over several weeks, balancing therapeutic benefit with doxazosin-induced postural hypotension.

BPH: Goal: 4-8 mg/day; maximum dose: 8 mg/day

Hypertension: Maximum dose: 16 mg/day

Reinitiation of therapy: If therapy is discontinued for several days, restart at 1 mg dose and titrate as before

Extended release: BPH: 4 mg once daily with breakfast; titrate based on response and tolerability every 3-4 weeks to maximum recommended dose of 8 mg/day

Reinitiation of therapy: If therapy is discontinued for several days, restart at 4 mg dose and titrate as before.

Conversion to extended release from immediate release: Omit final evening dose of immediate release prior to starting morning dosing with extended release product; initiate extended release product using 4 mg once daily

Dosage Forms

Tablet: 1 mg, 2 mg, 4 mg, 8 mg

Cardura®: 1 mg, 2 mg, 4 mg, 8 mg

Tablet, extended release:

Cardura® XL: 4 mg, 8 mg

doxazosin mesylate *see* doxazosin *on page* 333

doxepin (DOKS e pin)

Sound-Alike/Look-Alike Issues

doxepin may be confused with digoxin, doxapram, doxazosin, Doxidan®, doxycycline
Sinequan® may be confused with saquinavir, Serentil®, Seroquel®, Singulair®
Zonalon® may be confused with Zone-A Forte®

Synonyms doxepin hydrochloride

U.S./Canadian Brand Names Apo-Doxepin® [Can]; Novo-Doxepin [Can]; Prudoxin™ [US]; Sinequan® [Can]; Zonalon® [US/Can]

Therapeutic Category Antidepressant, Tricyclic (Tertiary Amine); Topical Skin Product

Use

Oral: Depression
Topical: Short-term (<8 days) management of moderate pruritus in adults with atopic dermatitis or lichen simplex chronicus

Usual Dosage

Oral: Topical: Burning mouth syndrome (dental use): Cream: Apply 3-4 times daily
Oral (entire daily dose may be given at bedtime):
Depression or anxiety:
Adolescents: Initial: 25-50 mg/day in single or divided doses; gradually increase to 100 mg/day
Adults: Initial: 25-150 mg/day at bedtime or in 2-3 divided doses; may gradually increase up to 300 mg/day; single dose should not exceed 150 mg; select patients may respond to 25-50 mg/day
Chronic urticaria, angioedema, nocturnal pruritus: Adults: 10-30 mg/day
Topical: Pruritus: Adults: Apply a thin film 4 times/day with at least 3- to 4-hour interval between applications; not recommended for use >8 days. **Note:** Low-dose (25-50 mg) oral administration has also been used to treat pruritus, but systemic effects are increased.

Dosage Forms

Capsule: 10 mg, 25 mg, 50 mg, 75 mg, 100 mg, 150 mg
Cream:
Prudoxin™: 5% (45 g)
Zonalon®: 5% (30 g, 45 g)
Solution, oral concentrate: 10 mg/mL

doxepin hydrochloride *see* doxepin *on page* 334

doxercalciferol (doks er kal si fe FEER ole)

Synonyms 1α-hydroxyergocalciferol

U.S./Canadian Brand Names Hectorol® [US/Can]

Therapeutic Category Vitamin D Analog

Use Treatment of secondary hyperparathyroidism in patients with chronic kidney disease

Usual Dosage

Oral:
Dialysis patients: Dose should be titrated to lower iPTH to 150-300 pg/mL; dose is adjusted at 8-week intervals (maximum dose: 20 mcg 3 times/week)
Initial dose: iPTH >400 pg/mL: 10 mcg 3 times/week at dialysis
Dose titration:
iPTH level decreased by 50% and >300 pg/mL: Dose can be increased to 12.5 mcg 3 times/week for 8 more weeks; this titration process can continue at 8-week intervals; each increase should be by 2.5 mcg/dose
iPTH level 150-300 pg/mL: Maintain current dose
iPTH level <100 pg/mL: Suspend doxercalciferol for 1 week; resume at a reduced dose; decrease each dose (not weekly dose) by at least 2.5 mcg
Predialysis patients: Dose should be titrated to lower iPTH to 35-70 pg/mL with stage 3 disease or to 70-110 pg/mL with stage 4 disease: Dose may be adjusted at 2-week intervals (maximum dose: 3.5 mcg/day)
Initial dose: 1 mcg/day
Dose titration:
iPTH level >70 pg/mL with stage 3 disease or >110 pg/mL with stage 4 disease: Increase dose by 0.5 mcg every 2 weeks as necessary
iPTH level 35-70 pg/mL with stage 3 disease or 70-110 pg/mL with stage 4 disease: Maintain current dose

iPTH level is <35 pg/mL with stage 3 disease or <70 pg/mL with stage 4 disease: Suspend doxercalciferol for 1 week, then resume at a reduced dose (at least 0.5 mcg lower)

I.V.:

Dialysis patients: Dose should be titrated to lower iPTH to 150-300 pg/mL; dose is adjusted at 8-week intervals (maximum dose: 18 mcg/week)

Initial dose: iPTH level >400 pg/mL: 4 mcg 3 times/week after dialysis, administered as a bolus dose

Dose titration:

iPTH level decreased by <50% and >300 pg/mL: Dose can be increased by 1-2 mcg at 8-week intervals, as necessary

iPTH level decreased by >50% and >300 pg/mL: Maintain current dose

iPTH level 150-300 pg/mL: Maintain current dose

iPTH level <100 pg/mL: Suspend doxercalciferol for 1 week; resume at a reduced dose (at least 1 mcg lower)

Hypercalcemia, hyperphosphatemia, or serum calcium times phosphorus product >55 mg^2/dL^2: Decrease or suspend dose and/or adjust dose of phosphate binders; if dose is suspended, resume at a reduced dose (at least 1 mcg lower)

Dosage Forms

Capsule:

Hectorol®: 0.5 mcg, 1 mcg, 2.5 mcg

Injection, solution:

Hectorol®: 2 mcg/mL (2 mL)

Doxidan® [US-OTC] *see* bisacodyl *on page 142*

Doxil® [US] *see* doxorubicin (liposomal) *on page 336*

doxorubicin (doks oh ROO bi sin)

Sound-Alike/Look-Alike Issues

DOXOrubicin may be confused with dactinomycin, DAUNOrubicin, DAUNOrubicin liposomal, doxacurium, doxapram, doxazosin, DOXOrubicin liposomal, epirubicin, idarubicin

Adriamycin PFS® may be confused with achromycin, Aredia®, Idamycin®

ADR (error-prone abbreviation)

Conventional formulation (Adriamycin PFS®, Adriamycin RDF®) may be confused with the liposomal formulation (Doxil®)

Synonyms adria; doxorubicin hydrochloride; hydroxydaunomycin hydrochloride; hydroxyldaunorubicin hydrochloride; NSC-123127

Tall-Man **DOXO**rubicin

U.S./Canadian Brand Names Adriamycin® [US/Can]

Therapeutic Category Antineoplastic Agent

Use Treatment of leukemias, lymphomas, multiple myeloma, osseous and nonosseous sarcomas, mesotheliomas, germ cell tumors of the ovary or testis, and carcinomas of the head and neck, thyroid, lung, breast, stomach, pancreas, liver, ovary, bladder, prostate, uterus, neuroblastoma and Wilms tumor.

Usual Dosage I.V.: Refer to individual protocols. **Note:** Lower dosage should be considered for patients with inadequate marrow reserve (due to old age, prior treatment or neoplastic marrow infiltration)

Children:

35-75 mg/m^2/dose every 21 days **or**

20-30 mg/m^2/dose once weekly **or**

60-90 mg/m^2/dose given as a continuous infusion over 96 hours every 3-4 weeks

Adults: Usual or typical dose: 60-75 mg/m^2/dose every 21 days **or**

60 mg/m^2/dose every 2 weeks (dose dense) **or**

40-60 mg/m^2/dose every 3-4 weeks **or**

20-30 mg/m^2/day for 2-3 days every 4 weeks **or**

20 mg/m^2/dose once weekly

Dosage Forms

Injection, powder for reconstitution: 10 mg, 50 mg

Adriamycin®: 10 mg, 20 mg, 50 mg

Injection, solution: 2 mg/mL (5 mL, 10 mL, 25 mL, 100 mL)

Adriamycin®: 2 mg/mL (5 mL, 10 mL, 25 mL, 100 mL)

doxorubicin hydrochloride *see* doxorubicin *on page 335*

DOXOrubicin hydrochloride (liposomal) *see* doxorubicin (liposomal) *on page 336*

doxorubicin (liposomal) (doks oh ROO bi sin lip pah SOW mal)

Sound-Alike/Look-Alike Issues

DOXOrubicin liposomal may be confused with dactinomycin, DAUNOrubicin, DAUNOrubicin liposomal, doxacurium, doxapram, doxazosin, DOXOrubicin, epirubicin, idarubicin

DOXOrubicin liposomal may be confused with DAUNOrubicin liposomal

Doxil® may be confused with Doxy®, Paxil®

Liposomal formulation (Doxil®) may be confused with the conventional formulation (Adriamycin PFS®, Adriamycin RDF®)

Synonyms DOXOrubicin hydrochloride (liposomal); liposomal DOXOrubicin; NSC-712227; pegylated liposomal DOXOrubicin

Tall-Man DOXOrubicin (liposomal)

U.S./Canadian Brand Names Caelyx® [Can]; Doxil® [US]

Therapeutic Category Antineoplastic Agent

Use Treatment of ovarian cancer, multiple myeloma, and AIDS-related Kaposi sarcoma

Usual Dosage Details concerning dosing in combination regimens should also be consulted. **Liposomal formulations of doxorubicin should NOT be substituted for conventional doxorubicin hydrochloride on a mg-per-mg basis.**

AIDS-related Kaposi sarcoma: I.V.: 20 mg/m^2/dose once every 3 weeks

Multiple myeloma: I.V.: 30 mg/m^2/dose every 3 weeks (in combination with bortezomib)

Ovarian cancer: I.V.: 50 mg/m^2/dose every 4 weeks

Dosage Forms

Injection, solution:

Doxil®: 2 mg/mL (10 mL, 25 mL)

Doxy100™ [US] *see* doxycycline *on page* 336

Doxycin [Can] *see* doxycycline *on page* 336

doxycycline (doks i SYE kleen)

Sound-Alike/Look-Alike Issues

doxycycline may be confused with dicyclomine, doxepin, doxylamine

Doxy100™ may be confused with Doxil®

Monodox® may be confused with Maalox®

Oracea™ may be confused with Orencia®

Vibramycin® may be confused with vancomycin

Synonyms doxycycline calcium; doxycycline hyclate; doxycycline monohydrate

U.S./Canadian Brand Names Adoxa® [US]; Alodox™ [US]; Apo-Doxy Tabs® [Can]; Apo-Doxy® [Can]; Doryx® [US]; Doxy100™ [US]; Doxycin [Can]; Doxytec [Can]; Monodox® [US]; Novo-Doxylin [Can]; Nu-Doxycycline [Can]; Oracea™ [US]; Oraxyl™ [US]; Periostat® [US/Can]; Vibra-Tabs® [US/Can]; Vibramycin® [US]

Therapeutic Category Tetracycline Derivative

Use Principally in the treatment of infections caused by susceptible *Rickettsia*, *Chlamydia*, and *Mycoplasma*; alternative to mefloquine for malaria prophylaxis; treatment for syphilis, uncomplicated *Neisseria gonorrhoeae*, *Listeria*, *Actinomyces israelii*, and *Clostridium* infections in penicillin-allergic patients; used for community-acquired pneumonia and other common infections due to susceptible organisms; anthrax due to *Bacillus anthracis,* including inhalational anthrax (postexposure); treatment of infections caused by uncommon susceptible gram-negative and gram-positive organisms including *Borrelia recurrentis*, *Ureaplasma urealyticum*, *Haemophilus ducreyi*, *Yersinia pestis*, *Francisella tularensis*, *Vibrio cholerae*, *Campylobacter fetus*, *Brucella* spp, *Bartonella bacilliformis*, and *Calymmatobacterium granulomatis,* Q fever, Lyme disease; treatment of inflammatory lesions associated with rosacea; intestinal amebiasis; severe acne

Usual Dosage

Usual dosage range:

Children >8 years (<45 kg): Oral, I.V.: 2-5 mg/kg/day in 1-2 divided doses, not to exceed 200 mg/day

Children >8 years (>45 kg) and Adults: Oral, I.V.: 100-200 mg/day in 1-2 divided doses

Indication-specific dosing:

Children:

Anthrax: Doxycycline should be used in children if antibiotic susceptibility testing, exhaustion of drug supplies, or allergic reaction preclude use of penicillin or ciprofloxacin. For treatment, the consensus recommendation does not include a loading dose for doxycycline.

Inhalational (postexposure prophylaxis): Oral, I.V. (use oral route when possible):
≤8 years: 2.2 mg/kg every 12 hours for 60 days
>8 years and ≤45 kg: 2.2 mg/kg every 12 hours for 60 days
>8 years and >45 kg: 100 mg every 12 hours for 60 days

Cutaneous (treatment): Oral: See dosing for "Inhalational (postexposure prophylaxis)"

Note: In the presence of systemic involvement, extensive edema, and/or lesions on head/neck, doxycycline should initially be administered I.V.

Inhalational/gastrointestinal/oropharyngeal (treatment): I.V.: Refer to dosing for inhalational anthrax (postexposure prophylaxis); switch to oral therapy when clinically appropriate

Note: Initial treatment should include two or more agents predicted to be effective (per CDC recommendations). Agents suggested for use in conjunction with doxycycline or ciprofloxacin include rifampin, vancomycin, imipenem, penicillin, ampicillin, chloramphenicol, clindamycin, and clarithromycin. May switch to oral antimicrobial therapy when clinically appropriate. Continue combined therapy for 60 days

Children ≥8 years:

Malaria prophylaxis: Oral: 2 mg/kg/day (maximum: 100 mg/day). Start 1-2 days prior to travel to endemic area; continue daily during travel and for 4 weeks after leaving endemic area

Children ≥8 years (and >45 kg) and Adults:

Chlamydial infections, uncomplicated: Oral: 100 mg twice daily for ≥7 days

Lyme disease, Q fever, or tularemia: Oral: 100 mg twice daily for 14-21 days

Rickettsial disease or ehrlichiosis: Oral, I.V.: 100 mg twice daily for 7-14 days

Adults:

Anthrax:

Inhalational (postexposure prophylaxis): Oral, I.V. (use oral route when possible): 100 mg every 12 hours for 60 days

Cutaneous (treatment): Oral: 100 mg every 12 hours for 60 days. **Note:** In the presence of systemic involvement, extensive edema, lesions on head/neck, refer to I.V. dosing for treatment of inhalational/gastrointestinal/oropharyngeal anthrax

Inhalational/gastrointestinal/oropharyngeal (treatment): I.V.: Initial: 100 mg every 12 hours; switch to oral therapy when clinically appropriate; some recommend initial loading dose of 200 mg, followed by 100 mg every 8-12 hours. **Note:** Initial treatment should include two or more agents predicted to be effective (per CDC recommendations). Agents suggested for use in conjunction with doxycycline or ciprofloxacin include rifampin, vancomycin, imipenem, penicillin, ampicillin, chloramphenicol, clindamycin, and clarithromycin. May switch to oral antimicrobial therapy when clinically appropriate. Continue combined therapy for 60 days

Brucellosis: Oral: 100 mg twice daily for 6 weeks with rifampin or streptomycin

Community-acquired pneumonia, bronchitis: Oral, I.V.: 100 mg twice daily

Endometritis, salpingitis, parametritis, or peritonitis: I.V.: 100 mg twice daily with cefoxitin 2 g every 6 hours for 4 days and for ≥48 hours after patient improves; then continue with oral therapy 100 mg twice daily to complete a 10- to 14-day course of therapy

Gonococcal infection, acute (PID) in combination with another antibiotic: I.V.: 100 mg every 12 hours until improved, followed by 100 mg orally twice daily to complete 14 days

Malaria prophylaxis: 100 mg/day. Start 1-2 days prior to travel to endemic area; continue daily during travel and for 4 weeks after leaving endemic area

Nongonococcal urethritis: Oral: 100 mg twice daily for 7 days

Periodontitis: Oral (Periostat®): 20 mg twice daily as an adjunct following scaling and root planing; may be administered for up to 9 months. Safety beyond 12 months of treatment and efficacy beyond 9 months of treatment have not been established.

Rosacea: (Oracea™): Oral: 40 mg once daily in the morning

Syphilis:

Early syphilis: Oral, I.V.: 200 mg/day in divided doses for 14 days
Late syphilis: Oral, I.V.: 200 mg/day in divided doses for 28 days

***Yersinia pestis* (plague):** Oral: 100 mg twice daily for 7 days

Vibrio cholerae: Oral: 300 mg as a single dose

Dosage Forms

Capsule: 50 mg, 100 mg
Adoxa®: 150 mg
Monodox®: 50 mg, 75 mg, 100 mg
Oraxyl™: 20 mg
Vibramycin®: 100 mg

Capsule, variable release:
Oracea™: 40 mg [30 mg (immediate-release) and 10 mg (delayed-release)]

Injection, powder for reconstitution: 100 mg
Doxy100™: 100 mg
Powder for oral suspension: 25 mg/5 mL (60 mL)
Vibramycin®: 25 mg/5 mL
Syrup:
Vibramycin®: 50 mg/5 mL
Tablet: 20 mg, 50 mg, 75 mg, 100 mg, 150 mg
Adoxa®: 50 mg, 75 mg, 100 mg
Adoxa® Pak™ 1/75 [unit-dose pack]: 75 mg (31s)
Adoxa® Pak™ 1/150 [unit-dose pack]: 150 mg (30s)
Alodox™: 20 mg [kit includes Alodox™ tablets (60s), Ocusoft® Lid Scrub™ pads, eyelid cleanser, and goggles]
Periostat®: 20 mg
Vibra-Tabs®: 100 mg
Tablet, delayed-release coated pellets:
Doryx®: 75 mg, 100 mg, 150 mg [scored]

doxycycline calcium *see* doxycycline *on page* *336*
doxycycline hyclate *see* doxycycline *on page* *336*
doxycycline monohydrate *see* doxycycline *on page* *336*

doxylamine (dox IL a meen)

Sound-Alike/Look-Alike Issues
doxylamine may be confused with doxycycline
Synonyms doxylamine succinate
U.S./Canadian Brand Names Aldex® AN [US]; Good Sense Sleep Aid [US-OTC]; Unisom® SleepTabs® [US-OTC]; Unisom®-2 [Can]
Therapeutic Category Antihistamine
Use Treatment of short-term insomnia
Usual Dosage Oral: Adults: One tablet 30 minutes before bedtime; once daily or as instructed by healthcare professional
Dosage Forms
Tablet:
Good Sense Sleep Aid [OTC], Unisom® SleepTabs® [OTC]: 25 mg
Tablet, chewable:
Aldex® AN: 5 mg

doxylamine, acetaminophen, and dextromethorphan *see* acetaminophen, dextromethorphan, and doxylamine *on page* *26*
doxylamine, acetaminophen, dextromethorphan, and pseudoephedrine *see* acetaminophen, dextromethorphan, doxylamine, and pseudoephedrine *on page* *28*

doxylamine and pyridoxine *(Canada only)* (dox IL a meen & peer i DOX een)

Sound-Alike/Look-Alike Issues
doxylamine may be confused with doxycycline
Synonyms doxylamine succinate and pyridoxine hydrochloride; pyridoxine and doxylamine
U.S./Canadian Brand Names Diclectin® [Can]
Therapeutic Category Antihistamine; Vitamin
Use Treatment of pregnancy-associated nausea and vomiting
Usual Dosage Oral: Adults: Two delayed release tablets (a total of doxylamine 20 mg and pyridoxine 20 mg) at bedtime; in severe cases or in cases with nausea/vomiting during the day, dosage may be increased by 1 tablet in the morning and/or afternoon
Dosage Forms [CAN] = Canadian brand name
Tablet, delayed release:
Diclectin® [CAN]: Doxylamine 10 mg and pyridoxine 10 mg [not available in the U.S.]

doxylamine succinate *see* doxylamine *on page* *338*
doxylamine succinate and pyridoxine hydrochloride *see* doxylamine and pyridoxine *(Canada only) on page* *338*
doxylamine succinate, codeine phosphate, and acetaminophen *see* acetaminophen, codeine, and doxylamine *(Canada only) on page* *26*

Doxytec [Can] *see* doxycycline *on page 336*
DPA *see* valproic acid and derivatives *on page 1002*
D-Pan® *(Discontinued)* *see* dexpanthenol *on page 292*
DPE *see* dipivefrin *on page 323*
D-penicillamine *see* penicillamine *on page 759*
DPH *see* phenytoin *on page 780*
D-Phen 1000 [US] *see* guaifenesin and phenylephrine *on page 475*
DPM™ [US-OTC] *see* urea *on page 998*
Dramamine® [US-OTC] *see* dimenhydrinate *on page 312*
Dramamine® Less Drowsy Formula [US-OTC] *see* meclizine *on page 619*
Dramilin® Injection *(Discontinued)* *see* dimenhydrinate *on page 312*
Driminate® [US-OTC] *see* dimenhydrinate *on page 312*
Drinex [US-OTC] *see* acetaminophen, chlorpheniramine, and pseudoephedrine *on page 26*
Drinkables® Fruits and Vegetables [US-OTC] *see* vitamins (multiple/oral) *on page 1019*
Drinkables® MultiVitamins [US-OTC] *see* vitamins (multiple/oral) *on page 1019*
Drisdol® [US/Can] *see* ergocalciferol *on page 364*
Dristan™ 12-Hour [US-OTC] *see* oxymetazoline *on page 740*
Dristan® Long Lasting Nasal [Can] *see* oxymetazoline *on page 740*
Dristan® Long Lasting Nasal Solution *(Discontinued)* *see* oxymetazoline *on page 740*
Dristan® N.D. [Can] *see* acetaminophen and pseudoephedrine *on page 24*
Dristan® N.D., Extra Strength [Can] *see* acetaminophen and pseudoephedrine *on page 24*
Dristan® Saline Spray *(Discontinued)* *see* sodium chloride *on page 908*
Drithocreme® HP 1% *(Discontinued)* *see* anthralin *on page 80*
Dritho-Scalp® [US] *see* anthralin *on page 80*
Drixoral® [Can] *see* dexbrompheniramine and pseudoephedrine *on page 289*
Drixoral® Cough & Congestion Liquid Caps *(Discontinued)* *see* pseudoephedrine and dextromethorphan *on page 834*
Drixoral® Cough Liquid Caps *(Discontinued)* *see* dextromethorphan *on page 295*
Drixoral® Nasal [Can] *see* oxymetazoline *on page 740*
Drixoral® ND [Can] *see* pseudoephedrine *on page 833*
Drixoral® Non-Drowsy *(Discontinued)* *see* pseudoephedrine *on page 833*
Drize®-R *(Discontinued)* *see* chlorpheniramine, phenylephrine, and methscopolamine *on page 218*

dronabinol (droe NAB i nol)

Sound-Alike/Look-Alike Issues
dronabinol may be confused with droperidol

Synonyms delta-9 THC; delta-9-tetrahydro-cannabinol; tetrahydrocannabinol; THC

U.S./Canadian Brand Names Marinol® [US/Can]

Therapeutic Category Antiemetic

Controlled Substance C-III

Use Chemotherapy-associated nausea and vomiting refractory to other antiemetic(s); AIDS-related anorexia

Usual Dosage Refer to individual protocols. Oral:
Antiemetic: Children and Adults: 5 mg/m^2 1-3 hours before chemotherapy, then 5 mg/m^2/dose every 2-4 hours after chemotherapy for a total of 4-6 doses/day; increase doses in increments of 2.5 mg/m^2 to a maximum of 15 mg/m^2/dose.
Appetite stimulant: Adults: Initial: 2.5 mg twice daily (before lunch and dinner); titrate up to a maximum of 20 mg/day.

Dosage Forms
Capsule, soft gelatin: 2.5 mg, 5 mg, 10 mg
Marinol®: 2.5 mg, 5 mg, 10 mg

dronedarone (droe NE da rone)

Synonyms dronedarone hydrochloride; SR33589

U.S./Canadian Brand Names Multaq® [US]

Therapeutic Category Antiarrhythmic Agent, Miscellaneous

Use To reduce the risk of hospitalization related to paroxysmal or persistent atrial fibrillation (AF) or atrial flutter (AFl) in patients with a recent episode of AF/AFl and associated cardiovascular risk factors (eg, age >70 years, hypertension, diabetes, prior cerebrovascular accident, left atrial diameter ≥50 mm or left ventricular ejection fraction <40%), who are in normal sinus rhythm or will be cardioverted

Usual Dosage Oral: Adults: Atrial fibrillation/atrial flutter: 400 mg twice daily with morning and evening meals

Dosage Forms

Tablet:

Multaq®: 400 mg

dronedarone hydrochloride *see* dronedarone *on page* *339*

droperidol (droe PER i dole)

Sound-Alike/Look-Alike Issues

droperidol may be confused with dronabinol

Inapsine® may be confused with Nebcin®

Synonyms dehydrobenzperidol

U.S./Canadian Brand Names Droperidol Injection, USP [Can]

Therapeutic Category Antiemetic; Antipsychotic Agent, Butyrophenone

Use Prevention and/or treatment of nausea and vomiting from surgical and diagnostic procedures

Usual Dosage Titrate carefully to desired effect

Children 2-12 years: Nausea and vomiting: I.M., I.V.: 0.05-0.06 mg/kg (maximum initial dose: 0.1 mg/kg); additional doses may be repeated to achieve effect; administer additional doses with caution

Adults: Prevention of postoperative nausea and vomiting (PONV): I.M., I.V.: Initial: 0.625-2.5 mg; additional doses of 1.25 mg may be administered to achieve desired effect; administer additional doses with caution. Consensus guidelines recommend 0.625-1.25 mg I.V. administered after surgery

Dosage Forms

Injection, solution: 2.5 mg/mL (1 mL, 2 mL)

Droperidol Injection, USP [Can] *see* droperidol *on page* *340*

drospirenone and estradiol (droh SPYE re none & es tra DYE ole)

Synonyms E2 and DRSP; estradiol and drospirenone

U.S./Canadian Brand Names Angeliq® [US/Can]

Therapeutic Category Estrogen and Progestin Combination

Use Treatment of moderate-to-severe vasomotor symptoms associated with menopause; treatment of vulvar and vaginal atrophy associated with menopause

Usual Dosage Oral: Adults:

Moderate-to-severe vasomotor symptoms associated with menopause: One tablet daily; reevaluate patients at 3- and 6-month intervals to determine if treatment is still necessary.

Atrophic vaginitis in females with an intact uterus: One tablet daily; reevaluate patients at 3- and 6-month intervals to determine if treatment is still necessary.

Note: The lowest dose of estrogen/progestin that will control symptoms should be used; medication should be discontinued as soon as possible.

Dosage Forms

Tablet:

Angeliq®: Drospirenone 0.5 mg and estradiol 1 mg

drospirenone and ethinyl estradiol *see* ethinyl estradiol and drospirenone *on page* *384*

drotrecogin alfa (dro TRE coe jin AL fa)

Synonyms activated protein C, human, recombinant; drotrecogin alfa, activated; protein C (activated), human, recombinant

U.S./Canadian Brand Names Xigris® [US/Can]

Therapeutic Category Protein C (Activated)

Use Reduction of mortality from severe sepsis (associated with organ dysfunction) in adults at high risk of death (eg, APACHE II score ≥25)

Usual Dosage I.V.: Adults: Sepsis: 24 mcg/kg/hour for a total of 96 hours; stop infusion **immediately** if clinically-important bleeding is identified. **Note:** Use actual body weight for dosing.

Dosage Forms

Injection, powder for reconstitution [preservative free]:

Xigris®: 5 mg, 20 mg

drotrecogin alfa, activated *see* drotrecogin alfa *on page* *340*

DroTuss-CP [US] *see* phenylephrine, hydrocodone, and chlorpheniramine *on page* *778*

Droxia® [US] *see* hydroxyurea *on page* *510*

Dry Eye® Therapy Solution *(Discontinued)* *see* artificial tears *on page* *100*

Dryox® Gel *(Discontinued)* *see* benzoyl peroxide *on page* *132*

Dryox® Wash *(Discontinued)* *see* benzoyl peroxide *on page* *132*

Drysol™ [US] *see* aluminum chloride hexahydrate *on page* *54*

Dryvax® *(Discontinued)* *see* smallpox vaccine *on page* *906*

DSCG *see* cromolyn sodium *on page* *261*

D-ser(bu^{t})^{6},Azgly^{10}-LHRH *see* goserelin *on page* *471*

D-S-S® [US-OTC] *see* docusate *on page* *326*

DSS *see* docusate *on page* *326*

DT *see* diphtheria and tetanus toxoid *on page* *318*

D-Tann *(Discontinued)* *see* diphenhydramine and phenylephrine *on page* *317*

D-Tann HC *(Discontinued)*

DTaP *see* diphtheria, tetanus toxoids, and acellular pertussis vaccine *on page* *321*

DTap-HepB-IPV *see* diphtheria, tetanus toxoids, acellular pertussis, hepatitis B (recombinant), and poliovirus (inactivated) vaccine *on page* *320*

DTaP/Hib *see* diphtheria, tetanus toxoids, and acellular pertussis vaccine and *Haemophilus influenzae* b conjugate vaccine *on page* *323*

DTaP-IPV *see* diphtheria and tetanus toxoids, acellular pertussis, and poliovirus vaccine *on page* *319*

DTaP-IPV/Hib *see* diphtheria and tetanus toxoids, acellular pertussis, poliovirus and *Haemophilus* b conjugate vaccine *on page* *320*

DTIC® [Can] *see* dacarbazine *on page* *272*

DTIC *see* dacarbazine *on page* *272*

DTPA *see* diethylene triamine penta-acetic acid *on page* *306*

dTpa *see* diphtheria, tetanus toxoids, and acellular pertussis vaccine *on page* *321*

D-Trp(6)-LHRH *see* triptorelin *on page* *990*

Duac® CS [US] *see* clindamycin and benzoyl peroxide *on page* *240*

Duac® *(Discontinued)* *see* clindamycin and benzoyl peroxide *on page* *240*

Duet® [US] *see* vitamins (multiple/prenatal) *on page* *1020*

Duetact™ [US] *see* pioglitazone and glimepiride *on page* *785*

Duet® DHA [US] *see* vitamins (multiple/prenatal) *on page* *1020*

Duet® DHA^{ec} [US] *see* vitamins (multiple/prenatal) *on page* *1020*

Dukoral™ [Can] *see* traveler's diarrhea and cholera vaccine *(Canada only) on page* *978*

Dulcolax® [US-OTC/Can] *see* bisacodyl *on page* *142*

Dulcolax® Stool Softener [US-OTC] *see* docusate *on page* *326*

Dull-C® [US-OTC] *see* ascorbic acid *on page* *100*

duloxetine (doo LOX e teen)

Sound-Alike/Look-Alike Issues

DULoxetine may be confused with FLUoxetine

Synonyms (+)-(*S*)-*N*-methyl-γ-(1-naphthyloxy)-2-thiophenepropylamine hydrochloride; duloxetine hydrochloride; LY248686

Tall-Man DULoxetine

U.S./Canadian Brand Names Cymbalta® [US/Can]

Therapeutic Category Antidepressant, Serotonin/Norepinephrine Reuptake Inhibitor

Use Acute and maintenance treatment of major depressive disorder (MDD); treatment of generalized anxiety disorder (GAD); management of pain associated with diabetic neuropathy; management of fibromyalgia

Usual Dosage Oral: Adults:

Major depressive disorder: Initial: 40-60 mg/day; dose may be divided (ie, 20 or 30 mg twice daily) or given as a single daily dose of 60 mg; maintenance: 60 mg once daily; for doses >60 mg/day, titrate dose in increments of 30 mg/day over 1 week as tolerated to a maximum dose: 120 mg/day. **Note:** Doses >60 mg/day have not been demonstrated to be more effective.

Diabetic neuropathy: 60 mg once daily; lower initial doses may be considered in patients where tolerability is a concern and/or renal impairment is present. **Note:** Doses up to 120 mg/day administered in clinical trials offered no additional benefit and were less well tolerated than dose of 60 mg/day.

Fibromyalgia: Initial: 30 mg/day for 1 week, then increase to 60 mg/day as tolerated. **Note:** Doses up to 120 mg/day administered in clinical trials offered no additional benefit and were less well tolerated than dose of 60 mg/day.

Generalized anxiety disorder: Initial: 30-60 mg/day as a single daily dose; patients initiated at 30 mg/day should be titrated to 60 mg/day after 1 week; maximum dose: 120 mg/day. **Note:** Doses >60 mg/day have not been demonstrated to be more effective than 60 mg/day.

Dosage Forms

Capsule, delayed release, enteric coated pellets:

Cymbalta®: 20 mg, 30 mg, 60 mg

duloxetine hydrochloride *see* duloxetine *on page* *341*

Duocaine™ ***(Discontinued)***

DuoCet™ ***(Discontinued)*** *see* hydrocodone and acetaminophen *on page* *501*

Duodote™ [US] *see* atropine and pralidoxime *on page* *112*

Duofilm® [Can] *see* salicylic acid *on page* *884*

Duoforte® 27 [Can] *see* salicylic acid *on page* *884*

Duomax [US] *see* guaifenesin and phenylephrine *on page* *475*

DuoNeb® [US] *see* ipratropium and albuterol *on page* *545*

DuoPlant® ***(Discontinued)*** *see* salicylic acid *on page* *884*

Duotan PD ***(Discontinued)*** *see* dexchlorpheniramine and pseudoephedrine *on page* *290*

Duo-Trach® Injection ***(Discontinued)*** *see* lidocaine *on page* *584*

DuoTrav™ [CAN] *see* travoprost and timolol *(Canada only) on page* *979*

DuP 753 *see* losartan *on page* *600*

Duphalac® ***(Discontinued)*** *see* lactulose *on page* *565*

Duraclon® [US] *see* clonidine *on page* *245*

Duradrin® ***(Discontinued)*** *see* acetaminophen, isometheptene, and dichloralphenazone *on page* *29*

Duradyl® [US] *see* chlorpheniramine, phenylephrine, and methscopolamine *on page* *218*

Duradyne DHC® ***(Discontinued)*** *see* hydrocodone and acetaminophen *on page* *501*

Duragesic® [US/Can] *see* fentanyl *on page* *410*

Dura-Gest® ***(Discontinued)***

Durahist™ [US] *see* chlorpheniramine, pseudoephedrine, and methscopolamine *on page* *221*

Durahist™ PE [US] *see* chlorpheniramine, phenylephrine, and methscopolamine *on page* *218*

Duralith® [Can] *see* lithium *on page* *594*

Duralone® Injection ***(Discontinued)*** *see* methylprednisolone *on page* *647*

Duramist® Plus [US-OTC] *see* oxymetazoline *on page* *740*

Duramorph® [US] *see* morphine sulfate *on page* *667*

Duraphen™ II DM [US] *see* guaifenesin, dextromethorphan, and phenylephrine *on page* *478*

Duraphen™ DM ***(Discontinued)*** *see* guaifenesin, dextromethorphan, and phenylephrine *on page* *478*

Duraphen™ Forte [US] *see* guaifenesin, dextromethorphan, and phenylephrine *on page* *478*

DuraTan™ Forte [US] *see* chlorpheniramine, pseudoephedrine, and dextromethorphan *on page* *220*

Duratest® Injection ***(Discontinued)*** *see* testosterone *on page* *947*

Durathate® Injection ***(Discontinued)*** *see* testosterone *on page* *947*

Duration® ***(Discontinued)*** *see* oxymetazoline *on page* *740*

Duratuss® [US] *see* guaifenesin and phenylephrine *on page* *475*

Duratuss® DA [US] *see* chlorpheniramine and pseudoephedrine *on page* *215*

Duratuss® DM [US] *see* guaifenesin and dextromethorphan *on page* *474*

Duratuss GP® [US] *see* guaifenesin and phenylephrine *on page* *475*

Duratuss® HD *(Discontinued)*
Dura-Vent®/DA *(Discontinued)* *see* chlorpheniramine, phenylephrine, and methscopolamine *on page 218*
Dura-Vent® *(Discontinued)*
Durezol™ [US] *see* difluprednate *on page 308*
Duricef® *(Discontinued)* *see* cefadroxil *on page 191*
Duricef® Oral Suspension 125 mg/5 mL *(Discontinued)* *see* cefadroxil *on page 191*
Durolane® [Can] *see* hyaluronate and derivatives *on page 496*
Durrax® Oral *(Discontinued)* *see* hydroxyzine *on page 511*

dutasteride (doo TAS teer ide)

U.S./Canadian Brand Names Avodart® [US/Can]

Therapeutic Category Antineoplastic Agent, Anthracenedione

Use Treatment of symptomatic benign prostatic hyperplasia (BPH) as monotherapy or combination therapy with tamsulosin

Usual Dosage Oral: Adults: Males: BPH: 0.5 mg once daily alone or in combination with tamsulosin

Dosage Forms

Capsule, softgel:
Avodart®: 0.5 mg

Duvoid® [Can] *see* bethanechol *on page 139*
Duvoid® *(Discontinued)* *see* bethanechol *on page 139*
D-Vi-Sol® [Can] *see* cholecalciferol *on page 224*
DW286 *see* gemifloxacin *on page 458*
Dwelle® Ophthalmic Solution *(Discontinued)* *see* artificial tears *on page 100*
Dyazide® [US] *see* hydrochlorothiazide and triamterene *on page 500*
Dycill® [Can] *see* dicloxacillin *on page 304*
Dycill® *(Discontinued)* *see* dicloxacillin *on page 304*
Dyclone® *(Discontinued)* *see* dyclonine *on page 343*

dyclonine (DYE kloe neen)

Sound-Alike/Look-Alike Issues
dyclonine may be confused with dicyclomine

Synonyms dyclonine hydrochloride

U.S./Canadian Brand Names Cēpacol® Dual Action Maximum Strength [US-OTC]; Sucrets® [US-OTC]

Therapeutic Category Local Anesthetic

Use Temporary relief of pain associated with oral mucosa

Usual Dosage Oral:

Lozenge: Children ≥2 years and Adults: One lozenge every 2 hours as needed (maximum: 10 lozenges/day)

Spray:
Children ≥3-12 years: 1-3 sprays, up to 4 times a day
Children ≥12 years and Adults: 1-4 sprays, up to 4 times a day

Dosage Forms

Lozenge:
Sucrets® [OTC]: 1.2 mg, 2 mg, 3 mg

Spray, oral:
Cēpacol® Dual Action Maximum Strength [OTC]: 0.1%

dyclonine hydrochloride *see* dyclonine *on page 343*
Dygase *(Discontinued)* *see* pancreatin *on page 746*
Dylix [US] *see* dyphylline *on page 344*
Dymenate® Injection *(Discontinued)* *see* dimenhydrinate *on page 312*
Dynabac® *(Discontinued)*
Dynacin® [US] *see* minocycline *on page 659*
DynaCirc® [Can] *see* isradipine *on page 552*
DynaCirc® CR [US] *see* isradipine *on page 552*

DynaCirc® *(Discontinued)* *see* isradipine *on page* 552
Dyna-Hex® [US-OTC] *see* chlorhexidine gluconate *on page* 210
Dynahist-ER Pediatric® *(Discontinued)* *see* chlorpheniramine and pseudoephedrine *on page* 215
Dynapen® *(Discontinued)* *see* dicloxacillin *on page* 304
Dynatuss-EX *(Discontinued)* *see* guaifenesin, dextromethorphan, and phenylephrine *on page* 478
Dynex *(Discontinued)* *see* guaifenesin and pseudoephedrine *on page* 477

dyphylline (DYE fi lin)

Synonyms dihydroxypropyl theophylline
U.S./Canadian Brand Names Dilor® [Can]; Dylix [US]; Lufyllin® [US/Can]
Therapeutic Category Theophylline Derivative
Use Bronchodilator in reversible airway obstruction due to asthma, chronic bronchitis, or emphysema
Usual Dosage Oral: Adults: Up to 15 mg/kg 4 times/day, individualize dosage
Dosage Forms
Elixir:
Dylix: 100 mg/15 mL
Tablet:
Lufyllin®: 200 mg, 400 mg

dyphylline and guaifenesin (DYE fi lin & gwye FEN e sin)

Synonyms guaifenesin and dyphylline
U.S./Canadian Brand Names COPD [US]; Difil-G [US]; Difil®-G Forte [US]; Dilex-G [US]; Dilor-G® [US]; Lufyllin®-GG [US]
Therapeutic Category Expectorant; Theophylline Derivative
Use Treatment of bronchial asthma and reversible bronchospasm associated with chronic bronchitis and emphysema
Usual Dosage Oral:
Children 6-12 years:
Elixir: Lufyllin®-GG: 15-30 mL 3 or 4 times/day
Syrup: Dilex-G:
18-27 kg: 1.25-1.6 mL 4 times/day
27-36 kg: 2.5-3.3 mL 4 times/day
36.5-45 kg: 3.3-3.7 mL 4 times/day
Tablet: Lufyllin®-GG: 1/2 -1 tablet 3 or 4 times/day
Children >12 years and Adults:
Elixir: Lufyllin®-GG: 30 mL 4 times/day
Syrup:
Dilex-G: 5-10 mL 4 times/day
Difil®-G Forte: 5-10 mL 3 or 4 times/day; may double or triple (in severe cases) according to patient response
Tablet: Difil-G, Dilex-G, Lufyllin®-GG: One tablet 3 or 4 times/day
Dosage Forms
Elixir: Dyphylline 100 mg and guaifenesin 100 mg per 15 mL
Lufyllin®-GG: Dyphylline 100 mg and guaifenesin 100 mg per 15 mL
Liquid: Dyphylline 100 mg and guaifenesin 100 mg per 5 mL
Difil®-G Forte: Dyphylline 100 mg and guaifenesin 100 mg per 5 mL
Syrup:
Dilex-G: Dyphylline 100 mg and guaifenesin 200 mg per 5 mL
Tablet: Dyphylline 200 mg and guaifenesin 200 mg
COPD, Lufyllin®-GG: Dyphylline 200 mg and guaifenesin 200 mg
Difil-G: Dyphylline 200 mg and guaifenesin 300 mg
Dilex-G: Dyphylline 200 mg and guaifenesin 400 mg

Dyrenium® [US] *see* triamterene *on page* 984
Dyrexan-OD® *(Discontinued)* *see* phendimetrazine *on page* 770
Dysport™ [US] *see* abobotulinumtoxinA *on page* 17
Dytan™ [US] *see* diphenhydramine *on page* 315
E2 and DRSP *see* drospirenone and estradiol *on page* 340
7E3 *see* abciximab *on page* 17

E2020 *see* donepezil *on page* *330*
E 2080 *see* rufinamide *on page* *882*
EACA *see* aminocaproic acid *on page* *63*
EarSol® HC [US] *see* hydrocortisone (topical) *on page* *505*
Easprin® [US] *see* aspirin *on page* *103*
Ebixa® [Can] *see* memantine *on page* *623*

echothiophate iodide (ek oh THYE oh fate EYE oh dide)

Synonyms ecostigmine iodide

U.S./Canadian Brand Names Phospholine Iodide® [US]

Therapeutic Category Cholinesterase Inhibitor

Use Used as miotic in treatment of chronic, open-angle glaucoma; may be useful in specific cases of angle-closure glaucoma (postiridectomy or where surgery refused/contraindicated); postcataract surgery-related glaucoma; accommodative esotropia

Usual Dosage Ophthalmic:

Children: Accommodative esotropia:

Diagnosis: Instill 1 drop (0.125%) once daily into both eyes at bedtime for 2-3 weeks

Treatment: Usual dose: Instill 1 drop of 0.06% once daily or 0.125% every other day (maximum: 0.125% daily). **Note:** Use lowest concentration and frequency which gives satisfactory response; if necessary, doses >0.125% daily may be used for short periods of time.

Adults: Open-angle or secondary glaucoma:

Initial: Instill 1 drop (0.03%) twice daily into eyes with 1 dose just prior to bedtime

Maintenance: Some patients have been treated with 1 dose daily or every other day

Conversion from other ophthalmic agents: If IOP control was unsatisfactory, patients may be expected to require higher doses of echothiophate (eg, ≥0.06%); however, patients should be initially started on the 0.03% strength for a short period to better tolerance.

Dosage Forms

Powder for reconstitution, ophthalmic:

Phospholine Iodide®: 6.25 mg (5 mL) [0.125%]

EC-Naprosyn® [US] *see* naproxen *on page* *681*
***E. coli* asparaginase** *see* asparaginase *on page* *102*

econazole (e KONE a zole)

Synonyms econazole nitrate

Therapeutic Category Antifungal Agent

Use Topical treatment of tinea pedis (athlete's foot), tinea cruris (jock itch), tinea corporis (ringworm), tinea versicolor, and cutaneous candidiasis

Usual Dosage Topical: Children and Adults:

Tinea pedis: Apply sufficient amount to cover affected areas once daily for 1 month

Tinea cruris, tinea corporis, tinea versicolor: Apply sufficient amount to cover affected areas once daily for 2 weeks

Cutaneous candidiasis: Apply sufficient quantity twice daily (morning and evening) for 2 weeks

Dosage Forms

Cream, topical: 1% (15 g, 30 g, 85 g)

econazole nitrate *see* econazole *on page* *345*
Econopred® Plus [US] *see* prednisolone (ophthalmic) *on page* *813*
ecostigmine iodide *see* echothiophate iodide *on page* *345*
Ecotrin® [US-OTC] *see* aspirin *on page* *103*
Ecotrin® Low Strength [US-OTC] *see* aspirin *on page* *103*
Ecotrin® Maximum Strength [US-OTC] *see* aspirin *on page* *103*
Ectosone [Can] *see* betamethasone (topical) *on page* *138*

eculizumab (e kue LIZ oo mab)

Sound-Alike/Look-Alike Issues

eculizumab may be confused with efalizumab

U.S./Canadian Brand Names Soliris™ [US]

Therapeutic Category Monoclonal Antibody; Monoclonal Antibody, Complement Inhibitor

Use Treatment of paroxysmal nocturnal hemoglobinuria (PNH) to reduce hemolysis

Usual Dosage Note: Patients must receive meningococcal vaccine at least 2 weeks prior to treatment initiation; revaccinate according to current guidelines.

I.V.: Adults: PNH: 600 mg once weekly (±2 days) for 4 weeks, followed by 900 mg 1 week (±2 days) later; then maintenance: 900 mg every 2 weeks (±2 days) thereafter

Treatment should be administered at the recommended time interval, however, the administration day may be varied by ±2 days if serum LDH levels suggest increased hemolysis before the end of the dosing interval.

Dosage Forms

Injection, solution [preservative free]:

Soliris™: 10 mg/mL (30 mL)

Ed A-Hist™ [US] *see* chlorpheniramine and phenylephrine *on page* 214

Ed A-Hist DM [US] *see* chlorpheniramine, phenylephrine, and dextromethorphan *on page* 217

edathamil disodium *see* edetate disodium *on page* 347

Ed Chlorped [US] *see* chlorpheniramine *on page* 213

Ed ChlorPed D [US] *see* chlorpheniramine and phenylephrine *on page* 214

Ed-Chlor-Tan [US] *see* chlorpheniramine *on page* 213

Edecrin® [US/Can] *see* ethacrynic acid *on page* 382

edetate CALCIUM disodium (ED e tate KAL see um dye SOW dee um)

Sound-Alike/Look-Alike Issues

edetate CALCIUM disodium (CaEDTA) may be confused with edetate disodium (Na_2EDTA). To avoid potentially serious errors, the abbreviation "EDTA" should **never** be used. CDC recommends that edetate disodium should **never** be used for chelation therapy in children. Fatal hypocalcemia may result if edetate disodium is used for chelation therapy instead of edetate calcium disodium. ISMP recommends confirming the diagnosis to help distinguish between the two drugs prior to dispensing and/or administering either drug.

edetate CALCIUM disodium may be confused with etomidate

Synonyms CaEDTA ; calcium disodium edetate; edetate disodium CALCIUM

U.S./Canadian Brand Names Calcium Disodium Versenate® [US]

Therapeutic Category Chelating Agent

Use Treatment of symptomatic acute and chronic lead poisoning or for symptomatic patients with high blood lead levels

Usual Dosage

Treatment of lead poisoning: Children and Adults: **Note:** For the treatment of high blood lead levels in children, the CDC recommends chelation treatment when blood lead levels are >45 mcg/dL. In adults, available guidelines recommend chelation therapy with blood lead levels >50 mcg/dL and significant symptoms; chelation therapy may also be indicated with blood lead levels ≥100 mcg/dL and/or symptoms. Depending upon the blood lead level, additional courses may be necessary; at least 2-4 days, and preferably 2-4 weeks, should elapse before repeat treatment is initiated.

Asymptomatic lead poisoning with blood lead level >20 mcg/dL and <70 mcg/dL (manufacturer labeling): I.M., I.V.: 1000 mg/m^2/day (25-50 mg/kg/day) for 5 days. **Note:** The AAP recommends succimer as the drug used for initial management in asymptomatic children when blood lead levels are >45 mcg/dL and <70 mcg/dL. Edetate CALCIUM disodium can be used in children allergic to succimer.

Symptomatic lead poisoning or blood lead levels ≥70 mcg/dL (manufacturer labeling): I.M., I.V.: 1000 mg/m^2/day (25-50 mg/kg/day) for 5 days. Edetate CALCIUM disodium should be administered 4 hours after the initial dimercaprol dose. Edetate CALCIUM disodium should be used in conjunction with dimercaprol when blood lead levels are >70 mcg/dL or when symptoms of lead poisoning are present.

Lead encephalopathy: I.M., I.V.: 1500 mg/m^2/day (50-75 mg/kg/day). Edetate CALCIUM disodium should be administered 4 hours after the initial dimercaprol dose. Edetate CALCIUM disodium should be used in conjunction with dimercaprol when blood lead levels are >70 mcg/dL or when symptoms of lead poisoning are present.

Lead nephropathy: Adults: An alternative dosing regimen reflecting the reduction in renal clearance is based upon the serum creatinine. Dose of edetate CALCIUM disodium based on serum creatinine: **Note:** Repeat regimen monthly until lead levels are reduced to an acceptable level:

S_{cr} 2-3 mg/dL / Cl_{cr} 30-50 mL/minute: Reduce recommended dose by 50% and administer daily

S_{cr} 3-4 mg/dL / Cl_{cr} 20-30 mL/minute: Reduce recommended dose by 50% and administer every 48 hours

S_{cr} >4 mg/dL / Cl_{cr} <20 mL/minute: Reduce recommended dose by 50% and administer once weekly

Dosage Forms

Injection, solution:

Calcium Disodium Versenate®: 200 mg/mL (5 mL)

edetate disodium (ED e tate dye SOW dee um)

Sound-Alike/Look-Alike Issues

edetate disodium (Na_2EDTA) may be confused with edetate calcium disodium (CaEDTA). To avoid potentially serious errors, the abbreviation "EDTA" should **never** be used. CDC recommends that edetate disodium should **never** be used for chelation therapy in children. Fatal hypocalcemia may result if edetate disodium is used for chelation therapy instead of edetate calcium disodium. ISMP recommends confirming the diagnosis to help distinguish between the two drugs prior to dispensing and/or administering either drug.

edetate disodium may be confused with etomidate

Synonyms edathamil disodium; Na_2EDTA; sodium edetate

U.S./Canadian Brand Names Endrate [US]

Therapeutic Category Chelating Agent

Use Emergency treatment of hypercalcemia in adults

Usual Dosage Note: Confirm the diagnosis prior to dispensing.

I.V.: Adults: Hypercalcemia: 50 mg/kg/day over 3 or more hours to a maximum of 3 g/24 hours; a suggested regimen of 5 days followed by 2 days without drug and repeated courses up to 15 total doses

Dosage Forms

Injection, solution: 150 mg/mL (20 mL)

edetate disodium CALCIUM *see* edetate CALCIUM disodium *on page* 346

Edex® [US] *see* alprostadil *on page* 51

Edluar™ [US] *see* zolpidem *on page* 1033

edrophonium (ed roe FOE nee um)

Synonyms edrophonium chloride

U.S./Canadian Brand Names Enlon® [US/Can]; Tensilon® [Can]

Therapeutic Category Cholinergic Agent

Use Diagnosis of myasthenia gravis; differentiation of cholinergic crises from myasthenia crises; reversal of nondepolarizing neuromuscular blockers

Usual Dosage Usually administered I.V., however, if not possible, I.M. or SubQ may be used:

Infants:

I.M.: 0.5-1 mg

I.V.: Initial: 0.1 mg, followed by 0.4 mg if no response; total dose = 0.5 mg

Children:

Diagnosis: Initial: 0.04 mg/kg over 1 minute followed by 0.16 mg/kg if no response, to a maximum total dose of 5 mg for children <34 kg, or 10 mg for children >34 kg **or**

Alternative dosing (manufacturer's recommendation):

≤34 kg: 1 mg; if no response after 45 seconds, repeat dosage in 1 mg increments every 30-45 seconds, up to a total of 5 mg

>34 kg: 2 mg; if no response after 45 seconds, repeat dosage in 1 mg increments every 30-45 seconds, up to a total of 10 mg

I.M.:

<34 kg: 1 mg

>34 kg: 5 mg

Titration of oral anticholinesterase therapy: 0.04 mg/kg once given 1 hour after oral intake of the drug being used in treatment; if strength improves, an increase in neostigmine or pyridostigmine dose is indicated

Adults:

Diagnosis:

I.V.: 2 mg test dose administered over 15-30 seconds; 8 mg given 45 seconds later if no response is seen; test dose may be repeated after 30 minutes

I.M.: Initial: 10 mg; if no cholinergic reaction occurs, administer 2 mg 30 minutes later to rule out false-negative reaction

Titration of oral anticholinesterase therapy: 1-2 mg given 1 hour after oral dose of anticholinesterase; if strength improves, an increase in neostigmine or pyridostigmine dose is indicated

Reversal of nondepolarizing neuromuscular blocking agents (neostigmine with atropine usually preferred): I.V.: 10 mg over 30-45 seconds; may repeat every 5-10 minutes up to 40 mg

Termination of paroxysmal atrial tachycardia: I.V. rapid injection: 5-10 mg

Differentiation of cholinergic from myasthenic crisis: I.V.: 1 mg; may repeat after 1 minute. **Note:** Intubation and controlled ventilation may be required if patient has cholinergic crisis

Dosage Forms

Injection, solution:

Enlon®: 10 mg/mL (15 mL)

edrophonium and atropine (ed roe FOE nee um & A troe peen)

Synonyms atropine sulfate and edrophonium chloride; edrophonium chloride and atropine sulfate

U.S./Canadian Brand Names Enlon-Plus® [US]

Therapeutic Category Anticholinergic Agent; Antidote; Cholinergic Agonist

Use Reversal of nondepolarizing neuromuscular blockers; adjunct treatment of respiratory depression caused by curare overdose

Usual Dosage I.V.: Adults: Reversal of neuromuscular blockade: 0.05-0.1 mL/kg given over 45-60 seconds. The dose delivered is 0.5-1 mg/kg of edrophonium and 0.007-0.014 mg/kg of atropine. An edrophonium dose of 1 mg/kg should rarely be exceeded. **Note:** Monitor closely for bradyarrhythmias.

Dosage Forms

Injection, solution:

Enlon-Plus®: Edrophonium 10 mg/mL and atropine 0.14 mg/mL (5 mL, 15 mL)

edrophonium chloride *see* edrophonium *on page* 347

edrophonium chloride and atropine sulfate *see* edrophonium and atropine *on page* 348

ED-SPAZ® *(Discontinued)* *see* hyoscyamine *on page* 512

ED-TLC [US] *see* phenylephrine, hydrocodone, and chlorpheniramine *on page* 778

ED-Tuss HC [US] *see* phenylephrine, hydrocodone, and chlorpheniramine *on page* 778

EEMT™ [US] *see* estrogens (esterified) and methyltestosterone *on page* 380

EEMT™ HS [US] *see* estrogens (esterified) and methyltestosterone *on page* 380

E.E.S.® [US/Can] *see* erythromycin *on page* 368

efalizumab (e fa li ZOO mab)

Sound-Alike/Look-Alike Issues

efalizumab may be confused with eculizumab

Raptiva® maybe confused with Rapaflo™

Synonyms anti-CD11a; hu1124

Therapeutic Category Immunosuppressant Agent; Monoclonal Antibody

Use Treatment of chronic moderate-to-severe plaque psoriasis in patients who are candidates for systemic therapy or phototherapy

Usual Dosage SubQ: Adults: Psoriasis: Initial: 0.7 mg/kg, followed by weekly dose of 1 mg/kg (maximum: 200 mg/dose)

efavirenz (e FAV e renz)

U.S./Canadian Brand Names Sustiva® [US/Can]

Therapeutic Category Antiretroviral Agent, Nonnucleoside Reverse Transcriptase Inhibitor (NNRTI)

Use Treatment of HIV-1 infections in combination with at least two other antiretroviral agents

Usual Dosage Oral:

Children ≥3 years: Dosage is based on body weight:

10 kg to <15 kg: 200 mg once daily

15 kg to <20 kg: 250 mg once daily

20 kg to <25 kg: 300 mg once daily

25 kg to <32.5 kg: 350 mg once daily

32.5 kg to <40 kg: 400 mg once daily

≥40 kg: 600 mg once daily

Adults: 600 mg once daily

Dosage Forms

Capsule:

Sustiva®: 50 mg, 200 mg

Tablet:

Sustiva®: 600 mg

efavirenz, emtricitabine, and tenofovir

(e FAV e renz, em trye SYE ta been, & te NOE fo veer)

Synonyms emtricitabine, efavirenz, and tenofovir; FTC, TDF, and EFV; tenofovir disoproxil fumarate, efavirenz, and emtricitabine

U.S./Canadian Brand Names Atripla® [US/Can]

Therapeutic Category Antiretroviral Agent, Nonnucleoside Reverse Transcriptase Inhibitor (NNRTI); Antiretroviral Agent, Nucleoside Reverse Transcriptase Inhibitor (NRTI); Antiretroviral Agent, Reverse Transcriptase Inhibitor (Nucleotide)

Use Treatment of HIV infection

Usual Dosage Oral: Adults: One tablet once daily

Dosage Forms

Tablet:

Atripla®: Efavirenz 600 mg, emtricitabine 200 mg, and tenofovir disoproxil fumarate 300 mg

Effer-K™ [US] *see* potassium bicarbonate and potassium citrate *on page 802*

Effer-Syllium® *(Discontinued)* *see* psyllium *on page 837*

Effexor® [US] *see* venlafaxine *on page 1009*

Effexor XR® [US/Can] *see* venlafaxine *on page 1009*

Effient™ [US] *see* prasugrel *on page 810*

Eflone® *(Discontinued)* *see* fluorometholone *on page 431*

eflornithine (ee FLOR ni theen)

Sound-Alike/Look-Alike Issues

Vaniqa™ may be confused with Viagra®

Synonyms DFMO; eflornithine hydrochloride

U.S./Canadian Brand Names Vaniqa™ [US/Can]

Therapeutic Category Antiprotozoal; Topical Skin Product

Use Cream: Females ≥12 years: Reduce unwanted hair from face and adjacent areas under the chin

Orphan status: Injection: Treatment of meningoencephalitic stage of *Trypanosoma brucei gambiense* infection (sleeping sickness)

Usual Dosage

Children ≥12 years and Adults: Females: Topical: Apply thin layer of cream to affected areas of face and adjacent chin twice daily, at least 8 hours apart

Adults: I.V. infusion: 100 mg/kg/dose given every 6 hours (over at least 45 minutes) for 14 days

Dosage Forms

Cream, topical:

Vaniqa™: 13.9% (30 g)

Injection, solution:

Vaniqa™: 200 mg/mL (100 mL) [orphan drug status]

eflornithine hydrochloride *see* eflornithine *on page 349*

Efodine® *(Discontinued)* *see* povidone-iodine *on page 807*

eformoterol and budesonide *see* budesonide and formoterol *on page 155*

Efudex® [US/Can] *see* fluorouracil *on page 431*

E-Gems® [US-OTC] *see* vitamin E *on page 1018*

E-Gems Elite® [US-OTC] *see* vitamin E *on page 1018*

E-Gems Plus® [US-OTC] *see* vitamin E *on page 1018*

EHDP *see* etidronate disodium *on page 397*

Elaprase™ [US/Can] *see* idursulfase *on page 518*

Elavil® *(Discontinued)* *see* amitriptyline *on page 65*

Eldepryl® [US] *see* selegiline *on page 895*

Eldopaque® [US-OTC/Can] *see* hydroquinone *on page 508*

Eldopaque Forte® [US] *see* hydroquinone *on page 508*
Eldoquin® [US-OTC/Can] *see* hydroquinone *on page 508*
Eldoquin Forte® [US] *see* hydroquinone *on page 508*
electrolyte lavage solution *see* polyethylene glycol-electrolyte solution *on page 797*
electrolyte lavage solution *see* polyethylene glycol-electrolyte solution and bisacodyl *on page 798*

electrolyte solution, renal replacement

(ee LEK trow lite soe LOO shun REE nil ree PLASE ment)

Synonyms continuous renal replacement therapy; CRRT; renal replacement solution

U.S./Canadian Brand Names Normocarb HF™ [US]; PrismaSol [US]

Therapeutic Category Alkalinizing Agent; Electrolyte Supplement

Use Used as a replacement solution to replenish water, correct electrolytes, and adjust acid-base balance depleted by hemofiltration or hemodiafiltration (continuous renal replacement therapy [CRRT])

Usual Dosage Note: If using PrismaSol, ensure that compartment A and B are mixed.

Continuous renal replacement circuit: Children and Adults: Pre- or post-filter: Volume of solution administered depends upon the patient's fluid balance, target fluid balance, body weight, and amount of fluid removed during hemofiltration process.

Post-filter replacement: Volume infused/hour should not be greater than 1/3 of blood flow rate (eg, blood flow rate 100 mL/minute [6000 mL/hour], post-filter replacement rate ≤2000 mL/hour)

Dosage Forms

Injection, solution [concentrate; preservative free]:

Normocarb HF™ 25: Bicarbonate 25 mEq/L, chloride 116.5 mEq/L, magnesium 1.5 mEq/L, sodium 140 mEq/L (240 mL) [strength represents final solution after mixing; when diluted as directed, makes 3240 mL of infusate]

Normocarb HF™ 35: Bicarbonate 35 mEq/L, chloride 106.5 mEq/L, magnesium 1.5 mEq/L, sodium 140 mEq/L (240 mL) [strength represents final solution after mixing; when diluted as directed, makes 3240 mL of infusate]

Injection, solution [preservative free]:

PrismaSol BGK 0/2.5: Bicarbonate 32 mEq/L, calcium 2.5 mEq/L, chloride 109 mEq/L, dextrose 100 mg/dL, lactate 3 mEq/L, magnesium 1.5 mEq/L, sodium 140 mEq/L (5000 mL) [strength represents final solution after mixing]

PrismaSol BGK 2/0: Bicarbonate 32 mEq/L, chloride 108 mEq/L, dextrose 100 mg/dL, lactate 3 mEq/L, magnesium 1 mEq/L, potassium 2 mEq/L, sodium 140 mEq/L (5000 mL) [strength represents final solution after mixing]

PrismaSol BGK 2/3.5: Bicarbonate 32 mEq/L, calcium 3.5 mEq/L, chloride 111.5 mEq/L, dextrose 100 mg/dL, lactate 3 mEq/L, magnesium 1 mEq/L, potassium 2 mEq/L, sodium 140 mEq/L (5000 mL) [strength represents final solution after mixing]

PrismaSol BGK 4/2.5: Bicarbonate 32 mEq/L, calcium 2.5 mEq/L, chloride 113 mEq/L, dextrose 100 mg/dL, lactate 3 mEq/L, magnesium 1.5 mEq/L, potassium 4 mEq/L, sodium 140 mEq/L (5000 mL) [strength represents final solution after mixing]

PrismaSol BK 0/3.5: Bicarbonate 32 mEq/L, calcium 3.5 mEq/L, chloride 109.5 mEq/L, lactate 3 mEq/L, magnesium 1 mEq/L, sodium 140 mEq/L (5000 mL) [strength represents final solution after mixing]

Elestat™ [US] *see* epinastine *on page 357*
Elestrin™ [US] *see* estradiol *on page 373*

eletriptan (el e TRIP tan)

Synonyms eletriptan hydrobromide

U.S./Canadian Brand Names Relpax® [US/Can]

Therapeutic Category Serotonin 5-$HT_{1B,\ 1D}$ Receptor Agonist

Use Acute treatment of migraine, with or without aura

Usual Dosage Oral: Adults: Acute migraine: 20-40 mg; if the headache improves but returns, dose may be repeated after 2 hours have elapsed since first dose; maximum 80 mg/day.

Note: If the first dose is ineffective, diagnosis needs to be reevaluated. Safety of treating >3 headaches/month has not been established.

Dosage Forms

Tablet:

Relpax®: 20 mg, 40 mg

eletriptan hydrobromide *see* eletriptan *on page 350*

Elidel® [US/Can] *see* pimecrolimus *on page 784*
Eligard® [US/Can] *see* leuprolide *on page 575*
Elimite® [US] *see* permethrin *on page 769*
Elitek™ [US] *see* rasburicase *on page 854*
Elixomin® ***(Discontinued)*** *see* theophylline *on page 953*
Elixophyllin® [US] *see* theophylline *on page 953*
Elixophyllin-GG® ***(Discontinued)***
ElixSure™ Fever/Pain ***(Discontinued)*** *see* acetaminophen *on page 19*
Ellence® [US/Can] *see* epirubicin *on page 360*
Elmiron® [US/Can] *see* pentosan polysulfate sodium *on page 766*
Elocom® [Can] *see* mometasone *on page 665*
Elocon® [US] *see* mometasone *on page 665*
Eloxatin® [US/Can] *see* oxaliplatin *on page 733*
Elspar® [US] *see* asparaginase *on page 102*
Eltor® [Can] *see* pseudoephedrine *on page 833*

eltrombopag (el TROM boe pag)

Synonyms eltrombopag olamine; Revolade®; SB-497115; SB-497115-GR

U.S./Canadian Brand Names Promacta® [US]

Therapeutic Category Colony Stimulating Factor; Thrombopoietic Agent

Use Treatment of thrombocytopenia in patients with chronic immune (idiopathic) thrombocytopenic purpura (ITP) at risk for bleeding who have had insufficient response to corticosteroids, immune globulin, or splenectomy

Usual Dosage **Note:** Discontinue if platelet count does not respond to a level that avoids clinically important bleeding after 4 weeks at the maximum daily dose of 75 mg.

Oral: Adults: ITP: Initial: 50 mg once daily; adjust dose to achieve and maintain platelet count ≥50,000/mm^3 to reduce the risk of bleeding; maximum dose: 75 mg once daily

Dosage Forms

Tablet:

Promacta®: 25 mg, 50 mg

eltrombopag olamine *see* eltrombopag *on page 351*
Eltroxin® [Can] *see* levothyroxine *on page 583*
Emadine® [US] *see* emedastine *on page 351*
Embeda™ [US] *see* morphine sulfate *on page 667*
Embeline™ ***(Discontinued)*** *see* clobetasol *on page 242*
Embeline™ E ***(Discontinued)*** *see* clobetasol *on page 242*
Emcyt® [US/Can] *see* estramustine *on page 377*
Emecheck® ***(Discontinued)***

emedastine (em e DAS teen)

Synonyms emedastine difumarate

U.S./Canadian Brand Names Emadine® [US]

Therapeutic Category Antihistamine, H_1 Blocker, Ophthalmic

Use Treatment of allergic conjunctivitis

Usual Dosage Ophthalmic: Children ≥3 years and Adults: Instill 1 drop in affected eye up to 4 times/day

Dosage Forms

Solution, ophthalmic:

Emadine®: 0.05% (5 mL)

emedastine difumarate *see* emedastine *on page 351*
Emend® [US/Can] *see* aprepitant *on page 94*
Emend® for Injection [US] *see* fosaprepitant *on page 445*
Emetrol® [US-OTC] *see* fructose, dextrose, and phosphoric acid *on page 448*
Emitrip® ***(Discontinued)*** *see* amitriptyline *on page 65*
Emko® ***(Discontinued)*** *see* nonoxynol 9 *on page 703*
EMLA® [US/Can] *see* lidocaine and prilocaine *on page 588*

Emo-Cort® [Can] *see* hydrocortisone (topical) *on page* 505
Emsam® [US] *see* selegiline *on page* 895

emtricitabine (em trye SYE ta been)

Synonyms BW524W91; coviracil; FTC

U.S./Canadian Brand Names Emtriva® [US/Can]

Therapeutic Category Antiretroviral Agent, Nucleoside Reverse Transcriptase Inhibitor (NRTI)

Use Treatment of HIV infection in combination with at least two other antiretroviral agents

Usual Dosage Oral:

Children:
- 0-3 months: Solution: 3 mg/kg/day
- 3 months to 17 years:
  - Capsule: Children >33 kg: 200 mg once daily
  - Solution: 6 mg/kg once daily; maximum: 240 mg/day

Adults:
- Capsule: 200 mg once daily
- Solution: 240 mg once daily

Dosage Forms

Capsule:
Emtriva®: 200 mg

Solution:
Emtriva®: 10 mg/mL

emtricitabine and tenofovir (em trye SYE ta been & te NOE fo veer)

Synonyms tenofovir and emtricitabine

U.S./Canadian Brand Names Truvada® [US/Can]

Therapeutic Category Antiretroviral Agent, Nucleoside Reverse Transcriptase Inhibitor (NRTI); Antiretroviral Agent, Reverse Transcriptase Inhibitor (Nucleotide)

Use Treatment of HIV infection in combination with other antiretroviral agents

Usual Dosage Oral: Adults: One tablet (emtricitabine 200 mg and tenofovir 300 mg) once daily

Note: Concurrent use with adefovir, emtricitabine, lamivudine, and/or tenofovir alone or as a combination product should be avoided.

Dosage Forms

Tablet:
Truvada®: Emtricitabine 200 mg and tenofovir 300 mg

emtricitabine, efavirenz, and tenofovir *see* efavirenz, emtricitabine, and tenofovir *on page* 349
Emtriva® [US/Can] *see* emtricitabine *on page* 352
Emulsoil® ***(Discontinued)*** *see* castor oil *on page* 190
E-Mycin® ***(Discontinued)***
E-Mycin-E® ***(Discontinued)***
ENA 713 *see* rivastigmine *on page* 873
Enablex® [US/Can] *see* darifenacin *on page* 277

enalapril (e NAL a pril)

Sound-Alike/Look-Alike Issues

enalapril may be confused with Anafranil®, Elavil®, Eldepryl®, nafarelin, ramipril

Synonyms enalapril maleate; enalaprilat

U.S./Canadian Brand Names Apo-Enalapril® [Can]; CO Enalapril [Can]; Gen-Enalapril [Can]; Novo-Enalapril [Can]; PMS-Enalapril [Can]; Pro-Enalapril [Can]; ratio-Enalapril [Can]; Riva-Enalapril [Can]; Sandoz-Enalapril [Can]; Taro-Enalapril [Can]; Vasotec® I.V. [Can]; Vasotec® [US/Can]

Therapeutic Category Angiotensin-Converting Enzyme (ACE) Inhibitor

Use Treatment of hypertension; treatment of symptomatic heart failure; treatment of asymptomatic left ventricular dysfunction

Usual Dosage Use lower listed initial dose in patients with hyponatremia, hypovolemia, severe congestive heart failure, decreased renal function, or in those receiving diuretics.

Children 1 month to 17 years: Oral: **Enalapril**: Hypertension: Initial: 0.08 mg/kg/day (up to 5 mg) in 1-2 divided doses; adjust dosage based on patient response; doses >0.58 mg/kg (40 mg) have not been evaluated in pediatric patients

Adults:

Oral: **Enalapril:**

Asymptomatic left ventricular dysfunction: 2.5 mg twice daily, titrated as tolerated to 20 mg/day

Heart failure: Initial: 2.5 mg once or twice daily (usual range: 5-40 mg/day in 2 divided doses); titrate slowly at 1- to 2-week intervals. Target dose: 10-20 mg twice daily

Hypertension: 2.5-5 mg/day then increase as required, usually at 1- to 2-week intervals; usual dose range (JNC 7): 2.5-40 mg/day in 1-2 divided doses. **Note:** Initiate with 2.5 mg if patient is taking a diuretic which cannot be discontinued. May add a diuretic if blood pressure cannot be controlled with enalapril alone.

I.V.: **Enalaprilat:**

Heart failure: Avoid I.V. administration in patients with unstable heart failure or those suffering acute myocardial infarction.

Hypertension: 1.25 mg/dose, given over 5 minutes every 6 hours; doses as high as 5 mg/dose every 6 hours have been tolerated for up to 36 hours. **Note:** If patients are concomitantly receiving diuretic therapy, begin with 0.625 mg I.V. over 5 minutes; if the effect is not adequate after 1 hour, repeat the dose and administer 1.25 mg at 6-hour intervals thereafter; if adequate, administer 0.625 mg I.V. every 6 hours.

Conversion from I.V. to oral therapy if not concurrently on diuretics: 5 mg once daily; subsequent titration as needed; if concurrently receiving diuretics and responding to 0.625 mg I.V. every 6 hours, initiate with 2.5 mg/day.

Dosage Forms

Injection, solution: 1.25 mg/mL (1 mL, 2 mL)

Tablet: 2.5 mg, 5 mg, 10 mg, 20 mg

Vasotec®: 2.5 mg, 5 mg, 10 mg, 20 mg

enalapril and felodipine (e NAL a pril & fe LOE di peen)

Synonyms enalapril maleate and felodipine; felodipine and enalapril

U.S./Canadian Brand Names Lexxel® [Can]

Therapeutic Category Antihypertensive Agent, Combination

Use Treatment of hypertension, however, not indicated for initial treatment of hypertension; replacement therapy in patients receiving separate dosage forms (for patient convenience); when monotherapy with one component fails to achieve desired antihypertensive effect, or when dose-limiting adverse effects limit upward titration of monotherapy

Usual Dosage Oral: Adults: Enalapril 5-20 mg and felodipine 2.5-10 mg once daily

enalapril and hydrochlorothiazide (e NAL a pril & hye droe klor oh THYE a zide)

Synonyms enalapril maleate and hydrochlorothiazide; hydrochlorothiazide and enalapril

U.S./Canadian Brand Names Vaseretic® [US/Can]

Therapeutic Category Antihypertensive Agent, Combination

Use Treatment of hypertension

Usual Dosage Oral: Adults: Enalapril 5-10 mg and hydrochlorothiazide 12.5-25 mg once daily (maximum: 40 mg/day [enalapril]; 50 mg/day [hydrochlorothiazide])

Dosage Forms

Tablet: 5/12.5: Enalapril 5 mg and hydrochlorothiazide 12.5 mg; 10/25: Enalapril 10 mg and hydrochlorothiazide 25 mg

Vaseretic®: 10/25: enalapril 10 mg and hydrochlorothiazide 25 mg

enalaprilat *see* enalapril *on page 352*

enalapril maleate *see* enalapril *on page 352*

enalapril maleate and felodipine *see* enalapril and felodipine *on page 353*

enalapril maleate and hydrochlorothiazide *see* enalapril and hydrochlorothiazide *on page 353*

Enbrel® [US/Can] *see* etanercept *on page 381*

Encare® [US-OTC] *see* nonoxynol 9 *on page 703*

Encora® [US] *see* vitamins (multiple/oral) *on page 1019*

Encort™ [US] *see* hydrocortisone (rectal) *on page 503*

EndaCof *(Discontinued)*

EndaCof-DM [US] *see* brompheniramine, pseudoephedrine, and dextromethorphan *on page 152*
EndaCof-PD [US] *see* brompheniramine, pseudoephedrine, and dextromethorphan *on page 152*
EndaCof-XP *(Discontinued)*
Endagen™-HD *(Discontinued)* *see* phenylephrine, hydrocodone, and chlorpheniramine *on page 778*
Endantadine® [Can] *see* amantadine *on page 57*
EndoAvitene® [US] *see* collagen hemostat *on page 255*
Endocet® [US/Can] *see* oxycodone and acetaminophen *on page 738*
Endocodone® *(Discontinued)* *see* oxycodone *on page 737*
Endodan® [US/Can] *see* oxycodone and aspirin *on page 739*
Endo®-Levodopa/Carbidopa [Can] *see* carbidopa and levodopa *on page 184*
Endolor® *(Discontinued)*
Endometrin® [US] *see* progesterone *on page 822*
Endrate [US] *see* edetate disodium *on page 347*
Enduron® *(Discontinued)* *see* methyclothiazide *on page 642*
Enduronyl® Forte *(Discontinued)*
Enemeez® [US-OTC] *see* docusate *on page 326*
Enemeez® Plus [US-OTC] *see* docusate *on page 326*
Ener-B® *(Discontinued)* *see* cyanocobalamin *on page 263*
Enerjets [US-OTC] *see* caffeine *on page 165*
Enfamil® Glucose [US] *see* dextrose *on page 298*

enflurane (EN floo rane)

Sound-Alike/Look-Alike Issues
enflurane may be confused with isoflurane

U.S./Canadian Brand Names Compound 347™ [US]; Ethrane® [US]

Therapeutic Category General Anesthetic

Use Induction and maintenance of general anesthesia; **Note:** Use for induction of general anesthesia is not recommended due to its irritant properties and unpleasant odor which causes breath-holding and coughing.

Usual Dosage Minimum alveolar concentration (MAC), the concentration at which 50% of patients do not respond to surgical incision, is 1.6% for enflurane. The concentration at which amnesia and loss of awareness occur (MAC - awake) is 0.4%. Surgical levels of anesthesia are achieved with concentrations between 0.5% to 3%.

Dosage Forms

Liquid, for inhalation:
Compound 347™, Ethrane®: >99.9% (250 mL)

enfuvirtide (en FYOO vir tide)

Synonyms T-20

U.S./Canadian Brand Names Fuzeon® [US/Can]

Therapeutic Category Antiretroviral Agent, Fusion Protein Inhibitor

Use Treatment of HIV-1 infection in combination with other antiretroviral agents in treatment-experienced patients with evidence of HIV-1 replication despite ongoing antiretroviral therapy

Usual Dosage SubQ:
Children 6-16 years: 2 mg/kg twice daily (maximum dose: 90 mg twice daily)
Adolescents ≥16 years and Adults: 90 mg twice daily

Dosage Forms

Injection, powder for reconstitution [preservative free]:
Fuzeon®: 108 mg

ENG *see* etonogestrel *on page 398*
Engerix-B® [US/Can] *see* hepatitis B vaccine (recombinant) *on page 490*
Engerix-B® and Havrix® *see* hepatitis A and hepatitis B recombinant vaccine *on page 488*
enhanced-potency inactivated poliovirus vaccine *see* poliovirus vaccine (inactivated) *on page 796*
Enhancer [US] *see* barium *on page 122*
Enisyl® *(Discontinued)* *see* l-lysine *on page 595*

Enjuvia™ [US] *see* estrogens (conjugated B/synthetic) *on page 378*

Enlon® [US/Can] *see* edrophonium *on page 347*

Enlon-Plus® [US] *see* edrophonium and atropine *on page 348*

Enomine® ***(Discontinued)***

Enovil® ***(Discontinued)*** *see* amitriptyline *on page 65*

enoxaparin (ee noks a PA rin)

Sound-Alike/Look-Alike Issues

Lovenox® may be confused with Lasix®, Levaquin®, Lotronex®, Protonix®

Synonyms enoxaparin sodium

U.S./Canadian Brand Names Enoxaparin Injection [Can]; Lovenox® HP [Can]; Lovenox® [US/Can]

Therapeutic Category Anticoagulant (Other)

Use

Acute coronary syndromes: Unstable angina (UA), non-ST-elevation (NSTEMI), and ST-elevation myocardial infarction (STEMI)

DVT prophylaxis: Following hip or knee replacement surgery, abdominal surgery, or in medical patients with severely-restricted mobility during acute illness who are at risk for thromboembolic complications

DVT treatment (acute): Inpatient treatment (patients with and without pulmonary embolism) and outpatient treatment (patients without pulmonary embolism)

Note: High-risk patients include those with one or more of the following risk factors: >40 years of age, obesity, general anesthesia lasting >30 minutes, malignancy, history of deep vein thrombosis or pulmonary embolism

Usual Dosage SubQ: Adults:

DVT prophylaxis:

Hip replacement surgery:

Twice-daily dosing: 30 mg every 12 hours, with initial dose within 12-24 hours after surgery, and every 12 hours for at least 10 days or until risk of DVT has diminished or the patient is adequately anticoagulated on warfarin.

Once-daily dosing: 40 mg once daily, with initial dose within 9-15 hours before surgery, and daily for at least 10 days (or up to 35 days postoperatively) or until risk of DVT has diminished or the patient is adequately anticoagulated on warfarin.

Knee replacement surgery: 30 mg every 12 hours, with initial dose within 12-24 hours after surgery, and every 12 hours for at least 10 days or until risk of DVT has diminished or the patient is adequately anticoagulated on warfarin.

Abdominal surgery: 40 mg once daily, with initial dose given 2 hours prior to surgery; continue until risk of DVT has diminished (usually 7-10 days).

Bariatric surgery: Roux-en-Y gastric bypass: Appropriate dosing strategies have not been clearly defined:

BMI ≤50 kg/m^2: 40 mg every 12 hours

BMI >50 kg/m^2: 60 mg every 12 hours

Note: Bariatric surgery guidelines suggest initiation 30-120 minutes before surgery and postoperatively until patient is fully mobile. Alternatively, limiting administration to the postoperative period may reduce perioperative bleeding.

Medical patients with severely-restricted mobility during acute illness: 40 mg once daily; continue until risk of DVT has diminished (usually 6-11 days).

DVT treatment (acute): **Note:** Start warfarin on the first treatment day and continue enoxaparin until INR is between 2 and 3 (usually 5-7 days).

Inpatient treatment (with or without pulmonary embolism): 1 mg/kg/dose every 12 hours or 1.5 mg/kg once daily.

Outpatient treatment (without pulmonary embolism): 1 mg/kg/dose every 12 hours.

Percutaneous coronary intervention (PCI), adjunctive therapy: In enoxaparin-treated patients undergoing PCI, if balloon inflation occurs ≤8 hours after the last SubQ enoxaparin dose, no additional dosing is needed. If balloon inflation occurs 8-12 hours after the last SubQ enoxaparin dose, a single I.V. dose of 0.3 mg/kg should be administered

ST-elevation myocardial infarction (STEMI):

Patients <75 years of age: Initial: 30 mg I.V. single bolus plus 1 mg/kg (maximum 100 mg for the first 2 doses only) SubQ every 12 hours. The first SubQ dose should be administered with the I.V. bolus. Maintenance: After first 2 doses, administer 1 mg/kg SubQ every 12 hours.

Patients ≥75 years of age: Initial: SubQ: 0.75 mg/kg every 12 hours (**Note:** No I.V. bolus is administered in this population); a maximum dose of 75 mg is recommended for the first 2 doses. Maintenance: After first 2 doses, administer 0.75 mg/kg SubQ every 12 hours

Obesity: Use weight-based dosing; a maximum dose of 100 mg is recommended for the first 2 doses

Additional notes on STEMI treatment: Therapy was continued for 8 days or until hospital discharge; optimal duration not defined. Unless contraindicated, all patients received aspirin (75-325 mg daily) in clinical trials. In patients with STEMI receiving thrombolytics, initiate enoxaparin dosing between 15 minutes before and 30 minutes after fibrinolytic therapy. In patients undergoing PCI, if balloon inflation occurs ≤8 hours after the last SubQ enoxaparin dose, no additional dosing is needed. If balloon inflation occurs 8-12 hours after last SubQ enoxaparin dose, a single I.V. dose of 0.3 mg/kg should be administered.

Unstable angina or non-ST-elevation myocardial infarction (NSTEMI): 1 mg/kg every 12 hours in conjunction with oral aspirin therapy (100-325 mg once daily); continue until clinical stabilization (a minimum of at least 2 days)

Dosage Forms

Injection, solution [graduated prefilled syringe; preservative free]:

Lovenox®: 60 mg/0.6 mL (0.6 mL); 80 mg/0.8 mL (0.8 mL); 100 mg/mL (1 mL); 120 mg/0.8 mL (0.8 mL); 150 mg/mL (1 mL)

Injection, solution [multidose vial]:

Lovenox®: 100 mg/mL (3 mL)

Injection, solution [prefilled syringe; preservative free]:

Lovenox®: 30 mg/0.3 mL (0.3 mL); 40 mg/0.4 mL (0.4 mL)

Enoxaparin Injection [Can] *see* enoxaparin *on page* 355

enoxaparin sodium *see* enoxaparin *on page* 355

Enpresse™ [US] *see* ethinyl estradiol and levonorgestrel *on page* 387

Ensure® [US-OTC] *see* nutritional formula, enteral/oral *on page* 715

Ensure Plus® [US-OTC] *see* nutritional formula, enteral/oral *on page* 715

entacapone (en TA ka pone)

U.S./Canadian Brand Names Comtan® [US/Can]

Therapeutic Category Anti-Parkinson Agent; Reverse COMT Inhibitor

Use Adjunct to levodopa/carbidopa therapy in patients with idiopathic Parkinson disease who experience "wearing-off" symptoms at the end of a dosing interval

Usual Dosage Oral: Adults: 200 mg with each dose of levodopa/carbidopa, up to a maximum of 8 times/day (maximum daily dose: 1600 mg/day). To optimize therapy, the dosage of levodopa may need reduced or the dosing interval may need extended. Patients taking levodopa ≥800 mg/day or who had moderate-to-severe dyskinesias prior to therapy required an average decrease of 25% in the daily levodopa dose.

Dosage Forms

Tablet:

Comtan®: 200 mg

entacapone, carbidopa, and levodopa *see* levodopa, carbidopa, and entacapone *on page* 579

entecavir (en TE ka veer)

U.S./Canadian Brand Names Baraclude® [US/Can]

Therapeutic Category Antiretroviral Agent, Reverse Transcriptase Inhibitor (Nucleoside)

Use Treatment of chronic hepatitis B infection in adults with evidence of active viral replication and either evidence of persistent transaminase elevations or histologically-active disease

Usual Dosage Oral: Adolescents ≥16 years and Adults:

Nucleoside treatment naive: 0.5 mg daily

Lamivudine-resistant viremia (or known lamivudine- or telbivudine-resistant mutations): 1 mg daily

Note: Usual treatment duration is at least 1 year and varies with HBeAg status; consult current guidelines and literature.

Dosage Forms

Oral solution:

Baraclude®: 0.05 mg/mL

Tablet:

Baraclude®: 0.5 mg, 1 mg

Entereg® [US] *see* alvimopan *on page* *57*

enterotoxigenic *Escherichia coli* and *Vibrio cholera* vaccine *see* traveler's diarrhea and cholera vaccine *(Canada only) on page* *978*

Entero Vu™ [US] *see* barium *on page* *122*

Entertainer's Secret® [US-OTC] *see* saliva substitute *on page* *887*

Entex® *(Discontinued)* *see* guaifenesin and phenylephrine *on page* *475*

Entex® ER *(Discontinued)* *see* guaifenesin and phenylephrine *on page* *475*

Entex® HC *(Discontinued)*

Entex® LA [Can] *see* guaifenesin and pseudoephedrine *on page* *477*

Entex® LA *(Discontinued)* *see* guaifenesin and phenylephrine *on page* *475*

Entex® PSE *(Discontinued)* *see* guaifenesin and pseudoephedrine *on page* *477*

Entocort® [Can] *see* budesonide *on page* *153*

Entocort® EC [US] *see* budesonide *on page* *153*

Entrobar® [US] *see* barium *on page* *122*

EntroEase® [US] *see* barium *on page* *122*

Entrophen® [Can] *see* aspirin *on page* *103*

Entsol® [US-OTC] *see* sodium chloride *on page* *908*

Entuss-D® Liquid *(Discontinued)*

Enulose [US] *see* lactulose *on page* *565*

Eovist® [US] *see* gadoxetate *on page* *453*

Eperbel-S *(Discontinued)*

ephedrine (e FED rin)

Sound-Alike/Look-Alike Issues

ePHEDrine may be confused with Epifrin®, EPINEPHrine

Synonyms ephedrine sulfate

Tall-Man e**PHED**rine

Therapeutic Category Adrenergic Agonist Agent

Use Treatment of bronchial asthma, acute bronchospasm, idiopathic orthostatic hypotension, anesthesia-induced hypotension

Usual Dosage

Children:

Oral, SubQ: 3 mg/kg/day or 25-100 mg/m^2/day in 4-6 divided doses every 4-6 hours

I.M., slow I.V. push: 0.2-0.3 mg/kg/dose every 4-6 hours

Adults:

Oral: 25-50 mg every 3-4 hours as needed

I.M., SubQ: 25-50 mg, parenteral adult dose should not exceed 150 mg in 24 hours

I.V.: 5-25 mg/dose slow I.V. push repeated after 5-10 minutes as needed, then every 3-4 hours not to exceed 150 mg/24 hours

Dosage Forms

Capsule: 25 mg

Injection, solution: 50 mg/mL (1 mL, 10 mL)

ephedrine, chlorpheniramine, phenylephrine, and carbetapentane *see* chlorpheniramine, ephedrine, phenylephrine, and carbetapentane *on page* *216*

ephedrine sulfate *see* ephedrine *on page* *357*

EpiClenz™ [US-OTC] *see* alcohol (ethyl) *on page* *42*

epidermal thymocyte activating factor *see* aldesleukin *on page* *43*

Epidrin [US] *see* acetaminophen, isometheptene, and dichloralphenazone *on page* *29*

Epiduo™ [US] *see* adapalene and benzoyl peroxide *on page* *36*

Epifoam® [US] *see* pramoxine and hydrocortisone *on page* *810*

Epifrin® *(Discontinued)* *see* epinephrine *on page* *358*

epinastine (ep i NAS teen)

Synonyms epinastine hydrochloride

U.S./Canadian Brand Names Elestat™ [US]

Therapeutic Category Antihistamine, H_1 Blocker, Ophthalmic

Use Treatment of allergic conjunctivitis

Usual Dosage Ophthalmic: Children ≥3 years and Adults: Allergic conjunctivitis: Instill 1 drop into each eye twice daily; continue throughout period of exposure, even in the absence of symptoms

Dosage Forms

Solution, ophthalmic:

Elestat™: 0.05% (5 mL)

epinastine hydrochloride *see* epinastine *on page* 357

epinephrine (ep i NEF rin)

Sound-Alike/Look-Alike Issues

EPINEPHrine may be confused with ePHEDrine

Epifrin® may be confused with ephedrine, EpiPen®

EpiPen® may be confused with Epifrin®

Synonyms adrenaline; epinephrine bitartrate; epinephrine hydrochloride; racemic epinephrine; racepinephrine

Tall-Man **EPINEPH**rine

U.S./Canadian Brand Names Adrenalin® [US/Can]; EpiPen® Jr [US/Can]; EpiPen® [US/Can]; Primatene® Mist [US-OTC]; S2® [US-OTC]; Twinject® [US/Can]

Therapeutic Category Adrenergic Agonist Agent

Use Treatment of bronchospasms, bronchial asthma, nasal congestion, viral croup, anaphylactic reactions, cardiac arrest; added to local anesthetics to decrease systemic absorption of intraspinal and local anesthetics and increase duration of action; decrease superficial hemorrhage

Usual Dosage

Neonates: Cardiac arrest:

I.V.: 0.01-0.03 mg/kg (0.1-0.3 mL/kg of **1:10,000** solution) every 3-5 minutes until return of spontaneous circulation

Intratracheal: Although I.V. route is preferred, may consider administration of doses up to 0.1 mg/kg (1 mL/kg of **1:10,000** solution) every 3-5 minutes until I.V. access established or return of spontaneous circulation

Infants and Children:

Asystole/pulseless arrest, pulseless VT/VF (after failed defibrillations):

I.V., I.O.: 0.01 mg/kg (0.1 mL/kg of **1:10,000** solution) (maximum single dose: 1 mg) every 3-5 minutes until return of spontaneous circulation

Intratracheal: 0.1 mg/kg (0.1 mL/kg of **1:1000** solution) (maximum single dose: 10 mg) every 3-5 minutes until I.V./I.O access established or return of spontaneous circulation

Bradycardia (symptomatic; unresponsive to atropine or pacing):

I.V., I.O.: 0.01 mg/kg (0.1 mL/kg of **1:10,000** solution) (maximum single dose: 1 mg) every 3-5 minutes as needed

Intratracheal: 0.1 mg/kg or (0.1 mL/kg of **1:1000** solution) (maximum single dose: 10 mg) every 3-5 minutes as needed until I.V./I.O access established

Continuous I.V. infusion: 0.1-1 mcg/kg/minute; doses <0.3 mcg/kg/minute generally produce beta-adrenergic effects and higher doses generally produce alpha-adrenergic vasoconstriction; titrate dosage to desired effect

Bronchodilator:

SubQ: 0.01 mg/kg (0.01 mL/kg of **1:1000** solution) (maximum single dose: 0.5 mg) every 20 minutes for 3 doses

Nebulization: S2® (racepinephrine, OTC labeling):

Children <4 years: Jet nebulizer: Croup: 0.05 mL/kg (maximum dose: 0.5 mL); dilute in 3 mL of NS. Administer over ~15 minutes; do not administer more frequently than every 2 hours

Children ≥4 years: Refer to adult dosing.

Inhalation: Children ≥4 years: Primatene® Mist: Refer to adult dosing.

Decongestant: Children ≥6 years: Refer to adult dosing

Hypersensitivity reaction: **Note:** SubQ administration results in slower absorption and is less reliable. I.M. administration in the anterolateral aspect of the thigh is preferred in the setting of anaphylaxis.

I.M., SubQ: 0.01 mg/kg (0.01 mL/kg of **1:1000** solution) (maximum single dose: 0.5 mg) every 5-20 minutes; larger I.M. or SubQ doses, use of I.V. route, or continuous infusion may be needed for severe anaphylactic reactions

Self-administration following severe allergic reactions (eg, insect stings, food): **Note:** World Health Organization (WHO) and Anaphylaxis Canada recommend the availability of 1 dose for every 10-20 minutes of travel time to a medical emergency facility:

EpiPen® Jr: I.M., SubQ: Children 15-29 kg: 0.15 mg; if anaphylactic symptoms persist, dose may be repeated in 5-15 minutes using an additional EpiPen® Jr

EpiPen®: I.M., SubQ: Children ≥30 kg: 0.3 mg; if anaphylactic symptoms persist, dose may be repeated in 5-15 minutes using an additional EpiPen®

Twinject®: I.M. SubQ:

Children 15-29 kg: 0.15 mg; if anaphylactic symptoms persist, dose may be repeated in 5-15 minutes using the same device after partial disassembly

Children ≥30 kg: 0.3 mg; if anaphylactic symptoms persist, dose may be repeated in 5-15 minutes using the same device after partial disassembly

Adults:

Asystole/pulseless arrest, pulseless VT/VF:

I.V., I.O.: 1 mg every 3-5 minutes until return of spontaneous circulation; if this approach fails, higher doses of epinephrine (up to 0.2 mg/kg) have been used for treatment of specific problems (eg, beta-blocker or calcium channel blocker overdose)

Intratracheal: 2-2.5 mg every 3-5 minutes until I.V./I.O access established or return of spontaneous circulation; dilute in 5-10 mL NS or distilled water. **Note:** Absorption is greater with distilled water, but causes more adverse effects on PaO_2.

Bradycardia (symptomatic; unresponsive to atropine or pacing): I.V. infusion: 1-10 mcg/minute; titrate to desired effect

Bronchodilator:

SubQ: 0.3-0.5 mg (**1:1000** solution) every 20 minutes for 3 doses

Nebulization: S2® (racepinephrine, OTC labeling):

Hand-bulb nebulizer: Add 0.5 mL (~10 drops) to nebulizer; 1-3 inhalations up to every 3 hours if needed

Jet nebulizer: Add 0.5 mL (~10 drops) to nebulizer and dilute with 3 mL of NS; administer over ~15 minutes every 3-4 hours as needed

Inhalation: Primatene® Mist (OTC labeling): One inhalation, wait at least 1 minute; if not relieved, may use once more. Do not use again for at least 3 hours.

Decongestant: Intranasal: Apply **1:1000** solution locally as drops or spray or with sterile swab

Hypersensitivity reaction: **Note:** SubQ administration results in slower absorption and is less reliable. I.M. administration in the anterolateral aspect of the thigh is preferred in the setting of anaphylaxis.

I.M., SubQ: 0.3-0.5 mg (**1:1000** solution) every 15-20 minutes if condition requires

I.V.: 0.1 mg (**1:10,000** solution) over 5 minutes; may infuse at 1-4 mcg/minute to prevent the need to repeat injections frequently

Self-administration following severe allergic reactions (eg, insect stings, food): **Note:** The World Health Organization (WHO) and Anaphylaxis Canada recommend the availability of one dose for every 10-20 minutes of travel time to a medical emergency facility. More than 2 doses should only be administered under direct medical supervision.

Twinject®: I.M., SubQ: 0.3 mg; if anaphylactic symptoms persist, dose may be repeated in 5-15 minutes using the same device after partial disassembly

EpiPen®: I.M., SubQ: 0.3 mg; if anaphylactic symptoms persist, dose may be repeated in 5-15 minutes using an additional EpiPen®

Dosage Forms

Aerosol for oral inhalation:

Primatene® Mist [OTC]: 0.22 mg/inhalation (15 mL)

Injection, solution [prefilled auto injector]:

EpiPen®: 0.3 mg/0.3 mL (2 mL) [1:1000; delivers 0.3 mg per injection; available as single unit or in double-unit pack with training unit]

EpiPen® Jr: 0.15 mg/0.3 mL (2 mL) [1:2000 solution; delivers 0.15 mg per injection; available as single unit or in double-unit pack with training unit]

Twinject®: 0.15 mg/0.15 mL (1.1 mL) [1:1000 solution; delivers 0.15 mg per injection; two 0.15 mg doses per injector]; 0.3 mg/0.3 mL (1.1 mL) [1:1000 solution; delivers 0.3 mg per injection; two 0.3 mg doses per injector]

Injection, solution: 0.1 mg/mL (10 mL) [1:10,000 solution]; 1 mg/mL (1 mL) [1:1000 solution]

Adrenalin®: 1 mg/mL (1 mL, 30 mL) [1:1000 solution]

Solution for oral inhalation [racepinephrine; preservative free]:

S2® [OTC]: 2.25% (0.5 mL)

Solution, intranasal [drops, spray]:

Adrenalin®: 1 mg/mL (30 mL) [1:1000 solution]

epinephrine and articaine hydrochloride *see* articaine and epinephrine *on page 99*

epinephrine and chlorpheniramine (ep i NEF rin & klor fen IR a meen)

Synonyms insect sting kit

U.S./Canadian Brand Names Ana-Kit® [US]

Therapeutic Category Antidote

Use Anaphylaxis emergency treatment of insect bites or stings by the sensitive patient that may occur within minutes of insect sting or exposure to an allergic substance

Usual Dosage I.M. or SubQ: Children and Adults:

Epinephrine:
- <2 years: 0.05-0.1 mL
- 2-6 years: 0.15 mL
- 6-12 years: 0.2 mL
- >12 years: 0.3 mL

Chlorpheniramine:
- <6 years: 1 tablet
- 6-12 years: 2 tablets
- >12 years: 4 tablets

Dosage Forms

Kit:

Ana-Kit®: Epinephrine 1:1000 (1 mL), chlorpheniramine chewable tablet 2 mg (4), sterile alcohol pads (2), tourniquet (1)

epinephrine and lidocaine *see* lidocaine and epinephrine *on page 586*
epinephrine bitartrate *see* epinephrine *on page 358*
epinephrine bitartrate and bupivacaine hydrochloride *see* bupivacaine and epinephrine *on page 157*
epinephrine hydrochloride *see* epinephrine *on page 358*
EpiPen® [US/Can] *see* epinephrine *on page 358*
EpiPen® Jr [US/Can] *see* epinephrine *on page 358*
epipodophyllotoxin *see* etoposide *on page 398*
EpiQuin™ Micro [US] *see* hydroquinone *on page 508*

epirubicin (ep i ROO bi sin)

Sound-Alike/Look-Alike Issues

epirubicin may be confused with DAUNOrubicin, DOXOrubicin, idarubicin
Ellence® may be confused with Elase®

Synonyms epirubicin hydrochloride; NSC-256942; pidorubicin; pidorubicin hydrochloride

U.S./Canadian Brand Names Ellence® [US/Can]; Pharmorubicin® [Can]

Therapeutic Category Antineoplastic Agent, Anthracycline; Antineoplastic Agent, Antibiotic

Use Adjuvant therapy for primary breast cancer

Usual Dosage I.V.: Adults: 100-120 mg/m^2 once every 3-4 weeks **or** 50-60 mg/m^2 days 1 and 8 every 3-4 weeks

Breast cancer:

CEF-120: 60 mg/m^2 on days 1 and 8 every 28 days for 6 cycles

FEC-100: 100 mg/m^2 on day 1 every 21 days for 6 cycles

Note: Patients receiving 120 mg/m^2/cycle as part of combination therapy should also receive prophylactic therapy with sulfamethoxazole/trimethoprim or a fluoroquinolone.

Dosage modifications:

Delay day 1 dose until platelets are ≥100,000/mm^3, ANC ≥1500/mm^3, and nonhematologic toxicities have recovered to ≤grade 1

Reduce day 1 dose in subsequent cycles to 75% of previous day 1 dose if patient experiences nadir platelet counts <50,000/mm^3, ANC <250/mm^3, neutropenic fever, or grade 3/4 nonhematologic toxicity during the previous cycle

For divided doses (day 1 and day 8), reduce day 8 dose to 75% of day 1 dose if platelet counts are 75,000-100,000/mm^3 and ANC is 1000-1499/mm^3; omit day 8 dose if platelets are <75,000/mm^3, ANC <1000/mm^3, or grade 3/4 nonhematologic toxicity

Dosage adjustment in bone marrow dysfunction: Heavily-treated patients, patients with preexisting bone marrow depression or neoplastic bone marrow infiltration: Lower starting doses (75-90 mg/mm^2) should be considered.

Dosage Forms

Injection, powder for reconstitution [preservative free]: 50 mg, 200 mg

Injection, solution [preservative free]: 2 mg/mL (5 mL, 25 mL, 75 mL, 100 mL)

Ellence®: 2 mg/mL (25 mL, 100 mL)

epirubicin hydrochloride *see* epirubicin *on page 360*

Epitol® [US] *see* carbamazepine *on page 180*

Epival® I.V. [Can] *see* valproic acid and derivatives *on page 1002*

Epivir® [US] *see* lamivudine *on page 566*

Epivir-HBV® [US] *see* lamivudine *on page 566*

eplerenone (e PLER en one)

Sound-Alike/Look-Alike Issues

Inspra™ may be confused with Spiriva®

U.S./Canadian Brand Names Inspra™ [US]

Therapeutic Category Antihypertensive Agent; Selective Aldosterone Blocker

Use Treatment of hypertension (may be used alone or in combination with other antihypertensive agents); treatment of heart failure (HF) following acute MI

Usual Dosage Oral: Adults:

Hypertension: Initial: 50 mg once daily; may increase to 50 mg twice daily if response is not adequate; may take up to 4 weeks for full therapeutic response. Doses >100 mg/day are associated with increased risk of hyperkalemia and no greater therapeutic effect.

Concurrent use with moderate CYP3A4 inhibitors: Initial: 25 mg once daily

Heart failure (post-MI): Initial: 25 mg once daily; dosage goal: Titrate to 50 mg once daily within 4 weeks, as tolerated

Dosage Forms

Tablet: 25 mg, 50 mg

Inspra™: 25 mg, 50 mg

EPO *see* epoetin alfa *on page 361*

epoetin alfa (e POE e tin AL fa)

Sound-Alike/Look-Alike Issues

epoetin alfa may be confused with darbepoetin alfa, epoetin beta

Epogen® may be confused with Neupogen®

Synonyms *r*HuEPO-α; EPO; erythropoiesis-stimulating agent (ESA); erythropoietin; NSC-724223

U.S./Canadian Brand Names Epogen® [US]; Eprex® [Can]; Procrit® [US]

Therapeutic Category Colony-Stimulating Factor

Use Treatment of anemia (elevate/maintain red blood cell level and decrease the need for transfusions) associated with HIV (zidovudine) therapy, chronic renal failure (including patients on dialysis and not on dialysis); reduction of allogeneic blood transfusion for elective, noncardiac, nonvascular surgery; treatment of anemia due to concurrent chemotherapy in patients with metastatic cancer (nonmyeloid malignancies)

Note: Erythropoietin is **not** indicated for use in cancer patients under the following conditions:

- receiving hormonal therapy, therapeutic biologic products, or radiation therapy unless also receiving concurrent myelosuppressive chemotherapy
- receiving myelosuppressive therapy when the expected outcome is curative
- anemia due to other factors (eg, iron deficiency, folate deficiency, or gastrointestinal bleed)

Usual Dosage Note: Hemoglobin levels should not exceed 12 g/dL and should not rise >1 g/dL per 2-week time period during therapy in any patient.

Chronic renal failure patients: Individualize dosing to achieve and maintain hemoglobin levels between 10-12 g/dL. Hemoglobin levels should not exceed 12 g/dL. **Note:** I.V. route is preferred for hemodialysis patients.

Children: I.V., SubQ: Initial dose: 50 units/kg 3 times/week

Adults: I.V., SubQ: Initial dose: 50-100 units/kg 3 times/week

Dosage adjustment in Children and Adults: SubQ, I.V.:

Decrease dose by 25%: If hemoglobin approaches 12 g/dL **or** hemoglobin increases >1 g/dL in any 2-week period. If hemoglobin continues to increase, temporarily discontinue therapy until hemoglobin begins to decrease, then resume therapy with a ~25% reduction from previous dose.

Increase dose by 25%: If hemoglobin <10 g/dL and does not increase by 1 g/dL after 4 weeks of therapy (with adequate iron stores) **or** hemoglobin decreases below 10 g/dL. If transferrin saturation >20%, may increase epoetin dose. Do not increase dose more frequently than at 4-week intervals, unless clinically indicated (hemoglobin response time for dose increases may be 2-6 weeks).

Inadequate or lack of response: If patient does not attain target hemoglobin range of 10-12 g/dL after appropriate dose titrations over 12 weeks:

Do not continue to increase dose and use the minimum effective dose that will maintain a hemoglobin level sufficient to avoid red blood cell transfusions **and** evaluate patient for other causes of anemia.

Monitor hemoglobin closely thereafter, and if responsiveness improves, may resume making dosage adjustments as recommended above. If responsiveness does not improve and recurrent red blood cell transfusions continue to be needed, discontinue therapy.

Maintenance dose: Individualize to target hemoglobin range of 10-12 g/dL; limit additional dosage increases to every 4 weeks (or longer)

Dialysis patients: Median dose:

Children: 167 units/kg/week (hemodialysis) **or** 76 units/kg/week (peritoneal dialysis), in 2-3 divided doses per week

Adults: 75 units/kg 3 times/week

Nondialysis patients:

Children: Dosing range: 50-250 units/kg 1-3 times/week

Adults: Dosing range: 75-150 units/kg/week

Zidovudine-treated, HIV-infected patients (patients with erythropoietin levels >500 mU/mL are **unlikely** to respond): Titrate dosage to use the minimum effective dose that will maintain a hemoglobin level sufficient to avoid red blood cell transfusions. Hemoglobin levels should not exceed 12 g/dL.

Children: SubQ, I.V.: Limited data available; reported dosing range: 50-400 units/kg 2-3 times/week

Adults (with serum erythropoietin levels ≤500 and zidovudine doses ≤4200 mg/week): SubQ, I.V.: 100 units/kg 3 times/week for 8 weeks

Dosage adjustment:

Increase dose by 50-100 units/kg 3 times/week: If response is not satisfactory in terms of reducing transfusion requirements **or** increasing hemoglobin after 8 weeks of therapy. Evaluate response every 4-8 weeks thereafter, and adjust the dose accordingly by 50-100 units/kg increments 3 times/week. If patients has not responded satisfactorily to 300 units/kg/dose 3 times/week, a response to higher doses is unlikely.

Withhold dose: If hemoglobin exceeds 12 g/dL. Resume treatment with a 25% dose reduction when hemoglobin drops below 11 g/dL

Cancer patient on chemotherapy: Treatment of patients with erythropoietin levels >200 mU/mL is **not recommended by the manufacturer.** Titrate dosage to use the minimum effective dose that will maintain a hemoglobin level sufficient to avoid red blood cell transfusions. Do not initiate therapy if hemoglobin ≥10 g/dL. Discontinue erythropoietin following completion of chemotherapy.

Children: I.V.: 600 units/kg once weekly (maximum: 40,000 units)

Dosage adjustment:

Increase dose: If response is not satisfactory after a sufficient period of evaluation (no increase in hemoglobin by ≥1 g/dL after 4 weeks of once-weekly therapy), the dose may be increased every 4 weeks (or longer) to 900 units/kg/week; maximum 60,000 units. If patient does not respond, a response to higher doses is unlikely.

Withhold dose: If hemoglobin exceeds a level needed to avoid red blood cell transfusion. Resume treatment with a 25% dose reduction when hemoglobin approaches a level where transfusions may be required.

Reduce dose by 25%: If hemoglobin increases >1 g/dL in any 2-week period **or** hemoglobin reaches a level sufficient to avoid red blood cell transfusion.

Discontinue: If after 8 weeks of therapy there is no response (ie, increased hemoglobin levels) or transfusions still required.

Adults: SubQ: Initial dose: 150 units/kg 3 times/week or 40,000 units once weekly; commonly used doses range from 10,000 units 3 times/week to 40,000-60,000 units once weekly.

Dosage adjustment:

Increase dose: If response is not satisfactory after a sufficient period of evaluation (no reduction in transfusion requirements or increase in hemoglobin after 8 weeks of 3 times/week therapy) **or** (no increase in hemoglobin by ≥1 g/dL after 4 weeks of once-weekly therapy), the dose may be increased every 4 weeks (or longer) to 300 units/kg 3 times/week, **or** when dosed weekly, increased all at once to 60,000 units weekly. If patient does not respond, a response to higher doses is unlikely.

Withhold dose: If hemoglobin exceeds a level needed to avoid red blood cell transfusion. Resume treatment with a 25% dose reduction when hemoglobin approaches a level where transfusions may be required.

Reduce dose by 25%: If hemoglobin increases >1 g/dL in any 2-week period **or** hemoglobin reaches a level sufficient to avoid red blood cell transfusion.

Discontinue: If after 8 weeks of therapy there is no response (ie, increased hemoglobin levels) or transfusions still required.

Surgery patients: Prior to initiating treatment, obtain a hemoglobin to establish that it is >10 g/dL and ≤13 g/dL: Adults: SubQ: Initial dose: 300 units/kg/day for 10 days before surgery, on the day of surgery, and for 4 days after surgery

Alternative dose: 600 units/kg in once weekly doses (21, 14, and 7 days before surgery) plus a fourth dose on the day of surgery

Dosage Forms

Injection, solution [preservative free]:

Epogen®, Procrit®: 2000 units/mL (1 mL); 3000 units/mL (1 mL); 4000 units/mL (1 mL); 10,000 units/mL (1 mL); 40,000 units/mL (1 mL)

Injection, solution [with preservative]:

Epogen®, Procrit®: 10,000 units/mL (2 mL); 20,000 units/mL (1 mL)

Epogen® [US] *see* epoetin alfa *on page 361*

epoprostenol (e poe PROST en ole)

Synonyms epoprostenol sodium; PGI_2; PGX; prostacyclin

U.S./Canadian Brand Names Flolan® [US/Can]

Therapeutic Category Platelet Inhibitor

Use Treatment of idiopathic pulmonary arterial hypertension (IPAH); pulmonary hypertension associated with the scleroderma spectrum of disease (SSD) in NYHA Class III and Class IV patients who do not respond adequately to conventional therapy

Usual Dosage I.V.: Adults:

Pulmonary arterial hypertension (PAH): Initial: 1-2 ng/kg/minute, increase dose in increments of 1-2 ng/kg/minute every 15 minutes or longer until dose-limiting side effects are noted or tolerance limit to epoprostenol is observed. Significant patient variability in optimal dose exists. Maximum dose with chronic therapy has not been defined; however, doses as high as 195 ng/kg/minute have been described in children.

Note: The need for increased doses should be expected with chronic use; incremental increases occur more frequently during the first few months after the drug is initiated.

Dose adjustment:

Increase dose in 1-2 ng/kg/minute increments at intervals of at least 15 minutes if symptoms persist or recur following improvement. In clinical trials, dosing increases occurred at intervals of 24-48 hours.

Decrease dose in 2 ng/kg/minute decrements at intervals of at least 15 minutes in case of dose-limiting pharmacologic events. Avoid abrupt withdrawal or sudden large dose reductions.

Lung transplant: In patients receiving lung transplants, epoprostenol may be tapered after the initiation of cardiopulmonary bypass.

Dosage Forms

Injection, powder for reconstitution: 0.5 mg, 1.5 mg

Flolan®: 0.5 mg, 1.5 mg

epoprostenol sodium *see* epoprostenol *on page 363*

epothilone B lactam *see* ixabepilone *on page 554*

Eprex® [Can] *see* epoetin alfa *on page 361*

eprosartan (ep roe SAR tan)

U.S./Canadian Brand Names Teveten® [US/Can]

Therapeutic Category Angiotensin II Receptor Antagonist

Use Treatment of hypertension; may be used alone or in combination with other antihypertensives

Usual Dosage Oral: Adults: Dosage must be individualized; can administer once or twice daily with total daily doses of 400-800 mg. Usual starting dose is 600 mg once daily as monotherapy in patients who are euvolemic. Limited clinical experience with doses >800 mg.

Dosage Forms

Tablet:

Teveten®: 400 mg, 600 mg

eprosartan and hydrochlorothiazide (ep roe SAR tan & hye droe klor oh THYE a zide)

Synonyms eprosartan mesylate and hydrochlorothiazide; hydrochlorothiazide and eprosartan

U.S./Canadian Brand Names Teveten® HCT [US/Can]; Teveten® Plus [Can]

Therapeutic Category Angiotensin II Antagonist Combination; Antihypertensive Agent, Combination; Diuretic, Thiazide

Use Treatment of hypertension (not indicated for initial treatment)

Usual Dosage Oral: Adults: Dose is individualized (combination substituted for individual components)

Usual recommended dose: Eprosartan 600 mg/hydrochlorothiazide 12.5 mg once daily (maximum dose: Eprosartan 600 mg/hydrochlorothiazide 25 mg once daily)

Dosage Forms

Tablet:

Teveten® HCT: 600 mg/12.5 mg: Eprosartan 600 mg and hydrochlorothiazide 12.5 mg; 600 mg/25 mg: Eprosartan 600 mg and hydrochlorothiazide 25 mg

eprosartan mesylate and hydrochlorothiazide *see* eprosartan and hydrochlorothiazide *on page 364*

epsilon aminocaproic acid *see* aminocaproic acid *on page 63*

epsom salts *see* magnesium sulfate *on page 611*

EPT *see* teniposide *on page 944*

eptacog alfa (activated) *see* factor VIIa (recombinant) *on page 402*

eptifibatide (ep TIF i ba tide)

Synonyms intrifiban

U.S./Canadian Brand Names Integrilin® [US/Can]

Therapeutic Category Antiplatelet Agent

Use Treatment of patients with acute coronary syndrome (unstable angina/non-Q wave myocardial infarction [UA/NQMI]), including patients who are to be managed medically and those undergoing percutaneous coronary intervention (PCI including angioplasty, intracoronary stenting)

Usual Dosage I.V.: Adults:

Acute coronary syndrome: Bolus of 180 mcg/kg (maximum: 22.6 mg) over 1-2 minutes, begun as soon as possible following diagnosis, followed by a continuous infusion of 2 mcg/kg/minute (maximum: 15 mg/hour) until hospital discharge or initiation of CABG surgery, up to 72 hours. Concurrent aspirin and heparin therapy (target aPTT 50-70 seconds) are recommended.

Percutaneous coronary intervention (PCI) with or without stenting: Bolus of 180 mcg/kg (maximum: 22.6 mg) administered immediately before the initiation of PCI, followed by a continuous infusion of 2 mcg/kg/minute (maximum: 15 mg/hour). A second 180 mcg/kg bolus (maximum: 22.6 mg) should be administered 10 minutes after the first bolus. Infusion should be continued until hospital discharge or for up to 18-24 hours, whichever comes first. Concurrent aspirin (160-325 mg 1-24 hours before PCI and daily thereafter) and heparin therapy (ACT 200-300 seconds during PCI) are recommended. Heparin infusion after PCI is discouraged. In patients who undergo coronary artery bypass graft surgery, discontinue infusion prior to surgery.

Dosage Forms

Injection, solution:

Integrilin®: 0.75 mg/mL (100 mL); 2 mg/mL (10 mL, 100 mL)

Epzicom® [US] *see* abacavir and lamivudine *on page 16*

Equagesic® [US] *see* meprobamate and aspirin *on page 629*

Equalactin® [US-OTC] *see* polycarbophil *on page 797*

Equalizer Gas Relief [US-OTC] *see* simethicone *on page 901*

Equanil® *(Discontinued)* *see* meprobamate *on page 629*

Equetro® [US] *see* carbamazepine *on page 180*

Equilet® *(Discontinued)* *see* calcium carbonate *on page 170*

Eraxis™ [US/Can] *see* anidulafungin *on page 80*

Erbitux® [US/Can] *see* cetuximab *on page 205*

ergocalciferol (er goe kal SIF e role)

Sound-Alike/Look-Alike Issues

Calciferol™ may be confused with calcitriol

Drisdol® may be confused with Drysol™

Synonyms activated ergosterol; viosterol; vitamin D_2

U.S./Canadian Brand Names Drisdol® [US/Can]; Ostoforte® [Can]

Therapeutic Category Vitamin D Analog

Use Treatment of refractory rickets, hypophosphatemia, hypoparathyroidism; dietary supplement

Usual Dosage Oral: **Note:** 1 mcg = 40 int. units

Dietary Intake Reference: Note: DIR is currently being reviewed:

Infants and Children: 5 mcg (200 int. units)/day

Adults:

18-50 years: 5 mcg/day (200 int. units/day)

51-70 years: 10 mcg/day (400 int. units/day)

Adequate intake:

Infants and Children: 10 mcg/day (400 int. units/day)

Breast-fed (fully or partially) Infants: 10 mcg/day (400 int. units/day) beginning in the first few days of life; continue supplementation until infant is weaned to ≥1 L/day or 1 quart/day of vitamin D-fortified formula or whole milk (after 12 months of age)

Nonbreast-fed Infants, Older Children ingesting <1000 mL of vitamin D-fortified formula or milk: 10 mcg/day (400 int. units/day)

Adolescents without adequate intake: 10 mcg/day (400 int. units/day)

Children with increased risk of vitamin D deficiency (chronic fat malabsorption, maintained on chronic antiseizure medications): Higher doses may be required; use laboratory testing (25 (OH)D, PTH, bone mineral status) to evaluate

Osteoporosis prevention and treatment: Adults ≥50 years: 10 mcg/day (800-1000 int. units/day)

Vitamin D deficiency/insufficiency in patients with CKD stages 3-4 (K/DOQI guidelines): **Note:** Dose is based on 25-hydroxyvitamin D serum level [25(OH) D]:

Children (treatment duration should be a total of 3 months):

Serum 25(OH)D <5 ng/mL:

8000 int. units/day for 4 weeks, then 4000 int. units/day for 2 months **or**

50,000 int. units/week for 4 weeks, then 50,000 int. units twice a month for 2 months

Serum 25(OH)D 5-15 ng/mL:

4000 int units/day **or**

50,000 int units every other week

Serum 25(OH)D 16-30 ng/mL:

2000 int. units/day **or**

50,000 int. units every 4 weeks

Adults (treatment duration should be a total of 6 months):

Serum 25(OH)D <5 ng/mL:

50,000 int. units/week for 12 weeks, then 50,000 int. units/month

Serum 25(OH)D 5-15 ng/mL:

50,000 int. units/week for 4 weeks, then 50,000 int. units/month

Serum 25(OH)D 16-30 ng/mL:

50,000 int. units/month

Hypoparathyroidism:

Children: 1.25-5 mg/day (50,000-200,000 int. units) and calcium supplements

Adults: 625 mcg to 5 mg/day (25,000-200,000 int. units) and calcium supplements

Nutritional rickets and osteomalacia:

Children and Adults (with normal absorption): 25-125 mcg/day (1000-5000 int. units)

Children with malabsorption: 250-625 mcg/day (10,000-25,000 int. units)

Adults with malabsorption: 250-7500 mcg (10,000-300,000 int. units)

Vitamin D-*dependent* rickets:

Children: 75-125 mcg/day (3000-5000 int. units); maximum: 1500 mcg/day

Adults: 250 mcg to 1.5 mg/day (10,000-60,000 int. units)

Vitamin D-*resistant* rickets: Children and Adults: 12,000-500,000 int. units/day

Familial hypophosphatemia:

Children: 40,000-80,000 int. units plus phosphate supplements; dose may be reduced once growth is complete

Adults: 10,000-60,000 int. units plus phosphate supplements

Dosage Forms

Capsule:

Drisdol®: 50,000 int. units

Liquid, oral [drops]:

Drisdol®: 8000 int. units/mL [OTC]

Tablet: 400 int. units [OTC]

ergoloid mesylates (ER goe loid MES i lates)

Synonyms dihydroergotoxine; dihydrogenated ergot alkaloids

U.S./Canadian Brand Names Hydergine® [Can]

Therapeutic Category Ergot Alkaloid and Derivative

Use Treatment of cerebrovascular insufficiency in primary progressive dementia, Alzheimer dementia, and senile onset

Usual Dosage Oral: Adults: 1 mg 3 times/day up to 4.5-12 mg/day; up to 6 months of therapy may be necessary

Dosage Forms

Tablet: 1 mg

Tablet, sublingual: 1 mg

Ergomar® [US] *see* ergotamine *on page 366*

ergometrine maleate *see* ergonovine *on page 366*

ergonovine (er goe NOE veen)

Synonyms ergometrine maleate; ergonovine maleate

U.S./Canadian Brand Names Ergotrate® [US]

Therapeutic Category Ergot Alkaloid and Derivative

Use Prevention and treatment of postpartum and postabortion hemorrhage caused by uterine atony or subinvolution

Usual Dosage Adults:

I.M., I.V. (I.V. should be reserved for emergency use only): 0.2 mg, may repeat dose in 2-4 hours if needed

Oral, SL:

Immediate postpartum: 0.2 mg (usually given I.M. or I.V)

Late postpartum: 0.2-0.4 mg every 6-12 hours until danger of uterine atony has passed (usually ~48 hours)

Dosage Forms

Injection:

Ergotrate®: 0.2 mg/mL (1 mL)

Tablet:

Ergotrate®: 0.2 mg

ergonovine maleate *see* ergonovine *on page 366*

ergotamine (er GOT a meen)

Synonyms ergotamine tartrate

U.S./Canadian Brand Names Ergomar® [US]

Therapeutic Category Ergot Alkaloid and Derivative

Use Abort or prevent vascular headaches, such as migraine, migraine variants, or so-called "histaminic cephalalgia"

Usual Dosage Sublingual: One tablet under tongue at first sign, then 1 tablet every 30 minutes if needed; maximum dose: 3 tablets/24 hours, 5 tablets/week

Dosage Forms

Tablet, sublingual:

Ergomar®: 2 mg

ergotamine and caffeine (er GOT a meen & KAF een)

Sound-Alike/Look-Alike Issues

Cafergot® may be confused with Carafate®

Synonyms caffeine and ergotamine; ergotamine tartrate and caffeine

U.S./Canadian Brand Names Cafergor® [Can]; Cafergot® [US]; Migergot [US]

Therapeutic Category Antimigraine Agent; Ergot Derivative; Stimulant

Use Abort or prevent vascular headaches, such as migraine, migraine variants, or so-called "histaminic cephalalgia"

Usual Dosage Adults:

Oral: Two tablets at onset of attack; then 1 tablet every 30 minutes as needed; maximum: 6 tablets per attack; do not exceed 10 tablets/week.

Rectal: One suppository rectally at first sign of an attack; follow with second dose after 1 hour, if needed; maximum: 2 per attack; do not exceed 5/week.

Dosage Forms

Suppository, rectal:

Migergot: Ergotamine tartrate 2 mg and caffeine 100 mg (12s)

Tablet: Ergotamine tartrate 1 mg and caffeine 100 mg

Cafergot®: Ergotamine tartrate 1 mg and caffeine 100 mg

ergotamine tartrate *see* ergotamine *on page* 366

ergotamine tartrate and caffeine *see* ergotamine and caffeine *on page* 366

Ergotamine Tartrate and Caffeine Cafatine® *(Discontinued)* *see* ergotamine *on page* 366

Ergotrate® [US] *see* ergonovine *on page* 366

erlotinib (er LOE tye nib)

Sound-Alike/Look-Alike Issues

erlotinib may be confused with gefitinib, imatinib

Synonyms CP358774; erlotinib hydrochloride; OSI-774

U.S./Canadian Brand Names Tarceva® [US/Can]

Therapeutic Category Antineoplastic Agent, Tyrosine Kinase Inhibitor

Use Treatment of locally advanced or metastatic nonsmall cell lung cancer (NSCLC) refractory to at least 1 prior chemotherapy regimen (as monotherapy); locally advanced, unresectable or metastatic pancreatic cancer (first-line therapy in combination with gemcitabine)

Usual Dosage Oral: Adults: **Note:** Details concerning dosing in combination regimens should also be consulted. Dose adjustments are likely to be needed when erlotinib is administered concomitantly with strong CYP3A4 inducers or inhibitors. A dose increase to a maximum dose of 300 mg may be required in patients who continue to smoke.

NSCLC (refractory): 150 mg once daily

Pancreatic cancer: 100 mg once daily in combination with gemcitabine

Dosage Forms

Tablet:

Tarceva®: 25 mg, 100 mg, 150 mg

erlotinib hydrochloride *see* erlotinib *on page* 367

Errin™ [US] *see* norethindrone *on page* 704

Ertaczo® [US] *see* sertaconazole *on page* 897

ertapenem (er ta PEN em)

Sound-Alike/Look-Alike Issues

ertapenem may be confused with imipenem, meropenem

Invanz® may be confused with Avinza™

Synonyms ertapenem sodium; L-749,345; MK0826

U.S./Canadian Brand Names Invanz® [US/Can]

Therapeutic Category Antibiotic, Carbapenem

Use Treatment of the following moderate-to-severe infections: Complicated intraabdominal infections, complicated skin and skin structure infections (including diabetic foot infections without osteomyelitis), complicated UTI (including pyelonephritis), acute pelvic infections (including postpartum endomyometritis, septic abortion, postsurgical gynecologic infections), and community-acquired pneumonia. Prophylaxis of surgical site infection following elective colorectal surgery. Antibacterial coverage includes aerobic gram-positive organisms, aerobic gram-negative organisms, anaerobic organisms.

Note: Methicillin-resistant *Staphylococcus*, *Enterococcus* spp, penicillin-resistant strains of *Streptococcus pneumoniae*, beta-lactamase-positive strains of *Haemophilus influenzae* are **resistant** to ertapenem, as are most *Pseudomonas aeruginosa*.

Usual Dosage Note: I.V. therapy may be administered for up to 14 days; I.M. therapy for up to 7 days

Usual dosage ranges:

Children 3 months to 12 years: I.M., I.V.: 15 mg/kg twice daily (maximum: 1 g/day)

Children ≥13 years and Adults: I.M., I.V.: 1 g/day

Indication-specific dosing:

Children 3 months to 12 years: I.M., I.V.:

Community-acquired pneumonia, complicated urinary tract infections (including pyelonephritis): 15 mg/kg twice daily (maximum: 1 g/day); duration of total antibiotic treatment: 10-14 days (**Note:** Duration includes possible switch to appropriate oral therapy after at least 3 days of parenteral treatment, once clinical improvement demonstrated.)

Intraabdominal infection: 15 mg/kg twice daily (maximum: 1 g/day) for 5-14 days

Pelvic infections (acute): 15 mg/kg twice daily (maximum: 1 g/day) for 3-10 days

Skin and skin structure infections: 15 mg/kg twice daily (maximum: 1 g/day) for 7-14 days

Children ≥13 years and Adults: I.M., I.V.:

Community-acquired pneumonia, complicated urinary tract infections (including pyelonephritis): 1 g/day; duration of total antibiotic treatment: 10-14 days (**Note:** Duration includes possible switch to appropriate oral therapy after at least 3 days of parenteral treatment, once clinical improvement demonstrated.)

Intraabdominal infection: 1 g/day for 5-14 days

Pelvic infections (acute): 1 g/day for 3-10 days

Skin and skin structure infections (including diabetic foot infections): 1 g/day for 7-14 days

Adults: I.V.: **Prophylaxis of surgical site following colorectal surgery:** 1 g given 1 hour preoperatively

Dosage Forms

Injection, powder for reconstitution:

Invanz®: 1 g

ertapenem sodium *see* ertapenem *on page 367*

***Erwinia* asparaginase** *see* asparaginase *on page 102*

Erybid™ [Can] *see* erythromycin *on page 368*

Eryc® [Can] *see* erythromycin *on page 368*

Eryc® *(Discontinued)* *see* erythromycin *on page 368*

Eryderm® *(Discontinued)* *see* erythromycin *on page 368*

Erygel® *(Discontinued)* *see* erythromycin *on page 368*

EryPed® [US] *see* erythromycin *on page 368*

Ery-Tab® [US] *see* erythromycin *on page 368*

Erythrocin® [US] *see* erythromycin *on page 368*

erythromycin (er ith roe MYE sin)

Sound-Alike/Look-Alike Issues

erythromycin may be confused with azithromycin, clarithromycin, Ethmozine®

Akne-Mycin® may be confused with AK-Mycin®

E.E.S.® may be confused with DES®

Eryc® may be confused with Emcyt®, Ery-Tab®

Ery-Tab® may be confused with Eryc®

Erythrocin® may be confused with Ethmozine®

Synonyms erythromycin base; erythromycin ethylsuccinate; erythromycin lactobionate; erythromycin stearate

U.S./Canadian Brand Names Akne-Mycin® [US]; Apo-Erythro Base® [Can]; Apo-Erythro E-C® [Can]; Apo-Erythro-ES® [Can]; Apo-Erythro-S® [Can]; Diomycin® [Can]; E.E.S.® [US/Can]; Ery-Tab® [US]; Erybid™ [Can]; Eryc® [Can]; EryPed® [US]; Erythro-RX [US]; Erythrocin® [US]; Novo-Rythro Estolate [Can]; Novo-Rythro Ethylsuccinate [Can]; Nu-Erythromycin-S [Can]; PCE® [US/Can]; PMS-Erythromycin [Can]; Romycin® [US]; Sans Acne® [Can]

Therapeutic Category Acne Products; Antibiotic, Ophthalmic; Antibiotic, Topical; Macrolide (Antibiotic)

Use

Systemic: Treatment of susceptible bacterial infections including *S. pyogenes*, some *S. pneumoniae*, some *S. aureus*, *M. pneumoniae*, *Legionella pneumophila*, diphtheria, pertussis, *Chlamydia*, erythrasma, *N. gonorrhoeae*, *E. histolytica*, syphilis and nongonococcal urethritis, and *Campylobacter* gastroenteritis; used in conjunction with neomycin for decontaminating the bowel

Ophthalmic: Treatment of superficial eye infections involving the conjunctiva or cornea; neonatal ophthalmia

Topical: Treatment of acne vulgaris

Usual Dosage Note: Due to differences in absorption, 400 mg erythromycin ethylsuccinate produces the same serum levels as 250 mg erythromycin base or stearate.

Usual dosage range:

Neonates: Ophthalmic: Prophylaxis of neonatal gonococcal or chlamydial conjunctivitis: 0.5-1 cm ribbon of ointment should be instilled into each conjunctival sac

Infants and Children:

Oral:

Base: 30-50 mg/kg/day in 2-4 divided doses; maximum: 2 g/day

Ethylsuccinate: 30-50 mg/kg/day in 2-4 divided doses; maximum: 3.2 g/day

Stearate: 30-50 mg/kg/day in 2-4 divided doses; maximum: 2 g/day

I.V.: Lactobionate: 15-50 mg/kg/day divided every 6 hours, not to exceed 4 g/day

Children and Adults:

Ophthalmic: Instill 1/2" (1.25 cm) 2-6 times/day depending on the severity of the infection

Topical: Acne: Apply over the affected area twice daily after the skin has been thoroughly washed and patted dry

Adults:

Oral:

Base: 250-500 mg every 6-12 hours; maximum 4 g/day

Ethylsuccinate: 400-800 mg every 6-12 hours; maximum: 4 g/day

I.V.: Lactobionate: 15-20 mg/kg/day divided every 6 hours or 500 mg to 1 g every 6 hours, or given as a continuous infusion over 24 hours; maximum: 4 g/24 hours

Indication-specific dosing:

Children:

Conjunctivitis, neonatal *(C. trachomatis):* Oral: 50 mg/kg/day (base or ethylsuccinate) in 4 divided doses for 14 days

Mild/moderate infection: Oral: 30-50 mg/kg/day in divided doses every 6-12 hours

Pertussis: Oral: 40-50 mg/kg/day in 4 divided doses for 14 days; maximum 2 g/day (not preferred agent for infants <1 month due to IHPS)

Pharyngitis, tonsillitis (streptococcal): Oral: 20 mg (base)/kg/day or 40 mg (ethylsuccinate)/kg/day in 2 divided doses for 10 days. **Note:** No longer preferred therapy due to increased organism resistance.

Pneumonia *(C. trachomatis):* Oral: 50 mg/kg/day (base or ethylsuccinate) in 4 divided doses for 14-21 days

Preop bowel preparation: Oral: 20 mg (base)/kg at 1, 2, and 11 PM on the day before surgery combined with mechanical cleansing of the large intestine and oral neomycin

Severe infection: I.V.: 15-50 mg/kg/day; maximum: 4 g/day

Adults:

Legionnaires disease: Oral: 1.6-4 g (ethylsuccinate)/day or 1-4 g (base)/day in divided doses for 21 days. **Note:** No longer preferred therapy and only used in nonhospitalized patients.

Lymphogranuloma venereum: Oral: 500 mg (base) 4 times/day for 21 days

Nongonococcal urethritis (including coinfection with *C. trachomatis*): Oral: 500 mg (base) 4 times/day for 7 days or 800 mg (ethylsuccinate) 4 times/day for 7 days. **Note:** May use 250 mg (base) or 400 mg (ethylsuccinate) 4 times/day for 14 days if gastrointestinal intolerance.

Pelvic inflammatory disease: I.V.: 500 mg every 6 hours for 3 days, followed by 1000 mg (base)/day orally in 2-4 divided doses for 7 days. **Note:** Not recommended therapy per current treatment guidelines.

Pertussis: Oral: 500 mg (base) every 6 hours for 14 days

Syphilis, primary: Oral: 48-64 g (ethylsuccinate) or 30-40 g (base) in divided doses over 10-15 days. **Note:** Not recommended therapy per current treatment guidelines.

Dosage Forms [CAN] = Canadian brand name

Capsule, delayed release, enteric-coated pellets: 250 mg

Gel, topical: 2% (30 g, 60 g)

Granules for oral suspension:

E.E.S.®: 200 mg/5 mL

Injection, powder for reconstitution:

Erythrocin®: 500 mg, 1 g

Ointment, ophthalmic: 0.5% [5 mg/g] (1 g, 3.5 g)

Romycin®: 0.5% [5 mg/g] (3.5 g)

Ointment, topical:

Akne-Mycin®: 2% (25 g)

Powder for oral suspension:

EryPed®: 200 mg/5 mL, 400 mg/5 mL

Powder, for prescription compounding:

Erythro-RX: USP (50 g)

Solution, topical: 2% (60 mL)
Sans Acne® [CAN]: 2% (60 mL) [not available in the U.S.]
Suspension, oral:
E.E.S.®: 400 mg/5 mL
Tablet: 250 mg, 400 mg, 500 mg
Erythrocin®: 250 mg, 500 mg
Tablet, delayed release, enteric coated:
Ery-Tab®: 250 mg, 333 mg, 500 mg
Tablet [polymer-coated particles]:
PCE®: 333 mg, 500 mg

erythromycin and benzoyl peroxide (er ith roe MYE sin & BEN zoe il per OKS ide)

Synonyms benzoyl peroxide and erythromycin

U.S./Canadian Brand Names Benzamycin® Pak [US]; Benzamycin® [US]

Therapeutic Category Acne Products

Use Topical control of acne vulgaris

Usual Dosage Adolescents ≥12 years and Adults: Apply twice daily, morning and evening

Dosage Forms
Gel, topical: Erythromycin 30 mg and benzoyl peroxide 50 mg per g (23 g, 47g)
Benzamycin®: Erythromycin 30 mg and benzoyl peroxide 50 mg per g (47 g)
Benzamycin® Pak: Erythromycin 30 mg and benzoyl peroxide 50 mg per 0.8 g packet (60s)

erythromycin and sulfisoxazole (er ith roe MYE sin & sul fi SOKS a zole)

Sound-Alike/Look-Alike Issues
Pediazole® may be confused with Pediapred®

Synonyms sulfisoxazole and erythromycin

U.S./Canadian Brand Names E.S.P.® [US]; Pediazole® [Can]

Therapeutic Category Macrolide (Antibiotic); Sulfonamide

Use Treatment of susceptible bacterial infections of the upper and lower respiratory tract, otitis media in children caused by susceptible strains of *Haemophilus influenzae*, and many other infections in patients allergic to penicillin

Usual Dosage Oral (dosage recommendation is based on the product's erythromycin content):
Children ≥2 months: 50 mg/kg/day erythromycin and 150 mg/kg/day sulfisoxazole in divided doses every 6 hours; not to exceed 2 g erythromycin/day or 6 g sulfisoxazole/day for 10 days
Adults >45 kg: 400 mg erythromycin and 1200 mg sulfisoxazole every 6 hours

Dosage Forms
Powder for oral suspension: Erythromycin 200 mg and sulfisoxazole 600 mg per 5 mL
E.S.P.®: Erythromycin 200 mg and sulfisoxazole 600 mg per 5 mL

erythromycin base *see* erythromycin *on page* 368
erythromycin ethylsuccinate *see* erythromycin *on page* 368
erythromycin lactobionate *see* erythromycin *on page* 368
erythromycin stearate *see* erythromycin *on page* 368
erythropoiesis-stimulating agent (ESA) *see* darbepoetin alfa *on page* 277
erythropoiesis-stimulating agent (ESA) *see* epoetin alfa *on page* 361
erythropoiesis-stimulating protein *see* darbepoetin alfa *on page* 277
erythropoietin *see* epoetin alfa *on page* 361
Erythro-RX [US] *see* erythromycin *on page* 368

escitalopram (es sye TAL oh pram)

Sound-Alike/Look-Alike Issues
Lexapro® may be confused with Loxitane®

Synonyms escitalopram oxalate; Lu-26-054; S-citalopram

U.S./Canadian Brand Names Cipralex® [Can]; Lexapro® [US]

Therapeutic Category Antidepressant, Selective Serotonin Reuptake Inhibitor

Use Treatment of major depressive disorder; generalized anxiety disorders (GAD)

Usual Dosage Oral:

Children ≥12 years: Major depressive disorder: Initial: 10 mg once daily; dose may be increased to 20 mg once daily after at least 3 weeks

Adults: Major depressive disorder, generalized anxiety disorder: Initial: 10 mg once daily; dose may be increased to 20 mg once daily after at least 1 week

Dosage Forms

Solution, oral:

Lexapro®: 1 mg/mL (240 mL)

Tablet:

Lexapro®: 5 mg, 10 mg, 20 mg

Note: Cipralex® [CAN] is available only in 10 mg and 20 mg strengths.

escitalopram oxalate *see* escitalopram *on page 370*

Eserine® [Can] *see* physostigmine *on page 782*

eserine salicylate *see* physostigmine *on page 782*

Esgic® [US] *see* butalbital, acetaminophen, and caffeine *on page 161*

Esgic-Plus™ [US] *see* butalbital, acetaminophen, and caffeine *on page 161*

Esidrix Tablets *(Discontinued)* *see* hydrochlorothiazide *on page 499*

Eskalith CR® *(Discontinued)* *see* lithium *on page 594*

Eskalith® *(Discontinued)* *see* lithium *on page 594*

esmolol (ES moe lol)

Sound-Alike/Look-Alike Issues

esmolol may be confused with Osmitrol®

Brevibloc® may be confused with bretylium, Brevital®, Bumex®, Buprenex®

Synonyms esmolol hydrochloride

U.S./Canadian Brand Names Brevibloc® [US/Can]

Therapeutic Category Antiarrhythmic Agent, Class II; Beta-Adrenergic Blocker

Use Treatment of supraventricular tachycardia (SVT) and atrial fibrillation/flutter (control ventricular rate); treatment of tachycardia and/or hypertension; treatment of noncompensatory sinus tachycardia

Usual Dosage **I.V. infusion requires an infusion pump** (must be adjusted to individual response and tolerance):

Adults:

Intraoperative tachycardia and/or hypertension (immediate control): Initial bolus: 80 mg (~1 mg/kg) over 30 seconds, followed by a 150 mcg/kg/minute infusion, if necessary. Adjust infusion rate as needed to maintain desired heart rate and/or blood pressure, up to 300 mcg/kg/minute.

For control of postoperative hypertension, as many as one-third of patients may require higher doses (250-300 mcg/kg/minute) to control blood pressure; the safety of doses >300 mcg/kg/minute has not been studied.

Supraventricular tachycardia or gradual control of postoperative tachycardia/hypertension: Loading dose: 500 mcg/kg over 1 minute; follow with a 50 mcg/kg/minute infusion for 4 minutes; response to this initial infusion rate may be a rough indication of the responsiveness of the ventricular rate.

Infusion may be continued at 50 mcg/kg/minute or, if the response is inadequate, titrated upward in 50 mcg/kg/minute increments (increased no more frequently than every 4 minutes) to a maximum of 200 mcg/kg/minute.

To achieve more rapid response, following the initial loading dose and 50 mcg/kg/minute infusion, rebolus with a second 500 mcg/kg loading dose over 1 minute, and increase the maintenance infusion to 100 mcg/kg/minute for 4 minutes. If necessary, a third (and final) 500 mcg/kg loading dose may be administered, prior to increasing to an infusion rate of 150 mcg/kg/minute. After 4 minutes of the 150 mcg/kg/minute infusion, the infusion rate may be increased to a maximum rate of 200 mcg/kg/minute (without a bolus dose).

Usual dosage range (SVT): 50-200 mcg/kg/minute with average dose of 100 mcg/kg/minute.

Guidelines for transfer to oral therapy (beta-blocker, calcium channel blocker):

Infusion should be reduced by 50% 30 minutes following the first dose of the alternative agent

Manufacturer suggests following the second dose of the alternative drug, patient's response should be monitored and if control is adequate for the first hours, esmolol may be discontinued.

Dosage Forms

Infusion [premixed in sodium chloride; preservative free]:

Brevibloc®: 2000 mg (100 mL) [20 mg/mL; double strength]; 2500 mg (250 mL) [10 mg/mL]

Injection, solution: 10 mg/mL (10 mL)

Brevibloc®:
10 mg/mL (10 mL)
20 mg/mL (5 mL, 100 mL)

esmolol hydrochloride *see* esmolol *on page* 371

E-Solve-2® Topical ***(Discontinued)***

esomeprazole (es oh ME pray zol)

Sound-Alike/Look-Alike Issues

esomeprazole may be confused with aripiprazole
Nexium® may be confused with Nexavar®

Synonyms esomeprazole magnesium; esomeprazole sodium

U.S./Canadian Brand Names Nexium® [US/Can]

Therapeutic Category Proton Pump Inhibitor

Use

Oral: Short-term (4-8 weeks) treatment of erosive esophagitis; maintaining symptom resolution and healing of erosive esophagitis; treatment of symptomatic gastroesophageal reflux disease (GERD); as part of a multidrug regimen for *Helicobacter pylori* eradication in patients with duodenal ulcer disease (active or history of within the past 5 years); prevention of gastric ulcers in patients at risk (age ≥60 years and/or history of gastric ulcer) associated with continuous NSAID therapy; long-term treatment of pathological hypersecretory conditions including Zollinger-Ellison syndrome

Canadian labeling: Additional use (not in U.S. labeling): Oral: Treatment of nonerosive reflux disease (NERD)

I.V.: Short-term (≤10 days) treatment of gastroesophageal reflux disease (GERD) when oral therapy is not possible or appropriate

Usual Dosage

Children 1-11 years: Oral: **Note:** Safety and efficacy of doses >1 mg/kg/day and/or therapy beyond 8 weeks have not been established.

Symptomatic GERD: 10 mg once daily for up to 8 weeks

Erosive esophagitis (healing):

<20 kg: 10 mg once daily for 8 weeks

≥20 kg: 10-20 mg once daily for 8 weeks

Nonerosive reflux disease (NERD) (Canadian labeling): 10 mg once daily for up to 8 weeks

Adolescents 12-17 years: Oral:

GERD: 20-40 mg once daily for up to 8 weeks

NERD (Canadian labeling): 20 mg once daily for 2-4 weeks; lack of symptom control after 4 weeks warrants further evaluation

Adults:

Oral:

Erosive esophagitis (healing): Initial: 20-40 mg once daily for 4-8 weeks; if incomplete healing, may continue for an additional 4-8 weeks; maintenance: 20 mg once daily (controlled studies did not extend beyond 6 months)

NERD (Canadian labeling): Initial: 20 mg once daily for 2-4 weeks; lack of symptom control after 4 weeks warrants further evaluation; maintenance (in patients with successful initial therapy): 20 mg once daily as needed

Symptomatic GERD: 20 mg once daily for 4 weeks; may continue an additional 4 weeks if symptoms persist

Helicobacter pylori eradication:

Manufacturer labeling: 40 mg once daily administered with amoxicillin 1000 mg *and* clarithromycin 500 mg twice daily for 10 days

American College of Gastroenterology guidelines:

Nonpenicillin allergy: 40 mg once daily administered with amoxicillin 1000 mg *and* clarithromycin 500 mg twice daily for 10-14 days

Penicillin allergy: 40 mg once daily administered with clarithromycin 500 mg *and* metronidazole 500 mg twice daily for 10-14 days **or** 40 mg once daily administered with bismuth subsalicylate 525 mg *and* metronidazole 250 mg *plus* tetracycline 500 mg 4 times/day for 10-14 days

Canadian labeling: 20 mg twice daily for 7 days; requires combination therapy

Prevention of NSAID-induced gastric ulcers: 20-40 mg once daily for up to 6 months

Treatment of NSAID-induced gastric ulcers (Canadian labeling): 20 mg once daily for 4-8 weeks.

Pathological hypersecretory conditions (Zollinger-Ellison syndrome): 40 mg twice daily; adjust regimen to individual patient needs; doses up to 240 mg/day have been administered

I.V.: Treatment of GERD (short-term): 20 mg or 40 mg once daily for ≤10 days; change to oral therapy as soon as appropriate

Dosage Forms Note: Strength expressed as base. [CAN] = Canadian availability

Capsule, delayed release:

Nexium®: 20 mg, 40 mg

Granules, for oral suspension, delayed release, as magnesium:

Nexium®: 10 mg/packet (30s); 20 mg/packet (30s); 40 mg/packet (30s)

Nexium® [CAN]: 10 mg/packet (28s)

Injection, powder for reconstitution:

Nexium®: 20 mg, 40 mg

Tablet, extended release, as magnesium:

Nexium® [CAN]: 20 mg, 40 mg [not available in U.S.]

esomeprazole magnesium *see* esomeprazole *on page 372*

esomeprazole sodium *see* esomeprazole *on page 372*

Esopho-Cat® [US] *see* barium *on page 122*

Esoterica® Daytime [US-OTC] *see* hydroquinone *on page 508*

Esoterica® Nighttime [US-OTC] *see* hydroquinone *on page 508*

E.S.P.® [US] *see* erythromycin and sulfisoxazole *on page 370*

Especol® [US-OTC] *see* fructose, dextrose, and phosphoric acid *on page 448*

Estalis® [Can] *see* estradiol and norethindrone *on page 376*

Estalis-Sequi® [Can] *see* estradiol and norethindrone *on page 376*

Estar® [Can] *see* coal tar *on page 250*

estazolam (es TA zoe lam)

Sound-Alike/Look-Alike Issues

ProSom® may be confused with PhosLo®, Proscar®, Pro-Sof® Plus, Prozac®, Psorcon®

Therapeutic Category Benzodiazepine

Controlled Substance C-IV

Use Short-term management of insomnia

Usual Dosage Oral: Adults: 1 mg at bedtime, some patients may require 2 mg; start at doses of 0.5 mg in debilitated patients

Dosage Forms

Tablet: 1 mg, 2 mg

Ester-E™ [US-OTC] *see* vitamin E *on page 1018*

esterified estrogen and methyltestosterone *see* estrogens (esterified) and methyltestosterone *on page 380*

esterified estrogens *see* estrogens (esterified) *on page 380*

Estivin® II Ophthalmic *(Discontinued)* *see* naphazoline *on page 680*

Estra-L® Injection *(Discontinued)* *see* estradiol *on page 373*

Estrace® [US/Can] *see* estradiol *on page 373*

Estraderm® [US/Can] *see* estradiol *on page 373*

estradiol (es tra DYE ole)

Sound-Alike/Look-Alike Issues

Alora® may be confused with Aldara®

Elestrin™ may be confused with alosetron

Estraderm® may be confused with Testoderm®

Synonyms estradiol acetate; estradiol cypionate; estradiol hemihydrate; estradiol transdermal; estradiol valerate

U.S./Canadian Brand Names Alora® [US]; Climara® [US/Can]; Delestrogen® [US]; Depo®-Estradiol [US/Can]; Divigel® [US]; Elestrin™ [US]; Estrace® [US/Can]; Estraderm® [US/Can]; Estradot® [Can]; Estrasorb™ [US]; Estring® [US/Can]; EstroGel® [US/Can]; Evamist™ [US]; Femring® [US]; Femtrace® [US]; Menostar® [US/Can]; Oesclim® [Can]; Sandoz-Estradiol Derm 100 [Can]; Sandoz-Estradiol Derm 50 [Can]; Sandoz-Estradiol Derm 75 [Can]; Vagifem® [US/Can]; Vivelle-Dot® [US]

Therapeutic Category Estrogen Derivative

Use Treatment of moderate-to-severe vasomotor symptoms associated with menopause; treatment of vulvar and vaginal atrophy; hypoestrogenism (due to hypogonadism, castration, or primary ovarian failure); prostatic cancer (palliation), breast cancer (palliation), osteoporosis (prophylaxis); abnormal uterine bleeding due to hormonal imbalance; postmenopausal urogenital symptoms of the lower urinary tract (urinary urgency, dysuria)

Usual Dosage All dosage needs to be adjusted based upon the patient's response

Oral:

Prostate cancer (androgen-dependent, inoperable, progressing): 10 mg 3 times/day for at least 3 months

Breast cancer (inoperable, progressing in appropriately selected patients): 10 mg 3 times/day for at least 3 months

Osteoporosis prophylaxis in postmenopausal females: 0.5 mg/day in a cyclic regimen (3 weeks on and 1 week off)

Female hypoestrogenism (due to hypogonadism, castration, or primary ovarian failure): 1-2 mg/day; titrate as necessary to control symptoms using minimal effective dose for maintenance therapy

Moderate-to-severe vasomotor symptoms associated with menopause: 1-2 mg/day, adjusted as necessary to limit symptoms; administration should be cyclic (3 weeks on, 1 week off). Patients should be re-evaluated at 3- to 6-month intervals to determine if treatment is still necessary.

I.M.:

Prostate cancer: Valerate: ≥30 mg or more every 1-2 weeks

Moderate-to-severe vasomotor symptoms associated with menopause:

Cypionate: 1-5 mg every 3-4 weeks

Valerate: 10-20 mg every 4 weeks

Female hypoestrogenism (due to hypogonadism):

Cypionate: 1.5-2 mg monthly

Valerate: 10-20 mg every 4 weeks

Topical:

Emulsion: Moderate-to-severe vasomotor symptoms associated with menopause: 3.84 g applied once daily in the morning

Gel:

Moderate-to-severe vasomotor symptoms associated with menopause:

Divigel®: 0.25 g/day; adjust dose based on patient response. Dosing range: 0.25-1 g/day

Elestrin™: 0.87g/day applied at the same time each day

EstroGel®: 1.25 g/day applied at the same time each day

Vulvar and vaginal atrophy:

Elestrin™: 0.87g/day applied at the same time each day

EstroGel®: 1.25 g/day applied at the same time each day

Spray: Moderate-to-severe vasomotor symptoms associated with menopause (Evamist™): Initial: One spray (1.53 mg) per day. Adjust dose based on patient response. Dosing range: 1-3 sprays per day.

Transdermal: Indicated dose may be used continuously in patients without an intact uterus. May be given continuously or cyclically (3 weeks on, 1 week off) in patients with an intact uterus **(exception - Menostar®, see specific dosing instructions).** When changing patients from oral to transdermal therapy, start transdermal patch 1 week after discontinuing oral hormone (may begin sooner if symptoms reappear within 1 week):

Once-weekly patch:

Moderate-to-severe vasomotor symptoms associated with menopause, vulvar and vaginal atrophy associated with menopause, female hypoestrogenism (Climara®): Apply 0.025 mg/day patch once weekly. Adjust dose as necessary to control symptoms. Patients should be re-evaluated at 3- to 6-month intervals to determine if treatment is still necessary.

Osteoporosis prophylaxis in postmenopausal women:

Climara®: Apply patch once weekly; minimum effective dose 0.025 mg/day; adjust response to therapy by biochemical markers and bone mineral density

Menostar®: Apply patch once weekly. In women with a uterus, also administer a progestin for 14 days every 6-12 months

Twice-weekly patch:

Moderate-to-severe vasomotor symptoms associated with menopause, vulvar/vaginal atrophy, female hypogonadism: Titrate to lowest dose possible to control symptoms, adjusting initial dose after the first month of therapy; reevaluate therapy at 3- to 6-month intervals to taper or discontinue medication:

Alora®, Estraderm®, Vivelle-Dot®: Apply 0.05 mg patch twice weekly

Vivelle®: Apply 0.0375 mg patch twice weekly

Prevention of osteoporosis in postmenopausal women:

Alora®, Vivelle®, Vivelle-Dot®: Apply 0.025 mg patch twice weekly, increase dose as necessary

Estraderm®: Apply 0.05 mg patch twice weekly

Vaginal cream: Vulvar and vaginal atrophy: Insert 2-4 g/day intravaginally for 2 weeks, then gradually reduce to 1/2 the initial dose for 2 weeks, followed by a maintenance dose of 1 g 1-3 times/week

Vaginal ring:

Postmenopausal vaginal atrophy, urogenital symptoms: Estring®: 2 mg intravaginally; following insertion, ring should remain in place for 90 days

Moderate-to-severe vasomotor symptoms associated with menopause; vulvar/vaginal atrophy: Femring®: 0.05 mg intravaginally; following insertion, ring should remain in place for 3 months; dose may be increased to 0.1 mg if needed

Vaginal tablets: Atrophic vaginitis: Vagifem®: Initial: Insert 1 tablet once daily for 2 weeks; maintenance: Insert 1 tablet twice weekly; attempts to discontinue or taper medication should be made at 3- to 6-month intervals

Dosage Forms

Cream, vaginal:

Estrace®: 0.1 mg/g (42.5 g)

Emulsion, topical:

Estrasorb™: 2.5 mg/g (56s) [each pouch contains 4.35 mg estradiol hemihydrate; contents of two pouches delivers estradiol 0.05 mg/day]

Gel, topical:

Divigel®: 0.1% (0.25 g) [delivers estradiol 0.25 mg/packet]; (0.5 g) [delivers 0.5 mg estradiol/packet]; (1 g) [delivers estradiol 1 mg/packet]

Elestrin™: 0.06% (144 g) [delivers estradiol 0.52 mg/0.87 g; 100 actuations]

EstroGel®: 0.06% (50 g) [delivers estradiol 0.75 mg/1.25 g; 32 actuations]

Injection, oil:

Depo®-Estradiol: 5 mg/mL (5 mL)

Injection, oil: 10 mg/mL (5 mL); 20 mg/mL (5 mL); 40 mg/mL (5 mL)

Delestrogen®: 10 mg/mL (5 mL); 20 mg/mL (5 mL); 40 mg/mL (5 mL)

Ring, vaginal:

Estring®: 2 mg (1s) [total estradiol 2 mg; releases 7.5 mcg/day over 90 days]

Femring®: 0.05 mg/day (1s) [total estradiol 12.4 mg; releases 0.05 mg/day over 3 months]; 0.1 mg/day (1s) [total estradiol 24.8 mg; releases 0.1 mg/day over 3 months]

Solution, topical [spray]:

Evamist™: 1.53 mg/spray (8.1 mL)

Tablet, oral: 0.45 mg, 0.9 mg, 1.8 mg

Femtrace®: 0.45 mg, 0.9 mg, 1.8 mg

Tablet, oral, micronized: 0.5 mg, 1 mg, 2 mg

Estrace®: 0.5 mg, 1 mg, 2 mg

Tablet, vaginal:

Vagifem®: 25 mcg

Transdermal system: 0.025 mg/24 hours (4s) [once-weekly patch]; 0.0375 mg/24 hours (4s) [once weekly patch]; 0.05 mg/24 hours (4s) [once-weekly patch]; 0.06 mg/24 hours (4s) [once weekly patch]; 0.075 mg/24 hours [once-weekly patch]; 0.1 mg/24 hours (4s) [once-weekly patch]

Brands:

Alora® [twice-weekly patch]:

0.025 mg/24 hours (8s) [9 cm^2, total estradiol 0.77 mg]

0.05 mg/24 hours (8s) [18 cm^2, total estradiol 1.5 mg]

0.075 mg/24 hours (8s) [27 cm^2, total estradiol 2.3 mg]

0.1 mg/24 hours (8s) [36 cm^2, total estradiol 3.1 mg]

Climara® [once-weekly patch]:

0.025 mg/24 hours (4s) [6.5 cm^2, total estradiol 2.04 mg]

0.0375 mg/24 hours (4s) [9.375 cm^2, total estradiol 2.85 mg]

0.05 mg/24 hours (4s) [12.5 cm^2, total estradiol 3.8 mg]

0.06 mg/24 hours (4s) [15 cm^2, total estradiol 4.55 mg]

0.075 mg/24 hours (4s) [18.75 cm^2, total estradiol 5.7 mg]

0.1 mg/24 hours (4s) [25 cm^2, total estradiol 7.6 mg]

Estraderm® [twice-weekly patch]:

0.05 mg/24 hours (8s) [10 cm^2, total estradiol 4 mg]

0.1 mg/24 hours (8s) [20 cm^2, total estradiol 8 mg]

Menostar® [once-weekly patch]: 0.014 mg/24 hours (4s) [3.25 cm^2, total estradiol 1 mg]

Vivelle-Dot® [twice-weekly patch]:
0.025 mg/day (24s) [2.5 cm^2, total estradiol 0.39 mg]
0.0375 mg/day (24s) [3.75 cm^2, total estradiol 0.585 mg]
0.05 mg/day (24s) [5 cm^2, total estradiol 0.78 mg]
0.075 mg/day (24s) [7.5 cm^2, total estradiol 1.17 mg]
0.1 mg/day (24s) [10 cm^2, total estradiol 1.56 mg]

estradiol acetate *see* estradiol *on page 373*

estradiol and drospirenone *see* drospirenone and estradiol *on page 340*

estradiol and levonorgestrel (es tra DYE ole & LEE voe nor jes trel)

Synonyms levonorgestrel and estradiol

U.S./Canadian Brand Names ClimaraPro® [US]

Therapeutic Category Estrogen and Progestin Combination

Use Women with an intact uterus: Treatment of moderate-to-severe vasomotor symptoms associated with menopause; prevention of postmenopausal osteoporosis

Usual Dosage Topical: Adult females with an intact uterus: Treatment of moderate-to-severe vasomotor symptoms associated with menopause or prevention of postmenopausal osteoporosis:
Estradiol 0.045 mg/levonorgestrel 0.015 mg: Apply one patch weekly

Dosage Forms

Transdermal system:
ClimaraPro®: Estradiol 0.045 mg/24 hours and levonorgestrel 0.015 mg/24 hours (4s) [once-weekly patch]

estradiol and NGM *see* estradiol and norgestimate *on page 377*

estradiol and norethindrone (es tra DYE ole & nor eth IN drone)

Synonyms norethindrone and estradiol

U.S./Canadian Brand Names Activella® [US]; CombiPatch® [US]; Estalis-Sequi® [Can]; Estalis® [Can]

Therapeutic Category Estrogen and Progestin Combination

Use Women with an intact uterus:
Tablet: Treatment of moderate-to-severe vasomotor symptoms associated with menopause; treatment of vulvar and vaginal atrophy; prophylaxis for postmenopausal osteoporosis
Transdermal patch: Treatment of moderate-to-severe vasomotor symptoms associated with menopause; treatment of vulvar and vaginal atrophy; treatment of hypoestrogenism due to hypogonadism, castration, or primary ovarian failure

Usual Dosage Note: Patients should be treated with the lowest effective dose and for the shortest duration, consistent with treatment goals. Adults:
Oral (Activella®): One tablet daily
Transdermal patch (CombiPatch®):
Continuous combined regimen: Apply 1 patch twice weekly
Continuous sequential regimen: Apply estradiol-only patch for first 14 days of cycle, followed by one CombiPatch® applied twice weekly for the remaining 14 days of a 28-day cycle
Transdermal patch, combination pack (product-specific dosing for Canadian formulation):
Estalis®: Continuous combined regimen: Apply a new patch twice weekly during a 28-day cycle
Estalis-Sequi®: Continuous sequential regimen: Apply estradiol-only patch (Vivelle®) for first 14 days, followed by one Estalis® patch applied twice weekly during the last 14 days of a 28-day cycle
Note: In women previously receiving oral estrogens, initiate upon reappearance of menopausal symptoms following discontinuation of oral therapy.

Dosage Forms [CAN] = Canadian brand name

Combination pack:
Estalis-Sequi® 140/50 [CAN; not available in U.S.]:
Transdermal system (Vivelle®): Estradiol 50 mcg per day (4s) [14.5 sq cm; total estradiol 4.33 mg]
Transdermal system (Estalis®): Norethindrone 140 mcg and estradiol 50 mcg per day (4s) [9 sq cm; total norethindrone 2.7 mg, total estradiol 0.62 mg; not available in the U.S.]
Estalis-Sequi® 250/50 [CAN; not available in U.S.]:
Transdermal system (Vivelle®): Estradiol 50 mcg per day (4s) [14.5 sq cm; total estradiol 4.33 mg]
Transdermal system (Estalis®): Norethindrone250 mcg and estradiol 50 mcg per day (4s) [16 sq cm; total norethindrone 4.8 mg, total estradiol 0.51 mg; not available in the U.S.]

Tablet:
Activella® 0.5/0.1: Estradiol 0.5 mg and norethindrone acetate 0.1mg (28s)
Activella® 1/0.5: Estradiol 1 mg and norethindrone acetate 0.5 mg (28s)
Transdermal system:
CombiPatch®:
0.05/0.14: Estradiol 0.05 mg and norethindrone 0.14 mg per day (8s) [9 sq cm]
0.05/0.25: Estradiol 0.05 mg and norethindrone 0.25 mg per day (8s) [16 sq cm]
Estalis® [CAN]:
140/50: Norethindrone 140 mcg and estradiol 50 mcg per day (8s) [9 sq cm; total norethindrone 2.7 mg, total estradiol 0.62 mg; not available in the U.S.]
250/50 Norethindrone 250 mcg and estradiol 50 mcg per day (8s) [16 sq cm; total norethindrone 4.8 mg, total estradiol 0.51 mg; not available in U.S.]

estradiol and norgestimate (es tra DYE ole & nor JES ti mate)

Synonyms estradiol and NGM; norgestimate and estradiol; ortho prefest

U.S./Canadian Brand Names Prefest™ [US]

Therapeutic Category Estrogen and Progestin Combination

Use Women with an intact uterus: Treatment of moderate-to-severe vasomotor symptoms associated with menopause; treatment of atrophic vaginitis; prevention of osteoporosis

Usual Dosage Oral: Adults: Females with an intact uterus: Treatment of menopausal symptoms, atrophic vaginitis, prevention of osteoporosis: Treatment is cyclical and consists of the following: One tablet of estradiol 1 mg (pink tablet) once daily for 3 days, followed by 1 tablet of estradiol 1 mg and norgestimate 0.09 mg (white tablet) once daily for 3 days; repeat sequence continuously. **Note:** This dose may not be the lowest effective combination for these indications. In case of a missed tablet, restart therapy with next available tablet in sequence (taking only 1 tablet each day).

Dosage Forms
Tablet:
Prefest™: Estradiol 1 mg [15 pink tablets] and estradiol 1 mg and norgestimate 0.09 mg [15 white tablets] (supplied in blister card of 30)

estradiol cypionate *see* estradiol *on page 373*
estradiol hemihydrate *see* estradiol *on page 373*
estradiol transdermal *see* estradiol *on page 373*
estradiol valerate *see* estradiol *on page 373*
Estradot® [Can] *see* estradiol *on page 373*

estramustine (es tra MUS teen)

Sound-Alike/Look-Alike Issues
estramustine may be confused with exemestane
Emcyt® may be confused with Eryc®

Synonyms estramustine phosphate; estramustine phosphate sodium; NSC-89199

U.S./Canadian Brand Names Emcyt® [US/Can]

Therapeutic Category Antineoplastic Agent

Use Palliative treatment of progressive or metastatic prostate cancer

Usual Dosage Details concerning dosing in combination regimens should also be consulted.
Oral: Adults: Males: Prostate cancer: 14 mg/kg/day (range: 10-16 mg/kg/day) in 3 or 4 divided doses

Dosage Forms
Capsule:
Emcyt®: 140 mg

estramustine phosphate *see* estramustine *on page 377*
estramustine phosphate sodium *see* estramustine *on page 377*
Estrasorb™ [US] *see* estradiol *on page 373*
Estratab® [Can] *see* estrogens (esterified) *on page 380*
Estratab® *(Discontinued)* *see* estrogens (esterified) *on page 380*
Estratest® [Can] *see* estrogens (esterified) and methyltestosterone *on page 380*
Estratest® *(Discontinued)* *see* estrogens (esterified) and methyltestosterone *on page 380*
Estratest® H.S. *(Discontinued)* *see* estrogens (esterified) and methyltestosterone *on page 380*
Estring® [US/Can] *see* estradiol *on page 373*

Estro-Cyp® Injection ***(Discontinued)*** *see* estradiol *on page* 373
EstroGel® [US/Can] *see* estradiol *on page* 373
estrogenic substances, conjugated *see* estrogens (conjugated/equine) *on page* 378

estrogens (conjugated A/synthetic) (ES troe jenz, KON joo gate ed, aye, sin THET ik)

Sound-Alike/Look-Alike Issues

Cenestin® may be confused with Senexon®

U.S./Canadian Brand Names Cenestin® [US/Can]

Therapeutic Category Estrogen Derivative

Use Treatment of moderate-to-severe vasomotor symptoms of menopause; treatment of vulvar and vaginal atrophy

Usual Dosage The lowest dose that will control symptoms should be used; medication should be discontinued as soon as possible. Oral: Adults:

Moderate-to-severe vasomotor symptoms: 0.45 mg/day; may be titrated up to 1.25 mg/day. Attempts to discontinue medication should be made at 3- to 6-month intervals.

Vulvar and vaginal atrophy: 0.3 mg/day

Dosage Forms

Tablet:

Cenestin®: 0.3 mg, 0.45 mg, 0.625 mg, 0.9 mg, 1.25 mg

estrogens (conjugated B/synthetic) (ES troe jenz, KON joo gate ed, bee, sin THET ik)

Sound-Alike/Look-Alike Issues

Enjuvia™ may be confused with Januvia™

U.S./Canadian Brand Names Enjuvia™ [US]

Therapeutic Category Estrogen Derivative

Use Treatment of moderate-to-severe vasomotor symptoms of menopause; treatment of vulvar and vaginal atrophy associated with menopause; treatment of moderate-to-severe vaginal dryness and pain with intercourse associated with menopause

Usual Dosage The lowest dose that will control symptoms should be used; medication should be discontinued as soon as possible. Oral:

Adults:

Moderate-to-severe vasomotor symptoms associated with menopause: 0.3 mg/day; may be titrated up to 1.25 mg/day. Attempts to discontinue medication should be made at 3- to 6-month intervals.

Vaginal dryness/vulvar and vaginal atrophy associated with menopause: 0.3 mg/day. Attempts to discontinue medication should be made at 3- to 6-month intervals.

Dosage Forms

Tablet:

Enjuvia™: 0.3 mg, 0.45 mg, 0.625 mg, 0.9 mg, 1.25 mg

estrogens (conjugated/equine) (ES troe jenz KON joo gate ed, EE kwine)

Sound-Alike/Look-Alike Issues

Premarin® may be confused with Primaxin®, Provera®, Remeron®

Synonyms C.E.S.; CE; CEE; conjugated estrogen; estrogenic substances, conjugated

U.S./Canadian Brand Names C.E.S.® [Can]; Premarin® [US/Can]

Therapeutic Category Estrogen Derivative

Use Treatment of moderate-to-severe vasomotor symptoms associated with menopause; treatment of vulvar and vaginal atrophy; hypoestrogenism (due to hypogonadism, castration, or primary ovarian failure); prostatic cancer (palliation); breast cancer (palliation); osteoporosis (prophylaxis, postmenopausal women at significant risk only); abnormal uterine bleeding; moderate-to-severe dyspareunia (pain during intercourse) due to vaginal/vulvar atrophy of menopause

Usual Dosage Adults:

Male: Androgen-dependent prostate cancer palliation: Oral: 1.25-2.5 mg 3 times/day

Female:

Prevention of postmenopausal osteoporosis: Oral: Initial: 0.3 mg/day cyclically* or daily, depending on medical assessment of patient. Dose may be adjusted based on bone mineral density and clinical response. The lowest effective dose should be used.

Moderate-to-severe vasomotor symptoms associated with menopause: Oral: Initial: 0.3 mg/day, cyclically* or daily, depending on medical assessment of patient. The lowest dose that will control symptoms should be used. Medication should be discontinued as soon as possible.
Moderate-to-severe dyspareunia: Intravaginal: Vaginal cream: 0.5 g twice weekly (eg, Monday and Thursday) or once daily cyclically*
Vulvar and vaginal atrophy:
Oral: Initial: 0.3 mg/day; the lowest dose that will control symptoms should be used. May be given cyclically* or daily, depending on medical assessment of patient. Medication should be discontinued as soon as possible.
Vaginal cream: Intravaginal: 0.5-2 g/day given cyclically*
Abnormal uterine bleeding:
Acute/heavy bleeding:
I.M., I.V.: 25 mg, may repeat in 6-12 hours if needed
Note: Treatment should be followed by a low-dose oral contraceptive; medroxyprogesterone acetate along with or following estrogen therapy can also be given
Female hypogonadism: Oral: 0.3-0.625 mg/day given cyclically*; dose may be titrated in 6- to 12-month intervals; progestin treatment should be added to maintain bone mineral density once skeletal maturity is achieved.
Female castration, primary ovarian failure: Oral: 1.25 mg/day given cyclically*; adjust according to severity of symptoms and patient response. For maintenance, adjust to the lowest effective dose.
***Cyclic administration:** Either 3 weeks on, 1 week off **or** 25 days on, 5 days off

Male and Female:
Breast cancer palliation, metastatic disease in selected patients: Oral: 10 mg 3 times/day for at least 3 months

Dosage Forms

Cream, vaginal:
Premarin®: 0.625 mg/g (42.5 g)
Injection, powder for reconstitution:
Premarin®: 25 mg
Tablet:
Premarin®: 0.3 mg, 0.45 mg, 0.625 mg, 0.9 mg, 1.25 mg

estrogens (conjugated/equine) and medroxyprogesterone

(ES troe jenz KON joo gate ed/EE kwine & me DROKS ee proe JES te rone)

Sound-Alike/Look-Alike Issues
Premphase® may be confused with Prempro™
Prempro™ may be confused with Premphase®

Synonyms medroxyprogesterone and estrogens (conjugated); MPA and estrogens (conjugated)

U.S./Canadian Brand Names Premphase® [US/Can]; Premplus® [Can]; Prempro™ [US/Can]

Therapeutic Category Estrogen and Progestin Combination

Use Women with an intact uterus: Treatment of moderate-to-severe vasomotor symptoms associated with menopause; treatment of atrophic vaginitis; osteoporosis (prophylaxis)

Usual Dosage Oral: Adults:
Treatment of moderate-to-severe vasomotor symptoms associated with menopause or treatment of atrophic vaginitis in females with an intact uterus. (The lowest dose that will control symptoms should be used; medication should be discontinued as soon as possible):
Premphase®: One maroon conjugated estrogen 0.625 mg tablet daily on days 1 through 14 and one light blue conjugated estrogen 0.625 mg/MPA 5 mg tablet daily on days 15 through 28; reevaluate patients at 3- and 6-month intervals to determine if treatment is still necessary; monitor patients for signs of endometrial cancer; rule out malignancy if unexplained vaginal bleeding occurs
Prempro™: One conjugated estrogen 0.3 mg/MPA 1.5 mg tablet daily; reevaluate at 3-and 6-month intervals to determine if therapy is still needed; dose may be increased to a maximum of one conjugated estrogen 0.625 mg/MPA 5 mg tablet daily in patients with bleeding or spotting, once malignancy has been ruled out
Osteoporosis prophylaxis in females with an intact uterus:
Premphase®: One maroon conjugated estrogen 0.625 tablet daily on days 1 through 14 and one light blue conjugated estrogen 0.625 mg/MPA 5 mg tablet daily on days 15 through 28; monitor patients for signs of endometrial cancer; rule out malignancy if unexplained vaginal bleeding occurs
Prempro™: One conjugated estrogen 0.3 mg/MPA 1.5 mg tablet daily; dose may be increased to one conjugated estrogen 0.625 mg/MPA 5 mg tablet daily; in patients with bleeding or spotting, once malignancy has been ruled out

Dosage Forms

Tablet:

Premphase® [therapy pack contains two separate tablet formulations]: Conjugated estrogens 0.625 mg [14 maroon tablets] and conjugated estrogen 0.625 mg/medroxyprogesterone 5 mg [14 light blue tablets] (28s)

Prempro™:

0.3/1.5: Conjugated estrogens 0.3 mg and medroxyprogesterone 1.5 mg (28s)

0.45/1.5: Conjugated estrogens 0.45 mg and medroxyprogesterone 1.5 mg (28s)

0.625/2.5: Conjugated estrogens 0.625 mg and medroxyprogesterone 2.5 mg (28s)

0.625/5: Conjugated estrogens 0.625 mg and medroxyprogesterone 5 mg (28s)

estrogens (esterified) (ES troe jenz, es TER i fied)

Sound-Alike/Look-Alike Issues

Estratab® may be confused with Estratest®, Estratest® H.S.

Synonyms esterified estrogens

U.S./Canadian Brand Names Estratab® [Can]; Menest® [US/Can]

Therapeutic Category Estrogen Derivative

Use Treatment of moderate-to-severe vasomotor symptoms associated with menopause; treatment of vulvar and vaginal atrophy; hypoestrogenism (due to hypogonadism, castration, or primary ovarian failure); prostatic cancer (palliation); breast cancer (palliation); osteoporosis (prophylaxis, in women at significant risk only)

Usual Dosage Oral: Adults:

Prostate cancer (palliation): 1.25-2.5 mg 3 times/day

Female hypogonadism: 2.5-7.5 mg of estrogen daily for 20 days followed by a 10-day rest period. Administer cyclically (3 weeks on and 1 week off). If bleeding does not occur by the end of the 10-day period, repeat the same dosing schedule; the number of courses is dependent upon the responsiveness of the endometrium. If bleeding occurs before the end of the 10-day period, begin an estrogen-progestin cyclic regimen of 2.5-7.5 mg esterified estrogens daily for 20 days. During the last 5 days of estrogen therapy, give an oral progestin. If bleeding occurs before regimen is concluded, discontinue therapy and resume on the fifth day of bleeding.

Moderate-to-severe vasomotor symptoms associated with menopause: 1.25 mg/day administered cyclically (3 weeks on and 1 week off). If patient has not menstruated within the last 2 months or more, cyclic administration is started arbitrary. If the patient is menstruating, cyclical administration is started on day 5 of the bleeding. For short-term use only and should be discontinued as soon as possible. Reevaluate at 3- to 6-month intervals for tapering or discontinuation of therapy.

Atopic vaginitis and kraurosis vulvae: 0.3 to ≥1.25 mg/day, depending on the tissue response of the individual patient. Administer cyclically. For short-term use only and should be discontinued as soon as possible. Reevaluate at 3- to 6-month intervals for tapering or discontinuation of therapy.

Breast cancer (palliation): 10 mg 3 times/day for at least 3 months

Osteoporosis in postmenopausal women: Initial: 0.3 mg/day and increase to a maximum daily dose of 1.25 mg/day; initiate therapy as soon as possible after menopause; cyclically or daily, depending on medical assessment of patient. Monitor patients with an intact uterus for signs of endometrial cancer; rule out malignancy if unexplained vaginal bleeding occurs

Female castration and primary ovarian failure: 1.25 mg/day, cyclically. Adjust dosage upward or downward, according to the severity of symptoms and patient response. For maintenance, adjust dosage to lowest level that will provide effective control.

Dosage Forms

Tablet:

Menest®: 0.3 mg, 0.625 mg, 1.25 mg, 2.5 mg

estrogens (esterified) and methyltestosterone

(ES troe jenz es TER i fied & meth il tes TOS te rone)

Sound-Alike/Look-Alike Issues

Estratest® may be confused with Eskalith®, Estratab®, Estratest® H.S.

Estratest® H.S. may be confused with Eskalith®, Estratab®, Estratest®

Synonyms conjugated estrogen and methyltestosterone; esterified estrogen and methyltestosterone

U.S./Canadian Brand Names Covaryx™ HS [US]; Covaryx™ [US]; EEMT™ HS [US]; EEMT™ [US]; Estratest® [Can]

Therapeutic Category Estrogen and Androgen Combination

Use Vasomotor symptoms of menopause

Usual Dosage Oral: Adults: Females: Lowest dose that will control symptoms should be chosen, normally given 3 weeks on and 1 week off

Dosage Forms

Tablet: Esterified estrogens 1.25 mg and methyltestosterone 2.5 mg; esterified estrogen 0.625 mg and methyltestosterone 1.25 mg

Covaryx™, EEMT™: Esterified estrogen 1.25 mg and methyltestosterone 2.5 mg

Covaryx™ H.S., EEMT™ HS: Esterified estrogen 0.625 mg and methyltestosterone 1.25 mg

estropipate (ES troe pih pate)

Synonyms piperazine estrone sulfate

U.S./Canadian Brand Names Ogen® [US/Can]; Ortho-Est® [US]

Therapeutic Category Estrogen Derivative

Use Treatment of moderate-to-severe vasomotor symptoms associated with menopause; treatment of vulvar and vaginal atrophy; hypoestrogenism (due to hypogonadism, castration, or primary ovarian failure); osteoporosis (prophylaxis, in women at significant risk only)

Usual Dosage Oral: Adults:

Moderate-to-severe vasomotor symptoms associated with menopause: Usual dosage range: 0.75-6 mg estropipate daily; use the lowest dose and regimen that will control symptoms, and discontinue as soon as possible. Attempt to discontinue or taper medication at 3- to 6-month intervals. If a patient with vasomotor symptoms has not menstruated within the last ≥2 months, start the cyclic administration arbitrarily. If the patient has menstruated, start cyclic administration on day 5 of bleeding.

Female hypogonadism: 1.5-9 mg estropipate daily for the first 3 weeks, followed by a rest period of 8-10 days; use the lowest dose and regimen that will control symptoms. Repeat if bleeding does not occur by the end of the rest period. The duration of therapy necessary to product the withdrawal bleeding will vary according to the responsiveness of the endometrium. If satisfactory withdrawal bleeding does not occur, give an oral progestin in addition to estrogen during the third week of the cycle.

Female castration or primary ovarian failure: 1.5-9 mg estropipate daily for the first 3 weeks of a theoretical cycle, followed by a rest period of 8-10 days; use the lowest dose and regimen that will control symptoms

Osteoporosis prophylaxis: 0.75 mg estropipate daily for 25 days of a 31-day cycle

Atrophic vaginitis or kraurosis vulvae: 0.75-6 mg estropipate daily; administer cyclically. Use the lowest dose and regimen that will control symptoms; discontinue as soon as possible.

Dosage Forms

Tablet: 0.625 mg [estropipate 0.75 mg]; 1.25 mg [estropipate 1.5 mg]; 2.5 mg [estropipate 3 mg]

Ortho-Est®: 0.625 mg [estropipate 0.75 mg]; 1.25 mg [estropipate 1.5 mg]

Estrostep® 21 *(Discontinued)* *see* ethinyl estradiol and norethindrone *on page 390*

Estrostep® Fe [US] *see* ethinyl estradiol and norethindrone *on page 390*

eszopiclone (es zoe PIK lone)

Sound-Alike/Look-Alike Issues

Lunesta® may be confused with Neulasta®

U.S./Canadian Brand Names Lunesta® [US]

Therapeutic Category Hypnotic, Nonbenzodiazepine

Controlled Substance C-IV

Use Treatment of insomnia

Usual Dosage Oral: Adults: Insomnia: Initial: 2 mg immediately before bedtime (maximum dose: 3 mg)

Concurrent use with strong CYP3A4 inhibitor: 1 mg immediately before bedtime; if needed, dose may be increased to 2 mg

Dosage Forms

Tablet:

Lunesta®: 1 mg, 2 mg, 3 mg

etanercept (et a NER sept)

Sound-Alike/Look-Alike Issues

Enbrel® may be confused with Levbid®

U.S./Canadian Brand Names Enbrel® [US/Can]

Therapeutic Category Antirheumatic, Disease Modifying

Use Treatment of moderately- to severely-active rheumatoid arthritis (RA); moderately- to severely-active polyarticular juvenile idiopathic arthritis (JIA); psoriatic arthritis; active ankylosing spondylitis (AS); moderate-to-severe chronic plaque psoriasis

Usual Dosage SubQ:

Children 2-17 years: Juvenile idiopathic arthritis:

Once-weekly dosing: 0.8 mg/kg (maximum: 50 mg/dose) once weekly

Twice-weekly dosing: 0.4 mg/kg (maximum: 25 mg/dose) twice weekly (individual doses should be separated by 72-96 hours)

Adults:

Rheumatoid arthritis, psoriatic arthritis, ankylosing spondylitis:

Once-weekly dosing: 50 mg once weekly

Twice weekly dosing: 25 mg given twice weekly (individual doses should be separated by 72-96 hours)

Plaque psoriasis:

Initial: 50 mg twice weekly, 3-4 days apart (starting doses of 25 or 50 mg once weekly have also been used successfully); maintain initial dose for 3 months

Maintenance dose: 50 mg once weekly

Dosage Forms

Injection, powder for reconstitution:

Enbrel®: 25 mg

Injection, solution [preservative free]:

Enbrel®: 50 mg/mL (0.51 mL, 0.98 mL)

ethacrynate sodium *see* ethacrynic acid *on page 382*

ethacrynic acid (eth a KRIN ik AS id)

Sound-Alike/Look-Alike Issues

Edecrin® may be confused with Eulexin®, Ecotrin®

Synonyms ethacrynate sodium

U.S./Canadian Brand Names Edecrin® [US/Can]; Sodium Edecrin® [US]

Therapeutic Category Diuretic, Loop

Use Management of edema associated with congestive heart failure; hepatic cirrhosis or renal disease; short-term management of ascites due to malignancy, idiopathic edema, and lymphedema

Usual Dosage I.V. formulation should be diluted in D_5W or NS (1 mg/mL) and infused over several minutes.

Children: Oral: 1 mg/kg/dose once daily; increase at intervals of 2-3 days as needed, to a maximum of 3 mg/kg/day.

Adults:

Oral: 50-200 mg/day in 1-2 divided doses; may increase in increments of 25-50 mg at intervals of several days; doses up to 200 mg twice daily may be required with severe, refractory edema.

I.V.: 0.5-1 mg/kg/dose (maximum: 100 mg/dose); repeat doses not routinely recommended; however, if indicated, repeat doses every 8-12 hours.

Dosage Forms

Injection, powder for reconstitution:

Sodium Edecrin®: 50 mg

Tablet:

Edecrin®: 25 mg [scored]

ethambutol (e THAM byoo tole)

Sound-Alike/Look-Alike Issues

Myambutol® may be confused with Nembutal®

Synonyms ethambutol hydrochloride

U.S./Canadian Brand Names Etibi® [Can]; Myambutol® [US]

Therapeutic Category Antimycobacterial Agent

Use Treatment of pulmonary tuberculosis in conjunction with other antituberculosis agents

Usual Dosage

Usual dosage range: Oral:

Children: 15-20 mg/kg/day (maximum: 1 g/day) **or** 50 mg/kg/dose twice weekly (maximum: 2.5 g/dose)

Adults: 15-25 mg/kg daily **or** 25-30 mg/kg/dose 3 times/week (maximum: 2.5 g/dose) **or** 50 mg/kg/dose twice weekly (maximum: 4 g/dose)

Indication-specific dosing: Oral:

Tuberculosis, active: Note: Used as part of a multidrug regimen; treatment regimens consist of an initial 2 month phase, followed by a continuation phase of 4 or 7 additional months; frequency of dosing may differ depending on phase of therapy.

FDA-approved labeling: Children ≥13 years and Adults: Initial: 15 mg/kg once daily; Retreatment (previous antituberculosis therapy): 25 mg/kg once daily

Dosage Forms

Tablet: 100 mg, 400 mg

Myambutol®: 100 mg, 400 mg

ethambutol hydrochloride *see* ethambutol *on page 382*

Ethamolin® [US] *see* ethanolamine oleate *on page 383*

ethanoic acid *see* acetic acid *on page 30*

ethanol *see* alcohol (ethyl) *on page 42*

ethanolamine oleate (ETH a nol a meen OH lee ate)

Sound-Alike/Look-Alike Issues

Ethamolin® may be confused with ethanol

Synonyms monoethanolamine

U.S./Canadian Brand Names Ethamolin® [US]

Therapeutic Category Sclerosing Agent

Use Orphan drug: Sclerosing agent used for bleeding esophageal varices

Usual Dosage Adults: 1.5-5 mL per varix, up to 20 mL total or 0.4 mL/kg for a 50 kg patient; doses should be decreased in patients with severe hepatic dysfunction and should receive less than recommended maximum dose

Dosage Forms

Injection, solution:

Ethamolin®: 5% [50 mg/mL] (2 mL)

EtheDent™ [US] *see* fluoride *on page 430*

EthexDERM™ BPW-5 *(Discontinued)* *see* benzoyl peroxide *on page 132*

EthexDERM™ BPW-10 *(Discontinued)* *see* benzoyl peroxide *on page 132*

Ethezyme™ 650 *(Discontinued)* *see* papain and urea *on page 749*

Ethezyme™ 830 *(Discontinued)* *see* papain and urea *on page 749*

Ethezyme™ *(Discontinued)* *see* papain and urea *on page 749*

ethinyl estradiol and cyproterone acetate *see* cyproterone and ethinyl estradiol *(Canada only) on page 268*

ethinyl estradiol and desogestrel (ETH in il es tra DYE ole & des oh JES trel)

Sound-Alike/Look-Alike Issues

Apri® may be confused with Apriso™

Ortho-Cept® may be confused with Ortho-Cyclen®

Synonyms desogestrel and ethinyl estradiol

U.S./Canadian Brand Names Apri® [US]; Cesia™ [US]; Cyclessa® [US/Can]; Desogen® [US]; Kariva™ [US]; Linessa® [Can]; Marvelon® [Can]; Mircette® [US]; Ortho-Cept® [US/Can]; Reclipsen™ [US]; Solia™ [US]; Velivet™ [US]

Therapeutic Category Contraceptive, Oral

Use Prevention of pregnancy

Usual Dosage Oral: Adults: Females: Contraception:

Schedule 1 (Sunday starter): Dose begins on first Sunday after onset of menstruation; if the menstrual period starts on Sunday, take first tablet that very same day. **With a Sunday start, an additional method of contraception should be used until after the first 7 days of consecutive administration.**

For 21-tablet package: Dosage is 1 tablet daily for 21 consecutive days, followed by 7 days off of the medication; a new course begins on the 8th day after the last tablet is taken.

For 28-tablet package: Dosage is 1 tablet daily without interruption.

Schedule 2 (Day 1 starter): Dose starts on first day of menstrual cycle taking 1 tablet daily.

For 21-tablet package: Dosage is 1 tablet daily for 21 consecutive days, followed by 7 days off of the medication; a new course begins on the 8th day after the last tablet is taken.

For 28-tablet package: Dosage is 1 tablet daily without interruption.

If all doses have been taken on schedule and one menstrual period is missed, continue dosing cycle. If two consecutive menstrual periods are missed, pregnancy test is required before new dosing cycle is started.

Missed doses **monophasic formulations** (refer to package insert for complete information):

One dose missed: Take as soon as remembered or take 2 tablets next day

Two consecutive doses missed in the first 2 weeks: Take 2 tablets as soon as remembered or 2 tablets next 2 days. **An additional method of contraception should be used for 7 days after missed dose.**

Two consecutive doses missed in week 3 or three consecutive doses missed at any time:

Schedule 1 (Sunday starter): Continue to take 1 tablet daily until Sunday, then discard the rest of the pack, and a new pack is started that same day.

Schedule 2 (Day 1 starter): Current pack should be discarded, and a new pack started that same day. **An additional method of contraception should be used for 7 days after missed dose.**

Missed doses **biphasic/triphasic formulations** (refer to package insert for complete information):

One dose missed: Take as soon as remembered or take 2 tablets next day.

Two consecutive doses missed in week 1 or week 2 of the pack: Take 2 tablets as soon as remembered and 2 tablets the next day. Resume taking 1 tablet daily until the pack is empty. **An additional method of contraception should be used for 7 days after a missed dose.**

Two consecutive doses missed in week 3 of the pack; **an additional method of contraception must be used for 7 days after a missed dose**:

Schedule 1 (Sunday starter): Take 1 tablet every day until Sunday. Discard the remaining pack and start a new pack of pills on the same day.

Schedule 2 (Day 1 starter): Discard the remaining pack and start a new pack the same day.

Three or more consecutive doses missed; **an additional method of contraception must be used for 7 days after a missed dose**:

Schedule 1 (Sunday starter): Take 1 tablet every day until Sunday; on Sunday, discard the pack and start a new pack.

Schedule 2 (Day 1 starter): Discard the remaining pack and begin new pack of tablets starting on the same day.

Dosage Forms

Tablet, low-dose formulations:

Kariva™:

Day 1-21: Ethinyl estradiol 0.02 mg and desogestrel 0.15 mg [21 white tablets]

Day 22-23: 2 inactive light green tablets

Day 24-28: Ethinyl estradiol 0.01 mg [5 light blue tablets] (28s)

Mircette®:

Day 1-21: Ethinyl estradiol 0.02 mg and desogestrel 0.15 mg [21 white tablets]

Day 22-23: 2 inactive green tablets

Day 24-28: Ethinyl estradiol 0.01 mg [5 yellow tablets] (28s)

Tablet, monophasic formulations:

Apri® 28: Ethinyl estradiol 0.03 mg and desogestrel 0.15 mg (28s) [21 rose tablets and 7 white inactive tablets]

Desogen®, Reclipsen™, Solia™: Ethinyl estradiol 0.03 mg and desogestrel 0.15 mg (28s) [21 white tablets and 7 green inactive tablets]

Ortho-Cept® 28: Ethinyl estradiol 0.03 mg and desogestrel 0.15 mg (28s) [21 orange tablets and 7 green inactive tablets]

Tablet, triphasic formulations:

Cesia™, Cyclessa®:

Day 1-7: Ethinyl estradiol 0.025 mg and desogestrel 0.1 mg [7 light yellow tablets]

Day 8-14: Ethinyl estradiol 0.025 mg and desogestrel 0.125 mg [7 orange tablets]

Day 14-21: Ethinyl estradiol 0.025 mg and desogestrel 0.15 mg [7 red tablets]

Day 21-28: 7 green inactive tablets (28s)

Velivet™:

Day 1-7: Ethinyl estradiol 0.025 mg and desogestrel 0.1 mg [7 beige tablets]

Day 8-14: Ethinyl estradiol 0.025 mg and desogestrel 0.125 mg [7 orange tablets]

Day 14-21: Ethinyl estradiol 0.025 mg and desogestrel 0.15 mg [7 pink tablets]

Day 21-28: 7 white inactive tablets (28s)

ethinyl estradiol and drospirenone (ETH in il es tra DYE ole & droh SPYE re none)

Sound-Alike/Look-Alike Issues

Yasmin® may be confused with Yaz®

Yaz® may be confused with Yasmin®

Synonyms drospirenone and ethinyl estradiol

U.S./Canadian Brand Names Ocella™ [US]; Yasmin® [US/Can]; Yaz® [US/Can]

Therapeutic Category Contraceptive, Oral

Use Females: Prevention of pregnancy; treatment of premenstrual dysphoric disorder (PMDD); treatment of acne

Usual Dosage Oral:

Children ≥14 years and Adults: Females: Acne (Yaz®): Refer to dosing for contraception

Adults: Females: Contraception (Yasmin®, Yaz®), PMDD (Yaz®): Dosage is 1 tablet daily for 28 consecutive days. Dose should be taken at the same time each day, either after the evening meal or at bedtime. Dosing may be started on the first day of menstrual period (Day 1 starter) or on the first Sunday after the onset of the menstrual period (Sunday starter).

Day 1 starter: Dose starts on first day of menstrual cycle taking 1 tablet daily.

Sunday starter: Dose begins on first Sunday after onset of menstruation; if the menstrual period starts on Sunday, take first tablet that very same day. **With a Sunday start, an additional method of contraception should be used until after the first 7 days of consecutive administration.**

If all doses have been taken on schedule and one menstrual period is missed, continue dosing cycle. If two consecutive menstrual periods are missed, pregnancy test is required before new dosing cycle is started.

If doses have been missed during the first 3 weeks and the menstrual period is missed, pregnancy should be ruled out prior to continuing treatment.

Missed doses (monophasic formulations) (refer to package insert for complete information):

One dose missed: Take as soon as remembered or take 2 tablets next day

Two consecutive doses missed in the first 2 weeks: Take 2 tablets as soon as remembered or 2 tablets next 2 days. **An additional method of contraception should be used for 7 days after missed dose.**

Two consecutive doses missed in week 3 or three consecutive doses missed at any time: **An additional method of contraception must be used for 7 days after a missed dose.**

Day 1 starter: Current pack should be discarded, and a new pack should be started that same day.

Sunday starter: Continue dose of 1 tablet daily until Sunday, then discard the rest of the pack, and a new pack should be started that same day.

Any number of doses missed in week 4: Continue taking one pill each day until pack is empty; no back-up method of contraception is needed

Dosage Forms

Tablet:

Ocella™, Yasmin®: Ethinyl estradiol 0.03 mg and drospirenone 3 mg [21 yellow active tablets and 7 white inactive tablets] (28s)

Yaz®: Ethinyl estradiol 0.02 mg and drospirenone 3 mg [24 light pink tablets and 4 white inactive tablets] (28s)

ethinyl estradiol and ethynodiol diacetate

(ETH in il es tra DYE ole & e thye noe DYE ole dye AS e tate)

Sound-Alike/Look-Alike Issues

Demulen® may be confused with Dalmane®, Demerol®

Synonyms ethynodiol diacetate and ethinyl estradiol

U.S./Canadian Brand Names Demulen® 30 [Can]; Kelnor™ [US]; Zovia® [US]

Therapeutic Category Contraceptive, Oral

Use Prevention of pregnancy

Usual Dosage Oral: Adults: Females: Contraception:

Schedule 1 (Sunday starter): Dose begins on first Sunday after onset of menstruation; if the menstrual period starts on Sunday, take first tablet that very same day. **With a Sunday start, an additional method of contraception should be used until after the first 7 days of consecutive administration.**

For 21-tablet package: 1 tablet/day for 21 consecutive days, followed by 7 days off of the medication; a new course begins on the 8th day after the last tablet is taken.

For 28-tablet package: 1 tablet/day without interruption.

Schedule 2 (Day 1 starter): Dose starts on first day of menstrual cycle taking 1 tablet daily.

For 21-tablet package: 1 tablet/day for 21 consecutive days, followed by 7 days off of the medication; a new course begins on the 8th day after the last tablet is taken.

For 28-tablet package: 1 tablet/day without interruption.

If all doses have been taken on schedule and one menstrual period is missed, continue dosing cycle. If two consecutive menstrual periods are missed, pregnancy test is required before new dosing cycle is started.

Missed doses **monophasic formulations** (refer to package insert for complete information):

One dose missed: Take as soon as remembered or take 2 tablets next day

Two consecutive doses missed in the first 2 weeks: Take 2 tablets as soon as remembered or 2 tablets next 2 days. **An additional method of contraception should be used for 7 days after missed dose.**

Two consecutive doses missed in week 3 or three consecutive doses missed at any time: **An additional method of contraception should be used for 7 days after missed dose:**

Schedule 1 (Sunday starter): Continue dose of 1 tablet daily until Sunday, then discard the rest of the pack, and a new pack should be started that same day.

Schedule 2 (Day 1 starter): Current package should be discarded, and a new pack should be started that same day.

Dosage Forms

Tablet, monophasic formulations:

Kelnor™ 1/35: Ethinyl estradiol 0.035 mg and ethynodiol diacetate 1 mg [21 light yellow tablets and 7 white inactive tablets] (28s)

Zovia® 1/35-28: Ethinyl estradiol 0.035 mg and ethynodiol diacetate 1 mg [21 light pink tablets and 7 white inactive tablets] (28s)

Zovia® 1/50-28: Ethinyl estradiol 0.05 mg and ethynodiol diacetate 1 mg [21 pink tablets and 7 white inactive tablets] (28s)

ethinyl estradiol and etonogestrel (ETH in il es tra DYE ole & et oh noe JES trel)

Synonyms etonogestrel and ethinyl estradiol

U.S./Canadian Brand Names NuvaRing® [US/Can]

Therapeutic Category Contraceptive, Oral; Estrogen and Progestin Combination

Use Prevention of pregnancy

Usual Dosage Vaginal: Adults: Females: Contraception: One ring, inserted vaginally and left in place for 3 consecutive weeks, then removed for 1 week. A new ring is inserted 7 days after the last was removed (even if bleeding is not complete) and should be inserted at approximately the same time of day the ring was removed the previous week.

Initial treatment should begin as follows (pregnancy should always be ruled out first):

No hormonal contraceptive use in the past month: Insert ring on the first day of menstrual cycle ("Day 1"). May also insert on days 2-5 even if bleeding is not complete, however, **a spermicide or barrier method of contraception should be used for the following 7 days.***

Switching from combination oral contraceptive: Ring can be inserted on any day within 7 days after the last **active** tablet in the cycle was taken and no later than the first day a new cycle of tablets would begin. Additional forms of contraception are not needed.

Switching from progestin-only contraceptive: **A spermicide or barrier method of contraception should be used for the following 7 days with any of the following.***

If previously using a progestin-only mini-pill, insert the ring on any day of the month; do not skip days between the last pill and insertion of the ring.

If previously using an implant, insert the ring on the same day of implant removal.

If previously using a progestin-containing IUD, insert the ring on day of IUD removal.

If previously using a progestin injection, insert the ring on the day the next injection would be given.

Following complete 1st trimester abortion: Insert ring within the first 5 days of abortion. If not inserted within 5 days, follow instructions for "No hormonal contraceptive use within the past month" and instruct patient to use a nonhormonal contraceptive in the interim.

Following delivery or 2nd trimester abortion: Insert ring 4 weeks postpartum (in women who are not breast-feeding) or following 2nd trimester abortion. **A spermicide or barrier method of contraception should be used for the following 7 days.***

If the ring is accidentally removed from the vagina at anytime during the 3-week period of use, it may be rinsed with cool or lukewarm water (not hot) and reinserted as soon as possible. If the ring is not reinserted within 3 hours, contraceptive effectiveness will be decreased. **A spermicide or barrier method of contraception should be used until the ring has been in place for 7 consecutive days.***

If the ring has been removed for longer than 1 week, pregnancy must be ruled out prior to restarting therapy. **A spermicide or barrier method of contraception should be used for the following 7 days.***

If the ring has been left in place for >3 weeks, a new ring should be inserted following a 1-week (ring-free) interval. Protection continues during week 4, however, if the ring is left in place >4 weeks, pregnancy must be ruled out prior to insertion and **a spermicide or barrier method of contraception should be used for the following 7 days.***

Disconnected ring: In the event the ring disconnects at the weld joint, discard and replace with a new ring.

***Note:** Diaphragms may interfere with proper ring placement, and therefore, are not recommended for use as an additional form of contraception.

Dosage Forms

Ring, vaginal:

NuvaRing®: Ethinyl estradiol 0.015 mg/day and etonogestrel 0.12 mg/day (1s) [3-week duration]

ethinyl estradiol and levonorgestrel (ETH in il es tra DYE ole & LEE voe nor jes trel)

Sound-Alike/Look-Alike Issues

Alesse® may be confused with Aleve®
Nordette® may be confused with Nicorette®
Seasonale® may be confused with Seasonique™
Seasonique™ may be confused with Seasonale®
Tri-Levlen® may be confused with Trilafon®
Triphasil® may be confused with Tri-Norinyl®

Synonyms levonorgestrel and ethinyl estradiol

U.S./Canadian Brand Names Alesse® [US/Can]; Aviane™ [US/Can]; Enpresse™ [US]; Jolessa™ [US]; Lessina™ [US]; Levlen® [US]; Levlite™ [US]; Levora® [US]; LoSeasonique™ [US]; Lutera™ [US]; Lybrel™ [US]; Min-Ovral® [Can]; Nordette® [US]; Portia™ [US]; Quasense™ [US]; Seasonale® [US/Can]; Seasonique™ [US]; Sronyx™ [US]; Triphasil® [US/Can]; Triquilar® [Can]; Trivora® [US]

Therapeutic Category Contraceptive, Oral

Use Prevention of pregnancy; postcoital contraception

Usual Dosage Oral: Adults: Females:

Contraception, 28-day cycle:

Schedule 1 (Sunday starter): Dose begins on first Sunday after onset of menstruation; if the menstrual period starts on Sunday, take first tablet that very same day. With a Sunday start, an additional method of contraception should be used until after the first 7 days of consecutive administration:

For 21-tablet package: 1 tablet/day for 21 consecutive days, followed by 7 days off of the medication; a new course begins on the 8th day after the last tablet is taken

For 28-tablet package: 1 tablet/day without interruption

Schedule 2 (Day 1 starter): Dose starts on first day of menstrual cycle taking 1 tablet/day:

For 21-tablet package: 1 tablet/day for 21 consecutive days, followed by 7 days off of the medication; a new course begins on the 8th day after the last tablet is taken

For 28-tablet package: 1 tablet/day without interruption

If all doses have been taken on schedule and one menstrual period is missed, continue dosing cycle. If two consecutive menstrual periods are missed, pregnancy test is required before new dosing cycle is started.

Missed doses **monophasic formulations** (refer to package insert for complete information):

One dose missed: Take as soon as remembered or take 2 tablets next day

Two consecutive doses missed in the first 2 weeks: Take 2 tablets as soon as remembered or 2 tablets next 2 days. An additional method of contraception should be used for 7 days after missed dose.

Two consecutive doses missed in week 3 or three consecutive doses missed at any time: An additional method of contraception must be used for 7 days after a missed dose:

Schedule 1 (Sunday starter): Continue dose of 1 tablet daily until Sunday, then discard the rest of the pack, and a new pack should be started that same day.

Schedule 2 (Day 1 starter): Current pack should be discarded, and a new pack should be started that same day.

Missed doses **biphasic/triphasic formulations** (refer to package insert for complete information):

One dose missed: Take as soon as remembered or take 2 tablets next day.

Two consecutive doses missed in week 1 or week 2 of the pack: Take 2 tablets as soon as remembered and 2 tablets the next day. Resume taking 1 tablet daily until the pack is empty. An additional method of contraception should be used for 7 days after a missed dose.

Two consecutive doses missed in week 3 of the pack: An additional method of contraception must be used for 7 days after a missed dose.

Schedule 1 (Sunday starter): Take 1 tablet every day until Sunday. Discard the remaining pack and start a new pack of pills on the same day.

Schedule 2 (Day 1 starter): Discard the remaining pack and start a new pack the same day.

Three or more consecutive doses missed: An additional method of contraception must be used for 7 days after a missed dose.

Schedule 1 (Sunday starter): Take 1 tablet every day until Sunday; on Sunday, discard the pack and start a new pack.

Schedule 2 (Day 1 starter): Discard the remaining pack and begin new pack of tablets starting on the same day.

Contraception, 91-day cycle (extended cycle regimen): Dose begins on first Sunday after onset of menstruation; if the menstrual period starts on Sunday, take first tablet that very same day. An additional method of contraception should be used until after the first 7 days of consecutive administration:

Seasonale®: One active tablet/day for 84 consecutive days, followed by 1 inactive tablet/day for 7 days; if all doses have been taken on schedule and one menstrual period is missed, pregnancy should be ruled out prior to continuing therapy.

Seasonique™, LoSeasonique™: One active tablet/day for 84 consecutive days, followed by 1 low dose estrogen tablet/day for 7 days; if all doses have been taken on schedule and one menstrual period is missed, pregnancy should be ruled out prior to continuing therapy.

Missed doses:

One dose missed: Take as soon as remembered or take 2 tablets the next day

Two consecutive doses missed: Take 2 tablets as soon as remembered or 2 tablets the next 2 days. An additional nonhormonal method of contraception should be used for 7 consecutive days after the missed dose.

Three or more consecutive doses missed: Do not take the missed doses; continue taking 1 tablet/day until pack is complete. Bleeding may occur during the following week. An additional nonhormonal method of contraception should be used for 7 consecutive days after the missed dose.

Any number of pills during week 13: Throw away the missed pills and keep taking scheduled pills until the pack is finished. A back-up method of contraception is not needed

Contraception, continuous use (extended cycle regimen): Lybrel™: Take one tablet daily, at the same time each day, without a tablet-free interval. Therapy should be initiated as follows:

No previous contraception: Begin on the first day of menstrual cycle. Back-up contraception is not needed.

Previously taking a 21-day or 28-day combination hormonal contraceptive: Begin on day 1 of the withdrawal bleed (at the latest, 7 days after the last active tablet). Back-up contraception is not needed.

Previously using a progestin-only pill: Begin the day after taking a progestin only pill. Back-up contraception is needed for the first 7 days of therapy.

Previously using contraceptive implant: Begin the day of implant removal. Back-up contraception is needed for the first 7 days of therapy.

Previously using contraceptive injection: Begin when the next injection is due. Back-up contraception is needed for the first 7 days of therapy.

Missed doses:

One dose missed: Take as soon as remembered then take the next tablet at the regular time (2 tablets in 1 day). An additional nonhormonal method of contraception should also be used for 7 consecutive days.

Two consecutive doses missed: If remembered the day of the second missed tablet, take 2 tablets as soon as remembered, then 1 tablet the next day. If remembered the day after the second tablet is missed, take 2 tablets the day remembered, then 2 tablets the next day. An additional nonhormonal method of contraception should also be used for 7 consecutive days.

Three or more consecutive doses missed: Take 1 tablet daily and contact healthcare provider; do not take the missed pills. An additional nonhormonal method of contraception should also be used for 7 consecutive days.

Product Availability LoSeasonique™: FDA approved October 2008; availability anticipated May 2009

Dosage Forms

Tablet, oral [low-dose formulation]:

Alesse® 28: Ethinyl estradiol 0.02 mg and levonorgestrel 0.1 mg (28s) [21 pink tablets and 7 light green inactive tablets]

Aviane™ 28: Ethinyl estradiol 0.02 mg and levonorgestrel 0.1 mg (28s) [21 orange tablets and 7 light green inactive tablets]

Lessina™ 28, Levlite™ 28: Ethinyl estradiol 0.02 mg and levonorgestrel 0.1 mg (28s) [21 pink tablets and 7 white inactive tablets]

Lutera™, Sronyx™: Ethinyl estradiol 0.02 mg and levonorgestrel 0.1 mg (28s) [21 white tablets and 7 peach inactive tablets]

Tablet, oral [monophasic formulation]:

Levlen® 28: Ethinyl estradiol 0.03 mg and levonorgestrel 0.15 mg (28s) [21 light orange tablets and 7 pink inactive tablets]

Levora® 28: Ethinyl estradiol 0.03 mg and levonorgestrel 0.15 mg (28s) [21 white tablets and 7 peach inactive tablets]

Nordette® 28: Ethinyl estradiol 0.03 mg and levonorgestrel 0.15 mg (28s) [21 light orange tablets and 7 pink inactive tablets]

Portia™ 28: Ethinyl estradiol 0.03 mg and levonorgestrel 0.15 mg (28s) [21 pink tablets and 7 white inactive tablets]

Tablet, oral [extended cycle regimen]:

Jolessa™, Seasonale®: Ethinyl estradiol 0.03 mg and levonorgestrel 0.15 mg (91s) [84 pink tablets and 7 white inactive tablets]

LoSeasonique™: Ethinyl estradiol 0.02 mg and levonorgestrel 0.1 mg (91s) [84 orange tablets] and ethinyl estradiol 0.01 mg [7 yellow tablets]

Quasense™: Ethinyl estradiol 0.03 mg and levonorgestrel 0.15 mg] (91s) [84 white tablets and 7 peach inactive tablets]

Seasonique™: Ethinyl estradiol 0.03 mg and levonorgestrel 0.15 mg (91s) [84 light blue-green tablets] and ethinyl estradiol 0.01 mg [7 yellow tablets]

Tablet, oral [noncyclic regimen]:

Lybrel™: Ethinyl estradiol 0.02 mg and levonorgestrel 0.09 mg (28s) [28 yellow tablets]

Tablet, oral [triphasic formulation]:

Enpresse™ 28:
- Day 1-6: Ethinyl estradiol 0.03 mg and levonorgestrel 0.05 mg [6 pink tablets]
- Day 7-11: Ethinyl estradiol 0.04 mg and levonorgestrel 0.075 mg [5 white tablets]
- Day 12-21: Ethinyl estradiol 0.03 mg and levonorgestrel 0.125 mg [10 orange tablets]
- Day 22-28: 7 light green inactive tablets (28s)

Triphasil® 28:
- Day 1-6: Ethinyl estradiol 0.03 mg and levonorgestrel 0.05 mg [6 brown tablets]
- Day 7-11: Ethinyl estradiol 0.04 mg and levonorgestrel 0.075 mg [5 white tablets]
- Day 12-21: Ethinyl estradiol 0.03 mg and levonorgestrel 0.125 mg [10 light yellow tablets]
- Day 22-28: 7 light green inactive tablets (28s)

Trivora® 28:
- Day 1-6: Ethinyl estradiol 0.03 mg and levonorgestrel 0.05 mg [6 blue tablets]
- Day 7-11: Ethinyl estradiol 0.04 mg and levonorgestrel 0.075 mg [5 white tablets]
- Day 12-21: Ethinyl estradiol 0.03 mg and levonorgestrel 0.125 mg [10 pink tablets]
- Day 22-28: 7 peach inactive tablets (28s)

ethinyl estradiol and NGM *see* ethinyl estradiol and norgestimate *on page* 393

ethinyl estradiol and norelgestromin (ETH in il es tra DYE ole & nor el JES troe min)

Synonyms norelgestromin and ethinyl estradiol

U.S./Canadian Brand Names Evra® [Can]; Ortho Evra® [US]

Therapeutic Category Contraceptive, Oral; Estrogen and Progestin Combination

Use Prevention of pregnancy

Usual Dosage Topical: Adults: Females:

Contraception: Apply one patch each week for 3 weeks (21 total days); followed by one week that is patch-free. Each patch should be applied on the same day each week ("patch change day") and only one patch should be worn at a time. No more than 7 days should pass during the patch-free interval.

Schedule 1 (Sunday starter): Dose begins on first Sunday after onset of menstruation; if the menstrual period starts on Sunday, apply one patch that very same day. **With a Sunday start, an additional method of contraception (nonhormonal) should be used until after the first 7 days of consecutive administration.** Each patch change will then occur on Sunday.

Schedule 2 (Day 1 starter): Dose starts on first day of menstrual cycle, applying one patch during the first 24 hours of menstrual cycle. No backup method of contraception is needed as long as the patch is applied on the first day of cycle. Each patch change will then occur on that same day of the week.

Additional dosing considerations:

No bleeding during patch-free week/missed menstrual period: If patch has been applied as directed, continue treatment on usual "patch change day". If used correctly, no bleeding during patch-free week does not necessarily indicate pregnancy. However, if no withdrawal bleeding occurs for 2 consecutive cycles, pregnancy should be ruled out. If patch has not been applied as directed, and one menstrual period is missed, pregnancy should be ruled out prior to continuing treatment.

If a patch becomes partially or completely detached for <24 hours: Try to reapply to same place, or replace with a new patch immediately. Do not reapply if patch is no longer sticky, if it is sticking to itself or another surface, or if it has material sticking to it.

If a patch becomes partially or completely detached for >24 hours (or time period is unknown): Apply a new patch and use this day of the week as the new "patch change day" from this point on. **An additional method of contraception (nonhormonal) should be used until after the first 7 days of consecutive administration.**

Switching from oral contraceptives: Apply first patch on the first day of withdrawal bleeding. If there is no bleeding within 5 days of taking the last active tablet, pregnancy must first be ruled out. If patch is applied later than the first day of bleeding, **an additional method of contraception (nonhormonal) should be used until after the first 7 days of consecutive administration**

Use after childbirth: Therapy should not be started <4 weeks after childbirth. Pregnancy should be ruled out prior to treatment if menstrual periods have not restarted. **An additional method of contraception (nonhormonal) should be used until after the first 7 days of consecutive administration.**

Use after abortion or miscarriage: Therapy may be started immediately if abortion/miscarriage occur within the first trimester. If therapy is not started within 5 days, follow instructions for first time use. If abortion/miscarriage occur during the second trimester, therapy should not be started for at least 4 weeks. Follow directions for use after childbirth.

Dosage Forms The Canadian formulation differs from the U.S. product in both composition and manufacturing process (although delivery rates appear similar). [CAN] = Canadian brand name.

Patch, transdermal:

Evra® [CAN]: Ethinyl estradiol 0.6 mg and norelgestromin 6 mg [releases ethinyl estradiol 20 mcg and norelgestromin 150 mcg per day] (1s, 3s) [not available in the U.S.]

Ortho Evra®: Ethinyl estradiol 0.75 mg and norelgestromin 6 mg [releases ethinyl estradiol 20 mcg and norelgestromin 150 mcg per day] (1s, 3s)

ethinyl estradiol and norethindrone (ETH in il es tra DYE ole & nor eth IN drone)

Sound-Alike/Look-Alike Issues

femhrt® may be confused with Femara®
Modicon® may be confused with Mylicon®
Norinyl® may be confused with Nardil®
Tri-Norinyl® may be confused with Triphasil®

Synonyms norethindrone acetate and ethinyl estradiol

U.S./Canadian Brand Names Aranelle™ [US]; Balziva™ [US]; Brevicon® 0.5/35 [Can]; Brevicon® 1/35 [Can]; Brevicon® [US]; Estrostep® Fe [US]; Femcon® Fe [US]; femhrt® [US/Can]; Junel™ Fe [US]; Junel™ [US]; Leena™ [US]; Loestrin® 24 Fe [US]; Loestrin® Fe [US]; Loestrin® [US]; Loestrin™ 1.5/30 [Can]; Microgestin™ Fe [US]; Microgestin™ [US]; Minestrin™ 1/20 [Can]; Modicon® [US]; Necon® 0.5/35 [US]; Necon® 1/35 [US]; Necon® 10/11 [US]; Necon® 7/7/7 [US]; Norinyl® 1+35 [US]; Nortrel™ 7/7/7 [US]; Nortrel™ [US]; Ortho-Novum® 7/7/7 [US]; Ortho-Novum® [US]; Ortho® 0.5/35 [Can]; Ortho® 1/35 [Can]; Ortho® 7/7/7 [Can]; Ovcon® [US]; Select™ 1/35 [Can]; Synphasic® [Can]; Tilia™ Fe [US]; Tri-Legest™ Fe [US]; Tri-Norinyl® [US]; Zenchent™ [US]

Therapeutic Category Contraceptive, Oral

Use Prevention of pregnancy; treatment of acne; moderate-to-severe vasomotor symptoms associated with menopause; prevention of osteoporosis (in women at significant risk only)

Usual Dosage Oral:

Adolescents ≥15 years and Adults: Females: Acne: Estrostep® Fe: Refer to dosing for contraception

Adults: Females:

Moderate-to-severe vasomotor symptoms associated with menopause: Initial: femhrt® 0.5/2.5: 1 tablet daily; patient should be re-evaluated at 3- to 6-month intervals to determine if treatment is still necessary; patient should be maintained at the lowest effective dose

Prevention of osteoporosis: Initial: femhrt® 0.5/2.5: 1 tablet daily; patient should be maintained on the lowest effective dose

Contraception:

Schedule 1 (Sunday starter): Dose begins on first Sunday after onset of menstruation; if the menstrual period starts on Sunday, take first tablet that very same day. With a Sunday start, an additional method of contraception should be used until after the first 7 days of consecutive administration.

For 21-tablet package: Dosage is 1 tablet daily for 21 consecutive days, followed by 7 days off of the medication; a new course begins on the 8th day after the last tablet is taken.

For 28-tablet package: Dosage is 1 tablet daily without interruption.

Schedule 2 (Day 1 starter): Dose starts on first day of menstrual cycle taking 1 tablet daily.

For 21-tablet package: Dosage is 1 tablet daily for 21 consecutive days, followed by 7 days off the medication; a new course begins on the 8th day after the last tablet is taken.

For 28-tablet package: Dosage is 1 tablet daily without interruption.

If all doses have been taken on schedule and one menstrual period is missed, continue dosing cycle. If two consecutive menstrual periods are missed, pregnancy test is required before new dosing cycle is started.

Missed doses **monophasic formulations** (refer to package insert for complete information):

One dose missed: Take as soon as remembered or take 2 tablets next day Two consecutive doses missed in the first 2 weeks: Take 2 tablets as soon as remembered or 2 tablets next 2 days. An additional method of contraception should be used for 7 days after missed dose.

Two consecutive doses missed in week 3 or three consecutive doses missed at any time: An additional method of contraception must be used for 7 days after a missed dose.

Schedule 1 (Sunday starter): Continue dose of 1 tablet daily until Sunday, then discard the rest of the pack, and a new pack should be started that same day.

Schedule 2 (Day 1 starter): Current pack should be discarded, and a new pack should be started that same day.

Missed doses **biphasic/triphasic formulations** (refer to package insert for complete information):

One dose missed: Take as soon as remembered or take 2 tablets next day.

Two consecutive doses missed in week 1 or week 2 of the pack: Take 2 tablets as soon as remembered and 2 tablets the next day. Resume taking 1 tablet daily until the pack is empty. An additional method of contraception should be used for 7 days after a missed dose.

Two consecutive doses missed in week 3 of the pack: An additional method of contraception must be used for 7 days after a missed dose.

Schedule 1 (Sunday Starter): Take 1 tablet every day until Sunday. Discard the remaining pack and start a new pack of pills on the same day.

Schedule 2 (Day 1 starter): Discard the remaining pack and start a new pack the same day.

Three or more consecutive doses missed: An additional method of contraception must be used for 7 days after a missed dose.

Schedule 1 (Sunday Starter): Take 1 tablet every day until Sunday; on Sunday, discard the pack and start a new pack.

Schedule 2 (Day 1 Starter): Discard the remaining pack and begin new pack of tablets starting on the same day.

Dosage Forms

Tablet:

femhrt®: 1/5: Ethinyl estradiol 5 mcg and norethindrone 1 mg [white tablets]; 0.5/2.5: Ethinyl estradiol 2.5 mcg and norethindrone 0.5 mg [white tablets]

Tablet, monophasic formulations:

Balziva™: Ethinyl estradiol 0.035 mg and norethindrone 0.4 mg (28s) [21 light peach tablets and 7 white inactive tablets]

Brevicon®: Ethinyl estradiol 0.035 mg and norethindrone 0.5 mg (28s) [21 blue tablets and 7 orange inactive tablets]

Junel™ 21 1/20: Ethinyl estradiol 0.02 mg and norethindrone 1 mg (21s) [yellow tablets]

Junel™ 21 1.5/30: Ethinyl estradiol 0.03 mg and norethindrone 1.5 mg (21s) [pink tablets]

Junel™ Fe 1/20: Ethinyl estradiol 0.02 mg and norethindrone 1 mg (28s) [21 yellow tablets] and ferrous fumarate 75 mg [7 brown tablets]

Junel™ Fe 1.5/30: Ethinyl estradiol 0.03 mg and norethindrone 1.5 mg (28s) [21 pink tablets] and ferrous fumarate 75 mg [7 brown tablets]

Loestrin® 21 1/20, Microgestin™ 1/20: Ethinyl estradiol 0.02 mg and norethindrone 1 mg (21s) [white tablets]

Loestrin® 21 1.5/30, Microgestin™ 1.5/30: Ethinyl estradiol 0.03 mg and norethindrone 1.5 mg (21s) [green tablets]

Loestrin® 24 Fe: 1/20: Ethinyl estradiol 0.02 mg and norethindrone acetate 1 mg (28s) [24 white tablets] and ferrous fumarate 75 mg [4 brown tablets]

Loestrin® Fe 1/20, Microgestin™ Fe 1/20: Ethinyl estradiol 0.02 mg and norethindrone 1 mg (28s) [21 white tablets] and ferrous fumarate 75 mg [7 brown tablets]

Loestrin® Fe 1.5/30, Microgestin™ Fe 1.5/30: Ethinyl estradiol 0.03 mg and norethindrone 1.5 mg (28s) [21 green tablets] and ferrous fumarate 75 mg [7 brown tablets]

Modicon® 28: Ethinyl estradiol 0.035 mg and norethindrone 0.5 mg (28s) [21 white tablets and 7 green inactive tablets]

Necon® 0.5/35-28: Ethinyl estradiol 0.035 mg and norethindrone 0.5 mg (28s) [21 light yellow tablets and 7 white inactive tablets]

Necon® 1/35-28: Ethinyl estradiol 0.035 mg and norethindrone 1 mg (28s) [21 dark yellow tablets and 7 white inactive tablets]

Norinyl® 1+35: Ethinyl estradiol 0.035 mg and norethindrone 1 mg (28s) [21 yellow-green tablets and 7 orange inactive tablets]

Nortrel™ 0.5/35 mg:

Ethinyl estradiol 0.035 mg and norethindrone 0.5 mg (21s) [light yellow tablets]

Ethinyl estradiol 0.035 mg and norethindrone 0.5 mg (28s) [21 light yellow tablets and 7 white inactive tablets]

Nortrel™ 1/35 mg:

Ethinyl estradiol 0.035 mg and norethindrone 1 mg (21s) [yellow tablets]

Ethinyl estradiol 0.035 mg and norethindrone 1 mg (21s) [21 yellow tablets and 7 white inactive tablets]

Ortho-Novum® 1/35 28: Ethinyl estradiol 0.035 mg and norethindrone 1 mg (28s) [21 peach tablets and 7 green inactive tablets]

Ovcon® 35 28-day: Ethinyl estradiol 0.035 mg and norethindrone 0.4 mg (28s) [21 peach tablets and 7 green inactive tablets]

Ovcon® 50: Ethinyl estradiol 0.05 mg and norethindrone 1 mg (28s) [21 yellow tablets and 7 green inactive tablets]

Zenchent™: Ethinyl estradiol 0.035 mg and norethindrone 0.4 mg (28s) [21 light peach tablets and 7 white inactive tablets]

Tablet, chewable, monophasic formulations:

Femcon® Fe: Ethinyl estradiol 0.035 mg and norethindrone 0.4 mg (28s) [21 white tablets and 7 brown ferrous fumarate 75 mg tablets] [spearmint flavor]

Tablet, biphasic formulations:

Necon® 10/11-28:

Day 1-10: Ethinyl estradiol 0.035 mg and norethindrone 0.5 mg [10 light yellow tablets]

Day 11-21: Ethinyl estradiol 0.035 mg and norethindrone 1 mg [11 dark yellow tablets]

Day 22-28: 7 white inactive tablets (28s)

Ortho-Novum® 10/11-28:

Day 1-10: Ethinyl estradiol 0.035 mg and norethindrone 0.5 mg [10 white tablets]

Day 11-21: Ethinyl estradiol 0.035 mg and norethindrone 1 mg [11 peach tablets]

Day 22-28: 7 green inactive tablets (28s)

Tablet, triphasic formulations:

Aranelle™:

Day 1-7: Ethinyl estradiol 0.035 mg and norethindrone 0.5 mg [7 light yellow tablets]

Day 8-16: Ethinyl estradiol 0.035 mg and norethindrone 1 mg [9 white tablets]

Day 17-21: Ethinyl estradiol 0.035 mg and norethindrone 0.5 mg [5 light yellow tablets]

Day 22-28: 7 peach inactive tablets (28s)

Estrostep® Fe:

Day 1-5: Ethinyl estradiol 0.02 mg and norethindrone 1 mg [5 white triangular tablets]

Day 6-12: Ethinyl estradiol 0.03 mg and norethindrone 1 mg [7 white square tablets]

Day 13-21: Ethinyl estradiol 0.035 mg and norethindrone 1 mg [9 white round tablets]

Day 22-28: Ferrous fumarate 75 mg [7 brown tablets] (28s)

Leena™:

Day 1-7: Ethinyl estradiol 0.035 mg and norethindrone 0.5 mg [7 light blue tablets]

Day 8-16: Ethinyl estradiol 0.035 mg and norethindrone 1 mg [9 light yellow-green tablets]

Day 17-21: Ethinyl estradiol 0.035 mg and norethindrone 0.5 mg [5 light blue tablets]

Day 22-28: 7 orange inactive tablets (28s)

Necon® 7/7/7, Ortho-Novum® 7/7/7 28:

Day 1-7: Ethinyl estradiol 0.035 mg and norethindrone 0.5 mg [7 white tablets]

Day 8-14: Ethinyl estradiol 0.035 mg and norethindrone 0.75 mg [7 light peach tablets]

Day 15-21: Ethinyl estradiol 0.035 mg and norethindrone 1 mg [7 peach tablets]

Day 22-28: 7 green inactive tablets (28s)

Nortrel™ 7/7/7 28:

Day 1-7: Ethinyl estradiol 0.035 mg and norethindrone 0.5 mg [7 light yellow tablets]

Day 8-14: Ethinyl estradiol 0.035 mg and norethindrone 0.75 mg [7 blue tablets]

Day 15-21: Ethinyl estradiol 0.035 mg and norethindrone 1 mg [7 peach tablets]

Day 22-28: 7 white inactive tablets (28s)

Ortho-Novum® 7/7/7 28:

Day 1-7: Ethinyl estradiol 0.035 mg and norethindrone 0.5 mg [7 white tablets]

Day 8-14: Ethinyl estradiol 0.035 mg and norethindrone 0.75 mg [7 light peach tablets]

Day 15-21: Ethinyl estradiol 0.035 mg and norethindrone 1 mg [7 peach tablets]

Day 22-28: 7 green inactive tablets (28s)

Tilia™ Fe:
Day 1-5: Ethinyl estradiol 0.02 mg and norethindrone acetate 1 mg [5 white triangular tablets]
Day 6-12: Ethinyl estradiol 0.03 mg and norethindrone acetate 1 mg [7 white square tablets]
Day 13-21: Ethinyl estradiol 0.035 mg and norethindrone acetate 1 mg [9 white round tablets]
Day 22-28: Ferrous fumarate 75 mg [7 brown tablets] (28s)
Tri-Legest™ Fe:
Day 1-5: Ethinyl estradiol 0.02 mg and norethindrone acetate 1 mg [5 light pink tablets]
Day 6-12: Ethinyl estradiol 0.03 mg and norethindrone acetate 1 mg [7 light yellow tablets]
Day 13-21: Ethinyl estradiol 0.035 mg and norethindrone acetate 1 mg [9 light blue tablets]
Day 22-28: Ferrous fumarate 75 mg [7 brown tablets] (28s)
Tri-Norinyl® 28:
Day 1-7: Ethinyl estradiol 0.035 mg and norethindrone 0.5 mg [7 blue tablets]
Day 8-16: Ethinyl estradiol 0.035 mg and norethindrone 1 mg [9 yellow-green tablets]
Day 17-21: Ethinyl estradiol 0.035 mg and norethindrone 0.5 mg [5 blue tablets]
Day 22-28: 7 orange inactive tablets (28s)

ethinyl estradiol and norgestimate (ETH in il es tra DYE ole & nor JES ti mate)

Sound-Alike/Look-Alike Issues
Ortho-Cyclen® may be confused with Ortho-Cept®
Ortho Tri-Cyclen® may be confused with Ortho Tri-Cyclen® Lo
Ortho Tri-Cyclen® Lo may be confused with Ortho Tri-Cyclen®

Synonyms ethinyl estradiol and NGM; norgestimate and ethinyl estradiol

U.S./Canadian Brand Names Cyclen® [Can]; MonoNessa® [US]; Ortho Tri-Cyclen® Lo [US]; Ortho Tri-Cyclen® [US]; Ortho-Cyclen® [US]; Previfem® [US]; Sprintec® [US]; Tri-Cyclen® Lo [Can]; Tri-Cyclen® [Can]; Tri-Lo-Sprintec™ [US]; Tri-Previfem® [US]; Tri-Sprintec® [US]; TriNessa® [US]

Therapeutic Category Contraceptive, Oral

Use Prevention of pregnancy; treatment of acne

Usual Dosage Oral:
Children ≥15 years and Adults: Females: Acne (Ortho Tri-Cyclen®): Refer to dosing for contraception

Adults: Females:
Contraception:
Schedule 1 (Sunday starter): Dose begins on first Sunday after onset of menstruation; if the menstrual period starts on Sunday, take first tablet that very same day. **With a Sunday start, an additional method of contraception should be used until after the first 7 days of consecutive administration.**
For 21-tablet package: Dosage is 1 tablet daily for 21 consecutive days, followed by 7 days off of the medication; a new course begins on the 8th day after the last tablet is taken.
For 28-tablet package: Dosage is 1 tablet daily without interruption.
Schedule 2 (Day 1 starter): Dose starts on first day of menstrual cycle taking 1 tablet daily.
For 21-tablet package: Dosage is 1 tablet daily for 21 consecutive days, followed by 7 days off of the medication; a new course begins on the 8th day after the last tablet is taken.
For 28-tablet package: Dosage is 1 tablet daily without interruption.
If all doses have been taken on schedule and one menstrual period is missed, continue dosing cycle. If two consecutive menstrual periods are missed, pregnancy test is required before new dosing cycle is started.
Missed doses **monophasic formulations** (refer to package insert for complete information):
One dose missed: Take as soon as remembered or take 2 tablets next day
Two consecutive doses missed in the first 2 weeks: Take 2 tablets as soon as remembered or 2 tablets next 2 days. **An additional method of contraception should be used for 7 days after missed dose.**
Two consecutive doses missed in week 3 or three consecutive doses missed at any time: **An additional method of contraception must be used for 7 days after a missed dose:**
Schedule 1 (Sunday starter): Continue dose of 1 tablet daily until Sunday, then discard the rest of the pack, and a new pack should be started that same day.
Schedule 2 (Day 1 starter): Current pack should be discarded, and a new pack should be started that same day.
Missed doses **biphasic/triphasic formulations** (refer to package insert for complete information):
One dose missed: Take as soon as remembered or take 2 tablets next day.
Two consecutive doses missed in week 1 or week 2 of the pack: Take 2 tablets as soon as remembered and 2 tablets the next day. Resume taking 1 tablet daily until the pack is empty. **An additional method of contraception must be used for 7 days after a missed dose.**

Two consecutive doses missed in week 3 of the pack. **An additional method of contraception must be used for 7 days after a missed dose.**

Schedule 1 (Sunday starter): Take 1 tablet every day until Sunday. Discard the remaining pack and start a new pack of pills on the same day.

Schedule 2 (Day 1 starter): Discard the remaining pack and start a new pack the same day.

Three or more consecutive doses missed. **An additional method of contraception must be used for 7 days after a missed dose.**

Schedule 1 (Sunday starter): Take 1 tablet every day until Sunday; on Sunday, discard the pack and start a new pack.

Schedule 2 (Day 1 starter): Discard the remaining pack and begin new pack of tablets starting on the same day.

Dosage Forms

Tablet, monophasic formulations:

MonoNessa®, Ortho-Cyclen®: Ethinyl estradiol 0.035 mg and norgestimate 0.25 mg (28s) [21 blue tablets and 7 green inactive tablets]

Previfem®: Ethinyl estradiol 0.035 mg and norgestimate 0.25 mg (28s) [21 blue tablets and 7 teal inactive tablets]

Sprintec®: Ethinyl estradiol 0.035 mg and norgestimate 0.25 mg (28s) [21 blue tablets and 7 white inactive tablets]

Tablet, triphasic formulations:

Ortho Tri-Cyclen®, TriNessa®:

Day 1-7: Ethinyl estradiol 0.035 mg and norgestimate 0.18 mg [7 white tablets]
Day 8-14: Ethinyl estradiol 0.035 mg and norgestimate 0.215 mg [7 light blue tablets]
Day 15-21: Ethinyl estradiol 0.035 mg and norgestimate 0.25 mg [7 blue tablets]
Day 22-28: 7 green inactive tablets (28s)

Tri-Lo-Sprintec™:

Day 1-7: Ethinyl estradiol 0.025 mg and norgestimate 0.18 mg [7 white tablets]
Day 8-14: Ethinyl estradiol 0.025 mg and norgestimate 0.215 mg [7 light blue tablets]
Day 15-21: Ethinyl estradiol 0.025 mg and norgestimate 0.25 mg [7 blue tablets]
Day 22-28: 7 white inactive tablets (28s)

Tri-Previfem®:

Day 1-7: Ethinyl estradiol 0.035 mg and norgestimate 0.18 mg [7 white tablets]
Day 8-14: Ethinyl estradiol 0.035 mg and norgestimate 0.215 mg [7 light blue tablets]
Day 15-21: Ethinyl estradiol 0.035 mg and norgestimate 0.25 mg [7 blue tablets]
Day 22-28: 7 teal inactive tablets (28s)

Tri-Sprintec®:

Day 1-7: Ethinyl estradiol 0.035 mg and norgestimate 0.18 mg [7 gray tablets]
Day 8-14: Ethinyl estradiol 0.035 mg and norgestimate 0.215 mg [7 light blue tablets]
Day 15-21: Ethinyl estradiol 0.035 mg and norgestimate 0.25 mg [7 blue tablets]
Day 22-28: 7 white inactive tablets (28s)

Ortho Tri-Cyclen® Lo:

Day 1-7: Ethinyl estradiol 0.025 mg and norgestimate 0.18 mg [7 white tablets]
Day 8-14: Ethinyl estradiol 0.025 mg and norgestimate 0.215 mg [7 light blue tablets]
Day 15-21: Ethinyl estradiol 0.025 mg and norgestimate 0.25 mg [7 dark blue tablets]
Day 22-28: 7 green inactive tablets (28s)

ethinyl estradiol and norgestrel (ETH in il es tra DYE ole & nor JES trel)

Synonyms morning after pill; norgestrel and ethinyl estradiol

U.S./Canadian Brand Names Cryselle® 28 [US]; Lo/Ovral®-28 [US]; Low-Ogestrel® [US]; Ogestrel® [US]; Ovral® [Can]

Therapeutic Category Contraceptive, Oral

Use Prevention of pregnancy; postcoital contraceptive or "morning after" pill

Usual Dosage Oral: Adults: Females:

Contraception:

Schedule 1 (Sunday starter): Dose begins on first Sunday after onset of menstruation; if the menstrual period starts on Sunday, take first tablet that very same day. **With a Sunday start, an additional method of contraception should be used until after the first 7 days of consecutive administration.**

For 21-tablet package: Dosage is 1 tablet daily for 21 consecutive days, followed by 7 days off of the medication; a new course begins on the 8th day after the last tablet is taken.

For 28-tablet package: Dosage is 1 tablet daily without interruption.

Schedule 2 (Day 1 starter): Dose starts on first day of menstrual cycle taking 1 tablet daily.

For 21-tablet package: Dosage is 1 tablet daily for 21 consecutive days, followed by 7 days off of the medication; a new course begins on the 8th day after the last tablet is taken.

For 28-tablet package: Dosage is 1 tablet daily without interruption.

If all doses have been taken on schedule and one menstrual period is missed, continue dosing cycle. If two consecutive menstrual periods are missed, pregnancy test is required before new dosing cycle is started.

Missed doses **monophasic formulations** (refer to package insert for complete information):

One dose missed: Take as soon as remembered or take 2 tablets next day

Two consecutive doses missed in the first 2 weeks: Take 2 tablets as soon as remembered or 2 tablets next 2 days. **An additional method of contraception should be used for 7 days after missed dose.**

Two consecutive doses missed in week 3 or three consecutive doses missed at any time:

Schedule 1 (Sunday starter): Continue to take 1 tablet daily until Sunday, then discard the rest of the pack, and a new pack is started that same day.

Schedule 2 (Day 1 starter): Current pack should be discarded, and a new pack started that same day. **An additional method of contraception should be used for 7 days after missed dose.**

Postcoital contraception:

Ethinyl estradiol 0.03 mg and norgestrel 0.3 mg formulation: 4 tablets within 72 hours of unprotected intercourse and 4 tablets 12 hours after first dose

Ethinyl estradiol 0.05 mg and norgestrel 0.5 mg formulation: 2 tablets within 72 hours of unprotected intercourse and 2 tablets 12 hours after first dose

Dosage Forms

Tablet, monophasic formulations:

Cryselle® 28: Ethinyl estradiol 0.03 mg and norgestrel 0.3 mg [21 white tablets and 7 light green inactive tablets] (28s)

Low-Ogestrel®: Ethinyl estradiol 0.03 mg and norgestrel 0.3 mg [21 white tablets and 7 peach inactive tablets] (28s)

Lo/Ovral®-28: Ethinyl estradiol 0.03 mg and norgestrel 0.3 mg [21 white tablets and 7 pink inactive tablets] (28s)

Ogestrel®: Ethinyl estradiol 0.05 mg and norgestrel 0.5 mg [21 white tablets and 7 peach inactive tablets] (28s)

ethiofos *see* amifostine *on page 60*

ethionamide (e thye on AM ide)

U.S./Canadian Brand Names Trecator® [US/Can]

Therapeutic Category Antimycobacterial Agent

Use Treatment of tuberculosis and other mycobacterial diseases, in conjunction with other antituberculosis agents, when first-line agents have failed or resistance has been demonstrated

Usual Dosage Oral:

Children: 15-20 mg/kg/day in 2-3 divided doses, not to exceed 1 g/day

Adults: 15-20 mg/kg/day; initiate dose at 250 mg/day for 1-2 days, then increase to 250 mg twice daily for 1-2 days, with gradual increases to highest tolerated dose; average adult dose: 750 mg/day (maximum: 1 g/day in 3-4 divided doses)

Dosage Forms

Tablet:

Trecator®: 250 mg

Ethmozine® ***(Discontinued)***

ethosuximide (eth oh SUKS i mide)

Sound-Alike/Look-Alike Issues

ethosuximide may be confused with methsuximide

Zarontin® may be confused with Xalatan®, Zantac®, Zaroxolyn®

U.S./Canadian Brand Names Zarontin® [US/Can]

Therapeutic Category Anticonvulsant

Use Management of absence (petit mal) seizures

Usual Dosage Oral:

Children 3-6 years: Initial: 250 mg/day; increase every 4-7 days; usual maintenance dose: 20 mg/kg/day; maximum dose: 1.5 g/day in divided doses

Children >6 years and Adults: Initial: 500 mg/day; increase by 250 mg as needed every 4-7 days, up to 1.5 g/day in divided doses; usual maintenance dose for most pediatric patients is 20 mg/kg/day.

Dosage Forms
Capsule: 250 mg
Zarontin®: 250 mg
Syrup: 250 mg/5 mL
Zarontin®: 250 mg/5 mL

ethotoin (ETH oh toyn)

Synonyms ethylphenylhydantoin
U.S./Canadian Brand Names Peganone® [US/Can]
Therapeutic Category Hydantoin
Use Generalized tonic-clonic or complex-partial seizures
Usual Dosage Oral: **Note:** Administer in 4-6 divided doses daily; titrate over several days based on patient response
Children ≥1 year: Maximum initial dose: 750 mg/day; usual maintenance dose: 0.5-1 g/day; maximum dose: 3 g/day
Adults: Initial dose: ≤1 g/day; usual maintenance dose: 2-3 g/day
Dosage Forms
Tablet:
Peganone®: 250 mg

ETH-Oxydose™ *(Discontinued)* *see* oxycodone *on page 737*
ethoxynaphthamido penicillin sodium *see* nafcillin *on page 677*
Ethrane® [US] *see* enflurane *on page 354*
ethyl alcohol *see* alcohol (ethyl) *on page 42*
ethyl aminobenzoate *see* benzocaine *on page 129*

ethyl chloride (ETH il KLOR ide)

Synonyms chloroethane
U.S./Canadian Brand Names Gebauer's Ethyl Chloride® [US]
Therapeutic Category Local Anesthetic
Use Local anesthetic in minor operative procedures and to relieve pain caused by insect stings and burns, and irritation caused by myofascial and visceral pain syndromes
Usual Dosage Dosage varies with use
Dosage Forms
Aerosol:
Gebauer's Ethyl Chloride®: 100% (103 mL)

ethyl chloride and dichlorotetrafluoroethane

(ETH il KLOR ide & dye klor oh te tra floo or oh ETH ane)
Synonyms dichlorotetrafluoroethane and ethyl chloride
Therapeutic Category Local Anesthetic
Use Topical refrigerant anesthetic to control pain associated with minor surgical procedures, dermabrasion, injections, contusions, and minor strains
Usual Dosage Press gently on side of spray valve allowing the liquid to emerge as a fine mist approximately 2" to 4" from site of application

ethyl esters of omega-3 fatty acids *see* omega-3-acid ethyl esters *on page 723*
ethylphenylhydantoin *see* ethotoin *on page 396*
ethynodiol diacetate and ethinyl estradiol *see* ethinyl estradiol and ethynodiol diacetate *on page 385*
Ethyol® [US/Can] *see* amifostine *on page 60*
Etibi® [Can] *see* ethambutol *on page 382*

etidronate and calcium *(Canada only)* (e ti DROE nate & KAL see um)

Synonyms calcium carbonate and etidronate disodium
U.S./Canadian Brand Names CO-Etidrocal [Can]; Didrocal™ [Can]; GEN-ETI-CAL CAREPAC [Can]; Novo-Etidronatecal [Can]
Therapeutic Category Bisphosphonate Derivative; Calcium Salt

Use Treatment and prevention of postmenopausal osteoporosis; prevention of corticosteroid-induced osteoporosis

Usual Dosage Note: 90-day treatment regimen involves sequential administration of two products within the packaging; not to be taken concurrently. The first blister card contains white tablets containing etidronate disodium, while the remaining four blister cards contains blue, capsule-shaped tablets containing calcium carbonate.

Oral: Adults: Etidronate disodium 400 mg once daily for 14 days, followed by calcium carbonate 1250 mg (500 mg elemental calcium) once daily for 76 days

Dosage Forms [CAN] = Canadian brand name

Combination package [each package contains five blister cards (90-day supply)]:

Didrocal™ [CAN; not available in the U.S.]

Tablet, etidronate: 400 mg (14s) [first card (white tablets)]

Tablet, calcium: 1250 mg (76s) [remaining cards (blue tablets)]

etidronate disodium (e ti DROE nate dye SOW dee um)

Sound-Alike/Look-Alike Issues

etidronate may be confused with etidocaine, etomidate, etretinate

Synonyms EHDP; sodium etidronate

U.S./Canadian Brand Names Didronel® [US/Can]; Gen-Etidronate [Can]

Therapeutic Category Bisphosphonate Derivative

Use Symptomatic treatment of Paget disease; prevention and treatment of heterotopic ossification due to spinal cord injury or after total hip replacement

Usual Dosage Oral: Adults:

Paget disease:

Initial: 5-10 mg/kg/day (not to exceed 6 months) or 11-20 mg/kg/day (not to exceed 3 months). Doses >20 mg/kg/day are **not** recommended.

Retreatment: Initiate only after etidronate-free period ≥90 days. Monitor patients every 3-6 months. Retreatment regimens are the same as for initial treatment.

Heterotopic ossification:

Caused by spinal cord injury: 20 mg/kg/day for 2 weeks, then 10 mg/kg/day for 10 weeks; total treatment period: 12 weeks

Complicating total hip replacement: 20 mg/kg/day for 1 month preoperatively then 20 mg/kg/day for 3 months postoperatively; total treatment period is 4 months

Dosage Forms

Tablet:

Didronel®: 400 mg

etodolac (ee toe DOE lak)

Sound-Alike/Look-Alike Issues

Lodine® may be confused with codeine, iodine, lopidine®, Lopid®

Synonyms etodolic acid

U.S./Canadian Brand Names Apo-Etodolac® [Can]; Utradol™ [Can]

Therapeutic Category Analgesic, Nonnarcotic; Nonsteroidal Antiinflammatory Drug (NSAID)

Use Acute and long-term use in the management of signs and symptoms of osteoarthritis; rheumatoid arthritis and juvenile rheumatoid arthritis; management of acute pain

Usual Dosage Note: For chronic conditions, response is usually observed within 2 weeks.

Children 6-16 years: Oral: Juvenile rheumatoid arthritis: Extended release formulation:

20-30 kg: 400 mg once daily

31-45 kg: 600 mg once daily

46-60 kg: 800 mg once daily

>60 kg: 1000 mg once daily

Adults: Oral:

Acute pain: Immediate release formulation: 200-400 mg every 6-8 hours, as needed, not to exceed total daily doses of 1000 mg

Rheumatoid arthritis, osteoarthritis:

Immediate release formulation: 400 mg 2 times/day **or** 300 mg 2-3 times/day **or** 500 mg 2 times/day (doses >1000 mg/day have not been evaluated)

Extended release formulation: 400-1000 mg once daily

Dosage Forms
Capsule: 200 mg, 300 mg
Tablet: 400 mg, 500 mg
Tablet, extended release: 400 mg, 500 mg, 600 mg

etodolic acid *see* etodolac *on page* 397

EtOH *see* alcohol (ethyl) *on page* 42

etomidate (e TOM i date)

Sound-Alike/Look-Alike Issues
etomidate may be confused with etidronate

U.S./Canadian Brand Names Amidate® [US/Can]

Therapeutic Category General Anesthetic

Use Induction and maintenance of general anesthesia

Usual Dosage I.V.: Children >10 years and Adults: Initial: 0.2-0.6 mg/kg over 30-60 seconds for induction of anesthesia; maintenance: 5-20 mcg/kg/minute

Dosage Forms
Injection, solution: 2 mg/mL (10 mL, 20 mL)
Amidate®: 2 mg/mL (10 mL, 20 mL)

etonogestrel (e toe noe JES trel)

Synonyms 3-keto-desogestrel; ENG

U.S./Canadian Brand Names Implanon™ [US]

Therapeutic Category Contraceptive; Progestin

Use Prevention of pregnancy; for use in women who request long-acting (up to 3 years) contraception

Usual Dosage
Children: Not for use prior to menarche.
Adults: Contraception: Subdermal: Implant 1 rod in the inner side of the upper, nondominant arm. Remove no later than 3 years after the date of insertion. After ruling out pregnancy, timing of insertion is based on the patient's contraceptive history:
No hormonal contraceptives within the past month: Insert between days 1 through 5 of menstruation, even if woman is still bleeding
Switching from combination hormonal contraceptive:
Oral tablet: Insert anytime within 7 days after the last active tablet
Vaginal ring: Insert anytime during the 7-day ring-free period
Transdermal system: Insert anytime during the 7-day patch-free period
Switching from a progestin-only contraceptive:
Oral pill: Any day during the month; do not skip days between the last pill and implant insertion
Implant: Insert on same day as removal of implant
IUD: Insert on same day as removal of IUD
Injection: Insert on day next injection is due
First trimester abortion or miscarriage: Insert immediately. If not inserted within first 5 days follow directions for "no hormonal contraception within the past month"
Following delivery or second trimester abortion: May insert between 21 and 28 days (if not exclusively breast-feeding) or after 4 weeks (if exclusively breast-feeding). Patients should use a second form of contraception for the first 7 days if insertion occurs at >4 weeks.
Note: If following above insertion schedule, no backup contraception needed. If deviating, use back-up method for 7 days postinsertion.

Dosage Forms
Rod, subdermal:
Implanon™: 68 mg

etonogestrel and ethinyl estradiol *see* ethinyl estradiol and etonogestrel *on page* 386

Etopophos® [US] *see* etoposide phosphate *on page* 399

etoposide (e toe POE side)

Sound-Alike/Look-Alike Issues
etoposide may be confused with teniposide
VePesid® may be confused with Versed

Synonyms epipodophyllotoxin; VP-16; VP-16-213

U.S./Canadian Brand Names Toposar™ [US]

Therapeutic Category Antineoplastic Agent

Use Treatment of refractory testicular tumors; treatment of small cell lung cancer

Usual Dosage Refer to individual protocols: Adults:

Small cell lung cancer (in combination with other approved chemotherapeutic drugs):

Oral: Due to poor bioavailability, oral doses should be twice the I.V. dose, rounded to the nearest 50 mg given once daily

I.V.: 35 mg/m²/day for 4 days or 50 mg/m²/day for 5 days every 3-4 weeks

IVPB: 60-100 mg/m²/day for 3 days (with cisplatin)

CIV: 500 mg/m² over 24 hours every 3 weeks

Testicular cancer (in combination with other approved chemotherapeutic drugs):

IVPB: 50-100 mg/m²/day for 5 days repeated every 3-4 weeks

I.V.: 100 mg/m² every other day for 3 doses repeated every 3-4 weeks

Dosage Forms

Capsule, softgel: 50 mg

Injection, solution: 20 mg/mL (5 mL, 25 mL, 50 mL)

Toposar™: 20 mg/mL (5 mL, 25 mL, 50 mL)

etoposide phosphate (e toe POE side FOS fate)

Sound-Alike/Look-Alike Issues

etoposide may be confused with teniposide

U.S./Canadian Brand Names Etopophos® [US]

Therapeutic Category Antineoplastic Agent

Use Treatment of refractory testicular tumors; treatment of small cell lung cancer

Usual Dosage Refer to individual protocols. Adults: **Note:** Etoposide phosphate is a prodrug of etoposide, doses should be expressed as the desired **ETOPOSIDE** dose; **not** as the etoposide phosphate dose. (eg, etoposide phosphate equivalent to ____ mg etoposide).

Small cell lung cancer (in combination with other approved chemotherapeutic drugs): I.V.: Etoposide 35 mg/m²/day for 4 days to 50 mg/m²/day for 5 days. Courses are repeated at 3- to 4-week intervals after adequate recovery from any toxicity.

Testicular cancer (in combination with other approved chemotherapeutic agents): I.V.: Etoposide 50-100 mg/m²/day on days 1-5 to 100 mg/m²/day on days 1, 3, and 5. Courses are repeated at 3- to 4-week intervals after adequate recovery from any toxicity.

Dosage Forms

Injection, powder for reconstitution:

Etopophos®: 100 mg

Etrafon® [Can] *see* amitriptyline and perphenazine *on page* 66

etravirine (et ra VIR een)

Synonyms TMC125

U.S./Canadian Brand Names Intelence™ [US/Can]

Therapeutic Category Antiretroviral Agent, Nonnucleoside Reverse Transcriptase Inhibitor (NNRTI)

Use Treatment of HIV-1 infection in combination with at least two additional antiretroviral agents in treatment-experienced patients exhibiting viral replication with documented nonnucleoside reverse transcriptase inhibitor (NNRTI) resistance

Usual Dosage Oral: Adults: 200 mg twice daily after meals

Dosage Forms

Tablet:

Intelence™: 100 mg

ETS-2% Topical *(Discontinued)*

Eudal®-SR [US] *see* guaifenesin and pseudoephedrine *on page* 477

Euflex® [Can] *see* flutamide *on page* 436

Euflexxa™ [US] *see* hyaluronate and derivatives *on page* 496

Euglucon® [Can] *see* glyburide *on page* 467

Eulexin® [Can] *see* flutamide *on page* 436

Eurax® [US] *see* crotamiton *on page* 262

Euro-Lithium [Can] *see* lithium *on page* 594

Euthyrox [Can] *see* levothyroxine *on page 583*
Evac-Q-Mag® ***(Discontinued)*** *see* magnesium citrate *on page 607*
Evac-U-Gen [US-OTC] *see* senna *on page 896*
Evalose® ***(Discontinued)*** *see* lactulose *on page 565*
Evamist™ [US] *see* estradiol *on page 373*

everolimus (e ver OH li mus)

Sound-Alike/Look-Alike Issues
everolimus may be confused with sirolimus, tacrolimus, temsirolimus

Synonyms RAD001

U.S./Canadian Brand Names Afinitor® [US]

Therapeutic Category Antineoplastic Agent, mTOR Kinase Inhibitor; mTOR Kinase Inhibitor

Use Treatment of advanced renal cell cancer (RCC), after sunitinib or sorafenib failure

Usual Dosage Oral: Adults: RCC: 10 mg once daily

Dosage Forms
Tablet:
Afinitor®: 5 mg, 10 mg

Everone® 200 [Can] *see* testosterone *on page 947*
Everone® Injection ***(Discontinued)*** *see* testosterone *on page 947*
Evicel™ [US] *see* fibrin sealant kit *on page 417*
Evista® [US/Can] *see* raloxifene *on page 849*
Evithrom™ [US] *see* thrombin (topical) *on page 957*
Evoclin® [US] *see* clindamycin *on page 239*
Evoxac® [US/Can] *see* cevimeline *on page 206*
Evra® [Can] *see* ethinyl estradiol and norelgestromin *on page 389*
Exactacain™ [US] *see* benzocaine, butamben, and tetracaine *on page 131*
Excedrin® Extra Strength [US-OTC] *see* acetaminophen, aspirin, and caffeine *on page 24*
Excedrin® IB ***(Discontinued)*** *see* ibuprofen *on page 515*
Excedrin® Migraine [US-OTC] *see* acetaminophen, aspirin, and caffeine *on page 24*
Excedrin PM® [US-OTC] *see* acetaminophen and diphenhydramine *on page 21*
Excedrin® Sinus Headache [US-OTC] *see* acetaminophen and phenylephrine *on page 22*
Excedrin® Tension Headache [US-OTC] *see* acetaminophen *on page 19*
ExeClear ***(Discontinued)***
ExeCof [US] *see* guaifenesin, dextromethorphan, and phenylephrine *on page 478*
ExeCof-XP ***(Discontinued)***
ExeFen [US] *see* guaifenesin and pseudoephedrine *on page 477*
ExeFen-DMX [US] *see* guaifenesin, pseudoephedrine, and dextromethorphan *on page 479*
ExeFen-PD [US] *see* guaifenesin and phenylephrine *on page 475*
Exelderm® [US/Can] *see* sulconazole *on page 926*
Exelon® [US/Can] *see* rivastigmine *on page 873*

exemestane (ex e MES tane)

Sound-Alike/Look-Alike Issues
exemestane may be confused with estramustine
Aromasin® may be confused with Arimidex®

U.S./Canadian Brand Names Aromasin® [US/Can]

Therapeutic Category Antineoplastic Agent, Miscellaneous

Use Treatment of advanced breast cancer in postmenopausal women whose disease has progressed following tamoxifen therapy; adjuvant treatment of postmenopausal estrogen receptor-positive early breast cancer following 2-3 years of tamoxifen (for a total of 5 years of adjuvant therapy)

Usual Dosage Oral: Adults: 25 mg once daily

Dosage Forms
Tablet:
Aromasin®: 25 mg

exenatide (ex EN a tide)

Synonyms AC 2993; AC002993; exendin-4; LY2148568

U.S./Canadian Brand Names Byetta® [US]

Therapeutic Category Antidiabetic Agent, Incretin Mimetic

Use Management (adjunctive) of type 2 diabetes mellitus (noninsulin-dependent, NIDDM) in patients receiving a sulfonylurea, thiazolidinedione, or metformin (or a combination of these agents)

Usual Dosage SubQ: Adults: Initial: 5 mcg twice daily within 60 minutes prior to a meal; after 1 month, may be increased to 10 mcg twice daily (based on response)

Dosage Forms

Injection, solution:

Byetta®: 250 mcg/mL (1.2 mL [5 mcg/0.02 mL; 60-dose pen]); (2.4 mL [10 mcg/0.04 mL; 60-dose pen])

exendin-4 *see* exenatide *on page* *401*

ExeTuss ***(Discontinued)*** *see* guaifenesin and phenylephrine *on page* *475*

ExeTuss-DM [US] *see* guaifenesin, dextromethorphan, and phenylephrine *on page* *478*

ExeTuss-GP [US] *see* guaifenesin and phenylephrine *on page* *475*

ExeTuss HC ***(Discontinued)***

Exforge® [US] *see* amlodipine and valsartan *on page* *68*

Exforge HCT® [US] *see* amlodipine, valsartan, and hydrochlorothiazide *on page* *69*

Exidine® Scrub ***(Discontinued)*** *see* chlorhexidine gluconate *on page* *210*

Exjade® [US/Can] *see* deferasirox *on page* *280*

ex-lax® [US-OTC] *see* senna *on page* *896*

ex-lax® Maximum Strength [US-OTC] *see* senna *on page* *896*

ex-lax® Ultra [US-OTC] *see* bisacodyl *on page* *142*

Exorex® [US] *see* coal tar *on page* *250*

Exsel® ***(Discontinued)*** *see* selenium sulfide *on page* *895*

Extendryl® ***(Discontinued)*** *see* chlorpheniramine, phenylephrine, and methscopolamine *on page* *218*

Extendryl® GCP [US] *see* carbetapentane, guaifenesin, and phenylephrine *on page* *182*

Extendryl® HC ***(Discontinued)***

Extendryl® JR ***(Discontinued)*** *see* chlorpheniramine, phenylephrine, and methscopolamine *on page* *218*

Extendryl PSE [US] *see* pseudoephedrine and methscopolamine *on page* *835*

Extendryl® SR ***(Discontinued)*** *see* chlorpheniramine, phenylephrine, and methscopolamine *on page* *218*

Extina® [US] *see* ketoconazole *on page* *557*

Extra Action Cough Syrup ***(Discontinued)*** *see* guaifenesin and dextromethorphan *on page* *474*

Extraneal® [US] *see* icodextrin *on page* *517*

EYE001 *see* pegaptanib *on page* *755*

Eye-Lube-A® Solution ***(Discontinued)*** *see* artificial tears *on page* *100*

Eye-Sed® Ophthalmic ***(Discontinued)*** *see* zinc sulfate *on page* *1031*

Eye-Sine™ ***(Discontinued)*** *see* tetrahydrozoline *on page* *951*

Eyestil [Can] *see* hyaluronate and derivatives *on page* *496*

Eye-Stream® [Can] *see* balanced salt solution *on page* *121*

E-Z-Cat® [US] *see* barium *on page* *122*

E-Z-Cat® Dry [US] *see* barium *on page* *122*

EZ-Char™ [US-OTC] *see* charcoal *on page* *206*

E-Z-Disk™ [US] *see* barium *on page* *122*

ezetimibe (ez ET i mibe)

Sound-Alike/Look-Alike Issues

Zetia® may be confused with Zebeta®, Zestril®

U.S./Canadian Brand Names Ezetrol® [Can]; Zetia® [US]

Therapeutic Category Antilipemic Agent, 2-Azetidinone

Use Use in combination with dietary therapy for the treatment of primary hypercholesterolemia (as monotherapy or in combination with HMG-CoA reductase inhibitors); homozygous sitosterolemia; homozygous familial hypercholesterolemia (in combination with atorvastatin or simvastatin); mixed hyperlipidemia (in combination with fenofibrate)

Usual Dosage Oral: Children ≥10 years and Adults: 10 mg/day

Dosage Forms

Tablet:

Zetia®: 10 mg

ezetimibe and simvastatin (ez ET i mibe & SIM va stat in)

Sound-Alike/Look-Alike Issues

Vytorin® may be confused with Vyvanse™

Synonyms simvastatin and ezetimibe

U.S./Canadian Brand Names Vytorin® [US]

Therapeutic Category Antilipemic Agent, 2-Azetidinone

Use Used in combination with dietary modification for the treatment of primary hypercholesterolemia and homozygous familial hypercholesterolemia

Usual Dosage Oral: Adults:

Homozygous familial hypercholesterolemia: Ezetimibe 10 mg and simvastatin 40 mg once daily or ezetimibe 10 mg and simvastatin 80 mg once daily in the evening. Dosing range: Ezetimibe 10 mg and simvastatin 10-80 mg once daily.

Hyperlipidemias: Initial: Ezetimibe 10 mg and simvastatin 20 mg once daily in the evening

Dosage Forms

Tablet:

Vytorin®:

10/10: Ezetimibe 10 mg and simvastatin 10 mg
10/20: Ezetimibe 10 mg and simvastatin 20 mg
10/40: Ezetimibe 10 mg and simvastatin 40 mg
10/80: Ezetimibe 10 mg and simvastatin 80 mg

Ezetrol® [Can] *see* ezetimibe *on page 401*

Ezide® ***(Discontinued)*** *see* hydrochlorothiazide *on page 499*

E•R•O [US-OTC] *see* carbamide peroxide *on page 181*

F_3T *see* trifluridine *on page 986*

fabAV *see* crotalidae polyvalent immune FAB (ovine) *on page 262*

Fabrazyme® [US/Can] *see* agalsidase beta *on page 38*

Factive® [US/Can] *see* gemifloxacin *on page 458*

factor VIIa (recombinant) (FAK ter SEV en aye ree KOM be nant)

Sound-Alike/Look-Alike Issues

NovoSeven® may be confused with Novacet®

Synonyms coagulation factor VIIa; eptacog alfa (activated); rFVIIa

U.S./Canadian Brand Names Niastase® [Can]; NovoSeven® RT [US]

Therapeutic Category Antihemophilic Agent; Blood Product Derivative

Use Treatment of bleeding episodes and prevention of bleeding in surgical interventions in patients with hemophilia A or B with inhibitors to factor VIII or factor IX, acquired hemophilia, and in patients with congenital factor VII deficiency

Usual Dosage Children and Adults: I.V. administration only: Hemophilia A or B with inhibitors:

Bleeding episodes: 90 mcg/kg every 2 hours until hemostasis is achieved or until the treatment is judged ineffective. The dose and interval may be adjusted based upon the severity of bleeding and the degree of hemostasis achieved. For patients experiencing severe bleeds, dosing should be continued at 3- to 6-hour intervals after hemostasis has been achieved and the duration of dosing should be minimized.

Surgical interventions: 90 mcg/kg immediately before surgery; repeat at 2-hour intervals for the duration of surgery. Continue every 2 hours for 48 hours, then every 2-6 hours until healed for minor surgery; continue every 2 hours for 5 days, then every 4 hours until healed for major surgery.

Congenital factor VII deficiency: Bleeding episodes and surgical interventions: 15-30 mcg/kg every 4-6 hours until hemostasis. Doses as low as 10 mcg/kg have been effective.

Acquired hemophilia: 70-90 mcg/kg every 2-3 hours until hemostasis is achieved

Product Availability

Novoseven® RT: FDA approved May 2008; formulation is currently available.

Novo Nordisk® is replacing Novoseven® with Novoseven® RT, a room temperature formulation that allows the product to be stored either refrigerated or at room temperature (2°C to 25°C/36°F to 77°F) prior to reconstitution. The previously available Novoseven® required refrigeration prior to reconstitution.

Dosage Forms

Injection, powder for reconstitution [preservative free]:

NovoSeven® RT: 1 mg, 2 mg, 5 mg

factor VIII (human) *see* antihemophilic factor (human) *on page 81*

factor VIII (human) *see* antihemophilic factor/von Willebrand factor complex (human) *on page 83*

factor VIII (recombinant) *see* antihemophilic factor (recombinant) *on page 82*

factor IX (FAK ter nyne)

Synonyms factor IX concentrate

U.S./Canadian Brand Names AlphaNine® SD [US]; BeneFix® [US/Can]; Immunine® VH [Can]; Mononine® [US/Can]

Therapeutic Category Antihemophilic Agent

Use Control bleeding in patients with factor IX deficiency (hemophilia B or Christmas disease)

Usual Dosage Dosage is expressed in int. units of factor IX activity; dosing must be individualized based on severity of factor IX deficiency, extent and location of bleeding, and clinical status of patient. I.V.:

Formula for int. units required to raise blood level %:

AlphaNine® SD, Mononine®: Children and Adults:

Number of factor IX int. units required = body weight (in kg) x desired factor IX level increase (int. units/dL or % of normal) x 1 int. unit/kg

For example, for a 100% level a 70 kg patient who has an actual level of 20%: Number of factor IX int. units needed = 70 kg x 80% x 1 int. unit/kg = 5600 int. units

BeneFix®:

Children <15 years:

Number of factor IX int. units required = body weight (in kg) x desired factor IX level increase (int. units/dL or % of normal) x 1.4 int. units/kg

Children ≥15 years and Adults:

Number of factor IX int. units required = body weight (in kg) x desired factor IX level increase (int. units/dL or % of normal) x 1.3 int. units/kg

Guidelines: As a general rule, the level of factor IX required for treatment of different conditions is listed below:

Minor spontaneous hemorrhage, prophylaxis:

Desired levels of factor IX for hemostasis: 15% to 25%

Initial loading dose to achieve desired level: 20-30 int. units/kg

Frequency of dosing: Every 12-24 hours if necessary

Duration of treatment: 1-2 days

Moderate hemorrhage:

Desired levels of factor IX for hemostasis: 25% to 50%

Initial loading dose to achieve desired level: 25-50 int. units/kg

Frequency of dosing: Every 12-24 hours

Duration of treatment: 2-7 days

Major hemorrhage:

Desired levels of factor IX for hemostasis: >50%

Initial loading dose to achieve desired level: 30-50 int. units/kg

Frequency of dosing: Every 12-24 hours, depending on half-life and measured factor IX levels (after 3-5 days, maintain at least 20% activity)

Duration of treatment: 7-10 days, depending upon nature of insult

Surgery or major trauma:

Desired levels of factor IX for hemostasis: 50% to 100%

Initial loading dose to achieve desired level: 50-100 int. units/kg

Frequency of dosing: Every 12-24 hours or every 18-30 hours, depending on half-life and measured factor IX levels

Duration of treatment: 7-10 days, depending upon nature of insult

Dosage Forms

Injection, powder for reconstitution (exact potency labeled on each vial):
AlphaNine® SD, BeneFix®, Mononine®

factor IX complex (human) (FAK ter nyne KOM pleks HYU man)

U.S./Canadian Brand Names Bebulin® VH [US]; Profilnine® SD [US]

Therapeutic Category Antihemophilic Agent

Use Prevention and control of bleeding in patients with factor IX deficiency (hemophilia B or Christmas disease)

Usual Dosage Children and Adults: Dosage is expressed in units of factor IX activity and must be individualized. When multiple doses are required, administer at 24-hour intervals unless otherwise specified. Administer I.V. only:

Formula for units required to raise blood level %:

Bebulin® VH: In general, Factor IX 1 int. unit/kg will increase the plasma factor IX level by 0.8%
Number of Factor IX int. units required = body weight (kg) x desired factor IX increase (% of normal) x 1.2 int. units/kg

Profilnine® SD: In general, Factor IX 1 int. unit/kg will increase the plasma factor IX level by 1%:
Number of Factor IX int. units required = bodyweight (kg) x desired factor IX increase (% of normal) x 1 int. unit/kg

As a general rule, the level of factor IX required for treatment of different conditions is listed below:

Minor bleeding (early hemarthrosis, minor epistaxis, gingival bleeding, mild hematuria: Raise Factor IX level to 20% of normal; generally a single dose required.

Moderate bleeding (severe joint bleeding, early hematoma, major open bleeding, minor trauma, minor hemoptysis, hematemesis, melena, major hematuria): Raise Factor IX level to 40% of normal; average duration of treatment is 2 days or until adequate wound healing.

Major bleeding (severe hematoma, major trauma, severe hemoptysis, hematemesis, melena): Raise Factor IX level to 50 to ≥60% of normal; average duration of treatment is 2-3 days or until adequate wound healing. Do not raise ≥50% in patients who may be predisposed to thrombosis.

Minor surgery: Raise Factor IX level to 40% to 60% of normal on day of surgery then decrease from 40% of normal to 20% of normal during initial postoperative period (1-2 weeks or until adequate wound healing). The preoperative dose should be given 1 hour prior to surgery. The average dosing interval may be every 12 hours initially, then every 24 hours later in the postoperative period.

Dental surgery: Raise Factor IX level to 40% to 60% of normal on day of surgery. One infusion is generally sufficient for the extraction of one tooth; for the extraction of multiple teeth replacement therapy may be required for up to 1 week (See dosing guidelines for Minor Surgery).

Major surgery: Raise Factor IX level to ≥60% of normal on day of surgery; do not raise ≥50% in patients who may be predisposed to thrombosis. Decrease from 60% of normal to 20% of normal during initial post operative period (1-2 weeks), and late postoperative period (≥3 weeks) continuing until adequate wound healing is achieved. The preoperative dose should be given 1 hour prior to surgery. The average dosing interval may be every 12 hours initially, then every 24 hours later in the postoperative period.

Long-term prophylactic treatment: 20-30 int. units/kg once or twice a week may reduce frequency of spontaneous hemorrhage; dosing should be individualized.

Dosage Forms

Injection, powder for reconstitution [single-dose vial; exact potency labeled on each vial]:
Bebulin® VH, Profilnine® SD

factor IX concentrate *see* factor IX *on page 403*

Factrel® ***(Discontinued)***

famciclovir (fam SYE kloe veer)

Sound-Alike/Look-Alike Issues

Famvir® may be confused with Femara®

U.S./Canadian Brand Names Apo-Famciclovir [Can]; CO Famciclovir [Can]; Famvir® [US/Can]; PMS-Famciclovir [Can]; Sandoz-Famciclovir [Can]

Therapeutic Category Antiviral Agent

Use Treatment of acute herpes zoster (shingles); treatment and suppression of recurrent episodes of genital herpes in immunocompetent patients; treatment of herpes labialis (cold sores) in immunocompetent patients; treatment of recurrent mucocutaneous/genital herpes simplex in HIV-infected patients

Usual Dosage Oral: Adults:

Acute herpes zoster: 500 mg every 8 hours for 7 days (**Note:** Initiate therapy within 72 hours of rash onset.)

Recurrent genital herpes simplex in immunocompetent patients:

Initial: 1000 mg twice daily for 1 day (**Note:** initiate therapy within 6 hours of symptoms/lesions.)

Suppressive therapy: 250 mg twice daily for up to 1 year

Recurrent herpes labialis (cold sores): 1500 mg as a single dose; initiate therapy at first sign or symptom such as tingling, burning, or itching (initiated within 1 hour in clinical studies)

Recurrent mucocutaneous/genital herpes simplex in HIV patients: 500 mg twice daily for 7 days

Dosage Forms

Tablet: 125 mg, 250 mg, 500 mg

Famvir®: 125 mg, 250 mg, 500 mg

famotidine (fa MOE ti deen)

Sound-Alike/Look-Alike Issues

famotidine may be confused with FLUoxetine, furosemide

U.S./Canadian Brand Names Apo-Famotidine® Injectable [Can]; Apo-Famotidine® [Can]; Famotidine Omega [Can]; Gen-Famotidine [Can]; Novo-Famotidine [Can]; Nu-Famotidine [Can]; Pepcid® AC Maximum Strength [US-OTC]; Pepcid® AC [US-OTC/Can]; Pepcid® I.V. [Can]; Pepcid® [US/Can]; ratio-Famotidine [Can]; Riva-Famotidine [Can]; Ulcidine [Can]

Therapeutic Category Histamine H_2 Antagonist

Use Maintenance therapy and treatment of duodenal ulcer; treatment of gastroesophageal reflux, active benign gastric ulcer, and pathological hypersecretory conditions

OTC labeling: Relief of heartburn, acid indigestion, and sour stomach

Usual Dosage

Children: Treatment duration and dose should be individualized

Peptic ulcer: 1-16 years:

Oral: 0.5 mg/kg/day at bedtime or divided twice daily (maximum dose: 40 mg/day); doses of up to 1 mg/kg/day have been used in clinical studies

I.V.: 0.25 mg/kg every 12 hours (maximum dose: 40 mg/day); doses of up to 0.5 mg/kg have been used in clinical studies

GERD: Oral:

<3 months: 0.5 mg/kg once daily

3-12 months: 0.5 mg/kg twice daily

1-16 years: 1 mg/kg/day divided twice daily (maximum dose: 40 mg twice daily); doses of up to 2 mg/kg/day have been used in clinical studies

Children ≥12 years and Adults: Heartburn, indigestion, sour stomach: OTC labeling: Oral: 10-20 mg every 12 hours; dose may be taken 15-60 minutes before eating foods known to cause heartburn

Adults:

Duodenal ulcer: Oral: Acute therapy: 40 mg/day at bedtime for 4-8 weeks; maintenance therapy: 20 mg/day at bedtime

Gastric ulcer: Oral: Acute therapy: 40 mg/day at bedtime

Hypersecretory conditions: Oral: Initial: 20 mg every 6 hours, may increase in increments up to 160 mg every 6 hours

GERD: Oral: 20 mg twice daily for 6 weeks

Esophagitis and accompanying symptoms due to GERD: Oral: 20 mg or 40 mg twice daily for up to 12 weeks

Patients unable to take oral medication: I.V.: 20 mg every 12 hours

Dosage Forms

Infusion [premixed in NS]:

Injection, solution: 10 mg/mL (4 mL, 20 mL, 50 mL)

Injection, solution [preservative free]: 10 mg/mL (2 mL)

Powder for oral suspension:

Pepcid®: 40 mg/5 mL

Tablet: 10 mg [OTC], 20 mg, 40 mg

Pepcid®: 20 mg, 40 mg

Pepcid® AC [OTC]: 10 mg, 20 mg

Pepcid® AC Maximum Strength [OTC]: 20 mg

famotidine, calcium carbonate, and magnesium hydroxide

(fa MOE ti deen, KAL see um KAR bun ate, & mag NEE zhum hye DROKS ide)

Synonyms calcium carbonate, magnesium hydroxide, and famotidine; magnesium hydroxide, famotidine, and calcium carbonate

U.S./Canadian Brand Names Pepcid® Complete [US-OTC/Can]

Therapeutic Category Antacid; Histamine H_2 Antagonist

Use Relief of heartburn due to acid indigestion

Usual Dosage Oral: Children ≥12 years and Adults: Relief of heartburn due to acid indigestion: Pepcid® Complete: 1 tablet as needed; no more than 2 tablets in 24 hours; do **not** swallow whole, chew tablet completely before swallowing; do not use for longer than 14 days

Dosage Forms

Tablet, chewable:

Pepcid® Complete [OTC]: Famotidine 10 mg, calcium carbonate 800 mg, and magnesium hydroxide 165 mg

Famotidine Omega [Can] *see* famotidine *on page 405*

Famvir® [US/Can] *see* famciclovir *on page 404*

Fanapt™ [US] *see* iloperidone *on page 519*

Fansidar® [US] *see* sulfadoxine and pyrimethamine *on page 928*

2F-ara-AMP *see* fludarabine *on page 425*

Fareston® [US/Can] *see* toremifene *on page 971*

Faslodex® [US] *see* fulvestrant *on page 448*

Fasturtec® [Can] *see* rasburicase *on page 854*

fat emulsion (fat e MUL shun)

Synonyms intravenous fat emulsion

U.S./Canadian Brand Names Intralipid® [US/Can]; Liposyn® II [US/Can]; Liposyn® III [US]

Therapeutic Category Intravenous Nutritional Therapy

Use Source of calories and essential fatty acids for patients requiring parenteral nutrition of extended duration; prevention and treatment of essential fatty acid deficiency (EFAD)

Usual Dosage I.V.: **Note:** At the onset of therapy, the patient should be observed for any immediate allergic reactions.

Nutrition:

Premature infants: Initial dose: 0.25-0.5 g/kg/day, increase by 0.25-0.5 g/kg/day to a maximum of 3 g/kg/day depending on needs/nutritional goals; limit to 1 g/kg/day if on phototherapy; should be administered over 24 hours (A.S.P.E.N. guidelines)

Infants and Children: Initial dose: 0.5-1 g/kg/day, increase by 0.5 g/kg/day to a maximum of 3 g/kg/day depending on needs/nutritional goals; may administer over 24 hours (A.S.P.E.N. guidelines)

Note: Pediatric patients: Monitor triglycerides while receiving intralipids. If serum triglyceride levels >200 mg/dL, stop infusion and restart at 0.5-1g/kg/day. Intravenous heparin (1 unit/mL of parenteral nutrition) may enhance the clearance of lipid emulsions.

Adults: Initial dose: 1 g/kg/day, increase by 0.5-1 g/kg/day to a maximum of 2.5-3 g/kg/day

Prevention of essential fatty acid deficiency (EFAD): Adults: Administer 8% to 10% of total caloric intake as fat emulsion (may be higher in stressed patients with EFAD); may be given 2-3 times weekly to meet essential fatty acid requirements

Dosage Forms

Injection, emulsion [soybean oil]:

Intralipid®: 20% [200 mg/mL] (50 mL, 100 mL, 250 mL, 500 mL, 1000 mL); 30% [300 mg/mL] (500 mL)

Liposyn® II: 10% (500 mL); 20% (500 mL)

Liposyn® III: 10% [100 mg/mL] (200 mL, 500 mL); 20% [200 mg/mL] (200 mL, 500 mL); 30% [300 mg/mL] (500 mL)

Father John's® [US-OTC] *see* dextromethorphan *on page 295*

Father John's® Plus [US-OTC] *see* chlorpheniramine, phenylephrine, and dextromethorphan *on page 217*

FazaClo® [US] *see* clozapine *on page 249*

5-FC *see* flucytosine *on page 425*

FC1157a *see* toremifene *on page 971*

FE200486 *see* degarelix *on page 281*

febuxostat (feb UX oh stat)

Synonyms TEI-6720; TMX-67

U.S./Canadian Brand Names Uloric® [US]

Therapeutic Category Xanthine Oxidase Inhibitor

Use Chronic management of hyperuricemia in patients with gout

Usual Dosage Oral: Adults: Initial: 40 mg once daily; may increase to 80 mg once daily in patients who do not achieve a serum uric acid level <6 mg/dL after 2 weeks

Note: It is recommended to take an NSAID or colchicine with initiation of therapy and may continue for up to 6 months to help prevent gout flares. If a gout flare occurs, febuxostat does not need to be discontinued.

Dosage Forms

Tablet:

Uloric®: 40 mg, 80 mg

Fedahist® Expectorant *(Discontinued)* *see* guaifenesin and pseudoephedrine *on page 477*

Fedahist® Expectorant Pediatric *(Discontinued)* *see* guaifenesin and pseudoephedrine *on page 477*

Fedahist® Tablet *(Discontinued)* *see* chlorpheniramine and pseudoephedrine *on page 215*

Feen-A-Mint® *(Discontinued)* *see* bisacodyl *on page 142*

Feiba VH [US] *see* antiinhibitor coagulant complex *on page 85*

Feiba VH Immuno [Can] *see* antiinhibitor coagulant complex *on page 85*

felbamate (FEL ba mate)

U.S./Canadian Brand Names Felbatol® [US]

Therapeutic Category Anticonvulsant

Use Not as a first-line antiepileptic treatment; only in those patients who respond inadequately to alternative treatments and whose epilepsy is so severe that a substantial risk of aplastic anemia and/or liver failure is deemed acceptable in light of the benefits conferred by its use. Patient must be fully advised of risk and provide signed written informed consent. Felbamate can be used as either monotherapy or adjunctive therapy in the treatment of partial seizures (with and without generalization) and in adults with epilepsy. Used as adjunctive therapy in the treatment of partial and generalized seizures associated with Lennox-Gastaut syndrome in children.

Usual Dosage Anticonvulsant:

Monotherapy: Children >14 years and Adults:

Initial: 1200 mg/day in divided doses 3 or 4 times/day; titrate previously untreated patients under close clinical supervision, increasing the dosage in 600 mg increments every 2 weeks to 2400 mg/day based on clinical response and thereafter to 3600 mg/day as clinically indicated

Conversion to monotherapy: Initiate at 1200 mg/day in divided doses 3 or 4 times/day, reduce the dosage of the concomitant anticonvulsant(s) by 20% to 33% at the initiation of felbamate therapy; at week 2, increase the felbamate dosage to 2400 mg/day while reducing the dosage of the other anticonvulsant(s) up to an additional 33% of their original dosage; at week 3, increase the felbamate dosage up to 3600 mg/day and continue to reduce the dosage of the other anticonvulsant(s) as clinically indicated

Adjunctive therapy: **Note:** Dose of concomitant carbamazepine, phenobarbital, phenytoin, or valproic acid should be decreased by 20% to 33% when initiating felbamate therapy. Further dosage reductions may be necessary as dose of felbamate is increased.

Children 2-14 years with Lennox-Gastaut syndrome: Initial: 15 mg/kg/day in divided doses 3 or 4 times/day; may increase once per week by 15 mg/kg/day increments up to 45 mg/kg/day in divided doses 3 or 4 times/day.

Children >14 years and Adults: Initial: 1200 mg/day in divided doses 3 or 4 times/day; may increase once per week by 1200 mg/day increments up to 3600 mg/day in divided doses 3 or 4 times/day.

Dosage Forms

Suspension, oral:

Felbatol®: 600 mg/5 mL

Tablet:

Felbatol®: 400 mg, 600 mg

Felbatol® [US] *see* felbamate *on page 407*

Feldene® [US] *see* piroxicam *on page 788*

felodipine (fe LOE di peen)

Sound-Alike/Look-Alike Issues

Plendil® may be confused with Isordil®, pindolol, Pletal®, Prilosec®, Prinivil®

U.S./Canadian Brand Names Plendil® [Can]; Renedil® [Can]

Therapeutic Category Calcium Channel Blocker

Use Treatment of hypertension

Usual Dosage Oral: Adults: Hypertension: 2.5-10 mg once daily; usual initial dose: 5 mg; increase by 5 mg at 2-week intervals, as needed, to a maximum of 20 mg/day

Usual dose range (JNC 7) for hypertension: 2.5-20 mg once daily

felodipine and enalapril *see* enalapril and felodipine *on page 353*

felodipine and ramipril *see* ramipril and felodipine *(Canada only) on page 850*

Femara® [US/Can] *see* letrozole *on page 575*

Fematrol [US-OTC] *see* bisacodyl *on page 142*

Femcet® *(Discontinued)*

Femcon® Fe [US] *see* ethinyl estradiol and norethindrone *on page 390*

Femguard® *(Discontinued)* *see* sulfabenzamide, sulfacetamide, and sulfathiazole *on page 926*

femhrt® [US/Can] *see* ethinyl estradiol and norethindrone *on page 390*

Femilax™ [US-OTC] *see* bisacodyl *on page 142*

Femiron® [US-OTC] *see* ferrous fumarate *on page 413*

Fem-Prin® [US-OTC] *see* acetaminophen, aspirin, and caffeine *on page 24*

Femring® [US] *see* estradiol *on page 373*

Femstat® One [Can] *see* butoconazole *on page 163*

Femtrace® [US] *see* estradiol *on page 373*

Fenesin DM IR [US] *see* guaifenesin and dextromethorphan *on page 474*

Fenesin IR [US] *see* guaifenesin *on page 473*

Fenesin PE IR [US] *see* guaifenesin and phenylephrine *on page 475*

fenofibrate (fen oh FYE brate)

Sound-Alike/Look-Alike Issues

TriCor® may be confused with Tracleer®

Synonyms procetofene; proctofene

U.S./Canadian Brand Names Antara® [US]; Apo-Feno-Micro® [Can]; Apo-Fenofibrate® [Can]; Dom-Fenofibrate Supra [Can]; Feno-Micro-200 [Can]; Fenoglide™ [US]; Fenomax [Can]; Gen-Fenofibrate Micro [Can]; Lipidil EZ® [Can]; Lipidil Micro® [Can]; Lipidil Supra® [Can]; Lipofen® [US]; Lofibra® [US]; Novo-Fenofibrate [Can]; Novo-Fenofibrate-S [Can]; Nu-Fenofibrate [Can]; PHL-Fenofibrate Supra [Can]; PMS-Fenofibrate Micro [Can]; Pro-Feno-Super [Can]; ratio-Fenofibrate MC [Can]; Riva-Fenofibrate Micro [Can]; Sandoz Fenofibrate S [Can]; TriCor® [US]; Triglide™ [US]

Therapeutic Category Antihyperlipidemic Agent, Miscellaneous

Use Adjunct to dietary therapy for the treatment of adults with elevations of serum triglyceride levels (types IV and V hyperlipidemia); adjunct to dietary therapy for the reduction of low density lipoprotein cholesterol (LDL-C), total cholesterol (total-C), triglycerides, and apolipoprotein B (apo B) in adult patients with primary hypercholesterolemia or mixed dyslipidemia (Fredrickson types IIa and IIb)

Usual Dosage Oral: Adults:

Hypertriglyceridemia: Initial:

Antara® (micronized): 43-130 mg/day; maximum dose: 130 mg/day
Fenoglide™: 40-120 mg/day; maximum dose: 120 mg/day
Lipidil EZ® [CAN; not available in U.S.]: 145 mg/day; maximum dose: 145 mg/day
Lipidil Micro® [CAN; not available in U.S.]: 200 mg/day; maximum dose: 200 mg/day
Lipidil Supra® [CAN; not available in U.S.]: 160 mg/day; maximum dose: 200 mg/day
Lipofen®: 50-150 mg/day; maximum dose: 150 mg/day
Lofibra® (micronized): 67-200 mg/day with meals; maximum dose: 200 mg/day
Lofibra® (tablets): 54-160 mg/day; maximum dose: 160 mg/day
TriCor®: 48-145 mg/day; maximum dose: 145 mg/day
Triglide™: 50-160 mg/day; maximum dose: 160 mg/day

Hypercholesterolemia or mixed hyperlipidemia:

Antara® (micronized): 130 mg/day
Fenoglide™: 120 mg/day

Lipidil EZ® [CAN; not available in U.S.]: 145 mg/day; maximum dose: 145 mg/day
Lipidil Micro® [CAN; not available in U.S.]: 200 mg/day; maximum dose: 200 mg/day
Lipidil Supra® [CAN; not available in U.S.]: 160 mg/day; maximum dose: 200 mg/day
Lipofen®: 150 mg/day
Lofibra® (micronized): 200 mg/day
Lofibra® (tablets): 160 mg/day
TriCor®: 145 mg/day
Triglide™: 160 mg/day

Dosage Forms

Capsule:
Lipofen®: 50 mg, 150 mg
Capsule [micronized]: 67 mg, 134 mg, 200 mg
Antara®: 43 mg, 130 mg
Lofibra®: 67 mg, 134 mg, 200 mg
Tablet: 54 mg, 160 mg
Fenoglide™: 40 mg, 120 mg
Lofibra®: 54 mg, 160 mg
TriCor®: 48 mg, 145 mg
Triglide™: 50 mg, 160 mg

fenofibric acid (fen oh FYE brik AS id)

Sound-Alike/Look-Alike Issues
TriLipix™ may be confused with Trileptal®, TriLyte®

Synonyms ABT-335; choline fenofibrate

U.S./Canadian Brand Names TriLipix™ [US]

Therapeutic Category Antilipemic Agent, Fibric Acid

Use Adjunct to dietary therapy for the treatment of severely elevated serum triglyceride levels; adjunct to dietary therapy for the reduction of low density lipoprotein cholesterol (LDL-C), total cholesterol (total-C), triglycerides, and apolipoprotein B (apo B) and to increase high density lipoprotein cholesterol (HDL-C) in patients with primary hypercholesterolemia or mixed dyslipidemia

TriLipix™ is also indicated as adjunct to dietary therapy concomitantly with a statin to reduce triglyceride levels and increase HDL-C levels in patients with mixed dyslipidemia and coronary heart disease (CHD) or at risk for CHD

Usual Dosage Oral: Adults:
Mixed dyslipidemia (coadministered with a statin): 135 mg once daily (maximum: 135 mg/day)
Hypertriglyceridemia: Initial: 45-135 mg once daily; Maintenance: Individualize according to patient response (maximum: 135 mg/day)
Primary hypercholesterolemia or mixed dyslipidemia: 135 mg once daily (maximum: 135 mg/day)

Dosage Forms

Capsule, delayed release:
TriLipix™: 45 mg, 135 mg
Tablet:
Fibricor™: 35 mg, 105 mg

Fenoglide™ [US] *see* fenofibrate *on page* 408

fenoldopam (fe NOL doe pam)

Synonyms fenoldopam mesylate

U.S./Canadian Brand Names Corlopam® [US/Can]

Therapeutic Category Antihypertensive Agent

Use Treatment of severe hypertension (up to 48 hours in adults), including in patients with renal compromise; short-term (up to 4 hours) blood pressure reduction in pediatric patients

Usual Dosage I.V.: Hypertension, severe:
Children: Initial: 0.2 mcg/kg/minute; may be increased to dosages of 0.3-0.5 mcg/kg/minute every 20-30 minutes (maximum dose: 0.8 mcg/kg/minute); limited to short-term (4 hours) use
Adults: Initial: 0.1-0.3 mcg/kg/minute (lower initial doses may be associated with less reflex tachycardia); may be increased in increments of 0.05-0.1 mcg/kg/minute every 15 minutes until target blood pressure is reached; the maximal infusion rate reported in clinical studies was 1.6 mcg/kg/minute

Dosage Forms

Injection, solution: 10 mg/mL (1 mL, 2 mL)
Corlopam®: 10 mg/mL (1 mL, 2 mL)

fenoldopam mesylate *see* fenoldopam *on page 409*

Fenomax [Can] *see* fenofibrate *on page 408*

Feno-Micro-200 [Can] *see* fenofibrate *on page 408*

fenoprofen (fen oh PROE fen)

Sound-Alike/Look-Alike Issues

fenoprofen may be confused with flurbiprofen

Nalfon® may be confused with Naldecon®

Synonyms fenoprofen calcium

U.S./Canadian Brand Names Nalfon® [US/Can]

Therapeutic Category Analgesic, Nonnarcotic; Nonsteroidal Antiinflammatory Drug (NSAID)

Use Symptomatic treatment of acute and chronic rheumatoid arthritis and osteoarthritis; relief of mild-to-moderate pain

Usual Dosage Oral: Adults:

Rheumatoid arthritis, osteoarthritis: 300-600 mg 3-4 times/day; maximum dose: 3.2 g/day

Mild-to-moderate pain: 200 mg every 4-6 hours as needed; maximum dose: 3.2 g/day

Dosage Forms

Capsule:

Nalfon®: 200 mg

Tablet: 600 mg

fenoprofen calcium *see* fenoprofen *on page 410*

fenoterol *(Canada only)* (fen oh TER ole)

Synonyms fenoterol hydrobromide

U.S./Canadian Brand Names Berotec® [Can]

Therapeutic Category Beta$_2$-Adrenergic Agonist Agent

Use Treatment and prevention of symptoms of reversible obstructive pulmonary disease (including asthma and acute bronchospasm), chronic bronchitis, emphysema

Usual Dosage Inhalation: Children ≥12 years of age and Adults:

MDI:

Acute treatment: 1 puff initially; may repeat in 5 minutes; if relief is not evident, additional doses and/or other therapy may be necessary

Intermittent/long-term treatment: 1-2 puffs 3-4 times/day (maximum of 8 puffs/24 hours)

Solution: 0.5-1 mg (up to maximum of 2.5 mg)

Dosage Forms [CAN] = Canadian brand name

Aerosol for inhalation: MDI:

Berotec® [CAN]: 100 mcg/dose [not available in the U.S.]

Solution for inhalation:

Berotec® [CAN] 0.625 mg/mL (2 mL); 0.25 mg/mL (2 mL) [not available in the U.S.]

fenoterol hydrobromide *see* fenoterol *(Canada only) on page 410*

fentanyl (FEN ta nil)

Sound-Alike/Look-Alike Issues

fentaNYL may be confused with alfentanil, SUFentanil

Synonyms fentanyl citrate; fentanyl hydrochloride; OTFC (oral transmucosal fentanyl citrate)

Tall-Man fenta**NYL**

U.S./Canadian Brand Names Actiq® [US/Can]; Duragesic® [US/Can]; Fentanyl Citrate Injection, USP [Can]; Fentora® [US]; Novo-Fentanyl [Can]; Onsolis™ [US]; RAN™-Fentanyl Transdermal System [Can]; ratio-Fentanyl [Can]; Sublimaze® [US]

Therapeutic Category Analgesic, Narcotic; General Anesthetic

Controlled Substance C-II

Use

Injection: Relief of pain, preoperative medication, adjunct to general or regional anesthesia

Iontophoretic transdermal system (Ionsys™): Short-term, in-hospital management of acute postoperative pain

Transdermal patch (eg, Duragesic®): Management of persistent moderate-to-severe chronic pain

Transmucosal lozenge (eg, Actiq®), buccal tablet (Fentora®): Management of breakthrough cancer pain in opioid-tolerant patients

Usual Dosage Note: These are guidelines and do not represent the maximum doses that may be required in all patients. Doses and dosage intervals should be titrated to pain relief/prevention. Monitor vital signs routinely. Single I.M. doses have a duration of 1-2 hours, single I.V. doses last 0.5-1 hour.

Surgery:

Children ≥2 years: Adjunct to anesthesia (induction and maintenance): Slow I.V.: 2-3 mcg/kg/dose every 1-2 hours as needed

Adults:

Premedication: I.M., slow I.V.: 50-100 mcg/dose 30-60 minutes prior to surgery

Adjunct to regional anesthesia: Slow I.V.: 25-100 mcg/dose over 1-2 minutes. **Note:** An I.V. should be in place with regional anesthesia so the I.M. route is rarely used but still maintained as an option in the package labeling.

Adjunct to general anesthesia: Slow I.V.:

Low dose: 0.5-2 mcg/kg/dose depending on the indication

Moderate dose: Initial: 2-20 mcg/kg/dose; Maintenance (bolus or infusion): 1-2 mcg/kg/hour. Discontinuing fentanyl infusion 30-60 minutes prior to the end of surgery will usually allow adequate ventilation upon emergence from anesthesia. For "fast-tracking" and early extubation following major surgery, total fentanyl doses are limited to 10-15 mcg/kg.

High dose: 20-50 mcg/kg/dose; **Note:** Fentanyl is rarely used, but is still maintained in the package labeling.

Breakthrough cancer pain: For patients who are tolerant to and currently receiving opioid therapy for persistent cancer pain; dosing should be individually titrated to provide adequate analgesia with minimal side effects. Dose titration should be done if patient requires more than 1 dose/breakthrough pain episode for several consecutive episodes. Patients experiencing >4 breakthrough pain episodes/day should have the dose of their long-term opioid reevaluated.

Children ≥16 years and Adults: Lozenge: Initial dose: 200 mcg; the second dose may be started 15 minutes after completion of the first dose. Consumption should be limited to ≤4 units/day. Additional requirements suggest need for improved baseline therapy.

Adults: Buccal tablet (Fentora®): Initial dose: 100 mcg; a second 100 mcg dose, if needed, may be started 30 minutes after the start of the first dose. **Note:** For patients previously using the transmucosal lozenge (Actiq®), the initial dose should be selected using the conversions listed below (maximum: 2 doses per breakthrough pain episode every 4 hours).

Dose titration, if required, should be done using multiples of the 100 mcg tablets. Patient can take two 100 mcg tablets (one on each side of mouth). If that dose is not successful, can use four 100 mcg tablets (two on each side of mouth). If titration requires >400 mcg/dose, then use 200 mcg tablets.

Conversion from lozenge to buccal tablet (Fentora®):

Lozenge dose 200-400 mcg, then buccal tablet 100 mcg

Lozenge dose 600-800 mcg, then buccal tablet 200 mcg

Lozenge dose 1200-1600 mcg, then buccal tablet 400 mcg

Note: Four 100 mcg buccal tablets deliver approximately 12% and 13% higher values of C_{max} and AUC, respectively, compared to one 400 mcg buccal tablet. To prevent confusion, patient should only have one strength available at a time. Using more than four buccal tablets at a time has not been studied.

Chronic pain management: Children ≥2 years and Adults (opioid-tolerant patients): Transdermal patch (eg, Duragesic®):

Initial: To convert patients from oral or parenteral opioids to transdermal patch, a 24-hour analgesic requirement should be calculated (based on prior opiate use). Using the tables, the appropriate initial dose can be determined. The initial fentanyl dosage may be approximated from the 24-hour morphine dosage equivalent and titrated to minimize adverse effects and provide analgesia. With the initial application, the absorption of transdermal fentanyl requires several hours to reach plateau; therefore transdermal fentanyl is inappropriate for management of acute pain. Change patch every 72 hours.

Conversion from continuous infusion of fentanyl: In patients who have adequate pain relief with a fentanyl infusion, fentanyl may be converted to transdermal dosing at a rate equivalent to the intravenous rate. A two-step taper of the infusion to be completed over 12 hours has been recommended after the patch is applied. The infusion is decreased to 50% of the original rate six hours after the application of the first patch, and subsequently discontinued twelve hours after application.

Titration: Short-acting agents may be required until analgesic efficacy is established and/or as supplements for "breakthrough" pain. The amount of supplemental doses should be closely monitored. Appropriate dosage increases may be based on daily supplemental dosage using the ratio of 45 mg/24 hours of oral morphine to a 12.5 mcg/hour increase in fentanyl dosage.

Frequency of adjustment: The dosage should not be titrated more frequently than every 3 days after the initial dose or every 6 days thereafter. Patients should wear a consistent fentanyl dosage through two applications (6 days) before dosage increase based on supplemental opiate dosages can be estimated. **Note:** Upon discontinuation, ~17 hours are required for a 50% decrease in fentanyl levels.

Frequency of application: The majority of patients may be controlled on every 72-hour administration; however, a small number of patients require every 48-hour administration.

Product Availability

Onsolis™: FDA approved July 2009; availability expected in the fourth quarter of 2009

Onsolis™ (fentanyl buccal soluble film) is approved for the management of breakthrough pain in adult patients with cancer. It will only be available through a restricted distribution program called the FOCUS program.

Dosage Forms

Injection, solution [preservative free]: 0.05 mg/mL (2 mL, 5 mL, 10 mL, 20 mL, 50 mL)

Sublimaze®: 0.05 mg/mL (2 mL, 5 mL, 20 mL)

Lozenge, oral [transmucosal]: 200 mcg, 400 mcg, 600 mcg, 800 mcg, 1200 mcg, 1600 mcg

Actiq®: 200 mcg, 400 mcg, 600 mcg, 800 mcg, 1200 mcg, 1600 mcg

Powder, for prescription compounding: USP (1 g)

Tablet, for buccal application:

Fentora®: 100 mcg, 200 mcg, 300 mcg, 400 mcg, 600 mcg, 800 mcg

Transdermal system, topical: 12 (5s) [delivers 12.5 mcg/hour; 3.13 cm^2]; 12 (5s) [delivers 12.5 mcg/hour; 5 cm^2]; 25 (5s) [delivers 25 mcg/hour; 10 cm^2]; 25 (5s) [delivers 25 mcg/hour; 6.25 cm^2]; 50 (5s) [delivers 50 mcg/hour; 12.5 cm^2]; 50 (5s) [delivers 50 mcg/hour; 20 cm^2]; 75 (5s) [delivers 75 mcg/hour; 18.75 cm^2]; 75 (5s) [delivers 75 mcg/hour; 30 cm^2]; 75 (5s) [delivers 75 mcg/hour; 32.1 cm^2]; 100 (5s) [delivers 100 mcg/hour; 25 cm^2]; 100 (5s) [delivers 100 mcg/hour; 40 cm^2]; 100 (5s) [delivers 100 mcg/hour; 42.8 cm^2]

Duragesic®: 12 [delivers 12.5 mcg/hour; 5 cm^2] (5s); 25 [delivers 25 mcg/hour; 10 cm^2] (5s); 50 [delivers 50 mcg/hour; 20 cm^2] (5s); 75 [delivers 75 mcg/hour; 30 cm^2]; 100 [delivers 100 mcg/hour; 40 cm^2] (5s)

fentanyl citrate *see* fentanyl *on page 410*

Fentanyl Citrate Injection, USP [Can] *see* fentanyl *on page 410*

fentanyl hydrochloride *see* fentanyl *on page 410*

Fentanyl Oralet® *(Discontinued)* *see* fentanyl *on page 410*

Fentora® [US] *see* fentanyl *on page 410*

Feosol® [US-OTC] *see* ferrous sulfate *on page 414*

Feosol® Elixir *(Discontinued)* *see* ferrous sulfate *on page 414*

Feostat® *(Discontinued)* *see* ferrous fumarate *on page 413*

Feraheme™ [US] *see* ferumoxytol *on page 416*

Ferancee® *(Discontinued)* *see* ferrous sulfate and ascorbic acid *on page 415*

Feratab® [US-OTC] *see* ferrous sulfate *on page 414*

Fer-Gen-Sol [US-OTC] *see* ferrous sulfate *on page 414*

Fergon® [US-OTC] *see* ferrous gluconate *on page 414*

Feridex I.V.® *(Discontinued)* *see* ferumoxides *on page 416*

Fer-In-Sol® [US-OTC/Can] *see* ferrous sulfate *on page 414*

Fer-In-Sol® Syrup *(Discontinued)* *see* ferrous sulfate *on page 414*

Fer-iron® [US-OTC] *see* ferrous sulfate *on page 414*

Fermalac [Can] *see* Lactobacillus *on page 564*

Ferodan™ [Can] *see* ferrous sulfate *on page 414*

Fero-Grad 500® [US-OTC] *see* ferrous sulfate and ascorbic acid *on page 415*

Fero-Gradumet® *(Discontinued)* *see* ferrous sulfate *on page 414*

Ferospace® *(Discontinued)* *see* ferrous sulfate *on page 414*

Ferralet® *(Discontinued)* *see* ferrous gluconate *on page 414*

Ferralyn® Lanacaps® *(Discontinued)* *see* ferrous sulfate *on page 414*

Ferra-TD® *(Discontinued)* *see* ferrous sulfate *on page 414*

Ferretts [US-OTC] *see* ferrous fumarate *on page 413*

Ferrex 150 [US-OTC] *see* polysaccharide-iron complex *on page 799*

ferric (III) hexacyanoferrate (II) *see* ferric hexacyanoferrate *on page 413*

ferric gluconate (FER ik GLOO koe nate)

Sound-Alike/Look-Alike Issues

ferric gluconate may be confused with ferumoxytol

Ferrlecit® may be confused with Ferralet®

Synonyms sodium ferric gluconate

U.S./Canadian Brand Names Ferrlecit® [US/Can]

Therapeutic Category Iron Salt

Use Repletion of total body iron content in patients with iron-deficiency anemia who are undergoing hemodialysis in conjunction with erythropoietin therapy

Usual Dosage I.V.: Repletion of iron in hemodialysis patients:

Children ≥6 years: 1.5 mg/kg of elemental iron (maximum: 125 mg/dose) diluted in NS 25 mL, administered over 60 minutes at 8 sequential dialysis sessions

Adults: 125 mg elemental iron per 10 mL (either by I.V. infusion or slow I.V. injection). Most patients will require a cumulative dose of 1 g elemental iron over approximately 8 sequential dialysis treatments to achieve a favorable response.

Note: A test dose of 2 mL diluted in NS 50 mL administered over 60 minutes was previously recommended (not in current manufacturer labeling). Doses >125 mg are associated with increased adverse events.

Dosage Forms

Injection, solution:

Ferrlecit®: Elemental iron 12.5 mg/mL (5 mL)

ferric hexacyanoferrate (FER ik hex a SYE an oh fer ate)

Synonyms ferric (III) hexacyanoferrate (II); insoluble prussian blue; prussian blue

U.S./Canadian Brand Names Radiogardase® [US]

Therapeutic Category Antidote

Use Treatment of known or suspected internal contamination with radioactive cesium and/or radioactive or nonradioactive thallium

Usual Dosage Oral: Internal contamination with radioactive cesium and/or radioactive or nonradioactive thallium:

Children 2-12 years: 1 g 3 times/day; treatment should begin as soon as possible following exposure, but is also effective if therapy is delayed

Children >12 years and Adults: 3 g 3 times/day; treatment should begin as soon as possible following exposure, but is also effective if therapy is delayed

Note: Cesium exposure: Once internal radioactivity is substantially decreased, dosage may be reduced to 1-2 g 3 times/day to improve gastrointestinal tolerance

Dosage Forms

Capsule:

Radiogardase®: 0.5 g

Ferrlecit® [US/Can] *see* ferric gluconate *on page 413*

Ferro-Sequels® [US-OTC] *see* ferrous fumarate *on page 413*

ferrous fumarate (FER us FYOO ma rate)

Sound-Alike/Look-Alike Issues

Feostat® may be confused with Feosol®

Synonyms iron fumarate

U.S./Canadian Brand Names Femiron® [US-OTC]; Ferretts [US-OTC]; Ferro-Sequels® [US-OTC]; Hemocyte® [US-OTC]; Ircon® [US-OTC]; Nephro-Fer® [US-OTC]; Palafer® [Can]

Therapeutic Category Electrolyte Supplement, Oral

Use Prevention and treatment of iron-deficiency anemias

Usual Dosage

Dietary Reference Intake: Dose is RDA presented as elemental iron unless otherwise noted:

0-6 months: 0.27 mg/day (adequate intake)

7-12 months: 11 mg/day

1-3 years: 7 mg/day

4-8 years: 10 mg/day

9-13 years: 8 mg/day

14-18 years: Male: 11 mg/day; Female: 15 mg/day; Pregnant female: 27 mg/day; Lactating female: 10 mg/day
19-50 years: Male: 8 mg/day; Female: 18 mg/day; Pregnant female: 27 mg/day; Lactating female: 9 mg/day
≥50 years: 8 mg/day

Doses expressed in terms of elemental iron; elemental iron content of ferrous fumarate is 33%.
Oral:
Children:
Severe iron-deficiency anemia: 4-6 mg elemental iron/kg/day in 3 divided doses
Mild-to-moderate iron-deficiency anemia: 3 mg elemental iron/kg/day in 1-2 divided doses
Prophylaxis: 1-2 mg elemental iron/kg/day
Adults:
Iron deficiency: Usual range: 150-200 mg elemental iron/day in divided doses; 60-100 mg elemental iron twice daily, up to 60 mg elemental iron 4 times/day
Prophylaxis: 60-100 mg elemental iron/day
To avoid GI upset, start with a single daily dose and increase by 1 tablet/day each week or as tolerated until desired daily dose is achieved

Dosage Forms
Tablet: 324 mg
Femiron® [OTC]: 63 mg
Ferretts [OTC]: 325 mg
Hemocyte® [OTC]: 324 mg
Ircon® [OTC]: 200 mg
Nephro-Fer® [OTC]: 350 mg
Tablet, timed release:
Ferro-Sequels® [OTC]: 150 mg

ferrous gluconate (FER us GLOO koe nate)

Synonyms iron gluconate
U.S./Canadian Brand Names Apo-Ferrous Gluconate® [Can]; Fergon® [US-OTC]; Novo-Ferrogluc [Can]
Therapeutic Category Electrolyte Supplement, Oral
Use Prevention and treatment of iron-deficiency anemias
Usual Dosage Oral:
Dietary Reference Intake: Dose is RDA presented as elemental iron unless otherwise noted:
0-6 months: 0.27 mg/day (adequate intake)
7-12 months: 11 mg/day
1-3 years: 7 mg/day
4-8 years: 10 mg/day
9-13 years: 8 mg/day
14-18 years: Male: 11 mg/day; Female: 15 mg/day; Pregnant female: 27 mg/day; Lactating female: 10 mg/day
19-50 years: Male: 8 mg/day; Female: 18 mg/day; Pregnant female: 27 mg/day; Lactating female: 9 mg/day
≥50 years: 8 mg/day

Dose expressed in terms of elemental iron:
Children:
Severe iron-deficiency anemia: 4-6 mg Fe/kg/day in 3 divided doses
Mild-to-moderate iron-deficiency anemia: 3 mg Fe/kg/day in 1-2 divided doses
Prophylaxis: 1-2 mg Fe/kg/day
Adults:
Iron deficiency: 60 mg twice daily up to 60 mg 4 times/day
Prophylaxis: 60 mg/day

Dosage Forms
Tablet: 325 mg
Fergon® [OTC]: 240 mg

ferrous sulfate (FER us SUL fate)

Sound-Alike/Look-Alike Issues
Feosol® may be confused with Feostat®, Fer-In-Sol®

Fer-In-Sol® may be confused with Feosol®
Slow FE® may be confused with Slow-K®

Synonyms $FeSO_4$; iron sulfate

U.S./Canadian Brand Names Apo-Ferrous Sulfate® [Can]; Feosol® [US-OTC]; Fer-Gen-Sol [US-OTC]; Fer-In-Sol® [US-OTC/Can]; Fer-iron® [US-OTC]; Feratab® [US-OTC]; Ferodan™ [Can]; MyKidz Iron 10™ [US-OTC]; Slow FE® [US-OTC]

Therapeutic Category Electrolyte Supplement, Oral

Use Prevention and treatment of iron-deficiency anemias

Usual Dosage Oral: **Note:** Multiple concentrations of ferrous sulfate oral liquid exist; close attention must be paid to the concentration when ordering and administering ferrous sulfate; incorrect selection or substitution of one ferrous sulfate liquid for another without proper dosage volume adjustment may result in serious over- or underdosing.

Dietary Reference Intake: Dose is RDA presented as elemental iron unless otherwise noted:
0-6 months: 0.27 mg/day (adequate intake)
7-12 months: 11 mg/day
1-3 years: 7 mg/day
4-8 years: 10 mg/day
9-13 years: 8 mg/day
14-18 years: Male: 11 mg/day; Female: 15 mg/day; Pregnant female: 27 mg/day; Lactating female: 10 mg/day
19-50 years: Male: 8 mg/day; Female: 18 mg/day; Pregnant female: 27 mg/day; Lactating female: 9 mg/day
≥50 years: 8 mg/day

Children **(dose expressed in terms of elemental iron)**:
Severe iron-deficiency anemia: 4-6 mg Fe/kg/day in 3 divided doses
Mild-to-moderate iron-deficiency anemia: 3 mg Fe/kg/day in 1-2 divided doses
Prophylaxis: 1-2 mg Fe/kg/day up to a maximum of 15 mg/day
Adults **(dose expressed in terms of ferrous sulfate)**:
Iron deficiency: 300 mg twice daily up to 300 mg 4 times/day or 250 mg (extended release) 1-2 times/day
Prophylaxis: 300 mg/day

Dosage Forms [CAN] = Canadian brand-specific information
Elixir, oral: 220 mg/5 mL
Liquid, oral: 300 mg/5 mL (5 mL)
Liquid, oral [drops]: 75 mg/0.6 mL
Fer-Gen-Sol [OTC], Fer-iron® [OTC]: 75 mg/0.6 mL
Fer-In-Sol® [OTC]: 75 mg/1 mL
Suspension, oral [drops]:
MyKidz Iron 10™ [OTC]: 75 mg/1.5 mL
Tablet, oral: 324 mg, 325 mg
Feratab® [OTC]: 300 mg
Tablet, oral [exsiccated]: 200 mg
Feosol® [OTC]: 200 mg
Tablet, oral [exsiccated, timed release]: 160 mg
Slow FE® [OTC]: 160 mg
Tablet, oral, slow release: 160 mg

ferrous sulfate and ascorbic acid (FER us SUL fate & a SKOR bik AS id)

Synonyms ascorbic acid and ferrous sulfate; iron sulfate and vitamin C

U.S./Canadian Brand Names Fero-Grad 500® [US-OTC]

Therapeutic Category Vitamin

Use Treatment of iron deficiency in nonpregnant adults; treatment and prevention of iron deficiency in pregnant adults

Usual Dosage Oral: Adults: 1 tablet daily

Dosage Forms
Tablet, controlled release:
Fero-Grad 500® [OTC]: Ferrous sulfate 525 mg and ascorbic acid 500 mg

Fertinorm® H.P. [Can] *see* urofollitropin *on page 999*

ferumoxides (fer yoo MOX ides)

Sound-Alike/Look-Alike Issues

Feridex I.V.® may be confused with Fertinex®

Therapeutic Category Radiopaque Agents

Use For I.V. administration as an adjunct to MRI (in adult patients) to enhance the T2 weighted images used in the detection and evaluation of lesions of the liver

Usual Dosage Adults: 0.56 mg of iron (0.05 mL)/kg body weight diluted in 100 mL of 5% dextrose and infused over 30 minutes; a 5-micron filter is recommended; do not administer undiluted

ferumoxytol (fer ue MOX i tol)

Sound-Alike/Look-Alike Issues

ferumoxytol may be confused with ferric gluconate, iron dextran complex, iron sucrose

U.S./Canadian Brand Names Feraheme™ [US]

Therapeutic Category Iron Salt

Use Treatment of iron-deficiency anemia in chronic kidney disease

Usual Dosage Doses expressed in mg of **elemental** iron. **Note:** Test dose: Product labeling does not indicate need for a test dose.

I.V.: Adults: Iron-deficiency anemia in chronic kidney disease: 510 mg (17 mL) as a single dose, followed by a second 510 mg dose 3-8 days after initial dose. Recommended dose may be readministered in patients with persistent or recurrent iron-deficiency anemia.

Dosage Forms

Injection, solution:

Feraheme™: Elemental iron 30 mg/mL (17 mL)

FESO *see* fesoterodine *on page* 416

FeSO$_4$ *see* ferrous sulfate *on page* 414

fesoterodine (fes oh TER oh deen)

Sound-Alike/Look-Alike Issues

fesoterodine may be confused with fexofenadine, tolterodine

Synonyms FESO; fesoterodine fumarate

U.S./Canadian Brand Names Toviaz™ [US]

Therapeutic Category Anticholinergic Agent

Use Treatment of patients with an overactive bladder with symptoms of urinary frequency, urgency, or urge incontinence.

Usual Dosage Oral: Adults: Overactive bladder: 4 mg once daily; dose may be increased to 8 mg once daily based on individual response and tolerability

Dosage Forms

Tablet, extended release, oral:

Toviaz™: 4 mg, 8 mg

fesoterodine fumarate *see* fesoterodine *on page* 416

Fe-Tinic™ 150 ***(Discontinued)*** *see* polysaccharide-iron complex *on page* 799

FeverAll® [US-OTC] *see* acetaminophen *on page* 19

Fexmid® [US] *see* cyclobenzaprine *on page* 264

fexofenadine (feks oh FEN a deen)

Sound-Alike/Look-Alike Issues

fexofenadine may be confused with fesoterodine

Allegra® may be confused with Viagra®

Synonyms fexofenadine hydrochloride

U.S./Canadian Brand Names Allegra® ODT [US]; Allegra® [US/Can]

Therapeutic Category Antihistamine

Use Relief of symptoms associated with seasonal allergic rhinitis; treatment of chronic idiopathic urticaria

Usual Dosage Oral:

Chronic idiopathic urticaria: Children 6 months to <2 years: 15 mg twice daily

Chronic idiopathic urticaria, seasonal allergic rhinitis:
Children 2-11 years: 30 mg twice daily
Children ≥12 years and Adults: 60 mg twice daily **or** 180 mg once daily

Dosage Forms

Suspension:
Allegra®: 6 mg/mL

Tablet: 30 mg, 60 mg, 180 mg
Allegra®: 60 mg, 180 mg

Tablet, orally disintegrating:
Allegra® ODT: 30 mg

fexofenadine and pseudoephedrine (feks oh FEN a deen & soo doe e FED rin)

Sound-Alike/Look-Alike Issues
Allegra-D® may be confused with Viagra®

Synonyms pseudoephedrine and fexofenadine

U.S./Canadian Brand Names Allegra-D® 12 Hour [US]; Allegra-D® 24 Hour [US]; Allegra-D® [Can]

Therapeutic Category Antihistamine/Decongestant Combination

Use Relief of symptoms associated with seasonal allergic rhinitis in adults and children ≥12 years of age

Usual Dosage Oral: Children ≥12 years and Adults:
Allegra-D® 12 Hour: One tablet twice daily
Allegra-D® 24 Hour: One tablet once daily

Dosage Forms

Tablet, extended release:
Allegra-D® 12 Hour: Fexofenadine 60 mg [immediate release] and pseudoephedrine 120 mg [extended release]
Allegra-D® 24 Hour: Fexofenadine 180 mg [immediate release] and pseudoephedrine 240 mg [extended release]

fexofenadine hydrochloride *see* fexofenadine *on page* 416
Fiberall® [US] *see* psyllium *on page* 837
FiberCon® [US-OTC] *see* polycarbophil *on page* 797
Fiber-Lax® [US-OTC] *see* polycarbophil *on page* 797
Fiber-Tabs™ [US-OTC] *see* polycarbophil *on page* 797

fibrinogen concentrate (human) (fi BRIN o gin KON suhn trate HYU man)

Synonyms coagulation factor I

U.S./Canadian Brand Names RiaSTAP™ [US]

Therapeutic Category Blood Product Derivative

Use Treatment of acute bleeding episodes in patients with congenital fibrinogen deficiency (afibrinogenemia and hypofibrinogenemia)

Usual Dosage I.V.: Children and Adults: Congenital fibrinogen deficiency: **Note:** Adjust dose based on laboratory values and condition of patient. Maintain a target fibrinogen level of 100 mg/dL until hemostasis is achieved.
When baseline fibrinogen level is known:
Dose (mg/kg) = [Target level (mg/dL) - measured level (mg/dL)] **divided by** 1.7 (mg/dL per mg/kg body weight)
When baseline fibrinogen level is not known: 70 mg/kg

Dosage Forms

Injection, powder for reconstitution:
RiaSTAP™: 900-1300 mg [contains albumin (human); exact potency labeled on vial]

fibrin sealant (human) *see* fibrin sealant kit *on page* 417

fibrin sealant kit (FI brin SEEL ent kit)

Synonyms fibrin sealant (human); FS; FS VH S/D

U.S./Canadian Brand Names Artiss™ [US]; Crosseal™ [US]; Evicel™ [US]; Tisseel® VH S/D [US]; Tisseel® VH [Can]

Therapeutic Category Hemostatic Agent

Use

Artiss™: Aid in adhering autologous skin grafts in burn patients (not indicated for hemostasis)

Evicel™: Adjunct to hemostasis in surgery when control of bleeding by conventional surgical techniques is ineffective or impractical

Tisseel® VH: Adjunct to hemostasis in cardiopulmonary bypass surgery and splenic injury (due to blunt or penetrating trauma to the abdomen) when the control of bleeding by conventional surgical techniques is ineffective or impractical; adjunctive sealant for closure of colostomies; hemostatic agent in heparinized patients undergoing cardiopulmonary bypass

Usual Dosage

Adjunct to hemostasis: Apply topically in an even, thin layer (do not inject directly into circulatory system); actual dose is based on size of surface to be covered:

Evicel™: Children and Adults: Spray or drop onto surface of bleeding tissue in short bursts (0.1-0.2 mL); if hemostatic effect is not complete, apply a second layer. To cover a layer of 1 mm thickness:

Maximum area to be sealed: 20 cm^2
Required size of Evicel™ kit: 2 mL
Maximum area to be sealed: 40 cm^2
Required size of Evicel™ kit: 4 mL
Maximum area to be sealed: 100 cm^2
Required size of Evicel™ kit: 10 mL

Tisseel® VH: Adults: Apply in thin layers to avoid excess formation of granulation tissue and slow absorption of the sealant. Following application, hold the sealed parts in the desired position for 3-5 minutes. To prevent sealant from adhering to gloves or surgical instruments, wet them with saline prior to contact.

Maximum area to be sealed: 8 cm^2
Required package size of Tisseel® VH: 2 mL
Maximum area to be sealed: 16 cm^2
Required package size of Tisseel® VH: 4 mL
Maximum area to be sealed: 40 cm^2
Required package size of Tisseel® VH: 10 mL

Autologous skin graft adherence: *Artiss™:* Children ≥1 year and Adults: Apply by spraying topically in an even, thin layer over the wound bed immediately prior to applying graft (do not inject directly into circulatory system); actual dose is based on size of surface to be covered:

Approximate graft fixation area: 100 cm^2
Required size of Artiss™ kit: 2 mL
Approximate graft fixation area: 200 cm^2
Required size of Artiss™ kit: 4 mL
Approximate graft fixation area: 500 cm^2
Required size of Artiss™ kit: 10 mL

Dosage Forms

Kit [each 2 mL kit contains]: Tisseel® VH S/D:
Powder for solution, topical:
Fibrinogen 67-106 mg/mL
Thrombin 400-625 int. units/mL
Solution, topical:
Aprotinin 2250-3750 KIU/mL
Calcium chloride 36-44 μmol/mL

Kit [each 2 mL kit contains, preservative free]: Evicel™: Solution, topical:
Fibrinogen 55-85 mg/mL (1 mL)
Thrombin 800-1200 int. units/mL
Calcium chloride 5.6-6.2 mg/mL (1 mL)

Kit [each 4 mL kit contains]:
Artiss™:
Powder for solution, topical:
Fibrinogen 67-106 mg/mL
Thrombin 2.5-6.5 int. units/mL
Solution, topical:
Aprotinin 2250-3750 KIU/mL
Calcium chloride 36-44 μmol/mL

Tisseel® VH S/D:
Powder for solution, topical:
Fibrinogen 67-106 mg/mL
Thrombin 400-625 int. units/mL
Solution, topical:
Aprotinin 2250-3750 KIU/mL
Calcium chloride 36-44 µmol/mL

Kit [each 4 mL kit contains, preservative free]: Evicel™: Solution, topical:
Calcium chloride 5.6-6.2 mg/mL (2 mL)
Fibrinogen 55-85 mg/mL (2 mL)
Thrombin 800-1200 int. units/mL

Kit [each 10 mL kit contains]:
Artiss™:
Powder, for solution, topical:
Fibrinogen 67-106 mg/mL
Thrombin 2.5-6.5 int. units/mL
Solution, topical:
Calcium chloride 36-44 µmol/mL
Aprotinin 2250-3750 KIU/mL
Tisseel® VH S/D:
Powder for solution, topical:
Fibrinogen 67-106 mg/mL
Thrombin 400-625 int. units/mL
Solution, topical:
Aprotinin 2250-3750 KIU/mL
Calcium chloride 36-44 µmol/mL

Kit [each 10 mL kit contains, preservative free]: Evicel™:
Solution, topical:
Fibrinogen 55-85 mg/mL (5 mL)
Thrombin 800-1200 int. units/mL
Calcium chloride 5.6-6.2 mg/mL (5 mL)

Kit, topical [each kit contains]: Crosseal™:
Calcium chloride 5.6-6.0 mg/mL
Fibrinogen 40-60 mg/mL
Spray application device: Thrombin 800-1200 int. units/mL (1 mL, 2 mL, 5 mL)

Solution, topical [each dual-chamber 2 mL prefilled syringe contains]: Tisseel™ VH S/D:
Sealer protein chamber:
Aprotinin 2250-3750 KIU/mL
Fibrinogen 67-106 mg/mL
Thrombin chamber:
Calcium chloride 36-44 µmol/mL
Thrombin 400-625 int. units/mL

Solution, topical [each dual-chamber 4 mL prefilled syringe contains]: Tisseel™ VH S/D:
Sealer protein chamber:
Aprotinin 2250-3750 KIU/mL
Fibrinogen 67-106 mg/mL
Thrombin chamber:
Calcium chloride 36-44 µmol/mL
Thrombin 400-625 int. units/mL

Solution, topical [each dual-chamber 10 mL prefilled syringe contains]: Tisseel™ VH S/D:
Sealer protein chamber:
Aprotinin 2250-3750 KIU/mL
Fibrinogen 67-106 mg/mL
Thrombin chamber:
Calcium chloride 36-44 µmol/mL
Thrombin 400-625 int. units/mL

Fibro-XL [US-OTC] *see* psyllium *on page 837*

Fibro-Lax [US-OTC] *see* psyllium *on page 837*

filgrastim (fil GRA stim)

Sound-Alike/Look-Alike Issues

Neupogen® may be confused with Epogen®, Neulasta®, Neumega®, Neupro®, Nutramigen®

Synonyms G-CSF; granulocyte colony-stimulating factor; NSC-614629

U.S./Canadian Brand Names Neupogen® [US/Can]

Therapeutic Category Colony-Stimulating Factor

Use Stimulation of granulocyte production in chemotherapy-induced neutropenia (nonmyeloid malignancies, acute myeloid leukemia, and bone marrow transplantation); severe chronic neutropenia (SCN); moblilization of hematopoietic progenitor cells in patients undergoing peripheral blood progenitor cell (PBPC) collection

Usual Dosage Details concerning dosing in combination regimens and institution protocols should also be consulted.

Dosing, even in morbidly obese patients, should be based on actual body weight. Rounding doses to the nearest vial size often enhances patient convenience and reduces costs without compromising clinical response.

Children and Adults:

Chemotherapy-induced neutropenia: SubQ, I.V.: 5 mcg/kg/day; doses may be increased by 5 mcg/kg according to the duration and severity of the neutropenia; continue for up to 14 days or until the ANC reaches 10,000/mm^3

Bone marrow transplantation: SubQ, I.V.: 10 mcg/kg/day; adjust the dose according to the duration and severity of neutropenia; recommended steps based on neutrophil response:

When ANC >1000/mm^3 for 3 consecutive days: Reduce filgrastim dose to 5 mcg/kg/day

If ANC remains >1000/mm^3 for 3 more consecutive days: Discontinue filgrastim

If ANC decreases to <1000/mm^3: Resume at 5 mcg/kg/day

If ANC decreases <1000/mm^3 during the 5 mcg/kg/day dose, increase filgrastim to 10 mcg/kg/day and follow the above steps

Peripheral blood progenitor cell (PBPC) collection: SubQ: 10 mcg/kg daily in donors, usually for 6-7 days. Begin at least 4 days before the first leukopheresis and continue until the last leukopheresis; consider dose adjustment for WBC >100,000/mm^3

Hematopoietic stem cell mobilization (in combination with plerixafor, for autologous transplantation in patients with non-Hodgkin lymphoma and multiple myeloma): SubQ: 10 mcg/kg once daily; begin 4 days before initiation of plerixafor; continue G-CSF on each day prior to apheresis

Severe chronic neutropenia: SubQ:

Congenital: 6 mcg/kg twice daily; adjust the dose based on ANC and clinical response

Idiopathic/cyclic: 5 mcg/kg/day; adjust the dose based on ANC and clinical response

Anemia in myelodysplastic syndrome (unlabeled use - in combination with epoetin): SubQ: 0.3-3 mcg/kg daily **or** 30-150 mcg daily **or** 1-2 mcg/kg 2-3 times weekly

Dosage Forms

Injection, solution [preservative free]:

Neupogen®: 300 mcg/mL (1 mL, 1.6 mL) [vial]; 600 mcg/mL (0.5 mL, 0.8 mL) [prefilled Singleject® syringe]

Finacea® [US/Can] *see* azelaic acid *on page* 115

finasteride (fi NAS teer ide)

Sound-Alike/Look-Alike Issues

finasteride may be confused with furosemide

Proscar® may be confused with ProSom®, Prozac®, Psorcon®

U.S./Canadian Brand Names Propecia® [US/Can]; Proscar® [US/Can]

Therapeutic Category Antiandrogen

Use

Propecia®: Treatment of male pattern hair loss in **men only**. Safety and efficacy were demonstrated in men between 18-41 years of age.

Proscar®: Treatment of symptomatic benign prostatic hyperplasia (BPH); can be used in combination with an alpha-blocker, doxazosin

Usual Dosage Oral: Adults: Male:

Benign prostatic hyperplasia (Proscar®): 5 mg once daily as a single dose; clinical responses occur within 12 weeks to 6 months of initiation of therapy; long-term administration is recommended for maximal response

Male pattern baldness (Propecia®): 1 mg daily

Dosage Forms
Tablet: 5 mg
Propecia®: 1 mg
Proscar®: 5 mg

Fiorgen PF® ***(Discontinued)***
Fioricet® [US] *see* butalbital, acetaminophen, and caffeine *on page 161*
Fioricet® with Codeine [US] *see* butalbital, acetaminophen, caffeine, and codeine *on page 162*
Fiorinal® [US/Can] *see* butalbital, aspirin, and caffeine *on page 162*
Fiorinal®-C 1/2 [Can] *see* butalbital, aspirin, caffeine, and codeine *on page 163*
Fiorinal®-C 1/4 [Can] *see* butalbital, aspirin, caffeine, and codeine *on page 163*
Fiorinal® with Codeine [US] *see* butalbital, aspirin, caffeine, and codeine *on page 163*
Firmagon® [US] *see* degarelix *on page 281*
First™-Progesterone VGS [US] *see* progesterone *on page 822*
First® Testosterone [US] *see* testosterone *on page 947*
First® Testosterone MC [US] *see* testosterone *on page 947*
fisalamine *see* mesalamine *on page 631*
fish oil *see* omega-3-acid ethyl esters *on page 723*
FK506 *see* tacrolimus *on page 935*
Flagyl® [US/Can] *see* metronidazole *on page 651*
Flagyl® 375 [US] *see* metronidazole *on page 651*
Flagyl ER® [US] *see* metronidazole *on page 651*
Flagystatin® [Can] *see* metronidazole and nystatin *(Canada only) on page 652*
Flamazine® [Can] *see* silver sulfadiazine *on page 901*
Flarex® [US/Can] *see* fluorometholone *on page 431*
flavan *see* flavocoxid *on page 421*

flavocoxid (fla vo KOKS id)

Synonyms flavan; flavonoid
U.S./Canadian Brand Names Limbrel 250™ [US]; Limbrel 500™ [US]
Therapeutic Category Antiinflammatory Agent
Use Clinical dietary management of osteoarthritis, including associated inflammation
Usual Dosage Oral: 250 mg every 8-12 hours
Dosage Forms
Capsule, oral [new formulation]:
Limbrel 250™: 250 mg
Limbrel 500™: 500 mg

flavonoid *see* flavocoxid *on page 421*
Flavorcee® ***(Discontinued)*** *see* ascorbic acid *on page 100*

flavoxate (fla VOKS ate)

Sound-Alike/Look-Alike Issues
flavoxate may be confused with fluvoxamine
Urispas® may be confused with Urised®
Synonyms flavoxate hydrochloride
U.S./Canadian Brand Names Apo-Flavoxate® [Can]; Urispas® [US/Can]
Therapeutic Category Antispasmodic Agent, Urinary
Use Antispasmodic to provide symptomatic relief of dysuria, nocturia, suprapubic pain, urgency, and incontinence due to detrusor instability and hyperreflexia in elderly with cystitis, urethritis, urethrocystitis, urethrotrigonitis, and prostatitis
Usual Dosage Oral: Children >12 years and Adults: 100-200 mg 3-4 times/day; reduce the dose when symptoms improve
Dosage Forms
Tablet: 100 mg
Urispas®: 100 mg

flavoxate hydrochloride *see* flavoxate *on page 421*

Flebogamma® [US] *see* immune globulin (intravenous) *on page* 523

flecainide (fle KAY nide)

Sound-Alike/Look-Alike Issues

flecainide may be confused with fluconazole

Tambocor™ may be confused with Pamelor®, Temodar®, tamoxifen

Synonyms flecainide acetate

U.S./Canadian Brand Names Apo-Flecainide® [Can]; Tambocor™ [US/Can]

Therapeutic Category Antiarrhythmic Agent, Class I-C

Use Prevention and suppression of documented life-threatening ventricular arrhythmias (eg, sustained ventricular tachycardia); controlling symptomatic, disabling supraventricular tachycardias in patients without structural heart disease in whom other agents fail

Usual Dosage Oral:

Children:

Initial: 3 mg/kg/day or 50-100 mg/m^2/day in 3 divided doses

Usual: 3-6 mg/kg/day or 100-150 mg/m^2/day in 3 divided doses; up to 11 mg/kg/day or 200 mg/m^2/day for uncontrolled patients with subtherapeutic levels

Adults:

Life-threatening ventricular arrhythmias:

Initial: 100 mg every 12 hours

Increase by 50-100 mg/day (given in 2 doses/day) every 4 days; maximum: 400 mg/day

Use of higher initial doses and more rapid dosage adjustments have resulted in an increased incidence of proarrhythmic events and congestive heart failure, particularly during the first few days. Do not use a loading dose. Use very cautiously in patients with history of congestive heart failure or myocardial infarction.

Prevention of paroxysmal supraventricular arrhythmias in patients with disabling symptoms but no structural heart disease: Initial: 50 mg every 12 hours; increase by 50 mg twice daily at 4-day intervals; maximum: 300 mg/day

Dosage Forms

Tablet: 50 mg, 100 mg, 150 mg

Tambocor™: 50 mg, 100 mg, 150 mg

flecainide acetate *see* flecainide *on page* 422
Flector® [US] *see* diclofenac *on page* 303
Fleet® Babylax® ***(Discontinued)*** *see* glycerin *on page* 468
Fleet® Bisacodyl [US-OTC] *see* bisacodyl *on page* 142
Fleet® Enema [US-OTC/Can] *see* sodium phosphates *on page* 912
Fleet® Enema Extra® [US-OTC] *see* sodium phosphates *on page* 912
Fleet® Flavored Castor Oil ***(Discontinued)*** *see* castor oil *on page* 190
Fleet® Glycerin Suppositories [US-OTC] *see* glycerin *on page* 468
Fleet® Glycerin Suppositories Maximum Strength [US-OTC] *see* glycerin *on page* 468
Fleet® Laxative ***(Discontinued)*** *see* bisacodyl *on page* 142
Fleet® Liquid Glycerin Suppositories [US-OTC] *see* glycerin *on page* 468
Fleet® Pedia-Lax™ Chewable Tablet [US-OTC] *see* magnesium hydroxide *on page* 608
Fleet® Pedia-Lax™ Enema [US-OTC] *see* sodium phosphates *on page* 912
Fleet® Pedia-Lax™ Glycerin Suppositories [US-OTC] *see* glycerin *on page* 468
Fleet® Pedia-Lax™ Liquid Glycerin Suppositories [US-OTC] *see* glycerin *on page* 468
Fleet® Pedia-Lax™ Liquid Stool Softener [US-OTC] *see* docusate *on page* 326
Fleet® Pedia-Lax™ Quick Dissolve [US-OTC] *see* senna *on page* 896
Fleet® Phospho-soda® ***(Discontinued)*** *see* sodium phosphates *on page* 912
Fleet® Phospho-soda® EZ-Prep™ ***(Discontinued)*** *see* sodium phosphates *on page* 912
Fleet® Sof-Lax® [US-OTC] *see* docusate *on page* 326
Fleet® Stimulant Laxative [US-OTC] *see* bisacodyl *on page* 142
Fletcher's® [US-OTC] *see* senna *on page* 896
Flexaphen® ***(Discontinued)*** *see* chlorzoxazone *on page* 223
Flexbumin [US] *see* albumin *on page* 40
Flexeril® [US/Can] *see* cyclobenzaprine *on page* 264

Flexitec [Can] *see* cyclobenzaprine *on page 264*
Flex-Power [US-OTC] *see* trolamine *on page 991*
Flextra-650 [US] *see* acetaminophen and phenyltoloxamine *on page 23*
Flextra-DS [US] *see* acetaminophen and phenyltoloxamine *on page 23*
Flintstones™ Complete [US-OTC] *see* vitamins (multiple/pediatric) *on page 1020*
Flintstones™ Gummies [US-OTC] *see* vitamins (multiple/pediatric) *on page 1020*
Flintstones™ Gummies Vita-Packs [US-OTC] *see* vitamins (multiple/pediatric) *on page 1020*
Flintstones™ Plus Bone Building Support [US-OTC] *see* vitamins (multiple/pediatric) *on page 1020*
Flintstones™ Plus Immunity Support [US-OTC] *see* vitamins (multiple/pediatric) *on page 1020*
Flintstones™ Plus Iron [US-OTC] *see* vitamins (multiple/pediatric) *on page 1020*
Flintstones™ Sour Gummies [US-OTC] *see* vitamins (multiple/pediatric) *on page 1020*
floctafenina *see* floctafenine *(Canada only) on page 423*

floctafenine *(Canada only)* (flok ta FEN een)

Synonyms floctafenina; floctafeninum

U.S./Canadian Brand Names Apo-Floctafenine® [Can]

Therapeutic Category Nonsteroidal Antiinflammatory Drug (NSAID), Oral

Use Short-term management of acute, mild-to-moderate pain

Usual Dosage Oral: Adults: 200-400 mg every 6-8 hours as needed, up to a maximum of 1200 mg/day

Dosage Forms [CAN] = Canadian brand name

Tablet:
Apo-Floctafenine® [CAN]: 200 mg, 400 mg [not available in the U.S.]

floctafeninum *see* floctafenine *(Canada only) on page 423*
Flolan® [US/Can] *see* epoprostenol *on page 363*
Flomax® [US/Can] *see* tamsulosin *on page 938*
Flomax® CR [Can] *see* tamsulosin *on page 938*
Flonase® [US/Can] *see* fluticasone (nasal) *on page 437*
Floranex™ [US-OTC] *see* Lactobacillus *on page 564*
Flora-Q™ [US-OTC] *see* Lactobacillus *on page 564*
Florastor® [US-OTC] *see Saccharomyces boulardii on page 883*
Florastor® Kids [US-OTC] *see Saccharomyces boulardii on page 883*
Florazole® ER [Can] *see* metronidazole *on page 651*
Florical® [US-OTC] *see* calcium carbonate *on page 170*
Florinef® [Can] *see* fludrocortisone *on page 426*
Florinef® *(Discontinued)* *see* fludrocortisone *on page 426*
Florone E® *(Discontinued)* *see* diflorasone *on page 307*
Flovent® Diskus® [Can] *see* fluticasone (oral inhalation) *on page 437*
Flovent® HFA [US/Can] *see* fluticasone (oral inhalation) *on page 437*
Floxin® [US/Can] *see* ofloxacin *on page 718*

floxuridine (floks YOOR i deen)

Sound-Alike/Look-Alike Issues
floxuridine may be confused with Fludara®, fludarabine
FUDR® may be confused with Fludara®

Synonyms fluorodeoxyuridine; FUDR

U.S./Canadian Brand Names FUDR® [US/Can]

Therapeutic Category Antineoplastic Agent

Use Management of hepatic metastases of colorectal and gastric cancers

Usual Dosage Refer to individual protocols. Intraarterial:
0.1-0.6 mg/kg/day
4-20 mg/day

Dosage Forms

Injection, powder for reconstitution: 500 mg
FUDR®: 500 mg

Fluanxol® [Can] *see* flupenthixol *(Canada only) on page 433*
Fluarix® [US] *see* influenza virus vaccine *on page 528*
flubenisolone *see* betamethasone (topical) *on page 138*
Flucaine® [US] *see* proparacaine and fluorescein *on page 826*

fluconazole (floo KOE na zole)

Sound-Alike/Look-Alike Issues
fluconazole may be confused with flecainide, FLUoxetine, furosemide, itraconazole
Diflucan® may be confused with diclofenac, Diprivan®, disulfiram

U.S./Canadian Brand Names Apo-Fluconazole® [Can]; CO Fluconazole [Can]; Diflucan® [US/Can]; Dom-Fluconazole [Can]; Fluconazole Injection [Can]; Fluconazole Omega [Can]; Gen-Fluconazole [Can]; GMD-Fluconazole [Can]; Novo-Fluconazole [Can]; PHL-Fluconazole [Can]; PMS-Fluconazole [Can]; Pro-Fluconazole [Can]; Riva-Fluconazole [Can]; Taro-Fluconazole [Can]; Zym-Fluconazole [Can]

Therapeutic Category Antifungal Agent

Use Treatment of candidiasis (vaginal, oropharyngeal, esophageal, urinary tract infections, peritonitis, pneumonia, and systemic infections); cryptococcal meningitis; antifungal prophylaxis in allogeneic bone marrow transplant recipients

Usual Dosage The daily dose of fluconazole is the same for oral and I.V. administration

Usual dosage range:

Neonates: First 2 weeks of life, especially premature neonates: Same dose as older children every 72 hours

Children: Loading dose: 6-12 mg/kg; maintenance: 3-12 mg/kg/day; duration and dosage depends on severity of infection

Adults: 200-800 mg/day; duration and dosage depends on severity of infection

Indication-specific dosing:

Children:

Candidiasis:

Oropharyngeal: Loading dose: 6 mg/kg; maintenance: 3 mg/kg/day for 2 weeks

Esophageal: Loading dose: 6 mg/kg; maintenance: 3-12 mg/kg/day for 21 days and at least 2 weeks following resolution of symptoms

Systemic infection: 6 mg/kg every 12 hours for 28 days

Meningitis, cryptococcal: Loading dose: 12 mg/kg; maintenance: 6-12 mg/kg/day for 10-12 weeks following negative CSF culture; relapse suppression (HIV-positive): 6 mg/kg/day

Adults:

Candidiasis:

Candidemia (neutropenic and nonneutropenic): Loading dose: 800 mg on first day, then 400 mg/day for 14 days after last positive blood culture and resolution of signs/symptoms; **Note:** Not recommended for neutropenic patients with recent azole exposure and critical illness

Chronic, disseminated: 400 mg/day until calcification or lesion resolution

CNS Candidemia: 400-800 mg/day until CSF/radiological abnormalities resolved; **Note:** Recommended as alternative therapy in patients intolerant of amphotericin B

Oropharyngeal (long-term suppression): 100-200 mg/day for 7-14 days; chronic therapy of 100 mg 3 times weekly is recommended in immunocompromised patients with history of oropharyngeal candidiasis (OPC)

Osteoarticular: 400 mg/day for 6-12 months (osteomyelitis) or 6 weeks (septic arthritis)

Esophageal: 200-400 mg/day for 14-21 days

Prophylaxis:

Solid organ: 200-400 mg/day fo 7-14 days

Neutropenic patients: 400 mg/day for duration of neutropenia

Urinary tract:

Fungus balls: 200-400 mg/day

Pyelonephritis: 200-400 mg/day for 2 weeks

Symptomatic cystitis: 200 mg/day for 2 weeks

Vaginal: 150 mg as a single dose

Endophthalmitis: 400-800 mg/day for 4-6 weeks until examination indicates resolution

Meningitis, cryptococcal: Amphotericin 0.7-1 mg/kg +/- 5-FC for 2 weeks then fluconazole 400 mg/day for at least 10 weeks (consider life-long in HIV-positive); maintenance (HIV-positive): 200-400 mg/day life-long

Pericarditis or myocarditis: 400-800 mg/day

Dosage Forms

Infusion [premixed in sodium chloride or dextrose]: 200 mg (100 mL); 400 mg (200 mL)
Diflucan® [premixed in sodium chloride or dextrose]: 200 mg (100 mL); 400 mg (200 mL)
Powder for oral suspension: 10 mg/mL, 40 mg/mL
Diflucan®: 10 mg/mL, 40 mg/mL
Tablet: 50 mg, 100 mg, 150 mg, 200 mg
Diflucan®: 50 mg, 100 mg, 150 mg, 200 mg

Fluconazole Injection [Can] *see* fluconazole *on page 424*
Fluconazole Omega [Can] *see* fluconazole *on page 424*

flucytosine (floo SYE toe seen)

Sound-Alike/Look-Alike Issues
flucytosine may be confused with fluorouracil
Ancobon® may be confused with Oncovin®

Synonyms 5-FC; 5-fluorocytosine; 5-flurocytosine

U.S./Canadian Brand Names Ancobon® [US/Can]

Therapeutic Category Antifungal Agent

Use Adjunctive treatment of systemic fungal infections (eg, septicemia, endocarditis, UTI, meningitis, or pulmonary) caused by susceptible strains of *Candida* or *Cryptococcus*

Usual Dosage

Usual dosage ranges:
Oral: Adults: 50-150 mg/kg/day in divided doses every 6 hours

Indication-specific dosing:
Oral: Adults:
Endocarditis: 25-37.5 mg/kg every 6 hours (with amphotericin B) for at least 6 weeks after valve replacement
Meningoencephalitis, cryptococcal: Induction: 25 mg/kg/dose (with amphotericin B) every 6 hours for 2 weeks; if clinical improvement, may discontinue both amphotericin and flucytosine and follow with an extended course of fluconazole (400 mg/day); alternatively, may continue flucytosine for 6-10 weeks (with amphotericin B) without conversion to fluconazole treatment

Dosage Forms

Capsule:
Ancobon®: 250 mg, 500 mg

Fludara® [US/Can] *see* fludarabine *on page 425*

fludarabine (floo DARE a been)

Sound-Alike/Look-Alike Issues
fludarabine may be confused with cladribine, floxuridine, Flumadine®
Fludara® may be confused with FUDR®

Synonyms 2F-ara-AMP; fludarabine phosphate; NSC-312887

U.S./Canadian Brand Names Fludara® [US/Can]

Therapeutic Category Antineoplastic Agent

Use
U.S. labeling: Treatment of progressive or refractory B-cell chronic lymphocytic leukemia (CLL)
Canadian labeling: Second-line treatment of chronic lymphocytic leukemia (CLL); second-line treatment of low-grade, refractory non-Hodgkin lymphoma (NHL)

Usual Dosage Details concerning dosing in combination regimens should also be consulted.
Oral: Adults: CLL: 40 mg/m^2 once daily for 5 days every 28 days
I.V.: Adults: CLL: 25 mg/m^2/day for 5 days every 28 days

Product Availability Fludarabine oral formulation (brand name pending): FDA approved December 2008; availability currently undetermined

Dosage Forms [CAN] = Canadian brand name

Injection, powder for reconstitution: 50 mg
Fludara®: 50 mg
Injection, solution [preservative free]: 25 mg/mL (2 mL)
Tablet: 10 mg
Fludara® [CAN]: 10 mg

fludarabine phosphate *see* fludarabine *on page 425*

fludrocortisone (floo droe KOR ti sone)

Sound-Alike/Look-Alike Issues

Florinef® may be confused with Fioricet®, Fiorinal®

Synonyms 9α-fluorohydrocortisone acetate; fludrocortisone acetate; fluohydrisone acetate; fluohydrocortisone acetate

U.S./Canadian Brand Names Florinef® [Can]

Therapeutic Category Adrenal Corticosteroid (Mineralocorticoid)

Use Partial replacement therapy for primary and secondary adrenocortical insufficiency in Addison disease; treatment of salt-losing adrenogenital syndrome

Usual Dosage Oral:

Infants and Children: 0.05-0.1 mg/day

Adults: 0.1-0.2 mg/day with ranges of 0.1 mg 3 times/week to 0.2 mg/day

Addison disease: Initial: 0.1 mg/day; if transient hypertension develops, reduce the dose to 0.05 mg/day. Preferred administration with cortisone (10-37.5 mg/day) or hydrocortisone (10-30 mg/day).

Salt-losing adrenogenital syndrome: 0.1-0.2 mg/day

Dosage Forms

Tablet: 0.1 mg

fludrocortisone acetate *see* fludrocortisone *on page* 426

FluLaval® [US] *see* influenza virus vaccine *on page* 528

Flumadine® [US/Can] *see* rimantadine *on page* 868

flumazenil (FLOO may ze nil)

Sound-Alike/Look-Alike Issues

flumazenil may be confused with influenza virus vaccine

U.S./Canadian Brand Names Anexate® [Can]; Flumazenil Injection [Can]; Flumazenil Injection, USP [Can]; Romazicon® [US/Can]

Therapeutic Category Antidote

Use Benzodiazepine antagonist; reverses sedative effects of benzodiazepines used in conscious sedation and general anesthesia; treatment of benzodiazepine overdose

Usual Dosage I.V.:

Children: Reversal of conscious sedation and general anesthesia:

Initial dose: 0.01 mg/kg over 15 seconds (maximum: 0.2 mg)

Repeat doses (maximum: 4 doses): 0.005-0.01 mg/kg (maximum: 0.2 mg) repeated at 1-minute intervals

Maximum total cumulative dose: 1 mg or 0.05 mg/kg (whichever is lower)

Adults:

Reversal of conscious sedation and general anesthesia:

Initial dose: 0.2 mg over 15 seconds

Repeat doses (maximum: 4 doses): If desired level of consciousness is not obtained, 0.2 mg may be repeated at 1-minute intervals.

Maximum total cumulative dose: 1 mg (usual dose: 0.6-1 mg). In the event of resedation: Repeat doses may be given at 20-minute intervals with maximum of 1 mg/dose and 3 mg/hour

Suspected benzodiazepine overdose:

Initial dose: 0.2 mg over 30 seconds; if the desired level of consciousness is not obtained, 0.3 mg can be given over 30 seconds

Repeat doses: 0.5 mg over 30 seconds repeated at 1-minute intervals

Maximum total cumulative dose: 3 mg (usual dose: 1-3 mg). Patients with a partial response at 3 mg may require additional titration up to a total dose of 5 mg. If a patient has not responded 5 minutes after cumulative dose of 5 mg, the major cause of sedation is not likely due to benzodiazepines. In the event of resedation: May repeat doses at 20-minute intervals with maximum of 1 mg/dose and 3 mg/hour.

Resedation: Repeated doses may be given at 20-minute intervals as needed; repeat treatment doses of 1 mg (at a rate of 0.5 mg/minute) should be given at any time and no more than 3 mg should be given in any hour. After intoxication with high doses of benzodiazepines, the duration of a single dose of flumazenil is not expected to exceed 1 hour; if desired, the period of wakefulness may be prolonged with repeated low intravenous doses of flumazenil, or by an infusion of 0.1-0.4 mg/hour. Most patients with benzodiazepine overdose will respond to a cumulative dose of 1-3 mg and doses >3 mg do not reliably produce additional effects. Rarely, patients with a partial response at 3 mg may require additional titration up to a total dose of 5 mg. **If a patient has not responded 5 minutes after receiving a cumulative dose of 5 mg, the major cause of sedation is not likely to be due to benzodiazepines.**

Dosage Forms

Injection, solution: 0.1 mg/mL (5 mL, 10 mL)

Romazicon®: 0.1 mg/mL (5 mL, 10 mL)

Flumazenil Injection [Can] *see* flumazenil *on page 426*

Flumazenil Injection, USP [Can] *see* flumazenil *on page 426*

flumethasone and clioquinol *see* clioquinol and flumethasone *(Canada only) on page 241*

FluMist® [US] *see* influenza virus vaccine *on page 528*

flunarizine *(Canada only)* (floo NAR i zeen)

Synonyms flunarizine hydrochloride

U.S./Canadian Brand Names Apo-Flunarizine® [Can]; Novo-Flunarizine [Can]; Sibelium® [Can]

Therapeutic Category Calcium-Entry Blocker (Selective)

Use Prophylaxis of classic (with aura) or common (without aura) migraine; symptomatic treatment of vestibular vertigo (due to a diagnosed functional disorder of the vestibular system)

Usual Dosage Oral: Adults (<65 years): Usual dose: 5-10 mg/day, usually administered at bedtime

Migraine prophylaxis: Initial dose: 10 mg at bedtime

Maintenance dose (following initial control of symptoms): 10 mg at bedtime administered 5 consecutive days, followed by 2 consecutive medication-free days each week.

Duration of therapy: In nonresponders, discontinue if no response occurs within 2 months. If response is noted, discontinue after 6 months; restart if patient relapses.

Vertigo: Initial dose: 10 mg at bedtime until symptoms are controlled

Duration of therapy:

Chronic vertigo: Discontinue if no response within 1 month.

Paroxysmal vertigo: Discontinue if no response is noted within 2 months.

Dosage Forms [CAN] = Canadian brand name

Capsule:

Apo-Flunarizine® [CAN], Novo-Flunarizine [CAN], Sibelium® [CAN]: 5 mg [not available in the U.S.]

flunarizine hydrochloride *see* flunarizine *(Canada only) on page 427*

flunisolide (floo NISS oh lide)

Sound-Alike/Look-Alike Issues

flunisolide may be confused with Flumadine®, fluocinonide

Nasarel® may be confused with Nizoral®

U.S./Canadian Brand Names AeroBid® [US]; AeroBid®-M [US]; Alti-Flunisolide [Can]; Apo-Flunisolide® [Can]; Nasalide® [Can]; PMS-Flunisolide [Can]; Rhinalar® [Can]

Therapeutic Category Adrenal Corticosteroid

Use Steroid-dependent asthma; nasal solution is used for seasonal or perennial rhinitis

Usual Dosage

Oral inhalation: Asthma (AeroBid®, AeroBid®-M):

Children 6-15 years: 2 inhalations twice daily (morning and evening); up to 4 inhalations/day

Children ≥16 years and Adults: 2 inhalations twice daily (morning and evening); up to 8 inhalations/day maximum

NIH Asthma Guidelines (administer in divided doses twice daily):

Children 5-11 years:

"Low" dose: 500-750 mcg/day

"Medium" dose: 1000-1250 mcg/day

"High" dose: >1250 mcg/day

Children ≥12 years and Adults:

"Low" dose: 500-1000 mcg/day

"Medium" dose: >1000-2000 mcg/day

"High" dose: >2000 mcg/day

Intranasal: Rhinitis:

Children 6-14 years: 1 spray each nostril 3 times daily **or** 2 sprays in each nostril twice daily; not to exceed 4 sprays/day in each nostril

Children ≥15 years and Adults: 2 sprays each nostril twice daily (morning and evening); may increase to 2 sprays 3 times daily; maximum dose: 8 sprays/day in each nostril

Dosage Forms

Aerosol for oral inhalation:

AeroBid®, AeroBid®-M: 250 mcg/actuation (7 g)

Solution, intranasal [spray]: 25 mcg/actuation (25 mL); 29 mcg/actuation (25 mL)

fluocinolone (floo oh SIN oh lone)

Sound-Alike/Look-Alike Issues

fluocinolone may be confused with fluocinonide

Synonyms fluocinolone acetonide

U.S./Canadian Brand Names Capex® [US/Can]; Derma-Smoothe/FS® [US/Can]; DermOtic® [US]; Retisert® [US]; Synalar® [Can]

Therapeutic Category Corticosteroid, Topical

Use Relief of susceptible inflammatory dermatosis [low, medium corticosteroid]; dermatitis or psoriasis of the scalp; atopic dermatitis in adults and children ≥3 months of age

Ocular implant (Retisert®): Treatment of chronic, noninfectious uveitis affecting the posterior segment of the eye

Otic (DermOtic® Oil): Relief of chronic eczematous external otitis in adults and children ≥2 years of age.

Usual Dosage

Ocular implant: Chronic uveitis: Children ≥12 years and Adults: One silicone-encased tablet (0.59 mg) surgically implanted into the posterior segment of the eye is designed to initially release 0.6 mcg/day, decreasing over 30 days to a steady-state release rate of 0.3-0.4 mcg/day for 30 months. Recurrence of uveitis denotes depletion of tablet, requiring reimplantation.

Otic: Chronic eczematous external otitis: Children ≥2 years and Adults: 5 drops into the affected ear twice daily for 1-2 weeks

Topical:

Atopic dermatitis (Derma-Smoothe/FS® body oil):

Children ≥3 months: Moisten skin; apply a thin film to affected area twice daily; do not use for longer than 4 weeks

Adults: Apply a thin film to affected area 3 times/day

Corticosteroid-responsive dermatoses: Children and Adults: Cream, ointment, solution: Apply a thin layer to affected area 2-4 times/day; may use occlusive dressings to manage psoriasis or recalcitrant conditions

Inflammatory and pruritic manifestations (dental use): Adults: Apply to oral lesion 4 times/day, after meals and at bedtime

Scalp psoriasis (Derma-Smoothe/FS® scalp oil): Adults: Massage thoroughly into wet or dampened hair/scalp; cover with shower cap. Leave on overnight (or for at least 4 hours). Remove by washing hair with shampoo and rinsing thoroughly.

Seborrheic dermatitis of the scalp (Capex®): Adults: Apply no more than 1 ounce to scalp once daily; work into lather and allow to remain on scalp for ~5 minutes. Remove from hair and scalp by rinsing thoroughly with water.

Dosage Forms

Cream: 0.01% (15 g, 60 g); 0.025% (15 g, 60 g)

Implant, intravitreal:

Retisert®: 0.59 mg

Oil:

Derma-Smoothe/FS® [body oil]: 0.01% (120 mL)

Derma-Smoothe/FS® [scalp oil]: 0.01% (120 mL)

DermaOtic® [otic drops]: 0.01% (20 mL)

Ointment: 0.025% (15 g, 60 g)

Shampoo:

Capex®: 0.01% (120 mL)

Solution: 0.01% (60 mL)

fluocinolone acetonide *see* fluocinolone *on page 428*

fluocinolone, hydroquinone, and tretinoin

(floo oh SIN oh lone, HYE droe kwin one, & TRET i noyn)

Synonyms hydroquinone, fluocinolone acetonide, and tretinoin; tretinoin, fluocinolone acetonide, and hydroquinone

U.S./Canadian Brand Names Tri-Luma™ [US]

Therapeutic Category Corticosteroid, Topical; Depigmenting Agent; Retinoic Acid Derivative

Use Short-term treatment of moderate-to-severe melasma of the face

Usual Dosage Topical: Adults: Melasma: Apply a thin film once daily to hyperpigmented areas of melasma (including 1/2 inch of normal-appearing surrounding skin). Apply 30 minutes prior to bedtime; not indicated for use beyond 8 weeks. Do not use occlusive dressings.

Dosage Forms

Cream, topical:

Tri-Luma™: Hydroquinone 4%, tretinoin 0.05%, fluocinolone 0.01% (30 g)

fluocinonide (floo oh SIN oh nide)

Sound-Alike/Look-Alike Issues

fluocinonide may be confused with flunisolide, fluocinolone

Lidex® may be confused with Lasix®, Videx®, Wydase®

U.S./Canadian Brand Names Lidemol® [Can]; Lidex® [Can]; Lyderm® [Can]; Tiamol® [Can]; Topactin [Can]; Topsyn® [Can]; Vanos™ [US]

Therapeutic Category Corticosteroid, Topical

Use Antiinflammatory, antipruritic; treatment of plaque-type psoriasis (up to 10% of body surface area) [high-potency topical corticosteroid]

Usual Dosage

Children and Adults: Pruritus and inflammation: Topical (0.5% cream): Apply thin layer to affected area 2-4 times/day depending on the severity of the condition. Therapy should be discontinued when control is achieved; if no improvement is seen, reassessment of diagnosis may be necessary.

Children ≥12 years and Adults: Plaque-type psoriasis (Vanos™): Topical (0.1% cream): Apply a thin layer once or twice daily to affected areas (limited to <10% of body surface area). **Note:** Not recommended for use >2 consecutive weeks or >60 g/week total exposure. Discontinue when control is achieved.

Dosage Forms

Cream: 0.1% (30 g, 60 g)

Vanos™: 0.1% (30 g, 60 g)

Cream, anhydrous, emollient: 0.05% (15 g, 30 g, 60 g, 120 g)

Cream, aqueous, emollient: 0.05% (15 g, 30 g, 60 g)

Gel: 0.05% (15 g, 30 g, 60 g)

Ointment: 0.05% (15 g, 30 g, 60 g)

Solution: 0.05% (20 mL, 60 mL)

fluohydrisone acetate *see* fludrocortisone *on page* *426*

fluohydrocortisone acetate *see* fludrocortisone *on page* *426*

Fluonid® Topical *(Discontinued)* *see* fluocinolone *on page* *428*

Fluor-I-Strip® *(Discontinued)* *see* fluorescein *on page* *429*

Fluoracaine® *(Discontinued)* *see* proparacaine and fluorescein *on page* *826*

Fluor-A-Day [US/Can] *see* fluoride *on page* *430*

FluorCare® Neutral *(Discontinued)* *see* fluoride *on page* *430*

fluorescein (FLURE e seen)

Synonyms fluorescein sodium; sodium fluorescein; soluble fluorescein

U.S./Canadian Brand Names AK-Fluor® [US]; Angiofluor™ Lite [US]; Angiofluor™ [US]; Fluorescite® [US/Can]; Fluorets® [US]; Ful-Glo® [US]

Therapeutic Category Diagnostic Agent

Use

Injection: Diagnostic aid in ophthalmic angiography and angioscopy

Topical: To stain the anterior segment of the eye for procedures (such as fitting contact lenses), disclosing corneal injury, and in applanation tonometry

Usual Dosage

Ophthalmic: Strips: Children and Adults: Moisten strip with sterile water, saline or ophthalmic fluid. Touch conjunctiva or fornix with tip of strip until adequately stained. For best results, patient should blink several times after application.

Injection:

Children: 3.5 mg/lb (7.7 mg/kg) injected rapidly into antecubital vein

Adults: 500-750 mg injected rapidly into antecubital vein

Note: Prior to use, an intradermal test dose of 0.05 mL may be used if an allergy is suspected. Evaluate 30-60 minutes following intradermal injection.

Oral: Adults: 1 g of injection solution has been administered orally in patients with inaccessible veins and when early phases of an angiogram are not needed.

Dosage Forms

Injection, solution: 10% (5 mL); 25% (2 mL)
AK-Fluor®, Angiofluor™, Angiofluor™ Lite, Fluorescite®: 10% (5 mL); 25% (2 mL)

Strip, ophthalmic: 1 mg
Fluorets®: 1 mg (100)
Ful-Glo®: 0.6 mg (300); 1 mg (300)

fluorescein and proparacaine *see* proparacaine and fluorescein *on page 826*

fluorescein sodium *see* fluorescein *on page 429*

Fluorescite® [US/Can] *see* fluorescein *on page 429*

Fluorets® [US] *see* fluorescein *on page 429*

fluoride (FLOR ide)

Sound-Alike/Look-Alike Issues

Luride® may be confused with Lortab®
Phos-Flur® may be confused with PhosLo®
Thera-Flur-N® may be confused with Thera-Flu®

Synonyms acidulated phosphate fluoride; sodium fluoride; stannous fluoride

U.S./Canadian Brand Names ACT® Plus [US-OTC]; ACT® x2™ [US-OTC]; ACT® [US-OTC]; CaviRinse™ [US]; ControlRx® [US]; Denta 5000 Plus [US]; DentaGel [US]; EtheDent™ [US]; Fluor-A-Day [US/Can]; Fluorigard® [US-OTC]; Fluorinse® [US]; Flura-Drops® [US]; Gel-Kam® Rinse [US]; Gel-Kam® [US-OTC]; Just for Kids™ [US-OTC]; Lozi-Flur™ [US]; Luride® Lozi-Tab® [US]; NeutraCare® [US]; NeutraGard® Advanced [US]; NeutraGard® Plus [US]; NeutraGard® [US-OTC]; Omnii Gel™ [US-OTC]; PerioMed™ [US]; Phos-Flur® Rinse [US-OTC]; Phos-Flur® [US]; PreviDent® 5000 Plus™ [US]; PreviDent® [US]; StanGard® Perio [US]; StanGard® [US]; Stop® [US]

Therapeutic Category Mineral, Oral

Use Prevention of dental caries

Usual Dosage Oral:

The recommended daily dose of oral fluoride supplement (mg), based on fluoride ion content (ppm) in drinking water (2.2 mg of sodium fluoride is equivalent to 1 mg of fluoride ion): Adapted from Recommeded Dosage Schedule of The American Dental Association, The American Academy of Pediatric Dentistry, and The American Academy of Pediatrics:

Less than 0.3 ppm:
- Birth to 6 months: 0 mg
- 6 months to 3 years: 0.25 mg
- 3-6 years: 0.5 mg
- 6-16 years: 1 mg

0.3-0.6 ppm:
- Birth to 3 years: 0 mg
- 3-6 years: 0.25 mg
- 6-16 years: 0.5 mg

Cream: Children ≥6 years and Adults: Brush teeth with cream once daily regardless of fluoride content of drinking water

Dental rinse or gel:

Children 6-12 years: 5-10 mL rinse or apply to teeth and spit daily after brushing
Adults: 10 mL rinse or apply to teeth and spit daily after brushing
PreviDent® rinse: Children >6 years and Adults: Once weekly, rinse 10 mL vigorously around and between teeth for 1 minute, then spit; this should be done preferably at bedtime, after thoroughly brushing teeth; for maximum benefit, do not eat, drink, or rinse mouth for at least 30 minutes after treatment; do not swallow
Fluorinse®: Children >6 years and Adults: Once weekly, vigorously swish 5-10 mL in mouth for 1 minute, then spit

Lozenge (Lozi-Flur™): Adults: One lozenge daily regardless of fluoride content of drinking water

Dosage Forms

Cream, oral [toothpaste]: 1.1% (51 g)
Denta 5000 Plus, EtheDent™, PreviDent® 5000 Plus®: 1.1% (51g)

Gel, topical: 1.1% (56 g)
DentaGel, EtheDent™: 1.1% (56 g)
Gel-Kam® [OTC]: 0.4% (129 g)

Just for Kids™ [OTC], Omnii Gel™ [OTC], StanGard®: 0.4% (122 g)
NeutraCare®, NeutraGard® Advanced, Phos-Flur®, PreviDent®: 1.1% (60 g)
Stop®: 0.4% (120 g)

Lozenge:
Lozi-Flur™: 2.21 mg

Paste, oral [toothpaste]: 1.1% (56 g)
ControlRx®: 1.1% (56 g)

Solution, oral drops: 1.1 mg/mL
Flura-Drops®: 0.55 mg/drop

Solution, oral rinse: 0.05%, 0.2%, 0.44%, 0.5%
ACT® [OTC], ACT® Plus [OCT], Fluorigard® [OTC], NeutraGard® [OTC]: 0.05%
ACT® x2™ [OTC]: 0.5%
CaviRinse™, Fluorinse®, NeutraGard® Plus, PreviDent®: 0.2%
Phos-Flur®: 0.044%

Solution, oral rinse concentrate: 0.63%
Gel-Kam® [OTC], PerioMed™, StanGard® Perio: 0.63%

Tablet, chewable: 0.5 mg, 1.1 mg, 2.2 mg
Fluor-A-Day: 0.56 mg, 1.1 mg, 2.21 mg
Luride® Lozi-Tab®: 0.55 mg, 1.1 mg

Fluorigard® [US-OTC] *see* fluoride *on page* 430
Fluori-Methane® [US] *see* dichlorodifluoromethane and trichloromonofluoromethane *on page* 303
Fluorinse® [US] *see* fluoride *on page* 430
Fluoritab® *(Discontinued)* *see* fluoride *on page* 430
5-fluorocytosine *see* flucytosine *on page* 425
fluorodeoxyuridine *see* floxuridine *on page* 423
9α-fluorohydrocortisone acetate *see* fludrocortisone *on page* 426

fluorometholone (flure oh METH oh lone)

U.S./Canadian Brand Names Flarex® [US/Can]; FML® Forte [US/Can]; FML® [US/Can]; PMS-Fluorometholone [Can]

Therapeutic Category Adrenal Corticosteroid

Use Treatment of steroid-responsive inflammatory conditions of the eye

Usual Dosage Ophthalmic:

Children >2 years and Adults: Reevaluate therapy if improvement is not seen within 2 days; use care not to discontinue prematurely; in chronic conditions, gradually decrease dosing frequency prior to discontinuing treatment

Ointment (FML®): Apply small amount (~1/2 inch ribbon) to conjunctival sac 1-3 times/day; may increase application to every 4 hours during the initial 24-48 hours

Suspension:

FML®: Instill 1 drop into conjunctival sac 2-4 times/day; may instill 1 drop every 4 hours during initial 24-48 hours

FML® Forte: Instill 1 drop into conjunctival sac 2-4 times/day

Adults: Suspension (Flarex®): Instill 1-2 drops into conjunctival sac 4 times/day; may increase application to 2 drops every 2 hours during initial 24-48 hours. Consult prescriber if no improvement after 14 days.

Dosage Forms

Ointment, ophthalmic:
FML®: 0.1% (3.5 g)

Suspension, ophthalmic: 0.1% (5 mL, 10 mL, 15 mL)
Flarex®: 0.1% (5 mL)
FML®: 0.1% (5 mL, 10 mL, 15 mL)
FML® Forte: 0.25% (2 mL, 5 mL, 10 mL, 15 mL)

Fluor-Op® *(Discontinued)* *see* fluorometholone *on page* 431
Fluoroplex® [US] *see* fluorouracil *on page* 431

fluorouracil (flure oh YOOR a sil)

Sound-Alike/Look-Alike Issues

fluorouracil may be confused with flucytosine
Carac® may be confused with Kuric™
Efudex® may be confused with Efidac (Efidac 24®), Eurax®

Synonyms 5-fluorouracil; 5-FU; FU

U.S./Canadian Brand Names Adrucil® [US]; Carac® [US]; Efudex® [US/Can]; Fluoroplex® [US]

Therapeutic Category Antineoplastic Agent

Use Treatment of carcinomas of the breast, colon, rectum, pancreas, or stomach; topically for the management of actinic or solar keratoses and superficial basal cell carcinomas

Usual Dosage Adults:

Refer to individual protocols:

I.V. bolus: 500-600 mg/m^2 every 3-4 weeks **or** 425 mg/m^2 on days 1-5 every 4 weeks

Continuous I.V. infusion: 1000 mg/m^2/day for 4-5 days every 3-4 weeks **or**

2300-2600 mg/m^2 on day 1 every week **or**

300-400 mg/m^2/day **or**

225 mg/m^2/day for 5-8 weeks (with radiation therapy)

Actinic keratoses: Topical:

Carac®: Apply thin film to lesions once daily for up to 4 weeks, as tolerated

Efudex®: Apply to lesions twice daily for 2-4 weeks; complete healing may not be evident for 1-2 months following treatment

Fluoroplex®: Apply to lesions twice daily for 2-6 weeks

Superficial basal cell carcinoma: Topical: Efudex® 5%: Apply to affected lesions twice daily for 3-6 weeks; treatment may be continued for up to 10-12 weeks

Dosage Forms

Cream, topical:

Carac®: 0.5% (30 g)

Efudex®: 5% (40 g)

Fluoroplex®: 1% (30 g)

Injection, solution: 50 mg/mL (10 mL, 20 mL, 50 mL, 100 mL)

Adrucil®: 50 mg/mL (10 mL, 50 mL, 100 mL)

Solution, topical: 2% (10 mL); 5% (10 mL)

Efudex®: 5% (10 mL)

5-fluorouracil *see* fluorouracil *on page* 431

Fluorouracil® ***(Discontinued)*** *see* fluorouracil *on page* 431

Fluothane® ***(Discontinued)*** *see* halothane *on page* 485

fluoxetine (floo OKS e teen)

Sound-Alike/Look-Alike Issues

FLUoxetine may be confused with DULoxetine, famotidine, Feldene®, fluconazole, fluvastatin, fluvoxamine, fosinopril, furosemide, PARoxetine, thiothixene

Prozac® may be confused with Paxil®, Prelone®, Prilosec®, Prograf®, Proscar®, ProSom®, ProStep®, Provera®

Sarafem® may be confused with Serophene®

Synonyms fluoxetine hydrochloride

Tall-Man **FLU**oxetine

U.S./Canadian Brand Names Apo-Fluoxetine® [Can]; CO Fluoxetine [Can]; Dom-Fluoxetine [Can]; Fluoxetine [Can]; FXT 40 [Can]; Gen-Fluoxetine [Can]; Novo-Fluoxetine [Can]; Nu-Fluoxetine [Can]; PHL-Fluoxetine [Can]; PMS-Fluoxetine [Can]; PRO-Fluoxetine [Can]; Prozac® Weekly™ [US]; Prozac® [US/Can]; ratio-Fluoxetine [Can]; Riva-Fluoxetine [Can]; Sandoz-Fluoxetine [Can]; Sarafem® [US]; Selfemra™ [US]; ZYM-Fluoxetine [Can]

Therapeutic Category Antidepressant, Selective Serotonin Reuptake Inhibitor

Use Treatment of major depressive disorder (MDD); treatment of binge-eating and vomiting in patients with moderate-to-severe bulimia nervosa; obsessive-compulsive disorder (OCD); premenstrual dysphoric disorder (PMDD); panic disorder with or without agoraphobia; in combination with olanzapine for treatment-resistant or bipolar I depression

Usual Dosage Oral: **Note:** Upon discontinuation of fluoxetine therapy, gradually taper dose. If intolerable symptoms occur following a dose reduction, consider resuming the previously prescribed dose and/or decrease dose at a more gradual rate.

Children:

Depression: 8-18 years: 10-20 mg/day; lower-weight children can be started at 10 mg/day, may increase to 20 mg/day after 1 week if needed

Obsessive-compulsive disorder: 7-17 years: Initial: 10 mg/day; may increase after 2 weeks if inadequate clinical response to 20 mg/day; further increases may be considered after several weeks to recommended range of 20-30 mg/day (lower weight children) or 20-60 mg/day (adolescents and higher weight children)

Adults: 20 mg/day in the morning; may increase after several weeks by 20 mg/day increments; maximum: 80 mg/day; doses >20 mg may be given once daily or divided twice daily. **Note:** Lower doses of 5-10 mg/day have been used for initial treatment.

Indication-specific dosing:

Bulimia nervosa: 60 mg/day

Depression: Initial: 20 mg/day; may increase after several weeks if inadequate response (maximum: 80 mg/day). Patients maintained on Prozac® 20 mg/day may be changed to Prozac® Weekly™ 90 mg/week, starting dose 7 days after the last 20 mg/day dose

Depression associated with bipolar disorder (in combination with olanzapine): Initial: 20 mg in the evening; adjust as tolerated to usual range of 20-50 mg/day. See "Note."

Obsessive-compulsive disorder: Initial: 20 mg/day; may increase after several weeks if inadequate response; recommended range: 20-60 mg/day (maximum: 80 mg/day)

Panic disorder: Initial: 10 mg/day; after 1 week, increase to 20 mg/day; may increase after several weeks; doses >60 mg/day have not been evaluated

Premenstrual dysphoric disorder (Sarafem®): 20 mg/day continuously, **or** 20 mg/day starting 14 days prior to menstruation and through first full day of menses (repeat with each cycle)

Treatment-resistant depression (in combination with olanzapine): Initial: 20 mg in the evening; adjust as tolerated to usual range of 20-50 mg/day. See "Note."

Note: When using individual components of fluoxetine with olanzapine rather than fixed dose combination product (Symbyax®), approximate dosage correspondence is as follows:

Olanzapine 2.5 mg + fluoxetine 20 mg = Symbyax® 3/25
Olanzapine 5 mg + fluoxetine 20 mg = Symbyax® 6/25
Olanzapine 12.5 mg + fluoxetine 20 mg = Symbyax® 12/25
Olanzapine 5 mg + fluoxetine 50 mg = Symbyax® 6/50
Olanzapine 12.5 mg + fluoxetine 50 mg = Symbyax® 12/50

Dosage Forms

Capsule: 10 mg, 20 mg, 40 mg
Prozac®: 10 mg, 20 mg, 40 mg
Selfemra™: 10 mg, 20 mg

Capsule, delayed release:
Prozac® Weekly™: 90 mg

Solution, oral: 20 mg/5 mL
Prozac®: 20 mg/5 mL

Tablet: 10 mg, 20 mg
Sarafem®: 10 mg, 20 mg

Fluoxetine [Can] *see* fluoxetine *on page 432*

fluoxetine and olanzapine *see* olanzapine and fluoxetine *on page 720*

fluoxetine hydrochloride *see* fluoxetine *on page 432*

fluoxymesterone (floo oks i MES te rone)

U.S./Canadian Brand Names Androxy™ [US]

Therapeutic Category Androgen

Controlled Substance C-III

Use Replacement of endogenous testicular hormone; in females, palliative treatment of breast cancer

Usual Dosage Oral: Adults:

Male:
Hypogonadism: 5-20 mg/day
Delayed puberty: 2.5-20 mg/day for 4-6 months

Female: Inoperable breast carcinoma: 10-40 mg/day in divided doses for 1-3 months

Dosage Forms

Tablet: 10 mg
Androxy™: 10 mg

flupenthixol *(Canada only)* (floo pen THIKS ol)

Synonyms flupenthixol decanoate; flupenthixol dihydrochloride

U.S./Canadian Brand Names Fluanxol® [Can]

Therapeutic Category Antipsychotic Agent; Thioxanthene Derivative

Use Maintenance therapy of chronic schizophrenic patients whose main manifestations do **not** include excitement, agitation, or hyperactivity

Usual Dosage

I.M. (depot): Flupenthixol is administered by deep I.M. injection, preferably in the gluteus maximus, **NOT for I.V. use**; maintenance dosages are given at 2- to 3-week intervals

Patients not previously treated with long-acting depot neuroleptics should be given an initial test dose of 5-20 mg. An initial dose of 20 mg is usually well tolerated; however, a 5 mg test dose is recommended in elderly, frail, and cachectic patients, and in patients whose individual or family history suggests a predisposition to extrapyramidal reactions. In the subsequent 5-10 days, the therapeutic response and the appearance of extrapyramidal symptoms should be carefully monitored. Oral neuroleptic drugs may be continued, but dosage should be reduced during this overlapping period and eventually discontinued.

Oral: Initial: 1 mg 3 times/day; dose must be individualized. May be increased by 1 mg every 2-3 days based on tolerance and control of symptoms. Usual maintenance dosage: 3-6 mg/day in divided doses (doses ≥12 mg/day used in some patients).

Dosage Forms [CAN] = Canadian brand name

Injection, solution [depot]:

Fluanxol® [CAN]: 20 mg/mL (10 mL); 100 mg/mL (2 mL) [not available in the U.S.]

Tablet:

Fluanxol® [CAN]: 0.5 mg, 3 mg [not available in the U.S.]

flupenthixol decanoate *see* flupenthixol *(Canada only) on page 433*

flupenthixol dihydrochloride *see* flupenthixol *(Canada only) on page 433*

fluphenazine (floo FEN a zeen)

Sound-Alike/Look-Alike Issues

Prolixin® may be confused with Proloprim®

Synonyms fluphenazine decanoate

U.S./Canadian Brand Names Apo-Fluphenazine Decanoate® [Can]; Apo-Fluphenazine® [Can]; Modecate® Concentrate [Can]; Modecate® [Can]; PMS-Fluphenazine Decanoate [Can]

Therapeutic Category Phenothiazine Derivative

Use Management of manifestations of psychotic disorders and schizophrenia; depot formulation may offer improved outcome in individuals with psychosis who are nonadherent with oral antipsychotics

Usual Dosage Adults: Psychoses:

Oral: 0.5-10 mg/day in divided doses at 6- to 8-hour intervals; some patients may require up to 40 mg/day

I.M.: 2.5-10 mg/day in divided doses at 6- to 8-hour intervals (parenteral dose is 1/3 to 1/2 the oral dose for the hydrochloride salts)

I.M. (decanoate): 12.5-37.5 mg every 2 weeks

Conversion from hydrochloride to decanoate I.M. 0.5 mL (12.5 mg) decanoate every 3 weeks is approximately equivalent to 10 mg hydrochloride/day; **Note:** Clinically, an every-2-week interval is frequently utilized

Dosage Forms

Injection, oil: 25 mg/mL (5 mL)

Injection, solution: 2.5 mg/mL (10 mL)

Tablet: 1 mg, 2.5 mg, 5 mg, 10 mg

fluphenazine decanoate *see* fluphenazine *on page 434*

Flura® ***(Discontinued)*** *see* fluoride *on page 430*

Flura-Drops® [US] *see* fluoride *on page 430*

flurandrenolide (flure an DREN oh lide)

Sound-Alike/Look-Alike Issues

Cordran® may be confused with Cardura®, codeine, Cordarone®

Synonyms flurandrenolone

U.S./Canadian Brand Names Cordran® SP [US]; Cordran® [US/Can]

Therapeutic Category Corticosteroid, Topical

Use Inflammation of corticosteroid-responsive dermatoses [medium potency topical corticosteroid]

Usual Dosage Topical: Therapy should be discontinued when control is achieved; if no improvement is seen, reassessment of diagnosis may be necessary.
Children:
Cream: Apply sparingly 1-2 times/day
Tape: Apply once daily
Adults: Cream, lotion: Apply sparingly 2-3 times/day

Dosage Forms
Cream, emulsified:
Cordran® SP: 0.05% (15 g, 30 g, 60 g)
Lotion:
Cordran®: 0.05% (15 mL, 60 mL)
Tape, topical [roll]:
Cordran®: 4 mcg/cm^2 (24 inch, 80 inch)

flurandrenolone *see* flurandrenolide *on page 434*

Flurate® Ophthalmic Solution *(Discontinued)* *see* fluorescein *on page 429*

flurazepam (flure AZ e pam)

Sound-Alike/Look-Alike Issues
flurazepam may be confused with temazepam
Dalmane® may be confused with Demulen®, Dialume®

Synonyms flurazepam hydrochloride

U.S./Canadian Brand Names Apo-Flurazepam® [Can]; Dalmane® [Can]; Som Pam [Can]

Therapeutic Category Benzodiazepine

Controlled Substance C-IV

Use Short-term treatment of insomnia

Usual Dosage Oral: Insomnia:
Children: ≥15 years: 15 mg at bedtime
Adults: 15-30 mg at bedtime

Dosage Forms
Capsule: 15 mg, 30 mg

flurazepam hydrochloride *see* flurazepam *on page 435*

flurbiprofen (flure BI proe fen)

Sound-Alike/Look-Alike Issues
flurbiprofen may be confused with fenoprofen
Ansaid® may be confused with Asacol®, Axid®
Ocufen® may be confused with Ocuflox®, Ocupress®

Synonyms flurbiprofen sodium

U.S./Canadian Brand Names Alti-Flurbiprofen [Can]; Ansaid® [Can]; Apo-Flurbiprofen® [Can]; Froben-SR® [Can]; Froben® [Can]; Novo-Flurprofen [Can]; Nu-Flurprofen [Can]; Ocufen® [US/Can]

Therapeutic Category Analgesic, Nonnarcotic; Nonsteroidal Antiinflammatory Drug (NSAID)

Use
Oral: Treatment of rheumatoid arthritis and osteoarthritis
Ophthalmic: Inhibition of intraoperative miosis

Usual Dosage
Oral:
Rheumatoid arthritis and osteoarthritis: 200-300 mg/day in 2-, 3-, or 4 divided doses; do not administer more than 100 mg for any single dose; maximum: 300 mg/day
Dental: Management of postoperative pain: 100 mg every 12 hours
Ophthalmic: Instill 1 drop every 30 minutes, beginning 2 hours prior to surgery (total of 4 drops in each affected eye)

Dosage Forms
Solution, ophthalmic: 0.03% (2.5 mL)
Ocufen®: 0.03% (2.5 mL)
Tablet: 50 mg, 100 mg

flurbiprofen sodium *see* flurbiprofen *on page 435*

5-flurocytosine *see* flucytosine *on page 425*

Fluro-Ethyl® *(Discontinued)* *see* ethyl chloride and dichlorotetrafluoroethane *on page 396*

Flurosyn® Topical *(Discontinued)* *see* fluocinolone *on page* 428
FluShield® *(Discontinued)* *see* influenza virus vaccine *on page* 528

flutamide (FLOO ta mide)

Sound-Alike/Look-Alike Issues
flutamide may be confused with Flumadine®, thalidomide
Eulexin® may be confused with Edecrin®, Eurax®

Synonyms 4′-nitro-3′-trifluoromethylisobutyrantide; niftolid; NSC-147834; SCH 13521

U.S./Canadian Brand Names Apo-Flutamide® [Can]; Euflex® [Can]; Eulexin® [Can]; Novo-Flutamide [Can]

Therapeutic Category Antiandrogen

Use Treatment of metastatic prostatic carcinoma in combination therapy with LHRH agonist analogues

Usual Dosage Oral: Adults: Prostatic carcinoma: 250 mg 3 times/day

Dosage Forms
Capsule: 125 mg

fluticasone and salmeterol (floo TIK a sone & sal ME te role)

Sound-Alike/Look-Alike Issues
Advair® may be confused with Adcirca™, Advicor®

Synonyms fluticasone propionate and salmeterol xinafoate; salmeterol and fluticasone

U.S./Canadian Brand Names Advair Diskus® [US/Can]; Advair® HFA [US]; Advair® [Can]

Therapeutic Category $Beta_2$-Adrenergic Agonist Agent; Corticosteroid, Inhalant

Use Maintenance treatment of asthma; maintenance treatment of COPD

Usual Dosage Oral inhalation: **Note:** Do not use to transfer patients from systemic corticosteroid therapy.

COPD: Adults:
Advair Diskus®: Fluticasone 250 mcg/salmeterol 50 mcg twice daily, 12 hours apart. **Note:** This is the maximum dose.
Advair Diskus® [Canadian labeling; not in approved U.S. labeling]: Fluticasone 250 mcg/salmeterol 50 mcg **or** fluticasone 500 mcg/salmeterol 50 mcg twice daily, 12 hours apart.
Maximum dose: Fluticasone 500 mcg/salmeterol 50 mcg per inhalation (2 inhalations/day)

Asthma:
Children 4-11 years: Advair Diskus®: Fluticasone 100 mcg/salmeterol 50 mcg twice daily, 12 hours apart. **Note:** This is the maximum dose.
Children ≥12 and Adults:
Advair Diskus®: One inhalation twice daily, morning and evening, 12 hours apart
Maximum dose: Fluticasone 500 mcg/salmeterol 50 mcg per inhalation (2 inhalations/day)
Advair® HFA: Two inhalations twice daily, morning and evening, 12 hours apart
Maximum dose: Fluticasone 230 mcg/salmeterol 21 mcg per inhalation (4 inhalations/day)
Advair® 125 or Advair® 250 [Canadian labeling; not in approved U.S. labeling]: Two inhalations twice daily, morning and evening, 12 hours apart
Maximum dose: Fluticasone 250 mcg/salmeterol 25 mcg per inhalation (4 inhalations/day)

Note: Initial dose prescribed should be based upon previous dose of inhaled-steroid asthma therapy. Dose should be increased after 2 weeks if adequate response is not achieved. Patients should be titrated to lowest effective dose once stable. Each suggestion below specifies the product strength to use; remember to **use 1 inhalation for Diskus® and 2 inhalations for HFA.**

Dosage Forms Excipient information presented when available (limited, particularly for generics); consult specific product labeling. [DSC] = Discontinued product; [CAN] = Canadian brand name/formulation

Aerosol, for oral inhalation:
Advair® HFA:
45/21: Fluticasone propionate 45 mcg and salmeterol 21 mcg (12 g)
115/21: Fluticasone propionate 115 mcg and salmeterol 21 mcg (12 g)
230/21: Fluticasone propionate 230 mcg and salmeterol 21 mcg (12 g)
Advair® [CAN]:
125/25: Fluticasone propionate 125 mcg and salmeterol 25 mcg (12 g) [not available in the U.S.]
250/25: Fluticasone propionate 250 mcg and salmeterol 25 mcg (12 g) [not available in the U.S.]

Powder, for oral inhalation:
Advair Diskus®:
100/50: Fluticasone propionate 100 mcg and salmeterol 50 mcg (14s, 60s)
250/50: Fluticasone propionate 250 mcg and salmeterol 50 mcg (60s)
500/50: Fluticasone propionate 500 mcg and salmeterol 50 mcg (60s)

fluticasone (nasal) (floo TIK a sone NAY sal)

U.S./Canadian Brand Names Flonase® [US/Can]

Therapeutic Category Adrenal Corticosteroid

Use Intranasal: Management of seasonal and perennial allergic rhinitis and nonallergic rhinitis in patients ≥4 years of age

Usual Dosage Intranasal: Rhinitis:

Children ≥4 years and Adolescents: Initial: 1 spray (50 mcg/spray) per nostril once daily; patients not adequately responding or patients with more severe symptoms may use 2 sprays (100 mcg) per nostril. Depending on response, dosage may be reduced to 100 mcg daily. Total daily dosage should not exceed 2 sprays in each nostril (200 mcg)/day. Dosing should be at regular intervals.

Adults: Initial: 2 sprays (50 mcg/spray) per nostril once daily; may also be divided into 100 mcg twice a day. After the first few days, dosage may be reduced to 1 spray per nostril once daily for maintenance therapy. Dosing should be at regular intervals.

Dosage Forms

Suspension, intranasal, as furoate [spray]:

Veramyst™: 27.5 mcg/inhalation (10 g)

Suspension, intranasal, as propionate [spray]: 50 mcg/inhalation (16 g)

Flonase®: 50 mcg/inhalation (16 g)

fluticasone (oral inhalation) (floo TIK a sone or al in ha LAY shun)

U.S./Canadian Brand Names Flovent® Diskus® [Can]; Flovent® HFA [US/Can]

Therapeutic Category Adrenal Corticosteroid

Use Inhalation: Maintenance treatment of asthma as prophylactic therapy. It is also indicated for patients requiring oral corticosteroid therapy for asthma to assist in total discontinuation or reduction of total oral dose. NOT indicated for the relief of acute bronchospasm.

Usual Dosage Inhalation, oral: Asthma:

Flovent® HFA: Children ≥12 years: Refer to adult dosing.

Flovent® Diskus® [Can]:

Children 4-16 years: Usual starting dose: 50-100 mcg twice daily; may increase to 200 mcg twice daily in patients not adequately controlled; titrate to the lowest effective dose once asthma stability is achieved

Children ≥16 years: Refer to adult dosing.

Adults: **Note:** Titrate to the lowest effective dose once asthma stability is achieved

Flovent® HFA: Manufacturers labeling: Dosing based on previous therapy

Bronchodilator alone: Recommended starting dose: 88 mcg twice daily; highest recommended dose: 440 mcg twice daily

Inhaled corticosteroids: Recommended starting dose: 88-220 mcg twice daily; highest recommended dose: 440 mcg twice daily; a higher starting dose may be considered in patients previously requiring higher doses of inhaled corticosteroids

Oral corticosteroids: Recommended starting dose:

Flovent® HFA: 440 mcg twice daily

Highest recommended dose: 880 mcg twice daily; starting dose is patient dependent. In patients on chronic oral corticosteroids therapy, reduce prednisone dose no faster than 2.5-5 mg/day on a weekly basis; begin taper after 1 week of fluticasone therapy

NIH Asthma Guidelines (administer in divided doses twice daily).

"Low" dose: 88-264 mcg/day

"Medium" dose: 264-660 mcg/day

"High" dose: >660 mcg/day

Flovent® Diskus® [CAN]:

Mild asthma: 100-250 mcg twice daily

Moderate asthma: 250-500 mcg twice da

Severe asthma: 500 mcg twice daily; may increase to 1000 mcg twice daily in very severe patients requiring high doses of corticosteroids

Dosage Forms [CAN] = Canadian brand name

Aerosol for oral inhalation [CFC free]:

Flovent® HFA: 44 mcg/inhalation (10.6 g); 110 mcg/inhalation (12 g); 220 mcg/inhalation (12 g)

Powder for oral inhalation [prefilled blister pack]:

Flovent® Diskus® [U.S.]: 50 mcg (60s)

Flovent® Diskus®) [CAN]: 50 mcg (28s, 60s); 100 mcg (28s, 60s); 250 mcg (28s, 60s); 500 mcg (28s, 60s) [not available in the U.S.]

fluticasone propionate and salmeterol xinafoate *see* fluticasone and salmeterol *on page 436*

fluticasone (topical) (floo TIK a sone TOP i kal)

Sound-Alike/Look-Alike Issues

Cutivate® may be confused with Ultravate®

U.S./Canadian Brand Names Cutivate® [US/Can]

Therapeutic Category Adrenal Corticosteroid; Corticosteroid, Topical

Use Relief of inflammation and pruritus associated with corticosteroid-responsive dermatoses; atopic dermatitis

Usual Dosage Topical:

Corticosteroid-responsive dermatoses:

Children ≥3 months: Cream: Apply sparingly to affected area twice daily. If no improvement is seen within 2 weeks, reassessment of diagnosis may be necessary

Adults: Cream, lotion, ointment: Apply sparingly to affected area twice daily. If no improvement is seen within 2 weeks, reassessment of diagnosis may be necessary.

Atopic dermatitis:

Children ≥3 months: Cream: Apply sparingly to affected area twice daily. If no improvement is seen within 2 weeks, reassessment of diagnosis may be necessary.

Children ≥1 year: Lotion: Apply sparingly to affected area twice daily

Adults: Cream, lotion: Apply sparingly to affected area once or twice daily. If no improvement is seen within 2 weeks, reassessment of diagnosis may be necessary

Dosage Forms

Cream: 0.05% (15 g, 30 g, 60 g)

Cutivate®: 0.05% (30 g, 60 g)

Lotion:

Cutivate®: 0.05% (60 mL)

Ointment: 0.005% (15 g, 30 g, 60 g)

Cutivate®: 0.005% (30 g, 60 g)

fluvastatin (FLOO va sta tin)

Sound-Alike/Look-Alike Issues

fluvastatin may be confused with fluoxetine, nystatin

U.S./Canadian Brand Names Lescol® XL [US/Can]; Lescol® [US/Can]

Therapeutic Category HMG-CoA Reductase Inhibitor

Use To be used as a component of multiple risk factor intervention in patients at risk for atherosclerosis vascular disease due to hypercholesterolemia

Adjunct to dietary therapy to reduce elevated total cholesterol (total-C), LDL-C, triglyceride, and apolipoprotein B (apo-B) levels and to increase HDL-C in primary hypercholesterolemia and mixed dyslipidemia (Fredrickson types IIa and IIb); to slow the progression of coronary atherosclerosis in patients with coronary heart disease; reduce risk of coronary revascularization procedures in patients with coronary heart disease

Usual Dosage Oral:

Adolescents 10-16 years: Heterozygous familial hypercholesterolemia: Initial: 20 mg once daily; may increase every 6 weeks based on tolerability and response to a maximum recommended dose of 80 mg/day, given in 2 divided doses (immediate release capsule) or as a single daily dose (extended release tablet)

Note: Indicated only for adjunctive therapy when diet alone cannot reduce LDL-C below 190 mg/dL, or 160 mg/dL (with cardiovascular risk factors). Female patients must be 1 year postmenarche.

Adults:

Patients requiring ≥25% decrease in LDL-C: 40 mg capsule once daily in the evening, 80 mg extended release tablet once daily (anytime), or 40 mg capsule twice daily

Patients requiring <25% decrease in LDL-C: Initial: 20 mg capsule once daily in the evening; may increase based on tolerability and response to a maximum recommended dose of 80 mg/day, given in 2 divided doses (immediate release capsule) or as a single daily dose (extended release tablet)

Dosage Forms

Capsule:

Lescol®: 20 mg, 40 mg

Tablet, extended release:

Lescol® XL: 80 mg

Fluviral S/F® [Can] *see* influenza virus vaccine *on page* 528

Fluvirin® [US] *see* influenza virus vaccine *on page* 528

fluvoxamine (floo VOKS a meen)

Sound-Alike/Look-Alike Issues

fluvoxamine may be confused with flavoxate, fluoxetine

Luvox may be confused with Lasix®, Levoxyl®, Lovenox®

U.S./Canadian Brand Names Alti-Fluvoxamine [Can]; Apo-Fluvoxamine® [Can]; Luvox® CR [US]; Luvox® [Can]; Novo-Fluvoxamine [Can]; Nu-Fluvoxamine [Can]; PMS-Fluvoxamine [Can]; Rhoxal-fluvoxamine [Can]; Riva-Fluvox [Can]; Sandoz-Fluvoxamine [Can]

Therapeutic Category Antidepressant, Selective Serotonin Reuptake Inhibitor

Use Treatment of obsessive-compulsive disorder (OCD); treatment of social anxiety disorder

Usual Dosage Oral:

Obsessive-compulsive disorder:

Children 8-17 years: Immediate release: Initial: 25 mg once daily at bedtime; may be increased in 25 mg increments at 4- to 7-day intervals, as tolerated, to maximum therapeutic benefit; usual dose range: 50-200 mg/day. **Note:** When total daily dose exceeds 50 mg, the dose should be given in 2 divided doses with larger portion administered at bedtime.

Maximum: Children: 8-11 years: 200 mg/day, adolescents: 300 mg/day; lower doses may be effective in female versus male patients

Adults:

Immediate release: Initial: 50 mg once daily at bedtime; may be increased in 50 mg increments at 4- to 7-day intervals, as tolerated; usual dose range: 100-300 mg/day; maximum dose: 300 mg/day. **Note:** When total daily dose exceeds 100 mg, the dose should be given in 2 divided doses with larger portion administered at bedtime.

Extended release: Initial: 100 mg once daily at bedtime; may be increased in 50 mg increments at intervals of at least 1 week; usual dosage range: 100-300 mg/day; maximum dose: 300 mg/day

Social anxiety disorder: Adults: Extended release: Initial: 100 mg once daily at bedtime; may be increased in 50 mg increments at intervals of at least 1 week; usual dosage range: 100-300 mg/day; maximum dose: 300 mg/day

Dosage Forms

Tablet:

25 mg, 50 mg, 100 mg

Capsule, extended release:

Luvox® CR: 100 mg, 150 mg

Fluzone® [US] *see* influenza virus vaccine *on page 528*

FML® [US/Can] *see* fluorometholone *on page 431*

FML® Forte [US/Can] *see* fluorometholone *on page 431*

FML-S® ***(Discontinued)***

Focalin® [US] *see* dexmethylphenidate *on page 291*

Focalin® XR [US] *see* dexmethylphenidate *on page 291*

Foille® [US-OTC] *see* benzocaine *on page 129*

folacin *see* folic acid *on page 439*

Folacin-800 [US-OTC] *see* folic acid *on page 439*

folacin, vitamin B_{12}, and vitamin B_6 *see* folic acid, cyanocobalamin, and pyridoxine *on page 440*

Folamin™ [US] *see* folic acid, cyanocobalamin, and pyridoxine *on page 440*

folate *see* folic acid *on page 439*

Folbee [US] *see* folic acid, cyanocobalamin, and pyridoxine *on page 440*

Folbic [US] *see* folic acid, cyanocobalamin, and pyridoxine *on page 440*

Folex® PFS™ ***(Discontinued)*** *see* methotrexate *on page 639*

Folgard® [US-OTC] *see* folic acid, cyanocobalamin, and pyridoxine *on page 440*

Folgard RX® [US] *see* folic acid, cyanocobalamin, and pyridoxine *on page 440*

Folgard RX 2.2® ***(Discontinued)*** *see* folic acid, cyanocobalamin, and pyridoxine *on page 440*

folic acid (FOE lik AS id)

Sound-Alike/Look-Alike Issues

folic acid may be confused with folinic acid

Synonyms folacin; folate; pteroylglutamic acid

U.S./Canadian Brand Names Apo-Folic® [Can]; Folacin-800 [US-OTC]

Therapeutic Category Vitamin, Water Soluble

Use Treatment of megaloblastic and macrocytic anemias due to folate deficiency; dietary supplement to prevent neural tube defects

Usual Dosage

Oral, I.M., I.V., SubQ: Anemia:
 Infants: 0.1 mg/day
 Children <4 years: Up to 0.3 mg/day
 Children >4 years and Adults: 0.4 mg/day
 Pregnant and lactating women: 0.8 mg/day
Oral:
 RDA: Expressed as dietary folate equivalents:
  Children:
   1-3 years: 150 mcg/day
   4-8 years: 200 mcg/day
   9-13 years: 300 mcg/day
  Children ≥14 years and Adults: 400 mcg/day
 Prevention of neural tube defects:
  Females of childbearing potential: 400-800 mcg/day (USPSTF)
  Females at high risk or with family history of neural tube defects: 4 mg/day

Dosage Forms

Injection, solution: 5 mg/mL (10 mL)
Tablet: 0.4 mg, 0.8 mg, 1 mg
 Folacin-800 [OTC]: 0.8 mg

folic acid, cyanocobalamin, and pyridoxine

(FOE lik AS id, sye an oh koe BAL a min, & peer i DOKS een)

Synonyms cyanocobalamin, folic acid, and pyridoxine; folacin, vitamin B_{12}, and vitamin B_6; pyridoxine, folic acid, and cyanocobalamin

U.S./Canadian Brand Names Folamin™ [US]; Folbee [US]; Folbic [US]; Folgard RX® [US]; Folgard® [US-OTC]; Foltx® [US]; Tricardio B [US]

Therapeutic Category Vitamin

Use Nutritional supplement in end-stage renal failure, dialysis, hyperhomocysteinemia, homocystinuria, malabsorption syndromes, dietary deficiencies

Usual Dosage Oral: Adults: 1 tablet daily

Dosage Forms

Tablet: Folic acid 0.8 mg, cyanocobalamin 1000 mcg, and pyridoxine 50 mg
 Folamin™, Folbic, Foltx®: Folic acid 2.5 mg, cyanocobalamin 2000 mcg, and pyridoxine 25 mg
 Folbee: Folic acid 2.5 mg, cyanocobalamin 1000 mcg, and pyridoxine 25 mg
 Folgard® [OTC]: Folic acid 0.8 mg, cyanocobalamin 115 mcg, and pyridoxine 10 mg
 Folgard RX®: Folic acid 2.2 mg, cyanocobalamin 1000 mcg, and pyridoxine 25 mg
 Tricardio B: Folic acid 0.4 mg, cyanocobalamin 250 mcg, and pyridoxine 25 mg

follicle-stimulating hormone, human *see* urofollitropin *on page 999*
follicle stimulating hormone, recombinant *see* follitropin alfa *on page 440*
follicle stimulating hormone, recombinant *see* follitropin beta *on page 441*
Follistim® AQ [US] *see* follitropin beta *on page 441*
Follistim® AQ Cartridge [US] *see* follitropin beta *on page 441*

follitropin alfa (foe li TRO pin AL fa)

Synonyms follicle stimulating hormone, recombinant; FSH; rFSH-alpha; rhFSH-alpha

U.S./Canadian Brand Names Gonal-f® Pen [Can]; Gonal-f® RFF [US]; Gonal-f® [US/Can]

Therapeutic Category Ovulation Stimulator

Use

Gonal-f®: Ovulation induction in patients in whom the cause of infertility is functional and not caused by primary ovarian failure; development of multiple follicles with Assisted Reproductive Technology (ART); spermatogenesis induction

Gonal-f® RFF: Ovulation induction in patients in whom the cause of infertility is functional and not caused by primary ovarian failure; development of multiple follicles with ART

Usual Dosage Adults: **Note:** Dose should be individualized. Use the lowest dose consistent with the expectation of good results. Over the course of treatment, doses may vary depending on individual patient response.

Gonal-f®, Gonal-f® RFF: Females:

Ovulation induction: SubQ: Initial: 75 int. units/day; incremental dose adjustments of up to 37.5 int. units may be considered after 14 days; further dose increases of the same magnitude can be made, if necessary, every 7 days (maximum dose: 300 int. units/day). If response to follitropin is appropriate, hCG is given 1 day following the last dose. Withhold hCG if serum estradiol is >2000 pg/mL, if the ovaries are abnormally enlarged, or if abdominal pain occurs. In general, therapy should not exceed 35 days.

ART: SubQ: Initiate therapy with follitropin alfa in the early follicular phase (cycle day 2 or day 3) at a dose of 150 int. units/day, until sufficient follicular development is attained. In most cases, therapy should not exceed 10 days. In patients ≥35 years whose endogenous gonadotropin levels are suppressed, initiate follitropin alfa at a dose of 225 int. units/day. Continue treatment until adequate follicular development is indicated as determined by ultrasound in combination with measurement of serum estradiol levels. Consider adjustments to dose after 5 days based on the patient's response; adjust subsequent dosage every 3-5 days by ≤75-150 int. units additionally at each adjustment. Doses >450 int. units/day are not recommended. Once adequate follicular development is evident, administer hCG to induce final follicular maturation in preparation for oocyte. Withhold hCG if the ovaries are abnormally enlarged.

Gonal-f®: Males: Spermatogenesis induction: SubQ: Therapy should begin with hCG pretreatment until serum testosterone is in normal range, then 150 int. units 3 times/week with hCG 3 times/week; continue with lowest dose needed to induce spermatogenesis (maximum dose: 300 int. units 3 times/week); may be given for up to 18 months

Dosage Forms

Injection, powder for reconstitution [rDNA origin]:

Gonal-f®: 450 int. units

Gonal-f® RFF: 75 int. units

Injection, solution [rDNA origin]:

Gonal-f® RFF: 300 int. units/0.5 mL (0.5 mL); 450 int. units/0.75 mL (0.75 mL); 900 int. units/1.5 mL (1.5 mL)

follitropin beta (foe li TRO pin BAY ta)

Synonyms follicle stimulating hormone, recombinant; rFSH-beta; rhFSH-beta

U.S./Canadian Brand Names Follistim® AQ Cartridge [US]; Follistim® AQ [US]; Puregon® [Can]

Therapeutic Category Ovulation Stimulator

Use Ovulation induction in patients in whom the cause of infertility is functional and not caused by primary ovarian failure; development of multiple follicles with Assisted Reproductive Technology (ART)

Usual Dosage Adults: Females: **Note:** Dose should be individualized. Use the lowest dose consistent with the expectation of good results. Over the course of treatment, doses may vary depending on individual patient response.

Ovulation induction:

Follistim® AQ: I.M., SubQ: Stepwise approach: Initiate therapy with 75 int. units/day for up to 14 days. Increase by 37.5 int. units at weekly intervals until follicular growth or serum estradiol levels indicate an adequate response. The maximum (individualized) daily dose that has been safely used for ovulation induction in patients during clinical trials is 300 int. units. If response to follitropin is appropriate, hCG is given 1 day following the last dose. Withhold hCG if the ovaries are abnormally enlarged, or if abdominal pain occurs.

Follistim® AQ Cartridge: SubQ: Stepwise approach: Initiate therapy with 75 int. units/day for up to 7 days. Increase by 25 or 50 int. units at weekly intervals until follicular growth or serum estradiol levels indicate an adequate response. The maximum (individualized) daily dose that has been safely used for ovulation induction in patients during clinical trials is 175 int. units. If response to follitropin is appropriate, hCG is given 1 day following the last dose. Withhold hCG if the ovaries are abnormally enlarged, or if abdominal pain occurs.

ART:

Follistim® AQ: I.M., SubQ: A starting dose of 150-225 int. units is recommended for at least the first 4 days of treatment. The dose may be adjusted for the individual patient based upon their ovarian response. The usual maintenance dose was 75-300 int. units for 6-12 days; 375-600 int. units in patients who were poor responders. The maximum daily dose used in clinical studies is 600 int. units. When a sufficient number of follicles of adequate size are present, the final maturation of the follicles is induced by administering hCG. Oocyte retrieval is performed 34-36 hours later. Withhold hCG in cases where the ovaries are abnormally enlarged on the last day of follitropin beta therapy.

Follistim® AQ Cartridge: SubQ: A starting dose of 150-225 int. units is recommended for at least the first 5 days of treatment. The dose may be adjusted for the individual patient based upon their ovarian response. The maximum daily dose used in clinical studies is 450 int. units. When a sufficient number of follicles of adequate size are present, the final maturation of the follicles is induced by administering hCG. Oocyte retrieval is performed 34-36 hours later. Withhold hCG in cases where the ovaries are abnormally enlarged on the last day of follitropin beta therapy.

Dosage Forms

Injection, solution [rDNA origin]:

Follistim® AQ Cartridge: 175 int. units/0.21 mL (0.21 mL); 350 int. units/0.42 mL (0.42 mL); 650 int. units/0.78 mL (0.78 mL); 975 int. units/1.17 mL (1.17 mL)

Injection, solution [rDNA origin; single-dose]:

Follistim® AQ: 75 int. units/0.5 mL (0.5 mL); 150 int. units/0.5 mL (0.5 mL)

Foltrin® [US] *see* vitamins (multiple/oral) *on page 1019*

Foltx® [US] *see* folic acid, cyanocobalamin, and pyridoxine *on page 440*

Folvite® *(Discontinued)* *see* folic acid *on page 439*

fomepizole (foe ME pi zole)

Sound-Alike/Look-Alike Issues

fomepizole may be confused with omeprazole

Synonyms 4-methylpyrazole; 4-MP

U.S./Canadian Brand Names Antizol® [US]

Therapeutic Category Antidote

Use Treatment of methanol or ethylene glycol poisoning alone or in combination with hemodialysis

Usual Dosage Note: Fomepizole therapy should begin immediately upon suspicion of ethylene glycol or methanol ingestion.

Adults: Ethylene glycol and methanol toxicity: I.V.: A loading dose of 15 mg/kg should be administered, followed by doses of 10 mg/kg every 12 hours for 4 doses, then 15 mg/kg every 12 hours thereafter until ethylene glycol levels have been reduced <20 mg/dL and patient is asymptomatic with normal pH

Dosage Forms

Injection, solution [preservative free]: 1 g/mL (1.5 mL)

Antizol®: 1 g/mL (1.5 mL)

fondaparinux (fon da PARE i nuks)

Synonyms fondaparinux sodium

U.S./Canadian Brand Names Arixtra® [US/Can]

Therapeutic Category Factor Xa Inhibitor

Use Prophylaxis of deep vein thrombosis (DVT) in patients undergoing surgery for hip replacement, knee replacement, hip fracture (including extended prophylaxis following hip fracture surgery), or abdominal surgery (in patients at risk for thromboembolic complications); treatment of acute pulmonary embolism (PE); treatment of acute DVT without PE

Note: Additional Canadian approvals (not approved in U.S.): Unstable angina or non-ST segment elevation myocardial infarction (UA/NSTEMI) for the prevention of death and subsequent MI; ST segment elevation MI (STEMI) for the prevention of death and myocardial reinfarction

Usual Dosage SubQ: Adults:

DVT prophylaxis: Adults ≥50 kg: 2.5 mg once daily. **Note:** Initiate dose after hemostasis has been established, 6-8 hours postoperatively.

Usual duration: 5-9 days (up to 10 days following abdominal surgery or up to 11 days following hip replacement or knee replacement)

Extended prophylaxis is recommended following hip fracture surgery (has been tolerated for up to 32 days total).

Acute DVT/PE treatment: **Note:** Start warfarin on the first treatment day and continue fondaparinux until INR is between 2 and 3 (usually 5-7 days):

<50 kg: 5 mg once daily

50-100 kg: 7.5 mg once daily

>100 kg: 10 mg once daily

Usual duration: 5-9 days (has been administered up to 26 days)

Canadian labeling only: Adults:

UA/NSTEMI: SubQ: 2.5 mg once daily; initiate as soon as possible after diagnosis; treat for up to 8 days or until hospital discharge.

STEMI: I.V.: 2.5 mg once; subsequent doses: SubQ: 2.5 mg once daily; treat for up to 8 days or until hospital discharge

Dosage Forms

Injection, solution:

Arixtra®: 2.5 mg/0.5 mL (0.5 mL); 5 mg/0.4 mL (0.4 mL); 7.5 mg/0.6 mL (0.6 mL); 10 mg/0.8 mL (0.8 mL)

fondaparinux sodium *see* fondaparinux *on page 442*

Foradil® [Can] *see* formoterol *on page 443*

Foradil® Aerolizer® [US] *see* formoterol *on page 443*

Forane® [US/Can] *see* isoflurane *on page 548*

formoterol (for MOH te rol)

Sound-Alike/Look-Alike Issues

Foradil® may be confused with Toradol®

Synonyms formoterol fumarate; formoterol fumarate dihydrate

U.S./Canadian Brand Names Foradil® Aerolizer® [US]; Foradil® [Can]; Oxeze® Turbuhaler® [Can]; Perforomist™ [US]

Therapeutic Category $Beta_2$-Adrenergic Agonist Agent

Use Maintenance treatment of asthma and prevention of bronchospasm in patients ≥5 years of age with reversible obstructive airway disease, including patients with symptoms of nocturnal asthma, who require regular treatment with inhaled, short-acting $beta_2$-agonists; maintenance treatment of bronchoconstriction in patients with COPD; prevention of exercise-induced bronchospasm in patients ≥5 years of age

Note:

Oxeze® is also approved in Canada for acute relief of symptoms ("on demand" treatment) in patients ≥6 years of age.

Perforomist™ is only indicated for maintenance treatment of bronchoconstriction in patients with COPD.

Usual Dosage

Asthma maintenance treatment: Children ≥5 years and Adults: Inhalation: **Note:** For long-term asthma control, long-acting $beta_2$-agonists (LABAs) should be used in combination with inhaled corticosteroids and **not** as monotherapy

Foradil®: 12 mcg capsule inhaled every 12 hours via Aerolizer™ device

Oxeze® (CAN): **Note:** Not labeled for use in the U.S.: Children ≥6 years and Adults: Inhalation: 6 mcg or 12 mcg every 12 hours. Maximum dose: Children: 24 mcg/day; Adults: 48 mcg/day

Prevention of exercise-induced bronchospasm: Children ≥5 years and Adults: Inhalation:

Foradil®:12 mcg capsule inhaled via Aerolizer™ device at least 15 minutes before exercise on an "as needed" basis; additional doses should not be used for another 12 hours. **Note:** If already using for asthma maintenance, then should not use additional doses for exercise-induced bronchospasm. Because LABAs may disguise poorly controlled persistent asthma, frequent or chronic use of LABAs for exercise-induced bronchospasm is discouraged by the NIH Asthma Guidelines.

Oxeze® (CAN): **Note:** Not labeled for use in the U.S.: Children ≥6 years and Adults: Inhalation: 6 mcg or 12 mcg at least 15 minutes before exercise.

COPD maintenance treatment: Adults: Inhalation:

Foradil®: 12 mcg capsule inhaled every 12 hours via Aerolizer™ device

Perforomist™: 20 mcg unit-dose vial twice daily (maximum dose: 40 mcg/day)

Additional indication for Oxeze® (approved in Canada): Acute ("on demand") relief of bronchoconstriction: Children ≥12 years and Adults: 6 mcg or 12 mcg as a single dose (maximum dose: 72 mcg in any 24-hour period). The prolonged use of high dosages (48 mcg/day for ≥3 consecutive days) may be a sign of suboptimal control, and should prompt the reevaluation of therapy.

Dosage Forms [CAN] = Canadian brand name

Powder for oral inhalation:

Foradil® Aerolizer®: 12 mcg/capsule (12s, 60s)

Oxeze® Turbuhaler® [CAN]: 6 mcg/inhalation, 12 mcg/inhalation [not available in the U.S.]

Solution for nebulization:

Perforomist™: 20 mcg/2 mL (2 mL)

formoterol and budesonide *see* budesonide and formoterol *on page 155*

formoterol fumarate *see* formoterol *on page* *443*
formoterol fumarate dihydrate *see* formoterol *on page* *443*
formoterol fumarate dihydrate and budesonide *see* budesonide and formoterol *on page* *155*
Formula EM [US-OTC] *see* fructose, dextrose, and phosphoric acid *on page* *448*
Formula Q® *(Discontinued)* *see* quinine *on page* *846*
Formulation R™ [US-OTC] *see* phenylephrine *on page* *774*
Formulex® [Can] *see* dicyclomine *on page* *305*
5-formyl tetrahydrofolate *see* leucovorin calcium *on page* *575*
Fortamet® [US] *see* metformin *on page* *633*
Fortaz® [US/Can] *see* ceftazidime *on page* *196*
Forteo® [US/Can] *see* teriparatide *on page* *946*
Fortical® [US] *see* calcitonin *on page* *167*
Fortovase® *(Discontinued)* *see* saquinavir *on page* *890*
Fosamax® [US/Can] *see* alendronate *on page* *44*
Fosamax Plus D™ [US] *see* alendronate and cholecalciferol *on page* *45*

fosamprenavir (FOS am pren a veer)

Sound-Alike/Look-Alike Issues
Lexiva® may be confused with Levitra®

Synonyms fosamprenavir calcium; GW433908G

U.S./Canadian Brand Names Lexiva® [US]; Telzir® [Can]

Therapeutic Category Antiretroviral Agent, Protease Inhibitor

Use Treatment of HIV infections in combination with at least two other antiretroviral agents

Usual Dosage Oral: HIV infection:

Children:

Antiretroviral therapy-naive patients:

Children 2-5 years of age: Fosamprenavir 30 mg/kg/dose twice daily (not to exceed adult dosage of 1400 mg twice daily without ritonavir)

Children ≥6 years of age:

Unboosted regimen: Fosamprenavir 30 mg/kg/dose twice daily (not to exceed adult dosage of 1400 mg twice daily without ritonavir)

Ritonavir-boosted regimen: Fosamprenavir 18 mg/kg/dose twice daily plus ritonavir 3 mg/kg/dose twice daily (not to exceed the adult dose of fosamprenavir 700 mg plus ritonavir 100 mg twice daily)

Protease inhibitor (PI)-experienced patients: Children ≥6 years of age: Fosamprenavir 18 mg/kg/dose plus ritonavir 3 mg/kg/dose twice daily (not to exceed the adult dose of fosamprenavir 700 mg plus ritonavir 100 mg twice daily)

Notes: The adult regimen of 1400 mg twice daily may be used for pediatric patients who weigh ≥47 kg. When combined with ritonavir, the adult regimen of fosamprenavir 700 mg plus ritonavir 100 mg twice daily can be used in children who weigh ≥39 kg while ritonavir capsules may be used for pediatric patients who weigh ≥33 kg.

Adults:

Antiretroviral therapy-naive patients:

Unboosted regimen: 1400 mg twice daily (without ritonavir)

Ritonavir-boosted regimens:

Once-daily regimen: Fosamprenavir 1400 mg plus ritonavir 100-200 mg once daily

Twice-daily regimen: Fosamprenavir 700 mg plus ritonavir 100 mg twice daily

Protease inhibitor (PI)-experienced patients: Fosamprenavir 700 mg plus ritonavir 100 mg twice daily. **Note:** Once-daily administration is not recommended in protease inhibitor-experienced patients.

Combination therapy with efavirenz (ritonavir-boosted regimen):

Once-daily regimen (PI-naive patients only): Fosamprenavir 1400 mg plus ritonavir 300 mg plus efavirenz 600 mg once daily

Twice-daily regimen: Fosamprenavir 700 mg plus ritonavir 100 mg twice daily plus efavirenz 600 mg once daily

Combination therapy with maraviroc: Fosamprenavir 700 mg plus ritonavir 100 mg plus maraviroc 150 mg twice daily

Dosage Forms [CAN] = Canadian brand name

Tablet:

Lexiva®: 700 mg

Telzir® [CAN]: 700 mg [not available in the U.S.]

Suspension, oral:
Lexiva®: 50 mg/mL
Telzir® [CAN]: 50 mg/mL [not available in the U.S.]

fosamprenavir calcium *see* fosamprenavir *on page 444*

fosaprepitant (fos a PRE pi tant)

Sound-Alike/Look-Alike Issues
fosaprepitant may be confused with aprepitant, fosamprenavir, fospropofol
Emend® for injection (fosaprepitant) may be confused with Emend® (aprepitant) which is an oral capsule formulation.

Synonyms aprepitant injection; fosaprepitant dimeglumine; L-758,298; MK 0517

U.S./Canadian Brand Names Emend® for Injection [US]

Therapeutic Category Antiemetic; Substance P/Neurokinin 1 Receptor Antagonist

Use Prevention of acute and delayed nausea and vomiting associated with moderately- and highly-emetogenic chemotherapy (in combination with other antiemetics)

Usual Dosage I.V.: Adults: Prevention of chemotherapy-induced nausea/vomiting: 115 mg 30 minutes prior to chemotherapy on day 1 (followed by aprepitant 80 mg orally on days 2 and 3) in combination with other antiemetics

Dosage Forms
Injection, powder for reconstitution:
Emend® for Injection: 115 mg

fosaprepitant dimeglumine *see* fosaprepitant *on page 445*
Fosavance [Can] *see* alendronate and cholecalciferol *on page 45*

foscarnet (fos KAR net)

Synonyms PFA; phosphonoformate; phosphonoformic acid

U.S./Canadian Brand Names Foscavir® [Can]

Therapeutic Category Antiviral Agent

Use Treatment of acyclovir-resistant mucocutaneous herpes simplex virus (HSV) infections in immunocompromised persons (eg, with advanced AIDS); treatment of CMV retinitis in persons with HIV

Usual Dosage
CMV retinitis: I.V.:
Induction treatment: 60 mg/kg/dose every 8 hours **or** 90 mg/kg every 12 hours for 14-21 days
Maintenance therapy: 90-120 mg/kg/day as a single daily infusion
Herpes simplex infections (acyclovir-resistant): Induction: I.V.: 40 mg/kg/dose every 8-12 hours for 14-21 days

Dosage Forms
Injection, solution [preservative-free]: 24 mg/mL (250 mL, 500 mL)

Foscavir® [Can] *see* foscarnet *on page 445*
Foscavir® *(Discontinued)* *see* foscarnet *on page 445*

fosfomycin (fos foe MYE sin)

Sound-Alike/Look-Alike Issues
Monurol® may be confused with Monopril®

Synonyms fosfomycin tromethamine

U.S./Canadian Brand Names Monurol® [US/Can]

Therapeutic Category Antibiotic, Miscellaneous

Use Single oral dose in the treatment of uncomplicated urinary tract infections in women due to susceptible strains of *E. coli* and *Enterococcus faecalis*

Usual Dosage Oral: Adults: Females: Uncomplicated UTI: Single dose of 3 g in 3-4 oz (90-120 mL) of water

Dosage Forms
Powder for solution:
Monurol®: 3 g/sachet (3s)

fosfomycin tromethamine *see* fosfomycin *on page 445*

fosinopril (foe SIN oh pril)

Sound-Alike/Look-Alike Issues

fosinopril may be confused with FLUoxetine, Fosamax®, furosemide, lisinopril

Monopril® may be confused with Accupril®, minoxidil, moexipril, Monoket®, Monurol™, ramipril

Synonyms fosinopril sodium

U.S./Canadian Brand Names Apo-Fosinopril® [Can]; Gen-Fosinopril [Can]; Monopril® [US/Can]; Novo-Fosinopril [Can]; PMS-Fosinopril [Can]; RAN-Fosinopril [Can]; Riva-Fosinopril [Can]

Therapeutic Category Angiotensin-Converting Enzyme (ACE) Inhibitor

Use Treatment of hypertension, either alone or in combination with other antihypertensive agents; treatment of heart failure (HF)

Usual Dosage Oral:

Children ≥6 years and >50 kg: Hypertension: Initial: 5-10 mg once daily (maximum: 40 mg/day)

Adults:

Heart failure: Initial: 10 mg/day (5 mg if renal dysfunction present) and increase, as needed, to a maximum of 40 mg once daily over several weeks; usual dose: 20-40 mg/day. If hypotension, orthostasis, or azotemia occur during titration, consider decreasing concomitant diuretic dose, if any.

Hypertension: Initial: 10 mg/day; most patients are maintained on 20-40 mg/day (maximum: 80 mg/day). May need to divide the dose into two if trough effect is inadequate; discontinue the diuretic, if possible 2-3 days before initiation of therapy; resume diuretic therapy carefully, if needed.

Dosage Forms

Tablet: 10 mg, 20 mg, 40 mg

Monopril®: 40 mg

fosinopril and hydrochlorothiazide (foe SIN oh pril & hye droe klor oh THYE a zide)

Sound-Alike/Look-Alike Issues

Monopril® may be confused with Accupril®, minoxidil, moexipril, Monoket®, Monurol™, ramipril

Synonyms hydrochlorothiazide and fosinopril

U.S./Canadian Brand Names Monopril-HCT® [Can]

Therapeutic Category Angiotensin-Converting Enzyme (ACE) Inhibitor

Use Treatment of hypertension; not indicated for first-line treatment

Usual Dosage Note: A patient whose blood pressure is not adequately controlled with fosinopril or hydrochlorothiazide monotherapy may be switched to combination therapy; **not** for initial treatment.

Oral: Adults: Hypertension: Fosinopril 10-80 mg per day, hydrochlorothiazide 12.5-50 mg per day

Dosage Forms

Tablet: 0/12.5: Fosinopril 10 mg and hydrochlorothiazide 12.5 mg; 20/12.5: Fosinopril 20 mg and hydrochlorothiazide 12.5 mg

fosinopril sodium *see* fosinopril *on page 446*

fosphenytoin (FOS fen i toyn)

Sound-Alike/Look-Alike Issues

fosphenytoin may be confused with fospropofol

Cerebyx® may be confused with Celebrex®, Celexa™, Cerezyme®

Synonyms fosphenytoin sodium

U.S./Canadian Brand Names Cerebyx® [US/Can]

Therapeutic Category Hydantoin

Use Used for the control of generalized convulsive status epilepticus and prevention and treatment of seizures occurring during neurosurgery; indicated for short-term parenteral administration when other means of phenytoin administration are unavailable, inappropriate, or deemed less advantageous (the safety and effectiveness of fosphenytoin use for more than 5 days has not been systematically evaluated)

Usual Dosage The dose, concentration in solutions, and infusion rates for fosphenytoin are expressed as phenytoin sodium equivalents (PE); fosphenytoin should always be prescribed and dispensed in phenytoin sodium equivalents (PE)

Adults:

Status epilepticus: I.V.: Loading dose: 15-20 mg PE/kg I.V. administered at 100-150 mg PE/minute

Nonemergent loading and maintenance dosing: I.V. or I.M.:

Loading dose: 10-20 mg PE/kg I.V. or I.M. (maximum I.V. rate: 150 mg PE/minute)

Initial daily maintenance dose: 4-6 mg PE/kg/day I.V. or I.M.

I.M. or I.V. substitution for oral phenytoin therapy: May be substituted for oral phenytoin sodium at the same total daily dose; however, Dilantin® capsules are ~90% bioavailable by the oral route; phenytoin, supplied as fosphenytoin, is 100% bioavailable by both the I.M. and I.V. routes; for this reason, plasma phenytoin concentrations may increase when I.M. or I.V. fosphenytoin is substituted for oral phenytoin sodium therapy; in clinical trials I.M. fosphenytoin was administered as a single daily dose utilizing either 1 or 2 injection sites; some patients may require more frequent dosing

Dosage Forms

Injection, solution: 75 mg/mL (2 mL, 10 mL) [equivalent to phenytoin sodium 50 mg/mL]
Cerebyx®: 75 mg/mL (2 mL, 10 mL) [equivalent to phenytoin sodium 50 mg/mL]

fosphenytoin sodium *see* fosphenytoin *on page* 446

fospropofol (fos PROE po fole)

Sound-Alike/Look-Alike Issues

fospropofol may be confused with fosaprepitant, fosphenytoin, propofol

Synonyms aquavan; fospropofol disodium; GPI 15715

U.S./Canadian Brand Names Lusedra™ [US]

Therapeutic Category Sedative

Use Monitored anesthesia care (MAC) sedation in patients undergoing diagnostic or therapeutic procedures

Usual Dosage Monitored anesthesia care (MAC) sedation: I.V.: **Note: Onset of effect is delayed as compared to propofol-emulsion due to need for conversion to active component.** If <60 kg, base dosing on 60 kg; however, lower doses may be used to achieve lower levels of sedation. If >90 kg, base dosing on 90 kg.

Healthy adults <65 years or with mild systemic disease (ASA-PS1 or -PS2): *Standard dosing regimen:* Initial: 6.5 mg/kg (maximum initial dose: 577.5 mg or 16.5 mL), followed by supplemental doses of 1.6 mg/kg (maximum supplemental dose: 140 mg or 4 mL) no more frequently than every 4 minutes as needed to achieve desired level of sedation.

Product Availability Lusedra™: FDA approved December 2008; anticipated availability is currently undetermined

Dosage Forms

Injection [preservative-free]:
Lusedra™: 35 mg/mL (30 mL)

fospropofol disodium *see* fospropofol *on page* 447
Fosrenol® [US/Can] *see* lanthanum *on page* 572
Fototar® *(Discontinued)* *see* coal tar *on page* 250
Fragmin® [US/Can] *see* dalteparin *on page* 274
Fraxiparine™ [Can] *see* nadroparin *(Canada only) on page* 676
Fraxiparine™ Forte [Can] *see* nadroparin *(Canada only) on page* 676
FreAmine® [US] *see* amino acid injection *on page* 62
FreAmine® III [US] *see* amino acid injection *on page* 62
FreAmine® HBC® [US] *see* amino acid injection *on page* 62
Freedavite [US-OTC] *see* vitamins (multiple/oral) *on page* 1019
Freezone® [US-OTC] *see* salicylic acid *on page* 884
Frisium® [Can] *see* clobazam *(Canada only) on page* 241
Froben® [Can] *see* flurbiprofen *on page* 435
Froben-SR® [Can] *see* flurbiprofen *on page* 435
Frova® [US/Can] *see* frovatriptan *on page* 447

frovatriptan (froe va TRIP tan)

Synonyms frovatriptan succinate

U.S./Canadian Brand Names Frova® [US/Can]

Therapeutic Category Antimigraine Agent; Serotonin 5-$HT_{1B,\ 1D}$ Receptor Agonist

Use Acute treatment of migraine with or without aura

Usual Dosage Oral: Adults: Migraine:

U.S. labeling: 2.5 mg; if headache recurs, a second dose may be given if first dose provided relief and at least 2 hours have elapsed since the first dose (maximum daily dose: 7.5 mg)

Canadian labeling: 2.5 mg; if headache recurs, a second dose may be given if first dose provided relief and at least 4 hours have elapsed since the first dose (maximum daily dose: 5 mg)

Note: The safety of treating more than 4 migraines/month has not been established.

Dosage Forms

Tablet:

Frova®: 2.5 mg

frovatriptan succinate *see* frovatriptan *on page 447*

fructose, dextrose, and phosphoric acid (FRUK tose, DEKS trose, & foss FOR ik AS id)

Sound-Alike/Look-Alike Issues

Emetrol® may be confused with emetine

Synonyms dextrose, levulose and phosphoric acid; levulose, dextrose and phosphoric acid; phosphorated carbohydrate solution; phosphoric acid, levulose and dextrose

U.S./Canadian Brand Names Emetrol® [US-OTC]; Especol® [US-OTC]; Formula EM [US-OTC]; Kalmz [US-OTC]; Nausea Relief [US-OTC]; Nausetrol® [US-OTC]

Therapeutic Category Antiemetic

Use Relief of nausea associated with upset stomach that occurs with intestinal or stomach flu, and food indiscretions

Usual Dosage Oral: Nausea:

Children 2-12 years: 5-10 mL; repeat dose every 15 minutes until distress subsides; do not take for more than 1 hour (5 doses)

Children ≥12 years and Adults: 15-30 mL; repeat dose every 15 minutes until distress subsides; do not take for more than 1 hour (5 doses)

Dosage Forms

Liquid, oral: Fructose 1.87 g, dextrose 1.87 g, and phosphoric acid 21.5 mg per 5 mL

Emetrol® [OTC], Especol® [OTC], Formula EM [OTC], Kalmz [OTC], Nausea Relief [OTC], Nausetrol® [OTC]: Fructose 1.87 g, dextrose 1.87 g, and phosphoric acid 21.5 mg per 5 mL

frusemide *see* furosemide *on page 449*

FS *see* fibrin sealant kit *on page 417*

FSH *see* follitropin alfa *on page 440*

FSH *see* urofollitropin *on page 999*

FS Shampoo® Topical *(Discontinued)* *see* fluocinolone *on page 428*

FS VH S/D *see* fibrin sealant kit *on page 417*

FTC *see* emtricitabine *on page 352*

FTC, TDF, and EFV *see* efavirenz, emtricitabine, and tenofovir *on page 349*

FU *see* fluorouracil *on page 431*

5-FU *see* fluorouracil *on page 431*

Fucidin® [Can] *see* fusidic acid *(Canada only) on page 450*

Fucithalmic® [Can] *see* fusidic acid *(Canada only) on page 450*

FUDR® [US/Can] *see* floxuridine *on page 423*

FUDR *see* floxuridine *on page 423*

Ful-Glo® [US] *see* fluorescein *on page 429*

fulvestrant (fool VES trant)

Synonyms ICI-182,780; zeneca 182,780; ZM-182,780

U.S./Canadian Brand Names Faslodex® [US]

Therapeutic Category Antineoplastic Agent, Estrogen Receptor Antagonist

Use Treatment of hormone receptor positive metastatic breast cancer in postmenopausal women with disease progression following antiestrogen therapy

Usual Dosage I.M.: Adults (postmenopausal women): 250 mg at 1-month intervals

Dosage Forms

Injection, solution [prefilled syringe]:

Faslodex®: 50 mg/mL (2.5 mL, 5 mL)

Fumasorb® *(Discontinued)* *see* ferrous fumarate *on page 413*

Fumerin® *(Discontinued)* *see* ferrous fumarate *on page 413*

Funduscein® Injection *(Discontinued)* *see* fluorescein *on page 429*

FungiGuard [US-OTC] *see* tolnaftate *on page 968*
Fungi-Nail® [US-OTC] *see* undecylenic acid and derivatives *on page 997*
Fungizone® [Can] *see* amphotericin B (conventional) *on page 73*
Fung-O® [US-OTC] *see* salicylic acid *on page 884*
Fungoid® [US-OTC] *see* miconazole *on page 654*
Furacin® Topical *(Discontinued)*
Furadantin® [US] *see* nitrofurantoin *on page 700*
Furalan® *(Discontinued)* *see* nitrofurantoin *on page 700*
Furan® *(Discontinued)* *see* nitrofurantoin *on page 700*
Furanite® *(Discontinued)* *see* nitrofurantoin *on page 700*
furazosin *see* prazosin *on page 812*

furosemide (fyoor OH se mide)

Sound-Alike/Look-Alike Issues

furosemide may be confused with famotidine, finasteride, fluconazole, FLUoxetine, fosinopril, loperamide, torsemide

Lasix® may be confused with Esidrix®, Lanoxin®, Lidex®, Lomotil®, Lovenox®, Luvox®, Luxiq®

Synonyms frusemide

U.S./Canadian Brand Names Apo-Furosemide® [Can]; Dom-Furosemide [Can]; Furosemide Injection, USP [Can]; Furosemide Special [Can]; Lasix® Special [Can]; Lasix® [US/Can]; Novo-Semide [Can]; Nu-Furosemide [Can]; PMS-Furosemide [Can]

Therapeutic Category Diuretic, Loop

Use Management of edema associated with heart failure and hepatic or renal disease; acute pulmonary edema; treatment of hypertension (alone or in combination with other antihypertensives)

Usual Dosage

Infants and Children: Edema, heart failure:

Oral: Initial: 2 mg/kg/dose increased in increments of 1-2 mg/kg/dose with each succeeding dose at intervals of 6-8 hours until a satisfactory response is achieved; maximum dose: 6 mg/kg/dose

I.M., I.V.: Initial: 1 mg/kg/dose; if response not adequate, may increase dose in increments of 1 mg/kg/dose and administer not sooner than 2 hours after previous dose, until a satisfactory response is achieved; may administer maintenance dose at intervals of every 6-12 hours; maximum dose: 6 mg/kg/dose

Adults:

Edema, heart failure:

Oral: Initial: 20-80 mg/dose; if response not adequate, may repeat the same dose or increase dose in increments of 20-40 mg/dose at intervals of 6-8 hours; usual maintenance dose interval is once or twice daily; may be titrated up to 600 mg/day with severe edematous states. **Note:** May also be given on 2-4 consecutive days every week.

I.M., I.V.: Initial: 20-40 mg/dose; if response not adequate, may repeat the same dose or increase dose in increments of 20 mg/dose and administer 1-2 hours after previous dose (maximum dose: 200 mg/dose). Individually determined dose should then be given once or twice daily although some patients may initially require dosing as frequent as every 6 hours. **Note:** ACC/AHA 2009 guidelines for heart failure recommend a maximum single dose of 160-200 mg.

Continuous I.V. infusion: Initial: I.V. bolus dose 20-40 mg over 1-2 minutes, followed by continuous I.V. infusion doses of 10-40 mg/hour. If urine output is <1 mL/kg/hour, double as necessary to a maximum of 80-160 mg/hour. The risk associated with higher infusion rates (80-160 mg/hour) must be weighed against alternative strategies. **Note:** ACC/AHA 2009 guidelines for heart failure recommend 40 mg I.V. load, then 10-40 mg/hour infusion.

Acute pulmonary edema: I.V.: 40 mg over 1-2 minutes. If response not adequate within 1 hour, may increase dose to 80 mg. **Note:** ACC/AHA 2009 guidelines for heart failure recommend a maximum single dose of 160-200 mg.

Hypertension, resistant (JNC 7): Oral: 20-80 mg/day in 2 divided doses

Refractory heart failure: Oral, I.V.: Doses up to 8 g/day have been used.

Dosage Forms

Injection, solution: 10 mg/mL (2 mL, 4 mL, 10 mL)
Injection, solution [preservative free]: 10 mg/mL (2 mL, 4 mL, 10 mL)
Solution, oral: 10 mg/mL, 40 mg/5 mL
Tablet: 20 mg, 40 mg, 80 mg
Lasix®: 20 mg
Lasix®: 40 mg, 80 mg [scored]

Furosemide Injection, USP [Can] *see* furosemide *on page* 449

Furosemide Special [Can] *see* furosemide *on page* 449

fusidic acid *(Canada only)* (fyoo SI dik AS id)

Synonyms sodium fusidate

U.S./Canadian Brand Names Fucidin® [Can]; Fucithalmic® [Can]

Therapeutic Category Antifungal Agent, Systemic

Use

Systemic: Treatment of skin and soft tissue infections, or osteomyelitis, caused by susceptible organisms, including *Staphylococcus aureus* (penicillinase-producing or nonpenicillinase strains); may be used in the treatment of pneumonia, septicemia, endocarditis, burns, and cystic fibrosis caused by susceptible organisms when other antibiotics have failed

Topical: Treatment of primary and secondary skin infections caused by susceptible organisms

Ophthalmic: Treatment of superficial infections of the eye and conjunctiva caused by susceptible organisms

Usual Dosage

I.V.:

Children ≤12 years: 20 mg/kg/day in 3 divided doses

Children >12 years and Adults: 500 mg sodium fusidate 3 times/day

Ophthalmic: Children ≥2 years and Adults: Instill 1 drop in each eye every 12 hours for 7 days

Topical: Children and Adults: Apply to affected area 3-4 times/day until favorable results are achieved. If a gauze dressing is used, frequency of application may be reduced to 1-2 times/day.

Oral: Adults: 500 mg sodium fusidate 3 times/day. (**Note:** Oral dosage may be increased to 1000 mg 3 times/day in fulminating infections.)

Dosage Forms [CAN] = Canadian brand name

Cream:

Fucidin® [CAN]: 2% (15 g, 30 g) [not available in the U.S.]

Injection, powder for reconstitution:

Fucidin® [CAN]: 500 mg [not available in the U.S.]

Ointment, topical:

Fucidin® [CAN]: 2% (15 g, 30 g) [not available in the U.S.]

Suspension, ophthalmic:

Fucithalmic® [CAN]: 10 mg/g [1%] (0.2 g) [unit-dose, without preservative]; (3 g, 5 g) [multidose, contains benzalkonium chloride] [not available in the U.S.]

Tablet:

Fucidin® [CAN]: 250 mg [not available in the U.S.]

Fusilev™ [US] *see* LEVOleucovorin *on page* 581

Fuzeon® [US/Can] *see* enfuvirtide *on page* 354

FVIII/vWF *see* antihemophilic factor/von Willebrand factor complex (human) *on page* 83

FXT 40 [Can] *see* fluoxetine *on page* 432

GAA *see* alglucosidase alfa *on page* 46

gabapentin (GA ba pen tin)

Sound-Alike/Look-Alike Issues

Neurontin® may be confused with Motrin®, Neoral®, nitrofurantoin, Noroxin®, Zarontin®

U.S./Canadian Brand Names Apo-Gabapentin® [Can]; CO Gabapentin [Can]; Dom-Gabapentin [Can]; Gen-Gabapentin [Can]; Neurontin® [US/Can]; Novo-Gabapentin [Can]; Nu-Gabapentin [Can]; PHL-Gabapentin [Can]; PMS-Gabapentin [Can]; ratio-Gabapentin [Can]; Riva-Gabapentin [Can]

Therapeutic Category Anticonvulsant

Use Adjunct for treatment of partial seizures with and without secondary generalized seizures in patients >12 years of age with epilepsy; adjunct for treatment of partial seizures in pediatric patients 3-12 years of age; management of postherpetic neuralgia (PHN) in adults

Usual Dosage Oral:

Children: Anticonvulsant:

3-12 years: Initial: 10-15 mg/kg/day in 3 divided doses; titrate to effective dose over ~3 days; dosages of up to 50 mg/kg/day have been tolerated in clinical studies

3-4 years: Effective dose: 40 mg/kg/day in 3 divided doses

≥5-12 years: Effective dose: 25-35 mg/kg/day in 3 divided doses

See **"Note"** in Adults dosing.

Children >12 years and Adults:

Anticonvulsant: Initial: 300 mg 3 times/day; if necessary the dose may be increased up to 1800 mg/day. Doses of up to 2400 mg/day have been tolerated in long-term clinical studies; up to 3600 mg/day has been tolerated in short-term studies.

Note: If gabapentin is discontinued or if another anticonvulsant is added to therapy, it should be done slowly over a minimum of 1 week

Adults: Postherpetic neuralgia or neuropathic pain: Day 1: 300 mg, Day 2: 300 mg twice daily, Day 3: 300 mg 3 times/day; dose may be titrated as needed for pain relief (range: 1800-3600 mg/day, daily doses >1800 mg do not generally show greater benefit)

Dosage Forms

Capsule: 100 mg, 300 mg, 400 mg

Neurontin®: 100 mg, 300 mg, 400 mg

Solution, oral:

Neurontin®: 250 mg/5 mL

Tablet: 100 mg, 300 mg, 400 mg, 600 mg, 800 mg

Neurontin®: 600 mg, 800 mg

Gabitril® [US/Can] *see* tiagabine *on page 958*

gadobenate dimeglumine (gad oh BEN ate dye MEG loo meen)

Synonyms gadolinum-BOPTA; Gd-BOPTA

U.S./Canadian Brand Names Multihance® Multipak™ [US]; Multihance® [US]

Therapeutic Category Diagnostic Agent; Radiological/Contrast Media, Nonionic

Use Contrast medium for magnetic resonance imaging (MRI) to visualize CNS lesions with abnormal vascularity in the brain, spine, and associated tissues

Usual Dosage I.V.: Adults: CNS lesions: 0.1 mmol/kg (0.2 mL/kg)

Dosage Forms

Injection, solution [preservative free]:

Multihance®: 529 mg/mL (5 mL, 10 mL, 15 mL, 20 mL)

Multihance® Multipack™: 529 mg/mL (50 mL, 100 mL)

gadobutrol *(Canada only)* (gad oh BYOO trol)

Sound-Alike/Look-Alike Issues

Gadovist® may be confused with Magnevist®, Vasovist™

Synonyms gadovist 1.0

U.S./Canadian Brand Names Gadovist® [Can]

Therapeutic Category Gadolinium-Containing Contrast Agent; Radiological/Contrast Media, Nonionic

Use Contrast medium for magnetic resonance imaging (MRI) of CNS lesions (brain, spine, and associated tissues); perfusion studies to diagnose stroke, or to detect focal cerebral ischemia or tumor perfusion; contrast-enhanced magnetic resonance angiography (CE-MRA)

Usual Dosage I.V.: Adults:

General CNS imaging: 0.1 mmol/kg (0.1 mL/kg); if needed, a second dose of 0.1-0.2 mmol/kg (0.1-0.2 mL/kg) may be repeated once within 30 minutes of the first dose

Exclusion of metastatic or recurrent tumors: 0.3 mmol/kg (0.3 mL/kg)

Perfusion studies: 0.3 mmol/kg (0.3 mL/kg)

CE-MRA:

Imaging of a single field of view (FOV):

Patient weight <75 kg: 7.5 mL

Patient weight ≥75 kg: 10 mL

Imaging >1 FOV:

Patient weight <75 kg: 15 mL

Patient weight ≥75 kg: 20 mL

Dosage Forms [CAN] = Canadian brand name

Injection, solution [preservative free]:

Gadovist® [CAN]: 604.72 mg/mL (15 mL) [not available in U.S.]

gadodiamide (gad oh DYE a mide)

Synonyms gadolinium-DTPA-BMA; Gd-DTPA-BMA

U.S./Canadian Brand Names Omniscan™ [US]

Therapeutic Category Radiological/Contrast Media, Nonionic

Use Contrast medium for magnetic resonance imaging (MRI) to visualize CNS lesions with abnormal vascularity in the brain, spine, and associated tissues, and to visualize body lesions with abnormal vascularity within the thoracic (noncardiac), abdominal, pelvic cavities, and retroperitoneal space

Usual Dosage I.V.:

Children ≥2 years:

Body imaging:

Kidney: 0.05 mmol/kg (0.1 mL/kg); the safety of additional doses has not been studied

Intrathoracic (noncardiac), intraabdominal, pelvic cavities: 0.1 mmol/kg (0.2 mL/kg)

CNS imaging: 0.1 mmol/kg (0.2 mL/kg); the safety of additional doses has not been studied

Adults:

Body imaging:

Kidney: 0.05 mmol/kg (0.1 mL/kg); the safety of additional doses has not been studied

Intrathoracic (noncardiac), intraabdominal, pelvic cavities: 0.1 mmol/kg (0.2 mL/kg); the safety of additional doses has not been studied

CNS imaging: 0.1 mmol/kg (0.2 mL/kg); if needed, a second dose of 0.2 mmol/kg (0.4 mL/kg) may be repeated once within 20 minutes of the first dose

Dosage Forms

Injection, solution [preservative free]:

Omniscan™: 287 mg/mL (5 mL, 10 mL, 15 mL, 20 mL, 50 mL)

gadofosveset *(Canada only)* (gad oh FOS ve set)

Sound-Alike/Look-Alike Issues

Vasovist® may be confused with Magnevist®, Gadovist®

Synonyms gadofosveset trisodium

U.S./Canadian Brand Names Vasovist® [Can]

Therapeutic Category Gadolinium-Containing Contrast Agent; Radiological/Contrast Media, Paramagnetic Agent

Use Contrast medium used to enhance visualization of abdominal or limb vasculature in magnetic resonance angiography (MRA)

Usual Dosage I.V.: Adults: MRA: 0.03 mmol/kg (0.12 mL/kg); doses >0.03 mmol/kg are not recommended

Dosage Forms [CAN] = Canadian brand name

Injection, solution [preservative free]:

Vasovist® [CAN]: 0.25 mmoL/mL (10 mL, 15 mL, 20 mL) [not available in U.S.]

gadofosveset trisodium *see* gadofosveset *(Canada only) on page 452*

gadolinium-DTPA *see* gadopentetate dimeglumine *on page 452*

gadolinium-DTPA-BMA *see* gadodiamide *on page 451*

gadolinium-DTPA-BMEA *see* gadoversetamide *on page 453*

gadolinium-HP-DO3A *see* gadoteridol *on page 452*

gadolinum-BOPTA *see* gadobenate dimeglumine *on page 451*

gadopentetate dimeglumine (gad oh PEN te tate dye MEG loo meen)

Synonyms gadolinium-DTPA; Gd-DTPA

U.S./Canadian Brand Names Magnevist® [US/Can]

Therapeutic Category Radiological/Contrast Media, Paramagnetic Agent

Use Contrast medium for magnetic resonance imaging (MRI) to visualize lesions with abnormal vascularity in the brain, spine and associated tissues, head and neck, and body (excluding the heart)

Usual Dosage I.V.: Children ≥2 years and Adults: MRI: 0.1 mmol/kg (0.2 mL/kg)

Note: Dosing for patients >130 kg (286 pounds) has not been studied.

Dosage Forms

Injection, solution [preservative free]:

Magnevist®: Gadopentetate dimeglumine 469.01 mg/mL (5 mL, 10 mL, 15 mL, 20 mL, 50 mL, 100 mL)

gadoteridol (gad oh TER i dol)

Synonyms gadolinium-HP-DO3A; Gd-HP-DO3A

U.S./Canadian Brand Names ProHance® [US]

Therapeutic Category Radiological/Contrast Media, Nonionic

Use Contrast medium for magnetic resonance imaging (MRI) to visualize CNS lesions with abnormal vascularity in the brain, spine, and associated tissues and to visualize extracranial/extraspinal tissues in the head and neck

Usual Dosage I.V.:

Children ≥2 years: CNS imaging: 0.1 mmol/kg (0.2 mL/kg); the safety of additional doses has not been studied

Adults:

CNS imaging: 0.1 mmol/kg (0.2 mL/kg); if needed, a second dose of 0.2 mmol/kg (0.4 mL/kg) may be repeated once within 30 minutes of the first dose

Extracranial/extraspinal tissue: 0.1 mmol/kg (0.2 mL/kg)

Dosage Forms

Injection, solution [preservative free]:

ProHance®: 279.3 mg/mL (5 mL, 10 mL, 15 mL, 17 mL, 20 mL, 50 mL) [contains calteridol calcium 0.23 mg/mL and tromethamine 1.21 mg/mL]

ProHance® Multipack™: 279.3 mg/mL (50 mL) [contains calteridol calcium 0.23 mg/mL and tromethamine 1.21 mg/mL; pharmacy bulk package]

gadoversetamide (gad oh ver SET a mide)

Synonyms gadolinium-DTPA-BMEA; Gd-DTPA-BMEA

U.S./Canadian Brand Names OptiMARK® [US]

Therapeutic Category Radiological/Contrast Media, Nonionic

Use Contrast medium for magnetic resonance imaging (MRI) to visualize lesions with abnormal vascularity in the liver or CNS (brain, spine, and associated tissues)

Usual Dosage I.V.: Adults: CNS or liver lesions: 0.1 mmol/kg (0.2 mL/kg)

Dosage Forms

Injection, solution [preservative free]:

OptiMARK®: 330.9 mg/mL (5 mL, 10 mL, 15 mL, 20 mL, 30 mL, 50 mL)

Gadovist® [Can] *see* gadobutrol *(Canada only) on page 451*

gadovist 1.0 *see* gadobutrol *(Canada only) on page 451*

gadoxetate (gad OX e tate)

Sound-Alike/Look-Alike Issues

Eovist® may be confused with Evista®

Synonyms gadoxetate disodium; Gd-EOB-DTPA

U.S./Canadian Brand Names Eovist® [US]

Therapeutic Category Gadolinium-Containing Contrast Agent; Radiological/Contrast Media, Ionic (Low Osmolality); Radiological/Contrast Media, Paramagnetic Agent

Use Contrast medium for magnetic resonance imaging (MRI) to detect and characterize lesions within focal liver disease

Usual Dosage I.V.: Adults: Visualization of liver lesions: 0.025 mmol/kg (0.1 mL/kg)

Dosage Forms

Injection, solution [preservative free]:

Eovist®: 181.43 mg/mL (10 mL)

gadoxetate disodium *see* gadoxetate *on page 453*

galantamine (ga LAN ta meen)

Sound-Alike/Look-Alike Issues

Razedyne™ may be confused with Rozerem™

Reminyl® may be confused with Amaryl®, Robinul®

Synonyms galantamine hydrobromide

U.S./Canadian Brand Names Razadyne™ ER [US]; Razadyne™ [US]; Reminyl® ER [Can]; Reminyl® [Can]

Therapeutic Category Acetylcholinesterase Inhibitor (Central)

Use Treatment of mild-to-moderate dementia of Alzheimer disease

Usual Dosage Oral: Adults:

Note: Oral solution and tablet should be taken with breakfast and dinner; capsule should be taken with breakfast. If therapy is interrupted for ≥3 days, restart at the lowest dose and increase to current dose.

Immediate release tablet or solution: Mild-to-moderate dementia of Alzheimer's: Initial: 4 mg twice a day for 4 weeks; if tolerated, increase to 8 mg twice daily for ≥4 weeks; if tolerated, increase to 12 mg twice daily
Range: 16-24 mg/day in 2 divided doses
Extended-release capsule: Initial: 8 mg once daily for 4 weeks; if tolerated, increase to 16 mg once daily for ≥4 weeks; if tolerated, increase to 24 mg once daily
Range: 16-24 mg once daily
Conversion to galantamine from other cholinesterase inhibitors: Patients experiencing poor tolerability with donepezil or rivastigmine should wait until side effects subside or allow a 7-day washout period prior to beginning galantamine. Patients not experiencing side effects with donepezil or rivastigmine may begin galantamine therapy the day immediately following discontinuation of previous therapy.

Dosage Forms
Capsule, extended release, oral: 8 mg, 16 mg, 24 mg
Razadyne® ER: 8 mg, 16 mg, 24 mg
Solution, oral: 4 mg/mL (100 mL)
Razadyne®: 4 mg/mL
Tablet: 4 mg, 8 mg, 12 mg
Razadyne®: 4 mg, 8 mg, 12 mg

galantamine hydrobromide *see* galantamine *on page* 453

galsulfase (gal SUL fase)

Synonyms recombinant N-acetylgalactosamine 4-sulfatase; rhASB
U.S./Canadian Brand Names Naglazyme™ [US]
Therapeutic Category Enzyme
Use Replacement therapy in mucopolysaccharidosis VI (MPS VI; Maroteaux-Lamy Syndrome) for improvement of walking and stair-climbing capacity
Usual Dosage Note: Premedicate with antihistamines with/without antipyretics 30-60 minutes prior to infusion. MPS VI: Children >5 years and Adults: I.V.: 1 mg/kg once weekly
Dosage Forms
Injection, solution [preservative free]:
Naglazyme™: 5 mg/5 mL (5 mL)

Gamimune® N [Can] *see* immune globulin (intravenous) *on page* 523
Gamimune® N Injection *(Discontinued)* *see* immune globulin (intravenous) *on page* 523
gamma benzene hexachloride *see* lindane *on page* 590
Gamma E-Gems® [US-OTC] *see* vitamin E *on page* 1018
Gamma-E Plus [US-OTC] *see* vitamin E *on page* 1018
Gammagard Liquid [US/Can] *see* immune globulin (intravenous) *on page* 523
Gammagard S/D [US/Can] *see* immune globulin (intravenous) *on page* 523
gamma globulin *see* immune globulin (intramuscular) *on page* 522
gamma hydroxybutyric acid *see* sodium oxybate *on page* 911
gammaphos *see* amifostine *on page* 60
Gammar®-P I.V. *(Discontinued)* *see* immune globulin (intravenous) *on page* 523
GammaSTAN™ S/D [US] *see* immune globulin (intramuscular) *on page* 522
Gamulin® Rh *(Discontinued)*
Gamunex® [US/Can] *see* immune globulin (intravenous) *on page* 523

ganciclovir (gan SYE kloe veer)

Sound-Alike/Look-Alike Issues
ganciclovir may be confused with acyclovir
Cytovene® may be confused with Cytosar®, Cytosar-U®
Synonyms DHPG sodium; GCV sodium; nordeoxyguanosine
U.S./Canadian Brand Names Cytovene® [US/Can]; Vitrasert® [US/Can]
Therapeutic Category Antiviral Agent
Use
Parenteral: Treatment of CMV retinitis in immunocompromised individuals, including patients with acquired immunodeficiency syndrome; prophylaxis of CMV infection in transplant patients

Oral: Alternative to the I.V. formulation for maintenance treatment of CMV retinitis in immunocompromised patients, including patients with AIDS, in whom retinitis is stable following appropriate induction therapy and for whom the risk of more rapid progression is balanced by the benefit associated with avoiding daily I.V. infusions.

Implant: Treatment of CMV retinitis

Usual Dosage

CMV retinitis: Slow I.V. infusion (dosing is based on total body weight):

Children >3 months and Adults:

Induction therapy: 5 mg/kg/dose every 12 hours for 14-21 days followed by maintenance therapy

Maintenance therapy: 5 mg/kg/day as a single daily dose for 7 days/week or 6 mg/kg/day for 5 days/week

CMV retinitis: Oral: 1000 mg 3 times/day with food **or** 500 mg 6 times/day with food

Prevention of CMV disease in patients with advanced HIV infection and normal renal function: Oral: 1000 mg 3 times/day with food

Prevention of CMV disease in transplant patients: Same initial and maintenance dose as CMV retinitis except duration of initial course is 7-14 days, duration of maintenance therapy is dependent on clinical condition and degree of immunosuppression

Intravitreal implant: One implant for 5- to 8-month period; following depletion of ganciclovir, as evidenced by progression of retinitis, implant may be removed and replaced

Product Availability

Zirgan™: FDA approved September 2009; availability expected in early 2010

Zirgan™ is an ophthalmic gel indicated for the treatment of acute herpetic keratitis.

Dosage Forms

Capsule: 250 mg, 500 mg

Implant, intravitreal:

Vitrasert®: 4.5 mg [released gradually over 5-8 months]

Injection, powder for reconstitution:

Cytovene®: 500 mg

Ganidin NR [US] *see* guaifenesin *on page 473*

ganirelix (ga ni REL ix)

Synonyms antagon; ganirelix acetate

U.S./Canadian Brand Names Orgalutran® [Can]

Therapeutic Category Antigonadotropic Agent

Use Inhibits premature luteinizing hormone (LH) surges in women undergoing controlled ovarian hyperstimulation

Usual Dosage SubQ: Adults: 250 mcg/day during the mid-to-late phase after initiating follicle-stimulating hormone on day 2 or 3 of cycle. Treatment should be continued daily until the day of chorionic gonadotropin administration.

Dosage Forms

Injection, solution: 250 mcg/0.5 mL

ganirelix acetate *see* ganirelix *on page 455*

Gani-Tuss DM NR [US] *see* guaifenesin and dextromethorphan *on page 474*

Gani-Tuss® NR [US] *see* guaifenesin and codeine *on page 473*

Gantrisin® [US] *see* sulfisoxazole *on page 931*

GAR-936 *see* tigecycline *on page 960*

Garamycin® [Can] *see* gentamicin *on page 461*

Garamycin® *(Discontinued)* *see* gentamicin *on page 461*

Gardasil® [US/Can] *see* papillomavirus (types 6, 11, 16, 18) vaccine (human, recombinant) *on page 750*

Gas-X® [US-OTC] *see* simethicone *on page 901*

Gas-X®, Children's Tongue Twisters™ [US-OTC] *see* simethicone *on page 901*

Gas-X® Extra Strength [US-OTC] *see* simethicone *on page 901*

Gas-X® Infant [US-OTC] *see* simethicone *on page 901*

Gas-X® Maximum Strength [US-OTC] *see* simethicone *on page 901*

Gas-X® Thin Strips™ [US-OTC] *see* simethicone *on page 901*

Gas Ban™ [US-OTC] *see* calcium carbonate and simethicone *on page 171*

Gas-Ban DS® ***(Discontinued)*** *see* aluminum hydroxide, magnesium hydroxide, and simethicone *on page* *56*

Gastrocrom® [US] *see* cromolyn sodium *on page* *261*

Gastrografin® [US] *see* diatrizoate meglumine and diatrizoate sodium *on page* *300*

Gastrosed™ ***(Discontinued)*** *see* hyoscyamine *on page* *512*

gatifloxacin (gat i FLOKS a sin)

U.S./Canadian Brand Names Zymar® [US/Can]

Therapeutic Category Antibiotic, Quinolone

Use Treatment of bacterial conjunctivitis

Usual Dosage Ophthalmic: Children ≥1 year and Adults: Bacterial conjunctivitis:

Days 1 and 2: Instill 1 drop into affected eye(s) every 2 hours while awake (maximum: 8 times/day)

Days 3-7: Instill 1 drop into affected eye(s) up to 4 times/day while awake

Dosage Forms

Solution, ophthalmic:

Zymar®: 0.3% (5 mL)

Gaviscon® Extra Strength [US-OTC] *see* aluminum hydroxide and magnesium carbonate *on page* *55*

Gaviscon® Liquid [US-OTC] *see* aluminum hydroxide and magnesium carbonate *on page* *55*

Gaviscon® Tablet [US-OTC] *see* aluminum hydroxide and magnesium trisilicate *on page* *56*

G-CSF *see* filgrastim *on page* *420*

G-CSF (PEG conjugate) *see* pegfilgrastim *on page* *755*

GCV sodium *see* ganciclovir *on page* *454*

GD-Amlodipine [Can] *see* amlodipine *on page* *66*

Gd-BOPTA *see* gadobenate dimeglumine *on page* *451*

GD-Celecoxib [Can] *see* celecoxib *on page* *201*

Gd-DTPA *see* gadopentetate dimeglumine *on page* *452*

Gd-DTPA-BMA *see* gadodiamide *on page* *451*

Gd-DTPA-BMEA *see* gadoversetamide *on page* *453*

Gd-EOB-DTPA *see* gadoxetate *on page* *453*

Gd-HP-DO3A *see* gadoteridol *on page* *452*

GD-Quinapril [Can] *see* quinapril *on page* *844*

Gebauer's Ethyl Chloride® [US] *see* ethyl chloride *on page* *396*

Gee Gee® ***(Discontinued)*** *see* guaifenesin *on page* *473*

gefitinib (ge FI tye nib)

Sound-Alike/Look-Alike Issues

gefitinib may be confused with erlotinib

Synonyms NSC-715055; ZD1839

U.S./Canadian Brand Names IRESSA® [US]

Therapeutic Category Antineoplastic Agent, Tyrosine Kinase Inhibitor

Use

U.S. labeling: Treatment of locally advanced or metastatic nonsmall cell lung cancer after failure of platinum-based and docetaxel therapies. Treatment is limited to patients who are benefiting or have benefited from treatment with gefitinib.

Note: Due to the lack of improved survival data from clinical trials of gefitinib, and in response to positive survival data with another EGFR inhibitor, physicians are advised to use other treatment options in advanced nonsmall cell lung cancer patients following one or two prior chemotherapy regimens when they are refractory/intolerant to their most recent regimen.

Canada labeling: Approved indication is limited to NSCLC patients with epidermal growth factor receptor (EGFR) expression status positive or unknown.

Usual Dosage Note: In response to the lack of improved survival data from the ISEL trial, AstraZeneca has temporarily suspended promotion of this drug.

Oral: Adults: 250 mg/day; consider 500 mg/day in patients receiving effective CYP3A4 inducers (eg, rifampin, phenytoin)

Dosage Forms
Tablet:
IRESSA®: 250 mg

gelatin (absorbable) (JEL a tin, ab SORB a ble)

Synonyms absorbable gelatin sponge
U.S./Canadian Brand Names Gelfilm® [US]; Gelfoam® [US]
Therapeutic Category Hemostatic Agent
Use Adjunct to provide hemostasis in surgery; open prostatic surgery
Usual Dosage Hemostasis: Apply packs or sponges dry or saturated with sodium chloride. When applied dry, hold in place with moderate pressure. When applied wet, squeeze to remove air bubbles. The powder is applied as a paste prepared by adding approximately 4 mL of sterile saline solution to the powder.
Dosage Forms
Film, ophthalmic:
Gelfilm®: 25 mm x 50 mm (6s)
Film, topical:
Gelfilm®: 100 mm x 125 mm (1s)
Powder, topical:
Gelfoam®: 1 g
Sponge, dental:
Gelfoam®: Size 4 (12s)
Sponge, topical:
Gelfoam®:
Size 50 (4s)
Size 100 (6s)
Size 200 (6s)
Size 2 cm (1s)
Size 6 cm (6s)
Size 12-7 mm (12s)

gelatin, pectin, and methylcellulose (JEL a tin, PEK tin, & meth il SEL yoo lose)

Synonyms methylcellulose, gelatin, and pectin; pectin, gelatin, and methylcellulose
Therapeutic Category Protectant, Topical
Use Temporary relief from minor oral irritations
Usual Dosage Press small dabs into place until the involved area is coated with a thin film; do not try to spread onto area; may be used as often as needed

Gelclair® [US] *see* mucosal barrier gel, oral *on page 671*
Gelfilm® [US] *see* gelatin (absorbable) *on page 457*
Gelfoam® [US] *see* gelatin (absorbable) *on page 457*
Gel-Kam® [US-OTC] *see* fluoride *on page 430*
Gel-Kam® Rinse [US] *see* fluoride *on page 430*
Gelnique™ [US] *see* oxybutynin *on page 736*
GelRite [US-OTC] *see* alcohol (ethyl) *on page 42*
Gel-Stat™ [US-OTC] *see* alcohol (ethyl) *on page 42*
Gel-Tin® *(Discontinued)* *see* fluoride *on page 430*
Gelucast® [US] *see* zinc gelatin *on page 1030*
Gelusil® [US-OTC/Can] *see* aluminum hydroxide, magnesium hydroxide, and simethicone *on page 56*
Gelusil® Extra Strength [Can] *see* aluminum hydroxide and magnesium hydroxide *on page 55*

gemcitabine (jem SITE a been)

Sound-Alike/Look-Alike Issues
gemcitabine may be confused with gemtuzumab
Gemzar® may be confused with Zinecard®
Synonyms gemcitabine hydrochloride; NSC-613327
U.S./Canadian Brand Names Gemzar® [US/Can]
Therapeutic Category Antineoplastic Agent

Use Treatment of metastatic breast cancer; locally-advanced or metastatic nonsmall cell lung cancer (NSCLC) or pancreatic cancer; advanced, relapsed ovarian cancer

Usual Dosage Refer to individual protocols. **Note**: Prolongation of the infusion time >60 minutes and administration more frequently than once weekly have been shown to increase toxicity. I.V.:

Pancreatic cancer: Initial: 1000 mg/m^2 weekly for up to 7 weeks followed by 1 week rest; then weekly for 3 weeks out of every 4 weeks.

Dose adjustment: Patients who complete an entire cycle of therapy may have the dose in subsequent cycles increased by 25% as long as the absolute granulocyte count (AGC) nadir is >1500 x 10^6/L, platelet nadir is >100,000 x 10^6/L, and nonhematologic toxicity is less than WHO Grade 1. If the increased dose is tolerated (with the same parameters) the dose in subsequent cycles may again be increased by 20%.

Nonsmall cell lung cancer:

1000 mg/m^2 days 1, 8, and 15; repeat cycle every 28 days

or

1250 mg/m^2 days 1 and 8; repeat cycle every 21 days

Breast cancer: 1250 mg/m^2 days 1 and 8; repeat cycle every 21 days

Ovarian cancer: 1000 mg/m^2 days 1 and 8; repeat cycle every 21 days

Dosage Forms

Injection, powder for reconstitution:

Gemzar®: 200 mg, 1 g

gemcitabine hydrochloride *see* gemcitabine *on page 457*

gemfibrozil (jem FI broe zil)

Sound-Alike/Look-Alike Issues

Lopid® may be confused with Levbid®, Lodine®, Lorabid®, Slo-bid™

Synonyms CI-719

U.S./Canadian Brand Names Apo-Gemfibrozil® [Can]; Gen-Gemfibrozil [Can]; GMD-Gemfibrozil [Can]; Lopid® [US/Can]; Novo-Gemfibrozil [Can]; Nu-Gemfibrozil [Can]; PMS-Gemfibrozil [Can]

Therapeutic Category Antihyperlipidemic Agent, Miscellaneous

Use Treatment of hypertriglyceridemia in Fredrickson types IV and V hyperlipidemia for patients who are at greater risk for pancreatitis and who have not responded to dietary intervention; to reduce the risk of CHD development in Fredrickson type IIb patients without a history or symptoms of existing CHD who have not responded to dietary and other interventions (including pharmacologic treatment) and who have decreased HDL, increased LDL, and increased triglycerides

Usual Dosage Oral: Adults: 1200 mg/day in 2 divided doses, 30 minutes before breakfast and dinner

Dosage Forms

Tablet, oral: 600 mg

Lopid®: 600 mg

gemifloxacin (je mi FLOKS a sin)

Synonyms DW286; gemifloxacin mesylate; LA 20304a; SB-265805

U.S./Canadian Brand Names Factive® [US/Can]

Therapeutic Category Antibiotic, Quinolone

Use Treatment of acute exacerbation of chronic bronchitis; treatment of community-acquired pneumonia (CAP), including pneumonia caused by multidrug-resistant strains of *S. pneumoniae* (MDRSP)

Usual Dosage

Usual dosage range:

Oral: Adults: 320 mg once daily

Indication-specific dosing:

Oral: Adults:

Acute exacerbations of chronic bronchitis: 320 mg once daily for 5 days

Community-acquired pneumonia (mild-to-moderate): 320 mg once daily for 5 or 7 days (decision to use 5- or 7-day regimen should be guided by initial sputum culture; 7 days are recommended for MDRSP, *Klebsiella*, or *M. catarrhalis* infection)

Dosage Forms

Tablet:

Factive®: 320 mg

gemifloxacin mesylate *see* gemifloxacin *on page 458*

gemtuzumab ozogamicin (gem TOO zoo mab oh zog a MY sin)

Sound-Alike/Look-Alike Issues
gemtuzumab may be confused with gemcitabine

Synonyms CMA-676; NSC-720568

U.S./Canadian Brand Names Mylotarg® [US/Can]

Therapeutic Category Antineoplastic Agent, Natural Source (Plant) Derivative

Use Treatment of relapsed CD33 positive acute myeloid leukemia (AML) in patients ≥60 years of age who are not candidates for cytotoxic chemotherapy

Usual Dosage I.V.:

Children: **Note:** Patients should receive diphenhydramine (1 mg/kg) 1 hour prior to infusion and acetaminophen 15 mg/kg 1 hour prior to infusion and every 4 hours for 2 additional doses.

Adults: **Note:** Patients should receive diphenhydramine 50 mg orally and acetaminophen 650-1000 mg orally 1 hour prior to administration of each dose. Acetaminophen dosage should be repeated as needed every 4 hours for 2 additional doses. Pretreatment with methylprednisolone may ameliorate infusion-related symptoms.

AML: ≥60 years: 9 mg/m^2 infused over 2 hours. A full treatment course is a total of 2 doses administered with 14 days between doses. Full hematologic recovery is not necessary for administration of the second dose. There has been only limited experience with repeat courses of gemtuzumab ozogamicin.

Dosage Forms

Injection, powder for reconstitution [preservative free]:
Mylotarg®: 5 mg

Gemzar® [US/Can] *see* gemcitabine *on page 457*

Genabid® *(Discontinued)*

Genac™ [US-OTC] *see* triprolidine and pseudoephedrine *on page 989*

Gen-Acebutolol [Can] *see* acebutolol *on page 19*

Genaced™ [US-OTC] *see* acetaminophen, aspirin, and caffeine *on page 24*

Genacote™ [US-OTC] *see* aspirin *on page 103*

Gen-Acyclovir [Can] *see* acyclovir *on page 33*

Genahist™ [US-OTC] *see* diphenhydramine *on page 315*

Gen-Alendronate [Can] *see* alendronate *on page 44*

Gen-Alprazolam [Can] *see* alprazolam *on page 51*

Gen-Amilazide [Can] *see* amiloride and hydrochlorothiazide *on page 61*

Genamin® Expectorant *(Discontinued)*

Gen-Amiodarone [Can] *see* amiodarone *on page 64*

Gen-Amlodipine [Can] *see* amlodipine *on page 66*

Gen-Amoxicillin [Can] *see* amoxicillin *on page 70*

Gen-Anagrelide [Can] *see* anagrelide *on page 78*

Genapap™ Children [US-OTC] *see* acetaminophen *on page 19*

Genapap™ *(Discontinued)* *see* acetaminophen *on page 19*

Genapap™ Extra Strength [US-OTC] *see* acetaminophen *on page 19*

Genapap™ Infant *(Discontinued)* *see* acetaminophen *on page 19*

Genapap™ Sinus Maximum Strength *(Discontinued)* *see* acetaminophen and pseudoephedrine *on page 24*

Genaphed® [US-OTC] *see* pseudoephedrine *on page 833*

Genasal [US-OTC] *see* oxymetazoline *on page 740*

Genasoft® [US-OTC] *see* docusate *on page 326*

Genasyme® [US-OTC] *see* simethicone *on page 901*

Gen-Atenolol [Can] *see* atenolol *on page 107*

Genaton™ [US-OTC] *see* aluminum hydroxide and magnesium carbonate *on page 55*

Genaton Tablet [US-OTC] *see* aluminum hydroxide and magnesium trisilicate *on page 56*

Genatuss® *(Discontinued)* *see* guaifenesin *on page 473*

Genatuss DM® [US-OTC] *see* guaifenesin and dextromethorphan *on page 474*

Gen-Azathioprine [Can] *see* azathioprine *on page 115*

GEN-Azithromycin [Can] *see* azithromycin *on page 116*

Gen-Baclofen [Can] *see* baclofen *on page 120*

Gen-Lisinopril/Hctz [Can] *see* lisinopril and hydrochlorothiazide *on page 594*
Gen-Lovastatin [Can] *see* lovastatin *on page 602*
Gen-Medroxy [Can] *see* medroxyprogesterone *on page 620*
Gen-Meloxicam [Can] *see* meloxicam *on page 622*
Gen-Metformin [Can] *see* metformin *on page 633*
Gen-Metoprolol [Can] *see* metoprolol *on page 650*
Gen-Minocycline [Can] *see* minocycline *on page 659*
Gen-Mirtazapine [Can] *see* mirtazapine *on page 661*
Gen-Nabumetone [Can] *see* nabumetone *on page 675*
Gen-Naproxen EC [Can] *see* naproxen *on page 681*
GEN-Nifedipine XL [Can] *see* nifedipine *on page 697*
Gen-Nitro [Can] *see* nitroglycerin *on page 700*
Gen-Nizatidine [Can] *see* nizatidine *on page 702*
Gen-Nortriptyline [Can] *see* nortriptyline *on page 706*
Gen-Ondansetron [Can] *see* ondansetron *on page 726*
Genoptic® *(Discontinued)* *see* gentamicin *on page 461*
Genora® 0.5/35 *(Discontinued)* *see* ethinyl estradiol and norethindrone *on page 390*
Genora® 1/35 *(Discontinued)* *see* ethinyl estradiol and norethindrone *on page 390*
Genora® 1/50 *(Discontinued)* *see* norethindrone and mestranol *on page 704*
Genotropin® [US] *see* somatropin *on page 916*
Genotropin Miniquick® [US] *see* somatropin *on page 916*
Gen-Oxybutynin [Can] *see* oxybutynin *on page 736*
Gen-Pantoprazole [Can] *see* pantoprazole *on page 748*
Gen-Paroxetine [Can] *see* paroxetine *on page 752*
Gen-Pindolol [Can] *see* pindolol *on page 785*
Gen-Pioglitazone [Can] *see* pioglitazone *on page 785*
Gen-Piroxicam [Can] *see* piroxicam *on page 788*
GEN-Pravastatin [Can] *see* pravastatin *on page 811*
Genpril® *(Discontinued)* *see* ibuprofen *on page 515*
Gen-Quetiapine [Can] *see* quetiapine *on page 844*
GEN-Ramipril [Can] *see* ramipril *on page 850*
Gen-Ranidine [Can] *see* ranitidine *on page 852*
Gen-Risperidone [Can] *see* risperidone *on page 870*
Gen-Salbutamol [Can] *see* albuterol *on page 41*
Gen-Selegiline [Can] *see* selegiline *on page 895*
Gen-Sertraline [Can] *see* sertraline *on page 898*
Gen-Simvastatin [Can] *see* simvastatin *on page 902*
Gen-Sotalol [Can] *see* sotalol *on page 919*
Gen-Sumatriptan [Can] *see* sumatriptan *on page 932*
Gentacidin® *(Discontinued)* *see* gentamicin *on page 461*
Gentak® [US] *see* gentamicin *on page 461*

gentamicin (jen ta MYE sin)

Sound-Alike/Look-Alike Issues

gentamicin may be confused with gentian violet, kanamycin, vancomycin
Garamycin® may be confused with kanamycin, Terramycin®

Synonyms gentamicin sulfate

U.S./Canadian Brand Names Alcomicin® [Can]; Diogent® [Can]; Garamycin® [Can]; Gentak® [US]; Gentamicin Injection, USP [Can]; Gentasol™ [US]; SAB-Gentamicin [Can]

Therapeutic Category Aminoglycoside (Antibiotic); Antibiotic, Ophthalmic; Antibiotic, Topical

Use Treatment of susceptible bacterial infections, normally gram-negative organisms, including *Pseudomonas*, *Proteus*, *Serratia*, and gram-positive *Staphylococcus*; treatment of bone infections, respiratory tract infections, skin and soft tissue infections, as well as abdominal and urinary tract infections, and septicemia; treatment of infective endocarditis; used topically to treat superficial infections of the skin or ophthalmic infections caused by susceptible bacteria

Usual Dosage Note: Dosage Individualization is **critical** because of the low therapeutic index.

Use of ideal body weight (IBW) for determining the mg/kg/dose appears to be more accurate than dosing on the basis of total body weight (TBW). In morbid obesity, dosage requirement may best be estimated using a dosing weight of IBW + 0.4 (TBW - IBW).

Initial and periodic plasma drug levels (eg, peak-and-trough with conventional dosing) should be determined, particularly in critically-ill patients with serious infections or in disease states known to significantly alter aminoglycoside pharmacokinetics (eg, cystic fibrosis, burns, or major surgery).

Usual dosage range:

Infants and Children <5 years: I.M., I.V.: 2.5 mg/kg/dose every 8 hours*

Children ≥5 years: I.M., I.V.: 2-2.5 mg/kg/dose every 8 hours*

***Note:** Higher individual doses and/or more frequent intervals (eg, every 6 hours) may be required in selected clinical situations (cystic fibrosis) or serum levels document the need

Children and Adults:

Ophthalmic:

Ointment: Instill 1/2" (1.25 cm) 2-3 times/day to every 3-4 hours

Solution: Instill 1-2 drops every 2-4 hours, up to 2 drops every hour for severe infections

Topical: Apply 3-4 times/day to affected area

Adults:

I.M., I.V.:

Conventional: 1-2.5 mg/kg/dose every 8-12 hours; to ensure adequate peak concentrations early in therapy, higher initial dosage may be considered in selected patients when extracellular water is increased (edema, septic shock, postsurgical, or trauma)

Once daily: 4-7 mg/kg/dose once daily; some clinicians recommend this approach for all patients with normal renal function; this dose is at least as efficacious with similar, if not less, toxicity than conventional dosing

Intrathecal: 4-8 mg/day

Indication-specific dosing:

Neonates: I.V.:

Meningitis:

0-7 days of age: <2000 g: 2.5 mg/kg every 18-24 hours; >2000 g: 2.5 mg/kg every 12 hours

8-28 days of age: <2000 g: 2.5 mg/kg every 8-12 hours; >2000 g: 2.5 mg/kg every 8 hours

Children and Adults: I.M., I.V.:

Brucellosis: 240 mg (I.M.) daily or 5 mg/kg (I.V.) daily for 7 days; either regimen recommended in combination with doxycycline

Cholangitis: 4-6 mg/kg once daily with ampicillin

Diverticulitis (complicated): 1.5-2 mg/kg every 8 hours (with ampicillin and metronidazole)

Endocarditis: Treatment: 3 mg/kg/day in 1-3 divided doses

Meningitis:

(Enterococcus sp or *Pseudomonas aeruginosa)*: Loading dose 2 mg/kg, then 1.7 mg/kg/dose every 8 hours (administered with another bacteriocidal drug)

Listeria: 5-7 mg/kg/day (with penicillin) for 1 week

Pelvic inflammatory disease: Loading dose: 2 mg/kg, then 1.5 mg/kg every 8 hours

Alternate therapy: 4.5 mg/kg once daily

Plague *(Yersinia pestis)*: Treatment: 5 mg/kg/day, followed by postexposure prophylaxis with doxycycline

Pneumonia, hospital- or ventilator-associated: 7 mg/kg/day (with antipseudomonal beta-lactam or carbapenem)

Synergy (for gram-positive infections): 3 mg/kg/day in 1-3 divided doses (with ampicillin)

Tularemia: 5 mg/kg/day divided every 8 hours for 1-2 weeks

Urinary tract infection: 1.5 mg/kg/dose every 8 hours

Dosage Forms

Cream, topical: 0.1% (15 g, 30 g)

Infusion [premixed in NS]: 40 mg (50 mL); 60 mg (50 mL, 100 mL); 70 mg (50 mL); 80 mg (50 mL, 100 mL); 90 mg (100 mL); 100 mg (50 mL, 100 mL); 120 mg (100 mL)

Injection, solution: 10 mg/mL (6 mL, 8 mL, 10 mL); 40 mg/mL (2 mL, 20 mL)

Injection, solution [pediatric]: 10 mg/mL (2 mL)

Injection, solution [pediatric; preservative free]: 10 mg/mL (2 mL)

Ointment, ophthalmic: 0.3% [3 mg/g] (3.5 g)

Gentak®: 0.3% [3 mg/g] (3.5 g)

Ointment, topical: 0.1% (15 g, 30 g)
Solution, ophthalmic: 0.3% (5 mL, 15 mL)
Gentak®: 0.3% (5 mL)
Gentasol™: 0.3% (5 mL)

glargine insulin *see* insulin glargine *on page 531*

glatiramer acetate (gla TIR a mer AS e tate)

Sound-Alike/Look-Alike Issues

Copaxone® may be confused with Compazine®

Synonyms copolymer-1

U.S./Canadian Brand Names Copaxone® [US/Can]

Therapeutic Category Biological, Miscellaneous

Use Management of relapsing-remitting type multiple sclerosis, including patients with a first clinical episode with MRI features consistent with multiple sclerosis

Usual Dosage SubQ: Adults: 20 mg daily

Dosage Forms

Injection, solution [preservative free]:

Copaxone®: 20 mg/mL (1 mL)

Glaucon® ***(Discontinued)*** *see* epinephrine *on page 358*
Gleevec® [US/Can] *see* imatinib *on page 519*
Gliadel® [US] *see* carmustine *on page 187*
Gliadel Wafer® [Can] *see* carmustine *on page 187*
glibenclamide *see* glyburide *on page 467*
Gliclazide-80 [Can] *see* gliclazide *(Canada only) on page 464*

gliclazide *(Canada only)* (GLYE kla zide)

U.S./Canadian Brand Names Apo-Gliclazide® [Can]; Diamicron® MR [Can]; Diamicron® [Can]; Gen-Gliclazide [Can]; Gliclazide-80 [Can]; Novo-Gliclazide [Can]; PMS-Gliclazide [Can]; Sandoz-Gliclazide [Can]

Therapeutic Category Antidiabetic Agent; Hypoglycemic Agent, Oral; Sulfonylurea Agent

Use Management of type 2 diabetes mellitus (noninsulin-dependent, NIDDM)

Usual Dosage Oral: Adults:

Immediate release tablet: Initial: 80-160 mg/day; typical dose range 80-320 mg/day; dosage of ≥160 mg should be divided into 2 equal parts for twice-daily administration; maximum dose: 320 mg/day; should be taken with meals

Sustained release tablet: 30-120 mg once daily

Note: There is no fixed dosage regimen for the management of diabetes mellitus with gliclazide or any other hypoglycemic agent. Dose must be individualized based on frequent determinations of blood glucose during dose titration and throughout maintenance.

Dosage Forms [CAN] = Canadian brand name

Tablet: 80 mg [not available in the U.S.]

Diamicron® [CAN]: 80 mg [not available in the U.S.]

Tablet, sustained release:

Diamicron® MR [CAN]: 30 mg [not available in the U.S.]

glimepiride (GLYE me pye ride)

Sound-Alike/Look-Alike Issues

glimepiride may be confused with glipiZIDE

Amaryl® may be confused with Altace®, Amerge®, Reminyl®

U.S./Canadian Brand Names Amaryl® [US/Can]; Apo-Glimepiride [Can]; CO Glimepiride [Can]; Novo-Glimepiride [Can]; PMS-Glimepiride [Can]; ratio-Glimepiride [Can]; Rhoxal-glimepiride [Can]; Sandoz-Glimepiride [Can]

Therapeutic Category Antidiabetic Agent, Oral

Use Management of type 2 diabetes mellitus (noninsulin-dependent, NIDDM) as an adjunct to diet and exercise to lower blood glucose; may be used in combination with metformin or insulin in patients whose hyperglycemia cannot be controlled by diet and exercise in conjunction with a single oral hypoglycemic agent

Usual Dosage Oral: Adults: Initial: 1-2 mg once daily, administered with breakfast or the first main meal; usual maintenance dose: 1-4 mg once daily; after a dose of 2 mg once daily, increase in increments of 2 mg at 1- to 2-week intervals based upon the patient's blood glucose response to a maximum of 8 mg once daily. If inadequate response to maximal dose, combination therapy with metformin may be considered.

Combination with insulin therapy (fasting glucose level for instituting combination therapy is in the range of >150 mg/dL in plasma or serum depending on the patient): Initial recommended dose: 8 mg once daily with the first main meal

After starting with low-dose insulin, upward adjustments of insulin can be done approximately weekly as guided by frequent measurements of fasting blood glucose. Once stable, combination-therapy patients should monitor their capillary blood glucose on an ongoing basis, preferably daily.

Conversion from therapy with long half-life agents: Observe patient carefully for 1-2 weeks when converting from a longer half-life agent (eg, chlorpropamide) to glimepiride due to overlapping hypoglycemic effects.

Dosage Forms

Tablet: 1 mg, 2 mg, 4 mg

Amaryl®: 1 mg, 2 mg, 4 mg

glimepiride and pioglitazone *see* pioglitazone and glimepiride *on page 785*

glimepiride and pioglitazone hydrochloride *see* pioglitazone and glimepiride *on page 785*

glimepiride and rosiglitazone maleate *see* rosiglitazone and glimepiride *on page 879*

glipizide (GLIP i zide)

Sound-Alike/Look-Alike Issues

glipiZIDE may be confused with glimepiride, glyBURIDE

Glucotrol® may be confused with Glucophage®, Glucotrol® XL, glyBURIDE

Glucotrol® XL may be confused with Glucotrol®

Synonyms glydiazinamide

Tall-Man glipi**ZIDE**

U.S./Canadian Brand Names Glucotrol XL® [US]; Glucotrol® [US]

Therapeutic Category Antidiabetic Agent, Oral

Use Management of type 2 diabetes mellitus (noninsulin-dependent, NIDDM)

Usual Dosage Oral (allow several days between dose titrations): Adults: Initial: 5 mg/day; adjust dosage at 2.5-5 mg daily increments as determined by blood glucose response at intervals of several days.

Immediate release tablet: Maximum recommended once-daily dose: 15 mg; maximum recommended total daily dose: 40 mg. Doses >15 mg/day should be administered in divided doses.

Extended release tablet (Glucotrol XL®): Maximum recommended dose: 20 mg

When transferring from insulin to glipizide:

Current insulin requirement ≤20 units: Discontinue insulin and initiate glipizide at usual dose

Current insulin requirement >20 units: Decrease insulin by 50% and initiate glipizide at usual dose; gradually decrease insulin dose based on patient response. Several days should elapse between dosage changes.

Dosage Forms

Tablet: 5 mg, 10 mg

Glucotrol®: 5 mg, 10 mg

Tablet, extended release: 2.5 mg, 5 mg, 10 mg

Glucotrol XL®: 2.5 mg, 5 mg, 10 mg

glipizide and metformin (GLIP i zide & met FOR min)

Synonyms glipizide and metformin hydrochloride; metformin and glipizide

U.S./Canadian Brand Names Metaglip™ [US]

Therapeutic Category Antidiabetic Agent (Biguanide); Antidiabetic Agent (Sulfonylurea)

Use Indicated as an adjunct to diet and exercise to improve glycemic control in adults with type 2 diabetes mellitus (noninsulin-dependent, NIDDM)

Usual Dosage Oral: Adults: Type 2 diabetes:

Patients inadequately controlled on diet and exercise alone: Initial dose: Glipizide 2.5 mg/metformin 250 mg once daily with a meal. In patients with fasting plasma glucose (FPG) 280-320 mg/dL, initiate therapy with glipizide 2.5 mg/metformin 500 mg twice daily.

Note: Increase dose by 1 tablet/day every 2 weeks (maximum daily dose: Glipizide 10 mg/metformin 2000 mg in divided doses)

Patients inadequately controlled on a sulfonylurea and/or metformin: Initial dose: Glipizide 2.5 mg/metformin 500 mg or glipizide 5 mg/metformin 500 mg twice daily with morning and evening meals; starting dose should not exceed current daily dose of glipizide (or sulfonylurea equivalent) and/or metformin.

Note: Increase dose in increments of no more than glipizide 5 mg/metformin 500 mg (maximum daily dose: Glipizide 20 mg/metformin 2000 mg)

Dosage Forms

Tablet: 2.5/250: Glipizide 2.5 mg and metformin 250 mg; 2.5/500: Glipizide 2.5 mg and metformin 500 mg; 5/500: Glipizide 5 mg and metformin 500 mg

Metaglip™: 2.5/250: Glipizide 2.5 mg and metformin 250 mg; 2.5/500: Glipizide 2.5 mg and metformin 500 mg; 5/500: Glipizide 5 mg and metformin 500 mg

glipizide and metformin hydrochloride *see* glipizide and metformin *on page 465*

glivec *see* imatinib *on page 519*

GlucaGen® [US] *see* glucagon *on page 466*

GlucaGen® Diagnostic Kit [US] *see* glucagon *on page 466*

GlucaGen® HypoKit™ [US] *see* glucagon *on page 466*

glucagon (GLOO ka gon)

Sound-Alike/Look-Alike Issues

glucagon may be confused with Glaucon®

Synonyms glucagon hydrochloride

U.S./Canadian Brand Names GlucaGen® Diagnostic Kit [US]; GlucaGen® HypoKit™ [US]; GlucaGen® [US]; Glucagon Emergency Kit [US]

Therapeutic Category Antihypoglycemic Agent

Use Management of hypoglycemia; diagnostic aid in radiologic examinations to temporarily inhibit GI tract movement

Usual Dosage

Hypoglycemia or insulin shock therapy: I.M., I.V., SubQ:

Children <20 kg: 0.5 mg or 20-30 mcg/kg/dose; repeated in 20 minutes as needed

Children ≥20 kg and Adults: 1 mg; may repeat in 20 minutes as needed

Note: I.V. dextrose should be administered as soon as it is available; if patient fails to respond to glucagon, I.V. dextrose must be given.

Diagnostic aid: Adults: I.M., I.V.: 0.25-2 mg 10 minutes prior to procedure

Dosage Forms

Injection, powder for reconstitution:

GlucaGen®, GlucaGen® Diagnostic Kit, GlucaGen® HypoKit™, Glucagon Emergency Kit: 1 mg

Glucagon Diagnostic Kit *(Discontinued)* *see* glucagon *on page 466*

Glucagon Emergency Kit [US] *see* glucagon *on page 466*

glucagon hydrochloride *see* glucagon *on page 466*

Glucobay™ [Can] *see* acarbose *on page 18*

GlucoBurst® [US-OTC] *see* dextrose *on page 298*

glucocerebrosidase *see* alglucerase *on page 46*

GlucoNorm® [Can] *see* repaglinide *on page 858*

Glucophage® [US/Can] *see* metformin *on page 633*

Glucophage® XR [US] *see* metformin *on page 633*

glucose *see* dextrose *on page 298*

glucose monohydrate *see* dextrose *on page 298*

glucose polymers (GLOO kose POL i merz)

U.S./Canadian Brand Names Moducal® [US-OTC]; Polycose® [US-OTC]

Therapeutic Category Nutritional Supplement

Use Supplies calories for those persons not able to meet the caloric requirement with usual food intake

Usual Dosage Oral: Adults: Add to foods or beverages or mix in water

Dosage Forms

Powder:

Moducal® [OTC]: 368 g

Polycose® [OTC]: 350 g

Glucotrol® [US] *see* glipizide *on page 465*

Glucotrol XL® [US] *see* glipizide *on page 465*

Glucovance® [US] *see* glyburide and metformin *on page 467*

glulisine insulin *see* insulin glulisine *on page 531*
Glumetza™ [US/Can] *see* metformin *on page 633*

glutamic acid (gloo TAM ik AS id)

Synonyms glutamic acid hydrochloride

Therapeutic Category Gastrointestinal Agent, Miscellaneous

Use Treatment of hypochlorhydria and achlorhydria

Usual Dosage Oral: Adults: 500-1000 mg/day before meals or food

Dosage Forms

Tablet: 500 mg

glutamic acid hydrochloride *see* glutamic acid *on page 467*
Glutofac®-MX [US] *see* vitamins (multiple/oral) *on page 1019*
Glutofac®-ZX [US] *see* vitamins (multiple/oral) *on page 1019*
Glutol™ [US-OTC] *see* dextrose *on page 298*
Glutose 15™ [US-OTC] *see* dextrose *on page 298*
Glutose 45™ [US-OTC] *see* dextrose *on page 298*
Glyate® ***(Discontinued)*** *see* guaifenesin *on page 473*
glybenclamide *see* glyburide *on page 467*
glybenzcyclamide *see* glyburide *on page 467*

glyburide (GLYE byoor ide)

Sound-Alike/Look-Alike Issues

glyBURIDE may be confused with glipiZIDE, Glucotrol®
Diaβeta® may be confused with Diabinese®, Zebeta®
Micronase® may be confused with microK®, miconazole, Micronor®, Microzide™

Synonyms glibenclamide; glybenclamide; glybenzcyclamide

Tall-Man gly**BURIDE**

U.S./Canadian Brand Names Albert® Glyburide [Can]; Apo-Glyburide® [Can]; Diaβeta® [US/Can]; Euglucon® [Can]; Gen-Glybe [Can]; Glynase® PresTab® [US]; Novo-Glyburide [Can]; Nu-Glyburide [Can]; PMS-Glyburide [Can]; PRO-Glyburide [Can]; ratio-Glyburide [Can]; Sandoz-Glyburide [Can]

Therapeutic Category Antidiabetic Agent, Oral

Use Adjunct to diet and exercise for the management of type 2 diabetes mellitus (noninsulin-dependent, NIDDM)

Usual Dosage Oral: Adults:

Diaβeta®, Micronase®:

Initial: 2.5-5 mg/day, administered with breakfast or the first main meal of the day. In patients who are more sensitive to hypoglycemic drugs, start at 1.25 mg/day.

Increase in increments of no more than 2.5 mg/day at weekly intervals based on the patient's blood glucose response

Maintenance: 1.25-20 mg/day given as single or divided doses; maximum: 20 mg/day

Micronized tablets (Glynase® PresTab®): Adults:

Initial: 1.5-3 mg/day, administered with breakfast or the first main meal of the day in patients who are more sensitive to hypoglycemic drugs, start at 0.75 mg/day. Increase in increments of no more than 1.5 mg/day in weekly intervals based on the patient's blood glucose response.

Maintenance: 0.75-12 mg/day given as a single dose or in divided doses. Some patients (especially those receiving >6 mg/day) may have a more satisfactory response with twice-daily dosing. Maximum: 12 mg/day

Dosage Forms

Tablet: 1.25 mg, 2.5 mg, 5 mg

Diaβeta®: 1.25 mg, 2.5 mg, 5 mg

Tablet, micronized: 1.5 mg, 3 mg, 6 mg

Glynase® PresTab®: 1.5 mg, 3 mg, 6 mg

glyburide and metformin (GLYE byoor ide & met FOR min)

Sound-Alike/Look-Alike Issues

Glucovance® may be confused with Vyvanse™

Synonyms glyburide and metformin hydrochloride; metformin and glyburide

U.S./Canadian Brand Names Glucovance® [US]

Therapeutic Category Antidiabetic Agent (Sulfonylurea); Antidiabetic Agent, Oral

Use Adjunct to diet and exercise for the management of type 2 diabetes mellitus (noninsulin-dependent, NIDDM)

Usual Dosage **Note:** Dose must be individualized. Dosages expressed as glyburide/metformin components.

Oral: Adults:

Initial therapy (no prior treatment with sulfonylurea or metformin): 1.25 mg/250 mg once daily with a meal; patients with Hb A_{1c} >9% or fasting plasma glucose (FPG) >200 mg/dL may start with 1.25 mg/250 mg twice daily with meals. **Note:** Doses of 5 mg /500 mg should not be used as initial therapy, due to risk of hypoglycemia.

Dosage may be increased in increments of 1.25 mg/250 mg, at intervals of not less than 2 weeks; maximum daily dose: 10 mg/2000 mg (limited experience with higher doses)

Previously treated with a sulfonylurea or metformin alone: Initial: 2.5 mg/500 mg or 5 mg/500 mg twice daily with meals; increase in increments no greater than 5 mg/500 mg; maximum daily dose: 20 mg/2000 mg

When switching patients previously on a sulfonylurea and metformin together, do not exceed the daily dose of glyburide (or glyburide equivalent) or metformin.

Note: May combine with a thiazolidinedione in patients with an inadequate response to glyburide/metformin therapy (risk of hypoglycemia may be increased). When adding thiazolidinedione, continue glyburide and metformin at current dose and initiate thiazolidinedione at recommended starting dose.

Dosage Forms

Tablet: Glyburide 1.25 mg and metformin 250 mg; glyburide 2.5 mg and metformin 500 mg; glyburide 5 mg and metformin 500 mg

Glucovance®: 1.25 mg/250 mg: Glyburide 1.25 mg and metformin 250 mg; 2.5 mg/500 mg: Glyburide 2.5 mg and metformin 500 mg; 5 mg/500 mg: Glyburide 5 mg and metformin 500 mg

glyburide and metformin hydrochloride *see* glyburide and metformin *on page 467*

glycerin (GLIS er in)

Synonyms glycerol

U.S./Canadian Brand Names Bausch & Lomb® Computer Eye Drops [US-OTC]; Colace® Adult/Children Suppositories [US-OTC]; Colace® Infant/Children Suppositories [US-OTC]; Fleet® Glycerin Suppositories Maximum Strength [US-OTC]; Fleet® Glycerin Suppositories [US-OTC]; Fleet® Liquid Glycerin Suppositories [US-OTC]; Fleet® Pedia-Lax™ Glycerin Suppositories [US-OTC]; Fleet® Pedia-Lax™ Liquid Glycerin Suppositories [US-OTC]; Sani-Supp® [US-OTC]

Therapeutic Category Laxative; Ophthalmic Agent, Miscellaneous

Use Constipation; reduction of intraocular pressure; reduction of corneal edema; glycerin has been administered orally to reduce intracranial pressure

Usual Dosage

Constipation: Rectal:

Children <6 years: 1 infant suppository 1-2 times/day as needed or 2-5 mL as an enema

Children >6 years and Adults: 1 adult suppository 1-2 times/day as needed or 5-15 mL as an enema

Children and Adults:

Reduction of intraocular pressure: Oral: 1-1.8 g/kg 1-1½ hours preoperatively; additional doses may be administered at 5-hour intervals

Reduction of intracranial pressure: Oral: 1.5 g/kg/day divided every 4 hours; 1 g/kg/dose every 6 hours has also been used

Reduction of corneal edema: Ophthalmic solution: Instill 1-2 drops in eye(s) prior to examination OR for lubricant effect, instill 1-2 drops in eye(s) every 3-4 hours

Dosage Forms

Solution, ophthalmic, sterile:

Bausch & Lomb® Computer Eye Drops [OTC]: 1% (15 mL)

Solution, rectal:

Fleet® Liquid Glycerin Suppositories [OTC]: 5.6 g/5.5 mL (7.5 mL)

Fleet® Pedia-Lax™ Liquid Glycerin Suppositories [OTC]: 2.3 mg/2.3 mL (4 mL)

Suppository, rectal [adult]: 82.5% (12s, 24s, 25s, 50s, 100s)

Colace® Adult/Children [OTC]: 2.1 g (12s, 24s, 48s, 100s)

Fleet® Glycerin Suppositories [OTC]: 2 g (12s, 24s, 50s)

Fleet® Glycerin Suppositories Maximum Strength [OTC]: 3 g (18s)

Sani-Supp® [OTC]: 82.5% (10s, 25s, 50s)

Suppository, rectal [pediatric]: 82.5% (12s, 25s)
Colace® Infant/Children [OTC]: 1.2 g (12s, 24s)
Fleet® Pedia-Lax™ Glycerin Suppositories [OTC]: 1 g (12s)
Sani-Supp® [OTC]: 82.5% (10s, 25s)

glycerol *see* glycerin *on page 468*
glycerol guaiacolate *see* guaifenesin *on page 473*
Glycerol-T® ***(Discontinued)***
glycerol triacetate *see* triacetin *on page 981*
glyceryl trinitrate *see* nitroglycerin *on page 700*
Glycofed® ***(Discontinued)*** *see* guaifenesin and pseudoephedrine *on page 477*
GlycoLax® [US] *see* polyethylene glycol 3350 *on page 797*
Glycon [Can] *see* metformin *on page 633*

glycopyrrolate (glye koe PYE roe late)

Sound-Alike/Look-Alike Issues
Robinul® may be confused with Reminyl®

Synonyms glycopyrronium bromide

U.S./Canadian Brand Names Glycopyrrolate Injection, USP [Can]; Robinul® Forte [US]; Robinul® [US]

Therapeutic Category Anticholinergic Agent

Use Inhibit salivation and excessive secretions of the respiratory tract preoperatively; control of upper airway secretions; adjunct in treatment of peptic ulcer (currently replaced by more effective agents); prevention and treatment of bradycardia

Usual Dosage
Children:
Reduction of secretions (preanesthetic):
Oral: 40-100 mcg/kg/dose 3-4 times/day
I.M., I.V.: 4-10 mcg/kg/dose every 3-4 hours; maximum: 0.2 mg/dose or 0.8 mg/24 hours
Intraoperative: I.V.: 4 mcg/kg not to exceed 0.1 mg; repeat at 2- to 3-minute intervals as needed
Preoperative: I.M.:
<2 years: 4-9 mcg/kg 30-60 minutes before procedure
>2 years: 4 mcg/kg 30-60 minutes before procedure
Children and Adults: Reverse neuromuscular blockade: I.V.: 0.2 mg for each 1 mg of neostigmine or 5 mg of pyridostigmine administered or 5-15 mcg/kg glycopyrrolate with 25-70 mcg/kg of neostigmine or 0.1-0.3 mg/kg of pyridostigmine (agents usually administered simultaneously, but glycopyrrolate may be administered first if bradycardia is present)
Adults:
Reduction of secretions:
Intraoperative: I.V.: 0.1 mg repeated as needed at 2- to 3-minute intervals
Preoperative: I.M.: 4 mcg/kg 30-60 minutes before procedure
Peptic ulcer:
Oral: 1-2 mg 2-3 times/day
I.M., I.V.: 0.1-0.2 mg 3-4 times/day

Dosage Forms
Injection, solution: 0.2 mg/mL (1 mL, 2 mL, 5 mL, 20 mL)
Robinul®: 0.2 mg/mL (1 mL, 2 mL, 5 mL)
Tablet:
Robinul®: 1 mg
Robinul® Forte: 2 mg

Glycopyrrolate Injection, USP [Can] *see* glycopyrrolate *on page 469*
glycopyrronium bromide *see* glycopyrrolate *on page 469*
glycosum *see* dextrose *on page 298*
Glycotuss® ***(Discontinued)*** *see* guaifenesin *on page 473*
Glycotuss-dM® ***(Discontinued)*** *see* guaifenesin and dextromethorphan *on page 474*
glydiazinamide *see* glipizide *on page 465*
Glynase® PresTab® [US] *see* glyburide *on page 467*
Gly-Oxide® [US-OTC] *see* carbamide peroxide *on page 181*
Glyquin® ***(Discontinued)*** *see* hydroquinone *on page 508*
Glyquin® XM [Can] *see* hydroquinone *on page 508*

Glyquin-XM™ ***(Discontinued)*** *see* hydroquinone *on page 508*
Glyset® [US/Can] *see* miglitol *on page 658*
GM-CSF *see* sargramostim *on page 891*
GMD-Fluconazole [Can] *see* fluconazole *on page 424*
GMD-Gemfibrozil [Can] *see* gemfibrozil *on page 458*
GMD-Sertraline [Can] *see* sertraline *on page 898*
G-myticin® ***(Discontinued)*** *see* gentamicin *on page 461*
Gold Bond® Antifungal ***(Discontinued)*** *see* tolnaftate *on page 968*

gold sodium thiomalate (gold SOW dee um thye oh MAL ate)

Synonyms sodium aurothiomalate

U.S./Canadian Brand Names Myochrysine® [US/Can]

Therapeutic Category Gold Compound

Use Treatment of progressive rheumatoid arthritis

Usual Dosage I.M.:

Children: Initial: Test dose of 10 mg is recommended, followed by 1 mg/kg/week for 20 weeks; maintenance: 1 mg/kg/dose at 2- to 4-week intervals thereafter for as long as therapy is clinically beneficial and toxicity does not develop. Administration for 2-4 months is usually required before clinical improvement is observed.

Adults: 10 mg first week; 25 mg second week; then 25-50 mg/week until 1 g cumulative dose has been given; if improvement occurs without adverse reactions, administer 25-50 mg every 2-3 weeks for 2-20 weeks, then every 3-4 weeks indefinitely

Dosage Forms

Injection, solution:

Myochrysine®: 50 mg/mL (1 mL, 10 mL)

golimumab (goe LIM ue mab)

Synonyms CNTO-148

U.S./Canadian Brand Names Simponi™ [US]

Therapeutic Category Antipsoriatic Agent; Antirheumatic, Disease Modifying; Monoclonal Antibody; Tumor Necrosis Factor (TNF) Blocking Agent

Use Treatment of active rheumatoid arthritis (moderate-to-severe), active psoriatic arthritis, and active ankylosing spondylitis

Usual Dosage Note: Should be administered in conjunction with methotrexate in rheumatoid arthritis; may administer with or without methotrexate or other nonbiologic disease-modifying antirheumatic drugs (DMARDs) in psoriatic arthritis or ankylosing spondylitis.

SubQ: Adults: Rheumatoid arthritis, psoriatic arthritis, ankylosing spondylitis: 50 mg once per month

Dosage Forms

Injection, solution [preservative free]:

Simponi™: 50 mg/0.5 mL (0.5 mL)

GoLYTELY® [US] *see* polyethylene glycol-electrolyte solution *on page 797*
gonadorelin ***(Discontinued)***
Gonak™ [US-OTC] *see* hydroxypropyl methylcellulose *on page 510*
Gonal-f® [US/Can] *see* follitropin alfa *on page 440*
Gonal-f® Pen [Can] *see* follitropin alfa *on page 440*
Gonal-f® RFF [US] *see* follitropin alfa *on page 440*
gonioscopic ophthalmic solution *see* hydroxypropyl methylcellulose *on page 510*
Goniosoft™ [US] *see* hydroxypropyl methylcellulose *on page 510*
Goniosol® ***(Discontinued)*** *see* hydroxypropyl methylcellulose *on page 510*
Good Sense Sleep Aid [US-OTC] *see* doxylamine *on page 338*
Goody's® Extra Strength Headache Powder [US-OTC] *see* acetaminophen, aspirin, and caffeine *on page 24*
Goody's® Extra Strength Pain Relief [US-OTC] *see* acetaminophen, aspirin, and caffeine *on page 24*
Goody's PM® [US-OTC] *see* acetaminophen and diphenhydramine *on page 21*
Gordofilm® [US-OTC] *see* salicylic acid *on page 884*

Gordon Boro-Packs [US-OTC] *see* aluminum sulfate and calcium acetate *on page 57*
Gormel® [US-OTC] *see* urea *on page 998*

goserelin (GOE se rel in)

Synonyms D-ser(bu^t)^6,Azgly^{10}-LHRH; goserelin acetate; ICI-118630; NSC-606864

U.S./Canadian Brand Names Zoladex® LA [Can]; Zoladex® [US/Can]

Therapeutic Category Gonadotropin-Releasing Hormone Analog

Use Palliative treatment of advanced breast cancer and carcinoma of the prostate; treatment of endometriosis, including pain relief and reduction of endometriotic lesions; endometrial thinning agent as part of treatment for dysfunctional uterine bleeding

Usual Dosage SubQ: Adults:

Prostate cancer:

Monthly implant: 3.6 mg injected into upper abdomen every 28 days

3-month implant: 10.8 mg injected into the upper abdominal wall every 12 weeks

Breast cancer, endometriosis, endometrial thinning: Monthly implant: 3.6 mg injected into upper abdomen every 28 days

Note: For breast cancer, treatment may continue indefinitely; for endometriosis, it is recommended that duration of treatment not exceed 6 months. Only 1-2 doses are recommended for endometrial thinning.

Dosage Forms

Implant, subcutaneous:

Zoladex®: 3.6 mg [1-month implant packaged with 16-gauge hypodermic needle]; 10.8 mg [3-month implant packaged with 14-gauge hypodermic needle]

goserelin acetate *see* goserelin *on page 471*
GP 47680 *see* oxcarbazepine *on page 734*
GPI 15715 *see* fospropofol *on page 447*
GR38032R *see* ondansetron *on page 726*
gramicidin, neomycin, and polymyxin B *see* neomycin, polymyxin B, and gramicidin *on page 688*

granisetron (gra NI se tron)

Sound-Alike/Look-Alike Issues

granisetron may be confused with dolasetron, ondansetron, palonosetron

Synonyms BRL 43694

U.S./Canadian Brand Names Apo-Granisetron [Can]; Granisol™ [US]; Kytril® [US/Can]; Sancuso® [US]

Therapeutic Category Selective 5-HT_3 Receptor Antagonist

Use Prophylaxis of nausea and vomiting associated with emetogenic chemotherapy and radiation therapy; prophylaxis and treatment of postoperative nausea and vomiting (PONV)

Usual Dosage

Oral: Adults:

Prophylaxis of chemotherapy-related emesis: 2 mg once daily up to 1 hour before chemotherapy or 1 mg twice daily; the first 1 mg dose should be given up to 1 hour before chemotherapy.

Prophylaxis of radiation therapy-associated emesis: 2 mg once daily given 1 hour before radiation therapy.

I.V.:

Children ≥2 years and Adults: Prophylaxis of chemotherapy-related emesis:

Within U.S.: 10 mcg/kg/dose (maximum: 1 mg/dose) given 30 minutes prior to chemotherapy; for some drugs (eg, carboplatin, cyclophosphamide) with a later onset of emetic action, 10 mcg/kg every 12 hours may be necessary

Outside U.S.: 40 mcg/kg/dose (or 3 mg/dose); maximum: 9 mg/24 hours

Breakthrough: Granisetron has not been shown to be effective in terminating nausea or vomiting once it occurs and should not be used for this purpose.

Adults: PONV:

Prevention: 1 mg given undiluted over 30 seconds; the manufacturer recommends administration before induction of anesthesia or immediately before reversal of anesthesia.

Treatment: 1 mg given undiluted over 30 seconds

Transdermal patch: Adults: Prophylaxis of chemotherapy-related emesis: Apply 1 patch at least 24 hours prior to chemotherapy; do not apply ≥48 hours before chemotherapy. Remove patch a minimum of 24 hours after chemotherapy completion. Maximum duration: Patch may be worn up to 7 days, depending on chemotherapy regimen duration.

Dosage Forms
Injection, solution: 1 mg/mL (1 mL, 4 mL)
Granisol™: 2 mg/10 mL (30 mL)
Kytril®: 1 mg/mL (1 mL, 4 mL)
Injection, solution [preservative free]: 0.1 mg/mL (1 mL); 1 mg/mL (1 mL)
Kytril®: 0.1 mg/mL (1 mL)
Tablet: 1 mg
Kytril®: 1 mg
Transdermal system, topical:
Sancuso®: 3.1 mg/24 hours (1s)

Granisol™ [US] *see* granisetron *on page* 471

Granulex® [US] *see* trypsin, balsam Peru, and castor oil *on page* 993

granulocyte colony-stimulating factor *see* filgrastim *on page* 420

granulocyte colony stimulating factor (PEG conjugate) *see* pegfilgrastim *on page* 755

granulocyte-macrophage colony-stimulating factor *see* sargramostim *on page* 891

Gravol® [Can] *see* dimenhydrinate *on page* 312

green tea extract *see* sinecatechins *on page* 903

Grifulvin® V [US] *see* griseofulvin *on page* 472

Grifulvin® V Tablet 250 mg and 500 mg *(Discontinued)* *see* griseofulvin *on page* 472

Grisactin® Ultra *(Discontinued)* *see* griseofulvin *on page* 472

griseofulvin (gri see oh FUL vin)

Synonyms griseofulvin microsize; griseofulvin ultramicrosize
U.S./Canadian Brand Names Grifulvin® V [US]; Gris-PEG® [US]
Therapeutic Category Antifungal Agent
Use Treatment of susceptible tinea infections of the skin, hair, and nails
Usual Dosage Oral:
Children >2 years:
Microsize: 10-20 mg/kg/day in single or 2 divided doses.
Ultramicrosize: Usual: 7.3 mg/kg/day in single dose or 2 divided doses; range: 5-15 mg/kg/day in single dose or 2 divided doses (maximum: 750 mg/day)
Adults:
Microsize: 500-1000 mg/day in single or divided doses
Ultramicrosize: 375 mg/day in single or divided doses; doses up to 750 mg/day have been used for infections more difficult to eradicate such as tinea unguium and tinea pedis
Duration of therapy depends on the site of infection:
Tinea corporis: 2-4 weeks
Tinea capitis: 4-6 weeks or longer (up to 8-12 weeks)
Tinea pedis: 4-8 weeks
Tinea unguium: 3-6 months or longer
Dosage Forms
Suspension, oral [microsize]: 125 mg/5 mL
Tablet, oral [microsize]:
Grifulvin® V: 500 mg
Tablet, oral [ultramicrosize]:
Gris-PEG®: 125 mg, 250 mg

griseofulvin microsize *see* griseofulvin *on page* 472

griseofulvin ultramicrosize *see* griseofulvin *on page* 472

Gris-PEG® [US] *see* griseofulvin *on page* 472

growth hormone, human *see* somatropin *on page* 916

Guaicon DM [US-OTC] *see* guaifenesin and dextromethorphan *on page* 474

Guaifed® [US] *see* guaifenesin and phenylephrine *on page* 475

Guaifed-PD® [US] *see* guaifenesin and phenylephrine *on page* 475

Guaifen™ DM *(Discontinued)* *see* guaifenesin, dextromethorphan, and phenylephrine *on page* 478

guaifenesin (gwye FEN e sin)

Sound-Alike/Look-Alike Issues

guaiFENesin may be confused with guanFACINE
Mucinex® may be confused with Mucomyst®
Naldecon® may be confused with Nalfon®

Synonyms GG; glycerol guaiacolate

Tall-Man guai**FEN**esin

U.S./Canadian Brand Names Allfen [US-OTC]; Balminil Expectorant [Can]; Benylin® E Extra Strength [Can]; Diabetic Tussin® EX [US-OTC]; Fenesin IR [US]; Ganidin NR [US]; Guiatuss™ [US-OTC]; Koffex Expectorant [Can]; Mucinex® Maximum Strength [US-OTC]; Mucinex® [US-OTC]; Mucinex®, Children's Mini-Melts™ [US-OTC]; Mucinex®, Children's [US-OTC]; Mucinex®, Junior Mini-Melts™ [US-OTC]; Organidin® NR [US]; Phanasin® Diabetic Choice [US-OTC]; Phanasin® [US-OTC]; Refenesen™ 400 [US-OTC]; Refenesen™ [US-OTC]; Robitussin® [US-OTC/Can]; Scot-Tussin® Expectorant [US-OTC]; Siltussin DAS [US-OTC]; Siltussin SA [US-OTC]; Vicks® Casero™ Chest Congestion Relief [US-OTC]; XPECT™ [US-OTC]

Therapeutic Category Expectorant

Use Help loosen phlegm and thin bronchial secretions to make coughs more productive

Usual Dosage Oral:

Children:

6 months to 2 years: 25-50 mg every 4 hours, not to exceed 300 mg/day
2-5 years: 50-100 mg every 4 hours, not to exceed 600 mg/day
6-11 years: 100-200 mg every 4 hours, not to exceed 1.2 g/day

Children >12 years and Adults: 200-400 mg every 4 hours to a maximum of 2.4 g/day

Extended release tablet: 600-1200 mg every 12 hours, not to exceed 2.4 g/day

Dosage Forms

Caplet, oral:

Fenesin IR, Refenesen™ 400 [OTC]: 400 mg

Granules, oral:

Mucinex® Children's Mini-Melts™ [OTC]: 50 mg/packet (12s)
Mucinex® Junior Mini-Melts™ [OTC]: 100 mg/packet (12s)

Liquid, oral: 100 mg/5 mL

Diabetic Tussin EX® [OTC], Ganidin NR, Mucinex® Children's [OTC], Organidin® NR, Siltussin DAS [OTC]: 100 mg/5 mL

Syrup, oral: 100 mg/5 mL

Guiatuss™ [OTC], Phanasin® [OTC], Phanasin® Diabetic Choice [OTC], Robitussin® [OTC], Scot-Tussin® Expectorant [OTC], Siltussin SA [OTC]: 100 mg/5 mL
Vicks® Casero™ [OTC]: 100 mg/6.25 mL

Tablet, oral: 200 mg

Allfen [OTC]: 400 mg
Organidin® NR: 200 mg
Refenesen™ [OTC]: 200 mg
XPECT™ [OTC]: 400 mg

Tablet, extended release, oral:

Mucinex® [OTC]: 600 mg
Mucinex® Maximum Strength [OTC]: 1200 mg

Guaifenesin AC [US] *see* guaifenesin and codeine *on page* 473

guaifenesin and codeine (gwye FEN e sin & KOE deen)

Synonyms codeine and guaifenesin

U.S./Canadian Brand Names Cheracol® Syrup [US]; Diabetic Tussin C® [US]; Gani-Tuss® NR [US]; Guaifenesin AC [US]; Guaituss AC [US]; Kolephrin® #1 [US]; Mytussin® AC [US]; Robafen® AC [US]; Romilar® AC [US]; Tussi-Organidin® NR [US]; Tussi-Organidin® S-NR [US]; Tusso-C™ [US]

Therapeutic Category Antitussive/Expectorant

Controlled Substance C-V

Use Temporary control of cough due to minor throat and bronchial irritation

Usual Dosage Oral: **Note:** Also refer to specific product labeling:

Children:

2-6 years (Diabetic Tussin C® liquid, Tussi-Organidin® NR): Codeine 1 mg/kg/day in 4 divided doses

6-12 years (Diabetic Tussin C®, Kolephrin® #1, Romilar® AC, Tussi-Organidin® NR liquid): 5 mL every 4 hours; maximum: 30 mL/24 hours

Children ≥12 years and Adults: Diabetic Tussin C®, Kolephrin® #1, Romilar® AC, Tussi-Organidin® NR liquid: 10 mL every 4 hours; maximum: 60 mL/24 hours

Dosage Forms

Liquid: Guaifenesin 300 mg and codeine 10 mg per 5 mL

Diabetic Tussin C®, Tusso-C™: Guaifenesin 200 mg and codeine 10 mg per 5 mL

Gani-Tuss® NR, Guaifenesin AC, Kolephrin® #1: Guaifenesin 100 mg and codeine 10 mg per 5 mL

Tussi-Organidin® NR, Tussi-Organidin® S-NR: Guaifenesin 300 mg and codeine 10 mg per 5 mL

Syrup:

Cheracol®, Guaituss AC, Mytussin® AC, Robafen® AC, Romilar® AC, Tusso-C™: Guaifenesin 100 mg and codeine 10 mg per 5 mL

guaifenesin and dextromethorphan (gwye FEN e sin & deks troe meth OR fan)

Sound-Alike/Look-Alike Issues

Benylin® may be confused with Benadryl®, Ventolin®

Synonyms dextromethorphan and guaifenesin

U.S./Canadian Brand Names Allfen DM [US-OTC]; Balminil DM E [Can]; Benylin® DM-E [Can]; Cheracol® D [US-OTC]; Cheracol® Plus [US-OTC]; Coricidin HBP® Chest Congestion and Cough [US-OTC]; Diabetic Tussin® DM Maximum Strength [US-OTC]; Diabetic Tussin® DM [US-OTC]; Double Tussin DM [US-OTC]; Duratuss® DM [US]; Fenesin DM IR [US]; Gani-Tuss DM NR [US]; Genatuss DM® [US-OTC]; Guaicon DM [US-OTC]; Guia-D [US]; Guiacon DMS [US-OTC]; Guiatuss-DM® [US-OTC]; Koffex DM-Expectorant [Can]; Kolephrin® GG/DM [US-OTC]; Mintab DM [US]; Mucinex® Children's Cough [US-OTC]; Mucinex® DM Maximum Strength [US-OTC]; Mucinex® DM [US-OTC]; Phanatuss® DM [US-OTC]; Phlemex [US]; Refenesen™ DM [US-OTC]; Respa-DM® [US]; Robafen DM Clear [US-OTC]; Robafen DM [US-OTC]; Robitussin® Cough and Congestion [US-OTC]; Robitussin® DM [US-OTC/Can]; Robitussin® Sugar Free Cough [US-OTC]; Safe Tussin® DM [US-OTC]; Scot-Tussin® Senior [US-OTC]; Silexin [US-OTC]; Siltussin DM DAS [US-OTC]; Siltussin DM [US-OTC]; Simuc-DM [US]; Su-Tuss DM [US]; Touro® DM [US]; Tussi-Bid® [US]; Tussi-Organidin® DM NR [US]; Tussi-Organidin® DM-S NR [US]; Vicks® 44E [US-OTC]; Vicks® Pediatric Formula 44E [US-OTC]; Z-Cof LA™ [US]

Therapeutic Category Antitussive/Expectorant

Use Temporary control of cough due to minor throat and bronchial irritation

Usual Dosage Oral:

Children 2-6 years:

General dosing guidelines: Guaifenesin 50-100 mg and dextromethorphan 2.5-5 mg every 4 hours (maximum dose: Guaifenesin 600 mg and dextromethorphan 30 mg per day)

Product-specific labeling:

Touro® DM: 1/2 tablet every 12 hours (maximum: 1 tablet/24 hour)

Robitussin® DM, Robitussin® Sugar Free Cough: 2.5 mL every 4 hours (maximum: 6 doses/24 hours)

Vicks® Pediatric Formula 44E: 7.5 mL every 4 hours (maximum: 6 doses/24 hours)

Children: 6-12 years:

General dosing guidelines: Guaifenesin 100-200 mg and dextromethorphan 5-10 mg every 4 hours (maximum dose: Guaifenesin 1200 mg and dextromethorphan 60 mg per day)

Product-specific labeling:

Touro® DM: 1 tablet every 12 hours (maximum: 2 tablets/24 hours)

Robitussin® DM, Robitussin® Sugar Free Cough: 5 mL every 4 hours (maximum: 6 doses/24 hours)

Vicks® 44E: 7.5 mL every 4 hours (maximum: 6 doses/24 hours)

Vicks® Pediatric Formula 44E: 15 mL every 4 hours (maximum: 6 doses/24 hours)

Z-Cof LA™: 1/2 tablet very 12 hours

Children ≥12 years and Adults:

General dosing guidelines: Guaifenesin 200-400 mg and dextromethorphan 10-20 mg every 4 hours (maximum dose: Guaifenesin 2400 mg and dextromethorphan 120 mg per day)

Product-specific labeling:

Mucinex® DM, Touro® DM: 1-2 tablets every 12 hours (maximum: 4 tablets/24 hours)

Robitussin® DM, Robitussin® Sugar Free Cough: 10 mL every 4 hours (maximum: 6 doses/24 hours)

Vicks® 44E: 15 mL every 4 hours (maximum: 6 doses/24 hours)

Vicks® Pediatric Formula 44E: 30 mL every 4 hours (maximum: 6 doses/24 hours)

Z-Cof LA™: 1 tablet every 12 hours

Dosage Forms

Caplet:

Fenesin DM IR: Guaifenesin 400 mg and dextromethorphan 15 mg

Refenesen™ DM [OTC]: Guaifenesin 400 mg and dextromethorphan 20 mg

Capsule, softgel:

Coricidin HBP® Chest Congestion and Cough [OTC]: Guaifenesin 200 mg and dextromethorphan 10 mg

Elixir:

Duratuss® DM, Simuc-DM: Guaifenesin 225 mg and dextromethorphan 25 mg per 5 mL

Su-Tuss DM: Guaifenesin 200 mg and dextromethorphan 20 mg per 5 mL

Liquid: Guaifenesin 100 mg and dextromethorphan 10 mg per 5 mL; guaifenesin 300 mg and dextromethorphan 10 mg per 5 mL

Diabetic Tussin® DM [OTC], Gani-Tuss DM NR: Guaifenesin 100 mg and dextromethorphan 10 mg per 5 mL

Diabetic Tussin® DM Maximum Strength [OTC]: Guaifenesin 200 mg and dextromethorphan 10 mg per 5 mL

Double Tussin DM [OTC]: Guaifenesin 300 mg and dextromethorphan 200 mg per 5 mL

Kolephrin® GG/DM [OTC]: Guaifenesin 150 mg and dextromethorphan 10 mg per 5 mL

Mucinex® Children's Cough [OTC]: Guaifenesin 100 mg and dextromethorphan 5 mg per 5 mL

Safe Tussin® DM [OTC]: Guaifenesin 100 mg and dextromethorphan 15 mg per 5 mL

Scot-Tussin® Senior [OTC]: Guaifenesin 200 mg and dextromethorphan 15 mg per 5 mL

Tussi-Organidin® DM NR: Guaifenesin 300 mg and dextromethorphan 10 mg per 5 mL

Tussi-Organidin® DM-S NR: Guaifenesin 300 mg and dextromethorphan 10 mg per 5 mL

Vicks® 44E [OTC]: Guaifenesin 200 mg and dextromethorphan hydrobromide 20 mg per 15 mL

Vicks® Pediatric Formula 44E [OTC]: Guaifenesin 100 mg and dextromethorphan hydrobromide 10 mg per 15 mL

Syrup: Guaifenesin 100 mg and dextromethorphan 10 mg per 5 mL

Cheracol® D [OTC], Cheracol® Plus [OTC], Genatuss DM® [OTC], Guiatuss® DM [OTC], Guaicon DM [OTC], Guaicon DMS [OTC], Phanatuss® DM [OTC], Robafen DM [OTC], Robafen DM Clear [OTC], Robitussin® Cough and Congestion [OTC], Robitussin®-DM [OTC], Robitussin® Sugar Free Cough [OTC], Silexin [OTC], Siltussin DM [OTC], Siltussin DM DAS [OTC]: Guaifenesin 100 mg and dextromethorphan 10 mg per 5 mL

Mintab DM: Guaifenesin 200 mg and dextromethorphan hydrobromide 10 mg per 5 mL

Tablet: Guaifenesin 1000 mg and dextromethorphan hydrobromide 60 mg; guaifenesin 1200 mg and dextromethorphan hydrobromide 60 mg

Allfen DM [OTC]: Guaifenesin 400 mg and dextromethorphan 20 mg

Silexin [OTC]: Guaifenesin 100 mg and dextromethorphan hydrobromide 10 mg

Tablet, extended release: 800/30: Guaifenesin 800 mg and dextromethorphan 30 mg; 1200/20: Guaifenesin 1200 mg and dextromethorphan 20 mg

Mucinex® DM [OTC], Respa-DM®: Guaifenesin 600 mg and dextromethorphan 30 mg

Mucinex® DM Maximum Strength [OTC]: Guaifenesin 1200 mg and dextromethorphan 60 mg

Phlemex: Guaifenesin 1200 mg and dextromethorphan 20 mg

Touro® DM: Guaifenesin 575 mg and dextromethorphan 30 mg

Tablet, long-acting: Guaifenesin 1000 mg and dextromethorphan 60 mg

Z-Cof LA™ [scored]: Guaifenesin 650 mg and dextromethorphan 30 mg

Tablet, sustained release:

Tussi-Bid®: Guaifenesin 1200 mg and dextromethorphan 60 mg

Tablet, timed release [scored]: Guaifenesin 1200 mg and dextromethorphan 60 mg

Guia-D: Guaifenesin 1000 mg and dextromethorphan 60 mg

guaifenesin and dyphylline *see* dyphylline and guaifenesin *on page* 344

guaifenesin and phenylephrine (gwye FEN e sin & fen il EF rin)

Sound-Alike/Look-Alike Issues

Entex® may be confused with Tenex®

Entex® LA brand name represents a different product in the U.S. than it does in Canada. In the U.S., Entex® LA contains guaifenesin and phenylephrine, while in Canada the product bearing this brand name contains guaifenesin and pseudoephedrine.

Synonyms guaifenesin and phenylephrine tannate; phenylephrine hydrochloride and guaifenesin

U.S./Canadian Brand Names Aldex™ [US]; Crantex LA [US]; D-Phen 1000 [US]; Deconsal® II [US]; Donatussin Drops [US]; Duomax [US]; Duratuss GP® [US]; Duratuss® [US]; ExeFen-PD [US]; ExeTuss-GP [US]; Fenesin PE IR [US]; Guaifed-PD® [US]; Guaifed® [US]; Guaiphen-D 1200 [US]; Guaiphen-D [US]; Guaiphen-PD [US]; Liquibid-D® [US]; MyDex [US]; Nexphen PD [US]; norel® EX [US]; Pendex [US]; Refenesen™ PE [US-OTC]; Rescon GG [US-OTC]; Sil-Tex [US]; Sina-12X [US]; SINUvent® PE [US]

Therapeutic Category Cold Preparation

Use Temporary relief of nasal congestion, sinusitis, rhinitis, and hay fever; temporary relief of cough associated with upper respiratory tract conditions, especially when associated with dry, nonproductive cough

Usual Dosage Oral:

Children 3-6 months (Donatussin): 0.3-0.6 mL; may repeat every 4-6 hours as needed; maximum 4 doses/24 hours

Children 6 months to 1 year (Donatussin): 0.6-1 mL; may repeat every 4-6 hours as needed; maximum: 4 doses/24 hours

Children 1-2 years (Donatussin): 1-2 mL; may repeat every 4-6 hours as needed; maximum: 4 doses/24 hours

Children 2-6 years:

Rescon GG, Sil-Tex: 2.5 mL every 4-6 hours; maximum: 10 mL/24 hours

Sina-12X suspension: 2.5-5 mL every 12 hours

Children 6-12 years:

Aldex™, Crantex LA, Duomax, Liquibid-D®, Sina-12X tablet: One-half tablet every 12 hours; maximum: 1 tablet/24 hours

Deconsal® II: One capsule daily

Rescon GG: 5 mL every 4-6 hours; maximum: 20 mL/24 hours

ExeFen-PD: One-half to 1 tablet every 12 hours

Guaifed-PD®: One capsule every 12 hours

SINUvent® PE: One tablet every 12 hours; maximum: 2 tablets/24 hours

Sina-12X suspension: Refer to adult dosing.

Children ≥12 years: Aldex™, Crantex LA, Deconsal® II, Duomax, ExeFen-PD, ExeTuss-GP, Guaifed®, Guaifed-PD®, Liquibid-D®, Rescon GG, Sil-Tex, Sina-12X, SINUvent® PE: Refer to adult dosing

Adults:

Aldex™, Crantex LA, Duomax, ExeTuss-GP, Liquibid-D®: One tablet every 12 hours

Deconsal® II: 1-2 capsules every 12 hours; maximum: 3 capsules/24 hours

Sil-Tex: 5-10 mL every 4-6 hours; maximum: 40 mL/24 hours

Guaifed-PD®: 1-2 capsules every 12 hours

Guaifed®: One capsule every 12 hours; maximum: 2 capsules/24 hours

ExeFen-PD: 1-2 tablets every 12 hours

SINUvent® PE: Two tablets every 12 hours

Rescon GG: 10 mL every 4-6 hours; maximum: 40 mL/24 hours

Sina-12X suspension: 5-10 mL every 12 hours

Sina-12X tablet: 1-2 tablets every 12 hours; maximum: 4 tablets/24 hours

Dosage Forms

Caplet:

Fenesin PE IR, Refenesen™ PE [OTC]: Guaifenesin 400 mg and phenylephrine 10 mg

Capsule:

Nexphen PD: Guaifenesin 200 mg and phenylephrine hydrochloride 7 mg

Capsule, variable release:

Deconsal® II: Guaifenesin 375 mg [immediate release] and phenylephrine 20 mg [extended release]

Guaifed®: Guaifenesin 400 mg [immediate release] and phenylephrine 15 mg [extended release]

Guaifed-PD®: Guaifenesin 200 mg [immediate release] and phenylephrine 7.5 mg [extended release]

Liquid: Guaifenesin 100 mg and phenylephrine 7.5 mg per 5 mL

Rescon GG [OTC]: Guaifenesin 100 mg and phenylephrine 5 mg per 5 mL

Sil-Tex: Guaifenesin 100 mg and phenylephrine 7.5 mg per 5 mL

Liquid [drops]:

Donatussin: Guaifenesin 20 mg and phenylephrine hydrochloride 1.5 mg

Suspension:

Sina-12X: Guaifenesin 100 mg and phenylephrine 5 mg per 5 mL

Tablet: Guaifenesin 900 mg and phenylephrine 30 mg

Sina-12X: Guaifenesin 200 mg and phenylephrine 25 mg

Tablet, extended release: Guaifenesin 600 mg and phenylephrine 20 mg; guaifenesin 600 mg and phenylephrine 40 mg; guaifenesin 1200 mg and phenylephrine 40 mg
Aldex™: Guaifenesin 650 mg and phenylephrine 25 mg
D-Phen 1000: Guaifenesin 1000 mg and phenylephrine 30 mg
ExeFen-PD: Guaifenesin 600 mg and phenylephrine 10 mg
SINUvent® PE: Guaifenesin 600 mg and phenylephrine 15 mg
Tablet, long acting: Guaifenesin 900 mg and phenylephrine 25 mg; guaifenesin 1200 mg and phenylephrine hydrochloride 25 mg
Tablet, prolonged release: Guaifenesin 600 mg and phenylephrine 15 mg
Tablet, sustained release: Guaifenesin 600 mg and phenylephrine 30 mg; guaifenesin 1200 mg and phenylephrine 30 mg
Crantex LA: Guaifenesin 600 mg and phenylephrine 30 mg
Duratuss®: Guaifenesin 1200 mg and phenylephrine 25 mg
Duratuss GP®, ExeTuss-GP: Guaifenesin 1200 mg and phenylephrine hydrochloride 25 mg
MyDex: Guaifenesin 900 mg and phenylephrine hydrochloride 30 mg
Pendex: Guaifenesin 600 mg and phenylephrine hydrochloride 10 mg
Tablet, timed release:
Guaiphen-D: Guaifenesin 600 mg and phenylephrine hydrochloride 40 mg
Guaiphen-D 1200: Guaifenesin 1200 mg and phenylephrine hydrochloride 40 mg
Guaiphen-PD: Guaifenesin 275 mg and phenylephrine hydrochloride 25 mg
Tablet, variable release:
Liquibid-D®: Guaifenesin 400 mg and phenylephrine 10 mg [immediate release] and guaifenesin 800 mg and phenylephrine 30 mg [sustained release]
norel® EX: Guaifenesin 400 mg [immediate release] and guaifenesin 400 mg and phenylephrine hydrochloride 40 mg [extended release]

guaifenesin and phenylephrine tannate *see* guaifenesin and phenylephrine *on page 475*

guaifenesin and potassium guaiacolsulfonate *(Discontinued)*

guaifenesin and pseudoephedrine (gwye FEN e sin & soo doe e FED rin)

Sound-Alike/Look-Alike Issues
Entex® may be confused with Tenex®
Entex® LA brand name represents a different product in the U.S. than it does in Canada. In the U.S., Entex® LA contains guaifenesin and phenylephrine, while in Canada the product bearing this brand name contains guaifenesin and pseudoephedrine.
Profen II® may be confused with Profen II DM®, Profen Forte®, Profen Forte™ DM

Synonyms pseudoephedrine and guaifenesin

U.S./Canadian Brand Names Ambifed-G [US]; Congestac® [US-OTC]; Contac® Cold-Chest Congestion, Non Drowsy, Regular Strength [Can]; Entex® LA [Can]; Eudal®-SR [US]; ExeFen [US]; Guaimax-D® [US]; Levall G [US]; Maxifed-G® [US]; Maxifed® [US]; Medent LD [US]; Mucinex® D Maximum Strength [US-OTC]; Mucinex®-D [US-OTC]; Nasatab® LA [US]; Novahistex® Expectorant with Decongestant [Can]; Pseudo GG TR [US]; Pseudo Max [US]; Refenesen Plus [US-OTC]; Respa®-1st [US]; Rutuss Jr [US]; Sinutab® Non-Drying [US-OTC]; SudaTex-G [US]; Touro LA® [US]

Therapeutic Category Expectorant/Decongestant

Use Temporary relief of nasal congestion and to help loosen phlegm and thin bronchial secretions in the treatment of cough

Usual Dosage Oral:
Children 2-6 years: Maxifed-G®: One-third to 1/2 tablet every 12 hours (maximum: 1 tablet/12 hours)
Children 6-12 years:
Ambifed-G, Eudal®-SR, Guaimax-D®, Maxifed®, Nasatab® LA: One-half caplet or tablet every 12 hours (maximum: 1 tablet/24 hours)
Congestac®: One-half caplet every 4-6 hours (maximum: 2 caplets/24 hours)
Levall G: One capsule every 24 hours
Maxifed-G®: One-half to 1 tablet every 12 hours (maximum: 2 tablets/24 hours)
Children >12 years and Adults:
Ambifed-G, Eudal®- SR, Guaimax-D®, Levall G, Mucinex® D 1200/120, Nasatab® LA, Touro LA®: One tablet or capsule every 12 hours (maximum: 2 tablets or capsules in 24 hours)
Congestac®: One caplet every 4-6 hours (maximum: 4 caplets in 24 hours)
Maxifed®: One to 1 1/2 tablets every 12 hours (maximum: 3 tablets/24 hours)

Dosage Forms
Caplet:
Congestac® [OTC], Refenesen Plus [OTC]: Guaifenesin 400 mg and pseudoephedrine 60 mg

Caplet, long-acting:
Touro LA®: Guaifenesin 500 mg and pseudoephedrine 120 mg
Caplet, prolonged release:
Ambifed-G: Guaifenesin 1000 mg and pseudoephedrine 60 mg
Capsule, liquicap:
Sinutab® Non-Drying [OTC]: Guaifenesin 200 mg and pseudoephedrine 30 mg
Capsule, variable release:
Levall G: Guaifenesin 400 mg [immediate release] and pseudoephedrine 90 mg [extended release]
Syrup: Guaifenesin 200 mg and pseudoephedrine 40 mg per 5 mL
Tablet:
ExeFen: Guaifenesin 780 mg and pseudoephedrine 80 mg
Rutuss Jr: 600/45: Guaifenesin 600 mg and pseudoephedrine 45 mg
Tablet, extended release:
Mucinex® D Maximum Strength [OTC]: Guaifenesin 1200 mg and pseudoephedrine 120 mg
Guaimax-D®: Guaifenesin 600 mg and pseudoephedrine 120 mg
Maxifed®: Guaifenesin 780 mg and pseudoephedrine 80 mg
Maxifed-G®: Guaifenesin 580 mg and pseudoephedrine 60 mg
Mucinex®-D [OTC] 600/60: Guaifenesin 600 mg and pseudoephedrine 60 mg
Pseudo Max: Guaifenesin 700 mg and pseudoephedrine 80 mg
Tablet, long acting:
Medent LD: Guaifenesin 800 mg and pseudoephedrine 60 mg
Tablet, sustained release:
Nasatab® LA: Guaifenesin 500 mg and pseudoephedrine 120 mg
Respa®-1st: Guaifenesin 600 mg and pseudoephedrine 58 mg
SudaTex-G: Guaifenesin 580 mg and pseudoephedrine 60 mg

guaifenesin, carbetapentane citrate, and phenylephrine hydrochloride *see* carbetapentane, guaifenesin, and phenylephrine *on page* 182

guaifenesin, chlorpheniramine, phenylephrine, and dextromethorphan *see* dextromethorphan, chlorpheniramine, phenylephrine, and guaifenesin *on page* 297

guaifenesin, dextromethorphan, and phenylephrine

(gwye FEN e sin, deks troe meth OR fan, & fen il EF rin)

Synonyms guaifenesin, dextromethorphan hydrobromide, and phenylephrine hydrochloride; phenylephrine hydrochloride, guaifenesin, and dextromethorphan hydrobromide

U.S./Canadian Brand Names Certuss-D® [US]; Dacex-DM [US]; Dexcon-PE [US]; Duraphen™ Forte [US]; Duraphen™ II DM [US]; ExeCof [US]; ExeTuss-DM [US]; Giltuss Pediatric® [US]; Giltuss TR® [US]; Giltuss® [US]; Maxiphen DM [US]; Robitussin® Cold and Cough CF [US-OTC]; Robitussin® Pediatric Cold and Cough CF [US-OTC]; SINUtuss® DM [US]; TriTuss® ER [US]; TriTuss® [US]; Tusso™-DMR [US]

Therapeutic Category Antitussive; Decongestant

Use Symptomatic relief of dry nonproductive coughs and upper respiratory symptoms associated with hay fever, colds, or the flu

Usual Dosage Also refer to specific product labeling. Oral:
Children 6-12 years (Certuss-D®, Duraphen™ Forte, Duraphen™ II DM, Maxiphen DM): One-half tablet every 12 hours, not to exceed 1 tablet/24 hours
Children ≥12 years and Adults:
Certuss-D®, Duraphen™ Forte, Maxiphen DM: One tablet every 12 hours, not to exceed 2 tablets/24 hours
Duraphen™ II DM: 1-1½ tablets twice daily, not to exceed 3 tablets/24 hours

Dosage Forms
Caplet:
Dexcon-PE: Guaifenesin 550 mg, dextromethorphan 25 mg, and phenylephrine 20 mg
Caplet, extended release:
TriTuss®-ER: Guaifenesin 600 mg, dextromethorphan 30 mg, and phenylephrine 10 mg
Capsule:
Tusso™-DMR: Guaifenesin 288 mg, dextromethorphan 14 mg, and phenylephrine 7 mg
Liquid:
Giltuss®: Guaifenesin 300 mg, dextromethorphan 15 mg, and phenylephrine 10 mg per 5 mL
Giltuss Pediatric®: Guaifenesin 50 mg, dextromethorphan 5 mg, and phenylephrine 2.5 mg per mL

Liquid, oral [drops]: Guaifenesin 50 mg, dextromethorphan 5 mg, and phenylephrine 2.5 mg per mL
Robitussin® Pediatric Cold and Cough CF: Guaifenesin 100 mg, dextromethorphan 5 mg, and phenylephrine 2.5 mg per 2.5 mL

Syrup: Guaifenesin 200 mg, dextromethorphan 30 mg, and phenylephrine 10 mg
Dacex-DM, TriTuss®: Guaifenesin 175 mg, dextromethorphan 25 mg, and phenylephrine 12.5 mg per 5 mL
Robitussin® Cold and Cough CF: Guaifenesin 100 mg, dextromethorphan 10 mg, and phenylephrine 5 mg per 5 mL

Tablet [scored]:
SINUtuss™ DM: Guaifenesin 600 mg, dextromethorphan hydrobromide 30 mg, and phenylephrine hydrochloride 15 mg

Tablet, extended release [scored]:
Duraphen™ II DM: Guaifenesin 800 mg, dextromethorphan 20 mg, and phenylephrine 20 mg
Duraphen™ Forte: Guaifenesin 1200 mg, dextromethorphan 30 mg, and phenylephrine 30 mg

Tablet, prolonged release [scored]:
Maxiphen DM: Guaifenesin 1000 mg, dextromethorphan 60 mg, and phenylephrine 40 mg

Tablet, sustained release: Guaifenesin 1200 mg, dextromethorphan 20 mg, and phenylephrine 40 mg
Certuss-D® [scored]: Guaifenesin 600 mg, dextromethorphan 60 mg, and phenylephrine 40 mg
ExeCof: Guaifenesin 100 mg, dextromethorphan 60 mg, and phenylephrine 40 mg
ExeTuss-DM: Guaifenesin 600 mg, dextromethorphan 25 mg, and phenylephrine 20 mg

Tablet, timed release [scored]:
Giltuss TR®: Guaifenesin 600 mg, dextromethorphan 30 mg, and phenylephrine 20 mg

guaifenesin, dextromethorphan hydrobromide, and phenylephrine hydrochloride *see* guaifenesin, dextromethorphan, and phenylephrine *on page* 478

guaifenesin, dihydrocodeine, and pseudoephedrine *see* dihydrocodeine, pseudoephedrine, and guaifenesin *on page* 310

guaifenesin, phenylephrine, and chlorpheniramine *see* chlorpheniramine, phenylephrine, and guaifenesin *on page* 218

guaifenesin, phenylephrine tannate, and pyrilamine tannate *see* phenylephrine, pyrilamine, and guaifenesin *on page* 779

guaifenesin, pseudoephedrine, and codeine

(gwye FEN e sin, soo doe e FED rin, & KOE deen)

Synonyms codeine, guaifenesin, and pseudoephedrine; pseudoephedrine, guaifenesin, and codeine

U.S./Canadian Brand Names Benylin® 3.3 mg-D-E [Can]; Calmylin with Codeine [Can]; Mytussin® DAC [US]

Therapeutic Category Antitussive/Decongestant/Expectorant

Controlled Substance C-III; C-V

Use Temporarily relieves nasal congestion and controls cough associated with upper respiratory infections and related conditions (common cold, sinusitis, bronchitis, influenza)

Usual Dosage Oral:
Children 6-12 years: 5 mL every 4 hours (maximum: 20 mL/24 hours)
Children >12 years and Adults: 10 mL every 4 hours (maximum: 40 mL/24 hours)

Dosage Forms

Syrup:
Mytussin® DAC: Guaifenesin 100 mg, pseudoephedrine 30 mg, and codeine 10 mg per 5 mL

guaifenesin, pseudoephedrine, and dextromethorphan

(gwye FEN e sin, soo doe e FED rin, & deks troe meth OR fan)

Sound-Alike/Look-Alike Issues
Profen II DM® may be confused with Profen II®, Profen Forte®, Profen Forte™ DM
Profen Forte™ DM may be confused with Profen II®, Profen II DM®, Profen Forte®

Synonyms dextromethorphan, guaifenesin, and pseudoephedrine; pseudoephedrine, dextromethorphan, and guaifenesin

U.S./Canadian Brand Names Ambifed-G DM [US]; Balminil DM + Decongestant + Expectorant [Can]; Benylin® DM-D-E [Can]; ExeFen-DMX [US]; Koffex DM + Decongestant + Expectorant [Can]; Maxifed DM [US]; Maxifed DMX [US]; Medent-DM [US]; Novahistex® DM Decongestant Expectorant [Can]; Novahistine® DM Decongestant Expectorant [Can]; Profen Forte™ DM [US]; Profen II DM® [US]; Pseudo Max DMX [US]; Relacon-DM NR [US]; Robitussin® Cough and Cold CF [US-OTC]; Robitussin® Cough and Cold Infant CF [US-OTC]; Robitussin® Cough and Cold [US-OTC/Can]; Ru-Tuss DM [US];

SudaTex-DM [US]; Touro® CC [US]; Touro® CC-LD [US]; Tusnel Liquid® [US]; Tusnel Pediatric® [US]; Tusnel-DM Pediatric® [US]; Z-Cof™ 12DM [US]

Therapeutic Category Cold Preparation

Use Temporarily relieves nasal congestion and controls cough due to minor throat and bronchial irritation; helps loosen phlegm and thin bronchial secretions to make coughs more productive

Usual Dosage Note: Also refer to specific product labeling.

Children 2-6 years:

Maxifed DM: 1/3 to 1/2 tablet every 12 hours, not to exceed 1 tablet/24 hours

Profen II DM® (syrup): 1.25-2.5 mL every 4 hours, not to exceed 15 mL/24 hours

Robitussin® Cough and Cold Infant CF: 2.5 mL every 4-6 hours, not to exceed 4 doses/24 hours

Touro® CC: 1/2 tablet every 12 hour, not to exceed 1 tablet/24 hours

Z-Cof™ 12DM: 2.5 mL 2-3 times/day, not to exceed 7.5 mL/24 hours

Children 6-12 years:

Ambifed-G DM, Profen Forte™ DM, Profen II DM®: 1/2 tablet every 12 hours not to exceed 1 tablet/24 hours

Maxifed DM: 1/2 to 1 tablet every 12 hours, not to exceed 2 tablets/24 hours

Touro® CC: 1 tablet every 12 hours, not to exceed 2 tablets/24 hours

Profen II DM® (syrup): 2.5-5 mL every 4 hours, not to exceed 30 mL/24 hours

Z-Cof™ 12DM: 5 mL 2-3 times/day, not to exceed 15 mL/24 hours

Children ≥12 years and Adults:

Ambifed-G DM, Profen Forte™ DM: 1 tablet every 12 hours not to exceed 2 tablets/24 hours

Maxifed DM, Touro® CC: 1-2 tablets every 12 hours, not to exceed 4 tablets/24 hours

Profen II DM® (tablet): 1 to 1 1/2 tablets every 12 hours, not to exceed 3 tablets/24 hours

Profen II DM® (syrup): 5-10 mL every 4 hours, not to exceed 60 mL/24 hours

Z-Cof™ 12DM: 10 mL 2-3 times/day, not to exceed 30 mL/24 hours

Dosage Forms

Caplet, prolonged release:

Ambifed-G DM: Guaifenesin 1000 mg, pseudoephedrine 60 mg, and dextromethorphan 30 mg

Caplet, sustained release:

Touro® CC: Guaifenesin 575 mg, pseudoephedrine 60 mg, and dextromethorphan 30 mg

Touro® CC-LD: Guaifenesin 575 mg, pseudoephedrine 25 mg, and dextromethorphan 30 mg

Capsule, softgel:

Robitussin® Cough and Cold [OTC]: Guaifenesin 200 mg, pseudoephedrine 30 mg, and dextromethorphan 10 mg

Liquid: Guaifenesin 100 mg, pseudoephedrine 30 mg, and dextromethorphan 10 mg per 5 mL

Profen II DM®: Guaifenesin 200 mg, pseudoephedrine 15 mg, and dextromethorphan 10 mg per 5 mL

Relacon-DM NR, Z-Cof™ 12DM: Guaifenesin 200 mg, pseudoephedrine 40 mg, and dextromethorphan 15 mg

Tusnel Liquid®: Guaifenesin 200 mg, pseudoephedrine 30 mg, and dextromethorphan 15 mg per 5 mL

Tusnel Pediatric®: Guaifenesin 50 mg, pseudoephedrine 15 mg, and dextromethorphan 5 mg per 5 mL

Liquid, oral [drops]:

Robitussin® Cough and Cold Infant CF [OTC]: Guaifenesin 100 mg, pseudoephedrine 15 mg, and dextromethorphan 5 mg per 2.5 mL

Tusnel-DM Pediatric®: Guaifenesin 25 mg, pseudoephedrine 5 mg, and dextromethorphan 5 mg per 1 mL

Suspension:

Z-Cof™ 12DM: Guaifenesin 175 mg, pseudoephedrine 30 mg, and dextromethorphan 15 mg per 5 mL

Syrup: Guaifenesin 100 mg, pseudoephedrine 45 mg, and dextromethorphan 15 mg per 5 mL

Robitussin® Cough and Cold CF [OTC]: Guaifenesin 100 mg, pseudoephedrine 30 mg, and dextromethorphan 10 mg per 5 mL

Ru-Tuss DM: Guaifenesin 100 mg, pseudoephedrine 45 mg, and dextromethorphan 15 mg per 5 mL

Tablet, extended release: Guaifenesin 100 mg, pseudoephedrine hydrochloride 30 mg, and dextromethorphan hydrobromide 10 mg; guaifenesin 800 mg, pseudoephedrine 60 mg, and dextromethorphan30 mg; guaifenesin 1200 mg, pseudoephedrine 60 mg, and dextromethorphan 60 mg; guaifenesin 1200 mg, pseudoephedrine 120 mg, and dextromethorphan 60 mg; guaifenesin 800 mg, pseudoephedrine90 mg, and dextromethorphan 60 mg; guaifenesin 550 mg, pseudoephedrine 60 mg, and dextromethorphan 30 mg; guaifenesin 595 mg, pseudoephedrine 48 mg, and dextromethorphan 32 mg; guaifenesin 600 mg, pseudoephedrine 60 mg, and dextromethorphan 30 mg

Profen Forte™ DM: Guaifenesin 800 mg, pseudoephedrine 90 mg, and dextromethorphan 60 mg

Profen II DM®: Guaifenesin 800 mg, pseudoephedrine 45 mg, and dextromethorphan 30 mg

Tablet, long acting: Guaifenesin 800 mg, pseudoephedrine 60 mg, and dextromethorphan 30 mg

Medent-DM: Guaifenesin 800 mg, pseudoephedrine 60 mg, and dextromethorphan 30 mg

Tablet, sustained release:
ExeFen-DMX, Maxifed DM: Guaifenesin 780 mg, pseudoephedrine 80 mg, and dextromethorphan 40 mg
Maxifed DM, SudaTex-DM: Guaifenesin 580 mg, pseudoephedrine 60 mg, and dextromethorphan 30 mg
Pseudo Max DMX: Guaifenesin 700 mg, pseudoephedrine 80 mg, and dextromethorphan 40 mg

Guaifenex® *(Discontinued)*
Guaifenex® DM *(Discontinued)* *see* guaifenesin and dextromethorphan *on page 474*
Guaifenex® GP *(Discontinued)* *see* guaifenesin and pseudoephedrine *on page 477*
Guaifenex® PPA 75 *(Discontinued)*
Guaifenex® PSE *(Discontinued)* *see* guaifenesin and pseudoephedrine *on page 477*
Guaifenex™-Rx *(Discontinued)* *see* guaifenesin and pseudoephedrine *on page 477*
Guaifenex™-Rx DM *(Discontinued)* *see* guaifenesin, pseudoephedrine, and dextromethorphan *on page 479*
Guaimax-D® [US] *see* guaifenesin and pseudoephedrine *on page 477*
Guaipax® *(Discontinued)*
Guaiphen-D [US] *see* guaifenesin and phenylephrine *on page 475*
Guaiphen-D 1200 [US] *see* guaifenesin and phenylephrine *on page 475*
Guaiphen-PD [US] *see* guaifenesin and phenylephrine *on page 475*
Guaitab® *(Discontinued)* *see* guaifenesin and pseudoephedrine *on page 477*
Guaituss AC [US] *see* guaifenesin and codeine *on page 473*
Guaituss CF® *(Discontinued)*
Guaivent® *(Discontinued)* *see* guaifenesin and pseudoephedrine *on page 477*

guanabenz (GWAHN a benz)

Sound-Alike/Look-Alike Issues
guanabenz may be confused with guanadrel, guanfacine

Synonyms guanabenz acetate

U.S./Canadian Brand Names Wytensin® [Can]

Therapeutic Category Alpha-Adrenergic Agonist

Use Management of hypertension

Usual Dosage Oral: Adults: Initial: 4 mg twice daily; increase in increments of 4-8 mg/day every 1-2 weeks to a maximum of 32 mg twice daily

Dosage Forms
Tablet: 4 mg, 8 mg

guanabenz acetate *see* guanabenz *on page 481*

guanfacine (GWAHN fa seen)

Sound-Alike/Look-Alike Issues
guanFACINE may be confused with guaiFENesin, guanabenz, guanidine
Tenex® may be confused with Entex®, Ten-K®, Xanax®

Synonyms guanfacine hydrochloride

Tall-Man guan**FACINE**

U.S./Canadian Brand Names Tenex® [US/Can]

Therapeutic Category Alpha-Adrenergic Agonist

Use Management of hypertension

Usual Dosage Oral: Adults: Hypertension: 1 mg usually at bedtime, may increase if needed at 3- to 4-week intervals; usual dose range (JNC 7): 0.5-2 mg once daily

Product Availability
Intuniv™: FDA approved August 2009; availability expected November 2009
Intuniv™ extended-release tablets are approved for the treatment of attention-deficit/hyperactivity disorder (ADHD) in children and adolescents 6-17 years of age.

Dosage Forms
Tablet: 1 mg, 2 mg
Tenex®: 1 mg, 2 mg

guanfacine hydrochloride *see* guanfacine *on page 481*

guanidine (GWAHN i deen)

Sound-Alike/Look-Alike Issues

guanidine may be confused with guanfacine, guanethidine

Synonyms guanidine hydrochloride

Therapeutic Category Cholinergic Agent

Use Reduction of the symptoms of muscle weakness associated with the myasthenic syndrome of Eaton-Lambert, not for myasthenia gravis

Usual Dosage Oral: Adults: Eaton-Lambert syndrome: Initial: 10-15 mg/kg/day in 3-4 divided doses, gradually increase to 35 mg/kg/day or up to development of side effects

Dosage Forms

Tablet: 125 mg

guanidine hydrochloride *see* guanidine *on page* *482*

Guia-D [US] *see* guaifenesin and dextromethorphan *on page* *474*

Guiacon DMS [US-OTC] *see* guaifenesin and dextromethorphan *on page* *474*

GuiaCough® *(Discontinued)* *see* guaifenesin and dextromethorphan *on page* *474*

GuiaCough® Expectorant *(Discontinued)* *see* guaifenesin *on page* *473*

Guiaplex™ HC *(Discontinued)*

Guiatex® *(Discontinued)*

Guiatuss™ [US-OTC] *see* guaifenesin *on page* *473*

Guiatuss DAC *(Discontinued)* *see* guaifenesin, pseudoephedrine, and codeine *on page* *479*

Guiatuss-DM® [US-OTC] *see* guaifenesin and dextromethorphan *on page* *474*

gum benjamin *see* benzoin *on page* *132*

GW506U78 *see* nelarabine *on page* *685*

GW-1000-02 *see* tetrahydrocannabinol and cannabidiol *(Canada only) on page* *951*

GW433908G *see* fosamprenavir *on page* *444*

GW572016 *see* lapatinib *on page* *572*

G-well® *(Discontinued)* *see* lindane *on page* *590*

Gynazole-1® [US/Can] *see* butoconazole *on page* *163*

Gyne-Lotrimin® 3 [US-OTC] *see* clotrimazole *on page* *248*

Gyne-Lotrimin® 7 [US-OTC] *see* clotrimazole *on page* *248*

Gyne-Sulf® *(Discontinued)* *see* sulfabenzamide, sulfacetamide, and sulfathiazole *on page* *926*

Gynodiol® *(Discontinued)* *see* estradiol *on page* *373*

Gynogen L.A.® Injection *(Discontinued)* *see* estradiol *on page* *373*

Gynol II® [US-OTC] *see* nonoxynol 9 *on page* *703*

Gynol II® Extra Strength [US-OTC] *see* nonoxynol 9 *on page* *703*

Gynovite® Plus [US-OTC] *see* vitamins (multiple/oral) *on page* *1019*

H5N1 influenza vaccine *see* influenza virus vaccine (H5N1) *on page* *529*

Habitrol® [Can] *see* nicotine *on page* *695*

Haemophilus B conjugate and hepatitis B vaccine

(he MOF i lus bee KON joo gate & hep a TYE tis bee vak SEEN)

Sound-Alike/Look-Alike Issues

Comvax® may be confused with Recombivax [Recombivax HB®]

Synonyms *Haemophilus* b (meningococcal protein conjugate) conjugate vaccine; hepatitis B vaccine (recombinant); hib conjugate vaccine; hib-hepB

U.S./Canadian Brand Names Comvax® [US]

Therapeutic Category Vaccine, Inactivated Virus

Use

Immunization against invasive disease caused by *H. influenzae* type b and against infection caused by all known subtypes of hepatitis B virus in infants 6 weeks to 15 months of age born of hepatitis B surface antigen (HB_sAg) negative mothers

Infants born of HB_sAg-positive mothers or mothers of unknown HB_sAg status should receive hepatitis B immune globulin and hepatitis B vaccine (recombinant) at birth and should complete the hepatitis B vaccination series given according to a particular schedule

Usual Dosage I.M.: Infants: 0.5 mL at 2, 4, and 12-15 months of age (total of 3 doses)

If the recommended schedule cannot be followed, the interval between the first two doses should be at least 6 weeks and the interval between the second and third dose should be as close as possible to 8-11 months. Minimum age for first dose is 6 weeks.

Modified Schedule: Children who receive one dose of hepatitis B vaccine at or shortly after birth may receive Comvax® on a schedule of 2, 4, and 12-15 months of age

Dosage Forms

Injection, suspension [preservative free]:

Comvax®: *Haemophilus* b capsular polysaccharide 7.5 mcg and hepatitis B surface antigen 5 mcg per 0.5 mL (0.5 mL)

***Haemophilus* B conjugate (Hib)** *see* diphtheria and tetanus toxoids, acellular pertussis, poliovirus and *Haemophilus* b conjugate vaccine *on page 320*

Haemophilus B conjugate vaccine (he MOF fi lus bee KON joo gate vak SEEN)

Synonyms *Haemophilus* b oligosaccharide conjugate vaccine; *Haemophilus* b polysaccharide vaccine; diphtheria toxoid conjugate; HbCV; hib; hib conjugate vaccine; hib polysaccharide conjugate; PRP-OMP; PRP-T

U.S./Canadian Brand Names ActHIB® [US/Can]; PedvaxHIB® [US/Can]

Therapeutic Category Vaccine, Inactivated Bacteria

Use Routine immunization of children against invasive disease caused by *H. influenzae* type b

The Advisory Committee on Immunization Practices (ACIP) recommends routine vaccination of all children through age 59 months. Efficacy data is not available for use in older children and adults with chronic conditions associated with an increased risk of Hib disease. However, a single dose may also be considered for older children, adolescents, and adults who did not receive the childhood series and who have had splenectomies or who have sickle cell disease, leukemia or HIV infection.

Usual Dosage Children: I.M.: 0.5 mL as a single dose should be administered to previously unvaccinated children according to one of the following "brand-specific" schedules; number of doses in series is dependent upon age at first dose

ActHIB®: *Age at first dose:*

2 months of age: Immunization consists of 3 doses (0.5 mL/dose) administered at 2-, 4- and 6 months of age (may reconstitute with provided diluent or DTP vaccine). A booster dose is given at 15-18 months of age (may reconstitute with provided diluent or Tripedia® vaccine).

7-11 months of age: Two doses (0.5 mL/dose) administered 8 months apart, with a booster dose at 15-18 months of age

12-14 months of age: One dose (0.5 mL) followed by a booster dose 2 months later

PedvaxHIB®: *Age at first dose:*

2-10 months of age: Two doses (0.5 mL/dose) administered 2 months apart; booster dose at 12-15 months of age

11-14 months of age: Two doses (0.5 mL/dose) administered 1 months apart

15-71 months of age: One 0.5 mL dose

Dosage Forms

Injection, powder for reconstitution [preservative free]:

ActHIB® *Haemophilus* b capsular polysaccharide 10 mcg per 0.5 mL

Hiberix®: *Haemophilus* b capsular polysaccharide 10 mcg per 0.5 mL

Injection, suspension:

PedvaxHIB®: *Haemophilus* b capsular polysaccharide 7.5 mcg

***Haemophilus* b (meningococcal protein conjugate) conjugate vaccine** *see Haemophilus* B conjugate and hepatitis B vaccine *on page 482*

***Haemophilus* b oligosaccharide conjugate vaccine** *see Haemophilus* B conjugate vaccine *on page 483*

***Haemophilus* B polysaccharide** *see* diphtheria and tetanus toxoids, acellular pertussis, poliovirus and *Haemophilus* b conjugate vaccine *on page 320*

***Haemophilus* b polysaccharide vaccine** *see Haemophilus* B conjugate vaccine *on page 483*

***Haemophilus influenzae* b conjugate vaccine and diphtheria, tetanus toxoids, and acellular pertussis vaccine** *see* diphtheria, tetanus toxoids, and acellular pertussis vaccine and *Haemophilus influenzae* b conjugate vaccine *on page 323*

halcinonide (hal SIN oh nide)

Sound-Alike/Look-Alike Issues

halcinonide may be confused with Halcion®

Halog® may be confused with Haldol®, Mycolog®

U.S./Canadian Brand Names Halog® [US/Can]

Therapeutic Category Corticosteroid, Topical

Use Inflammation of corticosteroid-responsive dermatoses [high potency topical corticosteroid]

Usual Dosage Topical: Children and Adults: Steroid-responsive dermatoses: Apply sparingly 1-3 times/day, occlusive dressing may be used for severe or resistant dermatoses; a thin film is effective; do not overuse. Therapy should be discontinued when control is achieved; if no improvement is seen, reassessment of diagnosis may be necessary.

Dosage Forms

Cream:

Halog®: 0.1% (30 g, 60 g)

Ointment:

Halog®: 0.1% (30 g, 60 g)

Halcion® [US/Can] *see* triazolam *on page 984*

Haldol® [US] *see* haloperidol *on page 484*

Haldol® Decanoate [US] *see* haloperidol *on page 484*

Haley's M-O *see* magnesium hydroxide and mineral oil *on page 609*

HalfLytely® and Bisacodyl [US] *see* polyethylene glycol-electrolyte solution and bisacodyl *on page 798*

Halfprin® [US-OTC] *see* aspirin *on page 103*

halobetasol (hal oh BAY ta sol)

Sound-Alike/Look-Alike Issues

Ultravate® may be confused with Cutivate®

Synonyms halobetasol propionate

U.S./Canadian Brand Names Ultravate® [US/Can]

Therapeutic Category Corticosteroid, Topical

Use Relief of inflammatory and pruritic manifestations of corticosteroid-response dermatoses [super high potency topical corticosteroid]

Usual Dosage Topical: Children ≥12 years and Adults:

Inflammatory and pruritic manifestations (dental use): Cream: Apply sparingly to lesion twice daily. Treatment should not exceed 2 consecutive weeks and total dosage should not exceed 50 g/week. Therapy should be discontinued when control is achieved; if no improvement is seen, reassessment of diagnosis may be necessary.

Steroid-responsive dermatoses: Apply sparingly to skin twice daily, rub in gently and completely; treatment should not exceed 2 consecutive weeks and total dosage should not exceed 50 g/week. Therapy should be discontinued when control is achieved; if no improvement is seen, reassessment of diagnosis may be necessary.

Dosage Forms

Cream: 0.05% (15 g, 50 g)

Ultravate®: 0.05% (15 g, 50 g)

Ointment: 0.05% (15 g, 50 g)

Ultravate®: 0.05% (15 g, 50 g)

halobetasol propionate *see* halobetasol *on page 484*

Halog® [US/Can] *see* halcinonide *on page 483*

Halog®-E *(Discontinued)* *see* halcinonide *on page 483*

haloperidol (ha loe PER i dole)

Sound-Alike/Look-Alike Issues

haloperidol may be confused Halotestin®

Haldol® may be confused with Halcion®, Halenol®, Halog®, Halotestin®, Stadol®

Synonyms haloperidol decanoate; haloperidol lactate

U.S./Canadian Brand Names Apo-Haloperidol LA® [Can]; Apo-Haloperidol® [Can]; Haldol® Decanoate [US]; Haldol® [US]; Haloperidol Injection, USP [Can]; Haloperidol Long Acting [Can]; Haloperidol-LA Omega [Can]; Haloperidol-LA [Can]; Novo-Peridol [Can]; Peridol [Can]; PMS-Haloperidol LA [Can]

Therapeutic Category Antipsychotic Agent, Butyrophenone

Use Management of schizophrenia; control of tics and vocal utterances of Tourette disorder in children and adults; severe behavioral problems in children

Usual Dosage

Children: 3-12 years (15-40 kg): Oral:

Initial: 0.05 mg/kg/day or 0.25-0.5 mg/day given in 2-3 divided doses; increase by 0.25-0.5 mg every 5-7 days; maximum: 0.15 mg/kg/day

Usual maintenance:

Agitation or hyperkinesia: 0.01-0.03 mg/kg/day once daily

Nonpsychotic disorders: 0.05-0.075 mg/kg/day in 2-3 divided doses

Psychotic disorders: 0.05-0.15 mg/kg/day in 2-3 divided doses

Children 6-12 years: Sedation/psychotic disorders: I.M. (as lactate): 1-3 mg/dose every 4-8 hours to a maximum of 0.15 mg/kg/day; change over to oral therapy as soon as able

Adults: Psychosis:

Oral: 0.5-5 mg 2-3 times/day; usual maximum: 30 mg/day

I.M. (as lactate): 2-5 mg every 4-8 hours as needed

I.M. (as decanoate): Initial: 10-20 times the daily oral dose administered at 4-week intervals

Maintenance dose: 10-15 times initial oral dose; used to stabilize psychiatric symptoms

Dosage Forms

Injection, oil: 50 mg/mL (1 mL, 5 mL); 100 mg/mL (1 mL, 5 mL)

Injection, solution: 5 mg/mL (1 mL, 10 mL)

Haldol®: 5 mg/mL (1 mL)

Solution, oral concentrate: 2 mg/mL

Tablet: 0.5 mg, 1 mg, 2 mg, 5 mg, 10 mg, 20 mg

haloperidol decanoate *see* haloperidol *on page 484*

Haloperidol Injection, USP [Can] *see* haloperidol *on page 484*

Haloperidol-LA [Can] *see* haloperidol *on page 484*

haloperidol lactate *see* haloperidol *on page 484*

Haloperidol-LA Omega [Can] *see* haloperidol *on page 484*

Haloperidol Long Acting [Can] *see* haloperidol *on page 484*

halothane (HA loe thane)

Sound-Alike/Look-Alike Issues

halothane may be confused with Halotestin®

Therapeutic Category General Anesthetic

Use Induction and maintenance of general anesthesia

Usual Dosage Minimum alveolar concentration (MAC), the concentration at which 50% of patients do not respond to surgical incision, is 0.74% for halothane. The concentration at which amnesia and loss of awareness occur (MAC - awake) is 0.41%. Surgical levels of anesthesia are maintained with concentrations between 0.5% to 2%; inspired concentrations of up to 3% required for induction of anesthesia.

Dosage Forms

Liquid: 99.9% (250 mL)

Halotussin® *(Discontinued)* *see* guaifenesin *on page 473*

Halotussin® DM *(Discontinued)* *see* guaifenesin and dextromethorphan *on page 474*

Halotussin® PE *(Discontinued)* *see* guaifenesin and pseudoephedrine *on page 477*

Haltran® *(Discontinued)* *see* ibuprofen *on page 515*

hamamelis water *see* witch hazel *on page 1023*

HandClens® [US-OTC] *see* benzalkonium chloride *on page 129*

harkoseride *see* lacosamide *on page 563*

HAVRIX® [US/Can] *see* hepatitis A vaccine *on page 489*

Havrix® and Engerix-B® *see* hepatitis A and hepatitis B recombinant vaccine *on page 488*

HbCV *see Haemophilus* B conjugate vaccine *on page 483*

HBIG *see* hepatitis B immune globulin (human) *on page 489*

hBNP *see* nesiritide *on page 690*

hCG *see* chorionic gonadotropin (human) *on page 225*

HD 200® Plus [US] *see* barium *on page 122*

HDA® Toothache [US-OTC] *see* benzocaine *on page 129*

HDCV *see* rabies vaccine *on page* 848
Head & Shoulders® Citrus Breeze [US-OTC] *see* pyrithione zinc *on page* 842
Head & Shoulders® Citrus Breeze 2-in-1 [US-OTC] *see* pyrithione zinc *on page* 842
Head & Shoulders® Classic Clean [US-OTC] *see* pyrithione zinc *on page* 842
Head & Shoulders® Classic Clean 2-In-1 [US-OTC] *see* pyrithione zinc *on page* 842
Head & Shoulders® Dry Scalp Care [US-OTC] *see* pyrithione zinc *on page* 842
Head & Shoulders® Dry Scalp Care 2-in-1 [US-OTC] *see* pyrithione zinc *on page* 842
Head & Shoulders® Extra Volume [US-OTC] *see* pyrithione zinc *on page* 842
Head & Shoulders® intensive solutions 2-in-1 [US-OTC] *see* pyrithione zinc *on page* 842
Head & Shoulders® intensive solutions for dry/damaged hair [US-OTC] *see* pyrithione zinc *on page* 842
Head & Shoulders® intensive solutions for fine/oily hair [US-OTC] *see* pyrithione zinc *on page* 842
Head & Shoulders® intensive solutions for normal hair [US-OTC] *see* pyrithione zinc *on page* 842
Head & Shoulders® Intensive Treatment [US-OTC] *see* selenium sulfide *on page* 895
Head & Shoulders® Ocean Lift [US-OTC] *see* pyrithione zinc *on page* 842
Head & Shoulders® Ocean Lift 2-in-1 [US-OTC] *see* pyrithione zinc *on page* 842
Head & Shoulders® Refresh [US-OTC] *see* pyrithione zinc *on page* 842
Head & Shoulders® Refresh 2-in-1 [US-OTC] *see* pyrithione zinc *on page* 842
Head & Shoulders® Restoring Shine [US-OTC] *see* pyrithione zinc *on page* 842
Head & Shoulders® Restoring Shine 2-in-1 [US-OTC] *see* pyrithione zinc *on page* 842
Head & Shoulders® Sensitive Care [US-OTC] *see* pyrithione zinc *on page* 842
Head & Shoulders® Sensitive Care 2-in-1 [US-OTC] *see* pyrithione zinc *on page* 842
Head & Shoulders® Smooth & Silky [US-OTC] *see* pyrithione zinc *on page* 842
Head & Shoulders® Smooth & Silky 2-In-1 [US-OTC] *see* pyrithione zinc *on page* 842
Healon® [US/Can] *see* hyaluronate and derivatives *on page* 496
Healon®5 [US] *see* hyaluronate and derivatives *on page* 496
Healon GV® [US/Can] *see* hyaluronate and derivatives *on page* 496
Hectorol® [US/Can] *see* doxercalciferol *on page* 334
Helidac® [US] *see* bismuth, metronidazole, and tetracycline *on page* 143
Helistat® [US] *see* collagen hemostat *on page* 255
Helitene® [US] *see* collagen hemostat *on page* 255
Helixate® FS [US/Can] *see* antihemophilic factor (recombinant) *on page* 82
Hemabate® [US/Can] *see* carboprost tromethamine *on page* 186
hematin *see* hemin *on page* 486
hemiacidrin *see* citric acid, magnesium carbonate, and glucono-delta-lactone *on page* 234

hemin (HEE min)

Synonyms hematin

U.S./Canadian Brand Names Panhematin® [US]

Therapeutic Category Blood Modifiers

Use Treatment of recurrent attacks of acute intermittent porphyria (AIP)

Usual Dosage I.V.: Children ≥16 years and Adults: 1-4 mg/kg/day administered over 10-15 minutes for 3-14 days; may be repeated no earlier than every 12 hours; not to exceed 6 mg/kg in any 24-hour period

Dosage Forms

Injection, powder for reconstitution [preservative free]:
Panhematin®: 313 mg

Hemocyte® [US-OTC] *see* ferrous fumarate *on page* 413
Hemocyte Plus® [US] *see* vitamins (multiple/oral) *on page* 1019
Hemofil M [US/Can] *see* antihemophilic factor (human) *on page* 81
Hemril®-30 [US] *see* hydrocortisone (rectal) *on page* 503
HepA *see* hepatitis A vaccine *on page* 489
HepaGam B™ [US/Can] *see* hepatitis B immune globulin (human) *on page* 489

HepA-HepB *see* hepatitis A and hepatitis B recombinant vaccine *on page 488*
Hepalean® [Can] *see* heparin *on page 487*
Hepalean® Leo [Can] *see* heparin *on page 487*
Hepalean®-LOK [Can] *see* heparin *on page 487*

heparin (HEP a rin)

Sound-Alike/Look-Alike Issues
heparin may be confused with Hespan®

Synonyms heparin calcium; heparin lock flush; heparin sodium

U.S./Canadian Brand Names Hep-Lock U/P [US]; Hep-Lock® [US]; Hepalean® Leo [Can]; Hepalean® [Can]; Hepalean®-LOK [Can]; HepFlush®-10 [US]

Therapeutic Category Anticoagulant (Other)

Use Prophylaxis and treatment of thromboembolic disorders; as an anticoagulant for extracorporeal and dialysis procedures

Note: Heparin lock flush solution is intended only to maintain patency of I.V. devices and is **not** to be used for anticoagulant therapy.

Usual Dosage

Children:

Intermittent I.V.: Initial: 50-100 units/kg, then 50-100 units/kg every 4 hours

I.V. infusion: Initial: 50 units/kg, then 15-25 units/kg/hour; increase dose by 2-4 units/kg/hour every 6-8 hours as required

Adults:

Prophylaxis (low-dose heparin): SubQ: 5000 units every 8-12 hours

Intermittent I.V.: Initial: 10,000 units, then 50-70 units/kg (5000-10,000 units) every 4-6 hours

I.V. infusion (weight-based dosing per institutional nomogram recommended):

Acute coronary syndromes: MI: Fibrinolytic therapy:

Full-dose alteplase, reteplase, or tenecteplase with dosing as follows: Concurrent bolus of 60 units/kg (maximum: 4000 units), then 12 units/kg/hour (maximum: 1000 units/hour) as continuous infusion. Check aPTT every 4-6 hours; adjust to target of 1.5-2 times the upper limit of control (50-70 seconds in clinical trials); usual range 10-30 units/kg/hour. Duration of heparin therapy depends on concurrent therapy and the specific patient risks for systemic or venous thromboembolism.

Streptokinase: Heparin use optional depending on concurrent therapy and specific patient risks for systemic or venous thromboembolism (anterior MI, CHF, previous embolus, atrial fibrillation, LV thrombus): If heparin is administered, start when aPTT <2 times the upper limit of control; do not use a bolus, but initiate infusion adjusted to a target aPTT of 1.5-2 times the upper limit of control (50-70 seconds in clinical trials). If heparin is not administered by infusion, 7500-12,500 units SubQ every 12 hours (when aPTT <2 times the upper limit of control) is recommended.

Percutaneous coronary intervention: Heparin bolus and infusion may be administered to an activated clotting time (ACT) of 300-350 seconds if no concurrent GPIIb/IIIa receptor antagonist is administered or 200-250 seconds if a GPIIb/IIIa receptor antagonist is administered.

Treatment of unstable angina (high-risk and some intermediate-risk patients): Initial bolus of 60-70 units/kg (maximum: 5000 units), followed by an initial infusion of 12-15 units/kg/hour (maximum: 1000 units/hour). The American College of Chest Physicians consensus conference has recommended dosage adjustments to correspond to a therapeutic range equivalent to heparin levels of 0.3-0.7 units/mL by antifactor Xa determinations.

Treatment of venous thromboembolism:

DVT/PE: I.V. push: 80 units/kg followed by continuous infusion of 18 units/kg/hour

DVT: SubQ: 17,500 units every 12 hours

Line flushing: When using daily flushes of heparin to maintain patency of single and double lumen central catheters, 10 units/mL is commonly used for younger infants (eg, <10 kg) while 100 units/mL is used for older infants, children, and adults. Capped PVC catheters and peripheral heparin locks require flushing more frequently (eg, every 6-8 hours). Volume of heparin flush is usually similar to volume of catheter (or slightly greater). Additional flushes should be given when stagnant blood is observed in catheter, after catheter is used for drug or blood administration, and after blood withdrawal from catheter.

Addition of heparin (0.5-3 unit/mL) to peripheral and central parenteral nutrition has not been shown to decrease catheter-related thrombosis. The final concentration of heparin used for TPN solutions may need to be decreased to 0.5 units/mL in small infants receiving larger amounts of volume in order to avoid approaching therapeutic amounts. Arterial lines are heparinized with a final concentration of 1 unit/mL.

Dosage Forms

Infusion [premixed in NaCl 0.45%; porcine intestinal mucosa source]: 12,500 units (250 mL); 25,000 units (250 mL, 500 mL)

Infusion [preservative free; premixed in D_5W; porcine intestinal mucosa source]: 10,000 units (100 mL); 12,500 units (250 mL); 20,000 units (500 mL); 25,000 units (250 mL, 500 mL)

Infusion [preservative free; premixed in NaCl 0.9%; porcine intestinal mucosa source]: 1000 units (500 mL); 2000 units (1000 mL)

Injection, solution [lock flush preparation; porcine intestinal mucosa source; multidose vial]: 10 units/mL (1 mL, 10 mL, 30 mL); 100 units/mL (1 mL, 5 mL, 10 mL, 30 mL)

Hep-Lock®: 10 units/mL (1 mL, 2 mL, 10 mL, 30 mL); 100 units/mL (1 mL, 2 mL, 10 mL, 30 mL)

Injection, solution [lock flush preparation; porcine intestinal mucosa source; prefilled syringe]: 10 units/mL (1 mL, 2 mL, 3 mL, 5 mL); 100 units/mL (1 mL, 2 mL, 3 mL, 5 mL)

Injection, solution [preservative free; lock flush preparation; porcine intestinal mucosa source; prefilled syringe]: 1 unit/mL (2 mL, 3 mL, 5 mL); 2 units/mL (3 mL); 10 units/mL (2.5 mL, 3 mL, 5 mL, 10 mL); 100 units/mL (3 mL, 5 mL, 10 mL)

Injection, solution [preservative free; lock flush preparation; porcine intestinal mucosa source; vial]: 10 units/mL (10 mL)

HepFlush®-10: 10 units/mL (10 mL)

Hep-Lock U/P: 10 units/mL (1 mL); 100 units/mL (1 mL)

Injection, solution [porcine intestinal mucosa source; multidose vial]: 1000 units/mL (1 mL, 10 mL, 30 mL); 5000 units/mL (1 mL, 10 mL); 10,000 units/mL (1 mL, 4 mL, 5 mL); 20,000 units/mL (1 mL)

Injection, solution [porcine intestinal mucosa source; prefilled syringe]: 5000 units/mL (1 mL)

Injection, solution [preservative free; porcine intestinal mucosa source; prefilled syringe]: 10,000 units/mL (0.5 mL)

Injection, solution [preservative free; porcine intestinal mucosa source; vial]: 1000 units/mL (2 mL); 2000 units/mL (5 mL); 2500 units/mL (10 mL)

heparin calcium *see* heparin *on page 487*

heparin cofactor I *see* antithrombin III *on page 85*

heparin lock flush *see* heparin *on page 487*

heparin sodium *see* heparin *on page 487*

HepatAmine® [US] *see* amino acid injection *on page 62*

Hepatasol® [US] *see* amino acid injection *on page 62*

hepatitis A and hepatitis B recombinant vaccine

(hep a TYE tis aye & hep a TYE tis bee ree KOM be nant vak SEEN)

Synonyms Engerix-B® and Havrix®; Havrix® and Engerix-B®; HepA-HepB; hepatitis B and hepatitis A vaccine

U.S./Canadian Brand Names Twinrix® [US/Can]

Therapeutic Category Vaccine

Use Active immunization against disease caused by hepatitis A virus and hepatitis B virus (all known subtypes) in populations desiring protection against or at high risk of exposure to these viruses.

Populations include travelers to areas of intermediate/high endemicity for **both** HAV and HBV; those at increased risk of HBV infection due to behavioral or occupational factors; patients with chronic liver disease; laboratory workers who handle live HAV and HBV; healthcare workers, police, and other personnel who render first-aid or medical assistance; workers who come in contact with sewage; employees of day care centers and correctional facilities; patients/staff of hemodialysis units; male homosexuals; patients frequently receiving blood products; military personnel; users of injectable illicit drugs; close household contacts of patients with hepatitis A and hepatitis B infection; residents of drug and alcohol treatment centers

Usual Dosage I.M.: Adults: Primary immunization: Three doses (1 mL each) given on a 0-, 1-, and 6-month schedule

Alternative regimen: Accelerated regimen: Four doses (1 mL each) on day 0, 7, and 21-30, followed by a booster at 12 months

Dosage Forms

Injection, suspension [preservative free]:

Twinrix®: Hepatitis A virus antigen 720 ELISA units and hepatitis B surface antigen 20 mcg per mL (1 mL)

hepatitis A vaccine (hep a TYE tis aye vak SEEN)

Synonyms HepA

U.S./Canadian Brand Names Avaxim® [Can]; Avaxim®-Pediatric [Can]; HAVRIX® [US/Can]; VAQTA® [US/Can]

Therapeutic Category Vaccine, Inactivated Virus

Use

Active immunization against disease caused by hepatitis A virus (HAV)

The Advisory Committee on Immunization Practices (ACIP) recommends routine vaccination for:

- All children ≥12 months of age
- Travelers to countries with intermediate to high endemicity of HAV (a list of countries is available at http://wwwn.cdc.gov/travel/contentdiseases.aspx)
- Persons who anticipate close personal contact with international adoptee from a country of intermediate to high endemicity of HAV, during their first 60 days of arrival into the United States (eg, household contacts, babysitters)
- Men who have sex with men
- Illegal drug users
- Patients with chronic liver disease
- Patients who receive clotting-factor concentrates
- Persons who work with HAV-infected primates or with HAV in a research laboratory setting

Usual Dosage I.M.: **Note:** When used for primary immunization, the vaccine should be given at least 2 weeks prior to expected HAV exposure. When used for post-exposure prophylaxis, the vaccine should be given as soon as possible.

HAVRIX®:

Children 12 months to 18 years: 720 ELISA units (0.5 mL) with a booster dose of 720 ELISA units to be given 6-12 months following primary immunization

Adults: 1440 ELISA units (1 mL) with a booster dose of 1440 ELISA units to be given 6-12 months following primary immunization

VAQTA®:

Children 12 months to 18 years: 25 units (0.5 mL) with 25 units (0.5 mL) booster dose of 25 units to be given 6-18 months after primary immunization (6-12 months if initial dose was with HAVRIX®)

Adults: 50 units (1 mL) with 50 units (1 mL) booster dose of 50 units to be given 6-18 months after primary immunization (6-12 months if initial dose was with HAVRIX®)

Dosage Forms

Injection, suspension [adult formulation; preservative free]:

HAVRIX®: Hepatitis A virus antigen 1440 ELISA units/mL (1 mL)

VAQTA®: Hepatitis A virus antigen 50 units/mL (1 mL)

Injection, suspension [pediatric formulation; preservative free]:

HAVRIX®: Hepatitis A virus antigen 720 ELISA units/0.5 mL (0.5 mL)

Injection, suspension [pediatric/adolescent formulation; preservative free]:

VAQTA®: Hepatitis A virus antigen 25 units/0.5 mL (0.5 mL)

hepatitis B and hepatitis A vaccine *see* hepatitis A and hepatitis B recombinant vaccine *on page 488*

hepatitis B immune globulin (human) (hep a TYE tis bee i MYUN GLOB yoo lin YU man)

Sound-Alike/Look-Alike Issues

HBIG may be confused with BabyBIG

Synonyms HBIG

U.S./Canadian Brand Names HepaGam B™ [US/Can]; HyperHep B® [Can]; HyperHEP B™ S/D [US]; Nabi-HB® [US]

Therapeutic Category Immune Globulin

Use

Passive prophylactic immunity to hepatitis B following: Acute exposure to blood containing hepatitis B surface antigen (HBsAg); perinatal exposure of infants born to HBsAg-positive mothers; sexual exposure to HBsAg-positive persons; household exposure to persons with acute HBV infection

Prevention of hepatitis B virus recurrence after liver transplantation in HBsAg-positive transplant patients

Note: Hepatitis B immune globulin is not indicated for treatment of active hepatitis B infection and is ineffective in the treatment of chronic active hepatitis B infection.

Usual Dosage

I.M.:

Newborns: Perinatal exposure of infants born to HBsAg-positive mothers: 0.5 mL as soon after birth as possible (within 12 hours); active vaccination with hepatitis B vaccine may begin at the same time in a different site (if not contraindicated). If first dose of hepatitis B vaccine is delayed for as long as 3 months, dose may be repeated. If hepatitis B vaccine is refused, dose may be repeated at 3 and 6 months.

Infants <12 months: Household exposure prophylaxis: 0.5 mL (to be administered if mother or primary caregiver has acute HBV infection)

Children ≥12 months and Adults: Postexposure prophylaxis: 0.06 mL/kg as soon as possible after exposure (ie, within 24 hours of needlestick, ocular, or mucosal exposure or within 14 days of sexual exposure); usual dose: 3-5 mL; repeat at 28-30 days after exposure in nonresponders to hepatitis B vaccine or in patients who refuse vaccination

Note: HBIG may be administered at the same time (but at a different site) or up to 1 month preceding hepatitis B vaccination without impairing the active immune response

I.V.: Adults: Prevention of hepatitis B virus recurrence after liver transplantation (HepaGam B™): 20,000 int. units/dose according to the following schedule:

Anhepatic phase (Initial dose): One dose given with the liver transplant

Week 1 postop: One dose daily for 7 days (days 1-7)

Weeks 2-12 postop: One dose every 2 weeks starting day 14

Month 4 onward: One dose monthly starting on month 4

Dose adjustment: Adjust dose to reach anti-HBs levels of 500 int. units/L within the first week after transplantation. In patients with surgical bleeding, abdominal fluid drainage >500 mL or those undergoing plasmapheresis, administer 10,000 int. units/dose every 6 hours until target anti-HBs levels are reached.

Dosage Forms Note: Potency expressed in international units (as compared to the WHO standard) is noted by individual lot on the vial label.

Injection, solution [preservative free]:

HyperHEP B™ S/D: Anti-HBs ≥220 int. units/mL (0.5 mL, 1 mL, 5 mL)

Nabi-HB®: Anti-HBs >312 int. units/mL (1 mL, 5 mL)

HepaGam B™: Anti-HBs 312 int. units/mL (1 mL, 5 mL)

hepatitis B inactivated virus vaccine (recombinant DNA) *see* hepatitis B vaccine (recombinant) *on page 490*

hepatitis B vaccine (recombinant) (hep a TYE tis bee vak SEEN ree KOM be nant)

Sound-Alike/Look-Alike Issues

Engerix-B® adult may be confused with Engerix-B® pediatric/adolescent

Recombivax HB® may be confused with Comvax®

Synonyms hepatitis B inactivated virus vaccine (recombinant DNA); HepB

U.S./Canadian Brand Names Engerix-B® [US/Can]; Recombivax HB® [US/Can]

Therapeutic Category Vaccine, Inactivated Virus

Use Immunization against infection caused by all known subtypes of hepatitis B virus (HBV), in individuals seeking protection from HBV infection and/or in the following individuals considered at high risk of potential exposure to hepatitis B virus or HBsAg-positive materials:

Workplace Exposure:

- Healthcare workers[1] (including students, custodial staff, lab personnel, etc)
- Police and fire personnel
- Military personnel
- Morticians and embalmers
- Clients/staff of institutions for the developmentally disabled

Lifestyle Factors:

- Homosexual men
- Heterosexually-active persons with multiple partners in a 6-month period or those with recently acquired sexually-transmitted disease
- Intravenous drug users

Specific Patient Groups:

- Those on hemodialysis[2], receiving transfusions[3], or in hematology/oncology units
- Adolescents
- Infants born of HBsAG-positive mothers

- Individuals with chronic liver disease
- Individual with HIV infection

Others:

- Prison inmates and staff of correctional facilities
- Household and sexual contacts of HBV carriers
- Residents, immigrants, adoptees, and refugees from areas with endemic HBV infection (eg, Alaskan Eskimos, Pacific Islanders, Indochinese, and Haitian descent)
- International travelers to areas of endemic HBV
- Children born after 11/21/1991

[1]The risk of hepatitis B virus (HBV) infection for healthcare workers varies both between hospitals and within hospitals. Hepatitis B vaccination is recommended for all healthcare workers with blood exposure.
[2]Hemodialysis patients often respond poorly to hepatitis B vaccination; higher vaccine doses or increased number of doses are required. A special formulation of one vaccine is now available for such persons (Recombivax HB®, 40 mcg/mL). The anti-HB_s (antibody to hepatitis B surface antigen) response of such persons should be tested after they are vaccinated, and those who have not responded should be revaccinated with 1-3 additional doses. Patients with chronic renal disease should be vaccinated as early as possible, ideally before they require hemodialysis. In addition, their anti-HB_s levels should be monitored at 6- to 12-month intervals to assess the need for revaccination.
[3]Patients with hemophilia should be immunized subcutaneously, not intramuscularly.

In addition, the Advisory Committee on Immunization Practices (ACIP) recommends vaccination for any persons who are wounded in bombings or similar mass casualty events who have penetrating injuries or nonintact skin exposure, or who have contact with mucous membranes (exception - superficial contact with intact skin), and who cannot confirm receipt of a hepatitis B vaccination.

Usual Dosage I.M.:

Immunization regimen: Regimen consists of 3 doses (0, 1, and 6 months): First dose given on the elected date, second dose given 1 month later, third dose given 6 months after the first dose.

When used for immediate prophylactic intervention (eg, administration to persons who are wounded in bombings or similar mass casualty events), vaccination should begin within 24 hours and no later than 7 days following the event.

Note: Infants born to mothers whose HB_sAg status is unknown should follow the regimen for HB_sAg-positive mothers, omitting the dose of HBIG.

Note: Preterm infants <2000 g and born to HB_sAg-negative mothers should have the first dose delayed until 1 month after birth or hospital discharge due to decreased immune response in underweight infants.

Initial dose:

Birth (infants born of HB_s Ag-negative mothers) to 19 years:
Recombivax HB®: 0.5 mL (5 mcg/0.5 mL pediatric/adolescent formulation) **or**
Engerix-B®: 0.5 mL (10 mcg/0.5 mL formulation)

20 years and older:
Recombivax HB®: 1 mL (10 mcg/mL adult formulation) **or**
Engerix-B®: 1 mL (20 mcg/mL formulation)

Dialysis or immunocompromised patients (revaccinate if anti-HB_s <10 mIU/mL ≥1-2 months after third dose):
Recombivax HB®: 1 mL (40 mcg/mL dialysis formulation) **or**
Engerix-B®: 2 mL (two 1 mL doses given at different sites using the 20 mcg/mL formulation)

1-month dose:

Birth (infants born of HB_sAg-negative mothers) to 19 years:
Recombivax HB®: 0.5 mL (5 mcg/0.5 mL pediatric/adolescent formulation) **or**
Engerix-B®: 0.5 mL (10 mcg/0.5 mL formulation)

20 years and older:
Recombivax HB®: 1 mL (10 mcg/mL adult formulation) **or**
Engerix-B®: 1 mL (20 mcg/mL formulation)

Dialysis or immunocompromised patients (revaccinate if anti-HB_s <10 mIU/mL ≥1-2 months after third dose):
Recombivax HB®: 1 mL (40 mcg/mL dialysis formulation) **or**
Engerix-B®: 2 mL (two 1 mL doses given at different sites using the 20 mcg/mL formulation)

2-month dose:

Dialysis or immunocompromised patients (revaccinate if anti-HB_s <10 mIU/mL ≥1-2 months after third dose):
Engerix-B®: 2 mL (two 1 mL doses given at different sites using the 20 mcg/mL formulation)

6-month dose (final dose in series should not be administered before age of 24 weeks):

Birth (infants born of HB_sAg-negative mothers) to 19 years:

Recombivax HB®: 0.5 mL (5 mcg/0.5 mL pediatric/adolescent formulation)

Engerix-B®: 0.5 mL (10 mcg/0.5 mL formulation)

20 years and older:

Recombivax HB®: 1 mL (10 mcg/mL adult formulation) **or**

Engerix-B®: 1 mL (20 mcg/mL formulation)

Dialysis or immunocompromised patients (revaccinate if anti-HB_s <10 mIU/mL ≥1-2 months after third dose):

Recombivax HB®: 1 mL (40 mcg/mL dialysis formulation) **or**

Engerix-B®: 2 mL (two 1 mL doses given at different sites using the 20 mcg/mL formulation)

Alternative dosing schedule for **Recombivax HB®:**

Children 11-15 years (10 mcg/mL adult formulation): First dose of 1 mL given on the elected date, second dose given 4-6 months later

Adults ≥20 years: Doses may be administered at 0, 1, and 4 months **or** at 0, 2, and 4 months

Alternative dosing schedules for **Engerix-B®:**

Children ≤10 years (10 mcg/0.5 mL formulation): High-risk children: 0.5 mL at 0, 1, 2, and 12 months; lower-risk children ages 5-10 who are candidates for an extended administration schedule may receive an alternative regimen of 0.5 mL at 0, 12, and 24 months. If booster dose is needed, revaccinate with 0.5 mL.

Adolescents 11-19 years (20 mcg/mL formulation): 1 mL at 0, 1, and 6 months. High-risk adolescents: 1 mL at 0, 1, 2, and 12 months; lower-risk adolescents 11-16 years who are candidates for an extended administration schedule may receive an alternative regimen of 0.5 mL (using the 10 mcg/ 0.5 mL) formulation at 0, 12, and 24 months. If booster dose is needed, revaccinate with 20 mcg.

Adults ≥20 years:

Doses may be administered at 0, 1, and 4 months **or** at 0, 2, and 4 months

High-risk adults (20 mcg/mL formulation): 1 mL at 0, 1, 2, and 12 months. If booster dose is needed, revaccinate with 1 mL.

Postexposure prophylaxis: **Note:** High-risk individuals may include children born of hepatitis B-infected mothers, those who have been or might be exposed or those who have traveled to high-risk areas.

Postexposure prophylaxis recommended dosage for infants born to HB_sAg-positive mothers (by product/age):

Engerix-B® (pediatric formulation 10 mcg/0.5 mL):

Give 0.5 mL at birth (≤12 hours); repeat 0.5 mL at 1 month and 6 months.

The first dose may be given at birth at the same time as HBIG, but give in the opposite anterolateral thigh. This may better ensure vaccine absorption.

An alternate regimen is administration of the vaccine at birth, and at 1, 2, and 12 months later.

Recombivax HB® (pediatric/adolescent formulation 5 mcg/0.5 mL):

Give 0.5 mL at birth (≤12 hours); repeat 0.5 mL at 1 month and 6 months

The first dose may be given at birth at the same time as HBIG, but give in the opposite anterolateral thigh. This may better ensure vaccine absorption.

Hepatitis B immune globulin: Give 0.5 mL at birth (or within 7 days of birth).

Dosage Forms

Injection, suspension [adult; preservative free]:

Engerix-B®: Hepatitis B surface antigen 20 mcg/mL (1 mL)

Recombivax HB®: Hepatitis B surface antigen 10 mcg/mL (1 mL, 3 mL)

Injection, suspension [pediatric/adolescent; preservative free]:

Engerix-B®: Hepatitis B surface antigen 10 mcg/0.5 mL (0.5 mL)

Recombivax HB®: Hepatitis B surface antigen 5 mcg/0.5 mL (0.5 mL)

Injection, suspension [dialysis formulation; preservative free]:

Recombivax HB®: Hepatitis B surface antigen 40 mcg/mL (1 mL)

hepatitis B vaccine (recombinant) *see Haemophilus* B conjugate and hepatitis B vaccine *on page 482*

HepB *see* hepatitis B vaccine (recombinant) *on page 490*

HepFlush®-10 [US] *see* heparin *on page 487*

Hep-Lock® [US] *see* heparin *on page 487*

Hep-Lock U/P [US] *see* heparin *on page 487*

Hepsera™ [US/Can] *see* adefovir *on page 36*

Heptalac® ***(Discontinued)*** *see* lactulose *on page 565*

Heptovir® [Can] *see* lamivudine *on page 566*

Herceptin® [US/Can] *see* trastuzumab *on page* 977
HES *see* hetastarch *on page* 493
Hespan® [US] *see* hetastarch *on page* 493

hetastarch (HET a starch)

Sound-Alike/Look-Alike Issues
Hespan® may be confused with heparin

Synonyms HES; hydroxyethyl starch

U.S./Canadian Brand Names Hespan® [US]; Hextend® [US/Can]; Voluven® [US/Can]

Therapeutic Category Plasma Volume Expander

Use Blood volume expander used in treatment of hypovolemia; prevention of hypovolemia (Voluven®); adjunct in leukapheresis to improve harvesting and increase the yield of granulocytes by centrifugation (Hespan®)

Usual Dosage I.V. infusion (requires an infusion pump):
Plasma volume expansion:
Children:
<2 years: Voluven®: Average dose: 7-25 mL/kg; titrate to individual colloid needs, hemodynamic and hydration status
2-12 years: Not studied
>12 years: Voluven®: Up to 50 mL/kg/day
Adults: 500-1000 mL (up to 1500 mL/day) or 20 mL/kg/day (up to 1500 mL/day); larger volumes (15,000 mL/24 hours) have been used safely in small numbers of patients
Voluven®: Up to 50 mL/kg/day
Leukapheresis (Hextend®): 250-700 mL; **Note:** Citrate anticoagulant is added before use.

Dosage Forms
Infusion [premixed in lactated electrolyte injection]:
Hextend®: 6% (500 mL)
Infusion, solution [premixed in NaCl 0.9%]: 6% (500 mL)
Hespan®, Voluven®: 6% (500 mL)

Hexabrix™ [US] *see* ioxaglate meglumine and ioxaglate sodium *on page* 543
hexachlorocyclohexane *see* lindane *on page* 590

hexachlorophene (heks a KLOR oh feen)

Sound-Alike/Look-Alike Issues
pHisoHex® may be confused with Fostex®, pHisoDerm®

U.S./Canadian Brand Names pHisoHex® [US/Can]

Therapeutic Category Antibacterial, Topical

Use Surgical scrub and as a bacteriostatic skin cleanser; control an outbreak of gram-positive infection when other procedures have been unsuccessful

Usual Dosage Topical: Children and Adults: Apply 5 mL cleanser and water to area to be cleansed; lather and rinse thoroughly under running water

Dosage Forms
Liquid, topical:
pHisoHex®: 3% (150 mL, 500 mL, 3840 mL)

Hexalen® [US/Can] *see* altretamine *on page* 54
hexamethylenetetramine *see* methenamine *on page* 637
hexamethylmelamine *see* altretamine *on page* 54
Hexit™ [Can] *see* lindane *on page* 590
HEXM *see* altretamine *on page* 54
Hextend® [US/Can] *see* hetastarch *on page* 493

hexylresorcinol (heks il re ZOR si nole)

U.S./Canadian Brand Names S.T. 37® [US-OTC]; Sucrets® Original [US-OTC]

Therapeutic Category Local Anesthetic

Use Minor antiseptic and local anesthetic for sore throat; topical antiseptic for minor cuts or abrasions

Usual Dosage Children ≥2 years and Adults:
Antiseptic: Topical: Solution: Apply to affected area 1-3 times/day

Sore throat: Oral:

Lozenge: May be used as needed, allow to dissolve slowly in mouth (maximum: 10 lozenges/day)

Solution: Gargle or swish in mouth up to 4 times/day

Dosage Forms

Lozenge:

Sucrets® Original [OTC]: 2.4 mg

Solution:

S.T. 37® [OTC]: 0.1%

hFSH *see* urofollitropin *on page 999*

hGH *see* somatropin *on page 916*

hib *see Haemophilus* B conjugate vaccine *on page 483*

hib conjugate vaccine *see Haemophilus* B conjugate and hepatitis B vaccine *on page 482*

hib conjugate vaccine *see Haemophilus* B conjugate vaccine *on page 483*

hib-hepB *see Haemophilus* B conjugate and hepatitis B vaccine *on page 482*

Hibiclens® [US-OTC] *see* chlorhexidine gluconate *on page 210*

Hibidil® 1:2000 [Can] *see* chlorhexidine gluconate *on page 210*

Hibistat® [US-OTC] *see* chlorhexidine gluconate *on page 210*

hib polysaccharide conjugate *see Haemophilus* B conjugate vaccine *on page 483*

HibTITER® ***(Discontinued)*** *see Haemophilus* B conjugate vaccine *on page 483*

High Gamma Vitamin E Complete™ [US-OTC] *see* vitamin E *on page 1018*

high-molecular-weight iron dextran (DexFerrum®) *see* iron dextran complex *on page 546*

Hi-Kovite [US-OTC] *see* vitamins (multiple/oral) *on page 1019*

Hiprex® [US/Can] *see* methenamine *on page 637*

hirulog *see* bivalirudin *on page 144*

Histacol™ BD [US] *see* brompheniramine, pseudoephedrine, and dextromethorphan *on page 152*

Histade™ ***(Discontinued)*** *see* chlorpheniramine and pseudoephedrine *on page 215*

Histalet® X ***(Discontinued)*** *see* guaifenesin and pseudoephedrine *on page 477*

Histantil [Can] *see* promethazine *on page 823*

Histaprin [US-OTC] *see* diphenhydramine *on page 315*

Histatab PH [US] *see* chlorpheniramine, phenylephrine, and methscopolamine *on page 218*

Histatab® Plus ***(Discontinued)*** *see* chlorpheniramine and phenylephrine *on page 214*

Hista-Vent® DA ***(Discontinued)*** *see* chlorpheniramine, phenylephrine, and methscopolamine *on page 218*

Hista-Vent® PSE ***(Discontinued)*** *see* chlorpheniramine, pseudoephedrine, and methscopolamine *on page 221*

Histerone® Injection ***(Discontinued)*** *see* testosterone *on page 947*

Histex™ I/E ***(Discontinued)*** *see* carbinoxamine *on page 185*

Histex™ ***(Discontinued)*** *see* chlorpheniramine and pseudoephedrine *on page 215*

Histex® SR [US] *see* brompheniramine and pseudoephedrine *on page 150*

Histinex® D Liquid ***(Discontinued)***

Histinex® HC [US] *see* phenylephrine, hydrocodone, and chlorpheniramine *on page 778*

Histinex® PV ***(Discontinued)***

Histor-D® Syrup ***(Discontinued)*** *see* chlorpheniramine and phenylephrine *on page 214*

Histor-D® Timecelles® ***(Discontinued)*** *see* chlorpheniramine, phenylephrine, and methscopolamine *on page 218*

Histrodrix® ***(Discontinued)*** *see* dexbrompheniramine and pseudoephedrine *on page 289*

Histussin D® ***(Discontinued)***

Histussin® HC ***(Discontinued)*** *see* phenylephrine, hydrocodone, and chlorpheniramine *on page 778*

Hi-Vegi-Lip [US-OTC] *see* pancreatin *on page 746*

Hivid® ***(Discontinued)***

hMG *see* menotropins *on page 625*

HMM *see* altretamine *on page 54*

HMR 3647 *see* telithromycin *on page 941*

HMS Liquifilm® ***(Discontinued)***

HN_2 *see* mechlorethamine *on page 618*

Hold® DM [US-OTC] *see* dextromethorphan *on page* 295

homatropine (hoe MA troe peen)

Sound-Alike/Look-Alike Issues
homatropine may be confused with Humatrope®, somatropin

Synonyms homatropine hydrobromide

U.S./Canadian Brand Names Isopto® Homatropine [US]

Therapeutic Category Anticholinergic Agent

Use Producing cycloplegia and mydriasis for refraction; treatment of acute inflammatory conditions of the uveal tract; optical aid in axial lens opacities

Usual Dosage Ophthalmic:
Children:
Mydriasis and cycloplegia for refraction: Instill 1 drop of 2% solution immediately before the procedure; repeat at 10-minute intervals as needed
Uveitis: Instill 1 drop of 2% solution 2-3 times/day
Adults:
Mydriasis and cycloplegia for refraction: Instill 1-2 drops of 2% solution or 1 drop of 5% solution before the procedure; repeat at 5- to 10-minute intervals as needed; maximum of 3 doses for refraction
Uveitis: Instill 1-2 drops of 2% or 5% 2-3 times/day up to every 3-4 hours as needed

Dosage Forms
Solution, ophthalmic:
Isopto® Homatropine: 2% (5 mL); 5% (5 mL, 15 mL)

homatropine and hydrocodone *see* hydrocodone and homatropine *on page* 502
homatropine hydrobromide *see* homatropine *on page* 495
horse antihuman thymocyte gamma globulin *see* antithymocyte globulin (equine) *on page* 86
H.P. Acthar® Gel [US] *see* corticotropin *on page* 258
Hp-PAC® [Can] *see* lansoprazole, amoxicillin, and clarithromycin *on page* 571
HPV4 *see* papillomavirus (types 6, 11, 16, 18) vaccine (human, recombinant) *on page* 750
HPV vaccine *see* papillomavirus (types 6, 11, 16, 18) vaccine (human, recombinant) *on page* 750
HTF919 *see* tegaserod *on page* 940
hu1124 *see* efalizumab *on page* 348
Humalog® [US/Can] *see* insulin lispro *on page* 531
Humalog® Mix 25 [Can] *see* insulin lispro protamine and insulin lispro *on page* 532
Humalog® Mix 50/50™ [US] *see* insulin lispro protamine and insulin lispro *on page* 532
Humalog® Mix 50/50 Insulin *(Discontinued)*
Humalog® Mix 75/25™ [US] *see* insulin lispro protamine and insulin lispro *on page* 532
human antitumor necrosis factor alpha *see* adalimumab *on page* 35
human C1 inhibitor *see* C1 inhibitor (human) *on page* 165
human corticotrophin-releasing hormone, analogue *see* corticorelin *on page* 258
human diploid cell cultures rabies vaccine *see* rabies vaccine *on page* 848
human growth hormone *see* somatropin *on page* 916
humanized IgG1 anti-CD52 monoclonal antibody *see* alemtuzumab *on page* 44
human LFA-3/IgG(1) fusion protein *see* alefacept *on page* 44
human menopausal gonadotropin *see* menotropins *on page* 625
human papillomavirus vaccine *see* papillomavirus (types 6, 11, 16, 18) vaccine (human, recombinant) *on page* 750
human rotavirus vaccine, attenuated (HRV) *see* rotavirus vaccine *on page* 880
human thyroid stimulating hormone *see* thyrotropin alpha *on page* 958
Humate-P® [US/Can] *see* antihemophilic factor/von Willebrand factor complex (human) *on page* 83
Humatin® [Can] *see* paromomycin *on page* 752
Humatin® *(Discontinued)* *see* paromomycin *on page* 752
Humatrope® [US/Can] *see* somatropin *on page* 916
Humegon® [Can] *see* chorionic gonadotropin (human) *on page* 225
Humegon® *(Discontinued)* *see* menotropins *on page* 625
Humibid® CS *(Discontinued)* *see* guaifenesin and dextromethorphan *on page* 474

Humibid® DM ***(Discontinued)*** *see* guaifenesin and dextromethorphan *on page* *474*
Humibid® *e* ***(Discontinued)*** *see* guaifenesin *on page* *473*
Humibid® LA ***(Discontinued)*** *see* guaifenesin *on page* *473*
Humibid® LA ***(reformulation) (Discontinued)***
Humibid® Pediatric ***(Discontinued)*** *see* guaifenesin *on page* *473*
Humibid® Sprinkle ***(Discontinued)*** *see* guaifenesin *on page* *473*
Humira® [US/Can] *see* adalimumab *on page* *35*
Humist® [US-OTC] *see* sodium chloride *on page* *908*
Humist® for Kids [US-OTC] *see* sodium chloride *on page* *908*
Humulin® 20/80 [Can] *see* insulin NPH and insulin regular *on page* *532*
Humulin® 50/50 ***(Discontinued)*** *see* insulin NPH and insulin regular *on page* *532*
Humulin® L ***(Discontinued)***
Humulin® 70/30 [US/Can] *see* insulin NPH and insulin regular *on page* *532*
Humulin® N [US/Can] *see* insulin NPH *on page* *532*
Humulin® R [US/Can] *see* insulin regular *on page* *533*
Humulin® R U-500 [US] *see* insulin regular *on page* *533*
Humulin® U ***(Discontinued)***
Hurricaine® [US-OTC] *see* benzocaine *on page* *129*
HXM *see* altretamine *on page* *54*
Hyalgan® [US] *see* hyaluronate and derivatives *on page* *496*
hyaluronan *see* hyaluronate and derivatives *on page* *496*

hyaluronate and derivatives (hye al yoor ON ate & dah RIV ah tives)

Sound-Alike/Look-Alike Issues

Healon® may be confused with Hyalgan®
Hyalgan® may be confused with Healon®
Synvisc® may be confused with Synagis®

Synonyms hyaluronan; hyaluronic acid; hylan polymers; sodium hyaluronate

U.S./Canadian Brand Names Bionect® [US]; Cystistat® [Can]; Durolane® [Can]; Euflexxa™ [US]; Eyestil [Can]; Healon GV® [US/Can]; Healon® [US/Can]; Healon®5 [US]; Hyalgan® [US]; Hylaform® Plus [US]; Hylaform® [US]; Hylira™ [US]; IPM Wound Gel™ [US-OTC]; Juvederm™ 24HV [US]; Juvederm™ 30 [US]; Juvederm™ 30HV [US]; Orthovisc® [US/Can]; Perlane® [US]; Provisc® [US]; Restylane® [US]; Supartz™ [US]; Suplasyn® [Can]; Synvisc® [US]; Vitrax® [US]

Therapeutic Category Antirheumatic Miscellaneous; Ophthalmic Agent, Viscoelastic; Skin and Mucous Membrane Agent

Use

Intraarticular injection: Treatment of pain in osteoarthritis in knee in patients who have failed nonpharmacologic treatment and simple analgesics
Intradermal: Correction of moderate-to-severe facial wrinkles or folds
Ophthalmic: Surgical aid in cataract extraction, intraocular implantation, corneal transplant, glaucoma filtration, and retinal attachment surgery
Topical cream, gel, spray: Management of skin ulcers and wounds
Topical lotion: Treatment of xerosis (dry, scaly skin)

Usual Dosage Adults:

Osteoarthritis of the knee: Intraarticular:

Eulexxa™: Inject 20 mg (2 mL) once weekly for 3 weeks
Hyalgan®: Inject 20 mg (2 mL) once weekly for 5 weeks; some patients may benefit with a total of 3 injections
Orthovisc®: Inject 30 mg (2 mL) once weekly for 3-4 weeks
Supartz™: Inject 25 mg (2.5 mL) once weekly for 5 weeks
Synvisc®: Inject 16 mg (2 mL) once weekly for 3 weeks (total of 3 injections)

Facial wrinkles: Intradermal:

Note: Formulations differ in terms of recommended injection depth: Juvederm™, Hylaform®, and Restylane® are intended for mid to deep intradermal injection; Perlane® is intended for injection into the deep dermis to superficial subcutis

Hylaform®, Hylaform® Plus: Inject as required for cosmetic result; typical treatment regimen requires <2 mL; limit injection to ≤1.5 mL per injection site; maximum: 20 mL/60 kg/year

Juvederm™ (all formulations): Inject as required for cosmetic result; typical treatment regimen requires <2 mL; limit injection to 1.6 mL per injection site; maximum: 20 mL/60 kg/year

Perlane®: Inject as required into deep dermis/superficial subcutis for cosmetic result; typical treatment regimen requires 1.9-4.6 mL; maximum 6 mL per treatment

Restylane®: Inject as required for cosmetic result; typical treatment regimen requires <2 mL; limit injection to ≤1.5 mL per injection site

Ophthalmic (Healon®, Provisc®, Vitrax®): Depends upon procedure (slowly introduce a sufficient quantity into eye)

Topical: Note: Formulations are used for different indications:

Bionect® cream, gel, and spray: Apply a thin layer to clean and disinfected wound or ulcer 2-3 times/day, and cover with sterile gauze pad. If needed, cover with elastic or compressive bandage.

IPM Wound Gel™: Apply to clean dry ulcer or wound, and cover with nonstick dressing; repeat daily. Discontinue if wound size increase after 3-4 applications.

Hylira™ lotion: Apply to affected area and rub in thoroughly 2-3 times daily. Discontinue if condition worsens.

Dosage Forms

Hylan B:

Injection, gel:

Hylaform® [500 micron particle]: 5.5 mg/mL (0.75 mL)

Hylaform® Plus [700 micron particle]: 5.5 mg/mL (0.75 mL)

Hylan Polymers A and B (Hylan G-F 20):

Injection, solution, intraarticular:

Synvisc®: 8 mg/mL (2 mL)

Hyaluronate:

Cream, topical:

Bionect®: 0.2% (25 g)

Gel, topical:

Bionect®: 0.2% (30 g, 60 g)

IPM Wound Gel™ [OTC]: 2.5% (10 g)

Lotion, topical: 0.1% (340 g, 1000 g)

Hylira™ Lotion: 0.1% (340 g, 1000 g)

Injection, gel, intradermal:

Juvederm™ 24HV, Juvederm™ 30, Juvederm™ 30HV: 24 mg/mL [prefilled syringe]

Perlane®: 20 mg/mL (1mL) [prefilled syringe]

Restylane®: 20 mg/mL

Injection, solution, intraarticular:

Euflexxa™, Hyalgan®: 10 mg/mL (2 mL)

Orthovisc®: 15 mg/mL (2 mL)

Supartz™: 10 mg/mL (2.5 mL)

Synvisc®: 8 mg/mL (2 mL)

Injection, solution, intraocular:

Healon®: 10 mg/mL (0.4 mL, 0.55 mL, 0.85 mL, 2 mL)

Healon®5: 23 mg/mL

Healon GV®: 14 mg/mL (0.55 mL, 0.85 mL)

Provisc®: 10 mg/mL (0.4 mL, 0.55 mL, 0.8 mL)

Vitrax®: 30 mg/mL (0.65 mL)

hyaluronic acid *see* hyaluronate and derivatives *on page 496*

hyaluronidase (hye al yoor ON i dase)

Sound-Alike/Look-Alike Issues

Wydase® may be confused with Lidex®, Wyamine®

U.S./Canadian Brand Names Amphadase™ [US]; Hydase™ [US]; Hylenex™ [US]; Vitrase® [US]

Therapeutic Category Enzyme

Use Increase the dispersion and absorption of other injected drugs; increase rate of absorption of parenteral fluids given by subcutaneous administration (hypodermoclysis)

Usual Dosage Note: A preliminary skin test for hypersensitivity can be performed.

Skin test: Intradermal: 0.02 mL (3 units) of a 150 units/mL solution. Positive reaction consists of a wheal with pseudopods appearing within 5 minutes and persisting for 20-30 minutes with localized itching.

Hypodermoclysis: SubQ: Infants and Children: 150 units followed by subcutaneous isotonic fluid administration at a rate appropriate for age, weight, and clinical condition of the patient; 150 units ▶

facilitates absorption of >1000 mL of solution **or** add 15 units to each 100 mL of I.V. fluid to be administered subcutaneously

Premature Infants and Neonates: Volume of a single clysis should not exceed 25 mL/kg and the rate of administration should not exceed 2 mL/minute

Children <3 years (Amphadase™, Hydase™, Vitrase®): Volume of a single clysis should not exceed 200 mL

Children ≥3 years and Adults: Rate and volume of a single clysis should not exceed those used for infusion of I.V. fluids

Dosage Forms

Injection, powder for reconstitution:
Vitrase®: 6200 units

Injection, solution:
Amphadase™: 150 units/mL (1 mL)

Injection, solution [preservative free]:
Hydase™: 150 units/mL (1 mL)
Hylenex™: 150 units/mL (1 mL, 2 mL)
Vitrase®: 200 units/mL (2 mL)

hycamptamine *see* topotecan *on page* *970*
Hycamtin® [US/Can] *see* topotecan *on page* *970*
hycet™ [US] *see* hydrocodone and acetaminophen *on page* *501*
HycoClear Tuss® *(Discontinued)*
Hycodan® *(Discontinued)* *see* hydrocodone and homatropine *on page* *502*
Hycomine® Compound *(Discontinued)*
Hycomine® *(Discontinued)*
Hycomine® Pediatric *(Discontinued)*
Hycort™ [Can] *see* hydrocortisone (topical) *on page* *505*
Hycotuss® *(Discontinued)*
Hydase™ [US] *see* hyaluronidase *on page* *497*
Hydeltra T.B.A.® [Can] *see* prednisolone (systemic) *on page* *813*
Hydergine® [Can] *see* ergoloid mesylates *on page* *366*
Hydergine® *(Discontinued)* *see* ergoloid mesylates *on page* *366*
Hyderm [Can] *see* hydrocortisone (topical) *on page* *505*

hydralazine (hye DRAL a zeen)

Sound-Alike/Look-Alike Issues
hydrALAZINE may be confused with hydrOXYzine

Synonyms hydralazine hydrochloride

Tall-Man hydr**ALAZINE**

U.S./Canadian Brand Names Apo-Hydralazine® [Can]; Apresoline® [Can]; Novo-Hylazin [Can]; Nu-Hydral [Can]

Therapeutic Category Vasodilator

Use Management of moderate-to-severe hypertension

Usual Dosage

Children:

Oral: Initial: 0.75-1 mg/kg/day in 2-4 divided doses; increase over 3-4 weeks to maximum of 7.5 mg/kg/day in 2-4 divided doses; maximum daily dose: 200 mg/day

I.M., I.V.: 0.1-0.2 mg/kg/dose (not to exceed 20 mg) every 4-6 hours as needed, up to 1.7-3.5 mg/kg/day in 4-6 divided doses

Adults:

Oral:

Hypertension:

Initial dose: 10 mg 4 times/day for first 2-4 days; increase to 25 mg 4 times/day for the balance of the first week

Increase by 10-25 mg/dose gradually to 50 mg 4 times/day (maximum: 300 mg/day); usual dose range (JNC 7): 25-100 mg/day in 2 divided doses

Congestive heart failure:

Initial dose: 10-25 mg 3-4 times/day

Adjustment: Dosage must be adjusted based on individual response

Target dose: 225-300 mg/day in divided doses; use in combination with isosorbide dinitrate

I.M., I.V.:

Hypertension: Initial: 10-20 mg/dose every 4-6 hours as needed, may increase to 40 mg/dose; change to oral therapy as soon as possible.

Preeclampsia/eclampsia: 5 mg/dose then 5-10 mg every 20-30 minutes as needed.

Dosage Forms

Injection, solution: 20 mg/mL (1 mL)

Tablet: 10 mg, 25 mg, 50 mg, 100 mg

hydralazine and hydrochlorothiazide (hye DRAL a zeen & hye droe klor oh THYE a zide)

Synonyms hydrochlorothiazide and hydralazine

Therapeutic Category Antihypertensive Agent, Combination

Use Management of moderate-to-severe hypertension and treatment of congestive heart failure

Usual Dosage Oral: Adults: Hydralazine 25-100 mg/day and hydrochlorothiazide 25-50 mg/day in 2 divided doses (maximum: hydrochlorothiazide: 50 mg/day)

Dosage Forms

Capsule: 25/25: Hydralazine 25 mg and hydrochlorothiazide 25 mg; 50/50: Hydralazine 50 mg and hydrochlorothiazide 50 mg; 100/50: Hydralazine 100 mg and hydrochlorothiazide 50 mg

hydralazine and isosorbide dinitrate *see* isosorbide dinitrate and hydralazine *on page 550*

hydralazine hydrochloride *see* hydralazine *on page 498*

Hydramine [US-OTC] *see* diphenhydramine *on page 315*

hydrated chloral *see* chloral hydrate *on page 208*

Hydrate® *(Discontinued)* *see* dimenhydrinate *on page 312*

Hydrea® [US/Can] *see* hydroxyurea *on page 510*

Hydrisalic™ [US-OTC] *see* salicylic acid *on page 884*

Hydro 40™ [US] *see* urea *on page 998*

Hydrocet® *(Discontinued)* *see* hydrocodone and acetaminophen *on page 501*

hydrochlorothiazide (hye droe klor oh THYE a zide)

Sound-Alike/Look-Alike Issues

hydrochlorothiazide may be confused with hydrocortisone, hydroflumethiazide

Esidrix may be confused with Lasix®

HCTZ is an error-prone abbreviation (mistaken as hydrocortisone)

Microzide™ may be confused with Maxzide®, Micronase®

U.S./Canadian Brand Names Apo-Hydro® [Can]; Microzide® [US]; Novo-Hydrazide [Can]; PMS-Hydrochlorothiazide [Can]

Therapeutic Category Diuretic, Thiazide

Use Management of mild-to-moderate hypertension; treatment of edema in heart failure and nephrotic syndrome

Usual Dosage Oral (effect of drug may be decreased when used every day):

Children (in pediatric patients, chlorothiazide may be preferred over hydrochlorothiazide as there are more dosage formulations [eg, suspension] available): Edema, hypertension:

<6 months: 1-3 mg/kg/day in 2 divided doses

>6 months to 2 years: 1-3 mg/kg/day in 2 divided doses; maximum: 37.5 mg/day

>2-17 years: Initial: 1 mg/kg/day; maximum: 3 mg/kg/day (50 mg/day)

Adults:

Edema: 25-100 mg/day in 1-2 doses; maximum: 200 mg/day

Hypertension: 12.5-50 mg/day; minimal increase in response and more electrolyte disturbances are seen with doses >50 mg/day

Dosage Forms

Capsule: 12.5 mg

Microzide®: 12.5 mg

Tablet: 25 mg, 50 mg

hydrochlorothiazide, amlodipine, and valsartan *see* amlodipine, valsartan, and hydrochlorothiazide *on page 69*

hydrochlorothiazide and aliskiren *see* aliskiren and hydrochlorothiazide *on page 47*

hydrochlorothiazide and amiloride *see* amiloride and hydrochlorothiazide *on page 61*

hydrochlorothiazide and benazepril *see* benazepril and hydrochlorothiazide *on page 127*

hydrochlorothiazide and bisoprolol *see* bisoprolol and hydrochlorothiazide *on page 144*
hydrochlorothiazide and captopril *see* captopril and hydrochlorothiazide *on page 179*
hydrochlorothiazide and cilazapril *see* cilazapril and hydrochlorothiazide *(Canada only) on page 228*
hydrochlorothiazide and enalapril *see* enalapril and hydrochlorothiazide *on page 353*
hydrochlorothiazide and eprosartan *see* eprosartan and hydrochlorothiazide *on page 364*
hydrochlorothiazide and fosinopril *see* fosinopril and hydrochlorothiazide *on page 446*
hydrochlorothiazide and hydralazine *see* hydralazine and hydrochlorothiazide *on page 499*
hydrochlorothiazide and irbesartan *see* irbesartan and hydrochlorothiazide *on page 545*
hydrochlorothiazide and lisinopril *see* lisinopril and hydrochlorothiazide *on page 594*
hydrochlorothiazide and losartan *see* losartan and hydrochlorothiazide *on page 601*
hydrochlorothiazide and methyldopa *see* methyldopa and hydrochlorothiazide *on page 643*
hydrochlorothiazide and metoprolol *see* metoprolol and hydrochlorothiazide *on page 651*
hydrochlorothiazide and metoprolol tartrate *see* metoprolol and hydrochlorothiazide *on page 651*
hydrochlorothiazide and moexipril *see* moexipril and hydrochlorothiazide *on page 664*
hydrochlorothiazide and olmesartan medoxomil *see* olmesartan and hydrochlorothiazide *on page 721*
hydrochlorothiazide and propranolol *see* propranolol and hydrochlorothiazide *on page 829*
hydrochlorothiazide and quinapril *see* quinapril and hydrochlorothiazide *on page 845*
hydrochlorothiazide and ramipril *see* ramipril and hydrochlorothiazide *(Canada only) on page 851*

hydrochlorothiazide and spironolactone

(hye droe klor oh THYE a zide & speer on oh LAK tone)

Sound-Alike/Look-Alike Issues
Aldactazide® may be confused with Aldactone®

Synonyms spironolactone and hydrochlorothiazide

U.S./Canadian Brand Names Aldactazide 25® [Can]; Aldactazide 50® [Can]; Aldactazide® [US]; Novo-Spirozine [Can]

Therapeutic Category Antihypertensive Agent, Combination

Use Management of mild-to-moderate hypertension; treatment of edema in congestive heart failure and nephrotic syndrome, and cirrhosis of the liver accompanied by edema and/or ascites

Usual Dosage Oral:
Children: 1.5-3 mg/kg/day in 2-4 divided doses (maximum: 200 mg/day)
Adults: Hydrochlorothiazide 12.5-50 mg/day and spironolactone 12.5-50 mg/day; manufacturer labeling states hydrochlorothiazide maximum 200 mg/day; however, usual dose in JNC-7 is 12.5-50 mg/day

Dosage Forms
Tablet: Hydrochlorothiazide 25 mg and spironolactone 25 mg
Aldactazide®: 25/25: Hydrochlorothiazide 25 mg and spironolactone 25 mg; 50/50: Hydrochlorothiazide 50 mg and spironolactone 50 mg

hydrochlorothiazide and telmisartan *see* telmisartan and hydrochlorothiazide *on page 942*

hydrochlorothiazide and triamterene

(hye droe klor oh THYE a zide & trye AM ter een)

Sound-Alike/Look-Alike Issues
Dyazide® may be confused with diazoxide, Dynacin®
Maxzide® may be confused with Maxidex®, Microzide®

Synonyms triamterene and hydrochlorothiazide

U.S./Canadian Brand Names Apo-Triazide® [Can]; Dyazide® [US]; Maxzide® [US]; Maxzide®-25 [US]; Novo-Triamzide [Can]; Nu-Triazide [Can]; Penta-Triamterene HCTZ [Can]; Riva-Zide [Can]

Therapeutic Category Antihypertensive Agent, Combination

Use Treatment of hypertension or edema (not recommended for initial treatment) when hypokalemia has developed on hydrochlorothiazide alone or when the development of hypokalemia must be avoided

Usual Dosage Oral: Adults:
Hydrochlorothiazide 25 mg and triamterene 37.5 mg: 1-2 tablets/capsules once daily
Hydrochlorothiazide 50 mg and triamterene 75 mg: 1/2-1 tablet daily

Dosage Forms
Capsule: Hydrochlorothiazide 25 mg and triamterene 37.5 mg; hydrochlorothiazide 25 mg and triamterene 50 mg

Dyazide®: Hydrochlorothiazide 25 mg and triamterene 37.5 mg

Tablet: Hydrochlorothiazide 25 mg and triamterene 37.5 mg; hydrochlorothiazide 50 mg and triamterene 75 mg

Maxzide®: Hydrochlorothiazide 50 mg and triamterene 75 mg [scored]

Maxzide®-25: Hydrochlorothiazide 25 mg and triamterene 37.5 mg [scored]

hydrochlorothiazide and valsartan *see* valsartan and hydrochlorothiazide *on page 1004*

Hydrocil® Instant [US-OTC] *see* psyllium *on page 837*

hydrocodone and acetaminophen (hye droe KOE done & a seet a MIN oh fen)

Sound-Alike/Look-Alike Issues

Lorcet® may be confused with Fioricet®

Lortab® may be confused with Cortef®, Lorabid®, Luride®

Vicodin® may be confused with Hycodan®, Hycomine®, Indocin®, Uridon®

Zydone® may be confused with Vytone®

Synonyms acetaminophen and hydrocodone

U.S./Canadian Brand Names hycet™ [US]; Lorcet® 10/650 [US]; Lorcet® Plus [US]; Lortab® [US]; Margesic® H [US]; Maxidone® [US]; Norco® [US]; Stagesic™ [US]; Vicodin® ES [US]; Vicodin® HP [US]; Vicodin® [US]; Xodol® 10/300 [US]; Xodol® 5/300 [US]; Xodol® 7.5/300 [US]; Zamicet™ [US]; Zydone® [US]

Therapeutic Category Analgesic, Narcotic

Controlled Substance C-III

Use Relief of moderate-to-severe pain

Usual Dosage Oral (doses should be titrated to appropriate analgesic effect): Analgesic:

Children 2-13 years or <50 kg: Hydrocodone 0.1-0.2 mg/kg/dose every 4-6 hours; do not exceed 6 doses/day or the maximum recommended dose of acetaminophen

Children and Adults ≥50 kg: Average starting dose in opioid naive patients: Hydrocodone 5-10 mg 4 times/day; the dosage of acetaminophen should be limited to ≤4 g/day (and possibly less in patients with hepatic impairment or ethanol use).

Dosage ranges (based on specific product labeling): Hydrocodone 2.5-10 mg every 4-6 hours; maximum: 60 mg hydrocodone/day (maximum dose of hydrocodone may be limited by the acetaminophen content of specific product)

Dosage Forms

Capsule: Hydrocodone 5 mg and acetaminophen 500 mg

Margesic® H, Stagesic™: Hydrocodone 5 mg and acetaminophen 500 mg

Elixir: Hydrocodone 7.5 mg and acetaminophen 500 mg per 15 mL

Lortab®: Hydrocodone 7.5 mg and acetaminophen 500 mg per 15 mL

Solution, oral: Hydrocodone 7.5 mg and acetaminophen 500 mg per 15 mL

hycet™: Hydrocodone 7.5 mg and acetaminophen 325 mg per 15 mL

Zamicet™: Hydrocodone 10 mg and acetaminophen 325 mg per 15 mL

Tablet:

Generics:

Hydrocodone 2.5 mg and acetaminophen 500 mg
Hydrocodone 5 mg and acetaminophen 325 mg
Hydrocodone 5 mg and acetaminophen 500 mg
Hydrocodone 7.5 mg and acetaminophen 325 mg
Hydrocodone 7.5 mg and acetaminophen 500 mg
Hydrocodone 7.5 mg and acetaminophen 650 mg
Hydrocodone 7.5 mg and acetaminophen 750 mg
Hydrocodone 10 mg and acetaminophen 325 mg
Hydrocodone 10 mg and acetaminophen 500 mg
Hydrocodone 10 mg and acetaminophen 650 mg
Hydrocodone 10 mg and acetaminophen 660 mg
Hydrocodone 10 mg and acetaminophen 750 mg

Brands:

Lorcet® 10/650: Hydrocodone 10 mg and acetaminophen 650 mg

Lorcet® Plus: Hydrocodone 7.5 mg and acetaminophen 650 mg

Lortab®: /500: Hydrocodone 5 mg and acetaminophen 500 mg; 7.5/500: Hydrocodone 7.5 mg and acetaminophen 500 mg; 10/500: Hydrocodone 10 mg and acetaminophen 500 mg

Maxidone®: Hydrocodone 10 mg and acetaminophen 750 mg

Norco®: Hydrocodone 5 mg and acetaminophen 325 mg; hydrocodone 7.5 mg and acetaminophen 325 mg; hydrocodone 10 mg and acetaminophen 325 mg
Vicodin®: Hydrocodone 5 mg and acetaminophen 500 mg
Vicodin® ES: Hydrocodone 7.5 mg and acetaminophen 750 mg
Vicodin® HP: Hydrocodone 10 mg and acetaminophen 660 mg
Xodol®: 5/300: Hydrocodone 5 mg and acetaminophen 300 mg; 7.5/300: Hydrocodone 7.5 mg and acetaminophen 300 mg; 10/300: Hydrocodone 10 mg and acetaminophen 300 mg
Zydone®: Hydrocodone 5 mg and acetaminophen 400 mg; hydrocodone 7.5 mg and acetaminophen 400 mg; hydrocodone 10 mg and acetaminophen 400 mg

hydrocodone and aspirin *(Discontinued)*

hydrocodone and chlorpheniramine (hye droe KOE done & klor fen IR a meen)

Sound-Alike/Look-Alike Issues

Tussionex® represents a different product in the U.S. than it does in Canada. In the U.S., Tussionex® contains hydrocodone and chlorpheniramine, while in Canada the product bearing this name contains hydrocodone and phenyltoloxamine.

Synonyms chlorpheniramine maleate and hydrocodone bitartrate; hydrocodone polistirex and chlorpheniramine polistirex

U.S./Canadian Brand Names TussiCaps® [US]; Tussionex® [US]

Therapeutic Category Antihistamine/Antitussive

Controlled Substance C-III

Use Symptomatic relief of cough and upper respiratory symptoms associated with cold and allergy

Usual Dosage Oral:

Children 6-12 years
TussiCaps®: 5 mg/4 mg: One capsule every 12 hours (maximum: 2 capsules/24 hours)
Tussionex®: 2.5 mL every 12 hours; do not exceed 5 mL/24 hours
Children >12 years and Adults:
TussiCaps® 10 mg/8 mg: One capsule every 12 hours (maximum: 2 capsules/24 hours)
Tussionex®: 5 mL every 12 hours; do not exceed 10 mL/24 hours

Dosage Forms

Capsule, extended release:
TussiCaps® 5/4: Hydrocodone bitartrate 5 mg and chlorpheniramine maleate 4 mg
TussiCaps® 10/8: Hydrocodone bitartrate 10 mg and chlorpheniramine maleate 8 mg
Suspension, extended release:
Tussionex®: Hydrocodone bitartrate 10 mg and chlorpheniramine maleate 8 mg per 5 mL

hydrocodone and guaifenesin *(Discontinued)*

hydrocodone and homatropine (hye droe KOE done & hoe MA troe peen)

Sound-Alike/Look-Alike Issues

Hycodan® may be confused with Hycomine®, Vicodin®

Synonyms homatropine and hydrocodone; hydrocodone bitartrate and homatropine methylbromide

U.S./Canadian Brand Names Hydromet® [US]; Tussigon® [US]

Therapeutic Category Antitussive

Controlled Substance C-III

Use Symptomatic relief of cough

Usual Dosage Oral:

Children 6-11 years: 1/2 tablet or 2.5 mL every 4-6 hours as needed (maximum: 3 tablets or 15 mL/24 hours)
Children ≥12 years and Adults: 1 tablet or 5 mL every 4-6 hours as needed (maximum: 6 tablets/24 hours or 30 mL/24 hours)

Dosage Forms

Syrup: Hydrocodone 5 mg and homatropine 1.5 mg per 5 mL
Hydromet®: Hydrocodone 5 mg and homatropine 1.5 mg per 5 mL
Tablet:
Tussigon®: Hydrocodone 5 mg and homatropine 1.5 mg

hydrocodone and ibuprofen (hye droe KOE done & eye byoo PROE fen)

Sound-Alike/Look-Alike Issues

Reprexain® may be confused with Zyprexa®

Synonyms hydrocodone bitartrate and ibuprofen; ibuprofen and hydrocodone

U.S./Canadian Brand Names Ibudone™ [US]; Reprexain® [US]; Vicoprofen® [US/Can]

Therapeutic Category Analgesic, Narcotic

Controlled Substance C-III

Use Short-term (generally <10 days) management of moderate-to-severe acute pain; is not indicated for treatment of such conditions as osteoarthritis or rheumatoid arthritis

Usual Dosage Oral:

Adults: 1 tablet every 4-6 hours as needed for pain; maximum: 5 tablets/day. **Note:** Short-term use is recommended (<10 days).

Dosage Forms

Tablet: Hydrocodone 5 mg and ibuprofen 200 mg; hydrocodone 7.5 mg and ibuprofen 200 mg

Ibudone™: 5/200: Hydrocodone bitartrate 5 mg and ibuprofen 200 mg; 10/200: Hydrocodone bitartrate 10 mg and ibuprofen 200 mg

Reprexain®: Hydrocodone 5 mg and ibuprofen 200 mg; hydrocodone 7.5 mg and ibuprofen 200 mg

Vicoprofen®: Hydrocodone 7.5 mg and ibuprofen 200 mg

hydrocodone and pseudoephedrine ***(Discontinued)***

hydrocodone bitartrate and homatropine methylbromide *see* hydrocodone and homatropine *on page 502*

hydrocodone bitartrate and ibuprofen *see* hydrocodone and ibuprofen *on page 503*

hydrocodone, carbinoxamine, and pseudoephedrine ***(Discontinued)***

hydrocodone, chlorpheniramine, phenylephrine, acetaminophen, and caffeine ***(Discontinued)***

Hydrocodone PA® Syrup ***(Discontinued)***

hydrocodone, phenylephrine, and chlorpheniramine *see* phenylephrine, hydrocodone, and chlorpheniramine *on page 778*

hydrocodone, phenylephrine, and diphenhydramine ***(Discontinued)***

hydrocodone, phenylephrine, and guaifenesin ***(Discontinued)***

hydrocodone polistirex and chlorpheniramine polistirex *see* hydrocodone and chlorpheniramine *on page 502*

hydrocodone, pseudoephedrine, and guaifenesin ***(Discontinued)***

hydrocortisone acetate *see* hydrocortisone (rectal) *on page 503*

hydrocortisone, acetic acid, and propylene glycol diacetate *see* acetic acid, propylene glycol diacetate, and hydrocortisone *on page 30*

hydrocortisone and benzoyl peroxide *see* benzoyl peroxide and hydrocortisone *on page 134*

hydrocortisone and ciprofloxacin *see* ciprofloxacin and hydrocortisone *on page 232*

hydrocortisone and iodoquinol *see* iodoquinol and hydrocortisone *on page 539*

hydrocortisone and lidocaine *see* lidocaine and hydrocortisone *on page 587*

hydrocortisone and pramoxine *see* pramoxine and hydrocortisone *on page 810*

hydrocortisone and urea *see* urea and hydrocortisone *on page 999*

hydrocortisone, bacitracin, neomycin, and polymyxin B *see* bacitracin, neomycin, polymyxin B, and hydrocortisone *on page 120*

hydrocortisone butyrate *see* hydrocortisone (topical) *on page 505*

hydrocortisone, neomycin, and polymyxin B *see* neomycin, polymyxin B, and hydrocortisone *on page 688*

hydrocortisone, neomycin, colistin, and thonzonium *see* neomycin, colistin, hydrocortisone, and thonzonium *on page 687*

hydrocortisone probutate *see* hydrocortisone (topical) *on page 505*

hydrocortisone (rectal) (hye droe KOR ti sone REK tal)

Sound-Alike/Look-Alike Issues

hydrocortisone may be confused with hydrocodone, hydroxychloroquine, hydrochlorothiazide

Anusol-HC® may be confused with Anusol®

Anusol® may be confused with Anusol-HC®, Aplisol®, Aquasol®

Proctocort® may be confused with ProctoCream®
ProctoCream® may be confused with Proctocort®
HCT (occasional abbreviation for hydrocortisone) is an error-prone abbreviation (mistaken as hydrochlorothiazide)

Synonyms hydrocortisone acetate

U.S./Canadian Brand Names Anucort-HC® [US]; Anusol-HC® [US]; Anusol® HC-1 [US-OTC]; Colocort® [US]; Cortenema® [Can]; Cortifoam® [US/Can]; Encort™ [US]; Hemril®-30 [US]; Nupercainal® Hydrocortisone Cream [US-OTC]; Preparation H® Hydrocortisone [US-OTC]; Procto-Kit™ [US]; Procto-Pak™ [US]; Proctocort® [US]; ProctoCream® HC [US]; Proctosert [US]; Proctosol-HC® [US]; Proctozone-HC™ [US]; Tucks® Anti-Itch [US-OTC]

Therapeutic Category Adrenal Corticosteroid

Use Adjunctive treatment of ulcerative colitis; rectal itching; hemorrhoids

Usual Dosage Rectal: Adults: Ulcerative colitis: 10-100 mg 1-2 times/day for 2-3 weeks

Dosage Forms

Aerosol, rectal:
Cortifoam®: 10% (15 g)

Cream, rectal: 1% (30 g)
Cortizone®-10 [OTC]: 1% (30 g)
Nupercainal® Hydrocortisone Cream [OTC]: 1% (27 g, 30 g)
Preparation H® Hydrocortisone [OTC]: 1% (27 g)

Suppository, rectal: 25 mg (12s, 24s, 100s)
Anucort-HC®, Tucks® Anti-Itch [OTC]: 25 mg (12s, 24s, 100s)
Anusol-HC®, Proctosol-HC®: 25 mg (12s, 24s)
Encort™, Proctocort®: 30 mg (12s)
Hemril®-30, Proctosert: 30 mg (12s, 24s)

Suspension, rectal: 100 mg/60 mL (7s)
Colocort®: 100 mg/60 mL (1s, 7s)

hydrocortisone sodium succinate *see* hydrocortisone (systemic) *on page 504*

hydrocortisone (systemic) (hye droe KOR ti sone sis TEM ik)

Sound-Alike/Look-Alike Issues
hydrocortisone may be confused with hydrocodone, hydroxychloroquine, hydrochlorothiazide
Cortef® may be confused with Lortab®
HCT (occasional abbreviation for hydrocortisone) is an error-prone abbreviation (mistaken as hydrochlorothiazide)

Synonyms compound F; cortisol; hydrocortisone sodium succinate

U.S./Canadian Brand Names Cortef® [US/Can]; Solu-Cortef® [US/Can]

Therapeutic Category Adrenal Corticosteroid

Use Management of adrenocortical insufficiency

Usual Dosage Dose should be based on severity of disease and patient response

Acute adrenal insufficiency: I.M., I.V.:
Infants and young Children: Succinate: 1-2 mg/kg/dose bolus, then 25-150 mg/day in divided doses every 6-8 hours
Older Children: Succinate: 1-2 mg/kg bolus then 150-250 mg/day in divided doses every 6-8 hours
Adults: Succinate: 100 mg I.V. bolus, then 300 mg/day in divided doses every 8 hours or as a continuous infusion for 48 hours; once patient is stable change to oral, 50 mg every 8 hours for 6 doses, then taper to 30-50 mg/day in divided doses

Chronic adrenal corticoid insufficiency: Adults: Oral: 20-30 mg/day

Antiinflammatory or immunosuppressive:
Infants and Children:
Oral: 2.5-10 mg/kg/day **or** 75-300 mg/m^2/day every 6-8 hours
I.M., I.V.: Succinate: 1-5 mg/kg/day **or** 30-150 mg/m^2/day divided every 12-24 hours
Adolescents and Adults: Oral, I.M., I.V.: Succinate: 15-240 mg every 12 hours

Congenital adrenal hyperplasia: Oral: Initial: 10-20 mg/m^2/day in 3 divided doses; a variety of dosing schedules have been used. **Note:** Inconsistencies have occurred with liquid formulations; tablets may provide more reliable levels. Doses must be individualized by monitoring growth, bone age, and hormonal levels. Mineralocorticoid and sodium supplementation may be required based upon electrolyte regulation and plasma renin activity.

Physiologic replacement: Children:
Oral: 0.5-0.75 mg/kg/day **or** 20-25 mg/m^2/day every 8 hours
I.M.: Succinate: 0.25-0.35 mg/kg/day **or** 12-15 mg/m^2/day once daily
Shock: I.M., I.V.: Succinate:
Children: Initial: 50 mg/kg, then repeated in 4 hours and/or every 24 hours as needed
Adolescents and Adults: 500 mg to 2 g every 2-6 hours
Status asthmaticus: Children and Adults: I.V.: Succinate: 1-2 mg/kg/dose every 6 hours for 24 hours, then maintenance of 0.5-1 mg/kg every 6 hours
Adults:
Rheumatic diseases:
Intralesional, intraarticular, soft tissue injection: Acetate:
Large joints: 25 mg (up to 37.5 mg)
Small joints: 10-25 mg
Tendon sheaths: 5-12.5 mg
Soft tissue infiltration: 25-50 mg (up to 75 mg)
Bursae: 25-37.5 mg
Ganglia: 12.5-25 mg
Stress dosing (surgery) in patients known to be adrenally-suppressed or on chronic systemic steroids: I.V.:
Minor stress (ie, inguinal herniorrhaphy): 25 mg/day for 1 day
Moderate stress (ie, joint replacement, cholecystectomy): 50-75 mg/day (25 mg every 8-12 hours) for 1-2 days
Major stress (pancreatoduodenectomy, esophagogastrectomy, cardiac surgery): 100-150 mg/day (50 mg every 8-12 hours) for 2-3 days

Dosage Forms

Injection, powder for reconstitution:
Solu-Cortef®: 100 mg, 250 mg, 500 mg, 1 g
Tablet: 20 mg
Cortef®: 5 mg, 10 mg, 20 mg

hydrocortisone (topical) (hye droe KOR ti sone TOP i kal)

Sound-Alike/Look-Alike Issues

hydrocortisone may be confused with hydrocodone, hydroxychloroquine, hydrochlorothiazide
Cortizone® may be confused with cortisone
HCT (occasional abbreviation for hydrocortisone) is an error-prone abbreviation (mistaken as hydrochlorothiazide)
Hytone® may be confused with Vytone®

Synonyms hydrocortisone butyrate; hydrocortisone probutate; hydrocortisone valerate

U.S./Canadian Brand Names Aquacort® [Can]; Aquanil™ HC [US-OTC]; Beta-HC® [US]; Caldecort® [US-OTC]; Cetacort® [US]; Cortaid® Intensive Therapy [US-OTC]; Cortaid® Maximum Strength [US-OTC]; Cortaid® Sensitive Skin [US-OTC]; Cortamed® [Can]; Corticool® [US-OTC]; Cortizone®-10 Maximum Strength [US-OTC]; Cortizone®-10 Plus Maximum Strength [US-OTC]; Cortizone®-10 Quick Shot [US-OTC]; Dermarest Dricort® [US-OTC]; Dermtex® HC [US-OTC]; EarSol® HC [US]; Emo-Cort® [Can]; Hycort™ [Can]; Hyderm [Can]; HydroVal® [Can]; HydroZone Plus [US-OTC]; Hytone® [US]; IvySoothe® [US-OTC]; Locoid Lipocream® [US]; Locoid® [US/Can]; Nutracort® [US]; Pandel® [US]; Post Peel Healing Balm [US-OTC]; Prevex® HC [Can]; Sarna® HC [Can]; Sarnol®-HC [US-OTC]; Texacort® [US]; Westcort® [US/Can]

Therapeutic Category Corticosteroid, Topical

Use Relief of inflammation of corticosteroid-responsive dermatoses (low and medium potency topical corticosteroid)

Usual Dosage Topical: Children >2 years and Adults: Dermatosis: Apply to affected area 2-4 times/day (Buteprate: Apply once or twice daily). Therapy should be discontinued when control is achieved; if no improvement is seen, reassessment of diagnosis may be necessary.

Dosage Forms

Cream, topical: 0.2% (15 g, 45 g, 60 g); 0.5% (9 g, 30 g, 60 g); 1% (1.5 g, 30 g, 114 g, 454 g); 2.5% (20 g, 30 g, 454 g)
Caldecort® [OTC], HydroZone Plus [OTC], IvySoothe® [OTC], Proctocort®, Procto-Pak™, Procto-Kit™: 1% (30 g)
Cortaid® Intensive Therapy [OTC]: 1% (60 g)
Cortaid® Maximum Strength [OTC]: 1% (15 g, 30 g, 40 g, 60 g)
Cortaid® Sensitive Skin [OTC]: 0.5% (15 g)

Cortizone®-10 Maximum Strength [OTC]: 1% (15 g, 30 g, 60 g)
Cortizone®-10 Plus Maximum Strength [OTC]: 1% (30 g, 60 g)
Dermarest® Dricort® [OTC]: 1% (15 g, 30 g)
Hytone®: 2.5% (30 g, 60 g)
Locoid®, Locoid Lipocream®: 0.1% (15 g, 45 g)
Pandel®: 0.1% (15 g, 45 g, 80 g)
Post Peel Healing Balm [OTC]: 1% (23 g)
Westcort®: 0.2% (15 g, 45 g, 60 g)

Gel, topical:
Corticool®: 1% (45 g)

Lotion, topical: 1% (120 mL); 2.5% (60 mL)
Aquanil™ HC [OTC], HydroZone Plus: 1% (120 mL)
Beta-HC®, Sarnol®-HC [OTC]: 1% (60 mL)
Hytone®: 2.5% (60 mL)
Nutracort®: 1% (60 mL, 120 mL); 2.5% (60 mL, 120 mL)

Ointment, topical: 0.2% (15 g, 45 g, 60 g); 0.5% (30 g); 1% (30 g, 454 g); 2.5% (20 g, 30 g, 454 g)
Cortaid® Maximum Strength [OTC]: 1% (15 g, 30 g)
Cortizone®-10 Maximum Strength [OTC]: 1% (30 g, 60 g)
Locoid®: 0.1% (15 g, 45 g)
Westcort®: 0.2% (15 g, 45 g, 60 g)

Solution, otic:
EarSol® HC: 1% (30 mL)

Solution, topical: 0.1% (20 mL, 60 mL); 2.5% (30 mL)
Texacort®: 2.5% (30 mL)
Locoid®: 0.1% (20 mL, 60 mL)

Solution, topical spray:
Cortaid® Intensive Therapy [OTC]: 1% (60 mL)
Cortizone®-10 Quick Shot [OTC]: 1% (44 mL)
Dermtex® HC [OTC]: 1% (52 mL)

hydrocortisone valerate *see* hydrocortisone (topical) *on page 505*

HydroDIURIL® ***(Discontinued)*** *see* hydrochlorothiazide *on page 499*

Hydro DP ***(Discontinued)***

HydroFed ***(Discontinued)***

Hydrogesic® ***(Discontinued)*** *see* hydrocodone and acetaminophen *on page 501*

Hydro-GP ***(Discontinued)***

Hydromet® [US] *see* hydrocodone and homatropine *on page 502*

Hydromorph Contin® [Can] *see* hydromorphone *on page 506*

Hydromorph-IR® [Can] *see* hydromorphone *on page 506*

hydromorphone (hye droe MOR fone)

Sound-Alike/Look-Alike Issues

Dilaudid® may be confused with Demerol®, Dilantin®

HYDROmorphone may be confused with morphine; significant overdoses have occurred when hydromorphone products have been inadvertently administered instead of morphine sulfate. Commercially available prefilled syringes of both products looks similar and are often stored in close proximity to each other. **Note:** Hydromorphone 1 mg oral is approximately equal to morphine 4 mg oral; hydromorphone 1 mg I.V. is approximately equal to morphine 5 mg I.V.

Dilaudid®, Dilaudid-HP®: Extreme caution should be taken to avoid confusing the highly-concentrated (Dilaudid-HP®) injection with the less-concentrated (Dilaudid®) injectable product.

Synonyms dihydromorphinone; hydromorphone hydrochloride

Tall-Man HYDROmorphone

U.S./Canadian Brand Names Dilaudid-HP-Plus® [Can]; Dilaudid-HP® [US/Can]; Dilaudid-XP® [Can]; Dilaudid® Sterile Powder [Can]; Dilaudid® [US/Can]; Hydromorph Contin® [Can]; Hydromorph-IR® [Can]; Hydromorphone HP [Can]; Hydromorphone HP® 10 [Can]; Hydromorphone HP® 20 [Can]; Hydromorphone HP® 50 [Can]; Hydromorphone HP® Forte [Can]; Hydromorphone Hydrochloride Injection, USP [Can]; PMS-Hydromorphone [Can]

Therapeutic Category Analgesic, Narcotic

Controlled Substance C-II

Use Management of moderate-to-severe pain

Usual Dosage

Acute pain (moderate-to-severe): **Note:** These are guidelines and do not represent the maximum doses that may be required in all patients. Doses should be titrated to pain relief/prevention.

Children ≥6 months and <50 kg:

Oral: 0.03-0.08 mg/kg/dose every 3-4 hours as needed

I.V.: 0.015 mg/kg/dose every 3-6 hours as needed

Children >50 kg and Adults:

Oral: Initial: Opiate-naive: 2-4 mg every 3-6 hours as needed; elderly/debilitated patients may require lower doses; patients with prior opiate exposure may require higher initial doses; usual dosage range: 2-8 mg every 3-4 hours as needed

I.V.: Initial: Opiate-naive: 0.2-0.6 mg every 2-3 hours as needed; patients with prior opiate exposure may tolerate higher initial doses

Patient-controlled analgesia (PCA): (Opiate-naive: Consider lower end of dosing range)

Usual concentration: 0.2 mg/mL

Demand dose: Usual: 0.1-0.2 mg; range: 0.05-0.5 mg

Lockout interval: 5-15 minutes

4-hour limit: 4-6 mg

Epidural:

Bolus dose: 1-1.5 mg

Infusion concentration: 0.05-0.075 mg/mL

Infusion rate: 0.04-0.4 mg/hour

Demand dose: 0.15 mg

Lockout interval: 30 minutes

I.M., SubQ: **Note:** I.M. use may result in variable absorption and a lag time to peak effect.

Initial: Opiate-naive: 0.8-1 mg every 4-6 hours as needed; patients with prior opiate exposure may require higher initial doses; usual dosage range: 1-2 mg every 3-6 hours as needed

Rectal: 3 mg every 4-8 hours as needed

Chronic pain: Adults: Oral: **Note:** Patients taking opioids chronically may become tolerant and require doses higher than the usual dosage range to maintain the desired effect. Tolerance can be managed by appropriate dose titration. There is no optimal or maximal dose for hydromorphone in chronic pain. The appropriate dose is one that relieves pain throughout its dosing interval without causing unmanageable side effects.

Controlled release formulation (Hydromorph Contin®, not available in U.S.): 3-30 mg every 12 hours. **Note:** A patient's hydromorphone requirement should be established using prompt release formulations; conversion to long acting products may be considered when chronic, continuous treatment is required. Higher dosages should be reserved for use only in opioid-tolerant patients.

Dosage Forms [CAN] = Canadian brand name

Capsule, controlled release:

Hydromorph Contin® [CAN]: 3 mg, 6 mg, 12 mg, 18 mg, 24 mg, 30 mg [not available in U.S.]

Injection, powder for reconstitution:

Dilaudid-HP®: 250 mg

Injection, solution: 1 mg/mL (1 mL); 2 mg/mL (1 mL, 20 mL); 4 mg/mL (1 mL)

Dilaudid®: 1 mg/mL (1 mL); 2 mg/mL (1 mL); 4 mg/mL (1 mL)

Dilaudid-HP®: 10 mg/mL (1 mL, 5 mL)

Dilaudid-HP®: 10 mg/mL (50 mL)

Injection, solution [preservative free]: 10 mg/mL (1 mL, 5 mL, 50 mL)

Liquid, oral:

Dilaudid®: 1 mg/mL (480 mL)

Powder, for prescription compounding: 100% (15 grain)

Suppository, rectal: 3 mg

Tablet: 2 mg, 4 mg, 8 mg

Dilaudid®: 2 mg, 4 mg, 8 mg

Hydromorphone HP [Can] *see* hydromorphone *on page* 506

Hydromorphone HP® 10 [Can] *see* hydromorphone *on page* 506

Hydromorphone HP® 20 [Can] *see* hydromorphone *on page* 506

Hydromorphone HP® 50 [Can] *see* hydromorphone *on page* 506

Hydromorphone HP® Forte [Can] *see* hydromorphone *on page* 506

hydromorphone hydrochloride *see* hydromorphone *on page* 506

Hydromorphone Hydrochloride Injection, USP [Can] *see* hydromorphone *on page* 506

Hydromox® *(Discontinued)*

Hydron CP [US] *see* phenylephrine, hydrocodone, and chlorpheniramine *on page 778*
Hydron PSC ***(Discontinued)***
Hydro-Par® ***(Discontinued)*** *see* hydrochlorothiazide *on page 499*
Hydro-PC II [US] *see* phenylephrine, hydrocodone, and chlorpheniramine *on page 778*
Hydro PC II Plus [US] *see* phenylephrine, hydrocodone, and chlorpheniramine *on page 778*
hydroquinol *see* hydroquinone *on page 508*

hydroquinone (HYE droe kwin one)

Sound-Alike/Look-Alike Issues

Eldopaque® may be confused with Eldoquin®
Eldoquin® may be confused with Eldopaque®
Eldopaque Forte® may be confused with Eldoquin Forte®
Eldoquin Forte® may be confused with Eldopaque Forte®

Synonyms hydroquinol; quinol

U.S./Canadian Brand Names Aclaro PD™ [US]; Alphaquin HP® [US]; Dermarest® Skin Correction Cream Plus [US-OTC]; Eldopaque Forte® [US]; Eldopaque® [US-OTC/Can]; Eldoquin Forte® [US]; Eldoquin® [US-OTC/Can]; EpiQuin™ Micro [US]; Esoterica® Daytime [US-OTC]; Esoterica® Nighttime [US-OTC]; Glyquin® XM [Can]; Lustra-AF® [US]; Lustra-Ultra™ [US]; Lustra® [US/Can]; Melanex® [US]; Melpaque HP® [US]; Melquin HP® [US]; Melquin-3® [US]; NeoStrata® AHA [US-OTC]; NeoStrata® HQ [Can]; Nuquin HP® [US]; Palmer's® Skin Success Eventone® Fade Cream [US-OTC]; Solaquin Forte® [Can]; Solaquin® [Can]; Ultraquin™ [Can]

Therapeutic Category Topical Skin Product

Use Gradual bleaching of hyperpigmented skin conditions

Usual Dosage Topical: Children >12 years and Adults: Apply thin layer and rub in twice daily

Dosage Forms

Cream, topical: 4% (30 g)
Alphaquin HP®: 4% (30 g, 60 g)
Eldoquin® [OTC]: 2% (30 g)
Eldoquin Forte®, EpiQuin™ Micro, Lustra®: 4% (30 g)
Esoterica® Nighttime [OTC]: 2% (70 g)
Melquin HP®: 4% (15 g, 30 g)

Cream, topical [with sunscreen]: 4% (30 g)
Dermarest® Skin Correcting Cream Plus [OTC]: 2% (85 g)
Eldopaque® [OTC]: 2% (15 g, 30 g)
Eldopaque Forte®: 4% (30 g)
Esoterica® Daytime [OTC]: 2% (70 g)
Lustra-AF®, Lustra-Ultra™: 4% (30 g, 60 g)
Melpaque HP®: 4% (15 g, 30 g)
Nuquin HP®: 4% (15 g, 30 g, 60 g)
Palmer's® Skin Success Eventone® Fade Cream [OTC]: 2% (81 g, 132 g)

Emulsion, topical:
Aclaro PD™: 4% (42.5 g)

Gel, topical:
NeoStrata® AHA [OTC]: 2% (45 g)

Gel, topical [with sunscreen]: 4% (30 g)
Nuquin HP®: 4% (15 g, 30 g)

Solution, topical:
Melanex®, Melquin-3®: 3% (30 mL)

hydroquinone, fluocinolone acetonide, and tretinoin *see* fluocinolone, hydroquinone, and tretinoin *on page 428*
Hydrotropine® ***(Discontinued)*** *see* hydrocodone and homatropine *on page 502*
Hydro-Tussin™-CBX ***(Discontinued)***
Hydro-Tussin™ DHC ***(Discontinued)*** *see* pseudoephedrine, dihydrocodeine, and chlorpheniramine *on page 836*
Hydro-Tussin™ DM ***(Discontinued)*** *see* guaifenesin and dextromethorphan *on page 474*
Hydro-Tussin™ EXP ***(Discontinued)*** *see* dihydrocodeine, pseudoephedrine, and guaifenesin *on page 310*
Hydro-Tussin™ HC ***(Discontinued)***
Hydro-Tussin™ HD ***(Discontinued)***

Hydro-Tussin™ XP ***(Discontinued)***

HydroVal® [Can] *see* hydrocortisone (topical) *on page 505*

hydroxyamphetamine and tropicamide (hye droks ee am FET a meen & troe PIK a mide)

Synonyms hydroxyamphetamine hydrobromide and tropicamide; tropicamide and hydroxyamphetamine

U.S./Canadian Brand Names Paremyd® [US]

Therapeutic Category Adrenergic Agonist Agent, Ophthalmic

Use Short-term pupil dilation for diagnostic procedures and exams

Usual Dosage Ophthalmic: Adults: Instill 1-2 drops into conjunctival sac(s)

Dosage Forms

Solution, ophthalmic:

Paremyd®: Hydroxyamphetamine 1% and tropicamide 0.25% (15 mL)

hydroxyamphetamine hydrobromide and tropicamide *see* hydroxyamphetamine and tropicamide *on page 509*

4-hydroxybutyrate *see* sodium oxybate *on page 911*

hydroxycarbamide *see* hydroxyurea *on page 510*

hydroxychloroquine (hye droks ee KLOR oh kwin)

Sound-Alike/Look-Alike Issues

hydroxychloroquine may be confused with hydrocortisone

Plaquenil® may be confused with Platinol®

Synonyms hydroxychloroquine sulfate

U.S./Canadian Brand Names Apo-Hydroxyquine® [Can]; Gen-Hydroxychloroquine [Can]; Plaquenil® [US/Can]; Pro-Hydroxyquine [Can]

Therapeutic Category Aminoquinoline (Antimalarial)

Use Suppression and treatment of acute attacks of malaria; treatment of systemic lupus erythematosus (SLE) and rheumatoid arthritis

Usual Dosage Note: Hydroxychloroquine sulfate 200 mg is equivalent to 155 mg hydroxychloroquine base and 250 mg chloroquine phosphate. All doses below expressed as hydroxychloroquine sulfate. Second-line alternative treatment for malaria (chloroquine is preferred).

Oral:

Children:

Malaria, chemoprophylaxis: 6.5 mg/kg once weekly (not to exceed 400 mg/dose); begin 2 weeks before exposure; continue for 4 weeks (per CDC guidelines) after leaving endemic area; if suppressive therapy is not begun prior to the exposure, double the initial dose and give in 2 doses, 6 hours apart and continue treatment for 8 weeks

Malaria, acute attack: 13 mg/kg initially (not to exceed 800 mg/dose), followed by 6.5 mg/kg (not to exceed 400 mg/dose) at 6, 24, and 48 hours

Adults:

Malaria, chemoprophylaxis: 400 mg weekly on same day each week; begin 2 weeks before exposure; continue for 4 weeks (per CDC guidelines) after leaving endemic area; if suppressive therapy is not begun prior to the exposure, double the initial dose and give in 2 doses, 6 hours apart and continue treatment for 8 weeks

Malaria, acute attack: 800 mg initially, followed by 400 mg at 6, 24, and 48 hours

Rheumatoid arthritis: Initial: 400-600 mg/day taken with food or milk; increase dose gradually until optimum response level is reached; usually after 4-12 weeks dose should be reduced by 1/2 to a maintenance dose of 200-400 mg/day

Lupus erythematosus: 400 mg every day or twice daily for several weeks-months depending on response; 200-400 mg/day for prolonged maintenance therapy

Dosage Forms

Tablet: 200 mg

Plaquenil®: 200 mg

hydroxychloroquine sulfate *see* hydroxychloroquine *on page 509*

hydroxydaunomycin hydrochloride *see* doxorubicin *on page 335*

hydroxyethylcellulose *see* artificial tears *on page 100*

hydroxyethyl starch *see* hetastarch *on page 493*

hydroxyldaunorubicin hydrochloride *see* doxorubicin *on page 335*

hydroxypropyl cellulose (hye droks ee PROE pil SEL yoo lose)

U.S./Canadian Brand Names Lacrisert® [US/Can]

Therapeutic Category Ophthalmic Agent, Miscellaneous

Use Dry eyes (moderate-to-severe)

Usual Dosage Ophthalmic: Adults: Apply once daily into the inferior cul-de-sac beneath the base of tarsus, not in apposition to the cornea nor beneath the eyelid at the level of the tarsal plate

Dosage Forms

Insert, ophthalmic [preservative free]:
Lacrisert®: 5 mg

hydroxypropyl methylcellulose (hye droks ee PROE pil meth il SEL yoo lose)

Sound-Alike/Look-Alike Issues
Isopto® Tears may be confused with Isoptin®

Synonyms gonioscopic ophthalmic solution; hypromellose

U.S./Canadian Brand Names Cellugel® [US]; GenTeal® Mild [US-OTC]; GenTeal® [US-OTC/Can]; Gonak™ [US-OTC]; Goniosoft™ [US]; Isopto® Tears [US-OTC/Can]; Tearisol® [US-OTC]; Tears Again® MC [US-OTC]

Therapeutic Category Ophthalmic Agent, Miscellaneous

Use Relief of burning and minor irritation due to dry eyes; diagnostic agent in gonioscopic examination

Usual Dosage Ophthalmic: Adults: Dry eyes: Instill 1-2 drops in affected eye(s) as needed

Dosage Forms

Gel, ophthalmic:
GenTeal® [OTC]: 0.3% (10 mL)

Solution, ophthalmic: 0.4% (15 mL)
GenTeal® [OTC]: 0.3% (15 mL, 25 mL)
GenTeal® Mild [OTC]: 0.2% (15 mL, 25 mL)
Gonak™ [OTC], Goniosoft™: 2.5% (15 mL)
Isopto® Tears [OTC], Tearisol® [OTC]: 0.5% (15 mL)
Tears Again® MC [OTC]: 0.3% (15 mL)

Solution, ophthalmic [for injection]:
Cellugel®: 2% (1 mL)

9-hydroxy-risperidone *see* paliperidone *on page* 743

hydroxyurea (hye droks ee yoor EE a)

Sound-Alike/Look-Alike Issues
hydroxyurea may be confused with hydrOXYzine

Synonyms hydroxycarbamide

U.S./Canadian Brand Names Apo-Hydroxyurea® [Can]; Droxia® [US]; Gen-Hydroxyurea [Can]; Hydrea® [US/Can]; Mylocel™ [US]

Therapeutic Category Antineoplastic Agent

Use Treatment of melanoma, refractory chronic myelocytic leukemia (CML), relapsed and refractory metastatic ovarian cancer; radiosensitizing agent in the treatment of squamous cell head and neck cancer (excluding lip cancer); adjunct in the management of sickle cell patients who have had at least three painful crises in the previous 12 months (to reduce frequency of these crises and the need for blood transfusions)

Usual Dosage Oral (refer to individual protocols): All doses should be based on ideal or actual body weight, whichever is less:

Adults: Dose should always be titrated to patient response and WBC counts; usual oral doses range from 10-30 mg/kg/day or 500-3000 mg/day; if WBC count falls to <2500 cells/mm^3, or the platelet count to <100,000/mm^3, therapy should be stopped for at least 3 days and resumed when values rise toward normal

Solid tumors:
Intermittent therapy: 80 mg/kg as a single dose every third day
Continuous therapy: 20-30 mg/kg/day given as a single dose/day

Concomitant therapy with irradiation: 80 mg/kg as a single dose every third day starting at least 7 days before initiation of irradiation

Resistant chronic myelocytic leukemia: Continuous therapy: 20-30 mg/kg once daily

Sickle cell anemia (moderate/severe disease): Initial: 15 mg/kg/day, increased by 5 mg/kg every 12 weeks if blood counts are in an acceptable range until the maximum tolerated dose of 35 mg/kg/day is achieved or the dose that does not produce toxic effects

Acceptable range:

Neutrophils ≥2500 cells/mm^3

Platelets ≥95,000/mm^3

Hemoglobin >5.3 g/dL, and

Reticulocytes ≥95,000/mm^3 if the hemoglobin concentration is <9 g/dL

Toxic range:

Neutrophils <2000 cells/mm^3

Platelets <80,000/mm^3

Hemoglobin <4.5 g/dL

Reticulocytes <80,000/mm^3 if the hemoglobin concentration is <9 g/dL

Monitor for toxicity every 2 weeks; if toxicity occurs, stop treatment until the bone marrow recovers; restart at 2.5 mg/kg/day less than the dose at which toxicity occurs; if no toxicity occurs over the next 12 weeks, then the subsequent dose should be increased by 2.5 mg/kg/day; reduced dosage of hydroxyurea alternating with erythropoietin may decrease myelotoxicity and increase levels of fetal hemoglobin in patients who have not been helped by hydroxyurea alone

Dosage Forms

Capsule: 500 mg

Droxia®: 200 mg, 300 mg, 400 mg

Hydrea®: 500 mg

Tablet:

Mylocel™: 1000 mg

hydroxyzine (hye DROKS i zeen)

Sound-Alike/Look-Alike Issues

hydrOXYzine may be confused with hydrALAZINE, hydroxyurea

Atarax® may be confused with amoxicillin, Ativan®

Vistaril® may be confused with Restoril®, Versed, Zestril®

Synonyms hydroxyzine hydrochloride; hydroxyzine pamoate

Tall-Man hydro**OXY**zine

U.S./Canadian Brand Names Apo-Hydroxyzine® [Can]; Atarax® [Can]; Hydroxyzine Hydrochloride Injection, USP [Can]; Novo-Hydroxyzin [Can]; PMS-Hydroxyzine [Can]; Vistaril® [US/Can]

Therapeutic Category Antiemetic; Antihistamine

Use Treatment of anxiety; preoperative sedative; antipruritic

Usual Dosage

Children:

Preoperative sedation:

Oral: 0.6 mg/kg/dose

I.M.: 0.5-1 mg/kg/dose

Pruritus, anxiety: Oral:

<6 years: 50 mg daily in divided doses

≥6 years: 50-100 mg daily in divided doses

Adults:

Anxiety: Oral, I.M.: 50-100 mg 4 times/day

Preoperative sedation:

Oral: 50-100 mg

I.M.: 25-100 mg

Pruritus: Oral, I.M.: 25 mg 3-4 times/day

Dosage Forms

Capsule: 25 mg, 50 mg, 100 mg

Vistaril®: 25 mg, 50 mg

Injection, solution: 25 mg/mL (1 mL); 50 mg/mL (1 mL, 2 mL, 10 mL)

Syrup: 10 mg/5 mL

Tablet: 10 mg, 25 mg, 50 mg

hydroxyzine hydrochloride *see* hydroxyzine *on page 511*

Hydroxyzine Hydrochloride Injection, USP [Can] *see* hydroxyzine *on page 511*

hydroxyzine pamoate *see* hydroxyzine *on page 511*

HydroZone Plus [US-OTC] *see* hydrocortisone (topical) *on page 505*

Hyflex-DS® ***(Discontinued)*** *see* acetaminophen and phenyltoloxamine *on page 23*
Hygroton® ***(Discontinued)*** *see* chlorthalidone *on page 223*
Hylaform® [US] *see* hyaluronate and derivatives *on page 496*
Hylaform® Plus [US] *see* hyaluronate and derivatives *on page 496*
hylan polymers *see* hyaluronate and derivatives *on page 496*
Hylenex™ [US] *see* hyaluronidase *on page 497*
Hylira™ [US] *see* hyaluronate and derivatives *on page 496*
Hylutin Injection ***(Discontinued)***
HyoMax™-DT [US] *see* hyoscyamine *on page 512*
HyoMax™-FT [US] *see* hyoscyamine *on page 512*
hyoscine butylbromide *see* scopolamine derivatives *on page 892*
hyoscine hydrobromide *see* scopolamine derivatives *on page 892*

hyoscyamine (hye oh SYE a meen)

Sound-Alike/Look-Alike Issues

Anaspaz® may be confused with Anaprox®, Antispas®
Levbid® may be confused with Enbrel®, Lithobid®, Lopid®, Lorabid®
Levsin®/SL maybe confused with Levaquin®

Synonyms *l*-hyoscyamine sulfate; hyoscyamine sulfate

U.S./Canadian Brand Names Anaspaz® [US]; HyoMax™-DT [US]; HyoMax™-FT [US]; Hyosyne [US]; Levbid® [US]; Levsin® [US/Can]; Levsin®/SL [US]; Symax® DuoTab [US]; Symax® FasTab [US]; Symax® SL [US]; Symax® SR [US]

Therapeutic Category Anticholinergic Agent

Use

Oral: Adjunctive therapy for peptic ulcers, irritable bowel, neurogenic bladder/bowel; treatment of infant colic, GI tract disorders caused by spasm; to reduce rigidity, tremors, sialorrhea, and hyperhidrosis associated with parkinsonism; as a drying agent in acute rhinitis

Injection: Preoperative antimuscarinic to reduce secretions and block cardiac vagal inhibitory reflexes; to improve radiologic visibility of the kidneys; symptomatic relief of biliary and renal colic; reduce GI motility to facilitate diagnostic procedures (ie, endoscopy, hypotonic duodenography); reduce pain and hypersecretion in pancreatitis, certain cases of partial heart block associated with vagal activity; reversal of neuromuscular blockade

Usual Dosage

Oral: Children: Gastrointestinal disorders: Dose as listed, based on age and weight (kg) using 0.125 mg/mL drops; repeat dose every 4 hours as needed:

Children <2 years:
3.4 kg: 4 drops; maximum: 24 drops/24 hours
5 kg: 5 drops; maximum: 30 drops/24 hours
7 kg: 6 drops; maximum: 36 drops/24 hours
10 kg: 8 drops; maximum: 48 drops/24 hours

Oral, S.L.:

Children 2-12 years: Gastrointestinal disorders: Dose as listed, based on age and weight (kg); repeat dose every 4 hours as needed:
10 kg: 0.031-0.033 mg; maximum: 0.75 mg/24 hours
20 kg: 0.0625 mg; maximum: 0.75 mg/24 hours
40 kg: 0.0938 mg; maximum: 0.75 mg/24 hours
50 kg: 0.125 mg; maximum: 0.75 mg/24 hours

Children >12 years and Adults: Gastrointestinal disorders: 0.125-0.25 mg every 4 hours or as needed (before meals or food); maximum: 1.5 mg/24 hours
Cystospaz®: 0.15-0.3 mg up to 4 times/day

Oral (timed release): Children >12 years and Adults: Gastrointestinal disorders: 0.375-0.75 mg every 12 hours; maximum: 1.5 mg/24 hours

I.M., I.V., SubQ: Children >12 years and Adults: Gastrointestinal disorders: 0.25-0.5 mg; may repeat as needed up to 4 times/day, at 4-hour intervals

I.V.: Children >2 year and Adults: I.V.: Preanesthesia: 5 mcg/kg given 30-60 minutes prior to induction of anesthesia or at the time preoperative narcotics or sedatives are administered

I.V.: Adults: Diagnostic procedures: 0.25-0.5 mg given 5-10 minutes prior to procedure
To reduce drug-induced bradycardia during surgery: 0.125 mg; repeat as needed

To reverse neuromuscular blockade: 0.2 mg for every 1 mg neostigmine (or the physostigmine/pyridostigmine equivalent)

Dosage Forms

Elixir, oral: 0.125 mg/5 mL (473 mL)
Hyosyne: 0.125 mg/5 mL (473 mL)

Injection, solution:
Levsin®: 0.5 mg/mL (1 mL)

Solution, oral [drops]: 0.125 mg/mL
Hyosyne: 0.125 mg/mL

Tablet, chewable/disintegrating, oral:
HyoMax™-FT, Symax® FasTab: 0.125 mg

Tablet, oral:
Levsin®: 0.125 mg

Tablet, sublinual:
Levsin®/SL, Symax® SL: 0.125 mg

Tablet, extended release, oral:
Levbid®: 0.375 mg

Tablet, orally disintegrating, oral: 0.125 mg
Anaspaz®: 0.125 mg [scored]

Tablet, sustained release, oral:
Symax® SR: 0.375 mg

Tablet, variable release, oral:
HyoMax™-DT, Symax® DuoTab: Hyoscyamine 0.125 mg [immediate release] and hyoscyamine 0.25 mg [sustained release]

hyoscyamine, atropine, scopolamine, and phenobarbital

(hye oh SYE a meen, A troe peen, skoe POL a meen, & fee noe BAR bi tal)

Sound-Alike/Look-Alike Issues

Donnatal® may be confused with Donnagel®

Synonyms atropine, hyoscyamine, scopolamine, and phenobarbital; belladonna alkaloids with phenobarbital; phenobarbital, hyoscyamine, atropine, and scopolamine; scopolamine, hyoscyamine, atropine, and phenobarbital

U.S./Canadian Brand Names Donnatal Extentabs® [US]; Donnatal® [US]

Therapeutic Category Anticholinergic Agent

Use Adjunct in treatment of irritable bowel syndrome, acute enterocolitis, duodenal ulcer

Usual Dosage Oral:

Children: Donnatal® elixir: To be given every 4-6 hours; initial dose based on weight:
4.5 kg: 0.5 mL every 4 hours **or** 0.75 mL every 6 hours
10 kg: 1 mL every 4 hours **or** 1.5 mL every 6 hours
14 kg: 1.5 mL every 4 hours **or** 2 mL every 6 hours
23 kg: 2.5 mL every 4 hours **or** 3.8 mL every 6 hours
34 kg: 3.8 mL every 4 hours **or** 5 mL every 6 hours
≥45 kg: 5 mL every 4 hours **or** 7.5 mL every 6 hours

Adults:
Donnatal®: 1-2 tablets or 5-10 mL of elixir 3-4 times/day
Donnatal Extentabs®: 1 tablet every 12 hours; may increase to 1 tablet every 8 hours if needed

Dosage Forms

Elixir:
Donnatal®: Hyoscyamine 0.1037 mg, atropine 0.0194 mg, scopolamine 0.0065 mg, and phenobarbital 16.2 mg per 5 mL

Tablet: Hyoscyamine 0.1037 mg, atropine 0.0194 mg, scopolamine 0.0065 mg, and phenobarbital 16.2 mg
Donnatal®: Hyoscyamine 0.1037 mg, atropine 0.0194 mg, scopolamine 0.0065 mg, and phenobarbital 16.2 mg

Tablet, extended release:
Donnatal Extentabs®: Hyoscyamine 0.3111 mg, atropine 0.0582 mg, scopolamine 0.0195 mg, and phenobarbital 48.6 mg

hyoscyamine, methenamine, benzoic acid, phenyl salicylate, and methylene blue *see* methenamine, phenyl salicylate, methylene blue, benzoic acid, and hyoscyamine *on page 637*

hyoscyamine sulfate *see* hyoscyamine *on page 512*

Hyosyne [US] *see* hyoscyamine *on page 512*
Hy-Pam® Oral *(Discontinued)* *see* hydroxyzine *on page 511*
Hypaque™ Sodium [US] *see* diatrizoate sodium *on page 301*
Hyperab® *(Discontinued)* *see* rabies immune globulin (human) *on page 848*
hyperal *see* total parenteral nutrition *on page 972*
hyperalimentation *see* total parenteral nutrition *on page 972*
Hypercare™ [US] *see* aluminum chloride hexahydrate *on page 54*
HyperHep B® [Can] *see* hepatitis B immune globulin (human) *on page 489*
HyperHEP B™ S/D [US] *see* hepatitis B immune globulin (human) *on page 489*
HyperRAB™ S/D [US/Can] *see* rabies immune globulin (human) *on page 848*
HyperRHO™ S/D Full Dose [US] *see* $Rh_o(D)$ immune globulin *on page 862*
HyperRHO™ S/D Mini Dose [US] *see* $Rh_o(D)$ immune globulin *on page 862*
Hyper-Sal™ [US] *see* sodium chloride *on page 908*
Hyperstat® *(Discontinued)* *see* diazoxide *on page 302*
HyperTET™ S/D [US/Can] *see* tetanus immune globulin (human) *on page 948*
Hyphed *(Discontinued)*
Hy-Phen® *(Discontinued)* *see* hydrocodone and acetaminophen *on page 501*
HypoTears [US-OTC] *see* artificial tears *on page 100*
HypoTears PF [US-OTC] *see* artificial tears *on page 100*
HypRho®-D *(Discontinued)*
HypRho®-D Mini-Dose *(Discontinued)*
Hyprogest® 250 *(Discontinued)*
hypromellose *see* hydroxypropyl methylcellulose *on page 510*
Hytakerol® *(Discontinued)*
HyTan™ *(Discontinued)* *see* hydrocodone and chlorpheniramine *on page 502*
Hytone® [US] *see* hydrocortisone (topical) *on page 505*
Hytrin® [Can] *see* terazosin *on page 945*
Hytrin® *(Discontinued)* *see* terazosin *on page 945*
Hyzaar® [US/Can] *see* losartan and hydrochlorothiazide *on page 601*
Hyzaar® DS [Can] *see* losartan and hydrochlorothiazide *on page 601*
Hyzine® *(Discontinued)* *see* hydroxyzine *on page 511*
I^{123} iobenguane *see* iobenguane I 123 *on page 537*
I-123 MIBG *see* iobenguane I 123 *on page 537*

ibandronate (eye BAN droh nate)

Synonyms ibandronate sodium; ibandronic acid

U.S./Canadian Brand Names Bondronat® [Can]; Boniva® [US]

Therapeutic Category Bisphosphonate Derivative

Use Treatment and prevention of osteoporosis in postmenopausal females

Usual Dosage

Oral:

Treatment of postmenopausal osteoporosis: 2.5 mg once daily **or** 150 mg once a month

Prevention of postmenopausal osteoporosis: 2.5 once daily **or** 150 mg once a month

I.V.: Treatment of postmenopausal osteoporosis: 3 mg every 3 months

Dosage Forms

Injection, solution:

Boniva®: 1 mg/mL (3 mL)

Tablet:

Boniva®: 2.5 mg [once-daily formulation]; 150 mg [once-monthly formulation]

ibandronate sodium *see* ibandronate *on page 514*
ibandronic acid *see* ibandronate *on page 514*
Iberet®-500 *(Discontinued)* *see* vitamins (multiple/oral) *on page 1019*
ibidomide hydrochloride *see* labetalol *on page 562*

ibritumomab (ib ri TYOO mo mab)

Synonyms ibritumomab tiuxetan; IDEC-Y2B8; In-111 ibritumomab; In-111 zevalin; Y-90 ibritumomab; Y-90 zevalin

U.S./Canadian Brand Names Zevalin® [US/Can]

Therapeutic Category Antineoplastic Agent, Monoclonal Antibody; Radiopharmaceutical

Use Treatment of relapsed or refractory low-grade, follicular, or transformed B-cell non-Hodgkin lymphoma

Usual Dosage I.V.: Adults: **Note:** Premedication with acetaminophen and diphenhydramine is recommended for rituximab infusions. Ibritumomab is administered **only** as part of the Zevalin® therapeutic regimen (a combined treatment regimen with rituximab). The regimen consists of two steps:

Day 1:

Rituximab infusion: 250 mg/m^2 at an initial rate of 50 mg/hour. If hypersensitivity or infusion-related events do not occur, increase infusion in increments of 50 mg/hour every 30 minutes, to a maximum of 400 mg/hour. Discontinue for severe infusion reaction. For less severe infusion reactions, temporarily slow or interrupt; the infusion may be resumed at one-half the previous rate upon improvement of symptoms.

In-111 ibritumomab infusion: Within 4 hours of the completion of rituximab infusion, inject 5 mCi (1.6 mg total antibody dose) over 10 minutes.

Biodistribution of In-111 ibritumomab should be assessed by imaging at 48-72 hours postinjection. Optional additional imaging may be performed to resolve ambiguities. If biodistribution is not acceptable, the patient should not proceed to Step 2.

Day 7, 8, or 9:

Rituximab infusion: 250 mg/m^2 at an initial rate of 100 mg/hour (50 mg/hour if infusion-related events occurred with the first infusion). If hypersensitivity or infusion-related events do not occur, increase infusion in increments of 100 mg/hour every 30 minutes, to a maximum of 400 mg/hour, as tolerated.

Y-90 ibritumomab infusion: Within 4 hours of the completion of rituximab infusion:

Platelet count ≥150,000 cells/mm^3: Inject 0.4 mCi/kg (14.8 MBq/kg actual body weight) over 10 minutes; maximum dose: 32 mCi (1184 MBq)

Platelet count between 100,000-149,000 cells/mm^3: Inject 0.3 mCi/kg (11.1 MBq/kg actual body weight) over 10 minutes; maximum dose: 32 mCi (1184 MBq)

Platelet count <100,000 cells/mm^3: Do **not** administer

Maximum dose: The prescribed, measured, and administered dose of Y-90 ibritumomab must not exceed 32 mCi (1184 MBq), regardless of the patient's body weight

Dosage Forms Each kit contains 4 vials for preparation of either In-111 or Y-90 conjugate (as indicated on container label)

Injection, solution:

Zevalin®: 1.6 mg/mL (2 mL)

ibritumomab tiuxetan *see* ibritumomab *on page 515*

Ibu® [US] *see* ibuprofen *on page 515*

Ibu-200 [US-OTC] *see* ibuprofen *on page 515*

Ibudone™ [US] *see* hydrocodone and ibuprofen *on page 503*

Ibuprin® *(Discontinued)* *see* ibuprofen *on page 515*

ibuprofen (eye byoo PROE fen)

Sound-Alike/Look-Alike Issues

Haltran® may be confused with Halfprin®

Motrin® may be confused with Neurontin®

Synonyms *p*-isobutylhydratropic acid; ibuprofen lysine

U.S./Canadian Brand Names Addaprin [US-OTC]; Advil® Children's [US-OTC]; Advil® Infants' [US-OTC]; Advil® Migraine [US-OTC]; Advil® [US-OTC/Can]; Apo-Ibuprofen® [Can]; Caldolor™ [US]; I-Prin [US-OTC]; Ibu-200 [US-OTC]; Ibu® [US]; Midol® Cramp and Body Aches [US-OTC]; Motrin® Children's [US-OTC/Can]; Motrin® IB [US-OTC/Can]; Motrin® Infants' [US-OTC]; Motrin® Junior [US-OTC]; NeoProfen® [US]; Novo-Profen [Can]; Nu-Ibuprofen [Can]; Proprinal [US-OTC]; Ultraprin [US-OTC]

Therapeutic Category Analgesic, Nonnarcotic; Antipyretic; Nonsteroidal Antiinflammatory Drug (NSAID)

Use

Oral: Inflammatory diseases and rheumatoid disorders including juvenile rheumatoid arthritis, mild-to-moderate pain, fever, dysmenorrhea, osteoarthritis

Ibuprofen injection (Caldolor™): Management of mild-to-moderate pain; management moderate-to-severe pain when used concurrently with an opioid analgesic; reduction of fever

Ibuprofen lysine injection (NeoProfen®): To induce closure of a clinically-significant patent ductus arteriosus (PDA) in premature infants weighing between 500-1500 g and who are ≤32 weeks gestational age (GA) when usual treatments are ineffective

Usual Dosage

I.V.: Infants between 500-1500 g and ≤32 weeks GA: Patent ductus arteriosus: Initial dose: Ibuprofen 10 mg/kg, followed by two doses of 5 mg/kg at 24 and 48 hours. Dose should be based on birth weight.

Oral:

Children:

Antipyretic: 6 months to 12 years: Temperature <102.5°F (39°C): 5 mg/kg/dose; temperature >102.5°F: 10 mg/kg/dose given every 6-8 hours (maximum daily dose: 40 mg/kg/day)

Juvenile rheumatoid arthritis: 30-50 mg/kg/24 hours divided every 8 hours; start at lower end of dosing range and titrate upward (maximum: 2.4 g/day)

Analgesic: 4-10 mg/kg/dose every 6-8 hours

OTC labeling (analgesic, antipyretic): **Note:** Treatment for >10 days is not recommended unless directed by healthcare provider:

Children 6 months to 11 years: See below; use of weight to select dose is preferred; doses may be repeated every 6-8 hours (maximum: 4 doses/day)

Children ≥12 years: 200 mg every 4-6 hours as needed (maximum: 1200 mg/24 hours)

Ibuprofen Dosing:

Weight 12-17 lbs (6-11 months of age): 50 mg
Weight 18-23 lbs (12-23 months of age): 75 mg
Weight 24-35 lbs (2-3 years of age): 100 mg
Weight 35-47 lbs (4-5 years of age): 150 mg
Weight 48-59 lbs (6-8 years of age): 200 mg
Weight 60-71 lbs (9-10 years of age): 250 mg
Weight 72-95 lbs (11 years of age): 300 mg

Adults:

Inflammatory disease: 400-800 mg/dose 3-4 times/day (maximum dose: 3.2 g/day)

Analgesia/pain/fever/dysmenorrhea: 200-400 mg/dose every 4-6 hours (maximum daily dose: 1.2 g, unless directed by physician; under physician supervision daily doses ≤2.4 g may be used)

OTC labeling (analgesic, antipyretic): 200 mg every 4-6 hours as needed (maximum: 1200 mg/24 hours); treatment for >10 days is not recommended unless directed by healthcare provider

Migraine: 2 capsules at onset of symptoms (maximum: 400 mg/24 hours unless directed by healthcare provider)

Dosage Forms

Caplet: 200 mg [OTC]
Advil® [OTC], Ibu-200 [OTC], Motrin® IB [OTC]: 200 mg
Motrin® Junior [OTC]: 100 mg [scored]

Capsule, liquid-filled:
Advil® [OTC], Advil® Migraine [OTC]: 200 mg

Gelcap:
Advil® [OTC]: 200 mg

Injection, solution:
Caldolor™: 100 mg/mL (4 mL, 8 mL)

Injection, solution, as lysine [preservative free]:
NeoProfen®: 17.1 mg/mL (2 mL) [equivalent to ibuprofen 10 mg/mL]

Suspension, oral: 100 mg/5 mL
Advil® Children's [OTC], Motrin® Children's [OTC]: 100 mg/5 mL

Suspension, oral [concentrate, drops]: 40 mg/mL
Advil® Infants' [OTC], Motrin® Infants' [OTC]: 40 mg/mL

Tablet: 200 mg [OTC], 400 mg, 600 mg, 800 mg
Addaprin [OTC], Advil® [OTC], Ibu-200 [OTC], I-Prin [OTC], Midol® Cramp and Body Aches [OTC], Motrin® IB [OTC], Proprinal [OTC], Ultraprin [OTC]: 200 mg
Ibu®: 400 mg, 600 mg, 800 mg

Tablet, chewable:
Advil® Children's [OTC]: 50 mg
Motrin® Junior [OTC]: 100 mg

ibuprofen and hydrocodone *see* hydrocodone and ibuprofen *on page* 503
ibuprofen and oxycodone *see* oxycodone and ibuprofen *on page* 739
ibuprofen and pseudoephedrine *see* pseudoephedrine and ibuprofen *on page* 835
ibuprofen lysine *see* ibuprofen *on page* 515

ibuprofen, pseudoephedrine, and chlorpheniramine

(eye byoo PROE fen, soo doe e FED rin, & klor fen IR a meen)

Synonyms chlorpheniramine maleate, ibuprofen, and pseudoephedrine; ibuprofen, pseudoephedrine, and chlorpheniramine maleate; pseudoephedrine, chlorpheniramine, and ibuprofen

U.S./Canadian Brand Names Advil® Allergy Sinus [US]; Advil® Cold and Sinus Plus [Can]; Advil® Multi-Symptom Cold [US]

Therapeutic Category Antihistamine/Decongestant/Analgesic

Use Temporary relief of symptoms associated with the common cold, hay fever, or other respiratory allergies

Usual Dosage Oral: Children ≥12 years and Adults: One caplet every 4-6 hours while symptoms persist (maximum: 6 caplets/24 hours); treatment for >10 days is not recommended unless directed by healthcare provider

Dosage Forms

Caplet:

Advil® Allergy Sinus, Advil® Multi-Symptom Cold: Ibuprofen 200 mg, pseudoephedrine 30 mg, and chlorpheniramine 2 mg

ibuprofen, pseudoephedrine, and chlorpheniramine maleate *see* ibuprofen, pseudoephedrine, and chlorpheniramine *on page* 517

ibutilide (i BYOO ti lide)

Synonyms ibutilide fumarate

U.S./Canadian Brand Names Corvert® [US]

Therapeutic Category Antiarrhythmic Agent, Class III

Use Acute termination of atrial fibrillation or flutter of recent onset; the effectiveness of ibutilide has not been determined in patients with arrhythmias >90 days in duration

Usual Dosage I.V.: Initial: Adults:

<60 kg: 0.01 mg/kg over 10 minutes

≥60 kg: 1 mg over 10 minutes

If the arrhythmia does not terminate within 10 minutes after the end of the initial infusion, a second infusion of equal strength may be infused over a 10-minute period

Dosage Forms

Injection, solution:

Corvert®: 0.1 mg/mL (10 mL)

ibutilide fumarate *see* ibutilide *on page* 517

IC51 *see* Japanese encephalitis virus vaccine (inactivated) *on page* 555

IC-Green™ [US] *see* indocyanine green *on page* 526

ICI-182,780 *see* fulvestrant *on page* 448

ICI-204,219 *see* zafirlukast *on page* 1026

ICI-46474 *see* tamoxifen *on page* 937

ICI-118630 *see* goserelin *on page* 471

ICI-176334 *see* bicalutamide *on page* 141

ICI-D1033 *see* anastrozole *on page* 79

ICI-D1694 *see* raltitrexed *(Canada only) on page* 849

ICL670 *see* deferasirox *on page* 280

icodextrin (eye KOE dex trin)

U.S./Canadian Brand Names Adept® [US]; Extraneal® [US]

Therapeutic Category Adhesiolytic; Peritoneal Dialysate, Osmotic

Use

Adept®: Reduction of postsurgical adhesions in gynecologic laparoscopic procedures

Extraneal®: Daily exchange for the long dwell (8- to 16-hour) during continuous ambulatory peritoneal dialysis (CAPD) or automated peritoneal dialysis (APD) for the management of end-stage renal disease (ESRD); improvement of long-dwell ultrafiltration and clearance of creatinine and urea nitrogen (compared to 4.25% dextrose) in patients with high/average or greater transport characteristics as measured by peritoneal equilibration test (PET)

Usual Dosage Intraperitoneal: Adults:
CAPD or APD (Extraneal®): Given as a single daily exchange in CAPD or APD; dwell time of 8-16 hours is suggested
Laparoscopic gynecologic surgery (Adept®): Irrigate with at least 100 mL every 30 minutes during surgery; aspirate remaining fluid after surgery is completed, then instill 1 L into the cavity

Dosage Forms
Solution, intraperitoneal:
Adept®: 4% (1.5 L) [for laparoscopic surgery]
Extraneal®: 7.5% (1.5 L, 2 L, 2.5 L) [for peritoneal dialysis]

ICRF-187 *see* dexrazoxane *on page* *292*
Idamycin® [Can] *see* idarubicin *on page* *518*
Idamycin® *(Discontinued)* *see* idarubicin *on page* *518*
Idamycin PFS® [US] *see* idarubicin *on page* *518*

idarubicin (eye da ROO bi sin)

Sound-Alike/Look-Alike Issues
IDArubicin may be confused with DOXOrubicin, DAUNOrubicin, epirubicin
Idamycin PFS® may be confused with Adriamycin

Synonyms 4-demethoxydaunorubicin; 4-DMDR; idarubicin hydrochloride; IDR; IMI 30; NSC-256439; SC 33428

Tall-Man **IDA**rubicin

U.S./Canadian Brand Names Idamycin PFS® [US]; Idamycin® [Can]

Therapeutic Category Antineoplastic Agent

Use Treatment of acute leukemias (AML, ANLL, ALL), accelerated phase or blast crisis of chronic myelogenous leukemia (CML), breast cancer

Usual Dosage I.V. (refer to individual protocols):
Children:
Leukemia: 10-12 mg/m^2/day for 3 days every 3 weeks
Solid tumors: 5 mg/m^2/day for 3 days every 3 weeks
Adults:
Leukemia induction: 12 mg/m^2/day for 3 days
Leukemia consolidation: 10-12 mg/m^2/day for 2 days

Dosage Forms
Injection, solution [preservative free]: 1 mg/mL (5 mL, 10 mL, 20 mL)
Idamycin PFS®: 1 mg/mL (5 mL, 10 mL, 20 mL)

idarubicin hydrochloride *see* idarubicin *on page* *518*
IDEC-C2B8 *see* rituximab *on page* *872*
IDEC-Y2B8 *see* ibritumomab *on page* *515*
IDR *see* idarubicin *on page* *518*

idursulfase (eye dur SUL fase)

Sound-Alike/Look-Alike Issues
Elaprase™ may be confused with Elspar®

U.S./Canadian Brand Names Elaprase™ [US/Can]

Therapeutic Category Enzyme

Use Replacement therapy in mucopolysaccharidosis II (MPS II, Hunter syndrome) for improvement of walking capacity

Usual Dosage I.V.: Children ≥5 years and Adults: MPS II: 0.5 mg/kg once weekly

Dosage Forms
Injection, solution [preservative free]:
Elaprase™: 2 mg/mL (5 mL)

Ifex® [Can] *see* ifosfamide *on page* *518*
Ifex® *(Discontinued)* *see* ifosfamide *on page* *518*

ifosfamide (eye FOSS fa mide)

Sound-Alike/Look-Alike Issues
ifosfamide may be confused with cyclophosphamide

Synonyms isophosphamide; NSC-109724; Z4942

U.S./Canadian Brand Names Ifex® [Can]

Therapeutic Category Antineoplastic Agent

Use Treatment of testicular cancer

Usual Dosage Refer to individual protocols. To prevent bladder toxicity, ifosfamide should be given with the urinary protector mesna and hydration of at least 2 L of oral or I.V. fluid per day.

I.V.: Adults: Testicular cancer: 1200 mg/m^2/day for 5 days every 3 weeks

Dosage Forms

Injection, powder for reconstitution: 1 g

Injection, solution: 50 mg/mL (20 mL, 60 mL)

IG *see* immune globulin (intramuscular) *on page 522*

IgG4-kappa monoclonal antibody *see* natalizumab *on page 683*

IGIM *see* immune globulin (intramuscular) *on page 522*

IGIV *see* immune globulin (intravenous) *on page 523*

IGIVnex® [Can] *see* immune globulin (intravenous) *on page 523*

IL-1Ra *see* anakinra *on page 78*

IL-2 *see* aldesleukin *on page 43*

IL-11 *see* oprelvekin *on page 728*

Ilaris® [US] *see* canakinumab *on page 176*

Ilopan-Choline® Oral *(Discontinued)* *see* dexpanthenol *on page 292*

Ilopan® Injection *(Discontinued)* *see* dexpanthenol *on page 292*

iloperidone (eye loe PER i done)

U.S./Canadian Brand Names Fanapt™ [US]

Therapeutic Category Antipsychotic Agent, Atypical

Use Acute treatment of schizophrenia

Product Availability Fanapt™: FDA approved May 2009; availability expected by year-end; consult prescribing information for additional information

iloprost (EYE loe prost)

Synonyms iloprost tromethamine; prostacyclin PGI_2

U.S./Canadian Brand Names Ventavis® [US]

Therapeutic Category Prostaglandin

Use Treatment of idiopathic pulmonary arterial hypertension in patients with NYHA Class III or IV symptoms

Usual Dosage Inhalation: Adults: Initial: 2.5 mcg/dose; if tolerated, increase to 5 mcg/dose; administer 6-9 times daily (dosing at intervals ≥2 hours while awake according to individual need and tolerability); maintenance dose: 2.5-5 mcg/dose; maximum daily dose: 45 mcg

Dosage Forms

Solution for oral inhalation [preservative-free]:

Ventavis®: 10 mcg/mL (1 mL, 2 mL)

iloprost tromethamine *see* iloprost *on page 519*

Ilozyme® *(Discontinued)* *see* pancrelipase *on page 746*

imatinib (eye MAT eh nib)

Sound-Alike/Look-Alike Issues

imatinib may be confused with dasatinib, erlotinib, nilotinib, sorafenib, sunitinib

Synonyms CGP-57148B; glivec; imatinib mesylate; STI-571

U.S./Canadian Brand Names Gleevec® [US/Can]

Therapeutic Category Antineoplastic Agent, Tyrosine Kinase Inhibitor

Use Treatment of:

Gastrointestinal stromal tumors (GIST) kit-positive (CD117), including unresectable and/or metastatic malignant and adjuvant treatment following complete resection

Philadelphia chromosome-positive (Ph+) chronic myeloid leukemia (CML) in chronic phase (newly-diagnosed)

Ph+ CML in chronic phase in pediatric patients recurring following stem cell transplant or who are resistant to interferon-alpha therapy (**not** an approved use in Canada)
Ph+ CML in blast crisis, accelerated phase, or chronic phase after failure of interferon therapy
Ph+ acute lymphoblastic leukemia (ALL) (relapsed or refractory)
Aggressive systemic mastocytosis (ASM) without D816V c-Kit mutation (or c-Kit mutation status unknown)
Dermatofibrosarcoma protuberans (DFSP) (unresectable, recurrent and/or metastatic)
Hypereosinophilic syndrome (HES) and/or chronic eosinophilic leukemia (CEL)
Myelodysplastic/myeloproliferative disease (MDS/MPD) associated with platelet-derived growth factor receptor (PDGFR) gene rearrangements

Note: The following use is approved in Canada (not an approved indication in the U.S.):
Ph+ ALL induction therapy (newly diagnosed)

Usual Dosage Adults: **Note:** Doses ≤600 mg should be administered once daily, 800 mg doses should be administered as 400 mg twice a day.

Ph+ CML:

Chronic phase: 400 mg once daily; may be increased to 600 mg/day, if tolerated, for disease progression, lack of hematologic response after 3 months, lack of cytogenetic response after 6-12 months, or loss of previous hematologic or cytogenetic response

Canadian labeling and NCCN CML guidelines (v.1.2010): Includes range up to 800 mg/day (400 mg twice daily)

Accelerated phase or blast crisis: 600 mg once daily; may be increased to 800 mg/day (400 mg twice daily), if tolerated, for disease progression, lack of hematologic response after 3 months, lack of cytogenetic response after 6-12 months, or loss of previous hematologic or cytogenetic response

Dosage Forms

Tablet:

Gleevec®: 100 mg; 400 mg

imatinib mesylate *see* imatinib *on page 519*

IMC-C225 *see* cetuximab *on page 205*

Imdur® [US/Can] *see* isosorbide mononitrate *on page 551*

123I-metaiodobenzylguanidine (MIBG) *see* iobenguane I 123 *on page 537*

imferon *see* iron dextran complex *on page 546*

IMI 30 *see* idarubicin *on page 518*

IMid-1 *see* lenalidomide *on page 574*

imidazole carboxamide *see* dacarbazine *on page 272*

imidazole carboxamide dimethyltriazene *see* dacarbazine *on page 272*

imiglucerase (i mi GLOO ser ace)

Sound-Alike/Look-Alike Issues

Cerezyme® may be confused with Cerebyx®, Ceredase®

U.S./Canadian Brand Names Cerezyme® [US/Can]

Therapeutic Category Enzyme

Use Long-term enzyme replacement therapy for patients with Type 1 Gaucher disease

Usual Dosage I.V.: Children ≥2 years and Adults: Initial: 30-60 units/kg every 2 weeks; dosing is individualized based on disease severity. Dosing range: 2.5 units/kg 3 times/week up to as much as 60 units/kg administered as frequently as once a week or as infrequently as every 4 weeks. Average dose: 60 units/kg administered every 2 weeks

Dosage Forms

Injection, powder for reconstitution:

Cerezyme®: 200 units, 400 units

imipemide *see* imipenem and cilastatin *on page 520*

imipenem and cilastatin (i mi PEN em & sye la STAT in)

Sound-Alike/Look-Alike Issues

imipenem may be confused with ertapenem, meropenem
Primaxin® may be confused with Premarin®, Primacor®

Synonyms imipemide

U.S./Canadian Brand Names Primaxin® I.V. [Can]; Primaxin® [US/Can]

Therapeutic Category Carbapenem (Antibiotic)

Use Treatment of lower respiratory tract, urinary tract, intraabdominal, gynecologic, bone and joint, skin and skin structure, and polymicrobic infections as well as bacterial septicemia and endocarditis. Antibacterial activity includes resistant gram-negative bacilli (*Pseudomonas aeruginosa* and *Enterobacter* sp), gram-positive bacteria (methicillin-sensitive *Staphylococcus aureus* and *Streptococcus* sp) and anaerobes.

Usual Dosage

Usual dosage ranges: Note: Dosage based on **imipenem** content:

Neonates ≤3 months and weight ≥1500 g: Non-CNS infections: I.V.:
- <1 week: 25 mg/kg every 12 hours
- 1-4 weeks: 25 mg/kg every 8 hours
- 4 weeks to 3 months: 25 mg/kg every 6 hours

Children >3 months: Non-CNS infections: I.V.: 15-25 mg/kg every 6 hours; maximum dosage: Susceptible infections: 2 g/day; moderately-susceptible organisms: 4 g/day

Adults:
- I.M.: 500-750 mg every 12 hours; maximum: 1500 mg/day
- I.V.: Weight ≥70 kg: 250-1000 mg every 6-8 hours; maximum: 4 g/day

Indication-specific dosing: Note: Doses based on imipenem content. I.M. administration is not intended for severe or life-threatening infections (eg, septicemia, endocarditis, shock), UTI, bone/joint or polymicrobic infections:

Children: I.V.: **Cystic fibrosis:** Doses up to 90 mg/kg/day have been used

Adults:

Intraabdominal infections:
- I.V.: Mild infection: 250-500 mg every 6 hours; severe: 500 mg every 6 hours
- I.M.: Mild-to-moderate infection: 750 mg every 12 hours

Lower respiratory tract, skins/skin structure, gynecologic infections: I.M.: Mild/moderate: 500-750 mg every 12 hours

Mild infection: Note: Rarely a suitable option in mild infections; normally reserved for moderate-to-severe cases:
- I.M.: 500 mg every 12 hours
- I.V.:
  - *Fully-susceptible organisms:* 250 mg every 6 hours
  - *Moderately-susceptible organisms:* 500 mg every 6 hours

Moderate infection:
- I.M.: 750 mg every 12 hours
- I.V.:
  - *Fully-susceptible organisms:* 500 mg every 6-8 hours
  - *Moderately-susceptible organisms:* 500 mg every 6 hours or 1 g every 8 hours

***Pseudomonas* infections:** I.V.: 500 mg every 6 hours; **Note:** Higher doses may be required based on organism sensitivity.

Severe infection: I.V.:
- *Fully-susceptible organisms:* 500 mg every 6 hours
- *Moderately-susceptible organisms:* 1 g every 6-8 hours
- Maximum daily dose should not exceed 50 mg/kg or 4 g/day, whichever is lower

Urinary tract infection: I.V.:
- *Uncomplicated:* 250 mg every 6 hours
- *Complicated:* 500 mg every 6 hours

Dosage Forms

Injection, powder for reconstitution [I.M.]:
Primaxin®: Imipenem 500 mg and cilastatin 500 mg

Injection, powder for reconstitution [I.V.]:
Primaxin®: Imipenem 250 mg and cilastatin 250 mg; imipenem 500 mg and cilastatin 500 mg

imipramine (im IP ra meen)

Sound-Alike/Look-Alike Issues
imipramine may be confused with amitriptyline, desipramine, Norpramin®

Synonyms imipramine hydrochloride; imipramine pamoate

U.S./Canadian Brand Names Apo-Imipramine® [Can]; Novo-Pramine [Can]; Tofranil-PM® [US]; Tofranil® [US/Can]

Therapeutic Category Antidepressant, Tricyclic (Tertiary Amine)

Use Treatment of depression; treatment of nocturnal enuresis in children

Usual Dosage Oral:

Children: Enuresis: ≥6 years: Initial: 25 mg at bedtime, if inadequate response still seen after 1 week of therapy, increase by 25 mg/day; dose should not exceed 2.5 mg/kg/day or 50 mg at bedtime if 6-12 years of age or 75 mg at bedtime if ≥12 years of age

Adolescents: Depression: Initial: 25-50 mg/day; increase gradually; maximum: 100 mg/day in single or divided doses

Adults: Depression:

Outpatients: Initial: 75 mg/day; may increase gradually to 150 mg/day. May be given in divided doses or as a single bedtime dose; maximum: 200 mg/day

Inpatients: Initial: 100-150 mg/day; may increase gradually to 200 mg/day; if no response after 2 weeks, may further increase to 250-300 mg/day. May be given in divided doses or as a single bedtime dose; maximum: 300 mg/day.

Dosage Forms

Capsule: 75 mg, 100 mg, 125 mg, 150 mg

Tofranil-PM®: 75 mg, 100 mg, 125 mg, 150 mg

Tablet: 10 mg, 25 mg, 50 mg

Tofranil®: 10 mg, 25 mg, 50 mg

imipramine hydrochloride *see* imipramine *on page* 521

imipramine pamoate *see* imipramine *on page* 521

imiquimod (i mi KWI mod)

Sound-Alike/Look-Alike Issues

Aldara® may be confused with Alora®, Lialda™

U.S./Canadian Brand Names Aldara® [US/Can]

Therapeutic Category Immune Response Modifier

Use Treatment of external genital and perianal warts/condyloma acuminata; nonhyperkeratotic, nonhypertrophic actinic keratosis on face or scalp; superficial basal cell carcinoma (sBCC) with a maximum tumor diameter of 2 cm located on the trunk, neck, or extremities (excluding hands or feet)

Usual Dosage Topical: **Note:** A rest period of several days may be taken if required by the patient's discomfort or severity of the local skin reaction. Treatment may resume once the reaction subsides.

Children ≥12 years and Adults: Perianal warts/condyloma acuminata: Apply a thin layer 3 times/week prior to bedtime and leave on skin for 6-10 hours. Remove with mild soap and water. Examples of 3 times/week application schedules are: Monday, Wednesday, Friday; or Tuesday, Thursday, Saturday. Continue imiquimod treatment until there is total clearance of the genital/perianal warts for ≤16 weeks.

Adults:

Actinic keratosis: Apply twice weekly for 16 weeks to a treatment area on face or scalp (but not both concurrently); apply prior to bedtime and leave on skin for 8 hours. Remove with mild soap and water.

Common oral warts (dental use): Apply once daily prior to bedtime

Superficial basal cell carcinoma: Apply once daily prior to bedtime, 5 days/week for 6 weeks. Treatment area should include a 1 cm margin of skin around the tumor. Leave on skin for 8 hours. Remove with mild soap and water.

Dosage Forms

Cream:

Aldara®: 5% (12s, 24s)

Imitrex® [US/Can] *see* sumatriptan *on page* 932

Imitrex® DF [Can] *see* sumatriptan *on page* 932

Imitrex® Nasal Spray [Can] *see* sumatriptan *on page* 932

ImmuCyst® [Can] *see* BCG vaccine *on page* 124

immune globulin (intramuscular) (i MYUN GLOB yoo lin, IN tra MUS kyoo ler)

Synonyms gamma globulin; IG; IGIM; immune serum globulin; ISG

U.S./Canadian Brand Names BayGam® [Can]; GammaSTAN™ S/D [US]

Therapeutic Category Immune Globulin

Use To provide passive immunity in susceptible individuals under the following circumstances:

Hepatitis A: Within 14 days of exposure and prior to manifestation of disease

Measles: For use within 6 days of exposure in an unvaccinated person, who has not previously had measles

Varicella: When Varicella Zoster Immune Globulin is not available

Rubella: Postexposure prophylaxis (within 72 hours) to reduce the risk of infection in exposed pregnant women who will not consider therapeutic abortion

Immunoglobulin deficiency: To help prevent serious infections

Usual Dosage I.M.: Children and Adults:

Hepatitis A:

Preexposure prophylaxis upon travel into endemic areas (hepatitis A vaccine preferred):

0.02 mL/kg for anticipated risk of exposure <3 months

0.06 mL/kg for anticipated risk of exposure ≥3 months

Repeat approximate dose every 5 months if exposure continues

Postexposure prophylaxis: 0.02 mL/kg given within 14 days of exposure. IG is not needed if at least 1 dose of hepatitis A vaccine was given at ≥1 month before exposure

Measles:

Prophylaxis, immunocompetent: 0.25 mL/kg/dose (maximum dose: 15 mL) given within 6 days of exposure followed by live attenuated measles vaccine in 5-6 months when indicated

Prophylaxis, immunocompromised: 0.5 mL/kg (maximum dose: 15 mL) immediately following exposure

Rubella: Prophylaxis during pregnancy: 0.55 mL/kg/dose within 72 hours of exposure

Varicella: Prophylaxis: 0.6-1.2 mL/kg (varicella zoster immune globulin preferred) within 72 hours of exposure

IgG deficiency: 0.66 mL/kg/dose every 3-4 weeks. A double dose may be given at onset of therapy; some patients may require more frequent injections.

Dosage Forms

Injection, solution [preservative free; solvent detergent-treated]:

GamaSTAN™ S/D: 15% to 18% (2 mL, 10 mL)

immune globulin (intravenous) (i MYUN GLOB yoo lin, IN tra VEE nus)

Sound-Alike/Look-Alike Issues

immune globulin (intravenous) may be confused with hepatitis B immune globulin

Gamimune® N may be confused with CytoGam®

Synonyms IGIV; IV immune globulin; IVIG

U.S./Canadian Brand Names Carimune® NF [US]; Flebogamma® [US]; Gamimune® N [Can]; Gammagard Liquid [US/Can]; Gammagard S/D [US/Can]; Gamunex® [US/Can]; IGIVnex® [Can]; Octagam® [US]; Privigen™ [US]

Therapeutic Category Immune Globulin

Use

Treatment of primary immunodeficiency syndromes (congenital agammaglobulinemia, severe combined immunodeficiency syndromes [SCIDS], common variable immunodeficiency, X-linked immunodeficiency, Wiskott-Aldrich syndrome) (Carimune® NF, Flebogamma®, Gammagard Liquid, Gammagard S/D, Gamunex®, Octagam®, Privigen™)

Treatment of immune (idiopathic) thrombocytopenic purpura (ITP) (Carimune® NF, Gammagard S/D, Gamunex®, Privigen™)

Treatment of chronic inflammatory demyelinating polyneuropathy (CIDP) (Gamunex®)

Prevention of coronary artery aneurysms associated with Kawasaki disease (in combination with aspirin) (Gammagard S/D)

Prevention of bacterial infection in B-cell chronic lymphocytic leukemia (CLL) (Gammagard S/D)

Usual Dosage Approved doses and regimens may vary between brands; check manufacturer guidelines.

Note: Some clinicians dose IVIG on ideal body weight or an adjusted ideal body weight in morbidly-obese patients.

Children: I.V.: Pediatric HIV, prevention of infection (CDC guidelines): 400 mg/kg every 2-4 weeks

Children and Adults: I.V.:

Primary immunodeficiency disorders: **Note:** Adjust dose/frequency based desired IgG levels and clinical response:

General dosing range: 200-800 mg/kg per month

Carimune® NF: 200 mg/kg every 4 weeks. May increase dose to 300 mg/kg every 4 weeks or may increase frequency based on patient response.

Flebogamma®, Gammagard Liquid, Gammagard S/D, Gamunex®, Octagam®: 300-600 mg/kg every 3-4 weeks; adjusted based on dosage and interval in conjunction with monitored serum IgG concentrations

Privigen™: 200-800 mg/kg every 3-4 weeks; adjusted based on dosage and interval in conjunction with monitored serum IgG concentrations

B-cell chronic lymphocytic leukemia (CLL) (Gammagard S/D): 400 mg/kg/dose every 3-4 weeks

Immune (idiopathic) thrombocytopenic purpura (ITP):
Carimune® NF:
Acute: 400 mg/kg/day for 2-5 days
Chronic: 400 mg/kg as needed to maintain platelet count ≥30,000/mm^3 or to control significant bleeding; may increase dose if needed (range: 800-1000 mg/kg)
Gammagard S/D: 1000 mg/kg; adjust additional doses based on patient response or platelet count. Up to 3 separate doses may be administered on alternate days if required.
Gamunex®: 1000 mg/kg/day for 1-2 days, **or** 400 mg/kg/day for 5 days
Privigen™: 1000 mg/kg/day for 2 consecutive days
Chronic inflammatory demyelinating polyneuropathy (CIDP): Gamunex®: Loading dose: 2000 mg/kg divided over 2-4 consecutive days; Maintenance: 1000 mg/kg/day for 1 day every 3 weeks **or** 500 mg/kg/day for 2 consecutive days every 3 weeks
Kawasaki disease: Initiate IVIG therapy within 10 days of disease onset: Must be used in combination with aspirin: 80-100 mg/kg/day in 4 divided doses for 14 days; when fever subsides, dose aspirin at 3-5 mg/kg once daily for ≥6-8 weeks
AHA guidelines: 2000 mg/kg as a single dose
Gammagard S/D: 1000 mg/kg as a single dose administered over 10 hours, **or** 400 mg/kg/day for 4 days. Begin within 7 days of onset of fever.

Dosage Forms

Injection, powder for reconstitution [preservative free, nanofiltered]:
Carimune® NF: 3 g, 6 g, 12 g
Injection, powder for reconstitution [preservative free, solvent detergent-treated]:
Gammagard S/D: 2.5 g, 5 g, 10 g
Injection, solution [preservative free; solvent detergent-treated]:
Gammagard Liquid: 10% (10 mL, 25 mL, 50 mL, 100 mL, 200 mL)
Injection, solution [preservative free]:
Flebogamma®: 5% (10 mL, 50 mL, 100 mL, 200 mL)
Gamunex®: 10% (10 mL, 25 mL, 50 mL, 100 mL, 200 mL)
Privigen™: 10% (50 mL, 100 mL, 200 mL)

immune globulin (subcutaneous) (i MYUN GLOB yoo lin sub kyoo TAY nee us)

Synonyms immune globulin subcutaneous (human); SCIG

U.S./Canadian Brand Names Vivaglobin® [US]

Therapeutic Category Immune Globulin

Use Treatment of primary immune deficiency (PID)

Usual Dosage Note: Consider premedicating with acetaminophen and diphenhydramine.
SubQ infusion: Children ≥2 years and Adults: 100-200 mg/kg weekly (maximum rate: 20 mL/hour; doses >15 mL should be divided between sites); adjust the dose over time to achieve desired clinical response or target IgG levels
Conversion from I.V. to SubQ: Multiply previous I.V. dose by 1.37, then divide into a weekly regimen by dividing by the previous I.V. dosing interval (eg, if the dosing interval was every 3 weeks, divide by 3); adjust the dose over time to achieve desired clinical response or target IgG levels. SubQ infusion administration should begin 1 week after the last I.V. dose.

Dosage Forms

Injection, solution [preservative free]:
Vivaglobin®: IgG 160 mg/mL (3 mL, 10 mL, 20 mL)

immune globulin subcutaneous (human) *see* immune globulin (subcutaneous) *on page 524*
immune serum globulin *see* immune globulin (intramuscular) *on page 522*
Immunine® VH [Can] *see* factor IX *on page 403*
Imodium® [Can] *see* loperamide *on page 597*
Imodium® A-D [US-OTC] *see* loperamide *on page 597*
Imodium® Advanced *(Discontinued)* *see* loperamide and simethicone *on page 598*
Imodium® Multi-Symptom Relief [US-OTC] *see* loperamide and simethicone *on page 598*
Imogam® Rabies-HT [US] *see* rabies immune globulin (human) *on page 848*
Imogam® Rabies Pasteurized [Can] *see* rabies immune globulin (human) *on page 848*
Imovane® [Can] *see* zopiclone *(Canada only) on page 1034*
Imovax® Rabies [US/Can] *see* rabies vaccine *on page 848*
Implanon™ [US] *see* etonogestrel *on page 398*
Imuran® [US/Can] *see* azathioprine *on page 115*

In-111 ibritumomab *see* ibritumomab *on page 515*
In-111 zevalin *see* ibritumomab *on page 515*

inamrinone (eye NAM ri none)

Sound-Alike/Look-Alike Issues
amrinone may be confused with aMILoride, amiodarone
Synonyms amrinone lactate
Therapeutic Category Adrenergic Agonist Agent
Use Short-term therapy in patients with intractable heart failure
Usual Dosage Dosage is based on clinical response (**Note:** Dose should not exceed 10 mg/kg/24 hours).
Adults: 0.75 mg/kg I.V. bolus over 2-3 minutes followed by maintenance infusion of 5-10 mcg/kg/minute; I.V. bolus may need to be repeated in 30 minutes.
Dosage Forms
Injection, solution: 5 mg/mL (20 mL)

I-Naphline® Ophthalmic ***(Discontinued)*** *see* naphazoline *on page 680*
Inapsine® ***(Discontinued)*** *see* droperidol *on page 340*
Increlex™ [US] *see* mecasermin *on page 618*

indapamide (in DAP a mide)

Sound-Alike/Look-Alike Issues
indapamide may be confused with Iopidine®
U.S./Canadian Brand Names Apo-Indapamide® [Can]; Dom-Indapamide [Can]; Gen-Indapamide [Can]; Lozide® [Can]; Lozol® [Can]; Novo-Indapamide [Can]; Nu-Indapamide [Can]; PHL-Indapamide [Can]; PMS-Indapamide [Can]; Pro-Indapamide [Can]; Riva-Indapamide [Can]
Therapeutic Category Diuretic, Miscellaneous
Use Management of mild-to-moderate hypertension; treatment of edema in heart failure and nephrotic syndrome
Usual Dosage Oral: Adults:
Edema: 2.5-5 mg/day. **Note:** There is little therapeutic benefit to increasing the dose >5 mg/day; there is, however, an increased risk of electrolyte disturbances
Hypertension: 1.25 mg in the morning, may increase to 5 mg/day by increments of 1.25-2.5 mg; consider adding another antihypertensive and decreasing the dose if response is not adequate
Dosage Forms
Tablet: 1.25 mg, 2.5 mg

indapamide and perindopril erbumine *see* perindopril erbumine and indapamide *(Canada only) on page 768*
Inderal® [Can] *see* propranolol *on page 828*
Inderal® ***(Discontinued)*** *see* propranolol *on page 828*
Inderal® LA [US/Can] *see* propranolol *on page 828*
Inderide® ***(Discontinued)*** *see* propranolol and hydrochlorothiazide *on page 829*
indigo carmine *see* indigotindisulfonate sodium *on page 525*

indigotindisulfonate sodium (in di goe tin dye SUL foe nate SOW dee um)

Synonyms indigo carmine
Therapeutic Category Diagnostic Agent, Kidney Function
Use Localizing ureteral orifices during cystoscopy and ureteral catheterization
Usual Dosage I.M., I.V. (preferred): Localizing ureteral orifices:
Infants and Children: Doses <5 mL preferred to avoid skin discoloration (usual adult dose: 5 mL)
Adults: Usually 5 mL; doses <5 mL preferred in underweight adults to avoid skin discoloration
Dosage Forms Injection, solution: 8 mg/mL (5 mL)

indinavir (in DIN a veer)

Sound-Alike/Look-Alike Issues
indinavir may be confused with Denavir™
Synonyms indinavir sulfate
U.S./Canadian Brand Names Crixivan® [US/Can]

Therapeutic Category Antiviral Agent

Use Treatment of HIV infection; should always be used as part of a multidrug regimen (at least three antiretroviral agents)

Usual Dosage Oral: Adults: Unboosted regimen: 800 mg every 8 hours

Ritonavir-boosted regimens:

Ritonavir 100-200 mg twice daily plus indinavir 800 mg twice daily **or**

Ritonavir 400 mg twice daily plus indinavir 400 mg twice daily

Dosage Forms

Capsule:

Crixivan®: 100 mg, 200 mg, 333 mg, 400 mg

indinavir sulfate *see* indinavir *on page* 525

Indocid® P.D.A. [Can] *see* indomethacin *on page* 526

Indocin® [US/Can] *see* indomethacin *on page* 526

Indocin® I.V. [US] *see* indomethacin *on page* 526

indocyanine green (in doe SYE a neen green)

U.S./Canadian Brand Names IC-Green™ [US]

Therapeutic Category Diagnostic Agent

Use Determining hepatic function, cardiac output, and liver blood flow; ophthalmic angiography

Usual Dosage Adults:

Ophthalmic angiography: Use doses of up to 40 mg of dye in 2 mL of aqueous solvent, in some patients, half the volume (1 mL) has been found to produce angiograms of comparable resolution; immediately following the bolus dose of dye, a bolus of sodium chloride 0.9% 5 mL is given; this regimen will deliver a spatially limited dye bolus of optimal concentration to the choroidal vasculature following I.V. injection into the antecubital vein.

Cardiac output determination: Dye is injected as rapidly as possible through a cardiac catheter; the usual dose is 1.25 mg for infants, 2.5 mg for children, and 5 mg for adults; total dose should not exceed 2 mg/kg; the dye should be flushed from the catheter with sodium chloride 0.9% to prevent hemolysis

Dosage Forms

Injection, powder for reconstitution: 25 mg

IC-Green™: 25 mg

Indo-Lemmon [Can] *see* indomethacin *on page* 526

indometacin *see* indomethacin *on page* 526

indomethacin (in doe METH a sin)

Sound-Alike/Look-Alike Issues

Indocin® may be confused with Imodium®, Lincocin®, Minocin®, Vicodin®

Synonyms indometacin; indomethacin sodium trihydrate

U.S./Canadian Brand Names Apo-Indomethacin® [Can]; Indo-Lemmon [Can]; Indocid® P.D.A. [Can]; Indocin® I.V. [US]; Indocin® [US/Can]; Indotec [Can]; Novo-Methacin [Can]; Nu-Indo [Can]; Rhodacine® [Can]

Therapeutic Category Analgesic, Nonnarcotic; Nonsteroidal Antiinflammatory Drug (NSAID)

Use Acute gouty arthritis, acute bursitis/tendonitis, moderate-to-severe osteoarthritis, rheumatoid arthritis, ankylosing spondylitis; I.V. form used as alternative to surgery for closure of patent ductus arteriosus in neonates

Usual Dosage

Patent ductus arteriosus:

Neonates: I.V.: Initial: 0.2 mg/kg, followed by 2 doses depending on postnatal age (PNA):

PNA **at time of first dose** <48 hours: 0.1 mg/kg at 12- to 24-hour intervals

PNA **at time of first dose** 2-7 days: 0.2 mg/kg at 12- to 24-hour intervals

PNA **at time of first dose** >7 days: 0.25 mg/kg at 12- to 24-hour intervals

In general, may use 12-hour dosing interval if urine output >1 mL/kg/hour after prior dose; use 24-hour dosing interval if urine output is <1 mL/kg/hour but >0.6 mL/kg/hour; doses should be withheld if patient has oliguria (urine output <0.6 mL/kg/hour) or anuria

Inflammatory/rheumatoid disorders: Oral: Use lowest effective dose.

Children ≥2 years: 1-2 mg/kg/day in 2-4 divided doses; maximum dose: 4 mg/kg/day; not to exceed 150-200 mg/day

Adults: 25-50 mg/dose 2-3 times/day; maximum dose: 200 mg/day; extended release capsule should be given on a 1-2 times/day schedule (maximum dose for extended release: 150 mg/day). In patients with arthritis and persistent night pain and/or morning stiffness may give the larger portion (up to 100 mg) of the total daily dose at bedtime.

Bursitis/tendonitis: Oral: Adults: Initial dose: 75-150 mg/day in 3-4 divided doses **or** 1-2 divided doses for extended release; usual treatment is 7-14 days

Acute gouty arthritis: Oral: Adults: 50 mg 3 times daily until pain is tolerable then reduce dose; usual treatment <3-5 days

Dosage Forms

Capsule: 25 mg, 50 mg

Capsule, extended release, oral: 75 mg

Injection, powder for reconstitution:

Indocin® I.V.: 1 mg

Suppository, rectal: 50 mg (30s)

Suspension, oral: 25 mg/5 mL

Indocin®: 25 mg/5 mL

indomethacin sodium trihydrate *see* indomethacin *on page 526*

Indotec [Can] *see* indomethacin *on page 526*

INF-alpha 2 *see* interferon alfa-2b *on page 534*

Infanrix® [US] *see* diphtheria, tetanus toxoids, and acellular pertussis vaccine *on page 321*

Infantaire [US-OTC] *see* acetaminophen *on page 19*

Infantaire Gas Drops [US-OTC] *see* simethicone *on page 901*

Infants' Tylenol® Cold Plus Cough Concentrated Drops *(Discontinued)*

Infasurf® [US] *see* calfactant *on page 175*

INFeD® [US] *see* iron dextran complex *on page 546*

Infergen® [US] *see* interferon alfacon-1 *on page 535*

Inflamase® Mild [Can] *see* prednisolone (ophthalmic) *on page 813*

infliximab (in FLIKS e mab)

Sound-Alike/Look-Alike Issues

inFLIXimab may be confused with riTUXimab

Remicade® may be confused with Renacidin®, Rituxan®

Synonyms avakine; infliximab, recombinant

Tall-Man in**FLIX**imab

U.S./Canadian Brand Names Remicade® [US/Can]

Therapeutic Category Monoclonal Antibody

Use

Treatment of moderately- to severely-active rheumatoid arthritis (with methotrexate)

Treatment of moderately- to severely-active Crohn disease with inadequate response to conventional therapy (to reduce signs/symptoms and induce and maintain clinical remission) or to reduce the number of draining enterocutaneous and rectovaginal fistulas and maintain fistula closure

Treatment of psoriatic arthritis (to reduce signs/symptoms of active arthritis and inhibit progression of structural damage and improve physical function)

Treatment of chronic severe plaque psoriasis

Treatment of active ankylosing spondylitis (reduce signs/symptoms)

Treatment of moderately- to severely-active ulcerative colitis with inadequate response to conventional therapy (reduce signs/symptoms and induce and maintain clinical remission, mucosal healing and eliminate corticosteroid use)

Usual Dosage I.V.: **Note:** Premedication with antihistamines (H_1-antagonist and/or H_2-antagonist), acetaminophen and/or corticosteroids may be considered to prevent and/or manage infusion-related reactions:

Children: U.S. labeling ≥6 years, Canadian labeling ≥9 years: Crohn disease: 5 mg/kg at 0, 2, and 6 weeks, followed by a maintenance dose of 5 mg/kg every 8 weeks; if no response by week 14, consider discontinuing therapy

Adults:

Crohn disease: Induction regimen: 5 mg/kg at 0, 2, and 6 weeks, followed by 5 mg/kg every 8 weeks thereafter; dose may be increased to 10 mg/kg in patients who respond but then lose their response. If no response by week 14, consider discontinuing therapy.

Psoriatic arthritis (with or without methotrexate): 5 mg/kg at 0, 2, and 6 weeks, then every 8 weeks

Rheumatoid arthritis (in combination with methotrexate therapy): 3 mg/kg at 0, 2, and 6 weeks, then every 8 weeks thereafter; doses have ranged from 3-10 mg/kg intravenous infusion repeated at 4- to 8-week intervals

Ankylosing spondylitis: 5 mg/kg at 0, 2, and 6 weeks, followed by 5 mg/kg every 6 weeks thereafter

Plaque psoriasis: 5 mg/kg at 0, 2, and 6 weeks, then every 8 weeks thereafter

Ulcerative colitis: 5 mg/kg at 0, 2, and 6 weeks, followed by 5 mg/kg every 8 weeks thereafter

Dosage Forms

Injection, powder for reconstitution [preservative free]:

Remicade®: 100 mg

infliximab, recombinant *see* infliximab *on page* *527*

influenza virus vaccine (in floo EN za VYE rus vak SEEN)

Sound-Alike/Look-Alike Issues

influenza virus vaccine may be confused with flumazenil

influenza virus vaccine (human strain) may be confused with the avian strain (H5N1) of influenza virus vaccine

Influenza virus vaccine may be confused with tetanus toxoid and tuberculin products. Medication errors have occurred when tuberculin skin tests (PPD) have been inadvertently administered instead of tetanus toxoid products and influenza virus vaccine. These products are refrigerated and often stored in close proximity to each other.

Fluarix® may be confused with Flarex®

Synonyms influenza virus vaccine (purified surface antigen); influenza virus vaccine (split-virus); influenza virus vaccine (trivalent, live); live attenuated influenza vaccine (LAIV); trivalent inactivated influenza vaccine (TIV)

U.S./Canadian Brand Names Afluria® [US]; Fluarix® [US]; FluLaval® [US]; FluMist® [US]; Fluviral S/F® [Can]; Fluvirin® [US]; Fluzone® [US]; Vaxigrip® [Can]

Therapeutic Category Vaccine, Inactivated Virus

Use Provide active immunity to influenza virus strains contained in the vaccine

Advisory Committee on Immunization Practices (ACIP) recommends annual vaccination for all children (6 months to 18 years) and adults. Target groups for vaccination (those at higher risk of complications from influenza infection and their close contacts) include the following:

- Persons ≥50 years of age
- Residents of nursing homes and other chronic-care facilities that house persons of any age with chronic medical conditions
- Adults and children with chronic disorders of the pulmonary or cardiovascular systems (except hypertension), including asthma
- Adults and children who have chronic metabolic diseases (including diabetes mellitus), hepatic disease, renal dysfunction, hematologic disorders, hemoglobinopathies, or immunosuppression (including immunosuppression caused by medications or HIV)
- Adults and children with conditions which may compromise respiratory function, the handling of respiratory secretions, or that can increase the risk of aspiration (eg, cognitive dysfunction, spinal; cord injuries, seizure disorders, other neuromuscular disorders)
- Children and adolescents (6 months to 18 years of age) who are receiving long-term aspirin therapy and therefore, may be at risk for developing Reye syndrome after influenza
- Women who will be pregnant during the influenza season
- Children 6-59 months of age
- Healthcare personnel
- Household contacts and caregivers of children <5 years (particularly children <6 months) and adults ≥50 years
- Household contacts and caregivers of persons with medical conditions which put them at high risk of complications from influenza infection

Usual Dosage It is important to note that influenza seasons vary in their timing and duration from year to year. In general, vaccination should begin soon after the vaccine becomes available and if possible, prior to October. However, vaccination should continue throughout the influenza season as long as vaccine is available.

Note: Children <9 years who are not previously vaccinated or who received only 1 dose of vaccine during the previous season (if it was their first year of vaccination) should receive 2 doses separated by ≥4 weeks, in order to achieve satisfactory antibody response per ACIP recommendations.

I.M.:
Fluzone®:
Children 6-35 months: 0.25 mL/dose (1 or 2 doses per season; see **Note**)
Children 3-8 years: 0.5 mL/dose (1 or 2 doses per season; see **Note**)
Children ≥9 years and Adults: 0.5 mL/dose (1 dose per season)
Fluvirin®:
Children 4-8 years: 0.5 mL/dose (1 or 2 doses per season; see **Note**)
Children ≥9 years and Adults: 0.5 mL/dose (1 dose per season)
Afluria®, Fluarix®, FluLaval®: Adults: 0.5 mL/dose (1 dose per season)
Intranasal (FluMist®):
Children 2-8 years, previously **not vaccinated** with influenza vaccine: Two doses (0.2 mL/dose) separated by at least 4 weeks (see **Note**)
Children 2-8 years, previously **vaccinated** with influenza vaccine: 0.2 mL/dose (1 dose per season; see **Note**)
Children ≥9 years and Adults ≤49 years: 0.2 mL/dose (1 dose per season)

Dosage Forms
Injection, suspension [purified split-virus]:
Afluria®, FluLaval®, Fluvirin®, Fluzone®: 5 mL
Injection, suspension [purified split-virus; preservative free]:
Afluria®, Fluarix®, Fluvirin®: 0.5 mL
Fluzone®: 0.25 mL, 0.5 mL
Solution, intranasal [preservative free; spray]:
FluMist®: 0.2 mL

influenza virus vaccine (H5N1) (in floo EN za VYE rus vak SEEN H5N1)

Sound-Alike/Look-Alike Issues
influenza virus vaccine (H5N1) may be confused with the nonavian strain of influenza virus vaccine

Synonyms avian influenza virus vaccine; bird flu vaccine; H5N1 influenza vaccine; influenza virus vaccine (monovalent)

Therapeutic Category Vaccine

Use Active immunization of adults at increased risk of exposure to the H5N1 viral subtype of influenza

Usual Dosage I.M.: Adults 18-64 years: 1 mL, followed by second 1 mL dose given 28 days later (acceptable range: 21-35 days)

Dosage Forms
Injection, suspension [monovalent]: Hemagglutinin (H5N1 strain) 90 mcg/1 mL (5 mL)

influenza virus vaccine (monovalent) *see* influenza virus vaccine (H5N1) *on page 529*
influenza virus vaccine (purified surface antigen) *see* influenza virus vaccine *on page 528*
influenza virus vaccine (split-virus) *see* influenza virus vaccine *on page 528*
influenza virus vaccine (trivalent, live) *see* influenza virus vaccine *on page 528*
Infufer® [Can] *see* iron dextran complex *on page 546*
Infumorph® 200 [US] *see* morphine sulfate *on page 667*
Infumorph® 500 [US] *see* morphine sulfate *on page 667*
Infuvite® Adult [US] *see* vitamins (multiple/injectable) *on page 1019*
Infuvite® Pediatric [US] *see* vitamins (multiple/injectable) *on page 1019*
INH *see* isoniazid *on page 548*
Inhibace® [Can] *see* cilazapril *(Canada only) on page 228*
Inhibace® Plus [Can] *see* cilazapril and hydrochlorothiazide *(Canada only) on page 228*
Innohep® [US/Can] *see* tinzaparin *on page 962*
InnoPran XL™ [US] *see* propranolol *on page 828*
Inocor® *(Discontinued)*
INOmax® [US/Can] *see* nitric oxide *on page 699*
Inova™ [US] *see* benzoyl peroxide *on page 132*
insect sting kit *see* epinephrine and chlorpheniramine *on page 360*
insoluble prussian blue *see* ferric hexacyanoferrate *on page 413*
Inspra™ [US] *see* eplerenone *on page 361*
Insta-Glucose® [US-OTC] *see* dextrose *on page 298*
Instat™ [US] *see* collagen hemostat *on page 255*

Instat™ MCH [US] *see* collagen hemostat *on page* 255

insulin aspart (IN soo lin AS part)

Sound-Alike/Look-Alike Issues

NovoLog® may be confused with Humalog®, Novolin®

NovoLog® Mix 70/30 may be confused with NovoLog®

Synonyms aspart insulin

U.S./Canadian Brand Names NovoLog® [US]; NovoRapid® [Can]

Therapeutic Category Antidiabetic Agent, Insulin

Use Treatment of type 1 diabetes mellitus (insulin-dependent, IDDM) and type 2 diabetes mellitus (noninsulin-dependent, NIDDM) to improve glycemic control

Usual Dosage Note: When compared to insulin regular, insulin aspart has a more rapid onset and shorter duration of activity.

SubQ: Diabetes mellitus: Type 1: Children ≥2 years and Adults: Refer to insulin regular on page 533

I.V.: Glycemic control in selected clinical situations and under appropriate medical supervision: Adults: Refer to insulin regular on page 533

Dosage Forms

Injection, solution:

NovoLog®: 100 units/mL (3 mL) [FlexPen® prefilled syringe or PenFill® prefilled cartridge]; (10 mL)

insulin aspart and insulin aspart protamine *see* insulin aspart protamine and insulin aspart *on page* 530

insulin aspart protamine and insulin aspart

(IN soo lin AS part PROE ta meen & IN soo lin AS part)

Sound-Alike/Look-Alike Issues

NovoLog® Mix 70/30 may be confused with Novolin® 70/30

Synonyms insulin aspart and insulin aspart protamine

U.S./Canadian Brand Names NovoLog® Mix 70/30 [US]; NovoMix® 30 [Can]

Therapeutic Category Antidiabetic Agent, Insulin

Use Treatment of type 1 diabetes mellitus (insulin-dependent, IDDM) and type 2 diabetes mellitus (noninsulin-dependent, NIDDM) to improve glycemic control

Usual Dosage Note: Insulin aspart protamine and insulin aspart combination products are approximately equipotent to insulin NPH and insulin regular combination products but with a more rapid onset and similar duration of activity.

SubQ: Diabetes mellitus, type 1 and type 2: Adults: Refer to insulin regular on page 533

Dosage Forms

Injection, suspension:

NovoLog® Mix 70/30: Insulin aspart protamine suspension 70% [intermediate acting] and insulin aspart solution 30% [rapid acting]: 100 units/mL (3 mL) [FlexPen® prefilled syringe]; (10 mL) [vial]

insulin detemir (IN soo lin DE te mir)

Synonyms detemir insulin

U.S./Canadian Brand Names Levemir® [US/Can]

Therapeutic Category Antidiabetic Agent, Insulin

Use Treatment of type 1 diabetes mellitus (insulin-dependent, IDDM) and type 2 diabetes mellitus (noninsulin-dependent, NIDDM) to improve glycemic control

Usual Dosage Also refer to insulin regular on page 533.

Note: Duration is dose-dependent. Dosage must be carefully titrated (adjustment of dose and timing. Adjustment of concomitant antidiabetic treatment (short-acting insulins or oral antidiabetic agents) may be required. In Canada, insulin detemir is not approved for use in children.

SubQ: Children ≥6 years and Adults:

Basal insulin or basal-bolus (Type 1 or type 2 diabetes): May be substituted on a unit-per-unit basis. Adjust dose to achieve glycemic targets.

Insulin-naive patients (type 2 diabetes only): 0.1-0.2 units/kg once daily in the evening or 10 units once or twice daily. Adjust dose to achieve glycemic targets. **Note:** Canadian labeling recommends 10 units once daily (twice daily dosing is not included).

Dosage Forms

Injection, solution:

Levemir®: 100 units/mL (3 mL) [FlexPen® prefilled syringe]; (10 mL) [vial]

insulin glargine (IN soo lin GLAR jeen)

Sound-Alike/Look-Alike Issues

insulin glargine may be confused with insulin glulisine
Lantus® may be confused with Lente®

Synonyms glargine insulin

U.S./Canadian Brand Names Lantus® OptiSet® [Can]; Lantus® [US/Can]

Therapeutic Category Antidiabetic Agent, Insulin

Use Treatment of type 1 diabetes mellitus (insulin-dependent, IDDM) and type 2 diabetes mellitus (noninsulin-dependent, NIDDM) requiring basal (long-acting) insulin to improve glycemic control

Usual Dosage SubQ: Children ≥6 years and Adults:

Type 1 diabetes: As a basal component of combination insulin regimen, normally 50% to 75% of daily insulin requirement is administered as a long-acting form. More rapid acting forms are usually used in association with meals. Refer to insulin regular on page 533.

Type 2 diabetes:

Patient not already on insulin: 10 units once daily, adjusted according to patient response (range in clinical study: 2-100 units/day)

Patient already receiving insulin: In clinical studies, when changing to insulin glargine from once-daily NPH or Ultralente® insulin, the initial dose was not changed; when changing from twice-daily NPH to once-daily insulin glargine, the total daily dose was reduced by 20% and adjusted according to patient response

Dosage Forms

Injection, solution:

Lantus®: 100 units/mL (3 mL) [OptiClik® prefilled cartridge or SoloStar® disposable insulin device]; (10 mL) [vial]

insulin glulisine (IN soo lin gloo LIS een)

Sound-Alike/Look-Alike Issues

insulin glulisine may be confused with insulin glargine

Synonyms glulisine insulin

U.S./Canadian Brand Names Apidra® [US/Can]

Therapeutic Category Antidiabetic Agent, Insulin

Use Treatment of type 1 diabetes mellitus (insulin-dependent, IDDM) and type 2 diabetes mellitus (noninsulin-dependent, NIDDM) to improve glycemic control

Usual Dosage Refer to insulin regular on page 533. Insulin glulisine is equipotent to insulin regular, but has a more rapid onset. Insulin glulisine is normally administered as a premeal component of the insulin regimen. It is normally used along with a long-acting (basal) form of insulin or continuous basal administration of insulin via a SubQ infusion pump.

SubQ: When used in a meal-related treatment regimen, 50% to 70% of total daily insulin requirement may be provided by insulin glulisine (in divided doses) and the remainder provided by an intermediate- or long-acting insulin. Insulin glulisine may also be administered by external subcutaneous infusion pumps.

I.V.: Under close medical supervision, insulin glulisine may be administered by infusion.

Dosage Forms

Injection, solution:

Apidra®: 100 units/mL (3 mL [cartridge], 3 mL [SoloStar® prefilled pen], 10 mL [vial])

insulin lispro (IN soo lin LYE sproe)

Sound-Alike/Look-Alike Issues

Humalog® may be confused with Humulin®, Humira®, Novolog®

Synonyms lispro insulin

U.S./Canadian Brand Names Humalog® [US/Can]

Therapeutic Category Antidiabetic Agent, Insulin

Use Treatment of type 1 diabetes mellitus (insulin-dependent, IDDM) and type 2 diabetes mellitus (noninsulin-dependent, NIDDM) to improve glycemic control

Usual Dosage Refer to insulin regular monograph on page 533. Insulin lispro is equipotent to insulin regular, but has a more rapid onset.

Dosage Forms

Injection, solution:

Humalog®: 100 units/mL (3 mL) [prefilled cartridge or prefilled disposable pen]; (10 mL) [vial]

insulin lispro and insulin lispro protamine *see* insulin lispro protamine and insulin lispro *on page 532*

insulin lispro protamine and insulin lispro

(IN soo lin LYE sproe PROE ta meen & IN soo lin LYE sproe)

Sound-Alike/Look-Alike Issues

Humalog® Mix 75/25™ may be confused with Humulin® 70/30.

Synonyms insulin lispro and insulin lispro protamine

U.S./Canadian Brand Names Humalog® Mix 25 [Can]; Humalog® Mix 50/50™ [US]; Humalog® Mix 75/25™ [US]

Therapeutic Category Antidiabetic Agent, Insulin

Use Treatment of type 1 diabetes mellitus (insulin-dependent, IDDM) and type 2 diabetes mellitus (noninsulin-dependent, NIDDM) to improve glycemic control

Usual Dosage Refer to insulin regular monograph on page 533. Fixed ratio insulins (such as insulin lispro protamine and insulin lispro) are normally administered in 2 daily doses.

Dosage Forms

Injection, suspension:

Humalog® Mix 50/50™: Insulin lispro protamine suspension 50% [intermediate acting] and insulin lispro solution 50% [rapid acting]: 100 units/mL (3 mL) [disposable pen]; (10 mL) [vial]

Humalog® Mix 75/25™: Insulin lispro protamine suspension 75% [intermediate acting] and insulin lispro solution 25% [rapid acting]: 100 units/mL (3 mL) [disposable pen]; (10 mL) [vial]

insulin NPH (IN soo lin N P H)

Sound-Alike/Look-Alike Issues

Humulin® may be confused with Humalog®, Humira®, Novolin®

Novolin® may be confused with Humulin®, NovoLog®

Synonyms isophane insulin; NPH insulin

U.S./Canadian Brand Names Humulin® N [US/Can]; Novolin® ge NPH [Can]; Novolin® N [US]

Therapeutic Category Insulin, Intermediate-Acting

Use Treatment of type 1 diabetes mellitus (insulin-dependent, IDDM) and type 2 diabetes mellitus (noninsulin-dependent, NIDDM) to improve glycemic control

Usual Dosage Note: When compared to insulin regular, insulin NPH has a slower onset and longer duration of activity.

SubQ: Diabetes mellitus, type 1 and type 2: Children and Adults: Refer to insulin regular on page 533

Dosage Forms [CAN] = Canadian brand name

Injection, suspension:

Humulin® N, Novolin® N: 100 units/mL (3 mL, 10 mL)

Novolin® ge NPH [CAN]: 100 units/mL (3 mL, 10 mL) [not available in the U.S.]

insulin NPH and insulin regular (IN soo lin N P H & IN soo lin REG yoo ler)

Sound-Alike/Look-Alike Issues

Humulin® 70/30 may be confused with Humalog® Mix 75/25, Novolin® 70/30

Novolin® 70/30 may be confused with Humulin® 70/30, NovoLog® Mix 70/30

Synonyms insulin regular and insulin NPH; isophane insulin and regular insulin; NPH insulin and regular insulin

U.S./Canadian Brand Names Humulin® 20/80 [Can]; Humulin® 70/30 [US/Can]; Novolin® 70/30 [US]; Novolin® ge 30/70 [Can]; Novolin® ge 40/60 [Can]; Novolin® ge 50/50 [Can]

Therapeutic Category Antidiabetic Agent, Insulin

Use Treatment of type 1 diabetes mellitus (insulin-dependent, IDDM) and type 2 diabetes mellitus (noninsulin-dependent, NIDDM) to improve glycemic control

Usual Dosage Note: When compared to insulin NPH, the combination product (insulin NPH and insulin regular) has a more rapid onset of action and a similar duration of action.

SubQ: Diabetes mellitus, type 1 and type 2: Children and Adults: Refer to insulin regular on page 533

Dosage Forms

Injection, suspension:

Humulin® 70/30: Insulin NPH suspension 70% [intermediate acting] and insulin regular solution 30% [short acting]: 100 units/mL (3 mL, 10 mL)

Novolin® 70/30: Insulin NPH suspension 70% [intermediate acting] and insulin regular solution 30% [short acting]: 100 units/mL (3 mL, 10 mL)

Additional formulations available in Canada [not available in the U.S.]:

Injection, suspension:

Humulin® 20/80: Insulin regular solution 20% [short acting] and insulin NPH suspension 80% [intermediate acting]: 100 units/mL (3 mL)

Novolin® ge 30/70: Insulin regular solution 30% [short acting] and insulin NPH suspension 70% [intermediate acting]: 100 units/mL (3 mL)

Novolin® ge 40/60: Insulin regular solution 40% [short acting] and insulin NPH suspension 60% [intermediate acting]: 100 units/mL (3 mL)

Novolin® ge 50/50: Insulin regular solution 50% [short acting] and insulin NPH suspension 50% [intermediate acting]: 100 units/mL (3 mL)

insulin regular (IN soo lin REG yoo ler)

Sound-Alike/Look-Alike Issues

Humulin® may be confused with Humalog®, Humira®, Novolin®

Novolin® may be confused with Humulin®, NovoLog®

Synonyms regular insulin

U.S./Canadian Brand Names Humulin® R U-500 [US]; Humulin® R [US/Can]; Novolin® ge Toronto [Can]; Novolin® R [US]

Therapeutic Category Antidiabetic Agent, Insulin; Antidote

Use Treatment of type 1 diabetes mellitus (insulin-dependent, IDDM); type 2 diabetes mellitus (noninsulin-dependent, NIDDM) unresponsive to treatment with diet and/or oral hypoglycemics, to improve glycemic control; adjunct to parenteral nutrition; diabetic ketoacidosis (DKA)

Usual Dosage

Diabetes mellitus: SubQ: **Note:** Insulin requirements vary dramatically between patients and therapy requires dosage adjustments with careful medical supervision. Specific formulations may require distinct administration procedures; please see individual agents.

Type 1: Children and Adults: **Note:** Multiple daily injections (MDI) guided by blood glucose monitoring or the use of continuous subcutaneous insulin infusions (CSII) is the standard of care for patients with type 1 diabetes. Combinations of insulin formulations are commonly used.

Initial dose: 0.5-1.0 units/kg/day in divided doses. Conservative initial doses of 0.2-0.4 units/kg/day may be recommended to avoid the potential for hypoglycemia.

Division of daily insulin requirement: Generally, 50% to 75% of the total daily dose (TDD) is given as an intermediate- or long-acting form of insulin (in 1-2 daily injections). The remaining portion of the TDD is then divided and administered before or at mealtimes (depending on the formulation) as a rapid-acting or short-acting form of insulin. Premixed combinations are available that deliver the rapid- or short-acting component at the same time as the intermediate- or long-acting component. Some patients may benefit from the use of CSII which delivers rapid-acting insulin as a continuous infusion throughout the day and as boluses at mealtimes via an external pump device.

Adjustment of dose: Dosage must be titrated to achieve glucose control and avoid hypoglycemia. Adjust dose to maintain preprandial plasma glucose between 70-130 mg/dL for most patients. Since treatment regimens often consist of multiple formulations, dosage adjustments must address the specific phase of insulin release that is primarily contributing to the patient's impaired glycemic control. Treatment and monitoring regimens must be individualized.

Usual maintenance range: 0.5-1.2 units/kg/day in divided doses. Insulin requirements are patient-specific and may vary based on age, body weight, and/or activity factors:

Adolescents: May require as much as 1.5 units/kg/day during puberty

Prepuberty: 0.7-1 unit/kg/day

Type 2: Children and Adults: The goal of therapy is to achieve an Hb A_{1c} <7% as quickly as possible using the safe titration of medications. According to a consensus statement by the ADA and European Association for the Study of Diabetes (EASD), basal insulin therapy (eg, intermediate- or long-acting insulin) should be considered in patients with type 2 diabetes who fail to achieve glycemic goals with lifestyle interventions and metformin ± a sulfonylurea. Pioglitazone or a GLP-1 agonist may also be considered prior to initiation of basal insulin therapy. In patients who continue to fail to achieve glycemic goals despite the addition of basal insulin, intensification of insulin therapy should be considered; this generally consists of multiple daily injections with a combination of insulin formulations.

Initial basal insulin dose: 0.2 units/kg or 10 units/day. **Note:** Current guidelines recommend that insulin therapy begin with intermediate- or long-acting insulin given at bedtime or long-acting insulin given in the morning.

Adjustment of basal insulin dose: Increase dose by 2 units/day every 3 days until fasting glucose levels are consistently within target range (70-130 mg/dL); may increase dose in larger increments (eg, 4 units/day) if fasting glucose levels are >180 mg/dL

Note: If the patient experiences hypoglycemia following adjustment, reduce dose by 4 units/day or 10% of total daily dose, whichever is greater. Additional algorithms, such as the "1-1-100", "2-4-6-8", "3-0-3", and "3-2-1" algorithms, exist to aid in the titration of basal insulin; therapy should be individualized and based on patient-specific details.

Intensification of therapy: Add a second injection of a short-, rapid-, or intermediate-acting insulin as needed based on blood glucose monitoring; the timing of administration and type of insulin added for intensification of therapy depends on the blood glucose level that is consistently out of the target range (eg, preprandial glucose levels before lunch or dinner, postprandial glucose levels, and/or bedtime glucose levels). Additional injections and subsequent dosage adjustments must address the specific phase of insulin release that is primarily contributing to the patient's impaired glycemic control. Intensification of therapy can usually begin with a second injection of ~4 units/day followed by adjustments of ~2 units/day every 3 days until the targeted blood glucose is within range.

In the setting of glucose toxicity (loss of beta-cell sensitivity to glucose concentrations), insulin therapy may be used for short-term management to restore sensitivity of beta-cells; in these cases, the dose may need to be rapidly reduced/withdrawn when sensitivity is re-established.

Dosage Forms

Injection, solution:

Humulin® R: 100 units/mL (10 mL)

Novolin® R: 100 units/mL (3 mL) [InnoLet® prefilled syringe or PenFill® prefilled cartridge]; (10 mL) [vial]

Injection, solution [concentrate]:

Humulin® R U-500: 500 units/mL (20 mL vial)

insulin regular and insulin NPH *see* insulin NPH and insulin regular *on page 532*

Intal® [Can] *see* cromolyn sodium *on page 261*

Intal® *(Discontinued)* *see* cromolyn sodium *on page 261*

Integrilin® [US/Can] *see* eptifibatide *on page 364*

Intelence™ [US/Can] *see* etravirine *on page 399*

Intensol® Solution *(Discontinued)* *see* metoclopramide *on page 649*

interferon alfa-2a *(Discontinued)*

interferon alfa-2a (PEG conjugate) *see* peginterferon alfa-2a *on page 756*

interferon alfa-2b (PEG conjugate) *see* peginterferon alfa-2b *on page 756*

interferon alfa-2b (in ter FEER on AL fa too bee)

Sound-Alike/Look-Alike Issues

interferon alfa-2b may be confused with interferon alfa-2a, interferon alfa-n3, pegylated interferon alfa-2b

Intron® A may be confused with PEG-Intron®

Synonyms INF-alpha 2; interferon alpha-2b; NSC-377523; rLFN-α2; α-2-interferon

U.S./Canadian Brand Names Intron® A [US/Can]

Therapeutic Category Biological Response Modulator

Use

Patients ≥1 year of age: Chronic hepatitis B

Patients ≥3 years of age: Chronic hepatitis C (in combination with ribavirin)

Patients ≥18 years of age: Condyloma acuminata, chronic hepatitis B, chronic hepatitis C, hairy cell leukemia, malignant melanoma, AIDS-related Kaposi sarcoma, follicular non-Hodgkin lymphoma

Usual Dosage Details concerning dosing in combination regimens should also be consulted. **Note:** Withhold treatment for ANC <500/mm^3 or platelets <25,000/mm^3. Consider premedication with acetaminophen prior to administration to reduce the incidence of some adverse reactions. Not all dosage forms and strengths are appropriate for all indications; refer to product labeling for details.

Children 1-17 years: Chronic hepatitis B: SubQ: 3 million units/m^2 3 times/week for 1 week; then 6 million units/m^2 3 times/week; maximum: 10 million units 3 times/week; total duration of therapy 16-24 weeks

Children ≥3 years: Chronic hepatitis C: In combination with ribavirin

Adults:

Hairy cell leukemia: I.M., SubQ: 2 million units/m^2 3 times/week for up to 6 months (may continue treatment with continued treatment response)

Lymphoma (follicular): SubQ: 5 million units 3 times/week for up to 18 months

Malignant melanoma: Induction: 20 million units/m^2 I.V. for 5 consecutive days per week for 4 weeks, followed by maintenance dosing of 10 million units/m^2 SubQ 3 times/week for 48 weeks

AIDS-related Kaposi sarcoma: I.M., SubQ: 30 million units/m^2 3 times/week

Chronic hepatitis B: I.M., SubQ: 5 million units/day or 10 million units 3 times/week for 16 weeks

Chronic hepatitis C: I.M., SubQ: 3 million units 3 times/week for 16 weeks. In patients with normalization of ALT at 16 weeks, continue treatment for 18-24 months; consider discontinuation if normalization does not occur at 16 weeks. **Note:** May be used in combination therapy with ribavirin in previously untreated patients or in patients who relapse following alpha interferon therapy.

Condyloma acuminata: Intralesionally: 1 million units/lesion (maximum: 5 lesions/treatment) 3 times/week (on alternate days) for 3 weeks; may administer a second course at 12-16 weeks

Dosage Forms

Injection, powder for reconstitution [preservative free]:

Intron® A: 10 million int. units; 18 million int. units; 50 million int. units

Injection, solution:

Intron® A:

6 million int. units/mL (3 mL); 10 million int. units/1 mL (2.5 mL) [contains edetate disodium, polysorbate 80]

3 million int. units/0.2 mL (1.2 mL) [contains edetate disodium, polysorbate 80; delivers 6 doses of 0.2 mL each; 18 million int. units total per pen]

5 million int. units/0.2 mL (1.2 mL) [contains edetate disodium, polysorbate 80; delivers 6 doses of 0.2 mL each; 30 million int. units total per pen]

10 million int. units/0.2 mL (1.2 mL) [contains edetate disodium, polysorbate 80; delivers 6 doses of 0.2 mL each; 60 million int. units total per pen]

interferon alfacon-1 (in ter FEER on AL fa con one)

Sound-Alike/Look-Alike Issues

interferon alfacon-1 may be confused with interferon alfa-2a, interferon alfa-2b, interferon alfa-n3, peginterferon alfa-2b

U.S./Canadian Brand Names Infergen® [US]

Therapeutic Category Interferon

Use Treatment of chronic hepatitis C virus (HCV) infection in patients ≥18 years of age with compensated liver disease and anti-HCV serum antibodies or HCV RNA.

Usual Dosage SubQ: Adults ≥18 years:

Chronic HCV infection: 9 mcg 3 times/week for 24 weeks; allow 48 hours between doses

Patients who have previously tolerated interferon therapy but did not respond or relapsed: 15 mcg 3 times/week for up to 48 weeks

Dose reduction for toxicity: Dose should be held in patients who experience a severe adverse reaction, and treatment should be stopped or decreased if the reaction does not become tolerable.

Doses were reduced from 9 mcg to 7.5 mcg in the pivotal study.

For patients receiving 15 mcg/dose, doses were reduced in 3 mcg decrements. Efficacy is decreased with doses <7.5 mcg

Dosage Forms

Injection, solution [preservative free]:

Infergen®: 30 mcg/mL (0.3 mL, 0.5 mL)

interferon alfa-n3 (in ter FEER on AL fa en three)

Sound-Alike/Look-Alike Issues

Alferon® may be confused with Alkeran®

U.S./Canadian Brand Names Alferon® N [US/Can]

Therapeutic Category Biological Response Modulator

Use Patients ≥18 years of age: Intralesional treatment of refractory or recurring genital or venereal warts (condylomata acuminata)

Usual Dosage Adults: Inject 250,000 units (0.05 mL) in each wart twice weekly for a maximum of 8 weeks; therapy should not be repeated for at least 3 months after the initial 8-week course of therapy

Dosage Forms

Injection, solution:

Alferon® N: 5 million int. units (1 mL)

interferon alpha-2b *see* interferon alfa-2b *on page* 534

interferon beta-1a (in ter FEER on BAY ta won aye)

Sound-Alike/Look-Alike Issues

Avonex® may be confused with Avelox®

Synonyms rIFN beta-1a

U.S./Canadian Brand Names Avonex® [US/Can]; Rebif® [US/Can]

Therapeutic Category Biological Response Modulator

Use Treatment of relapsing forms of multiple sclerosis (MS)

Usual Dosage Adults: **Note:** Analgesics and/or antipyretics may help decrease flu-like symptoms on treatment days:

I.M. (Avonex®): 30 mcg once weekly

SubQ (Rebif®): Doses should be separated by at least 48 hours:

Target dose 44 mcg 3 times/week:

Initial: 8.8 mcg (20% of final dose) 3 times/week for 2 weeks

Titration: 22 mcg (50% of final dose) 3 times/week for 2 weeks

Final dose: 44 mcg 3 times/week

Target dose 22 mcg 3 times/week:

Initial: 4.4 mcg (20% of final dose) 3 times/week for 2 weeks

Titration: 11 mcg (50% of final dose) 3 times/week for 2 weeks

Final dose: 22 mcg 3 times/week

Dosage Forms

Combination package [preservative free]:

Rebif® Titration Pack:

Injection, solution: 8.8 mcg/0.2 mL (0.2 mL) [6 prefilled syringes]

Injection, solution: 22 mcg/0.5 mL (0.5 mL) [6 prefilled syringes]

Injection, powder for reconstitution:

Avonex®: 33 mcg [6.6 million units; provides 30 mcg/mL following reconstitution]

Injection, solution:

Avonex®: 30 mcg/0.5 mL (0.5 mL)

Injection, solution [preservative free]:

Rebif®: 22 mcg/0.5 mL (0.5 mL) [prefilled syringe]; 44 mcg/0.5 mL (0.5 mL) [prefilled syringe]

interferon beta-1b (in ter FEER on BAY ta won bee)

Synonyms rIFN beta-1b

U.S./Canadian Brand Names Betaseron® [US/Can]

Therapeutic Category Biological Response Modulator

Use Treatment of relapsing forms of multiple sclerosis (MS); treatment of first clinical episode with MRI features consistent with MS

Usual Dosage SubQ: **Note:** Gradual dose-titration, analgesics, and/or antipyretics may help decrease flu-like symptoms on treatment days:

Adults: Initial: 0.0625 mg (2 million units; 0.25 mL) every other day; gradually increase dose by 0.0625 every 2 weeks

Target dose: 0.25 mg (8 million units; 1 mL) every other day

Dosage Forms

Injection, powder for reconstitution [preservative free]:

Betaseron®: 0.3 mg [9.6 million units] [prefilled syringe]

interferon gamma-1b (in ter FEER on GAM ah won bee)

U.S./Canadian Brand Names Actimmune® [US/Can]

Therapeutic Category Biological Response Modulator

Use Reduce frequency and severity of serious infections associated with chronic granulomatous disease; delay time to disease progression in patients with severe, malignant osteopetrosis

Usual Dosage If severe reactions occur, reduce dose by 50% or therapy should be interrupted until adverse reaction abates.

Children: Severe, malignant osteopetrosis: SubQ:

BSA ≤0.5 m^2: 1.5 mcg/kg/dose 3 times/week

BSA >0.5 m^2: 50 mcg/m^2 (1 million int. units/m^2) 3 times/week

Children and Adults: Chronic granulomatous disease: SubQ:

BSA ≤0.5 m^2: 1.5 mcg/kg/dose 3 times/week

BSA >0.5 m^2: 50 mcg/m^2 (1 million int. units/m^2) 3 times/week

Note: Previously expressed as 1.5 million units/m^2; 50 mcg is equivalent to 1 million int. units/m^2.

Dosage Forms
Injection, solution [preservative free]:
Actimmune®: 100 mcg [2 million int. units] (0.5 mL)

iobenguane I 123 (eye oh BEN gwane eye one TWEN tee three)

Synonyms 123 meta-iodobenzlyguanidine sulfate; 123I-metaiodobenzylguanidine (MIBG); I-123 MIBG; I^{123} iobenguane; iobenguane sulfate I 123

U.S./Canadian Brand Names AdreView™ [US]

Therapeutic Category Radiopharmaceutical

Use As an adjunct to other diagnostic tests, in the detection of primary or metastatic pheochromocytoma or neuroblastoma

Usual Dosage Note: Thyroid protective agents (SSKI, Lugol's solution or potassium iodide), should be given at least 1 hour prior to administration. Perform whole body planar scintigraphy imaging 18-30 hours after Iobenguane I 123 administration.

Radioimaging: I.V.:
Children 1 month to 16 years and <70 kg: Dose according to body weight
Children <16 years and ≥70 kg: 10 mCi (370 MBq)
Children ≥16 years and Adults: 10 mCi (370 MBq)

Pediatric dosing by body weight: Children 1 month to <16 years and <70 kg:
3 kg: 1 mCi (37 MBq)
4 kg: 1.4 mCi (52 MBq)
6 kg: 1.9 mCi (70 MBq)
8 kg: 2.3 mCi (85.1 MBq)
10 kg: 2.7 mCi (99.9 MBq)
12 kg: 3.2 mCi (118.4 MBq)
14 kg: 3.6 mCi (133.2 MBq)
16 kg: 4 mCi (148 MBq)
18 kg: 4.4 mCi (162.8 MBq)
20 kg: 4.6 mCi (170.2 MBq)
22 kg: 5 mCi (185 MBq)
24 kg: 5.3 mCi (196.1 MBq)
26 kg: 5.6 mCi (207.2 MBq)
28 kg: 5.8 mCi (214.6 MBq)
30 kg: 6.2 mCi (229.4 MBq)
32 kg: 6.5 mCi (240.5 MBq)
34 kg: 6.8 mCi (251.6 MBq)
36 kg: 7.1 mCi (262.7 MBq)
38 kg: 7.3 mCi (270.1 MBq)
40 kg: 7.6 mCi (281.2 MBq)
42 kg: 7.8 mCi (288.6 MBq)
44 kg: 8 mCi (296 MBq)
46 kg: 8.2 mCi (303.4 MBq)
48 kg: 8.5 mCi (314.5 MBq)
50 kg: 8.8 mCi (325.6 MBq)

52-54 kg: 9 mCi (333 MBq)
56-58 kg: 9.2 mCi (340.4 MBq)
60-62 kg: 9.6 mCi (355.2 MBq)
64-66 kg: 9.8 mCi (362.6 MBq)
68 kg: 9.9 mCi (366.3 MBq)

Dosage Forms

Injection, solution:
AdreView™: Iobenguane sulfate 0.08 mg and I 123 74 MBq (2 mCi) per mL (5 mL)

iobenguane sulfate I 123 *see* iobenguane I 123 *on page 537*

Iodex [US-OTC] *see* iodine *on page 538*

Iodex-p® ***(Discontinued)*** *see* povidone-iodine *on page 807*

iodine (EYE oh dyne)

Sound-Alike/Look-Alike Issues
iodine may be confused with codeine, Iopidine®, Lodine®

U.S./Canadian Brand Names Iodex [US-OTC]; Iodoflex™ [US]; Iodosorb® [US]

Therapeutic Category Topical Skin Product

Use Used topically as an antiseptic in the management of minor, superficial skin wounds and has been used to disinfect the skin preoperatively

Usual Dosage

Topical:
- Cleaning wet ulcers and wounds (Iodosorb®, Iodoflex™): Apply to clean wound; maximum: 50 g/application and 150 g/week. Change dressing ~3 times/week; reduce applications as exudate decreases. Do not use for >3 months; discontinue when wound is free of exudate.
- Antiseptic for minor cuts, scrapes, burns: Apply small amount to affected area 1-3 times/day

Oral: RDA:
- Children:
  - 1-8 years: 90 mcg/day
  - 9-13 years: 120 mcg/day
  - ≥14 years: Refer to adult dosing
- Adults: 150 mcg/day
  - Pregnancy: 220 mcg/day
  - Breast-feeding: 290 mcg/day

Dosage Forms

Dressing, topical [gel pad]:
Iodoflex™: 0.9% (5 g, 10 g)

Gel, topical:
Iodosorb®: 0.9% (40 g)

Ointment, topical:
Iodex [OTC]: 4.7% (30 g, 720 g)

Tincture, topical: 2% (30 mL, 480 mL); 7% (30 mL, 480 mL)

iodine *see* trace metals *on page 974*

iodine I 131 tositumomab and tositumomab *see* tositumomab and iodine I 131 tositumomab *on page 971*

iodipamide meglumine (eye oh DI pa mide MEG loo meen)

U.S./Canadian Brand Names Cholografin® Meglumine [US]

Therapeutic Category Iodinated Contrast Media; Radiological/Contrast Media, Ionic

Use Contrast medium for intravenous cholangiography and cholecystography

Usual Dosage Note: Do not repeat for 24 hours

I.V.: Cholangiography and cholecystography:
- Infants and Children: 0.3-0.6 mL/kg (maximum: 20 mL)
- Adults: 20 mL

Dosage Forms

Injection, solution:
Cholografin® Meglumine: 520 mg/mL (20 mL)

iodipamide meglumine and diatrizoate meglumine *see* diatrizoate meglumine and iodipamide meglumine *on page 300*

iodixanol (EYE oh dix an ole)

U.S./Canadian Brand Names Visipaque™ [US]

Therapeutic Category Iodinated Contrast Media; Radiological/Contrast Media, Nonionic

Use

Intraarterial: Digital subtraction angiography, angiocardiography, peripheral arteriography, visceral arteriography, cerebral arteriography

Intravenous: Contrast enhanced computed tomography imaging, excretory urography, and peripheral venography

Usual Dosage

Children >1 year: **Note:** Maximum recommended total dose of iodine: Not been established

Intraarterial (cerebral, cardiac chambers, and related major arteries and visceral studies): Iodixanol 320 mg iodine/mL: 1-2 mL/kg; maximum dose: 4 mL/kg

I.V. (contrast-enhanced computer tomography or excretory urography): Iodixanol 270 mg iodine /mL: 1-2 mL/kg; maximum dose: 2 mL/kg

Children >12 years and Adults: **Note:** Maximum recommended total dose of iodine: 80 g

Intraarterial: Iodixanol 320 mg iodine/mL: Dose individualized based on injection site and study type; refer to product labeling

I.V.: Iodixanol 270 mg and 320 mg iodine/mL: concentration and dose vary based on study type; refer to product labeling.

Dosage Forms

Injection, solution [preservative free]:

Visipaque™ 270: 550 mg/mL (50 mL, 100 mL, 125 mL, 150 mL, 200 mL)

Visipaque™ 320: 652 mg/mL (50 mL, 100 mL, 125 mL, 150 mL, 200 mL)

iodochlorhydroxyquin and flumethasone *see* clioquinol and flumethasone *(Canada only) on page 241*

Iodoflex™ [US] *see* iodine *on page 538*

iodoquinol (eye oh doe KWIN ole)

Synonyms diiodohydroxyquin

U.S./Canadian Brand Names Diodoquin® [Can]; Yodoxin® [US]

Therapeutic Category Amebicide

Use Treatment of acute and chronic intestinal amebiasis; asymptomatic cyst passers; *Blastocystis hominis* infections; ineffective for amebic hepatitis or hepatic abscess

Usual Dosage Oral:

Children: 30-40 mg/kg/day (maximum: 650 mg/dose) in 3 divided doses for 20 days; not to exceed 1.95 g/day

Adults: 650 mg 3 times/day after meals for 20 days; not to exceed 1.95 g/day

Dosage Forms

Tablet:

Yodoxin®: 210 mg, 650 mg

iodoquinol and hydrocortisone (eye oh doe KWIN ole & hye droe KOR ti sone)

Sound-Alike/Look-Alike Issues

Vytone® may be confused with Hytone®, Zydone®

Synonyms hydrocortisone and iodoquinol

U.S./Canadian Brand Names Alcortin™ [US]; Dermazene® [US]; Vytone® [US]

Therapeutic Category Antifungal/Corticosteroid

Use Treatment of eczema (including impetiginized, nuchal, and nummular); acne urticaria; anogenital pruritus, atopic dermatitis, chronic infectious dermatitis; chronic eczematoid otitis externa; folliculitis, intertrigo; lichen simplex chronicus; moniliasis; mycotic dermatoses; neurodermatitis (localized or systemic); pyoderma, stasis dermatitis

Usual Dosage Topical: Children ≥12 years and Adults: Apply 3-4 times/day

Dosage Forms

Cream: Iodoquinol 1% and hydrocortisone 1% (30 g)

Dermazene®: Iodoquinol 1% and hydrocortisone 1% (30 g, 45 g)

Vytone®: Iodoquinol 1% and hydrocortisone 1% (30 g)

Gel:

Alcortin™: Iodoquinol 1% and hydrocortisone 2% (2 g)

Iodosorb® [US] *see* iodine *on page 538*

iohexol (eye oh HEX ole)

U.S./Canadian Brand Names Omnipaque™ [US]

Therapeutic Category Polypeptide Hormone; Radiological/Contrast Media, Nonionic

Use

Intrathecal: Myelography; contrast enhancement for computerized tomography

Intravascular: Angiocardiography, aortography, digital subtraction angiography, peripheral arteriography, excretory urography; contrast enhancement for computed tomographic imaging

Oral/body cavity: Arthrography, GI tract examination, hysterosalpingography, pancreatography, cholangiopancreatography, herniography, cystourethrography; enhanced computed tomography of the abdomen

Usual Dosage Dosing is based numerous variables including: Type of examination, route of administration, patient age/weight, and product. Consult specific product information for detailed dosing.

Dosage Forms

Solution, injection [preservative free]:

Omnipaque™:

140: 302 mg/mL (50 mL)
180: 388 mg/mL (10 mL, 20 mL)
240: 518 mg/mL (10 mL, 20 mL, 100 mL, 150 mL, 200 mL)
300: 647 mg/mL (10 mL, 30 mL, 50 mL, 75 mL, 100 mL, 125 mL, 150 mL, 200 mL)
350: 755 mg/mL (50 mL, 75 mL, 100 mL, 125 mL, 150 mL, 200 mL, 250 mL)

Solution, oral [preservative free]:

Omnipaque™:

240: 518 mg/mL (50 mL)
350: 755 mg/mL (50 mL)

Ionamin® [Can] *see* phentermine *on page 773*

Ionil® [US-OTC] *see* salicylic acid *on page 884*

Ionil Plus® [US-OTC] *see* salicylic acid *on page 884*

Ionil T® Plus *(Discontinued)* *see* coal tar *on page 250*

iopamidol (eye oh PA mi dole)

U.S./Canadian Brand Names Isovue Multipack® [US]; Isovue-M® [US]; Isovue® [US]

Therapeutic Category Iodinated Contrast Media; Radiological/Contrast Media, Nonionic

Use

Intrathecal (Isovue-M®): Myelography contrast enhancement of computed tomographic cisternography and ventriculography; thoracolumbar myelography

Intravascular (Isovue®, Isovue Multipack®): Angiography (eg, coronary, cerebral, peripheral arteriogram), pediatric angiocardiography, excretory urography; contrast enhancement of computed tomographic imaging (in adults and children); evaluation of certain malignancies; image enhancement of non-neoplastic lesions

Usual Dosage Dosing is based numerous variables including: Type of examination, route of administration, patient age/weight, and product. Consult specific product information for detailed dosing.

Dosage Forms

Injection, solution:

Isovue Multipack®: 51% (200 mL)
Isovue Multipack®: 61% (200 mL, 500 mL)
Isovue Multipack®: 76% (200 mL, 500 mL)
Isovue®: 51% (50 mL, 100 mL, 150 mL, 200 mL)
Isovue® 200: 41% (50 mL, 200 mL)
Isovue® 300: 61% (30 mL, 50 mL, 75 mL, 100 mL, 125 mL, 150 mL)

Injection, solution, intrathecal:

Isovue-M®: 41% (10 mL, 20 mL)
Isovue-M®: 61% (15 mL)

Iopidine® [US/Can] *see* apraclonidine *on page 94*

iopromide (eye oh PROE mide)

U.S./Canadian Brand Names Ultravist® [US]

Therapeutic Category Radiological/Contrast Media, Nonionic

Use Enhance imaging in cerebral arteriography and peripheral arteriography; coronary arteriography and left ventriculography, visceral angiography and aortography; contrast-enhanced computed tomographic imaging of the head and body, excretory urography, intraarterial digital subtraction angiography, peripheral venography

Usual Dosage

Children >2 years: I.V.:

Cardiac chambers and related arteries (370 mg iodine/mL): 1-2 mL/kg; maximum dose for procedure: 4 mL/kg

Contrast-enhanced CT (300 mg iodine/mL): 1-2 mL/kg; maximum dose for procedure: 3 mL/kg

Adults: **Note:** Maximum recommended total dose of iodine is 86 g. Individualize dose based upon patient's age, body weight, size of the vessel, and the rate of blood flow within the vessel.

Intravascular:

Aortography and visceral angiography (370 mg iodine/mL): Volume and rate of administration based on blood flow and specific characteristics of vessels being studied; maximum dose for procedure: 225 mL

Cerebral arteriography (300 mg iodine/mL): Maximum dose for procedure: 150 mL

Carotid artery visualization: 3-12 mL

Vertebral artery visualization: 4-12 mL

Aortic arch injection: 20-50 mL

Coronary arteriography and left ventriculography (370 mg iodine/mL): Maximum dose for procedure: 225 mL

Left coronary: 3-14 mL

Right coronary: 3-14 mL

Left ventricle: 30-60 mL

Intraarterial digital subtraction angiography (150 mg iodine/mL): Maximum dose for procedure: 250 mL

Carotid arteries: 6-10 mL

Vertebral: 4-8 mL

Aorta: 20-50 mL

Major branches of the abdominal aorta: 2-20 mL

Peripheral arteriography (300 mg iodine/mL): Maximum dose for procedure: 250 mL. **Note:** The artery needs a pulse to be injected.

Subclavian or femoral artery: 5-40 mL

Aortic bifurcation for distal runoff 25-50 mL

I.V.:

Contrast-enhanced CT (300 mg iodine/mL):

Head: 50-200 mL; maximum dose for procedure: 200 mL

Body: 50-200 mL (usual dose for infusion is 100-200 mL); **Note:** Can be given by bolus injection, by rapid infusion, or both; maximum dose for procedure: 200 mL

Excretory urography (normal renal function; 300 mg iodine/mL): 1 mL/kg; maximum dose for procedure: 100 mL

Peripheral venography (240 mg iodine/mL): Minimum amount to clearly visualize the structure under examination; maximum dose for procedure: 250 mL

Dosage Forms

Injection, solution:

Ultravist®:

Iodine 150 mg/mL (provides iopromide 311.7 mg/mL) (50 mL)

Iodine 240 mg/mL (provides iopromide 498.72 mg/mL) (50 mL, 100 mL, 200 mL)

Iodine 300 mg/mL (provides iopromide 623.4 mg/mL) (50 mL, 100 mL, 150 mL, 500 mL)

Iodine 370 mg/mL (provides iopromide 768.86 mg/mL) (50 mL, 100 mL, 150 mL, 200 mL, 500 mL)

Iosat™ [US-OTC] *see* potassium iodide *on page* 805

iothalamate meglumine (eye oh thal A mate MEG loo meen)

U.S./Canadian Brand Names Conray® 30 [US]; Conray® 43 [US]; Conray® [US]; Cysto-Conray® II [US]

Therapeutic Category Iodinated Contrast Media; Radiological/Contrast Media, Ionic

Use

Solution for injection: Arthrography, cerebral angiography, cranial computerized angiotomography, digital subtraction angiography, direct cholangiography, endoscopic retrograde cholangiopancreatography, excretory urography, peripheral arteriography, urography, venography; contrast enhancement of computed tomographic images

Solution for instillation: Retrograde cystography and cystourethrography

Dosage Forms

Injection, solution:

Conray®: 60% (30 mL, 50 mL, 100 mL, 150 mL)

Conray® 30: 30% (50 mL, 150 mL)

Conray® 43: 43% (50 mL, 100 mL, 200 mL, 250 mL)

Injection, solution for instillation:

Cysto-Conray® II: 17.2% (250 mL, 500 mL)

iothalamate sodium (eye oh thal A mate SOW dee um)

U.S./Canadian Brand Names Conray® 400 [US]

Therapeutic Category Iodinated Contrast Media; Radiological/Contrast Media, Ionic

Use Excretory urography, angiocardiography, aortography; contrast enhancement of computed tomographic brain images

Dosage Forms

Injection, solution:

Conray® 400: 66.8% (50 mL)

iotrolan *(Canada only)* (eye OH troe lan)

Sound-Alike/Look-Alike Issues

Osmovist® may be confused with Gadovist®, Magnevist®, Vasovist®

U.S./Canadian Brand Names Osmovist® [Can]

Therapeutic Category Iodinated Contrast Media; Radiological/Contrast Media, Nonionic (Iso-Osmolality)

Use Myelography (lumbar, cervical, total columnar); computerized tomography (CT) of spinal and subarachnoid spaces

Usual Dosage Note: The minimum concentration and volume necessary to obtain adequate visualization should be employed. Repositioning of patients creates turbulence and a rapid dilution of contrast medium. Higher concentrations may be necessary in these patients. If needed, repeat administration should take place no sooner than 72 hours after previous administration (recommended interval between repeat administrations is 5-7 days).

Intrathecal: Adults:

- Radiculography excluding medullary cone: 7-10 mL
- Lumbar myelography: 7-10 mL
- Lumbar myelography with thoracic transition: 7-12 mL
- Thoracic myelography:
  - 240 mg iodine/mL: 10-15 mL
  - 300 mg iodine/mL: 8-12 mL
- Total columnar myelography: 10-15 mL
- Cervical myelography:
  - Direct, lateral access between C1/C2:
    - 240 mg iodine/mL: 8-12 mL
    - 300 mg iodine/mL: 7-10 mL
  - Indirect instillation, lumbar region:
    - 240 mg iodine/mL: 15 mL
    - 300 mg iodine/mL: 8-15 mL
- Ventriculography: Indirect instillation, lumbar region: 3-5 mL
- Cisternography: Indirect instillation, lumbar region:
  - 240 mg iodine/mL: 4-12 mL
  - 300 mg iodine/mL: 4-10 mL

Dosage Forms

Injection, solution, intrathecal [preservative free]:

Osmovist® [CAN; not available in U.S.]:

240 [contains iotrolan 513 mg equivalent to iodine 240 mg/mL] (10 mL)

300 [contains iotrolan 641 mg equivalent to iodine 300 mg /mL] (10 mL)

ioversol (EYE oh ver sole)

U.S./Canadian Brand Names Optiray® [US]

Therapeutic Category Iodinated Contrast Media; Radiological/Contrast Media, Nonionic

Use Arteriography, angiography, angiocardiography, ventriculography, excretory urography, and venography procedures; contrast enhanced tomographic imaging

Dosage Forms

Injection, solution [preservative free]:

Optiray®:

160: 34% (50 mL)
240: 51% (50 mL, 100 mL, 125 mL, 200 mL, 500 mL)
300: 64% (50 mL, 100 mL, 150 mL, 200 mL)
320: 68% (20 mL, 30 mL, 50 mL, 75 mL, 100 mL, 125 mL, 150 mL, 200 mL, 250 mL)
350: 74% (50 mL, 75 mL, 100 mL, 150 mL, 200 mL, 250 mL, 500 mL)

ioxaglate meglumine and ioxaglate sodium

(eye ox AG late MEG loo meen & eye ox AG late SOW dee um)

Synonyms ioxaglate sodium and ioxaglate meglumine

U.S./Canadian Brand Names Hexabrix™ [US]

Therapeutic Category Iodinated Contrast Media; Radiological/Contrast Media, Ionic

Use Angiocardiography, arteriography, aortography, arthrography, angiography, hysterosalpingography, venography, and urography procedures; contrast enhancement of computed tomographic imaging

Dosage Forms

Injection, solution:

Hexabrix™: Ioxaglate meglumine 39.3% and ioxaglate sodium 19.6% (20 mL, 50 mL, 100 mL, 150 mL, 200 mL)

ioxaglate sodium and ioxaglate meglumine *see* ioxaglate meglumine and ioxaglate sodium *on page 543*

ioxilan (eye OKS ee lan)

U.S./Canadian Brand Names Oxilan® 300 [Can]; Oxilan® 350 [Can]; Oxilan® [US]

Therapeutic Category Iodinated Contrast Media; Radiological/Contrast Media, Nonionic

Use

Intraarterial: Ioxilan 300 mgI/mL is indicated for cerebral arteriography. Ioxilan 350 mgI/mL is indicated for coronary arteriography and left ventriculography, visceral angiography, aortography, and peripheral arteriography

Intravenous: Both products are indicated for excretory urography and contrast-enhanced computed tomographic (CECT) imaging of the head and body

Usual Dosage Adults:

Intraarterial: Coronary arteriography and left ventriculography: For visualization of coronary arteries and left ventricle, ioxilan injection with a concentration of 350 mg iodine/mL is recommended

Usual injection volumes:

Left and right coronary: 2-10 mL (0.7-3.5 g iodine)
Left ventricle: 25-50 mL (8.75-17.5 g iodine)

Total doses should not exceed 250 mL; the injection rate of ioxilan should approximate the flow rate in the vessel injected

Cerebral arteriography: For evaluation of arterial lesions of the brain, a concentration of 300 mg iodine/mL is indicated

Recommended doses: 8-12 mL (2.4-3.6 g iodine)

Total dose should not exceed 150 mL

Dosage Forms

Injection, solution [preservative free]:

Oxilan®: 300: 62% (50 mL, 100 mL, 150 mL, 200 mL); 350: 73% (50 mL, 100 mL, 150 mL, 200 mL)

ipecac syrup (IP e kak SIR up)

Synonyms syrup of ipecac

Therapeutic Category Antidote

Use Treatment of acute oral drug overdosage and in certain poisonings

Usual Dosage Oral:

Children:

6-12 months: 5-10 mL followed by 10-20 mL/kg of water; repeat dose one time if vomiting does not occur within 20 minutes

1-12 years: 15 mL followed by 10-20 mL/kg of water; repeat dose one time if vomiting does not occur within 20 minutes

If emesis does not occur within 30 minutes after second dose, ipecac must be removed from stomach by gastric lavage

Adults: 15-30 mL followed by 200-300 mL of water; repeat dose one time if vomiting does not occur within 20 minutes

Dosage Forms

Syrup: 70 mg/mL (30 mL)

I-Pentolate® *(Discontinued)* *see* cyclopentolate *on page 265*

IPG-Citalopram [Can] *see* citalopram *on page 234*

I-Phrine® Ophthalmic Solution *(Discontinued)* *see* phenylephrine *on page 774*

I-Picamide® *(Discontinued)* *see* tropicamide *on page 992*

Iplex™ *(Discontinued)* *see* mecasermin *on page 618*

IPM Wound Gel™ [US-OTC] *see* hyaluronate and derivatives *on page 496*

IPOL® [US/Can] *see* poliovirus vaccine (inactivated) *on page 796*

ipratropium (i pra TROE pee um)

Sound-Alike/Look-Alike Issues

ipratropium may be confused with tiotropium

Atrovent® may be confused with Alupent®, Serevent®

Synonyms ipratropium bromide

U.S./Canadian Brand Names Alti-Ipratropium [Can]; Apo-Ipravent® [Can]; Atrovent® HFA [US/Can]; Atrovent® [US/Can]; Gen-Ipratropium [Can]; Novo-Ipramide [Can]; Nu-Ipratropium [Can]; PMS-Ipratropium [Can]

Therapeutic Category Anticholinergic Agent

Use

Oral inhalation: Anticholinergic bronchodilator used in bronchospasm associated with COPD, bronchitis, and emphysema

Nasal spray: Symptomatic relief of rhinorrhea associated with the common cold and allergic and nonallergic rhinitis

Usual Dosage

Nebulization:

Children ≤12 years: Asthma exacerbation, acute: 250-500 mcg every 20 minutes for 3 doses, then as needed. **Note:** Should be given in combination with a short-acting beta-adrenergic agonist.

Children >12 years and Adults:

Bronchodilator for COPD: 500 mcg (one unit-dose vial) 3-4 times/day with doses 6-8 hours apart

Asthma exacerbation, acute: 500 mcg every 20 minutes for 3 doses, then as needed. **Note:** Should be given in combination with a short-acting beta-adrenergic agonist.

Oral inhalation: MDI:

Children ≤12 years: Asthma exacerbation, acute: 4-8 inhalations every 20 minutes as needed for up to 3 hours. **Note:** Should be given in combination with a short-acting beta-adrenergic agonist.

Children >12 years and Adults:

Bronchodilator for COPD: 2 inhalations 4 times/day, up to 12 inhalations/24 hours

Asthma exacerbation, acute: 8 inhalations every 20 minutes as needed for up to 3 hours. **Note:** Should be given in combination with a short-acting beta-adrenergic agonist.

Intranasal: Nasal spray:

Symptomatic relief of rhinorrhea associated with the common cold (safety and efficacy of use beyond 4 days in patients with the common cold have not been established):

Children 5-11 years: 0.06%: 2 sprays in each nostril 3 times/day

Children ≥12 years and Adults: 0.06%: 2 sprays in each nostril 3-4 times/day

Symptomatic relief of rhinorrhea associated with allergic/nonallergic rhinitis: Children ≥6 years and Adults: 0.03%: 2 sprays in each nostril 2-3 times/day

Symptomatic relief of rhinorrhea associated with seasonal allergic rhinitis (safety and efficacy of use beyond 3 weeks in patients with seasonal allergic rhinitis has not been established): Children ≥5 years and Adults: 0.06%: 2 sprays in each nostril 4 times/day

Dosage Forms

Aerosol for oral inhalation:

Atrovent® HFA: 17 mcg/actuation (12.9 g)

Solution for nebulization: 0.02% (2.5 mL)

Solution, intranasal [spray]:

Atrovent®: 0.03% (30 mL); 0.06% (15 mL)

ipratropium and albuterol (i pra TROE pee um & al BYOO ter ole)

Sound-Alike/Look-Alike Issues

Combivent® may be confused with Combivir®, Serevent®

Synonyms albuterol and ipratropium; salbutamol and ipratropium

U.S./Canadian Brand Names CO Ipra-Sal [Can]; Combivent UDV [Can]; Combivent® [US]; DuoNeb® [US]; Gen-Combo Sterinebs [Can]; ratio-Ipra Sal UDV [Can]

Therapeutic Category Bronchodilator

Use Treatment of COPD in those patients who are currently on a regular bronchodilator who continue to have bronchospasms and require a second bronchodilator

Usual Dosage Adults:

Aerosol for inhalation: 2 inhalations 4 times/day (maximum: 12 inhalations/24 hours)

Solution for nebulization: Initial: 3 mL every 6 hours (maximum: 3 mL every 4 hours)

Dosage Forms

Aerosol for oral inhalation:

Combivent®: Ipratropium 18 mcg and albuterol 103 mcg per actuation (14.7 g) [200 metered actuations]

Solution for nebulization: Ipratropium 0.5 mg and albuterol 2.5 mg per 3 mL (30s, 60s)

DuoNeb®: Ipratropium 0.5 mg and albuterol 2.5 mg per 3 mL (30s, 60s)

ipratropium bromide *see* ipratropium *on page* 544

I-Prin [US-OTC] *see* ibuprofen *on page* 515

iproveratril hydrochloride *see* verapamil *on page* 1010

IPV *see* poliovirus vaccine (inactivated) *on page* 796

Iquix® [US] *see* levofloxacin *on page* 580

irbesartan (ir be SAR tan)

Sound-Alike/Look-Alike Issues

Avapro® may be confused with Anaprox®

U.S./Canadian Brand Names Avapro® [US/Can]

Therapeutic Category Angiotensin II Receptor Antagonist

Use Treatment of hypertension alone or in combination with other antihypertensives; treatment of diabetic nephropathy in patients with type 2 diabetes mellitus (noninsulin-dependent, NIDDM) and hypertension

Usual Dosage Oral:

Hypertension:

Children: ≥6-12 years: Initial: 75 mg once daily; may be titrated to a maximum of 150 mg once daily

Children ≥13 years and Adults: 150 mg once daily; patients may be titrated to 300 mg once daily

Note: Starting dose in volume-depleted patients should be 75 mg

Nephropathy in patients with type 2 diabetes and hypertension: Adults: Target dose: 300 mg once daily

Dosage Forms

Tablet:

Avapro®: 75 mg, 150 mg, 300 mg

irbesartan and hydrochlorothiazide (ir be SAR tan & hye droe klor oh THYE a zide)

Sound-Alike/Look-Alike Issues

Avalide® may be confused with Avandia®

Synonyms Avapro® HCT; hydrochlorothiazide and irbesartan

U.S./Canadian Brand Names Avalide® [US/Can]

Therapeutic Category Antihypertensive Agent, Combination

Use Combination therapy for the management of hypertension; may be used as initial therapy in patients likely to need multiple drugs to achieve blood pressure goals

Note: In Canada, this combination product is approved for initial therapy in severe, essential hypertension (sitting diastolic blood pressure [DBP] ≥110 mm Hg).

Usual Dosage Oral: Adults:

Add-on therapy: Dose must be individualized. A patient who is not controlled with either agent alone may be switched to the combination product. Mean effect increases with the dose of each component. The lowest dosage available is irbesartan 150 mg/hydrochlorothiazide 12.5 mg. Dose increases should be made not more frequently than every 2-4 weeks.

Initial therapy: Irbesartan 150 mg/hydrochlorothiazide 12.5 mg once daily. If initial response is inadequate, may titrate dose after 2-4 weeks, to a maximum dose of irbesartan 300 mg/ hydrochlorothiazide 25 mg once daily.

Dosage Forms

Tablet:

Avalide®: Irbesartan 150 mg and hydrochlorothiazide 12.5 mg; irbesartan 300 mg and hydrochlorothiazide 12.5 mg; irbesartan 300 mg and hydrochlorothiazide 25 mg

Ircon® [US-OTC] *see* ferrous fumarate *on page* 413

IRESSA® [US] *see* gefitinib *on page* 456

irinotecan (eye rye no TEE kan)

Synonyms camptothecin-11; CPT-11; NSC-616348

U.S./Canadian Brand Names Camptosar® [US/Can]; Irinotecan Hydrochloride Trihydrate [Can]

Therapeutic Category Antineoplastic Agent

Use Treatment of metastatic carcinoma of the colon or rectum

Usual Dosage I.V. (Refer to individual protocols): **Note:** A reduction in the starting dose by one dose level should be considered for patients ≥65 years of age, prior pelvic/abdominal radiotherapy, performance status of 2, homozygosity for UGT1A1*28 allele, or increased bilirubin (dosing for patients with a bilirubin >2 mg/dL cannot be recommended based on lack of data per manufacturer).

Single-agent therapy:

125 mg/m^2 over 90 minutes on days 1, 8, 15, and 22 of a 6-week treatment cycle

Adjusted dose level -1: 100 mg/m^2

Adjusted dose level -2: 75 mg/m^2

Once-every-3-week regimen: 350 mg/m^2 over 90 minutes, once every 3 weeks

Adjusted dose level -1: 300 mg/m^2

Adjusted dose level -2: 250 mg/m^2

Depending on the patient's ability to tolerate therapy, doses should be adjusted in increments of 25-50 mg/m^2. Irinotecan doses may range from 50-150 mg/m^2 for the weekly regimen. Patients may be dosed as low as 200 mg/m^2 (in 50 mg/m^2 decrements) for the once-every-3-week regimen.

Combination therapy with fluorouracil and leucovorin: Six-week (42-day) cycle:

Regimen 1: 125 mg/m^2 over 90 minutes on days 1, 8, 15, and 22; to be given in combination with bolus leucovorin and fluorouracil (leucovorin administered immediately following irinotecan; fluorouracil immediately following leucovorin)

Adjusted dose level -1: 100 mg/m^2

Adjusted dose level -2: 75 mg/m^2

Regimen 2: 180 mg/m^2 over 90 minutes on days 1, 15, and 29; to be given in combination with infusional leucovorin and bolus/infusion fluorouracil (leucovorin administered immediately following irinotecan; fluorouracil immediately following leucovorin)

Adjusted dose level -1: 150 mg/m^2

Adjusted dose level -2: 120 mg/m^2

Note: For all regimens: It is recommended that new courses begin only after the granulocyte count recovers to ≥1500/mm^3, the platelet count recovers to ≥100,000/mm^3, and treatment-related diarrhea has fully resolved. Treatment should be delayed 1-2 weeks to allow for recovery from treatment-related toxicities. If the patient has not recovered after a 2-week delay, consideration should be given to discontinuing irinotecan.

Dosage Forms

Injection, solution: 20 mg/mL (2 mL, 5 mL, 25 mL)

Camptosar®: 20 mg/mL (2 mL, 5 mL)

Irinotecan Hydrochloride Trihydrate [Can] *see* irinotecan *on page* 546

iron dextran *see* iron dextran complex *on page* 546

iron dextran complex (EYE ern DEKS tran KOM pleks)

Sound-Alike/Look-Alike Issues

iron dextran complex may be confused with ferumoxytol

Dexferrum® may be confused with Desferal®

Synonyms high-molecular-weight iron dextran (DexFerrum®); imferon; iron dextran; low-Molecular-weight iron dextran (INFeD®)

U.S./Canadian Brand Names Dexferrum® [US]; Dexiron™ [Can]; INFeD® [US]; Infufer® [Can]

Therapeutic Category Electrolyte Supplement, Oral

Use Treatment of iron deficiency in patients in whom oral administration is infeasible or ineffective

Usual Dosage I.M. (INFeD®; Z-track method should be used for I.M. injection), I.V. (Dexferrum®, INFeD®):

A 0.5 mL test dose (0.25 mL in infants) should be given prior to starting iron dextran therapy; total dose should be divided into a daily schedule for I.M., total dose may be given as a single continuous infusion. Individual doses of ≤2 mL may be administered daily until calculated total dose is received.

Iron-deficiency anemia:

Children 5-15 kg: Should not normally be given in the first 4 months of life:

Dose (mL) = 0.0442 (desired hemoglobin - observed hemoglobin) x W + (0.26 x W)

Desired hemoglobin: Usually 12 g/dL

W = Total body weight in kg

Children >15 kg and Adults:

Dose (mL) = 0.0442 (desired hemoglobin - observed hemoglobin) x LBW + (0.26 x LBW)

Desired hemoglobin: Usually 14.8 g/dL

LBW = Lean body weight in kg

Iron replacement therapy for blood loss: Replacement iron (mg) = blood loss (mL) x hematocrit

Cancer-associated anemia (NCCN guidelines v.3.2009): Adults: I.V.: Test dose: 25 mg slow I.V. slow push, followed 1 hour later by 100 mg over 5 minutes; larger doses (unlabeled), up to total dose infusion (over several hours) may be administered

Maximum daily dosage: Manufacturer's labeling: **Note:** Replacement of larger estimated iron deficits may be achieved by serial administration of smaller incremental dosages. Daily dosages should be limited to:

Children:

<5 kg: 25 mg iron (0.5 mL)

5-10 kg: 50 mg iron (1 mL)

Children ≥10 kg and Adults: 100 mg iron (2 mL)

Dosage Forms

Injection, solution:

Dexferrum®: 50 mg/mL (1 mL, 2 mL)

INFeD®: 50 mg/mL (2 mL)

iron fumarate *see* ferrous fumarate *on page 413*

iron gluconate *see* ferrous gluconate *on page 414*

iron-polysaccharide complex *see* polysaccharide-iron complex *on page 799*

iron sucrose (EYE ern SOO krose)

Sound-Alike/Look-Alike Issues

iron sucrose may be confused with ferumoxytol

U.S./Canadian Brand Names Venofer® [US/Can]

Therapeutic Category Iron Salt

Use Treatment of iron-deficiency anemia in chronic renal failure, including nondialysis-dependent patients (with or without erythropoietin therapy) and dialysis-dependent patients receiving erythropoietin therapy

Usual Dosage Doses expressed in mg of **elemental** iron. **Note:** Test dose: Product labeling does not indicate need for a test dose in product-naive patients.

I.V.: Adults: Iron-deficiency anemia in chronic renal disease:

Hemodialysis-dependent patient: 100 mg over 2-5 minutes administered 1-3 times/week during dialysis; administer no more than 3 times/week to a cumulative total dose of 1000 mg (10 doses); may continue to administer at lowest dose necessary to maintain target hemoglobin, hematocrit, and iron storage parameters

Peritoneal dialysis-dependent patient: Slow intravenous infusion at the following schedule: Two infusions of 300 mg each over 1 1/2 hours 14 days apart followed by a single 400 mg infusion over 2 1/2 hours 14 days later (total cumulative dose of 1000 mg in 3 divided doses)

Nondialysis-dependent patient: 200 mg slow injection (over 2-5 minutes) on 5 different occasions within a 14-day period. Total cumulative dose: 1000 mg in 14-day period. **Note:** Dosage has also been administered as two infusions of 500 mg in a maximum of 250 mL 0.9% NaCl infused over 3.5-4 hours on day 1 and day 14 (limited experience)

Dosage Forms

Injection, solution [preservative free]:

Venofer®: 20 mg of elemental iron/mL (5 mL, 10 mL)

iron sulfate *see* ferrous sulfate *on page 414*

iron sulfate and vitamin C *see* ferrous sulfate and ascorbic acid *on page 415*

Isagel® [US-OTC] *see* alcohol (ethyl) *on page 42*

ISD *see* isosorbide dinitrate *on page 550*

ISDN *see* isosorbide dinitrate *on page 550*

Isentress® [US/Can] *see* raltegravir *on page 849*

ISG *see* immune globulin (intramuscular) *on page 522*

ISMN *see* isosorbide mononitrate *on page 551*

Ismo® [US] *see* isosorbide mononitrate *on page 551*

isoamyl nitrite *see* amyl nitrite *on page 78*

isobamate *see* carisoprodol *on page 187*

Isocal® [US-OTC] *see* nutritional formula, enteral/oral *on page 715*

isocarboxazid (eye soe kar BOKS a zid)

U.S./Canadian Brand Names Marplan® [US]

Therapeutic Category Antidepressant, Monoamine Oxidase Inhibitor

Use Treatment of depression

Usual Dosage Oral: Adults: Initial: 10 mg 2-4 times/day; may increase by 10 mg/day every 2-4 days to 40 mg/day by the end of the first week (divided into 2-4 doses). After first week, may increase by up to 20 mg/week to a maximum of 60 mg/day. May take 3-6 weeks to see effects. Dose should be reduced once maximum clinical effect is seen. If no response obtained within 6 weeks, additional titration is unlikely to be beneficial. **Note:** Use caution in patients on >40 mg/day; experience is limited.

Dosage Forms

Tablet:

Marplan®: 10 mg

Isochron™ [US] *see* isosorbide dinitrate *on page 550*

isoflurane (eye soe FLURE ane)

Sound-Alike/Look-Alike Issues

isoflurane may be confused with enflurane, isoflurophate

U.S./Canadian Brand Names Forane® [US/Can]; Terrell™ [US]

Therapeutic Category General Anesthetic

Use Induction and maintenance of general anesthesia

Note: Use of isoflurane for induction of general anesthesia is not recommended due to its irritant properties and unpleasant odor, which causes breath-holding or coughing.

Usual Dosage Inhalation: Adults:

Anesthesia: Minimum alveolar concentration (MAC), the concentration at which 50% of patients do not respond to surgical incision, is 1.15% (44 years of age) for isoflurane.

Induction: 1.5% to 3%

Maintenance: In nitrous oxide: 1% to 2.5%; in oxygen: 1.5% to 3.5%

Dosage Forms

Liquid, for inhalation: >99.9% (100 mL, 250 mL)

Forane®, Terrell™: >99.9% (100 mL, 250 mL)

isometheptene, acetaminophen, and dichloralphenazone *see* acetaminophen, isometheptene, and dichloralphenazone *on page 29*

isometheptene, dichloralphenazone, and acetaminophen *see* acetaminophen, isometheptene, and dichloralphenazone *on page 29*

IsonaRif™ [US] *see* rifampin and isoniazid *on page 867*

isoniazid (eye soe NYE a zid)

Synonyms INH; isonicotinic acid hydrazide

U.S./Canadian Brand Names Isotamine® [Can]; PMS-Isoniazid [Can]

Therapeutic Category Antitubercular Agent

Use Treatment of susceptible tuberculosis infections; treatment of latent tuberculosis infection (LTBI)

Usual Dosage

Usual dosage ranges: Oral, I.M.:

Infants and Children: 10-15 mg/kg/day in 1-2 divided doses (maximum: 300 mg/day) or 20-40 mg/kg given 2-3 times per week (maximum: 900 mg/dose)

Adults: 5 mg/kg/day (usual: 300 mg/day) as a single daily dose or 15 mg/kg (maximum: 900 mg/dose) given 2-3 times per week

Indication-specific dosing: Oral, I.M.: Recommendations often change due to resistant strains and newly-developed information; consult *MMWR* for current CDC recommendations. Intramuscular injection is available for patients who are unable to either take or absorb oral therapy.

Infants and Children:

Tuberculosis, active:

Daily therapy: 10-15 mg/kg/day in 1-2 divided doses (maximum: 300 mg/day)

Twice weekly or 3 times/week directly observed therapy (DOT): 20-40 mg/kg (maximum: 900 mg)

Tuberculosis, latent infection (LTBI): 10 mg/kg/day as a single dose (maximum: 300 mg/day) **or** 20-30 mg/kg (maximum: 900 mg/dose) twice weekly for 9 months

Adults: **Note:** Concomitant administration of 10-50 mg/day pyridoxine is recommended in malnourished patients or those prone to neuropathy (eg, alcoholics, patients with diabetes).

Tuberculosis, active:

Daily therapy: 5 mg/kg/day given daily (usual dose: 300 mg/day)

Twice weekly or 3 times/week directly observed therapy (DOT): 15 mg/kg (maximum: 900 mg). **Note:** CDC guidelines state that once-weekly therapy (15 mg/kg/dose) may be considered, but only after the first 2 months of initial therapy in HIV-negative patients, and only in combination with rifapentine.

Note: Treatment may be defined by the number of doses administered (eg, "six-month" therapy involves 182 doses of INH and rifampin, and 56 doses of pyrazinamide). Six months is the shortest interval of time over which these doses may be administered, assuming no interruption of therapy.

Tuberculosis, latent infection (LTBI): 300 mg/day or 900 mg twice weekly for 6-9 months in patients who do not have HIV infection (9 months is optimal, 6 months may be considered to reduce costs of therapy) and 9 months in patients who have HIV infection. Extend to 12 months of therapy if interruptions in treatment occur.

Dosage Forms

Oral solution: 50 mg/5 mL

Tablet: 100 mg, 300 mg

isoniazid and rifampin *see* rifampin and isoniazid *on page 867*

isoniazid, pyrazinamide, and rifampin *see* rifampin, isoniazid, and pyrazinamide *on page 867*

isonicotinic acid hydrazide *see* isoniazid *on page 548*

isonipecaine hydrochloride *see* meperidine *on page 626*

isophane insulin *see* insulin NPH *on page 532*

isophane insulin and regular insulin *see* insulin NPH and insulin regular *on page 532*

isophosphamide *see* ifosfamide *on page 518*

isoproterenol (eye soe proe TER e nole)

Sound-Alike/Look-Alike Issues

Isuprel® may be confused with Disophrol®, Ismelin®, Isordil®

Synonyms isoproterenol hydrochloride

U.S./Canadian Brand Names Isuprel® [US]

Therapeutic Category Adrenergic Agonist Agent

Use Manufacturer's labeled indications (see **"Note"**): Mild or transient episodes of heart block that do not require electric shock or pacemaker therapy; serious episodes of heart block and Adams-Stokes attacks (except when caused by ventricular tachycardia or fibrillation); cardiac arrest until electric shock or pacemaker therapy is available; bronchospasm during anesthesia; adjunct to fluid and electrolyte replacement therapy and other drugs and procedures in the treatment of hypovolemic or septic shock and low cardiac output states (eg, decompensated heart failure, cardiogenic shock)

Note: The use of isoproterenol in advanced cardiac life support (ACLS) has largely been supplanted by the use of other adrenergic agents (eg, epinephrine and dopamine). The use of isoproterenol for bronchospasm during anesthesia and cardiogenic, hypovolemic, or septic shock is no longer recommended.

Usual Dosage Continuous I.V. infusion:

Bradyarrhythmias, AV nodal block, or refractory torsade de pointes:

Children: 0.05-2 mcg/kg/minute; titrate to patient response

Adults: 2-10 mcg/minute; titrate to patient response

Tilt table testing for syncope: Adults: Initial: 1 mcg/minute; increase as necessary based on response to a maximum dose of 5 mcg/minute. **Note:** Timing of initiation and dose adjustment during test may be institution specific.

Dosage Forms

Injection, solution:

Isuprel®: 0.2 mg/mL (1:5000) (1 mL, 5 mL)

isoproterenol hydrochloride *see* isoproterenol *on page 549*

Isoptin® ***(Discontinued)*** *see* verapamil *on page 1010*

Isoptin® SR [US/Can] *see* verapamil *on page 1010*

Isopto® Atropine [US/Can] *see* atropine *on page 110*

Isopto® Carbachol [US/Can] *see* carbachol *on page 180*

Isopto® Carpine [US/Can] *see* pilocarpine *on page 783*

Isopto® Cetapred® ***(Discontinued)***

Isopto® Eserine [Can] *see* physostigmine *on page 782*

Isopto® Eserine ***(Discontinued)*** *see* physostigmine *on page 782*

Isopto® Frin Ophthalmic Solution ***(Discontinued)*** *see* phenylephrine *on page 774*

Isopto® Homatropine [US] *see* homatropine *on page 495*

Isopto® Hyoscine [US] *see* scopolamine derivatives *on page 892*

Isopto® Plain Solution ***(Discontinued)*** *see* artificial tears *on page 100*

Isopto® Tears [US-OTC/Can] *see* hydroxypropyl methylcellulose *on page 510*

Isordil® [US] *see* isosorbide dinitrate *on page 550*

isosorbide dinitrate (eye soe SOR bide dye NYE trate)

Sound-Alike/Look-Alike Issues

Isordil® may be confused with Inderal®, Isuprel®, Plendil®

Synonyms ISD; ISDN

U.S./Canadian Brand Names Apo-ISDN® [Can]; Cedocard®-SR [Can]; Coronex® [Can]; Dilatrate®-SR [US]; Isochron™ [US]; Isordil® [US]; Novo-Sorbide [Can]; PMS-Isosorbide [Can]

Therapeutic Category Vasodilator

Use Prevention and treatment of angina pectoris; for congestive heart failure; to relieve pain, dysphagia, and spasm in esophageal spasm with GE reflux

Usual Dosage Oral: Adults:

Angina: 5-40 mg 4 times/day or 40 mg every 8-12 hours in sustained-release dosage form

Sublingual: 2.5-5 mg every 5-10 minutes for maximum of 3 doses in 15-30 minutes; may also use prophylactically 15 minutes prior to activities which may provoke an attack

Congestive heart failure:

Initial dose: 20 mg 3-4 times per day

Target dose: 120-160 mg/day in divided doses; use in combination with hydralazine

Tolerance to nitrate effects develops with chronic exposure: Dose escalation does not overcome this effect. Tolerance can only be overcome by short periods of nitrate absence from the body. Short periods (10-12 hours) of nitrate withdrawal help minimize tolerance. General recommendations are to take the last dose of short-acting agents no later than 7 PM; administer 2-3 times/day rather than 4 times/day. Sustained release preparations could be administered at times to allow a 15- to 17-hour interval between first and last daily dose. Example: Administer sustained release at 8 AM and 2 PM for a twice daily regimen.

Dosage Forms

Capsule, sustained release:

Dilatrate®-SR: 40 mg

Tablet: 5 mg, 10 mg, 20 mg, 30 mg

Isordil®: 5 mg, 40 mg

Tablet, extended release:

Isochron™: 40 mg

Tablet, sublingual: 2.5 mg, 5 mg

isosorbide dinitrate and hydralazine

(eye soe SOR bide dye NYE trate & hye DRAL a zeen)

Synonyms hydralazine and isosorbide dinitrate

U.S./Canadian Brand Names BiDil® [US]

Therapeutic Category Vasodilator

Use Treatment of heart failure, adjunct to standard therapy, in self-identified African-Americans

Usual Dosage Oral: Adults: Initial: 1 tablet 3 times/day; titrate to a maximum dose of 2 tablets 3 times/day

Dosage Forms

Tablet:

BiDil®: Isosorbide 20 mg and hydralazine 37.5 mg

isosorbide mononitrate (eye soe SOR bide mon oh NYE trate)

Sound-Alike/Look-Alike Issues

Imdur® may be confused with Imuran®, Inderal LA®, K-Dur®

Monoket® may be confused with Monopril®

Synonyms ISMN

U.S./Canadian Brand Names Apo-ISMN® [Can]; Imdur® [US/Can]; Ismo® [US]; Monoket® [US]; PMS-ISMN [Can]; Pro-ISMN [Can]

Therapeutic Category Vasodilator

Use Long-acting metabolite of the vasodilator isosorbide dinitrate used for the prophylactic treatment of angina pectoris

Usual Dosage Oral: Adults and Geriatrics (start with lowest recommended dose):

Regular tablet: 5-20 mg twice daily with the two doses given 7 hours apart (eg, 8 AM and 3 PM) to decrease tolerance development; then titrate to 10 mg twice daily in first 2-3 days.

Extended release tablet: Initial: 30-60 mg given in morning as a single dose; titrate upward as needed, giving at least 3 days between increases; maximum daily single dose: 240 mg

Tolerance to nitrate effects develops with chronic exposure. Dose escalation does not overcome this effect. Tolerance can only be overcome by short periods of nitrate absence from the body. Short periods (10-12 hours) of nitrate withdrawal help minimize tolerance. Recommended dosage regimens incorporate this interval. General recommendations are to take the last dose of short-acting agents no later than 7 PM; administer 2 times/day rather than 4 times/day. Administer sustained release tablet once daily in the morning.

Dosage Forms

Tablet: 10 mg, 20 mg

Ismo®: 20 mg

Monoket®: 10 mg, 20 mg

Tablet, extended release: 30 mg, 60 mg, 120 mg

Imdur®: 30 mg, 60 mg, 120 mg

isosulfan blue (eye soe SUL fan bloo)

U.S./Canadian Brand Names Lymphazurin™ [US]

Therapeutic Category Contrast Agent

Use Adjunct to lymphography for visualization of the lymphatic system; sentinel node identification

Usual Dosage SubQ: Adults: Inject 0.5 mL into 3 interdigital spaces of each extremity per study; maximum: 3 mL (30 mg)

Dosage Forms

Injection, solution [preservative-free]:

Lymphazurin™: 1% (5 mL)

Isotamine® [Can] *see* isoniazid *on page* 548

isotretinoin (eye soe TRET i noyn)

Sound-Alike/Look-Alike Issues

isotretinoin may be confused with tretinoin

Accutane® may be confused with Accolate®, Accupril®

Claravis™ may be confused with Cleviprex™

Synonyms 13-*cis*-retinoic acid

U.S./Canadian Brand Names Accutane® [Can]; Amnesteem™ [US]; Claravis™ [US]; Clarus™ [Can]; Isotrex® [Can]; Sotret® [US]

Therapeutic Category Retinoic Acid Derivative

Use Treatment of severe recalcitrant nodular acne unresponsive to conventional therapy

Usual Dosage Oral: Children 12-17 years and Adults: Severe recalcitrant nodular acne: 0.5-1 mg/kg/day in 2 divided doses (dosages as low as 0.05 mg/kg/day have been reported to be beneficial) for 15-20 weeks or until the total cyst count decreases by 70%, whichever is sooner. Adults with very severe disease/scarring or primarily involves the trunk may require dosage adjustment up to 2 mg/kg/day. A second course of therapy may be initiated after a period of ≥2 months off therapy.

Dosage Forms

Capsule:

Amnesteem™, Claravis™: 10 mg, 20 mg, 40 mg

Sotret®: 10 mg, 20 mg, 30 mg, 40 mg

Isotrex® [Can] *see* isotretinoin *on page* 551

Isovue® [US] *see* iopamidol *on page* 540

Isovue-M® [US] *see* iopamidol *on page* 540

Isovue Multipack® [US] *see* iopamidol *on page* 540

isoxsuprine (eye SOKS syoo preen)

Sound-Alike/Look-Alike Issues

Vasodilan® may be confused with Vasocidin®

Synonyms isoxsuprine hydrochloride

Therapeutic Category Vasodilator

Use Treatment of peripheral vascular diseases, such as arteriosclerosis obliterans and Raynaud disease

Usual Dosage Oral: Adults: 10-20 mg 3-4 times/day

Dosage Forms

Tablet: 10 mg, 20 mg

isoxsuprine hydrochloride *see* isoxsuprine *on page* 552

isradipine (iz RA di peen)

Sound-Alike/Look-Alike Issues

DynaCirc® may be confused with Dynabac®, Dynacin®

U.S./Canadian Brand Names DynaCirc® CR [US]; DynaCirc® [Can]

Therapeutic Category Calcium Channel Blocker

Use Treatment of hypertension

Usual Dosage Oral: Adults:

Capsule: 2.5 mg twice daily; antihypertensive response occurs in 2-3 hours; maximal response in 2-4 weeks; increase dose at 2- to 4-week intervals at 2.5-5 mg increments; usual dose range (JNC 7): 2.5-10 mg/day in 2 divided doses. **Note:** Most patients show no improvement with doses >10 mg/day except adverse reaction rate increases; therefore, maximal dose in older adults should be 10 mg/day.

Controlled release tablet: 5 mg once daily; antihypertensive response occurs in 2 hours. Adjust dose in increments of 5 mg at 2-4 week intervals. Maximum dose: 20 mg/day; adverse events are increased at doses >10 mg/day.

Dosage Forms

Capsule: 2.5 mg, 5 mg

Tablet, controlled release:

DynaCirc® CR: 5 mg, 10 mg

Istalol® [US] *see* timolol *on page* 961

Isuprel® [US] *see* isoproterenol *on page* 549

Itch-X® [US-OTC] *see* pramoxine *on page* 809

itraconazole (i tra KOE na zole)

Sound-Alike/Look-Alike Issues

itraconazole may be confused with fluconazole

Sporanox® may be confused with Suprax®, Topamax®

U.S./Canadian Brand Names Sporanox® [US/Can]

Therapeutic Category Antifungal Agent

Use

Oral capsules: Treatment of susceptible fungal infections in immunocompromised and immunocompetent patients including blastomycosis and histoplasmosis; indicated for aspergillosis (in patients intolerant/refractory to amphotericin B), and onychomycosis of the toenail and fingernail (in nonimmunocompromised patients)

Oral solution: Treatment of oral and esophageal candidiasis

Usual Dosage Oral:

Usual dosage range:

Adults: 100-400 mg/day; doses >200 mg/day are given in 2 divided doses; length of therapy varies from 1 day to >6 months depending on the condition and mycological response

Indication-specific dosing:

Adults:

Aspergillosis, invasive (salvage therapy): Duration of therapy should be a minimum of 6-12 weeks or throughout period of immunosuppression: Oral: 200-400 mg/day; **Note:** 2008 IDSA guidelines recommend 600 mg/day for 3 days, followed by 400 mg/day

Appropriate use: Itraconazole should **NOT** be used for voriconazole-refractory aspergillosis since the same antifungal and/or resistance mechanism(s) may be shared by both agents. Itraconazole oral solution and capsule formulations are not bioequivalent or interchangeable. Due to variable bioavailability of oral preparations, therapeutic drug monitoring advisable.

Aspergillosis, allergic (ABPA, sinusitis): 200 mg/day; may be used in conjunction with corticosteroids

Blastomycosis: 200 mg 3 times/day for 3 days, then 200 mg twice daily for 6-12 months; in moderately-severe to severe infection, therapy should be initiated with ~2 weeks of amphotericin B

Brain abscess: Cerebral phaeohyphomycosis (dematiaceous): 200 mg twice daily for at least 6 months with amphotericin

Candidiasis:

Oropharyngeal: Oral solution: 200 mg once daily for 1-2 weeks; in patients unresponsive or refractory to fluconazole: 100 mg twice daily (clinical response expected in 1-2 weeks)

Esophageal: Oral solution: 100-200 mg once daily for a minimum of 3 weeks; continue dosing for 2 weeks after resolution of symptoms

Coccidioidomycosis: 200 mg twice daily

Histoplasmosis: 200 mg 3 times/day for 3 days, then 200 mg twice daily (or once daily in mild-to-moderate disease) for 6-12 weeks in mild-to-moderate disease or ≥12 months in progressive disseminated or chronic cavitary pulmonary histoplasmosis; in moderately-severe to severe infection, therapy should be initiated with ~2 weeks of a lipid formation of amphotericin B

Long-term suppression therapy: 200 mg/day

Meningitis:

Coccidioides: 400-800 mg/day

Appropriate use: Fluconazole is preferred for meningeal infections.

Onychomycosis: 200 mg once daily for 12 consecutive weeks; alternative "pulse-dosing" may be considering for fingernail involvement only: 200 mg twice daily for 1 week; repeat 1-week course after 3-week off-time

Pneumonia:

Coccidioides: Mild-to-moderate: 200 mg twice daily

Coccidioides, HIV-positive (focal pneumonia): 200 mg 3 times/day for 3 days, then 200 mg twice daily

Protothecal infection: 200 mg once daily for 2 months

Sporotrichosis:

Lymphocutaneous: 100-200 mg/day for 3-6 months

Osteoarticular and pulmonary: 200 mg twice daily for 1-2 years (may use amphotericin B initially for stabilization)

Dosage Forms

Capsule: 100 mg

Sporanox®: 100 mg

Solution, oral:

Sporanox®: 100 mg/10 mL

I-Tropine® *(Discontinued)* *see* atropine *on page 110*

ivermectin (eye ver MEK tin)

U.S./Canadian Brand Names Stromectol® [US]

Therapeutic Category Antibiotic, Miscellaneous

Use Treatment of the following infections: Strongyloidiasis of the intestinal tract due to the nematode parasite *Strongyloides stercoralis*. Onchocerciasis due to the nematode parasite *Onchocerca volvulus*. Ivermectin is only active against the immature form of *Onchocerca volvulus*, and the intestinal forms of *Strongyloides stercoralis*.

Usual Dosage Oral: Children ≥15 kg and Adults:

Onchocerciasis: 150 mcg/kg as a single dose; retreatment may be required every 3-12 months until the adult worms die

Weight-based dosage to provide ~150 mcg/kg:

15-25 kg: 3 mg
26-44 kg: 6 mg
45-64 kg: 9 mg
65-84 kg: 12 mg
≥85 kg: 150 mcg/kg

Strongyloidiasis: 200 mcg/kg as a single dose; perform follow-up stool examinations; CDC recommendations: 200 mcg/kg/day for 2 days

Weight-based dosage to provide ~200 mcg/kg:

15-24 kg: 3 mg
25-35 kg: 6 mg
36-50 kg: 9 mg
51-65 kg: 12 mg
66-79 kg: 15 mg
≥80 kg: 200 mcg/kg

Dosage Forms

Tablet [scored]:
Stromectol®: 3 mg

IVIG *see* immune globulin (intravenous) *on page* 523
IV immune globulin *see* immune globulin (intravenous) *on page* 523
IvyBlock® [US-OTC] *see* bentoquatam *on page* 128
Ivy-Rid® [US-OTC] *see* benzocaine *on page* 129
IvySoothe® [US-OTC] *see* hydrocortisone (topical) *on page* 505

ixabepilone (ix ab EP i lone)

Synonyms azaepothilone B; BMS-247550; epothilone B lactam

U.S./Canadian Brand Names Ixempra® [US]

Therapeutic Category Antineoplastic Agent, Antimicrotubular; Antineoplastic Agent, Epothilone B Analog

Use Treatment of metastatic or locally-advanced breast cancer (refractory or resistant)

Usual Dosage Details concerning dosing in combination regimens should also be consulted. **Note:** Premedicate with an H_1-antagonist (eg, oral diphenhydramine 50 mg) and H_2-antagonist (eg, oral ranitidine 150-300 mg) 1 hour prior to infusion. Patients with a history of hypersensitivity should also be premedicated with corticosteroids (orally 1 hour before or I.V. 30 minutes before infusion). Body surface area (BSA) is capped at a maximum of 2.2 m^2.

I.V.: Adults: Breast cancer (metastatic or locally advanced): 40 mg/m^2/dose over 3 hours every 3 weeks (maximum dose: 88 mg) either as monotherapy or in combination with capecitabine

Dosage Forms

Injection, powder for reconstitution:
Ixempra®: 15 mg, 45 mg

Ixempra® [US] *see* ixabepilone *on page* 554
Ixiaro® [US] *see* Japanese encephalitis virus vaccine (inactivated) *on page* 555
JAMP-Citalopram [Can] *see* citalopram *on page* 234
JAMP-Ondansetron [Can] *see* ondansetron *on page* 726
Janimine® ***(Discontinued)*** *see* imipramine *on page* 521
Jantoven® [US] *see* warfarin *on page* 1022
Janumet™ [US] *see* sitagliptin and metformin *on page* 905
Januvia™ [US] *see* sitagliptin *on page* 904

Japanese encephalitis virus vaccine (inactivated)

(jap a NEESE en sef a LYE tis VYE rus vak SEEN, in ak ti VAY ted)

Synonyms IC51

U.S./Canadian Brand Names Ixiaro® [US]; JE-VAX® [US/Can]

Therapeutic Category Vaccine, Inactivated Virus

Use Active immunization against Japanese encephalitis

Japanese encephalitis vaccine is not recommended for all persons traveling to or residing in Asia. The Advisory Committee on Immunization Practices (ACIP) recommends vaccination for:

- Persons spending ≥1 month in endemic areas during transmission season
- Research laboratory workers who may be exposed to the Japanese encephalitis virus

Vaccination may also be considered for persons spending <30 days in endemic areas, such as:

- Travel to areas with an ongoing outbreak
- Travelers planning to go outside of urban areas and have an increased risk of exposure. For example, high-risk activities include extensive outdoor activity in rural areas especially at night; extensive outdoor activities such as camping, hiking, etc; staying in accommodations without air conditioning, screens or bed nets.
- Travelers to endemic areas who are unsure of specific destination, activities, or duration of travel

Usual Dosage U.S. recommended primary immunization schedule:

Ixiaro®: Adults ≥17 years: I.M.: 0.5 mL/dose; a total of 2 doses given on days 0 and 28

Je-Vax®:

Children 1-3 years: SubQ: 0.5 mL/dose; a total of 3 doses given on days 0, 7, and 30

Children >3 years and Adults: SubQ: 1 mL/dose; a total of 3 doses given on days 0, 7, and 30

Booster dose: Give after 2 years, or according to current recommendation

Abbreviated dosing schedule: Three recommended doses, given on days 0, 7, and 14 with the last dose given at least 10 days before travel. Alternately, two doses given 1 week apart provide immunity in ~80% of patients. Abbreviated schedules should be used only when necessary due to time constraints.

Dosage Forms

Injection, powder for reconstitution:

JE-VAX®

Injection, suspension:

Ixiaro®: Inactivated JEV proteins 6 mcg/0.5 mL (0.5 mL)

Jenamicin® ***(Discontinued)*** *see* gentamicin *on page 461*

Jenest™-28 ***(Discontinued)*** *see* ethinyl estradiol and norethindrone *on page 390*

JE-VAX® [US/Can] *see* Japanese encephalitis virus vaccine (inactivated) *on page 555*

Jolessa™ [US] *see* ethinyl estradiol and levonorgestrel *on page 387*

Jolivette™ [US] *see* norethindrone *on page 704*

Junel™ [US] *see* ethinyl estradiol and norethindrone *on page 390*

Junel™ Fe [US] *see* ethinyl estradiol and norethindrone *on page 390*

Just for Kids™ [US-OTC] *see* fluoride *on page 430*

Just Tears® Solution ***(Discontinued)*** *see* artificial tears *on page 100*

Juvederm™ 24HV [US] *see* hyaluronate and derivatives *on page 496*

Juvederm™ 30 [US] *see* hyaluronate and derivatives *on page 496*

Juvederm™ 30HV [US] *see* hyaluronate and derivatives *on page 496*

K-10® [Can] *see* potassium chloride *on page 803*

Kabikinase® ***(Discontinued)***

Kadian® [US/Can] *see* morphine sulfate *on page 667*

Kala® [US-OTC] *see* Lactobacillus *on page 564*

Kalcinate® ***(Discontinued)*** *see* calcium gluconate *on page 173*

Kaletra® [US/Can] *see* lopinavir and ritonavir *on page 598*

Kalexate [US] *see* sodium polystyrene sulfonate *on page 914*

Kalmz [US-OTC] *see* fructose, dextrose, and phosphoric acid *on page 448*

kanamycin (kan a MYE sin)

Sound-Alike/Look-Alike Issues

kanamycin may be confused with Garamycin®, gentamicin

Synonyms kanamycin sulfate

U.S./Canadian Brand Names Kantrex® [US/Can]

Therapeutic Category Aminoglycoside (Antibiotic)

Use Treatment of serious infections caused by susceptible strains of *E. coli*, *Proteus* species, *Enterobacter aerogenes*, *Klebsiella pneumoniae*, *Serratia marcescens*, and *Acinetobacter* species; second-line treatment of *Mycobacterium tuberculosis*

Usual Dosage Note: Dosing should be based on ideal body weight

Children: Infections: I.M., I.V.: 15 mg/kg/day in divided doses every 8-12 hours

Adults:

Infections: I.M., I.V.: 5-7.5 mg/kg/dose in divided doses every 8-12 hours (<15 mg/kg/day)

Intraperitoneal: After contamination in surgery: 500 mg

Irrigating solution: 0.25%; maximum 1.5 g/day (via all administration routes)

Aerosol: 250 mg 2-4 times/day

Dosage Forms

Injection, solution:

Kantrex®: 1 g/3 mL (3 mL)

kanamycin sulfate *see* kanamycin *on page* 555

Kank-A® Soft Brush™ [US-OTC] *see* benzocaine *on page* 129

Kantrex® [US/Can] *see* kanamycin *on page* 555

Kaochlor-Eff® ***(Discontinued)***

Kaochlor® SF ***(Discontinued)*** *see* potassium chloride *on page* 803

Kaodene® ***(Discontinued)***

Kaodene® NN ***(Discontinued)***

Kaon-Cl-10® [US] *see* potassium chloride *on page* 803

Kao-Paverin® [US-OTC] *see* loperamide *on page* 597

Kaopectate® [US-OTC] *see* bismuth *on page* 142

Kaopectate® II ***(Discontinued)*** *see* loperamide *on page* 597

Kaopectate® Advanced Formula ***(Discontinued)***

Kaopectate® Extra Strength [US-OTC] *see* bismuth *on page* 142

Kaopectate® Maximum Strength Caplets ***(Discontinued)***

Kao-Spen® ***(Discontinued)***

Kao-Tin [US-OTC] *see* bismuth *on page* 142

Kapectolin ***(Discontinued)*** *see* bismuth *on page* 142

Kapidex™ [US] *see* dexlansoprazole *on page* 290

Karidium® ***(Discontinued)*** *see* fluoride *on page* 430

Karigel® ***(Discontinued)*** *see* fluoride *on page* 430

Karigel®-N ***(Discontinued)*** *see* fluoride *on page* 430

Kariva™ [US] *see* ethinyl estradiol and desogestrel *on page* 383

Kasof® ***(Discontinued)*** *see* docusate *on page* 326

Kaybovite-1000® ***(Discontinued)*** *see* cyanocobalamin *on page* 263

Kay Ciel® ***(Discontinued)*** *see* potassium chloride *on page* 803

Kayexalate® [US/Can] *see* sodium polystyrene sulfonate *on page* 914

K-Citra® [Can] *see* potassium citrate *on page* 804

KCl *see* potassium chloride *on page* 803

K-Dur® [Can] *see* potassium chloride *on page* 803

kdur *see* potassium chloride *on page* 803

Keflex® [US] *see* cephalexin *on page* 202

Keftab® [Can] *see* cephalexin *on page* 202

Kefurox® Injection ***(Discontinued)*** *see* cefuroxime *on page* 199

Kefzol® ***(Discontinued)*** *see* cefazolin *on page* 191

K-Electrolyte® Effervescent ***(Discontinued)*** *see* potassium bicarbonate *on page* 802

Kelnor™ [US] *see* ethinyl estradiol and ethynodiol diacetate *on page* 385

Kemadrin® ***(Discontinued)*** *see* procyclidine *on page* 822

Kemsol® [Can] *see* dimethyl sulfoxide *on page* 314

Kenacort® Oral ***(Discontinued)***

ketamine (KEET a meen)

Sound-Alike/Look-Alike Issues
Ketalar® may be confused with Kenalog®, ketorolac

Synonyms ketamine hydrochloride

U.S./Canadian Brand Names Ketalar® [US/Can]; Ketamine Hydrochloride Injection, USP [Can]

Therapeutic Category General Anesthetic

Controlled Substance C-III

Use Induction and maintenance of general anesthesia

Usual Dosage May be used in combination with anticholinergic agents to decrease hypersalivation.
Children ≥16 years and Adults:
Induction of anesthesia:
I.M.: 6.5-13 mg/kg; usual dose to produce 12-25 minutes of anesthesia: 10 mg/kg
I.V.: 1-4.5 mg/kg; usual dose to produce 5-10 minutes of anesthesia: 2 mg/kg
I.V. infusion: 1-2 mg/kg infuse over 0.5 mg/kg/minute; may administer with diazepam to prevent emergence reactions
Maintenance of anesthesia: Supplemental doses of 1/2 to the full induction dose; may also be maintained with a continuous infusion of 0.1-5 mg/minute

Dosage Forms
Injection, solution: 10 mg/mL (20 mL); 50 mg/mL (10 mL); 100 mg/mL (5 mL)
Ketalar®: 10 mg/mL (20 mL); 50 mg/mL (10 mL); 100 mg/mL (5 mL)

ketoconazole (kee toe KOE na zole)

Sound-Alike/Look-Alike Issues
Kuric™ may be confused with Carac®
Nizoral® may be confused with Nasarel®, Neoral®, Nitrol®

U.S./Canadian Brand Names Apo-Ketoconazole® [Can]; Extina® [US]; Ketoderm® [Can]; Kuric™ [US]; Nizoral® A-D [US-OTC]; Nizoral® [US]; Novo-Ketoconazole [Can]; Xolegel® [US/Can]

Therapeutic Category Antifungal Agent

Use
Systemic: Treatment of susceptible fungal infections, including candidiasis, oral thrush, blastomycosis, histoplasmosis, paracoccidioidomycosis, coccidioidomycosis, chromomycosis, candiduria, chronic mucocutaneous candidiasis, as well as certain recalcitrant cutaneous dermatophytoses

Topical:
Cream: Treatment of tinea corporis, tinea cruris, tinea versicolor, cutaneous candidiasis, seborrheic dermatitis
Foam, gel: Treatment of seborrheic dermatitis
Shampoo: Treatment of dandruff, seborrheic dermatitis, tinea versicolor

Usual Dosage
Oral:
Fungal infections:
Children ≥2 years: 3.3-6.6 mg/kg/day as a single dose for 1-2 weeks for candidiasis, for at least 4 weeks in recalcitrant dermatophyte infections, and for up to 6 months for other systemic mycoses
Adults: 200-400 mg/day as a single daily dose for durations as stated above
Shampoo: Seborrheic dermatitis, tinea versicolor: Children ≥12 years and Adults: Apply twice weekly for 4 weeks with at least 3 days between each shampoo
Topical:
Tinea infections: Adults: Cream: Rub gently into the affected area once daily. Duration of treatment: Tinea corporis, cruris: 2 weeks; tinea pedis: 6 weeks
Seborrheic dermatitis: Children ≥12 years and Adults:
Cream: Rub gently into the affected area twice daily for 4 weeks or until clinical response is noted
Foam: Apply to affected area twice daily for 4 weeks
Gel: Rub gently into the affected area once daily for 2 weeks

Dosage Forms
Aerosol, topical [foam]:
Extina®: 2% (50 g, 100 g)
Cream, topical: 2% (15 g, 30 g, 60 g)
Kuric™: 2%: (75 g)
Gel, topical:
Xolegel®: 2% (15 g, 45 g)
Shampoo, topical: 1% (120 mL), 2% (120 mL)
Nizoral®: 2% (120 mL)
Nizoral® A-D [OTC]: 1% (120 mL, 210 mL)
Tablet: 200 mg

Ketoderm® [Can] *see* ketoconazole *on page 557*
3-keto-desogestrel *see* etonogestrel *on page 398*

ketoprofen (kee toe PROE fen)

Sound-Alike/Look-Alike Issues
ketoprofen may be confused with ketotifen
Oruvail® may be confused with Clinoril®, Elavil®

U.S./Canadian Brand Names Apo-Keto SR® [Can]; Apo-Keto-E® [Can]; Apo-Keto® [Can]; Novo-Keto [Can]; Novo-Keto-EC [Can]; Nu-Ketoprofen [Can]; Nu-Ketoprofen-E [Can]; Oruvail® [Can]; Rhodis SR™ [Can]; Rhodis-EC™ [Can]; Rhodis™ [Can]

Therapeutic Category Analgesic, Nonnarcotic; Nonsteroidal Antiinflammatory Drug (NSAID)

Use Acute and long-term treatment of rheumatoid arthritis and osteoarthritis; primary dysmenorrhea; mild-to-moderate pain

Usual Dosage Note: The extended release formulation is not recommended for the treatment of acute pain.
Oral: Adults:
Rheumatoid arthritis, osteoarthritis (lower doses may be used in small patients or in the elderly, or debilitated):
Regular release: 50 mg 4 times/day **or** 75 mg 3 times/day; up to a maximum of 300 mg/day
Extended release: 200 mg once daily
Dysmenorrhea, mild-to-moderate pain: Regular release: 25-50 mg every 6-8 hours up to a maximum of 300 mg/day

Dosage Forms
Capsule, regular release: 50 mg, 75 mg
Capsule, extended release: 200 mg

ketorolac (KEE toe role ak)

Sound-Alike/Look-Alike Issues
ketorolac may be confused with Ketalar®

Acular® may be confused with Acthar®, Ocular®
Toradol® may be confused with Foradil®, Inderal®, Tegretol®, Torecan®, traMADol, tromethamine

Synonyms ketorolac tromethamine

U.S./Canadian Brand Names Acular LS® [US/Can]; Acular® PF [US]; Acular® [US/Can]; Apo-Ketorolac Injectable® [Can]; Apo-Ketorolac® [Can]; Ketorolac Tromethamine Injection, USP [Can]; Novo-Ketorolac [Can]; ratio-Ketorolac [Can]; Toradol® IM [Can]; Toradol® [Can]

Therapeutic Category Analgesic, Nonnarcotic; Nonsteroidal Antiinflammatory Drug (NSAID)

Use

Oral, injection: Short-term (≤5 days) management of moderate-to-severe acute pain requiring analgesia at the opioid level

Ophthalmic: Temporary relief of ocular itching due to seasonal allergic conjunctivitis; postoperative inflammation following cataract extraction; reduction of ocular pain and photophobia following incisional refractive surgery; reduction of ocular pain, burning, and stinging following corneal refractive surgery

Usual Dosage

Children ≥16 years and Adults (pain relief usually begins within 10 minutes with parenteral forms): **Note:** The maximum combined duration of treatment (for parenteral and oral) is 5 days; do not increase dose or frequency; supplement with low-dose opioids if needed for breakthrough pain.

I.M.: 60 mg as a single dose or 30 mg every 6 hours (maximum daily dose: 120 mg)

I.V.: 30 mg as a single dose or 30 mg every 6 hours (maximum daily dose: 120 mg)

Children ≥17 years and Adults: Oral: 20 mg, followed by 10 mg every 4-6 hours; do not exceed 40 mg/day; oral dosing is intended to be a continuation of I.M. or I.V. therapy only

Note: The maximum combined duration of treatment (for parenteral and oral) is 5 days; do not increase dose or frequency; supplement with low-dose opioids if needed for breakthrough pain. Therapy should not be initiated with oral formulation.

Ophthalmic: Children ≥3 years and Adults:

Allergic conjunctivitis (relief of ocular itching) (Acular®): Instill 1 drop (0.25 mg) 4 times/day

Inflammation following cataract extraction (Acular®): Instill 1 drop (0.25 mg) to affected eye(s) 4 times/day beginning 24 hours after surgery; continue for 2 weeks

Pain and photophobia following incisional refractive surgery (Acular® PF): Instill 1 drop (0.25 mg) 4 times/day to affected eye for up to 3 days

Pain following corneal refractive surgery (Acular LS®): Instill 1 drop 4 times/day as needed to affected eye for up to 4 days

Dosage Forms

Injection, solution: 15 mg/mL (1 mL); 30 mg/mL (1 mL, 2 mL, 10 mL)

Solution, ophthalmic:

Acular®: 0.5% (3 mL, 5 mL, 10 mL)

Acular LS®: 0.4% (5 mL)

Acular® P.F. [preservative free]: 0.5% (0.4 mL)

Tablet: 10 mg

ketorolac tromethamine *see* ketorolac *on page* 558

Ketorolac Tromethamine Injection, USP [Can] *see* ketorolac *on page* 558

ketotifen (kee toe TYE fen)

Sound-Alike/Look-Alike Issues

ketotifen may be confused with ketoprofen

Synonyms ketotifen fumarate

U.S./Canadian Brand Names Alaway™ [US-OTC]; Claritin™ Eye [US-OTC]; Novo-Ketotifen® [Can]; Nu-Ketotifen® [Can]; Zaditen® [Can]; Zaditor® [US-OTC/Can]; Zyrtec® Itchy Eye [US-OTC]

Therapeutic Category Antihistamine, H_1 Blocker, Ophthalmic

Use

Ophthalmic: Temporary relief of eye itching due to allergic conjunctivitis

Oral (Canadian use; not approved in U.S.): Adjunctive therapy in the chronic treatment of pediatric patients ≥6 months of age with mild, atopic asthma

Usual Dosage

Ophthalmic: Allergic conjunctivitis: Children ≥3 years and Adults: Instill 1 drop into the affected eye(s) twice daily, every 8-12 hours

Oral (not approved in U.S.): Atopic asthma (**Note:** Not for acute attacks):

Children 6 months to 3 years: Initial: 0.025 mg/kg once daily or in 2 divided doses for 5 days; Maintenance: 0.05 mg/kg twice daily

Children >3 years: Initial: 0.5 mg once daily or in 2 divided doses for 5 days; Maintenance: 1 mg twice daily

Dosage Forms [CAN] = Canadian brand name
Solution, ophthalmic [drops]: 0.025% (5 mL)
Alaway™ [OTC]: 0.025% (10 mL)
Claritin™ Eye [OTC], Zaditor® [OTC], Zyrtec® Itchy Eye [OTC]: 0.025% (5 mL)
Syrup: 1 mg/5 mL (250 mL) [not available in U.S.]
Novo-Ketotifen® [CAN]: 1 mg/5 mL (250 mL) [not available in U.S.]
Nu-Ketotifen® [CAN]: 1 mg/5 mL (250 mL) [not available in U.S.]
Zaditen® [CAN]: 1 mg/5 mL (250 mL) [not available in U.S.]
Tablet: 1 mg [not available in U.S.]
Novo-ketotifen® [CAN]: 1 mg [not available in U.S.]
Zaditen® [CAN]: 1 mg [not available in U.S.]

ketotifen fumarate *see* ketotifen *on page* 559
Key-E® [US-OTC] *see* vitamin E *on page* 1018
Key-E® Kaps [US-OTC] *see* vitamin E *on page* 1018
Keygesic [US-OTC] *see* magnesium salicylate *on page* 610
Key-Pred® *(Discontinued)*
Key-Pred-SP® *(Discontinued)*
K-G® *(Discontinued)* *see* potassium gluconate *on page* 805
K-Gen® Effervescent *(Discontinued)* *see* potassium bicarbonate *on page* 802
khlōditan *see* mitotane *on page* 662
KI *see* potassium iodide *on page* 805
K-Ide® *(Discontinued)*
Kidkare Children's Cough and Cold [US-OTC] *see* chlorpheniramine, pseudoephedrine, and dextromethorphan *on page* 220
Kidkare Decongestant [US-OTC] *see* pseudoephedrine *on page* 833
Kidrolase® [Can] *see* asparaginase *on page* 102
Kinerase® *(Discontinued)* *see* hyaluronidase *on page* 497
Kineret® [US/Can] *see* anakinra *on page* 78
Kinesed® *(Discontinued)* *see* hyoscyamine, atropine, scopolamine, and phenobarbital *on page* 513
Kinevac® [US] *see* sincalide *on page* 903
Kinlytic™ [US] *see* urokinase *on page* 999
Kinrix™ [US] *see* diphtheria and tetanus toxoids, acellular pertussis, and poliovirus vaccine *on page* 319
Kionex® [US] *see* sodium polystyrene sulfonate *on page* 914
Kivexa™ [Can] *see* abacavir and lamivudine *on page* 16
Klaron® [US] *see* sulfacetamide *on page* 927
Klean-Prep® [Can] *see* polyethylene glycol-electrolyte solution *on page* 797
K-Lease® *(Discontinued)* *see* potassium chloride *on page* 803
Klerist-D® Tablet *(Discontinued)* *see* chlorpheniramine and pseudoephedrine *on page* 215
Klonopin® [US/Can] *see* clonazepam *on page* 245
Klonopin® Wafers *(Discontinued)* *see* clonazepam *on page* 245
K-Lor® [US/Can] *see* potassium chloride *on page* 803
Klor-Con® [US] *see* potassium chloride *on page* 803
Klor-Con® 8 [US] *see* potassium chloride *on page* 803
Klor-Con® 10 [US] *see* potassium chloride *on page* 803
Klor-Con®/25 [US] *see* potassium chloride *on page* 803
Klor-Con® M [US] *see* potassium chloride *on page* 803
Klor-Con®/EF [US] *see* potassium bicarbonate and potassium citrate *on page* 802
Kloromin® Oral *(Discontinued)* *see* chlorpheniramine *on page* 213
Klorvess® *(Discontinued)* *see* potassium chloride *on page* 803
Klorvess® Effervescent *(Discontinued)*
K-Lyte® [US] *see* potassium bicarbonate and potassium citrate *on page* 802
K-Lyte® [Can] *see* potassium citrate *on page* 804

L-M-X™ 5 [US-OTC] *see* lidocaine *on page 584*
L 754030 *see* aprepitant *on page 94*
LA 20304a *see* gemifloxacin *on page 458*

labetalol (la BET a lole)

Sound-Alike/Look-Alike Issues

labetalol may be confused with betaxolol, Hexadrol®, lamoTRIgine
Normodyne® may be confused with Norpramin®
Trandate® may be confused with traMADol, Trendar®, Trental®, Tridrate®

Synonyms ibidomide hydrochloride; labetalol hydrochloride

U.S./Canadian Brand Names Apo-Labetalol® [Can]; Labetalol Hydrochloride Injection, USP [Can]; Normodyne® [Can]; Trandate® [US/Can]

Therapeutic Category Alpha-/Beta- Adrenergic Blocker

Use Treatment of mild-to-severe hypertension; I.V. for severe hypertension (eg, hypertensive emergencies)

Usual Dosage

Children: Due to limited documentation of its use, labetalol should be initiated cautiously in pediatric patients with careful dosage adjustment and blood pressure monitoring.

I.V., intermittent bolus doses of 0.3-1 mg/kg/dose have been reported.

For treatment of pediatric hypertensive emergencies, initial continuous infusions of 0.4-1 mg/kg/hour with a maximum of 3 mg/kg/hour have been used. Administration requires the use of an infusion pump.

Adults:

Oral: Initial: 100 mg twice daily, may increase as needed every 2-3 days by 100 mg twice daily (titration increments not to exceed 200 mg twice daily) until desired response is obtained; usual dose: 200-400 mg twice daily; may require up to 2.4 g/day.

Usual dose range (JNC 7): 200-800 mg/day in 2 divided doses

I.V.: 20 mg (0.25 mg/kg for an 80 kg patient) I.V. push over 2 minutes; may administer 40-80 mg at 10-minute intervals, up to 300 mg total dose.

I.V. infusion (acute loading): Initial: 2 mg/minute; titrate to response up to 300 mg total dose, if needed. Administration requires the use of an infusion pump.

I.V. infusion (500 mg/250 mL D_5W) rates:

1 mg/minute: 30 mL/hour
2 mg/minute: 60 mL/hour
3 mg/minute: 90 mL/hour
4 mg/minute: 120 mL/hour
5 mg/minute: 150 mL/hour
6 mg/minute: 180 mL/hour

Note: Although loading infusions are well described in the product labeling, the labeling is silent in specific clinical situations, such as in the patient who has an initial response to labetalol infusions but cannot be converted to an oral route for subsequent dosing. There is limited documentation of prolonged continuous infusions. In rare clinical situations, higher continuous infusion dosages (up to 6 mg/minute) have been used in the critical care setting (eg, aortic dissection). At the other extreme, continuous infusions at relatively low doses (0.03-0.1 mg/minute) have been used in some settings (following loading infusion in patients who are unable to be converted to oral regimens or in some cases as a continuation of outpatient oral regimens). These prolonged infusions should not be confused with loading infusions. Because of wide variation in the use of infusions, an awareness of institutional policies and practices is extremely important. Careful clarification of orders and specific infusion rates/units is required to avoid confusion. Due to the prolonged duration of action, careful monitoring should be extended for the duration of the infusion and for several hours after the infusion. Excessive administration may result in prolonged hypotension and/or bradycardia.

Dosage Forms

Injection, solution: 5 mg/mL (4 mL, 8 mL, 20 mL, 40 mL)
Trandate®: 5 mg/mL (20 mL, 40 mL)
Tablet: 100 mg, 200 mg, 300 mg
Trandate®: 100 mg, 200 mg, 300 mg

labetalol hydrochloride *see* labetalol *on page 562*
Labetalol Hydrochloride Injection, USP [Can] *see* labetalol *on page 562*
Lac-Dose [US-OTC] *see* lactase *on page 563*
Lac-Hydrin® [US] *see* lactic acid and ammonium hydroxide *on page 564*
Lac-Hydrin® Five [US-OTC] *see* lactic acid and ammonium hydroxide *on page 564*

LAClotion™ [US] *see* lactic acid and ammonium hydroxide *on page 564*

lacosamide (la KOE sa mide)

Sound-Alike/Look-Alike Issues

lacosamide may be confused with zonisamide

Synonyms ADD 234037; harkoseride; LCM; SPM 927

U.S./Canadian Brand Names Vimpat® [US]

Therapeutic Category Anticonvulsant, Miscellaneous

Use Adjunctive therapy in the treatment of partial-onset seizures

Usual Dosage Oral, I.V.: Adolescents ≥17 years and Adults: Partial onset seizure:

Initial: 50 mg twice daily; may be increased at weekly intervals by 100 mg/day

Maintenance dose: 200-400 mg/day

Note: When switching from oral to I.V. formulations, the total daily dose and frequency should be the same; I.V. therapy should only be used temporarily.

Dosage Forms

Injection, solution:

Vimpat®: 10 mg/mL (20 mL)

Tablet:

Vimpat®: 50 mg, 100 mg, 150 mg, 200 mg

Lacril® Ophthalmic Solution *(Discontinued)* *see* artificial tears *on page 100*

Lacrisert® [US/Can] *see* hydroxypropyl cellulose *on page 510*

LaCrosse Complete [US-OTC] *see* sodium phosphates *on page 912*

Lactaid® Extra Strength *(Discontinued)* *see* lactase *on page 563*

Lactaid® Fast Act [US-OTC] *see* lactase *on page 563*

Lactaid® Original [US-OTC] *see* lactase *on page 563*

Lactaid® Ultra *(Discontinued)* *see* lactase *on page 563*

lactase (LAK tase)

U.S./Canadian Brand Names Dairyaid® [Can]; Lac-Dose [US-OTC]; Lactaid® Fast Act [US-OTC]; Lactaid® Original [US-OTC]; Lactrase® [US-OTC]

Therapeutic Category Nutritional Supplement

Use Help digest lactose in milk for patients with lactose intolerance

Usual Dosage Oral:

Capsule: 1-2 capsules taken with milk or meal; pretreat milk with 1-2 capsules/quart of milk

Liquid: 5-15 drops/quart of milk

Tablet: 1-3 tablets with meals

Dosage Forms

Caplet:

Lactaid® Original [OTC]: 3000 FCC lactase units

Lactaid® Fast Act [OTC]: 9000 FCC lactase units

Capsule:

Lactrase® [OTC]: 250 mg standardized enzyme lactase

Tablet, oral, chewable:

Lactaid® Fast Act [OTC]: 9000 FCC lactase units

Tablet, oral:

Lac-Dose [OTC]: 3000 FCC lactase units

lactic acid (LAK tik AS id)

Synonyms sodium-PCA and lactic acid

U.S./Canadian Brand Names LactiCare® [US-OTC]; Lactinol-E® [US]; Lactinol® [US]

Therapeutic Category Topical Skin Product

Use Lubricate and moisturize the skin counteracting dryness and itching

Usual Dosage Topical: Adults: Lubricant/moisturizer: Apply twice daily

Dosage Forms

Cream: 10% (120 g)

Lactinol-E®: 10% (120 g)

Lotion: 10% (360 mL)

LactiCare® [OTC]: 5% (222 mL, 340 mL)

Lactinol®: 10% (360 mL)

lactic acid and ammonium hydroxide (LAK tik AS id & a MOE nee um hye DROKS ide)

Synonyms ammonium hydroxide and lactic acid; ammonium lactate

U.S./Canadian Brand Names AmLactin® [US-OTC]; Geri-Hydrolac™ [US-OTC]; Geri-Hydrolac™-12 [US-OTC]; Lac-Hydrin® Five [US-OTC]; Lac-Hydrin® [US]; LAClotion™ [US]

Therapeutic Category Topical Skin Product

Use Treatment of moderate-to-severe xerosis and ichthyosis vulgaris

Usual Dosage Topical:

Cream: Children ≥2 years and Adults: Apply twice daily to affected area; rub in well

Lotion: Children and Adults: Apply twice daily to affected area; rub in well

Dosage Forms

Cream, topical: Lactic acid 12% with ammonium hydroxide (140 g, 280 g, 385 g)

AmLactin® [OTC]: Lactic acid 12% with ammonium hydroxide (140 g)

Lac-Hydrin®: Lactic acid 12% with ammonium hydroxide (280 g, 385 g)

Lotion, topical: Lactic acid 12% with ammonium hydroxide (225 g, 400 g)

AmLactin® [OTC], Lac-Hydrin®, LAClotion™: Lactic acid 12% with ammonium hydroxide (225 g, 400 g)

Geri-Hydrolac™ [OTC], Lac-Hydrin® Five: Lactic acid 5% with ammonium hydroxide (120 mL, 240 mL)

Geri-Hydrolac™-12 [OTC]: Lactic acid 12% with ammonium hydroxide (120 mL, 240 mL)

LactiCare® [US-OTC] *see* lactic acid *on page* 563

Lactinex™ [US-OTC] *see* Lactobacillus *on page* 564

Lactinol® [US] *see* lactic acid *on page* 563

Lactinol-E® [US] *see* lactic acid *on page* 563

Lactobacillus (lak toe ba SIL us)

Synonyms *Lactobacillus acidophilus*; *Lactobacillus bifidus*; *Lactobacillus bulgaricus*; *Lactobacillus casei*; *Lactobacillus paracasei*; *Lactobacillus reuteri*; *Lactobacillus rhamnosus* GG

U.S./Canadian Brand Names Bacid® [US-OTC/Can]; Culturelle® [US-OTC]; Dofus [US-OTC]; Fermalac [Can]; Flora-Q™ [US-OTC]; Floranex™ [US-OTC]; Kala® [US-OTC]; Lactinex™ [US-OTC]; Lacto-Bifidus [US-OTC]; Lacto-Key [US-OTC]; Lacto-Pectin [US-OTC]; Lacto-TriBlend [US-OTC]; Megadophilus® [US-OTC]; MoreDophilus® [US-OTC]; Superdophilus® [US-OTC]

Therapeutic Category Gastrointestinal Agent, Miscellaneous

Use Promote normal bacterial flora of the intestinal tract

Usual Dosage Dietary supplement: Oral: Dosing varies by manufacturer; consult product labeling

Children (Culturelle®): 1 capsule daily

Adults:

Bacid®: 2 caplets/day

Culturelle®: 1 capsule daily; may increase to twice daily

Flora-Q™: 1 capsule/day

Lacto-Key 100 or 600: 1-2 capsules/day

Lactinex™: 1 packet or 4 tablets 3-4 times/day

Dosage Forms

Capsule:

Culturelle® [OTC]: *L. rhamnosus* GG 10 billion colony-forming units

Dofus [OTC]: *L. acidophilus* and *L. bifidus* 10:1 ratio

Flora-Q™ [OTC]: *L. acidophilus* and *L. paracasei* ≥8 billion colony-forming units

Lacto-Key [OTC]:

100: *L. acidophilus* 1 billion colony-forming units

600: *L. acidophilus* 6 billion colony-forming units

Lacto-Bifidus [OTC]:

100: *L. bifidus* 1 billion colony-forming units

600: *L. bifidus* 6 billion colony-forming units

Lacto-Pectin [OTC]: *L. acidophilus* and *L. casei* ≥5 billion colony-forming units

Lacto-TriBlend [OTC]:

100: *L. acidophilus, L. bifidus,* and *L. bulgaricus* 1 billion colony-forming units

600: *L. acidophilus, L. bifidus,* and *L. bulgaricus* 6 billion colony-forming units

Megadophilus® [OTC], Superdophilus® [OTC]: *L. acidophilus* 2 billion units

Capsule, softgel: *L. acidophilus* 100 active units

Caplet:
Bacid® [OTC]: *L. acidophilus 80%* and *L. bulgaricus* 10%
Granules:
Lactinex™ [OTC]: *L. acidophilus* and *L. bulgaricus* 100 million live cells per 1 g packet (12s)
Powder:
Lacto-TriBlend [OTC]: *L. acidophilus, L. bifidus,* and *L. bulgaricus* 10 billion colony-forming units per ¼ teaspoon
Megadophilus® [OTC], Superdophilus® [OTC]: *L. acidophilus* 2 billion units per half-teaspoon
MoreDophilus® [OTC]: *L. acidophilus* 12.4 billion units per teaspoon
Tablet:
Kala® [OTC]: *L. acidophilus* 200 million units
Lactinex™ [OTC]: *L. acidophilus* and *L. bulgaricus* 1 million live cells
Tablet, chewable: *L. reuteri* 100 million organisms
Floranex™ [OTC]: *L. acidophilus* and *L. bulgaricus* 1 million colony-forming units
Wafer: *L. acidophilus* 90 mg and *L. bifidus* 25 mg (100s)

Lactobacillus acidophilus *see* Lactobacillus *on page 564*
Lactobacillus bifidus *see* Lactobacillus *on page 564*
Lactobacillus bulgaricus *see* Lactobacillus *on page 564*
Lactobacillus casei *see* Lactobacillus *on page 564*
Lactobacillus paracasei *see* Lactobacillus *on page 564*
Lactobacillus reuteri *see* Lactobacillus *on page 564*
***Lactobacillus rhamnosus* GG** *see* Lactobacillus *on page 564*
Lacto-Bifidus [US-OTC] *see* Lactobacillus *on page 564*
lactoflavin *see* riboflavin *on page 865*
Lacto-Key [US-OTC] *see* Lactobacillus *on page 564*
Lacto-Pectin [US-OTC] *see* Lactobacillus *on page 564*
Lacto-TriBlend [US-OTC] *see* Lactobacillus *on page 564*
Lactrase® [US-OTC] *see* lactase *on page 563*

lactulose (LAK tyoo lose)

Sound-Alike/Look-Alike Issues
lactulose may be confused with lactose

U.S./Canadian Brand Names Acilac [Can]; Apo-Lactulose® [Can]; Constulose [US]; Enulose [US]; Generlac [US]; Kristalose® [US]; Laxilose [Can]; PMS-Lactulose [Can]

Therapeutic Category Ammonium Detoxicant; Laxative

Use Adjunct in the prevention and treatment of portal-systemic encephalopathy; treatment of chronic constipation

Usual Dosage Diarrhea may indicate overdosage and responds to dose reduction
Prevention of portal systemic encephalopathy (PSE): Oral:
Infants: 2.5-10 mL/day divided 3-4 times/day; adjust dosage to produce 2-3 stools/day
Older Children: Daily dose of 40-90 mL divided 3-4 times/day; if initial dose causes diarrhea, then reduce it immediately; adjust dosage to produce 2-3 stools/day
Constipation: Oral:
Children: 5 g/day (7.5 mL) after breakfast
Adults: 15-30 mL/day increased to 60 mL/day in 1-2 divided doses if necessary
Acute PSE: Adults:
Oral: 20-30 g (30-45 mL) every 1-2 hours to induce rapid laxation; adjust dosage daily to produce 2-3 soft stools; doses of 30-45 mL may be given hourly to cause rapid laxation, then reduce to recommended dose; usual daily dose: 60-100 g (90-150 mL) daily
Rectal administration: 200 g (300 mL) diluted with 700 mL of H_2O or NS; administer rectally via rectal balloon catheter and retain 30-60 minutes every 4-6 hours

Dosage Forms
Crystals for solution, oral:
Kristalose®: 10 g/packet (30s), 20 g/packet (30s)
Solution, oral: 10 g/15 mL
Constulose, Enulose, Generlac: 10 g/15 mL
Solution, oral/rectal: 10 g/15 mL (237 mL, 473 mL, 946 mL)

Lactulose PSE® *(Discontinued)* *see* lactulose *on page 565*

Iadakamycin *see* azacitidine *on page 114*
Lagesic™ [US] *see* acetaminophen and phenyltoloxamine *on page 23*
L-All 12 *(Discontinued)* *see* carbetapentane and phenylephrine *on page 182*
L-AmB *see* amphotericin B liposomal *on page 75*
Lamictal® [US/Can] *see* lamotrigine *on page 567*
Lamictal® ODT™ [US] *see* lamotrigine *on page 567*
Lamictal® XR™ [US] *see* lamotrigine *on page 567*
Lamisil® Oral [US/Can] *see* terbinafine (oral) *on page 945*
Lamisil® Topical [US/Can] *see* terbinafine (topical) *on page 945*

lamivudine (la MI vyoo deen)

Sound-Alike/Look-Alike Issues
lamiVUDine may be confused with lamoTRIgine
Epivir® may be confused with Combivir®

Synonyms 3TC

Tall-Man lami**VUD**ine

U.S./Canadian Brand Names 3TC® [Can]; Epivir-HBV® [US]; Epivir® [US]; Heptovir® [Can]

Therapeutic Category Antiviral Agent

Use
Epivir®: Treatment of HIV infection when antiretroviral therapy is warranted; should always be used as part of a multidrug regimen (at least three antiretroviral agents)
Epivir-HBV®: Treatment of chronic hepatitis B associated with evidence of hepatitis B viral replication and active liver inflammation

Usual Dosage Oral: **Note:** The formulation and dosage of Epivir-HBV® are not appropriate for patients infected with both HBV and HIV. Use with at least two other antiretroviral agents when treating HIV.

HIV:
Neonates <30 days (AIDS*info* guidelines): 2 mg/kg/dose twice daily
Infants 1-3 months (AIDS*info* guidelines): 4 mg/kg/dose twice daily
Infants and Children 3 months to 16 years: 4 mg/kg/dose twice daily (maximum: 150 mg/dose twice daily)
Alternate weight-based dosing using scored 150 mg tablets (AIDSinfo guidelines):
14-21 kg: 75 mg/dose twice daily (150 mg/day)
22-29 kg: 75 mg in the morning, 150 mg in the evening (225 mg/day)
≥30 kg: 150 mg/dose twice daily (300 mg/day)
Adults: 150 mg twice daily or 300 mg once daily
<50 kg (AIDS*info* guidelines): 4 mg/kg/dose twice daily (maximum: 150 mg/dose twice daily)

Treatment of hepatitis B (Epivir-HBV®): Note: Usual treatment duration is at least 1 year and varies with HBeAg status, consult current guidelines and literature.
Children 2-17 years: 3 mg/kg/dose once daily (maximum: 100 mg/day)
Adults: 100 mg/day

Prevention of maternal-fetal HIV transmission (AIDSinfo guidelines): Note: Lamivudine may be used in combination with zidovudine and nevirapine in select situations (eg, infants born to mothers with suboptimal viral suppression at delivery, infants born to mothers with only intrapartum therapy or no therapy, or infants born to mothers with known antiretroviral drug-resistant virus). Lamivudine is used in this situation to reduce the development of nevirapine resistant virus:
Mother: 150 mg twice daily starting at onset of labor and continuing through 1 week postpartum
Neonate: 2 mg/kg/dose twice daily given at birth through 1 week of age

Dosage Forms

Solution, oral:
Epivir®: 10 mg/mL
Epivir-HBV®: 5 mg/mL

Tablet:
Epivir®: 150 mg [scored], 300 mg
Epivir-HBV®: 100 mg

lamivudine, abacavir, and zidovudine *see* abacavir, lamivudine, and zidovudine *on page 16*
lamivudine and abacavir *see* abacavir and lamivudine *on page 16*
lamivudine and zidovudine *see* zidovudine and lamivudine *on page 1029*

lamotrigine (la MOE tri jeen)

Sound-Alike/Look-Alike Issues

lamoTRIgine may be confused with labetalol, Lamisil®, lamiVUDine, levothyroxine, Lomotil®, ludiomil
Lamictal® may be confused with Lamisil®, Lomotil®, ludiomil

Synonyms BW-430C; LTG

Tall-Man lamo**TRI**gine

U.S./Canadian Brand Names Apo-Lamotrigine® [Can]; Lamictal® ODT™ [US]; Lamictal® XR™ [US]; Lamictal® [US/Can]; Mylan-Lamotrigine [Can]; Novo-Lamotrigine [Can]; PMS-Lamotrigine [Can]; ratio-Lamotrigine [Can]

Therapeutic Category Anticonvulsant

Use Adjunctive therapy in the treatment of generalized seizures of Lennox-Gastaut syndrome, primary generalized tonic-clonic seizures, and partial seizures in adults and children ≥2 years of age; conversion to monotherapy in adults (≥16 years of age) with partial seizures who are receiving treatment with valproic acid or a single enzyme-inducing antiepileptic drug (specifically carbamazepine, phenytoin, phenobarbital or primidone); maintenance treatment of bipolar I disorder in adults

Usual Dosage Note: Only whole tablets should be used for dosing, round calculated dose down to the nearest whole tablet. Extended release formulation not approved for children ≤12 years of age. Enzyme-inducing regimens specifically refer to those containing carbamazepine, phenytoin, phenobarbital, or primidone. Oral:

Children 2-12 years: Lennox-Gastaut (adjunctive), primary generalized tonic-clonic seizures (adjunctive), or partial seizures (adjunctive): **Note:** Children <30 kg will likely require maintenance doses to be increased as much as 50% based on clinical response regardless of regimen below:

Immediate release formulations: Initial: 0.3 mg/kg/day in 1-2 divided doses for weeks 1 and 2, then increase to 0.6 mg/kg/day in 2 divided doses for weeks 3 and 4. Maintenance: Titrate dose to effect; after week 4, increase daily dose every 1-2 weeks by 0.6 mg/kg/day; usual maintenance: 4.5-7.5 mg/kg/day in 2 divided doses; maximum: 300 mg/day in 2 divided doses

Adjustment for AED regimens **containing** valproic acid (see **"Note"** below): Immediate release formulations: Initial: 0.15 mg/kg/day in 1-2 divided doses for weeks 1 and 2, then increase to 0.3 mg/kg/day in 1-2 divided doses for weeks 3 and 4. Maintenance: Titrate dose to effect; after week 4, increase daily dose every 1-2 weeks by 0.3 mg/kg/day; usual maintenance: 1-5 mg/kg/day in 2 divided doses; maximum: 200 mg/day in 1-2 divided doses

Note: For patients >6.7 kg and <14 kg, initial dosing should be 2 mg every other day for first 2 weeks, then increased to 2 mg daily for weeks 3-4. For patients taking lamotrigine with valproic acid alone, the usual maintenance dose is 1-3 mg/kg/day in 2 divided doses

Adjustment for **enzyme-inducing** AED regimens **without** valproic acid: Immediate release formulations: Initial: 0.6 mg/kg/day in 2 divided doses for weeks 1 and 2, then increase to 1.2 mg/kg/day in 2 divided doses for weeks 3 and 4. Maintenance: Titrate dose to effect; after week 4, increase daily dose every 1-2 weeks by 1.2 mg/kg/day; usual maintenance: 5-15 mg/kg/day in 2 divided doses; maximum: 400 mg/day in 2 divided doses

Children >12 years: Lennox-Gastaut (adjunctive), primary generalized tonic-clonic seizures (adjunctive), or partial seizures (adjunctive): Refer to adult dosing.

Children ≥16 years: Conversion from adjunctive therapy with valproic acid or a single enzyme-inducing AED regimen to monotherapy with lamotrigine: Refer to adult dosing.

Adults:

Lennox-Gastaut (adjunctive), primary generalized tonic-clonic seizures (adjunctive) or partial seizures (adjunctive): Immediate release formulations: Initial: 25 mg/day for weeks 1 and 2, then increase to 50 mg/day for weeks 3 and 4. Maintenance: Titrate dose to effect; after week 4 increase daily dose every 1-2 weeks by 50 mg/day; usual maintenance: 225-375 mg/day in 2 divided doses

Adjustment for AED regimens **containing** valproic acid (see **"Note"** below): Initial: 25 mg every other day for weeks 1 and 2, then increase to 25 mg every day for weeks 3 and 4. Maintenance: Titrate dose to effect; after week 4 increase daily dose every 1-2 weeks by 25-50 mg/day; usual maintenance: 100-400 mg/day in 1 or 2 divided doses

Note: For patients taking lamotrigine with valproic acid alone, the usual maintenance dose is 100-200 mg/day

Adjustment for **enzyme-inducing** AED regimens **without** valproic acid: Initial: 50 mg/day for weeks 1 and 2, then increase to 100 mg/day in 2 divided doses for weeks 3 and 4. Maintenance: titrate dose to effect; after week 4 increase daily dose every 1-2 weeks by 100 mg/day; usual maintenance: 300-500 mg/day in 2 divided doses. Doses as high as 700 mg/day have been used, though additional benefit has not been established.

Conversion to monotherapy with lamotrigine:

Conversion from adjunctive therapy with valproic acid: Initiate and titrate as per recommendations to a lamotrigine dose of 200 mg/day. Then taper valproic acid dose in decrements of not >500 mg/day at intervals of 1 week (or longer) to a valproic acid dosage of 500 mg/day; this dosage should be maintained for 1 week. The lamotrigine dosage should then be increased to 300 mg/day while valproic acid is decreased to 250 mg/day; this dosage should be maintained for 1 week. Valproic acid may then be discontinued, while the lamotrigine dose is increased by 100 mg/day at weekly intervals to achieve a lamotrigine maintenance dose of 500 mg/day.

Conversion from adjunctive therapy with carbamazepine, phenytoin, phenobarbital, or primidone: Initiate and titrate as per recommendations to a lamotrigine dose of 500 mg/day. Concomitant enzyme-inducing AED should then be withdrawn by 20% decrements each week over a 4-week period. Patients should be monitored for rash.

Conversion from adjunctive therapy with AED other than carbamazepine, phenytoin, phenobarbital, primidone or valproic acid: No specific guidelines available

Partial seizures (adjunctive): Extended release formulation: **Note:** Dose increases after week 8 should not exceed 100 mg/day at weekly intervals

Regimens **containing** valproic acid: Initial: Week 1 and 2: 25 mg every other day; Week 3 and 4: 25 mg every day; Week 5: 50 mg every day; Week 6: 100 mg every day; Week 7: 150 mg every day; Maintenance: 200-250 mg every day

Regimens **containing** carbamazepine, phenytoin, phenobarbital, or primidone and **without** valproic acid: Initial: Week 1 and 2: 50 mg every day; Week 3 and 4: 100 mg every day; Week 5: 200 mg every day; Week 6: 300 mg every day; Week 7: 400 mg every day; Maintenance: 400-600 mg every day

Regimens **not containing** carbamazepine, phenytoin, phenobarbital, primidone, or valproic acid: Initial: Week 1 and 2: 25 mg every day; Week 3 and 4: 50 mg every day; Week 5: 100 mg every day; Week 6: 150 mg every day; Week 7: 200 mg every day; Maintenance: 300-400 mg every day

Bipolar disorder:

Initial: 25 mg/day for weeks 1 and 2, then increase to 50 mg/day for weeks 3 and 4, then increase to 100 mg/day for week 5; maintenance: increase dose to 200 mg/day beginning week 6

Adjustment for regimens **containing** valproic acid: Initial: 25 mg every other day for weeks 1 and 2, then increase to 25 mg every day for weeks 3 and 4, then increase to 50 mg/day for week 5; maintenance: 100 mg/day beginning week 6

Adjustment for **enzyme-inducing** regimens **without** valproic acid: Initial: 50 mg/day for weeks 1 and 2, then increase to 100 mg/day in divided doses for weeks 3 and 4, then increase to 200 mg/day in divided doses for week 5, then increase to 300 mg/day in divided dose for week 6; maintenance: 400 mg/day in divided doses beginning week 7

Adjustment following discontinuation of psychotropic medication:

Discontinuing valproic acid with current dose of lamotrigine 100 mg/day: 150 mg/day for week 1, then increase to 200 mg/day beginning week 2

Discontinuing carbamazepine, phenytoin, phenobarbital, primidone, or rifampin with current dose of lamotrigine 400 mg/day: 400 mg/day for week 1, then decrease to 300 mg/day for week 2, then decrease to 200 mg/day beginning week 3

Conversion from immediate release to extended release (Lamictal® XR™): Initial dose of the extended release tablet should match the total daily dose of the immediate-release formulation; monitor for seizure control, especially in patients on AED agents. Adjust dose as needed within the recommended dosing guidelines.

Discontinuing therapy: Children and Adults: Decrease dose by ~50% per week, over at least 2 weeks unless safety concerns require a more rapid withdrawal. Discontinuing carbamazepine, phenytoin, phenobarbital, or primidone should prolong the half-life of lamotrigine; discontinuing valproic acid should shorten the half-life of lamotrigine

Restarting therapy after discontinuation: If lamotrigine has been withheld for >5 half-lives, consider restarting according to initial dosing recommendations.

Dosage adjustment with estrogen-containing hormonal contraceptives: Follow initial lamotrigine dosing guidelines, maintenance dose should be adjusted as follows:

Patients taking concomitant carbamazepine, phenytoin, phenobarbital, primidone or rifampin: No dosing adjustment required

Patients **not** taking concomitant carbamazepine, phenytoin, phenobarbital, primidone or rifampin: Lamotrigine maintenance dose may need increased by twofold over target dose. If already taking a stable dose of lamotrigine and starting contraceptive, maintenance dose may need increased by twofold. Dose increases should start when contraceptive is started and titrated to clinical response increasing no more rapidly than 50-100 mg/day every week. Gradual increases of lamotrigine plasma levels may occur during the inactive "pill-free" week and will be greater when dose increases are made the week before. If increased adverse events consistently occur during "pill-free" week, overall maintenance dose adjustments may be required. When discontinuing estrogen-containing hormonal contraceptive, dose of lamotrigine may need decreased by as much as 50%; do not decrease by more than 25% of total daily dose over a 2-week period unless clinical response or plasma levels indicate otherwise. Dose adjustments during "pill-free" week are not recommended.

Dosage Forms

Table, oralt: 25 mg, 100 mg, 150 mg, 200 mg
Lamictal®: 25 mg, 100 mg, 150 mg, 200 mg

Tablet, oral [combination package; each unit-dose starter kit contains]:
Lamictal® [blue kit; for patients taking valproic acid]:
25 mg (35s)
Lamictal® [green kit; for patients taking carbamazepine, phenytoin, phenobarbital, primidone, or rifampin and **not** taking valproic acid]:
25 mg (84s)
100 mg (14s)
Lamictal® [orange kit; for patients **not** taking carbamazepine, phenytoin, phenobarbital, primidone, rifampin, or valproic acid]:
25 mg (42s)
100 mg (7s)

Tablet, dispersible/chewable, oral: 5 mg, 25 mg
Lamictal®: 2 mg, 25 mg
Lamictal®: 5 mg [scored]

Tablet, extended release, oral:
Lamictal® XR™: 25 mg, 50 mg, 100 mg, 200 mg

Tablet, extended release, oral [combination packge; each patient titration kit contains]:
Lamictal® XR™ [blue XR kit; for patients taking valproic acid]:
25 mg (21s)
50 mg (7s)
Lamictal® XR™ [green XR kit; for patients taking carbamazepine, phenytoin, phenobarbital, or primidone and **not** taking valproic acid]:
50 mg (14s)
100 mg (14s)
200 mg (7s)
Lamictal® XR™ [orange XR kit; for patients **not** taking carbamazepine, phenytoin, phenobarbital, primidone, or valproic acid]:
25 mg (14s)
50 mg (14s)
100 mg (7s)

Tablet, orally disintegrating, oral:
Lamictal® ODT™: 25 mg, 50 mg, 100 mg, 200 mg

Tablet, orally disintegrating, oral [combination package; each patient titration kit contains]:
Lamictal® ODT™ [blue ODT kit; for patients taking valproic acid]:
25 mg (21s)
50 mg (7s)
Lamictal® ODT™ [green ODT kit; for patients taking carbamazepine, phenytoin, phenobarbital, primidone, or rifampin and **not** taking valproic acid]:
50 mg (42s)
100 mg (14s)
Lamictal® ODT™ [orange ODT kit; for patients **not** taking carbamazepine, phenytoin, phenobarbital, primidone, rifampin, or valproic acid]:
25 mg (14s)
50 mg (14s)
100 mg (7s)

Lanacane® [US-OTC] *see* benzocaine *on page 129*

Lanacane® Maximum Strength [US-OTC] *see* benzocaine *on page 129*

Lanaphilic® [US-OTC] *see* urea *on page 998*

lanolin, cetyl alcohol, glycerin, petrolatum, and mineral oil

(LAN oh lin, SEE til AL koe hol, GLIS er in, pe troe LAY tum, & MIN er al oyl)

Synonyms cetyl alcohol, glycerin, lanolin, mineral oil, and petrolatum; mineral oil, petrolatum, lanolin, cetyl alcohol, and glycerin

U.S./Canadian Brand Names Lubriderm® Fragrance Free [US-OTC]; Lubriderm® [US-OTC]

Therapeutic Category Topical Skin Product

Use Treatment of dry skin

Usual Dosage Topical: Apply to skin as necessary

Dosage Forms

Lotion, topical [bottle]: 180 mL, 300 mL, 480 mL

Lubriderm® Fragrance Free [OTC], Lubriderm® [OTC]: 180 mL, 300 mL, 480 mL

Lotion, topical [tube]: 100 mL

Lubriderm® Fragrance Free [OTC], Lubriderm® [OTC]: 100 mL

Lanorinal® ***(Discontinued)***

Lanoxicaps® [Can] *see* digoxin *on page 308*

Lanoxicaps® ***(Discontinued)*** *see* digoxin *on page 308*

Lanoxin® [US/Can] *see* digoxin *on page 308*

lanreotide (lan REE oh tide)

Sound-Alike/Look-Alike Issues

Somatuline® may be confused with somatropin, SUMAtriptan

Synonyms lanreotide acetate

U.S./Canadian Brand Names Somatuline® Autogel® [Can]; Somatuline® Depot [US]

Therapeutic Category Somatostatin Analog

Use Long-term treatment of acromegaly in patients who are not candidates for or are unresponsive to surgery and/or radiotherapy

Canadian labeling: Also approved in Canada for relief of symptoms of acromegaly

Usual Dosage SubQ: **Note: Differences in U.S. and Canadian labeled dosing:**

U.S. labeling: Adults: Acromegaly: 90 mg once every 4 weeks for 3 months; after initial 90 days of therapy, adjust dose based on clinical response of patient, growth hormone (GH) levels, and/or insulin-like growth factor 1 (IGF-1) levels as follows:

GH ≤1 ng/mL, IGF-1 normal, symptoms stable: 60 mg once every 4 weeks

GH >1-2.5 ng/mL, IGF-1 normal, symptoms stable: 90 mg once every 4 weeks

GH >2.5 ng/mL, IGF-1 elevated and/or uncontrolled symptoms: 120 mg once every 4 weeks

Canadian labeling: Children ≥16 years and Adults: Acromegaly: 90 mg once every 4 weeks for 3 months; after initial 90 days of therapy, adjust dose based on clinical response of patient, growth hormone (GH) levels, and/or insulin-like growth factor 1 (IGF-1) levels as follows:

GH = 1 ng/mL, IGF-1 normal, symptoms stable: 60 mg once every 4 weeks

GH >1-2.5 ng/mL, IGF-1 normal, symptoms stable: 90 mg once every 4 weeks

GH >2.5 ng/mL, IGF-1 elevated and/or uncontrolled symptoms: 120 mg once every 4 weeks

Dosage Forms Excipient information presented when available (limited, particularly for generics); consult specific product labeling. [CAN] = Canadian brand name

Injection, solution:

Somatuline® Autogel® [CAN]: 60 mg/ 0.3 mL (0.3 mL); 90 mg/ 0.3 mL (0.3 mL); 120 mg/0.5 mL (0.5 mL)

Somatuline® Depot: 60 mg/0.3 mL (0.3 mL); 90 mg/0.3 mL (0.3 mL); 120 mg/0.5 mL (0.5 mL)

lanreotide acetate *see* lanreotide *on page 570*

lansoprazole (lan SOE pra zole)

Sound-Alike/Look-Alike Issues

lansoprazole may be confused with aripiprazole, dexlansoprazole

Prevacid® may be confused with Pravachol®, Prevpac®, Prilosec®, Prinivil®

U.S./Canadian Brand Names Apo-Lansoprazole® [Can]; Prevacid® SoluTab™ [US]; Prevacid® [US/Can]

Therapeutic Category Gastric Acid Secretion Inhibitor

Use Short-term treatment of active duodenal ulcers; maintenance treatment of healed duodenal ulcers; as part of a multidrug regimen for *H. pylori* eradication to reduce the risk of duodenal ulcer recurrence; short-term treatment of active benign gastric ulcer; treatment of NSAID-associated gastric ulcer; to reduce the risk of NSAID-associated gastric ulcer in patients with a history of gastric ulcer who require an NSAID; short-term treatment of symptomatic GERD; short-term treatment for all grades of erosive esophagitis; to maintain healing of erosive esophagitis; long-term treatment of pathological hypersecretory conditions, including Zollinger-Ellison syndrome

Usual Dosage Oral:

Children 1-11 years: GERD, erosive esophagitis:

≤30 kg: 15 mg once daily

>30 kg: 30 mg once daily

Note: Doses were increased in some pediatric patients if still symptomatic after 2 or more weeks of treatment (maximum dose: 30 mg twice daily)

Children 12-17 years:

Nonerosive GERD: 15 mg once daily for up to 8 weeks

Erosive esophagitis: 30 mg once daily for up to 8 weeks

Adults:

Duodenal ulcer: Short-term treatment: 15 mg once daily for 4 weeks; maintenance therapy: 15 mg once daily

Gastric ulcer: Short-term treatment: 30 mg once daily for up to 8 weeks

NSAID-associated gastric ulcer (healing): 30 mg once daily for 8 weeks; controlled studies did not extend past 8 weeks of therapy

NSAID-associated gastric ulcer (to reduce risk): 15 mg once daily for up to 12 weeks; controlled studies did not extend past 12 weeks of therapy

Symptomatic GERD: Short-term treatment: 15 mg once daily for up to 8 weeks

Erosive esophagitis: Short-term treatment: 30 mg once daily for up to 8 weeks; continued treatment for an additional 8 weeks may be considered for recurrence or for patients who do not heal after the first 8 weeks of therapy; maintenance therapy: 15 mg once daily

Hypersecretory conditions: Initial: 60 mg once daily; adjust dose based upon patient response and to reduce acid secretion to <10 mEq/hour (5 mEq/hour in patients with prior gastric surgery); doses of 90 mg twice daily have been used; administer doses >120 mg/day in divided doses

Helicobacter pylori eradication:

Manufacturer labeling: 30 mg 3 times/day administered with amoxicillin 1000 mg 3 times/day for 14 days **or** 30 mg twice daily administered with amoxicillin 1000 mg *and* clarithromycin 500 mg twice daily for 10-14 days

American College of Gastroenterology guidelines:

Nonpenicillin allergy: 30 mg twice daily administered with amoxicillin 1000 mg *and* clarithromycin 500 mg twice daily for 10-14 days

Penicillin allergy: 30 mg twice daily administered with clarithromycin 500 mg *and* metronidazole 500 mg twice daily for 10-14 days **or** 30 mg once or twice daily administered with bismuth subsalicylate 525 mg *and* metronidazole 250 mg *plus* tetracycline 500 mg 4 times/day for 10-14 days

Dosage Forms

Capsule, delayed release:

Prevacid®: 15 mg, 30 mg

Tablet, delayed release, orally disintegrating:

Prevacid® SoluTab™: 15 mg, 30 mg

lansoprazole, amoxicillin, and clarithromycin

(lan SOE pra zole, a moks i SIL in, & kla RITH roe mye sin)

Sound-Alike/Look-Alike Issues

Prevpac® may be confused with Prevacid®

Synonyms amoxicillin, clarithromycin, and lansoprazole; clarithromycin, lansoprazole, and amoxicillin; lansoprazole, amoxicillin, and clarithromycin

U.S./Canadian Brand Names Hp-PAC® [Can]; Prevpac® [US]

Therapeutic Category Antibiotic, Macrolide Combination; Antibiotic, Penicillin; Gastrointestinal Agent, Miscellaneous

Use Eradication of *H. pylori* to reduce the risk of recurrent duodenal ulcer

Usual Dosage Oral: Adults: Lansoprazole 30 mg, amoxicillin 1 g, and clarithromycin 500 mg taken together twice daily for 10 or 14 days

Dosage Forms

Combination package [each administration card contains]:

Prevpac®:

Capsule: Amoxicillin 500 mg (4 capsules/day)

Capsule, delayed release (Prevacid®): Lansoprazole 30 mg (2 capsules/day)

Tablet (Biaxin®): Clarithromycin 500 mg (2 tablets/day)

lansoprazole, amoxicillin, and clarithromycin *see* lansoprazole, amoxicillin, and clarithromycin *on page* 571

lansoprazole and naproxen (lan SOE pra zole & na PROKS en)

Sound-Alike/Look-Alike Issues

Prevacid® may be confused with Pravachol®, Prevpac®, Prilosec®, Prinivil®

Synonyms NapraPAC®; naproxen and lansoprazole

U.S./Canadian Brand Names Prevacid® NapraPAC® [US]

Therapeutic Category Gastric Acid Secretion Inhibitor; Nonsteroidal Antiinflammatory Drug (NSAID)

Use Reduction of the risk of NSAID-associated gastric ulcers in patients with history of gastric ulcer who require an NSAID for the treatment of rheumatoid arthritis, osteoarthritis, and ankylosing spondylitis

Usual Dosage Oral: Adults: Reduce NSAID-associated gastric ulcers during treatment for arthritis: Lansoprazole 15 mg once daily in the morning; naproxen 500 mg twice daily

Dosage Forms

Combination package:

Prevacid® NapraPAC® 500 [each administration card contains]:

Capsule, delayed release (Prevacid®): Lansoprazole 15 mg (7 capsules per card)

Tablet (Naprosyn®): Naproxen 500 mg (14 tablets per card)

lanthanum (LAN tha num)

Sound-Alike/Look-Alike Issues

lanthanum may be confused with lithium

Synonyms lanthanum carbonate

U.S./Canadian Brand Names Fosrenol® [US/Can]

Therapeutic Category Phosphate Binder

Use Reduction of serum phosphate in patients with stage 5 chronic kidney disease (end-stage renal disease [ESRD]; kidney failure: GFR <15 mL/minute/1.73 m^2 or dialysis)

Usual Dosage Oral: Adults: Initial: 1500 mg/day divided and taken with meals; typical increases of 750 mg/day every 2-3 weeks are suggested as needed to bring the serum phosphate level <6 mg/dL; usual dosage range: 1500-3000 mg; doses of up to 3750 mg have been used

Dosage Forms

Tablet, chewable:

Fosrenol®: 500 mg, 750 mg, 1000 mg

lanthanum carbonate *see* lanthanum *on page* 572

Lantus® [US/Can] *see* insulin glargine *on page* 531

Lantus® OptiSet® [Can] *see* insulin glargine *on page* 531

Lanvis® [Can] *see* thioguanine *on page* 955

Lapase *(Discontinued)* *see* pancreatin *on page* 746

lapatinib (la PA ti nib)

Sound-Alike/Look-Alike Issues

lapatinib may be confused with dasatinib, erlotinib, imatinib

Synonyms GW572016; lapatinib ditosylate; NSC-727989

U.S./Canadian Brand Names Tykerb® [US/Can]

Therapeutic Category Antineoplastic Agent, Tyrosine Kinase Inhibitor; Epidermal Growth Factor Receptor (EGFR) Inhibitor

Use Treatment (in combination with capecitabine) of HER2/neu overexpressing advanced or metastatic breast cancer, in patients who have received prior therapy (with an anthracycline, a taxane, and trastuzumab)

Usual Dosage Details concerning dosing in combination regimens should also be consulted. **Note:** Dose reductions are likely to be needed when lapatinib is administered concomitantly with a strong CYP3A4 inhibitor (an alternate medication for CYP3A4 enzyme inhibitors should be investigated first).
Oral: Adults: 1250 mg once daily (in combination with capecitabine)

Dosage Forms

Tablet:
Tykerb®: 250 mg

lapatinib ditosylate *see* lapatinib *on page 572*

Largactil® [Can] *see* chlorpromazine *on page 222*

Lariam® [Can] *see* mefloquine *on page 621*

Lariam® *(Discontinued)* *see* mefloquine *on page 621*

laronidase (lair OH ni days)

Synonyms recombinant α-L-iduronidase (glycosaminoglycan α-L-iduronohydrolase)

U.S./Canadian Brand Names Aldurazyme® [US/Can]

Therapeutic Category Enzyme

Use Treatment of Hurler and Hurler-Scheie forms of mucopolysaccharidosis I (MPS I); treatment of Scheie form of MPS I in patients with moderate-to-severe symptoms

Usual Dosage Note: Premedicate with antipyretic and/or antihistamines 1 hour prior to start of infusion.
I.V.: Children ≥5 years and Adults: 0.58 mg/kg once weekly; dose should be rounded up to the nearest whole vial

Dosage Forms

Injection, solution [preservative free]:
Aldurazyme®: 2.9 mg/5 mL (5 mL)

Lasix® [US/Can] *see* furosemide *on page 449*

Lasix® Special [Can] *see* furosemide *on page 449*

L-asparaginase *see* asparaginase *on page 102*

L-asparaginase with polyethylene glycol *see* pegaspargase *on page 755*

lassar's zinc paste *see* zinc oxide *on page 1030*

latanoprost (la TA noe prost)

Sound-Alike/Look-Alike Issues
Xalatan® may be confused with Travatan®, Zarontin®

U.S./Canadian Brand Names Xalatan® [US/Can]

Therapeutic Category Prostaglandin

Use Reduction of elevated intraocular pressure in patients with open-angle glaucoma or ocular hypertension

Usual Dosage Ophthalmic: Adults: 1 drop (1.5 mcg) in the affected eye(s) once daily in the evening; do not exceed the once daily dosage because it has been shown that more frequent administration may decrease the IOP lowering effect
Note: A medication delivery device (Xal-Ease™) is available for use with Xalatan®.

Dosage Forms

Solution, ophthalmic:
Xalatan®: 0.005% (2.5 mL)

Latisse™ [US] *see* bimatoprost *on page 141*

***Latrodectus mactans* antivenin** *see* antivenin *(Latrodectus mactans) on page 87*

Lavacol® [US-OTC] *see* alcohol (ethyl) *on page 42*

Laxilose [Can] *see* lactulose *on page 565*

***l*-bunolol hydrochloride** *see* levobunolol *on page 578*

L-Carnitine® [US-OTC] *see* levocarnitine *on page 578*

L-carnitine *see* levocarnitine *on page 578*

LCD *see* coal tar *on page 250*

LCM *see* lacosamide *on page 563*

L-deoxythymidine *see* telbivudine *on page 941*

L-deprenyl *see* selegiline *on page 895*

LDP-341 *see* bortezomib *on page 146*

Lectopam® [Can] *see* bromazepam *(Canada only) on page 148*
Leena™ [US] *see* ethinyl estradiol and norethindrone *on page 390*

leflunomide (le FLOO noh mide)

U.S./Canadian Brand Names Apo-Leflunomide® [Can]; Arava® [US/Can]; DOM-Leflunomide [Can]; GEN-Leflunomide [Can]; NOVO-Leflunomide [Can]; PHL-Leflunomide [Can]; PMS-Leflunomide [Can]; SANDOZ-Leflunomide [Can]

Therapeutic Category Antiinflammatory Agent

Use Treatment of active rheumatoid arthritis; indicated to reduce signs and symptoms, and to inhibit structural damage and improve physical function

Usual Dosage Oral: Adults: Rheumatoid arthritis: Loading dose: 100 mg/day for 3 days, followed by 20 mg/day; **Note:** The loading dose may be omitted in patients at increased risk of hepatic or hematologic toxicity (eg, recent concomitant methotrexate). Dosage may be decreased to 10 mg/day in patients who have difficulty tolerating the 20 mg dose. Due to the long half-life of the active metabolite, serum concentrations may require a prolonged period to decline after dosage reduction.

Dosage Forms

Tablet: 10 mg, 20 mg
Arava®: 10 mg, 20 mg

Legatrin PM® [US-OTC] *see* acetaminophen and diphenhydramine *on page 21*

lenalidomide (le na LID oh mide)

Synonyms CC-5013; IMid-1

U.S./Canadian Brand Names Revlimid® [US/Can]

Therapeutic Category Angiogenesis Inhibitor; Immunosuppressant Agent; Tumor Necrosis Factor (TNF) Blocking Agent

Use Treatment of myelodysplastic syndrome (MDS) in patients with deletion 5q (del 5q) cytogenetic abnormality with transfusion-dependent anemia; treatment of multiple myeloma

Usual Dosage Oral: Adults:
Multiple myeloma: 25 mg once daily for 21 days of a 28-day treatment cycle (in combination with dexamethasone)
Myelodysplastic syndrome (MDS) with deletion 5q: 10 mg once daily

Dosage Forms

Capsule:
Revlimid®: 5 mg, 10 mg, 15 mg, 25 mg

Lente® Iletin® II *(Discontinued)*

lepirudin (leh puh ROO din)

Synonyms lepirudin (rDNA); recombinant hirudin

U.S./Canadian Brand Names Refludan® [US/Can]

Therapeutic Category Anticoagulant (Other)

Use Indicated for anticoagulation in patients with heparin-induced thrombocytopenia (HIT) and associated thromboembolic disease in order to prevent further thromboembolic complications

Usual Dosage Note: Maximum infusion dose: Do not exceed 0.21 mg/kg/hour unless an evaluation of coagulation abnormalities limiting response has been completed.

Heparin-induced thrombocytopenia: Bolus dose: 0.4 mg/kg IVP (over 15-20 seconds), followed by continuous infusion at 0.15 mg/kg/hour (maximum initial bolus dose: 44 mg; maximum initial infusion dose: 16.5 mg/hour); bolus and infusion must be reduced in renal insufficiency

Dosage Forms

Injection, powder for reconstitution:
Refludan®: 50 mg

lepirudin (rDNA) *see* lepirudin *on page 574*
Lescol® [US/Can] *see* fluvastatin *on page 438*
Lescol® XL [US/Can] *see* fluvastatin *on page 438*
Lessina™ [US] *see* ethinyl estradiol and levonorgestrel *on page 387*
Letairis™ [US] *see* ambrisentan *on page 59*

letrozole (LET roe zole)

Sound-Alike/Look-Alike Issues

letrozole may be confused with anastrozole

Femara® may be confused with Famvir®, femhrt®, Provera®

Synonyms CGS-20267; NSC-719345

U.S./Canadian Brand Names Femara® [US/Can]

Therapeutic Category Antineoplastic Agent, Hormone (Antiestrogen)

Use For use in postmenopausal women in the adjuvant treatment of hormone receptor positive early breast cancer, extended adjuvant treatment of early breast cancer after 5 years of tamoxifen, advanced breast cancer with disease progression following antiestrogen therapy, hormone receptor positive or hormone receptor unknown, locally-advanced, or metastatic breast cancer

Usual Dosage Oral: Adults: Females: Breast cancer: 2.5 mg once daily

Dosage Forms

Tablet:

Femara®: 2.5 mg

leucovorin calcium (loo koe VOR in KAL see um)

Sound-Alike/Look-Alike Issues

leucovorin may be confused with Leukeran®, Leukine®, LEVOleucovorin

folinic acid may be confused with folic acid

folinic acid is an error prone synonym and should not be used

Synonyms 5-formyl tetrahydrofolate; calcium leucovorin; citrovorum factor

Therapeutic Category Folic Acid Derivative

Use Antidote for folic acid antagonists (methotrexate, trimethoprim, pyrimethamine) and rescue therapy following high-dose methotrexate; in combination with fluorouracil in the treatment of colon cancer; treatment of megaloblastic anemias when folate is deficient as in infancy, sprue, pregnancy, and nutritional deficiency when oral folate therapy is not possible

Usual Dosage

Children and Adults:

Treatment of folic acid antagonist overdosage: Oral: 5-15 mg/day

Folate-deficient megaloblastic anemia: I.M.: ≤1 mg/day

High-dose methotrexate-rescue dose: Initial: Oral, I.M., I.V.: 15 mg (~10 mg/m^2); start 24 hours after beginning methotrexate infusion; continue every 6 hours for 10 doses, until methotrexate level is <0.05 micromole/L. Adjust dose as follows:

Normal methotrexate elimination: Oral, I.M., I.V.: 15 mg every 6 hours

Delayed early methotrexate elimination: I.V.: 150 mg every 3 hours until methotrexate level is <1 micromole/L, then 15 mg every 3 hours until methotrexate level is <0.05 micromole/L

Adults:

Colorectal cancer (also refer to Combination Regimens):

I.V.: 200 mg/m^2 over at least 3 minutes (used in combination with fluorouracil 370 mg/m^2)

or

I.V.: 20 mg/m^2 (used in combination with fluorouracil 425 mg/m^2)

Dosage Forms Note: Strength expressed as base

Injection, powder for reconstitution: 50 mg, 100 mg, 200 mg, 350 mg

Injection, solution [preservative free]: 10 mg/mL (50 mL)

Tablet: 5 mg, 10 mg, 15 mg, 25 mg

Leukeran® [US/Can] *see* chlorambucil *on page 208*

Leukine® [US/Can] *see* sargramostim *on page 891*

leuprolide (loo PROE lide)

Sound-Alike/Look-Alike Issues

Lupron® may be confused with Nuprin®

Lupron Depot®-3 Month may be confused with Lupron Depot-Ped®

Synonyms abbott-43818; leuprolide acetate; leuprorelin acetate; TAP-144

U.S./Canadian Brand Names Eligard® [US/Can]; Lupron Depot-Ped® [US]; Lupron Depot® [US/Can]; Lupron® [US/Can]

Therapeutic Category Antineoplastic Agent; Luteinizing Hormone-Releasing Hormone Analog

Use Palliative treatment of advanced prostate cancer; management of endometriosis; treatment of anemia caused by uterine leiomyomata (fibroids); central precocious puberty

Usual Dosage

Children: Precocious puberty (consider discontinuing by age 11 for females and by age 12 for males):

SubQ (Lupron®): Initial: 50 mcg/kg/day (per manufacturer, doses of 20-45 mcg/kg/day have also been reported); titrate dose upward by 10 mcg/kg/day if down-regulation is not achieved

I.M. (Lupron Depot-Ped®): 0.3 mg/kg/dose given every 28 days (minimum dose: 7.5 mg)

≤25 kg: 7.5 mg

>25-37.5 kg: 11.25 mg

>37.5 kg: 15 mg

Titrate dose upward in increments of 3.75 mg every 4 weeks if down-regulation is not achieved.

Adults:

Advanced prostate cancer:

SubQ:

Eligard®: 7.5 mg monthly **or** 22.5 mg every 3 months **or** 30 mg every 4 months **or** 45 mg every 6 months

Lupron®: 1 mg/day

I.M.:

Lupron Depot®: 7.5 mg/dose given monthly (every 28-33 days) **or**

Lupron Depot®-3: 22.5 mg every 3 months **or**

Lupron Depot®-4: 30 mg every 4 months

Endometriosis: I.M.: Initial therapy may be with leuprolide alone or in combination with norethindrone; if retreatment for an additional 6 months is necessary, norethindrone should be used. Retreatment is not recommended for longer than one additional 6-month course.

Lupron Depot®: 3.75 mg/month for up to 6 months **or**

Lupron Depot®-3: 11.25 mg every 3 months for up to 2 doses (6 months total duration of treatment)

Uterine leiomyomata (fibroids): I.M. (in combination with iron):

Lupron Depot®: 3.75 mg/month for up to 3 months **or**

Lupron Depot®-3: 11.25 mg as a single injection

Dosage Forms

Injection, solution: 5 mg/mL (2.8 mL)

Lupron®: 5 mg/mL (2.8 mL)

Injection, powder for reconstitution [depot formulation]:

Eligard®:

7.5 mg [released over 1 month]

22.5 mg [released over 3 months]

30 mg [released over 4 months]

45 mg [released over 6 months]

Lupron Depot®: 3.75 mg, 7.5 mg [released over 1 month]

Lupron Depot®-3 Month: 11.25 mg, 22.5 mg [released over 3 months]

Lupron Depot®-4 Month: 30 mg [released over 4 months]

Lupron Depot-Ped®: 7.5 mg, 11.25 mg, 15 mg [released over 1 month]

leuprolide acetate *see* leuprolide *on page* 575

leuprorelin acetate *see* leuprolide *on page* 575

leurocristine sulfate *see* vincristine *on page* 1014

Leustatin® [US/Can] *see* cladribine *on page* 235

levalbuterol (leve al BYOO ter ole)

Sound-Alike/Look-Alike Issues

Xopenex® may be confused with Xanax®

Synonyms levalbuterol hydrochloride; levalbuterol tartrate; R-albuterol

U.S./Canadian Brand Names Xopenex HFA™ [US]; Xopenex® [US/Can]

Therapeutic Category Adrenergic Agonist Agent; $Beta_2$-Adrenergic Agonist Agent; Bronchodilator

Use Treatment or prevention of bronchospasm in children and adults with reversible obstructive airway disease

Usual Dosage

Metered-dose inhaler (45 mcg/puff):

Children 5-11 years:

Bronchospasm, quick relief: 1-2 puffs every 4-6 hours as needed

Exacerbation of asthma (acute, severe): 4-8 puffs every 20 minutes for 3 doses, then every 1-4 hours as needed

Children ≥12 years and Adults:

Bronchospasm, quick relief: 1-2 puffs every 4-6 hours

Exacerbation of asthma (acute, severe): 4-8 puffs every 20 minutes for up to 4 hours, then every 1-4 hours as needed

Solution for nebulization:

Children: ≤4 years:

Bronchospasm, quick relief: 0.31-1.25 mg every 4-6 hours as needed

Exacerbation of asthma (acute, severe): 0.075 mg/kg (minimum: 1.25 mg) every 20 minutes for 3 doses, then 0.075-0.15 mg/kg (maximum: 5 mg) every 1-4 hours as needed

Children 5-11 years:

Bronchospasm, quick relief: 0.31-0.63 mg every 8 hours as needed

Exacerbation of asthma (acute, severe): 0.075 mg/kg (minimum: 1.25 mg) every 20 minutes for 3 doses, then 0.075-0.15 mg/kg (maximum: 5 mg) every 1-4 hours as needed

Children ≥12 years and Adults:

Bronchospasm, quick relief: 0.63-1.25 mg every 8 hours as needed

Exacerbation of asthma (acute, severe): 1.25-2.5 mg every 20 minutes for 3 doses, then 1.25-5 mg every 1-4 hours as needed

Dosage Forms

Aerosol, oral:

Xopenex®, Xopenex HFA™: 45 mcg/actuation (15 g)

Solution for nebulization [preservative free]:

Xopenex®, Xopenex HFA™: 0.31 mg/3 mL (24s); 0.63 mg/3 mL (24s); 1.25 mg/3 mL (24s)

Solution for nebulization [concentrate; preservative free]: 1.25 mg/0.5 mL (30s)

Xopenex®, Xopenex HFA™: 1.25 mg/0.5 mL (30s)

levalbuterol hydrochloride *see* levalbuterol *on page 576*

levalbuterol tartrate *see* levalbuterol *on page 576*

Levall 5.0 *(Discontinued)*

Levall™ *(Discontinued)* *see* carbetapentane, guaifenesin, and phenylephrine *on page 182*

Levall G [US] *see* guaifenesin and pseudoephedrine *on page 477*

Levaquin® [US/Can] *see* levofloxacin *on page 580*

levarterenol bitartrate *see* norepinephrine *on page 704*

Levate® [Can] *see* amitriptyline *on page 65*

Levatol® [US/Can] *see* penbutolol *on page 759*

Levbid® [US] *see* hyoscyamine *on page 512*

Levemir® [US/Can] *see* insulin detemir *on page 530*

levetiracetam (lee va tye RA se tam)

Sound-Alike/Look-Alike Issues

levetiracetam may be confused with levofloxacin

Keppra® may be confused with Keflex®, Keppra XR™

Potential for dispensing errors between Keppra® and Kaletra® (lopinavir/ritonavir)

U.S./Canadian Brand Names Apo-Levetiracetam [Can]; CO Levetiracetam [Can]; DOM-Levetiracetam [Can]; Keppra XR™ [US]; Keppra® [US/Can]; PHL-Levetiracetam [Can]; PMS-Levetiracetam [Can]

Therapeutic Category Anticonvulsant

Use Adjunctive therapy in the treatment of partial onset, myoclonic, and/or primary generalized tonic-clonic seizures

Usual Dosage

Oral:

Children 4-15 years: Partial onset seizures: Immediate release: 10 mg/kg/dose given twice daily; may increase every 2 weeks by 10 mg/kg/dose to a maximum of 30 mg/kg/dose twice daily

Children 6-15 years: Tonic-clonic seizures: Immediate release: Initial: 10 mg/kg dose given twice daily; may increase every 2 weeks by 10 mg/kg/dose to the recommended dose of 30 mg/kg twice daily. Efficacy of doses >60 mg/kg/day has not been established.

Children ≥12 years and Adults: Myoclonic seizures: Immediate release: Initial: 500 mg twice daily; may increase every 2 weeks by 500 mg/dose to the recommended dose of 1500 mg twice daily. Efficacy of doses >3000 mg/day has not been established.

Children ≥16 years and Adults:

Partial onset seizure:

Immediate release: Initial: 500 mg twice daily; may increase every 2 weeks by 500 mg/dose to a maximum of 1500 mg twice daily. Doses >3000 mg/day have been used in trials; however, there is no evidence of increased benefit.

Extended release: Initial: 1000 mg once daily; may increase every 2 weeks by 1000 mg/day to a maximum of 3000 mg once daily.

Tonic-clonic seizures: Immediate release: Initial: 500 mg twice daily; may increase every 2 weeks by 500 mg/dose to the recommended dose of 1500 mg twice daily. Efficacy of doses >3000 mg/day has not been established.

I.V.: Children ≥16 years and Adults: Partial onset seizure: Initial: 500 mg twice daily; may increase every 2 weeks by 500 mg/dose to a maximum of 1500 mg twice daily. Doses >3000 mg/day have been used in trials; however, there is no evidence of increased benefit.

Note: When switching from oral to I.V. formulations, the total daily dose should be the same.

Dosage Forms

Injection, solution:

Keppra®: 100 mg/mL (5 mL)

Solution, oral: 100 mg/mL

Keppra®: 100 mg/mL

Tablet: 250 mg, 500 mg, 750 mg, 1000 mg

Keppra®: 250 mg, 500 mg, 750 mg, 1000 mg

Tablet, extended release:

Keppra XR™: 500 mg, 750 mg

Levitra® [US/Can] *see* vardenafil *on page* *1006*

Levlen® [US] *see* ethinyl estradiol and levonorgestrel *on page* *387*

Levlite™ [US] *see* ethinyl estradiol and levonorgestrel *on page* *387*

levobunolol (lee voe BYOO noe lole)

Sound-Alike/Look-Alike Issues

levobunolol may be confused with levocabastine

Betagan® may be confused with Betadine®, Betoptic® S

Synonyms *l*-bunolol hydrochloride; levobunolol hydrochloride

U.S./Canadian Brand Names Apo-Levobunolol® [Can]; Betagan® [US/Can]; Novo-Levobunolol [Can]; Optho-Bunolol® [Can]; PMS-Levobunolol [Can]; Sandoz-Levobunolol [Can]

Therapeutic Category Beta-Adrenergic Blocker

Use To lower intraocular pressure in chronic open-angle glaucoma or ocular hypertension

Usual Dosage Ophthalmic: Adults: Instill 1 drop in the affected eye(s) 1-2 times/day

Dosage Forms

Solution, ophthalmic: 0.25% (5 mL, 10 mL); 0.5% (5 mL, 10 mL, 15 mL)

Betagan®: 0.25% (5 mL, 10 mL); 0.5% (2 mL, 5 mL, 10 mL, 15 mL)

levobunolol hydrochloride *see* levobunolol *on page* *578*

levocarnitine (lee voe KAR ni teen)

Sound-Alike/Look-Alike Issues

levocarnitine may be confused with levocabastine

Synonyms L-carnitine

U.S./Canadian Brand Names Carnitine-300 [US-OTC]; Carnitor® SF [US]; Carnitor® [US/Can]; L-Carnitine® [US-OTC]

Therapeutic Category Dietary Supplement

Use

Oral: Primary systemic carnitine deficiency; acute and chronic treatment of patients with an inborn error of metabolism which results in secondary carnitine deficiency

I.V.: Acute and chronic treatment of patients with an inborn error of metabolism which results in secondary carnitine deficiency; prevention and treatment of carnitine deficiency in patients with end-stage renal disease (ESRD) who are undergoing hemodialysis.

Usual Dosage

Carnitine deficiency:

Oral:

Infants/Children: Initial: 50 mg/kg/day; titrate to 50-100 mg/kg/day in divided doses with a maximum dose of 3 g/day

Adults: 990 mg (tablet) 2-3 times/day or 1-3 g/day (solution)

I.V.: Children and Adults: 50 mg/kg/day in divided doses; titrate based on patient response. Maximum reported dose: 300 mg/kg. An equivalent loading dose may be used in patients in severe metabolic crisis.

ESRD patients on hemodialysis: I.V.: Adults: 20 mg/kg dry body weight as a slow 2- to 3-minute bolus after each dialysis session

Note: Safety and efficacy of oral carnitine have not been established in ESRD. Chronic administration of high **oral** doses to patients with severely compromised renal function or ESRD patients on dialysis may result in accumulation of **potentially toxic** metabolites.

Dosage Forms

Capsule, oral:

Carnitine-300 [OTC]: 300 mg

L-Carnitine® [OTC]: 250 mg

Injection, solution [preservative free]: 200 mg/mL (5 mL, 12.5 mL)

Carnitor®: 200 mg/mL (5 mL)

Solution, oral: 100 mg/mL

Carnitor®, Carnitor® SF: 100 mg/mL

Tablet, oral: 330 mg

Carnitor®: 330 mg

L-Carnitine® [OTC]: 500 mg

levocetirizine (LEE vo se TI ra zeen)

Sound-Alike/Look-Alike Issues

levocetirizine may be confused with cetirizine

Synonyms levocetirizine dihydrochloride

U.S./Canadian Brand Names Xyzal® [US]

Therapeutic Category Antihistamine

Use Relief of symptoms of perennial and seasonal allergic rhinitis; treatment of skin manifestations (uncomplicated) of chronic idiopathic urticaria

Usual Dosage Oral: Allergic rhinitis, chronic urticaria:

Children 6-11 years: 2.5 mg once daily (in the evening); maximum: 2.5 mg/day

Children ≥12 years and Adults: 5 mg once daily (in the evening); some patients may experience relief of symptoms with 2.5 mg once daily

Dosage Forms

Solution, oral, as dihydrochloride:

Xyzal®: 0.5 mg/mL (150 mL)

Tablet, as dihydrochloride [scored]:

Xyzal®: 5 mg

levocetirizine dihydrochloride *see* levocetirizine *on page 579*

levodopa and benserazide *see* benserazide and levodopa *(Canada only) on page 128*

levodopa and carbidopa *see* carbidopa and levodopa *on page 184*

levodopa, carbidopa, and entacapone (lee voe DOE pa, kar bi DOE pa, & en TA ka pone)

Synonyms carbidopa, entacapone, and levodopa; carbidopa, levodopa, and entacapone; entacapone, carbidopa, and levodopa

U.S./Canadian Brand Names Stalevo® [US/Can]

Therapeutic Category Anti-Parkinson Agent (Dopamine Agonist); Anti-Parkinson Agent, COMT Inhibitor

Use Treatment of idiopathic Parkinson disease

Usual Dosage Oral: Adults: Parkinson disease:

Note: All strengths of Stalevo® contain a carbidopa/levodopa ratio of 1:4 plus entacapone 200 mg.

Dose should be individualized based on therapeutic response; doses may be adjusted by changing strength or adjusting interval. Fractionated doses are not recommended and only 1 tablet should be given at each dosing interval; maximum daily dose: 8 tablets of Stalevo® 50, 75, 100, 125, or 150, **or** 6 tablets of Stalevo® 200.

Patients previously treated with carbidopa/levodopa immediate release tablets (ratio of 1:4):
With current entacapone therapy: May switch directly to corresponding strength of combination tablet. No data available on transferring patients from controlled release preparations or products with a 1:10 ratio of carbidopa/levodopa.
Without entacapone therapy:
If current levodopa dose is >600 mg/day: Levodopa dose reduction may be required when adding entacapone to therapy; therefore, titrate dose using individual products first (carbidopa/levodopa immediate release with a ratio of 1:4 plus entacapone 200 mg); then transfer to combination product once stabilized.
If current levodopa dose is <600 mg without dyskinesias: May transfer to corresponding dose of combination product; monitor, dose reduction of levodopa may be required.
Patients previously treated with benserazide/levodopa immediate release tablets (Canadian labeling, not in U.S. labeling): With current entacapone therapy: Prior to switching to combination product (carbidopa/levodopa/entacapone), withhold treatment for 1 night, then initiate (carbidopa/levodopa/entacapone) therapy the following morning at a dose that provides either an equivalent amount or ~5% to 10% more levodopa.

Dosage Forms

Tablet:
Stalevo®: 50: Levodopa 50 mg, carbidopa 12.5 mg, and entacapone 200 mg; 75: Levodopa 75 mg, carbidopa 18.75 mg, and entacapone 200 mg; 100: Levodopa 100 mg, carbidopa 25 mg, and entacapone 200 mg; 125: Levodopa 125 mg, carbidopa 31.25 mg, and entacapone 200 mg; 150: Levodopa 150 mg, carbidopa 37.5 mg, and entacapone 200 mg; 200: Levodopa 200 mg, carbidopa 50 mg, and entacapone 200 mg

Levo-Dromoran® [US] *see* levorphanol *on page* 582

levofloxacin (lee voe FLOKS a sin)

Sound-Alike/Look-Alike Issues
levofloxacin may be confused with levetiracetam, levodopa, levothyroxine
Levaquin® may be confused with Levoxyl®, Levsin/SL®, Lovenox®

U.S./Canadian Brand Names Apo-Levofloxacin [Can]; Gen-Levofloxacin [Can]; Iquix® [US]; Levaquin® [US/Can]; Novo-Levofloxacin [Can]; PMS-Levofloxacin [Can]; Quixin® [US]

Therapeutic Category Antibiotic, Ophthalmic; Antibiotic, Quinolone

Use
Systemic: Treatment of community-acquired pneumonia, including multidrug resistant strains of *S. pneumoniae* (MDRSP); nosocomial pneumonia; chronic bronchitis (acute bacterial exacerbation); acute bacterial sinusitis; prostatitis, urinary tract infection (uncomplicated or complicated); acute pyelonephritis; skin or skin structure infections (uncomplicated or complicated); reduce incidence or disease progression of inhalational anthrax (postexposure)
Ophthalmic: Treatment of bacterial conjunctivitis caused by susceptible organisms (Quixin® 0.5% ophthalmic solution); treatment of corneal ulcer caused by susceptible organisms (Iquix® 1.5% ophthalmic solution)

Usual Dosage Note: Sequential therapy (intravenous to oral) may be instituted based on prescriber's discretion.

Usual dosage range:
Children ≥1 year: Ophthalmic: 1-2 drops every 2-6 hours
Adults:
Ophthalmic: 1-2 drops every 2-6 hours
Oral, I.V.: 250-500 mg every 24 hours; severe or complicated infections: 750 mg every 24 hours

Indication-specific dosing:
Children ≥1 year and Adults: Ophthalmic:
Conjunctivitis (0.5% ophthalmic solution):
Treatment day 1 and day 2: Instill 1-2 drops into affected eye(s) every 2 hours while awake, up to 8 times/day
Treatment day 3 through day 7: Instill 1-2 drops into affected eye(s) every 4 hours while awake, up to 4 times/day
Children ≥6 years and Adults: Ophthalmic:
Corneal ulceration (1.5% ophthalmic solution):
Treatment day 1 through day 3: Instill 1-2 drops into affected eye(s) every 30 minutes to 2 hours while awake and 4-6 hours after retiring
Treatment day 4 through completion: Instill 1-2 drops into affected eye(s) every 1-4 hours while awake

Children ≥6 months and Adults: Oral, I.V.:

Anthrax (inhalational, postexposure):

≤50 kg: 8 mg/kg every 12 hours for 60 days (do not exceed 250 mg/dose), beginning as soon as possible after exposure

>50 kg and Adults: 500 mg every 24 hours for 60 days, beginning as soon as possible after exposure

Adults: Oral, I.V.:

Chronic bronchitis (acute bacterial exacerbation): 500 mg every 24 hours for at least 7 days

Pneumonia:

Community-acquired: 500 mg every 24 hours for 7-14 days or 750 mg every 24 hours for 5 days (efficacy of 5-day regimen for MDRSP not established)

Nosocomial: 750 mg every 24 hours for 7-14 days

Prostatitis (chronic bacterial): 500 mg every 24 hours for 28 days

Sinusitis (acute bacterial): 500 mg every 24 hours for 10-14 days or 750 mg every 24 hours for 5 days

Skin and skin structure infections:

Uncomplicated: 500 mg every 24 hours for 7-10 days

Complicated: 750 mg every 24 hours for 7-14 days

Urinary tract infections:

Uncomplicated: 250 mg once daily for 3 days

Complicated, including pyelonephritis: 250 mg once daily for 10 days **or** 750 mg once daily for 5 days

Dosage Forms

Infusion, premixed in D_5W [preservative free]:

Levaquin®: 250 mg (50 mL); 500 mg (100 mL); 750 mg (150 mL)

Injection, solution [preservative free]:

Levaquin®: 25 mg/mL (20 mL, 30 mL)

Solution, ophthalmic [drops]:

Iquix®: 1.5% (5 mL)

Quixin®: 0.5% (5 mL)

Solution, oral:

Levaquin®: 25 mg/mL

levo-folinic acid *see* LEVOleucovorin *on page* 581

LEVOleucovorin (lee voe loo koe VOR in)

Sound-Alike/Look-Alike Issues

LEVOleucovorin may be confused with leucovorin calcium, Leukeran®, Leukine®

Synonyms 6S-leucovorin; calcium levoleucovorin; L-leucovorin; levo-folinic acid; levo-leucovorin; levoleucovorin calcium pentahydrate; S-leucovorin

U.S./Canadian Brand Names Fusilev™ [US]

Therapeutic Category Antidote; Rescue Agent (Chemotherapy)

Use Rescue agent after high-dose methotrexate therapy in osteosarcoma; antidote for impaired methotrexate elimination and for inadvertent overdosage of folic acid antagonists

Usual Dosage Note: Levoleucovorin is dosed at **one-half** the usual dose of the racemic form (leucovorin calcium):

High-dose methotrexate rescue: Children and Adults: I.V.: Usual dose: 7.5 mg (~5 mg/m^2) every 6 hours for 10 doses, beginning 24 hours after the start of the methotrexate infusion (based on a methotrexate dose of 12 g/m^2 I.V. over 4 hours). Levoleucovorin (and hydration and urinary alkalinization) should be continued and/or adjusted until the methotrexate level is <0.05 micromolar (5×10^{-8} M) as follows:

Normal methotrexate elimination (serum methotrexate levels ~10 micromolar at 24 hours post administration, 1 micromolar at 48 hours and <0.2 micromolar at 72 hours post infusion): 7.5 mg I.V. every 6 hours for 10 doses

Delayed late methotrexate elimination (serum methotrexate levels >0.2 micromolar at 72 hours and >0.05 micromolar at 96 hours post methotrexate infusion): Continue 7.5 mg I.V. every 6 hours until methotrexate level is <0.05 micromolar

Delayed early methotrexate elimination and/or evidence of acute renal injury (serum methotrexate level ≥50 micromolar at 24 hours, ≥5 micromolar at 48 hours or a doubling or more of the serum creatinine level at 24 hours post methotrexate infusion): 75 mg I.V. every 3 hours until methotrexate level is <1 micromolar, followed by 7.5 mg I.V. every 3 hours until methotrexate level is <0.05 micromolar

Significant clinical toxicity in the presence of less severe abnormalities in methotrexate elimination or renal function (as described above): Extend levoleucovorin treatment for an additional 24 hours (total of 14 doses) in subsequent treatment cycles.

Delayed methotrexate elimination due to third space fluid accumulation, renal insufficiency, or inadequate hydration: May require higher levoleucovorin doses or prolonged administration.

Methotrexate overdose (inadvertent): Children and Adults: I.V.: 7.5 mg (~5 mg/m^2) every 6 hours; continue until the methotrexate level is <0.01 micromolar (10^{-8} M). Initiate treatment as soon as possible after methotrexate overdose. Increase the levoleucovorin dose to 50 mg/m^2 I.V. every 3 hours if the 24 hour serum creatinine has increased 50% over baseline, or if the 24-hour methotrexate level is >5 micromolar (5×10^{-6} M), or if the 48-hour methotrexate level is >0.9 micromolar (9×10^{-7} M); continue levoleucovorin until the methotrexate level is <0.01 micromolar (10^{-8} M). Hydration (3 L/day) and urinary alkalinization (with sodium bicarbonate) should also be maintained.

Dosage Forms Note: Strength expressed as base

Injection, powder for reconstitution:

Fusilev™: 50 mg

levo-leucovorin *see* LEVOleucovorin *on page* 581

levoleucovorin calcium pentahydrate *see* LEVOleucovorin *on page* 581

levomepromazine *see* methotrimeprazine *(Canada only) on page* 640

levonordefrin and mepivacaine hydrochloride *see* mepivacaine and levonordefrin *on page* 628

levonorgestrel (LEE voe nor jes trel)

Synonyms LNg 20

U.S./Canadian Brand Names Mirena® [US/Can]; Next Choice™ [US-RX/OTC]; Norplant® Implant [Can]; Plan B® One-Step [US-RX/OTC]; Plan B® [US-RX/OTC/Can]

Therapeutic Category Contraceptive, Implant (Progestin); Contraceptive, Progestin Only

Use

Intrauterine device (IUD): Prevention of pregnancy

Oral: Emergency contraception following unprotected intercourse or possible contraceptive failure

Usual Dosage Adults: Females:

Long-term prevention of pregnancy: Intrauterine device: To be inserted into uterine cavity; should be inserted within 7 days of onset of menstruation or immediately after 1st trimester abortion; releases 20 mcg levonorgestrel/day over 5 years. May be removed and replaced with a new unit at anytime during menstrual cycle; do not leave any one system in place for >5 years

Emergency contraception: Oral: May be used at any time during menstrual cycle:

Plan B®, Next Choice™: One 0.75 mg tablet as soon as possible within 72 hours of unprotected sexual intercourse; a second 0.75 mg tablet should be taken 12 hours after the first dose

Plan B® One-Step: One 1.5 mg tablet as soon as possible within 72 hours of unprotected sexual intercourse

Dosage Forms

Intrauterine device:

Mirena®: 52 mg/unit

Tablet:

Next Choice™ [RX/OTC]: 0.75 mg

Plan B® [RX/OTC]: 0.75 mg

Plan B® One-Step [RX/OTC]: 1.5 mg

levonorgestrel and estradiol *see* estradiol and levonorgestrel *on page* 376

levonorgestrel and ethinyl estradiol *see* ethinyl estradiol and levonorgestrel *on page* 387

Levophed® [US/Can] *see* norepinephrine *on page* 704

Levora® [US] *see* ethinyl estradiol and levonorgestrel *on page* 387

levorphanol (lee VOR fa nole)

Synonyms levorphan tartrate; levorphanol tartrate

U.S./Canadian Brand Names Levo-Dromoran® [US]

Therapeutic Category Analgesic, Narcotic

Controlled Substance C-II

Use Relief of moderate-to-severe pain; preoperative sedation/analgesia; management of chronic pain (eg, cancer) requiring opioid therapy

Usual Dosage Adults: **Note:** These are guidelines and do not represent the maximum doses that may be required in all patients. Doses should be titrated to pain relief/prevention.

Acute pain (moderate-to-severe):

Oral: Initial: Opiate-naive: 2 mg every 6-8 hours as needed; patients with prior opiate exposure may require higher initial doses; usual dosage range: 2-4 mg every 6-8 hours as needed

I.M., SubQ: Initial: Opiate-naive: 1 mg every 6-8 hours as needed; patients with prior opiate exposure may require higher initial doses; usual dosage range: 1-2 mg every 6-8 hours as needed

Slow I.V.: Initial: Opiate-naive: Up to 1 mg/dose every 3-6 hours as needed; patients with prior opiate exposure may require higher initial doses

Chronic pain: Patients taking opioids chronically may become tolerant and require doses higher than the usual dosage range to maintain the desired effect. Tolerance can be managed by appropriate dose titration. **There is no optimal or maximal dose for levorphanol in chronic pain. The appropriate dose is one that relieves pain throughout its dosing interval without causing unmanageable side effects.**

Premedication: I.M., SubQ: 1-2 mg/dose 60-90 minutes prior to surgery; older or debilitated patients usually require less drug

Dosage Forms

Injection, solution:

Levo-Dromoran®: 2 mg/mL (1 mL, 10 mL)

Tablet: 2 mg

Levo-Dromoran®: 2 mg

levorphanol tartrate *see* levorphanol *on page* 582

levorphan tartrate *see* levorphanol *on page* 582

Levo-T™ *(Discontinued)* *see* levothyroxine *on page* 583

Levothroid® [US] *see* levothyroxine *on page* 583

levothyroxine (lee voe thye ROKS een)

Sound-Alike/Look-Alike Issues

levothyroxine may be confused with lamoTRIgine, Lanoxin®, levofloxacin, liothyronine

Levoxyl® may be confused with Lanoxin®, Levaquin®, Luvox®

Synthroid® may be confused with Symmetrel®

Synonyms *L*-thyroxine sodium; levothyroxine sodium; T_4

U.S./Canadian Brand Names Eltroxin® [Can]; Euthyrox [Can]; Levothroid® [US]; Levothyroxine Sodium [Can]; Levoxyl® [US]; Synthroid® [US/Can]; Unithroid® [US]

Therapeutic Category Thyroid Product

Use Replacement or supplemental therapy in hypothyroidism; pituitary TSH suppression

Usual Dosage Doses should be adjusted based on clinical response and laboratory parameters.

Oral:

Neonates, Infants, and Children: Hypothyroidism: Daily dosage based on body weight and age as listed below:

0-3 months: 10-15 mcg/kg/day; if the infant is at risk for development of cardiac failure, use a lower starting dose of 25 mcg/day; if the initial serum T_4 is very low (<5 mcg/dL) begin treatment at a higher dosage of 50 mcg/day

3-6 months: 8-10 mcg/kg/day **or** 25-50 mcg/day

6-12 months: 6-8 mcg/kg/day **or** 50-75 mcg/day

1-5 years: 5-6 mcg/kg/day **or** 75-100 mcg/day

6-12 years: 4-5 mcg/kg/day **or** 100-125 mcg/day

>12 years: 2-3 mcg/kg/day **or** ≥150 mcg/day

Growth and puberty complete: 1.7 mcg/kg/day; refer to Adult dosing.

Dosing modifications:

Hyperactivity in older children may be minimized by starting at 1/4 of the recommended dose and increasing each week by that amount until the full dose is achieved (4 weeks).

Children with severe or chronic hypothyroidism should be started at 25 mcg/day; adjust dose by 25 mcg every 2-4 weeks.

Adults (including children in whom growth and puberty are complete, healthy adults <50 years of age, and older adults who have been recently treated for hyperthyroidism or who have been hypothyroid for only a few months):

Hypothyroidism: ~1.7 mcg/kg/day; usual doses are ≤200 mcg/day (range: 100-125 mcg/day [70 kg adult]); doses ≥300 mcg/day are rare (consider poor compliance, malabsorption, and/or drug interactions). Titrate dose every 6 weeks.

Severe hypothyroidism: Initial: 12.5-25 mcg/day; adjust dose by 25 mcg/day every 2-4 weeks as appropriate

Myxedema: Oral agents are not recommended for myxedema: Refer to I.V. dosing.

Subclinical hypothyroidism (if treated): 1 mcg/kg/day

TSH suppression:

Well-differentiated thyroid cancer: Highly individualized; Doses >2 mcg/kg/day may be needed to suppress TSH to <0.1 mIU/mL. High-risk tumors may need a target level of <0.01 mIU/mL for TSH suppression.

Benign nodules and nontoxic multinodular goiter: Routine use of T_4 for TSH suppression is not recommended in patients with benign thyroid nodules. In patients deemed appropriate candidates, treatment should never be fully suppressive (TSH <0.1 mIU/mL). **Note:** Avoid use if TSH is already suppressed.

I.M., I.V.: Children, Adults: Hypothyroidism: 50% of the oral dose

I.V.: Adults: Myxedema coma or stupor: 200-500 mcg, then 100-300 mcg the next day if necessary; smaller doses should be considered in patients with cardiovascular disease

Dosage Forms

Injection, powder for reconstitution: 0.2 mg, 0.5 mg

Tablet: 25 mcg, 50 mcg, 75 mcg, 88 mcg, 100 mcg, 112 mcg, 125 mcg, 137 mcg, 150 mcg, 175 mcg, 200 mcg, 300 mcg

Levothroid®, Synthroid®: 25 mcg, 75 mcg, 88 mcg, 100 mcg, 112 mcg, 125 mcg, 137 mcg, 150 mcg, 175 mcg, 200 mcg, 300 mcg [scored]

Levothroid®, Levoxyl®, Synthroid®, Unithroid®: 50 mcg [scored]

Levoxyl®: 25 mcg, 75 mcg, 88 mcg, 100 mcg, 112 mcg, 125 mcg, 137 mcg, 150 mcg, 175 mcg, 200 mcg [scored]

Unithroid®: 25 mcg, 75 mcg, 88 mcg, 100 mcg, 112 mcg, 125 mcg, 150 mcg, 175 mcg, 200 mcg, 300 mcg [scored]

Levothyroxine Sodium [Can] *see* levothyroxine *on page* 583
levothyroxine sodium *see* levothyroxine *on page* 583
Levoxyl® [US] *see* levothyroxine *on page* 583
Levsin® [US/Can] *see* hyoscyamine *on page* 512
Levsin®/SL [US] *see* hyoscyamine *on page* 512
Levulan® [Can] *see* aminolevulinic acid *on page* 63
Levulan® Kerastick® [US] *see* aminolevulinic acid *on page* 63
levulose, dextrose and phosphoric acid *see* fructose, dextrose, and phosphoric acid *on page* 448
Lexapro® [US] *see* escitalopram *on page* 370
Lexiscan™ [US] *see* regadenoson *on page* 856
Lexiva® [US] *see* fosamprenavir *on page* 444
Lexxel® [Can] *see* enalapril and felodipine *on page* 353
Lexxel® *(Discontinued)* *see* enalapril and felodipine *on page* 353
LFA-3/IgG(1) fusion protein, human *see* alefacept *on page* 44
***l*-hyoscyamine sulfate** *see* hyoscyamine *on page* 512
Lialda™ [US] *see* mesalamine *on page* 631
Librax® *[original formulation]* [US/Can] *see* clidinium and chlordiazepoxide *on page* 238
Librax® *[reformulation] (Discontinued)*
Librium® [US] *see* chlordiazepoxide *on page* 209
Lice-Enz® Shampoo *(Discontinued)*
Licide® [US-OTC] *see* pyrethrins and piperonyl butoxide *on page* 839
LidaMantle® [US] *see* lidocaine *on page* 584
LidaMantle HC® [US] *see* lidocaine and hydrocortisone *on page* 587
LidaMantle HC® Relief Pad™ [US] *see* lidocaine and hydrocortisone *on page* 587
Lidemol® [Can] *see* fluocinonide *on page* 429
Lidex® [Can] *see* fluocinonide *on page* 429
Lidex® *(Discontinued)* *see* fluocinonide *on page* 429
Lidex-E® *(Discontinued)* *see* fluocinonide *on page* 429

lidocaine (LYE doe kane)

Synonyms lidocaine hydrochloride; lignocaine hydrochloride

U.S./Canadian Brand Names Akten™ [US]; Anestacon® [US]; Anestafoam™ [US-OTC]; Band-Aid® Hurt-Free™ Antiseptic Wash [US-OTC]; Betacaine® [Can]; Burn Jel® [US-OTC]; Burn-O-Jel [US-OTC]; BurnaMycin [US-OTC]; L-M-X™ 4 [US-OTC]; L-M-X™ 5 [US-OTC]; LidaMantle® [US]; Lidodan™ [Can]; Lidoderm® [US/Can]; LTA® 360 [US]; Premjact® [US-OTC]; Solarcaine® Aloe Extra Burn Relief [US-OTC]; Topicaine® [US-OTC]; Unburn® [US]; Xylocaine® Dental [US]; Xylocaine® MPF [US]; Xylocaine® Viscous [US]; Xylocaine® [US/Can]; Xylocard® [Can]; Zilactin-L® [US-OTC]; Zilactin® [Can]

Therapeutic Category Analgesic, Topical; Antiarrhythmic Agent, Class I-B; Local Anesthetic

Use Local and regional anesthesia by infiltration, nerve block, epidural, or spinal techniques; acute treatment of ventricular arrhythmias from myocardial infarction or cardiac manipulation

Ophthalmic: To provide local anesthesia to ocular surface during ophthalmologic procedures

Rectal: Temporary relief of pain and itching due to anorectal disorders

Topical: Local anesthetic for oral muscous membrane; use in laser/cosmetic surgeries; minor burns, cuts, and abrasions of the skin

Lidoderm® Patch: Relief of allodynia (painful hypersensitivity) and chronic pain in postherpetic neuralgia

Usual Dosage

Antiarrhythmic:

Children:

I.V., I.O.: **Note:** For use in pulseless VT or VF, give after defibrillation, CPR, and epinephrine:

Loading dose: 1 mg/kg (maximum 100 mg); follow with continuous infusion; may administer second bolus of 0.5-1 mg/kg if delay between bolus and start of infusion is >15 minutes

Continuous infusion: 20-50 mcg/kg/minute. Use 20 mcg/kg/minute in patients with shock, hepatic disease, cardiac arrest, mild CHF; moderate-to-severe CHF may require 1/2 loading dose and lower infusion rates to avoid toxicity.

E.T.: 2-3 mg/kg; flush with 5 mL of NS and follow with 5 assisted manual ventilations

Adults:

Ventricular fibrillation or pulseless ventricular tachycardia (after defibrillation, CPR, and vasopressor administration): I.V.: Initial: 1-1.5 mg/kg. Refractory ventricular tachycardia or ventricular fibrillation, a repeat 0.5-0.75 mg/kg bolus may be given every 5-10 minutes after initial dose for a maximum of 3 doses. Total dose should not exceed 3 mg/kg. Follow with continuous infusion (1-4 mg/minute) after return of perfusion. Reappearance of arrhythmia during constant infusion: 0.5 mg/kg bolus and reassessment of infusion.

E.T. (loading dose only): 2-2.5 times the recommended I.V. dose; dilute in 10 mL NS or distilled water. **Note:** Absorption is greater with distilled water, but causes more adverse effects on PaO_2.

Hemodynamically stable VT: 0.5-0.75 mg/kg followed by synchronized cardioversion

Note: Decrease dose in patients with CHF, shock, or hepatic disease.

Anesthetic, local injectable: Children and Adults: Varies with procedure, degree of anesthesia needed, vascularity of tissue, duration of anesthesia required, and physical condition of patient; maximum: 4.5 mg/kg/dose; do not repeat within 2 hours.

Anesthesia, ocular: Children and Adults: Apply 2 drops to ocular surface in area where procedure will occur; may reapply to maintain effect.

Anesthesia, topical: Unless otherwise noted, the following traditional pediatric guideline for topical lidocaine dosage may be observed: Apply to affected area as needed; maximum dose: 3 mg/kg/dose; do not repeat within 2 hours

Cream:

LidaMantle®: Skin irritation: Children and Adults: Apply to affected area 2-3 times/day as needed

L-M-X™ 4: Children ≥2 years and Adults: Apply 1/4 inch thick layer to intact skin. Leave on until adequate anesthetic effect is obtained. Remove cream and cleanse area before beginning procedure.

L-M-X™ 5: Relief of anorectal pain and itching: Children ≥12 years and Adults: Rectal: Apply topically to clean, dry area **or** using applicator, insert rectally, up to 6 times/day

Gel, ointment, solution: Adults: Apply to affected area ≤3 times/day as needed (maximum dose: 4.5 mg/kg, not to exceed 300 mg)

Jelly:

Children ≥10 years: Dose varies with age and weight (maximum dose: 4.5 mg/kg)

Adults (maximum dose: 30 mL [600 mg] in any 12-hour period):

Anesthesia of male urethra: 5-30 mL

Anesthesia of female urethra: 3-5 mL

Lubrication of endotracheal tube: Apply a moderate amount to external surface only

Liquid: Cold sores and fever blisters: Children ≥5 years and Adults: Apply to affected area every 6 hours as needed

Patch: Postherpetic neuralgia: Adults: Apply patch to most painful area. Up to 3 patches may be applied in a single application. Patch may remain in place for up to 12 hours in any 24-hour period.

Product Availability Zingo™: FDA approved August 2007; the product is not available following a non-safety recall and market withdrawal by the manufacturer, Anesiva, in November 2008

Dosage Forms

Aerosol, topical [foam]:
Anestafoam™ [OTC]: 4% (30 g)
Cream, rectal: 5% (15 g, 30 g)
L-M-X™ 5 [OTC]: 5% (15 g,30 g)
Cream, topical: 3% (30 g); 4% (5 g, 15 g, 30 g)
LidaMantle®: 3% (30 g, 85 g)
L-M-X™ 4 [OTC]: 4% (5g, 15 g,30 g)
Gel, ophthalmic [preservative free]:
Akten™: 3.5% (5 mL)
Gel, topical:
Burn Jel® [OTC]: 2% (3.5 g, 60 mL, 120 mL)
Burn-O-Jel [OTC]: 0.5% (90 g)
Solarcaine® Aloe Extra Burn Relief [OTC]: 0.5% (113 g, 226 g)
Topicaine® [OTC]: 4% (10 g, 30 g, 113 g)
Unburn®: 2.5% (3.5 g, 59 mL, 118 mL)
Infusion [premixed in D_5W]: 0.4% [4 mg/mL] (250 mL, 500 mL); 0.8% [8 mg/mL] (250 mL, 500 mL)
Injection, solution: 0.5% [5 mg/mL] (50 mL); 1% [10 mg/mL] (2 mL, 10 mL, 20 mL, 30 mL, 50 mL); 2% [20 mg/mL] (2 mL, 5 mL, 20 mL, 50 mL)
Xylocaine®: 0.5% [5 mg/mL] (50 mL); 1% [10 mg/mL] (10 mL, 20 mL, 50 mL); 2% [20 mg/mL] (10 mL, 20 mL, 50 mL)
Injection, solution [for dental use]:
Xylocaine® Dental: 2% (1.8 mL)
Injection, solution: [premixed in $D_{7.5}W$, preservative free]: 5% [50 mg/mL] (2 mL)
Injection, solution: [preservative free]: 0.5% [5 mg/mL] (50 mL); 1% [10 mg/mL] (2 mL, 5 mL, 30 mL); 1.5% [15 mg/mL] (20 mL); 2% [20 mg/mL] (2 mL, 5 mL, 10 mL); 4% [40 mg/mL] (5 mL)
Xylocaine®: 10% [100 mg/mL] (5 mL)
Xylocaine® MPF: 0.5% [5 mg/mL] (50 mL); 1% [10 mg/mL] (2 mL, 5 mL, 10 mL, 30 mL); 1.5% [15 mg/mL] (10 mL, 20 mL); 2% [20 mg/mL] (2 mL, 5 mL, 10 mL); 4% [40 mg/mL] (5 mL)
Jelly, topical: 2% (5 mL, 30 mL)
Anestacon®: 2% (15 mL)
Xylocaine®: 2% (5 mL, 30 mL)
Liquid, topical:
Zilactin®-L [OTC]: 2.5% (7.5 mL)
Lotion, topical: 3% (177 mL)
LidaMantle®: 3% (177 mL)
Ointment, topical: 5% (30 g, 37 g, 50 g)
Solution, topical: 4% [40 mg/mL] (50 mL)
Band-Aid® Hurt-Free™ Antiseptic Wash [OTC]: 2% (180 mL)
LTA® 360: 4% [40 mg/mL] (4 mL)
Xylocaine®: 4% [40 mg/mL] (50 mL)
Solution, topical [spray]:
BurnaMycin [OTC]: 0.5% (60 mL)
Premjact® [OTC]: 9.6% (13 mL)
Solarcaine® Aloe Extra Burn Relief [OTC]: 0.5% (127 g)
Solution, viscous, oral: 2% [20 mg/mL] (20 mL, 100 mL)
Xylocaine® Viscous: 2% [20 mg/mL] (100 mL, 450 mL)
Transdermal system, topical:
Lidoderm®: 5% (30s)

lidocaine and bupivacaine *(Discontinued)*

lidocaine and epinephrine (LYE doe kane & ep i NEF rin)

Synonyms epinephrine and lidocaine

U.S./Canadian Brand Names Lignospan® Forte [US]; Lignospan® Standard [US]; Xylocaine® MPF With Epinephrine [US]; Xylocaine® With Epinephrine [US/Can]

Therapeutic Category Local Anesthetic

Use Local infiltration anesthesia; AVS for nerve block; topical local analgesia for superficial dermatologic procedures

Usual Dosage Dosage varies with the anesthetic procedure, degree of anesthesia needed, vascularity of tissue, duration of anesthesia required, and physical condition of patient.

Dental anesthesia, infiltration, or conduction block:

Children <12 years: 20-30 mg (1-1.5 mL) of lidocaine hydrochloride as a 2% solution with epinephrine 1:100,000; maximum: 4.5 mg of lidocaine hydrochloride/kg of body weight or 100-150 mg as a single dose

Children ≥12 years and Adults: Do not exceed 7 mg/kg body weight up to a maximum range of 300 mg (usual dental practice) to 500 mg (approved product labeling) of lidocaine hydrochloride and 3 mcg (0.003 mg) of epinephrine/kg of body weight or 0.2 mg epinephrine per dental appointment. The effective anesthetic dose varies with procedure, intensity of anesthesia needed, duration of anesthesia required, and physical condition of the patient. Always use the lowest effective dose along with careful aspiration.

Note: For most routine dental procedures, lidocaine hydrochloride 2% with epinephrine 1:100,000 is preferred. When a more pronounced hemostasis is required, a 1:50,000 epinephrine concentration should be used.

Dermatologic procedure: Children ≥5 years and Adults: Topical: Place 1 transdermal patch over area requiring analgesia; attach patch to iontophoretic controller and leave on for 10 minutes. Remove patch and perform procedure within 10-20 minutes of patch removal. Do not use another patch for 30 minutes.

Dosage Forms

Injection, solution:

Generics:

0.5% / 1:200,000: Lidocaine hydrochloride 0.5% and epinephrine 1:200,000 (50 mL)
1% / 1:100,000: Lidocaine hydrochloride 1% and epinephrine 1:100,000 (20 mL, 30 mL, 50 mL)
2% / 1:100,000: Lidocaine hydrochloride 2% and epinephrine 1:100,000 (30 mL, 50 mL)

Brands:

Xylocaine® with Epinephrine:
0.5% / 1:200,000: Lidocaine hydrochloride 0.5% and epinephrine 1:200,000 (50 mL)
1% / 1:100,000: Lidocaine hydrochloride 1% and epinephrine 1:100,000 (10 mL, 20 mL, 50 mL)
2% / 1:100,000: Lidocaine hydrochloride 2% and epinephrine 1:100,000 (10 mL, 20 mL, 50 mL)

Injection, solution [preservative free]

Generics:

1% / 1:200,000: Lidocaine hydrochloride 1% and epinephrine 1:200,000 (30 mL)
1.5% / 1:200,000: Lidocaine hydrochloride 1.5% and epinephrine 1:200,000 (5 mL, 30 mL)
2% / 1:200,000: Lidocaine hydrochloride 2% and epinephrine 1:200,000 (20 mL)

Brands:

Xylocaine®-MPF with Epinephrine:
1% / 1:200,000: Lidocaine hydrochloride 1% and epinephrine 1:200,000 (5 mL, 10 mL, 30 mL)
1.5% / 1:200,000: Lidocaine hydrochloride 1.5% and epinephrine 1:200,000 (5 mL, 10 mL, 30 mL)
2% / 1:200,000: Lidocaine hydrochloride 2% and epinephrine 1:200,000 (5 mL, 10 mL, 20 mL)

Injection, solution [for dental use]

Generics:

2% / 1:50,000: Lidocaine hydrochloride 2% and epinephrine 1:50,000 (1.7 mL, 1.8 mL)
2% / 1:100,000: Lidocaine hydrochloride 2% and epinephrine 1:100,000 (1.7 mL, 1.8 mL)

Brands:

Lignospan® Forte: 2% / 1:50,000: Lidocaine hydrochloride 2% and epinephrine 1:50,000 (1.7 mL)
Lignospan® Standard: 2% / 1:100,000: Lidocaine hydrochloride 2% and epinephrine 1:100,000 (1.7 mL)

lidocaine and hydrocortisone (LYE doe kane & hye droe KOR ti sone)

Synonyms hydrocortisone and lidocaine

U.S./Canadian Brand Names AnaMantle HC® Cream [US]; AnaMantle HC® Forte [US]; AnaMantle HC® Gel [US]; LidaMantle HC® Relief Pad™ [US]; LidaMantle HC® [US]; LidoCort™ [US]; Peranex™ HC Medi-Pad [US]; Peranex™ HC [US]; RectaGel™ HC [US]

Therapeutic Category Anesthetic/Corticosteroid

Use Topical antiinflammatory and anesthetic for skin disorders; rectal for the treatment of hemorrhoids, anal fissures, pruritus ani, or similar conditions

Usual Dosage Adults:

Topical: Apply 2-3 times/day
Rectal: One applicatorful twice daily

Dosage Forms

Cream, rectal:

AnaMantle HC® Forte: Lidocaine 3% and hydrocortisone 1% (7 g)

AnaMantle HC®: Lidocaine 3% and hydrocortisone 0.5% (7 g)

Peranex™ HC: Lidocaine 2% and hydrocortisone 2% (7 g)

Cream, topical: Lidocaine 3% and hydrocortisone 0.5% (30 g)

LidaMantle HC®: Lidocaine 3% and hydrocortisone 0.5% (85 g)

Gel, rectal:

AnaMantle HC®, LidoCort™: Lidocaine 3% and hydrocortisone 2.5% (7 g)

RectaGel™ HC: Lidocaine 2.8% and hydrocortisone 0.55% (20 g)

Lotion, topical: Lidocaine 3% and hydrocortisone 0.5% (177 mL)

LidaMantle HC®: Lidocaine 3% and hydrocortisone 0.5% (177 mL)

Pad, topical:

LidaMantel HC® Relief Pad™: Lidocaine 2% and hydrocortisone 2% (60s)

Peranex™ HC Medi-Pad: Lidocaine 3% and hydrocortisone 1% (60s)

lidocaine and prilocaine (LYE doe kane & PRIL oh kane)

Synonyms prilocaine and lidocaine

U.S./Canadian Brand Names EMLA® [US/Can]; Oraquix® [US]

Therapeutic Category Analgesic, Topical

Use Topical anesthetic for use on normal intact skin to provide local analgesia for minor procedures such as I.V. cannulation or venipuncture; has also been used for painful procedures such as lumbar puncture and skin graft harvesting; for superficial minor surgery of genital mucous membranes and as an adjunct for local infiltration anesthesia in genital mucous membranes.

Usual Dosage Although the incidence of systemic adverse effects with EMLA® is very low, caution should be exercised, particularly when applying over large areas and leaving on for >2 hours

Children (intact skin): EMLA® should **not** be used in neonates with a gestation age <37 weeks nor in infants <12 months of age who are receiving treatment with methemoglobin-inducing agents

Dosing is based on child's age and weight:

Age 0-3 months or <5 kg: Apply a maximum of 1 g over no more than 10 cm^2 of skin; leave on for no longer than 1 hour

Age 3 months to 12 months and >5 kg: Apply no more than a maximum 2 g total over no more than 20 cm^2 of skin; leave on for no longer than 4 hours

Age 1-6 years and >10 kg: Apply no more than a maximum of 10 g total over no more than 100 cm^2 of skin; leave on for no longer than 4 hours.

Age 7-12 years and >20 kg: Apply no more than a maximum 20 g total over no more than 200 cm^2 of skin; leave on for no longer than 4 hours.

Note: If a patient greater than 3 months old does not meet the minimum weight requirement, the maximum total dose should be restricted to the corresponding maximum based on patient weight.

Adults (intact skin):

EMLA® cream and EMLA® anesthetic disc: A thick layer of EMLA® cream is applied to intact skin and covered with an occlusive dressing, or alternatively, an EMLA® anesthetic disc is applied to intact skin

Minor dermal procedures (eg, I.V. cannulation or venipuncture): Apply 2.5 g of cream (1/2 of the 5 g tube) over 20-25 cm of skin surface area, or 1 anesthetic disc (1 g over 10 cm^2) for at least 1 hour. **Note:** In clinical trials, 2 sites were usually prepared in case there was a technical problem with cannulation or venipuncture at the first site.

Major dermal procedures (eg, more painful dermatological procedures involving a larger skin area such as split thickness skin graft harvesting): Apply 2 g of cream per 10 cm^2 of skin and allow to remain in contact with the skin for at least 2 hours.

Adult male genital skin (eg, pretreatment prior to local anesthetic infiltration): Apply a thick layer of cream (1 g/10 cm^2) to the skin surface for 15 minutes. Local anesthetic infiltration should be performed immediately after removal of EMLA® cream.

Note: Dermal analgesia can be expected to increase for up to 3 hours under occlusive dressing and persist for 1-2 hours after removal of the cream

Adult females: Genital mucous membranes: Minor procedures (eg, removal of condylomata acuminata, pretreatment for local anesthetic infiltration): Apply 5-10 g (thick layer) of cream for 5-10 minutes

Periodontal gel (Oraqix®): Adults: Apply on gingival margin around selected teeth using the blunt-tipped applicator included in package. Wait 30 seconds, then fill the periodontal pockets using the blunt-tipped applicator until gel becomes visible at the gingival margin. Wait another 30 seconds before starting treatment. Maximum recommended dose: One treatment session: 5 cartridges (8.5 g)

Dosage Forms

Cream, topical: Lidocaine 2.5% and prilocaine 2.5% (5 g, 30 g)

EMLA®: Lidocaine 2.5% and prilocaine 2.5% (5 g, 30 g)

Disc, topical: Lidocaine 2.5% and prilocaine 2.5% per disc (2s, 10s)

Gel, periodontal:

Oraqix®: Lidocaine 2.5% and prilocaine 2.5% (1.7 g)

lidocaine and tetracaine (LYE doe kane & TET ra kane)

Synonyms tetracaine and lidocaine

U.S./Canadian Brand Names Pliaglis™ [US]; Synera™ [US]

Therapeutic Category Analgesic, Topical; Local Anesthetic

Use Topical anesthetic for use on normal intact skin for minor procedures (eg, I.V. cannulation or venipuncture) and superficial dermatologic procedures

Usual Dosage

Topical: Cream: Adults:

Superficial dermatological procedures (eg, dermal filler injection, facial laser ablation): Apply 20-30 minutes prior to procedure

Laser-assisted tattoo removal: Apply 60 minutes prior to procedure

Note: The amount of Pliaglis™ required is determined by the size of the treatment area. Use the ruler on the carton and in the packaging to measure out the proper amount (cm length of cream). Apply evenly and thinly (~1 mm or the thickness of a dime) over the area using a flat tool (eg, spatula, tongue depressor).

If surface area of treatment site:

10 cm^2: Apply 3 cm length Pliaglis™
20 cm^2: Apply 6 cm Pliaglis™
40 cm^2: Apply 12 cm Pliaglis™
80 cm^2: Apply 24 cm Pliaglis™
100 cm^2: Apply 30 cm Pliaglis™
150 cm^2: Apply 46 cm Pliaglis™
200 cm^2: Apply 61 cm Pliaglis™
250 cm^2: Apply 76 cm Pliaglis™
300 cm^2: Apply 91 cm Pliaglis™
350 cm^2: Apply 106 cm Pliaglis™
400 cm^2: Apply 121 cm Pliaglis™

After waiting the required application time, remove the Pliaglis™ by grasping a free edge and pulling it away from the skin.

Transdermal patch: Children ≥3 years and Adults:

Venipuncture or intravenous cannulation: Prior to procedure, apply to intact skin for 20-30 minutes; **Note:** Adults can use another patch at a new location to facilitate venous access after a failed attempt; remove previous patch.

Superficial dermatological procedures: Prior to procedure, apply to intact skin for 30 minutes

Dosage Forms

Cream, topical:

Pliaglis™: Lidocaine 7% and tetracaine 7% (30 g)

Transdermal system:

Synera™: Lidocaine 70 mg and tetracaine 70 mg (10s)

lidocaine hydrochloride *see* lidocaine *on page 584*

LidoCort™ [US] *see* lidocaine and hydrocortisone *on page 587*

Lidodan™ [Can] *see* lidocaine *on page 584*

Lidoderm® [US/Can] *see* lidocaine *on page 584*

LidoPen® I.M. Injection Auto-Injector *(Discontinued)* *see* lidocaine *on page 584*

LidoSite™ *(Discontinued)* *see* lidocaine and epinephrine *on page 586*

LID-Pack® [Can] *see* bacitracin and polymyxin B *on page 119*

lignocaine hydrochloride *see* lidocaine *on page 584*

Lignospan® Forte [US] *see* lidocaine and epinephrine *on page 586*

Lignospan® Standard [US] *see* lidocaine and epinephrine *on page 586*
Limbitrol® [US/Can] *see* amitriptyline and chlordiazepoxide *on page 66*
Limbitrol® DS *(Discontinued)* *see* amitriptyline and chlordiazepoxide *on page 66*
Limbrel 250™ [US] *see* flavocoxid *on page 421*
Limbrel 500™ [US] *see* flavocoxid *on page 421*
Limbrel™ *(Discontinued)* *see* flavocoxid *on page 421*
Lin-Amox [Can] *see* amoxicillin *on page 70*
Lin-Buspirone [Can] *see* buspirone *on page 160*
Lincocin® [US/Can] *see* lincomycin *on page 590*

lincomycin (lin koe MYE sin)

Sound-Alike/Look-Alike Issues
Lincocin® may be confused with Cleocin®, Indocin®, Minocin®

Synonyms lincomycin hydrochloride

U.S./Canadian Brand Names Lincocin® [US/Can]

Therapeutic Category Antibiotic, Lincosamide

Use Treatment of serious susceptible bacterial infections, mainly those caused by streptococci, pneumococci, and staphylococci resistant to other agents

Usual Dosage Note: Frequency may be increased if needed due to severity of infection

Children >1 month:
I.M.: 10 mg/kg every 12-24 hours
I.V.: 10-20 mg/kg/day in divided doses every 8-12 hours

Adults:
I.M.: 600 mg every 12-24 hours
I.V.: 600 mg to 1 g every 8-12 hours; maximum dose: 8 g/day
Subconjuctival injection: 75 mg (ocular fluid levels with sufficient MICs last for at least 5 hours)

Dosage Forms

Injection, solution:
Lincocin®: 300 mg/mL (2 mL, 10 mL)

lincomycin hydrochloride *see* lincomycin *on page 590*

lindane (LIN dane)

Synonyms benzene hexachloride; gamma benzene hexachloride; hexachlorocyclohexane

U.S./Canadian Brand Names Hexit™ [Can]; PMS-Lindane [Can]

Therapeutic Category Scabicides/Pediculicides

Use Treatment of *Sarcoptes scabiei* (scabies), *Pediculus capitis* (head lice), and *Phthirus pubis* (crab lice); FDA recommends reserving lindane as a second-line agent or with inadequate response to other therapies

Usual Dosage Topical: Children and Adults:

Scabies: Apply a thin layer of lotion and massage it on skin from the neck to the toes; after 8-12 hours, bathe and remove the drug

Head lice, crab lice: Apply shampoo to dry hair and massage into hair for 4 minutes; add small quantities of water to hair until lather forms, then rinse hair thoroughly and comb with a fine tooth comb to remove nits. Amount of shampoo needed is based on length and density of hair; most patients will require 30 mL (maximum: 60 mL).

Dosage Forms

Lotion, topical: 1% (60 mL)
Shampoo, topical: 1% (60 mL)

Linessa® [Can] *see* ethinyl estradiol and desogestrel *on page 383*

linezolid (li NE zoh lid)

Sound-Alike/Look-Alike Issues
Zyvox® may be confused with Ziox™, Zosyn®, Zovirax®

U.S./Canadian Brand Names Zyvoxam® [Can]; Zyvox® [US]

Therapeutic Category Antibiotic, Oxazolidinone

Use Treatment of vancomycin-resistant *Enterococcus faecium* (VRE) infections, nosocomial pneumonia caused by *Staphylococcus aureus* including MRSA or *Streptococcus pneumoniae* (including multidrug-resistant strains [MDRSP]), complicated and uncomplicated skin and skin structure infections (including diabetic foot infections without concomitant osteomyelitis), and community-acquired pneumonia caused by susceptible gram-positive organisms

Usual Dosage

VRE infections including concurrent bacteremia: Oral, I.V.:

Preterm neonates (<34 weeks gestational age): 10 mg/kg every 12 hours; neonates with a suboptimal clinical response can be advanced to 10 mg/kg every 8 hours. By day 7 of life, all neonates should receive 10 mg/kg every 8 hours.

Infants (excluding preterm neonates <1 week) and Children ≤11 years: 10 mg/kg every 8 hours for 14-28 days

Children ≥12 years and Adults: 600 mg every 12 hours for 14-28 days

MRSA: Adults: 600 mg every 12 hours

Nosocomial pneumonia, complicated skin and skin structure infections, community acquired pneumonia including concurrent bacteremia: Oral, I.V.:

Preterm neonates (<34 weeks gestational age): 10 mg/kg every 12 hours; neonates with a suboptimal clinical response can be advanced to 10 mg/kg every 8 hours. By day 7 of life, all neonates should receive 10 mg/kg every 8 hours.

Infants (excluding preterm neonates <1 week) and Children ≤11 years: 10 mg/kg every 8 hours for 10-14 days

Children ≥12 years and Adults: 600 mg every 12 hours for 10-14 days

Uncomplicated skin and skin structure infections: Oral:

Preterm neonates (<34 weeks gestational age): 10 mg/kg every 12 hours; neonates with a suboptimal clinical response can be advanced to 10 mg/kg every 8 hours. By day 7 of life, all neonates should receive 10 mg/kg every 8 hours.

Infants (excluding preterm neonates <1 week) and Children <5 years: 10 mg/kg every 8 hours for 10-14 days

Children 5-11 years: 10 mg/kg every 12 hours for 10-14 days

Children ≥12-18 years: 600 mg every 12 hours for 10-14 days

Adults: 400 mg every 12 hours for 10-14 days

Note: 400 mg dose is recommended in the product labeling; however, 600 mg dose is commonly employed clinically

Dosage Forms

Infusion [premixed]:

Zyvox®: 200 mg (100 mL); 600 mg (300 mL)

Powder for oral suspension:

Zyvox®: 20 mg/mL (150 mL)

Tablet:

Zyvox®: 600 mg

Lin-Sotalol [Can] *see* sotalol *on page 919*

Lioresal® [US/Can] *see* baclofen *on page 120*

Liotec [Can] *see* baclofen *on page 120*

liothyronine (lye oh THYE roe neen)

Sound-Alike/Look-Alike Issues

liothyronine may be confused with levothyroxine

T3 is an error-prone abbreviation (mistaken as acetaminophen and codeine [ie, Tylenol® #3])

Synonyms liothyronine sodium; sodium *L*-triiodothyronine

U.S./Canadian Brand Names Cytomel® [US/Can]; Triostat® [US]

Therapeutic Category Thyroid Product

Use

Oral: Replacement or supplemental therapy in hypothyroidism; management of nontoxic goiter; a diagnostic aid

I.V.: Treatment of myxedema coma/precoma

Usual Dosage Doses should be adjusted based on clinical response and laboratory parameters.

Children: Congenital hypothyroidism: Oral: 5 mcg/day increase by 5 mcg every 3-4 days until the desired response is achieved. Usual maintenance dose: 20 mcg/day for infants, 50 mcg/day for children 1-3 years of age, and adult dose for children >3 years.

Adults:

Hypothyroidism: Oral: 25 mcg/day increase by increments of 12.5-25 mcg/day every 1-2 weeks to a maximum of 100 mcg/day; usual maintenance dose: 25-75 mcg/day.

Patients with cardiovascular disease: Oral: 5 mcg/day; increase by 5 mcg/day every 2 weeks

T_3 suppression test: Oral: 75-100 mcg/day for 7 days

Myxedema: Oral: Initial: 5 mcg/day; increase in increments of 5-10 mcg/day every 1-2 weeks. When 25 mcg/day is reached, dosage may be increased at intervals of 5-25 mcg/day every 1-2 weeks. Usual maintenance dose: 50-100 mcg/day.

Myxedema coma: I.V.: 25-50 mcg

Patients with known or suspected cardiovascular disease: 10-20 mcg

Note: Normally, at least 4 hours should be allowed between doses to adequately assess therapeutic response and no more than 12 hours should elapse between doses to avoid fluctuations in hormone levels. Oral therapy should be resumed as soon as the clinical situation has been stabilized and the patient is able to take oral medication. If levothyroxine rather than liothyronine sodium is used in initiating oral therapy, the physician should bear in mind that there is a delay of several days in the onset of levothyroxine activity and that I.V. therapy should be discontinued gradually.

Simple (nontoxic) goiter: Oral: Initial: 5 mcg/day; increase by 5-10 mcg every 1-2 weeks; after 25 mcg/day is reached, may increase dose by 12.5-25 mcg. Usual maintenance dose: 75 mcg/day

Dosage Forms

Injection, solution: 10 mcg/mL (1 mL)

Triostat®: 10 mcg/mL (1 mL)

Tablet: 5 mcg, 25 mcg, 50 mcg

Cytomel®: 5 mcg, 25 mcg, 50 mcg

liothyronine sodium *see* liothyronine *on page* 591

liotrix (LYE oh triks)

Sound-Alike/Look-Alike Issues

liotrix may be confused with Klotrix®

Thyrolar® may be confused with Thyrogen®, Thytropar®

Synonyms T_3/T_4 liotrix

U.S./Canadian Brand Names Thyrolar® [US/Can]

Therapeutic Category Thyroid Product

Use Replacement or supplemental therapy in hypothyroidism (uniform mixture of T_4:T_3 in 4:1 ratio by weight); little advantage to this product exists and cost is not justified

Usual Dosage Oral:

Congenital hypothyroidism:

Children (dose of T_4 or levothyroxine/day):

0-6 months: 8-10 mcg/kg or 25-50 mcg/day

6-12 months: 6-8 mcg/kg or 50-75 mcg/day

1-5 years: 5-6 mcg/kg or 75-100 mcg/day

6-12 years: 4-5 mcg/kg or 100-150 mcg/day

>12 years: 2-3 mcg/kg or >150 mcg/day

Hypothyroidism (dose of thyroid equivalent): Adults: 30 mg/day (15 mg/day if cardiovascular impairment), increasing by increments of 15 mg/day at 2- to 3-week intervals to a maximum of 180 mg/day (usual maintenance dose: 60-120 mg/day)

Dosage Forms

Tablet:

Thyrolar®:

1/4 [levothyroxine 12.5 mcg and liothyronine 3.1 mcg]

1/2 [levothyroxine 25 mcg and liothyronine 6.25 mcg]

1 [levothyroxine 50 mcg and liothyronine 12.5 mcg]

2 [levothyroxine 100 mcg and liothyronine 25 mcg]

3 [levothyroxine 150 mcg and liothyronine 37.5 mcg]

lipancreatin *see* pancrelipase *on page* 746

lipase, protease, and amylase *see* pancrelipase *on page* 746

Lipidil EZ® [Can] *see* fenofibrate *on page* 408

Lipidil Micro® [Can] *see* fenofibrate *on page* 408

Lipidil Supra® [Can] *see* fenofibrate *on page* 408

Lipitor® [US/Can] *see* atorvastatin *on page* 108

Lipofen® [US] *see* fenofibrate *on page 408*
liposomal DAUNOrubicin *see* daunorubicin citrate (liposomal) *on page 278*
liposomal DOXOrubicin *see* doxorubicin (liposomal) *on page 336*
Liposyn® II [US/Can] *see* fat emulsion *on page 406*
Liposyn® III [US] *see* fat emulsion *on page 406*
Lipram 4500 *(Discontinued)* *see* pancrelipase *on page 746*
Lipram-CR *(Discontinued)* *see* pancrelipase *on page 746*
Lipram-PN *(Discontinued)* *see* pancrelipase *on page 746*
Lipram-UL *(Discontinued)* *see* pancrelipase *on page 746*
Liqua-Cal [US-OTC] *see* calcium and vitamin D *on page 169*
Liquadd™ [US] *see* dextroamphetamine *on page 293*
Liquaemin® *(Discontinued)* *see* heparin *on page 487*
Liquibid-D® [US] *see* guaifenesin and phenylephrine *on page 475*
Liquibid® 1200 *(Discontinued)* *see* guaifenesin *on page 473*
Liquibid® *(Discontinued)* *see* guaifenesin *on page 473*
Liquibid-PD 1200 *(Discontinued)* *see* guaifenesin and phenylephrine *on page 475*
Liquibid-PD *(Discontinued)* *see* guaifenesin and phenylephrine *on page 475*
Liqui-Char® *(Discontinued)* *see* charcoal *on page 206*
Liqui-Coat HD® [US] *see* barium *on page 122*
liquid antidote *see* charcoal *on page 206*
Liquid Barosperse® [US] *see* barium *on page 122*
Liquid Pred® *(Discontinued)* *see* prednisone *on page 814*
Liquifilm® Forte Solution *(Discontinued)* *see* artificial tears *on page 100*
Liquifilm® Tears [US-OTC] *see* artificial tears *on page 100*
Liquifilm® Tears Solution *(Discontinued)* *see* artificial tears *on page 100*

lisdexamfetamine (lis dex am FET a meen)

Sound-Alike/Look-Alike Issues
Vyvanse™ may be confused with Vytorin®, Glucovance®, Vivactil®

Synonyms lisdexamfetamine dimesylate; lisdexamphetamine; NRP104

U.S./Canadian Brand Names Vyvanse™ [US]

Therapeutic Category Stimulant

Controlled Substance C-II

Use Treatment of attention-deficit/hyperactivity disorder (ADHD)

Usual Dosage Oral: Individualize dosage based on patient need and response to therapy. Administer at the lowest effective dose.
Children: 6-12 years and Adults: Initial: 30 mg once daily in the morning; may increase in increments of 10 mg or 20 mg/day at weekly intervals until optimal response is obtained; maximum: 70 mg/day

Dosage Forms
Capsule:
Vyvanse™: 20 mg, 30 mg, 40 mg, 50 mg, 60 mg, 70 mg

lisdexamfetamine dimesylate *see* lisdexamfetamine *on page 593*
lisdexamphetamine *see* lisdexamfetamine *on page 593*

lisinopril (lyse IN oh pril)

Sound-Alike/Look-Alike Issues
lisinopril may be confused with fosinopril, Lioresal®, Risperdal®
Prinivil® may be confused with Plendil®, Pravachol®, Prevacid®, Prilosec®, Proventil®
Zestril® may be confused with Desyrel®, Restoril™, Vistaril®, Zegerid®, Zerit®, Zetia®, Zostrix®, Zyprexa®

U.S./Canadian Brand Names Apo-Lisinopril® [Can]; CO Lisinopril [Can]; Gen-Lisinopril [Can]; Novo-Lisinopril [Can]; PMS-Lisinopril [Can]; Prinivil® [US/Can]; Pro-Lisinopril [Can]; Ran-Lisinopril [Can]; ratio-Lisinopril [Can]; Riva-Lisinopril [Can]; Zestril® [US/Can]

Therapeutic Category Angiotensin-Converting Enzyme (ACE) Inhibitor

Use Treatment of hypertension, either alone or in combination with other antihypertensive agents; adjunctive therapy in treatment of heart failure (HF); treatment of acute myocardial infarction (MI) within 24 hours in hemodynamically-stable patients to improve survival

Usual Dosage Oral:

Heart failure: Adults: Initial: 2.5-5 mg once daily; then increase by no more than 10 mg increments at intervals no less than 2 weeks to a maximum daily dose of 40 mg. Usual maintenance: 5-40 mg/day as a single dose. Target dose: 20-40 mg once daily

Note: If patient has hyponatremia (serum sodium <130 meq/L) or renal impairment (Cl_{cr} <30 mL/minute or creatinine >3 mg/dL), then initial dose should be 2.5 mg/day

Hypertension:

Children ≥6 years: Initial: 0.07 mg/kg once daily (up to 5 mg); increase dose at 1- to 2-week intervals; doses >0.61 mg/kg or >40 mg have not been evaluated.

Adults: Usual dosage range (JNC 7): 10-40 mg/day

Not maintained on diuretic: Initial: 10 mg/day

Maintained on diuretic: Initial: 5 mg/day

Note: Antihypertensive effect may diminish toward the end of the dosing interval especially with doses of 10 mg/day. An increased dose may aid in extending the duration of antihypertensive effect. Doses up to 80 mg/day have been used, but do not appear to give greater effect.

Patients taking diuretics should have them discontinued 2-3 days prior to initiating lisinopril if possible. Restart diuretic after blood pressure is stable if needed. If diuretic cannot be discontinued prior to therapy, begin with 5 mg with close supervision until stable blood pressure. In patients with hyponatremia (<130 mEq/L), start dose at 2.5 mg/day

Acute myocardial infarction (within 24 hours in hemodynamically stable patients): Oral: 5 mg immediately, then 5 mg at 24 hours, 10 mg at 48 hours, and 10 mg every day thereafter for 6 weeks. Patients should continue to receive standard treatments such as thrombolytics, aspirin, and beta-blockers.

Dosage Forms

Tablet: 2.5 mg, 5 mg, 10 mg, 20 mg, 30 mg, 40 mg

Prinivil®: 5 mg, 10 mg, 20 mg

Zestril®: 2.5 mg, 5 mg, 10 mg, 20 mg, 30 mg, 40 mg

lisinopril and hydrochlorothiazide (lyse IN oh pril & hye droe klor oh THYE a zide)

Synonyms hydrochlorothiazide and lisinopril

U.S./Canadian Brand Names Apo-Lisinopril/Hctz [Can]; Gen-Lisinopril/Hctz [Can]; Novo-Lisinopril/Hctz [Can]; Prinzide® [US/Can]; Sandoz Lisinopril/Hctz [Can]; Zestoretic® [US/Can]

Therapeutic Category Antihypertensive Agent, Combination

Use Treatment of hypertension

Usual Dosage Oral: Adults: Dosage is individualized; see each component for appropriate dosing suggestions; doses >80 mg/day lisinopril or >50 mg/day hydrochlorothiazide are not recommended.

Dosage Forms

Tablet: 10/12.5: Lisinopril 10 mg and hydrochlorothiazide 12.5 mg; 20/12.5: Lisinopril 20 mg and hydrochlorothiazide 12.5 mg; 20/25: Lisinopril 20 mg and hydrochlorothiazide 25 mg

Prinzide®:

10/12.5: Lisinopril 10 mg and hydrochlorothiazide 12.5 mg

20/12.5: Lisinopril 20 mg and hydrochlorothiazide 12.5 mg

Zestoretic®:

10/12.5: Lisinopril 10 mg and hydrochlorothiazide 12.5 mg

20/12.5: Lisinopril 20 mg and hydrochlorothiazide 12.5 mg

20/25: Lisinopril 20 mg and hydrochlorothiazide 25 mg

lispro insulin *see* insulin lispro *on page* 531

Listermint® With Fluoride *(Discontinued)* *see* fluoride *on page* 430

Lithane™ [Can] *see* lithium *on page* 594

Lithane® *(Discontinued)* *see* lithium *on page* 594

lithium (LITH ee um)

Sound-Alike/Look-Alike Issues

lithium may be confused with lanthanum

Eskalith® may be confused with Estratest®

Lithobid® may be confused with Levbid®, Lithostat®

Synonyms lithium carbonate; lithium citrate

U.S./Canadian Brand Names Apo-Lithium® Carbonate SR [Can]; Apo-Lithium® Carbonate [Can]; Carbolith™ [Can]; Duralith® [Can]; Euro-Lithium [Can]; Lithane™ [Can]; Lithobid® [US]; PMS-Lithium Carbonate [Can]; PMS-Lithium Citrate [Can]

Therapeutic Category Antimanic Agent

Use Management of bipolar disorders; treatment of mania in individuals with bipolar disorder (maintenance treatment prevents or diminishes intensity of subsequent episodes)

Usual Dosage Oral: Monitor serum concentrations and clinical response (efficacy and toxicity) to determine proper dose. Adults: Bipolar disorder: 900-2400 mg/day in 3-4 divided doses or 900-1800 mg/day (sustained release) in 2 divided doses

Dosage Forms

Capsule, as carbonate: 150 mg, 300 mg, 600 mg
Solution: 300 mg/5 mL
Syrup: 300 mg/5 mL
Tablet: 300 mg
Tablet, controlled release: 450 mg
Tablet, slow release: 300 mg
Lithobid®: 300 mg

lithium carbonate *see* lithium *on page 594*
lithium citrate *see* lithium *on page 594*
Lithobid® [US] *see* lithium *on page 594*
Lithonate® *(Discontinued)* *see* lithium *on page 594*
Lithostat® [US/Can] *see* acetohydroxamic acid *on page 30*
Lithotabs® *(Discontinued)* *see* lithium *on page 594*
Little Colds® Multi-Symptom Cold Formula *(Discontinued)* *see* acetaminophen, dextromethorphan, and phenylephrine *on page 27*
Little Fevers™ [US-OTC] *see* acetaminophen *on page 19*
Little Noses® Decongestant [US-OTC] *see* phenylephrine *on page 774*
Little Noses® Saline [US-OTC] *see* sodium chloride *on page 908*
Little Noses® Stuffy Nose Kit [US-OTC] *see* sodium chloride *on page 908*
Little Phillips'® Milk of Magnesia [US-OTC] *see* magnesium hydroxide *on page 608*
Little Teethers® [US-OTC] *see* benzocaine *on page 129*
Little Tummys® Gas Relief [US-OTC] *see* simethicone *on page 901*
Little Tummys® Laxative [US-OTC] *see* senna *on page 896*
live attenuated influenza vaccine (LAIV) *see* influenza virus vaccine *on page 528*
live smallpox vaccine *see* smallpox vaccine *on page 906*
Livostin® *(Discontinued)*
L-leucovorin *see* LEVOleucovorin *on page 581*

l-lysine (el LYE seen)

Synonyms l-lysine hydrochloride

U.S./Canadian Brand Names Lysinyl [US-OTC]

Therapeutic Category Dietary Supplement

Use Improves utilization of vegetable proteins

Usual Dosage Oral: Adults:

Supplement: 334-1500 mg/day
Recurrent herpes simplex infection (dental use): 2000 mg every 4 hours until symptoms subside; begin treatment during early stage of recurrence

Dosage Forms

Capsule: 500 mg
Lysinyl [OTC]: 500 mg
Powder, oral: 100% (100 g)
Lysinyl [OTC]: 500 mg/ 1/4 teaspoon (150 g)
Tablet: 500 mg, 1000 mg

l-lysine hydrochloride *see* l-lysine *on page 595*
LM3100 *see* plerixafor *on page 789*
LMD® [US] *see* dextran *on page 292*

lodoxamide (loe DOKS a mide)

Synonyms lodoxamide tromethamine

U.S./Canadian Brand Names Alomide® [US/Can]

Therapeutic Category Mast Cell Stabilizer

Use Treatment of vernal keratoconjunctivitis, vernal conjunctivitis, and vernal keratitis

Usual Dosage Ophthalmic: Instill 1-2 drops in eye(s) 4 times/day for up to 3 months

Dosage Forms

Solution, ophthalmic:
Alomide®: 0.1% (10 mL)

lomustine (loe MUS teen)

Sound-Alike/Look-Alike Issues
lomustine may be confused with carmustine

Synonyms CCNU; lomustinum

U.S./Canadian Brand Names CeeNU® [US/Can]

Therapeutic Category Antineoplastic Agent

Use Treatment of brain tumors and Hodgkin disease

Usual Dosage Note: Repeat courses should only be administered after adequate recovery of leukocytes to >4000/mm^3 and platelets to >100,000/mm^3. Details concerning dosage in combination regimens should also be consulted.

Oral: Children and Adults: Brain tumors, Hodgkin lymphoma: 130 mg/m^2 as a single dose once every 6 weeks (dosage reductions may be recommended for combination chemotherapy regimens)

Compromised marrow function: Reduce dose to 100 mg/m^2 as a single dose once every 6 weeks

Dosage Forms

Capsule:

CeeNU®: 10 mg, 40 mg, 100 mg

lomustinum *see* lomustine *on page 596*

Loniten® [Can] *see* minoxidil *on page 660*

Loniten® 2.5 mg Tablet *(Discontinued)* *see* minoxidil *on page 660*

Lonox® [US] *see* diphenoxylate and atropine *on page 318*

Lo/Ovral®-28 [US] *see* ethinyl estradiol and norgestrel *on page 394*

Loperacap [Can] *see* loperamide *on page 597*

loperamide (loe PER a mide)

Sound-Alike/Look-Alike Issues

loperamide may be confused with furosemide

Imodium® A-D may be confused with Indocin®, Ionamin®

Synonyms loperamide hydrochloride

U.S./Canadian Brand Names Apo-Loperamide® [Can]; Diamode [US-OTC]; Diarr-Eze [Can]; Dom-Loperamide [Can]; Imodium® A-D [US-OTC]; Imodium® [Can]; K-Pek II [US-OTC]; Kao-Paverin® [US-OTC]; Loperacap [Can]; Novo-Loperamide [Can]; PMS-Loperamine [Can]; Rhoxal-loperamide [Can]; Rho®-Loperamine [Can]; Riva-Loperamine [Can]; Sandoz-Loperamide [Can]

Therapeutic Category Antidiarrheal

Use Treatment of chronic diarrhea associated with inflammatory bowel disease; acute nonspecific diarrhea; increased volume of ileostomy discharge

OTC labeling: Control of symptoms of diarrhea, including traveler's diarrhea

Usual Dosage Oral:

Children:

Acute diarrhea: Initial doses (in first 24 hours):

2-5 years (13-20 kg): 1 mg 3 times/day

6-8 years (20-30 kg): 2 mg twice daily

8-12 years (>30 kg): 2 mg 3 times/day

Maintenance: After initial dosing, 0.1 mg/kg doses after each loose stool, but not exceeding initial dosage

Traveler's diarrhea:

6-8 years: 2 mg after first loose stool, followed by 1 mg after each subsequent stool (maximum dose: 4 mg/day)

9-11 years: 2 mg after first loose stool, followed by 1 mg after each subsequent stool (maximum dose: 6 mg/day)

≥12 years: See adult dosing.

Adults:

Acute diarrhea: Initial: 4 mg, followed by 2 mg after each loose stool, up to 16 mg/day

Chronic diarrhea: Initial: Follow acute diarrhea; maintenance dose should be slowly titrated downward to minimum required to control symptoms (typically, 4-8 mg/day in divided doses)

Traveler's diarrhea: Initial: 4 mg after first loose stool, followed by 2 mg after each subsequent stool (maximum dose: 8 mg/day)

Dosage Forms

Caplet: 2 mg

Diamode [OTC], Imodium® A-D [OTC], Kao-Paverin® [OTC]: 2 mg

Capsule: 2 mg

Liquid, oral: 1 mg/5 mL

Imodium® A-D [OTC]: 1 mg/5 mL

Imodium® A-D [OTC] [*new formulation*]: 1 mg/7.5 mL

Tablet: 2 mg

K-Pek II [OTC]: 2 mg

loperamide and simethicone (loe PER a mide & sye METH i kone)

Synonyms simethicone and loperamide hydrochloride

U.S./Canadian Brand Names Imodium® Multi-Symptom Relief [US-OTC]

Therapeutic Category Antidiarrheal; Antiflatulent

Use Control of symptoms of diarrhea and gas (bloating, pressure, and cramps)

Usual Dosage Oral: Acute diarrhea (weight-based dosing is preferred):

Children:

6-8 years (48-59 lbs): 1 caplet or tablet after first loose stool, followed by 1/2 caplet/tablet with each subsequent loose stool (maximum: 2 caplets or tablets/24 hours)

9-11 years (60-95 lbs): 1 caplet or tablet after first loose stool, followed by 1/2 caplet or tablet with each subsequent loose stool (maximum: 3 caplets or tablets/24 hours)

Children >12 years and Adults: One caplet or tablet after first loose stool, followed by 1 caplet or tablet with each subsequent loose stool (maximum: 4 caplets or tablets/24 hours)

Dosage Forms

Caplet:

Imodium® Multi-Symptom Relief: Loperamide hydrochloride 2 mg and simethicone 125 mg [contains calcium 65 mg/caplet, sodium 4 mg/caplet]

Tablet, chewable:

Imodium® Muliti-Symptom Relief: Loperamide hydrochloride 2 mg and simethicone 125 mg [contains calcium 50 mg/tablet; mint flavor]

loperamide hydrochloride *see* loperamide *on page 597*

Lopid® [US/Can] *see* gemfibrozil *on page 458*

lopinavir and ritonavir (loe PIN a veer & rit ON uh veer)

Sound-Alike/Look-Alike Issues

Potential for dispensing errors between Kaletra™ and Keppra® (levetiracetam)

Synonyms ritonavir and lopinavir

U.S./Canadian Brand Names Kaletra® [US/Can]

Therapeutic Category Antiretroviral Agent, Nonnucleoside Reverse Transcriptase Inhibitor (NNRTI)

Use Treatment of HIV infection in combination with other antiretroviral agents

Usual Dosage Oral:

Children: Dosage based on weight or body surface area (BSA), **presented based on lopinavir component** (maximum dose: Lopinavir 400 mg/ritonavir 100 mg).

14 days to 6 months: 16 mg/kg or 300 mg/m^2 twice daily

6 months to 18 years: **Note:** FDA-approved dose is approximately equivalent to lopinavir 230 mg/m^2 per dose.

<15 kg: 12 mg/kg twice daily

15-40 kg: 10 mg/kg twice daily

>40 kg: Lopinavir 400 mg/ritonavir 100 mg twice daily

Note: For therapy-experienced patients with suspected reduced susceptibility to lopinavir, refer to adult dosing.

Children >12 years: Therapy-naive: Lopinavir 400 mg/ritonavir 100 mg twice daily (AIDS*info* guidelines). **Note:** For therapy-experienced patients with suspected reduced susceptibility to lopinavir, refer to adult dosing.

Adults:

Therapy-naive: Lopinavir 800 mg/ritonavir 200 mg once daily **or** lopinavir 400 mg/ritonavir 100 mg twice daily

Note: Once-daily dosing regimen should not be used with concurrent indinavir, maraviroc, saquinavir, phenytoin, carbamazepine, or phenobarbital therapy.

Therapy-experienced: Lopinavir 400 mg/ritonavir 100 mg twice daily

Note: For therapy-experienced patients receiving efavirenz or nevirapine, clinicians may use lopinavir 600 mg/ritonavir 150 mg twice daily **or** lopinavir 533 mg/ritonavir 133 mg solution twice daily (AIDS info guidelines)

Dosage Forms

Solution, oral:

Kaletra®: Lopinavir 80 mg and ritonavir 20 mg per mL

Tablet:

Kaletra®:

Lopinavir 100 mg and ritonavir 25 mg

Lopinavir 200 mg and ritonavir 50 mg

Lopressor® [US/Can] *see* metoprolol *on page 650*
Lopressor HCT® [US] *see* metoprolol and hydrochlorothiazide *on page 651*
Loprox® [US/Can] *see* ciclopirox *on page 227*
Loradamed [US-OTC] *see* loratadine *on page 599*

loratadine (lor AT a deen)

Sound-Alike/Look-Alike Issues
Claritin® may be confused with clarithromycin

U.S./Canadian Brand Names Alavert® Allergy 24 Hour [US-OTC]; Alavert® Children's Allergy [US-OTC]; Apo-Loratadine® [Can]; Claritin® 24 Hour Allergy [US-OTC]; Claritin® Children's Allergy [US-OTC]; Claritin® Kids [Can]; Claritin® Liqui-Gels® 24 Hour Allergy [US-OTC]; Claritin® RediTabs® 24 Hour Allergy [US-OTC]; Claritin® [Can]; Loradamed [US-OTC]; Tavist® ND Allergy [US-OTC]

Therapeutic Category Antihistamine

Use Relief of nasal and nonnasal symptoms of seasonal allergic rhinitis; treatment of chronic idiopathic urticaria

Usual Dosage Oral: Seasonal allergic rhinitis, chronic idiopathic urticaria:
Children 2-5 years: 5 mg once daily
Children ≥6 years and Adults: 10 mg once daily

Dosage Forms

Capsule, liquid gel, oral:
Claritin® Liqui-Gels® 24 Hour Allergy [OTC]: 10 mg

Solution, oral: 5 mg/5 mL (120 mL)

Syrup, oral: 5 mg/5 mL (120 mL)
Claritin® Children's Allergy [OTC]: 5 mg/5 mL (60 mL, 120 mL)

Tablet, oral: 10 mg
Alavert® Allergy 24 Hour [OTC], Claritin® 24 Hour Allergy [OTC], Loradamed [OTC], Tavist® ND Allergy [OTC]: 10 mg

Tablet, chewable, oral:
Claritin® Children's Allergy [OTC]: 5 mg

Tablet, orally disintegrating, oral:
Alavert® Allergy 24 Hour [OTC], Alavert® Children's Allergy [OTC], Claritin® RediTabs® 24 Hour Allergy [OTC]: 10 mg

loratadine and pseudoephedrine (lor AT a deen & soo doe e FED rin)

Sound-Alike/Look-Alike Issues
Claritin-D® may be confused with Claritin-D® 24
Claritin-D® 24 may be confused with Claritin-D®

Synonyms pseudoephedrine and loratadine

U.S./Canadian Brand Names Alavert™ Allergy and Sinus [US-OTC]; Chlor-Tripolon ND® [Can]; Claritin-D® 12 Hour Allergy & Congestion [US-OTC]; Claritin-D® 24 Hour Allergy & Congestion [US-OTC]; Claritin® Extra [Can]; Claritin® Liberator [Can]

Therapeutic Category Antihistamine/Decongestant Combination

Use Temporary relief of symptoms of seasonal allergic rhinitis, other upper respiratory allergies, or the common cold

Usual Dosage Oral: Children ≥12 years and Adults:
Claritin-D® 12-Hour: 1 tablet every 12 hours
Alavert™ Allergy and Sinus, Claritin-D® 24-Hour: 1 tablet daily

Dosage Forms

Tablet, extended release: Loratadine 10 mg and pseudoephedrine 240 mg
Alavert™ Allergy and Sinus [OTC]: Loratadine 5 mg and pseudoephedrine 120 mg
Claritin-D® 12 Hour Allergy & Congestion [OTC]: Loratadine 5 mg and pseudoephedrine 120 mg
Claritin-D® 24 Hour Allergy & Congestion [OTC]: Loratadine 10 mg and pseudoephedrine 240 mg

lorazepam (lor A ze pam)

Sound-Alike/Look-Alike Issues
LORazepam may be confused with ALPRAZolam, clonazePAM, diazepam, Lovaza®, temazepam, zolpidem
Ativan® may be confused with Ambien®, Atarax®, Atgam®, Avitene®

Tall-Man LORazepam

U.S./Canadian Brand Names Apo-Lorazepam® [Can]; Ativan® [US/Can]; Lorazepam Injection, USP [Can]; Lorazepam Intensol™ [US]; Novo-Lorazepam [Can]; Nu-Loraz [Can]; PHL-Lorazepam [Can]; PMS-Lorazepam [Can]; Riva-Lorazepam [Can]

Therapeutic Category Benzodiazepine

Controlled Substance C-IV

Use

Oral: Management of anxiety disorders or short-term (≤4 months) relief of the symptoms of anxiety or anxiety associated with depressive symptoms

I.V.: Status epilepticus, amnesia, sedation

Usual Dosage

Anxiety and sedation: Adults: Oral: 1-10 mg/day in 2-3 divided doses; usual dose: 2-6 mg/day in divided doses

Insomnia: Adults: Oral: 2-4 mg at bedtime

Preoperative: Adults:

I.M.: 0.05 mg/kg administered 2 hours before surgery (maximum: 4 mg/dose)

I.V.: 0.044 mg/kg 15-20 minutes before surgery (usual maximum: 2 mg/dose)

Preprocedural anxiety (dental use): Adults: Oral: 1-2 mg 1 hour before procedure

Operative amnesia: Adults: I.V.: Up to 0.05 mg/kg (maximum: 4 mg/dose)

Status epilepticus: I.V.: Adults: 4 mg/dose slow I.V. (maximum rate: 2 mg/minute); may repeat in 10-15 minutes; usual maximum dose: 8 mg

Rapid tranquilization of agitated patient (administer every 30-60 minutes): Adults:

Oral: 1-2 mg

I.M.: 0.5-1 mg

Average total dose for tranquilization: Oral, I.M.: 4-8 mg

Dosage Forms

Injection, solution: 2 mg/mL (1 mL, 10 mL); 4 mg/mL (1 mL, 10 mL)

Ativan®: 2 mg/mL (1 mL); 4 mg/mL (1 mL, 10 mL)

Injection, solution [preservative free]: 2 mg/mL (1 mL); 4 mg/mL (1 mL)

Solution, oral [concentrate]: 2 mg/mL (30 mL)

Lorazepam Intensol™: 2 mg/mL

Tablet: 0.5 mg, 1 mg, 2 mg

Ativan®: 0.5 mg

Ativan®: 1 mg, 2 mg [scored]

Lorazepam Injection, USP [Can] *see* lorazepam *on page 599*

Lorazepam Intensol™ [US] *see* lorazepam *on page 599*

Lorcet® 10/650 [US] *see* hydrocodone and acetaminophen *on page 501*

Lorcet®-HD *(Discontinued)* *see* hydrocodone and acetaminophen *on page 501*

Lorcet® Plus [US] *see* hydrocodone and acetaminophen *on page 501*

Lorsin® *(Discontinued)* *see* acetaminophen, chlorpheniramine, and pseudoephedrine *on page 26*

Lortab® [US] *see* hydrocodone and acetaminophen *on page 501*

Lortab® ASA *(Discontinued)*

losartan (loe SAR tan)

Sound-Alike/Look-Alike Issues

losartan may be confused with valsartan

Cozaar® may be confused with Colace®, Coreg®, Hyzaar®, Zocor®

Synonyms DuP 753; losartan potassium; MK594

U.S./Canadian Brand Names Cozaar® [US/Can]

Therapeutic Category Angiotensin II Receptor Antagonist

Use Treatment of hypertension (HTN); treatment of diabetic nephropathy in patients with type 2 diabetes mellitus (noninsulin-dependent, NIDDM) and a history of hypertension; stroke risk reduction in patients with HTN and left ventricular hypertrophy (LVH)

Usual Dosage Oral:

Hypertension:

Children 6-16 years:

U.S. labeling: 0.7 mg/kg once daily (maximum: 50 mg/day); doses >1.4 mg/kg (maximum: 100 mg) have not been studied

Canadian labeling:

≥20 kg to <50 kg: 25 mg once daily (maximum: 50 mg once daily)

≥50 kg: 50 mg once daily (maximum: 100 mg once daily)

Adults: Usual starting dose: 50 mg once daily; can be administered once or twice daily with total daily doses ranging from 25-100 mg

Patients receiving diuretics or with intravascular volume depletion: Usual initial dose: 25 mg once daily

Nephropathy in patients with type 2 diabetes and hypertension: Adults: Initial: 50 mg once daily; can be increased to 100 mg once daily based on blood pressure response

Stroke reduction (HTN with LVH): Adults: 50 mg once daily (maximum daily dose: 100 mg); may be used in combination with a thiazide diuretic

Dosage Forms

Tablet, oral:

Cozaar®: 25 mg, 50 mg, 100 mg

losartan and hydrochlorothiazide (loe SAR tan & hye droe klor oh THYE a zide)

Sound-Alike/Look-Alike Issues

Hyzaar® may be confused with Cozaar®

Synonyms hydrochlorothiazide and losartan

U.S./Canadian Brand Names Hyzaar® DS [Can]; Hyzaar® [US/Can]

Therapeutic Category Antihypertensive Agent, Combination

Use Treatment of hypertension; stroke risk reduction in patients with HTN and left ventricular hypertrophy (LVH)

Usual Dosage Oral: Adults: Dose is individualized (combination substituted for individual components); dose may be titrated after 2-4 weeks of therapy

Hypertension/stroke reduction in hypertension (with LVH): Usual recommended starting dose of losartan: 50 mg once daily when used as monotherapy in patients who are not volume depleted

Dosage Forms

Tablet:

Hyzaar®: 50/12.5: Losartan 50 mg and hydrochlorothiazide 12.5 mg; 100/12.5: Losartan 100 mg and hydrochlorothiazide 12.5 mg; 100/25: Losartan 100 mg and hydrochlorothiazide 25 mg

losartan potassium *see* losartan *on page* *600*

LoSeasonique™ [US] *see* ethinyl estradiol and levonorgestrel *on page* *387*

Losec® [Can] *see* omeprazole *on page* *723*

Losec MUPS® [Can] *see* omeprazole *on page* *723*

Losopan® *(Discontinued)* *see* magaldrate and simethicone *on page* *606*

Lotemax® [US/Can] *see* loteprednol *on page* *601*

Lotensin® [US/Can] *see* benazepril *on page* *126*

Lotensin® HCT [US] *see* benazepril and hydrochlorothiazide *on page* *127*

loteprednol (loe te PRED nol)

Synonyms loteprednol etabonate

U.S./Canadian Brand Names Alrex® [US/Can]; Lotemax® [US/Can]

Therapeutic Category Corticosteroid, Ophthalmic

Use

Suspension, 0.2% (Alrex®): Temporary relief of signs and symptoms of seasonal allergic conjunctivitis

Suspension, 0.5% (Lotemax®): Inflammatory conditions (treatment of steroid-responsive inflammatory conditions of the palpebral and bulbar conjunctiva, cornea, and anterior segment of the globe such as allergic conjunctivitis, acne rosacea, superficial punctate keratitis, herpes zoster keratitis, iritis, cyclitis, selected infective conjunctivitis, when the inherent hazard of steroid use is accepted to obtain an advisable diminution in edema and inflammation) and treatment of postoperative inflammation following ocular surgery

Usual Dosage Ophthalmic: Adults:

Suspension, 0.2% (Alrex®): Instill 1 drop into affected eye(s) 4 times/day

Suspension, 0.5% (Lotemax®):

Inflammatory conditions: Apply 1-2 drops into the conjunctival sac of the affected eye(s) 4 times/day. During the initial treatment within the first week, the dosing may be increased up to 1 drop every hour. Advise patients not to discontinue therapy prematurely. If signs and symptoms fail to improve after 2 days, reevaluate the patient.

Postoperative inflammation: Apply 1-2 drops into the conjunctival sac of the operated eye(s) 4 times/day beginning 24 hours after surgery and continuing throughout the first 2 weeks of the postoperative period

Dosage Forms

Suspension, ophthalmic:

Alrex®: 0.2% (5 mL, 10 mL)

Lotemax®: 0.5% (2.5 mL, 5 mL, 10 mL, 15 mL)

loteprednol and tobramycin (loe te PRED nol & toe bra MYE sin)

Synonyms loteprednol etabonate and tobramycin; tobramycin and loteprednol etabonate

U.S./Canadian Brand Names Zylet™ [US]

Therapeutic Category Antibiotic/Corticosteroid, Ophthalmic

Use Treatment of steroid-responsive ocular inflammatory conditions where either a superficial bacterial ocular infection or the risk of a superficial bacterial ocular infection exists

Usual Dosage Ophthalmic: Adults: Instill 1-2 drops into the affected eye(s) every 4-6 hours; may increase frequency during the first 24-48 hours to every 1-2 hours. Interval should increase as signs and symptoms improve. Further evaluation should occur for use of greater than 20 mL.

Dosage Forms

Suspension, ophthalmic:

Zylet™: Loteprednol 0.5% and tobramycin 0.3% (2.5 mL, 5 mL, 10 mL)

loteprednol etabonate *see* loteprednol *on page* 601

loteprednol etabonate and tobramycin *see* loteprednol and tobramycin *on page* 602

Lotrel® [US] *see* amlodipine and benazepril *on page* 67

Lotriderm® [Can] *see* betamethasone and clotrimazole *on page* 137

Lotrimin AF® [US-OTC] *see* miconazole *on page* 654

Lotrimin® AF Athlete's Foot Cream [US-OTC] *see* clotrimazole *on page* 248

Lotrimin® AF Cream *(Discontinued)* *see* clotrimazole *on page* 248

Lotrimin® AF for Her [US-OTC] *see* clotrimazole *on page* 248

Lotrimin® AF Jock Itch Cream [US-OTC] *see* clotrimazole *on page* 248

Lotrimin® AF Lotion *(Discontinued)* *see* clotrimazole *on page* 248

Lotrimin® AF Solution *(Discontinued)* *see* clotrimazole *on page* 248

Lotrimin® Ultra™ [US-OTC] *see* butenafine *on page* 163

Lotrisone® [US] *see* betamethasone and clotrimazole *on page* 137

Lotronex® [US] *see* alosetron *on page* 50

lovastatin (LOE va sta tin)

Sound-Alike/Look-Alike Issues

lovastatin may be confused with Leustatin®, Livostin®, Lotensin®, nystatin

Mevacor® may be confused with Benicar®, Mivacron®

Synonyms mevinolin; monacolin K

U.S./Canadian Brand Names Altoprev® [US]; Apo-Lovastatin® [Can]; CO Lovastatin [Can]; DOM-Lovastatin [Can]; Gen-Lovastatin [Can]; Mevacor® [US/Can]; Novo-Lovastatin [Can]; Nu-Lovastatin [Can]; PHL-Lovastatin [Can]; PMS-Lovastatin [Can]; PRO-Lovastatin [Can]; RAN™-Lovastatin [Can]; ratio-Lovastatin [Can]; Riva-Lovastatin [Can]; Sandoz-Lovastatin [Can]

Therapeutic Category HMG-CoA Reductase Inhibitor

Use

Adjunct to dietary therapy to decrease elevated serum total and LDL-cholesterol concentrations in primary hypercholesterolemia

Primary prevention of coronary artery disease (patients without symptomatic disease with average to moderately elevated total and LDL-cholesterol and below average HDL-cholesterol); slow progression of coronary atherosclerosis in patients with coronary heart disease

Adjunct to dietary therapy in adolescent patients (10-17 years of age, females >1 year postmenarche) with heterozygous familial hypercholesterolemia having LDL >189 mg/dL, **or** LDL >160 mg/dL with positive family history of premature cardiovascular disease (CVD), **or** LDL >160 mg/dL with the presence of at least two other CVD risk factors

Usual Dosage Oral:

Adolescents 10-17 years: Immediate release tablet:

LDL reduction <20%: Initial: 10 mg/day with evening meal

LDL reduction ≥20%: Initial: 20 mg/day with evening meal
Usual range: 10-40 mg with evening meal, then adjust dose at 4-week intervals
Adults: Initial: 20 mg with evening meal, then adjust at 4-week intervals; maximum dose: 80 mg/day immediate release tablet **or** 60 mg/day extended release tablet

Dosage Forms

Tablet: 10 mg, 20 mg, 40 mg
Mevacor®: 20 mg, 40 mg

Tablet, extended release:
Altoprev®: 20 mg, 40 mg, 60 mg

lovastatin and niacin *see* niacin and lovastatin *on page 694*

Lovaza® [US] *see* omega-3-acid ethyl esters *on page 723*

Lovenox® [US/Can] *see* enoxaparin *on page 355*

Lovenox® HP [Can] *see* enoxaparin *on page 355*

low-Molecular-weight iron dextran (INFeD®) *see* iron dextran complex *on page 546*

Low-Ogestrel® [US] *see* ethinyl estradiol and norgestrel *on page 394*

Loxapac® IM [Can] *see* loxapine *on page 603*

loxapine (LOKS a peen)

Sound-Alike/Look-Alike Issues
Loxitane® may be confused with Lexapro®, Soriatane®

Synonyms loxapine succinate; oxilapine succinate

U.S./Canadian Brand Names Apo-Loxapine® [Can]; Loxapac® IM [Can]; Loxitane® [US]; Nu-Loxapine [Can]; PMS-Loxapine [Can]

Therapeutic Category Antipsychotic Agent, Dibenzoxazepine

Use Management of psychotic disorders

Usual Dosage Oral: Adults: 10 mg twice daily, increase dose until psychotic symptoms are controlled; usual dose range: 20-100 mg/day in divided doses 2-4 times/day; dosages >250 mg/day are not recommended

Dosage Forms

Capsule: 5 mg, 10 mg, 25 mg, 50 mg
Loxitane®: 5 mg, 10 mg, 25 mg, 50 mg

loxapine succinate *see* loxapine *on page 603*

Loxitane® [US] *see* loxapine *on page 603*

Loxitane® I.M. *(Discontinued)* *see* loxapine *on page 603*

Lozide® [Can] *see* indapamide *on page 525*

Lozi-Flur™ [US] *see* fluoride *on page 430*

Lozi-Tab® *(Discontinued)* *see* fluoride *on page 430*

Lozol® [Can] *see* indapamide *on page 525*

Lozol® *(Discontinued)* *see* indapamide *on page 525*

L-PAM *see* melphalan *on page 622*

L-sarcolysin *see* melphalan *on page 622*

LTA® 360 [US] *see* lidocaine *on page 584*

LTG *see* lamotrigine *on page 567*

***L*-thyroxine sodium** *see* levothyroxine *on page 583*

Lu-26-054 *see* escitalopram *on page 370*

lubiprostone (loo bi PROS tone)

Synonyms RU 0211; SPI 0211

U.S./Canadian Brand Names Amitiza® [US]

Therapeutic Category Gastrointestinal Agent, Miscellaneous

Use Treatment of chronic idiopathic constipation; treatment of irritable bowel syndrome with constipation in adult women

Usual Dosage Oral:
Chronic idiopathic constipation: Adults: 24 mcg twice daily
Irritable bowel syndrome with constipation: Females ≥18 years: 8 mcg twice daily

Dosage Forms

Capsule, softgel:

Amitiza®: 8 mcg, 24 mcg

Lubriderm® [US-OTC] *see* lanolin, cetyl alcohol, glycerin, petrolatum, and mineral oil *on page 570*

Lubriderm® Fragrance Free [US-OTC] *see* lanolin, cetyl alcohol, glycerin, petrolatum, and mineral oil *on page 570*

LubriTears® Solution *(Discontinued)* *see* artificial tears *on page 100*

Lucentis® [US/Can] *see* ranibizumab *on page 851*

Ludiomil® *(Discontinued)* *see* maprotiline *on page 614*

Lufyllin® [US/Can] *see* dyphylline *on page 344*

Lufyllin®-GG [US] *see* dyphylline and guaifenesin *on page 344*

lumefantrine and artemether *see* artemether and lumefantrine *on page 99*

Lumigan® [US/Can] *see* bimatoprost *on page 141*

Luminal® Sodium [US] *see* phenobarbital *on page 771*

Lumitene™ [US] *see* beta-carotene *on page 136*

Lunesta® [US] *see* eszopiclone *on page 381*

LupiCare® Dandruff [US-OTC] *see* salicylic acid *on page 884*

LupiCare® Psoriasis [US-OTC] *see* salicylic acid *on page 884*

LupiCare® Psoriasis Scalp *(Discontinued)* *see* salicylic acid *on page 884*

Lupron® [US/Can] *see* leuprolide *on page 575*

Lupron Depot® [US/Can] *see* leuprolide *on page 575*

Lupron Depot-Ped® [US] *see* leuprolide *on page 575*

Luride® *(Discontinued)* *see* fluoride *on page 430*

Luride® Lozi-Tab® [US] *see* fluoride *on page 430*

Luride®-SF *(Discontinued)* *see* fluoride *on page 430*

Lusedra™ [US] *see* fospropofol *on page 447*

LuSonal™ [US] *see* phenylephrine *on page 774*

Lustra® [US/Can] *see* hydroquinone *on page 508*

Lustra-AF® [US] *see* hydroquinone *on page 508*

Lustra-Ultra™ [US] *see* hydroquinone *on page 508*

Lutera™ [US] *see* ethinyl estradiol and levonorgestrel *on page 387*

lutropin alfa (LOO troe pin AL fa)

Synonyms r-hLH; recombinant human luteinizing hormone

U.S./Canadian Brand Names Luveris® [US]

Therapeutic Category Gonadotropin; Ovulation Stimulator

Use Stimulation of follicular development in infertile hypogonadotropic hypogonadal (HH) women with profound luteinizing hormone (LH) deficiency; to be used in combination with follitropin alfa

Usual Dosage SubQ: Adults: Females: Infertility: 75 int. units daily until adequate follicular development is noted; maximum duration of treatment: 14 days; to be used concomitantly with follitropin alfa

Dosage Forms

Injection, powder for reconstitution:

Luveris®: 75 int. units

Luveris® [US] *see* lutropin alfa *on page 604*

Luvox® [Can] *see* fluvoxamine *on page 439*

Luvox® CR [US] *see* fluvoxamine *on page 439*

Luvox® *(Discontinued)* *see* fluvoxamine *on page 439*

Luxiq® [US] *see* betamethasone (topical) *on page 138*

LY139603 *see* atomoxetine *on page 108*

LY146032 *see* daptomycin *on page 276*

LY170053 *see* olanzapine *on page 719*

LY231514 *see* pemetrexed *on page 758*

LY246736 *see* alvimopan *on page 57*

LY248686 *see* duloxetine *on page 341*

LY303366 *see* anidulafungin *on page 80*
LY-640315 *see* prasugrel *on page 810*
LY2148568 *see* exenatide *on page 401*
Lybrel™ [US] *see* ethinyl estradiol and levonorgestrel *on page 387*
Lycolan® Elixir ***(Discontinued)*** *see* l-lysine *on page 595*
Lyderm® [Can] *see* fluocinonide *on page 429*
LYMErix™ ***(Discontinued)***
Lymphazurin™ [US] *see* isosulfan blue *on page 551*
lymphocyte immune globulin *see* antithymocyte globulin (equine) *on page 86*
lymphocyte mitogenic factor *see* aldesleukin *on page 43*
Lyphocin® Injection ***(Discontinued)*** *see* vancomycin *on page 1005*
Lyrica® [US/Can] *see* pregabalin *on page 815*
Lysinyl [US-OTC] *see* l-lysine *on page 595*
Lysodren® [US/Can] *see* mitotane *on page 662*
Maalox® [US-OTC] *see* aluminum hydroxide, magnesium hydroxide, and simethicone *on page 56*
Maalox® Anti-Gas ***(Discontinued)*** *see* aluminum hydroxide, magnesium hydroxide, and simethicone *on page 56*
Maalox® Anti-Gas Extra Strength ***(Discontinued)*** *see* aluminum hydroxide, magnesium hydroxide, and simethicone *on page 56*
Maalox® Extra Strength ***(Discontinued)*** *see* aluminum hydroxide and magnesium hydroxide *on page 55*
Maalox® Max [US-OTC] *see* aluminum hydroxide, magnesium hydroxide, and simethicone *on page 56*
Maalox® Plus ***(Discontinued)*** *see* aluminum hydroxide, magnesium hydroxide, and simethicone *on page 56*
Maalox® Regular Chewable [US-OTC] *see* calcium carbonate *on page 170*
Maalox® TC (Therapeutic Concentrate) ***(Discontinued)*** *see* aluminum hydroxide and magnesium hydroxide *on page 55*
Maalox® Total Stomach Relief® [US-OTC] *see* bismuth *on page 142*
MabCampath® [Can] *see* alemtuzumab *on page 44*
Macrobid® [US/Can] *see* nitrofurantoin *on page 700*
Macrodantin® [US/Can] *see* nitrofurantoin *on page 700*
Macrodex® ***(Discontinued)*** *see* dextran *on page 292*
Macugen® [US/Can] *see* pegaptanib *on page 755*

mafenide (MA fe nide)

Synonyms mafenide acetate

U.S./Canadian Brand Names Sulfamylon® [US]

Therapeutic Category Antibacterial, Topical

Use

Cream: Adjunctive antibacterial agent in the treatment of second- and third-degree burns

Solution: Adjunctive antibacterial agent for use under moist dressings over meshed autografts on excised burn wounds

Usual Dosage Topical: Children and Adults:

Cream: Apply once or twice daily with a sterile-gloved hand; apply to a thickness of approximately 1/16 inch; the burned area should be covered with cream at all times

Solution: Cover graft area with 1 layer of fine mesh gauze. Wet an 8-ply burn dressing with mafenide solution and cover graft area. Keep dressing wet using syringe or irrigation tubing every 4 hours (or as necessary), or by moistening dressing every 6-8 hours (or as necessary). Irrigation dressing should be secured with bolster dressing and wrapped as appropriate. May leave dressings in place for up to 5 days.

Dosage Forms

Cream, topical:

Sulfamylon®: 85 mg/g (60 g, 120 g, 454 g)

Powder, for topical solution, as acetate:

Sulfamylon®: 50 g/packet (5s)

mafenide acetate *see* mafenide *on page 605*

Mag 64™ [US-OTC] *see* magnesium chloride *on page 606*

magaldrate and simethicone (MAG al drate & sye METH i kone)

Sound-Alike/Look-Alike Issues

Riopan Plus® may be confused with Repan®

Synonyms simethicone and magaldrate

Therapeutic Category Antacid; Antiflatulent

Use Relief of hyperacidity associated with peptic ulcer, gastritis, peptic esophagitis, and hiatal hernia which are accompanied by symptoms of gas

Usual Dosage Oral: Adults: 5-10 mL (540-1080 mg magaldrate) between meals and at bedtime

Dosage Forms

Suspension, oral: Magaldrate 540 mg and simethicone 20 mg per 5 mL

Magalox Plus® ***(Discontinued)*** *see* aluminum hydroxide, magnesium hydroxide, and simethicone *on page 56*

Magan® ***(Discontinued)*** *see* magnesium salicylate *on page 610*

Mag Delay® [US-OTC] *see* magnesium chloride *on page 606*

Mag G® [US-OTC] *see* magnesium gluconate *on page 607*

MagGel™ 600 [US-OTC] *see* magnesium oxide *on page 610*

Maginex™ [US-OTC] *see* magnesium L-aspartate hydrochloride *on page 609*

Maginex™ DS [US-OTC] *see* magnesium L-aspartate hydrochloride *on page 609*

Magnacal® [US-OTC] *see* nutritional formula, enteral/oral *on page 715*

Magnacet™ [US] *see* oxycodone and acetaminophen *on page 738*

Magnelium® [Can] *see* magnesium glucoheptonate *on page 607*

magnesia magma *see* magnesium hydroxide *on page 608*

magnesium carbonate and aluminum hydroxide *see* aluminum hydroxide and magnesium carbonate *on page 55*

magnesium chloride (mag NEE zhum KLOR ide)

U.S./Canadian Brand Names Chloromag® [US]; Mag 64™ [US-OTC]; Mag Delay® [US-OTC]; Mag-SR with Calcium [US]; Mag-SR [US]; Slow-Mag® [US-OTC]

Therapeutic Category Electrolyte Supplement, Oral

Use Correction or prevention of hypomagnesemia; dietary supplement

Usual Dosage Note: Serum magnesium is poor reflection of repletional status as the majority of magnesium is intracellular; serum levels may be transiently normal for a few hours after a dose is given, therefore, aim for consistently high normal serum levels in patients with normal renal function for most efficient repletion.

Dietary supplement: Adults: Oral (Mag 64™, Mag Delay®, Slow-Mag®): 2 tablets once daily

Parenteral nutrition supplementation: I.V. (elemental magnesium):

- Children:
  - <50 kg: 0.3-0.5 mEq/kg/day
  - >50 kg: 10-30 mEq/day
- Adults: 8-24 mEq/day

RDA (elemental magnesium):

- Children:
  - 1-3 years: 80 mg/day
  - 4-8 years: 130 mg/day
  - 9-13 years: 240 mg/day
  - 14-18 years:
    - Female: 360 mg/day
    - Pregnant female: 400 mg/day
    - Male: 410 mg/day
- Adults:
  - 19-30 years:
    - Female: 310 mg/day
    - Pregnant female: 350 mg/day
    - Male: 400 mg/day
  - ≥31 years:
    - Female: 320 mg/day
    - Pregnant female: 360 mg/day
    - Male: 420 mg/day

Dosage Forms

Injection, solution, as hexahydrate: 200 mg/mL (50 mL)

Chloromag®: 200 mg/mL (50 mL)

Tablet, delayed release, enteric coated, oral:

Mag 64™ [OTC], Mag Delay® [OTC]: Elemental magnesium 64 mg

Tablet, enteric coated, oral:

Slow-Mag® [OTC]: Elemental magnesium 64 mg

Tablet, oral:

Mag SR: Elemental magnesium 64 mg

Mag SR with Calcium: Elemental magnesium 64 mg

magnesium citrate (mag NEE zhum SIT rate)

Synonyms citrate of magnesia

U.S./Canadian Brand Names Citro-Mag® [Can]; Citroma® [US-OTC]

Therapeutic Category Laxative

Use Evacuation of bowel prior to certain surgical and diagnostic procedures or overdose situations

Usual Dosage Oral: Cathartic:

Children:

<6 years: 0.5 mL/kg up to a maximum of 200 mL repeated every 4-6 hours until stools are clear

6-12 years: 100-150 mL

Children ≥12 years and Adults: 1/2 to 1 full bottle (120-300 mL)

Dosage Forms

Solution, oral: 290 mg/5 mL

Citroma® [OTC]: 290 mg/5 mL (300 mL)

Tablet: Elemental magnesium 100 mg

magnesium gluceptate *see* magnesium glucoheptonate *on page* 607

magnesium glucoheptonate (mag NEE zhum gloo koh HEP toh nate)

Synonyms magnesium gluceptate

U.S./Canadian Brand Names Magnelium® [Can]; Magnolex® [Can]; Magnorol® Sirop [Can]; ratio-Magnesium [Can]

Therapeutic Category Electrolyte Supplement, Parenteral; Magnesium Salt

Use Treatment and prevention of hypomagnesemia

Usual Dosage The recommended dietary allowance (RDA) of magnesium is 4.5 mg/kg which is a total daily allowance of 350-400 mg for adult men and 280-300 mg for adult women. During pregnancy the RDA is 300 mg and during lactation the RDA is 355 mg. Average daily intakes of dietary magnesium have declined in recent years due to processing of food.

Note: Serum magnesium is poor reflection of repletional status as the majority of magnesium is intracellular; serum levels may be transiently normal for a few hours after a dose is given, therefore, aim for consistently high normal serum levels in patients with normal renal function for most efficient repletion

Hypomagnesemia: Adults: Oral: 100-600 mg (5-30 mg elemental magnesium) 1-2 times/day with food.

Maintenance electrolyte requirements:

Daily requirements: 0.2-0.5 mEq/kg/24 hours or 3-10 mEq/1000 kcal/24 hours

Maximum: 8-16 mEq/24 hours

Dosage Forms [CAN] = Canadian brand name

Capsule: 20 mg, 300 mg [not available in the U.S.]

Magnelium® [CAN], Magnorol® [CAN]: 20 mg [not available in the U.S.]

Magnolex® [CAN]: 300 mg [not available in the U.S.]

Solution, oral: 100 mg/mL [not available in the U.S.]

ratio-Magnesium [CAN]: 100 mg/mL [not available in the U.S.]

Syrup: 90 mg/mL [not available in the U.S.]

Magnorol® Sirop [CAN]: 90 mg/mL [not available in the U.S.]

magnesium gluconate (mag NEE zhum GLOO koe nate)

U.S./Canadian Brand Names Mag G® [US-OTC]; Magonate® [US-OTC]; Magtrate® [US-OTC]

Therapeutic Category Electrolyte Supplement, Oral

Use Dietary supplement

Usual Dosage RDA (elemental magnesium):

Children:

1-3 years: 80 mg/day
4-8 years: 130 mg/day
9-13 years: 240 mg/day
14-18 years:
Female: 360 mg/day
Pregnant female: 400 mg/day
Male: 410 mg/day

Adults:

19-30 years:
Female: 310 mg/day
Pregnant female: 350 mg/day
Male: 400 mg/day
≥31 years:
Female: 320 mg/day
Pregnant female: 360 mg/day
Male: 420 mg/day

Dosage Forms

Liquid, oral:
Magonate® [OTC]: 1000 mg/5 mL

Tablet, oral: 500 mg, 550 mg
Mag G® [OTC], Magonate® [OTC], Magtrate® [OTC]: 500 mg

magnesium hydroxide (mag NEE zhum hye DROKS ide)

Synonyms magnesia magma; milk of magnesia; MOM

U.S./Canadian Brand Names Fleet® Pedia-Lax™ Chewable Tablet [US-OTC]; Little Phillips'® Milk of Magnesia [US-OTC]; Phillips'® Milk of Magnesia [US-OTC]

Therapeutic Category Antacid; Electrolyte Supplement, Oral; Laxative

Use Short-term treatment of occasional constipation and symptoms of hyperacidity, laxative; dietary supplement

Usual Dosage Oral:

Laxative:

Liquid:

Children: Magnesium hydroxide 400 mg/5 mL: 1-3 mL/kg/day; adjust dose to induce daily bowel movement

OTC labeling:

2-5 years: Magnesium hydroxide 400 mg/5 mL: 5-15 mL/day once daily at bedtime or in divided doses

6-11 years:
Magnesium hydroxide 400 mg/5 mL: 15-30 mL/day once daily at bedtime or in divided doses
Magnesium hydroxide 800 mg/5 mL: 7.5-15 mL/day once daily at bedtime or in divided doses

Children ≥12 years and Adults:
Magnesium hydroxide 400 mg/5 mL: 30-60 mL/day once daily at bedtime or in divided doses
Magnesium hydroxide 800 mg/5 mL: 15-30 mL/day once daily at bedtime or in divided doses

Tablet: OTC labeling:

Children:

3-5 years: Magnesium hydroxide 311 mg/tablet: 2 tablets/day once daily at bedtime or in divided doses

6-11 years: Magnesium hydroxide 311 mg/tablet: 4 tablets/day once daily at bedtime or in divided doses

Children ≥12 years and Adults: Magnesium hydroxide 311 mg/tablet: 8 tablets/day once daily at bedtime or in divided doses

Antacid: OTC labeling:

Liquid: Children ≥12 years and Adults: Magnesium hydroxide 400 mg/5 mL: 5-15 mL as needed up to 4 times/day

Tablet: Children ≥12 years and Adults: Magnesium hydroxide 311 mg/tablet: 2-4 tablets every 4 hours up to 4 times/day

Dietary supplement: OTC labeling (Phillips'® Chews): Children ≥12 years and Adults: Magnesium 500 mg: 2-4 tablets/day once daily at bedtime or in divided doses

Dosage Forms

Suspension, oral: 400 mg/5 mL

Milk of Magnesia [OTC], Phillips'® Milk of Magnesia [OTC]: 400 mg/5 mL

Suspension, oral [concentrate]: 2400 mg/10 mL

Little Phillips'® Milk of Magnesia [OTC], Milk of Magnesia [OTC], Phillips'® Milk of Magnesia [OTC]: 800 mg/5 mL

Tablet, chewable, oral:

Fleet® Pedia-Lax™ Chewable Tablet [OTC]: 400 mg

Phillips'® Milk of Magnesia [OTC]: 311 mg

magnesium hydroxide, aluminum hydroxide, and simethicone *see* aluminum hydroxide, magnesium hydroxide, and simethicone *on page 56*

magnesium hydroxide and aluminum hydroxide *see* aluminum hydroxide and magnesium hydroxide *on page 55*

magnesium hydroxide and calcium carbonate *see* calcium carbonate and magnesium hydroxide *on page 171*

magnesium hydroxide and mineral oil (mag NEE zhum hye DROKS ide & MIN er al oyl)

Synonyms Haley's M-O; MOM/mineral oil emulsion

U.S./Canadian Brand Names Phillips'® M-O [US-OTC]

Therapeutic Category Laxative

Use Short-term treatment of occasional constipation

Usual Dosage Oral: Laxative: OTC labeling:

Children 6-11 years: 20-30 mL at bedtime

Children ≥12 years and Adults: 45-60 mL at bedtime

Dosage Forms

Suspension, oral:

Phillips'® M-O [OTC]: Magnesium hydroxide 300 mg and mineral oil 1.25 mL per 5 mL

magnesium hydroxide, famotidine, and calcium carbonate *see* famotidine, calcium carbonate, and magnesium hydroxide *on page 406*

magnesium L-aspartate hydrochloride

(mag NEE zhum el as PAR tate hye droe KLOR ide)

Synonyms MAH

U.S./Canadian Brand Names Maginex™ DS [US-OTC]; Maginex™ [US-OTC]

Therapeutic Category Electrolyte Supplement, Oral

Use Dietary supplement

Usual Dosage

RDA (elemental magnesium):

Children:

1-3 years: 80 mg/day

4-8 years: 130 mg/day

9-13 years: 240 mg/day

14-18 years:

Female: 360 mg/day

Pregnant female: 400 mg/day

Male: 410 mg/day

Adults:

19-30 years:

Female: 310 mg/day

Pregnant female: 350 mg/day

Male: 400 mg/day

≥31 years:

Female: 320 mg/day

Pregnant female: 360 mg/day

Male: 420 mg/day

Dietary supplement: Adults: Oral: Magnesium-L-aspartate 1230 mg (magnesium 122 mg) up to 3 times/day

Dosage Forms

Granules, for solution, oral [preservative free]:
Maginex™ DS [OTC]: 1230 mg/packet (30s)
Tablet, enteric coated, oral [preservative free]:
Maginex™ [OTC]: 615 mg

magnesium oxide (mag NEE zhum OKS ide)

U.S./Canadian Brand Names Mag-Ox® 400 [US-OTC]; MagGel™ 600 [US-OTC]; MAGnesium-Oxide™ [US-OTC]; Phillips'® Laxative Dietary Supplement Cramp-Free [US-OTC]; Uro-Mag® [US-OTC]

Therapeutic Category Antacid; Electrolyte Supplement, Oral; Laxative

Use Electrolyte replacement

Usual Dosage

RDA (elemental magnesium):
Children:
- 1-3 years: 80 mg/day
- 4-8 years: 130 mg/day
- 9-13 years: 240 mg/day
- 14-18 years:
  - Female: 360 mg/day
  - Pregnant female: 400 mg/day
  - Male: 410 mg/day

Adults:
- 19-30 years:
  - Female: 310 mg/day
  - Pregnant female: 350 mg/day
  - Male: 400 mg/day
- ≥31 years:
  - Female: 320 mg/day
  - Pregnant female: 360 mg/day
  - Male: 420 mg/day

Dietary supplement: Adults: Oral:
Mag-Ox 400®: 2 tablets daily with food
Uro-Mag®: 4-5 capsules daily with food

Dosage Forms

Caplet, oral: Elemental magnesium 250 mg
Phillips'® Laxative Dietary Supplement Cramp-Free [OTC]: Elemental magnesium 500 mg
Capsule, oral:
Uro-Mag® [OTC]: 140 mg
Capsule, softgel, oral:
MagGel™ 600 [OTC]: 600 mg
Tablet, oral: 400 mg, elemental magnesium 250 mg, elemental magnesium 500 mg
Mag-Ox® 400 [OTC], MAGnesium-Oxide™ [OTC]: 400 mg

MAGnesium-Oxide™ [US-OTC] *see* magnesium oxide *on page 610*

magnesium salicylate (mag NEE zhum sa LIS i late)

U.S./Canadian Brand Names Doan's® Extra Strength [US-OTC]; Keygesic [US-OTC]; Momentum® [US-OTC]; MST 600 [US]

Therapeutic Category Nonsteroidal Antiinflammatory Drug (NSAID)

Use Mild-to-moderate pain, fever, various inflammatory conditions; relief of pain and inflammation of rheumatoid arthritis and osteoarthritis

Usual Dosage Oral: Children ≥12 years and Adults: Relief of mild-to-moderate pain:
Doan's® Extra Strength, Momentum®: Two caplets every 6 hours as needed (maximum: 8 caplets/24 hours)
Keygesic: One tablet every 4 hours as needed (maximum 4 tablets/24 hours)

Dosage Forms

Caplet, oral:
Doan's® Extra Strength [OTC]: 580 mg
Momentum® [OTC]: 580 mg
Tablet, oral, chelated:
Keygesic [OTC]: 650 mg

Tablet, oral:
MST 600: 600 mg

magnesium sulfate (mag NEE zhum SUL fate)

Sound-Alike/Look-Alike Issues
magnesium sulfate may be confused with manganese sulfate, morphine sulfate
$MgSO_4$ is an error-prone abbreviation (mistaken as morphine sulfate)

Synonyms epsom salts

Therapeutic Category Anticonvulsant; Electrolyte Supplement, Oral; Laxative

Use Treatment and prevention of hypomagnesemia; prevention and treatment of seizures in severe preeclampsia or eclampsia, pediatric acute nephritis; torsade de pointes; treatment of cardiac arrhythmias (VT/VF) caused by hypomagnesemia; soaking aid

Usual Dosage Dose represented as magnesium sulfate unless stated otherwise. **Note:** Serum magnesium is poor reflection of repletional status as the majority of magnesium is intracellular; serum levels may be transiently normal for a few hours after a dose is given, therefore, aim for consistently high normal serum levels in patients with normal renal function for most efficient repletion.

Note: 1 g of magnesium sulfate = 98.6 mg elemental magnesium = 8.12 mEq elemental magnesium
Hypomagnesemia: Note: Treatment depends on severity and clinical status:
Children: I.V., I.O.: 25-50 mg/kg/dose over 10-20 minutes (faster in cardiac arrest); maximum single dose: 2000 mg
Adults:
Mild deficiency: I.M.: 1 g every 6 hours for 4 doses, or as indicated by serum magnesium levels
Severe deficiency:
I.M.: Up to 250 mg/kg within a 4-hour period
I.V.: Severe, nonlife-threatening: 1-2 g/hour for 3-6 hours then 0.5-1 g/hour as needed to correct deficiency
Symptomatic deficiency: I.V.: 1-2 g over 5-60 minutes; maintenance infusion may be required to correct deficiency (0.5-1 g/hour).
Arrhythmia, hypomagnesemia-induced (life-threatening): 1-2 g over 5-20 minutes (torsades with cardiac arrest) or over 5-60 minutes (symptomatic arrhythmias without cardiac arrest)
Seizures, hypomagnesemia-induced: I.V.: 2 g over 10 minutes; calcium administration may also be appropriate as many patients are also hypocalcemic.
Eclampsia: Adults:
I.V.: 4-5 g infusion; followed by a 1-2 g/hour continous infusion; or may follow with I.M. doses of 4-5 g in each buttock every 4 hours. **Note:** Initial infusion may be given over 3-4 minutes if eclampsia is severe; maximum: 40 g/24 hours
ACOG Practice Bulletin 2002: 4-6 g over 15-20 minutes followed by 2 g/hour continuous infusion
Preeclampsia (severe): Adults: I.V. 4-5 g infusion; followed by a 1-2 g/hour continous infusion; or may follow with I.M. doses of 4-5 g in each buttock every 4 hours; maximum: 40 g/24 hour
Torsade de pointes: Adults: I.V.:
Pulseless: 1-2 g over 5-20 minutes
With pulse: 1-2 g over 5-60 minutes. **Note:** Slower administration preferable for stable patients.
Parenteral nutrition supplementation: I.V.:
Children:
<50 kg: 0.3-0.5 mEq elemental magnesium/kg/day
>50 kg: 10-30 mEq elemental magnesium/day
Adults: 8-24 mEq elemental magnesium/day
Soaking aid: Topical: Adults: Dissolve 2 cupfuls of powder per gallon of warm water
RDA:
Children:
1-3 years: 80 mg elemental magnesium/day
4-8 years: 130 mg elemental magnesium/day
9-13 years: 240 mg elemental magnesium/day
14-18 years:
Female: 360 mg elemental magnesium/day
Pregnant female: 400 mg elemental magnesium/day
Male: 410 mg elemental magnesium/day
Adults:
19-30 years:
Female: 310 mg elemental magnesium/day
Pregnant female: 350 mg elemental magnesium/day
Male: 400 mg elemental magnesium/day

≥31 years:
Female: 320 mg elemental magnesium/day
Pregnant female: 360 mg elemental magnesium/day
Male: 420 mg elemental magnesium/day

Dosage Forms

Infusion [premixed in D_5W]: 10 mg/mL (100 mL); 20 mg/mL (500 mL)
Infusion [premixed in water for injection]: 40 mg/mL (100 mL, 500 mL, 1000 mL); 80 mg/mL (50 mL)
Injection, solution: 500 mg/mL (2 mL, 10 mL, 20 mL, 50 mL)
Powder, oral/topical: Magnesium sulfate USP (227 g, 454 g, 480 g, 1810 g, 1920 g, 2720 g)

magnesium trisilicate and aluminum hydroxide *see* aluminum hydroxide and magnesium trisilicate *on page 56*

Magnevist® [US/Can] *see* gadopentetate dimeglumine *on page 452*
Magnolex® [Can] *see* magnesium glucoheptonate *on page 607*
Magnorol® Sirop [Can] *see* magnesium glucoheptonate *on page 607*
Magonate® [US-OTC] *see* magnesium gluconate *on page 607*
Magonate® Sport *(Discontinued)* *see* magnesium gluconate *on page 607*
Mag-Ox® 400 [US-OTC] *see* magnesium oxide *on page 610*
Magsal® *(Discontinued)* *see* magnesium salicylate *on page 610*
Mag-SR [US] *see* magnesium chloride *on page 606*
Mag-SR with Calcium [US] *see* magnesium chloride *on page 606*
Magtrate® [US-OTC] *see* magnesium gluconate *on page 607*
MAH *see* magnesium L-aspartate hydrochloride *on page 609*
Malarone® [US/Can] *see* atovaquone and proguanil *on page 109*
Malarone® Pediatric [Can] *see* atovaquone and proguanil *on page 109*

malathion (mal a THYE on)

U.S./Canadian Brand Names Ovide® [US]

Therapeutic Category Scabicides/Pediculicides

Use Treatment of head lice and their ova

Usual Dosage Sprinkle Ovide® lotion on dry hair and rub gently until the scalp is thoroughly moistened; pay special attention to the back of the head and neck. Allow to dry naturally - use no heat and leave uncovered. After 8-12 hours, the hair should be washed with a nonmedicated shampoo; rinse and use a fine-toothed comb to remove dead lice and eggs. If required, repeat with second application in 7-9 days. Further treatment is generally not necessary. Other family members should be evaluated to determine if infested and if so, receive treatment.

Dosage Forms

Lotion, topical: 0.5% (59 mL)
Ovide®: 0.5% (59 mL)

Mallisol® *(Discontinued)* *see* povidone-iodine *on page 807*

maltodextrin (mal toe DEK strin)

U.S./Canadian Brand Names Carrington® Oral Wound Rinse [US]; Multidex® [US-OTC]

Therapeutic Category Skin and Mucous Membrane Agent

Use Topical: Treatment of infected or noninfected wounds

Usual Dosage Adults:

Oral: Management of pain due to oral lesions: Carrington® Oral Wound Rinse: 1 tablespoonful, swish or gargle for ~1 minute, 4 times/day or more if needed

Topical: Wound dressing: Multidex®: After debridement and irrigation of wound, apply and cover with a nonadherent, nonocclusive dressing. May be applied to moist or dry, infected or noninfected wounds.

Dosage Forms

Gel, topical [preservative free]:
Multidex® [OTC]: (7 mL, 14 mL, 85 mL)
Powder, topical [preservative free]:
Multidex® [OTC]: 6 g, 12 g, 25 g, 45 g
Powder for suspension, oral:
Carrington® Oral Wound Rinse: 23 g

Solution, topical [spray, preservative free]:
Multidex® [OTC]: 45 mL

Mandelamine® [Can] *see* methenamine *on page 637*
Mandelamine® *(Discontinued)* *see* methenamine *on page 637*
mandrake *see* podophyllum resin *on page 795*
Manerix® [Can] *see* moclobemide *(Canada only) on page 663*
manganese *see* trace metals *on page 974*

mannitol (MAN i tole)

Sound-Alike/Look-Alike Issues
Osmitrol® may be confused with esmolol

Synonyms *D*-mannitol

U.S./Canadian Brand Names Osmitrol® [US/Can]; Resectisol® [US]

Therapeutic Category Diuretic, Osmotic

Use Reduction of increased intracranial pressure associated with cerebral edema; promotion of diuresis in the prevention and/or treatment of oliguria or anuria due to acute renal failure; reduction of increased intraocular pressure; promoting urinary excretion of toxic substances; genitourinary irrigant in transurethral prostatic resection or other transurethral surgical procedures

Usual Dosage
Children: I.V.:
Test dose (to assess adequate renal function): 200 mg/kg over 3-5 minutes to produce a urine flow of at least 1 mL/kg for 1-3 hours
Initial: 0.25-1 g/kg
Maintenance: 0.25-0.5 g/kg given every 4-6 hours
Adults:
I.V.:
Test dose (to assess adequate renal function): 12.5 g (200 mg/kg) over 3-5 minutes to produce a urine flow of at least 30-50 mL of urine per hour. If urine flow does not increase, a second test dose may be given. If test dose does not produce an acceptable urine output, then need to reassess management.
Initial: 0.5-1 g/kg
Maintenance: 0.25-0.5 g/kg every 4-6 hours; usual daily dose: 20-200 g/24 hours
Intracranial pressure: Cerebral edema: 0.25-1.5 g/kg/dose I.V. as a 15% to 20% solution over ≥30 minutes; maintain serum osmolality 310 to <320 mOsm/kg
Prevention of acute renal failure (oliguria): 50-100 g dose
Treatment of oliguria: 100 g dose
Preoperative for neurosurgery: 1.5-2 g/kg administered 1-1.5 hours prior to surgery
Reduction of intraocular pressure: 1.5-2 g/kg as a 15% to 20% solution; administer over 30 minutes
Topical: Transurethral irrigation: Use urogenital solution as required for irrigation

Dosage Forms
Injection, solution: 5% [50 mg/mL] (1000 mL); 10% [100 mg/mL] (500 mL, 1000 mL); 15% [150 mg/mL] (500 mL); 20% [200 mg/mL] (150 mL, 250 mL, 500 mL); 25% [250 mg/mL] (50 mL)
Osmitrol®: 5% [50 mg/mL] (1000 mL); 10% [100 mg/mL] (500 mL, 1000 mL); 15% [150 mg/mL] (500 mL); 20% [200 mg/mL] (250 mL, 500 mL)
Solution, urogenital: 5% [50 mg/mL] (2000 mL, 4000 mL)
Resectisol®: 5% [50 mg/mL] (2000 mL, 4000 mL)

mantoux *see* tuberculin tests *on page 993*
Maox® *(Discontinued)* *see* magnesium oxide *on page 610*
Mapap [US-OTC] *see* acetaminophen *on page 19*
Mapap Children's [US-OTC] *see* acetaminophen *on page 19*
Mapap Extra Strength [US-OTC] *see* acetaminophen *on page 19*
Mapap Infants [US-OTC] *see* acetaminophen *on page 19*
Mapap Jr. Strength [US-OTC] *see* acetaminophen *on page 19*
Mapap® Multi-Symptom Cold [US-OTC] *see* acetaminophen, dextromethorphan, and phenylephrine *on page 27*
Mapap PM [US-OTC] *see* acetaminophen and diphenhydramine *on page 21*
Mapap® Sinus Congestion and Pain Daytime [US-OTC] *see* acetaminophen and phenylephrine *on page 22*
Mapezine® [Can] *see* carbamazepine *on page 180*

maprotiline (ma PROE ti leen)

Sound-Alike/Look-Alike Issues
Ludiomil® may be confused with Lamictal®, lamotrigine, Lomotil®

Synonyms maprotiline hydrochloride

U.S./Canadian Brand Names Novo-Maprotiline [Can]

Therapeutic Category Antidepressant, Tetracyclic

Use Treatment of depression and anxiety associated with depression

Usual Dosage Oral: Adults: Depression/anxiety: 75 mg/day to start, increase by 25 mg every 2 weeks up to 150-225 mg/day; given in 3 divided doses or in a single daily dose

Dosage Forms
Tablet: 25 mg, 50 mg, 75 mg

maprotiline hydrochloride *see* maprotiline *on page 614*

maraviroc (mah RAV er rock)

Synonyms UK-427,857

U.S./Canadian Brand Names Celsentri™ [Can]; Selzentry™ [US]

Therapeutic Category Antiretroviral Agent, CCR5 Antagonist

Use Treatment of CCR5-tropic HIV-1 infection, in combination with other antiretroviral agents in treatment-experienced patients with evidence of viral replication and HIV-1 strains resistant to multiple antiretroviral therapy

Usual Dosage Oral: Adolescents ≥16 years and Adults: 300 mg twice daily

Dosage Forms
Tablet:
Selzentry™: 150 mg, 300 mg

Marcaine® [US/Can] *see* bupivacaine *on page 156*
Marcaine® Spinal [US] *see* bupivacaine *on page 156*
Marcaine® with Epinephrine [US] *see* bupivacaine and epinephrine *on page 157*
Margesic® H [US] *see* hydrocodone and acetaminophen *on page 501*
Marinol® [US/Can] *see* dronabinol *on page 339*
Mark 1™ *see* atropine and pralidoxime *on page 112*
Marmine® Injection *(Discontinued)* *see* dimenhydrinate *on page 312*
Marmine® Oral *(Discontinued)* *see* dimenhydrinate *on page 312*
Marplan® [US] *see* isocarboxazid *on page 548*
Marthritic® *(Discontinued)* *see* salsalate *on page 888*
Marvelon® [Can] *see* ethinyl estradiol and desogestrel *on page 383*
Matulane® [US/Can] *see* procarbazine *on page 820*
3M™ Avagard® *(Discontinued)* *see* chlorhexidine gluconate *on page 210*
Mavik® [US/Can] *see* trandolapril *on page 976*
Maxair™ Autohaler™ [US] *see* pirbuterol *on page 788*
Maxalt® [US/Can] *see* rizatriptan *on page 874*
Maxalt-MLT® [US] *see* rizatriptan *on page 874*
Maxalt RPD™ [Can] *see* rizatriptan *on page 874*
Maxaquin® *(Discontinued)*
Maxidex® [US/Can] *see* dexamethasone (ophthalmic) *on page 288*
Maxidone® [US] *see* hydrocodone and acetaminophen *on page 501*
Maxifed® [US] *see* guaifenesin and pseudoephedrine *on page 477*
Maxifed DM [US] *see* guaifenesin, pseudoephedrine, and dextromethorphan *on page 479*
Maxifed DMX [US] *see* guaifenesin, pseudoephedrine, and dextromethorphan *on page 479*
Maxifed-G® [US] *see* guaifenesin and pseudoephedrine *on page 477*
Maxiflor® *(Discontinued)* *see* diflorasone *on page 307*
Maximum D3® [US-OTC] *see* cholecalciferol *on page 224*
Maximum Strength Desenex® Antifungal Cream *(Discontinued)* *see* miconazole *on page 654*
Maximum Strength Dex-A-Diet® *(Discontinued)*
Maximum Strength Dexatrim® *(Discontinued)*

Maxiphen DM [US] *see* guaifenesin, dextromethorphan, and phenylephrine *on page 478*
Maxipime® [US/Can] *see* cefepime *on page 193*
Maxitrol® [US/Can] *see* neomycin, polymyxin B, and dexamethasone *on page 687*
Maxi-Tuss HC® [US] *see* phenylephrine, hydrocodone, and chlorpheniramine *on page 778*
Maxi-Tuss HCG *(Discontinued)*
Maxi-Tuss HCX [US] *see* phenylephrine, hydrocodone, and chlorpheniramine *on page 778*
Maxivate® [US] *see* betamethasone (topical) *on page 138*
Maxolon® *(Discontinued)* *see* metoclopramide *on page 649*
Maxzide® [US] *see* hydrochlorothiazide and triamterene *on page 500*
Maxzide®-25 [US] *see* hydrochlorothiazide and triamterene *on page 500*
may apple *see* podophyllum resin *on page 795*
3M™ Cavilon™ Skin Cleanser *(Discontinued)* *see* benzalkonium chloride *on page 129*
MCH *see* collagen hemostat *on page 255*

m-cresyl acetate (em-KREE sil AS e tate)

U.S./Canadian Brand Names Cresylate® [US]
Therapeutic Category Otic Agent, Antiinfective
Use Provides an acid medium; for external otitis infections caused by susceptible bacteria or fungus
Usual Dosage Otic: Instill 2-4 drops as required
Dosage Forms
Solution, otic:
Cresylate®: 25% (15 mL)

MCT *see* medium chain triglycerides *on page 620*
MCT Oil® [US-OTC/Can] *see* medium chain triglycerides *on page 620*
MCV *see* meningococcal polysaccharide (Groups A / C / Y and W-135) diphtheria toxoid conjugate vaccine *on page 624*
MCV4 *see* meningococcal polysaccharide (Groups A / C / Y and W-135) diphtheria toxoid conjugate vaccine *on page 624*
MD-76®R [US] *see* diatrizoate meglumine and diatrizoate sodium *on page 300*
MD-Gastroview® [US] *see* diatrizoate meglumine and diatrizoate sodium *on page 300*
MDL 73,147EF *see* dolasetron *on page 328*

measles, mumps, and rubella virus vaccine
(MEE zels, mumpz & roo BEL a VYE rus vak SEEN)

Sound-Alike/Look-Alike Issues
MMR (measles, mumps, and rubella virus vaccine) may be confused with MMRV (measles, mumps, rubella and varicella) vaccine
Synonyms MMR; mumps, measles, and rubella vaccines; rubella, measles, and mumps vaccines
U.S./Canadian Brand Names M-M-R® II [US/Can]; Priorix™ [Can]
Therapeutic Category Vaccine, Live Virus
Use Measles, mumps, and rubella prophylaxis
The Advisory Committee on Immunization Practices (ACIP) recommends routine vaccination for the following:
- All children (first dose given at 12-15 months of age)
- Adults born 1957 or later (without evidence of immunity or documentation of vaccination).
- Adults at higher risk for exposure to and transmission of measles mumps and rubella should receive special consideration for vaccination, unless an acceptable evidence of immunity exists. This includes international travelers, persons attending colleges and other post-high school education, persons working in healthcare facilities.

Usual Dosage SubQ:
Infants 6-11 months: *Measles outbreak:* If there is risk of exposure to measles, single-antigen measles vaccine should be administered. If single-antigen vaccine is not readily available, MMR is an acceptable alternative. Children should be revaccinated at ≥12 months with standard 2-dose series
Children ≥12 months: 0.5 mL
Primary immunization is recommended at 12-15 months of age and repeated at 4-6 years of age; the second dose is recommended prior to elementary school. If the second dose was not received, the

schedule should be completed by the 11- to 12-year old visit. For older children not previously vaccinated, at least 28 days should elapse between doses.

Mumps outbreak: During a mumps outbreak, children ages 1-4 years should consider a second dose of a live mumps virus vaccine; minimum interval between doses is 28 days

Measles outbreak: Revaccination with MMR is recommended for attendees and siblings of daycare facilities or schools if they cannot provide adequate documentation of 2 previous doses of a measles-containing vaccine after their first birthday or evidence of measles immunity.

Adults: 0.5 mL

Birth year in or after 1957 without evidence of immunity: 1 or 2 doses (0.5 mL/dose); minimum interval between doses is 28 days. Adults born in or after 1957 without documentation of vaccination on or after first birthday, without physician-diagnosed disease, or without laboratory evidence of immunity should be vaccinated (ideally) with 2 doses of vaccine separated by no less than 1 month. For those previously vaccinated with 1 dose of vaccine, revaccination is recommended for students entering colleges and other institutions of higher education, for healthcare workers at the time of employment, and for international travelers who visit endemic areas.

Persons vaccinated between 1963 and 1967 with a killed measles vaccine, followed by live vaccine within 3 months, or with a vaccine of unknown type should be revaccinated with live measles virus vaccine.

Women of childbearing potential, without documentation of rubella immunity, regardless of birth year, should also receive one dose of vaccine. Do not administer rubella to women who are or who may become pregnant within 1 month of receiving vaccine; administer following completion or termination of pregnancy

Mumps outbreak:

Healthcare workers born prior to 1957 without other evidence of immunity: Consider 2 doses of a live mumps virus vaccine; minimum interval between doses is 28 days

Low-risk adults: A second dose of a live mumps virus vaccine should be considered in adults who previously received 1 dose; minimum interval between doses is 28 days

Measles outbreak:

Students and personnel in affected schools and healthcare workers born prior to 1957 without evidence of measles immunity: One dose of MMR vaccine

Students and personnel in affected schools and healthcare workers born in or after 1957 without adequate documentation of 2 previous doses of a measles-containing vaccine after their first birthday or evidence of measles immunity: Two doses of MMR vaccine; minimum interval between doses is 28 days

Dosage Forms

Injection, powder for reconstitution [preservative free]:

M-M-R® II: Measles virus ≥1000 $TCID_{50}$, mumps virus ≥20,000 $TCID_{50}$, and rubella virus ≥1000 $TCID_{50}$

measles, mumps, rubella, and varicella virus vaccine

(MEE zels, mumpz, roo BEL a, & var i SEL a VYE rus vak SEEN)

Synonyms MMR-V; mumps, rubella, varicella, and measles vaccine; rubella, varicella, measles, and mumps vaccine; varicella, measles, mumps, and rubella vaccine

U.S./Canadian Brand Names ProQuad® [US]

Therapeutic Category Vaccine, Live Virus

Use To provide simultaneous active immunization against measles, mumps, rubella, and varicella

The Advisory Committee on Immunization Practices (ACIP) recommends routine vaccination against measles, mumps, rubella, and varicella in healthy children 12 months to 12 years of age. ACIP does not express a preference for use of MMRV vaccine over separate injections of equivalent component vaccines (ie, MMR vaccine and varicella vaccine).

Usual Dosage SubQ: Children 12 months to 12 years: One dose (0.5 mL)

Administer on or after the first birthday, as soon as child becomes eligible for vaccination. It may be used whenever all components of the vaccine are needed in children within this age group. (Refer to current CDC Recommended Immunization Schedule)

Dosage Forms

Injection, powder for reconstitution [preservative free]:

ProQuad®: Measles virus ≥3.00 $\log_{10}$ $TCID_{50}$, mumps virus ≥4.30 $\log_{10}$ $TCID_{50}$, rubella virus ≥3.00 $\log_{10}$ $TCID_{50}$, and varicella virus ≥3.99 $\log_{10}$ PFU

measles virus vaccine (live) (MEE zels VYE rus vak SEEN, live)

Sound-Alike/Look-Alike Issues

Attenuvax® may be confused with Meruvax®

Synonyms more attenuated enders strain; rubeola vaccine

U.S./Canadian Brand Names Attenuvax® [US]

Therapeutic Category Vaccine, Live Virus

Use Active immunization against measles (rubeola)

Note: Unless otherwise contraindicated, trivalent measles - mumps - rubella (MMR) is the vaccine of choice if recipients are likely to be susceptible to rubella and/or mumps as well as to measles.

The Advisory Committee on Immunization Practices (ACIP) recommends routine vaccination for the following:

- All children. For routine vaccination, the first dose given at 12-15 months of age
- Adults born 1957 or later (without evidence of immunity or documentation of vaccination)
- Adults at higher risk for exposure to and transmission of measles should receive special consideration for vaccination, unless an acceptable evidence of immunity exists. This includes international travelers, persons attending colleges and other post-high school education, persons working in healthcare facilities.

Usual Dosage Note: Trivalent measles - mumps - rubella (MMR) vaccine should be used unless contraindicated in adults and children ≥12 months of age.

Children ≥6 months:

SubQ: 0.5 mL in outer aspect of the upper arm. Primary vaccination recommended at 12-15 months of age and repeated at 4-6 years of age. For older children not previously vaccinated, at least 28 days should elapse between doses.

Children requiring vaccination with measles virus vaccine prior to 12 months of age (eg, during local outbreak, international travel to endemic area) should receive another dose between 12-15 months and again prior to elementary school. Vaccination with monovalent measles vaccine is preferred in children 6 to <12 months of age.

Measles outbreak: Revaccination with MMR is recommended for attendees and siblings of daycare facilities or schools if they cannot provide adequate documentation of 2 previous doses of a measles-containing vaccine after their first birthday or evidence of measles immunity.

Adults: SubQ: 0.5 mL.

Adults born in or after 1957 without documentation of live vaccine on or after first birthday, without physician-diagnosed measles, or without laboratory evidence of immunity should be vaccinated, ideally with 2 doses of vaccine separated by no less than 1 month. For those previously vaccinated with 1 dose of measles vaccine, revaccination is recommended for students entering colleges and other institutions of higher education, for healthcare workers at the time of employment, and for international travelers who visit endemic areas. Persons vaccinated between 1963 and 1967 with a killed measles vaccine, followed by live vaccine within 3 months, or with a vaccine of unknown type should be revaccinated with live measles virus vaccine.

Measles outbreak:

Students and personnel in affected schools and healthcare workers born before 1957 without evidence of measles immunity: Administer 1 dose of MMR vaccine

Students and personnel in affected schools and healthcare workers born in or after 1957 without adequate documentation of 2 previous doses of a measles-containing vaccine after their first birthday or evidence of measles immunity: Administer 2 doses of MMR vaccine; minimum interval between doses is 28 days

Dosage Forms

Injection, powder for reconstitution [preservative free]:

Attenuvax®: ≥1000 $TCID_{50}$

Measurin® ***(Discontinued)*** *see* aspirin *on page* 103

Mebaral® [US/Can] *see* mephobarbital *on page* 627

mebendazole (me BEN da zole)

U.S./Canadian Brand Names Vermox® [Can]

Therapeutic Category Anthelmintic

Use Treatment of pinworms (*Enterobius vermicularis*), whipworms (*Trichuris trichiura*), roundworms (*Ascaris lumbricoides*), and hookworms (*Ancylostoma duodenale*)

Usual Dosage Oral: Children ≥2 years and Adults:

Pinworms: 100 mg as a single dose; may need to repeat after 2 weeks; treatment should include family members in close contact with patient

Whipworms, roundworms, hookworms: One tablet twice daily, morning and evening on 3 consecutive days; if patient is not cured within 3-4 weeks, a second course of treatment may be administered

Capillariasis: 200 mg twice daily for 20 days

Dosage Forms
Tablet, chewable: 100 mg

mecamylamine (mek a MIL a meen)

Sound-Alike/Look-Alike Issues
mecamylamine may be confused with mesalamine

Synonyms mecamylamine hydrochloride

U.S./Canadian Brand Names Inversine® [US/Can]

Therapeutic Category Ganglionic Blocking Agent

Use Treatment of moderately severe to severe hypertension and in uncomplicated malignant hypertension

Usual Dosage Oral: Adults: 2.5 mg twice daily after meals for 2 days; increased by increments of 2.5 mg at intervals ≥2 days until desired blood pressure response is achieved; average daily dose: 25 mg (usually in 3 divided doses)

Note: Reduce dosage of other antihypertensives when combined with mecamylamine with exception of thiazide diuretics which may be maintained at usual dose while decreasing mecamylamine by 50%

Dosage Forms
Tablet:
Inversine®: 2.5 mg

mecamylamine hydrochloride *see* mecamylamine *on page* 618

mecasermin (mek a SER min)

Synonyms mecasermin (rDNA origin) ; mecasermin rinfabate; recombinant human insulin-like growth factor-1; rhIGF-1 (mecasermin [Increlex™]); rhIGF-1/rhIGFBP-3 (mecasermin rinfabate [Iplex™])

U.S./Canadian Brand Names Increlex™ [US]

Therapeutic Category Growth Hormone

Use Treatment of growth failure in children with severe primary insulin-like growth factor-1 deficiency (IGF-1 deficiency; primary IGFD), or with growth hormone (GH) gene deletions who have developed neutralizing antibodies to GH

Usual Dosage SubQ: Increlex™: Children ≥2 years: Primary IGFD: Initial: 0.04-0.08 mg/kg twice daily; if tolerated for 7 days, may increase by 0.04 mg/kg/dose (maximum dose: 0.12 mg/kg given twice daily). Must be administered within 20 minutes of a meal or snack; omit dose if patient is unable to eat. Reduce dose if hypoglycemia occurs despite adequate food intake.

Dosage Forms
Injection, solution:
Increlex™: 10 mg/mL (4 mL)

mecasermin (rDNA origin) *see* mecasermin *on page* 618

mecasermin rinfabate *see* mecasermin *on page* 618

mechlorethamine (me klor ETH a meen)

Synonyms chlorethazine; chlorethazine mustard; HN_2; mechlorethamine hydrochloride; mustine; nitrogen mustard; NSC-762

U.S./Canadian Brand Names Mustargen® [US/Can]

Therapeutic Category Antineoplastic Agent

Use Hodgkin disease; non-Hodgkin lymphoma; intracavitary injection for treatment of metastatic tumors; pleural and other malignant effusions; topical treatment of mycosis fungoides

Usual Dosage Refer to individual protocols.

Children and Adults: I.V.: 6 mg/m^2 on days 1 and 8 of a 28-day cycle (MOPP regimen)

Adults:

I.V.: 0.4 mg/kg **or** 12-16 mg/m^2 for one dose **or** divided into 0.1 mg/kg/day for 4 days, repeated at 4- to 6-week intervals

Intracavitary: 0.2-0.4 mg/kg (10-20 mg) as a single dose; may be repeated if fluid continues to accumulate.

Intrapericardially: 0.2-0.4 mg/kg as a single dose; may be repeated if fluid continues to accumulate.

Topical: 0.01% to 0.02% solution, lotion, or ointment

Dosage Forms
Injection, powder for reconstitution:
Mustargen®: 10 mg

mechlorethamine hydrochloride *see* mechlorethamine *on page* 618

meclizine (MEK li zeen)

Sound-Alike/Look-Alike Issues

Antivert® may be confused with Axert®

Synonyms meclizine hydrochloride; meclozine hydrochloride

U.S./Canadian Brand Names Antivert® [US]; Bonamine™ [Can]; Bonine® [US-OTC/Can]; Dramamine® Less Drowsy Formula [US-OTC]; Medi-Meclizine [US-OTC]; Trav-L-Tabs® [US-OTC]

Therapeutic Category Antihistamine

Use Prevention and treatment of symptoms of motion sickness; management of vertigo with diseases affecting the vestibular system

Usual Dosage Oral: Children >12 years and Adults:

Motion sickness: 12.5-25 mg 1 hour before travel, repeat dose every 12-24 hours if needed; doses up to 50 mg may be needed

Vertigo: 25-100 mg/day in divided doses

Dosage Forms

Caplet: 12.5 mg

Tablet: 12.5 mg, 25 mg

Antivert®: 12.5 mg, 25 mg, 50 mg

Dramamine® Less Drowsy Formula [OTC], Medi-Meclizine [OTC], Trav-L-Tabs® [OTC]: 25 mg

Tablet, chewable: 25 mg

Bonine® [OTC]: 25 mg

meclizine hydrochloride *see* meclizine *on page* 619

meclofenamate (me kloe fen AM ate)

Synonyms meclofenamate sodium

U.S./Canadian Brand Names Meclomen® [Can]

Therapeutic Category Analgesic, Nonnarcotic; Nonsteroidal Antiinflammatory Drug (NSAID)

Use Treatment of inflammatory disorders, arthritis, mild-to-moderate pain, dysmenorrhea

Usual Dosage Oral: Children >14 years and Adults:

Mild-to-moderate pain: 50 mg every 4-6 hours; increases to 100 mg may be required; maximum dose: 400 mg

Rheumatoid arthritis and osteoarthritis: 50 mg every 4-6 hours; increase, over weeks, to 200-400 mg/day in 3-4 divided doses; do not exceed 400 mg/day; maximal benefit for any dose may not be seen for 2-3 weeks

Dosage Forms

Capsule: 50 mg, 100 mg

meclofenamate sodium *see* meclofenamate *on page* 619

Meclomen® [Can] *see* meclofenamate *on page* 619

meclozine hydrochloride *see* meclizine *on page* 619

Med-Diltiazem [Can] *see* diltiazem *on page* 311

Medebar® Plus [US] *see* barium *on page* 122

Medent-DM [US] *see* guaifenesin, pseudoephedrine, and dextromethorphan *on page* 479

Medent LD [US] *see* guaifenesin and pseudoephedrine *on page* 477

medicinal carbon *see* charcoal *on page* 206

medicinal charcoal *see* charcoal *on page* 206

Medicone® Suppositories [US-OTC] *see* phenylephrine *on page* 774

Medidin® Liquid *(Discontinued)*

Medigesic® [US] *see* butalbital, acetaminophen, and caffeine *on page* 161

Medihaler-Iso® *(Discontinued)* *see* isoproterenol *on page* 549

Medi-Meclizine [US-OTC] *see* meclizine *on page* 619

Medipain 5® *(Discontinued)* *see* hydrocodone and acetaminophen *on page* 501

Medi-Phenyl [US-OTC] *see* phenylephrine *on page* 774

Medipren® *(Discontinued)* *see* ibuprofen *on page* 515

Mediproxen [US-OTC] *see* naproxen *on page* 681

Medi-Quick® Topical Ointment ***(Discontinued)*** *see* bacitracin, neomycin, and polymyxin B *on page 119*

Medispaz® ***(Discontinued)*** *see* hyoscyamine *on page 512*

Medi-Tuss® ***(Discontinued)*** *see* guaifenesin *on page 473*

medium chain triglycerides (mee DEE um chane trye GLIS er ides)

Synonyms MCT; triglycerides, medium chain

U.S./Canadian Brand Names MCT Oil® [US-OTC/Can]

Therapeutic Category Nutritional Supplement

Use Dietary supplement for those who cannot digest long chain fats; malabsorption associated with disorders such as pancreatic insufficiency, bile salt deficiency, short bowel syndrome, and bacterial overgrowth of the small bowel; induce ketosis as a prevention for seizures

Usual Dosage Oral:

Infants: Nutritional supplement: Initial: 0.5 mL every other feeding, then advance to every feeding, then increase in increments of 0.25-0.5 mL/feeding at intervals of 2-3 days as tolerated

Children: Seizures: About 40 mL with each meal or 50% to 70% (800-1120 kcal) of total calories (1600 kcal) as the oil will induce ketosis necessary for seizure control

Children and Adults: Cystic fibrosis: 3 tablespoons/day in divided doses

Adults: Malabsorption syndromes: 15 mL 3-4 times/day

Dosage Forms

Oil:

MCT Oil® [OTC]: 14 g/15 mL

MED-Metformin [Can] *see* metformin *on page 633*

Medralone® Injection ***(Discontinued)*** *see* methylprednisolone *on page 647*

Medrol® [US/Can] *see* methylprednisolone *on page 647*

medrol dose pack *see* methylprednisolone *on page 647*

medroxyprogesterone (me DROKS ee proe JES te rone)

Sound-Alike/Look-Alike Issues

medroxyPROGESTERone may be confused with hydroxyprogesterone, methylPREDNISolone, methylTESTOSTERone

Depo-Provera® may be confused with depo-subQ provera 104™

depo-subQ provera 104™ may be confused with Depo-Provera®

Provera® may be confused with Covera®, Femara®, Parlodel®, Premarin®, Proscar®, Prozac®

Synonyms acetoxymethylprogesterone; medroxyprogesterone acetate; methylacetoxyprogesterone

Tall-Man medroxy**PROGESTER**one

U.S./Canadian Brand Names Alti-MPA [Can]; Apo-Medroxy® [Can]; Depo-Prevera® [Can]; Depo-Provera® Contraceptive [US]; Depo-Provera® [US/Can]; depo-subQ provera 104™ [US]; Gen-Medroxy [Can]; Novo-Medrone [Can]; Provera-Pak [Can]; Provera® [US/Can]

Therapeutic Category Contraceptive, Progestin Only; Progestin

Use Endometrial carcinoma or renal carcinoma; secondary amenorrhea or abnormal uterine bleeding due to hormonal imbalance; reduction of endometrial hyperplasia in nonhysterectomized postmenopausal women receiving conjugated estrogens; prevention of pregnancy; management of endometriosis-associated pain

Usual Dosage

Adolescents and Adults:

Amenorrhea: Oral: 5-10 mg/day for 5-10 days

Abnormal uterine bleeding: Oral: 5-10 mg for 5-10 days starting on day 16 or 21 of cycle

Contraception:

Depo-Provera® Contraceptive: I.M.: 150 mg every 3 months

depo-subQ provera 104™: SubQ: 104 mg every 3 months (every 12-14 weeks)

Endometriosis: depo-subQ provera 104™: SubQ: 104 mg every 3 months (every 12-14 weeks)

Adults:

Endometrial or renal carcinoma (Depo-Provera®): I.M.: 400-1000 mg/week

Accompanying cyclic estrogen therapy, postmenopausal: Oral: 5-10 mg for 12-14 consecutive days each month, starting on day 1 or day 16 of the cycle; lower doses may be used if given with estrogen continuously throughout the cycle

Dosage Forms

Injection, suspension: 150 mg/mL (1 mL)

Depo-Provera®: 400 mg/mL (2.5 mL)

Depo-Provera® Contraceptive: 150 mg/mL (1 mL)

depo-subQ provera 104™: 104 mg/0.65 mL (0.65 mL)

Tablet: 2.5 mg, 5 mg, 10 mg

Provera®: 2.5 mg, 5 mg, 10 mg

medroxyprogesterone acetate *see* medroxyprogesterone *on page 620*

medroxyprogesterone and estrogens (conjugated) *see* estrogens (conjugated/equine) and medroxyprogesterone *on page 379*

medrysone *(Discontinued)*

MED-Sotalol [Can] *see* sotalol *on page 919*

Med-Verapamil [Can] *see* verapamil *on page 1010*

Mefenamic-250 [Can] *see* mefenamic acid *on page 621*

mefenamic acid (me fe NAM ik AS id)

Sound-Alike/Look-Alike Issues

Ponstel® may be confused with Pronestyl®

U.S./Canadian Brand Names Apo-Mefenamic® [Can]; Dom-Mefenamic Acid [Can]; Mefenamic-250 [Can]; Nu-Mefenamic [Can]; PMS-Mefenamic Acid [Can]; Ponstan® [Can]; Ponstel® [US]

Therapeutic Category Analgesic, Nonnarcotic; Nonsteroidal Antiinflammatory Drug (NSAID)

Use Short-term relief of mild-to-moderate pain including primary dysmenorrhea

Usual Dosage Oral: Children >14 years and Adults: 500 mg to start then 250 mg every 4 hours as needed; maximum therapy: 1 week

Dosage Forms

Capsule:

Ponstel®: 250 mg

mefloquine (ME floe kwin)

Synonyms mefloquine hydrochloride

U.S./Canadian Brand Names Apo-Mefloquine® [Can]; Lariam® [Can]

Therapeutic Category Antimalarial Agent

Use Treatment of mild-to-moderate acute malarial infections (including treatment of chloroquine-resistant malaria) and prevention of malaria caused by *Plasmodium falciparum* or *P. vivax*

Usual Dosage Oral (dose expressed as mg of mefloquine hydrochloride):

Children ≥6 months and >5 kg:

Malaria treatment: 20-25 mg/kg in 2 divided doses, taken 6-8 hours apart (maximum: 1250 mg). If clinical improvement is not seen within 48-72 hours, an alternative therapy should be used for retreatment.

Malaria prophylaxis: 5 mg/kg/once weekly (maximum dose: 250 mg) starting 1 week before arrival in endemic area, continuing weekly during travel and for 4 weeks after leaving endemic area.

Adults:

Malaria treatment (mild-to-moderate infection): 5 tablets (1250 mg) as a single dose. If clinical improvement is not seen within 48-72 hours, an alternative therapy should be used for retreatment.

Malaria prophylaxis: 1 tablet (250 mg) weekly starting 1 week before arrival in endemic area, continuing weekly during travel and for 4 weeks after leaving endemic area

Dosage Forms

Tablet: 250 mg

mefloquine hydrochloride *see* mefloquine *on page 621*

Megace® [US/Can] *see* megestrol *on page 621*

Megace® ES [US] *see* megestrol *on page 621*

Megace® OS [Can] *see* megestrol *on page 621*

Megadophilus® [US-OTC] *see* Lactobacillus *on page 564*

megestrol (me JES trole)

Sound-Alike/Look-Alike Issues

megestrol may be confused with mesalamine

Megace® may be confused with Reglan®

Synonyms 5071-1DL(6); megestrol acetate; NSC-71423

U.S./Canadian Brand Names Apo-Megestrol® [Can]; Megace® ES [US]; Megace® OS [Can]; Megace® [US/Can]; Nu-Megestrol [Can]

Therapeutic Category Antineoplastic Agent; Progestin

Use Palliative treatment of breast and endometrial carcinoma; treatment of anorexia, cachexia, or unexplained significant weight loss in patients with AIDS

Usual Dosage Oral: Adults: **Note:** Megace® ES suspension is not equivalent to other formulations on a mg-per-mg basis:

Tablet: Female (refer to individual protocols):

Breast carcinoma: 40 mg 4 times/day

Endometrial carcinoma: 40-320 mg/day in divided doses; use for 2 months to determine efficacy; maximum doses used have been up to 800 mg/day

Suspension: Male/Female: HIV-related cachexia:

Megace®: Initial dose: 800 mg/day; daily doses of 400 and 800 mg/day were found to be clinically effective

Megace® ES: 625 mg/day

Dosage Forms

Suspension, oral: 40 mg/mL

Megace®: 40 mg/mL

Megace® ES: 125 mg/mL

Tablet: 20 mg, 40 mg

megestrol acetate *see* megestrol *on page 621*

Melanex® [US] *see* hydroquinone *on page 508*

Melfiat® ***(Discontinued)*** *see* phendimetrazine *on page 770*

Mellaril® [Can] *see* thioridazine *on page 955*

Mellaril® (all products) ***(Discontinued)*** *see* thioridazine *on page 955*

Mellaril-S® ***(Discontinued)*** *see* thioridazine *on page 955*

meloxicam (mel OKS i kam)

U.S./Canadian Brand Names Apo-Meloxicam® [Can]; CO Meloxicam [Can]; Gen-Meloxicam [Can]; Mobicox® [Can]; Mobic® [US/Can]; Novo-Meloxicam [Can]; PMS-Meloxicam [Can]

Therapeutic Category Nonsteroidal Antiinflammatory Drug (NSAID)

Use Relief of signs and symptoms of osteoarthritis, rheumatoid arthritis, and juvenile rheumatoid arthritis (JRA)

Usual Dosage Oral:

Children ≥2 years: JRA: 0.125 mg/kg/day; maximum dose: 7.5 mg/day

Adults: Osteoarthritis, rheumatoid arthritis: Initial: 7.5 mg once daily; some patients may receive additional benefit from an increased dose of 15 mg once daily; maximum dose: 15 mg/day

Dosage Forms

Suspension:

Mobic®: 7.5 mg/5 mL

Tablet: 7.5 mg, 15 mg

Mobic®: 7.5 mg, 15 mg

Melpaque HP® [US] *see* hydroquinone *on page 508*

melphalan (MEL fa lan)

Sound-Alike/Look-Alike Issues

melphalan may be confused with Mephyton®, Myleran®

Alkeran® may be confused with Alferon®, Leukeran®, Myleran®

Synonyms L-PAM; L-sarcolysin; NSC-8806; phenylalanine mustard

U.S./Canadian Brand Names Alkeran® [US/Can]

Therapeutic Category Antineoplastic Agent

Use Palliative treatment of multiple myeloma and nonresectable epithelial ovarian carcinoma

Usual Dosage Refer to individual protocols.

Oral: Dose should always be adjusted to patient response and weekly blood counts: Adults:

Multiple myeloma (multiple regimens have been employed): **Note:** Response is gradual; may require repeated courses to realize benefit:

6 mg daily for 2-3 weeks initially, followed by up to 4 weeks rest, then a maintenance dose of 2 mg daily as hematologic recovery begins **or**

10 mg daily for 7-10 days; institute 2 mg daily maintenance dose after WBC >4000 cells/mm^3 and platelets >100,000 cells/mm^3 (~4-8 weeks); titrate maintenance dose to hematologic response **or**

0.15 mg/kg/day for 7 days, with a 2-6 week rest, followed by a maintenance dose of ≤0.05 mg/kg/day as hematologic recovery begins **or**

0.25 mg/kg/day for 4 days (or 0.2 mg/kg/day for 5 days); repeat at 4- to 6-week intervals as ANC and platelet counts return to normal

Ovarian carcinoma: 0.2 mg/kg/day for 5 days, repeat every 4-5 weeks.

I.V.: Adults: Multiple myeloma: 16 mg/m^2 administered at 2-week intervals for 4 doses, then administer at 4-week intervals after adequate hematologic recovery.

Dosage Forms

Injection, powder for reconstitution:

Alkeran®: 50 mg

Tablet:

Alkeran®: 2 mg

Melquin-3® [US] *see* hydroquinone *on page 508*

Melquin HP® [US] *see* hydroquinone *on page 508*

memantine (me MAN teen)

Sound-Alike/Look-Alike Issues

memantine may be confused with mesalamine

Synonyms memantine hydrochloride

U.S./Canadian Brand Names Ebixa® [Can]; Namenda™ [US]

Therapeutic Category N-Methyl-D-Aspartate Receptor Antagonist

Use Treatment of moderate-to-severe dementia of the Alzheimer type

Usual Dosage Oral: Adults:

Alzheimer disease: Initial: 5 mg/day; increase dose by 5 mg/day to a target dose of 20 mg/day; wait at least 1 week between dosage changes. Doses >5 mg/day should be given in 2 divided doses.

Suggested titration: 5 mg/day for ≥1 week; 5 mg twice daily for ≥1 week; 15 mg/day given in 5 mg and 10 mg separated doses for ≥1 week; then 10 mg twice daily

Dosage Forms

Solution, oral:

Namenda™: 2 mg/mL

Tablet:

Namenda™: 5 mg, 10 mg

Combination package [titration pack contains two separate tablet formulations]:

Namenda™: Memantine 5 mg (28s), 10 mg (21s)

memantine hydrochloride *see* memantine *on page 623*

Menactra® [US] *see* meningococcal polysaccharide (Groups A / C / Y and W-135) diphtheria toxoid conjugate vaccine *on page 624*

Menadol® ***(Discontinued)*** *see* ibuprofen *on page 515*

menCC *see* meningococcal group C-CRM197 conjugate vaccine *(Canada only) on page 623*

menC-CRM197 *see* meningococcal group C-CRM197 conjugate vaccine *(Canada only) on page 623*

Menest® [US/Can] *see* estrogens (esterified) *on page 380*

Meni-D® ***(Discontinued)*** *see* meclizine *on page 619*

meningococcal conjugate vaccine *see* meningococcal polysaccharide (Groups A / C / Y and W-135) diphtheria toxoid conjugate vaccine *on page 624*

meningococcal group C-CRM197 conjugate vaccine *(Canada only)*

(me NIN joe kok al groop see see ahr em wuhn nahyn tee sev uhn KON joo gate vak SEEN)

Synonyms menC-CRM197; menCC

U.S./Canadian Brand Names Menjugate® [Can]

Therapeutic Category Vaccine

Use To provide active immunization against invasive meningococcal disease caused by *N. meningitidis* serogroup C, in children ≥2 months and adults

The National Advisory Committee on Immunization (NACI) recommendations for persons considered at an increased risk for meningococcal disease:

Chemoprophylaxis and immunoprophylaxis: Selection of meningococcal vaccination to be based upon serogroup(s):

Individuals living in the same household or with close contact (eg, kissing, shared cigarettes, shared eating or drinking utensils) of infected patient

Employees and children of nursery schools or day care

Immunoprophylaxis: Selection of meningococcal vaccination to be based upon serogroup(s):

Adolescents and young adults

Laboratory workers routinely exposed to isolates of *N. meningitidis*

Military recruits

Persons traveling to or who reside in countries where *N. meningitidis* is hyperendemic or epidemic, particularly if contact with local population will be prolonged

Persons with terminal complement component deficiencies

Persons with anatomic or functional asplenia

Note: Use is also recommended during meningococcal outbreaks caused by serogroup C.

Chemoprophylaxis:

Healthcare workers with intensive unprotected contact with infected patients

Airline passengers sitting directly next to an infected patient for duration of at least 8 hours

See NACI guidelines for specific drug treatment at http://www.phac-aspc.gc.ca/naci-ccni

Usual Dosage I.M.:

Infants:

≥2-12 months: 0.5 mL as a single dose for a total of 3 doses administered at least 4 weeks apart

≥4-11 months without prior vaccination: 0.5 mL as a single dose for a total of 2 doses administered at least 4 weeks apart

Note: The NACI recommends at least 1 of the 3 sequential doses for infants ≥2-12 months be administered beyond 5 months of age.

Children ≥1 year and Adults: 0.5 mL as a single dose

Dosage Forms [CAN = Canadian brand name]

Injection, powder for reconstitution:

Menjugate® [CAN]: 10 mcg of oligosaccharide antigen group C [not available in U.S.]

meningococcal polysaccharide (Groups A / C / Y and W-135) diphtheria toxoid conjugate vaccine

(me NIN joe kok al pol i SAK a ride groops aye, see, why & dubl yoo won thur tee fyve dif THEER ee a TOKS oyds KON joo gate vak SEEN)

Synonyms MCV; MCV4; meningococcal conjugate vaccine

U.S./Canadian Brand Names Menactra® [US]

Therapeutic Category Vaccine

Use Provide active immunization of children and adults (2-55 years of age) against invasive meningococcal disease caused by *N. meningitidis* serogroups A, C, Y, and W-135

The Advisory Committee on Immunization Practices (ACIP) recommends routine vaccination of all persons 11-18 years of age at the earliest opportunity. Adolescents should be vaccinated at the 11-12 year visit. For adolescents not previously vaccinated, vaccine should be administered prior to high school entry (~15 years of age).

The ACIP also recommends vaccination for persons at increased risk for meningococcal disease. (Meningococcal conjugate vaccine [MCV] is preferred for persons aged 2-55 years; meningococcal polysaccharide vaccine [MPSV] may be used if MCV is not available). Persons at increased risk include:

College freshmen living in dormitories

Microbiologists routinely exposed to isolates of *N. meningitides*

Military recruits

Persons traveling to or who reside in countries where *N. meningitides* is hyperendemic or epidemic, particularly if contact with local population will be prolonged

Persons with terminal complement component deficiencies

Persons with anatomic or functional asplenia

Use is also recommended during meningococcal outbreaks caused by vaccine preventable serogroups.

Usual Dosage I.M.: Children ≥2 years and Adults ≤55 years: 0.5 mL

Note: Revaccination: May be indicated in patients previously vaccinated with MPSV who remain at increased risk for infection. The ACIP recommends the use of MCV for revaccination; however, use of MPSV is also acceptable. The need for revaccination in patients previously vaccinated with MCV is currently under study. Children 2-10 years who received MPSV ≥3 years previously, or older children and adults who received MPSV ≥5 years previously, and who are still at increased risk for meningococcal disease should be revaccinated with MCV.

Dosage Forms

Injection, solution [MCV; preservative free]:

Menactra®: 4 mcg each of polysaccharide antigen groups A, C, Y, and W-135 [bound to diphtheria toxoid 48 mcg] per 0.5 mL

meningococcal polysaccharide vaccine *see* meningococcal polysaccharide vaccine (groups A / C / Y and W-135) *on page 625*

meningococcal polysaccharide vaccine (groups A / C / Y and W-135)

(me NIN joe kok al pol i SAK a ride vak SEEN groops aye, see, why & dubl yoo won thur tee fyve)

Synonyms meningococcal polysaccharide vaccine; MPSV; MPSV4

U.S./Canadian Brand Names Menomune®-A/C/Y/W-135 [US]

Therapeutic Category Vaccine, Live Bacteria

Use Provide active immunity to meningococcal serogroups contained in the vaccine

The Advisory Committee on Immunization Practices (ACIP) recommends routine vaccination for persons at increased risk for meningococcal disease. (Meningococcal conjugate vaccine [MCV] is preferred for persons aged 2-55 years; meningococcal polysaccharide vaccine [MPSV] may be used if MCV is not available.) Persons at increased risk include:

College freshmen living in dormitories

Microbiologists routinely exposed to isolates of *N. meningitides*

Military recruits

Persons traveling to or who reside in countries where *N. meningitides* is hyperendemic or epidemic, particularly if contact with local population will be prolonged

Persons with terminal complement component deficiencies

Persons with anatomic or functional asplenia

Use is also recommended during meningococcal outbreaks caused by vaccine preventable serogroups.

Usual Dosage SubQ:

Children <2 years: Not usually recommended. Two doses (0.5 mL/dose), 3 months apart, may be considered in children 3-18 months to elicit short-term protection against serogroup A disease. A single dose may be considered in children 19-23 months. (ACIP recommendations)

Children ≥2 years and Adults: 0.5 mL

Note: Revaccination: May be indicated in patients previously vaccinated with MPSV who remain at increased risk for infection. The ACIP recommends the use of MCV for revaccination; however, use of MPSV is also acceptable. Children 2-10 years who received MPSV ≥3 years previously, or older children and adults who received MPSV ≥5 years previously, and who are still at increased risk for meningococcal disease should be revaccinated with MCV.

Dosage Forms

Injection, powder for reconstitution [MPSV]:

Menomune®-A/C/Y/W-135: 50 mcg each of polysaccharide antigen groups A, C, Y, and W-135 per 0.5 mL dose

Menjugate® [Can] *see* meningococcal group C-CRM197 conjugate vaccine *(Canada only)* *on page 623*

Menomune®-A/C/Y/W-135 [US] *see* meningococcal polysaccharide vaccine (groups A / C / Y and W-135) *on page 625*

Menopur® [US/Can] *see* menotropins *on page 625*

Menostar® [US/Can] *see* estradiol *on page 373*

menotropins (men oh TROE pins)

Sound-Alike/Look-Alike Issues

Repronex® may be confused with Regranex®

Synonyms hMG; human menopausal gonadotropin

U.S./Canadian Brand Names Menopur® [US/Can]; Repronex® [US/Can]

Therapeutic Category Gonadotropin

Use Female:

In conjunction with hCG to induce ovulation and pregnancy in infertile females experiencing oligoanovulation or anovulation when the cause of anovulation is functional and not caused by primary ovarian failure (Repronex®)

Stimulation of multiple follicle development in ovulatory patients as part of an assisted reproductive technology (ART) (Menopur®, Repronex®)

Usual Dosage Adults:

Repronex®: I.M., SubQ:

Induction of ovulation in patients with oligoanovulation (Female): Initial: 150 int. units daily for the first 5 days of treatment. Adjustments should not be made more frequently than once every 2 days and should not exceed 75-150 int. units per adjustment. Maximum daily dose should not exceed 450 int. units and dosing beyond 12 days is not recommended. If patient's response is appropriate, hCG 5000-10,000 units should be given one day following the last dose of Repronex®. Hold dose if serum estradiol is >2000 pg/mL, if the ovaries are abnormally enlarged, or if abdominal pain occurs; the patient should also be advised to refrain from intercourse. May repeat process if follicular development is inadequate or if pregnancy does not occur.

Assisted reproductive technologies (Female): Initial (in patients who have received GnRH agonist or antagonist pituitary suppression): 225 int. units; adjustments in dose should not be made more frequently than once every 2 days and should not exceed more than 75-150 int. units per adjustment. The maximum daily doses of Repronex® given should not exceed 450 int. units and dosing beyond 12 days is not recommended. Once adequate follicular development is evident, hCG (5000-10,000 units) should be administered to induce final follicular maturation in preparation for oocyte retrieval. Withhold treatment when ovaries are abnormally enlarged on last day of therapy (to reduce chance of developing OHSS).

Menopur®: SubQ: *Assisted reproductive technologies (ART):* Initial (in patients who have received GnRH agonist for pituitary suppression): 225 int. units; adjustments in dose should not be made more frequently than once every 2 days and should not exceed more than 150 int. units per adjustment. The maximum daily dose given should not exceed 450 int. units and dosing beyond 20 days is not recommended. Once adequate follicular development is evident, hCG should be administered to induce final follicular maturation in preparation for oocyte retrieval. Withhold treatment when ovaries are abnormally enlarged on last day of therapy (to reduce chance of developing OHSS).

Dosage Forms

Injection, powder for reconstitution:

Menopur®, Repronex®: Follicle stimulating hormone activity 75 int. units and luteinizing hormone activity 75 int. units

Mentax® [US] *see* butenafine *on page* 163

292 MEP® [Can] *see* meprobamate and aspirin *on page* 629

mepenzolate (me PEN zoe late)

Sound-Alike/Look-Alike Issues

Cantil® may be confused with Bentyl®

Synonyms mepenzolate bromide

U.S./Canadian Brand Names Cantil® [US/Can]

Therapeutic Category Anticholinergic Agent

Use Adjunctive treatment of peptic ulcer disease

Usual Dosage Oral: Adults: 25-50 mg 4 times/day with meals and at bedtime

Dosage Forms

Tablet:

Cantil®: 25 mg [contains tartrazine]

mepenzolate bromide *see* mepenzolate *on page* 626

mepergan *see* meperidine and promethazine *on page* 627

meperidine (me PER i deen)

Sound-Alike/Look-Alike Issues

meperidine may be confused with meprobamate

Demerol® may be confused with Demulen®, Desyrel®, dicumarol, Dilaudid®, Dymelor®, Pamelor®

Synonyms isonipecaine hydrochloride; meperidine hydrochloride; pethidine hydrochloride

U.S./Canadian Brand Names Demerol® [US/Can]

Therapeutic Category Analgesic, Narcotic

Controlled Substance C-II

Use Management of moderate-to-severe pain; adjunct to anesthesia and preoperative sedation

Usual Dosage **Note:** The American Pain Society (2003) and ISMP (2007) do not recommend meperidine's use as an analgesic.

Children: Pain: Oral, I.M., I.V., SubQ: 1-1.5 mg/kg/dose every 3-4 hours as needed; 1-2 mg/kg as a single dose preoperative medication may be used; maximum 100 mg/dose (**Note:** Oral route is not recommended for acute pain.)

Adults: Pain:

Oral: Initial: Opiate-naive: 50 mg every 3-4 hours as needed; usual dosage range: 50-150 mg every 2-4 hours as needed (manufacturers recommendation; oral route is not recommended for acute pain)

I.M., SubQ: Initial: Opiate-naive: 50-75 mg every 3-4 hours as needed; patients with prior opiate exposure may require higher initial doses

Slow I.V.: Initial: 5-10 mg every 5 minutes as needed

Preoperatively: 50-100 mg given 30-90 minutes before the beginning of anesthesia

Note: If use in acute pain (in patients without renal or CNS disease) cannot be avoided, treatment should be limited to ≤48 hours and doses should not exceed 600 mg/24 hours.

Dosage Forms

Injection, solution [ampul]: 25 mg/0.5 mL (0.5 mL); 25 mg/mL (1 mL); 50 mg/mL (1 mL, 1.5 mL, 2 mL); 75 mg/mL (1 mL); 100 mg/mL (1 mL)

Injection, solution [prefilled syringe]: 25 mg/mL (1 mL); 50 mg/mL (1 mL); 75 mg/mL (1 mL); 100 mg/mL (1 mL)

Injection, solution [for PCA pump]: 10 mg/mL (30 mL, 60 mL)

Injection, solution [vial]: 25 mg/mL (1 mL); 50 mg/mL (1 mL, 30 mL); 75 mg/mL (1 mL); 100 mg/mL (1 mL, 20 mL)

Solution, oral: 50 mg/5 mL (500 mL)

Tablet: 50 mg, 100 mg

Demerol®: 50 mg, 100 mg

meperidine and promethazine (me PER i deen & proe METH a zeen)

Sound-Alike/Look-Alike Issues

mepergan may be confused with meprobamate

Synonyms mepergan; promethazine and meperidine

Therapeutic Category Analgesic, Narcotic

Controlled Substance C-II

Use Management of moderate pain

Usual Dosage Oral: Adults: One capsule every 4-6 hours as needed

Dosage Forms

Capsule: Meperidine hydrochloride 50 mg and promethazine hydrochloride 25 mg

meperidine hydrochloride *see* meperidine *on page* 626

mephobarbital (me foe BAR bi tal)

Sound-Alike/Look-Alike Issues

mephobarbital may be confused with methocarbamol

Mebaral® may be confused with Medrol®, Mellaril®, Tegretol®

Synonyms methylphenobarbital

U.S./Canadian Brand Names Mebaral® [US/Can]

Therapeutic Category Barbiturate

Controlled Substance C-IV

Use Sedative; treatment of grand mal and petit mal epilepsy

Usual Dosage Oral:

Epilepsy:

Children: 6-12 mg/kg/day in 2-4 divided doses

Adults: 200-600 mg/day in 2-4 divided doses

Sedation:

Children:

<5 years: 16-32 mg 3-4 times/day

>5 years: 32-64 mg 3-4 times/day

Adults: 32-100 mg 3-4 times/day

Dosage Forms

Tablet:

Mebaral®: 32 mg, 50 mg, 100 mg

Mephyton® [US/Can] *see* phytonadione *on page* 782

mepivacaine (me PIV a kane)

Sound-Alike/Look-Alike Issues

mepivacaine may be confused with bupivacaine

Polocaine® may be confused with prilocaine

Synonyms mepivacaine hydrochloride

U.S./Canadian Brand Names Carbocaine® [US/Can]; Polocaine® Dental [US]; Polocaine® MPF [US]; Polocaine® [US/Can]; Scandonest® 3% Plain [US]

Therapeutic Category Local Anesthetic

Use Local or regional analgesia; anesthesia by local infiltration, peripheral and central neural techniques (epidural and caudal); **not** for use in spinal anesthesia

Usual Dosage

Injectable local anesthetic: Dose varies with procedure, degree of anesthesia needed, vascularity of tissue, duration of anesthesia required, and physical condition of patient. The smallest dose and concentration required to produce the desired effect should be used.

Children: Maximum dose: 5-6 mg/kg; only concentrations <2% should be used in children <3 years or <14 kg (30 lbs)

Adults: Maximum dose: 400 mg; do not exceed 1000 mg/24 hours

Cervical, brachial, intercostal, pudendal nerve block: 5-40 mL of a 1% solution (maximum: 400 mg) **or** 5-20 mL of a 2% solution (maximum: 400 mg). For pudendal block, inject 1/2 the total dose each side.

Transvaginal block (paracervical plus pudendal): Up to 30 mL (both sides) of a 1% solution (maximum: 300 mg). Inject 1/2 the total dose each side.

Paracervical block: Up to 20 mL (both sides) of a 1% solution (maximum: 200 mg). Inject 1/2 the total dose to each side. This is the maximum recommended dose per 90-minute procedure; inject slowly with 5 minutes between sides.

Caudal and epidural block (preservative free solutions only): 15-30 mL of a 1% solution (maximum: 300 mg) **or** 10-25 mL of a 1.5% solution (maximum: 375 mg) **or** 10-20 mL of a 2% solution (maximum: 400 mg)

Infiltration: Up to 40 mL of a 1% solution (maximum: 400 mg)

Therapeutic block (pain management): 1-5 mL of a 1% solution (maximum: 50 mg) **or** 1-5 mL of a 2% solution (maximum: 100 mg)

Dental anesthesia: Adults:

Single site in upper or lower jaw: 54 mg (1.8 mL) as a 3% solution

Infiltration and nerve block of entire oral cavity: 270 mg (9 mL) as a 3% solution. Manufacturer's maximum recommended dose is not more than 400 mg to normal healthy adults.

Dosage Forms

Injection, solution:

Carbocaine®, Polocaine®: 1% (50 mL); 2% (50 mL)

Injection, solution [for dental use]: 3% (1.8 mL)

Carbocaine®, Polocaine® Dental, Scandonest® 3% Plain: 3% (1.7 mL)

Injection, solution [preservative free]:

Carbocaine®, Polocaine® MPF: 1% (30 mL); 1.5% (30 mL); 2% (20 mL)

mepivacaine and levonordefrin (me PIV a kane & lee voe nor DEF rin)

Synonyms levonordefrin and mepivacaine hydrochloride

U.S./Canadian Brand Names Carbocaine® 2% with Neo-Cobefrin® [US]; Polocaine® 2% and Levonordefrin 1:20,000 [Can]; Polocaine® Dental with Levonordefrin [US]; Scandonest® 2% L [US]

Therapeutic Category Local Anesthetic

Use Amide-type anesthetic used for local infiltration anesthesia; injection near nerve trunks to produce nerve block

Usual Dosage

Children <10 years: Maximum pediatric dosage must be carefully calculated on the basis of patient's weight but should not exceed 6.6 mg/kg of body weight or 180 mg of mepivacaine hydrochloride as a 2% solution with levonordefrin 1:20,000

Children >10 years and Adults:

Dental infiltration and nerve block, single site: 36 mg (1.8 mL) of mepivacaine hydrochloride as a 2% solution with levonordefrin 1:20,000

Entire oral cavity: 180 mg (9 mL) of mepivacaine hydrochloride as a 2% solution with levonordefrin 1:20,000; up to a maximum of 6.6 mg/kg of body weight but not to exceed 400 mg of mepivacaine hydrochloride per appointment. The effective anesthetic dose varies with procedure, intensity of anesthesia needed, duration of anesthesia required, and physical condition of the patient. Always use the lowest effective dose along with careful aspiration.

Dosage Forms

Injection, solution [for dental use]:

Carbocaine® 2% with Neo-Cobefrin®: Mepivacaine 2% and levonordefrin 1:20,000 (1.7 mL)
Polocaine® Dental with Levonordefrin: Mepivacaine 2% and levonordefrin 1:20,000 (1.7 mL)
Scandonest® 2% L: Mepivacaine 2% and levonordefrin 1:20,000 (1.7 mL)

mepivacaine hydrochloride *see* mepivacaine *on page 628*

meprobamate (me proe BA mate)

Sound-Alike/Look-Alike Issues

meprobamate may be confused with Mepergan, meperidine

U.S./Canadian Brand Names Novo-Mepro [Can]

Therapeutic Category Antianxiety Agent

Controlled Substance C-IV

Use Management of anxiety disorders

Usual Dosage Oral: Anxiety:

Children 6-12 years: 100-200 mg 2-3 times/day
Adults: 400 mg 3-4 times/day, up to 2400 mg/day

Dosage Forms

Tablet: 200 mg, 400 mg

meprobamate and aspirin (me proe BA mate & AS pir in)

Synonyms aspirin and meprobamate

U.S./Canadian Brand Names 292 MEP® [Can]; Equagesic® [US]

Therapeutic Category Skeletal Muscle Relaxant

Controlled Substance C-IV

Use Adjunct to the short-term treatment of pain in patients with skeletal-muscular disease exhibiting tension and/or anxiety

Usual Dosage Oral: Children ≥12 years and Adults: 1-2 tablets 3-4 times/day for up to 10 days

Dosage Forms

Tablet:

Equagesic®: Meprobamate 200 mg and aspirin 325 mg

Mepron® [US/Can] *see* atovaquone *on page 109*

mequinol and tretinoin (ME kwi nole & TRET i noyn)

Synonyms tretinoin and mequinol

U.S./Canadian Brand Names Solagé® [US/Can]

Therapeutic Category Retinoic Acid Derivative; Vitamin A Derivative; Vitamin, Topical

Use Treatment of solar lentigines; the efficacy of using Solagé® daily for >24 weeks has not been established

Usual Dosage Solar lentigines: Topical: Apply twice daily to solar lentigines using the applicator tip while avoiding application to the surrounding skin. Separate application by at least 8 hours or as directed by physician.

Dosage Forms

Liquid, topical:

Solagé®: Mequinol 2% and tretinoin 0.01% (30 mL)

mercaptoethane sulfonate *see* mesna *on page 631*

mercaptopurine (mer kap toe PYOOR een)

Sound-Alike/Look-Alike Issues
Purinethol® may be confused with propylthiouracil
6-mercaptopurine (error-prone abbreviation)
6-MP (error-prone abbreviation)

Synonyms NSC-755

U.S./Canadian Brand Names Purinethol® [US/Can]

Therapeutic Category Antineoplastic Agent

Use Treatment (maintenance and induction) of acute lymphoblastic leukemia (ALL)

Usual Dosage Oral (refer to individual protocols):
Children: ALL:
Induction: 2.5-5 mg/kg/day **or** 70-100 mg/m^2/day given once daily
Maintenance: 1.5-2.5 mg/kg/day **or** 50-75 mg/m^2/day given once daily
Adults: ALL:
Induction: 2.5-5 mg/kg/day (100-200 mg)
Maintenance: 1.5-2.5 mg/kg/day **or** 80-100 mg/m^2/day given once daily
Note: In ALL, administration in the evening (vs morning administration) may lower the risk of relapse.

Dosage Forms
Tablet [scored]: 50 mg
Purinethol®: 50 mg

mercapturic acid *see* acetylcysteine *on page 31*

Meridia® [US/Can] *see* sibutramine *on page 899*

meropenem (mer oh PEN em)

Sound-Alike/Look-Alike Issues
meropenem may be confused with ertapenem, imipenem, metronidazole.

U.S./Canadian Brand Names Merrem® I.V. [US]; Merrem® [Can]

Therapeutic Category Carbapenem (Antibiotic)

Use Treatment of intraabdominal infections (complicated appendicitis and peritonitis); treatment of bacterial meningitis in pediatric patients ≥3 months of age caused by *S. pneumoniae*, *H. influenzae*, and *N. meningitidis*; treatment of complicated skin and skin structure infections caused by susceptible organisms

Usual Dosage
Usual dosage ranges:
Neonates: I.V.:
Postnatal age 0-7 days: 20 mg/kg/dose every 12 hours
Postnatal age >7 days:
Weight 1200-2000 g: 20 mg/kg/dose every 12 hours
Weight >2000 g: 20 mg/kg/dose every 8 hours
Children ≥3 months: I.V.: 30-120 mg/kg/day divided every 8 hours (maximum dose: 6 g/day)
Adults: I.V.: 1.5-6 g/day divided every 8 hours
Indication-specific dosing:
Children ≥3 months (<50 kg): I.V.:
Intraabdominal infections: 20 mg/kg every 8 hours (maximum dose: 1 g every 8 hours)
Meningitis: 40 mg/kg every 8 hours (maximum dose: 2 g every 8 hours)
Skin and skin structure infections (complicated): 10 mg/kg every 8 hours (maximum dose: 500 mg every 8 hours)
Children >50 kg and Adults: I.V.:
Cholangitis, intraabdominal infections: 1 g every 8 hours
Skin and skin structure infections (complicated): 500 mg every 8 hours; diabetic foot: 1 g every 8 hours

Dosage Forms
Injection, powder for reconstitution:
Merrem® I.V.: 500 mg, 1 g

Merrem® [Can] *see* meropenem *on page 630*

Merrem® I.V. [US] *see* meropenem *on page 630*

Mersyndol® With Codeine [Can] *see* acetaminophen, codeine, and doxylamine *(Canada only) on page 26*

Meruvax® II [US] *see* rubella virus vaccine (live) *on page 882*

mesalamine (me SAL a meen)

Sound-Alike/Look-Alike Issues

mesalamine may be confused with mecamylamine, megestrol, memantine, metaxalone, methenamine
Apriso™ may be confused with Apri®
Asacol® may be confused with Ansaid®, Os-Cal®, Visicol®
Lialda™ may be confused with Aldara®
Pentasa® may be confused with Pancrease®, Pangestyme™

Synonyms 5-aminosalicylic acid; 5-ASA; fisalamine; mesalazine

U.S./Canadian Brand Names Apriso™ [US]; Asacol® 800 [Can]; Asacol® HD [US]; Asacol® [US/Can]; Canasa® [US]; Lialda™ [US]; Mesasal® [Can]; Mezavant® [Can]; Novo-5 ASA [Can]; Pentasa® [US/Can]; Rowasa® [US]; Salofalk® [Can]

Therapeutic Category 5-Aminosalicylic Acid Derivative

Use

Oral: Treatment and maintenance of remission of mildly- to moderately-active ulcerative colitis
Asacol® HD: Treatment of moderately-active ulcerative colitis
Rectal: Treatment of active mild-to-moderate distal ulcerative colitis, proctosigmoiditis, or proctitis

Usual Dosage Adults:

Oral:
Treatment of ulcerative colitis (usual course of therapy is 3-8 weeks):
Capsule: 1 g 4 times/day
Tablet: Initial:
Asacol®: 800 mg 3 times/day for 6 weeks
Asacol® HD: 1.6 g 3 times/day for 6 weeks
Lialda™, Mezavant®: 2.4-4.8 g once daily for up to 8 weeks
Maintenance of remission of ulcerative colitis:
Capsule:
Apriso™: 1.5 g once daily in the morning
Pentasa®: 1 g 4 times/day
Tablet (Asacol®): 1.6 g/day in divided doses; **Note:** Asacol® HD, Lialda™, and Mezavant® tablets are approved for treatment only.
Rectal:
Retention enema: 60 mL (4 g) at bedtime, retained overnight, approximately 8 hours
Rectal suppository (Canasa®): Insert one 1000 mg suppository in rectum daily at bedtime
Note: Suppositories should be retained for at least 1-3 hours to achieve maximum benefit.
Note: Some patients may require rectal and oral therapy concurrently.

Dosage Forms [CAN] = Canadian brand name

Capsule, controlled release:
Pentasa®: 250 mg, 500 mg
Capsule, delayed and extended release:
Apriso™: 0.375 g
Suppository, rectal:
Canasa®: 1000 mg
Suspension, rectal: 4 g/60 mL (7s, 28s)
Rowasa®: 4 g/60 mL (7s, 28s)
Tablet, delayed release [enteric coated]:
Asacol®: 400 mg
Asacol® HD: 800 mg
Lialda™: 1.2 g
Tablet, delayed and extended release:
Mezavant® [CAN]: 1.2 g [not available in U.S.]

mesalazine *see* mesalamine *on page 631*
Mesasal® [Can] *see* mesalamine *on page 631*
M-Eslon® [Can] *see* morphine sulfate *on page 667*

mesna (MES na)

Synonyms mercaptoethane sulfonate; sodium 2-mercaptoethane sulfonate

U.S./Canadian Brand Names Mesnex® [US/Can]; Uromitexan [Can]

Therapeutic Category Antidote

Use Preventative agent to reduce the incidence of ifosfamide-induced hemorrhagic cystitis

Usual Dosage Children and Adults: **Note:** Details concerning dosing in combination regimens should also be consulted. Mesna dosing schedule should be repeated each day ifosfamide is received. If ifosfamide dose is adjusted, the mesna dose should also be modified to maintain the mesna-to-ifosfamide ratio.

I.V.: Prevention of ifosfamide-induced hemorrhagic cystitis:

Short infusion standard-dose ifosfamide (<2.5 g/m²/day): Mesna dose is equal to 60% of the ifosfamide dose given in 3 divided doses (0, 4, and 8 hours after the start of ifosfamide)

Continuous infusion standard-dose ifosfamide (<2.5 g/m²/day): ASCO guidelines: Mesna dose (as an I.V. bolus) is equal to 20% of the ifosfamide dose, followed by a continuous infusion of mesna at 40% of the ifosfamide dose, continue mesna infusion for 12-24 hours after completion of ifosfamide infusion

High-dose ifosfamide (>2.5 g/m²/day): ASCO guidelines: Evidence for use is inadequate; more frequent and prolonged mesna administration regimens may be required.

I.V. followed by oral (for ifosfamide doses ≤2 g/m²/day): Mesna dose is equal to 100% of the ifosfamide dose, given as 20% of the ifosfamide dose I.V. at hour 0, followed by 40% of the ifosfamide dose given orally 2- and 6 hours after start of ifosfamide

Dosage Forms

Injection, solution: 100 mg/mL (10 mL)

Mesnex®: 100 mg/mL (10 mL)

Tablet:

Mesnex®: 400 mg

Mesnex® [US/Can] *see* mesna *on page* *631*
Mestinon® [US/Can] *see* pyridostigmine *on page* *839*
Mestinon® Injection *(Discontinued)* *see* pyridostigmine *on page* *839*
Mestinon®-SR [Can] *see* pyridostigmine *on page* *839*
Mestinon® Timespan® [US] *see* pyridostigmine *on page* *839*
mestranol and norethindrone *see* norethindrone and mestranol *on page* *704*
metacortandralone *see* prednisolone (systemic) *on page* *813*
Metadate CD® [US] *see* methylphenidate *on page* *645*
Metadate® ER [US] *see* methylphenidate *on page* *645*
Metadol™ [Can] *see* methadone *on page* *635*
Metadol-D™ [Can] *see* methadone *on page* *635*
Metaglip™ [US] *see* glipizide and metformin *on page* *465*
123 meta-iodobenzlyguanidine sulfate *see* iobenguane I 123 *on page* *537*
Metamucil® [US-OTC/Can] *see* psyllium *on page* *837*
Metamucil® Plus Calcium [US-OTC] *see* psyllium *on page* *837*
Metamucil® Smooth Texture [US-OTC] *see* psyllium *on page* *837*
Metanx™ [US] *see* vitamin B complex combinations *on page* *1017*

metaproterenol (met a proe TER e nol)

Sound-Alike/Look-Alike Issues

metaproterenol may be confused with metipranolol, metoprolol

Alupent® may be confused with Atrovent®

Synonyms metaproterenol sulfate; orciprenaline sulfate

U.S./Canadian Brand Names Apo-Orciprenaline® [Can]; ratio-Orciprenaline® [Can]; Tanta-Orciprenaline® [Can]

Therapeutic Category Adrenergic Agonist Agent

Use Bronchodilator in reversible airway obstruction due to asthma or COPD

Usual Dosage

Oral:

Children:

<2 years: 0.4 mg/kg/dose given 3-4 times/day; in infants, the dose can be given every 8-12 hours

2-6 years: 1-2.6 mg/kg/day divided every 6 hours

6-9 years: 10 mg/dose 3-4 times/day

Children >9 years and Adults: 20 mg 3-4 times/day

Inhalation: Children >12 years and Adults: 2-3 inhalations every 3-4 hours, up to 12 inhalations in 24 hours

Nebulizer:

Infants and Children: 0.01-0.02 mL/kg of 5% solution; minimum dose: 0.1 mL; maximum dose: 0.3 mL diluted in 2-3 mL normal saline every 4-6 hours (may be given more frequently according to need)

Adolescents and Adults: 5-20 breaths of full strength 5% metaproterenol **or** 0.2 to 0.3 mL 5% metaproterenol in 2.5-3 mL normal saline until nebulized every 4-6 hours (can be given more frequently according to need)

Dosage Forms

Solution for nebulization [preservative free]: 0.4% [4 mg/mL] (2.5 mL); 0.6% [6 mg/mL] (2.5 mL)

Syrup: 10 mg/5 mL

Tablet: 10 mg, 20 mg

metaproterenol sulfate *see* metaproterenol *on page* 632

Metasep® ***(Discontinued)***

Metastron® [US/Can] *see* strontium-89 *on page* 923

metaxalone (me TAKS a lone)

Sound-Alike/Look-Alike Issues

metaxalone may be confused with mesalamine, metolazone

Skelaxin® may be confused with Robaxin®

U.S./Canadian Brand Names Skelaxin® [US/Can]

Therapeutic Category Skeletal Muscle Relaxant

Use Relief of discomfort associated with acute, painful musculoskeletal conditions

Usual Dosage Oral: Children >12 years and Adults: Muscle discomfort: 800 mg 3-4 times/day

Dosage Forms

Tablet:

Skelaxin®: 800 mg

metformin (met FOR min)

Sound-Alike/Look-Alike Issues

metFORMIN may be confused with metroNIDAZOLE

Glucophage® may be confused with Glucotrol®, Glutofac®

Synonyms metformin hydrochloride

Tall-Man met**FORMIN**

U.S./Canadian Brand Names Apo-Metformin® [Can]; CO Metformin [Can]; Dom-Metformin [Can]; Fortamet® [US]; Gen-Metformin [Can]; Glucophage® XR [US]; Glucophage® [US/Can]; Glumetza™ [US/Can]; Glycon [Can]; MED-Metformin [Can]; Novo-Metformin [Can]; Nu-Metformin [Can]; PHL-Metformin [Can]; PMS-Metformin [Can]; RAN™-Metformin [Can]; ratio-Metformin [Can]; Rhoxal-metformin [Can]; Riomet® [US]; Riva-Metformin [Can]; Sandoz-Metformin FC [Can]

Therapeutic Category Antidiabetic Agent, Oral

Use Management of type 2 diabetes mellitus (noninsulin-dependent, NIDDM) as monotherapy when hyperglycemia cannot be managed with diet and exercise alone. In adults, may be used concomitantly with a sulfonylurea or insulin to improve glycemic control.

Usual Dosage Type 2 diabetes management: **Note:** Allow 1-2 weeks between dose titrations: Generally, clinically significant responses are not seen at doses <1500 mg daily; however, a lower recommended starting dose and gradual increased dosage is recommended to minimize gastrointestinal symptoms.

Immediate release tablet or solution: Oral:

Children 10-16 years: Initial: 500 mg twice daily; increases in daily dosage should be made in increments of 500 mg at weekly intervals, given in divided doses, up to a maximum of 2000 mg/day

Chidlren ≥17 years and Adults: Initial: 500 mg twice daily **or** 850 mg once daily; increase dosage incrementally.

Incremental dosing recommendations based on dosage form:

500 mg tablet: One tablet/day at weekly intervals

850 mg tablet: One tablet/day every other week

Oral solution: 500 mg twice daily every other week

Doses of up to 2000 mg/day may be given twice daily. If a dose >2000 mg/day is required, it may be better tolerated in three divided doses. Maximum recommended dose 2550 mg/day.

Extended release tablet: Oral: **Note:** If glycemic control is not achieved at maximum dose, may divide dose and administer twice daily.

Children ≥17 years and Adults:

Fortamet®: Initial: 1000 mg once daily; dosage may be increased by 500 mg weekly; maximum dose: 2500 mg once daily

Glucophage® XR: Initial: 500 mg once daily; dosage may be increased by 500 mg weekly; maximum dose: 2000 mg once daily

Adults: Glumetza™: Initial: 1000 mg once daily; dosage may be increased by 500 mg weekly; maximum dose: 2000 mg once daily

Transfer from other antidiabetic agents: No transition period is generally necessary except when transferring from chlorpropamide. When transferring from chlorpropamide, care should be exercised during the first 2 weeks because of the prolonged retention of chlorpropamide in the body, leading to overlapping drug effects and possible hypoglycemia.

Concomitant metformin and oral sulfonylurea therapy: If patients have not responded to 4 weeks of the maximum dose of metformin monotherapy, consider a gradual addition of an oral sulfonylurea, even if prior primary or secondary failure to a sulfonylurea has occurred. Continue metformin at the maximum dose. If adequate response has not occurred following 3 months of metformin and sulfonylurea combination therapy, consider switching to insulin with or without metformin.

Failed sulfonylurea therapy: Patients with prior failure on glyburide may be treated by gradual addition of metformin. Initiate with glyburide 20 mg and metformin 500 mg daily. Metformin dosage may be increased by 500 mg/day at weekly intervals, up to a maximum metformin dose (dosage of glyburide maintained at 20 mg/day).

Concomitant metformin and insulin therapy: Initial: 500 mg metformin once daily, continue current insulin dose; increase by 500 mg metformin weekly until adequate glycemic control is achieved

Maximum daily dose: Immediate release and solution: 2550 mg metformin; Extended release: 2000-2500 mg (varies by product)

Decrease insulin dose 10% to 25% when FPG <120 mg/dL; monitor and make further adjustments as needed

Dosage Forms

Solution, oral:

Riomet®: 100 mg/mL

Tablet: 500 mg, 850 mg, 1000 mg

Glucophage®: 500 mg, 850 mg, 1000 mg

Tablet, extended release: 500 mg, 750 mg

Fortamet®: 500 mg, 1000 mg

Glucophage® XR: 500 mg

Glumetza™: 500 mg, 1000 mg

metformin and glipizide *see* glipizide and metformin *on page 465*

metformin and glyburide *see* glyburide and metformin *on page 467*

metformin and repaglinide *see* repaglinide and metformin *on page 859*

metformin and rosiglitazone *see* rosiglitazone and metformin *on page 879*

metformin and sitagliptin *see* sitagliptin and metformin *on page 905*

metformin hydrochloride *see* metformin *on page 633*

metformin hydrochloride and pioglitazone hydrochloride *see* pioglitazone and metformin *on page 786*

metformin hydrochloride and rosiglitazone maleate *see* rosiglitazone and metformin *on page 879*

methacholine (meth a KOLE leen)

Synonyms methacholine chloride

U.S./Canadian Brand Names Methacholine Omega [Can]; Provocholine® [US/Can]

Therapeutic Category Diagnostic Agent

Use Diagnosis of bronchial airway hyperactivity

Usual Dosage Note: For inhalation only: Children ≥5 years and Adults:

Before inhalation challenge, perform baseline pulmonary function tests; the patient must have an FEV_1 of at least 70% of the predicted value. The following is a suggested schedule for administration of methacholine challenge. Calculate cumulative units by multiplying number of breaths by concentration given. Total cumulative units is the sum of cumulative units for each concentration given. See table on next page.

Methacholine

Vial	Serial Concentration (mg/mL)	No. of Breaths	Cumulative Units per Concentration	Total Cumulative Units
E	0.025	5	0.125	0.125
D	0.25	5	1.25	1.375
C	2.5	5	12.5	13.88
B	10	5	50	63.88
A	25	5	125	188.88

Determine FEV_1 within 5 minutes of challenge, a positive challenge is a 20% reduction in FEV_1

Dosage Forms

Powder for reconstitution, for oral inhalation:

Provocholine®: 100 mg

methacholine chloride *see* methacholine *on page 634*

Methacholine Omega [Can] *see* methacholine *on page 634*

methadone (METH a done)

Sound-Alike/Look-Alike Issues

methadone may be confused with dexmethylphenidate, Mephyton®, methylphenidate, Metadate® CD, and Metadate® ER

Synonyms methadone hydrochloride

U.S./Canadian Brand Names Dolophine® [US]; Metadol-D™ [Can]; Metadol™ [Can]; Methadone Diskets® [US]; Methadone Intensol™ [US]; Methadose® [US]

Therapeutic Category Analgesic, Narcotic

Controlled Substance C-II

Use Management of moderate-to-severe pain; detoxification and maintenance treatment of opioid addiction as part of an FDA-approved program

Usual Dosage Regulations regarding methadone use may vary by state and/or country. Obtain advice from appropriate regulatory agencies and/or consult with pain management/palliative care specialists. **Note:** These are guidelines and do not represent the maximum doses that may be required in all patients. Methadone accumulates with repeated doses and dosage may need reduction after 3-5 days to prevent CNS depressant effects. Some patients may benefit from every 8-12 hour dosing interval for chronic pain management. Doses should be titrated to appropriate effects.

Adults:

Acute pain (moderate-to-severe):

Oral: Opioid-naive: Initial: 2.5-10 mg every 8-12 hours; more frequent administration may be required during initiation to maintain adequate analgesia. Dosage interval may range from 4-12 hours, since duration of analgesia is relatively short during the first days of therapy, but increases substantially with continued administration.

Chronic pain (opioid-tolerant): **Conversion from oral morphine to oral methadone:**

Daily oral morphine dose <100 mg: Estimated daily oral methadone dose: 20% to 30% of total daily morphine dose

Daily oral morphine dose 100-300 mg: Estimated daily oral methadone dose: 10% to 20% of total daily morphine dose

Daily oral morphine dose 300-600 mg: Estimated daily oral methadone dose: 8% to 12% of total daily morphine dose

Daily oral morphine dose 600-1000 mg: Estimated daily oral methadone dose: 5% to 10% of total daily morphine dose.

Daily oral morphine dose >1000 mg: Estimated daily oral methadone dose: <5% of total daily morphine dose.

Note: The total daily methadone dose should then be divided to reflect the intended dosing schedule.

I.V.: Manufacturers labeling: Initial: 2.5-10 mg every 8-12 hours in opioid-naive patients; titrate slowly to effect; may also be administered by SubQ or I.M. injection

Conversion from oral methadone to parenteral methadone dose: Initial dose: Parenteral:Oral ratio: 1:2 (eg, 5 mg parenteral methadone equals 10 mg oral methadone)

Detoxification: Oral:

Initial: A single dose of 20-30 mg is generally sufficient to suppress symptoms. Should not exceed 30 mg; lower doses should be considered in patients with low tolerance at initiation (eg, absence of opioids ≥5 days); an additional 5-10 mg of methadone may be provided if withdrawal symptoms have not been suppressed or if symptoms reappear after 2-4 hours; total daily dose on the first day should not exceed 40 mg, unless the program physician documents in the patient's record that 40 mg did not control opiate abstinence symptoms.

Maintenance: Titrate to a dosage which attenuates craving, blocks euphoric effects of other opiates, and tolerance to sedative effect of methadone. Usual range: 80-120 mg/day (titration should occur cautiously)

Withdrawal: Dose reductions should be <10% of the maintenance dose, every 10-14 days

Detoxification (short-term): Oral:

Initial: Titrate to ~40 mg/day in divided doses to achieve stabilization, may continue 40 mg dose for 2-3 days

Maintenance: Titrate to a dosage which prevents/attenuates euphoric effects of self-administered opioids, reduces drug craving, and withdrawal symptoms are prevented for 24 hours.

Withdrawal: Requires individualization. Decrease daily or every other day, keeping withdrawal symptoms tolerable; hospitalized patients may tolerate a 20% reduction/day; ambulatory patients may require a slower reduction

Dosage Forms

Injection, solution: 10 mg/mL (20 mL)

Solution, oral: 5 mg/5 mL, 10 mg/5 mL

Solution, oral, as hydrochloride [concentrate]: 10 mg/mL

Methadone Intensol™, Methadose®: 10 mg/mL

Tablet: 5 mg, 10 mg

Dolophine®: 5 mg, 10 mg

Methadose®: 5 mg, 10 mg [DSC]

Tablet, dispersible: 40 mg

Methadose®, Methadone Diskets®: 40 mg

Methadone Diskets® [US] *see* methadone *on page* 635

methadone hydrochloride *see* methadone *on page* 635

Methadone Intensol™ [US] *see* methadone *on page* 635

Methadose® [US] *see* methadone *on page* 635

methaminodiazepoxide hydrochloride *see* chlordiazepoxide *on page* 209

methamphetamine (meth am FET a meen)

Sound-Alike/Look-Alike Issues

Desoxyn® may be confused with digoxin

Synonyms desoxyephedrine hydrochloride; methamphetamine hydrochloride

U.S./Canadian Brand Names Desoxyn® [US/Can]

Therapeutic Category Amphetamine

Controlled Substance C-II

Use Treatment of attention-deficit/hyperactivity disorder (ADHD); exogenous obesity (short-term adjunct)

Usual Dosage Oral:

Children ≥6 years and Adults: ADHD: 5 mg 1-2 times/day; may increase by 5 mg increments at weekly intervals until optimum response is achieved, usually 20-25 mg/day

Children ≥12 years and Adults: Exogenous obesity: 5 mg 30 minutes before each meal; treatment duration should not exceed a few weeks

Dosage Forms

Tablet: 5 mg

Desoxyn®: 5 mg

methamphetamine hydrochloride *see* methamphetamine *on page* 636

methazolamide (meth a ZOE la mide)

Sound-Alike/Look-Alike Issues

methazolamide may be confused with methenamine, metolazone

Neptazane® may be confused with Nesacaine®

U.S./Canadian Brand Names Apo-Methazolamide® [Can]

Therapeutic Category Carbonic Anhydrase Inhibitor

Use Adjunctive treatment of open-angle or secondary glaucoma; short-term therapy of narrow-angle glaucoma when delay of surgery is desired

Usual Dosage Oral: Adults: 50-100 mg 2-3 times/day

Dosage Forms

Tablet: 25 mg, 50 mg

methenamine (meth EN a meen)

Sound-Alike/Look-Alike Issues

methenamine may be confused with mesalamine, methazolamide, methionine

Urex™ may be confused with Eurax®, Serax®

Synonyms hexamethylenetetramine; methenamine hippurate; methenamine mandelate

U.S./Canadian Brand Names Dehydral® [Can]; Hiprex® [US/Can]; Mandelamine® [Can]; Urasal® [Can]; Urex™ [US/Can]

Therapeutic Category Antibiotic, Miscellaneous

Use Prophylaxis or suppression of recurrent urinary tract infections; urinary tract discomfort secondary to hypermotility

Usual Dosage Oral:

Children:

>2-6 years: *Mandelate:* 50-75 mg/kg/day in 3-4 doses or 0.25 g/30 lb 4 times/day

6-12 years:

Hippurate: 0.5-1 g twice daily

Mandelate: 50-75 mg/kg/day in 3-4 doses or 0.5 g 4 times/day

>12 years and Adults:

Hippurate: 1 g twice daily

Mandelate: 1 g 4 times/day after meals and at bedtime

Dosage Forms

Tablet: 1 g

Hiprex®, Urex™: 1 g

methenamine hippurate *see* methenamine *on page* 637

methenamine mandelate *see* methenamine *on page* 637

methenamine, phenyl salicylate, methylene blue, benzoic acid, and hyoscyamine

(meth EN a meen, fen nil sa LIS i late, METH i leen bloo, ben ZOE ik AS id & hye oh SYE a meen)

Synonyms benzoic acid, hyoscyamine, methenamine, methylene blue, and phenyl salicylate; benzoic acid, methenamine, methylene blue, phenyl salicylate, and hyoscyamine; hyoscyamine, methenamine, benzoic acid, phenyl salicylate, and methylene blue; methylene blue, methenamine, benzoic acid, phenyl salicylate, and hyoscyamine; phenyl salicylate, methenamine, methylene blue, benzoic acid, and hyoscyamine

U.S./Canadian Brand Names Prosed®/DS [US]

Therapeutic Category Antibiotic, Miscellaneous

Use Urinary tract discomfort secondary to hypermotility resulting from infection or diagnostic procedures

Usual Dosage Oral:

Children >12 years: Dosage must be individualized

Adults: One tablet 4 times daily

Dosage Forms

Tablet, oral:

Prosed®/DS: Methenamine 81.6 mg, phenyl salicylate 36.2 mg, methylene blue 10.8 mg, benzoic acid 9 mg, hyoscyamine sulfate 0.12 mg

Methergine® [US/Can] *see* methylergonovine *on page* 644

methimazole (meth IM a zole)

Sound-Alike/Look-Alike Issues

methimazole may be confused with metolazone

Synonyms thiamazole

U.S./Canadian Brand Names Dom-Methimazole [Can]; Northyx™ [US]; PHL-Methimazole [Can]; Tapazole® [US/Can]

Therapeutic Category Antithyroid Agent

Use Palliative treatment of hyperthyroidism, return the hyperthyroid patient to a normal metabolic state prior to thyroidectomy, and to control thyrotoxic crisis that may accompany thyroidectomy

Usual Dosage Oral: Administer in 3 equally divided doses at approximately 8-hour intervals

Children: Initial: 0.4 mg/kg/day in 3 divided doses; maintenance: 0.2 mg/kg/day in 3 divided doses up to 30 mg/24 hours maximum

Alternatively: Initial: 0.5-0.7 mg/kg/day **or** 15-20 mg/m^2/day in 3 divided doses

Maintenance: 1/3 to 2/3 of the initial dose beginning when the patient is euthyroid

Maximum: 30 mg/24 hours

Adults: Initial: 15 mg/day in 3 divided doses (approximately every 8 hours) for mild hyperthyroidism; 30-40 mg/day in moderately-severe hyperthyroidism; 60 mg/day in severe hyperthyroidism; maintenance: 5-15 mg/day (may be given as a single daily dose in many cases)

Adjust dosage as required to achieve and maintain serum T_3, T_4, and TSH levels in the normal range. An elevated T_3 may be the sole indicator of inadequate treatment. An elevated TSH indicates excessive antithyroid treatment.

Thyrotoxic crisis (recommendations vary widely and have not been evaluated in comparative trials): Dosages of 20-30 mg every 6-12 hours have been recommended for short-term initial therapy, followed by gradual reduction to a maintenance dosage (5-15 mg/day). Rectal administration has been described.

Dosage Forms

Tablet: 5 mg, 10 mg, 20 mg

Northyx™: 5 mg, 10 mg, 15 mg, 20 mg

Tapazole®: 5 mg, 10 mg

Methitest™ [US] *see* methyltestosterone *on page* 648

methocarbamol (meth oh KAR ba mole)

Sound-Alike/Look-Alike Issues

methocarbamol may be confused with mephobarbital

Robaxin® may be confused with ribavirin, Rubex®, Skelaxin®

U.S./Canadian Brand Names Robaxin® [US/Can]

Therapeutic Category Skeletal Muscle Relaxant

Use Treatment of muscle spasm associated with acute painful musculoskeletal conditions; supportive therapy in tetanus

Usual Dosage

Tetanus: I.V.:

Children: Recommended **only** for use in tetanus: 15 mg/kg/dose or 500 mg/m^2/dose, may repeat every 6 hours if needed; maximum dose: 1.8 g/m^2/day for 3 days only

Adults: Initial dose: 1-3 g; may repeat dose every 6 hours until oral dosing is possible; injection should not be used for more than 3 consecutive days

Muscle spasm: Children ≥16 years and Adults:

Oral: 1.5 g 4 times/day for 2-3 days (up to 8 g/day may be given in severe conditions), then decrease to 4-4.5 g/day in 3-6 divided doses

I.M., I.V.: 1 g every 8 hours if oral not possible; injection should not be used for more than 3 consecutive days. If condition persists, may repeat course of therapy after a drug-free interval of 48 hours.

Dosage Forms

Injection, solution:

Robaxin®: 100 mg/mL (10 mL)

Tablet: 500 mg, 750 mg

Robaxin®: 500 mg, 750 mg

methohexital (meth oh HEKS i tal)

Sound-Alike/Look-Alike Issues

Brevital® may be confused with Brevibloc®

Synonyms methohexital sodium

U.S./Canadian Brand Names Brevital® Sodium [US]; Brevital® [Can]

Therapeutic Category Barbiturate

Controlled Substance C-IV

Use For induction of anesthesia prior to the use of other general anesthetic agents; as an adjunct to subpotent inhalational anesthetic agents for short surgical procedures; for short surgical, diagnostic, or therapeutic procedures associated with minimal painful stimuli

Additional indications for adults: For use with other parenteral agents, usually narcotic analgesics, to supplement subpotent inhalational anesthetic agents for longer surgical procedures; as an agent to induce a hypnotic state

Usual Dosage Doses must be titrated to effect.

Infants ≥1 month and Children: Anesthesia induction:

I.M.: 6.6-10 mg/kg of a 5% solution

Rectal: Usual: 25 mg/kg of a 1% solution

Adults: I.V.: Induction: 1-1.5 mg/kg; maintenance: 50-120 mcg/kg/minute (or 20-40 mg every 4-7 minutes)

Dosage Forms

Injection, powder for reconstitution:

Brevital® Sodium: 500 mg, 2.5 g

methohexital sodium *see* methohexital *on page* *638*

methotrexate (meth oh TREKS ate)

Sound-Alike/Look-Alike Issues

methotrexate may be confused with metolazone, mitoxantrone

MTX is an error-prone abbreviation (mistaken as mitoxantrone)

Synonyms amethopterin; methotrexate sodium; NSC-740

U.S./Canadian Brand Names Apo-Methotrexate® [Can]; ratio-Methotrexate [Can]; Rheumatrex® [US]; Trexall™ [US]

Therapeutic Category Antineoplastic Agent

Use Treatment of trophoblastic neoplasms; leukemias; psoriasis; rheumatoid arthritis (RA), including polyarticular-course juvenile rheumatoid arthritis (JRA); breast, head and neck, and lung carcinomas; osteosarcoma; soft-tissue sarcomas; carcinoma of gastrointestinal tract, esophagus, testes; lymphomas

Usual Dosage Refer to individual protocols.

Note: Doses between 100-500 mg/m^2 **may require** leucovorin rescue. Doses >500 mg/m^2 **require** leucovorin rescue: Oral, I.M., I.V.: Leucovorin 10-15 mg/m^2 every 6 hours for 8 or 10 doses, starting 24 hours after the start of methotrexate infusion. Continue until the methotrexate level is ≤0.1 micromolar (10^7M). Some clinicians continue leucovorin until the methotrexate level is <0.05 micromolar (5 x 10^8M) or 0.01 micromolar (10^8M).

If the 48-hour methotrexate level is >1 micromolar (10^7M) or the 72-hour methotrexate level is >0.2 micromolar (2 x 10^7M): I.V., I.M, Oral: Leucovorin 100 mg/m^2 every 6 hours until the methotrexate level is ≤0.1 micromolar (10^7M). Some clinicians continue leucovorin until the methotrexate level is <0.05 micromolar (5 x 10^8M) or 0.01 micromolar (10^8M).

Children:

Dermatomyositis: Oral: 15-20 mg/m^2/week as a single dose once weekly **or** 0.3-1 mg/kg/dose once weekly

Juvenile rheumatoid arthritis: Oral, I.M.: 10 mg/m^2 once weekly, then 5-15 mg/m^2/week as a single dose **or** as 3 divided doses given 12 hours apart

Antineoplastic dosage range:

Oral, I.M.: 7.5-30 mg/m^2/week **or** every 2 weeks

I.V.: 10-18,000 mg/m^2 bolus dosing **or** continuous infusion over 6-42 hours

Pediatric solid tumors (high-dose): I.V.:

<12 years: 12-25 g/m^2

≥12 years: 8 g/m^2

Acute lymphocytic leukemia (intermediate-dose): I.V.: Loading: 100 mg/m^2 bolus dose, followed by 900 mg/m^2/day infusion over 23-41 hours.

Meningeal leukemia: I.T.: 10-15 mg/m^2 (maximum dose: 15 mg) **or** an age-based dosing regimen; one possible system is:

≤3 months: 3 mg/dose

4-11 months: 6 mg/dose

1 year: 8 mg/dose

2 years: 10 mg/dose

≥3 years: 12 mg/dose

Adults: I.V.: Range is wide from 30-40 mg/m^2/week to 100-12,000 mg/m^2 with leucovorin rescue

Trophoblastic neoplasms:

Oral, I.M.: 15-30 mg/day for 5 days; repeat in 7 days for 3-5 courses

I.V.: 11 mg/m^2 days 1 through 5 every 3 weeks

Head and neck cancer: Oral, I.M., I.V.: 25-50 mg/m^2 once weekly

Mycosis fungoides (cutaneous T-cell lymphoma): Oral, I.M.: Initial (early stages):
5-50 mg once weekly **or**
15-37.5 mg twice weekly
Bladder cancer: I.V.:
30 mg/m^2 day 1 and 8 every 3 weeks **or**
30 mg/m^2 day 1, 15, and 22 every 4 weeks
Breast cancer: I.V.: 30-60 mg/m^2 days 1 and 8 every 3-4 weeks
Gastric cancer: I.V.: 1500 mg/m^2 every 4 weeks
Lymphoma, non-Hodgkin: I.V.:
30 mg/m^2 days 3 and 10 every 3 weeks **or**
120 mg/m^2 day 8 and 15 every 3-4 weeks **or**
200 mg/m^2 day 8 and 15 every 3 weeks **or**
400 mg/m^2 every 4 weeks for 3 cycles **or**
1 g/m^2 every 3 weeks **or**
1.5 g/m^2 every 4 weeks
Sarcoma: I.V.: 8-12 g/m^2 weekly for 2-4 weeks
Rheumatoid arthritis: Oral: 7.5 mg once weekly **or** 2.5 mg every 12 hours for 3 doses/week, not to exceed 20 mg/week
Psoriasis:
Oral: 2.5-5 mg/dose every 12 hours for 3 doses given weekly **or**
Oral, I.M.: 10-25 mg/dose given once weekly

Dosage Forms

Injection, powder for reconstitution: 1 g
Injection, solution: 25 mg/mL (2 mL, 10 mL)
Injection, solution [preservative free]: 25 mg/mL (2 mL, 4 mL, 8 mL, 10 mL, 40 mL)
Tablet: 2.5 mg
Trexall™: 5 mg, 7.5 mg, 10 mg, 15 mg
Tablet [dose pack]: 2.5 mg (4 cards with 2, 3, 4, 5, or 6 tablets each)
Rheumatrex®: 2.5 mg (4 cards with 2, 3, 4, 5, or 6 tablets each)

methotrexate sodium *see* methotrexate *on page* 639

methotrimeprazine *(Canada only)* (meth oh trye MEP ra zeen)

Synonyms levomepromazine; methotrimeprazine hydrochloride

U.S./Canadian Brand Names Apo-Methoprazine® [Can]; Novo-Meprazine [Can]; Nozinan® [Can]; PMS-Methotrimeprazine [Can]

Therapeutic Category Neuroleptic Agent

Use Treatment of schizophrenia or psychosis; management of pain, including pain caused by neuralgia or cancer; adjunct to general anesthesia; management of nausea and vomiting; sedation

Usual Dosage

Children >2 years:
Oral: 0.25 mg/kg/day in 2-3 divided doses; may increase gradually based on response.
Maximum dose: 40 mg/day in children <12 years
I.M.: 0.06-0.125 mg/kg/day in 1-3 divided doses
Adults:
Oral:
Anxiety, mild-to-moderate pain: 6-25 mg/day in 3 divided doses
Psychoses, severe pain: 50-75 mg/day in 2-3 divided doses; titrate to effect (doses up to 1000 mg/day or greater have been used in treatment of some patients with psychoses). If higher dosages are used to initiate therapy (100-200 mg/day), patients should be restricted to bed for the first few days of therapy.
Sedative: 10-25 mg at bedtime
I.M.:
Psychoses, severe pain: 75-100 mg (administered in 3-4 deep I.M. injections)
Analgesia (postoperative): 10-25 mg every 8 hours (2.5-7.5 mg every 4-6 hours is suggested postoperatively if residual effects of anesthetic may be present)
Premedication: 10-25 mg every 8 hours (final preoperative dose may be 25-50 mg administered ~1 hour prior to surgery)
I.V.: During surgical procedures/labor: 20-50 mcg/minute (some patients may require up to 100 mcg/minute)
SubQ (continuous infusion): Palliative care: 25-200 mcg/day (via syringe driver)

Dosage Forms [CAN] = Canadian brand name

Injection, solution:

Nozinan® [CAN]: 25 mg/mL (1 mL) [not available in the U.S.]

Solution, oral:

Nozinan® [CAN]: 5 mg/mL [not available in the U.S.]

Solution, oral drops:

Nozinan® [CAN]: 40 mg/mL [not available in the U.S.]

Tablet:

Apo-Methoprazine® [CAN]: 2 mg, 5 mg, 25 mg, 50 mg [not available in the U.S.]
Nozinan® [CAN]: 5 mg, 25 mg, 50 mg [not available in the U.S.]

methotrimeprazine hydrochloride *see* methotrimeprazine *(Canada only) on page* 640

methoxsalen (meth OKS a len)

Sound-Alike/Look-Alike Issues

methoxsalen soft gelatin capsules (Oxsoralen-Ultra®) may be confused with methoxsalen hard gelatin capsules (8-MOP®, Oxsoralen®); bioavailability and photosensitization onset differ between the two products.

Synonyms 8-methoxypsoralen; methoxypsoralen

U.S./Canadian Brand Names 8-MOP® [US]; Oxsoralen-Ultra® [US/Can]; Oxsoralen® [US/Can]; Ultramop™ [Can]; Uvadex® [US/Can]

Therapeutic Category Psoralen

Use

Oral: Symptomatic control of severe, recalcitrant disabling psoriasis; repigmentation of idiopathic vitiligo; palliative treatment of skin manifestations of cutaneous T-cell lymphoma (CTCL)

Topical: Repigmentation of idiopathic vitiligo

Extracorporeal: Palliative treatment of skin manifestations of CTCL

Usual Dosage Note: Refer to treatment protocols for UVA exposure guidelines.

Children >12 years and Adults: Vitiligo: Topical (Oxsoralen®): Lotion is applied prior to UVA light exposure, usually no more than once weekly

Adults:

Psoriasis: Oral:

Initial: 10-70 mg 1.5-2 hours (Oxsoralen-Ultra®) or 2 hours (8-MOP®) before exposure to UVA light; dose may be repeated 2-3 times per week, based on UVA exposure; doses must be given at least 48 hours apart. Dosage is based upon patient's body weight and skin type:

<30 kg: 10 mg
30-50 kg: 20 mg
51-65 kg: 30 mg
66-80 kg: 40 mg
81-90 kg: 50 mg
91-115 kg: 60 mg
>115 kg: 70 mg

Note: Dosage may be increased (one time) by 10 mg after 15th treatment if minimal or no response.

Maintenance: When 95% psoriasis clearing achieved, may begin 1 treatment every week for at least 2 treatments; followed by 1 treatment every 2 weeks for at least 2 treatments; then every 3 weeks for at least 2 treatments then as needed to maintain response while minimizing UVA exposure.

Vitiligo:

Oral (8-MOP®): 20 mg 2-4 hours before exposure to UVA light; dose may be repeated based on erythema and tenderness of skin; do not give on 2 consecutive days

CTCL: Extracorporeal (Uvadex®): 200 mcg injected into the photoactivation bag during the collection cycle using the UVAR® photopheresis system (consult user's guide). Treatment schedule: Two consecutive days every 4 weeks for a minimum of 7 treatment cycles, may accelerate to two consecutive days every 2 weeks if skin score worsens (eg, increases from baseline) after assessment during the fourth treatment cycle. If skin score improves by 25% after 4 consecutive weeks of accelerated therapy, may resume regular treatment schedule. Maximum: 20 accelerated therapy cycles.

Dosage Forms

Capsule:

8-MOP®, Oxsoralen-Ultra®: 10 mg

Lotion:

Oxsoralen®: 1% (30 mL)

Solution, for extracorporeal administration:
Uvadex®: 20 mcg/mL (10 mL) **[not for injection]**

methoxypsoralen *see* methoxsalen *on page 641*
8-methoxypsoralen *see* methoxsalen *on page 641*

methscopolamine (meth skoe POL a meen)

Synonyms methscopolamine bromide

U.S./Canadian Brand Names Pamine® Forte [US]; Pamine® [US/Can]

Therapeutic Category Anticholinergic Agent

Use Adjunctive therapy in the treatment of peptic ulcer

Usual Dosage Oral: Adults: 2.5 mg 30 minutes before meals or food and 2.5-5 mg at bedtime; may increase dose to 5 mg twice daily

Dosage Forms

Tablet: 2.5 mg, 5 mg
Pamine®: 2.5 mg
Pamine® Forte: 5 mg

methscopolamine and pseudoephedrine *see* pseudoephedrine and methscopolamine *on page 835*
methscopolamine bromide *see* methscopolamine *on page 642*
methscopolamine, chlorpheniramine, and pseudoephedrine *see* chlorpheniramine, pseudoephedrine, and methscopolamine *on page 221*
methscopolamine nitrate, chlorpheniramine maleate, and phenylephrine hydrochloride *see* chlorpheniramine, phenylephrine, and methscopolamine *on page 218*
methscopolamine, pseudoephedrine, and chlorpheniramine *see* chlorpheniramine, pseudoephedrine, and methscopolamine *on page 221*

methsuximide (meth SUKS i mide)

Sound-Alike/Look-Alike Issues
methsuximide may be confused with ethosuximide

U.S./Canadian Brand Names Celontin® [US/Can]

Therapeutic Category Anticonvulsant

Use Control of absence (petit mal) seizures that are refractory to other drugs

Usual Dosage Oral: Adults: Anticonvulsant: 300 mg/day for the first week; may increase by 300 mg/day at weekly intervals up to 1.2 g/day in 2-4 divided doses/day

Dosage Forms

Capsule:
Celontin®: 150 mg, 300 mg

methyclothiazide (meth i kloe THYE a zide)

Sound-Alike/Look-Alike Issues
Enduron® may be confused with Empirin®, Imuran®, Inderal®

Therapeutic Category Diuretic, Thiazide

Use Management of mild-to-moderate hypertension; treatment of edema in congestive heart failure and nephrotic syndrome

Usual Dosage Oral: Adults:
Edema: 2.5-10 mg/day
Hypertension: 2.5-5 mg/day; may add another antihypertensive if 5 mg is not adequate after a trial of 8-12 weeks of therapy

Dosage Forms

Tablet: 5 mg

methylacetoxyprogesterone *see* medroxyprogesterone *on page 620*

methylcellulose (meth il SEL yoo lose)

Sound-Alike/Look-Alike Issues
Citrucel® may be confused with Citracal®

U.S./Canadian Brand Names Citrucel® Fiber Shake [US-OTC]; Citrucel® Fiber Smoothie [US-OTC]; Citrucel® [US-OTC]; Soluble Fiber Therapy [US-OTC]

Therapeutic Category Laxative

Use Adjunct in treatment of constipation

Usual Dosage Oral:

Children 6-12 years:

Citrucel® caplet: 1 caplet up to 6 times/day; follow each dose with 8 oz of water

Citrucel® powder: Half the adult dose in 4 oz of cold water, 1-3 times/day

Children ≥12 years and Adults:

Citrucel® caplet: 2-4 caplets 1-3 times/day; follow each dose with 8 oz of water

Citrucel® powder: 1 heaping tablespoon (19 g) in 8 oz of cold water, 1-3 times/day

Dosage Forms

Caplet, oral:

Citrucel® [OTC]: 500 mg

Powder, oral: 2 g/level scoop (454 g)

Citrucel® Fiber Shake [OTC]: 2 g/level scoop (204 g, 413 g)

Citrucel® [OTC]: 2 g/level scoop (448 g, 840 g, 1418 g, 1843 g)

Soluble Fiber Therapy [OTC]: 2 g/level scoop (454 g)

Powder, oral [clear mix formula]:

Citrucel® Fiber Smoothie [OTC]: 2 g/level scoop (275 g, 539 g, 1021 g)

Powder, oral [sugar-free formulation]:

Citrucel® [OTC]: 2 g/level scoop (473 g, 907 g, 1190 g)

methylcellulose, gelatin, and pectin *see* gelatin, pectin, and methylcellulose *on page 457*

methylcobalamin, acetylcysteine, and methylfolate *see* methylfolate, methylcobalamin, and acetylcysteine *on page 644*

methyldopa (meth il DOE pa)

Sound-Alike/Look-Alike Issues

methyldopa may be confused with L-dopa, levodopa

Synonyms methyldopate hydrochloride

U.S./Canadian Brand Names Apo-Methyldopa® [Can]; Nu-Medopa [Can]

Therapeutic Category Alpha-Adrenergic Blocking Agent

Use Management of moderate-to-severe hypertension

Usual Dosage

Children:

Oral: Initial: 10 mg/kg/day in 2-4 divided doses; increase every 2 days as needed to maximum dose of 65 mg/kg/day; do not exceed 3 g/day.

I.V.: 5-10 mg/kg/dose every 6-8 hours up to a total dose of 65 mg/kg/24 hours or 3 g/24 hours

Adults:

Oral: Initial: 250 mg 2-3 times/day; increase every 2 days as needed (maximum dose: 3 g/day): usual dose range (JNC 7): 250-1000 mg/day in 2 divided doses

I.V.: 250-500 mg every 6-8 hours; maximum dose: 1 g every 6 hours

Dosage Forms

Injection, solution: 50 mg/mL (5 mL)

Tablet: 250 mg, 500 mg

methyldopa and hydrochlorothiazide (meth il DOE pa & hye droe klor oh THYE a zide)

Sound-Alike/Look-Alike Issues

Aldoril® may be confused with Aldoclor®, Aldomet®, Elavil®

Synonyms hydrochlorothiazide and methyldopa

U.S./Canadian Brand Names Apo-Methazide® [Can]

Therapeutic Category Antihypertensive Agent, Combination

Use Management of moderate-to-severe hypertension

Usual Dosage Oral: Dosage titrated on individual components, then switch to combination product; no more than methyldopa 3 g/day and/or hydrochlorothiazide 50 mg/day; maintain initial dose for first 48 hours, then decrease or increase at intervals of not less than 2 days until an adequate response is achieved

Methyldopa 250 mg and hydrochlorothiazide 15 mg: 2-3 times/day

Methyldopa 250 mg and hydrochlorothiazide 25 mg: Twice daily

Dosage Forms

Tablet: Methyldopa 250 mg and hydrochlorothiazide 15 mg; methyldopa 250 mg and hydrochlorothiazide 25 mg

methyldopate hydrochloride *see* methyldopa *on page 643*

methylene blue (METH i leen bloo)

Therapeutic Category Antidote

Use Antidote for cyanide poisoning and drug-induced methemoglobinemia, indicator dye

Usual Dosage

Children and Adults: Methemoglobinemia: I.V.: 1-2 mg/kg or 25-50 mg/m^2 over several minutes; may be repeated in 1 hour if necessary

Adults: Genitourinary antiseptic: Oral: 65-130 mg 3 times/day with a full glass of water (maximum: 390 mg/day)

Dosage Forms

Injection, solution: 10 mg/mL (1 mL, 10 mL)

methylene blue, methenamine, benzoic acid, phenyl salicylate, and hyoscyamine *see* methenamine, phenyl salicylate, methylene blue, benzoic acid, and hyoscyamine *on page 637*

methylergometrine maleate *see* methylergonovine *on page 644*

methylergonovine (meth il er goe NOE veen)

Sound-Alike/Look-Alike Issues

methylergonovine and terbutaline parenteral dosage forms look similar. Due to their contrasting indications, use care when administering these agents.

Methergine® may be confused with Brethine

Synonyms methylergometrine maleate; methylergonovine maleate

U.S./Canadian Brand Names Methergine® [US/Can]

Therapeutic Category Ergot Alkaloid and Derivative

Use Prevention and treatment of postpartum and postabortion hemorrhage caused by uterine atony or subinvolution

Usual Dosage Adults:

Oral: 0.2 mg 3-4 times/day in the puerperium for 2-7 days

I.M., I.V.: 0.2 mg after delivery of anterior shoulder, after delivery of placenta, or during puerperium; may be repeated as required at intervals of 2-4 hours

Dosage Forms

Injection, solution:

Methergine®: 0.2 mg/mL (1 mL)

Tablet:

Methergine®: 0.2 mg

methylergonovine maleate *see* methylergonovine *on page 644*

methylfolate (meth il FO late)

Synonyms 6(S)-5-methyltetrahydrofolate; 6(S)-5-MTHF; L-methylfolate

U.S./Canadian Brand Names Deplin™ [US]

Therapeutic Category Dietary Supplement

Use Medicinal food for management of patients with low plasma and/or low red blood cell folate

Usual Dosage Oral: Adults: One tablet (7.5 mg) daily

Dosage Forms

Tablet:

Deplin™: L-methylfolate 7.5 mg [gluten free, lactose free, sugar free, yeast free]

methylfolate, methylcobalamin, and acetylcysteine

(meth il FO late meth il koe BAL a min & a se teel SIS teen)

Synonyms acetylcysteine, methylcobalamin, and methylfolate; acetylcysteine, methylfolate, and methylcobalamin; L-methylfolate, methylcobalamin, and N-acetylcysteine; methylcobalamin, acetylcysteine, and methylfolate

U.S./Canadian Brand Names Cerefolin® NAC [US]

Therapeutic Category Dietary Supplement

Use Medicinal food for use in patients with neurovascular oxidative stress and/or hyperhomocysteinemia

Usual Dosage Oral: Children ≥12 years and Adults: One caplet daily

Dosage Forms

Caplet, oral:

Cerefolin® NAC: L-methylfolate 5.6 mg, methylcobalamin 2 mg, and N-acetylcysteine 600 mg [gluten free, sugar free]

Methylin® [US] *see* methylphenidate *on page 645*

Methylin® ER [US] *see* methylphenidate *on page 645*

methylmorphine *see* codeine *on page 252*

methylnaltrexone (meth il nal TREKS one)

Sound-Alike/Look-Alike Issues

methylnaltrexone may be confused with naltrexone

Synonyms methylnaltrexone bromide; N-methylnaltrexone bromide

U.S./Canadian Brand Names Relistor™ [US/Can]

Therapeutic Category Gastrointestinal Agent, Miscellaneous; Opioid Antagonist, Peripherally-Acting

Use Treatment of opioid-induced constipation in patients with advanced illness receiving palliative care with inadequate response to conventional laxative regimens

Usual Dosage SubQ: Adults: Opioid-induced constipation: Dosing is according to body weight: Administer 1 dose every other day as needed; maximum: 1 dose/24 hours

<38 kg: 0.15 mg/kg (round dose up to nearest 0.1 mL of volume)

38 to <62 kg: 8 mg

62-114 kg: 12 mg

>114 kg: 0.15 mg/kg (round dose up to nearest 0.1 mL of volume)

Dosage Forms

Injection, solution:

Relistor™: 12 mg/0.6 mL (0.6 mL) [contains edetate calcium disodium]

methylnaltrexone bromide *see* methylnaltrexone *on page 645*

methylphenidate (meth il FEN i date)

Sound-Alike/Look-Alike Issues

methylphenidate may be confused with methadone

Metadate CD® may be confused with Metadate® ER

Metadate® ER may be confused with Metadate CD®, methadone

Ritalin® may be confused with Ismelin®, Rifadin®, ritodrine

Ritalin LA® may be confused with Ritalin-SR®

Ritalin-SR® may be confused with Ritalin LA®

Synonyms methylphenidate hydrochloride

U.S./Canadian Brand Names Apo-Methylphenidate® SR [Can]; Apo-Methylphenidate® [Can]; Biphentin® [Can]; Concerta® [US/Can]; Daytrana™ [US]; Metadate CD® [US]; Metadate® ER [US]; Methylin® ER [US]; Methylin® [US]; PHL-Methylphenidate [Can]; PMS-Methylphenidate [Can]; ratio-Methylphenidate [Can]; Ritalin LA® [US]; Ritalin-SR® [US/Can]; Ritalin® [US/Can]; Sandoz® Methylphenidate SR [Can]

Therapeutic Category Central Nervous System Stimulant, Nonamphetamine

Controlled Substance C-II

Use Treatment of attention-deficit/hyperactivity disorder (ADHD); symptomatic management of narcolepsy

Usual Dosage

ADHD:

Oral:

Immediate release products Children ≥6 years and Adults: Initial: 5 mg/dose (~0.3 mg/kg/dose) given twice daily before breakfast and lunch; increase by 5-10 mg/day (0.2 mg/kg/day) at weekly intervals; maximum dose: 60 mg/day (2 mg/kg/day). **Note:** Discontinue periodically to reevaluate or if no improvement occurs within 1 month.

Extended release products:

Children ≥6 years and Adults:

Metadate® ER, Methylin® ER, Ritalin® SR: May be given in place of immediate release products, once the daily dose is titrated and the titrated 8-hour dosage corresponds to sustained or extended release tablet size; maximum: 60 mg/day

Metadate CD®, Ritalin LA®: Initial: 20 mg once daily; may be adjusted in 10-20 mg increments at weekly intervals; maximum: 60 mg/day

Children 6-12 years and Adolescents 13-17 years: *Concerta®:*

Patients not currently taking methylphenidate: Initial dose: 18 mg once daily in the morning

Patients currently taking methylphenidate: **Note:** Initial dose: Dosing based on current regimen and clinical judgment; suggested dosing listed below:

- Patients taking methylphenidate 5 mg 2-3 times/day: 18 mg once every morning
- Patients taking methylphenidate 10 mg 2-3 times/day: 36 mg once every morning
- Patients taking methylphenidate 15 mg 2-3 times/day: 54 mg once every morning

Dose adjustment: May increase dose in increments of 18 mg; dose may be adjusted at weekly intervals. A dosage strength of 27 mg is available for situations in which a dosage between 18-36 mg is desired. Maximum dose should not exceed 2 mg/kg/day **or** 54 mg/day in children 6-12 years or 72 mg/day in children 13-17 years.

Adults: *Concerta®:*

Patients not currently taking methylphenidate: Initial dose: 18-36 mg once daily in the morning

Patients currently taking methylphenidate: **Note:** Initial dose: Dosing based on current regimen and clinical judgment; suggested dosing listed below:

- Patients taking methylphenidate 5 mg 2-3 times/day: 18 mg once every morning
- Patients taking methylphenidate 10 mg 2-3 times/day: 36 mg once every morning
- Patients taking methylphenidate 15 mg 2-3 times/day: 54 mg once every morning
- Patients taking methylphenidate 20 mg 2-3 times/day: 72 mg once every morning

Dose adjustment: May increase dose in increments of 18 mg; dose may be adjusted at weekly intervals. A dosage strength of 27 mg is available for situations in which a dosage between 18-36 mg is desired. Maximum dose should not exceed 72 mg/day.

Transdermal (Daytrana™): Children ≥6 years: Initial: 10 mg patch once daily; remove up to 9 hours after application. Titrate based on response and tolerability; may increase to next transdermal dose no more frequently than every week. **Note:** Application should occur 2 hours prior to desired effect. Drug absorption may continue for a period of time after patch removal; patients converting from another formulation of methylphenidate should be initiated at 10 mg regardless of their previous dose and titrated as needed due to the differences in bioavailability of the transdermal formulation.

Narcolepsy: Oral: Adults: 10 mg 2-3 times/day, up to 60 mg/day

Dosage Forms

Capsule, extended release, oral, [bi-modal release]:

Metadate CD®: 10 mg [3 mg immediate release, 7 mg extended release]; 20 mg [6 mg immediate release, 14 mg extended release]; 30 mg [9 mg immediate release, 21 mg extended release]; 40 mg [12 mg immediate release, 28 mg extended release]; 50 mg [15 mg immediate release, 35 mg extended release]; 60 mg [18 mg immediate release, 42 mg extended release]

Ritalin LA®: 10 mg [5 mg immediate release, 5 mg extended release]; 20 mg [10 mg immediate release, 10 mg extended release]; 30 mg [15 mg immediate release, 15 mg extended release]; 40 mg [20 mg immediate release, 20 mg extended release]

Solution, oral:

Methylin®: 5 mg/5 mL, 10 mg/5 mL

Tablet: 5 mg, 10 mg, 20 mg

Methylin®, Ritalin®: 5 mg, 10 mg, 20 mg

Tablet, chewable:

Methylin®: 2.5 mg, 5 mg, 10 mg

Tablet, extended release:

Metadate® ER: 20 mg

Methylin® ER: 10 mg, 20 mg

Tablet, extended release [bi-modal release]:

Concerta®: 18 mg, 27 mg, 36 mg, 54 mg

Tablet, sustained release: 20 mg

Ritalin-SR®: 20 mg

Transdermal system [once-daily patch]:

Daytrana™: 10 mg/9 hours (30s); 15 mg/9 hours (30s); 20 mg/9 hours (30s); 30 mg/9 hours (30s)

methylphenidate hydrochloride *see* methylphenidate *on page* 645

methylphenobarbital *see* mephobarbital *on page* 627

methylphenoxy-benzene propanamine *see* atomoxetine *on page* 108

methylphenyl isoxazolyl penicillin *see* oxacillin *on page* 732

methylphytyl napthoquinone *see* phytonadione *on page* 782

methylprednisolone (meth il pred NIS oh lone)

Sound-Alike/Look-Alike Issues
methylPREDNISolone may be confused with medroxyPROGESTERone, predniSONE
Depo-Medrol® may be confused with Solu-Medrol®
Medrol® may be confused with Mebaral®
Solu-Medrol® may be confused with Depo-Medrol®, salmeterol, Solu-Cortef®

Synonyms 6-α-methylprednisolone; A-methapred; medrol dose pack; methylprednisolone acetate; methylprednisolone sodium succinate; solumedrol

Tall-Man methyl**PREDNIS**olone

U.S./Canadian Brand Names A-Methapred® [US]; Depo-Medrol® [US/Can]; Medrol® [US/Can]; Methylprednisolone Acetate [Can]; Solu-Medrol® [US/Can]

Therapeutic Category Adrenal Corticosteroid

Use Primarily as an antiinflammatory or immunosuppressant agent in the treatment of a variety of diseases including those of hematologic, allergic, inflammatory, neoplastic, and autoimmune origin. Prevention and treatment of graft-versus-host disease following allogeneic bone marrow transplantation.

Usual Dosage Dosing should be based on the lesser of ideal body weight or actual body weight

Only sodium succinate may be given I.V.; methylprednisolone sodium succinate is highly soluble and has a rapid effect by I.M. and I.V. routes. Methylprednisolone acetate has a low solubility and has a sustained I.M. effect.

Children:

Acute spinal cord injury: I.V. (sodium succinate): 30 mg/kg over 15 minutes, followed in 45 minutes by a continuous infusion of 5.4 mg/kg/hour for 23 hours

Antiinflammatory or immunosuppressive: Oral, I.M., I.V. (sodium succinate): 0.5-1.7 mg/kg/day **or** 5-25 mg/m^2/day in divided doses every 6-12 hours; "Pulse" therapy: 15-30 mg/kg/dose over ≥30 minutes given once daily for 3 days

Asthma exacerbations, including status asthmaticus (emergency medical care or hospital doses): Children <12 years: Oral, I.V.: 1-2 mg/kg/day in 2 divided doses (maximum: 60 mg/day) until peak expiratory flow is 70% of predicted or personal best

Lupus nephritis: I.V. (sodium succinate): 30 mg/kg over ≥30 minutes every other day for 6 doses

Status asthmaticus: I.V. (sodium succinate): Previous NAEPP guidelines still encountered in clinical practice: Loading dose: 2 mg/kg/dose, then 0.5-1 mg/kg/dose every 6 hours for up to 5 days; **Note:** See new dosing guidelines for asthma exacerbations above.

Adults: **Only sodium succinate may be given I.V.;** methylprednisolone sodium succinate is highly soluble and has a rapid effect by I.M. and I.V. routes. Methylprednisolone acetate has a low solubility and has a sustained I.M. effect.

Acute spinal cord injury: I.V. (sodium succinate): 30 mg/kg over 15 minutes, followed in 45 minutes by a continuous infusion of 5.4 mg/kg/hour for 23 hours

Allergic conditions: Oral: Tapered-dosage schedule:

Day 1: 24 mg on day 1 administered as 8 mg before breakfast, 4 mg after lunch, 4 mg after supper, and 8 mg at bedtime **OR** 24 mg as a single dose or divided into 2 or 3 doses upon initiation (regardless of time of day)

Day 2: 20 mg on day 2 administered as 4 mg before breakfast, 4 mg after lunch, 4 mg after supper, and 8 mg at bedtime

Day 3: 16 mg on day 3 administered as 4 mg before breakfast, 4 mg after lunch, 4 mg after supper, and 4 mg at bedtime

Day 4: 12 mg on day 4 administered as 4 mg before breakfast, 4 mg after lunch, and 4 mg at bedtime

Day 5: 8 mg on day 5 administered as 4 mg before breakfast and 4 mg at bedtime

Day 6: 4 mg on day 6 administered as 4 mg before breakfast

Antiinflammatory or immunosuppressive:

Oral: 2-60 mg/day in 1-4 divided doses to start, followed by gradual reduction in dosage to the lowest possible level consistent with maintaining an adequate clinical response.

I.M. (sodium succinate): 10-80 mg/day once daily

I.M. (acetate): 10-80 mg every 1-2 weeks

I.V. (sodium succinate): 10-40 mg over a period of several minutes and repeated I.V. or I.M. at intervals depending on clinical response; when high dosages are needed, give 30 mg/kg over a period ≥30 minutes and may be repeated every 4-6 hours for 48 hours.

Dermatitis, acute severe: I.M. (acetate): 80-120 mg as a single dose

Dermatitis, chronic: I.M. (acetate): 40-120 mg every 5-10 days

Status asthmaticus: I.V. (sodium succinate): Loading dose: 2 mg/kg/dose, then 0.5-1 mg/kg/dose every 6 hours for up to 5 days

Lupus nephritis: High-dose "pulse" therapy: I.V. (sodium succinate): 1 g/day for 3 days

Aplastic anemia: I.V. (sodium succinate): 1 mg/kg/day or 40 mg/day (whichever dose is higher), for 4 days. After 4 days, change to oral and continue until day 10 or until symptoms of serum sickness resolve, then rapidly reduce over approximately 2 weeks.

Pneumocystis pneumonia in AIDS patients: I.V.: 30 mg twice daily for 5 days, then 30 mg once daily for 5 days, then 15 mg once daily for 11 days

Intraarticular (acetate): Administer every 1-5 weeks.
- Large joints: 20-80 mg
- Small joints: 4-10 mg

Intralesional (acetate): 20-60 mg every 1-5 weeks

Dosage Forms

Injection, powder for reconstitution: 40 mg, 125 mg, 500 mg, 1 g
- A-Methapred®: 40 mg, 125 mg
- Solu-Medrol®: 40 mg, 125 mg, 500 mg, 1 g, 2 g
- Solu-Medrol®: 500 mg, 1 g

Injection, suspension: 40 mg/mL (1 mL, 5 mL, 10 mL); 80 mg/mL (1 mL, 5 mL)
- Depo-Medrol®: 20 mg/mL (5 mL); 40 mg/mL (5 mL, 10 mL); 80 mg/mL (5 mL)
- Depo-Medrol®: 40 mg/mL (1 mL); 80 mg/mL (1 mL)

Tablet, oral: 4 mg
- Medrol®: 2 mg, 4 mg, 8 mg, 16 mg, 32 mg

Tablet, oral [dose-pack]: 4 mg (21s)
- Medrol® Dosepak™: 4 mg (21s)

6-α-methylprednisolone *see* methylprednisolone *on page 647*

Methylprednisolone Acetate [Can] *see* methylprednisolone *on page 647*

methylprednisolone acetate *see* methylprednisolone *on page 647*

methylprednisolone sodium succinate *see* methylprednisolone *on page 647*

4-methylpyrazole *see* fomepizole *on page 442*

methyltestosterone (meth il tes TOS te rone)

Sound-Alike/Look-Alike Issues

methylTESTOSTERone may be confused with medroxyPROGESTERone

Virilon® may be confused with Verelan®

Tall-Man methyl**TESTOSTER**one

U.S./Canadian Brand Names Android® [US]; Methitest™ [US]; Testred® [US]; Virilon® [US]

Therapeutic Category Androgen

Controlled Substance C-III

Use

Male: Hypogonadism; delayed puberty; impotence and climacteric symptoms

Female: Palliative treatment of metastatic breast cancer

Usual Dosage Adults (buccal absorption produces twice the androgenic activity of oral tablets):

Male:
- Hypogonadism, male climacteric and impotence: Oral: 10-40 mg/day
- Androgen deficiency:
  - Oral: 10-50 mg/day
  - Buccal: 5-25 mg/day
- Postpubertal cryptorchidism: Oral: 30 mg/day

Female:
- Breast pain/engorgement:
  - Oral: 80 mg/day for 3-5 days
  - Buccal: 40 mg/day for 3-5 days
- Breast cancer:
  - Oral: 50-200 mg/day
  - Buccal: 25-100 mg/day

Dosage Forms

Capsule:
- Android®, Testred®, Virilon®: 10 mg

Tablet:
- Methitest™: 10 mg

Meticorten® ***(Discontinued)*** *see* prednisone *on page 814*

Metimyd Ophthalmic Ointment ***(Discontinued)***

metipranolol (met i PRAN oh lol)

Sound-Alike/Look-Alike Issues

metipranolol may be confused with metaproterenol

Synonyms metipranolol hydrochloride

U.S./Canadian Brand Names OptiPranolol® [US/Can]

Therapeutic Category Beta-Adrenergic Blocker

Use Agent for lowering intraocular pressure in patients with chronic open-angle glaucoma

Usual Dosage Ophthalmic: Adults: Instill 1 drop in the affected eye(s) twice daily

Dosage Forms

Solution, ophthalmic: 0.3% (5 mL, 10 mL)

OptiPranolol®: 0.3% (5 mL, 10 mL)

metipranolol hydrochloride *see* metipranolol *on page* 649

metoclopramide (met oh KLOE pra mide)

Sound-Alike/Look-Alike Issues

metoclopramide may be confused with metolazone

Reglan® may be confused with Megace®, Regonol®, Renagel®

U.S./Canadian Brand Names Apo-Metoclop® [Can]; Metoclopramide Hydrochloride Injection [Can]; Metoclopramide Omega [Can]; Nu-Metoclopramide [Can]; PMS-Metoclopramide [Can]; Reglan® [US]

Therapeutic Category Gastrointestinal Agent, Prokinetic

Use

Oral: Symptomatic treatment of diabetic gastroparesis; gastroesophageal reflux

I.V., I.M.: Symptomatic treatment of diabetic gastroparesis; postpyloric placement of enteral feeding tubes; prevention and/or treatment of nausea and vomiting associated with chemotherapy, or postsurgery; to stimulate gastric emptying and intestinal transit of barium during radiological examination of the stomach/small intestine

Usual Dosage

Children:

Postpyloric feeding tube placement: I.V.:

<6 years: 0.1 mg/kg

6-14 years: 2.5-5 mg

>14 years: Refer to adult dosing.

Adults:

Gastroesophageal reflux: Oral: 10-15 mg/dose up to 4 times/day 30 minutes before meals or food and at bedtime; single doses of 20 mg are occasionally needed for provoking situations. Treatment >12 weeks has not been evaluated.

Diabetic gastric stasis:

Oral: 10 mg 30 minutes before each meal and at bedtime

I.M., I.V. (for severe symptoms): 10 mg over 1-2 minutes; 10 days of I.V. therapy may be necessary for best response

Chemotherapy-induced emesis:

I.V.: 1-2 mg/kg 30 minutes before chemotherapy and repeated every 2 hours for 2 doses, then every 3 hours for 3 doses (manufacturer labeling)

Alternate dosing (with or without diphenhydramine):

Moderate emetic risk chemotherapy: 0.5 mg/kg every 6 hours on days 2-4

Low and minimal risk chemotherapy: 1-2 mg/kg every 3-4 hours

Breakthrough treatment: 1-2 mg/kg every 3-4 hours

Postoperative nausea and vomiting: I.M., I.V.: 10-20 mg near end of surgery

Postpyloric feeding tube placement, radiological exam: I.V.: 10 mg

Dosage Forms

Injection, solution [preservative free]: 5 mg/mL (2 mL)

Reglan®: 5 mg/mL (2 mL, 10 mL, 30 mL)

Solution, oral: 5 mg/5 mL (10 mL, 480 mL)

Tablet: 5 mg, 10 mg

Reglan®: 5 mg, 10 mg

Metoclopramide Hydrochloride Injection [Can] *see* metoclopramide *on page* 649

Metoclopramide Omega [Can] *see* metoclopramide *on page* 649

metolazone (me TOLE a zone)

Sound-Alike/Look-Alike Issues

metolazone may be confused with metaxalone, methazolamide, methimazole, methotrexate, metoclopramide, metoprolol, minoxidil

Zaroxolyn® may be confused with Zarontin®

U.S./Canadian Brand Names Zaroxolyn® [US/Can]

Therapeutic Category Diuretic, Miscellaneous

Use Management of mild-to-moderate hypertension; treatment of edema in heart failure and nephrotic syndrome, impaired renal function

Usual Dosage Oral: Adults:

Edema: Initial: 2.5-10 mg once daily; may increase as necessary to 20 mg once daily

Hypertension: 2.5-5 mg/dose every 24 hours

Dosage Forms

Tablet: 2.5 mg, 5 mg, 10 mg

Zaroxolyn®: 2.5 mg, 5 mg

Metopirone® [US] *see* metyrapone *on page* 653

metoprolol (me toe PROE lole)

Sound-Alike/Look-Alike Issues

metoprolol may be confused with metaproterenol, metolazone, misoprostol

Lopressor® may be confused with Lyrica®

Toprol-XL® may be confused with Tegretol®, Tegretol®-XR, Topamax®

Synonyms metoprolol succinate; metoprolol tartrate

U.S./Canadian Brand Names Apo-Metoprolol® [Can]; Betaloc® Durules® [Can]; Betaloc® [Can]; Dom-Metoprolol [Can]; Gen-Metoprolol [Can]; Lopressor® [US/Can]; Metoprolol Tartrate Injection, USP [Can]; Metoprolol-25 [Can]; Novo-Metoprolol [Can]; Nu-Metop [Can]; PHL-Metoprolol [Can]; PMS-Metoprolol [Can]; Riva-Metoprolol [Can]; Sandoz-Metoprolol [Can]; Toprol-XL® [US/Can]

Therapeutic Category Beta-Adrenergic Blocker

Use Treatment of angina pectoris, hypertension, or hemodynamically-stable acute myocardial infarction

Extended release: Treatment of angina pectoris or hypertension; to reduce mortality/hospitalization in patients with heart failure (stable NYHA Class II or III) already receiving ACE inhibitors, diuretics, and/or digoxin

Usual Dosage

Children: Hypertension: Oral:

1-17 years: Immediate release tablet: (National High Blood Pressure Education Program Working Group on High Blood Pressure in Children and Adolescents, 2004): Initial: 1-2 mg/kg/day; maximum 6 mg/kg/day (≤200 mg/day); administer in 2 divided doses

≥6 years: Extended release tablet: Initial: 1 mg/kg once daily (maximum initial dose: 50 mg/day). Adjust dose based on patient response (maximum: 2 mg/kg/day or 200 mg/day)

Adults:

Angina: Oral:

Immediate release: Initial: 50 mg twice daily; usual dosage range: 50-200 mg twice daily; maximum: 400 mg/day; increase dose at weekly intervals to desired effect

Extended release: Initial: 100 mg/day (maximum: 400 mg/day)

Maintenance: Oral (immediate release): 25-100 mg twice daily

Heart failure: Oral (extended release): Initial: 25 mg once daily (reduce to 12.5 mg once daily in NYHA class higher than class II); may double dosage every 2 weeks as tolerated (maximum: 200 mg/day)

Hypertension: Oral:

Immediate release: Initial: 50 mg twice daily; effective dosage range: 100-450 mg/day in 2-3 divided doses; increase dose at weekly intervals to desired effect; maximum: 450 mg/day; usual dosage range (JNC 7): 50-100 mg/day

Extended release: Initial: 25-100 mg once daily; increase doses at weekly (or longer) intervals to desired effect; maximum: 400 mg/day; usual dosage range (JNC 7): 50-100 mg/day

Hypertension/ventricular rate control: I.V. (in patients having nonfunctioning GI tract): Initial: 1.25-5 mg every 6-12 hours; titrate initial dose to response. Initially, low doses may be appropriate to establish response; however, up to 15 mg every 3-6 hours has been employed.

Myocardial infarction:

Acute: I.V.: 5 mg every 2 minutes for 3 doses in early treatment of myocardial infarction; thereafter, give 50 mg orally every 6 hours beginning 15 minutes after last I.V. dose and continue for 48 hours; then administer a maintenance dose of 100 mg twice daily. **Note:** If initial I.V. dosing is not tolerated, may give 25-50 mg orally (depending on degree of intolerance) every 6 hours beginning 15 minutes after the last I.V. dose or as soon as clinical condition permits.

Note: Switching dosage forms:

When switching from immediate release metoprolol to extended release, the same total daily dose of metoprolol should be used.

When switching between oral and intravenous dosage forms, equivalent beta-blocking effect is achieved when doses in a 2.5:1 (Oral:I.V.) ratio is used.

Dosage Forms

Injection, solution: 1 mg/mL (5 mL)

Lopressor®: 1 mg/mL (5 mL)

Tablet: 25 mg, 50 mg, 100 mg

Lopressor®: 50 mg, 100 mg

Tablet, extended release: 25 mg, 50 mg, 100 mg, 200 mg

Toprol-XL®: 25 mg, 50 mg, 100 mg, 200 mg

Metoprolol-25 [Can] *see* metoprolol *on page 650*

metoprolol and hydrochlorothiazide (me toe PROE lole & hye droe klor oh THYE a zide)

Synonyms hydrochlorothiazide and metoprolol; hydrochlorothiazide and metoprolol tartrate; metoprolol tartrate and hydrochlorothiazide

U.S./Canadian Brand Names Lopressor HCT® [US]

Therapeutic Category Beta Blocker, $Beta_1$ Selective; Diuretic, Thiazide

Use Treatment of hypertension (not recommended for initial treatment)

Usual Dosage Oral: Adults: Hypertension: Dosage should be determined by titration of the individual agents and the combination product substituted based upon the daily requirements.

Usual dose: Metoprolol 50-100 mg and hydrochlorothiazide 25-50 mg administered daily as single or divided doses (twice daily)

Note: Hydrochlorothiazide >50 mg/day is not recommended.

Concomitant therapy: It is recommended that if an additional antihypertensive agent is required, gradual titration should occur using 1/2 the usual starting dose of the other agent to avoid hypotension.

Dosage Forms

Tablet: 50/25: Metoprolol 50 mg and hydrochlorothiazide 25 mg; 100/25: Metoprolol 100 mg and hydrochlorothiazide 25 mg; 100/50: Metoprolol 100 mg and hydrochlorothiazide 50 mg

Lopressor HCT®: 50/25: Metoprolol 50 mg and hydrochlorothiazide 25 mg; 100/25: Metoprolol 100 mg and hydrochlorothiazide 25 mg; 100/50: Metoprolol 100 mg and hydrochlorothiazide 50 mg

metoprolol succinate *see* metoprolol *on page 650*

metoprolol tartrate *see* metoprolol *on page 650*

metoprolol tartrate and hydrochlorothiazide *see* metoprolol and hydrochlorothiazide *on page 651*

Metoprolol Tartrate Injection, USP [Can] *see* metoprolol *on page 650*

Metreton® ***(Discontinued)***

MetroCream® [US/Can] *see* metronidazole *on page 651*

MetroGel® [US/Can] *see* metronidazole *on page 651*

MetroGel-Vaginal® [US] *see* metronidazole *on page 651*

Metro I.V.® Injection ***(Discontinued)*** *see* metronidazole *on page 651*

MetroLotion® [US] *see* metronidazole *on page 651*

metronidazole (met roe NYE da zole)

Sound-Alike/Look-Alike Issues

metroNIDAZOLE may be confused with meropenem, metFORMIN

Synonyms metronidazole hydrochloride

Tall-Man metro**NIDAZOLE**

U.S./Canadian Brand Names Apo-Metronidazole® [Can]; Flagyl ER® [US]; Flagyl® 375 [US]; Flagyl® [US/Can]; Florazole® ER [Can]; MetroCream® [US/Can]; MetroGel-Vaginal® [US]; MetroGel® [US/Can]; MetroLotion® [US]; Nidagel™ [Can]; Noritate® [US/Can]; Trikacide [Can]; Vandazole® [US]

Therapeutic Category Amebicide; Antibiotic, Miscellaneous; Antibiotic, Topical; Antiprotozoal

Use Treatment of susceptible anaerobic bacterial and protozoal infections in the following conditions: Amebiasis, symptomatic and asymptomatic trichomoniasis; skin and skin structure infections; CNS infections; intraabdominal infections (as part of combination regimen); systemic anaerobic infections; treatment of antibiotic-associated pseudomembranous colitis (AAPC), bacterial vaginosis; as part of a multidrug regimen for *H. pylori* eradication to reduce the risk of duodenal ulcer recurrence

Topical: Treatment of inflammatory lesions and erythema of rosacea

Usual Dosage

Infants and Children:

Amebiasis: Oral: 35-50 mg/kg/day in divided doses every 8 hours for 10 days

Trichomoniasis: Oral: 15-30 mg/kg/day in divided doses every 8 hours for 7 days

Anaerobic infections:

Oral: 15-35 mg/kg/day in divided doses every 8 hours

I.V.: 30 mg/kg/day in divided doses every 6 hours

Clostridium difficile (antibiotic-associated colitis): Oral: 20 mg/kg/day divided every 6 hours

Maximum dose: 2 g/day

Adults:

Anaerobic infections (diverticulitis, intraabdominal, peritonitis, cholangitis, or abscess): Oral, I.V.: 500 mg every 6-8 hours, not to exceed 4 g/day

Acne rosacea: Topical:

0.75%: Apply and rub a thin film twice daily, morning and evening, to entire affected areas after washing. Significant therapeutic results should be noticed within 3 weeks. Clinical studies have demonstrated continuing improvement through 9 weeks of therapy.

1%: Apply thin film to affected area once daily

Amebiasis: Oral: 500-750 mg every 8 hours for 5-10 days

Antibiotic-associated pseudomembranous colitis: Oral: 250-500 mg 3-4 times/day for 10-14 days

Note: Due to the emergence of a new strain of *C. difficile*, some clinicians recommend converting to oral vancomycin therapy if the patient does not show a clear clinical response after 2 days of metronidazole therapy.

Giardiasis: 500 mg twice daily for 5-7 days

Helicobacter pylori eradication: Oral: 250-500 mg with meals and at bedtime for 14 days; requires combination therapy with at least one other antibiotic and an acid-suppressing agent (proton pump inhibitor or H_2 blocker)

Bacterial vaginosis or vaginitis due to *Gardnerella*, *Mobiluncus*:

Oral: 500 mg twice daily (regular release) or 750 mg once daily (extended release tablet) for 7 days

Vaginal: 1 applicatorful (~37.5 mg metronidazole) intravaginally once or twice daily for 5 days; apply once in morning and evening if using twice daily, if daily, use at bedtime

Trichomoniasis: Oral: 250 mg every 8 hours for 7 days **or** 375 mg twice daily for 7 days **or** 2 g as a single dose

Dosage Forms

Capsule, oral: 375 mg

Flagyl® 375: 375 mg

Cream, topical: 0.75% (45 g)

MetroCream®: 0.75% (45 g)

Noritate®: 1% (60 g)

Gel, topical: 1% (45 g)

MetroGel®: 1% (60 g)

Gel, vaginal: 0.75% (70 g)

MetroGel-Vaginal®, Vandazole®: 0.75% (70 g)

Infusion [premixed iso-osmotic sodium chloride solution]: 500 mg (100 mL)

Lotion, topical: 0.75% (60 mL)

MetroLotion®: 0.75% (60 mL)

Tablet, oral: 250 mg, 500 mg

Flagyl®: 250 mg, 500 mg

Tablet, extended release, oral:

Flagyl® ER: 750 mg

metronidazole and nystatin *(Canada only)* (met roe NYE da zole & nye STAT in)

Synonyms nystatin and metronidazole

U.S./Canadian Brand Names Flagystatin® [Can]

Therapeutic Category Antifungal Agent, Vaginal; Antiprotozoal, Nitroimidazole

Use Treatment of mixed vaginal infection due to *T. vaginalis* and *C. albicans*

Usual Dosage Intravaginal: Adults:

Vaginal tablet (ovule): Insert 1 tablet/day at bedtime for 10 consecutive days. May repeat for an additional 10 days if cure is not achieved.

Vaginal cream: Insert 1 applicatorful daily at bedtime for 10 consecutive days. May repeat for an additional 10 days if cure is not achieved.

Note: If *Trichomonas vaginalis* is not completely eliminated, oral (systemic) metronidazole (250 mg twice daily for 10 days) should be administered.

Dosage Forms [CAN] = Canadian brand name

Cream, vaginal:

Flagystatin® [CAN]: Metronidazole 500 mg and nystatin 100,000 units per applicatorful (55 g) [not available in the U.S.]

Tablet, vaginal:

Flagystatin® Ovule [CAN]: Metronidazole 500 mg and nystatin 100,000 units (10s) [not available in the U.S.]

metronidazole, bismuth subcitrate potassium, and tetracycline *see* bismuth, metronidazole, and tetracycline *on page 143*

metronidazole, bismuth subsalicylate, and tetracycline *see* bismuth, metronidazole, and tetracycline *on page 143*

metronidazole hydrochloride *see* metronidazole *on page 651*

metyrapone (me TEER a pone)

Sound-Alike/Look-Alike Issues

metyrapone may be confused with metyrosine

U.S./Canadian Brand Names Metopirone® [US]

Therapeutic Category Diagnostic Agent

Use Diagnostic test for hypothalamic-pituitary ACTH function

Usual Dosage Oral:

Children: 15 mg/kg every 4 hours for 6 doses; minimum dose: 250 mg

Adults: 750 mg every 4 hours for 6 doses

Dosage Forms

Capsule:

Metopirone®: 250 mg

metyrosine (me TYE roe seen)

Sound-Alike/Look-Alike Issues

metyrosine may be confused with metyrapone

Synonyms AMPT; OGMT

U.S./Canadian Brand Names Demser® [US/Can]

Therapeutic Category Tyrosine Hydroxylase Inhibitor

Use Short-term management of pheochromocytoma before surgery, long-term management when surgery is contraindicated or when chronic malignant pheochromocytoma exists

Usual Dosage Oral: Children >12 years and Adults: Initial: 250 mg 4 times/day, increased by 250-500 mg/day up to 4 g/day; maintenance: 2-3 g/day in 4 divided doses; for preoperative preparation, administer optimum effective dosage for 5-7 days

Dosage Forms

Capsule:

Demser®: 250 mg

Mevacor® [US/Can] *see* lovastatin *on page 602*

mevinolin *see* lovastatin *on page 602*

Mexar™ *(Discontinued)* *see* sulfacetamide *on page 927*

mexiletine (meks IL e teen)

U.S./Canadian Brand Names Novo-Mexiletine [Can]

Therapeutic Category Antiarrhythmic Agent, Class I-B

Use Management of serious ventricular arrhythmias; suppression of PVCs

Usual Dosage Oral: Adults: Initial: 200 mg every 8 hours (may load with 400 mg if necessary); adjust dose every 2-3 days; usual dose: 200-300 mg every 8 hours; maximum dose: 1.2 g/day (some patients respond to every 12-hour dosing). When switching from another antiarrhythmic, initiate a 200 mg dose 6-12 hours after stopping former agents, 3-6 hours after stopping procainamide.

Dosage Forms

Capsule: 150 mg, 200 mg, 250 mg

Mexitil® *(Discontinued)* *see* mexiletine *on page* 653

Mezavant® [Can] *see* mesalamine *on page* 631

MG 217® [US-OTC] *see* coal tar *on page* 250

MG 217® Medicated Tar [US-OTC] *see* coal tar *on page* 250

Miacalcin® [US] *see* calcitonin *on page* 167

Miacalcin® NS [Can] *see* calcitonin *on page* 167

Mi-Acid [US-OTC] *see* aluminum hydroxide, magnesium hydroxide, and simethicone *on page* 56

Mi-Acid™ Double Strength [US-OTC] *see* calcium carbonate and magnesium hydroxide *on page* 171

Mi-Acid Maximum Strength [US-OTC] *see* aluminum hydroxide, magnesium hydroxide, and simethicone *on page* 56

Micaderm® [US-OTC] *see* miconazole *on page* 654

micafungin (mi ka FUN gin)

Synonyms micafungin sodium

U.S./Canadian Brand Names Mycamine® [US/Can]

Therapeutic Category Antifungal Agent, Parenteral; Drug-induced Neuritis, Treatment Agent

Use Treatment of esophageal candidiasis; *Candida* prophylaxis in patients undergoing hematopoietic stem cell transplant (HSCT); treatment of candidemia, acute disseminated candidiasis, and other *Candida* infections (peritonitis and abscesses)

Usual Dosage I.V.: Adults:

Candidemia, acute disseminated candidiasis, and *Candida* peritonitis and abscesses: 100 mg daily; mean duration of therapy (from clinical trials) was 15 days (range: 10-47 days)

Esophageal candidiasis: 150 mg daily; mean duration of therapy (from clinical trials) was 15 days (range: 10-30 days)

Prophylaxis of *Candida* infection in hematopoietic stem cell transplantation: 50 mg daily

Dosage Forms

Injection, powder for reconstitution [preservative-free]:

Mycamine®: 50 mg, 100 mg [contains lactose]

micafungin sodium *see* micafungin *on page* 654

Micanol® [Can] *see* anthralin *on page* 80

Micardis® [US/Can] *see* telmisartan *on page* 941

Micardis® HCT [US] *see* telmisartan and hydrochlorothiazide *on page* 942

Micardis® Plus [Can] *see* telmisartan and hydrochlorothiazide *on page* 942

Micatin® [US/Can] *see* miconazole *on page* 654

miconazole (mi KON a zole)

Sound-Alike/Look-Alike Issues

miconazole may be confused with Micronase®, Micronor®

Lotrimin® may be confused with Lotrisone®, Otrivin®

Micatin® may be confused with Miacalcin®

Synonyms miconazole nitrate

U.S./Canadian Brand Names Aloe Vesta® Antifungal [US-OTC]; Baza® Antifungal [US-OTC]; Carrington Antifungal [US-OTC]; Critic-Aid® Clear AF [US-OTC]; DermaFungal [US-OTC]; Dermagran® AF [US-OTC]; Dermazole [Can]; DiabetAid™ Antifungal Foot Bath [US-OTC]; Fungoid® [US-OTC]; Lotrimin AF® [US-OTC]; Micaderm® [US-OTC]; Micatin® [US/Can]; Micozole [Can]; Micro-Guard® [US-OTC]; Miranel AF™ [US-OTC]; Mitrazol™ [US-OTC]; Monistat® 1 [US-OTC]; Monistat® 3 [US-OTC/Can]; Monistat® 7 [US-OTC]; Monistat® [Can]; Neosporin® AF [US-OTC]; Podactin Cream [US-OTC]; Secura® Antifungal Extra Thick [US-OTC]; Secura® Antifungal Greaseless [US-OTC]; Zeasorb®-AF [US-OTC]

Therapeutic Category Antifungal Agent

Use Treatment of vulvovaginal candidiasis and a variety of skin and mucous membrane fungal infections

Usual Dosage

Topical: Children and Adults: **Note:** Not for OTC use in children <2 years:
- Tinea corporis: Apply twice daily for 4 weeks
- Tinea pedis: Apply twice daily for 4 weeks
  - Effervescent tablet: Dissolve 1 tablet in ~1 gallon of water; soak feet for 15-30 minutes; pat dry
- Tinea cruris: Apply twice daily for 2 weeks

Vaginal: Children ≥12 years and Adults: Vulvovaginal candidiasis:
- Cream, 2%: Insert 1 applicatorful at bedtime for 7 days
- Cream, 4%: Insert 1 applicatorful at bedtime for 3 days
- Suppository, 100 mg: Insert 1 suppository at bedtime for 7 days
- Suppository, 200 mg: Insert 1 suppository at bedtime for 3 days
- Suppository, 1200 mg: Insert 1 suppository (a one-time dose); may be used at bedtime or during the day

Note: Many products are available as a combination pack, with a suppository for vaginal instillation and cream to relieve external symptoms. External cream may be used twice daily, as needed, for up to 7 days.

Dosage Forms

Aerosol, topical:
- Micatin® [OTC]: 2% (90 g)
- Micatin® [OTC], Neosporin® AF [OTC]: 2% (105 mL)

Aerosol, topical [powder]:
- Micatin® [OTC]: 2% (90 g)
- Neosporin® AF [OTC]: 2% (85 g)

Combination package, topical/vaginal: Cream, topical 2% (9 g); cream, vaginal 4% (3 x 5 g); cream, topical 2% (9 g); suppository, vaginal 200 mg (3s)
- Monistat® 1 [OTC], Monistat® 1 Day or Night [OTC]: Cream, topical 2% (9 g); insert, vaginal 1200 mg (1)
- Monistat® 3 [OTC]: Cream, topical 2% (9 g); insert, vaginal 200 mg (3)
- Monistat® 3 [OTC]: Cream, topical 2% (9 g); cream, vaginal 4% (25 g); cream, topical 2% (9 g); cream, vaginal 4% (3 x 5 g)
- Monistat® 7 [OTC]: Cream, topical 2% (9 g); cream, vaginal 2% (45 g); cream, topical 2% (9 g); cream, vaginal 2% (7 x 5 g)
- Monistat® 7 [OTC]: Cream, topical 2% (9 g); suppository, vaginal 100 mg (7)

Cream, topical: 2% (15 g, 30 g, 45 g)
- Baza® Antifungal [OTC]: 2% (4 g, 57 g, 142 g)
- Carrington Antifungal [OTC]: 2% (150 g)
- Micaderm® [OTC], Podactin [OTC]: 2% (30 g)
- Micatin® [OTC], Miranel AF™ [OTC], Neosporin® AF [OTC]: 2% (14 g)
- Micro-Guard® [OTC], Mitrazol™ [OTC], Secura® Antifungal Greaseless [OTC]: 2% (60 g)
- Secura® Antifungal Extra Thick [OTC]: 2% (97.5 g)

Cream, vaginal [prefilled or refillable applicator]: 2% (45 g)
- Monistat® 3 [OTC]: 4% (15 g, 25 g)
- Monistat® 7 [OTC]: 2% (45 g)

Gel, topical:
- Zeasorb®-AF [OTC]: 2% (24 g)

Ointment, topical:
- Aloe Vesta® Antifungal [OTC]: 2% (60 g, 150 g)
- Critic-Aid® Clear AF [OTC]: 2% (4 g, 57 g, 142 g)
- DermaFungal [OTC], Dermagran® AF [OTC]: 2% (120 g)

Powder, topical:
- Lotrimin AF® [OTC], Micro-Guard® [OTC]: 2% (90 g)
- Mitrazol™ [OTC]: 2% (30 g)
- Zeasorb®-AF [OTC]: 2% (70 g)

Suppository, vaginal: 100 mg (7s); 200 mg (3s)

Tablet, for solution, topical [effervescent]:
- DiabetAid™ Antifungal Foot Bath [OTC]: 2% (10s)

Tincture, topical: 2% (30 mL, 473 mL)
- Fungoid® [OTC]: 2% (30 mL, 473 mL)

miconazole and zinc oxide (mi KON a zole & zink OKS ide)

Synonyms zinc oxide and miconazole nitrate

U.S./Canadian Brand Names Vusion® [US]
Therapeutic Category Antifungal Agent, Topical
Use Adjunctive treatment of diaper dermatitis complicated by *Candida albicans* infection
Usual Dosage Topical: Children ≥4 weeks: Diaper dermatitis: Apply to affected area with each diaper change for 7 days. Treatment should continue for 7 days, even with initial improvement. Do not use for >7 days.
Dosage Forms
Ointment, topical:
Vusion®: Miconazole 0.25% and zinc oxide 15% (60 g)

miconazole nitrate *see* miconazole *on page* 654
Micozole [Can] *see* miconazole *on page* 654
MICRhoGAM® [US] *see* Rh_o(D) immune globulin *on page* 862
microfibrillar collagen hemostat *see* collagen hemostat *on page* 255
Microgestin™ [US] *see* ethinyl estradiol and norethindrone *on page* 390
Microgestin™ Fe [US] *see* ethinyl estradiol and norethindrone *on page* 390
Micro-Guard® [US-OTC] *see* miconazole *on page* 654
microK® [US] *see* potassium chloride *on page* 803
microK® 10 [US] *see* potassium chloride *on page* 803
Micro-K Extencaps® [Can] *see* potassium chloride *on page* 803
Micro-K® LS *(Discontinued)* *see* potassium chloride *on page* 803
Microlipid™ [US-OTC] *see* nutritional formula, enteral/oral *on page* 715
Micronase® *(Discontinued)* *see* glyburide *on page* 467
microNefrin® *(Discontinued)* *see* epinephrine *on page* 358
Micronor® [Can] *see* norethindrone *on page* 704
Microzide® [US] *see* hydrochlorothiazide *on page* 499
***Micrurus fulvius* antivenin** *see* antivenin *(Micrurus fulvius) on page* 87
Midamor® *(Discontinued)* *see* amiloride *on page* 61

midazolam (MID aye zoe lam)

Sound-Alike/Look-Alike Issues
Versed® may be confused with VePesid®, Vistaril®
Synonyms midazolam hydrochloride
U.S./Canadian Brand Names Apo-Midazolam® [Can]; Midazolam Injection [Can]
Therapeutic Category Benzodiazepine
Controlled Substance C-IV
Use Preoperative sedation; moderate sedation prior to diagnostic or radiographic procedures; ICU sedation (continuous infusion); induction and maintenance of general anesthesia
Usual Dosage The dose of midazolam needs to be individualized based on the patient's age, underlying diseases, and concurrent medications. Decrease dose (by ~30%) if narcotics or other CNS depressants are administered concomitantly. **Personnel and equipment needed for standard respiratory resuscitation should be immediately available during midazolam administration.**

Children <6 years may require higher doses and closer monitoring than older children; calculate dose on ideal body weight
Conscious sedation for procedures or preoperative sedation:
Oral: 0.25-0.5 mg/kg as a single dose preprocedure, up to a maximum of 20 mg; administer 30-45 minutes prior to procedure. Children <6 years or less cooperative patients may require as much as 1 mg/kg as a single dose; 0.25 mg/kg may suffice for children 6-16 years of age.
I.M.: 0.1-0.15 mg/kg 30-60 minutes before surgery or procedure; range 0.05-0.15 mg/kg; doses up to 0.5 mg/kg have been used in more anxious patients; maximum total dose: 10 mg
I.V.:
Infants <6 months: Limited information is available in nonintubated infants; dosing recommendations not clear; infants <6 months are at higher risk for airway obstruction and hypoventilation; titrate dose in small increments to desired effect; monitor carefully
Infants 6 months to Children 5 years: Initial: 0.05-0.1 mg/kg; titrate dose carefully; total dose of 0.6 mg/kg may be required; usual maximum total dose: 6 mg
Children 6-12 years: Initial: 0.025-0.05 mg/kg; titrate dose carefully; total doses of 0.4 mg/kg may be required; usual maximum total dose: 10 mg

Children 12-16 years: Dose as adults; usual maximum total dose: 10 mg

Conscious sedation during mechanical ventilation: Children: Loading dose: 0.05-0.2 mg/kg, followed by initial continuous infusion: 0.06-0.12 mg/kg/hour (1-2 mcg/kg/minute); titrate to the desired effect; usual range: 0.4-6 mcg/kg/minute

Adults:

Preoperative sedation:

I.M.: 0.07-0.08 mg/kg 30-60 minutes prior to surgery/procedure; usual dose: 5 mg; **Note:** Reduce dose in patients with COPD, high-risk patients, patients ≥60 years of age, and patients receiving other narcotics or CNS depressants

I.V.: 0.02-0.04 mg/kg; repeat every 5 minutes as needed to desired effect or up to 0.1-0.2 mg/kg

Conscious sedation: I.V.: Initial: 0.5-2 mg slow I.V. over at least 2 minutes; slowly titrate to effect by repeating doses every 2-3 minutes if needed; usual total dose: 2.5-5 mg

Healthy Adults <60 years: Some patients respond to doses as low as 1 mg; no more than 2.5 mg should be administered over a period of 2 minutes. Additional doses of midazolam may be administered after a 2-minute waiting period and evaluation of sedation after each dose increment. A total dose >5 mg is generally not needed. If narcotics or other CNS depressants are administered concomitantly, the midazolam dose should be reduced by 30%.

Anesthesia: I.V.:

Induction:

Unpremedicated patients: 0.3-0.35 mg/kg (up to 0.6 mg/kg in resistant cases)

Premedicated patients: 0.15-0.35 mg/kg

Maintenance: 0.05-0.3 mg/kg as needed, or continuous infusion 0.25-1.5 mcg/kg/minute

Sedation in mechanically-ventilated patients: I.V. continuous infusion: 100 mg in 250 mL D_5W or NS (if patient is fluid-restricted, may concentrate up to a maximum of 0.5 mg/mL); initial dose: 0.02-0.08 mg/kg (~1 mg to 5 mg in 70 kg adult) initially and repeated at 5- to 15-minute intervals until adequate sedation is achieved; may use continuous infusion to maintain sedation; usual dosage range for continuous infusion: 0.04-0.2 mg/kg/hour. Titrate to reach desired level of sedation.

Dosage Forms

Injection, solution: 1 mg/mL (2 mL, 5 mL, 10 mL); 5 mg/mL (1 mL, 2 mL, 5 mL, 10 mL)

Injection, solution [preservative free]: 1 mg/mL (2 mL, 5 mL); 5 mg/mL (1 mL, 2 mL)

Syrup: 2 mg/mL

midazolam hydrochloride *see* midazolam *on page* 656

Midazolam Injection [Can] *see* midazolam *on page* 656

midodrine (MI doe dreen)

Sound-Alike/Look-Alike Issues

midodrine may be confused with Midrin®

ProAmatine® may be confused with protamine

Synonyms midodrine hydrochloride

U.S./Canadian Brand Names Amatine® [Can]; Apo-Midodrine® [Can]; ProAmatine® [US]

Therapeutic Category Alpha-Adrenergic Agonist

Use Orphan drug: Treatment of symptomatic orthostatic hypotension

Usual Dosage Oral: Adults: 10 mg 3 times/day during daytime hours (every 3-4 hours) when patient is upright (maximum: 40 mg/day)

Dosage Forms

Tablet: 2.5 mg, 5 mg, 10 mg

ProAmatine®: 2.5 mg, 5 mg, 10 mg [scored]

midodrine hydrochloride *see* midodrine *on page* 657

Midol® Cramp and Body Aches [US-OTC] *see* ibuprofen *on page* 515

Midol® Extended Relief [US-OTC] *see* naproxen *on page* 681

Midol® Teen Formula [US-OTC] *see* acetaminophen and pamabrom *on page* 22

Midrin® [US] *see* acetaminophen, isometheptene, and dichloralphenazone *on page* 29

Mifeprex® [US] *see* mifepristone *on page* 657

mifepristone (mi FE pris tone)

Sound-Alike/Look-Alike Issues

mifepristone may be confused with misoprostol

Mifeprex® may be confused with Mirapex®

Synonyms RU-38486; RU-486

U.S./Canadian Brand Names Mifeprex® [US]

Therapeutic Category Abortifacient; Antineoplastic Agent, Hormone Antagonist; Antiprogestin

Use Medical termination of intrauterine pregnancy, through day 49 of pregnancy. Patients may need treatment with misoprostol and possibly surgery to complete therapy

Usual Dosage Oral: Adults:

Termination of pregnancy: Treatment consists of three office visits by the patient; the patient must read medication guide and sign patient agreement prior to treatment:

Day 1: 600 mg (three 200 mg tablets) taken as a single dose under physician supervision

Day 3: Patient must return to the healthcare provider 2 days following administration of mifepristone; unless abortion has occurred (confirmed using ultrasound or clinical examination): 400 mcg (two 200 mcg tablets) of misoprostol; patient may need treatment for cramps or gastrointestinal symptoms at this time

Day 14: Patient must return to the healthcare provider ~14 days after administration of mifepristone; confirm complete termination of pregnancy by ultrasound or clinical exam. Surgical termination is recommended to manage treatment failures.

Dosage Forms

Tablet:

Mifeprex®: 200 mg

Migergot [US] *see* ergotamine and caffeine *on page* 366

miglitol (MIG li tol)

Sound-Alike/Look-Alike Issues

Glyset® may be confused with Cycloset®

U.S./Canadian Brand Names Glyset® [US/Can]

Therapeutic Category Antidiabetic Agent, Oral

Use Type 2 diabetes mellitus (noninsulin-dependent, NIDDM):

Monotherapy as an adjunct to diet to improve glycemic control in patients with type 2 diabetes mellitus (noninsulin-dependent, NIDDM) whose hyperglycemia cannot be managed with diet alone

Combination therapy with a sulfonylurea when diet plus either miglitol or a sulfonylurea alone do not result in adequate glycemic control. The effect of miglitol to enhance glycemic control is additive to that of sulfonylureas when used in combination.

Usual Dosage Oral: Adults: 25 mg 3 times/day with the first bite of food at each meal; the dose may be increased to 50 mg 3 times/day after 4-8 weeks; maximum recommended dose: 100 mg 3 times/day

Dosage Forms

Tablet:

Glyset®: 25 mg, 50 mg, 100 mg

miglustat (MIG loo stat)

Synonyms OGT-918

U.S./Canadian Brand Names Zavesca® [US/Can]

Therapeutic Category Enzyme Inhibitor

Use Treatment of mild-to-moderate type 1 Gaucher disease when enzyme replacement therapy is not a therapeutic option

Usual Dosage Oral: Adults: Type 1 Gaucher disease: 100 mg 3 times/day; dose may be reduced to 100 mg 1-2 times/day in patients with adverse effects (ie, tremor, GI distress)

Dosage Forms

Capsule:

Zavesca®: 100 mg

Migquin *(Discontinued)* *see* acetaminophen, isometheptene, and dichloralphenazone *on page* 29

Migranal® [US/Can] *see* dihydroergotamine *on page* 310

Migrapap® *(Discontinued)* *see* acetaminophen, isometheptene, and dichloralphenazone *on page* 29

Migratine [US] *see* acetaminophen, isometheptene, and dichloralphenazone *on page* 29

Migrazone® *(Discontinued)* *see* acetaminophen, isometheptene, and dichloralphenazone *on page* 29

Migrin-A *(Discontinued)* *see* acetaminophen, isometheptene, and dichloralphenazone *on page* 29

Mild-C® [US-OTC] *see* ascorbic acid *on page* 100

milk of magnesia *see* magnesium hydroxide *on page* 608

milnacipran (mil NAY ci pran)

Sound-Alike/Look-Alike Issues
Savella™ may be confused with cevimeline, sevelamer

U.S./Canadian Brand Names Savella™ [US]

Therapeutic Category Antidepressant, Serotonin/Norepinephrine Reuptake Inhibitor

Use Management of fibromyalgia

Usual Dosage Oral: Adults: 50 mg twice daily (maximum dose: 200 mg/day)

Note: Recommended titration schedule: 12.5 mg once on day one, then 12.5 mg twice daily on days 2-3, 25 mg twice daily on days 4-7, then 50 mg twice daily thereafter.

Dosage Forms

Tablet, oral:
Savella™: 12.5 mg, 25 mg, 50 mg, 100 mg

Combination package, oral [titration pack contains three separate tablet formulations]:
Savella™: Tablet: 12.5 mg (5s); tablet: 25 mg (8s); tablet: 50 mg (42s)

Milontin® *(Discontinued)*

Milophene® [Can] *see* clomiphene *on page 244*

Milophene® *(Discontinued)* *see* clomiphene *on page 244*

milrinone (MIL ri none)

Sound-Alike/Look-Alike Issues
Primacor® may be confused with Primaxin®

Synonyms milrinone lactate

U.S./Canadian Brand Names Milrinone Lactate Injection [Can]; Primacor® [Can]

Therapeutic Category Cardiovascular Agent, Other

Use Short-term I.V. therapy of acutely-decompensated heart failure

Usual Dosage I.V.: Adults: Loading dose (optional): 50 mcg/kg administered over 10 minutes followed by a maintenance dose titrated according to the hemodynamic and clinical response; Maintenance dose: I.V. infusion: 0.375-0.75 mcg/kg/minute.

Dosage Forms

Infusion [premixed in D_5W]: 200 mcg/mL (100 mL, 200 mL)

Injection, solution: 1 mg/mL (10 mL, 20 mL, 50 mL)

milrinone lactate *see* milrinone *on page 659*

Milrinone Lactate Injection [Can] *see* milrinone *on page 659*

Miltown® *(Discontinued)* *see* meprobamate *on page 629*

Mindal DM *(Discontinued)* *see* guaifenesin and dextromethorphan *on page 474*

mineral oil, petrolatum, lanolin, cetyl alcohol, and glycerin *see* lanolin, cetyl alcohol, glycerin, petrolatum, and mineral oil *on page 570*

Minestrin™ 1/20 [Can] *see* ethinyl estradiol and norethindrone *on page 390*

Mini-Gamulin® Rh *(Discontinued)*

Mini-Prenatal [US-OTC] *see* vitamins (multiple/prenatal) *on page 1020*

Minipress® [US/Can] *see* prazosin *on page 812*

Minirin® [Can] *see* desmopressin acetate *on page 285*

Minitran™ [US/Can] *see* nitroglycerin *on page 700*

Minizide® *(Discontinued)*

Minocin® [US/Can] *see* minocycline *on page 659*

Minocin® PAC [US] *see* minocycline *on page 659*

minocycline (mi noe SYE kleen)

Sound-Alike/Look-Alike Issues
Dynacin® may be confused with Dyazide®, Dynabac®, DynaCirc®, Dynapen®
Minocin® may be confused with Indocin®, Lincocin®, Minizide®, Mithracin®, niacin

Synonyms minocycline hydrochloride

U.S./Canadian Brand Names Alti-Minocycline [Can]; Apo-Minocycline® [Can]; Dynacin® [US]; Gen-Minocycline [Can]; Minocin® PAC [US]; Minocin® [US/Can]; myrac™ [US]; Novo-Minocycline [Can]; PMS-Minocycline [Can]; Rhoxal-minocycline [Can]; Sandoz-Minocycline [Can]; Solodyn® [US]

Therapeutic Category Tetracycline Derivative

Use Treatment of susceptible bacterial infections of both gram-negative and gram-positive organisms; treatment of anthrax (inhalational, cutaneous, and gastrointestinal); moderate-to-severe acne; meningococcal (asymptomatic) carrier state; Rickettsial diseases (including Rocky Mountain spotted fever, Q fever); nongonococcal urethritis, gonorrhea; acute intestinal amebiasis

Extended release (Solodyn®): Only indicated for treatment of inflammatory lesions of non-nodular moderate-to-severe acne

Usual Dosage

Usual dosage range:

Capsule or immediate release tablet:

Children >8 years: Oral: Initial: 4 mg/kg, followed by 2 mg/kg/dose every 12 hours

Adults: Oral: Initial: 200 mg, followed by 100 mg every 12 hours; more frequent dosing intervals may be used (100-200 mg initially, followed by 50 mg 4 times daily)

Extended release tablet (Solodyn®): Children ≥12 years and Adults (≥45 kg): Oral: 45-135 mg once daily (weight based)

Indication-specific dosing:

Children ≥12 years: Oral: **Acne** *(inflammatory, non-nodular, moderate-to-severe)* (Solodyn®):

45-59 kg: 45 mg once daily

60-90 kg: 90 mg once daily

91-136 kg: 135 mg once daily

Note: Therapy should be continued for 12 weeks. Higher doses do not confer greater efficacy, and safety of use beyond 12 weeks has not been established.

Adults: Oral:

Acne: Capsule or immediate-release tablet: 50-100 mg twice daily

Inflammatory, non-nodular, moderate-to-severe (Solodyn®):

45-59 kg: 45 mg once daily

60-90 kg: 90 mg once daily

91-136 kg: 135 mg once daily

Note: Therapy should be continued for 12 weeks. Higher doses do not confer greater efficacy, and safety of use beyond 12 weeks has not been established.

Chlamydial or *Ureaplasma urealyticum* infection, uncomplicated: Urethral, endocervical, or rectal: 100 mg every 12 hours for at least 7 days

Gonococcal infection, uncomplicated (males):

Without urethritis or anorectal infection: Initial: 200 mg, followed by 100 mg every 12 hours for at least 4 days (cultures 2-3 days post-therapy)

Urethritis: 100 mg every 12 hours for 5 days

Meningococcal carrier state: 100 mg every 12 hours for 5 days

Mycobacterium marinum: 100 mg every 12 hours for 6-8 weeks

Nocardiosis, cutaneous (non-CNS): 100 mg every 12 hours

Syphilis: Initial: 200 mg, followed by 100 mg every 12 hours for 10-15 days

Dosage Forms

Capsule: 50 mg, 75 mg, 100 mg

Capsule, pellet filled:

Minocin®: 50 mg, 100 mg

Minocin® PAC: 50 mg, 100 mg

Tablet: 50 mg, 75 mg, 100 mg

Dynacin®: 50 mg, 75 mg, 100 mg

Myrac™: 50 mg, 75 mg

Myrac™: 100 mg [scored]

Tablet, extended release:

Solodyn®: 45 mg, 90 mg, 135 mg

minocycline hydrochloride *see* minocycline *on page 659*

Min-Ovral® [Can] *see* ethinyl estradiol and levonorgestrel *on page 387*

Minox [Can] *see* minoxidil *on page 660*

minoxidil (mi NOKS i dil)

Sound-Alike/Look-Alike Issues

minoxidil may be confused with metolazone, midodrine, Minipress®, Minocin®, Monopril®, Noxafil®

Loniten® may be confused with Lipitor®

U.S./Canadian Brand Names Apo-Gain® [Can]; Loniten® [Can]; Minox [Can]; Rogaine® Extra Strength for Men [US-OTC]; Rogaine® for Men [US-OTC]; Rogaine® for Women [US-OTC]; Rogaine® [Can]

Therapeutic Category Topical Skin Product; Vasodilator

Use Management of severe hypertension (usually in combination with a diuretic and beta-blocker); treatment (topical formulation) of alopecia androgenetica in males and females

Usual Dosage

Children <12 years: Hypertension: Oral: Initial: 0.1-0.2 mg/kg once daily; maximum: 5 mg/day; increase gradually every 3 days; usual dosage range: 0.25-1 mg/kg/day in 1-2 divided doses; maximum: 50 mg/day

Children ≥12 years and Adults: Hypertension: Oral: Initial: 5 mg once daily, increase gradually every 3 days (maximum: 100 mg/day); usual dosage range (JNC 7): 2.5-80 mg/day in 1-2 divided doses

Note: Dosage adjustment is needed when added to concomitant therapy.

Adults: Alopecia: Topical: Apply twice daily; 4 months of therapy may be necessary for hair growth.

Dosage Forms

Aerosol, topical [foam]:

Rogaine® for Men [OTC]: 5% (60 g)

Solution, topical: 2% (60 mL); 5% (60 mL)

Rogaine® for Women [OTC]: 2% (60 mL)

Rogaine® Extra Strength for Men [OTC]: 5% (60 mL)

Tablet: 2.5 mg, 10 mg

Mintab DM [US] *see* guaifenesin and dextromethorphan *on page* *474*

Mint-Ciprofloxacin [Can] *see* ciprofloxacin *on page* *229*

Mint-Citalopram [Can] *see* citalopram *on page* *234*

Mintezol® [US] *see* thiabendazole *on page* *954*

MINT-Ondansetron [Can] *see* ondansetron *on page* *726*

Mintox Extra Strength [US-OTC] *see* aluminum hydroxide, magnesium hydroxide, and simethicone *on page* *56*

Mintox Plus [US-OTC] *see* aluminum hydroxide, magnesium hydroxide, and simethicone *on page* *56*

Mint-Topiramate [Can] *see* topiramate *on page* *969*

Mintuss DR [US] *see* chlorpheniramine, phenylephrine, and dextromethorphan *on page* *217*

Mintuss G *(Discontinued)*

Mintuss HC [US] *see* phenylephrine, hydrocodone, and chlorpheniramine *on page* *778*

Mintuss MS [US] *see* phenylephrine, hydrocodone, and chlorpheniramine *on page* *778*

Minute-Gel® *(Discontinued)* *see* fluoride *on page* *430*

Miochol®-E [US/Can] *see* acetylcholine *on page* *31*

Miostat® [US/Can] *see* carbachol *on page* *180*

MiraLax® [US-OTC] *see* polyethylene glycol 3350 *on page* *797*

Miranel AF™ [US-OTC] *see* miconazole *on page* *654*

Mirapex® [US/Can] *see* pramipexole *on page* *808*

Mircette® [US] *see* ethinyl estradiol and desogestrel *on page* *383*

Mirena® [US/Can] *see* levonorgestrel *on page* *582*

mirtazapine (mir TAZ a peen)

Sound-Alike/Look-Alike Issues

Remeron® may be confused with Premarin®, ramelteon, Rozerem®, Zemuron®

U.S./Canadian Brand Names Apo-Mirtazapine [Can]; CO Mirtazapine [Can]; DOM-Mirtazapine [Can]; Gen-Mirtazapine [Can]; Novo-Mirtazapine [Can]; PHL-Mirtazapine [Can]; PMS-Mirtazapine [Can]; PRO-Mirtazapine [Can]; ratio-Mirtazapine [Can]; Remeron SolTab® [US]; Remeron® RD [Can]; Remeron® [US/Can]; Riva-Mirtazapine [Can]; Sandoz-Mirtazapine FC [Can]; Sandoz-Mirtazapine [Can]

Therapeutic Category Antidepressant, Alpha-2 Antagonist

Use Treatment of depression

Usual Dosage Oral: Adults: Treatment of depression: Initial: 15 mg nightly, titrate up to 15-45 mg/day with dose increases made no more frequently than every 1-2 weeks; there is an inverse relationship between dose and sedation

Dosage Forms

Tablet: 7.5 mg, 15 mg, 30 mg, 45 mg

Remeron®: 15 mg, 30 mg, 45 mg

Tablet, orally disintegrating: 15 mg, 30 mg, 45 mg

Remeron SolTab®: 15 mg, 30 mg, 45 mg

misoprostol (mye soe PROST ole)

Sound-Alike/Look-Alike Issues

misoprostol may be confused with metoprolol, mifepristone
Cytotec® may be confused with Cytoxan®, Sytobex®

U.S./Canadian Brand Names Apo-Misoprostol® [Can]; Cytotec® [US]; Novo-Misoprostol [Can]

Therapeutic Category Prostaglandin

Use Prevention of NSAID-induced gastric ulcers; medical termination of pregnancy of ≤49 days (in conjunction with mifepristone)

Usual Dosage Oral: Adults:

Prevention of NSAID-induced gastric ulcers: 200 mcg 4 times/day with food; if not tolerated, may decrease dose to 100 mcg 4 times/day with food or 200 mcg twice daily with food; last dose of the day should be taken at bedtime

Medical termination of pregnancy: Refer to mifepristone monograph.

Dosage Forms

Tablet: 100 mcg, 200 mcg
Cytotec®: 100 mcg, 200 mcg

misoprostol and diclofenac *see* diclofenac and misoprostol *on page* 304
Mito-Carn® ***(Discontinued)*** *see* levocarnitine *on page* 578

mitomycin (mye toe MYE sin)

Sound-Alike/Look-Alike Issues

mitomycin may be confused with mithramycin, mitotane, mitoxantrone

Synonyms mitomycin-C; mitomycin-X; MTC; NSC-26980

U.S./Canadian Brand Names Mutamycin® [Can]

Therapeutic Category Antineoplastic Agent

Use Treatment of adenocarcinoma of stomach or pancreas

Usual Dosage Refer to individual protocols. Adults:

Single agent therapy: I.V.: 20 mg/m^2 every 6-8 weeks
Combination therapy: I.V.: 10 mg/m^2 every 6-8 weeks
Bladder carcinoma: Intravesicular instillation (unapproved route): 20-40 mg instilled into the bladder and retained for 3 hours up to 3 times/week for up to 20 procedures per course

Dosage Forms

Injection, powder for reconstitution: 5 mg, 20 mg, 40 mg

mitomycin-X *see* mitomycin *on page* 662
mitomycin-C *see* mitomycin *on page* 662

mitotane (MYE toe tane)

Sound-Alike/Look-Alike Issues

mitotane may be confused with mitomycin, mitoxantrone

Synonyms chloditan; chlodithane; khloditan; mytotan; o,p′-DDD; ortho,para-DDD

U.S./Canadian Brand Names Lysodren® [US/Can]

Therapeutic Category Antineoplastic Agent

Use Treatment of inoperable adrenocortical carcinoma

Usual Dosage Oral: Adults: Adrenocortical carcinoma: Start at 2-6 g/day in 3-4 divided doses, then increase incrementally to 9-10 g/day in 3-4 divided doses (maximum tolerated range: 2-16 g/day, usually 9-10 g/day; maximum dose studied: 18-19 g/day)

Dosage Forms

Tablet [scored]:
Lysodren®: 500 mg

mitoxantrone (mye toe ZAN trone)

Sound-Alike/Look-Alike Issues

mitoxantrone may be confused with methotrexate, mitomycin, mitotane, Mutamycin®

Synonyms CL-232315; DHAD; DHAQ; dihydroxyanthracenedione; dihydroxyanthracenedione dihydrochloride; mitoxantrone dihydrochloride; mitoxantrone HCl; mitoxantrone hydrochloride; mitozantrone

U.S./Canadian Brand Names Mitoxantrone Injection® [Can]; Novantrone® [US/Can]

Therapeutic Category Antineoplastic Agent

Use Treatment of acute nonlymphocytic leukemias (ANLL [includes myelogenous, promyelocytic, monocytic and erythroid leukemias]); advanced hormone-refractory prostate cancer; secondary progressive or relapsing-remitting multiple sclerosis (MS)

Usual Dosage Details concerning dosing in combination regimens should also be consulted. I.V.: Adults:

Acute nonlymphocytic leukemias:

Induction: 12 mg/m^2 once daily for 3 days (in combination with cytarabine); for incomplete response, may repeat at 12 mg/m^2 once daily for 2 days

Consolidation: 12 mg/m^2 once daily for 2 days, repeat in 4 weeks

Multiple sclerosis: 12 mg/m^2 every 3 months (maximum lifetime cumulative dose: 140 mg/m^2; discontinue use with LVEF <50% or clinically significant reduction in LVEF)

Prostate cancer (advanced, hormone-refractory): 12-14 mg/m^2 every 3 weeks (in combination with corticosteroids)

Dosage Forms

Injection, solution [concentrate; preservative free]: 2 mg/mL (10 mL, 12.5 mL, 15 mL, 20 mL)

Novantrone®: 2 mg/mL (10 mL)

mitoxantrone dihydrochloride *see* mitoxantrone *on page 662*

mitoxantrone HCl *see* mitoxantrone *on page 662*

mitoxantrone hydrochloride *see* mitoxantrone *on page 662*

Mitoxantrone Injection® [Can] *see* mitoxantrone *on page 662*

mitozantrone *see* mitoxantrone *on page 662*

Mitran® Oral *(Discontinued)* *see* chlordiazepoxide *on page 209*

Mitrazol™ [US-OTC] *see* miconazole *on page 654*

Mivacron® *(Discontinued)*

mivacurium *(Discontinued)*

MK-191 *see* pivampicillin *(Canada only) on page 788*

MK-217 *see* alendronate *on page 44*

MK383 *see* tirofiban *on page 964*

MK-0431 *see* sitagliptin *on page 904*

MK462 *see* rizatriptan *on page 874*

MK 0517 *see* fosaprepitant *on page 445*

MK-0518 *see* raltegravir *on page 849*

MK594 *see* losartan *on page 600*

MK0826 *see* ertapenem *on page 367*

MK 869 *see* aprepitant *on page 94*

MLN341 *see* bortezomib *on page 146*

MMF *see* mycophenolate *on page 673*

MMR *see* measles, mumps, and rubella virus vaccine *on page 615*

M-M-R® II [US/Can] *see* measles, mumps, and rubella virus vaccine *on page 615*

MMR-V *see* measles, mumps, rubella, and varicella virus vaccine *on page 616*

Moban® [US/Can] *see* molindone *on page 665*

Mobic® [US/Can] *see* meloxicam *on page 622*

Mobicox® [Can] *see* meloxicam *on page 622*

Mobidin® *(Discontinued)* *see* magnesium salicylate *on page 610*

Mobisyl® [US-OTC] *see* trolamine *on page 991*

moclobemide *(Canada only)* (moe KLOE be mide)

U.S./Canadian Brand Names Apo-Moclobemide® [Can]; Dom-Moclobemide [Can]; Manerix® [Can]; Novo-Moclobemide [Can]; Nu-Moclobemide [Can]; PMS-Moclobemide [Can]

Therapeutic Category Antidepressant, Monoamine Oxidase Inhibitor

Use Symptomatic relief of depressive illness

Usual Dosage Oral: Adults: Initial: 300 mg/day in 2 divided doses; increase gradually to maximum of 600 mg/day; **Note:** Individual patient response may allow a reduction in daily dose in long-term therapy.

Dosage Forms [CAN] = Canadian brand name

Tablet: 150 mg, 300 mg [not available in the U.S.]

Alti-Moclobemide [CAN], Apo-Moclobemide® [CAN], Dom-Moclobemide® [CAN], Manerix®e [CAN], Novo-Moclobemidee [CAN], Nu-Moclobemidee [CAN], PMS-Moclobemide [CAN]: 150 mg, 300 mg [not available in the U.S.]

modafinil (moe DAF i nil)

U.S./Canadian Brand Names Alertec® [Can]; APO-Modafinil [Can]; Provigil® [US]

Therapeutic Category Central Nervous System Stimulant, Nonamphetamine

Controlled Substance C-IV

Use Improve wakefulness in patients with excessive daytime sleepiness associated with narcolepsy and shift work sleep disorder (SWSD); adjunctive therapy for obstructive sleep apnea/hypopnea syndrome (OSAHS)

Usual Dosage Oral: Adults:

Narcolepsy, obstructive sleep apnea/hypopnea syndrome (OSAHS): Initial: 200 mg as a single daily dose in the morning

Shift work sleep disorder (SWSD): Initial: 200 mg as a single dose taken ~1 hour prior to start of work shift

Note: Doses of 400 mg/day, given as a single dose, have been well tolerated, but there is no consistent evidence that this dose confers additional benefit

Dosage Forms

Tablet:

Provigil®: 100 mg, 200 mg

Modane® Soft *(Discontinued)* *see* docusate *on page 326*

Modecate® [Can] *see* fluphenazine *on page 434*

Modecate® Concentrate [Can] *see* fluphenazine *on page 434*

Modicon® [US] *see* ethinyl estradiol and norethindrone *on page 390*

modified Dakin's solution *see* sodium hypochlorite solution *on page 911*

Moducal® [US-OTC] *see* glucose polymers *on page 466*

Modulon® [Can] *see* trimebutine *(Canada only) on page 987*

Moduret [Can] *see* amiloride and hydrochlorothiazide *on page 61*

Moduretic® *(Discontinued)* *see* amiloride and hydrochlorothiazide *on page 61*

moexipril (mo EKS i pril)

Sound-Alike/Look-Alike Issues

moexipril may be confused with Monopril®

Synonyms moexipril hydrochloride

U.S./Canadian Brand Names Univasc® [US]

Therapeutic Category Angiotensin-Converting Enzyme (ACE) Inhibitor

Use Treatment of hypertension, alone or in combination with thiazide diuretics

Usual Dosage Oral: Adults: Initial: 7.5 mg once daily (in patients **not** receiving diuretics), 1 hour prior to a meal **or** 3.75 mg once daily (when combined with thiazide diuretics); maintenance dose: 7.5-30 mg/day in 1 or 2 divided doses 1 hour before meals

Dosage Forms

Tablet [scored]: 7.5 mg, 15 mg

Univasc®: 7.5 mg, 15 mg

moexipril and hydrochlorothiazide (mo EKS i pril & hye droe klor oh THYE a zide)

Synonyms hydrochlorothiazide and moexipril

U.S./Canadian Brand Names Uniretic® [US/Can]

Therapeutic Category Angiotensin-Converting Enzyme (ACE) Inhibitor; Diuretic, Thiazide

Use Treatment of hypertension; not indicated for initial treatment of hypertension

Usual Dosage Oral: Adults: 7.5-30 mg of moexipril, taken either in a single or divided dose 1 hour before meals; hydrochlorothiazide dose should be ≤50 mg/day

Dosage Forms

Tablet [scored]:

7.5/12.5: Moexipril 7.5 mg and hydrochlorothiazide 12.5

15/12.5: Moexipril 15 mg and hydrochlorothiazide 12.5

15/25: Moexipril 15 mg and hydrochlorothiazide 25

Uniretic®: 7.5/12.5: Moexipril 7.5 mg and hydrochlorothiazide 12.5 mg; 15/12.5: Moexipril 15 mg and hydrochlorothiazide 12.5 mg; 15/25: Moexipril 15 mg and hydrochlorothiazide 25 mg

moexipril hydrochloride *see* moexipril *on page 664*
Mogadon [Can] *see* nitrazepam *(Canada only) on page 699*
Moi-Stir® [US-OTC] *see* saliva substitute *on page 887*
Moisture® Eyes [US-OTC] *see* artificial tears *on page 100*
Moisture® Eyes PM [US-OTC] *see* artificial tears *on page 100*

molindone (moe LIN done)

Sound-Alike/Look-Alike Issues

molindone may be confused with Mobidin®

Moban® may be confused with Mobidin®, Modane®

Synonyms molindone hydrochloride

U.S./Canadian Brand Names Moban® [US/Can]

Therapeutic Category Antipsychotic Agent, Dihydroindoline

Use Management of schizophrenia

Usual Dosage Oral: Adults: Schizophrenia/psychoses:

Initial: 50-75 mg/day, may increase to 100 mg/day in 3-4 days; may further increase dose gradually to maximum of 225 mg/day

Maintenance: 5-15 mg (mild symptoms) or 10-25 mg (moderate symptoms) 3-4 times/day (up to 225 mg/day may be required in severe cases)

Dosage Forms

Tablet:

Moban®: 5 mg, 10 mg, 25 mg, 50 mg

molindone hydrochloride *see* molindone *on page 665*
molybdenum *see* trace metals *on page 974*
MOM *see* magnesium hydroxide *on page 608*
Momentum® [US-OTC] *see* magnesium salicylate *on page 610*

mometasone (moe MET a sone)

Sound-Alike/Look-Alike Issues

Elocon® lotion may be confused with ophthalmic solutions. Manufacturer's labeling emphasizes the product is **NOT** for use in the eyes.

Synonyms mometasone furoate

U.S./Canadian Brand Names Asmanex® Twisthaler® [US]; Elocom® [Can]; Elocon® [US]; Nasonex® [US/Can]; PMS-Mometasone [Can]; ratio-Mometasone [Can]; Taro-Mometasone [Can]

Therapeutic Category Corticosteroid, Intranasal; Corticosteroid, Topical

Use Relief of the inflammatory and pruritic manifestations of corticosteroid-responsive dermatoses (medium potency topical corticosteroid); treatment of nasal symptoms of seasonal and perennial allergic rhinitis; prevention of nasal symptoms associated with seasonal allergic rhinitis; treatment of nasal polyps in adults; maintenance treatment of asthma as prophylactic therapy or as a supplement in asthma patients requiring oral corticosteroids for the purpose of decreasing or eliminating the oral corticosteroid requirement

Usual Dosage

Oral inhalation:

Children 4-11 years: 110 mcg once daily in the evening (maximum: 110 mcg/day)

Children ≥12 years and Adults: Previous therapy:

Bronchodilators or inhaled corticosteroids: Initial: 1 inhalation (220 mcg) daily (maximum: 2 inhalations or 440 mcg/day); may be given in the evening or in divided doses twice daily

Oral corticosteroids: Initial: 440 mcg twice daily (maximum: 880 mcg/day); prednisone should be reduced no faster than 2.5 mg/day on a weekly basis, beginning after at least 1 week of mometasone furoate use

NIH Asthma Guidelines: Children ≥12 years and Adults:

"Low" dose: 220 mcg/day

"Medium" dose: 440 mcg/day

"High" dose: >440 mcg/day

Note: Maximum effects may not be evident for 1-2 weeks or longer; dose should be titrated to effect, using the lowest possible dose

Nasal spray:

Allergic rhinitis:

Children 2-11 years: 1 spray (50 mcg) in each nostril daily

Children ≥12 years and Adults: 2 sprays (100 mcg) in each nostril daily; when used for the prevention of allergic rhinitis, treatment should begin 2-4 weeks prior to pollen season

Nasal polyps: Adults: 2 sprays (100 mcg) in each nostril twice daily; 2 sprays (100 mcg) once daily may be effective in some patients

Topical: Apply sparingly, do not use occlusive dressings. Therapy should be discontinued when control is achieved; if no improvement is seen in 2 weeks, reassessment of diagnosis may be necessary.

Cream, ointment: Children ≥2 years and Adults: Apply a thin film to affected area once daily; do not use in pediatric patients for longer than 3 weeks

Lotion: Children ≥12 years and Adults: Apply a few drops to affected area once daily

Dosage Forms

Cream, topical: 0.1% (15 g, 45 g)

Elocon®: 0.1% (15 g, 45 g)

Lotion, topical: 0.1% (30 mL, 60 mL)

Elocon®: 0.1% (30 mL, 60 mL)

Ointment, topical: 0.1% (15 g, 45 g)

Elocon®: 0.1% (15 g, 45 g)

Powder for oral inhalation:

Asmanex® Twisthaler®: 110 mcg (30 units); 220 mcg (14 units, 30 units, 60 units, 120 units)

Suspension, intranasal [spray]:

Nasonex®: 50 mcg/spray (17 g)

mometasone furoate *see* mometasone *on page* 665

MOM/mineral oil emulsion *see* magnesium hydroxide and mineral oil *on page* 609

monacolin K *see* lovastatin *on page* 602

Monafed® ***(Discontinued)*** *see* guaifenesin *on page* 473

Monafed® DM ***(Discontinued)*** *see* guaifenesin and dextromethorphan *on page* 474

Monarc-M™ [US] *see* antihemophilic factor (human) *on page* 81

***Monilia* skin test** *see Candida albicans (Monilia) on page* 177

Monistat® [Can] *see* miconazole *on page* 654

Monistat® 1 [US-OTC] *see* miconazole *on page* 654

Monistat® 3 [US-OTC/Can] *see* miconazole *on page* 654

Monistat® 7 [US-OTC] *see* miconazole *on page* 654

Monistat-Derm® ***(Discontinued)*** *see* miconazole *on page* 654

Monistat i.v.™ Injection ***(Discontinued)*** *see* miconazole *on page* 654

Monitan® [Can] *see* acebutolol *on page* 19

monobenzone (mon oh BEN zone)

Therapeutic Category Topical Skin Product

Use Final depigmentation in extensive vitiligo

Usual Dosage Topical: Children ≥12 years and Adults: Apply 2-3 times daily; once depigmentation is obtained, may apply as needed (usually 2 times/week)

Monocaps [US-OTC] *see* vitamins (multiple/oral) *on page* 1019

Monoclate-P® [US] *see* antihemophilic factor (human) *on page* 81

monoclonal antibody *see* muromonab-CD3 *on page* 673

Monocor® [Can] *see* bisoprolol *on page* 144

Monodox® [US] *see* doxycycline *on page* 336

monoethanolamine *see* ethanolamine oleate *on page* 383

Monoket® [US] *see* isosorbide mononitrate *on page* 551

MonoNessa® [US] *see* ethinyl estradiol and norgestimate *on page* 393

Mononine® [US/Can] *see* factor IX *on page* 403

Monopril® [US/Can] *see* fosinopril *on page* 446

Monopril-HCT® [Can] *see* fosinopril and hydrochlorothiazide *on page* 446

Monopril-HCT® ***(Discontinued)*** *see* fosinopril and hydrochlorothiazide *on page* 446

montelukast (mon te LOO kast)

Sound-Alike/Look-Alike Issues

Singulair® may be confused with Sinequan®

Synonyms montelukast sodium

U.S./Canadian Brand Names Singulair® [US/Can]

Therapeutic Category Leukotriene Receptor Antagonist

Use Prophylaxis and chronic treatment of asthma; relief of symptoms of seasonal allergic rhinitis and perennial allergic rhinitis; prevention of exercise-induced bronchospasm

Usual Dosage Oral:

Children:

6-23 months: Perennial allergic rhinitis: 4 mg (oral granules) once daily

12-23 months: Asthma: 4 mg (oral granules) once daily, taken in the evening

2-5 years: Asthma, seasonal or perennial allergic rhinitis: 4 mg (chewable tablet or oral granules) once daily, taken in the evening

6-14 years: Asthma, seasonal or perennial allergic rhinitis: 5 mg (chewable tablet) once daily, taken in the evening

Children ≥15 years and Adults:

Asthma, seasonal or perennial allergic rhinitis: 10 mg/day, taken in the evening

Bronchoconstriction, exercise-induced (prevention): 10 mg at least 2 hours prior to exercise; additional doses should not be administered within 24 hours. Daily administration to prevent exercise-induced bronchoconstriction has not been evaluated.

Dosage Forms

Granules:

Singulair®: 4 mg/packet (30s)

Tablet:

Singulair®: 10 mg

Tablet, chewable:

Singulair®: 4 mg, 5 mg

montelukast sodium *see* montelukast *on page* 667

Monurol® [US/Can] *see* fosfomycin *on page* 445

8-MOP® [US] *see* methoxsalen *on page* 641

more attenuated enders strain *see* measles virus vaccine (live) *on page* 616

MoreDophilus® [US-OTC] *see* Lactobacillus *on page* 564

moricizine *(Discontinued)*

morning after pill *see* ethinyl estradiol and norgestrel *on page* 394

Morphine HP® [Can] *see* morphine sulfate *on page* 667

Morphine LP® Epidural [Can] *see* morphine sulfate *on page* 667

morphine sulfate (MOR feen SUL fate)

Sound-Alike/Look-Alike Issues

morphine may be confused with HYDROmorphone

morphine sulfate may be confused with magnesium sulfate

Avinza® may be confused with Evista®, Invanz®

MS Contin® may be confused with Oxycontin®

MSO_4 and MS are error-prone abbreviations (mistaken as magnesium sulfate)

Roxanol™ may be confused with OxyFast®, Roxicet™, Roxicodone®

U.S./Canadian Brand Names Astramorph/PF™ [US]; Avinza® [US]; DepoDur® [US]; Doloral [Can]; Duramorph® [US]; Embeda™ [US]; Infumorph® 200 [US]; Infumorph® 500 [US]; Kadian® [US/Can]; M-Eslon® [Can]; M.O.S.-SR® [Can]; M.O.S.-Sulfate® [Can]; M.O.S.® 10 [Can]; M.O.S.® 20 [Can]; M.O.S.® 30 [Can]; Morphine HP® [Can]; Morphine LP® Epidural [Can]; MS Contin® [US/Can]; MS-IR® [Can]; Novo-Morphine SR [Can]; Oramorph® SR [US]; PMS-Morphine Sulfate SR [Can]; ratio-Morphine SR [Can]; ratio-Morphine [Can]; Roxanol™ [US]; Statex® [Can]; Zomorph® [Can]

Therapeutic Category Analgesic, Narcotic

Controlled Substance C-II

Use Relief of moderate-to-severe acute and chronic pain; relief of pain of myocardial infarction; relief of dyspnea of acute left ventricular failure and pulmonary edema; preanesthetic medication

DepoDur®: Epidural (lumbar) single-dose management of surgical pain

Infumorph®: Used in continuous microinfusion devices for intrathecal or epidural administration in treatment of intractable chronic pain

Controlled, extended, or sustained release products: Only intended/indicated for use when repeated doses for an extended period of time are required. The 100 mg and 200 mg tablets or capsules of Kadian®, MS Contin®, and morphine sulfate controlled release tablets and the 60 mg, 90 mg, and 120 mg capsules of Avinza® should only be used in opioid-tolerant patients.

Usual Dosage Note: These are guidelines and do not represent the doses that may be required in all patients. Doses and dosage intervals should be titrated to pain relief/prevention.

Children >6 months and <50 kg: Acute pain (moderate-to-severe):

Oral (immediate release formulations): 0.15-0.3 mg/kg every 3-4 hours as needed

I.M., I.V.: 0.1-0.2 mg/kg every 3-4 hours as needed

I.V. infusion: Range: 10-60 mcg/kg/hour

Adults:

Acute pain (moderate-to-severe):

Oral (immediate release formulations): Opiate-naive: Initial: 10 mg every 4 hours as needed; patients with prior opiate exposure may require higher initial doses: usual dosage range: 10-30 mg every 4 hours as needed

I.M., SubQ: **Note:** Repeated SubQ administration causes local tissue irritation, pain, and induration.

Initial: Opiate-naive: 5-10 mg every 4 hours as needed; patients with prior opiate exposure may require higher initial doses; usual dosage range: 5-20 mg every 4 hours as needed

Rectal: 10-20 mg every 3-4 hours

I.V.: Initial: Opiate-naive: 2.5-5 mg every 3-4 hours; patients with prior opiate exposure may require higher initial doses. **Note:** Repeated doses (up to every 5 minutes if needed) in small increments (eg, 1-4 mg) may be preferred to larger and less frequent doses.

Acute myocardial infarction, analgesia: Initial management: 2-4 mg, give 2-8 mg every 5-15 minutes as needed.

I.V., SubQ continuous infusion: 0.8-10 mg/hour; usual range: Up to 80 mg/hour

Patient-controlled analgesia (PCA): (Opiate-naive: Consider lower end of dosing range):

Usual concentration: 1 mg/mL

Demand dose: Usual: 1 mg; range: 0.5-2.5 mg

Lockout interval: 5-10 minutes

Intrathecal (I.T.): **Note:** Administer with extreme caution and in reduced dosage to geriatric or debilitated patients. I.T. dose is usually 1/10 that of epidural dosage.

Opioid-naive: 0.2-1 mg/dose (may provide adequate relief for 24 hours); repeat doses are **not** recommended

Continuous microinfusion (Infumorph®): Initial: 0.2-1 mg/day

Opioid-tolerant: 1-10 mg/day

Continuous microinfusion (Infumorph®): Initial: 1-10 mg/day, titrate to effect; usual maximum is ~20 mg/day

Epidural: Pain management: **Note:** Administer with extreme caution and in reduced dosage to geriatric or debilitated patients. Vigilant monitoring is particularly important in these patients.

Single-dose (Astromorph/PF™, Duramorph®): Initial: 5 mg, if pain relief not achieved in 1 hour, careful administration of 1-2 mg at intervals sufficient to assess effectiveness may be given; maximum: 10 mg/24 hours

Infusion: Bolus dose: 1-6 mg; infusion rate: 0.1-0.2 mg/hour; maximum dose: 10 mg/24 hours

Continuous microinfusion (Infumorph®):

Opioid-naive: Initial: 0.2-1 mg/day

Opioid-tolerant: Initial: 1-10 mg/day, titrate to effect; usual maximum is ~20 mg/day

Surgical anesthesia: Epidural: Single-dose (extended release, DepoDur®): Lumbar epidural only; not recommended in patients <18 years of age:

Cesarean section: 10 mg (after clamping umbilical cord)

Lower abdominal/pelvic surgery: 10-15 mg

Major orthopedic surgery of lower extremity: 15 mg

For DepoDur®: To minimize the pharmacokinetic interaction resulting in higher peak serum concentrations of morphine, administer the test dose of the local anesthetic at least 15 minutes prior to DepoDur® administration. Use of DepoDur® with epidural local anesthetics has not been studied. Other medications should not be administered into the epidural space for at least 48 hours after administration of DepoDur®.

Note: Some patients may benefit from a 20 mg dose, however, the incidence of adverse effects may be increased.

Chronic pain: Note: Patients taking opioids chronically may become tolerant and require doses higher than the usual dosage range to maintain the desired effect. Tolerance can be managed by appropriate dose titration. There is no optimal or maximal dose for morphine in chronic pain. The appropriate dose is one that relieves pain throughout its dosing interval without causing unmanageable side effects.

Oral: Controlled, extended, or sustained release formulations: A patient's morphine requirement should be established using prompt-release formulations. Conversion to long-acting products may be considered when chronic, continuous treatment is required. Higher dosages should be reserved for use only in opioid-tolerant patients.

Capsules, extended release (Avinza®): Daily dose administered once daily (for best results, administer at same time each day)

Capsules, sustained release (Kadian®): Daily dose administered once daily or in 2 divided doses daily (every 12 hours)

Tablets, controlled release (MS Contin®), sustained release (Oramorph SR®), or extended release: Daily dose divided and administered every 8 or every 12 hours

Dosage Forms [CAN] Canadian brand name

Capsule, extended release, oral:
Avinza®: 30 mg, 45 mg, 60 mg, 75 mg, 90 mg, 120 mg
Kadian®: 10 mg, 20 mg, 30 mg, 50 mg, 60 mg, 80 mg, 100 mg, 200 mg

Infusion [premixed in D_5W]: 1 mg/mL (100 mL, 250 mL)

Injection, extended release liposomal suspension [lumbar epidural injection, preservative free]:
DepoDur®: 10 mg/mL (1 mL, 1.5 mL)

Injection, solution: 1 mg/mL (10 mL); 2 mg/mL (1 mL); 4 mg/mL (1 mL); 5 mg/mL (1 mL); 8 mg/mL (1 mL); 10 mg/0.7 mL (0.7 mL); 10 mg/mL (1 mL, 10 mL); 15 mg/mL (1 mL, 20 mL); 25 mg/mL (4 mL, 10 mL, 20 mL, 40 mL, 50 mL, 100 mL, 250 mL); 50 mg/mL (20 mL, 40 mL, 50 mL)

Injection, solution [epidural, intrathecal, or I.V. infusion; preservative free]:
Astramorph/PF™: 0.5 mg/mL (2 mL, 10 mL); 1 mg/mL (2 mL, 10 mL)
Duramorph®: 0.5 mg/mL (10 mL); 1 mg/mL (10 mL)

Injection, solution [epidural or intrathecal infusion via microinfusion device; preservative free]: 10 mg/mL (20 mL); 25 mg/mL (20 mL)
Infumorph® 200: 10 mg/mL (20 mL)
Infumorph® 500: 25 mg/mL (20 mL)

Injection, solution [for PCA pump]: 1 mg/mL (30 mL); 5 mg/mL (30 mL)

Injection, solution [for PCA pump, preservative free]: 1 mg/mL (30 mL)

Injection, solution [preservative free]: 0.5 mg/mL (10 mL); 1 mg/mL (10 mL); 25 mg/mL (10 mL)

Solution, oral: 10 mg/5 mL, 20 mg/5 mL
Doloral [CAN]: 1 mg/mL; 5 mg/mL [not available in U.S.]

Solution, oral [concentrate]: 20 mg/mL
Roxanol™: 20 mg/mL (30 mL, 120 mL); 100 mg/5 mL (240 mL)

Suppository, rectal: 5 mg (12s), 10 mg (12s), 20 mg (12s), 30 mg (12s)

Tablet, oral: 15 mg, 30 mg

Tablet, controlled release, oral: 15 mg, 30 mg, 60 mg, 100 mg, 200 mg
MS Contin®: 15 mg, 30 mg, 60 mg, 100 mg, 200 mg

Tablet, extended release, oral: 15 mg, 30 mg, 60 mg, 100 mg, 200 mg

Tablet, sustained release, oral:
Oramorph® SR: 15 mg, 30 mg, 60 mg, 100 mg

morrhuate sodium (MOR yoo ate SOW dee um)

U.S./Canadian Brand Names Scleromate® [US]

Therapeutic Category Sclerosing Agent

Use Treatment of small, uncomplicated varicose veins of the lower extremities

Usual Dosage I.V.: Adults: 50-250 mg, repeated at 5- to 7-day intervals (50-100 mg for small veins, 150-250 mg for large veins)

Dosage Forms

Injection, solution: 50 mg/mL (30 mL)
Scleromate®: 50 mg/mL (30 mL)

M.O.S.® 10 [Can] *see* morphine sulfate *on page 667*

M.O.S.® 20 [Can] *see* morphine sulfate *on page 667*

M.O.S.® 30 [Can] *see* morphine sulfate *on page 667*

Mosco® Callus & Corn Remover [US-OTC] *see* salicylic acid *on page 884*

M.O.S.-SR® [Can] *see* morphine sulfate *on page 667*

M.O.S.-Sulfate® [Can] *see* morphine sulfate *on page 667*
Motofen® [US] *see* difenoxin and atropine *on page 307*
Motrin® Children's [US-OTC/Can] *see* ibuprofen *on page 515*
Motrin® *(Discontinued)* *see* ibuprofen *on page 515*
Motrin® IB [US-OTC/Can] *see* ibuprofen *on page 515*
Motrin® IB Sinus *(Discontinued)* *see* pseudoephedrine and ibuprofen *on page 835*
Motrin® Infants' [US-OTC] *see* ibuprofen *on page 515*
Motrin® Junior [US-OTC] *see* ibuprofen *on page 515*
Mouthkote® [US-OTC] *see* saliva substitute *on page 887*
MoviPrep® [US] *see* polyethylene glycol-electrolyte solution *on page 797*
Moxatag™ [US] *see* amoxicillin *on page 70*

moxifloxacin (moxs i FLOKS a sin)

Sound-Alike/Look-Alike Issues
Avelox® may be confused with Avonex®

Synonyms moxifloxacin hydrochloride

U.S./Canadian Brand Names Avelox® I.V. [US/Can]; Avelox® [US/Can]; Vigamox® [US/Can]

Therapeutic Category Antibiotic, Quinolone

Use Treatment of mild-to-moderate community-acquired pneumonia, including multidrug-resistant *Streptococcus pneumoniae* (MDRSP); acute bacterial exacerbation of chronic bronchitis; acute bacterial sinusitis; complicated and uncomplicated skin and skin structure infections; complicated intraabdominal infections; bacterial conjunctivitis (ophthalmic formulation)

Usual Dosage

Usual dosage range:
Children ≥1 year and Adults: Ophthalmic: Instill 1 drop into affected eye(s) 3 times/day for 7 days
Adults: Oral, I.V.: 400 mg every 24 hours

Indication-specific dosing:
Children ≥1 year and Adults: Ophthalmic: **Bacterial conjunctivitis:** Instill 1 drop into affected eye(s) 3 times/day for 7 days
Adults: Oral, I.V.:
Acute bacterial sinusitis: 400 mg every 24 hours for 10 days
Chronic bronchitis, acute bacterial exacerbation: 400 mg every 24 hours for 5 days
Intraabdominal infections (complicated): 400 mg every 24 hours for 5-14 days (initiate with I.V.)
Pneumonia, community-acquired (including MDRSP): 400 mg every 24 hours for 7-14 days
Skin and skin structure infections:
Complicated: 400 mg every 24 hours for 7-21 days
Uncomplicated: 400 mg every 24 hours for 7 days

Dosage Forms

Infusion, premixed in sodium chloride 0.8% [preservative free]:
Avelox® I.V.: 400 mg (250 mL)

Solution, ophthalmic:
Vigamox®: 0.5% (3 mL)

Tablet:
Avelox®: 400 mg
Avelox® ABC Pack: 400 mg (5s)

moxifloxacin hydrochloride *see* moxifloxacin *on page 670*
Mozobil™ [US] *see* plerixafor *on page 789*
4-MP *see* fomepizole *on page 442*
MPA *see* mycophenolate *on page 673*
MPA and estrogens (conjugated) *see* estrogens (conjugated/equine) and medroxyprogesterone *on page 379*
M-Prednisol® Injection *(Discontinued)* *see* methylprednisolone *on page 647*
MPSV *see* meningococcal polysaccharide vaccine (groups A / C / Y and W-135) *on page 625*
MPSV4 *see* meningococcal polysaccharide vaccine (groups A / C / Y and W-135) *on page 625*
MS Contin® [US/Can] *see* morphine sulfate *on page 667*
MS-IR® [Can] *see* morphine sulfate *on page 667*
MST 600 [US] *see* magnesium salicylate *on page 610*

MTC *see* mitomycin *on page 662*
Mucinex® [US-OTC] *see* guaifenesin *on page 473*
Mucinex®-D [US-OTC] *see* guaifenesin and pseudoephedrine *on page 477*
Mucinex® D Maximum Strength [US-OTC] *see* guaifenesin and pseudoephedrine *on page 477*
Mucinex®, Children's [US-OTC] *see* guaifenesin *on page 473*
Mucinex® Children's Cough [US-OTC] *see* guaifenesin and dextromethorphan *on page 474*
Mucinex®, Children's Mini-Melts™ [US-OTC] *see* guaifenesin *on page 473*
Mucinex® DM [US-OTC] *see* guaifenesin and dextromethorphan *on page 474*
Mucinex® DM Maximum Strength [US-OTC] *see* guaifenesin and dextromethorphan *on page 474*
Mucinex® Full force™ [US-OTC] *see* oxymetazoline *on page 740*
Mucinex®, Junior Mini-Melts™ [US-OTC] *see* guaifenesin *on page 473*
Mucinex® Maximum Strength [US-OTC] *see* guaifenesin *on page 473*
Mucinex® moisture smart™ [US-OTC] *see* oxymetazoline *on page 740*
Mucomyst® [Can] *see* acetylcysteine *on page 31*

mucosal barrier gel, oral (myoo KOH sul BAR ee er GEL, OR al)

Synonyms mucosal bioadherent gel

U.S./Canadian Brand Names Gelclair® [US]

Therapeutic Category Gastrointestinal Agent, Miscellaneous

Use Management of oral mucosal pain caused by oral mucositis/stomatitis (resulting from chemotherapy or radiation therapy), irritation due to oral surgery, traumatic ulcers caused by braces/ill-fitting dentures or disease, diffuse aphthous ulcers (canker sores)

Usual Dosage Oral: Adults: Mucosal protection: Gargle and spit the mixture of 1 single-use packet (15 mL) and water 3 times daily, or as needed. May be used undiluted if water is unavailable.

Dosage Forms

Gel, oral [concentrate]:
Gelclair®: 15 mL/packet (15s)

mucosal bioadherent gel *see* mucosal barrier gel, oral *on page 671*
Mucosil™ *(Discontinued)* *see* acetylcysteine *on page 31*
Multaq® [US] *see* dronedarone *on page 339*
Multidex® [US-OTC] *see* maltodextrin *on page 612*
Multihance® [US] *see* gadobenate dimeglumine *on page 451*
Multihance® Multipak™ [US] *see* gadobenate dimeglumine *on page 451*
multiple vitamins *see* vitamins (multiple/oral) *on page 1019*
Multitest CMI® *(Discontinued)*
Multitrace®-4 [US] *see* trace metals *on page 974*
Multitrace®-4 Concentrate [US] *see* trace metals *on page 974*
Multitrace®-4 Neonatal [US] *see* trace metals *on page 974*
Multitrace®-4 Pediatric [US] *see* trace metals *on page 974*
Multitrace®-5 [US] *see* trace metals *on page 974*
Multitrace®-5 Concentrate [US] *see* trace metals *on page 974*
multivitamins/fluoride *see* vitamins (multiple/pediatric) *on page 1020*
mumps, measles, and rubella vaccines *see* measles, mumps, and rubella virus vaccine *on page 615*
mumps, rubella, varicella, and measles vaccine *see* measles, mumps, rubella, and varicella virus vaccine *on page 616*
Mumpsvax® [US] *see* mumps virus vaccine *on page 671*

mumps virus vaccine (mumpz VYE rus vak SEEN)

U.S./Canadian Brand Names Mumpsvax® [US]

Therapeutic Category Vaccine, Live Virus

Use Mumps prophylaxis by promoting active immunity

Note: Unless contraindicated, trivalent measles - mumps - rubella (MMR) is the vaccine of choice if recipients are likely to be susceptible to rubella and/or measles as well as to mumps.

The Advisory Committee on Immunization Practices (ACIP) recommends routine vaccination for the following:
- All children (first dose given at 12-15 months of age)
- Adults born 1957 or later (without evidence of immunity or documentation of vaccination)
- Adults at higher risk for exposure to and transmission of mumps should receive special consideration for vaccination, unless an acceptable evidence of immunity exists. This includes international travelers, persons attending colleges and other post-high school education, persons working in healthcare facilities.

Usual Dosage Note: Trivalent measles - mumps - rubella (MMR) vaccine should be used unless contraindicated in adults and children ≥12 months of age.Children ≥12 months: SubQ: 0.5 mL. Primary vaccination recommended at 12-15 months of age and repeated at 4-6 years of age. For older children not previously vaccinated, at least 28 days should elapse between doses.

Mumps outbreak: Children ages 1-4 years should be considered for receiving a second dose of a live mumps virus vaccine; minimum interval between doses is 28 days

Adults: SubQ: 0.5 mL

Adults born in or after 1957 without documentation of live vaccine on or after first birthday, without physician-diagnosed mumps, or without laboratory evidence of immunity should be vaccinated, ideally with 2 doses of vaccine separated by no less than 1 month. For those previously vaccinated with 1 dose of mumps vaccine, revaccination is recommended for students entering colleges and other institutions of higher education, for healthcare workers at the time of employment, and for international travelers who visit endemic areas. Unvaccinated healthcare providers born before 1957 and without evidence of mumps immunity, one dose of vaccine should be considered and a second dose should also be considered during an outbreak. During a mumps outbreak, vaccination may be considered for all persons born before 1957 who may be exposed to mumps and susceptible to infection.

Dosage Forms

Injection, powder for reconstitution [preservative free]:

Mumpsvax®: ≥20,000 $TCID_{50}$

mupirocin (myoo PEER oh sin)

Sound-Alike/Look-Alike Issues

Bactroban® may be confused with bacitracin, baclofen, Bactrim™

Synonyms mupirocin calcium; pseudomonic acid A

U.S./Canadian Brand Names Bactroban Cream® [US]; Bactroban Nasal® [US]; Bactroban® [US/Can]

Therapeutic Category Antibiotic, Topical

Use

Intranasal: Eradication of nasal colonization with MRSA in adult patients and healthcare workers

Topical: Treatment of impetigo or secondary infected traumatic skin lesions due to *S. aureus* and *S. pyogenes*

Usual Dosage

Intranasal: Children ≥12 years and Adults: Eradication of nasal MRSA: Approximately one-half of the ointment from the single-use tube should be applied into one nostril and the other half into the other nostril twice daily for 5 days

Topical:

Children ≥2 months and Adults: Impetigo: Ointment: Apply to affected area 3 times/day; reevaluate after 3-5 days if no clinical response

Children ≥3 months and Adults: Secondary skin infections: Cream: Apply to affected area 3 times/day for 10 days; reevaluate after 3-5 days if no clinical response

Dosage Forms

Cream, topical:

Bactroban Cream®: 2% (15 g, 30 g)

Ointment, intranasal:

Bactroban Nasal®: 2% (1 g)

Ointment, topical: 2% (0.9 g, 22 g)

Bactroban®: 2% (22 g)

mupirocin calcium *see* mupirocin *on page* *672*

Murine® Ear Wax Removal System [US-OTC] *see* carbamide peroxide *on page* *181*

Murine® Tears [US-OTC] *see* artificial tears *on page* *100*

Murine® Tears Plus [US-OTC] *see* tetrahydrozoline *on page* *951*

Muro 128® [US-OTC] *see* sodium chloride *on page* *908*

Murocel® [US-OTC] *see* artificial tears *on page* *100*

Murocoll-2® [US] *see* phenylephrine and scopolamine *on page 777*

muromonab-CD3 (myoo roe MOE nab see dee three)

Synonyms monoclonal antibody; OKT3

U.S./Canadian Brand Names Orthoclone OKT® 3 [US/Can]

Therapeutic Category Immunosuppressant Agent

Use Treatment of acute allograft rejection in renal transplant patients; treatment of acute hepatic, and kidney rejection episodes resistant to conventional treatment

Usual Dosage I.V. (refer to individual protocols):

Children <30 kg: 2.5 mg/day once daily for 7-14 days
Children >30 kg: 5 mg/day once daily for 7-14 days
OR
Children <12 years: 0.1 mg/kg/day once daily for 10-14 days
Children ≥12 years and Adults: 5 mg/day once daily for 10-14 days

Dosage Forms

Injection, solution:
Orthoclone OKT® 3: 1 mg/mL (5 mL)

Muroptic-5® ***(Discontinued)*** *see* sodium chloride *on page 908*
Muse® [US] *see* alprostadil *on page 51*
Muse® Pellet [Can] *see* alprostadil *on page 51*
Mustargen® [US/Can] *see* mechlorethamine *on page 618*
mustine *see* mechlorethamine *on page 618*
Mutamycin® [Can] *see* mitomycin *on page 662*
M.V.I.®-12 [US] *see* vitamins (multiple/injectable) *on page 1019*
M.V.I. Adult™ [US] *see* vitamins (multiple/injectable) *on page 1019*
M.V.I® Pediatric [US] *see* vitamins (multiple/injectable) *on page 1019*
Myadec® [US-OTC] *see* vitamins (multiple/oral) *on page 1019*
Myambutol® [US] *see* ethambutol *on page 382*
Mycamine® [US/Can] *see* micafungin *on page 654*
Mycelex® [US] *see* clotrimazole *on page 248*
Mycelex®-G ***(Discontinued)*** *see* clotrimazole *on page 248*
Mycifradin® Sulfate ***(Discontinued)*** *see* neomycin *on page 686*
Mycinaire™ ***(Discontinued)*** *see* sodium chloride *on page 908*
Mycinettes® [US-OTC] *see* benzocaine *on page 129*
Mycobutin® [US/Can] *see* rifabutin *on page 866*
Mycocide® NS [US-OTC] *see* tolnaftate *on page 968*
Mycolog®-II ***(Discontinued)*** *see* nystatin and triamcinolone *on page 716*
Myco-Nail [US-OTC] *see* triacetin *on page 981*
Myconel® Topical ***(Discontinued)*** *see* nystatin and triamcinolone *on page 716*

mycophenolate (mye koe FEN oh late)

Synonyms MMF; MPA; mycophenolate mofetil; mycophenolate sodium; mycophenolic acid

U.S./Canadian Brand Names CellCept® [US/Can]; Myfortic® [US/Can]

Therapeutic Category Immunosuppressant Agent

Use Prophylaxis of organ rejection concomitantly with cyclosporine and corticosteroids in patients receiving allogeneic renal (CellCept®, Myfortic®), cardiac (CellCept®), or hepatic (CellCept®) transplants

Usual Dosage

Children: Renal transplant: Oral:
CellCept® suspension: 600 mg/m^2/dose twice daily; maximum dose: 1 g twice daily
Alternatively, may use solid dosage forms according to BSA as follows:
BSA 1.25-1.5 m^2: 750 mg capsule twice daily
BSA >1.5 m^2: 1 g capsule or tablet twice daily
Myfortic®: 400 mg/m^2/dose twice daily; maximum dose: 720 mg twice daily
BSA <1.19 m^2: Use of this formulation is not recommended
BSA 1.19-1.58 m^2: 540 mg twice daily (maximum: 1080 mg/day)
BSA >1.58 m^2: 720 mg twice daily (maximum: 1440 mg/day)

Adults: **Note:** May be used I.V. for up to 14 days; transition to oral therapy as soon as tolerated.
Renal transplant:
CellCept®:
Oral: 1 g twice daily. Doses >2 g/day are not recommended.
I.V.: 1 g twice daily
Myfortic®: Oral: 720 mg twice daily (1440 mg/day)
Cardiac transplantation:
Oral (CellCept®): 1.5 g twice daily
I.V. (CellCept®): 1.5 g twice daily
Hepatic transplantation:
Oral (CellCept®): 1.5 g twice daily
I.V. (CellCept®): 1 g twice daily

Dosage Forms

Capsule, oral: 250 mg
CellCept®: 250 mg
Injection, powder for reconstitution:
CellCept®: 500 mg
Powder for suspension. oral:
CellCept®: 200 mg/mL
Tablet, oral: 500 mg
CellCept®: 500 mg
Tablet, delayed release, oral:
Myfortic®: 180 mg, 360 mg

mycophenolate mofetil *see* mycophenolate *on page 673*
mycophenolate sodium *see* mycophenolate *on page 673*
mycophenolic acid *see* mycophenolate *on page 673*
Mycostatin® [US] *see* nystatin *on page 715*
MyDex [US] *see* guaifenesin and phenylephrine *on page 475*
Mydfrin® [US/Can] *see* phenylephrine *on page 774*
Mydral™ [US] *see* tropicamide *on page 992*
Mydriacyl® [US/Can] *see* tropicamide *on page 992*
My First Flintstones™ [US-OTC] *see* vitamins (multiple/pediatric) *on page 1020*
Myfortic® [US/Can] *see* mycophenolate *on page 673*
MyHist-DM [US] *see* phenylephrine, pyrilamine, and dextromethorphan *on page 778*
MyHist-PD [US] *see* chlorpheniramine, pyrilamine, and phenylephrine *on page 221*
MyKidz Iron™ [US-OTC] *see* vitamins (multiple/pediatric) *on page 1020*
MyKidz Iron 10™ [US-OTC] *see* ferrous sulfate *on page 414*
MyKidz Iron FL™ [US] *see* vitamins (multiple/pediatric) *on page 1020*
Mykrox® *(Discontinued)* *see* metolazone *on page 650*
Mylan-Ciprofloxacin [Can] *see* ciprofloxacin *on page 229*
Mylan-Lamotrigine [Can] *see* lamotrigine *on page 567*
Mylan-Naproxen EC [Can] *see* naproxen *on page 681*
Mylanta™ [Can] *see* aluminum hydroxide and magnesium hydroxide *on page 55*
Mylanta®-II *(Discontinued)* *see* aluminum hydroxide, magnesium hydroxide, and simethicone *on page 56*
Mylanta AR® *(Discontinued)* *see* famotidine *on page 405*
Mylanta® Children's [US-OTC] *see* calcium carbonate *on page 170*
Mylanta® Double Strength [Can] *see* aluminum hydroxide, magnesium hydroxide, and simethicone *on page 56*
Mylanta® Extra Strength [Can] *see* aluminum hydroxide, magnesium hydroxide, and simethicone *on page 56*
Mylanta® Gas Maximum Strength [US-OTC] *see* simethicone *on page 901*
Mylanta® Gelcaps® [US-OTC] *see* calcium carbonate and magnesium hydroxide *on page 171*
Mylanta® Liquid [US-OTC] *see* aluminum hydroxide, magnesium hydroxide, and simethicone *on page 56*
Mylanta® Maximum Strength Liquid [US-OTC] *see* aluminum hydroxide, magnesium hydroxide, and simethicone *on page 56*

Mylan-Tamoxifen [Can] *see* tamoxifen *on page 937*
Mylan-Tamsulosin [Can] *see* tamsulosin *on page 938*
Mylanta® Regular Strength [Can] *see* aluminum hydroxide, magnesium hydroxide, and simethicone *on page 56*
Mylanta® Supreme [US-OTC] *see* calcium carbonate and magnesium hydroxide *on page 171*
Mylanta® Ultra [US-OTC] *see* calcium carbonate and magnesium hydroxide *on page 171*
Mylan-Topiramate [Can] *see* topiramate *on page 969*
Mylan-Venlafaxine XR [Can] *see* venlafaxine *on page 1009*
Mylan-Verapamil [Can] *see* verapamil *on page 1010*
Mylan-Verapamil SR [Can] *see* verapamil *on page 1010*
Myleran® [US/Can] *see* busulfan *on page 160*
Mylicon® Infants [US-OTC] *see* simethicone *on page 901*
Mylocel™ [US] *see* hydroxyurea *on page 510*
Mylotarg® [US/Can] *see* gemtuzumab ozogamicin *on page 459*
Myminic® Expectorant *(Discontinued)*
Myobloc® [US] *see* rimabotulinumtoxinB *on page 868*
Myochrysine® [US/Can] *see* gold sodium thiomalate *on page 470*
Myoflex® [US-OTC/Can] *see* trolamine *on page 991*
Myotonachol® *(Discontinued)* *see* bethanechol *on page 139*
Myozyme® [US] *see* alglucosidase alfa *on page 46*
Myphetane DX [US] *see* brompheniramine, pseudoephedrine, and dextromethorphan *on page 152*
myrac™ [US] *see* minocycline *on page 659*
Mysoline® [US] *see* primidone *on page 818*
Mytelase® [US/Can] *see* ambenonium *on page 58*
mytotan *see* mitotane *on page 662*
Mytrex *(Discontinued)* *see* nystatin and triamcinolone *on page 716*
Mytussin® AC [US] *see* guaifenesin and codeine *on page 473*
Mytussin® DAC [US] *see* guaifenesin, pseudoephedrine, and codeine *on page 479*
N-9 *see* nonoxynol 9 *on page 703*
Na_2EDTA *see* edetate disodium *on page 347*
NAAK *see* atropine and pralidoxime *on page 112*
Nabi-HB® [US] *see* hepatitis B immune globulin (human) *on page 489*
nab-paclitaxel *see* paclitaxel (protein bound) *on page 743*

nabumetone (na BYOO me tone)

U.S./Canadian Brand Names Apo-Nabumetone® [Can]; Gen-Nabumetone [Can]; Novo-Nabumetone [Can]; Relafen® [Can]; Rhoxal-nabumetone [Can]; Sandoz-Nabumetone [Can]

Therapeutic Category Analgesic, Nonnarcotic; Nonsteroidal Antiinflammatory Drug (NSAID)

Use Management of osteoarthritis and rheumatoid arthritis

Usual Dosage Oral: Adults: 1000 mg/day; an additional 500-1000 mg may be needed in some patients to obtain more symptomatic relief; may be administered once or twice daily (maximum dose: 2000 mg/day)
Note: Patients <50 kg are less likely to require doses >1000 mg/day.

Dosage Forms
Tablet: 500 mg, 750 mg

NAC *see* acetylcysteine *on page 31*
***N*-acetyl-L-cysteine** *see* acetylcysteine *on page 31*
***N*-acetylcysteine** *see* acetylcysteine *on page 31*
n-acetyl-p-aminophenol *see* acetaminophen *on page 19*
NaCl *see* sodium chloride *on page 908*

nadolol (NAY doe lol)

Sound-Alike/Look-Alike Issues
nadolol may be confused with Mandol®
Corgard® may be confused with Cognex®, Coreg®

U.S./Canadian Brand Names Alti-Nadolol [Can]; Apo-Nadol® [Can]; Corgard® [US/Can]; Novo-Nadolol [Can]

Therapeutic Category Beta-Adrenergic Blocker

Use Treatment of hypertension and angina pectoris; prophylaxis of migraine headaches

Usual Dosage Oral: Adults: Initial: 40 mg/day, increase dosage gradually by 40-80 mg increments at 3- to 7-day intervals until optimum clinical response is obtained with profound slowing of heart rate; doses up to 160-240 mg/day in angina and 240-320 mg/day in hypertension may be necessary.

Hypertension: Usual dosage range (JNC 7): 40-120 mg once daily

Dosage Forms

Tablet: 20 mg, 40 mg, 80 mg

Corgard®: 20 mg, 40 mg, 80 mg

nadolol and bendroflumethiazide (NAY doe lol & ben droe floo meth EYE a zide)

Synonyms bendroflumethiazide and nadolol

U.S./Canadian Brand Names Corzide® [US]

Therapeutic Category Antihypertensive Agent, Combination; Beta-Adrenergic Blocker, Nonselective; Diuretic, Thiazide

Use Treatment of hypertension; combination product should not be used for initial therapy

Usual Dosage Oral: Adults: Treatment of hypertension: Initial: Nadolol 40 mg and bendroflumethiazide 5 mg once daily. May increase dose to nadolol 80 mg and bendroflumethiazide 5 mg once daily if needed.

Dosage Forms

Tablet: Nadolol 40 mg and bendroflumethiazide 5 mg; nadolol 80 mg and bendroflumethiazide 5 mg

Corzide® 40/5: Nadolol 40 mg and bendroflumethiazide 5 mg [scored]

Corzide® 80/5: Nadolol 80 mg and bendroflumethiazide 5 mg [scored]

nadroparin calcium *see* nadroparin *(Canada only) on page 676*

nadroparin *(Canada only)* (nad roe PA rin)

Synonyms nadroparin calcium

U.S./Canadian Brand Names Fraxiparine™ Forte [Can]; Fraxiparine™ [Can]

Therapeutic Category Low Molecular Weight Heparin

Use Prophylaxis of thromboembolic disorders (particularly deep venous thrombosis and pulmonary embolism) in general and orthopedic surgery; treatment of deep venous thrombosis; prevention of clotting during hemodialysis

Usual Dosage SubQ: Adults:

Prophylaxis of thromboembolic disorders in general surgery: 2850 anti-Xa int. units once daily; begin 2-4 hours before surgery and continue for 7 days

Prophylaxis of thromboembolic disorders in hip replacement: 38 anti-Xa int. units/kg 12 hours before and 12 hours after surgery, **followed by** 38 anti-Xa int. units/kg/day up to and including day 3, **then** 57 anti-Xa int. units/kg/day for up to 10 days total therapy

Treatment of thromboembolic disorders: 171 anti-Xa int. units/kg/day to a maximum of 17,100 int. units; plasma anti-Xa levels should be 1.2-1.8 anti-Xa int. units/mL 3-4 hours postinjection

Patients at increased risk of bleeding: 86 anti-Xa int. units/kg twice daily; plasma anti-Xa levels should be 0.5-1.1 anti-Xa int. units/mL 3-4 hours postinjection

Prevention of clotting during hemodialysis: Single dose of 65 anti-Xa int. units/kg into arterial line at start of each dialysis session; may give additional dose if session lasts longer than 4 hours

Patients at risk of hemorrhage: Administer 50% of dose

Dosage Forms [CAN] = Canadian brand name

Injection, solution:

Fraxiparine™ [CAN]: 9500 anti-Xa int. units/mL (0.2 mL, 0.3 mL, 0.4 mL, 0.6 mL, 0.8 mL, 1 mL) [not available in the U.S.]

Fraxiparine™ Forte [CAN]: 19,000 anti-Xa int. units/mL (0.6 mL, 0.8 mL, 1 mL) [not available in the U.S.]

nafarelin (naf a REL in)

Sound-Alike/Look-Alike Issues

nafarelin may be confused with Anafranil®, enalapril

Synonyms nafarelin acetate

U.S./Canadian Brand Names Synarel® [US/Can]

Therapeutic Category Hormone, Posterior Pituitary

Use Treatment of endometriosis, including pain and reduction of lesions; treatment of central precocious puberty (CPP; gonadotropin-dependent precocious puberty) in children of both sexes

Usual Dosage Intranasal:

Endometriosis: Adults: Female: 1 spray (200 mcg) in 1 nostril each morning and the other nostril each evening starting on days 2-4 of menstrual cycle (total: 2 sprays/day). Dose may be increased to 2 sprays (400 mcg; 1 spray in each nostril) in the morning and evening if amenorrhea is not achieved (total: 8 sprays [1600 mcg]/day). Total duration of therapy should not exceed 6 months due to decreases in bone mineral density; retreatment is not recommended by the manufacturer.

Central precocious puberty: Children: Male/Female: 2 sprays (400 mcg) into each nostril in the morning and 2 sprays (400 mcg) into each nostril in the evening (total: 8 sprays [1600 mcg]/day). If inadequate suppression, may increase dose to 3 sprays (600 mcg) into alternating nostrils 3 times/day (total: 9 sprays [1800 mcg]/day).

Dosage Forms

Solution, intranasal [spray]:

Synarel®: 2 mg/mL (8 mL)

nafarelin acetate *see* nafarelin *on page 676*

Nafazair® Ophthalmic *(Discontinued)* *see* naphazoline *on page 680*

nafcillin (naf SIL in)

Synonyms ethoxynaphthamido penicillin sodium; nafcillin sodium; sodium nafcillin

U.S./Canadian Brand Names Nallpen® [Can]; Unipen® [Can]

Therapeutic Category Penicillin

Use Treatment of infections such as osteomyelitis, septicemia, endocarditis, and CNS infections caused by susceptible strains of staphylococci species

Usual Dosage

Usual dosage range:

Neonates: I.M., I.V.:

1200-2000 g, <7 days: 50 mg/kg/day divided every 12 hours
>2000 g, <7 days: 75 mg/kg/day divided every 8 hours
1200-2000 g, ≥7 days: 75 mg/kg/day divided every 8 hours
>2000 g, ≥7 days: 100-140 mg/kg/day divided every 6 hours

Children:

I.M.: 25 mg/kg twice daily
I.V.: 50-200 mg/kg/day in divided doses every 4-6 hours (maximum: 12 g/day)

Adults:

I.M.: 500 mg every 4-6 hours
I.V.: 500-2000 mg every 4-6 hours

Indication-specific dosing:

Children:

Mild-to-moderate infections: I.M., I.V.: 50-100 mg/kg/day in divided doses every 6 hours

Severe infections: I.M., I.V.: 100-200 mg/kg/day in divided doses every 4-6 hours (maximum dose: 12 g/day)

Staphylococcal endocarditis: I.V.:

Native valve: 200 mg/kg/day in divided doses every 4-6 hours for 6 weeks

Prosthetic valve: 200 mg/kg/day in divided doses every 4-6 hours for ≥6 weeks (use with rifampin and gentamicin)

Adults: I.V.:

Endocarditis: MSSA:

Native valve: 12 g/24 hours in 4-6 divided doses for 6 weeks

Prosthetic valve: 12 g/24 hours in 6 divided doses for ≥6 weeks (use with rifampin and gentamicin)

Joint:

Bursitis, septic: 2 g every 4 hours

Prosthetic: 2 g every 4-6 hours with rifampin for 6 weeks

***Staphylococcus aureus,* methicillin-susceptible infections, including brain abscess, empyema, erysipelas, mastitis, myositis, orbital cellulitis, osteomyelitis, pneumonia, splenic abscess, toxic shock, urinary tract (perinephric abscess):** 2 g every 4 hours

Dosage Forms

Infusion [premixed iso-osmotic dextrose solution]: 1 g (50 mL); 2 g (100 mL)

Injection, powder for reconstitution: 1 g, 2 g, 10 g

nafcillin sodium *see* nafcillin *on page* *677*

naftifine (NAF ti feen)

Synonyms naftifine hydrochloride

U.S./Canadian Brand Names Naftin® [US]

Therapeutic Category Antifungal Agent

Use Topical treatment of tinea cruris (jock itch), tinea corporis (ringworm), and tinea pedis (athlete's foot)

Usual Dosage Topical: Adults: Apply cream once daily and gel twice daily (morning and evening) for up to 4 weeks

Dosage Forms

Cream:

Naftin®: 1% (30 g, 60 g, 90 g)

Gel:

Naftin®: 1% (40 g, 60 g, 90 g)

naftifine hydrochloride *see* naftifine *on page* *678*

Naftin® [US] *see* naftifine *on page* *678*

Naglazyme™ [US] *see* galsulfase *on page* *454*

$NaHCO_3$ *see* sodium bicarbonate *on page* *907*

nalbuphine (NAL byoo feen)

Sound-Alike/Look-Alike Issues

Nubain® may be confused with Navane®, Nebcin®

Synonyms nalbuphine hydrochloride

U.S./Canadian Brand Names Nubain® [US]

Therapeutic Category Analgesic, Narcotic

Use Relief of moderate-to-severe pain; preoperative analgesia, postoperative and surgical anesthesia, and obstetrical analgesia during labor and delivery

Usual Dosage Adults:

Pain management: I.M., I.V., SubQ: 10 mg/70 kg every 3-6 hours; maximum single dose in nonopioid-tolerant patients: 20 mg; maximum daily dose: 160 mg

Surgical anesthesia supplement: I.V.: Induction: 0.3-3 mg/kg over 10-15 minutes; maintenance doses of 0.25-0.5 mg/kg may be given as required

Dosage Forms

Injection, solution: 10 mg/mL (10 mL); 20 mg/mL (10 mL)

Nubain®: 20 mg/mL (10 mL)

Injection, solution [preservative free]: 10 mg/mL (1 mL); 20 mg/mL (1 mL)

Nubain®: 10 mg/mL (1 mL); 20 mg/mL (1 mL)

nalbuphine hydrochloride *see* nalbuphine *on page* *678*

Nalcrom® [Can] *see* cromolyn sodium *on page* *261*

Naldecon® DX Adult Liquid *(Discontinued)*

Naldecon-EX® Children's Syrup *(Discontinued)*

Naldecon Senior EX® *(Discontinued)* *see* guaifenesin *on page* *473*

Nalex®-A [US] *see* chlorpheniramine, phenylephrine, and phenyltoloxamine *on page* *219*

Nalex A 12 [US] *see* chlorpheniramine, pyrilamine, and phenylephrine *on page* *221*

Nalfon® [US/Can] *see* fenoprofen *on page* *410*

Nallpen® [Can] *see* nafcillin *on page* *677*

Nallpen® *(Discontinued)* *see* nafcillin *on page* *677*

***N*-allylnoroxymorphine hydrochloride** *see* naloxone *on page* *678*

nalmefene *(Discontinued)*

naloxone (nal OKS one)

Sound-Alike/Look-Alike Issues

naloxone may be confused with Lanoxin®, naltrexone

Narcan® may be confused with Marcaine®, Norcuron®

Synonyms *N*-allylnoroxymorphine hydrochloride; naloxone hydrochloride

U.S./Canadian Brand Names Naloxone Hydrochloride Injection® [Can]

Therapeutic Category Antidote

Use Complete or partial reversal of opioid drug effects, including respiratory depression; management of known or suspected opioid overdose; diagnosis of suspected opioid dependence or acute opioid overdose

Usual Dosage **Note:** I.M., I.V. (preferred), and SubQ routes are available. Endotracheal administration is the least desirable and is supported by only anecdotal evidence (case report):

Infants and Children: Postoperative reversal: 0.01 mg/kg; may repeat every 2-3 minutes as needed based on response (adequate ventilation without significant pain)

Children:

Opioid intoxication: Respiratory depression:

I.V.:

Birth (including premature infants) to 5 years or <20 kg: Initial: 0.1 mg/kg (maximum dose: 2 mg); repeat every 2-3 minutes if needed

>5 years or ≥20 kg: 2 mg/dose; if no response, repeat every 2-3 minutes

Continuous infusion: I.V.: If continuous infusion is required, calculate dosage/hour based on effective intermittent dose used and duration of adequate response seen **or** use 2/3 of the initial effective naloxone bolus on an hourly basis; titrate dose (typically 0.04-0.16 mg/kg/hour for 2-5 days in children); 1/2 of the initial bolus dose should be readministered 15 minutes after initiation of the continuous infusion to prevent a drop in naloxone levels; increase infusion rate as needed to assure adequate ventilation and prevent withdrawal symptoms

Adults:

Opioid intoxication: Respiratory depression: I.V.: 0.4-2 mg; may need to repeat doses every 2-3 minutes; after reversal, may need to readminister dose(s) at a later interval (ie, 20-60 minutes) depending on type/duration of opioid. If no response is observed after 10 mg, consider other causes of respiratory depression. **Note:** Opioid-dependent patients may require lower doses (0.1 mg) titrated incrementally to avoid precipitating acute withdrawal.

Continuous infusion: I.V.: Calculate dosage/hour based on effective intermittent dose used and duration of adequate response seen **or** use 2/3 of the initial effective naloxone bolus on an hourly basis (typically 0.25-6.25 mg/hour); 1/2 of the initial bolus dose should be readministered 15 minutes after initiation of the continuous infusion to prevent a drop in naloxone levels; adjust infusion rate as needed to assure adequate ventilation and prevent withdrawal symptoms

Postoperative reversal: I.V.: 0.1-0.2 mg every 2-3 minutes until desired response (adequate ventilation and alertness without significant pain). **Note:** Repeat doses may be needed within 1-2 hour intervals depending on type, dose, and timing of the last dose of opioid administered.

Dosage Forms

Injection, solution, as hydrochloride: 0.4 mg/mL (1 mL, 10 mL)

Injection, solution, as hydrochloride [preservative free]: 0.4 mg/mL (1 mL); 1 mg/mL (2 mL)

naloxone and buprenorphine *see* buprenorphine and naloxone *on page 158*

naloxone hydrochloride *see* naloxone *on page 678*

naloxone hydrochloride and pentazocine hydrochloride *see* pentazocine *on page 764*

naloxone hydrochloride dihydrate and buprenorphine hydrochloride *see* buprenorphine and naloxone *on page 158*

Naloxone Hydrochloride Injection® [Can] *see* naloxone *on page 678*

naltrexone (nal TREKS one)

Sound-Alike/Look-Alike Issues

naltrexone may be confused with methylnaltrexone, naloxone

ReVia® may be confused with Revatio®, Revex®

Synonyms naltrexone hydrochloride

U.S./Canadian Brand Names Depade® [US]; ReVia® [US/Can]; Vivitrol™ [US]

Therapeutic Category Antidote

Use Treatment of ethanol dependence; blockade of the effects of exogenously administered opioids

Usual Dosage Adults: Do not give until patient is opioid-free for 7-10 days as determined by urinalysis

Oral: Alcohol dependence, opioid antidote: 25 mg; if no withdrawal signs within 1 hour give another 25 mg; maintenance regimen is flexible, variable and individualized (50 mg/day to 100-150 mg 3 times/week for 12 weeks); up to 800 mg/day has been tolerated in a small number of healthy adults without an adverse effect

I.M.: Alcohol dependence: 380 mg once every 4 weeks

Dosage Forms

Injection, microspheres for suspension, extended release:

Vivitrol™: 380 mg

Tablet: 50 mg

Depade®: 25 mg, 50 mg, 100 mg

ReVia®: 50 mg

naltrexone hydrochloride *see* naltrexone *on page 679*

Namenda™ [US] *see* memantine *on page 623*

nandrolone *(Canada only)* (NAN droe lone)

Synonyms nandrolone decanoate; nandrolone phenpropionate

U.S./Canadian Brand Names Deca-Durabolin® [Can]

Therapeutic Category Androgen

Use Adjunctive treatment in aplastic or sickle cell anemia, osteoporosis (senile and postmenopausal), pituitary dwarfism. Also demonstrates anabolic effects in chronic disease, inoperable breast cancer, decubitus ulcers, burns, corticoid-induced catabolic states, and myopathies.

Usual Dosage I.M.:

Children 2-13 years: 25-50 mg every 3-4 weeks for up to 12 weeks, then withhold for 4 weeks; if indicated, may resume treatment following 4-week rest period

Adults: General anabolic effects: 50–100 mg every 3-4 weeks for up to 12 weeks, then withhold for 4 weeks; if indicated, may resume treatment following 4-week rest period

Dosage Forms [CAN] = Canadian product

Injection, solution:

Deca-Durabolin® [CAN]: 100 mg/mL (2 mL) [not available in U.S.]

nandrolone decanoate *see* nandrolone *(Canada only) on page 680*

nandrolone phenpropionate *see* nandrolone *(Canada only) on page 680*

nanoparticle albumin-bound paclitaxel *see* paclitaxel (protein bound) *on page 743*

NAPA and NABZ *see* sodium phenylacetate and sodium benzoate *on page 912*

naphazoline (naf AZ oh leen)

Synonyms naphazoline hydrochloride

U.S./Canadian Brand Names AK-Con™ [US]; Clear eyes® for Dry Eyes and ACR Relief [US-OTC]; Clear eyes® for Dry Eyes and Redness Relief [US-OTC]; Clear eyes® Redness Relief [US-OTC]; Clear eyes® Seasonal Relief [US-OTC]; Naphcon Forte® [Can]; Privine® [US-OTC]; Vasocon® [Can]

Therapeutic Category Adrenergic Agonist Agent

Use Topical ocular vasoconstrictor; temporary relief of nasal congestion associated with the common cold, upper respiratory allergies, or sinusitis; relief of redness of the eye due to minor irritation

Usual Dosage

Nasal: Children ≥12 years and Adults: 0.05% instill 1-2 drops or sprays every 6 hours if needed; therapy should not exceed 3 days

Ophthalmic: Adults:

0.1% (prescription): 1-2 drops into conjuctival sac every 3-4 hours as needed

0.012% or 0.025% (OTC): 1-2 drops into affected eye(s) up to 4 times a day; therapy should not exceed 3 days

Dosage Forms

Solution, intranasal drops:

Privine® [OTC]: 0.05% (25 mL)

Solution, intranasal spray:

Privine® [OTC]: 0.05% (20 mL)

Solution, ophthalmic:

AK-Con™: 0.1% (15 mL)

Clear eyes® for Dry Eyes and ACR Relief [OTC]: 0.025% (15 mL)

Clear eyes® for Dry Eyes and Redness Relief [OTC]: 0.012% (15 mL)

Clear eyes® Redness Relief [OTC]: 0.012% (6 mL, 15 mL, 30 mL)

Clear eyes® Seasonal Relief [OTC]: 0.012% (15 mL, 30 mL)

naphazoline and pheniramine (naf AZ oh leen & fen NIR a meen)

Sound-Alike/Look-Alike Issues

Visine® may be confused with Visken®

Synonyms pheniramine and naphazoline

U.S./Canadian Brand Names Naphcon-A® [US-OTC/Can]; Opcon-A® [US-OTC]; Visine-A® [US-OTC]; Visine® Advanced Allergy [Can]

Therapeutic Category Antihistamine/Decongestant Combination

Use Treatment of ocular congestion, irritation, and itching

Usual Dosage Ophthalmic: Children ≥6 years and Adults: 1-2 drops up to 4 times/day

Dosage Forms

Solution, ophthalmic:

Naphcon-A® [OTC]: Naphazoline 0.025% and pheniramine 0.3%
Opcon-A® [OTC]: Naphazoline 0.027% and pheniramine 0.3%
Visine-A® [OTC]: Naphazoline 0.025% and pheniramine 0.3%

naphazoline hydrochloride *see* naphazoline *on page* 680
Naphcon-A® [US-OTC/Can] *see* naphazoline and pheniramine *on page* 681
Naphcon® *(Discontinued)* *see* naphazoline *on page* 680
Naphcon Forte® [Can] *see* naphazoline *on page* 680
Naphcon Forte® Ophthalmic *(Discontinued)* *see* naphazoline *on page* 680
NapraPAC® *see* lansoprazole and naproxen *on page* 572
Naprelan® [US] *see* naproxen *on page* 681
Naprosyn® [US/Can] *see* naproxen *on page* 681

naproxen (na PROKS en)

Sound-Alike/Look-Alike Issues

naproxen may be confused with Natacyn®, Nebcin®
Aleve® may be confused with Alesse®
Anaprox® may be confused with Anaspaz®, Avapro®
Naprelan® may be confused with Naprosyn®
Naprosyn® may be confused with Naprelan®, Natacyn®, Nebcin®

Synonyms naproxen sodium

U.S./Canadian Brand Names Aleve® [US-OTC]; Anaprox® DS [US/Can]; Anaprox® [US/Can]; Apo-Napro-Na DS® [Can]; Apo-Napro-Na® [Can]; Apo-Naproxen EC® [Can]; Apo-Naproxen SR® [Can]; Apo-Naproxen® [Can]; EC-Naprosyn® [US]; Gen-Naproxen EC [Can]; Mediproxen [US-OTC]; Midol® Extended Relief [US-OTC]; Mylan-Naproxen EC [Can]; Naprelan® [US]; Naprosyn® [US/Can]; Naxen® EC [Can]; Naxen® [Can]; Novo-Naproc EC [Can]; Novo-Naprox Sodium DS [Can]; Novo-Naprox Sodium [Can]; Novo-Naprox SR [Can]; Novo-Naprox [Can]; Nu-Naprox [Can]; Pamprin® Maximum Strength All Day Relief [US-OTC]; PMS-Naproxen EC [Can]; Pro-Naproxen EC [Can]; Riva-Naproxen [Can]; Sab-Naproxen [Can]

Therapeutic Category Analgesic, Nonnarcotic; Antipyretic; Nonsteroidal Antiinflammatory Drug (NSAID)

Use Management of ankylosing spondylitis, osteoarthritis, and rheumatoid disorders (including juvenile rheumatoid arthritis); acute gout; mild-to-moderate pain; tendonitis, bursitis; dysmenorrhea; fever

Usual Dosage **Note:** Dosage expressed as naproxen base; 200 mg naproxen base is equivalent to 220 mg naproxen sodium.

Oral:

Children >2 years: Juvenile arthritis: 10 mg/kg/day in 2 divided doses

Adults:

Gout, acute: Initial: 750 mg, followed by 250 mg every 8 hours until attack subsides. **Note:** EC-Naprosyn® is not recommended.

Pain (mild-to-moderate), dysmenorrhea, acute tendonitis, bursitis: Initial: 500 mg, then 250 mg every 6-8 hours; maximum: 1250 mg/day naproxen base

Rheumatoid arthritis, osteoarthritis, and ankylosing spondylitis: 500-1000 mg/day in 2 divided doses; may increase to 1.5 g/day of naproxen base for limited time period

OTC labeling: Pain/fever:

Children ≥12 years and Adults ≤65 years: 200 mg naproxen base every 8-12 hours; if needed, may take 400 mg naproxen base for the initial dose; maximum: 600 mg naproxen base/24 hours

Adults >65 years: 200 mg naproxen base every 12 hours

Dosage Forms

Caplet: 220 mg

Aleve® [OTC], Midol® Extended Relief [OTC], Pamprin® Maximum Strength All Day Relief [OTC]: 220 mg

Capsule, liquid gel: 220 mg

Aleve® [OTC]: 220 mg

Gelcap: 220 mg

Aleve® [OTC]: 220 mg

Suspension, oral: 125 mg/5 mL

Naprosyn®: 125 mg/5 mL

Tablet: 220 mg, 250 mg, 275 mg, 375 mg, 500 mg, 550 mg

Aleve® [OTC]: 220 mg

Anaprox®: 275 mg

Anaprox® DS: 550 mg

Mediproxen [OTC]: 220 mg

Naprosyn®: 250 mg, 375 mg, 500 mg

Tablet, controlled release:

Naprelan®: 412.5 mg, 550 mg, 825 mg

Tablet, delayed release: 375 mg, 500 mg

EC-Naprosyn®: 375 mg, 500 mg

naproxen and lansoprazole *see* lansoprazole and naproxen *on page 572*

naproxen and pseudoephedrine (na PROKS en & soo doe e FED rin)

Synonyms naproxen sodium and pseudoephedrine; pseudoephedrine and naproxen

U.S./Canadian Brand Names Aleve®-D Sinus & Cold [US-OTC]; Aleve®-D Sinus & Headache [US-OTC]

Therapeutic Category Decongestant/Analgesic

Use Temporary relief of cold, sinus, and flu symptoms (including nasal congestion, sinus congestion/pressure, headache, minor body aches and pains, and fever)

Usual Dosage Oral: Children ≥12 years and Adults: One caplet every 12 hours (maximum dose: 2 caplets/24 hours); treatment for >7 days is not recommended unless directed by healthcare provider.

Dosage Forms

Caplet, extended release:

Aleve®-D Sinus & Cold [OTC], Aleve®-D Sinus & Headache [OTC]: Naproxen sodium 220 mg [equivalent to naproxen 200 mg and sodium 20 mg] and pseudoephedrine hydrochloride 120 mg

naproxen and sumatriptan *see* sumatriptan and naproxen *on page 933*

naproxen sodium *see* naproxen *on page 681*

naproxen sodium and pseudoephedrine *see* naproxen and pseudoephedrine *on page 682*

naproxen sodium and sumatriptan *see* sumatriptan and naproxen *on page 933*

naproxen sodium and sumatriptan succinate *see* sumatriptan and naproxen *on page 933*

naratriptan (NAR a trip tan)

Sound-Alike/Look-Alike Issues

Amerge® may be confused with Altace®, Amaryl®

Synonyms naratriptan hydrochloride

U.S./Canadian Brand Names Amerge® [US/Can]

Therapeutic Category Antimigraine Agent; Serotonin Agonist

Use Treatment of acute migraine headache with or without aura

Usual Dosage Oral: Adults: 1-2.5 mg at the onset of headache; it is recommended to use the lowest possible dose to minimize adverse effects. If headache returns or does not fully resolve, the dose may be repeated after 4 hours; do not exceed 5 mg in 24 hours.

Dosage Forms

Tablet:

Amerge®: 1 mg, 2.5 mg

naratriptan hydrochloride *see* naratriptan *on page 682*

Narcan® *(Discontinued)* *see* naloxone *on page 678*

Nardil® [US/Can] *see* phenelzine *on page 771*

Naropin® [US/Can] *see* ropivacaine *on page* 877
Nasacort® AQ [US/Can] *see* triamcinolone (inhalation, nasal) *on page* 982
Nasacort® HFA [US] *see* triamcinolone (inhalation, nasal) *on page* 982
Nasahist B® *(Discontinued)* *see* brompheniramine *on page* 149
NasalCrom® [US-OTC] *see* cromolyn sodium *on page* 261
Nasalide® [Can] *see* flunisolide *on page* 427
Nasal Moist® Saline [US-OTC] *see* sodium chloride *on page* 908
Nasal Spray [US-OTC] *see* sodium chloride *on page* 908
Nasarel® *(Discontinued)* *see* flunisolide *on page* 427
Nasatab® LA [US] *see* guaifenesin and pseudoephedrine *on page* 477
Nascobal® [US] *see* cyanocobalamin *on page* 263
Nasofed™ *(Discontinued)* *see* pseudoephedrine *on page* 833
Nasonex® [US/Can] *see* mometasone *on page* 665
Nasop12™ *(Discontinued)* *see* phenylephrine *on page* 774
Natabec® *(Discontinued)*
Natabec® FA *(Discontinued)*
Natabec® Rx *(Discontinued)*
NataCaps™ [US] *see* vitamins (multiple/prenatal) *on page* 1020
NataChew® [US-OTC] *see* vitamins (multiple/prenatal) *on page* 1020
Natacyn® [US/Can] *see* natamycin *on page* 683
NataFort® [US-OTC] *see* vitamins (multiple/prenatal) *on page* 1020
NatalCare® CFe 60 *(Discontinued)* *see* vitamins (multiple/prenatal) *on page* 1020
NatalCare® GlossTabs™ [US] *see* vitamins (multiple/prenatal) *on page* 1020
NatalCare® PIC [US] *see* vitamins (multiple/prenatal) *on page* 1020
NatalCare® PIC Forte [US] *see* vitamins (multiple/prenatal) *on page* 1020
NatalCare® Plus [US] *see* vitamins (multiple/prenatal) *on page* 1020
NatalCare® Rx [US] *see* vitamins (multiple/prenatal) *on page* 1020
NatalCare® Three [US] *see* vitamins (multiple/prenatal) *on page* 1020
Natalins® Rx *(Discontinued)*

natalizumab (na ta LIZ u mab)

Synonyms AN100226; anti-4 alpha integrin; IgG4-kappa monoclonal antibody

U.S./Canadian Brand Names Tysabri® [US/Can]

Therapeutic Category Monoclonal Antibody, Selective Adhesion-Molecule Inhibitor

Use

U.S. labeling: Monotherapy for the treatment of relapsing forms of multiple sclerosis; treatment of moderately- to severely-active Crohn disease

Canada labeling: Treatment of relapsing forms of multiple sclerosis

Usual Dosage I.V.: Adults:

Multiple sclerosis: 300 mg infused over 1 hour every 4 weeks

Crohn disease: 300 mg infused over 1 hour every 4 weeks; discontinue if therapeutic benefit is not observed within initial 12 weeks of therapy

Dosage Forms

Injection, solution [preservative free]:

Tysabri®: 300 mg/15 mL (15 mL)

natamycin (na ta MYE sin)

Sound-Alike/Look-Alike Issues

Natacyn® may be confused with Naprosyn®

Synonyms pimaricin

U.S./Canadian Brand Names Natacyn® [US/Can]

Therapeutic Category Antifungal Agent

Use Treatment of blepharitis, conjunctivitis, and keratitis caused by susceptible fungi (*Aspergillus*, *Candida*, *Cephalosporium*, *Fusarium*, and *Penicillium*)

Usual Dosage Ophthalmic: Adults:

Fungal keratitis: Instill 1 drop in conjunctival sac every 1-2 hours, after 3-4 days reduce to one drop 6-8 times/day; usual course of therapy is 2-3 weeks or until resolution of active fungal keratitis (may be useful to gradually reduce dosage at 4-7 day intervals to assure elimination of organism)

Fungal blepharitis or conjunctivitis: Instill 1 drop in conjunctival sac every 4-6 hours

Dosage Forms

Suspension, ophthalmic:

Natacyn®: 5% (15 mL)

NataTab™ CFe [US] *see* vitamins (multiple/prenatal) *on page 1020*
NataTab™ FA [US] *see* vitamins (multiple/prenatal) *on page 1020*
NataTab™ Rx [US] *see* vitamins (multiple/prenatal) *on page 1020*

nateglinide (na te GLYE nide)

U.S./Canadian Brand Names Starlix® [US/Can]

Therapeutic Category Antidiabetic Agent

Use Management of type 2 diabetes mellitus (noninsulin-dependent, NIDDM) as monotherapy when hyperglycemia cannot be managed by diet and exercise alone; in combination with metformin or a thiazolidinedione to lower blood glucose in patients whose hyperglycemia cannot be controlled by exercise, diet, or a single agent alone

Usual Dosage Oral: Adults: Management of type 2 diabetes mellitus: Initial and maintenance dose: 120 mg 3 times/day, 1-30 minutes before meals; may be given alone or in combination with metformin or a thiazolidinedione; patients close to Hb A_{1c} goal may be started at 60 mg 3 times/day

Dosage Forms

Tablet:

Starlix®: 60 mg, 120 mg

Natrecor® [US/Can] *see* nesiritide *on page 690*
natriuretic peptide *see* nesiritide *on page 690*
Natulan® [Can] *see* procarbazine *on page 820*
Natural Fiber Therapy [US-OTC] *see* psyllium *on page 837*
Natural Fiber Therapy Smooth Texture [US-OTC] *see* psyllium *on page 837*
natural lung surfactant *see* beractant *on page 135*
Nature's Tears® [US-OTC] *see* artificial tears *on page 100*
Nature-Throid™ [US] *see* thyroid, desiccated *on page 957*
Naus-A-Way® ***(Discontinued)***
Nausea Relief [US-OTC] *see* fructose, dextrose, and phosphoric acid *on page 448*
Nauseatol [Can] *see* dimenhydrinate *on page 312*
Nausetrol® [US-OTC] *see* fructose, dextrose, and phosphoric acid *on page 448*
Navane® [US/Can] *see* thiothixene *on page 956*
Navelbine® [US/Can] *see* vinorelbine *on page 1014*
Navstel® [US] *see* balanced salt solution *on page 121*
Naxen® [Can] *see* naproxen *on page 681*
Naxen® EC [Can] *see* naproxen *on page 681*
Na-Zone® [US-OTC] *see* sodium chloride *on page 908*
***n*-docosanol** *see* docosanol *on page 326*
Nebcin® ***(Discontinued)*** *see* tobramycin *on page 965*

nebivolol (ne BIV oh lole)

Synonyms nebivolol hydrochloride

U.S./Canadian Brand Names Bystolic™ [US]

Therapeutic Category Beta Blocker, $Beta_1$ Selective

Use Treatment of hypertension, alone or in combination with other agents

Usual Dosage Oral: Adults: Hypertension: Initial: 5 mg once daily; if initial response is inadequate, may be increased at 2-week intervals to a maximum dose of 40 mg once daily

Dosage Forms

Tablet:

Bystolic™: 2.5 mg, 5 mg, 10 mg

nebivolol hydrochloride *see* nebivolol *on page* *684*
NebuPent® [US] *see* pentamidine *on page* *763*
Necon® 0.5/35 [US] *see* ethinyl estradiol and norethindrone *on page* *390*
Necon® 1/35 [US] *see* ethinyl estradiol and norethindrone *on page* *390*
Necon® 1/50 [US] *see* norethindrone and mestranol *on page* *704*
Necon® 7/7/7 [US] *see* ethinyl estradiol and norethindrone *on page* *390*
Necon® 10/11 [US] *see* ethinyl estradiol and norethindrone *on page* *390*

nedocromil (inhalation) (ne doe KROE mil in hil LA shun)

U.S./Canadian Brand Names Tilade® [US/Can]

Therapeutic Category Mast Cell Stabilizer

Use Maintenance therapy in patients with mild-to-moderate bronchial asthma

Usual Dosage Children >6 years and Adults: 2 inhalations 4 times/day; may reduce dosage to 2-3 times/day once desired clinical response to initial dose is observed

Dosage Forms

Aerosol for oral inhalation:
Tilade®: 1.75 mg/activation (16.2 g)

nedocromil (ophthalmic) (ne doe KROE mil op THAL mik)

U.S./Canadian Brand Names Alocril® [US/Can]

Therapeutic Category Mast Cell Stabilizer

Use Treatment of itching associated with allergic conjunctivitis

Usual Dosage Ophthalmic: Adults: 1-2 drops in eye(s) twice daily

Dosage Forms

Solution, ophthalmic:
Alocril®: 2% (5 mL)

nefazodone (nef AY zoe done)

Sound-Alike/Look-Alike Issues
Serzone® may be confused with selegiline, Serentil®, Seroquel®, sertraline

Synonyms nefazodone hydrochloride

Therapeutic Category Antidepressant, Miscellaneous

Use Treatment of depression

Usual Dosage Oral: Adults: Depression: 200 mg/day, administered in 2 divided doses initially, with a range of 300-600 mg/day in 2 divided doses thereafter

Dosage Forms

Tablet: 50 mg, 100 mg, 150 mg, 200 mg, 250 mg

nefazodone hydrochloride *see* nefazodone *on page* *685*

NegGram® ***(Discontinued)***

nelarabine (nel AY re been)

Synonyms 2-amino-6-methoxypurine arabinoside; 506U78; GW506U78

U.S./Canadian Brand Names Arranon® [US]; Atriance™ [Can]

Therapeutic Category Antineoplastic Agent, Antimetabolite

Use Treatment of relapsed or refractory T-cell acute lymphoblastic leukemia (ALL) and T-cell lymphoblastic lymphoma

Usual Dosage I.V.: T-cell ALL, T-cell lymphoblastic lymphoma:
Children: 650 mg/m^2/day on days 1 through 5; repeat every 21 days
Adults: 1500 mg/m^2/day on days 1, 3, and 5; repeat every 21 days

Dosage Forms [CAN] = Canadian brand name

Injection, solution:
Arranon®: 5 mg/mL (50 mL)
Atriance™ [CAN]: 5 mg/ml (50 mL)

nelfinavir (nel FIN a veer)

Sound-Alike/Look-Alike Issues
nelfinavir may be confused with nevirapine

Viracept® may be confused with Viramune®

Synonyms NFV

U.S./Canadian Brand Names Viracept® [US/Can]

Therapeutic Category Antiviral Agent

Use In combination with other antiretroviral therapy in the treatment of HIV infection

Usual Dosage Oral:

Children 2-13 years: 45-55 mg/kg twice daily **or** 25-35 mg/kg 3 times/day (maximum: 2500 mg/day). If tablets are unable to be taken, use oral powder in small amount of water, milk, formula, or dietary supplements; do not use acidic food/juice or store for >6 hours.

Adults: 750 mg 3 times/day or 1250 mg twice daily with meals in combination with other antiretroviral therapies

Dosage Forms

Powder, oral:

Viracept®: 50 mg/g

Tablet:

Viracept®: 250 mg, 625 mg

Nelova™ 0.5/35E *(Discontinued)* *see* ethinyl estradiol and norethindrone *on page 390*

Nelova™ 1/35E *(Discontinued)* *see* ethinyl estradiol and norethindrone *on page 390*

Nelova™ 1/50M *(Discontinued)* *see* norethindrone and mestranol *on page 704*

Nelova™ 10/11 *(Discontinued)* *see* ethinyl estradiol and norethindrone *on page 390*

Nembutal® [US] *see* pentobarbital *on page 765*

Nembutal® Sodium [Can] *see* pentobarbital *on page 765*

NeoBenz® Micro *(Discontinued)* *see* benzoyl peroxide *on page 132*

NeoBenz® Micro SD *(Discontinued)* *see* benzoyl peroxide *on page 132*

NeoBenz® Micro Wash [US] *see* benzoyl peroxide *on page 132*

Neo-Calglucon® *(Discontinued)* *see* calcium glubionate *on page 173*

Neo-Dexameth® Ophthalmic *(Discontinued)*

Neo DM [US] *see* chlorpheniramine, phenylephrine, and dextromethorphan *on page 217*

Neo-Durabolic® *(Discontinued)* *see* nandrolone *(Canada only) on page 680*

Neofed® *(Discontinued)* *see* pseudoephedrine *on page 833*

Neo-Fradin™ [US] *see* neomycin *on page 686*

Neofrin™ [US] *see* phenylephrine *on page 774*

Neomixin® Topical *(Discontinued)* *see* bacitracin, neomycin, and polymyxin B *on page 119*

neomycin (nee oh MYE sin)

Synonyms neomycin sulfate

U.S./Canadian Brand Names Neo-Fradin™ [US]; Neo-Rx [US]

Therapeutic Category Aminoglycoside (Antibiotic); Antibiotic, Topical

Use Orally to prepare GI tract for surgery; topically to treat minor skin infections; treatment of diarrhea caused by *E. coli*; adjunct in the treatment of hepatic encephalopathy; bladder irrigation; ocular infections

Usual Dosage

Children: Oral:

Preoperative intestinal antisepsis: 90 mg/kg/day divided every 4 hours for 2 days; or 25 mg/kg at 1 PM, 2 PM, and 11 PM on the day preceding surgery as an adjunct to mechanical cleansing of the intestine and in combination with erythromycin base

Hepatic encephalopathy: 50-100 mg/kg/day in divided doses every 6-8 hours or 2.5-7 g/m^2/day divided every 4-6 hours for 5-6 days not to exceed 12 g/day

Children and Adults: Topical: Topical solutions containing 0.1% to 1% neomycin have been used for irrigation

Adults: Oral:

Preoperative intestinal antisepsis: 1 g each hour for 4 doses then 1 g every 4 hours for 5 doses; or 1 g at 1 PM, 2 PM, and 11 PM on day preceding surgery as an adjunct to mechanical cleansing of the bowel and oral erythromycin; or 6 g/day divided every 4 hours for 2-3 days

Hepatic encephalopathy: 500-2000 mg every 6-8 hours or 4-12 g/day divided every 4-6 hours for 5-6 days

Chronic hepatic insufficiency: 4 g/day for an indefinite period

Dosage Forms

Powder, micronized [for prescription compounding]: (10 g, 100 g)
Neo-Rx: (10 g, 100 g)
Solution, oral: 125 mg/5 mL
Neo-Fradin™: 125 mg/5 mL
Tablet: 500 mg

neomycin and polymyxin B (nee oh MYE sin & pol i MIKS in bee)

Synonyms polymyxin B and neomycin

U.S./Canadian Brand Names Neosporin® G.U. Irrigant [US]; Neosporin® Irrigating Solution [Can]

Therapeutic Category Antibiotic, Topical; Genitourinary Irrigant

Use Short-term as a continuous irrigant or rinse in the urinary bladder to prevent bacteriuria and gram-negative rod septicemia associated with the use of indwelling catheters

Usual Dosage Children and Adults: Bladder irrigation: **Not for injection**; add 1 mL irrigant to 1 L isotonic saline solution and connect container to the inflow of lumen of 3-way catheter. Continuous irrigant or rinse in the urinary bladder for up to a maximum of 10 days with administration rate adjusted to patient's urine output; usually no more than 1 L of irrigant is used per day.

Dosage Forms

Solution, irrigation: Neomycin 40 mg and polymyxin B 200,000 units per mL (1 mL, 20 mL)
Neosporin® G.U. Irrigant: Neomycin 40 mg and polymyxin B 200,000 units per mL (1 mL, 20 mL)

neomycin, bacitracin, and polymyxin B *see* bacitracin, neomycin, and polymyxin B *on page 119*

neomycin, bacitracin, polymyxin B, and hydrocortisone *see* bacitracin, neomycin, polymyxin B, and hydrocortisone *on page 120*

neomycin, bacitracin, polymyxin B, and pramoxine *see* bacitracin, neomycin, polymyxin B, and pramoxine *on page 120*

neomycin, colistin, hydrocortisone, and thonzonium
(nee oh MYE sin, koe LIS tin, hye droe KOR ti sone, & thon ZOE nee um)

Synonyms colistin, hydrocortisone, neomycin, and thonzonium; hydrocortisone, neomycin, colistin, and thonzonium; thonzonium, neomycin, colistin, and hydrocortisone

U.S./Canadian Brand Names Coly-Mycin® S [US]; Cortisporin®-TC [US]

Therapeutic Category Antibiotic/Corticosteroid, Otic

Use Treatment of superficial and susceptible bacterial infections of the external auditory canal; for treatment of susceptible bacterial infections of mastoidectomy and fenestration cavities

Usual Dosage Otic:

Calibrated dropper:
Children: 4 drops in affected ear 3-4 times/day
Adults: 5 drops in affected ear 3-4 times/day
Dropper bottle:
Children: 3 drops in affected ear 3-4 times/day
Adults: 4 drops in affected ear 3-4 times/day

Note: Alternatively, a cotton wick may be inserted in the ear canal and saturated with suspension every 4 hours; wick should be replaced at least every 24 hours

Dosage Forms

Suspension, otic [drops]:
Coly-Mycin® S: Neomycin 0.33%, colistin 0.3%, hydrocortisone 1%, and thonzonium 0.05% (5 mL)
Cortisporin®-TC: Neomycin 0.33%, colistin 0.3%, hydrocortisone 1%, and thonzonium 0.05% (10 mL)

neomycin, polymyxin B, and dexamethasone
(nee oh MYE sin, pol i MIKS in bee, & deks a METH a sone)

Sound-Alike/Look-Alike Issues

AK-Trol® may be confused with AKTob®

Synonyms dexamethasone, neomycin, and polymyxin B; polymyxin B, neomycin, and dexamethasone

U.S./Canadian Brand Names Dioptrol® [Can]; Maxitrol® [US/Can]; Poly-Dex™ [US]

Therapeutic Category Antibiotic/Corticosteroid, Ophthalmic

Use Steroid-responsive inflammatory ocular conditions in which a corticosteroid is indicated and where bacterial infection or a risk of bacterial infection exists

Usual Dosage Ophthalmic: Children and Adults:

Ointment: Place a small amount (~1/2") in the affected eye 3-4 times/day or apply at bedtime as an adjunct with drops

Suspension: Instill 1-2 drops into affected eye(s) every 3-4 hours; in severe disease, drops may be used hourly and tapered to discontinuation

Dosage Forms

Ointment, ophthalmic: Neomycin 3.5 mg, polymyxin B 10,000 units, and dexamethasone 0.1% per g (3.5 g)

Maxitrol®, Poly-Dex™: Neomycin 3.5 mg, polymyxin B 10,000 units, and dexamethasone 0.1% per g (3.5 g)

Suspension, ophthalmic: Neomycin 3.5 mg, polymyxin B 10,000 units, and dexamethasone 0.1% per mL (5 mL)

Maxitrol®, Poly-Dex™: Neomycin 3.5 mg, polymyxin B10,000 units, and dexamethasone 0.1% per mL (5 mL)

neomycin, polymyxin B, and gramicidin

(nee oh MYE sin, pol i MIKS in bee, & gram i SYE din)

Synonyms gramicidin, neomycin, and polymyxin B; polymyxin B, neomycin, and gramicidin

U.S./Canadian Brand Names Neosporin® Ophthalmic Solution [US]; Neosporin® [Can]; Optimyxin Plus® [Can]

Therapeutic Category Antibiotic, Ophthalmic

Use Treatment of superficial ocular infection

Usual Dosage Ophthalmic: Children and Adults: Instill 1-2 drops 4-6 times/day or more frequently as required for severe infections

Dosage Forms

Solution, ophthalmic: Neomycin 1.75 mg, polymyxin B 10,000 units, and gramicidin 0.025 mg per 1 mL (10 mL)

Neosporin® Ophthalmic Solution: Neomycin 1.75 mg, polymyxin B 10,000 units, and gramicidin 0.025 mg per 1 mL (10 mL)

neomycin, polymyxin B, and hydrocortisone

(nee oh MYE sin, pol i MIKS in bee, & hye droe KOR ti sone)

Synonyms hydrocortisone, neomycin, and polymyxin B; polymyxin B, neomycin, and hydrocortisone

U.S./Canadian Brand Names Cortimyxin® [Can]; Cortisporin® Cream [US]; Cortisporin® Otic [US/Can]; PediOtic® [US]

Therapeutic Category Antibiotic/Corticosteroid, Ophthalmic; Antibiotic/Corticosteroid, Otic; Antibiotic/Corticosteroid, Topical

Use Steroid-responsive inflammatory condition for which a corticosteroid is indicated and where bacterial infection or a risk of bacterial infection exists

Usual Dosage Note: Duration of use of ophthalmic and otic preparations should be limited to 10 days unless otherwise directed by the healthcare provider.

Ophthalmic: Adults: Instill 1-2 drops 2-4 times/day, or more frequently as required for severe infections

Otic: Otic solution is used **only** for bacterial infections of external auditory canal (eg, swimmer's ear).

Children ≥2 years: Instill 3 drops into affected ear 3-4 times/day

Adults: Instill 4 drops into affected ear 3-4 times/day; otic suspension is the preferred otic preparation

Topical: Adults: Apply a thin layer 1-4 times/day. Therapy should be discontinued when control is achieved; if no improvement is seen, reassessment of diagnosis may be necessary.

Dosage Forms

Cream, topical: Neomycin 3.5 mg, polymyxin B 10,000 units, and hydrocortisone 5 mg per g (7.5 g)

Cortisporin®: Neomycin 3.5 mg, polymyxin B 10,000 units, and hydrocortisone 5 mg per g (7.5 g)

Solution, otic: Neomycin 3.5 mg, polymyxin B 10,000 units, and hydrocortisone 10 mg per mL (10 mL)

Cortisporin®: Neomycin 3.5 mg, polymyxin B 10,000 units, and hydrocortisone 10 mg per mL (10 mL)

Suspension, ophthalmic: Neomycin 3.5 mg, polymyxin B 10,000 units, and hydrocortisone 10 mg per mL (7.5 mL)

Suspension, otic: Neomycin 3.5 mg, polymyxin B 10,000 units, and hydrocortisone 10 mg per mL (10 mL)

Cortisporin®: Neomycin 3.5 mg, polymyxin B 10,000 units, and hydrocortisone 10 mg per mL (10 mL)

PediOtic®: Neomycin 3.5 mg, polymyxin B 10,000 units, and hydrocortisone 10 mg per mL (7.5 mL)

neomycin, polymyxin B, and prednisolone

(nee oh MYE sin, pol i MIKS in bee, & pred NIS oh lone)

Synonyms polymyxin B, neomycin, and prednisolone; prednisolone, neomycin, and polymyxin B

U.S./Canadian Brand Names Poly-Pred® [US]

Therapeutic Category Antibiotic/Corticosteroid, Ophthalmic

Use Steroid-responsive inflammatory ocular condition in which bacterial infection or a risk of bacterial ocular infection exists

Usual Dosage Ophthalmic: Children and Adults: Instill 1-2 drops every 3-4 hours; acute infections may require every 30-minute instillation initially with frequency of administration reduced as the infection is brought under control. To treat the lids: Instill 1-2 drops every 3-4 hours, close the eye and rub the excess on the lids and lid margins.

Dosage Forms

Suspension, ophthalmic:

Poly-Pred®: Neomycin 0.35%, polymyxin B 10,000 units per mL, and prednisolone 0.5% (5 mL)

neomycin sulfate *see* neomycin *on page 686*
neonatal trace metals *see* trace metals *on page 974*
NeoProfen® [US] *see* ibuprofen *on page 515*
Neoral® [US/Can] *see* cyclosporine *on page 266*
Neo-Rx [US] *see* neomycin *on page 686*
neosar *see* cyclophosphamide *on page 265*
Neosporin® [Can] *see* neomycin, polymyxin B, and gramicidin *on page 688*
Neosporin® AF [US-OTC] *see* miconazole *on page 654*
Neosporin® G.U. Irrigant [US] *see* neomycin and polymyxin B *on page 687*
Neosporin® Irrigating Solution [Can] *see* neomycin and polymyxin B *on page 687*
Neosporin® Neo To Go® [US-OTC] *see* bacitracin, neomycin, and polymyxin B *on page 119*
Neosporin® Ophthalmic Ointment *(Discontinued)* *see* bacitracin, neomycin, and polymyxin B *on page 119*
Neosporin® Ophthalmic Solution [US] *see* neomycin, polymyxin B, and gramicidin *on page 688*
Neosporin® + Pain Relief Ointment [US-OTC] *see* bacitracin, neomycin, polymyxin B, and pramoxine *on page 120*
Neosporin® Topical [US-OTC] *see* bacitracin, neomycin, and polymyxin B *on page 119*

neostigmine (nee oh STIG meen)

Sound-Alike/Look-Alike Issues

Prostigmin® may be confused with physostigmine

Synonyms neostigmine bromide; neostigmine methylsulfate

U.S./Canadian Brand Names Prostigmin® [US/Can]

Therapeutic Category Cholinergic Agent

Use Reversal of the effects of nondepolarizing neuromuscular-blocking agents; treatment of myasthenia gravis; prevention and treatment of postoperative bladder distention and urinary retention

Usual Dosage

Myasthenia gravis: Diagnosis: I.M.:
- Children: 0.04 mg/kg as a single dose
- Adults: 0.02 mg/kg as a single dose

Myasthenia gravis: Treatment:
- Children:
  - Oral: 2 mg/kg/day divided every 3-4 hours
  - I.M., I.V., SubQ: 0.01-0.04 mg/kg every 2-4 hours
- Adults:
  - Oral: 15 mg/dose every 3-4 hours up to 375 mg/day maximum; interval between doses must be individualized to maximal response
  - I.M., I.V., SubQ: 0.5-2.5 mg every 1-3 hours up to 10 mg/24 hours maximum

Reversal of nondepolarizing neuromuscular blockade after surgery in conjunction with atropine (must administer atropine several minutes prior to neostigmine): I.V.:
- Infants: 0.025-0.1 mg/kg/dose
- Children: 0.025-0.08 mg/kg/dose
- Adults: 0.5-2.5 mg; total dose not to exceed 5 mg

Bladder atony: Adults: I.M., SubQ:
Prevention: 0.25 mg every 4-6 hours for 2-3 days
Treatment: 0.5-1 mg every 3 hours for 5 doses after bladder has emptied

Dosage Forms

Injection, solution: 0.5 mg/mL (1 mL, 10 mL); 1 mg/mL (10 mL)
Prostigmin®: 0.5 mg/mL (1 mL, 10 mL); 1 mg/mL (10 mL)

Tablet:
Prostigmin®: 15 mg

neostigmine bromide *see* neostigmine *on page* *689*
neostigmine methylsulfate *see* neostigmine *on page* *689*
NeoStrata® AHA [US-OTC] *see* hydroquinone *on page* *508*
NeoStrata® HQ [Can] *see* hydroquinone *on page* *508*
Neo-Synephrine® [Can] *see* phenylephrine *on page* *774*
Neo-Synephrine® 12 Hour [US-OTC] *see* oxymetazoline *on page* *740*
Neo-Synephrine® 12 Hour Extra Moisturizing [US-OTC] *see* oxymetazoline *on page* *740*
Neo-Synephrine® Extra Strength [US-OTC] *see* phenylephrine *on page* *774*
Neo-Synephrine® Injection [US] *see* phenylephrine *on page* *774*
Neo-Synephrine® Mild [US-OTC] *see* phenylephrine *on page* *774*
Neo-Synephrine® Ophthalmic *(Discontinued)* *see* phenylephrine *on page* *774*
Neo-Synephrine® Regular Strength [US-OTC] *see* phenylephrine *on page* *774*
Neo-Tabs® *(Discontinued)* *see* neomycin *on page* *686*
NeoVadrin® *(Discontinued)*

nepafenac (ne pa FEN ak)

U.S./Canadian Brand Names Nevanac™ [US/Can]

Therapeutic Category Nonsteroidal Antiinflammatory Drug (NSAID), Ophthalmic

Use Treatment of pain and inflammation associated with cataract surgery

Usual Dosage Ophthalmic: Children ≥10 years and Adults: Instill 1 drop into affected eye(s) 3 times/day, beginning 1 day prior to surgery, the day of surgery, and through the first 2 weeks of the postoperative period

Dosage Forms

Suspension, ophthalmic:
Nevanac™: 0.1% (3 mL)

NephPlex® Rx [US] *see* vitamin B complex combinations *on page* *1017*
NephrAmine® [US] *see* amino acid injection *on page* *62*
Nephro-Calci® [US-OTC] *see* calcium carbonate *on page* *170*
Nephrocaps® [US] *see* vitamin B complex combinations *on page* *1017*
Nephro-Fer® [US-OTC] *see* ferrous fumarate *on page* *413*
Nephronex® [US] *see* vitamin B complex combinations *on page* *1017*
Nephron FA® [US] *see* vitamin B complex combinations *on page* *1017*
Nephro-Vite® [US-OTC] *see* vitamin B complex combinations *on page* *1017*
Nephro-Vite® Rx [US] *see* vitamin B complex combinations *on page* *1017*
Nephrox Suspension *(Discontinued)* *see* aluminum hydroxide *on page* *55*
Neptazane® *(Discontinued)* *see* methazolamide *on page* *636*
nerve agent antidote kit *see* atropine and pralidoxime *on page* *112*
Nervocaine® Injection *(Discontinued)* *see* lidocaine *on page* *584*
Nesacaine® [US] *see* chloroprocaine *on page* *212*
Nesacaine®-CE [Can] *see* chloroprocaine *on page* *212*
Nesacaine®-MPF [US] *see* chloroprocaine *on page* *212*

nesiritide (ni SIR i tide)

Synonyms B-type natriuretic peptide (human); hBNP; natriuretic peptide

U.S./Canadian Brand Names Natrecor® [US/Can]

Therapeutic Category Natriuretic Peptide, B-type, Human; Vasodilator

Use Treatment of acutely decompensated heart failure (HF) with dyspnea at rest or with minimal activity

Usual Dosage I.V.: Adults: Initial: 2 mcg/kg (bolus); followed by continuous infusion at 0.01 mcg/kg/minute.
Note: Should not be initiated at a dosage higher than initial recommended dose. There is limited experience with increasing the dose >0.01 mcg/kg/minute; in one trial, a limited number of patients received higher doses that were increased no faster than every 3 hours by 0.005 mcg/kg/minute (preceded by a bolus of 1 mcg/kg), up to a maximum of 0.03 mcg/kg/minute. Increases beyond the initial infusion rate should be limited to selected patients and accompanied by close hemodynamic and renal function monitoring.
Patients experiencing hypotension during the infusion: Infusion dose should be reduced or discontinued. Other measures to support blood pressure should be initiated (eg, I.V. fluids, Trendelenburg position). May attempt to restart at a lower dose (reduce previous infusion dose by 30% and omit bolus).

Dosage Forms
Injection, powder for reconstitution:
Natrecor®: 1.5 mg

Nestrex® ***(Discontinued)*** *see* pyridoxine *on page* *840*
Netromycin® ***(Discontinued)***
Neucalm-50® Injection ***(Discontinued)*** *see* hydroxyzine *on page* *511*
Neulasta® [US/Can] *see* pegfilgrastim *on page* *755*
Neuleptil® [Can] *see* periciazine *(Canada only) on page* *767*
Neumega® [US] *see* oprelvekin *on page* *728*
Neupogen® [US/Can] *see* filgrastim *on page* *420*
Neupro® ***(Discontinued)***
Neuramate® ***(Discontinued)*** *see* meprobamate *on page* *629*
Neurontin® [US/Can] *see* gabapentin *on page* *450*
Neut® [US] *see* sodium bicarbonate *on page* *907*
NeutraCare® [US] *see* fluoride *on page* *430*
NeutraGard® [US-OTC] *see* fluoride *on page* *430*
NeutraGard® Advanced [US] *see* fluoride *on page* *430*
NeutraGard® Plus [US] *see* fluoride *on page* *430*
Neutra-Phos® ***(Discontinued)*** *see* potassium phosphate and sodium phosphate *on page* *806*
Neutra-Phos®-K ***(Discontinued)*** *see* potassium phosphate *on page* *806*
NeuTrexin® ***(Discontinued)***
Neutrogena® Advanced Solutions™ [US-OTC] *see* salicylic acid *on page* *884*
Neutrogena® Blackhead Eliminating™ 2-in-1 Foaming Pads [US-OTC] *see* salicylic acid *on page* *884*
Neutrogena® Blackhead Eliminating™ Astringent ***(Discontinued)*** *see* salicylic acid *on page* *884*
Neutrogena® Blackhead Eliminating™ Daily Scrub [US-OTC] *see* salicylic acid *on page* *884*
Neutrogena® Blackhead Eliminating™ Treatment Mask ***(Discontinued)*** *see* salicylic acid *on page* *884*
Neutrogena® Body Clear® [US-OTC] *see* benzoyl peroxide *on page* *132*
Neutrogena® Body Clear® [US-OTC] *see* salicylic acid *on page* *884*
Neutrogena® Clear Pore™ [US-OTC] *see* benzoyl peroxide *on page* *132*
Neutrogena® Clear Pore™ Oil-Controlling Astringent [US-OTC] *see* salicylic acid *on page* *884*
Neutrogena® Oil-Free Acne Wash [US-OTC] *see* benzoyl peroxide *on page* *132*
Neutrogena® Oil-Free Acne Wash [US-OTC] *see* salicylic acid *on page* *884*
Neutrogena® Oil-Free Acne Wash 60 Second Mask Scrub [US-OTC] *see* salicylic acid *on page* *884*
Neutrogena® Oil-Free Acne Wash Cream Cleanser [US-OTC] *see* salicylic acid *on page* *884*
Neutrogena® Oil-Free Acne Wash Foam Cleanser [US-OTC] *see* salicylic acid *on page* *884*
Neutrogena® On The Spot® Acne Treatment [US-OTC] *see* benzoyl peroxide *on page* *132*
Neutrogena® Rapid Clear® Acne Defense [US-OTC] *see* salicylic acid *on page* *884*
Neutrogena® Rapid Clear® Acne Eliminating [US-OTC] *see* salicylic acid *on page* *884*
Neutrogena® T/Gel [US-OTC] *see* coal tar *on page* *250*
Neutrogena® T/Gel Extra Strength [US-OTC] *see* coal tar *on page* *250*
Neutrogena® T/Gel Stubborn Itch Control [US-OTC] *see* coal tar *on page* *250*

Nevanac™ [US/Can] *see* nepafenac *on page* 690

nevirapine (ne VYE ra peen)

Sound-Alike/Look-Alike Issues

nevirapine may be confused with nelfinavir
Viramune® may be confused with Viracept®

Synonyms NVP

U.S./Canadian Brand Names Viramune® [US/Can]

Therapeutic Category Antiviral Agent

Use In combination therapy with other antiretroviral agents for the treatment of HIV-1

Usual Dosage Oral:

HIV infection:

Infants ≥15 days and Children: 150 mg/m^2 once daily for first 14 days (maximum dose: 200 mg/day); increase dose to 150 mg/m^2 twice daily if no rash or untoward effects (maximum dose: ≤400 mg/day). Children ≤8 years of age: May require 200 mg/m^2 twice daily.

Adolescents and Adults: Initial: 200 mg once daily for first 14 days; maintenance: 200 mg twice daily (in combination with an additional antiretroviral agent) if there is no rash or other adverse event

Note: If patient experiences a rash during the 14-day lead-in period, dose should not be increased until the rash has resolved. Lead-in period should not exceed 28 days; alternative treatment should be considered at that point. Discontinue if severe rash, rash with constitutional symptoms, or rash with elevated hepatic transaminases is noted. Use of prednisone to prevent nevirapine-associated rash is not recommended. Permanently discontinue if symptomatic hepatic events occur. If therapy is interrupted for >7 days, restart with initial dose for 14 days.

Prevention of maternal-fetal HIV transmission (AIDS*info* guidelines): Note: Nevirapine is used in combination with zidovudine (and possibly lamivudine) in select situations (eg, infants born to mothers with suboptimal viral suppression at delivery, infants born to mothers with only intrapartum therapy or no therapy, or infants born to mothers with known antiretroviral drug-resistant virus)

Mother: 200 mg as a single dose at onset of labor

Neonate: 2 mg/kg as a single dose between birth and 72 hours if mother received intrapartum dose of nevirapine. If maternal dose was given ≤2 hours prior to delivery, administer infant dose as soon as possible following birth.

Dosage Forms

Suspension, oral:

Viramune®: 50 mg/5 mL

Tablet:

Viramune®: 200 mg

Nexavar® [US/Can] *see* sorafenib *on page* 918

Nexium® [US/Can] *see* esomeprazole *on page* 372

Nexphen PD [US] *see* guaifenesin and phenylephrine *on page* 475

Next Choice™ [US-RX/OTC] *see* levonorgestrel *on page* 582

NFV *see* nelfinavir *on page* 685

N.G.A.® Topical *(Discontinued)* *see* nystatin and triamcinolone *on page* 716

niacin (NYE a sin)

Sound-Alike/Look-Alike Issues

niacin may be confused with Minocin®, Niaspan®, Nispan®
Niaspan® may be confused with niacin
Nicobid® may be confused with Nitro-Bid®

Synonyms nicotinic acid; vitamin B_3

U.S./Canadian Brand Names Niacin-Time® [US]; Niacor® [US]; Niaspan® [US/Can]; Slo-Niacin® [US-OTC]

Therapeutic Category Vitamin, Water Soluble

Use Adjunctive treatment of dyslipidemias (types IIa and IIb or primary hypercholesterolemia) to lower the risk of recurrent MI and/or slow progression of coronary artery disease, including combination therapy with other antidyslipidemic agents when additional triglyceride-lowering or HDL-increasing effects are desired; treatment of hypertriglyceridemia in patients at risk of pancreatitis; treatment of peripheral vascular disease and circulatory disorders; treatment of pellagra; dietary supplement

Usual Dosage Note: Formulations of niacin (regular release versus extended release) are not interchangeable.

Children: Oral:

Pellagra: 50-100 mg/dose 3 times/day

Recommended daily allowances:

0-0.5 years: 5 mg/day

0.5-1 year: 6 mg/day

1-3 years: 9 mg/day

4-6 years: 12 mg/day

7-10 years: 13 mg/day

Children and Adolescents: Recommended daily allowances:

Male:

11-14 years: 17 mg/day

15-18 years: 20 mg/day

19-24 years: 19 mg/day

Female: 11-24 years: 15 mg/day

Adults: Oral:

Recommended daily allowances:

Male: 25-50 years: 19 mg/day; >51 years: 15 mg/day

Female: 25-50 years: 15 mg/day; >51 years: 13 mg/day

Hyperlipidemia: Usual target dose: Regular release: 1.5-6 g/day in 3 divided doses with or after meals using a dosage titration schedule. Extended release: 500 mg to 2 g once daily at bedtime.

Regular release formulation (Niacor®): Initial: 250 mg once daily (with evening meal); increase frequency and/or dose every 4-7 days to desired response or first-level therapeutic dose (1.5-2 g/day in 2-3 divided doses); after 2 months, may increase at 2- to 4-week intervals to 3 g/day in 3 divided doses (maximum dose: 6 g/day in 3 divided doses)

Extended release formulation (Niaspan®): Initial: 500 mg at bedtime for 4 weeks, then 1 g at bedtime for 4 weeks; adjust dose to response and tolerance; can increase to a maximum of 2 g/day, but only at 500 mg/day at 4-week intervals

With lovastatin: Recommended initial dose: 20 mg/day; Maximum lovastatin dose: 40 mg/day

Pellagra: 50-100 mg 3-4 times/day, maximum: 500 mg/day

Niacin deficiency: 10-20 mg/day, maximum: 100 mg/day

Dosage Forms

Caplet, timed release, oral: 500 mg

Capsule, oral: 50 mg, 250 mg

Capsule, extended release, oral: 250 mg, 500 mg

Capsule, timed release, oral: 250 mg, 400 mg, 500 mg

Tablet, oral: 50 mg, 100 mg, 250 mg, 500 mg

Niacor®: 500 mg [scored]

Tablet, controlled release, oral:

Slo-Niacin® [OTC]: 250 mg, 500 mg, 750 mg [scored]

Tablet, extended release, oral:

Niaspan®: 500 mg, 750 mg, 1000 mg

Tablet, timed release, oral: 250 mg, 500 mg, 750 mg, 1000 mg

Niacin-Time®: 500 mg

niacinamide (nye a SIN a mide)

Sound-Alike/Look-Alike Issues

niacinamide may be confused with niCARdipine

Synonyms nicotinamide; nicotinic acid amide; vitamin B_3

U.S./Canadian Brand Names Nicomide-T™ [US]

Therapeutic Category Vitamin, Water Soluble

Use

Oral: Prophylaxis and treatment of pellagra

Topical: Improve the appearance of acne and decrease visible inflammation and irritation caused by acne medications

Usual Dosage

Pellagra: Oral:

Children: 100-300 mg/day in divided doses

Adults: 300-500 mg/day

Acne: Topical: Adults: Apply to affected area on face twice daily

Dosage Forms

Cream:

Nicomide-T™: 4% (30 g)

Gel:

Nicomide-T™: 4% (30 g)

Tablet: 100 mg, 250 mg, 500 mg

niacin and lovastatin (NYE a sin & LOE va sta tin)

Sound-Alike/Look-Alike Issues

Advicor® may be confused with Adcirca™, Advair, Altocor™

Synonyms lovastatin and niacin

U.S./Canadian Brand Names Advicor® [US/Can]

Therapeutic Category HMG-CoA Reductase Inhibitor; Vitamin, Water Soluble

Use For use when treatment with both extended-release niacin and lovastatin is appropriate in combination with a standard cholesterol-lowering diet:

Extended-release niacin: Adjunctive treatment of dyslipidemias (types IIa and IIb or primary hypercholesterolemia) to lower the risk of recurrent MI and/or slow progression of coronary artery disease, including combination therapy with other antidyslipidemic agents when additional triglyceride-lowering or HDL-increasing effects are desired; treatment of hypertriglyceridemia in patients at risk of pancreatitis

Lovastatin: Treatment of primary hypercholesterolemia (Frederickson types IIa and IIb); primary and secondary prevention of cardiovascular disease

Usual Dosage Dosage forms are a fixed combination of niacin and lovastatin.

Oral: Adults: Lowest dose: Niacin 500 mg/lovastatin 20 mg; may increase by not more than 500 mg (niacin) at 4-week intervals (maximum dose: Niacin 2000 mg/lovastatin 40 mg daily); should be taken at bedtime with a low-fat snack. **Note:** If therapy is interrupted for >7 days, reinstitution of therapy should begin with the lowest dose followed by retitration as needed.

Not for use as initial therapy of dyslipidemias. May be substituted for equivalent dose of Niaspan®, however, manufacturer does not recommend direct substitution with other niacin products.

Dosage Forms

Tablet, variable release:

Advicor®: 500/20: Niacin 500 mg [extended release] and lovastatin 20 mg [immediate release]; 750/20: Niacin 750 mg [extended release] and lovastatin 20 mg [immediate release]; 1000/20: Niacin 1000 mg [extended release] and lovastatin 20 mg [immediate release]; 1000/40: Niacin 1000 mg [extended release] and lovastatin 40 mg [immediate release]

niacin and simvastatin (NYE a sin & sim va STAT in)

Synonyms simvastatin and niacin

U.S./Canadian Brand Names Simcor® [US]

Therapeutic Category Antilipemic Agent, HMG-CoA Reductase Inhibitor; Antilipemic Agent, Miscellaneous

Use Treatment of primary hypercholesterolemia, mixed dyslipidemia (types IIa and IIb), or hypertriglyceridemia (type IV hyperlipidemia) in combination with standard cholesterol-lowering diet when simvastatin or niacin monotherapy is inadequate

Usual Dosage Dosage forms are a fixed combination of niacin extended release and simvastatin.

Oral: Adults:

Lowest dose (initiate in patients naïve to niacin therapy or those currently receiving niacin immediate release): Niacin 500 mg/simvastatin 20 mg once daily at bedtime with a low-fat snack; may increase by not more than 500 mg (niacin) at 4-week intervals

Maintenance dose: Niacin 1000 mg/simvastatin 20 mg to niacin 2000 mg/simvastatin 40 mg once daily (maximum: Niacin 2000 mg/simvastatin 40 mg once daily)

Note: If therapy is interrupted for >7 days, reinstitution of therapy should begin with the lowest dose followed by retitration as tolerated. Not for use as initial therapy of dyslipidemias. May be substituted for equivalent dose of niacin extended release, however, manufacturer does not recommend direct substitution with immediate release preparations.

Dosage Forms

Tablet, variable release:

Simcor®: 500/20: Niacin 500 mg [extended release] and simvastatin 20 mg [immediate release]; 750/20: Niacin 750 mg [extended release] and simvastatin 20 mg [immediate release]; 1000/20: Niacin 1000 mg [extended release] and simvastatin 20 mg [immediate release]

Niacin-Time® [US] *see* niacin *on page* 692
Niacor® [US] *see* niacin *on page* 692
Niaspan® [US/Can] *see* niacin *on page* 692
Niastase® [Can] *see* factor VIIa (recombinant) *on page* 402

nicardipine (nye KAR de peen)

Sound-Alike/Look-Alike Issues
niCARdipine may be confused with niacinamide, NIFEdipine, niMODipine
Cardene® may be confused with Cardizem®, Cardura®, codeine

Synonyms nicardipine hydrochloride

Tall-Man ni**CAR**dipine

U.S./Canadian Brand Names Cardene® I.V. [US]; Cardene® SR [US]; Cardene® [US]

Therapeutic Category Calcium Channel Blocker

Use Chronic stable angina (immediate-release product only); management of hypertension (immediate and sustained release products); parenteral only for short-term use when oral treatment is not feasible

Usual Dosage Adults:
Oral:
Immediate release: Initial: 20 mg 3 times/day; usual: 20-40 mg 3 times/day (allow 3 days between dose increases)
Sustained release: Initial: 30 mg twice daily, titrate up to 60 mg twice daily
Note: The total daily dose of immediate-release product may not automatically be equivalent to the daily sustained-release dose; use caution in converting.
I.V.:
Acute hypertension: Initial: 5 mg/hour increased by 2.5 mg/hour every 15 minutes to a maximum of 15 mg/hour; consider reduction to 3 mg/hour after response is achieved. Monitor and titrate to lowest dose necessary to maintain stable blood pressure.
Substitution for oral therapy (approximate equivalents):
20 mg every 8 hours oral, equivalent to 0.5 mg/hour I.V. infusion
30 mg every 8 hours oral, equivalent to 1.2 mg/hour I.V. infusion
40 mg every 8 hours oral, equivalent to 2.2 mg/hour I.V. infusion

Dosage Forms
Capsule, oral: 20 mg, 30 mg
Cardene®: 20 mg, 30 mg
Capsule, sustained release, oral:
Cardene® SR: 30 mg, 45 mg, 60 mg
Infusion, premixed in iso-osmotic dextrose:
Cardene® I.V.: 20 mg (200 mL); 40 mg (200 mL)
Infusion, premixed in iso-osmotic sodium chloride:
Cardene® I.V.: 20 mg (200 mL); 40 mg (200 mL)
Injection, solution: 2.5 mg/mL (10 mL)
Cardene® I.V.: 2.5 mg/mL (10 mL)

nicardipine hydrochloride *see* nicardipine *on page* 695
N'ice® *(Discontinued)* *see* ascorbic acid *on page* 100
Nicobid® *(Discontinued)* *see* niacin *on page* 692
Nicoderm® [Can] *see* nicotine *on page* 695
NicoDerm® CQ® [US-OTC] *see* nicotine *on page* 695
Nicolar® *(Discontinued)* *see* niacin *on page* 692
Nicomide-T™ [US] *see* niacinamide *on page* 693
Nicorette® [US-OTC/Can] *see* nicotine *on page* 695
Nicorette® Plus [Can] *see* nicotine *on page* 695
nicotinamide *see* niacinamide *on page* 693

nicotine (nik oh TEEN)

Sound-Alike/Look-Alike Issues
NicoDerm® may be confused with Nitroderm
Nicorette® may be confused with Nordette®

U.S./Canadian Brand Names Commit® [US-OTC]; Habitrol® [Can]; NicoDerm® CQ® [US-OTC]; Nicoderm® [Can]; Nicorette® Plus [Can]; Nicorette® [US-OTC/Can]; Nicotrol® Inhaler [US]; Nicotrol® NS [US]; Nicotrol® [Can]; Thrive™ [US-OTC]

Therapeutic Category Smoking Deterrent

Use Treatment to aid smoking cessation for the relief of nicotine withdrawal symptoms (including nicotine craving)

Usual Dosage Smoking deterrent: Patients should be advised to completely stop smoking upon initiation of therapy.

Oral:

Gum: Chew 1 piece of gum when urge to smoke, up to 24 pieces/day. Patients who smoke <25 cigarettes/day should start with 2-mg strength; patients smoking ≥25 cigarettes/day should start with the 4-mg strength. Use according to the following 12-week dosing schedule:

Weeks 1-6: Chew 1 piece of gum every 1-2 hours; to increase chances of quitting, chew at least 9 pieces/day during the first 6 weeks

Weeks 7-9: Chew 1 piece of gum every 2-4 hours

Weeks 10-12: Chew 1 piece of gum every 4-8 hours

Inhaler: Usually 6 to 16 cartridges per day; best effect was achieved by frequent continuous puffing (20 minutes); recommended duration of treatment is 3 months, after which patients may be weaned from the inhaler by gradual reduction of the daily dose over 6-12 weeks

Lozenge: Patients who smoke their first cigarette within 30 minutes of waking should use the 4 mg strength; otherwise the 2 mg strength is recommended. Use according to the following 12-week dosing schedule:

Weeks 1-6: One lozenge every 1-2 hours

Weeks 7-9: One lozenge every 2-4 hours

Weeks 10-12: One lozenge every 4-8 hours

Note: Use at least 9 lozenges/day during first 6 weeks to improve chances of quitting; do not use more than one lozenge at a time (maximum: 5 lozenges every 6 hours, 20 lozenges/day)

Topical:

Transdermal patch: Apply new patch every 24 hours to nonhairy, clean, dry skin on the upper body or upper outer arm; each patch should be applied to a different site. **Note:** Adjustment may be required during initial treatment (move to higher dose if experiencing withdrawal symptoms; lower dose if side effects are experienced).

NicoDerm CQ®:

Patients smoking ≥10 cigarettes/day: Begin with **step 1** (21 mg/day) for 6 weeks, followed by **step 2** (14 mg/day) for 2 weeks; finish with **step 3** (7 mg/day) for 2 weeks

Patients smoking <10 cigarettes/day: Begin with **step 2** (14 mg/day) for 6 weeks, followed by **step 3** (7 mg/day) for 2 weeks

Note: Patients receiving >600 mg/day of cimetidine: Decrease to the next lower patch size

Note: Benefits of use of nicotine transdermal patches beyond 3 months have not been demonstrated.

Nasal: Spray: 1-2 sprays/hour; do not exceed more than 5 doses (10 sprays) per hour [maximum: 40 doses/day (80 sprays); each dose (2 sprays) contains 1 mg of nicotine]

Dosage Forms

Gum, chewing: 2 mg (20s, 40s, 50s, 100s, 110s); 4 mg (20s, 40s, 50s, 100s, 110s)

Nicorette® [OTC]: 2 mg (40s, 48s, 50s, 100s, 108s, 110s, 168s, 170s, 192s, 200s, 216s); 4 mg (40s, 48s, 50s, 100s, 108s, 110s, 168s, 170s, 192s, 200s, 216s)

Thrive™ [OTC]: 2 mg (40s); 4 mg (40s)

Lozenge:

Commit® [OTC]: 2 mg (48s, 72s, 84s, 108s, 168s); 4 mg (48s, 72s, 84s, 108s, 168s, 192s)

Oral inhalation system:

Nicotrol® Inhaler: 10 mg cartridge [cartridge delivers 4 mg nicotine] (168s)

Solution, intranasal spray:

Nicotrol® NS: 10 mg/mL (10 mL)

Transdermal system, topical: 7 mg/24 (30s); 14 mg/24 hours (30s); 21 mg/24 hours (30s)

NicoDerm® CQ® [OTC]: 7 mg/24 hours (14s); 14 mg/24 hours (14s); 21 mg/24 hours (14s)

nicotinic acid *see* niacin *on page* 692

nicotinic acid amide *see* niacinamide *on page* 693

Nicotrol® [Can] *see* nicotine *on page* 695

Nicotrol® Inhaler [US] *see* nicotine *on page* 695

Nicotrol® NS [US] *see* nicotine *on page* 695

Nico-Vert® *(Discontinued)* *see* meclizine *on page* 619

Nidagel™ [Can] *see* metronidazole *on page 651*
Nifediac CC® [US] *see* nifedipine *on page 697*
Nifedical XL® [US] *see* nifedipine *on page 697*

nifedipine (nye FED i peen)

Sound-Alike/Look-Alike Issues
NIFEdipine may be confused with niCARdipine, niMODipine, nisoldipine
Procardia XL® may be confused with Cartia® XT

Tall-Man **NIFE**dipine

U.S./Canadian Brand Names Adalat® CC [US]; Adalat® XL® [Can]; Afeditab® CR [US]; Apo-Nifed PA® [Can]; Apo-Nifed® [Can]; GEN-Nifedipine XL [Can]; Nifediac CC® [US]; Nifedical XL® [US]; Nifedipine PA [Can]; Nu-Nifed [Can]; Nu-Nifedipine-PA [Can]; PMS-Nifedipine [Can]; Procardia XL® [US]; Procardia® [US]

Therapeutic Category Calcium Channel Blocker

Use Management of chronic stable or vasospastic angina; treatment of hypertension (sustained release products only)

Usual Dosage Oral:
Children 1-17 years: Hypertension: Extended release tablet: Initial: 0.25-0.5 mg/kg/day once daily or in 2 divided doses; maximum: 3 mg/kg/day up to 120 mg/day
Adults: **Note:** Dosage adjustments should occur at 7- to 14-day intervals, to allow for adequate assessment of new dose; when switching from immediate release to sustained release formulations, use same total daily dose.
Chronic stable or vasospastic angina:
Immediate release: Initial: 10 mg 3 times/day; usual dose: 10-20 mg 3 times/day; maximum: 180 mg/day; **Note:** Do not use for acute anginal episodes; may precipitate myocardial infarction
Extended release: Initial: 30 or 60 mg once daily; maximum: 120-180 mg/day
Hypertension: Extended release: Initial: 30 or 60 mg once daily; maximum: 90-120 mg/day

Dosage Forms
Capsule, softgel: 10 mg, 20 mg
Procardia®: 10 mg
Tablet, extended release: 30 mg, 60 mg, 90 mg
Adalat® CC, Nifediac CC®, Procardia XL®: 30 mg, 60 mg, 90 mg
Afeditab® CR, Nifedical XL®: 30 mg, 60 mg

Nifedipine PA [Can] *see* nifedipine *on page 697*
Niferex® [US-OTC] *see* polysaccharide-iron complex *on page 799*
niftolid *see* flutamide *on page 436*
Nilandron® [US] *see* nilutamide *on page 697*

nilotinib (nye LOE ti nib)

Sound-Alike/Look-Alike Issues
nilotinib may be confused with imatinib, nilutamide

Synonyms AMN107; nilotinib hydrochloride monohydrate

U.S./Canadian Brand Names Tasigna® [US/Can]

Therapeutic Category Antineoplastic Agent, Tyrosine Kinase Inhibitor

Use Treatment of Philadelphia chromosome-positive chronic myelogenous leukemia (Ph+ CML) in chronic and accelerated phase (refractory or intolerant to prior therapy, including imatinib)

Usual Dosage Oral: Adults: 400 mg twice daily (continue treatment until disease progression or unacceptable toxicity)

Dosage Forms
Capsule:
Tasigna®: 200 mg

nilotinib hydrochloride monohydrate *see* nilotinib *on page 697*
Nilstat [Can] *see* nystatin *on page 715*
Nilstat® ***(Discontinued)*** *see* nystatin *on page 715*

nilutamide (ni LOO ta mide)

Sound-Alike/Look-Alike Issues
nilutamide may be confused with nilotinib

Synonyms NSC-684588; RU-23908
U.S./Canadian Brand Names Anandron® [Can]; Nilandron® [US]
Therapeutic Category Antineoplastic Agent
Use Treatment of metastatic prostate cancer
Usual Dosage Oral (refer to individual protocols): Adults: 300 mg daily for 30 days starting the same day or day after surgical castration, then 150 mg/day
Dosage Forms
Tablet:
Nilandron®: 150 mg

Nimbex® [US/Can] *see* cisatracurium *on page* 233

nimodipine (nye MOE di peen)

Sound-Alike/Look-Alike Issues
niMODipine may be confused with niCARdipine, NIFEdipine, nisoldipine
Tall-Man niMODipine
U.S./Canadian Brand Names Nimotop® [Can]
Therapeutic Category Calcium Channel Blocker
Use Vasospasm following subarachnoid hemorrhage from ruptured intracranial aneurysms
Usual Dosage **Note:** Capsules and contents are for oral administration **ONLY.** Oral: Adults: 60 mg every 4 hours for 21 days, start therapy within 96 hours after subarachnoid hemorrhage.
Dosage Forms
Capsule, liquid filled: 30 mg

Nimotop® [Can] *see* nimodipine *on page* 698
Nimotop® ***(Discontinued)*** *see* nimodipine *on page* 698
Nipent® [US/Can] *see* pentostatin *on page* 766
Niravam™ [US] *see* alprazolam *on page* 51

nisoldipine (nye SOL di peen)

Sound-Alike/Look-Alike Issues
nisoldipine may be confused with NIFEdipine, niMODipine
U.S./Canadian Brand Names Sular® [US]
Therapeutic Category Calcium Channel Blocker
Use Management of hypertension, alone or in combination with other antihypertensive agents
Usual Dosage Oral:
Sular® (Geomatrix® delivery system):
Adults: Initial: 17 mg once daily, then increase by 8.5 mg/week (or longer intervals) to attain adequate control of blood pressure
Usual dose range: 17-34 mg once daily; doses >34 mg once daily are not recommended
Nisoldipine extended-release tablet (original formulation):
Adults: Oral: Initial: 20 mg once daily, then increase by 10 mg/week (or longer intervals) to attain adequate control of blood pressure
Usual dose range (JNC 7): 10-40 mg once daily; doses >60 mg once daily are not recommended
Dosage Forms
Tablet, extended release [original formulation]: 20 mg, 30 mg, 40 mg
Tablet, extended release [Geomatrix® delivery system]:
Sular®: 8.5 mg, 17 mg, 25.5 mg, 34 mg

nitalapram *see* citalopram *on page* 234

nitazoxanide (nye ta ZOX a nide)

Synonyms NTZ
U.S./Canadian Brand Names Alinia® [US]
Therapeutic Category Antiprotozoal
Use Treatment of diarrhea caused by *Cryptosporidium parvum* or *Giardia lamblia*
Usual Dosage Oral:
Diarrhea caused by *Cryptosporidium parvum* or *Giardia lamblia*:
Children 1-3 years: 100 mg every 12 hours for 3 days

Children 4-11 years: 200 mg every 12 hours for 3 days
Children ≥12 years and Adults: 500 mg every 12 hours for 3 days

Dosage Forms

Powder for suspension, oral:
Alinia®: 100 mg/5 mL

Tablet:
Alinia®: 500 mg
Alinia® 3-Day Therapy Packs™ [unit-dose pack]: 500 mg (6s)

nitisinone (ni TIS i known)

U.S./Canadian Brand Names Orfadin® [US]

Therapeutic Category 4-Hydroxyphenylpyruvate Dioxygenase Inhibitor

Use Treatment of hereditary tyrosinemia type 1 (HT-1); to be used with dietary restriction of tyrosine and phenylalanine

Usual Dosage Oral: **Note:** Must be used in conjunction with a low-protein diet restricted in tyrosine and phenylalanine.

Infants: See dosing for Children and Adults; infants may require maximal dose once liver function has improved

Children and Adults: Initial: 1 mg/kg/day in divided doses, given in the morning and evening, 1 hour before meals; doses do not need to be divided evenly

Dosage Forms

Capsule:
Orfadin®: 2 mg, 5 mg, 10 mg

Nitoman™ [Can] *see* tetrabenazine *on page* 949
Nitrazadon [Can] *see* nitrazepam *(Canada only) on page* 699

nitrazepam *(Canada only)* (nye TRA ze pam)

Synonyms nitrozepamum

U.S./Canadian Brand Names Apo-Nitrazepam® [Can]; Mogadon [Can]; Nitrazadon [Can]; Nitrazepam (Pro-Doc) [Can]; Sandoz-Nitrazepam [Can]

Therapeutic Category Benzodiazepine

Controlled Substance CDSA IV

Use Short-term management of insomnia; treatment of myoclonic seizures

Usual Dosage Oral:

Children ≤30 kg: Myoclonic seizures: 0.3-1 mg/kg/day in 3 divided doses

Adults: Insomnia: 5-10 mg at bedtime; treatment should not exceed 7-10 consecutive days; use for more than 2-3 consecutive weeks requires complete reevaluation of patient

Dosage Forms [CAN] = Canadian brand name

Tablet:
Apo-Nitrazepam® [CAN], Mogadon [CAN], Nitrazadon [CAN], Nitrazepam [CAN], Sandoz-Nitrazepam [CAN]: 5 mg, 10 mg [not available in the U.S.]

Nitrazepam (Pro-Doc) [Can] *see* nitrazepam *(Canada only) on page* 699
Nitrek® *(Discontinued)* *see* nitroglycerin *on page* 700

nitric oxide (NYE trik OKS ide)

U.S./Canadian Brand Names INOmax® [US/Can]

Therapeutic Category Vasodilator, Pulmonary

Use Treatment of term and near-term (>34 weeks) neonates with hypoxic respiratory failure associated with pulmonary hypertension; used concurrently with ventilatory support and other agents

Usual Dosage Inhalation: Neonates (up to 14 days old): Hypoxic respiratory failure associated with pulmonary hypertension: 20 ppm. Treatment should be maintained up to 14 days or until the underlying oxygen desaturation has resolved and the neonate is ready to be weaned from therapy. In the CINRGI trial, patients whose oxygenation improved had their dose reduced to 5 ppm at the end of 4 hours of treatment. Doses above 20 ppm should not be used because of the risk of methemoglobinemia and elevated NO_2.

Dosage Forms

Gas, for inhalation:

INOmax®: 100 ppm [nitric oxide 0.01% and nitrogen 99.99%] (353 L, 1963 L); 800 ppm [nitric oxide 0.08% and nitrogen 99.92%] (353 L, 1963 L)

4′-nitro-3′-trifluoromethylisobutyrantide *see* flutamide *on page 436*

Nitro-Bid® [US] *see* nitroglycerin *on page 700*

Nitrodisc® Patch *(Discontinued)* *see* nitroglycerin *on page 700*

Nitro-Dur® [US/Can] *see* nitroglycerin *on page 700*

nitrofurantoin (nye troe fyoor AN toyn)

Sound-Alike/Look-Alike Issues

nitrofurantoin may be confused with Neurontin®, nitroglycerin

Macrobid® may be confused with microK®, Nitro-Bid®

U.S./Canadian Brand Names Apo-Nitrofurantoin® [Can]; Furadantin® [US]; Macrobid® [US/Can]; Macrodantin® [US/Can]; Novo-Furantoin [Can]

Therapeutic Category Antibiotic, Miscellaneous

Use Prevention and treatment of urinary tract infections caused by susceptible strains of *E. coli, S. aureus, Enterococcus, Klebsiella,* and *Enterobacter*

Usual Dosage Oral:

Children >1 month:

UTI treatment (Furadantin®, Macrodantin®): 5-7 mg/kg/day in divided doses every 6 hours; maximum: 400 mg/day. Administer for 7 days or at least 3 days after obtaining sterile urine

UTI prophylaxis (Furadantin®, Macrodantin®): 1-2 mg/kg/day in divided doses every 12-24 hours; maximum: 100 mg/day

Children >12 years: UTI treatment (Macrobid®): 100 mg twice daily for 7 days

Adults:

UTI treatment:

Furadantin®, Macrodantin®: 50-100 mg/dose every 6 hours; administer for 7 days or at least 3 days after obtaining sterile urine

Macrobid®: 100 mg twice daily for 7 days

UTI prophylaxis (Furadantin®, Macrodantin®): 50-100 mg/dose at bedtime

Dosage Forms

Capsule, macrocrystal: 50 mg, 100 mg

Macrodantin®: 25 mg, 50 mg, 100 mg

Capsule, macrocrystal/monohydrate: 100 mg

Macrobid®: 100 mg

Suspension, oral:

Furadantin®: 25 mg/5 mL

nitrogen mustard *see* mechlorethamine *on page 618*

nitroglycerin (nye troe GLI ser in)

Sound-Alike/Look-Alike Issues

nitroglycerin may be confused with nitrofurantoin, nitroprusside

Nitro-Bid® may be confused with Macrobid®, Nicobid®

Nitrol® may be confused with Nizoral®

Nitrostat® may be confused with Nilstat®, nystatin

Synonyms glyceryl trinitrate; nitroglycerol; NTG

U.S./Canadian Brand Names Gen-Nitro [Can]; Minitran™ [US/Can]; Nitro-Bid® [US]; Nitro-Dur® [US/Can]; Nitro-Time® [US]; Nitroglycerin Injection, USP [Can]; Nitrolingual® [US]; Nitrol® [Can]; Nitrostat® [US/Can]; Rho®-Nitro [Can]; Transderm-Nitro® [Can]; Trinipatch® 0.2 [Can]; Trinipatch® 0.4 [Can]; Trinipatch® 0.6 [Can]

Therapeutic Category Vasodilator

Use Treatment of angina pectoris; I.V. for congestive heart failure (especially when associated with acute myocardial infarction); pulmonary hypertension; perioperative hypertension (especially during cardiovascular surgery); induction of intraoperative hypotension

Usual Dosage Note: Hemodynamic and antianginal tolerance often develop within 24-48 hours of continuous nitrate administration. Nitrate-free interval (10-12 hours/day) is recommended to avoid tolerance development; gradually decrease dose in patients receiving NTG for prolonged period to avoid withdrawal reaction.

Children: Pulmonary hypertension: Continuous infusion: Start 0.25-0.5 mcg/kg/minute and titrate by 1 mcg/kg/minute at 20- to 60-minute intervals to desired effect; usual dose: 1-3 mcg/kg/minute; maximum: 5 mcg/kg/minute

Adults:

Oral: 2.5-9 mg 2-4 times/day (up to 26 mg 4 times/day)

I.V.: 5 mcg/minute, increase by 5 mcg/minute every 3-5 minutes to 20 mcg/minute; if no response at 20 mcg/minute increase by 10 mcg/minute every 3-5 minutes, up to 200 mcg/minute

Ointment: 1/2" upon rising and 1/2" 6 hours later; the dose may be doubled and even doubled again as needed

Patch, transdermal: Initial: 0.2-0.4 mg/hour, titrate to doses of 0.4-0.8 mg/hour; tolerance is minimized by using a patch-on period of 12-14 hours and patch-off period of 10-12 hours

Sublingual: 0.2-0.6 mg every 5 minutes for maximum of 3 doses in 15 minutes; may also use prophylactically 5-10 minutes prior to activities which may provoke an attack

Translingual: 1-2 sprays into mouth under tongue every 3-5 minutes for maximum of 3 doses in 15 minutes, may also be used 5-10 minutes prior to activities which may provoke an attack prophylactically

Dosage Forms

Capsule, extended release: 2.5 mg, 6.5 mg, 9 mg

Nitro-Time®: 2.5 mg, 6.5 mg, 9 mg

Infusion [premixed in D_5W]: 25 mg (250 mL) [0.1 mg/mL]; 50 mg (250 mL) [0.2 mg/mL]; 50 mg (500 mL) [0.1 mg/mL]; 100 mg (250 mL) [0.4 mg/mL]; 200 mg (500 mL) [0.4 mg/mL]

Injection, solution: 5 mg/mL (5 mL, 10 mL)

Ointment, topical:

Nitro-Bid®: 2% [20 mg/g] (1 g, 30 g, 60 g)

Solution, translingual [spray]:

Nitrolingual®: 0.4 mg/metered spray (4.9 g, 12 g, 16.9 g)

Tablet, sublingual: 0.3 mg, 0.4 mg, 0.6 mg

Nitrostat®: 0.3 mg, 0.4 mg, 0.6 mg

Transdermal system [once-daily patch]: 0.1 mg/hour (30s); 0.2 mg/hour (30s); 0.4 mg/hour (30s); 0.6 mg/hour (30s)

Minitran™: 0.1 mg/hour (30s); 0.2 mg/hour (30s); 0.4 mg/hour (30s); 0.6 mg/hour (30s)

Nitro-Dur®: 0.1 mg/hour (30s); 0.2 mg/hour (30s); 0.3 mg/hour (30s); 0.4 mg/hour (30s); 0.6 mg/hour (30s); 0.8 mg/hour (30s)

Nitroglycerin Injection, USP [Can] *see* nitroglycerin *on page 700*

nitroglycerol *see* nitroglycerin *on page 700*

Nitrol® [Can] *see* nitroglycerin *on page 700*

Nitrol® *(Discontinued)* *see* nitroglycerin *on page 700*

Nitrolingual® [US] *see* nitroglycerin *on page 700*

Nitrong® Oral Tablet *(Discontinued)* *see* nitroglycerin *on page 700*

Nitropress® [US] *see* nitroprusside *on page 701*

nitroprusside (nye troe PRUS ide)

Sound-Alike/Look-Alike Issues

nitroprusside may be confused with nitroglycerin

Synonyms nitroprusside sodium; sodium nitroferricyanide; sodium nitroprusside

U.S./Canadian Brand Names Nitropress® [US]

Therapeutic Category Vasodilator

Use Management of hypertensive crises; acute decompensated heart failure (HF); used for controlled hypotension to reduce bleeding during surgery

Usual Dosage Administration requires the use of an infusion pump. Average dose: 5 mcg/kg/minute.

Children: Pulmonary hypertension: I.V.: Initial: 1 mcg/kg/minute by continuous I.V. infusion; increase in increments of 1 mcg/kg/minute at intervals of 20-60 minutes; titrating to the desired response; usual dose: 3 mcg/kg/minute, rarely need >4 mcg/kg/minute; maximum: 5 mcg/kg/minute.

Adults: I.V. Initial: 0.3-0.5 mcg/kg/minute; increase in increments of 0.5 mcg/kg/minute, titrating to the desired hemodynamic effect or the appearance of headache or nausea; usual dose: 3 mcg/kg/minute; rarely need >4 mcg/kg/minute; maximum: 10 mcg/kg/minute. When administered by prolonged infusion faster than 2 mcg/kg/minute, cyanide is generated faster than an unaided patient can handle.

Dosage Forms

Injection, solution: 25 mg/mL (2 mL)

Nitropress®: 25 mg/mL (2 mL)

nitroprusside sodium *see* nitroprusside *on page* 701
NitroQuick® *(Discontinued)* *see* nitroglycerin *on page* 700
Nitrostat® [US/Can] *see* nitroglycerin *on page* 700
Nitro-Time® [US] *see* nitroglycerin *on page* 700

nitrous oxide (NYE trus OKS ide)

Therapeutic Category Anesthetic, Gas

Use Sedation, analgesia, and amnesia; principal adjunct to inhalation and intravenous general anesthesia

Usual Dosage Children and Adults:

Surgical: For sedation and analgesia: Concentrations of 25% to 50% nitrous oxide with oxygen. For general anesthesia, concentrations of 40% to 70% via mask or endotracheal tube. Minimal alveolar concentration (MAC), which can be considered the ED_{50} of inhalational anesthetics, is 105%; therefore delivery in a hyperbaric chamber is necessary to use as a complete anesthetic. When administered at 70%, reduces the MAC of other anesthetics by half.

Dental: For sedation and analgesia: Concentrations of 25% to 50% nitrous oxide with oxygen

Dosage Forms

Supplied in blue cylinders

nitrozepamum *see* nitrazepam *(Canada only) on page* 699
Nix® [US-OTC/Can] *see* permethrin *on page* 769

nizatidine (ni ZA ti deen)

Sound-Alike/Look-Alike Issues

Axid® may be confused with Ansaid®

U.S./Canadian Brand Names Apo-Nizatidine® [Can]; Axid® AR [US-OTC]; Axid® [US/Can]; Gen-Nizatidine [Can]; Novo-Nizatidine [Can]; Nu-Nizatidine [Can]; PMS-Nizatidine [Can]

Therapeutic Category Histamine H_2 Antagonist

Use Treatment and maintenance of duodenal ulcer; treatment of benign gastric ulcer; treatment of gastroesophageal reflux disease (GERD); OTC tablet used for the prevention of meal-induced heartburn, acid indigestion, and sour stomach

Usual Dosage Oral:

Children ≥12 years:
- GERD: Refer to adult dosing
- Meal-induced heartburn, acid indigestion and sour stomach: Refer to adult dosing

Adults:
- Duodenal ulcer:
  - Treatment of active ulcer: 300 mg at bedtime or 150 mg twice daily
  - Maintenance of healed ulcer: 150 mg/day at bedtime
- Gastric ulcer: 150 mg twice daily or 300 mg at bedtime
- GERD: 150 mg twice daily
- Meal-induced heartburn, acid indigestion, and sour stomach: 75 mg tablet [OTC] twice daily, 30 to 60 minutes prior to consuming food or beverages

Dosage Forms

Capsule: 150 mg, 300 mg

Solution, oral:

Axid®: 15 mg/mL

Tablet:

Axid® AR [OTC]: 75 mg

Nizoral® [US] *see* ketoconazole *on page* 557
Nizoral® A-D [US-OTC] *see* ketoconazole *on page* 557
N-methylhydrazine *see* procarbazine *on page* 820
N-methylnaltrexone bromide *see* methylnaltrexone *on page* 645
No Doz® Maximum Strength [US-OTC] *see* caffeine *on page* 165
NoHist [US] *see* chlorpheniramine and phenylephrine *on page* 214
NoHist-A [US] *see* chlorpheniramine, phenylephrine, and phenyltoloxamine *on page* 219
Nolahist® *(Discontinued)*
Nolex® LA *(Discontinued)*

Nolvadex®-D [Can] *see* tamoxifen *on page 937*
Nolvadex® ***(Discontinued)*** *see* tamoxifen *on page 937*

nonoxynol 9 (non OKS i nole nine)

Sound-Alike/Look-Alike Issues
Delfen® may be confused with Delsym®

Synonyms N-9

U.S./Canadian Brand Names Advantage-S® [US-OTC]; Conceptrol® [US-OTC]; Delfen® [US-OTC]; Encare® [US-OTC]; Gynol II® Extra Strength [US-OTC]; Gynol II® [US-OTC]; Today® [US-OTC]; VCF™ [US-OTC]

Therapeutic Category Spermicide

Use Prevention of pregnancy

Usual Dosage Adolescents and Adults: **Note:** Prior to use, refer to specific product labeling for complete instructions.
Prevention of pregnancy: Vaginal:
Advantage-S®, Conceptrol®: Insert 1 applicatorful vaginally up to 1 hour prior to intercourse
Encare®: Unwrap and insert 1 suppository vaginally at least 10 minutes prior to intercourse; effective for 1 hour
Today® Sponge: Insert 1 sponge vaginally prior to intercourse; allow to remain in place for 6 hours after intercourse before removing; effective for use up to 24 continuous hours. Do not leave in place for >30 hours.
VCF™:
Film: Insert 1 film vaginally at least 15 minutes, but no more than 3 hours, prior to intercourse. Insert new film for each act of intercourse or if more than 3 hours have elapsed.
Foam: Insert 1 applicatorful at least 15 minutes prior to intercourse; effective for up to 1 hour

Dosage Forms
Aerosol, vaginal [foam]:
Delfen® [OTC]: 12.5% (18 g) [contains benzoic acid]
VCF™ [OTC]: 12.5% (40 g)
Film, vaginal:
VCF™ [OTC]: 28% (3s, 6s,12s)
Gel, vaginal:
Advantage-S® [OTC]: 3.5% (1.5 g, 30 g)
Conceptrol® [OTC]: 4% (2.7 g)
Gynol II® [OTC]: 2% (108 g)
Gynol II® Extra Strength [OTC]: 3% (81 g)
Sponge, vaginal:
Today® [OTC]: 1 g (3s, 12s)
Suppository, vaginal:
Encare® [OTC]: 100 mg (12s, 18s)

No Pain-HP® ***(Discontinued)*** *see* capsaicin *on page 178*
Nora-BE™ [US] *see* norethindrone *on page 704*
noradrenaline *see* norepinephrine *on page 704*
noradrenaline acid tartrate *see* norepinephrine *on page 704*
Norcet® ***(Discontinued)*** *see* hydrocodone and acetaminophen *on page 501*
Norco® [US] *see* hydrocodone and acetaminophen *on page 501*
Norcuron® [Can] *see* vecuronium *on page 1008*
Norcuron® ***(Discontinued)*** *see* vecuronium *on page 1008*
nordeoxyguanosine *see* ganciclovir *on page 454*
Nordette® [US] *see* ethinyl estradiol and levonorgestrel *on page 387*
Norditropin® [US] *see* somatropin *on page 916*
Norditropin® NordiFlex® [US] *see* somatropin *on page 916*
Nordryl® Injection ***(Discontinued)*** *see* diphenhydramine *on page 315*
Nordryl® Oral ***(Discontinued)*** *see* diphenhydramine *on page 315*
Norel DM™ [US] *see* chlorpheniramine, phenylephrine, and dextromethorphan *on page 217*
norel® EX [US] *see* guaifenesin and phenylephrine *on page 475*
norelgestromin and ethinyl estradiol *see* ethinyl estradiol and norelgestromin *on page 389*

norepinephrine (nor ep i NEF rin)

Synonyms levarterenol bitartrate; noradrenaline; noradrenaline acid tartrate; norepinephrine bitartrate

U.S./Canadian Brand Names Levophed® [US/Can]

Therapeutic Category Adrenergic Agonist Agent

Use Treatment of shock which persists after adequate fluid volume replacement

Usual Dosage Administration requires the use of an infusion pump!

Note: Norepinephrine dosage is stated in terms of norepinephrine base.

Continuous I.V. infusion:

Children: Initial: 0.05-0.1 mcg/kg/minute; titrate to desired effect; maximum dose: 2 mcg/kg/minute

Adults: Initial: 0.5-1 mcg/minute and titrate to desired response; 8-30 mcg/minute is usual range

ACLS dosing range: 0.5-30 mcg/minute

Alternative weight-based dosing: 0.01-3 mcg/kg/minute

Dosage Forms Strength expressed as base:

Injection, solution: 1 mg/mL (4 mL)

Levophed®: 1 mg/mL (4 mL)

norepinephrine bitartrate *see* norepinephrine *on page 704*

Norethin™ 1/35E *(Discontinued)* *see* ethinyl estradiol and norethindrone *on page 390*

norethindrone (nor ETH in drone)

Sound-Alike/Look-Alike Issues

Micronor® may be confused with miconazole, Micronase®

Synonyms norethindrone acetate; norethisterone

U.S./Canadian Brand Names Aygestin® [US]; Camila™ [US]; Errin™ [US]; Jolivette™ [US]; Micronor® [Can]; Nor-QD® [US]; Nora-BE™ [US]; Norlutate® [Can]; Ortho Micronor® [US]

Therapeutic Category Contraceptive, Progestin Only; Progestin

Use Treatment of amenorrhea; abnormal uterine bleeding; endometriosis; prevention of pregnancy

Usual Dosage Oral: Adolescents and Adults: Female:

Contraception: Progesterone only: Norethindrone 0.35 mg every day (no missed days)

Initial dose: Start on first day of menstrual period or the day after a miscarriage or abortion. If switching from a combined oral contraceptive, begin the day after finishing the last active combined tablet.

Missed dose: Take as soon as remembered. A backup method of contraception should be used for 48 hours if dose is taken ≥3 hours late.

Amenorrhea and abnormal uterine bleeding: Norethindrone acetate: 2.5-10 mg/day for 5-10 days during the second half of the menstrual cycle

Endometriosis: Norethindrone acetate: 5 mg/day for 14 days; increase at increments of 2.5 mg/day every 2 weeks to reach 15 mg/day; continue for 6-9 months or until breakthrough bleeding demands temporary termination

Dosage Forms

Tablet: 0.35 mg, 5 mg

Aygestin®: 5 mg

Camila™, Errin™, Jolivette™, Ortho Micronor®, Nora-BE™, Nor-QD®: 0.35 mg

norethindrone acetate *see* norethindrone *on page 704*

norethindrone acetate and ethinyl estradiol *see* ethinyl estradiol and norethindrone *on page 390*

norethindrone and estradiol *see* estradiol and norethindrone *on page 376*

norethindrone and mestranol (nor eth IN drone & MES tra nole)

Sound-Alike/Look-Alike Issues

Norinyl® may be confused with Nardil®

Synonyms mestranol and norethindrone

U.S./Canadian Brand Names Necon® 1/50 [US]; Norinyl® 1+50 [US]; Ortho-Novum® 1/50 [Can]

Therapeutic Category Contraceptive, Oral

Use Prevention of pregnancy

Usual Dosage Oral: Adults: Female: Contraception:

Schedule 1 (Sunday starter): Dose begins on first Sunday after onset of menstruation; if the menstrual period starts on Sunday, take first tablet that very same day. **With a Sunday start, an additional method of contraception should be used until after the first 7 days of consecutive administration.**

For 21-tablet package: Dosage is 1 tablet daily for 21 consecutive days, followed by 7 days off of the medication; a new course begins on the 8th day after the last tablet is taken.
For 28-tablet package: Dosage is 1 tablet daily without interruption.
Schedule 2 (Day 1 starter): Dose starts on first day of menstrual cycle taking 1 tablet daily.
For 21-tablet package: Dosage is 1 tablet daily for 21 consecutive days, followed by 7 days off of the medication; a new course begins on the 8th day after the last tablet is taken.
For 28-tablet package: Dosage is 1 tablet daily without interruption.
If all doses have been taken on schedule and one menstrual period is missed, continue dosing cycle. If two consecutive menstrual periods are missed, pregnancy test is required before new dosing cycle is started.
Missed doses **monophasic formulations** (refer to package insert for complete information):
One dose missed: Take as soon as remembered or take 2 tablets next day
Two consecutive doses missed in the first 2 weeks: Take 2 tablets as soon as remembered or 2 tablets next 2 days. **An additional method of contraception should be used for 7 days after missed dose.**
Two consecutive doses missed in week 3 or three consecutive doses missed at any time: **An additional method of contraception must be used for 7 days after a missed dose:**
Schedule 1 (Sunday starter): Continue dose of 1 tablet daily until Sunday, then discard the rest of the pack, and a new pack should be started that same day.
Schedule 2 (Day 1 starter): Current pack should be discarded, and a new pack should be started that same day.

Dosage Forms

Tablet, monophasic formulations:
Necon® 1/50: Norethindrone 1 mg and mestranol 0.05 mg [21 light blue tablets and 7 white inactive tablets] (28s)
Norinyl® 1+50: Norethindrone 1 mg and mestranol 0.05 mg [21 white tablets and 7 orange inactive tablets] (28s)

norethisterone *see* norethindrone *on page 704*
Norflex™ [US/Can] *see* orphenadrine *on page 730*

norfloxacin (nor FLOKS a sin)

Sound-Alike/Look-Alike Issues
norfloxacin may be confused with Norflex™, Noroxin®
Noroxin® may be confused with Neurontin®, Norflex™, norfloxacin

U.S./Canadian Brand Names Apo-Norflox® [Can]; CO Norfloxacin [Can]; Norfloxacine® [Can]; Noroxin® [US/Can]; Novo-Norfloxacin [Can]; PMS-Norfloxacin [Can]; Riva-Norfloxacin [Can]

Therapeutic Category Quinolone

Use Uncomplicated and complicated urinary tract infections caused by susceptible gram-negative and gram-positive bacteria; sexually-transmitted disease (eg, uncomplicated urethral and cervical gonorrhea) caused by *N. gonorrhoeae*; prostatitis due to *E. coli*
Note: As of April 2007, the CDC no longer recommends the use of fluoroquinolones for the treatment of gonococcal disease.

Usual Dosage

Usual dosage range:
Adults: Oral: 400 mg every 12 hours (maximum: 800 mg/day)

Indication-specific dosing:
Adults: Oral:
Prostatitis: 400 mg every 12 hours for 4-6 weeks
Uncomplicated gonorrhea: 800 mg as a single dose. **Note:** As of April 2007, the CDC no longer recommends the use of fluoroquinolones for the treatment of uncomplicated gonococcal disease.
Urinary tract infections:
Uncomplicated due to *E. coli, K. pneumoniae, P. mirabilis*: 400 mg twice daily for 3 days
Uncomplicated due to other organisms: 400 mg twice daily for 7-10 days
Complicated: 400 mg twice daily for 10-21 days

Dosage Forms

Tablet:
Noroxin®: 400 mg

Norfloxacine® [Can] *see* norfloxacin *on page 705*
Norgesic™ *(Discontinued)* *see* orphenadrine, aspirin, and caffeine *on page 730*
Norgesic™ Forte *(Discontinued)* *see* orphenadrine, aspirin, and caffeine *on page 730*
norgestimate and estradiol *see* estradiol and norgestimate *on page 377*

norgestimate and ethinyl estradiol *see* ethinyl estradiol and norgestimate *on page 393*
norgestrel and ethinyl estradiol *see* ethinyl estradiol and norgestrel *on page 394*
Norinyl® 1+35 [US] *see* ethinyl estradiol and norethindrone *on page 390*
Norinyl® 1+50 [US] *see* norethindrone and mestranol *on page 704*
Noritate® [US/Can] *see* metronidazole *on page 651*
Norlutate® [Can] *see* norethindrone *on page 704*
normal human serum albumin *see* albumin *on page 40*
normal saline *see* sodium chloride *on page 908*
normal serum albumin (human) *see* albumin *on page 40*
Normiflo® ***(Discontinued)***
Normocarb HF™ [US] *see* electrolyte solution, renal replacement *on page 350*
Normodyne® [Can] *see* labetalol *on page 562*
Noroxin® [US/Can] *see* norfloxacin *on page 705*
Norpace® [US/Can] *see* disopyramide *on page 324*
Norpace® CR [US] *see* disopyramide *on page 324*
Norplant® Implant [Can] *see* levonorgestrel *on page 582*
Norplant® Implant ***(Discontinued)*** *see* levonorgestrel *on page 582*
Norpramin® [US/Can] *see* desipramine *on page 284*
Nor-QD® [US] *see* norethindrone *on page 704*
Nortemp Children's [US-OTC] *see* acetaminophen *on page 19*
North American antisnake-bite serum *see* crotalidae polyvalent immune FAB (ovine) *on page 262*
North American coral snake antivenin *see* antivenin *(Micrurus fulvius) on page 87*
Northyx™ [US] *see* methimazole *on page 637*
Nortrel™ [US] *see* ethinyl estradiol and norethindrone *on page 390*
Nortrel™ 7/7/7 [US] *see* ethinyl estradiol and norethindrone *on page 390*

nortriptyline (nor TRIP ti leen)

Sound-Alike/Look-Alike Issues
nortriptyline may be confused with amitriptyline, desipramine, Norpramin®
Aventyl® HCl may be confused with Bentyl®
Pamelor® may be confused with Demerol®, Dymelor®, Panlor® DC, Tambocor™

Synonyms nortriptyline hydrochloride

U.S./Canadian Brand Names Alti-Nortriptyline [Can]; Apo-Nortriptyline® [Can]; Aventyl® [Can]; Gen-Nortriptyline [Can]; Norventyl [Can]; Novo-Nortriptyline [Can]; Nu-Nortriptyline [Can]; Pamelor® [US]; PMS-Nortriptyline [Can]

Therapeutic Category Antidepressant, Tricyclic (Secondary Amine)

Use Treatment of symptoms of depression

Usual Dosage Oral: Adults:
Depression: 25 mg 3-4 times/day up to 150 mg/day; doses may be given once daily
Myofascial pain, neuralgia, burning mouth syndrome (dental use): Initial: 10-25 mg at bedtime; dosage may be increased by 25 mg/day weekly, if tolerated; usual maintenance dose: 75 mg as a single bedtime dose or 2 divided doses

Dosage Forms
Capsule: 10 mg, 25 mg, 50 mg, 75 mg
Pamelor®: 10 mg, 25 mg, 50 mg, 75 mg
Solution:
Pamelor®: 10 mg/5 mL

nortriptyline hydrochloride *see* nortriptyline *on page 706*
Norvasc® [US/Can] *see* amlodipine *on page 66*
Norventyl [Can] *see* nortriptyline *on page 706*
Norvir® [US/Can] *see* ritonavir *on page 871*
Norvir® SEC [Can] *see* ritonavir *on page 871*
Notuss®-DC [US] *see* pseudoephedrine and codeine *on page 834*
Novacet® ***(Discontinued)*** *see* sulfur and sulfacetamide *on page 931*
Novafed® A ***(Discontinued)*** *see* chlorpheniramine and pseudoephedrine *on page 215*

Nutralox® [US-OTC] *see* calcium carbonate *on page 170*
Nutraplus® [US-OTC] *see* urea *on page 998*
Nu-Trazodone [Can] *see* trazodone *on page 979*
Nu-Triazide [Can] *see* hydrochlorothiazide and triamterene *on page 500*
Nutrimin-Plus [US-OTC] *see* vitamins (multiple/oral) *on page 1019*
Nu-Trimipramine [Can] *see* trimipramine *on page 988*
NutriNate® [US] *see* vitamins (multiple/prenatal) *on page 1020*
NutriSpire™ [US] *see* vitamins (multiple/prenatal) *on page 1020*

nutritional formula, enteral/oral (noo TRISH un al FOR myoo la, EN ter al/OR al)

Synonyms dietary supplements

U.S./Canadian Brand Names Carnation Instant Breakfast® [US-OTC]; Citrotein® [US-OTC]; Criticare HN® [US-OTC]; Ensure Plus® [US-OTC]; Ensure® [US-OTC]; Isocal® [US-OTC]; Magnacal® [US-OTC]; Microlipid™ [US-OTC]; Osmolite® HN [US-OTC]; Pedialyte® [US-OTC]; Portagen® [US-OTC]; Pregestimil® [US-OTC]; Propac™ [US-OTC]; Soyalac® [US-OTC]; Vital HN® [US-OTC]; Vitaneed™ [US-OTC]; Vivonex® T.E.N. [US-OTC]; Vivonex® [US-OTC]

Therapeutic Category Nutritional Supplement

Dosage Forms

Liquid: Calcium and sodium caseinate, maltodextrin, sucrose, partially hydrogenated soy oil, soy lecithin
Powder: Amino acids, predigested carbohydrates, safflower oil

Nutropin® [US/Can] *see* somatropin *on page 916*
Nutropin AQ® [US/Can] *see* somatropin *on page 916*
NuvaRing® [US/Can] *see* ethinyl estradiol and etonogestrel *on page 386*
Nu-Verap [Can] *see* verapamil *on page 1010*
Nu-Verap SR [Can] *see* verapamil *on page 1010*
Nuvigil™ [US] *see* armodafinil *on page 98*
Nu-Zopiclone [Can] *see* zopiclone *(Canada only) on page 1034*
NVP *see* nevirapine *on page 692*
Nyaderm [Can] *see* nystatin *on page 715*
Nyamyc™ [US] *see* nystatin *on page 715*
Nycoff [US-OTC] *see* dextromethorphan *on page 295*
Nydrazid® *(Discontinued)* *see* isoniazid *on page 548*

nystatin (nye STAT in)

Sound-Alike/Look-Alike Issues

nystatin may be confused with HMG-CoA reductase inhibitors (also known as "statins"; eg, atorvastatin, fluvastatin, lovastatin, pravastatin, rosuvastatin, simvastatin), Nilstat®, Nitrostat®
Nilstat may be confused with Nitrostat®, nystatin

U.S./Canadian Brand Names Bio-Statin® [US]; Candistatin® [Can]; Mycostatin® [US]; Nilstat [Can]; Nyaderm [Can]; Nyamyc™ [US]; Nystat-Rx® [US]; Nystop® [US]; Paddock Nystatin™ [US]; Pedi-Dri® [US]; PMS-Nystatin [Can]

Therapeutic Category Antifungal Agent

Use Treatment of susceptible cutaneous, mucocutaneous, and oral cavity fungal infections normally caused by the *Candida* species

Usual Dosage

Oral candidiasis:
Suspension (swish and swallow orally):
Premature infants: 100,000 units 4 times/day
Infants: 200,000 units 4 times/day or 100,000 units to each side of mouth 4 times/day
Children and Adults: 400,000-600,000 units 4 times/day
Powder for compounding: Children and Adults: 1/8 teaspoon (500,000 units) to equal approximately 1/2 cup of water; give 4 times/day
Mucocutaneous infections: Children and Adults: Topical: Apply 2-3 times/day to affected areas; very moist topical lesions are treated best with powder
Intestinal infections: Adults: Oral: 500,000-1,000,000 units every 8 hours
Vaginal infections: Adults: Vaginal tablets: Insert 1 tablet/day at bedtime for 2 weeks

Dosage Forms

Capsule:
Bio-Statin®: 500,000 units, 1 million units
Cream: 100,000 units/g (15 g, 30 g)
Mycostatin®: 100,000 units/g (30 g)
Ointment, topical: 100,000 units/g (15 g, 30 g)
Powder, for prescription compounding: 50 million units (10 g); 150 million units (30 g); 500 million units (100 g); 2 billion units (400 g)
Nystat-Rx®: 50 million units (10 g); 150 million units (30 g); 500 million units (100 g); 1 billion units (190 g); 2 billion units (350 g)
Powder, for prescription compounding: 50 million units (10 g); 150 million units (30 g); 500 million units (100 g); 1 billion units (190 g); 2 billion units (350 g)
Bio-Statin®: 2 billion units (30 g)
Powder for suspension, oral [preservative free]:
Paddock Nystatin™: 50 million units (10 g); 150 million units (30 g); 500 million units (100 g); 2 billion units (400 g) [sugar free]
Powder, topical: 100,000 units/g (15 g, 30 g, 60 g)
Nyamyc™: 100,000 units/g (15 g, 30 g)
Nystop®: 100,000 units/g (15 g, 30 g, 60 g)
Pedi-Dri®: 100,000 units/g (56.7 g)
Suspension, oral: 100,000 units/mL
Tablet: 500,000 units
Tablet, vaginal: 100,000 units (15s)

nystatin and metronidazole *see* metronidazole and nystatin *(Canada only) on page* 652

nystatin and triamcinolone (nye STAT in & trye am SIN oh lone)

Sound-Alike/Look-Alike Issues
Mycolog®-II may be confused with Halog®

Synonyms triamcinolone and nystatin

Therapeutic Category Antifungal/Corticosteroid

Use Treatment of cutaneous candidiasis

Usual Dosage Topical: Children and Adults: Apply sparingly 2-4 times/day. Therapy should be discontinued when control is achieved; if no improvement is seen, reassessment of diagnosis may be necessary.

Dosage Forms
Cream: Nystatin 100,000 units and triamcinolone 0.1% (15 g, 30 g, 60 g)
Ointment: Nystatin 100,000 units and triamcinolone 0.1% (15 g, 30 g, 60 g)

Nystat-Rx® [US] *see* nystatin *on page* 715
Nystex® ***(Discontinued)*** *see* nystatin *on page* 715
Nystop® [US] *see* nystatin *on page* 715
Nytol® [Can] *see* diphenhydramine *on page* 315
Nytol® Extra Strength [Can] *see* diphenhydramine *on page* 315
Nytol® Quick Caps [US-OTC] *see* diphenhydramine *on page* 315
Nytol® Quick Gels [US-OTC] *see* diphenhydramine *on page* 315
Néevo® [US] *see* vitamins (multiple/prenatal) *on page* 1020
Néevo® DHA [US] *see* vitamins (multiple/prenatal) *on page* 1020
NāSal™ [US-OTC] *see* sodium chloride *on page* 908
NāSop™ ***(Discontinued)*** *see* phenylephrine *on page* 774
Nōstrilla® [US-OTC] *see* oxymetazoline *on page* 740
O-V Staticin® ***(Discontinued)*** *see* nystatin *on page* 715
Oasis® [US] *see* saliva substitute *on page* 887
Obezine® ***(Discontinued)*** *see* phendimetrazine *on page* 770
OCBZ *see* oxcarbazepine *on page* 734
Occlusal®-HP [US-OTC/Can] *see* salicylic acid *on page* 884
Ocean® [US-OTC] *see* sodium chloride *on page* 908
Ocean® for Kids [US-OTC] *see* sodium chloride *on page* 908
Ocella™ [US] *see* ethinyl estradiol and drospirenone *on page* 384

OCL® ***(Discontinued)*** *see* polyethylene glycol-electrolyte solution *on page* 797
Octagam® [US] *see* immune globulin (intravenous) *on page* 523
Octamide® ***(Discontinued)*** *see* metoclopramide *on page* 649
Octaplex® [Can] *see* prothrombin complex (human) [(factors II, VII, IX, X), protein C, and protein S] *(Canada only) on page* 832
Octicair® Otic ***(Discontinued)*** *see* neomycin, polymyxin B, and hydrocortisone *on page* 688
Octocaine® ***(Discontinued)*** *see* lidocaine and epinephrine *on page* 586
Octostim® [Can] *see* desmopressin acetate *on page* 285

octreotide (ok TREE oh tide)

Sound-Alike/Look-Alike Issues
Sandostatin® may be confused with Sandimmune®, Sandostatin LAR®, sargramostim, simvastatin

Synonyms NSC-671663; octreotide acetate

U.S./Canadian Brand Names Octreotide Acetate Injection [Can]; Octreotide Acetate Omega [Can]; Sandostatin LAR® [US/Can]; Sandostatin® [US/Can]

Therapeutic Category Somatostatin Analog

Use Control of symptoms in patients with metastatic carcinoid and vasoactive intestinal peptide-secreting tumors (VIPomas); treatment of acromegaly

Usual Dosage

Acromegaly: Adults:

SubQ, I.V.: Initial: 50 mcg 3 times/day; titrate to achieve growth hormone levels <5 ng/mL or IGF-I (somatomedin C) levels <1.9 units/mL in males and <2.2 units/mL in females. Usual effective dose 100-200 mcg 3 times/day; range 300-1500 mcg/day. **Note:** Should be withdrawn yearly for a 4-week interval (8 weeks for depot injection) in patients who have received irradiation. Resume if levels increase and signs/symptoms recur.

I.M. depot injection: Patients must be stabilized on subcutaneous octreotide for at least 2 weeks before switching to the long-acting depot. Upon switch: 20 mg I.M. intragluteally every 4 weeks for 3 months, then the dose may be modified based upon response.

Carcinoid tumors: Adults:

SubQ, I.V.: Initial 2 weeks: 100-600 mcg/day in 2-4 divided doses; usual range 50-750 mcg/day (some patients may require up to 1500 mcg/day)

I.M. depot injection: Patients must be stabilized on subcutaneous octreotide for at least 2 weeks before switching to the long-acting depot. Upon switch: 20 mg I.M. intragluteally every 4 weeks for 2 months, then the dose may be modified based upon response.

Note: Patients should continue to receive their SubQ injections for the first 2 weeks at the same dose in order to maintain therapeutic levels (some patients may require 3-4 weeks of continued SubQ injections). Patients who experience periodic exacerbations of symptoms may require temporary SubQ injections in addition to depot injections (at their previous SubQ dosing regimen) until symptoms have resolved.

VIPomas: Adults:

SubQ, I.V.: Initial 2 weeks: 200-300 mcg/day in 2-4 divided doses; titrate dose based on response/ tolerance. Range: 150-750 mcg/day (doses >450 mcg/day are rarely required)

I.M. depot injection: Patients must be stabilized on subcutaneous octreotide for at least 2 weeks before switching to the long-acting depot. Upon switch: 20 mg I.M. intragluteally every 4 weeks for 2 months, then the dose may be modified based upon response.

Note: Patients receiving depot injection should continue to receive their SubQ injections for the first 2 weeks at the same dose in order to maintain therapeutic levels (some patients may require 3-4 weeks of continued SubQ injections). Patients who experience periodic exacerbations of symptoms may require temporary SubQ injections in addition to depot injections (at their previous SubQ dosing regimen) until symptoms have resolved.

Dosage Forms

Injection, microspheres for suspension [depot formulation]:
Sandostatin LAR®: 10 mg, 20 mg, 30 mg

Injection, solution: 0.2 mg/mL (5 mL); 1 mg/mL (5 mL)
Sandostatin®: 0.2 mg/mL (5 mL); 1 mg/mL (5 mL)

Injection, solution [preservative free]: 0.05 mg/mL (1 mL); 0.1 mg/mL (1 mL); 0.5 mg/mL (1 mL)
Sandostatin®: 0.05 mg/mL (1 mL); 0.1 mg/mL (1 mL); 0.5 mg/mL (1 mL)

octreotide acetate *see* octreotide *on page* 717
Octreotide Acetate Injection [Can] *see* octreotide *on page* 717

Octreotide Acetate Omega [Can] *see* octreotide *on page 717*
OcuClear® *(Discontinued)* *see* oxymetazoline *on page 740*
Ocufen® [US/Can] *see* flurbiprofen *on page 435*
Ocuflox® [US/Can] *see* ofloxacin *on page 718*
OcuNefrin™ [US-OTC] *see* phenylephrine *on page 774*
Ocupress® *(Discontinued)* *see* carteolol *on page 188*
Ocupress® Ophthalmic [Can] *see* carteolol *on page 188*
Ocusert Pilo-20® *(Discontinued)* *see* pilocarpine *on page 783*
Ocusert Pilo-40® *(Discontinued)* *see* pilocarpine *on page 783*
Ocu-Sul® *(Discontinued)* *see* sulfacetamide *on page 927*
Ocutricin® Topical Ointment *(Discontinued)* *see* bacitracin, neomycin, and polymyxin B *on page 119*
Ocuvite® [US-OTC] *see* vitamins (multiple/oral) *on page 1019*
Ocuvite® Adult 50+ [US-OTC] *see* vitamins (multiple/oral) *on page 1019*
Ocuvite® Extra® [US-OTC] *see* vitamins (multiple/oral) *on page 1019*
Ocuvite® Lutein [US-OTC] *see* vitamins (multiple/oral) *on page 1019*
O-desmethylvenlafaxine *see* desvenlafaxine *on page 287*
ODV *see* desvenlafaxine *on page 287*
Oesclim® [Can] *see* estradiol *on page 373*
Off-Ezy® Wart Remover *(Discontinued)* *see* salicylic acid *on page 884*

ofloxacin (oh FLOKS a sin)

Sound-Alike/Look-Alike Issues

Floxin® may be confused with Flexeril®
Ocuflox® may be confused with Occlusal®-HP, Ocufen®

U.S./Canadian Brand Names Apo-Ofloxacin® [Can]; Apo-Oflox® [Can]; Floxin® [US/Can]; Novo-Ofloxacin [Can]; Ocuflox® [US/Can]; PMS-Ofloxacin [Can]

Therapeutic Category Antibiotic, Ophthalmic; Antibiotic, Otic; Quinolone

Use

Quinolone antibiotic for the treatment of acute exacerbations of chronic bronchitis, community-acquired pneumonia, skin and skin structure infections (uncomplicated), urethral and cervical gonorrhea (acute, uncomplicated), urethritis and cervicitis (nongonococcal), mixed infections of the urethra and cervix, pelvic inflammatory disease (acute), cystitis (uncomplicated), urinary tract infections (complicated), prostatitis

Note: As of April 2007, the CDC no longer recommends the use of fluoroquinolones for the treatment of gonococcal disease.

Ophthalmic: Treatment of superficial ocular infections involving the conjunctiva or cornea due to strains of susceptible organisms

Otic: Otitis externa, chronic suppurative otitis media, acute otitis media

Usual Dosage

Usual dosage range:

Children ≥6 months: Otic: 5 drops daily

Children >1 year: Ophthalmic: 1-2 drops every 30 minutes to 4 hours initially, decreasing to every 4-6 hours

Children >12 years: Otic: 10 drops once or twice daily

Adults:

Ophthalmic: 1-2 drops every 30 minutes to 4 hours initially, decreasing to every 4-6 hours
Oral: 200-400 mg every 12 hours
Otic: 10 drops once or twice daily

Indication-specific dosing:

Children 6 months to 13 years: Otic: **Otitis externa:** Instill 5 drops (or the contents of 1 single-dose container) into affected ear(s) once daily for 7 days

Children 1-12 years: Otic: **Acute otitis media with tympanostomy tubes:** Instill 5 drops (or the contents of 1 single-dose container) into affected ear(s) twice daily for 10 days

Children >1 year and Adults: Ophthalmic:

Conjunctivitis: Instill 1-2 drops in affected eye(s) every 2-4 hours for the first 2 days, then use 4 times/day for an additional 5 days

Corneal ulcer: Instill 1-2 drops every 30 minutes while awake and every 4-6 hours after retiring for the first 2 days; beginning on day 3, instill 1-2 drops every hour while awake for 4-6 additional days; thereafter, 1-2 drops 4 times/day until clinical cure.

Children >12 years and Adults: Otic: **Otitis media, chronic suppurative with perforated tympanic membranes:** Instill 10 drops (or the contents of 2 single-dose containers) into affected ear twice daily for 14 days

Children ≥13 years and Adults: Otic: **Otitis externa:** Instill 10 drops (or the contents of 2 single-dose containers) into affected ear(s) once daily for 7 days

Adults: Oral:

Cervicitis/urethritis:

Nongonococcal: 300 mg every 12 hours for 7 days

Gonococcal (acute, uncomplicated): 400 mg as a single dose; **Note:** As of April 2007, the CDC no longer recommends the use of fluoroquinolones for the treatment of uncomplicated gonococcal disease.

Chronic bronchitis (acute exacerbation), community-acquired pneumonia, skin and skin structure infections (uncomplicated): 400 mg every 12 hours for 10 days

Pelvic inflammatory disease (acute): 400 mg every 12 hours for 10-14 days with or without metronidazole; **Note:** The CDC recommends use only if standard cephalosporin therapy is not feasible and community prevalence of quinolone-resistant gonococcal organisms is low. Culture sensitivity must be confirmed.

Prostatitis:

Acute: 400 mg for 1 dose, then 300 mg twice daily for 10 days

Chronic: 200 mg every 12 hours for 6 weeks

UTI:

Uncomplicated: 200 mg every 12 hours for 3-7 days

Complicated: 200 mg every 12 hours for 10 days

Dosage Forms

Solution, ophthalmic [drops]: 0.3% (5 mL, 10 mL)

Ocuflox®: 0.3% (5 mL)

Solution, otic [drops]: 0.3% (5 mL, 10 mL)

Floxin®: 0.3% (5 mL, 10 mL)

Tablet: 200 mg, 300 mg, 400 mg

Ogen® [US/Can] *see* estropipate *on page 381*

Ogestrel® [US] *see* ethinyl estradiol and norgestrel *on page 394*

OGMT *see* metyrosine *on page 653*

OGT-918 *see* miglustat *on page 658*

9-OH-risperidone *see* paliperidone *on page 743*

OKT3 *see* muromonab-CD3 *on page 673*

olanzapine (oh LAN za peen)

Sound-Alike/Look-Alike Issues

OLANZapine may be confused with olsalazine, QUEtiapine

Zyprexa® may be confused with Celexa®, Reprexain®, Zestril®, Zyrtec®

Zyprexa® Zydis® may be confused with Zelapar™

Synonyms LY170053

Tall-Man OLANZapine

U.S./Canadian Brand Names Novo-Olanzapine [Can]; PMS-Olanzapine [Can]; Zyprexa® IntraMuscular [US]; Zyprexa® Zydis® [US/Can]; Zyprexa® [US/Can]

Therapeutic Category Antipsychotic Agent

Use Treatment of the manifestations of schizophrenia; treatment of acute or mixed mania episodes associated with bipolar I disorder (as monotherapy or in combination with lithium or valproate); maintenance treatment of bipolar disorder; acute agitation (patients with schizophrenia or bipolar mania); in combination with fluoxetine for treatment-resistant or bipolar I depression

Usual Dosage Adults:

Agitation (acute, associated with bipolar I mania or schizophrenia): I.M.: Initial dose: 5-10 mg (a lower dose of 2.5 mg may be considered when clinical factors warrant); additional doses (2.5-10 mg) may be considered; however, 2-4 hours should be allowed between doses to evaluate response (maximum total daily dose: 30 mg, per manufacturer's recommendation)

Bipolar I acute mixed or manic episodes: Oral:
Monotherapy: Initial: 10-15 mg once daily; increase by 5 mg/day at intervals of not less than 24 hours. Maintenance: 5-20 mg/day; recommended maximum dose: 20 mg/day.
Combination therapy (with lithium or valproate): Initial: 10 mg once daily; dosing range: 5-20 mg/day; recommended maximum dose: 20 mg/day.
Depression associated with bipolar disorder (in combination with fluoxetine): Oral: Initial: 5 mg in the evening; adjust as tolerated to usual range of 5-12.5 mg/day. See **"Note."**
Schizophrenia: Oral: Initial: 5-10 mg once daily (increase to 10 mg once daily within 5-7 days); thereafter, adjust by 5 mg/day at 1-week intervals, up to a recommended maximum of 20 mg/day. Maintenance: 10-20 mg once daily. Doses of 30-50 mg/day have been used; however, doses >10 mg/day have not demonstrated better efficacy, and safety and efficacy of doses >20 mg/day have not been evaluated.
Treatment-resistant depression (in combination with fluoxetine): Oral: Initial: 5 mg in the evening; adjust as tolerated to usual range of 5-12.5 mg/day. See **"Note."**
Note: When using individual components of fluoxetine with olanzapine rather than fixed dose combination product (Symbyax®), approximate dosage correspondence is as follows:
Olanzapine 2.5 mg + fluoxetine 20 mg = Symbyax® 3/25
Olanzapine 5 mg + fluoxetine 20 mg = Symbyax® 6/25
Olanzapine 12.5 mg + fluoxetine 20 mg = Symbyax® 12/25
Olanzapine 5 mg + fluoxetine 50 mg = Symbyax® 6/50
Olanzapine 12.5 mg + fluoxetine 50 mg = Symbyax® 12/50

Dosage Forms
Injection, powder for reconstitution:
Zyprexa® IntraMuscular: 10 mg
Tablet, oral:
Zyprexa®: 2.5 mg, 5 mg, 7.5 mg, 10 mg, 15 mg, 20 mg
Tablet, orally disintegrating:
Zyprexa® Zydis®: 5 mg, 10 mg, 15 mg, 20 mg

olanzapine and fluoxetine (oh LAN za peen & floo OKS e teen)

Sound-Alike/Look-Alike Issues
Symbyax® may be confused with Cymbalta®

Synonyms fluoxetine and olanzapine; olanzapine and fluoxetine hydrochloride

U.S./Canadian Brand Names Symbyax® [US]

Therapeutic Category Antidepressant, Selective Serotonin Reuptake Inhibitor; Antipsychotic Agent, Thienobenzodiaepine

Use Treatment of depressive episodes associated with bipolar I disorder; treatment-resistant depression (unresponsive to 2 trials of different antidepressants)

Usual Dosage Oral:
Adults: **Note:** Lower doses (olanzapine 3-6 mg/fluoxetine 25 mg) should be used in patients predisposed to hypotension, with hepatic impairment, with combined factors for reduced metabolism (females, the elderly, nonsmokers), or enhanced sensitivity to olanzapine; dose adjustments should be made with caution in this patient population.
Depression associated with bipolar I disorder: Initial: Olanzapine 6 mg/fluoxetine 25 mg once daily in the evening. Dosing range: Olanzapine 6-12 mg/fluoxetine 25-50 mg. Safety of daily doses of olanzapine >18 mg/fluoxetine >75 mg have not been evaluated.
Treatment-resistant depression: Initial: Olanzapine 6 mg/fluoxetine 25 mg once daily in the evening. Dosing range: Olanzapine 6-18 mg/fluoxetine 25-50 mg. Safety of daily doses of olanzapine >18 mg/fluoxetine >75 mg have not been evaluated.
Note: When using individual components of fluoxetine with olanzapine rather than fixed-dose combination product (Symbyax®), approximate dosage correspondence is as follows:
Olanzapine 2.5 mg + fluoxetine 20 mg = Symbyax® 3/25
Olanzapine 5 mg + fluoxetine 20 mg = Symbyax® 6/25
Olanzapine 12.5 mg + fluoxetine 20 mg = Symbyax® 12/25
Olanzapine 5 mg + fluoxetine 50 mg = Symbyax® 6/50
Olanzapine 12.5 mg + fluoxetine 50 mg = Symbyax® 12/50

Dosage Forms
Capsule:
Symbyax®:
3/25: Olanzapine 3 mg and fluoxetine 25 mg
6/25: Olanzapine 6 mg and fluoxetine 25 mg
6/50: Olanzapine 6 mg and fluoxetine 50 mg

12/25: Olanzapine 12 mg and fluoxetine 25 mg
12/50: Olanzapine 12 mg and fluoxetine 50 mg

olanzapine and fluoxetine hydrochloride *see* olanzapine and fluoxetine *on page 720*

oleovitamin A *see* vitamin A *on page 1016*

oleum ricini *see* castor oil *on page 190*

olmesartan (ole me SAR tan)

Sound-Alike/Look-Alike Issues

Benicar® may be confused with Mevacor®

Synonyms olmesartan medoxomil

U.S./Canadian Brand Names Benicar® [US]; Olmetec® [Can]

Therapeutic Category Angiotensin II Receptor Antagonist

Use Treatment of hypertension with or without concurrent use of other antihypertensive agents

Usual Dosage Oral: Adults: Initial: Usual starting dose is 20 mg once daily; if initial response is inadequate, may be increased to 40 mg once daily after 2 weeks. May administer with other antihypertensive agents if blood pressure inadequately controlled with olmesartan. Consider lower starting dose in patients with possible depletion of intravascular volume (eg, patients receiving diuretics).

Dosage Forms

Tablet:

Benicar®: 5 mg, 20 mg, 40 mg

olmesartan and amlodipine *see* amlodipine and olmesartan *on page 68*

olmesartan and hydrochlorothiazide (ole me SAR tan & hye droe klor oh THYE a zide)

Synonyms hydrochlorothiazide and olmesartan medoxomil; olmesartan medoxomil and hydrochlorothiazide

U.S./Canadian Brand Names Benicar HCT® [US]; Olmetec Plus® [Can]

Therapeutic Category Angiotensin II Receptor Antagonist; Diuretic, Thiazide

Use Treatment of hypertension (not recommended for initial treatment)

Usual Dosage Oral: Adults: One tablet daily; dosage must be individualized (see below). May be titrated at 2- to 4-week intervals.

Replacement therapy: May be substituted for previously titrated dosages of the individual components.

Patients not controlled with single-agent therapy: Initiate by adding the lowest available dose of the alternative component (hydrochlorothiazide 12.5 mg or olmesartan 20 mg). Titrate to effect (maximum daily hydrochlorothiazide dose: 25 mg; maximum daily olmesartan dose: 40 mg).

Dosage Forms

Tablet:

Benicar HCT®: 20/12.5: Olmesartan 20 mg and hydrochlorothiazide 12.5 mg; 40/12.5: Olmesartan 40 mg and hydrochlorothiazide 12.5 mg; 40/25: Olmesartan 40 mg and hydrochlorothiazide 25 mg

olmesartan medoxomil *see* olmesartan *on page 721*

olmesartan medoxomil and hydrochlorothiazide *see* olmesartan and hydrochlorothiazide *on page 721*

Olmetec® [Can] *see* olmesartan *on page 721*

Olmetec Plus® [Can] *see* olmesartan and hydrochlorothiazide *on page 721*

olopatadine (oh la PAT a deen)

Sound-Alike/Look-Alike Issues

Patanol® may be confused with Platinol®

Synonyms olopatadine hydrochloride

U.S./Canadian Brand Names Pataday™ [US]; Patanase® [US]; Patanol® [US/Can]

Therapeutic Category Antihistamine

Use

Nasal spray: Treatment of the symptoms of seasonal allergic rhinitis
Ophthalmic: Treatment of the signs and symptoms of allergic conjunctivitis

Usual Dosage
Intranasal (Patanase®): Children ≥12 years and Adults: 2 sprays into each nostril twice daily
Ophthalmic: Children ≥3 years and Adults:
Patanol®: Instill 1 drop into affected eye(s) twice daily (allowing 6-8 hours between doses); results from an environmental study demonstrated that olopatadine was effective when dosed twice daily for up to 6 weeks
Pataday™: Instill 1 drop into affected eye(s) once daily

Dosage Forms
Solution, intranasal [spray]:
Patanase®: 0.6% (30.5 g)
Solution, ophthalmic:
Patanol®: 0.1% (5 mL)
Pataday™: 0.2% (2.5 mL)

olopatadine hydrochloride *see* olopatadine *on page 721*

olsalazine (ole SAL a zeen)

Sound-Alike/Look-Alike Issues
olsalazine may be confused with OLANZapine
Dipentum® may be confused with Dilantin®

Synonyms olsalazine sodium

U.S./Canadian Brand Names Dipentum® [US/Can]

Therapeutic Category 5-Aminosalicylic Acid Derivative

Use Maintenance of remission of ulcerative colitis in patients intolerant to sulfasalazine

Usual Dosage Oral: Adults: 1 g/day in 2 divided doses

Dosage Forms
Capsule:
Dipentum®: 250 mg

olsalazine sodium *see* olsalazine *on page 722*
Olux® [US] *see* clobetasol *on page 242*
Olux-E™ [US] *see* clobetasol *on page 242*
Olux®/Olux-E™ CP [US] *see* clobetasol *on page 242*
Omacor® ***(Discontinued)*** *see* omega-3-acid ethyl esters *on page 723*

omalizumab (oh mah lye ZOO mab)

Synonyms rhuMAb-E25

U.S./Canadian Brand Names Xolair® [US/Can]

Therapeutic Category Monoclonal Antibody

Use Treatment of moderate-to-severe, persistent allergic asthma not adequately controlled with inhaled corticosteroids

Usual Dosage SubQ: Children ≥12 years and Adults: Asthma: Dose is based on pretreatment IgE serum levels and body weight. Dosing should not be adjusted based on IgE levels taken during treatment or <1 year following discontinuation of therapy; doses should be adjusted during treatment for significant changes in body weight
IgE ≥30-100 int. units/mL:
30-90 kg: 150 mg every 4 weeks
>90-150 kg: 300 mg every 4 weeks
IgE >100-200 int. units/mL:
30-90 kg: 300 mg every 4 weeks
>90-150 kg: 225 mg every 2 weeks
IgE >200-300 int. units/mL:
30-60 kg: 300 mg every 4 weeks
>60-90 kg: 225 mg every 2 weeks
>90-150 kg: 300 mg every 2 weeks
IgE >300-400 int. units/mL:
30-70 kg: 225 mg every 2 weeks
>70-90 kg: 300 mg every 2 weeks
>90 kg: Do not administer dose

IgE >400-500 int. units/mL:
30-70 kg: 300 mg every 2 weeks
>70-90 kg: 375 mg every 2 weeks
>90 kg: Do not administer dose
IgE >500-600 int. units/mL:
30-60 kg: 300 mg every 2 weeks
>60-70 kg: 375 mg every 2 weeks
>70 kg: Do not administer dose
IgE >600-700 int. units/mL:
30-60 kg: 375 mg every 2 weeks
>60 kg: Do not administer dose

Dosage Forms
Injection, powder for reconstitution [preservative free]:
Xolair®: 150 mg

omega-3-acid ethyl esters (oh MEG a three AS id ETH il ES ters)

Sound-Alike/Look-Alike Issues
Lovaza® may be confused with LORazepam
Omacor® may be confused with Amicar®

Synonyms ethyl esters of omega-3 fatty acids; fish oil

U.S./Canadian Brand Names Lovaza® [US]

Therapeutic Category Antilipemic Agent, Miscellaneous

Use Lovaza®: Adjunct to diet therapy in the treatment of hypertriglyceridemia (≥500 mg/dL)
Note: A number of OTC formulations containing omega-3 fatty acids are marketed as nutritional supplements; these do not have FDA-approved indications and may not contain the same amounts of the active ingredient.

Usual Dosage Oral: Adults: Hypertriglyceridemia: 4 g/day as a single daily dose or in 2 divided doses

Dosage Forms
Capsule, liquid gel, oral:
Lovaza®: 1 g

omeprazole (oh MEP ra zole)

Sound-Alike/Look-Alike Issues
omeprazole may be confused with aripiprazole, fomepizole
Prilosec® may be confused with Plendil®, Prevacid®, predniSONE, prilocaine, Prinivil®, Proventil®, Prozac®

Synonyms omeprazole magnesium

U.S./Canadian Brand Names Apo-Omeprazole® [Can]; Losec MUPS® [Can]; Losec® [Can]; PMS-Omeprazole DR [Can]; PMS-Omeprazole [Can]; Prilosec OTC™ [US-OTC]; Prilosec® [US]; ratio-Omeprazole [Can]; Sandoz Omeprazole [Can]

Therapeutic Category Gastric Acid Secretion Inhibitor

Use Short-term (4-8 weeks) treatment of active duodenal ulcer disease or active benign gastric ulcer; treatment of heartburn and other symptoms associated with gastroesophageal reflux disease (GERD); short-term (4-8 weeks) treatment of endoscopically-diagnosed erosive esophagitis; maintenance healing of erosive esophagitis; long-term treatment of pathological hypersecretory conditions; as part of a multidrug regimen for *H. pylori* eradication to reduce the risk of duodenal ulcer recurrence

OTC labeling: Short-term treatment of frequent, uncomplicated heartburn occurring ≥2 days/week

Usual Dosage Oral:
Children 1-16 years: GERD or other acid-related disorders:
5 kg to <10 kg: 5 mg once daily
10 kg to <20 kg: 10 mg once daily
≥20 kg: 20 mg once daily
Adults:
Active duodenal ulcer: 20 mg/day for 4-8 weeks
Gastric ulcers: 40 mg/day for 4-8 weeks
Symptomatic GERD (without esophageal lesions): 20 mg/day for up to 4 weeks
Erosive esophagitis: 20 mg/day for 4-8 weeks; maintenance of healing: 20 mg/day for up to 12 months total therapy (including treatment period of 4-8 weeks)

Helicobacter pylori eradication: Dose varies with regimen:

Manufacturer labeling: 40 mg once daily administered with clarithromycin 500 mg 3 times/day for 14 days **or** 20 mg twice daily administered with amoxicillin 1000 mg *and* clarithromycin 500 mg twice daily for 10 days. **Note:** Presence of ulcer at time of therapy initiation may necessitate an additional 14-18 days of omeprazole 20 mg/day (monotherapy) after completion of combination therapy.

American College of Gastroenterology guidelines:

Nonpenicillin therapy: 20 mg twice daily administered with amoxicillin 1000 mg *and* clarithromycin 500 mg twice daily for 10-14 days

Penicillin allergy: 20 mg twice daily administered with clarithromycin 500 mg *and* metronidazole 500 mg twice daily for 10-14 days **or** 20 mg once or twice daily administered with bismuth subsalicylate 525 mg *and* metronidazole 250 mg *plus* tetracycline 500 mg 4 times/day for 10-14 days

Pathological hypersecretory conditions: Initial: 60 mg once daily; doses up to 120 mg 3 times/day have been administered; administer daily doses >80 mg in divided doses

Frequent heartburn (OTC labeling): 20 mg/day for 14 days; treatment may be repeated after 4 months if needed

Dosage Forms

Capsule, delayed release: 10 mg, 20 mg, 40 mg

Prilosec®: 10 mg, 20 mg, 40 mg

Granules for suspension, delayed release, enteric coated, oral:

Prilosec®: 2.5 mg/packet; 10 mg/packet

Tablet, delayed release: 20 mg

Prilosec OTC™ [OTC]: 20 mg

omeprazole and sodium bicarbonate (oh MEP ra zole & SOW dee um bye KAR bun ate)

Sound-Alike/Look-Alike Issues

Zegerid® may be confused with Zestril®

Synonyms sodium bicarbonate and omeprazole

U.S./Canadian Brand Names Zegerid® [US]

Therapeutic Category Proton Pump Inhibitor; Substituted Benzimidazole

Use Short-term (4-8 weeks) treatment of active duodenal ulcer disease or active benign gastric ulcer; treatment of heartburn and other symptoms associated with gastroesophageal reflux disease (GERD); short-term (4-8 weeks) treatment of endoscopically-diagnosed erosive esophagitis; maintenance healing of erosive esophagitis; reduction of risk of upper gastrointestinal bleeding in critically-ill patients

Usual Dosage Oral: Adults:

Active duodenal ulcer: 20 mg/day for 4-8 weeks

Gastric ulcers: 40 mg/day for 4-8 weeks

Symptomatic GERD: 20 mg/day for up to 4 weeks

Erosive esophagitis: 20 mg/day for 4-8 weeks; maintenance of healing: 20 mg/day for up to 12 months total therapy (including treatment period of 4-8 weeks)

Risk reduction of upper GI bleeding in critically-ill patients (Zegerid® powder for oral suspension):

Loading dose: Day 1: 40 mg every 6-8 hours for two doses

Maintenance dose: 40 mg/day for up to 14 days; therapy >14 days has not been evaluated

Dosage Forms

Capsule, immediate release:

Zegerid®: 20 mg, 40 mg

Powder for oral suspension:

Zegerid®: 20 mg/packet, 40 mg/packet

omeprazole magnesium *see* omeprazole *on page* 723

Omnaris™ [US/Can] *see* ciclesonide *on page* 226

Omnicef® [US/Can] *see* cefdinir *on page* 192

OMNIhist® II L.A. [US] *see* chlorpheniramine, phenylephrine, and methscopolamine *on page* 218

Omnii Gel™ [US-OTC] *see* fluoride *on page* 430

Omnipaque™ [US] *see* iohexol *on page* 540

Omnipen® *(Discontinued)* *see* ampicillin *on page* 76

Omnipen®-N *(Discontinued)* *see* ampicillin *on page* 76

Omniscan™ [US] *see* gadodiamide *on page* 451

Omnitrope® [US] *see* somatropin *on page* 916

onabotulinumtoxinA (oh nuh BOT yoo lin num TOKS in aye)

Synonyms botulinum toxin type A; BTX-A

U.S./Canadian Brand Names Botox® Cosmetic [US/Can]; Botox® [US/Can]

Therapeutic Category Ophthalmic Agent, Toxin

Use Treatment of strabismus and blepharospasm associated with dystonia (including benign essential blepharospasm or VII nerve disorders) in patients ≥12 years of age; cervical dystonia (spasmodic torticollis) in patients ≥16 years of age; temporary improvement in the appearance of lines/wrinkles of the face (moderate-to-severe glabellar lines associated with corrugator and/or procerus muscle activity) in adult patients ≤65 years of age; treatment of severe primary axillary hyperhidrosis in adults not adequately controlled with topical treatments

Canadian labeling: Additional use (not in U.S. labeling): Focal spasticity, including treatment of stroke related upper limb spasticity; dynamic equines foot deformity in pediatric cerebral palsy patients

Usual Dosage

Cervical dystonia: Children ≥16 years and Adults: I.M.: For dosing guidance, the mean dose is 236 units (25th to 75th percentile range 198-300 units) divided among the affected muscles in patients previously treated with botulinum toxin. Initial dose in previously untreated patients should be lower. Sequential dosing should be based on the patient's head and neck position, localization of pain, muscle hypertrophy, patient response, and previous adverse reactions. The total dose injected into the sternocleidomastoid muscles should be ≤100 units to decrease the occurrence of dysphagia.

Canadian labeling (not in U.S. labeling): Effective range of 200-360 units has been used in clinical practice; maximum dose: 6 units/kg every 2 months

Blepharospasm: Children ≥12 years and Adults: I.M.: Initial dose: 1.25-2.5 units injected into the medial and lateral pretarsal orbicularis oculi of the upper lid and lateral pretarsal orbicularis oculi of lower lid; dose may be increased up to twice the previous dose if the response from the initial dose lasted ≤2 months; maximum dose per site: 5 units. Tolerance may occur if treatments are given more often than every 3 months, but the effect is not usually permanent. Cumulative dose:

U.S. labeling: ≤200 units in 30-day period

Canadian labeling (not in U.S. labeling): ≤200 units in 60-day period

Strabismus: Children ≥12 years and Adults: I.M.: **Note:** Several minutes prior to injection, administration of local anesthetic and ocular decongestant drops are recommended.

Initial dose:

Vertical muscles and for horizontal strabismus <20 prism diopters: 1.25-2.5 units in any one muscle

Horizontal strabismus of 20-50 prism diopters: 2.5-5 units in any one muscle

Persistent VI nerve palsy ≥1 month: 1.25-2.5 units in the medial rectus muscle

Reexamine patients 7-14 days after each injection to assess the effect of that dose. Subsequent doses for patients experiencing incomplete paralysis of the target may be increased up to twice the previous administered dose. The maximum recommended dose as a single injection for any one muscle is 25 units. Do not administer subsequent injections until the effects of the previous dose are gone.

Primary axillary hyperhidrosis: Adults ≥18 years: Intradermal: 50 units/axilla. Injection area should be defined by standard staining techniques. Injections should be evenly distributed into multiple sites (10-15), administered in 0.1-0.2 mL aliquots, ~1-2 cm apart. May repeat when clinical effect diminishes.

Reduction of glabellar lines: Adults ≤65 years: I.M.: An effective dose is determined by gross observation of the patient's ability to activate the superficial muscles injected. The location, size and use of muscles may vary markedly among individuals. Inject 0.1 mL (4 units) dose into each of five sites, two in each corrugator muscle and one in the procerus muscle for a total dose 0.5 mL (20 units) administered no more frequently than every 3-4 months.

Spasticity (cerebral palsy related; Canadian labeling [not approved in U.S. labeling]): Children ≥2 years: I.M.: 4 units/kg (total dose) divided into two injections into medial and lateral heads of the gastrocnemius of affected limb; if clinically indicated, may repeat every 2 months (maximum dose: 200 units)

Spasticity (focal; Canadian labeling [not approved in U.S. labeling]): Adults ≥18 years: I.M.: Individualize dose based on patient size, extent, and location of muscle involvement, degree of spasticity, local muscle weakness, and response to prior treatment. In clinical trials total doses up to 360 units were administered as separate injections typically divided among flexor muscles of the elbow, wrist, and fingers; may repeat therapy at 3-4 months with appropriate dosage based upon the clinical condition of patient at time of retreatment.

Suggested guidelines for the treatment of stroke-related upper limb spasticity: **Note:** Dose listed is total dose administered as individual or separate intramuscular injection(s):

Biceps brachii: 100-200 units (up to 4 sites)

Flexor digitorum profundus: 15-50 units (1-2 sites)

Flexor digitorum sublimes: 15-50 units (1-2 sites)

Flexor carpi radialis: 15-60 units (1-2 sites)

Flexor carpi ulnaris: 10-50 units (1-2 sites)
Adductor pollicis: 20 units (1-2 sites)
Flexor pollicis longus: 20 units (1-2 sites)

Dosage Forms

Injection, powder for reconstitution [preservative free]:
Botox®, Botox® Cosmetic: OnabotulinumtoxinA 100 units

Oncaspar® [US] *see* pegaspargase *on page* 755
Oncet® ***(Discontinued)*** *see* hydrocodone and homatropine *on page* 502
Oncotice™ [Can] *see* BCG vaccine *on page* 124
Oncovin® ***(Discontinued)*** *see* vincristine *on page* 1014

ondansetron (on DAN se tron)

Sound-Alike/Look-Alike Issues

ondansetron may be confused with dolasetron, granisetron, palonosetron
Zofran® may be confused with Zantac®, Zosyn®

Synonyms GR38032R; ondansetron hydrochloride

U.S./Canadian Brand Names Apo-Ondansetron® [Can]; DOM-Ondansetron [Can]; Gen-Ondansetron [Can]; JAMP-Ondansetron [Can]; MINT-Ondansetron [Can]; Novo-Ondansetron [Can]; Ondansetron Injection [Can]; Ondansetron-Omega [Can]; PHL-Ondansetron [Can]; PMS-Ondansetron [Can]; RAN-Ondansetron [Can]; ratio-Ondansetron [Can]; Sandoz-Ondansetron [Can]; Zofran® ODT [US/Can]; Zofran® [US/Can]

Therapeutic Category Selective 5-HT_3 Receptor Antagonist

Use Prevention of nausea and vomiting associated with moderately- to highly-emetogenic cancer chemotherapy; radiotherapy; prevention of postoperative nausea and vomiting (PONV); treatment of PONV if no prophylactic dose of ondansetron received

Usual Dosage Note: Studies in adults have shown a single daily dose of 8-12 mg I.V. or 8-24 mg orally to be as effective as mg/kg dosing, and should be considered for **all** patients whose mg/kg dose exceeds 8-12 mg I.V.; oral solution and ODT formulations are bioequivalent to corresponding doses of tablet formulation

Children:
I.V.:
Prevention of chemotherapy-induced emesis: 6 months to 18 years: 0.15 mg/kg/dose administered 30 minutes prior to chemotherapy, 4 and 8 hours after the first dose **or** 0.45 mg/kg/day as a single dose
Prevention of postoperative nausea and vomiting: 1 month to 12 years:
≤40 kg: 0.1 mg/kg as a single dose
>40 kg: 4 mg as a single dose
Oral: Prevention of chemotherapy-induced emesis:
4-11 years: 4 mg 30 minutes before chemotherapy; repeat 4 and 8 hours after initial dose, then 4 mg every 8 hours for 1-2 days after chemotherapy completed
≥12 years: Refer to adult dosing.

Adults:
I.V.: Prevention of chemotherapy-induced emesis:
0.15 mg/kg 3 times/day beginning 30 minutes prior to chemotherapy **or**
0.45 mg/kg once daily **or**
8-10 mg 1-2 times/day **or**
24 mg or 32 mg once daily
I.M., I.V.: Postoperative nausea and vomiting (PONV): 4 mg as a single dose approximately 30 minutes before the end of anesthesia (see Note below) or as treatment if vomiting occurs after surgery.
Note: The manufacturer recommends administration immediately before induction of anesthesia; however, this has been shown not to be as effective as administration at the end of surgery. Repeat doses given in response to inadequate control of nausea/vomiting from preoperative doses are generally ineffective.
Oral:
Chemotherapy-induced emesis:
Highly-emetogenic agents/single-day therapy: 24 mg given 30 minutes prior to the start of therapy
Moderately-emetogenic agents: 8 mg every 12 hours beginning 30 minutes before chemotherapy, continuously for 1-2 days after chemotherapy completed
Total body irradiation: 8 mg 1-2 hours before daily each fraction of radiotherapy
Single high-dose fraction radiotherapy to abdomen: 8 mg 1-2 hours before irradiation, then 8 mg every 8 hours after first dose for 1-2 days after completion of radiotherapy

Daily fractionated radiotherapy to abdomen: 8 mg 1-2 hours before irradiation, then 8 mg 8 hours after first dose for each day of radiotherapy

Postoperative nausea and vomiting: 16 mg given 1 hour prior to induction of anesthesia

Dosage Forms

Infusion, premixed in D_5 [preservative free]: 32 mg (50 mL)

Injection, solution: 2 mg/mL (2 mL, 20 mL)

Zofran®: 2 mg/mL (2 mL, 20 mL)

Injection, solution [preservative free]: 2 mg/mL (2 mL)

Solution, oral: 4 mg/5 mL (50 mL)

Zofran®: 4 mg/5 mL

Tablet: 4 mg; 8 mg

Zofran®: 4 mg, 8 mg

Tablet, orally disintegrating: 4 mg; 8 mg

Zofran® ODT: 4 mg, 8 mg

ondansetron hydrochloride *see* ondansetron *on page 726*

Ondansetron Injection [Can] *see* ondansetron *on page 726*

Ondansetron-Omega [Can] *see* ondansetron *on page 726*

One A Day® Cholesterol Plus [US-OTC] *see* vitamins (multiple/oral) *on page 1019*

One A Day® Energy [US-OTC] *see* vitamins (multiple/oral) *on page 1019*

One A Day® Essential [US-OTC] *see* vitamins (multiple/oral) *on page 1019*

One-A-Day® Kids Bugs Bunny and Friends Complete [US-OTC] *see* vitamins (multiple/pediatric) *on page 1020*

One-A-Day® Kids Scooby-Doo!™ Complete [US-OTC] *see* vitamins (multiple/pediatric) *on page 1020*

One A Day® Kids Scooby-Doo!™ Gummies [US-OTC] *see* vitamins (multiple/pediatric) *on page 1020*

One-A-Day® Kids Scooby-Doo!™ Plus Calcium [US-OTC] *see* vitamins (multiple/pediatric) *on page 1020*

One A Day® Maximum [US-OTC] *see* vitamins (multiple/oral) *on page 1019*

One A Day® Men's 50+ Advantage [US-OTC] *see* vitamins (multiple/oral) *on page 1019*

One A Day® Men's Health Formula [US-OTC] *see* vitamins (multiple/oral) *on page 1019*

One A Day® Teen Advantage for Her [US-OTC] *see* vitamins (multiple/oral) *on page 1019*

One A Day® Teen Advantage for Him [US-OTC] *see* vitamins (multiple/oral) *on page 1019*

One A Day® Weight Smart® Advanced [US-OTC] *see* vitamins (multiple/oral) *on page 1019*

One A Day® Women's 50+ Advantage [US-OTC] *see* vitamins (multiple/oral) *on page 1019*

One A Day® Women's [US-OTC] *see* vitamins (multiple/oral) *on page 1019*

One A Day® Women's Active Mind & Body [US-OTC] *see* vitamins (multiple/oral) *on page 1019*

One A Day® Women's Prenatal [US-OTC] *see* vitamins (multiple/prenatal) *on page 1020*

One Gram C [US-OTC] *see* ascorbic acid *on page 100*

Onglyza™ [US] *see* saxagliptin *on page 892*

Onsolis™ [US] *see* fentanyl *on page 410*

ONTAK® [US] *see* denileukin diftitox *on page 282*

Onxol® [US] *see* paclitaxel *on page 742*

Ony-Clear *(Discontinued)* *see* benzalkonium chloride *on page 129*

Opana® [US] *see* oxymorphone *on page 741*

Opana® ER [US] *see* oxymorphone *on page 741*

OPC-13013 *see* cilostazol *on page 228*

OPC-14597 *see* aripiprazole *on page 97*

OPC-41061 *see* tolvaptan *on page 969*

OP-CCK *see* sincalide *on page 903*

Opcon-A® [US-OTC] *see* naphazoline and pheniramine *on page 681*

Opcon® Ophthalmic *(Discontinued)* *see* naphazoline *on page 680*

o,p'-DDD *see* mitotane *on page 662*

Operand® [US-OTC] *see* povidone-iodine *on page 807*

Operand® Chlorhexidine Gluconate [US-OTC] *see* chlorhexidine gluconate *on page 210*

Ophthalgan® Ophthalmic *(Discontinued)* *see* glycerin *on page 468*

Ophthetic® ***(Discontinued)*** *see* proparacaine *on page* *826*
Ophthifluor® ***(Discontinued)*** *see* fluorescein *on page* *429*
Ophthochlor® Ophthalmic ***(Discontinued)*** *see* chloramphenicol *on page* *208*
Ophtho-Dipivefrin™ [Can] *see* dipivefrin *on page* *323*
Ophtho-Tate® [Can] *see* prednisolone (ophthalmic) *on page* *813*
opium and belladonna *see* belladonna and opium *on page* *126*

opium tincture (OH pee um TING chur)

Sound-Alike/Look-Alike Issues
opium tincture may be confused with camphorated tincture of opium (paregoric)
DTO is an error-prone abbreviation (mistaken as Diluted Tincture of Opium; dose equivalency of paregoric)

Synonyms opium tincture, deodorized

Therapeutic Category Analgesic, Narcotic

Controlled Substance C-II

Use Treatment of diarrhea or relief of pain

Usual Dosage Oral: **Note:** Opium tincture 10% contains morphine 10 mg/mL. use caution in ordering, dispensing, and/or administering.
Children:
Diarrhea: 0.005-0.01 mL/kg/dose every 3-4 hours for a maximum of 6 doses/24 hours
Analgesia: 0.01-0.02 mL/kg/dose every 3-4 hours
Adults:
Diarrhea: 0.3-1 mL/dose every 2-6 hours to maximum of 6 mL/24 hours
Analgesia: 0.6-1.5 mL/dose every 3-4 hours

Dosage Forms
Liquid: 10%

opium tincture, deodorized *see* opium tincture *on page* *728*

oprelvekin (oh PREL ve kin)

Sound-Alike/Look-Alike Issues
oprelvekin may be confused with aldesleukin, Proleukin®
Neumega® may be confused with Neulasta®, Neupogen®

Synonyms IL-11; interleukin-11; NSC-722848; recombinant human interleukin-11; recombinant interleukin-11; rhIL-11; rIL-11

U.S./Canadian Brand Names Neumega® [US]

Therapeutic Category Platelet Growth Factor

Use Prevention of severe thrombocytopenia; reduce the need for platelet transfusions following myelosuppressive chemotherapy

Usual Dosage SubQ: Administer first dose ~6-24 hours after the end of chemotherapy. Discontinue at least 48 hours before beginning the next cycle of chemotherapy.
Adults: 50 mcg/kg once daily for ~10-21 days (until postnadir platelet count ≥50,000 cells/μL)

Dosage Forms
Injection, powder for reconstitution:
Neumega®: 5 mg

Optase™ [US] *see* trypsin, balsam Peru, and castor oil *on page* *993*
Optho-Bunolol® [Can] *see* levobunolol *on page* *578*
Opti-Clear [US-OTC] *see* tetrahydrozoline *on page* *951*
Opticrom® [Can] *see* cromolyn sodium *on page* *261*
Optigene® 3 ***(Discontinued)*** *see* tetrahydrozoline *on page* *951*
OptiMARK® [US] *see* gadoversetamide *on page* *453*
Optimine® ***(Discontinued)***
Optimoist® Solution ***(Discontinued)*** *see* saliva substitute *on page* *887*
Optimyxin® [Can] *see* bacitracin and polymyxin B *on page* *119*
Optimyxin Plus® [Can] *see* neomycin, polymyxin B, and gramicidin *on page* *688*
OptiNate® [US] *see* vitamins (multiple/prenatal) *on page* *1020*
OptiPranolol® [US/Can] *see* metipranolol *on page* *649*

Optiray® [US] *see* ioversol *on page 542*
Optivar® [US] *see* azelastine *on page 115*
Optive™ [US-OTC] *see* carboxymethylcellulose *on page 186*
Optivite® P.M.T. [US-OTC] *see* vitamins (multiple/oral) *on page 1019*
Orabase® with Benzocaine [US-OTC] *see* benzocaine *on page 129*
Oracea™ [US] *see* doxycycline *on page 336*
Oracort [Can] *see* triamcinolone (systemic) *on page 982*
Oradex-C® ***(Discontinued)*** *see* dyclonine *on page 343*
Orajel® Baby Daytime and Nighttime [US-OTC] *see* benzocaine *on page 129*
Orajel® Baby Teething [US-OTC] *see* benzocaine *on page 129*
Orajel® Baby Teething Nighttime [US-OTC] *see* benzocaine *on page 129*
Orajel® Brace-Aid Oral Anesthetic ***(Discontinued)*** *see* benzocaine *on page 129*
Orajel® Denture Plus [US-OTC] *see* benzocaine *on page 129*
Orajel® Maximum Strength [US-OTC] *see* benzocaine *on page 129*
Orajel® Medicated Toothache [US-OTC] *see* benzocaine *on page 129*
Orajel® Mouth Sore [US-OTC] *see* benzocaine *on page 129*
Orajel® Multi-Action Cold Sore [US-OTC] *see* benzocaine *on page 129*
Orajel® Perioseptic® Spot Treatment [US-OTC] *see* carbamide peroxide *on page 181*
Orajel PM® Maximum Strength [US-OTC] *see* benzocaine *on page 129*
Orajel® Ultra Mouth Sore [US-OTC] *see* benzocaine *on page 129*
Oral Balance® [US-OTC] *see* saliva substitute *on page 887*
Oramorph® SR [US] *see* morphine sulfate *on page 667*
Oranyl [US-OTC] *see* pseudoephedrine *on page 833*
Orap® [US/Can] *see* pimozide *on page 784*
Orapred® [US] *see* prednisolone (systemic) *on page 813*
Oraquix® [US] *see* lidocaine and prilocaine *on page 588*
Orasone® ***(Discontinued)*** *see* prednisone *on page 814*
OraVerse™ [US] *see* phentolamine *on page 774*
Oraxyl™ [US] *see* doxycycline *on page 336*
Orazinc® [US-OTC] *see* zinc sulfate *on page 1031*
orciprenaline sulfate *see* metaproterenol *on page 632*
Orencia® [US/Can] *see* abatacept *on page 16*
Oreton® Methyl ***(Discontinued)*** *see* methyltestosterone *on page 648*
Orfadin® [US] *see* nitisinone *on page 699*
ORG 946 *see* rocuronium *on page 875*
Orgalutran® [Can] *see* ganirelix *on page 455*
Organidin® NR [US] *see* guaifenesin *on page 473*
Orgaran® [Can] *see* danaparoid *(Canada only) on page 275*
Orgaran® ***(Discontinued)*** *see* danaparoid *(Canada only) on page 275*
ORG NC 45 *see* vecuronium *on page 1008*
Orinase Diagnostic® ***(Discontinued)*** *see* tolbutamide *on page 967*
Orinase® Oral ***(Discontinued)*** *see* tolbutamide *on page 967*
ORLAAM® ***(Discontinued)***

orlistat (OR li stat)

Sound-Alike/Look-Alike Issues
Xenical® may be confused with Xeloda®

U.S./Canadian Brand Names Alli™ [US-OTC]; Xenical® [US/Can]

Therapeutic Category Lipase Inhibitor

Use Management of obesity, including weight loss and weight management, when used in conjunction with a reduced-calorie and low-fat diet; reduce the risk of weight regain after prior weight loss; indicated for obese patients with an initial body mass index (BMI) ≥30 kg/m^2 or ≥27 kg/m^2 in the presence of other risk factors (eg, diabetes, dyslipidemia, hypertension)

Usual Dosage Oral:
Children ≥12 years and Adults (Xenical®): 120 mg 3 times/day with each main meal containing fat (during or up to 1 hour after the meal); omit dose if meal is occasionally missed or contains no fat.
Adults (Alli™): OTC labeling: 60 mg 3 times/day with each main meal containing fat

Dosage Forms
Capsule:
Alli™ [OTC]: 60 mg
Xenical®: 120 mg

Ormazine® ***(Discontinued)*** *see* chlorpromazine *on page* 222
Ornex® [US-OTC] *see* acetaminophen and pseudoephedrine *on page* 24
Ornex® Maximum Strength [US-OTC] *see* acetaminophen and pseudoephedrine *on page* 24
Ornidyl® Injection ***(Discontinued)*** *see* eflornithine *on page* 349
ORO-Clense [Can] *see* chlorhexidine gluconate *on page* 210
Orphenace® [Can] *see* orphenadrine *on page* 730

orphenadrine (or FEN a dreen)

Sound-Alike/Look-Alike Issues
Norflex™ may be confused with norfloxacin, Noroxin®

Synonyms orphenadrine citrate

U.S./Canadian Brand Names Norflex™ [US/Can]; Orphenace® [Can]; Rhoxal-orphendrine [Can]

Therapeutic Category Skeletal Muscle Relaxant

Use Treatment of muscle spasm associated with acute painful musculoskeletal conditions

Usual Dosage Adults:
Oral: 100 mg twice daily
I.M., I.V.: 60 mg every 12 hours

Dosage Forms
Injection, solution: 30 mg/mL (2 mL)
Norflex™: 30 mg/mL (2 mL)
Tablet, extended release: 100 mg

orphenadrine, aspirin, and caffeine (or FEN a dreen, AS pir in, & KAF een)

Sound-Alike/Look-Alike Issues
Norgesic™ Forte may be confused with Norgesic 40®

Synonyms aspirin, caffeine, and orphenadrine; aspirin, orphenadrine, and caffeine; caffeine, orphenadrine, and aspirin

Therapeutic Category Analgesic, Nonnarcotic; Skeletal Muscle Relaxant

Use Relief of discomfort associated with skeletal muscular conditions

Usual Dosage Oral: 1-2 tablets 3-4 times/day

Dosage Forms
Tablet: Orphenadrine 25 mg, aspirin 385 mg, and caffeine 30 mg; orphenadrine 50 mg, aspirin 770 mg, and caffeine 60 mg

orphenadrine citrate *see* orphenadrine *on page* 730
Orphengesic ***(Discontinued)*** *see* orphenadrine, aspirin, and caffeine *on page* 730
Orphengesic Forte ***(Discontinued)*** *see* orphenadrine, aspirin, and caffeine *on page* 730
Ortho® 0.5/35 [Can] *see* ethinyl estradiol and norethindrone *on page* 390
Ortho® 1/35 [Can] *see* ethinyl estradiol and norethindrone *on page* 390
Ortho® 7/7/7 [Can] *see* ethinyl estradiol and norethindrone *on page* 390
Ortho-Cept® [US/Can] *see* ethinyl estradiol and desogestrel *on page* 383
Orthoclone OKT® 3 [US/Can] *see* muromonab-CD3 *on page* 673
Ortho-Cyclen® [US] *see* ethinyl estradiol and norgestimate *on page* 393
Ortho-Est® [US] *see* estropipate *on page* 381
Ortho Evra® [US] *see* ethinyl estradiol and norelgestromin *on page* 389
Ortho Micronor® [US] *see* norethindrone *on page* 704
Ortho-Novum® [US] *see* ethinyl estradiol and norethindrone *on page* 390
Ortho-Novum® 1/50 [Can] *see* norethindrone and mestranol *on page* 704
Ortho-Novum® 1/50 ***(Discontinued)*** *see* norethindrone and mestranol *on page* 704

oseltamivir (oh sel TAM i vir)

Sound-Alike/Look-Alike Issues

Tamiflu® may be confused with Thera-Flu®

U.S./Canadian Brand Names Tamiflu® [US/Can]

Therapeutic Category Antiviral Agent, Oral

Use Treatment of uncomplicated acute illness due to influenza (A or B) infection in children ≥1 year of age and adults who have been symptomatic for no more than 2 days; prophylaxis against influenza (A or B) infection in children ≥1 year of age and adults

The Advisory Committee on Immunization Practices (ACIP) recommends that **treatment** be considered for the following:

- Persons hospitalized with laboratory confirmed influenza (may also have benefit if started >48 hours after onset of illness).
- Persons with laboratory confirmed influenza pneumonia.
- Persons with laboratory confirmed influenza and bacterial infections.
- Persons with laboratory confirmed influenza and who are at higher risk for influenza complications.
- Persons presenting for care within 48 hours of laboratory confirmed influenza onset and who want to decrease duration and/or severity of their symptoms or decrease the risk of transmission to those at high risk for complications.

The ACIP recommends that **prophylaxis** be considered for the following:

- Persons at high risk for influenza infection during the first 2 weeks following vaccination (eg, children <9 years and not previously vaccinated) if the virus is circulating in the community.
- Persons at high risk for influenza infection, but the vaccination is contraindicated.
- Unvaccinated family members or healthcare providers with prolonged exposure to or close contact with high-risk persons, unvaccinated persons, or infants <6 months of age.
- Persons at high risk for influenza infection, their family members and close contacts, and healthcare workers when the circulating strain of influenza is not matched with the vaccine.
- Persons with immune deficiency or those who may not respond to vaccination.
- Unvaccinated staff and persons during response to an outbreak in a closed institutional setting that has patients at high risk for infection (eg, extended care facilities).

Usual Dosage Oral:

Treatment: Initiate treatment within 2 days of onset of symptoms; duration of treatment: 5 days:
 Children <1 year (interim recommendations for treatment of swine influenza):
  <3 months: 12 mg twice daily
  3-5 months: 20 mg twice daily
  6-11 months: 25 mg twice daily
 Children: 1-12 years:
  ≤15 kg: 30 mg twice daily
  >15 kg to ≤23 kg: 45 mg twice daily
  >23 kg to ≤40 kg: 60 mg twice daily
  >40 kg: 75 mg twice daily
 Adolescents ≥13 years and Adults: 75 mg twice daily
Prophylaxis: Initiate treatment within 2 days of contact with an infected individual; duration of treatment: 10 days

Children <1 year (interim recommendations for chemoprophylaxis of swine influenza):
- <3 months: Not recommended unless clinically critical
- 3-5 months: 20 mg once daily
- 6-11 months: 25 mg once daily

Children: 1-12 years:
- ≤15 kg: 30 mg once daily
- >15 kg to ≤23 kg: 45 mg once daily
- >23 kg to ≤40 kg: 60 mg once daily
- >40 kg: 75 mg once daily

Adolescents ≥13 years and Adults: 75 mg once daily. During community outbreaks, dosing is 75 mg once daily. May be used for up to 6 weeks; duration of protection lasts for length of dosing period

Dosage Forms

Capsule:
Tamiflu®: 30 mg, 45 mg, 75 mg

Powder for oral suspension:
Tamiflu®: 12 mg/mL

OSI-774 *see* erlotinib *on page* 367
Osmitrol® [US/Can] *see* mannitol *on page* 613
Osmoglyn® ***(Discontinued)*** *see* glycerin *on page* 468
Osmolite® HN [US-OTC] *see* nutritional formula, enteral/oral *on page* 715
OsmoPrep® [US] *see* sodium phosphates *on page* 912
Osmovist® [Can] *see* iotrolan *(Canada only) on page* 542
Osteocalcin® ***(Discontinued)*** *see* calcitonin *on page* 167
Osteocit® [Can] *see* calcium citrate *on page* 172
Ostoforte® [Can] *see* ergocalciferol *on page* 364
OTFC (oral transmucosal fentanyl citrate) *see* fentanyl *on page* 410
Otic-Care® Otic ***(Discontinued)*** *see* neomycin, polymyxin B, and hydrocortisone *on page* 688
Otix® [US-OTC] *see* carbamide peroxide *on page* 181
Otobiotic Otic Solution ***(Discontinued)***
Otocort® Otic ***(Discontinued)*** *see* neomycin, polymyxin B, and hydrocortisone *on page* 688
Otosporin® Otic ***(Discontinued)*** *see* neomycin, polymyxin B, and hydrocortisone *on page* 688
Otrivin® ***(Discontinued)***
Otrivin® Pediatric ***(Discontinued)***
Outgro® [US-OTC] *see* benzocaine *on page* 129
Ovace® [US] *see* sulfacetamide *on page* 927
Ovace® Plus [US] *see* sulfacetamide *on page* 927
Ovcon® [US] *see* ethinyl estradiol and norethindrone *on page* 390
Ovide® [US] *see* malathion *on page* 612
Ovidrel® [US/Can] *see* chorionic gonadotropin (recombinant) *on page* 225
ovine corticotrophin-releasing hormone *see* corticorelin *on page* 258
Ovol® [Can] *see* simethicone *on page* 901
Ovral® [Can] *see* ethinyl estradiol and norgestrel *on page* 394
Ovral® ***(Discontinued)*** *see* ethinyl estradiol and norgestrel *on page* 394
Ovrette® ***(Discontinued)***

oxacillin (oks a SIL in)

Synonyms methylphenyl isoxazolyl penicillin; oxacillin sodium

Therapeutic Category Penicillin

Use Treatment of infections such as osteomyelitis, septicemia, endocarditis, and CNS infections caused by susceptible strains of *Staphylococcus*

Usual Dosage

Usual dosage range:
Infants and Children: I.M., I.V.: 100-200 mg/kg/day in divided doses every 6 hours (maximum: 12 g/day)
Adults: I.M., I.V.: 250-2000 mg every 4-6 hours

Indication-specific dosing:

Children:

Arthritis (septic): I.V.: 37 mg/kg every 6 hours

Epiglottitis: I.V.: 150-200 mg/kg/day divided every 6 hours

Mild-to-moderate infections: I.M., I.V.: 100-150 mg/kg/day in divided doses every 6 hours (maximum: 4 g/day)

Severe infections: I.M., I.V.: 150-200 mg/kg/day in divided doses every 6 hours (maximum: 12 g/day)

Staphylococcal scalded-skin syndrome: I.V.: 150 mg/kg/day divided every 6 hours for 5-7 days

Adults:

Endocarditis: I.V.: 2 g every 4 hours with gentamicin

Mild-to-moderate infections: I.M., I.V.: 250-500 mg every 4-6 hours

Prosthetic joint infection: I.V.: 2 g every 4 hours with rifampin

Severe infections: I.M., I.V.: 1-2 g every 4-6 hours

***Staphylococcus aureus,* methicillin-susceptible infections, including brain abscess, bursitis, erysipelas, mastitis, mastoiditis, osteomyelitis, perinephric abscess, pneumonia, pyomyositis, scalded skin syndrome, toxic shock syndrome:** I.V.: 2 g every 4 hours

Dosage Forms

Infusion [premixed iso-osmotic dextrose solution]: 1 g (50 mL); 2 g (50 mL)

Injection, powder for reconstitution: 1 g, 2 g, 10 g

oxacillin sodium *see* oxacillin *on page 732*

oxalatoplatin *see* oxaliplatin *on page 733*

oxalatoplatinum *see* oxaliplatin *on page 733*

oxaliplatin (ox AL i pla tin)

Sound-Alike/Look-Alike Issues

oxaliplatin may be confused with Aloxi®, carboplatin, cisplatin

Synonyms diaminocyclohexane oxalatoplatinum; L-OHP; oxalatoplatin; oxalatoplatinum

U.S./Canadian Brand Names Eloxatin® [US/Can]

Therapeutic Category Antineoplastic Agent, Alkylating Agent

Use Treatment of stage III colon cancer (adjuvant) and advanced colorectal cancer

Usual Dosage Details concerning dosing in combination regimens should also be consulted. Delay dosage in subsequent cycles until recovery of neutrophils ≥1.5 x 10^9/L and platelets ≥75 x 10^9/L. I.V.:

Adults:

Advanced colorectal cancer: 85 mg/m^2 every 2 weeks until disease progression or unacceptable toxicity (in combination with fluorouracil/leucovorin)

Stage III colon cancer (adjuvant): 85 mg/m^2 every 2 weeks for 12 cycles (in combination with fluorouracil/leucovorin)

Dosage Forms [CAN] = Canadian availability; not available in U.S.

Injection, solution [preservative free; concentrate]: 5 mg/mL (10 mL, 20 mL)

Eloxatin®: 5 mg/mL (10 mL, 20 mL, 40 mL)

Injection, powder for reconstitution [preservative free]:

Eloxatin® [CAN]: 50 mg, 100 mg [not available in U.S.]

Oxandrin® [US] *see* oxandrolone *on page 733*

oxandrolone (oks AN droe lone)

U.S./Canadian Brand Names Oxandrin® [US]

Therapeutic Category Androgen

Controlled Substance C-III

Use Adjunctive therapy to promote weight gain after weight loss following extensive surgery, chronic infections, or severe trauma, and in some patients who, without definite pathophysiologic reasons, fail to gain or to maintain normal weight; to offset protein catabolism with prolonged corticosteroid administration; relief of bone pain associated with osteoporosis

Usual Dosage

Children: Total daily dose: ≤0.1 mg/kg **or** ≤0.045 mg/lb

Adults: 2.5-20 mg in divided doses 2-4 times/day based on individual response; a course of therapy of 2-4 weeks is usually adequate. This may be repeated intermittently as needed.

Dosage Forms

Tablet: 2.5 mg, 10 mg

Oxandrin®: 2.5 mg, 10 mg

oxaprozin (oks a PROE zin)

Sound-Alike/Look-Alike Issues

oxaprozin may be confused with oxazepam
Daypro® may be confused with Diupres®

U.S./Canadian Brand Names Apo-Oxaprozin® [Can]; Daypro® [US/Can]

Therapeutic Category Analgesic, Nonnarcotic; Nonsteroidal Antiinflammatory Drug (NSAID)

Use Acute and long-term use in the management of signs and symptoms of osteoarthritis and rheumatoid arthritis; juvenile rheumatoid arthritis

Usual Dosage Oral (individualize dosage to lowest effective dose to minimize adverse effects):

Children 6-16 years: Juvenile rheumatoid arthritis:
- 22-31 kg: 600 mg once daily
- 32-54 kg: 900 mg once daily
- ≥55 kg: 1200 mg once daily

Adults:
- Osteoarthritis: 600-1200 mg once daily; patients should be titrated to lowest dose possible; patients with low body weight should start with 600 mg daily
- Rheumatoid arthritis: 1200 mg once daily; a one-time loading dose of up to 1800 mg/day or 26 mg/kg (whichever is lower) may be given
- Maximum doses:
  - Patient <50 kg: Maximum: 1200 mg/day
  - Patient >50 kg with normal renal/hepatic function and low risk of peptic ulcer: Maximum: 1800 mg or 26 mg/kg (whichever is lower) in divided doses

Dosage Forms

Tablet: 600 mg
Daypro®: 600 mg

oxazepam (oks A ze pam)

Sound-Alike/Look-Alike Issues

oxazepam may be confused with oxaprozin, quazepam
Serax® may be confused with Eurax®, Urex®, Zyrtec®

U.S./Canadian Brand Names Apo-Oxazepam® [Can]; Bio-Oxazepam [Can]; Novoxapram® [Can]; Oxpam® [Can]; Oxpram® [Can]; PMS-Oxazepam [Can]; Riva-Oxazepam [Can]; Serax® [US]

Therapeutic Category Anticonvulsant; Benzodiazepine

Controlled Substance C-IV

Use Treatment of anxiety; management of ethanol withdrawal

Usual Dosage Oral: Adults:

Anxiety: 10-30 mg 3-4 times/day
Ethanol withdrawal: 15-30 mg 3-4 times/day
Hypnotic: 15-30 mg

Dosage Forms

Capsule: 10 mg, 15 mg, 30 mg
Serax®: 10 mg, 15 mg, 30 mg

Tablet:
Serax®: 15 mg

oxcarbazepine (ox car BAZ e peen)

Sound-Alike/Look-Alike Issues

OXcarbazepine may be confused with carBAMazepine
Trileptal® may be confused with TriLipix™

Synonyms GP 47680; OCBZ

Tall-Man OXcarbazepine

U.S./Canadian Brand Names Trileptal® [US/Can]

Therapeutic Category Anticonvulsant

Use Monotherapy or adjunctive therapy in the treatment of partial seizures in adults and children ≥4 years of age with epilepsy; adjunctive therapy in the treatment of partial seizures in children ≥2 years of age with epilepsy

Usual Dosage Oral:

Children 2-3 years:

Adjunctive therapy: 8-10 mg/kg/day, not to exceed 600 mg/day, given in 2 divided daily doses. Maintenance dose should be achieved over 2 weeks, and is dependent upon patient weight.

<20 kg: Consider initiating dose at 16-20 mg/kg/day; maximum maintenance dose should be achieved over 2-4 weeks and should not exceed 60 mg/kg/day

Children 4-16 years:

Adjunctive therapy: 8-10 mg/kg/day, not to exceed 600 mg/day, given in 2 divided daily doses. Maintenance dose should be achieved over 2 weeks, and is dependent upon patient weight, according to the following:

20-29 kg: 900 mg/day in 2 divided doses

29.1-39 kg: 1200 mg/day in 2 divided doses

>39 kg: 1800 mg/day in 2 divided doses

Children 4-16 years:

Conversion to monotherapy: Oxcarbazepine 8-10 mg/kg/day in twice daily divided doses, while simultaneously initiating the reduction of the dose of the concomitant antiepileptic drug; the concomitant drug should be withdrawn over 3-6 weeks. Oxcarbazepine dose may be increased by a maximum of 10 mg/kg/day at weekly intervals. See below for recommended total daily dose by weight.

Initiation of monotherapy: Oxcarbazepine should be initiated at 8-10 mg/kg/day in twice daily divided doses; doses may be titrated by 5 mg/kg/day every third day. See below for recommended total daily dose by weight.

Range of maintenance doses by weight during monotherapy:

20 kg: 600-900 mg/day

25-30 kg: 900-1200 mg/day

35-40 kg: 900-1500 mg/day

45 kg: 1200-1500 mg/day

50-55 kg: 1200-1800 mg/day

60-65 kg: 1200-2100 mg/day

70 kg: 1500-2100 mg/day

Adults:

Adjunctive therapy: Initial: 300 mg twice daily; dose may be increased by as much as 600 mg/day at weekly intervals; recommended daily dose: 1200 mg/day in 2 divided doses. Although daily doses >1200 mg/day were somewhat more efficacious, most patients were unable to tolerate 2400 mg/day (due to CNS effects).

Conversion to monotherapy: Oxcarbazepine 600 mg/day in twice daily divided doses while simultaneously initiating the reduction of the dose of the concomitant antiepileptic drug. The concomitant dosage should be withdrawn over 3-6 weeks, while the maximum dose of oxcarbazepine should be reached in about 2-4 weeks. Recommended daily dose: 2400 mg/day.

Initiation of monotherapy: Oxcarbazepine should be initiated at a dose of 600 mg/day in twice daily divided doses; doses may be titrated upward by 300 mg/day every third day to a final dose of 1200 mg/day given in 2 daily divided doses

Dosage Forms

Suspension, oral:

Trileptal®: 300 mg/5 mL

Tablet: 150 mg, 300 mg, 600 mg

Trileptal®: 150 mg, 300 mg, 600 mg

Oxeze® Turbuhaler® [Can] *see* formoterol *on page* 443

oxiconazole (oks i KON a zole)

Synonyms oxiconazole nitrate

U.S./Canadian Brand Names Oxistat® [US/Can]

Therapeutic Category Antifungal Agent

Use Treatment of tinea pedis (athlete's foot), tinea cruris (jock itch), tinea corporis (ringworm), and tinea (pityriasis) versicolor

Usual Dosage Topical: Children and Adults:

Tinea corporis/tinea cruris: Cream, lotion: Apply to affected areas 1-2 times daily for 2 weeks

Tinea pedis: Cream, lotion: Apply to affected areas 1-2 times daily for 1 month

Tinea versicolor: Cream: Apply to affected areas once daily for 2 weeks

Dosage Forms
Cream:
Oxistat®: 1% (15 g, 30 g, 60 g)
Lotion:
Oxistat®: 1% (30 mL)

oxiconazole nitrate *see* oxiconazole *on page* 735
oxidized regenerated cellulose *see* cellulose, oxidized regenerated *on page* 201
Oxilan® [US] *see* ioxilan *on page* 543
Oxilan® 300 [Can] *see* ioxilan *on page* 543
Oxilan® 350 [Can] *see* ioxilan *on page* 543
oxilapine succinate *see* loxapine *on page* 603
Oxipor® VHC [US-OTC] *see* coal tar *on page* 250
Oxistat® [US/Can] *see* oxiconazole *on page* 735
Oxpam® [Can] *see* oxazepam *on page* 734
oxpentifylline *see* pentoxifylline *on page* 766
Oxpram® [Can] *see* oxazepam *on page* 734

oxprenolol *(Canada only)* (ox PREN oh lole)

Synonyms oxprenolol hydrochloride
U.S./Canadian Brand Names Trasicor® [Can]
Therapeutic Category Beta-Adrenergic Blocker
Use Treatment of mild-or-moderate hypertension
Usual Dosage Oral: Adults:
Initial: 20 mg 3 times/day (regular-release formulation); increase by 60 mg/day (in 3 divided doses) at 1- to 2-week intervals until adequate control is obtained
Maintenance: 120-320 mg/day; do not exceed 480 mg
Dosage Forms [CAN] = Canadian brand name
Tablet:
Trasicor® [CAN]: 40 mg, 80 mg [not available in the U.S.]

oxprenolol hydrochloride *see* oxprenolol *(Canada only) on page* 736
Oxsoralen® [US/Can] *see* methoxsalen *on page* 641
Oxsoralen-Ultra® [US/Can] *see* methoxsalen *on page* 641
Oxy-5® ***(Discontinued)*** *see* benzoyl peroxide *on page* 132

oxybutynin (oks i BYOO ti nin)

Sound-Alike/Look-Alike Issues
oxybutynin may be confused with OxyContin®
Ditropan® may be confused with Detrol®, diazepam, Diprivan®, dithranol
Synonyms oxybutynin chloride
U.S./Canadian Brand Names Apo-Oxybutynin® [Can]; Ditropan XL® [US/Can]; Ditropan® [US/Can]; Gelnique™ [US]; Gen-Oxybutynin [Can]; Novo-Oxybutynin [Can]; Nu-Oxybutyn [Can]; Oxytrol® [US/Can]; PMS-Oxybutynin [Can]; Riva-Oxybutynin [Can]; Uromax® [Can]
Therapeutic Category Antispasmodic Agent, Urinary
Use Antispasmodic for neurogenic bladder (urgency, frequency, leakage, urge incontinence, dysuria); extended release formulation also indicated for treatment of symptoms associated with detrusor overactivity due to a neurological condition (eg, spina bifida)
Usual Dosage
Oral:
Children:
>5 years: 5 mg twice daily, up to 5 mg 3 times/day maximum
>6 years: Extended release: 5 mg once daily; adjust dose in 5 mg increments; maximum dose: 20 mg/day
Adults: 5 mg 2-3 times/day up to 5 mg 4 times/day maximum
Extended release: Initial: 5-10 mg once daily, adjust dose in 5 mg increments at weekly intervals; maximum: 30 mg daily
Topical gel: Adults: Apply contents of 1 sachet (100 mg/g) once daily
Transdermal: Adults: Apply one 3.9 mg/day patch twice weekly (every 3-4 days)

Note: Should be discontinued periodically to determine whether the patient can manage without the drug and to minimize resistance to the drug

Dosage Forms

Gel, topical:

Gelnique™: 10% (1 g)

Syrup: 5 mg/5 mL

Tablet: 5 mg

Ditropan®: 5 mg

Tablet, extended release: 5 mg, 10 mg, 15 mg

Ditropan XL®: 5 mg, 10 mg, 15 mg

Transdermal system:

Oxytrol®: 3.9 mg/day (8s)

oxybutynin chloride *see* oxybutynin *on page* *736*

oxychlorosene (oks i KLOR oh seen)

Synonyms oxychlorosene sodium

U.S./Canadian Brand Names Clorpactin® WCS-90 [US-OTC]

Therapeutic Category Antibiotic, Topical

Use Treatment of localized infections

Usual Dosage Topical (0.1% to 0.5% solutions): Apply by irrigation, instillation, spray, soaks, or wet compresses

Dosage Forms

Powder for solution:

Clorpactin® WCS-90 [OTC]: 2 g

oxychlorosene sodium *see* oxychlorosene *on page* *737*

Oxycocet® [Can] *see* oxycodone and acetaminophen *on page* *738*

Oxycodan® [Can] *see* oxycodone and aspirin *on page* *739*

oxycodone (oks i KOE done)

Sound-Alike/Look-Alike Issues

oxyCODONE may be confused with HYDROcodone, OxyContin®, oxymorphone

OxyContin® may be confused with MS Contin®, oxybutynin, oxycodone

Roxicodone® may be confused with Roxanol™

Synonyms dihydrohydroxycodeinone; oxycodone hydrochloride

Tall-Man oxy**CODONE**

U.S./Canadian Brand Names Oxy.IR® [Can]; OxyContin® [US/Can]; OxyIR® [US]; PMS-Oxycodone [Can]; Roxicodone® [US]; Supeudol® [Can]

Therapeutic Category Analgesic, Narcotic

Controlled Substance C-II

Use Management of moderate-to-severe pain, normally used in combination with nonopioid analgesics

OxyContin® is indicated for around-the-clock management of moderate-to-severe pain when an analgesic is needed for an extended period of time.

Usual Dosage Oral:

Children: Immediate release:

6-12 years: 1.25 mg every 6 hours as needed

>12 years: 2.5 mg every 6 hours as needed

Adults:

Immediate release: 5 mg every 6 hours as needed

Controlled release:

Opioid naive: 10 mg every 12 hours

Concurrent CNS depressants: Reduce usual dose by 1/3 to 1/2

Conversion from transdermal fentanyl: For each 25 mcg/hour transdermal dose, substitute 10 mg controlled release oxycodone every 12 hours; should be initiated 18 hours after the removal of the transdermal fentanyl patch

Currently on opioids: Use standard conversion chart to convert daily dose to oxycodone equivalent. Divide daily dose in 2 (for twice-daily dosing, usually every 12 hours) and round down to nearest dosage form.

Note: 60 mg, 80 mg, or 160 mg tablets are for use **only** in opioid-tolerant patients. Special safety considerations must be addressed when converting to OxyContin® doses ≥160 mg every 12 hours. Dietary caution must be taken when patients are initially titrated to 160 mg tablets. Using different strengths to obtain the same daily dose is equivalent (eg, four 40 mg tablets, two 80 mg tablets, one 160 mg tablet); all produce similar blood levels.

Multiplication factors for converting the daily dose of current oral opioid to the daily dose of oral oxycodone:

Current opioid mg/day dose x factor = Oxycodone mg/day dose

Codeine mg/day oral dose **x** 0.15 = Oxycodone mg/day dose
Hydrocodone mg/day oral dose **x** 0.9 = Oxycodone mg/day dose
Hydromorphone mg/day oral dose **x** 4 = Oxycodone mg/day dose
Levorphanol mg/day oral dose **x** 7.5 = Oxycodone mg/day dose
Meperidine mg/day oral dose **x** 0.1 = Oxycodone mg/day dose
Methadone mg/day oral dose **x** 1.5 = Oxycodone mg/day dose
Morphine mg/day oral dose **x** 0.5 = Oxycodone mg/day dose

Note: Divide the oxycodone mg/day dose into the appropriate dosing interval for the specific form being used.

Dosage Forms

Capsule, immediate release: 5 mg
OxyIR®: 5 mg
Liquid, oral, as hydrochloride [concentrate]:
Roxicodone®: 20 mg/mL (30 mL)
Solution, oral: 5 mg/5 mL
Roxicodone®: 5 mg/5 mL
Tablet: 5 mg, 10 mg, 15 mg, 20 mg, 30 mg
Roxicodone®: 5 mg, 15 mg, 30 mg
Tablet, controlled release:
OxyContin®: 10 mg, 15 mg, 20 mg, 30 mg, 40 mg, 60 mg, 80 mg
Tablet, extended release: 10 mg, 20 mg, 40 mg

oxycodone and acetaminophen (oks i KOE done & a seet a MIN oh fen)

Sound-Alike/Look-Alike Issues

Endocet® may be confused with Indocid®
Percocet® may be confused with Darvocet®, Fioricet®, Percodan®
Roxicet™ may be confused with Roxanol™
Tylox® may be confused with Trimox®, Tylenol®, Wymox®, Xanax®

Synonyms acetaminophen and oxycodone

U.S./Canadian Brand Names Endocet® [US/Can]; Magnacet™ [US]; Novo-Oxycodone Acet [Can]; Oxycocet® [Can]; Percocet® [US/Can]; Percocet®-Demi [Can]; PMS-Oxycodone-Acetaminophen [Can]; Primalev™ [US]; Roxicet™ 5/500 [US]; Roxicet™ [US]; Tylox® [US]

Therapeutic Category Analgesic, Narcotic

Controlled Substance C-II

Use Management of moderate-to-severe pain

Usual Dosage Oral: Doses should be given every 4-6 hours as needed and titrated to appropriate analgesic effects. **Note:** Initial dose is based on the **oxycodone** content; however, the maximum daily dose is based on the **acetaminophen** content.

Children: Maximum acetaminophen dose: Children <45 kg: 90 mg/kg/day; children >45 kg: 4 g/day
Mild-to-moderate pain: Initial dose, **based on oxycodone content:** 0.05-0.1 mg/kg/dose
Severe pain: Initial dose, **based on oxycodone content:** 0.3 mg/kg/dose
Adults:
Mild-to-moderate pain: Initial dose, **based on oxycodone content:** 2.5-5 mg
Severe pain: Initial dose, **based on oxycodone content:** 10-30 mg. Do not exceed acetaminophen 4 g/day.

Dosage Forms

Caplet: Oxycodone 5 mg and acetaminophen 500 mg
Roxicet™ 5/500: Oxycodone 5 mg and acetaminophen 500 mg
Capsule: Oxycodone 5 mg and acetaminophen 500 mg
Tylox®: Oxycodone 5 mg and acetaminophen 500 mg
Solution, oral: Oxycodone 5 mg and acetaminophen 325 mg per 5 mL
Roxicet™: Oxycodone 5 mg and acetaminophen 325 mg per 5 mL

Tablet:

Generics:

Oxycodone 2.5 mg and acetaminophen 325 mg
Oxycodone 5 mg and acetaminophen 325 mg
Oxycodone 7.5 mg and acetaminophen 325 mg
Oxycodone 7.5 mg and acetaminophen 500 mg
Oxycodone 10 mg and acetaminophen 325 mg
Oxycodone 10 mg and acetaminophen 650 mg

Brands:

Endocet®:
5/325 [scored]: Oxycodone 5 mg and acetaminophen 325 mg
7.5/325: Oxycodone 7.5 mg and acetaminophen 325 mg
7.5/500: Oxycodone 7.5 mg and acetaminophen 500 mg
10/325: Oxycodone 10 mg and acetaminophen 325 mg
10/650: Oxycodone 10 mg and acetaminophen 650 mg

Magnacet™
2.5/400: Oxycodone 2.5 mg and acetaminophen 400 mg
5/400: Oxycodone 5 mg and acetaminophen 400 mg
7.5/400: Oxycodone 7.5 mg and acetaminophen 400 mg
10/400: Oxycodone 10 mg and acetaminophen 400 mg

Percocet®:
2.5/325: Oxycodone 2.5 mg and acetaminophen 325 mg
5/325 [scored]: Oxycodone 5 mg and acetaminophen 325 mg
7.5/325: Oxycodone 7.5 mg and acetaminophen 325 mg
7.5/500: Oxycodone 7.5 mg and acetaminophen 500 mg
10/325: Oxycodone 10 mg and acetaminophen 325 mg
10/650: Oxycodone 10 mg and acetaminophen 650 mg

Primalev™:
2.5/300: Oxycodone 2.5 mg and acetaminophen 300 mg
5/300: Oxycodone 5 mg and acetaminophen 300 mg
7.5/300: Oxycodone 7.5 mg and acetaminophen 300 mg
10/300: Oxycodone 10 mg and acetaminophen 300 mg

Roxicet™ [scored]: Oxycodone 5 mg and acetaminophen 325 mg

oxycodone and aspirin (oks i KOE done & AS pir in)

Sound-Alike/Look-Alike Issues
Percodan® may be confused with Decadron®, Percocet®, Percogesic®, Periactin®

Synonyms aspirin and oxycodone

U.S./Canadian Brand Names Endodan® [US/Can]; Oxycodan® [Can]; Percodan® [US/Can]

Therapeutic Category Analgesic, Narcotic

Controlled Substance C-II

Use Management of moderate-to-severe pain

Usual Dosage Oral (based on oxycodone combined salts):

Children: Maximum oxycodone: 5 mg/dose; maximum aspirin dose should not exceed 4 g/day. Doses should be given every 6 hours as needed.
Mild-to-moderate pain: Initial dose, **based on oxycodone content:** 0.05-0.1 mg/kg/dose
Severe pain: Initial dose, **based on oxycodone content**: 0.3 mg/kg/dose

Adults: Percodan®: 1 tablet every 6 hours as needed for pain; maximum aspirin dose should not exceed 4 g/day.

Dosage Forms

Tablet: Oxycodone hydrochloride 4.5 mg, oxycodone terephthalate 0.38 mg, and aspirin 325 mg
Endodan®, Percodan®: Oxycodone hydrochloride 4.8355 mg and aspirin 325 mg

oxycodone and ibuprofen (oks i KOE done & eye byoo PROE fen)

Synonyms ibuprofen and oxycodone

U.S./Canadian Brand Names Combunox™ [US]

Therapeutic Category Analgesic, Opioid; Nonsteroidal Antiinflammatory Drug (NSAID), Oral

Controlled Substance C-II

Use Short-term (≤7 days) management of acute, moderate-to-severe pain

Usual Dosage Oral: Adults: Pain: Take 1 tablet every 6 hours as needed (maximum: 4 tablets/24 hours); do not take for longer than 7 days

Dosage Forms

Tablet: Oxycodone 5 mg and ibuprofen 400 mg

Combunox™: 5/400: Oxycodone 5 mg and ibuprofen 400 mg

oxycodone hydrochloride *see* oxycodone *on page* 737

OxyContin® [US/Can] *see* oxycodone *on page* 737

Oxyderm™ [Can] *see* benzoyl peroxide *on page* 132

Oxy.IR® [Can] *see* oxycodone *on page* 737

oxymetazoline (oks i met AZ oh leen)

Sound-Alike/Look-Alike Issues

oxymetazoline may be confused with oxymetholone

Afrin® may be confused with aspirin

Afrin® (oxymetazoline) may be confused with Afrin® (saline)

Neo-Synephrine® (oxymetazoline) may be confused with Neo-Synephrine® (phenylephrine)

Visine® may be confused with Visken®

Synonyms oxymetazoline hydrochloride

U.S./Canadian Brand Names 4-Way® 12 Hour [US-OTC]; Afrin® Extra Moisturizing [US-OTC]; Afrin® Original [US-OTC]; Afrin® Severe Congestion [US-OTC]; Afrin® Sinus [US-OTC]; Claritin® Allergic Decongestant [Can]; Dristan® Long Lasting Nasal [Can]; Dristan™ 12-Hour [US-OTC]; Drixoral® Nasal [Can]; Duramist® Plus [US-OTC]; Genasal [US-OTC]; Mucinex® Full force™ [US-OTC]; Mucinex® moisture smart™ [US-OTC]; Neo-Synephrine® 12 Hour Extra Moisturizing [US-OTC]; Neo-Synephrine® 12 Hour [US-OTC]; NRS® [US-OTC]; Nōstrilla® [US-OTC]; Vicks Sinex® 12 Hour Ultrafine Mist [US-OTC]; Vicks Sinex® 12 Hour [US-OTC]; Vicks® Early Defense™ [US-OTC]; Visine® L.R. [US-OTC]

Therapeutic Category Adrenergic Agonist Agent

Use Adjunctive therapy of middle ear infections, associated with acute or chronic rhinitis, the common cold, sinusitis, hay fever, or other allergies

Ophthalmic: Relief of redness of eye due to minor eye irritations

Usual Dosage

Intranasal (therapy should not exceed 3 days): Children ≥6 years and Adults: 0.05% solution: Instill 2-3 sprays into each nostril twice daily

Ophthalmic: Children ≥6 years and Adults: 0.025% solution: Instill 1-2 drops in affected eye(s) every 6 hours as needed or as directed by healthcare provider

Dosage Forms

Gel, intranasal [spray]:

Vicks® Early Defense™ [OTC]: 0.05% (14.7 mL)

Solution, intranasal [spray]: 0.05% (15 mL, 30 mL)

Afrin® Extra Moisturizing [OTC], Afrin® Severe Congestion [OTC], Afrin® Sinus [OTC], Dristan™ 12-Hour [OTC], Duramist® Plus [OTC], Neo-Synephrine® 12 Hour [OTC], Neo-Synephrine® 12 Hour Extra Moisturizing [OTC], Nōstrilla® [OTC], Vicks Sinex® 12 Hour Ultrafine Mist [OTC], Vicks Sinex® 12 Hour [OTC], 4-Way® 12 Hour [OTC]: 0.05% (15 mL)

Afrin® Original [OTC], Genasal [OTC], NRS® [OTC]: 0.05% (15 mL, 30 mL)

Mucinex® Full force™ [OTC], Mucinex® moisture smart™ [OTC]: 0.05% (22 mL)

Solution, ophthalmic:

Visine® L.R. [OTC]: 0.025% (15 mL, 30 mL)

oxymetazoline hydrochloride *see* oxymetazoline *on page* 740

oxymetholone (oks i METH oh lone)

Sound-Alike/Look-Alike Issues

oxymetholone may be confused with oxymetazoline, oxymorphone

U.S./Canadian Brand Names Anadrol®-50 [US]

Therapeutic Category Anabolic Steroid

Controlled Substance C-III

Use Treatment of anemias caused by deficient red cell production

Usual Dosage Oral: Children and Adults: Erythropoietic effects: 1-5 mg/kg/day in one daily dose; usual effective dose: 1-2 mg/kg/day; give for a minimum trial of 3-6 months because response may be delayed

Dosage Forms

Tablet:

Anadrol®-50: 50 mg

oxymorphone (oks i MOR fone)

Sound-Alike/Look-Alike Issues

oxymorphone may be confused with oxycodone, oxymetholone

Synonyms oxymorphone hydrochloride

U.S./Canadian Brand Names Opana® ER [US]; Opana® [US]

Therapeutic Category Analgesic, Narcotic

Controlled Substance C-II

Use

Parenteral: Management of moderate-to-severe pain

Oral, regular release: Management of moderate-to-severe pain

Oral, extended release: Management of moderate-to-severe pain in patients requiring around-the-clock opioid treatment for an extended period of time

Usual Dosage Adults: **Note:** Dosage must be individualized.

I.M., SubQ: Initial: 1-1.5 mg; may repeat every 4-6 hours as needed

Labor analgesia: I.M.: 0.5-1 mg

I.V.: Initial: 0.5 mg

Oral:

Immediate release:

Opioid-naive: 10-20 mg every 4-6 hours as needed. Initial dosages as low as 5 mg may be considered in selected patients and/or patients with renal impairment. Dosage adjustment should be based on level of analgesia, side effects, and pain intensity. Initiation of therapy with initial dose >20 mg is **not** recommended.

Currently on stable dose of parenteral oxymorphone: ~10 times the daily parenteral requirement. The calculated amount should be divided and given in 4-6 equal doses.

Currently on other opioids: Use standard conversion chart to convert daily dose to oxymorphone equivalent. Generally start with 1/2 the calculated daily oxymorphone dosage and administered in divided doses every 4-6 hours.

Extended release (Opana® ER):

Opioid-naive: Initial: 5 mg every 12 hours. Supplemental doses of immediate-release oxymorphone may be used as "rescue" medication as dosage is titrated.

Note: Continued requirement for supplemental dosing may be used to titrate the dose of extended-release continuous therapy. Adjust therapy incrementally, by 5-10 mg every 12 hours at intervals of every 3-7 days. Ideally, basal dosage may be titrated to generally mild pain or no pain with the regular use of fewer than 2 supplemental doses per 24 hours.

Currently on stable dose of parenteral oxymorphone: Approximately 10 times the daily parenteral requirement. The calculated amount should be given in 2 divided doses (every 12 hours).

Currently on opioids: Use conversion chart (see Note) to convert daily dose to oxymorphone equivalent. Generally start with 1/2 the calculated daily oxymorphone dosage. Divide daily dose in 2 (for every 12-hour dosing) and round down to nearest dosage form. **Note:** Per manufacturer, the following approximate oral dosages are equivalent to oxymorphone 10 mg:

Hydrocodone 20 mg

Oxycodone 20 mg

Methadone 20 mg

Morphine 30 mg

Conversion of stable dose of immediate-release oxymorphone to extended-release oxymorphone: Administer 1/2 of the daily dose of immediate-release oxymorphone (Opana®) as the extended-release formulation (Opana® ER) every 12 hours

Dosage Forms

Injection, solution:

Opana®: 1 mg/mL (1 mL)

Tablet:

Opana®: 5 mg, 10 mg

Tablet, extended release:

Opana® ER: 5 mg, 7.5 mg, 10 mg, 15 mg, 20 mg, 30 mg, 40 mg

oxymorphone hydrochloride *see* oxymorphone *on page* 741

oxytetracycline *(Discontinued)*

oxytocin (oks i TOE sin)

Sound-Alike/Look-Alike Issues

Pitocin® may be confused with Pitressin®

Synonyms pit

U.S./Canadian Brand Names Pitocin® [US/Can]; Syntocinon® [Can]

Therapeutic Category Oxytocic Agent

Use Induction of labor at term; control of postpartum bleeding; adjunctive therapy in management of abortion

Usual Dosage I.V. administration requires the use of an infusion pump. Adults:

Induction of labor: I.V.: 0.5-1 milliunits/minute; gradually increase dose in increments of 1-2 milliunits/minute until desired contraction pattern is established; dose may be decreased after desired frequency of contractions is reached and labor has progressed to 5-6 cm dilation. Infusion rates of 6 milliunits/minute provide oxytocin levels similar to those at spontaneous labor; rates >9-10 milliunits/minute are rarely required.

Postpartum bleeding:

I.M.: Total dose of 10 units after delivery

I.V.: 10-40 units by I.V. infusion in 1000 mL of intravenous fluid at a rate sufficient to control uterine atony

Adjunctive treatment of abortion: I.V.: 10-20 milliunits/minute; maximum total dose: 30 units/12 hours

Dosage Forms

Injection, solution: 10 units/mL (1 mL, 10 mL, 30 mL)

Pitocin®: 10 units/mL (1 mL, 10 mL)

Oxytrol® [US/Can] *see* oxybutynin *on page 736*

Oysco D [US-OTC] *see* calcium and vitamin D *on page 169*

Oysco 500 [US-OTC] *see* calcium carbonate *on page 170*

Oysco 500+D [US-OTC] *see* calcium and vitamin D *on page 169*

Oyst-Cal-D [US-OTC] *see* calcium and vitamin D *on page 169*

Oyst-Cal 500 [US-OTC] *see* calcium carbonate *on page 170*

Oyst-Cal-D 500 [US-OTC] *see* calcium and vitamin D *on page 169*

P2E1 *(Discontinued)*

P-V-Tussin® Syrup *(Discontinued)*

P-V Tussin Tablet *(Discontinued)*

P32 *see* chromic phosphate P 32 *on page 225*

P-071 *see* cetirizine *on page 204*

Pacerone® [US] *see* amiodarone *on page 64*

Pacis™ [Can] *see* BCG vaccine *on page 124*

paclitaxel (pac li TAKS el)

Sound-Alike/Look-Alike Issues

paclitaxel may be confused with paroxetine, Paxil®

paclitaxel (conventional) may be confused with paclitaxel (protein-bound)

Taxol® may be confused with Abraxane®, Paxil®, Taxotere®

Synonyms NSC-125973; NSC-673089

U.S./Canadian Brand Names Abraxane® For Injectable Suspension [Can]; Apo-Paclitaxel® [Can]; Onxol® [US]; Taxol® [Can]

Therapeutic Category Antineoplastic Agent

Use Treatment of breast, nonsmall cell lung, and ovarian cancers; treatment of AIDS-related Kaposi sarcoma (KS)

Usual Dosage Premedication with dexamethasone (20 mg orally or I.V. at 12 and 6 hours **or** 14 and 7 hours before the dose; reduce dexamethasone dose to 10 mg orally with advanced HIV disease), diphenhydramine (50 mg I.V. 30-60 minutes prior to the dose), and cimetidine, famotidine, or ranitidine (I.V. 30-60 minutes prior to the dose) is recommended.

Adults: I.V.: Refer to individual protocols

Ovarian carcinoma: 135-175 mg/m^2 over 3 hours every 3 weeks **or**

135 mg/m^2 over 24 hours every 3 weeks **or**

50-80 mg/m^2 over 1-3 hours weekly **or**

1.4-4 mg/m^2/day continuous infusion for 14 days every 4 weeks

Metastatic breast cancer: 175-250 mg/m^2 over 3 hours every 3 weeks **or**
50-80 mg/m^2 weekly **or**
1.4-4 mg/m^2/day continuous infusion for 14 days every 4 weeks
Nonsmall cell lung carcinoma: 135 mg/m^2 over 24 hours every 3 weeks
AIDS-related Kaposi sarcoma: 135 mg/m^2 over 3 hours every 3 weeks **or**
100 mg/m^2 over 3 hours every 2 weeks

Dosage Forms

Injection, solution: 6 mg/mL (5 mL, 16.7 mL, 25 mL, 50 mL)
Onxol®: 6 mg/mL (5 mL, 25 mL, 50 mL)

paclitaxel, albumin-bound *see* paclitaxel (protein bound) *on page 743*

paclitaxel (protein bound) (pac li TAKS el PROE teen bownd)

Sound-Alike/Look-Alike Issues

paclitaxel (protein bound) may be confused with paclitaxel (conventional)
Abraxane® may be confused with Paxil®, Taxol®, Taxotere®

Synonyms ABI-007; albumin-bound paclitaxel; albumin-stabilized nanoparticle paclitaxel; nab-paclitaxel; nanoparticle albumin-bound paclitaxel; paclitaxel, albumin-bound; protein-bound paclitaxel

U.S./Canadian Brand Names Abraxane® [US]

Therapeutic Category Antineoplastic Agent, Antimicrotubular; Antineoplastic Agent, Natural Source (Plant) Derivative

Use Treatment of refractory (metastatic) or relapsed (within 6 months of adjuvant therapy) breast cancer

Usual Dosage I.V.: Adults: Breast cancer: 260 mg/m^2 every 3 weeks

Dosage Forms

Injection, powder for reconstitution:
Abraxane®: 100 mg

Paddock Nystatin™ [US] *see* nystatin *on page 715*

Pain-A-Lay® [US-OTC] *see* phenol *on page 772*

Pain Eze [US-OTC] *see* acetaminophen *on page 19*

Pain-Off [US-OTC] *see* acetaminophen, aspirin, and caffeine *on page 24*

Palafer® [Can] *see* ferrous fumarate *on page 413*

Palcaps *(Discontinued)* *see* pancrelipase *on page 746*

Palgic® [US] *see* carbinoxamine *on page 185*

Palgic®-D *(Discontinued)*

Palgic®-DS *(Discontinued)*

palifermin (pal ee FER min)

Synonyms AMJ 9701; rhKGF; rhu keratinocyte growth factor; rHu-KGF

U.S./Canadian Brand Names Kepivance® [US]

Therapeutic Category Keratinocyte Growth Factor

Use Decrease the incidence and severity of severe oral mucositis associated with hematologic malignancies in patients receiving myelotoxic therapy requiring hematopoietic stem cell support

Usual Dosage I.V.: Adults: 60 mcg/kg/day for 3 consecutive days before and after myelotoxic therapy; total of 6 doses

Note: Administer first 3 doses prior to myelotoxic therapy, with the 3rd dose given 24-48 hours before therapy begins. The last 3 doses should be administered after myelotoxic therapy, with the first of these doses after but on the same day of hematopoietic stem cell infusion and at least 4 days after the most recent dose of palifermin.

Dosage Forms

Injection, powder for reconstitution [preservative free]:
Kepivance®: 6.25 mg

paliperidone (pal ee PER i done)

Synonyms 9-hydroxy-risperidone; 9-OH-risperidone

U.S./Canadian Brand Names Invega® Sustenna™ [US]; Invega® [US/Can]

Therapeutic Category Antipsychotic Agent, Atypical

Use Treatment of schizophrenia

Usual Dosage Oral: Adults: Schizophrenia: Usual: 6 mg once daily in the morning; titration not required, though some may benefit from higher or lower doses. If exceeding 6 mg/day, increases of 3 mg/day are recommended no more frequently than every 5 days, up to a maximum of 12 mg/day. Some patients may require only 3 mg/day.

Product Availability

Invega® Sustenna™ extended release injectable suspension: FDA approved July 2009; anticipated availability is currently undetermined

Dosage Forms

Tablet, extended-release:

Invega®: 3 mg, 6 mg, 9 mg

palivizumab (pah li VIZ u mab)

Sound-Alike/Look-Alike Issues

Synagis® may be confused with Synalgos®-DC, Synvisc®

U.S./Canadian Brand Names Synagis® [US/Can]

Therapeutic Category Monoclonal Antibody

Use Prevention of serious lower respiratory tract disease caused by respiratory syncytial virus (RSV) in infants and children at high risk of RSV disease

Usual Dosage I.M.: Infants and Children <2 years:

Prevention of RSV: 15 mg/kg of body weight, monthly throughout RSV season (first dose administered prior to commencement of RSV season)

Note: Cardiopulmonary bypass patients: Administer a dose as soon as possible after cardiopulmonary bypass procedure, even if <1 month from previous dose.

Dosage Forms

Injection, solution [preservative free]:

Synagis®: 100 mg/mL (0.5 mL, 1 mL)

Palladone™ *(Discontinued)* *see* hydromorphone *on page* 506

Palmer's® Skin Success Acne Cleanser [US-OTC] *see* salicylic acid *on page* 884

Palmer's® Skin Success Eventone® Fade Cream [US-OTC] *see* hydroquinone *on page* 508

Palmer's® Skin Success Invisible Acne [US-OTC] *see* benzoyl peroxide *on page* 132

Palmitate-A® [US-OTC] *see* vitamin A *on page* 1016

palonosetron (pal oh NOE se tron)

Sound-Alike/Look-Alike Issues

palonosetron may be confused with dolasetron, granisetron, ondansetron

Aloxi® may be confused with Eloxatin®, oxaliplatin

Synonyms palonosetron hydrochloride; RS-25259; RS-25259-197

U.S./Canadian Brand Names Aloxi® [US]

Therapeutic Category Antiemetic; Selective 5-HT_3 Receptor Antagonist

Use

I.V.: Prevention of chemotherapy-associated nausea and vomiting; indicated for prevention of acute (highly-emetogenic therapy) as well as acute and delayed (moderately-emetogenic therapy) nausea and vomiting; prevention of postoperative nausea and vomiting (PONV)

Oral: Prevention of chemotherapy-associated nausea and vomiting (moderately-emetogenic therapy)

Usual Dosage Adults:

Chemotherapy-associated nausea and vomiting:

I.V.: 0.25 mg 30 minutes prior to the start of chemotherapy administration

Oral: 0.5 mg 1 hour prior to the start of chemotherapy

Breakthrough: Palonosetron has not been shown to be effective in terminating nausea or vomiting once it occurs and should not be used for this purpose.

PONV: I.V.: 0.075 mg immediately prior to anesthesia induction

Product Availability Aloxi® capsules: FDA approved August 2008; anticipated availability currently undetermined

Dosage Forms

Capsule:

Aloxi®: 0.5 mg

Injection, solution:

Aloxi®: 0.05 mg/mL (1.5 mL, 5 mL)

palonosetron hydrochloride *see* palonosetron *on page* *744*
2-PAM *see* pralidoxime *on page* *808*

pamabrom (PAM a brom)

U.S./Canadian Brand Names Aqua-Ban® Maximum Strength [US-OTC]; diurex® Aquagels® [US-OTC]; diurex® Maximum Relief [US-OTC]; diurex® [US-OTC]

Therapeutic Category Diuretic

Use Temporary relief of symptoms associated with premenstrual and menstrual periods (eg, bloating, water-weight gain, swelling, full feeling)

Usual Dosage Oral: Adults: 50 mg after breakfast and then every 6 hours as needed (maximum: 200 mg/24 hours); should be taken 5-6 days prior to onset of menstrual period and continued until desired relief or end of period

Dosage Forms

Caplet, oral:
diurex® Maximum Relief [OTC]: 50 mg

Capsule, oral:
diurex® [OTC]: 50 mg

Capsule, soft gel, oral:
diurex® Aquagels® [OTC]: 50 mg

Tablet, oral:
Aqua-Ban® Maximum Strength [OTC]: 50 mg

pamabrom and acetaminophen *see* acetaminophen and pamabrom *on page* *22*
Pamelor® [US] *see* nortriptyline *on page* *706*

pamidronate (pa mi DROE nate)

Sound-Alike/Look-Alike Issues
pamidronate may be confused with papaverine
Aredia® may be confused with adriamycin, Meridia®

Synonyms pamidronate disodium

U.S./Canadian Brand Names Aredia® [US/Can]; Pamidronate Disodium Omega [Can]; Pamidronate Disodium® [Can]; PMS-Pamidronate [Can]; Rhoxal-pamidronate [Can]

Therapeutic Category Bisphosphonate Derivative

Use Treatment of moderate or severe hypercalcemia associated with malignancy; treatment of osteolytic bone lesions associated with multiple myeloma or metastatic breast cancer; moderate-to-severe Paget disease of bone

Usual Dosage Dilute prior to administration and infuse intravenously slowly over at least 2 hours. Single doses should not exceed 90 mg. I.V.: Adults:

Hypercalcemia of malignancy:

Moderate cancer-related hypercalcemia (corrected serum calcium: 12-13.5 mg/dL): 60-90 mg, as a single dose over 2-24 hours

Severe cancer-related hypercalcemia (corrected serum calcium: >13.5 mg/dL): 90 mg, as a single dose over 2-24 hours

A period of 7 days should elapse before the use of second course; repeat infusions every 2-3 weeks have been suggested, however, could be administered every 2-3 months according to the degree and of severity of hypercalcemia and/or the type of malignancy.

Osteolytic bone lesions with multiple myeloma: 90 mg over 2-4 hours monthly or every 3-4 weeks

Osteolytic bone lesions with metastatic breast cancer: 90 mg over 2 hours repeated every 3-4 weeks

Paget disease: 30 mg over 4 hours daily for 3 consecutive days

Dosage Forms

Injection, powder for reconstitution: 30 mg, 90 mg
Aredia®: 30 mg, 90 mg

Injection, solution: 3 mg/mL (10 mL); 6 mg/mL (10 mL); 9 mg/mL (10 mL)

Injection, solution [preservative free]: 3 mg/mL (10 mL)

Pamidronate Disodium® [Can] *see* pamidronate *on page* *745*
pamidronate disodium *see* pamidronate *on page* *745*
Pamidronate Disodium Omega [Can] *see* pamidronate *on page* *745*
Pamine® [US/Can] *see* methscopolamine *on page* *642*
Pamine® Forte [US] *see* methscopolamine *on page* *642*

p-aminoclonidine *see* apraclonidine *on page 94*
Pamprin IB® *(Discontinued)* *see* ibuprofen *on page 515*
Pamprin® Maximum Strength All Day Relief [US-OTC] *see* naproxen *on page 681*
Pan-2400™ [US-OTC] *see* pancreatin *on page 746*
Panadol® *(Discontinued)* *see* acetaminophen *on page 19*
Panafil® *(Discontinued)* *see* chlorophyllin, papain, and urea *on page 211*
Panafil® SE *(Discontinued)* *see* chlorophyllin, papain, and urea *on page 211*
Panasal® 5/500 *(Discontinued)*
Pancof® *(Discontinued)* *see* pseudoephedrine, dihydrocodeine, and chlorpheniramine *on page 836*
Pancof®-EXP [US] *see* dihydrocodeine, pseudoephedrine, and guaifenesin *on page 310*
Pancof-HC *(Discontinued)*
Pancof-XP *(Discontinued)*
Pancrease® [Can] *see* pancrelipase *on page 746*
Pancrease® MT [US/Can] *see* pancrelipase *on page 746*
pancreatic enzymes *see* pancrelipase *on page 746*

pancreatin (PAN kree a tin)

Sound-Alike/Look-Alike Issues
pancreatin may be confused with Panretin®

U.S./Canadian Brand Names Hi-Vegi-Lip [US-OTC]; Pan-2400™ [US-OTC]; Veg-Pancreatin 4X [US-OTC]

Therapeutic Category Enzyme

Use Relief of functional indigestion due to enzyme deficiency or imbalance

Usual Dosage Oral: Adults: Actual dose varies with condition of patient and is usually given with each meal or snack.

Dosage Forms

Capsule: Lipase 8500 units, protease 50,000 units, amylase 50,000 units
Pan-2400™ [OTC]: Lipase 9816 units, protease 60,214 units, amylase 75,900 units

Tablet: Lipase 565 units, protease 8200 units, amylase 8200 units [pancreatin 325 mg]; lipase 2400 units, protease 30,000 units, amylase 30,000 units
Hi-Vegi-Lip [OTC]: Lipase 4800 units, protease 60,000 units, amylase 60,000 units
Veg-Pancreatin 4X [OTC]: Lipase 5500 units, protease 69,000 units, amylase 69,000 units

Pancrecarb MS® [US] *see* pancrelipase *on page 746*

pancrelipase (pan kre LYE pase)

Sound-Alike/Look-Alike Issues
Pancrease® may be confused with Pentasa®
Pangestyme™ may be confused with Pentasa®
Viokase® may be confused with Viokase® 8
Viokase® 8 may be confused with Viokase®

Synonyms lipancreatin; lipase, protease, and amylase; pancreatic enzymes

U.S./Canadian Brand Names Cotazym® [Can]; Creon® [US/Can]; Pancrease® MT [US/Can]; Pancrease® [Can]; Pancrecarb MS® [US]; Ultrase® MT [US/Can]; Ultrase® [US/Can]; Viokase® [US/Can]

Therapeutic Category Enzyme

Use Treatment of exocrine pancreatic insufficiency (EPI) due to conditions such as cystic fibrosis

Usual Dosage Oral:

Malabsorption: Adjust dose based on body weight, clinical symptoms, and stool fat content. Allow several days between dose adjustments. Total daily dose reflects ~3 meals/day and 2-3 snacks/day, with half the mealtime dose given with a snack. Doses of lipase >2500 units/kg/meal should be used with caution and only with documentation of 3-day fecal fat measures. Doses of lipase >6000 units/kg/meal are associated with colonic stricture and should be decreased.

Children:
- ≤1 year: Lipase 2000-4000 units per 120 mL of formula or breast milk
- >1 and <4 years: Initial dose: Lipase 1000 units/kg/meal. Dosage range: Lipase 1000-2500 units/kg/meal. Maximum dose: Lipase 10,000 units/kg/day **or** lipase 4000 units/g of fat per day
- ≥4 years: Refer to adult dosing

Adults: Initial: Lipase 500 units/kg/meal. Dosage range: Lipase 500-2500 units/kg/meal. Maximum dose: Lipase 10,000 units/kg/day **or** lipase 4000 units/g of fat per day

Dosage Forms

Capsule, delayed release, enteric coated granules [porcine derived]:

Zenpep™: Lipase 5000 units, protease 17,000 units, amylase 27,000 units

Zenpep™: Lipase 10,000 units, protease 34,000 units, amylase 55,000 units

Zenpep™: Lipase 15,000 units, protease 51,000 units, amylase 82,000 units

Zenpep™: Lipase 20,000 units, protease 68,000 units, amylase 109,000 units

Capsule, delayed release, enteric coated microspheres [porcine derived]: Lipase 4500 units, protease 25,000 units, and amylase 20,000 units; Lipase 10,000 units, protease 30,000 units, and amylase 30,000 units; Lipase 16,000 units, protease 48,000 units, and amylase 48,000 units; Lipase 20,000 units, protease 44,000 units, and amylase 56,000 units

Pancrecarb MS-4®: Lipase 4000 units, protease 25,000 units, and amylase 25,000 units [buffered]

Pancrecarb MS-8®: Lipase 8000 units, protease 45,000 units, and amylase 40,000 units [buffered]

Pancrecarb MS-16® Lipase 16,000 units, protease 52,000 units, and amylase 52,000 units [buffered]

Capsule, delayed release, enteric coated microspheres [new formulation; porcine derived]:

Creon®: Lipase 6000 units, protease 19,000 units, and amylase 30,000 units

Creon®: Lipase 12000 units, protease 38,000 units, and amylase 60,000 units

Creon®: Lipase 24,000 units, protease 76,000 units, and amylase 120,000 units

Capsule, enteric coated microspheres [porcine derived]:

Ultrase®: Lipase 4500 units, protease 25,000 units, and amylase 20,000 units

Capsule, enteric coated microtablets [porcine derived]:

Pancrease® MT 4: Lipase 4000 units, protease 12,000 units, and amylase 12,000 units

Pancrease® MT 10: Lipase 10,000 units, protease 30,000 units, and amylase 30,000 units

Pancrease® MT 16: Lipase 16,000 units, protease 48,000 units, and amylase 48,000 units

Pancrease® MT 20: Lipase 20,000 units, protease 44,000 units, and amylase 56,000 units

Capsule, enteric coated minitablets [porcine derived]:

Ultrase® MT12: Lipase 12,000 units, protease 39,000 units, and amylase 39,000 units

Ultrase® MT18: Lipase 18,000 units, protease 58,500 units, and amylase 58,500 units

Ultrase® MT20: Lipase 20,000 units, protease 65,000 units, and amylase 65,000 units

Powder [porcine derived]:

Viokase®: Lipase 16,800 units, protease 70,000 units, and amylase 70,000 units per 0.7 g (227 g)

Tablet [porcine derived]:

Viokase® 8: Lipase 8000 units, protease 30,000 units, and amylase 30,000 units

Viokase® 16: Lipase 16,000 units, protease 60,000 units, and amylase 60,000 units

pancuronium (pan kyoo ROE nee um)

Sound-Alike/Look-Alike Issues

pancuronium may be confused with pipecuronium

Synonyms pancuronium bromide

U.S./Canadian Brand Names Pancuronium Bromide® [Can]

Therapeutic Category Skeletal Muscle Relaxant

Use Facilitation of endotracheal intubation and relaxation of skeletal muscles during surgery; facilitation of mechanical ventilation in ICU patients; does not relieve pain or produce sedation

Usual Dosage Administer I.V.; dose to effect; doses will vary due to interpatient variability; use ideal body weight for obese patients

Surgery:

Neonates <1 month:

Test dose: 0.02 mg/kg to measure responsiveness

Initial: 0.03 mg/kg/dose repeated twice at 5- to 10-minute intervals as needed; maintenance: 0.03-0.09 mg/kg/dose every 30 minutes to 4 hours as needed

Infants >1 month, Children, and Adults: Initial: 0.06-0.1 mg/kg or 0.05 mg/kg after initial dose of succinylcholine for intubation; maintenance dose: 0.01 mg/kg 60-100 minutes after initial dose and then 0.01 mg/kg every 25-60 minutes

Pretreatment/priming: 10% of intubating dose given 3-5 minutes before initial dose

ICU: 0.05-0.1 mg/kg bolus followed by 0.8-1.7 mcg/kg/minute once initial recovery from bolus observed or 0.1-0.2 mg/kg every 1-3 hours

Dosage Forms

Injection, solution: 1 mg/mL (10 mL); 2 mg/mL (2 mL, 5 mL)

Pancuronium Bromide® [Can] *see* pancuronium *on page* 747

pancuronium bromide *see* pancuronium *on page 747*
Pandel® [US] *see* hydrocortisone (topical) *on page 505*
Pangestyme™ CN *(Discontinued)* *see* pancrelipase *on page 746*
Pangestyme™ EC *(Discontinued)* *see* pancrelipase *on page 746*
Pangestyme™ MT *(Discontinued)* *see* pancrelipase *on page 746*
Pangestyme™ UL *(Discontinued)* *see* pancrelipase *on page 746*
Panglobulin® NF *(Discontinued)* *see* immune globulin (intravenous) *on page 523*
Panhematin® [US] *see* hemin *on page 486*

panitumumab (pan i TOOM yoo mab)

Synonyms ABX-EGF; NSC-742319; rHuMAb-EGFr

U.S./Canadian Brand Names Vectibix® [US/Can]

Therapeutic Category Antineoplastic Agent, Monoclonal Antibody; Epidermal Growth Factor Receptor (EGFR) Inhibitor

Use Monotherapy in treatment of refractory metastatic colorectal cancer

Note: Subset analyses (retrospective) in metastatic colorectal cancer trials have not shown a benefit with EGFR inhibitor treatment in patients whose tumors have codon 12 or 13 *KRAS* mutations; use is not recommended in these patients.

Usual Dosage I.V.: Adults: Metastatic colorectal cancer: 6 mg/kg every 2 weeks

Dosage Forms

Injection, solution [preservative free]:
Vectibix®: 20 mg/mL (5 mL, 10 mL, 20 mL)

Panixine DisperDose™ *(Discontinued)* *see* cephalexin *on page 202*
Panlor® DC [US] *see* acetaminophen, caffeine, and dihydrocodeine *on page 25*
Panlor® SS [US] *see* acetaminophen, caffeine, and dihydrocodeine *on page 25*
Panocaps *(Discontinued)* *see* pancrelipase *on page 746*
Panocaps MT *(Discontinued)* *see* pancrelipase *on page 746*
Panokase® 16 *(Discontinued)* *see* pancrelipase *on page 746*
Panokase® *(Discontinued)* *see* pancrelipase *on page 746*
PanOxyl® [Can] *see* benzoyl peroxide *on page 132*
PanOxyl® Aqua Gel [US] *see* benzoyl peroxide *on page 132*
PanOxyl® Bar [US-OTC] *see* benzoyl peroxide *on page 132*
Panretin® [US/Can] *see* alitretinoin *on page 47*
Panscol® Lotion *(Discontinued)* *see* salicylic acid *on page 884*
Panscol® Ointment *(Discontinued)* *see* salicylic acid *on page 884*
Panto-250 [US] *see* pantothenic acid *on page 749*
Panto™ I.V. [Can] *see* pantoprazole *on page 748*
Pantoloc® [Can] *see* pantoprazole *on page 748*
Pantopon® *(Discontinued)*

pantoprazole (pan TOE pra zole)

Sound-Alike/Look-Alike Issues

pantoprazole may be confused with aripiprazole
Protonix® may be confused with Lotronex®, Lovenox®, protamine

U.S./Canadian Brand Names Apo-Pantoprazole® [Can]; CO Pantoprazole [Can]; Gen-Pantoprazole [Can]; Novo-Pantoprazole [Can]; Pantoloc® [Can]; Panto™ I.V. [Can]; PMS-Pantoprazole [Can]; Protonix® [US/Can]; Ran-Pantoprazole [Can]; ratio-Pantoprazole [Can]; Riva-Pantoprazole [Can]; Sandoz-Pantoprazole [Can]; Tecta™ [Can]; ZYM-Pantoprazole [Can]

Therapeutic Category Proton Pump Inhibitor

Use

Oral: Treatment and maintenance of healing of erosive esophagitis associated with GERD; reduction in relapse rates of daytime and nighttime heartburn symptoms in GERD; hypersecretory disorders associated with Zollinger-Ellison syndrome or other GI hypersecretory disorders

I.V.: Short-term treatment (7-10 days) of patients with gastroesophageal reflux disease (GERD) and a history of erosive esophagitis; hypersecretory disorders associated with Zollinger-Ellison syndrome or other neoplastic disorders

Usual Dosage Adults:
Oral:
Erosive esophagitis associated with GERD:
Treatment: 40 mg once daily for up to 8 weeks; an additional 8 weeks may be used in patients who have not healed after an 8-week course
Maintenance of healing: 40 mg once daily
Note: Lower doses (20 mg once daily) have been used successfully in mild GERD treatment and maintenance of healing
Hypersecretory disorders (including Zollinger-Ellison): Initial: 40 mg twice daily; adjust dose based on patient needs; doses up to 240 mg/day have been administered
I.V.:
Erosive esophagitis associated with GERD: 40 mg once daily for 7-10 days
Hypersecretory disorders: 80 mg twice daily; adjust dose based on acid output measurements; 160-240 mg/day in divided doses has been used for a limited period (up to 7 days)

Dosage Forms
Granules for suspension, delayed release, enteric coated, as sodium, oral:
Protonix®: 40 mg/packet (30s)
Injection, powder for reconstitution:
Protonix®: 40 mg
Tablet, delayed release: 20 mg, 40 mg
Protonix®: 20 mg, 40 mg
Tablet, enteric coated:
Pantoloc® [CAN]: 40 mg [not available in the U.S.]

pantothenic acid (pan toe THEN ik AS id)

Synonyms calcium pantothenate; vitamin B_5
U.S./Canadian Brand Names Panto-250 [US]
Therapeutic Category Vitamin, Water Soluble
Use Pantothenic acid deficiency
Usual Dosage Oral: Adults: Recommended daily dose 4-7 mg/day
Dosage Forms
Capsule:
Panto-250: 250 mg [contains calcium 23 mg]
Liquid: 200 mg/5 mL (240 mL)
Tablet: 100 mg, 200 mg, 250 mg, 500 mg
Tablet, sustained release: 500 mg

pantothenyl alcohol *see* dexpanthenol *on page 292*

papain and urea (pa PAY in & yoor EE a)

Synonyms urea and papain
U.S./Canadian Brand Names Kovia® [US]
Therapeutic Category Enzyme, Topical Debridement; Topical Skin Product
Use Debridement of necrotic tissue and liquefaction of slough in acute and chronic lesions such as pressure ulcers, varicose and diabetic ulcers, burns, postoperative wounds, pilonidal cyst wounds, carbuncles, and miscellaneous traumatic or infected wounds
Usual Dosage Topical: Adults: Apply with each dressing change. Daily or twice daily dressing changes are preferred, but may be every 2-3 days. Cover with dressing following application.
Ointment: Apply 1/8-inch thickness over the wound with clean applicator.
Spray: Completely cover the wound site so that the wound is not visible.
Dosage Forms
Ointment, topical:
Kovia®: Papain 8.3 x 10^5 units/g and urea 10% (3.5 g) [single-dose packet]; 30 g

papain, urea, and chlorophyllin *see* chlorophyllin, papain, and urea *on page 211*

papaverine (pa PAV er een)

Sound-Alike/Look-Alike Issues
papaverine may be confused with pamidronate
Synonyms papaverine hydrochloride

Therapeutic Category Vasodilator

Use Oral: Relief of peripheral and cerebral ischemia associated with arterial spasm and myocardial ischemia complicated by arrhythmias

Usual Dosage

I.M., I.V.:

Children: 6 mg/kg/day in 4 divided doses

Adults: 30-65 mg (rarely up to 120 mg); may repeat every 3 hours

Oral, sustained release: Adults: 150-300 mg every 12 hours; in difficult cases: 150 mg every 8 hours

Dosage Forms

Capsule, sustained release: 150 mg

Injection, solution: 30 mg/mL (2 mL, 10 mL)

papaverine hydrochloride *see* papaverine *on page* 749

Papfyll™ ***(Discontinued)*** *see* chlorophyllin, papain, and urea *on page* 211

papillomavirus (types 6, 11, 16, 18) vaccine (human, recombinant)

(pap ih LO ma VYE rus typs six e LEV en SIX teen AYE teen vak SEEN YU man ree KOM be nant)

Synonyms HPV vaccine; HPV4; human papillomavirus vaccine; papillomavirus vaccine, recombinant; quadrivalent human papillomavirus vaccine

U.S./Canadian Brand Names Gardasil® [US/Can]

Therapeutic Category Vaccine

Use Females ≥9 years and ≤26 years of age: Prevention of cervical, vulvar, and vaginal cancer, genital warts, cervical adenocarcinoma *in situ*, and vulvar, vaginal, or cervical intraepithelial neoplasia caused by human papillomavirus (HPV) types 6, 11, 16, 18

The Advisory Committee on Immunization Practices (ACIP) recommends routine vaccination for females 11-12 years of age; catch-up vaccination is recommended for females 13-26 years of age

Usual Dosage I.M.: Females: Children ≥9 years and Adults ≤26 years: 0.5 mL followed by 0.5 mL at 2 and 6 months after initial dose

CDC recommended immunization schedule: Administer first dose to females at age 11-12 years; begin series in females aged 13-26 years if not previously vaccinated. Minimum interval between first and second doses is 4 weeks; the minimum interval between first and third doses is 24 weeks.

Dosage Forms

Injection, suspension [preservative free]:

Gardasil®: HPV 6 L1 protein 20 mcg, HPV 11 L1 protein 40 mcg, HPV 16 L1 protein 40 mcg, and HPV 18 L1 protein 20 mcg per 0.5 mL (0.5 mL)

papillomavirus vaccine, recombinant *see* papillomavirus (types 6, 11, 16, 18) vaccine (human, recombinant) *on page* 750

Paptase™ ***(Discontinued)*** *see* papain and urea *on page* 749

para-aminosalicylate sodium *see* aminosalicylic acid *on page* 64

paracetamol *see* acetaminophen *on page* 19

Paraflex® ***(Discontinued)*** *see* chlorzoxazone *on page* 223

Parafon Forte® [Can] *see* chlorzoxazone *on page* 223

Parafon Forte® ***(Discontinued)*** *see* chlorzoxazone *on page* 223

Parafon Forte® DSC [US] *see* chlorzoxazone *on page* 223

Paraplatin-AQ [Can] *see* carboplatin *on page* 185

Paraplatin® ***(Discontinued)*** *see* carboplatin *on page* 185

parathyroid hormone (1-34) *see* teriparatide *on page* 946

Para-Time SR® ***(Discontinued)*** *see* papaverine *on page* 749

Parcaine™ [US] *see* proparacaine *on page* 826

Parcopa™ [US] *see* carbidopa and levodopa *on page* 184

Paredrine® ***(Discontinued)***

paregoric (par e GOR ik)

Sound-Alike/Look-Alike Issues

paregoric may be confused with Percogesic®

camphorated tincture of opium is an error-prone synonym (mistaken as opium tincture)

Therapeutic Category Analgesic, Narcotic

Controlled Substance C-III

Use Treatment of diarrhea or relief of pain; neonatal opiate withdrawal

Usual Dosage Oral:

Neonatal opiate withdrawal: 3-6 drops every 3-6 hours as needed, or initially 0.2 mL every 3 hours; increase dosage by approximately 0.05 mL every 3 hours until withdrawal symptoms are controlled; it is rare to exceed 0.7 mL/dose. Stabilize withdrawal symptoms for 3-5 days, then gradually decrease dosage over a 2- to 4-week period.

Children: 0.25-0.5 mL/kg 1-4 times/day

Adults: 5-10 mL 1-4 times/day

Dosage Forms

Liquid, oral: Morphine equivalent 2 mg/5 mL

Paremyd® [US] *see* hydroxyamphetamine and tropicamide *on page* 509

parenteral nutrition *see* total parenteral nutrition *on page* 972

Parepectolin® ***(Discontinued)***

paricalcitol (pah ri KAL si tole)

Sound-Alike/Look-Alike Issues

paricalcitol may be confused with calcitriol

U.S./Canadian Brand Names Zemplar® [US/Can]

Therapeutic Category Vitamin D Analog

Use

I.V.: Prevention and treatment of secondary hyperparathyroidism associated with stage 5 chronic kidney disease (CKD)

Oral: Prevention and treatment of secondary hyperparathyroidism associated with stage 3 and 4 CKD and stage 5 CKD patients on hemodialysis or peritoneal dialysis

Usual Dosage Note: In stage 3-5 CKD maintain calcium phosphorus product (Ca x P) <55 mg^2/dL^2, reduce or interrupt dosing if recommended Ca x P is exceeded or hypercalcemia is observed.

Secondary hyperparathyroidism associated with chronic renal failure (stage 5 CKD):

Children ≥5 years and Adults: I.V.: 0.04-0.1 mcg/kg (2.8-7 mcg) given as a bolus dose no more frequently than every other day at any time during dialysis; dose may be increased by 2-4 mcg every 2-4 weeks; doses as high as 0.24 mcg/kg (16.8 mcg) have been administered safely; the dose of paricalcitol should be adjusted based on serum intact PTH (iPTH) levels, as follows:

Same or increasing iPTH level: Increase paricalcitol dose

iPTH level decreased by <30%: Increase paricalcitol dose

iPTH level decreased by >30% and <60%: Maintain paricalcitol dose

iPTH level decrease by >60%: Decrease paricalcitol dose

iPTH level 1.5-3 times upper limit of normal: Maintain paricalcitol dose

Adults: Oral: Initial dose, in mcg, based on baseline iPTH level divided by 80. Administered 3 times weekly, no more frequently than every other day. **Note:** To reduce the risk of hypercalcemia initiate only after baseline serum calcium has been adjusted to ≤9.5 mg/dL.

Dose titration:

Titration dose (mcg) = Most recent iPTH level (pg/mL) divided by 80

Dosage adjustment for hypercalcemia or elevated Ca x P: Decrease calculated dose by 2-4 mcg. If further adjustment is required, dose should be reduced or interrupted until these parameters are normalized. If applicable, phosphate binder dosing may also be adjusted or withheld, or switch to a noncalcium-based phosphate binder

Secondary hyperparathyroidism associated with stage 3 and 4 CKD: Adults: Oral: Initial dose based on baseline serum iPTH:

iPTH ≤500 pg/mL: 1 mcg/day or 2 mcg 3 times/week

iPTH >500 pg/mL: 2 mcg/day or 4 mcg 3 times/week

Dosage adjustment based on iPTH level relative to baseline, adjust dose at 2-4 week intervals:

iPTH same or increased: Increase paricalcitol dose by 1 mcg/day or 2 mcg 3 times/week

iPTH decreased by <30%: Increase paricalcitol dose by 1 mcg/day or 2 mcg 3 times//week

iPTH decreased by ≥30% or ≤60%: Maintain paricalcitol dose

iPTH decreased by >60%: Decrease paricalcitol dose by 1 mcg/day* or 2 mcg 3 times/week

iPTH <60 pg/mL: Decrease paricalcitol dose by 1 mcg/day* or 2 mcg 3 times/week

*If patient is taking the lowest dose on a once-daily regimen, but further dose reduction is needed, decrease dose to 1 mcg 3 times/week. If further dose reduction is required, withhold drug as needed and restart at a lower dose. If applicable, calcium-phosphate binder dosing may also be adjusted or withheld, or switch to noncalcium-based binder.

Dosage Forms

Capsule, gelatin:

Zemplar®: 1 mcg, 2 mcg, 4 mcg

Injection, solution:

Zemplar®: 2 mcg/mL (1 mL); 5 mcg/mL (1 mL, 2 mL)

Pariet® [Can] *see* rabeprazole *on page 847*

pariprazole *see* rabeprazole *on page 847*

Parlodel® [US/Can] *see* bromocriptine *on page 148*

Parlodel® SnapTabs® [US] *see* bromocriptine *on page 148*

Parnate® [US/Can] *see* tranylcypromine *on page 977*

paromomycin (par oh moe MYE sin)

Synonyms paromomycin sulfate

U.S./Canadian Brand Names Humatin® [Can]

Therapeutic Category Amebicide

Use Treatment of acute and chronic intestinal amebiasis; hepatic coma

Usual Dosage Oral:

Intestinal amebiasis: Children and Adults: 25-35 mg/kg/day in 3 divided doses for 5-10 days

Dientamoeba fragilis: Children and Adults: 25-30 mg/kg/day in 3 divided doses for 7 days

Tapeworm (fish, dog, bovine, porcine):

Children: 11 mg/kg every 15 minutes for 4 doses

Adults: 1 g every 15 minutes for 4 doses

Hepatic coma: Adults: 4 g/day in 2-4 divided doses for 5-6 days

Dwarf tapeworm: Children and Adults: 45 mg/kg/dose every day for 5-7 days

Dosage Forms

Capsule: 250 mg

paromomycin sulfate *see* paromomycin *on page 752*

paroxetine (pa ROKS e teen)

Sound-Alike/Look-Alike Issues

PARoxetine may be confused with FLUoxetine, paclitaxel, pyridoxine

Paxil® may be confused with Doxil®, paclitaxel, Plavix®, Prozac®, Taxol®

Synonyms paroxetine hydrochloride; paroxetine mesylate

Tall-Man PARoxetine

U.S./Canadian Brand Names Apo-Paroxetine® [Can]; CO Paroxetine [Can]; Gen-Paroxetine [Can]; Novo-Paroxetine [Can]; Paxil CR® [US/Can]; Paxil® [US/Can]; Pexeva® [US]; PMS-Paroxetine [Can]; ratio-Paroxetine [Can]; Rhoxal-paroxetine [Can]; Sandoz-Paroxetine [Can]

Therapeutic Category Antidepressant, Selective Serotonin Reuptake Inhibitor

Use Treatment of major depressive disorder (MDD); treatment of panic disorder with or without agoraphobia; obsessive-compulsive disorder (OCD); social anxiety disorder (social phobia); generalized anxiety disorder (GAD); posttraumatic stress disorder (PTSD); premenstrual dysphoric disorder (PMDD)

Usual Dosage Oral: Adults:

Major depressive disorder:

Paxil®, Pexeva®: Initial: 20 mg once daily, preferably in the morning; increase if needed by 10 mg/day increments at intervals of at least 1 week; maximum dose: 50 mg/day

Paxil CR®: Initial: 25 mg once daily; increase if needed by 12.5 mg/day increments at intervals of at least 1 week; maximum dose: 62.5 mg/day

Generalized anxiety disorder (Paxil®, Pexeva®): Initial: 20 mg once daily, preferably in the morning (if dose is increased, adjust in increments of 10 mg/day at 1-week intervals); doses of 20-50 mg/day were used in clinical trials, however, no greater benefit was seen with doses >20 mg.

Obsessive-compulsive disorder (Paxil®, Pexeva®): Initial: 20 mg once daily, preferably in the morning; increase if needed by 10 mg/day increments at intervals of at least 1 week; recommended dose: 40 mg/day; range: 20-60 mg/day; maximum dose: 60 mg/day

Panic disorder:

Paxil®, Pexeva®: Initial: 10 mg once daily, preferably in the morning; increase if needed by 10 mg/day increments at intervals of at least 1 week; recommended dose: 40 mg/day; range: 10-60 mg/day; maximum dose: 60 mg/day

Paxil CR®: Initial: 12.5 mg once daily; increase if needed by 12.5 mg/day at intervals of at least 1 week; maximum dose: 75 mg/day

Premenstrual dysphoric disorder (Paxil CR®): Initial: 12.5 mg once daily in the morning; may be increased to 25 mg/day; dosing changes should occur at intervals of at least 1 week. May be given daily throughout the menstrual cycle or limited to the luteal phase.

Posttraumatic stress disorder (Paxil®): Initial: 20 mg once daily, preferably in the morning; increase if needed by 10 mg/day increments at intervals of at least 1 week; range: 20-50 mg. Limited data suggest doses of 40 mg/day were not more efficacious than 20 mg/day.

Social anxiety disorder:

Paxil®: Initial: 20 mg once daily, preferably in the morning; recommended dose: 20 mg/day; range: 20-60 mg/day; doses >20 mg may not have additional benefit

Paxil CR®: Initial: 12.5 mg once daily, preferably in the morning; may be increased by 12.5 mg/day at intervals of at least 1 week; maximum dose: 37.5 mg/day

Dosage Forms Note: Strength expressed as base:

Suspension, oral: 10 mg/5 mL

Paxil®: 10 mg/5 mL (250 mL)

Tablet: 10 mg, 20 mg, 30 mg, 40 mg

Paxil®, Pexeva®: 10 mg, 20 mg, 30 mg, 40 mg

Tablet, controlled release, enteric coated: 37.5 mg

Paxil CR®: 12.5 mg, 25 mg, 37.5 mg

Tablet, extended release, enteric coated: 12.5 mg, 25 mg

paroxetine hydrochloride *see* paroxetine *on page* *752*

paroxetine mesylate *see* paroxetine *on page* *752*

Partuss® LA *(Discontinued)*

Parvolex® [Can] *see* acetylcysteine *on page* *31*

PAS *see* aminosalicylic acid *on page* *64*

Paser® [US] *see* aminosalicylic acid *on page* *64*

Pataday™ [US] *see* olopatadine *on page* *721*

Patanase® [US] *see* olopatadine *on page* *721*

Patanol® [US/Can] *see* olopatadine *on page* *721*

Pathilon® *(Discontinued)*

Pathocil® [Can] *see* dicloxacillin *on page* *304*

Pathocil® *(Discontinued)* *see* dicloxacillin *on page* *304*

Pavabid® *(Discontinued)* *see* papaverine *on page* *749*

Pavatine® *(Discontinued)*

Pavulon® *(Discontinued)* *see* pancuronium *on page* *747*

Paxene® *(Discontinued)* *see* paclitaxel *on page* *742*

Paxil® [US/Can] *see* paroxetine *on page* *752*

Paxil CR® [US/Can] *see* paroxetine *on page* *752*

PCE® [US/Can] *see* erythromycin *on page* *368*

PCEC *see* rabies vaccine *on page* *848*

P Chlor GG [US] *see* chlorpheniramine, phenylephrine, and guaifenesin *on page* *218*

PCM Allergy *(Discontinued)* *see* chlorpheniramine, phenylephrine, and methscopolamine *on page* *218*

PCM *(Discontinued)* *see* chlorpheniramine, phenylephrine, and methscopolamine *on page* *218*

PCV7 *see* pneumococcal conjugate vaccine (7-valent) *on page* *793*

PD-Cof [US] *see* chlorpheniramine, phenylephrine, and dextromethorphan *on page* *217*

PD-Hist-D [US] *see* chlorpheniramine and phenylephrine *on page* *214*

pectin, gelatin, and methylcellulose *see* gelatin, pectin, and methylcellulose *on page* *457*

Pedameth® *(Discontinued)*

PediaCare® Children's Long-Acting Cough [US-OTC] *see* dextromethorphan *on page* *295*

Pediacare® Children's Long Acting Cough Plus Cold *(Discontinued)* *see* pseudoephedrine and dextromethorphan *on page* *834*

PediaCare® Children's Medicated Freezer Pops Long Acting Cough *(Discontinued)* *see* dextromethorphan *on page* *295*

PediaCare® Children's Allergy [US-OTC] *see* diphenhydramine *on page* *315*

PediaCare® Children's Multi-Symptom Cold [US-OTC] *see* dextromethorphan and phenylephrine *on page 296*

PediaCare® Children's NightTime Cough [US-OTC] *see* diphenhydramine *on page 315*

PediaCare® Cold and Allergy *(Discontinued)* *see* chlorpheniramine and pseudoephedrine *on page 215*

PediaCare® Decongestant Infants *(Discontinued)* *see* pseudoephedrine *on page 833*

Pediacare® Infants' Decongestant & Cough *(Discontinued)* *see* pseudoephedrine and dextromethorphan *on page 834*

PediaCare® Infants' Long-Acting Cough *(Discontinued)* *see* dextromethorphan *on page 295*

PediaCare® Multi-Symptom Cold *(Discontinued)* *see* chlorpheniramine, pseudoephedrine, and dextromethorphan *on page 220*

PediaCare® NightRest Cough and Cold *(Discontinued)* *see* chlorpheniramine, pseudoephedrine, and dextromethorphan *on page 220*

Pediacof® *(Discontinued)* *see* chlorpheniramine, phenylephrine, codeine, and potassium iodide *on page 220*

Pediaflor® *(Discontinued)* *see* fluoride *on page 430*

PediaHist DM [US] *see* brompheniramine, pseudoephedrine, and dextromethorphan *on page 152*

Pedialyte® [US-OTC] *see* nutritional formula, enteral/oral *on page 715*

PediaPatch Transdermal Patch *(Discontinued)* *see* salicylic acid *on page 884*

Pediapred® [US/Can] *see* prednisolone (systemic) *on page 813*

Pedia-Profen™ *(Discontinued)* *see* ibuprofen *on page 515*

Pedia Relief™ [US-OTC] *see* chlorpheniramine, pseudoephedrine, and dextromethorphan *on page 220*

Pedia Relief Cough and Cold [US-OTC] *see* pseudoephedrine and dextromethorphan *on page 834*

Pedia Relief Infants [US-OTC] *see* pseudoephedrine and dextromethorphan *on page 834*

Pediarix® [US/Can] *see* diphtheria, tetanus toxoids, acellular pertussis, hepatitis B (recombinant), and poliovirus (inactivated) vaccine *on page 320*

PediaTan™ [US] *see* chlorpheniramine *on page 213*

PediaTan™ D [US] *see* chlorpheniramine and phenylephrine *on page 214*

Pediatex™ 12 *(Discontinued)* *see* carbinoxamine *on page 185*

Pediatex™-D *(Discontinued)*

Pediatex™ *(Discontinued)* *see* carbinoxamine *on page 185*

Pediatex™ DM *(Discontinued)*

Pediatex® TD [US] *see* triprolidine and pseudoephedrine *on page 989*

Pediatric Digoxin CSD [Can] *see* digoxin *on page 308*

Pediatric Triban® *(Discontinued)*

Pediatrix [Can] *see* acetaminophen *on page 19*

Pediazole® [Can] *see* erythromycin and sulfisoxazole *on page 370*

Pediazole® *(Discontinued)* *see* erythromycin and sulfisoxazole *on page 370*

Pedi-Boro® [US-OTC] *see* aluminum sulfate and calcium acetate *on page 57*

Pedi-Dri® [US] *see* nystatin *on page 715*

PediOtic® [US] *see* neomycin, polymyxin B, and hydrocortisone *on page 688*

Pedi-Pro® [US] *see* benzalkonium chloride *on page 129*

PedvaxHIB® [US/Can] *see Haemophilus* B conjugate vaccine *on page 483*

PEG *see* polyethylene glycol 3350 *on page 797*

PEG-L-asparaginase *see* pegaspargase *on page 755*

pegademase (bovine) (peg A de mase BOE vine)

U.S./Canadian Brand Names Adagen® [US/Can]

Therapeutic Category Enzyme

Use Enzyme replacement therapy for adenosine deaminase (ADA) deficiency in patients with severe combined immunodeficiency disease (SCID) who are not candidates for or who have failed bone marrow transplant

Usual Dosage Note: Dose should be individualized based on monitoring of plasma ADA activity levels and dATP content.

I.M.: Infants and Children: Dose given every 7 days, 10 units/kg the first dose, 15 units/kg the second dose, and 20 units/kg the third dose; maintenance dose: 20 units/kg/week is recommended depending on patient's ADA level; maximum single dose: 30 units/kg

Dosage Forms

Injection, solution [preservative free]:

Adagen®: 250 units/mL (1.5 mL)

Peganone® [US/Can] *see* ethotoin *on page 396*

pegaptanib (peg AP ta nib)

Synonyms EYE001; pegaptanib sodium

U.S./Canadian Brand Names Macugen® [US/Can]

Therapeutic Category Ophthalmic Agent; Vaccine, Recombinant

Use Treatment of neovascular (wet) age-related macular degeneration (AMD)

Usual Dosage Intravitreous injection: Adults: AMD: 0.3 mg into affected eye every 6 weeks

Dosage Forms

Injection, solution [preservative free; prefilled syringe]:

Macugen®: 0.3 mg/90 µL (90 µL)

pegaptanib sodium *see* pegaptanib *on page 755*

PEG-ASP *see* pegaspargase *on page 755*

PEG-asparaginase *see* pegaspargase *on page 755*

pegaspargase (peg AS par jase)

Sound-Alike/Look-Alike Issues

pegaspargase may be confused with asparaginase

Oncaspar® may be confused with Elspar®

Synonyms L-asparaginase with polyethylene glycol; PEG-ASP; PEG-asparaginase; PEG-L-asparaginase; PEGLA; polyethylene glycol-L-asparaginase

U.S./Canadian Brand Names Oncaspar® [US]

Therapeutic Category Antineoplastic Agent

Use Treatment of acute lymphocytic leukemia (ALL); treatment of ALL with previous hypersensitivity to native L-asparaginase

Usual Dosage Details concerning dosing in combinations regimens should also be consulted.

I.M., I.V.: Children and Adults: 2500 units/m^2 (as part of a combination chemotherapy regimen), not more frequently than every 14 days

Dosage Forms

Injection, solution [preservative free]:

Oncaspar®: 750 int. units/mL (5 mL)

Pegasys® [US/Can] *see* peginterferon alfa-2a *on page 756*

Pegetron® [Can] *see* peginterferon alfa-2b and ribavirin *(Canada only) on page 757*

pegfilgrastim (peg fil GRA stim)

Sound-Alike/Look-Alike Issues

Neulasta® may be confused with Neumega®, Neupogen®, and Lunesta®

Synonyms G-CSF (PEG conjugate); granulocyte colony stimulating factor (PEG conjugate); NSC-725961; pegylated G-CSF; SD/01

U.S./Canadian Brand Names Neulasta® [US/Can]

Therapeutic Category Colony-Stimulating Factor

Use To decrease the incidence of infection, by stimulation of granulocyte production, in patients with nonmyeloid malignancies receiving myelosuppressive therapy associated with a significant risk of febrile neutropenia

Usual Dosage SubQ: **Note:** Do not administer in the period between 14 days before and 24 hours after administration of cytotoxic chemotherapy. According to the NCCN guidelines, efficacy has been demonstrated with every-2-week chemotherapy regimens, however, benefit has not been demonstrated with regimens under a two-week duration

Adolescents >45 kg and Adults: 6 mg once per chemotherapy cycle, beginning 24-72 hours after completion of chemotherapy

Dosage Forms

Injection, solution [preservative free]:

Neulasta®: 10 mg/mL (0.6 mL)

peginterferon alfa-2a (peg in ter FEER on AL fa too aye)

Synonyms interferon alfa-2a (PEG conjugate); pegylated interferon alfa-2a

U.S./Canadian Brand Names Pegasys® [US/Can]

Therapeutic Category Interferon

Use Treatment of chronic hepatitis C (CHC), alone or in combination with ribavirin, in patients with compensated liver disease and not previously treated with alfa interferons (includes patients with histological evidence of cirrhosis [Child-Pugh class A] and patients with clinically-stable HIV disease); treatment of patients with HBeAg positive and HBeAg negative chronic hepatitis B with compensated liver disease and evidence of viral replication and liver inflammation

Usual Dosage SubQ: Adults:

Chronic hepatitis C (monoinfection or coinfection with HIV):

Monotherapy: 180 mcg once weekly for 48 weeks

Combination therapy with ribavirin: Recommended dosage: 180 mcg once/week with ribavirin (Copegus®)

Duration of therapy: Monoinfection (based on genotype):

Genotype 1,4: 48 weeks

Genotype 2,3: 24 weeks

Duration of therapy: Coinfection with HIV: 48 weeks

Note: *American Association for the Study of Liver Diseases (AASLD) guidelines recommendation:* Adults with chronic HCV infection: Treatment of choice: Ribavirin plus **peginterferon**; clinical condition and ability of patient to tolerate therapy should be evaluated to determine length and/or likely benefit of therapy. Recommended treatment duration (AASLD guidelines): Genotypes 1,4: 48 weeks; Genotypes 2,3: 24 weeks; Coinfection with HIV: 48 weeks.

Chronic hepatitis B: 180 mcg once weekly for 48 weeks

Dosage Forms

Injection, solution:

Pegasys®:

180 mcg/0.5 mL (0.5 mL) [prefilled syringe; contains benzyl alcohol and polysorbate 80; packaged with needles and alcohol swabs]

180 mcg/mL (1 mL) [vial; contains benzyl alcohol and polysorbate 80]

peginterferon alfa-2b (peg in ter FEER on AL fa too bee)

Sound-Alike/Look-Alike Issues

peginterferon alfa-2b may be confused with interferon alfa-2a, interferon alfa-2b, interferon alfa-n3, peginterferon alfa-2a

PegIntron™ may be confused with Intron® A

Synonyms interferon alfa-2b (PEG conjugate); pegylated interferon alfa-2b

U.S./Canadian Brand Names PegIntron™ Redipen® [Can]; PegIntron™ [US/Can]

Therapeutic Category Interferon

Use Treatment of chronic hepatitis C (in combination with ribavirin) in patients who have never received alfa interferons and have compensated liver disease; treatment of chronic hepatitis C (as monotherapy) in adult patients with compensated liver disease who have never received alfa interferons

Usual Dosage SubQ:

Children ≥3 years: Chronic hepatitis C:

Manufacturer labeling: Combination therapy with ribavirin: 60 mcg/m^2 once weekly (in combination with ribavirin 15 mg/kg/day in 2 divided doses); **Note:** Children who reach their 18th birthday during treatment should remain on the pediatric regimen. Treatment duration is 48 weeks for genotype 1, 24 weeks for genotypes 2 and 3. Discontinue combination therapy in patients with HCV (genotype 1) at 12 weeks if HCV-RNA decreases <2 log (compared to pretreatment) or if detectable HCV-RNA at 24 weeks.

American Association for the Study of Liver Diseases (AASLD) guideline recommendations: Children 2-17 years: Treatment of choice: **Peginterferon alfa-2b** 60 mcg/m^2 once weekly in combination with oral ribavirin 15 mg/kg/day for 48 weeks

Adults:

Chronic hepatitis C: Administer dose once weekly; **Note:** Treatment duration is 48 weeks for genotype 1, 24 weeks for genotypes 2 and 3, or 48 weeks for patients who previously failed therapy (regardless of genotype). Discontinue in patients with HCV (genotype 1) after 12 weeks if HCV RNA decreases <2 log (compared to pretreatment) or if detectable HCV RNA at 24 weeks.

Monotherapy: Initial: 1 mcg/kg/week

≤45 kg: 40 mcg once weekly
46-56 kg: 50 mcg once weekly
57-72 kg: 64 mcg once weekly
73-88 kg: 80 mcg once weekly
89-106 kg: 96 mcg once weekly
107-136 kg: 120 mcg once weekly
137-160 kg: 150 mcg once weekly

Combination therapy with ribavirin: Initial: 1.5 mcg/kg/week

<40 kg: 50 mcg once weekly (with ribavirin 800 mg/day)
40-50 kg: 64 mcg once weekly (with ribavirin 800 mg/day)
51-60 kg: 80 mcg once weekly (with ribavirin 800 mg/day)
61-65 kg: 96 mcg once weekly (with ribavirin 800 mg/day)
66-75 kg: 96 mcg once weekly (with ribavirin 1000 mg/day)
76-80 kg: 120 mcg once weekly (with ribavirin 1000 mg/day)
81-85 kg: 120 mcg once weekly (with ribavirin 1200 mg/day)
86-105 kg: 150 mcg once weekly (with ribavirin 1200 mg/day)
>105 kg: 1.5 mcg/kg once weekly (with ribavirin 1400 mg/day)

Note: *American Association for the Study of Liver Diseases (AASLD) guidelines recommendation:* Adults with chronic HCV infection: Treatment of choice: Ribavirin plus **peginterferon**; clinical condition and ability of patient to tolerate therapy should be evaluated to determine length and/or likely benefit of therapy. Recommended treatment duration (AASLD guidelines): Genotypes 1,4: 48 weeks; Genotypes 2,3: 24 weeks; Coinfection with HIV: 48 weeks.

Dosage Forms

Injection, powder for reconstitution [preservative free]:

PegIntron™: 50 mcg, 80 mcg, 120 mcg, 150 mcg
PegIntron™ Redipen®: 50 mcg, 80 mcg, 120 mcg, 150 mcg

peginterferon alfa-2b and ribavirin *(Canada only)*

(peg in ter FEER on AL fa too bee & rye ba VYE rin)

Synonyms ribavirin and peginterferon alfa-2b

U.S./Canadian Brand Names Pegetron® [Can]

Therapeutic Category Antiviral Agent; Interferon

Use Combination therapy for the treatment of chronic hepatitis C in patients with compensated liver disease

Usual Dosage Adults: **Note:** Canadian Consensus Guidelines recommend peginterferon plus ribavirin as treatment of choice for chronic hepatitis C.

Chronic hepatitis C: Recommended dosage of combination therapy:

Pegetron® peginterferon alfa-2b component: SubQ: 1.5 mcg/kg/week

and

Pegetron® ribavirin component: Oral:

≤64 kg: 800 mg/day (two 200 mg capsules in the morning and two 200 mg capsules in the evening)
64-84 kg: 1000 mg/day (two 200 mg capsules in the morning and three 200 mg capsules in the evening)
≥85 kg: 1200 mg/day (three 200 mg capsules in the morning and three 200 mg capsules in the evening)

Treatment duration: Canadian consensus guidelines:

HCV genotype 1: Treatment recommended for 48 weeks or may consider extended therapy up to 72 weeks in slow responders; may reduce treatment to 24 weeks in patients achieving RVR at 4 weeks **and** without poor response predictors (eg, high viral load, advanced fibrosis, elderly); discontinue therapy in patients failing to achieve EVR at 12 weeks or with detectable HCV RNA at 24 weeks; retreatment for 48 weeks is required in patients who relapse after discontinuing abbreviated therapy (24 weeks).

HCV genotypes 2,3: Treatment recommended for 24 weeks; may consider abbreviated therapy (12 or 16 weeks) in patients with weight-based ribavirin dosing and RVR; if relapse occurs following abbreviated therapy, retreat for 24 weeks

HCV genotype 4,5, and 6: Treatment recommended for 48 weeks; discontinue therapy in patients failing to achieve EVR at 12 weeks or with detectable HCV RNA at 24 weeks

Relapsing or nonresponding patients (regardless of genotype): Peginterferon/ribavirin therapy may be considered in patients that have relapsed or were nonresponsive to prior interferon monotherapy or interferon/ribavirin combination therapy; discontinue therapy if EVR not achieved after 12 weeks.

Dosage Forms [CAN] = Canadian product; not available in the U.S.

Combination package:

Pegetron® [CAN]:
Capsules: Ribavirin 200 mg (56s)
Injection, powder for reconstitution: Peginterferon alfa-2b: 50 mcg/0.5 mL

Pegetron® [CAN]:
Capsules: Ribavirin 200 mg (56s)
Injection, powder for reconstitution: Peginterferon alfa-2b: 80 mcg/0.5 mL

Pegetron® [CAN]:
Capsules: Ribavirin 200 mg (70s)
Injection, powder for reconstitution: Peginterferon alfa-2b: 100 mcg/0.5 mL

Pegetron® [CAN]:
Capsules: Ribavirin 200 mg (70s)
Injection, powder for reconstitution: Peginterferon alfa-2b: 120 mcg/0.5 mL

Pegetron® [CAN]:
Capsules: Ribavirin 200 mg (84s)
Injection, powder for reconstitution: Peginterferon alfa-2b: 150 mcg/0.5 mL

PegIntron™ [US/Can] *see* peginterferon alfa-2b *on page 756*
PegIntron™ Redipen® [Can] *see* peginterferon alfa-2b *on page 756*
PEGLA *see* pegaspargase *on page 755*
PegLyte® [Can] *see* polyethylene glycol-electrolyte solution *on page 797*

pegvisomant (peg VI soe mant)

Synonyms B2036-PEG

U.S./Canadian Brand Names Somavert® [US/Can]

Therapeutic Category Growth Hormone Receptor Antagonist

Use Treatment of acromegaly in patients resistant to or unable to tolerate other therapies

Usual Dosage SubQ: Adults: Initial loading dose: 40 mg; maintenance dose: 10 mg once daily; doses may be adjusted by 5 mg increments in 4- to 6-week intervals based on IGF-I concentrations (maximum maintenance dose: 30 mg/day)

Dosage Forms

Injection, powder for reconstitution [preservative free]:
Somavert®: 10 mg, 15 mg, 20 mg

pegylated G-CSF *see* pegfilgrastim *on page 755*
pegylated interferon alfa-2a *see* peginterferon alfa-2a *on page 756*
pegylated interferon alfa-2b *see* peginterferon alfa-2b *on page 756*
pegylated liposomal DOXOrubicin *see* doxorubicin (liposomal) *on page 336*
PE-Hist DM [US] *see* chlorpheniramine, phenylephrine, and dextromethorphan *on page 217*

pemetrexed (pem e TREKS ed)

Synonyms LY231514; pemetrexed disodium

U.S./Canadian Brand Names Alimta® [US/Can]

Therapeutic Category Antineoplastic Agent, Antimetabolite; Antineoplastic Agent, Antimetabolite (Antifolate)

Use Treatment of unresectable malignant pleural mesothelioma (in combination with cisplatin); treatment of locally advanced or metastatic nonsquamous nonsmall cell lung cancer (NSCLC; as initial treatment in combination with cisplatin, as single-agent maintenance treatment after 4 cycles of initial platinum-based doublet therapy, and single-agent treatment after prior chemotherapy)

Usual Dosage Details concerning dosing in combination regimens should also be consulted. **Note:** Start vitamin supplements 1 week before initial pemetrexed dose: Folic acid 350-1000 mcg/day orally (must be taken at least 5 out of 7 days prior to treatment initiation; continue during treatment and for 21 days after last pemetrexed dose) and vitamin B_{12} 1000 mcg I.M. during the week prior to treatment initiation and then every 3 cycles. Give dexamethasone 4 mg orally twice daily for 3 days, beginning the day before treatment to minimize cutaneous reactions. New treatment cycles should not begin unless ANC ≥1500/mm^3, platelets ≥100,000/mm^3, and Cl_{cr} ≥45 mL/minute.

I.V.: Adults:

Malignant pleural mesothelioma: 500 mg/m^2 on day 1 of each 21-day cycle (in combination with cisplatin)

Nonsmall cell lung cancer:

Initial treatment: 500 mg/m^2 on day 1 of each 21-day cycle (in combination with cisplatin)

Maintenance or second-line treatment: 500 mg/m^2 on day 1 of each 21-day cycle (as a single-agent)

Dosage Forms

Injection, powder for reconstitution:

Alimta®: 100 mg, 500 mg

pemetrexed disodium *see* pemetrexed *on page* 758

pemirolast (pe MIR oh last)

U.S./Canadian Brand Names Alamast® [US/Can]

Therapeutic Category Mast Cell Stabilizer; Ophthalmic Agent, Miscellaneous

Use Prevention of itching of the eye due to allergic conjunctivitis

Usual Dosage Children >3 years and Adults: 1-2 drops instilled in affected eye(s) 4 times/day

Dosage Forms

Solution, ophthalmic:

Alamast®: 0.1% (10 mL)

pemoline *(Discontinued)*

penbutolol (pen BYOO toe lole)

Sound-Alike/Look-Alike Issues

Levatol® may be confused with Lipitor®

Synonyms penbutolol sulfate

U.S./Canadian Brand Names Levatol® [US/Can]

Therapeutic Category Beta-Adrenergic Blocker

Use Treatment of mild-to-moderate arterial hypertension

Usual Dosage Oral: Adults: Initial: 20 mg once daily, full effect of a 20 or 40 mg dose is seen by the end of a 2-week period, doses of 40-80 mg have been tolerated but have shown little additional antihypertensive effects; usual dose range (JNC 7): 10-40 mg once daily

Dosage Forms

Tablet:

Levatol®: 20 mg

penbutolol sulfate *see* penbutolol *on page* 759

penciclovir (pen SYE kloe veer)

Sound-Alike/Look-Alike Issues

Denavir® may be confused with indinavir

U.S./Canadian Brand Names Denavir® [US]

Therapeutic Category Antiviral Agent

Use Topical treatment of herpes simplex labialis (cold sores)

Usual Dosage Topical: Children ≥12 years and Adults: Apply cream at the first sign or symptom of cold sore (eg, tingling, swelling); apply every 2 hours during waking hours for 4 days

Dosage Forms

Cream:

Denavir®: 1% (1.5 g)

Pendex [US] *see* guaifenesin and phenylephrine *on page* 475

Penetrex® *(Discontinued)*

penicillamine (pen i SIL a meen)

Sound-Alike/Look-Alike Issues

penicillamine may be confused with penicillin

Depen® may be confused with Endal®

Synonyms D-3-mercaptovaline; D-penicillamine; β,β-dimethylcysteine

U.S./Canadian Brand Names Cuprimine® [US/Can]; Depen® [US/Can]

Therapeutic Category Chelating Agent

Use Treatment of Wilson disease, cystinuria; adjunctive treatment of rheumatoid arthritis

Usual Dosage Oral:

Rheumatoid arthritis: Adults: 125-250 mg/day, may increase dose at 1- to 3-month intervals up to 1-1.5 g/day; maximum in older adults: 750 mg/day

Wilson disease (doses titrated to maintain urinary copper excretion >2 mg/day); decrease dose for surgery and during last trimester of pregnancy

Children <12 years: 20 mg/kg/day in 2-3 divided doses, round off to the nearest 250 mg dose; maximum: 1 g/day

Adults: 250 mg 4 times/day (maximum in older adults: 750 mg/day)

Cystinuria: **Note:** Adjust dose to limit cystine excretion to 100-200 mg/day (<100 mg/day with history of stone formation)

Children: 30 mg/kg/day in 4 divided doses

Dosage Forms

Capsule:

Cuprimine®: 250 mg

Tablet:

Depen®: 250 mg

penicillin G benzathine (pen i SIL in jee BENZ a theen)

Sound-Alike/Look-Alike Issues

penicillin may be confused with penicillamine

Bicillin® may be confused with Wycillin®

Bicillin® C-R (penicillin G benzathine and penicillin G procaine) may be confused with Bicillin® L-A (penicillin G benzathine). Penicillin G benzathine is the only product currently approved for the treatment of syphilis. Administration of penicillin G benzathine and penicillin G procaine combination instead of Bicillin® L-A may result in inadequate treatment response.

Synonyms benzathine benzylpenicillin; benzathine penicillin G; benzylpenicillin benzathine

U.S./Canadian Brand Names Bicillin® L-A [US/Can]

Therapeutic Category Penicillin

Use Active against some gram-positive organisms, few gram-negative organisms such as *Neisseria gonorrhoeae*, and some anaerobes and spirochetes; used in the treatment of syphilis; used only for the treatment of mild to moderately severe infections caused by organisms susceptible to low concentrations of penicillin G or for prophylaxis of infections caused by these organisms

Usual Dosage Note: Administer undiluted injection; higher doses result in more sustained rather than higher levels. Use a penicillin G benzathine-penicillin G procaine combination to achieve early peak levels in acute infections.

Usual dosage range:

Children: I.M.: 25,000-50,000 units/kg as a single dose (maximum: 2.4 million units)

Adults: I.M.: 1.2-2.4 million units as a single dose

Indication-specific dosing:

Neonates >1200 g: I.M.:

Congenital syphilis (asymptomatic): 50,000 units/kg as a single dose

Infants and Children: I.M.:

Group A streptococcal upper respiratory infection: 25,000-50,000 units/kg as a single dose (maximum: 1.2 million units)

Prophylaxis of recurrent rheumatic fever: 25,000-50,000 units/kg every 3-4 weeks (maximum: 1.2 million units/dose)

Syphilis:

Early: 50,000 units/kg as a single injection (maximum: 2.4 million units)

More than 1-year duration: 50,000 units/kg every week for 3 doses (maximum: 2.4 million units/dose)

Adults: I.M.:

Group A streptococcal upper respiratory infection: 1.2 million units as a single dose

Prophylaxis of recurrent rheumatic fever: 1.2 million units every 3-4 weeks or 600,000 units twice monthly

Syphilis:

Early: 2.4 million units as a single dose in 2 injection sites

More than 1-year duration: 2.4 million units in 2 injection sites once weekly for 3 doses

Neurosyphilis: Not indicated as single-drug therapy, but may be given once weekly for 3 weeks following I.V. treatment; refer to penicillin G (parenteral/aqueous) monograph for dosing

Dosage Forms

Injection, suspension [prefilled syringe]:

Bicillin® L-A: 600,000 units/mL (1 mL, 2 mL, 4 mL)

penicillin G benzathine and penicillin G procaine

(pen i SIL in jee BENZ a theen & pen i SIL in jee PROE kane)

Sound-Alike/Look-Alike Issues

penicillin may be confused with penicillamine

Bicillin® may be confused with Wycillin®

Bicillin® C-R (penicillin G benzathine and penicillin G procaine) may be confused with Bicillin® L-A (penicillin G benzathine). Penicillin G benzathine is the only product currently approved for the treatment of syphilis. Administration of penicillin G benzathine and penicillin G procaine combination instead of Bicillin® L-A may result in inadequate treatment response.

Synonyms penicillin G procaine and benzathine combined

U.S./Canadian Brand Names Bicillin® C-R 900/300 [US]; Bicillin® C-R [US]

Therapeutic Category Penicillin

Use May be used in specific situations in the treatment of streptococcal infections

Usual Dosage **Usual dosage range and indication-specific dosing:**

Streptococcal infections:

Children: I.M.:

<14 kg: 600,000 units in a single dose

14-27 kg: 900,000 units to 1.2 million units in a single dose

Children >27 kg and Adults: 2.4 million units in a single dose

Dosage Forms

Injection, suspension [prefilled syringe]:

Bicillin® C-R: 1,200,000 units: Penicillin G benzathine 600,000 units and penicillin G procaine 600,000 units per 2 mL (2 mL)

Bicillin® C-R 900/300: 1,200,000 units: Penicillin G benzathine 900,000 units and penicillin G procaine 300,000 units per 2 mL (2 mL)

penicillin G (parenteral/aqueous) (pen i SIL in jee, pa REN ter al, AYE kwee us)

Sound-Alike/Look-Alike Issues

penicillin may be confused with penicillamine

Synonyms benzylpenicillin potassium; benzylpenicillin sodium; crystalline penicillin; penicillin G potassium; penicillin G sodium

U.S./Canadian Brand Names Crystapen® [Can]; Pfizerpen® [US]

Therapeutic Category Penicillin

Use Treatment of infections (including sepsis, pneumonia, pericarditis, endocarditis, meningitis, anthrax) caused by susceptible organisms; active against some gram-positive organisms, generally not *Staphylococcus aureus*; some gram-negative organisms such as *Neisseria gonorrhoeae*, and some anaerobes and spirochetes

Usual Dosage

Usual dosage range:

Infants >1 month and Children: I.M., I.V.: 100,000-400,000 units/kg/day in divided doses every 4-6 hours (maximum dose: 24 million units/day)

Adults: I.M., I.V.: 2-30 million units/day in divided doses every 4-6 hours depending on sensitivity of the organism and severity of the infection

Indication-specific dosing:

Infants >1 month and Children:

Meningitis **(gonococcal):** I.V.: 250,000 units/kg/day in 4 divided doses

Moderate infections: I.M., I.V.: 100,000-250,000 units/kg/day in 4 divided doses

Severe infections: I.M., I.V.: 250,000-400,000 units/kg/day in divided doses every 4-6 hours (maximum dose: 24 million units/day)

Syphilis (congenital): Infants: I.V.: 50,000 units/kg every 4-6 hours for 10 days

Adults:

Actinomyces **species:** I.V.: 10-20 million units/day in divided doses every 4-6 hours for 4-6 weeks

Clostridium perfringens: I.V.: 24 million units/day in divided doses every 4-6 hours with clindamycin

Corynebacterium diphtheriae: I.V.: 2-3 million units/day in divided doses every 4-6 hours for 10-12 days
Erysipelas: I.V.: 1-2 million units every 4-6 hours
Erysipelothrix: I.V.: 2-4 million units every 4 hours
Fascial space infections: I.V.: 2-4 million units every 4-6 hours with metronidazole
Leptospirosis: I.V.: 1.5 million units every 6 hours for 7 days
Listeria: I.V.: 15-20 million units/day in divided doses every 4-6 hours for 2 weeks (meningitis) or 4 weeks (endocarditis)
Lyme disease (meningitis): I.V.: 20 million units/day in divided doses
Neurosyphilis: I.V.: 18-24 million units/day in divided doses every 4 hours (or by continuous infusion) for 10-14 days
Streptococcus:
Brain abscess: I.V.: 18-24 million units/day in divided doses every 4 hours with metronidazole
Endocarditis or osteomyelitis: I.V.: 3-4 million units every 4 hours for at least 4 weeks
Pregnancy (prophylaxis GBS): I.V.: 5 million units x 1 dose, then 2.5 million units every 4 hours until delivery
Skin and soft tissue: I.V.: 3-4 million units every 4 hours for 10 days
Toxic shock: I.V.: 24 million units/day in divided doses with clindamycin
Streptococcal pneumonia: I.V.: 2-3 million units every 4 hours
Whipple disease: I.V.: 2 million units every 4 hours for 2 weeks, followed by oral trimethoprim/sulfamethoxazole or doxycycline for 1 year
Relapse or CNS involvement: 4 million units every 4 hours for 4 weeks

Dosage Forms
Infusion, as potassium [premixed iso-osmotic dextrose solution, frozen]: 1 million units (50 mL), 2 million units (50 mL), 3 million units (50 mL)
Injection, powder for reconstitution: 5 million units, 20 million units
Pfizerpen®: 5 million units, 20 million units

penicillin G potassium *see* penicillin G (parenteral/aqueous) *on page 761*

penicillin G procaine (pen i SIL in jee PROE kane)

Sound-Alike/Look-Alike Issues
penicillin G procaine may be confused with penicillin V potassium
Wycillin® may be confused with Bicillin®

Synonyms APPG; aqueous procaine penicillin G; procaine benzylpenicillin; procaine penicillin G

U.S./Canadian Brand Names Pfizerpen-AS® [Can]; Wycillin® [Can]

Therapeutic Category Penicillin

Use Treatment of moderately-severe infections due to *Treponema pallidum* and other penicillin G-sensitive microorganisms that are susceptible to low, but prolonged serum penicillin concentrations; anthrax due to *Bacillus anthracis* (postexposure) to reduce the incidence or progression of disease following exposure to aerolized *Bacillus anthracis*

Usual Dosage
Usual dosage range:
Infants and Children: I.M.: 25,000-50,000 units/kg/day in divided doses 1-2 times/day; (maximum: 4.8 million units/day)
Adults: I.M.: 0.6-4.8 million units/day in divided doses every 12-24 hours
Indication-specific dosing:
Children: I.M.:
Anthrax, inhalational (postexposure prophylaxis): 25,000 units/kg every 12 hours (maximum: 1,200,000 units every 12 hours); see **"Note"** in Adults dosing
Syphilis (congenital): 50,000 units/kg/day for 10 days; if more than 1 day of therapy is missed, the entire course should be restarted
Adults: I.M.:
Anthrax:
Inhalational (postexposure prophylaxis): 1,200,000 units every 12 hours
Note: Overall treatment duration should be 60 days. Available safety data suggest continued administration of penicillin G procaine for longer than 2 weeks may incur additional risk for adverse reactions. Clinicians may consider switching to effective alternative treatment for completion of therapy beyond 2 weeks.
Cutaneous (treatment): 600,000-1,200,000 units/day; alternative therapy is recommended in severe cutaneous or other forms of anthrax infection

Endocarditis caused by susceptible viridans *Streptococcus* (when used in conjunction with an aminoglycoside): 1.2 million units every 6 hours for 2-4 weeks
Gonorrhea (uncomplicated): 4.8 million units as a single dose divided in 2 sites given 30 minutes after probenecid 1 g orally
Neurosyphilis: 2.4 million units/day with 500 mg probenecid by mouth 4 times/day for 10-14 days; **Note: Penicillin G aqueous I.V. is the preferred agent**
Whipple disease: 1.2 million units/day (with streptomycin) for 10-14 days, followed by oral trimethoprim/sulfamethoxazole or doxycycline for 1 year

Dosage Forms
Injection, suspension: 600,000 units/mL (1 mL, 2 mL)

penicillin G procaine and benzathine combined *see* penicillin G benzathine and penicillin G procaine *on page 761*

penicillin G sodium *see* penicillin G (parenteral/aqueous) *on page 761*

penicillin V potassium (pen i SIL in vee poe TASS ee um)

Sound-Alike/Look-Alike Issues
penicillin V procaine may be confused with penicillin G potassium

Synonyms pen VK; phenoxymethyl penicillin

U.S./Canadian Brand Names Apo-Pen VK® [Can]; Novo-Pen-VK [Can]; Nu-Pen-VK [Can]

Therapeutic Category Penicillin

Use Treatment of infections caused by susceptible organisms involving the respiratory tract, otitis media, sinusitis, skin, and urinary tract; prophylaxis in rheumatic fever

Usual Dosage
Usual dosage range:
Children <12 years: Oral: 25-50 mg/kg/day in divided doses every 6-8 hours (maximum dose: 3 g/day)
Children ≥12 years and Adults: Oral: 125-500 mg every 6-8 hours
Indication-specific dosing:
Children: Oral:
Pharyngitis (streptococcal): 250 mg 2-3 times/day for 10 days
Prophylaxis of pneumococcal infections:
Children <5 years: 125 mg twice daily
Children ≥5 years: 250 mg twice daily
Prophylaxis of recurrent rheumatic fever:
Children <5 years: 125 mg twice daily
Children ≥5 years: 250 mg twice daily
Adults: Oral:
Acintomycosis:
Mild: 2-4 g/day in 4 divided doses for 8 weeks
Surgical: 2-4 g/day in 4 divided doses for 6-12 months (after I.V. penicillin G therapy of 4-6 weeks)
Erysipelas: 500 mg 4 times/day
Periodontal infections: 250-500 mg every 6 hours for 5-7 days
Note: Efficacy of antimicrobial therapy in periapical abscess is questionable; the American Academy of Periodontology recommends use of antibiotic therapy only when systemic symptoms (eg, fever, lymphadenopathy) are present or in immunocompromised patients.
Pharyngitis (streptococcal): 500 mg 3-4 times/day for 10 days
Prophylaxis of pneumococcal or recurrent rheumatic fever infections: 250 mg twice daily

Dosage Forms 250 mg = 400,000 units
Powder for oral solution: 125 mg/5 mL, 250 mg/5 mL
Tablet: 250 mg, 500 mg

Penlac® [US/Can] *see* ciclopirox *on page 227*

Pennsaid® [Can] *see* diclofenac *on page 303*

Pentacarinat® Injection *(Discontinued)* *see* pentamidine *on page 763*

Pentacel® [US] *see* diphtheria and tetanus toxoids, acellular pertussis, poliovirus and *Haemophilus* b conjugate vaccine *on page 320*

pentahydrate *see* sodium thiosulfate *on page 915*

Pentam-300® [US] *see* pentamidine *on page 763*

pentamidine (pen TAM i deen)

Synonyms pentamidine isethionate

U.S./Canadian Brand Names NebuPent® [US]; Pentam-300® [US]; Pentamidine Isetionate for Injection [Can]

Therapeutic Category Antiprotozoal

Use Treatment and prevention of pneumonia caused by *Pneumocystis jiroveci* (PCP)

Usual Dosage

Children:

Treatment of PCP pneumonia: I.M., I.V. (I.V. preferred): 4 mg/kg/day once daily for 10-14 days

Prevention of PCP pneumonia:

I.M., I.V.: 4 mg/kg monthly or every 2 weeks

Inhalation (aerosolized pentamidine in children ≥5 years): 300 mg/dose given every 3-4 weeks via Respirgard® II inhaler (8 mg/kg dose has also been used in children <5 years)

Adults:

Treatment: I.M., I.V. (I.V. preferred): 4 mg/kg/day once daily for 14-21 days

Prevention: Inhalation: 300 mg every 4 weeks via Respirgard® II nebulizer

Dosage Forms

Injection, powder for reconstitution: [preservative free]:

Pentam-300®: 300 mg

Powder for solution, for nebulization: [preservative free]:

NebuPent®: 300 mg

pentamidine isethionate *see* pentamidine *on page* 763

Pentamidine Isetionate for Injection [Can] *see* pentamidine *on page* 763

Pentamycetin® [Can] *see* chloramphenicol *on page* 208

Pentasa® [US/Can] *see* mesalamine *on page* 631

pentasodium colistin methanesulfonate *see* colistimethate *on page* 254

Pentaspan® [US/Can] *see* pentastarch *on page* 764

pentastarch (PEN ta starch)

U.S./Canadian Brand Names Pentaspan® [US/Can]

Therapeutic Category Blood Modifiers

Use Orphan drug: Adjunct in leukapheresis to improve harvesting and increase yield of leukocytes by centrifugal means

Usual Dosage 250-700 mL to which citrate anticoagulant has been added is administered by adding to the input line of the centrifugation apparatus at a ratio of 1:8-1:13 to venous whole blood

Dosage Forms

Infusion [premixed in NS]:

Pentaspan®: 10% (500 mL)

Penta-Triamterene HCTZ [Can] *see* hydrochlorothiazide and triamterene *on page* 500

pentavalent human-bovine reassortant rotavirus vaccine (PRV) *see* rotavirus vaccine *on page* 880

pentazocine (pen TAZ oh seen)

Synonyms naloxone hydrochloride and pentazocine hydrochloride; pentazocine hydrochloride; pentazocine hydrochloride and naloxone hydrochloride; pentazocine lactate

U.S./Canadian Brand Names Talwin® Nx [US]; Talwin® [US/Can]

Therapeutic Category Analgesic, Narcotic

Controlled Substance C-IV

Use

Talwin®: Relief of moderate-to-severe pain; has also been used as a sedative prior to surgery and as a supplement to surgical anesthesia

Talwin® Nx: Relief of moderate-to-severe pain; indicated for oral use only

Usual Dosage

Preoperative/preanesthetic: Children 1-16 years: I.M.: 0.5 mg/kg

Analgesia:

Children: I.M.:

5-8 years: 15 mg

8-14 years: 30 mg

Children >12 years and Adults: Oral: 50 mg every 3-4 hours; may increase to 100 mg/dose if needed, but should not exceed 600 mg/day (maximum: 12 tablets/day)

Adults:
I.M., SubQ: 30-60 mg every 3-4 hours; do not exceed 60 mg/dose (maximum: 360 mg/day)
I.V.: 30 mg every 3-4 hours; do not exceed 30 mg/dose (maximum: 360 mg/day)

Dosage Forms

Injection, solution:
Talwin®: 30 mg/mL (1 mL, 10 mL)
Tablet: Pentazocine 50 mg and naloxone 0.5 mg
Talwin® Nx: Pentazocine 50 mg and naloxone 0.5 mg

pentazocine and acetaminophen (pen TAZ oh seen & a seet a MIN oh fen)

Sound-Alike/Look-Alike Issues
Talacen® may be confused with Tegison®, Timoptic®, Tinactin®

Synonyms acetaminophen and pentazocine; pentazocine hydrochloride and acetaminophen

U.S./Canadian Brand Names Talacen® [US]

Therapeutic Category Analgesic Combination (Opioid)

Controlled Substance C-IV

Use Relief of mild-to-moderate pain

Usual Dosage Oral: Adults: Analgesic: 1 caplet every 4 hours (maximum: 6 caplets/day)

Dosage Forms

Caplet: Pentazocine 25 mg and acetaminophen 650 mg
Talacen®: Pentazocine 25 mg and acetaminophen 650 mg
Tablet: Pentazocine 25 mg and acetaminophen 650 mg

pentazocine hydrochloride *see* pentazocine *on page 764*
pentazocine hydrochloride and acetaminophen *see* pentazocine and acetaminophen *on page 765*
pentazocine hydrochloride and naloxone hydrochloride *see* pentazocine *on page 764*
pentazocine lactate *see* pentazocine *on page 764*
pentetate calcium trisodium *see* diethylene triamine penta-acetic acid *on page 306*
pentetate zinc trisodium *see* diethylene triamine penta-acetic acid *on page 306*
Penthrane® ***(Discontinued)***

pentobarbital (pen toe BAR bi tal)

Sound-Alike/Look-Alike Issues
PENTobarbital may be confused with PHENobarbital
Nembutal® may be confused with Myambutol®

Synonyms pentobarbital sodium

Tall-Man PENTobarbital

U.S./Canadian Brand Names Nembutal® Sodium [Can]; Nembutal® [US]

Therapeutic Category Barbiturate

Controlled Substance C-II

Use Sedative/hypnotic; refractory status epilepticus

Usual Dosage

Children:
Hypnotic: I.M.: 2-6 mg/kg; maximum: 100 mg/dose
Preoperative/preprocedure sedation: ≥6 months:
Note: Limited information is available for infants <6 months of age.
I.M.: 2-6 mg/kg; maximum: 100 mg/dose
I.V.: 1-3 mg/kg to a maximum of 100 mg until asleep
Conscious sedation prior to a procedure: Children 5-12 years: I.V.: 2 mg/kg 5-10 minutes before procedures, may repeat one time
Adolescents: Conscious sedation: I.V.: 100 mg prior to a procedure
Status epilepticus: I.V.: **Note**: Intubation required; monitor hemodynamics
Children: Loading dose: 5-15 mg/kg given slowly over 1-2 hours; maintenance infusion: 0.5-5 mg/kg/hour
Adults: Loading dose: 10-20 mg/kg given slowly over 1-2 hours; maintenance infusion: 0.5-3 mg/kg/hour

Adults:
Hypnotic:
I.M.: 150-200 mg
I.V.: Initial: 100 mg, may repeat every 1-3 minutes up to 200-500 mg total dose
Preoperative sedation: I.M.: 150-200 mg
Refractory status epilepticus: I.V.: Loading dose: 10-20 mg/kg given slowly over 1-2 hours; maintenance infusion: 0.5-3 mg/kg/hour. **Note:** Intubation required; monitor hemodynamics.

Dosage Forms

Injection, solution:
Nembutal®: 50 mg/mL (20 mL, 50 mL)

pentobarbital sodium *see* pentobarbital *on page* *765*

pentosan polysulfate sodium (PEN toe san pol i SUL fate SOW dee um)

Sound-Alike/Look-Alike Issues
pentosan may be confused with pentostatin
Elmiron® may be confused with Imuran®

Synonyms PPS

U.S./Canadian Brand Names Elmiron® [US/Can]

Therapeutic Category Analgesic, Urinary

Use Relief of bladder pain or discomfort due to interstitial cystitis

Usual Dosage Oral: Children ≥16 years and Adults: 100 mg 3 times/day taken with water 1 hour before or 2 hours after meals

Note: Patients should be evaluated at 3 months and may be continued an additional 3 months if there has been no improvement and if there are no therapy-limiting side effects. **The risks and benefits of continued use beyond 6 months in patients who have not responded is not yet known**.

Dosage Forms

Capsule:
Elmiron®: 100 mg

pentostatin (pen toe STAT in)

Sound-Alike/Look-Alike Issues
pentostatin may be confused with pentamidine, pentosan

Synonyms 2′-deoxycoformycin; co-vidarabine; dCF; deoxycoformycin; NSC-218321

U.S./Canadian Brand Names Nipent® [US/Can]

Therapeutic Category Antineoplastic Agent

Use Treatment of hairy cell leukemia

Usual Dosage I.V.: Adults (refer to individual protocols): Hairy cell leukemia: 4 mg/m^2 every 2 weeks

Dosage Forms

Injection, powder for reconstitution [preservative free]: 10 mg
Nipent®: 10 mg

Pentothal® [US/Can] *see* thiopental *on page* *955*
Pentothal® Sodium Rectal Suspension *(Discontinued)* *see* thiopental *on page* *955*

pentoxifylline (pen toks IF i lin)

Sound-Alike/Look-Alike Issues
pentoxifylline may be confused with tamoxifen
Trental® may be confused with Bentyl®, Tegretol®, Trandate®

Synonyms oxpentifylline

U.S./Canadian Brand Names Albert® Pentoxifylline [Can]; Apo-Pentoxifylline SR® [Can]; Nu-Pentoxifylline SR [Can]; Pentoxil® [US]; ratio-Pentoxifylline [Can]; Trental® [US/Can]

Therapeutic Category Blood Viscosity Reducer Agent

Use Treatment of intermittent claudication on the basis of chronic occlusive arterial disease of the limbs; may improve function and symptoms, but not intended to replace more definitive therapy

Usual Dosage Oral: Adults: 400 mg 3 times/day with meals; maximal therapeutic benefit may take 2-4 weeks to develop; recommended to maintain therapy for at least 8 weeks. May reduce to 400 mg twice daily if GI or CNS side effects occur.

Dosage Forms

Tablet, controlled release:
Trental®: 400 mg

Tablet, extended release: 400 mg
Pentoxil®: 400 mg

Pentoxil® [US] *see* pentoxifylline *on page 766*
Pen.Vee® K *(Discontinued)* *see* penicillin V potassium *on page 763*
pen VK *see* penicillin V potassium *on page 763*
Pepcid® [US/Can] *see* famotidine *on page 405*
Pepcid® AC [US-OTC/Can] *see* famotidine *on page 405*
Pepcid® AC Maximum Strength [US-OTC] *see* famotidine *on page 405*
Pepcid® Complete [US-OTC/Can] *see* famotidine, calcium carbonate, and magnesium hydroxide *on page 406*
Pepcid® I.V. [Can] *see* famotidine *on page 405*
Pepcid RPD® *(Discontinued)* *see* famotidine *on page 405*
Peptic Relief [US-OTC] *see* bismuth *on page 142*
Pepto-Bismol® [US-OTC] *see* bismuth *on page 142*
Pepto-Bismol® Maximum Strength [US-OTC] *see* bismuth *on page 142*
Pepto® Diarrhea Control *(Discontinued)* *see* loperamide *on page 597*
Pepto Relief [US-OTC] *see* bismuth *on page 142*
Peranex™ HC [US] *see* lidocaine and hydrocortisone *on page 587*
Peranex™ HC Medi-Pad [US] *see* lidocaine and hydrocortisone *on page 587*
Perchloracap® *(Discontinued)*
Percocet® [US/Can] *see* oxycodone and acetaminophen *on page 738*
Percocet®-Demi [Can] *see* oxycodone and acetaminophen *on page 738*
Percodan® [US/Can] *see* oxycodone and aspirin *on page 739*
Percodan®-Demi *(Discontinued)* *see* oxycodone and aspirin *on page 739*
Percogesic® [US-OTC] *see* acetaminophen and phenyltoloxamine *on page 23*
Percogesic® Extra Strength [US-OTC] *see* acetaminophen and diphenhydramine *on page 21*
Percolone® *(Discontinued)* *see* oxycodone *on page 737*
Perdiem® Overnight Relief [US-OTC] *see* senna *on page 896*
Perfectoderm® Gel *(Discontinued)* *see* benzoyl peroxide *on page 132*

perflutren lipid microspheres (per FLOO tren LIP id MIKE roe sfeers)

U.S./Canadian Brand Names Definity® [US/Can]

Therapeutic Category Diagnostic Agent

Use Opacification of left ventricular chamber and improvement of delineation of the left ventricular endocardial border in patients with suboptimal echocardiograms

Usual Dosage Adults: Dose should be given following baseline noncontrast echocardiography. Imaging should begin immediately following dose and compared to noncontrast image. Mechanical index for the ultrasound device should be set at ≤0.8. **Note:** Maximum dose is either two I.V. bolus doses or one single I.V. infusion.

I.V. bolus: 10 microliters (µL)/kg of activated product, followed by 10 mL saline flush; may repeat in 30 minutes if needed

I.V. infusion: Initial: 4 mL/minute (or 240 mL/hour) of prepared infusion; titrate to achieve optimal image; maximum rate: 10 mL/minute (or 600 mL/hour)

Dosage Forms

Injection, solution [preservative free]:
Definity®: OFP 6.52 mg/mL and lipid blend 0.75 mg/mL (2 mL)

Perforomist™ [US] *see* formoterol *on page 443*
Pergonal® *(Discontinued)* *see* menotropins *on page 625*
Periactin® *(Discontinued)* *see* cyproheptadine *on page 268*

periciazine *(Canada only)* (per ee CYE ah zeen)

Synonyms pericyazine

U.S./Canadian Brand Names Neuleptil® [Can]

Therapeutic Category Phenothiazine Derivative

Use Adjunctive therapy in selected psychotic patients to control prevailing hostility, impulsivity, or aggression

Usual Dosage Oral:

Children >5 years: 2.5-10 mg in the morning, followed by 5-30 mg in the evening. In general, lower dosage should be used on initiation and gradually increased based on effect and tolerance.

Adults: 5-20 mg in the morning, followed by 10-40 mg in the evening. In dividing doses, it is suggested that the larger dose should be administered in the evening. In general, lower dosage should be used on initiation and gradually increased based on effect and tolerance.

Dosage Forms [CAN] = Canadian brand name

Capsule:

Neuleptil® [CAN]: 5 mg, 10 mg, 20 mg [not available in the U.S.]

Solution, oral drops:

Neuleptil® [CAN]: 10 mg/mL [not available in the U.S.]

Peri-Colace® [US-OTC] *see* docusate and senna *on page* 327

pericyazine *see* periciazine *(Canada only) on page* 767

Peridex® [US] *see* chlorhexidine gluconate *on page* 210

Peridex® Oral Rinse [Can] *see* chlorhexidine gluconate *on page* 210

Peridol [Can] *see* haloperidol *on page* 484

perindopril and indapamide *see* perindopril erbumine and indapamide *(Canada only) on page* 768

perindopril erbumine (per IN doe pril er BYOO meen)

U.S./Canadian Brand Names Aceon® [US]; Apo-Perindopril® [Can]; Coversyl® [Can]

Therapeutic Category Miscellaneous Product

Use Treatment of hypertension; reduction of cardiovascular mortality or nonfatal myocardial infarction in patients with stable coronary artery disease

Usual Dosage Oral: Adults:

Hypertension: Initial: 4 mg/day but may be titrated to response; usual range: 4-8 mg/day (may be given in 2 divided doses); increase at 1- to 2-week intervals (maximum: 16 mg/day)

Concomitant therapy with diuretics: To reduce the risk of hypotension, discontinue diuretic, if possible, 2-3 days prior to initiating perindopril. If unable to stop diuretic, initiate perindopril at 2-4 mg/day and monitor blood pressure closely for the first 2 weeks of therapy, and after any dose adjustment of perindopril or diuretic.

Stable coronary artery disease: Initial: 4 mg once daily for 2 weeks; increase as tolerated to 8 mg once daily.

Dosage Forms

Tablet:

Aceon®: 2 mg, 4 mg, 8 mg

perindopril erbumine and indapamide *(Canada only)*

(per IN doe pril er BYOO meen & in DAP a mide)

Synonyms indapamide and perindopril erbumine; perindopril and indapamide

U.S./Canadian Brand Names Coversyl® Plus [Can]

Therapeutic Category Angiotensin-Converting Enzyme (ACE) Inhibitor; Antihypertensive Agent, Combination; Diuretic, Thiazide-Related

Use Treatment of hypertension; not indicated for initial treatment of hypertension

Usual Dosage **Note: Not for initial therapy. Titration of individual components to an appropriate clinical response is required prior to converting to an equivalent dose of the combination product.**

Oral: Adults: Hypertension: Usual maintenance dose: Perindopril 4 mg/indapamide 1.25 mg once daily

Dosage Forms [CAN] = Canadian brand name

Tablet:

Coversyl® Plus [CAN]: Perindopril erbumine 4 mg and indapamide 1.25 mg [not available in the U.S.]

PerioChip® [US] *see* chlorhexidine gluconate *on page* 210

PerioGard® [US] *see* chlorhexidine gluconate *on page* 210

PerioMed™ [US] *see* fluoride *on page* 430

Periostat® [US/Can] *see* doxycycline *on page* 336

Perlane® [US] *see* hyaluronate and derivatives *on page* 496

permethrin (per METH rin)

U.S./Canadian Brand Names A200® Lice [US-OTC]; Acticin® [US]; Elimite® [US]; Kwellada-P™ [Can]; Nix® [US-OTC/Can]; Rid® Spray [US-OTC]

Therapeutic Category Scabicides/Pediculicides

Use Single-application treatment of infestation with *Pediculus humanus capitis* (head louse) and its nits or *Sarcoptes scabiei* (scabies); indicated for prophylactic use during epidemics of lice

Usual Dosage Topical:

Head lice: Children >2 months and Adults: After hair has been washed with shampoo, rinsed with water, and towel dried, apply a sufficient volume of topical liquid (lotion or cream rinse) to saturate the hair and scalp. Leave on hair for 10 minutes before rinsing off with water; remove remaining nits; may repeat in 1 week if lice or nits still present.

Scabies: Apply cream from head to toe; leave on for 8-14 hours before washing off with water; for infants, also apply on the hairline, neck, scalp, temple, and forehead; may reapply in 1 week if live mites appear

Permethrin 5% cream was shown to be safe and effective when applied to an infant <1 month of age with neonatal scabies; time of application was limited to 6 hours before rinsing with soap and water

Dosage Forms

Cream, topical: 5% (60 g)
Acticin®, Elimite®: 5% (60 g)

Lotion, topical: 1% (59 mL)

Liquid, topical [creme rinse formulation]: 1% (60 mL)
Nix® [OTC]: 1% (60 mL)

Solution, spray [for bedding and furniture]:
A200® Lice [OTC]: 0.5% (180 mL)
Nix® [OTC]: 0.25% (148 mL)
Rid® [OTC]: 0.5% (150 mL)

Permitil® Oral *(Discontinued)* *see* fluphenazine *on page* 434
Peroxin A5® *(Discontinued)* *see* benzoyl peroxide *on page* 132
Peroxin A10® *(Discontinued)* *see* benzoyl peroxide *on page* 132

perphenazine (per FEN a zeen)

Sound-Alike/Look-Alike Issues

Trilafon® may be confused with Tri-Levlen®

U.S./Canadian Brand Names Apo-Perphenazine® [Can]

Therapeutic Category Phenothiazine Derivative

Use Treatment of schizophrenia; severe nausea and vomiting

Usual Dosage Oral: Adults:

Schizophrenia/psychoses:

Nonhospitalized: Initial: 4-8 mg 3 times/day; reduce dose as soon as possible to minimum effective dosage (maximum: 64 mg/day)

Hospitalized: 8-16 mg 2-4 times/day (maximum: 64 mg/day)

Nausea/vomiting: 8-16 mg/day in divided doses (maximum: 24 mg/day)

Dosage Forms

Tablet: 2 mg, 4 mg, 8 mg, 16 mg

perphenazine and amitriptyline hydrochloride *see* amitriptyline and perphenazine *on page* 66
Persa-Gel® *(Discontinued)* *see* benzoyl peroxide *on page* 132
Persantine® [US/Can] *see* dipyridamole *on page* 324
Pertussin® CS *(Discontinued)* *see* dextromethorphan *on page* 295
Pertussin® ES *(Discontinued)* *see* dextromethorphan *on page* 295
pertussis, acellular (adsorbed) *see* diphtheria and tetanus toxoids, acellular pertussis, poliovirus and *Haemophilus* b conjugate vaccine *on page* 320
pethidine hydrochloride *see* meperidine *on page* 626
Pexeva® [US] *see* paroxetine *on page* 752
PFA *see* foscarnet *on page* 445
Pfizerpen® [US] *see* penicillin G (parenteral/aqueous) *on page* 761
Pfizerpen-AS® [Can] *see* penicillin G procaine *on page* 762
PGE_1 *see* alprostadil *on page* 51
PGE_2 *see* dinoprostone *on page* 314

PGI_2 *see* epoprostenol *on page 363*
PGX *see* epoprostenol *on page 363*
Phanasin® [US-OTC] *see* guaifenesin *on page 473*
Phanasin® Diabetic Choice [US-OTC] *see* guaifenesin *on page 473*
Phanatuss® DM [US-OTC] *see* guaifenesin and dextromethorphan *on page 474*
Phanatuss® HC *(Discontinued)*
Pharmaflur® 1.1 *(Discontinued)* *see* fluoride *on page 430*
Pharmaflur® *(Discontinued)* *see* fluoride *on page 430*
Pharmorubicin® [Can] *see* epirubicin *on page 360*
Phazyme™ [Can] *see* simethicone *on page 901*
Phazyme® *(Discontinued)* *see* simethicone *on page 901*
Phazyme® Ultra Strength [US-OTC] *see* simethicone *on page 901*
Phenabid® [US] *see* chlorpheniramine and phenylephrine *on page 214*
Phenabid DM® [US] *see* chlorpheniramine, phenylephrine, and dextromethorphan *on page 217*
Phenadex® Senior *(Discontinued)* *see* guaifenesin and dextromethorphan *on page 474*
Phenadoz™ [US] *see* promethazine *on page 823*
Phenagesic [US-OTC] *see* acetaminophen and phenyltoloxamine *on page 23*
Phenameth® DM *(Discontinued)* *see* promethazine and dextromethorphan *on page 824*
Phenaphen® *(Discontinued)* *see* acetaminophen *on page 19*
Phenaseptic [US-OTC] *see* phenol *on page 772*
PhenaVent™ D *(Discontinued)* *see* guaifenesin and phenylephrine *on page 475*
PhenaVent™ *(Discontinued)* *see* guaifenesin and phenylephrine *on page 475*
PhenaVent™ LA *(Discontinued)* *see* guaifenesin and phenylephrine *on page 475*
PhenaVent™ Ped *(Discontinued)* *see* guaifenesin and phenylephrine *on page 475*
Phenazine® Injection *(Discontinued)* *see* promethazine *on page 823*
Phenazo™ [Can] *see* phenazopyridine *on page 770*

phenazopyridine (fen az oh PEER i deen)

Sound-Alike/Look-Alike Issues
phenazopyridine may be confused with phenoxybenzamine
Pyridium® may be confused with Dyrenium®, Perdiem®, pyridoxine, pyrithione

Synonyms phenazopyridine hydrochloride; phenylazo diamino pyridine hydrochloride

U.S./Canadian Brand Names AZO-Gesic® [US-OTC]; AZO-Standard® Maximum Strength [US-OTC]; AZO-Standard® [US-OTC]; Baridium® [US-OTC]; Phenazo™ [Can]; Prodium® [US-OTC]; Pyridium® [US]; ReAzo [US-OTC]; UTI Relief® [US-OTC]

Therapeutic Category Analgesic, Urinary

Use Symptomatic relief of urinary burning, itching, frequency and urgency in association with urinary tract infection or following urologic procedures

Usual Dosage Oral:
Children: 12 mg/kg/day in 3 divided doses administered after meals for 2 days
Adults: 100-200 mg 3 times/day after meals for 2 days when used concomitantly with an antibacterial agent

Dosage Forms
Tablet: 100 mg, 200 mg
AZO-Gesic® [OTC], Prodium® [OTC], ReAzo [OTC]: 95 mg
AZO-Standard® [OTC]: 95 mg [gluten free]
AZO Standard® Maximum Strength [OTC]: 97.5 mg [gluten free]
Baridium® [OTC], UTI Relief® [OTC]: 97.2 mg
Pyridium®: 100 mg, 200 mg

phenazopyridine hydrochloride *see* phenazopyridine *on page 770*
Phencarb GG [US] *see* carbetapentane, guaifenesin, and phenylephrine *on page 182*

phendimetrazine (fen dye ME tra zeen)

Sound-Alike/Look-Alike Issues
Bontril® PDM may be confused with Bentyl®

Synonyms phendimetrazine tartrate

U.S./Canadian Brand Names Bontril® PDM [US]; Bontril® Slow Release [US]; Bontril® [Can]; Plegine® [Can]; Statobex® [Can]

Therapeutic Category Anorexiant

Controlled Substance C-III

Use Short-term (few weeks) adjunct in exogenous obesity

Usual Dosage Oral: Adults:

Capsule: 105 mg once daily in the morning before breakfast

Tablet: 17.5-35 mg 2 or 3 times daily, 1 hour before meals (maximum: 70 mg 3 times/day)

Dosage Forms

Capsule, slow release: 105 mg

Bontril® Slow Release: 105 mg

Tablet: 35 mg

Bontril® PDM: 35 mg

phendimetrazine tartrate *see* phendimetrazine *on page* *770*

Phendry® Oral *(Discontinued)* *see* diphenhydramine *on page* *315*

phenelzine (FEN el zeen)

Sound-Alike/Look-Alike Issues

phenelzine may be confused with phenytoin

Nardil® may be confused with Norinyl®

Synonyms phenelzine sulfate

U.S./Canadian Brand Names Nardil® [US/Can]

Therapeutic Category Antidepressant, Monoamine Oxidase Inhibitor

Use Symptomatic treatment of atypical, nonendogenous, or neurotic depression

Usual Dosage Oral: Adults: Depression: 15 mg 3 times/day; may increase to 60-90 mg/day during early phase of treatment, then reduce dose for maintenance therapy slowly after maximum benefit is obtained; takes 2-4 weeks for a significant response to occur

Dosage Forms

Tablet:

Nardil®: 15 mg

phenelzine sulfate *see* phenelzine *on page* *771*

Phenerbel-S® *(Discontinued)*

Phenergan® [US/Can] *see* promethazine *on page* *823*

Phenergan® VC With Codeine *(Discontinued)* *see* promethazine, phenylephrine, and codeine *on page* *825*

Phenergan® With Dextromethorphan *(Discontinued)* *see* promethazine and dextromethorphan *on page* *824*

pheniramine and naphazoline *see* naphazoline and pheniramine *on page* *681*

phenobarbital (fee noe BAR bi tal)

Sound-Alike/Look-Alike Issues

PHENobarbital may be confused with PENTobarbital, Phenergan®, phenytoin

Luminal® may be confused with Tuinal®

Synonyms phenobarbital sodium; phenobarbitone; phenylethylmalonylurea

Tall-Man **PHEN**obarbital

U.S./Canadian Brand Names Luminal® Sodium [US]; PMS-Phenobarbital [Can]

Therapeutic Category Anticonvulsant; Barbiturate

Controlled Substance C-IV

Use Management of generalized tonic-clonic (grand mal), status epilepticus, and partial seizures; sedative/hypnotic

Usual Dosage

Children:

Sedation: Oral: 2 mg/kg 3 times/day

Hypnotic: I.M., I.V.: 3-5 mg/kg at bedtime

Preoperative sedation: Oral, I.M., I.V.: 1-3 mg/kg 1-1.5 hours before procedure

Adults:
Sedation: Oral, I.M.: 30-120 mg/day in 2-3 divided doses
Hypnotic: Oral, I.M., I.V.: 100-320 mg at bedtime
Preoperative sedation: I.M.: 100-200 mg 1-1.5 hours before procedure

Anticonvulsant: Status epilepticus: **Loading dose:** I.V.:
Infants and Children: 15-20 mg/kg (maximum: 1000 mg/dose, maximum rate ≤30 mg/minute in children <60 kg); may repeat dose after 15 minutes as needed (maximum total dose: 40 mg/kg)
Adults: 10-20 mg/kg (maximum rate ≤60 mg/minute in patients ≥60 kg); may repeat dose in 20-minute intervals as needed (maximum total dose: 30 mg/kg)
Anticonvulsant maintenance dose: Oral, I.V.:
Infants: 5-8 mg/kg/day in 1-2 divided doses
Children:
1-5 years: 6-8 mg/kg/day in 1-2 divided doses
5-12 years: 4-6 mg/kg/day in 1-2 divided doses
Children >12 years and Adults: 1-3 mg/kg/day in divided doses or 50-100 mg 2-3 times/day

Dosage Forms
Elixir: 20 mg/5 mL
Injection, solution: 65 mg/mL (1 mL); 130 mg/mL (1 mL)
Luminal® Sodium: 60 mg/mL (1 mL); 130 mg/mL (1 mL)
Tablet: 15 mg, 30 mg, 60 mg, 100 mg

phenobarbital, hyoscyamine, atropine, and scopolamine *see* hyoscyamine, atropine, scopolamine, and phenobarbital *on page 513*

phenobarbital sodium *see* phenobarbital *on page 771*

phenobarbitone *see* phenobarbital *on page 771*

phenol (FEE nol)

Sound-Alike/Look-Alike Issues
Cēpastat® may be confused with Capastat®

Synonyms carbolic acid

U.S./Canadian Brand Names Castellani Paint Modified [US-OTC]; Cheracol® Spray [US-OTC]; Chloraseptic® Gargle [US-OTC]; Chloraseptic® Mouth Pain [US-OTC]; Chloraseptic® Pocket Pump [US-OTC]; Chloraseptic® Spray for Kids [US-OTC]; Chloraseptic® Spray [US-OTC]; Cēpastat® Extra Strength [US-OTC]; Cēpastat® [US-OTC]; P & S™ Liquid Phenol [Can]; Pain-A-Lay® [US-OTC]; Phenaseptic [US-OTC]; Phenol EZ® [US-OTC]; Ulcerease® [US-OTC]; Vicks® Formula 44® Sore Throat [US-OTC]

Therapeutic Category Pharmaceutical Aid

Use Relief of sore throat pain, mouth, gum, and throat irritations; antiseptic; topical anesthetic

Usual Dosage Sore throat:
Oral:
Children 2-12 years:
Chloraseptic®: Three sprays onto throat or affected area; may repeat every 2 hours
Chloraseptic® Spray for Kids: Five sprays onto throat or affected area; may repeat every 2 hours
Children >3 years (Ulcerease®): Refer to adult dosing.
Children 6-12 years:
Cēpastat®: Up to 1 lozenge every 2 hours as needed (maximum: 18 lozenges/24 hours)
Cēpastat® Extra Strength: Up to 1 lozenge every 2 hours as needed (maximum: 10 lozenges/24 hours)
Pain-A-Lay® Gargle: Using gauze pad, apply 10 mL to affected area, or gargle or swish for 15 seconds, then expectorate
Children ≥12 years and Adults:
Cēpastat® Extra Strength, Cēpastat®: Up to 2 lozenges every 2 hours as needed
Cheracol®, Pain-A-Lay® Spray: Spray directly in throat; rinse for 15 seconds then expectorate; may repeat every 2 hours
Chloraseptic®: Five sprays onto throat or affected area; may repeat every 2 hours
Chloraseptic® Gargle, Chloraseptic® Mouth Pain, Pain-A-Lay® Gargle, Ulcerease®: Gargle or swish for 15 seconds, then expectorate; may repeat every 2 hours
Topical: Antiseptic: Adults: Castellani Paint Modified: Apply small amount to affected area 1-3 times/day

Dosage Forms
Lozenge, oral:
Cēpastat® [OTC]: 14.5 mg (18s)
Cēpastat® Extra Strength [OTC]: 29 mg (18s)

Solution, oral [gargle]:
Chloraseptic® [OTC]: 1.4% (296 mL)
Pain-A-Lay® [OTC]: 1.4% (240 mL, 540 mL)
Ulcerease® [OTC]: 0.6% (180 mL)
Solution, oral [spray]:
Cheracol® [OTC], Chloraseptic® [OTC], Pain-A-Lay® [OTC], Phenaseptic [OTC], Vicks® Formula 44® Sore Throat [OTC]: 1.4% (180 mL)
Chloraseptic® for Kids [OTC]: 0.5% (177 mL)
Chloraseptic® Mouth Pain [OTC]: 1.4% (30 mL)
Chloraseptic® Pocket Pump [OTC]: 1.4% (20 mL)
Solution, topical:
Castellani Paint Modified [OTC]: Phenol 1.5% (30 mL)
Castellani Paint Modified [OTC] [colorless]: Phenol 1.5% (30 mL)
Swabs, topical:
Phenol EZ® [OTC]: 89% (30s) [~0.2 mL]

phenol and camphor *see* camphor and phenol *on page* *176*

Phenol EZ® [US-OTC] *see* phenol *on page* *772*

phenoptin *see* sapropterin *on page* *890*

Phenoxine® ***(Discontinued)***

phenoxybenzamine (fen oks ee BEN za meen)

Sound-Alike/Look-Alike Issues
phenoxybenzamine may be confused with phenazopyridine

Synonyms phenoxybenzamine hydrochloride

U.S./Canadian Brand Names Dibenzyline® [US/Can]

Therapeutic Category Alpha-Adrenergic Blocking Agent

Use Symptomatic management of pheochromocytoma

Usual Dosage Oral: Adults: Pheochromocytoma, hypertension: Initial: 10 mg twice daily; increase by 10 mg every other day until optimal blood pressure response is achieved; usual range: 20-40 mg 2-3 times/day. Doses up to 240 mg/day have been reported.

Dosage Forms
Capsule:
Dibenzyline®: 10 mg

phenoxybenzamine hydrochloride *see* phenoxybenzamine *on page* *773*

phenoxymethyl penicillin *see* penicillin V potassium *on page* *763*

phentermine (FEN ter meen)

Sound-Alike/Look-Alike Issues
phentermine may be confused with phentolamine, phenytoin

Synonyms phentermine hydrochloride

U.S./Canadian Brand Names Adipex-P® [US]; Ionamin® [Can]

Therapeutic Category Anorexiant

Controlled Substance C-IV

Use Short-term (few weeks) adjunct in exogenous obesity

Usual Dosage Oral: Children >16 years and Adults: Obesity:
Phentermine hydrochloride: 18.75-37.5 mg/day
Phentermine resin: 15-30 mg/day

Dosage Forms
Capsule: 15 mg, 30 mg, 37.5 mg
Adipex-P®: 37.5 mg
Tablet: 37.5 mg
Adipex-P®: 37.5 mg

phentermine hydrochloride *see* phentermine *on page* *773*

phentolamine (fen TOLE a meen)

Sound-Alike/Look-Alike Issues

phentolamine may be confused with phentermine, Ventolin®

Synonyms phentolamine mesylate

U.S./Canadian Brand Names OraVerse™ [US]; Regitine® [Can]; Rogitine® [Can]

Therapeutic Category Alpha-Adrenergic Blocking Agent; Diagnostic Agent

Use Diagnosis of pheochromocytoma and treatment of hypertension associated with pheochromocytoma or other forms of hypertension caused by excess sympathomimetic amines; treatment of dermal necrosis after extravasation of drugs with alpha-adrenergic effects (ie, dopamine, epinephrine, norepinephrine, phenylephrine)

OraVerse™: Reversal of soft tissue anesthesia and the associated functional deficits resulting from a local dental anesthetic containing a vasoconstrictor

Usual Dosage

Treatment of alpha-adrenergic agonist drug extravasation: SubQ:

Children: Infiltrate area with a small amount (eg, 1 mL given in 0.2 mL aliquots) of a 0.5-1 mg/mL solution (made by diluting 5-10 mg in 10 mL of NS) within 12 hours of extravasation; in general, do not exceed 0.1-0.2 mg/kg or 5 mg total

Adults: Infiltrate area with small amount of solution made by diluting 5-10 mg in 10 mL 0.9% sodium chloride within 12 hours of extravasation; in general, do not exceed 0.1-0.2 mg/kg (5 mg total); typically doses of ≤5 mg are effective; a case using 50 mg for a large extravasation has been reported.

If dose is effective, normal skin color should return to the blanched area within 1 hour

Diagnosis of pheochromocytoma: I.M., I.V.:

Children: 0.05-0.1 mg/kg/dose, maximum single dose: 5 mg

Adults: 5 mg

Surgery for pheochromocytoma: Hypertension: I.M., I.V.:

Children: 0.05-0.1 mg/kg/dose given 1-2 hours before procedure; repeat as needed every 2-4 hours until hypertension is controlled; maximum single dose: 5 mg

Adults: 5 mg given 1-2 hours before procedure and repeated as needed every 2-4 hours

Hypertensive crisis: Adults: 5-20 mg

Reversal of soft tissue (lip, tongue) anesthesia (OraVerse™): Infiltration or block technique: Submucosal oral injection:

Children: 15-30 kg: 0.2 mg maximum dose

Children >30 kg and <12 years: 0.4 mg maximum dose

Adults: **Note:** Dose is based upon the number of cartridges of local anesthetic administered. Infiltration or block injection:

0.2 mg if one-half cartridge of anesthesia was administered

0.4 mg if 1 cartridge of anesthesia was administered

0.8 mg if 2 cartridges of anesthesia were administered

Dosage Forms

Injection, powder for reconstitution: 5 mg

Injection, solution [preservative free]:

OraVerse™: 0.4 mg/1.7 mL [dental cartridge]

phentolamine mesylate *see* phentolamine *on page 774*

phenylalanine mustard *see* melphalan *on page 622*

phenylazo diamino pyridine hydrochloride *see* phenazopyridine *on page 770*

Phenyldrine® ***(Discontinued)***

phenylephrine (fen il EF rin)

Sound-Alike/Look-Alike Issues

Mydfrin® may be confused with Midrin®

Neo-Synephrine® (phenylephrine) may be confused with Neo-Synephrine® (oxymetazoline)

Sudafed PE™ may be confused with Sudafed®

Synonyms phenylephrine hydrochloride; phenylephrine tannate

U.S./Canadian Brand Names 4 Way® Fast Acting [US-OTC]; 4 Way® Menthol [US-OTC]; 4 Way® No Drip [US-OTC]; AK-Dilate® [US]; Altafrin [US]; Anu-Med [US-OTC]; Dimetapp® Toddler's [US-OTC]; Dionephrine® [Can]; Formulation R™ [US-OTC]; Little Noses® Decongestant [US-OTC]; LuSonal™ [US]; Medi-Phenyl [US-OTC]; Medicone® Suppositories [US-OTC]; Mydfrin® [US/Can]; Neo-Synephrine® Extra Strength [US-OTC]; Neo-Synephrine® Injection [US]; Neo-Synephrine® Mild [US-OTC]; Neo-Synephrine® Regular Strength [US-OTC]; Neo-Synephrine® [Can]; Neofrin™ [US-

OcuNefrin™ [US-OTC]; Preparation H® [US-OTC]; Rectacaine [US-OTC]; Rhinall [US-OTC]; Sudafed PE™ [US-OTC]; Triaminic® Thin Strips® Cold [US-OTC]; Tronolane® Suppository [US-OTC]; Vicks® Sinex® Nasal Spray [US-OTC]; Vicks® Sinex® UltraFine Mist [US-OTC]

Therapeutic Category Adrenergic Agonist Agent

Use Treatment of hypotension, vascular failure in shock; as a vasoconstrictor in regional analgesia; as a mydriatic in ophthalmic procedures and treatment of wide-angle glaucoma; supraventricular tachycardia

For OTC use as symptomatic relief of nasal and nasopharyngeal mucosal congestion, treatment of hemorrhoids, relief of redness of the eye due to irritation

Usual Dosage

Hemorrhoids: Children ≥12 years and Adults: Rectal:
- Cream/ointment: Apply to clean dry area, up to 4 times/day; may be used externally or inserted rectally using applicator.
- Suppository: Insert 1 suppository rectally, up to 4 times/day

Hypotension/shock:
- Children:
  - I.V. bolus: 5-20 mcg/kg/dose every 10-15 minutes as needed
  - I.V. infusion: 0.1-0.5 mcg/kg/minute
- Adults:
  - I.V. bolus: 0.1-0.5 mg/dose every 10-15 minutes as needed (initial dose should not exceed 0.5 mg)
  - I.V. infusion: Initial dose: 100-180 mcg/minute, **or alternatively**, 0.5 mcg/kg/minute; titrate to desired response. Dosing ranges between 0.4-9.1 mcg/kg/minute have been reported.

Nasal decongestant:
- Children:
  - 2-6 years: Intranasal: Instill 1 drop every 2-4 hours of 0.125% solution as needed. (**Note:** Therapy should not exceed 3 continuous days.)
  - 6-12 years:
    - Intranasal: Instill 1-2 sprays or instill 1-2 drops every 4 hours of 0.25% solution as needed. (**Note:** Therapy should not exceed 3 continuous days.)
    - Oral: Hydrochloride salt: 10 mg every 4 hours
- Children >12 years and Adults:
  - Intranasal: Instill 1-2 sprays or instill 1-2 drops every 4 hours of 0.25% to 0.5% solution as needed; 1% solution may be used in adult in cases of extreme nasal congestion; do not use nasal solutions more than 3 days
  - Oral: Hydrochloride salt: 10-20 mg every 4 hours

Ocular procedures:
- Infants <1 year: Instill 1 drop of 2.5% 15-30 minutes before procedures
- Children and Adults: Instill 1 drop of 2.5% or 10% solution, may repeat in 10-60 minutes as needed

Ophthalmic irritation (OTC formulation for relief of eye redness): Adults: Instill 1-2 drops 0.12% solution into affected eye, up to 4 times/day; do not use for >72 hours

Paroxysmal supraventricular tachycardia: I.V.:
- Children: 5-10 mcg/kg/dose over 20-30 seconds
- Adults: 0.25-0.5 mg/dose over 20-30 seconds

Dosage Forms

Cream, rectal:
- Formulation R™ [OTC]: 0.25% (54 g)

Filmstrip, orally disintegrating:
- Sudafed PE™ [OTC]: 10 mg (5s, 10s)
- Triaminic® Thin Strips® Cold [OTC]: 2.5 mg

Injection, solution: 1% [10 mg/mL] (1 mL, 5 mL, 10 mL)
- Neo-Synephrine®: 1% (1 mL)

Liquid, oral:
- LuSonal™: 7.5 mg/5 mL

Liquid, oral [drops]:
- Dimetapp® Toddler's [OTC]: 1.25 mg/0.8 mL

Ointment, rectal:
- Formulation R™ [OTC], Preparation H® [OTC]: 0.25% (30 g, 60 g)
- Rectacaine [OTC]: 0.25% (30 g)

Solution, intranasal [drops]:
- Little Noses® Decongestant [OTC]: 0.125% (15 mL)
- Neo-Synephrine® Extra Strength [OTC]: 1% (15 mL)
- Neo-Synephrine® Regular Strength [OTC]: 0.5% (15 mL)

Rhinall [OTC]: 0.25% (30 mL)

Solution, intranasal [spray]:

4 Way® Fast Acting [OTC]: 1% (15 mL, 30 mL) [contains benzalkonium chloride]

4 Way® Menthol [OTC], 4 Way® No Drip [OTC], Neo-Synephrine® Extra Strength [OTC]: 1% (15 mL)

Neo-Synephrine® Mild [OTC]: 0.25% (15 mL)

Neo-Synephrine® Regular Strength [OTC], Vicks® Sinex® [OTC], Vicks® Sinex® UltraFine Mist [OTC]: 0.5% (15 mL)

Rhinall [OTC]: 0.25% (40 mL)

Solution, ophthalmic: 2.5% (2 mL, 3 mL, 5 mL, 15 mL)

AK-Dilate®: 2.5% (2 mL, 15 mL); 10% (5 mL)

Altrafrin: 0.12% (15 mL) [OTC]; 2.5% (15 mL); 10% (5 mL)

Mydfrin®: 2.5% (3 mL, 5 mL)

Neofrin™: 2.5% (15 mL); 10% (15 mL)

OcuNefrin™ [OTC]: 0.12% (15 mL)

Suppository, rectal: 0.25% (12s)

Anu-Med [OTC]: 0.25% (12s)

Formulation R™ [OTC], Preparation H® [OTC]: 0.25% (12s, 24s, 48s)

Medicone® [OTC], Tronolane® [OTC]: 0.25% (12s, 24s)

Rectacaine [OTC]: 0.25% (12s)

Tablet: 10 mg

Medi-Phenyl [OTC]: 5 mg

Sudafed PE™ [OTC]: 10 mg

Phenylephrine CM [US] *see* chlorpheniramine, phenylephrine, and methscopolamine *on page 218*

phenylephrine, acetaminophen, and dextromethorphan *see* acetaminophen, dextromethorphan, and phenylephrine *on page 27*

phenylephrine and brompheniramine *see* brompheniramine and phenylephrine *on page 150*

phenylephrine and chlorpheniramine *see* chlorpheniramine and phenylephrine *on page 214*

phenylephrine and cyclopentolate *see* cyclopentolate and phenylephrine *on page 265*

phenylephrine and dextromethorphan *see* dextromethorphan and phenylephrine *on page 296*

phenylephrine and diphenhydramine *see* diphenhydramine and phenylephrine *on page 317*

phenylephrine and promethazine *see* promethazine and phenylephrine *on page 824*

phenylephrine and pyrilamine (fen il EF rin & peer IL a meen)

Synonyms pyrilamine tannate and phenylephrine tannate

U.S./Canadian Brand Names Aldex®D [US]; Deconsal® CT [US]; Ryna-12 S® [US]; Ryna®-12 [US]

Therapeutic Category Antihistamine; Antihistamine/Decongestant Combination; Sympathomimetic

Use Symptomatic relief of nasal congestion and discharge associated with the common cold, sinusitis, allergic rhinitis, and other respiratory tract conditions

Usual Dosage Oral: Relief of cough, congestion:

Aldex®D, Deconsal® CT:

Children 2-6 years: 2.5 mL of the suspension or 1/2 tablet every 12 hours

Children 6-12 years: 5 mL of the suspension or 1/2 to 1 tablet every 12 hours

Children >12 years and Adults: 5-10 mL of the suspension or 1-2 tablets every 12 hours

Ryna®-12:

Children 6-12 years: 1/2 to 1 tablet every 12 hours

Children >12 years and Adults: 1-2 tablets every 12 hours

Ryna-12 S®:

Children 2-6 years: 2.5-5 mL every 12 hours

Children >6 years: 5-10 mL every 12 hours

Dosage Forms

Suspension:

Aldex®D: Phenylephrine 5 mg and pyrilamine 16 mg

Ryna-12 S®: Phenylephrine 5 mg and pyrilamine 30 mg per 5 mL

Tablet:

Ryna®-12: Phenylephrine 25 mg and pyrilamine 60 mg

Tablet, chewable:

Deconsal® CT: Phenylephrine 10 mg and pyrilamine 16 mg

phenylephrine and scopolamine (fen il EF rin & skoe POL a meen)

Sound-Alike/Look-Alike Issues
Murocoll-2® may be confused with Murocel®

Synonyms scopolamine and phenylephrine

U.S./Canadian Brand Names Murocoll-2® [US]

Therapeutic Category Anticholinergic/Adrenergic Agonist

Use Mydriasis, cycloplegia, and to break posterior synechiae in iritis

Usual Dosage Ophthalmic: Instill 1-2 drops into eye(s); repeat in 5 minutes

Dosage Forms

Solution, ophthalmic:
Murocoll-2®: Phenylephrine 10% and scopolamine 0.3% (5 mL)

phenylephrine and zinc sulfate *(Canada only)* (fen il EF rin & zingk SUL fate)

Synonyms zinc sulfate and phenylephrine

U.S./Canadian Brand Names Zincfrin® [Can]

Therapeutic Category Adrenergic Agonist Agent

Use Soothe, moisturize, and remove redness due to minor eye irritation

Usual Dosage Ophthalmic: Instill 1-2 drops in eye(s) 2-4 times/day as needed

Dosage Forms

Solution, ophthalmic:
Zincfrin® [OTC; CAN]: Phenylephrine 0.12% and zinc sulfate 0.25% (15 mL)

phenylephrine, chlorpheniramine, and carbetapentane *see* carbetapentane, phenylephrine, and chlorpheniramine *on page 183*

phenylephrine, chlorpheniramine, and dextromethorphan *see* chlorpheniramine, phenylephrine, and dextromethorphan *on page 217*

phenylephrine, chlorpheniramine, and dihydrocodeine *see* dihydrocodeine, chlorpheniramine, and phenylephrine *on page 309*

phenylephrine, chlorpheniramine, and guaifenesin *see* chlorpheniramine, phenylephrine, and guaifenesin *on page 218*

phenylephrine, chlorpheniramine, and phenyltoloxamine *see* chlorpheniramine, phenylephrine, and phenyltoloxamine *on page 219*

phenylephrine, chlorpheniramine, and pyrilamine *see* chlorpheniramine, pyrilamine, and phenylephrine *on page 221*

phenylephrine, chlorpheniramine, codeine, and potassium iodide *see* chlorpheniramine, phenylephrine, codeine, and potassium iodide *on page 220*

phenylephrine, dextromethorphan, and acetaminophen *see* acetaminophen, dextromethorphan, and phenylephrine *on page 27*

phenylephrine, ephedrine, chlorpheniramine, and carbetapentane *see* chlorpheniramine, ephedrine, phenylephrine, and carbetapentane *on page 216*

phenylephrine hydrochloride *see* phenylephrine *on page 774*

phenylephrine hydrochloride, acetaminophen, and diphenhydramine *see* acetaminophen, diphenhydramine, and phenylephrine *on page 28*

phenylephrine hydrochloride and acetaminophen *see* acetaminophen and phenylephrine *on page 22*

phenylephrine hydrochloride and diphenhydramine hydrochloride *see* diphenhydramine and phenylephrine *on page 317*

phenylephrine hydrochloride and guaifenesin *see* guaifenesin and phenylephrine *on page 475*

phenylephrine hydrochloride, carbetapentane citrate, and guaifenesin *see* carbetapentane, guaifenesin, and phenylephrine *on page 182*

phenylephrine hydrochloride, chlorpheniramine maleate, dextromethorphan hydrobromide, and guaifenesin *see* dextromethorphan, chlorpheniramine, phenylephrine, and guaifenesin *on page 297*

phenylephrine hydrochloride, guaifenesin, and dextromethorphan hydrobromide *see* guaifenesin, dextromethorphan, and phenylephrine *on page 478*

phenylephrine hydrochloride, hydrocodone bitartrate, and chlorpheniramine Maleate *see* phenylephrine, hydrocodone, and chlorpheniramine *on page 778*

phenylephrine, hydrocodone, and chlorpheniramine

(fen il EF rin, hye droe KOE done, & klor fen IR a meen)

Synonyms chlorpheniramine, hydrocodone, and phenylephrine; dihydrocodeine bitartrate, phenylephrine hydrochloride, and chlorpheniramine maleate; hydrocodone, phenylephrine, and chlorpheniramine; phenylephrine hydrochloride, hydrocodone bitartrate, and chlorpheniramine Maleate

U.S./Canadian Brand Names B-Tuss™ [US]; Coughtuss [US]; Cytuss HC [US]; De-Chlor HC [US]; DroTuss-CP [US]; ED-TLC [US]; ED-Tuss HC [US]; Histinex® HC [US]; Hydro PC II Plus [US]; Hydro-PC II [US]; Hydron CP [US]; Maxi-Tuss HCX [US]; Maxi-Tuss HC® [US]; Mintuss HC [US]; Mintuss MS [US]; PolyTussin HD [US]; Rindal HD Plus [US]; Triant-HC™ [US]

Therapeutic Category Antihistamine; Antihistamine/Decongestant/Antitussive; Antitussive; Decongestant

Controlled Substance C-III

Use Symptomatic relief of cough and congestion associated with the common cold, sinusitis, or acute upper respiratory tract infections

Usual Dosage Oral:

Children 2-6 years: B-Tuss™: 1.25-2.5 mL every 6 hours (maximum: 10 mL/24 hours)

Children 6-12 years:

- B-Tuss™: 2.5-5 mL every 6 hours (maximum: 20 mL/24 hours)
- Histinex® HC, Cytuss HC: 5 mL every 4 hours (maximum: 20 mL/24 hours)
- Maxi-Tuss HC®, Maxi-Tuss HCX: 2.5 mL every 4 hours (maximum: 15 mL/24 hours)

Adults:

- B-Tuss™: 5-10 mL every 6 hours (maximum: 40 mL/24 hours)
- Histinex® HC, Cytuss HC: 10 mL every 4 hours (maximum: 40 mL/24 hours)
- Maxi-Tuss HC®, Maxi-Tuss HCX: 5 mL every 4 hours (maximum: 30 mL/24 hours)

Dosage Forms

Liquid:

- B-Tuss™: Phenylephrine 5 mg, hydrocodone 5 mg, and chlorpheniramine 2 mg per 5 mL
- Coughtuss, DroTuss-CP: Phenylephrine 5 mg, hydrocodone 5 mg, and chlorpheniramine 2 mg per 5 mL
- De-Chlor HC: Phenylephrine 10 mg, hydrocodone 2.5 mg, and chlorpheniramine 2 mg per 5 mL
- ED-Tuss HC: Phenylephrine 10 mg, hydrocodone 3.5 mg, and chlorpheniramine 4 mg per 5 mL
- ED-TLC: Phenylephrine 5 mg, hydrocodone 1.67 mg, and chlorpheniramine 2 mg per 5 mL
- Hydro PC II Plus: Phenylephrine 7.5 mg, hydrocodone 3.5 mg, and chlorpheniramine 2 mg per 5 mL
- Hydron CP: Phenylephrine 10 mg, hydrocodone 5 mg, and chlorpheniramine 2 mg per 5 mL
- Maxi-Tuss HCX: Phenylephrine 12 mg, hydrocodone 6 mg and chlorpheniramine 2 mg per 5 mL
- Triant-HC™: Phenylephrine 5 mg, hydrocodone 1.67 mg, and chlorpheniramine 2 mg per 5 mL

Syrup:

- Cytuss HC, Histinex® HC: Phenylephrine 5 mg, hydrocodone 2.5 mg, and chlorpheniramine 2 mg per 5 mL
- Hydro-PC II: Phenylephrine 7.5 mg, hydrocodone 2 mg, and chlorpheniramine 2 mg per 5 mL
- Maxi-Tuss HC®, Mintuss HD: Phenylephrine 10 mg, hydrocodone 2.5 mg, and chlorpheniramine 4 mg per 5 mL
- Mintuss HC: Phenylephrine 10 mg, hydrocodone 2.5 mg, and chlorpheniramine 2 mg per 5 mL
- Mintuss MS: Phenylephrine 10 mg, hydrocodone 5 mg, and chlorpheniramine 2 mg per 5 mL
- PolyTussin HD: Phenylephrine 5 mg, hydrocodone 6 mg, and chlorpheniramine 2 mg per 5 mL
- Rindal HD Plus: Phenylephrine 7.5 mg, hydrocodone 3.5 mg, and chlorpheniramine 2 mg per 5 mL

phenylephrine, promethazine, and codeine *see* promethazine, phenylephrine, and codeine *on page 825*

phenylephrine, pyrilamine, and dextromethorphan

(fen il EF rin, peer IL a meen, & deks troe meth OR fan)

Synonyms dextromethorphan tannate, pyrilamine tannate, and phenylephrine tannate; pyrilamine maleate, dextromethorphan hydrobromide, and phenylephrine hydrochloride

U.S./Canadian Brand Names Aldex® DM [US]; AllanVan-DM [US]; Codal-DM [US-OTC]; codimal® DM [US-OTC]; Codituss DM [US-OTC]; MyHist-DM [US]; Poly-Hist DM [US]; Viravan®-DM [US]

Therapeutic Category Antihistamine; Antihistamine/Decongestant/Antitussive; Antitussive; Sympathomimetic

Use Symptomatic relief of cough, nasal congestion, and discharge associated with the common cold, sinusitis, allergic rhinitis, and other respiratory tract conditions

Usual Dosage Oral: Relief of cough, congestion:

Children 2-6 years (Viravan®-DM): 2.5 mL of the suspension or 1/2 tablet every 12 hours
Children 6-12 years:
codimal® DM: 5 mL every 4 hours; maximum: 30 mL/24 hours
Viravan®-DM: 5 mL of the suspension or 1/2 to 1 tablet every 12 hours
Children >12 years and Adults:
codimal® DM: 10 mL every 4 hours; maximum: 60 mL/24 hours
Viravan®-DM: 5-10 mL of the suspension or 1-2 tablets every 12 hours

Dosage Forms

Liquid:
MyHist-DM: Phenylephrine 7.5 mg, pyrilamine 12.5 mg, and dextromethorphan 15 mg per 5 mL

Suspension:
AllanVan-DM, Viravan®-DM: Phenylephrine 12.5 mg, pyrilamine 30 mg, and dextromethorphan 25 mg per 5 mL
Aldex® DM: Phenylephrine 5 mg, pyrilamine 16 mg, and dextromethorphan 15 mg per 5 mL

Syrup:
Codal-DM [OTC], codimal® DM [OTC], Codituss DM [OTC]: Phenylephrine 5 mg, pyrilamine 8.33 mg, and dextromethorphan 10 mg
Poly Hist DM: Phenylephrine 7.5 mg, pyrilamine 8.33 mg, and dextromethorphan 10 mg

Tablet, chewable [scored]:
Deconsal® DM: Phenylephrine 10 mg, pyrilamine 16 mg, and dextromethorphan 15 mg
Viravan®-DM: Phenylephrine 25 mg, pyrilamine 30 mg, and dextromethorphan 25 mg

phenylephrine, pyrilamine, and guaifenesin

(fen il EF rin, peer IL a meen, & gwye FEN e sin)

Synonyms guaifenesin, phenylephrine tannate, and pyrilamine tannate; pyrilamine tannate, guaifenesin, and phenylephrine tannate

U.S./Canadian Brand Names Ryna-12X® [US]

Therapeutic Category Alpha/Beta Agonist; Decongestant; Expectorant; Histamine H_1 Antagonist; Histamine H_1 Antagonist, First Generation

Use Symptomatic relief of cough, nasal congestion, and discharge associated with the common cold, sinusitis, allergic rhinitis, and other respiratory tract conditions

Usual Dosage Oral: Relief of cough, congestion:

Children 2-6 years: 2.5-5 mL of the suspension every 12 hours
Children 6-11 years: 5-10 mL of the suspension **or** 1/2 to 1 tablet every 12 hours
Children ≥12 years and Adults: 1-2 tablets every 12 hours

Dosage Forms

Suspension:
Ryna-12X®: Phenylephrine 5 mg, pyrilamine 30 mg, and guaifenesin 100 mg per 5 mL

Tablet [scored]:
Ryna-12X®: Phenylephrine 25 mg, pyrilamine 60 mg, and guaifenesin 200 mg

phenylephrine tannate *see* phenylephrine *on page 774*

phenylephrine tannate and carbetapentane tannate *see* carbetapentane and phenylephrine *on page 182*

phenylephrine tannate and diphenhydramine tannate *see* diphenhydramine and phenylephrine *on page 317*

phenylephrine tannate, carbetapentane tannate, and pyrilamine tannate *see* carbetapentane, phenylephrine, and pyrilamine *on page 183*

phenylephrine tannate, chlorpheniramine tannate, and methscopolamine nitrate *see* chlorpheniramine, phenylephrine, and methscopolamine *on page 218*

phenylethylmalonylurea *see* phenobarbital *on page 771*

Phenylfenesin® L.A. *(Discontinued)*

Phenylgesic [US-OTC] *see* acetaminophen and phenyltoloxamine *on page 23*

phenyl salicylate, methenamine, methylene blue, benzoic acid, and hyoscyamine *see* methenamine, phenyl salicylate, methylene blue, benzoic acid, and hyoscyamine *on page 637*

phenyltoloxamine, chlorpheniramine, and phenylephrine *see* chlorpheniramine, phenylephrine, and phenyltoloxamine *on page 219*

phenyltoloxamine citrate and acetaminophen *see* acetaminophen and phenyltoloxamine *on page 23*

Phenytek® [US] *see* phenytoin *on page* 780

phenytoin (FEN i toyn)

Sound-Alike/Look-Alike Issues

phenytoin may be confused with phenelzine, phentermine, PHENobarbital
Dilantin® may be confused with Dilaudid®, diltiazem, Dipentum®

Synonyms diphenylhydantoin; DPH; phenytoin sodium; phenytoin sodium, extended; phenytoin sodium, prompt

U.S./Canadian Brand Names Dilantin® [US/Can]; Phenytek® [US]

Therapeutic Category Antiarrhythmic Agent, Class I-B; Hydantoin

Use Management of generalized tonic-clonic (grand mal), complex partial seizures; prevention of seizures following head trauma/neurosurgery

Usual Dosage

Status epilepticus: I.V.:

Infants and Children: Loading dose: 15-20 mg/kg in a single or divided dose; maintenance dose: Initial: 5 mg/kg/day in 2 divided doses; usual doses:

6 months to 3 years: 8-10 mg/kg/day
4-6 years: 7.5-9 mg/kg/day
7-9 years: 7-8 mg/kg/day
10-16 years: 6-7 mg/kg/day, some patients may require every 8 hours dosing

Adults: Loading dose: Manufacturer recommends 10-15 mg/kg, however, 15-20 mg/kg is generally recommended; maximum rate: 50 mg/minute

Anticonvulsant: Children and Adults: Oral:

Loading dose: 15-20 mg/kg; based on phenytoin serum concentrations and recent dosing history; administer oral loading dose in 3 divided doses given every 2-4 hours to decrease GI adverse effects and to ensure complete oral absorption; maintenance dose: same as I.V.

Neurosurgery (prophylactic): 100-200 mg at approximately 4-hour intervals during surgery and during the immediate postoperative period

Dosage Forms

Capsule, extended release: 100 mg
Dilantin®: 30 mg, 100 mg
Phenytek®: 200 mg, 300 mg

Capsule, prompt release: 100 mg

Injection, solution: 50 mg/mL (2 mL, 5 mL)

Suspension, oral: 100 mg/4 mL, 125 mg/5 mL
Dilantin®: 125 mg/5 mL

Tablet, chewable:
Dilantin®: 50 mg

phenytoin sodium *see* phenytoin *on page* 780
phenytoin sodium, extended *see* phenytoin *on page* 780
phenytoin sodium, prompt *see* phenytoin *on page* 780
Pherazine® VC With Codeine *(Discontinued)* *see* promethazine, phenylephrine, and codeine *on page* 825
Pherazine® With Codeine *(Discontinued)* *see* promethazine and codeine *on page* 824
Pherazine® With DM *(Discontinued)* *see* promethazine and dextromethorphan *on page* 824
Phillips'® M-O [US-OTC] *see* magnesium hydroxide and mineral oil *on page* 609
Phillips'® Laxative Dietary Supplement Cramp-Free [US-OTC] *see* magnesium oxide *on page* 610
Phillips'® Milk of Magnesia [US-OTC] *see* magnesium hydroxide *on page* 608
Phillips'® Stool Softener Laxative [US-OTC] *see* docusate *on page* 326
pHisoHex® [US/Can] *see* hexachlorophene *on page* 493
PHL-Alendronate [Can] *see* alendronate *on page* 44
PHL-Alendronate-FC [Can] *see* alendronate *on page* 44
PHL-Amiodarone [Can] *see* amiodarone *on page* 64
PHL-Amlodipine [Can] *see* amlodipine *on page* 66
PHL-Amoxicillin [Can] *see* amoxicillin *on page* 70
PHL-Anagrelide [Can] *see* anagrelide *on page* 78
PHL-Azithromycin [Can] *see* azithromycin *on page* 116

Phrenilin® [US] *see* butalbital and acetaminophen *on page 162*

Phrenilin® Forte [US] *see* butalbital and acetaminophen *on page 162*

Phrenilin® with Caffeine and Codeine *(Discontinued)* *see* butalbital, acetaminophen, caffeine, and codeine *on page 162*

***p*-hydroxyampicillin** *see* amoxicillin *on page 70*

Phyllocontin® [Can] *see* aminophylline *on page 63*

Phyllocontin®-350 [Can] *see* aminophylline *on page 63*

phylloquinone *see* phytonadione *on page 782*

physostigmine (fye zoe STIG meen)

Sound-Alike/Look-Alike Issues

physostigmine may be confused with Prostigmin®, pyridostigmine

Synonyms eserine salicylate; physostigmine salicylate; physostigmine sulfate

U.S./Canadian Brand Names Eserine® [Can]; Isopto® Eserine [Can]

Therapeutic Category Cholinesterase Inhibitor

Use Reverse toxic, life-threatening delirium caused by atropine, diphenhydramine, dimenhydrinate, *Atropa belladonna* (deadly nightshade), or jimsonweed (*Datura* spp)

Usual Dosage Reversal of toxic anticholinergic effects: **Note:** Administer slowly over 5 minutes to prevent respiratory distress and seizures. Continuous infusions of physostigmine should never be used.

Children: **Note:** Reserve for life-threatening situations only: I.V.: 0.01-0.03 mg/kg/dose; may repeat after 5-10 minutes to a maximum total dose of 2 mg or until response occurs or adverse cholinergic effects occur

Adults: I.M., I.V.: 0.5-2 mg to start, repeat every 20 minutes until response occurs or adverse effect occurs; repeat 1-4 mg every 30-60 minutes as life-threatening symptoms recur

Dosage Forms

Injection, solution: 1 mg/mL (2 mL)

physostigmine salicylate *see* physostigmine *on page 782*

physostigmine sulfate *see* physostigmine *on page 782*

phytomenadione *see* phytonadione *on page 782*

phytonadione (fye toe na DYE one)

Sound-Alike/Look-Alike Issues

Mephyton® may be confused with melphalan, methadone

Synonyms methylphytyl napthoquinone; phylloquinone; phytomenadione; vitamin K_1

U.S./Canadian Brand Names AquaMEPHYTON® [Can]; Konakion [Can]; Mephyton® [US/Can]

Therapeutic Category Vitamin, Fat Soluble

Use Prevention and treatment of hypoprothrombinemia caused by coumarin derivative-induced or other drug-induced vitamin K deficiency, hypoprothrombinemia caused by malabsorption or inability to synthesize vitamin K; hemorrhagic disease of the newborn

Usual Dosage Note: According to the manufacturer, SubQ is the preferred parenteral route; I.M. route should be avoided due to the risk of hematoma formation; I.V. route should be restricted for emergency use only. The American College of Chest Physicians recommends the I.V. route in patients with serious or life-threatening bleeding secondary to use of vitamin K antagonists.

Adequate intake:

- Children:
  - 1-3 years: 30 mcg/day
  - 4-8 years: 55 mcg/day
  - 9-13 years: 60 mcg/day
  - 14-18 years: 75 mcg/day
- Adults: Males: 120 mcg/day; Females: 90 mcg/day

Hemorrhagic disease of the newborn:

- Prophylaxis: I.M.: 0.5-1 mg within 1 hour of birth
- Treatment: I.M., SubQ: 1 mg/dose/day; higher doses may be necessary if mother has been receiving oral anticoagulants

Hypoprothrombinemia due to drugs (other than coumarin derivatives) or factors limiting absorption or synthesis: Adults: Oral, SubQ, I.M., I.V.: Initial: 2.5-25 mg (rarely up to 50 mg)

Vitamin K deficiency (supratherapeutic INR) secondary to coumarin derivative: Adults:

If INR above therapeutic range to <5 (no significant bleeding and rapid reversal unnecessary): Lower or hold next dose and monitor frequently; when INR approaches desired range, resume dosing with a lower dose.

If INR ≥5 and <9 (no significant bleeding): If no risk factors for bleeding exist, omit next 1 or 2 doses, monitor INR more frequently, and resume with an appropriately adjusted dose when INR in desired range.

Alternatively, if other risk factors for bleeding exist, omit next dose and administer vitamin K orally 1-2.5 mg; resume with an appropriately adjusted dose when INR in desired range.

If INR ≥5 and <9 (no significant bleeding and rapid reversal required for surgery): Administer vitamin K orally ≤5 mg and hold warfarin. Expect INR to be reduced within 24 hours; if INR still elevated, another 1-2 mg of vitamin K orally may be given.

If INR ≥9 (no significant bleeding): Hold warfarin, administer vitamin K orally 2.5-5 mg, expect INR to be reduced within 24-48 hours, monitor INR more frequently and give additional vitamin K at an appropriate dose if necessary. Resume warfarin at an appropriately adjusted dose when INR is in desired range.

If serious bleeding at any INR elevation: Hold warfarin, administer vitamin K 10 mg by slow I.V. infusion and supplement with FFP, PCC, or rFVIIa depending on the urgency of the situation; I.V. Vitamin K may be repeated every 12 hours.

If life-threatening bleeding: Hold warfarin, give FFP, PCC, or rFVIIa supplemented with vitamin K 10 mg slow I.V. infusion; repeat if necessary, depending on INR.

Notes:

If mild-to-moderate INR elevation without major bleeding occurs, administer vitamin K orally instead of subcutaneously.

Use of high doses of vitamin K (eg, 10-15 mg) may cause warfarin resistance for ≥1 week. During this period of resistance, heparin or low molecular weight heparin may be given until INR responds.

FFP=fresh frozen plasma; PCC=prothrombin complex concentrate; rFVIIa=recombinant factor VIIa

Dosage Forms

Injection, aqueous colloidal: 2 mg/mL (0.5 mL); 10 mg/mL (1 mL)

Injection, aqueous colloidal [preservative free]: 2 mg/mL (0.5 mL)

Tablet: 100 mcg [OTC]

Mephyton®: 5 mg

pidorubicin *see* epirubicin *on page* 360

pidorubicin hydrochloride *see* epirubicin *on page* 360

Pilagan® Ophthalmic *(Discontinued)* *see* pilocarpine *on page* 783

pilocarpine (pye loe KAR peen)

Sound-Alike/Look-Alike Issues

Isopto® Carpine may be confused with Isopto® Carbachol

Salagen® may be confused with Salacid®, selegiline

Synonyms pilocarpine hydrochloride

U.S./Canadian Brand Names Diocarpine [Can]; Isopto® Carpine [US/Can]; Pilopine HS® [US/Can]; Salagen® [US/Can]

Therapeutic Category Cholinergic Agent

Use

Ophthalmic: Management of chronic simple glaucoma, chronic and acute angle-closure glaucoma

Oral: Symptomatic treatment of xerostomia caused by salivary gland hypofunction resulting from radiotherapy for cancer of the head and neck or Sjögren syndrome

Usual Dosage Adults:

Ophthalmic: Glaucoma:

Solution: Instill 1-2 drops up to 6 times/day; adjust the concentration and frequency as required to control elevated intraocular pressure

Gel: Instill 0.5" ribbon into lower conjunctival sac once daily at bedtime

Oral: Xerostomia:

Following head and neck cancer: 5 mg 3 times/day, titration up to 10 mg 3 times/day may be considered for patients who have not responded adequately; do not exceed 2 tablets/dose

Sjögren syndrome: 5 mg 4 times/day

Dosage Forms

Gel, ophthalmic:

Pilopine HS®: 4% (4 g)

Solution, ophthalmic: 0.5% (15 mL); 1% (2 mL, 15 mL); 2% (2 mL, 15 mL); 3% (15 mL); 4% (2 mL, 15 mL); 6% (15 mL)
Isopto® Carpine: 1% (15 mL); 2% (15 mL); 4% (15 mL)
Tablet: 5 mg, 7.5 mg
Salagen®: 5 mg, 7.5 mg

pilocarpine hydrochloride *see* pilocarpine *on page* *783*
Pilopine HS® [US/Can] *see* pilocarpine *on page* *783*
Pilostat® Ophthalmic *(Discontinued)* *see* pilocarpine *on page* *783*
pimaricin *see* natamycin *on page* *683*

pimecrolimus (pim e KROE li mus)

Sound-Alike/Look-Alike Issues
pimecrolimus may be confused with tacrolimus

U.S./Canadian Brand Names Elidel® [US/Can]

Therapeutic Category Immunosuppressant Agent; Topical Skin Product

Use Short-term and intermittent long-term treatment of mild-to-moderate atopic dermatitis in patients not responsive to conventional therapy or when conventional therapy is not appropriate

Usual Dosage Topical: Children ≥2 years and Adults: Apply thin layer to affected area twice daily; rub in gently and completely. **Note:** Limit application to involved areas. Continue as long as signs and symptoms persist; discontinue if resolution occurs; reevaluate if symptoms persist >6 weeks.

Dosage Forms
Cream, topical:
Elidel®: 1% (30 g, 60 g, 100 g)

pimozide (PI moe zide)

U.S./Canadian Brand Names Apo-Pimozide® [Can]; Orap® [US/Can]; PMS-Pimozide [Can]

Therapeutic Category Neuroleptic Agent

Use Suppression of severe motor and phonic tics in patients with Tourette disorder who have failed to respond satisfactorily to standard treatment

Usual Dosage Oral: **Note:** An ECG should be performed baseline and periodically thereafter, especially during dosage adjustment:

Children ≤12 years: Tourette disorder: Initial: 0.05 mg/kg preferably once at bedtime; may be increased every third day; usual range: 2-4 mg/day; do not exceed 10 mg/day (0.2 mg/kg/day); maximum dose: 10 mg/day or 0.2 mg/kg/day (whichever is less)

Children >12 years and Adults: Tourette disorder: Initial: 1-2 mg/day in divided doses, then increase dosage as needed every other day; range is usually 7-10 mg/day, maximum dose: 10 mg/day or 0.2 mg/kg/day (whichever is less)

Dosage Forms
Tablet:
Orap®: 1 mg, 2 mg

Pin-X® [US-OTC] *see* pyrantel pamoate *on page* *838*
pinaverium bromide *see* pinaverium *(Canada only) on page* *784*

pinaverium *(Canada only)* (pin ah VEER ee um)

Synonyms pinaverium bromide

U.S./Canadian Brand Names Dicetel® [Can]

Therapeutic Category Calcium Antagonist; Gastrointestinal Agent, Miscellaneous

Use Treatment and relief of symptoms associated with irritable bowel syndrome (IBS); treatment of symptoms related to functional disorders of the biliary tract

Usual Dosage Oral: Adults: 50 mg 3 times/day; in exceptional cases, the dosage may be increased up to 100 mg 3 times/day (maximum dose: 300 mg/day). Tablets should be taken with a full glass of water during a meal/snack.

Dosage Forms [CAN] = Canadian brand name
Tablet:
Dicetel® [CAN]: 50 mg, 100 mg [not available in the U.S.]

pindolol (PIN doe lole)

Sound-Alike/Look-Alike Issues

pindolol may be confused with Parlodel®, Plendil®

Visken® may be confused with Visine®

U.S./Canadian Brand Names Apo-Pindol® [Can]; Gen-Pindolol [Can]; Novo-Pindol [Can]; Nu-Pindol [Can]; PMS-Pindolol [Can]; Visken® [Can]

Therapeutic Category Beta-Adrenergic Blocker

Use Treatment of hypertension, alone or in combination with other agents

Usual Dosage Oral: Adults: Hypertension: Initial: 5 mg twice daily, increase as necessary by 10 mg/day every 3-4 weeks (maximum daily dose: 60 mg); usual dose range (JNC 7): 10-40 mg twice daily

Dosage Forms

Tablet: 5 mg, 10 mg

pink bismuth *see* bismuth *on page 142*

Pin-Rid® ***(Discontinued)*** *see* pyrantel pamoate *on page 838*

pioglitazone (pye oh GLI ta zone)

Sound-Alike/Look-Alike Issues

Actos® may be confused with Actidose®, Actonel®

U.S./Canadian Brand Names Actos® [US/Can]; Apo-Pioglitazone [Can]; CO Pioglitazone [Can]; Gen-Pioglitazone [Can]; Novo-Pioglitazone [Can]; PMS-Pioglitazone [Can]; ratio-Pioglitazone [Can]; Sandoz-Pioglitazone [Can]; SPEF-Pioglitazone [Can]

Therapeutic Category Antidiabetic Agent; Thiazolidinedione Derivative

Use

Type 2 diabetes mellitus (noninsulin-dependent, NIDDM), monotherapy: Adjunct to diet and exercise, to improve glycemic control

Type 2 diabetes mellitus (noninsulin-dependent, NIDDM), combination therapy with sulfonylurea, metformin, or insulin: When diet, exercise, and a single agent alone does not result in adequate glycemic control

Usual Dosage Oral:

Adults:

Monotherapy: Initial: 15-30 mg once daily; if response is inadequate, the dosage may be increased in increments up to 45 mg once daily; maximum recommended dose: 45 mg once daily

Combination therapy: Maximum recommended dose: 45 mg/day

With sulfonylureas: Initial: 15-30 mg once daily; dose of sulfonylurea should be reduced if the patient reports hypoglycemia

With metformin: Initial: 15-30 mg once daily; it is unlikely that the dose of metformin will need to be reduced due to hypoglycemia

With insulin: Initial: 15-30 mg once daily; dose of insulin should be reduced by 10% to 25% if the patient reports hypoglycemia or if the plasma glucose falls to <100 mg/dL.

Dosage Forms

Tablet:

Actos®: 15 mg, 30 mg, 45 mg

pioglitazone and glimepiride (pye oh GLI ta zone & GLYE me pye ride)

Synonyms glimepiride and pioglitazone; glimepiride and pioglitazone hydrochloride

U.S./Canadian Brand Names Duetact™ [US]

Therapeutic Category Antidiabetic Agent, Sulfonylurea; Antidiabetic Agent, Thiazolidinedione; Hypoglycemic Agent, Oral

Use Management of type 2 diabetes mellitus (noninsulin-dependent, NIDDM) as an adjunct to diet and exercise

Usual Dosage Oral: Type 2 diabetes mellitus:

Adults: Initial dose should be based on current dose of pioglitazone and/or sulfonylurea.

Patients inadequately controlled on **glimepiride** alone: Initial dose: 30 mg/2 mg or 30 mg/4 mg once daily

Patients inadequately controlled on **pioglitazone** alone: Initial dose: 30 mg/2 mg once daily

Patients with systolic dysfunction (eg, NYHA Class I and II): Initiate only after patient has been safely titrated to 30 mg of pioglitazone. Initial dose: 30 mg/2 mg or 30 mg/4 mg once daily.

Note: No exact dosing relationship exists between glimepiride and other sulfonlyureas. Dosing should be limited to less than or equal to the maximum initial dose of glimepiride (2 mg). When converting patients from other sulfonylureas with longer half lives (eg, chlorpropamide) to glimepiride, observe patient carefully for 1-2 weeks due to overlapping hypoglycemic effects.

Dosing adjustment: Dosage may be increased up to max dose and formulation strengths available; tablet should not be given more than once daily; see individual agents for frequency of adjustments. Dosage adjustments in patients with systolic dysfunction should be done carefully and patient monitored for symptoms of worsening heart failure.

Maximum dose: Pioglitazone 45 mg/glimepiride 8 mg daily

Dosage Forms

Tablet:

Duetact™: 30 mg/2 mg: Pioglitazone 30 mg and glimepiride 2 mg; 30 mg/4 mg: Pioglitazone 30 mg and glimepiride 4 mg

pioglitazone and metformin (pye oh GLI ta zone & met FOR min)

Synonyms metformin hydrochloride and pioglitazone hydrochloride

U.S./Canadian Brand Names Actoplus Met® XR [US]; Actoplus Met® [US]

Therapeutic Category Antidiabetic Agent, Biguanide; Antidiabetic Agent, Thiazolidinedione

Use Management of type 2 diabetes mellitus (noninsulin-dependent, NIDDM)

Usual Dosage Oral: Type 2 diabetes mellitus:

Adults: Initial dose should be based on current dose of pioglitazone and/or metformin; daily dose should be divided and given with meals

Patients inadequately controlled on **metformin alone**: Initial dose: Pioglitazone 15-30 mg/day plus current dose of metformin

Patients inadequately controlled on **pioglitazone alone**: Initial dose: Metformin 1000-1700 mg/day plus current dose of pioglitazone

Note: When switching from combination pioglitazone and metformin as separate tablets: Use current dose.

Dosing adjustment: Doses may be increased as increments of pioglitazone 15 mg and/or metformin 500-850 mg, up to the maximum dose; doses should be titrated gradually. Guidelines for frequency of adjustment (adapted from rosiglitazone/metformin combination labeling):

After a change in the **metformin** dosage, titration can be done after 1-2 weeks

After a change in the **pioglitazone** dosage, titration can be done after 8-12 weeks

Maximum dose: Pioglitazone 45 mg/metformin 2550 mg daily

Product Availability Actoplus Met® XR: FDA approved May 2009; availability anticipated later in 2009

Dosage Forms

Tablet:

Actoplus Met®: 15/500: Pioglitazone 15 mg and metformin 500 mg; 15/850: Pioglitazone 15 mg and metformin 850 mg

piperacillin (pi PER a sil in)

Synonyms piperacillin sodium

U.S./Canadian Brand Names Piperacillin for Injection, USP [Can]

Therapeutic Category Penicillin

Use Treatment of susceptible infections such as septicemia, acute and chronic respiratory tract infections, skin and soft tissue infections, and urinary tract infections due to susceptible strains of *Pseudomonas*, *Proteus*, and *Escherichia coli* and *Enterobacter*; active against some streptococci and some anaerobic bacteria; febrile neutropenia (as part of combination regimen)

Usual Dosage

Usual dosage range:

Neonates: I.M., I.V.: 100 mg/kg every 12 hours

Infants and Children: I.M., I.V.: 200-300 mg/kg/day in divided doses every 4-6 hours

Adults: I.M., I.V.: 2-4 g/dose every 4-6 hours (maximum: 24 g/day)

Indication-specific dosing:

Children: I.M., I.V.: **Cystic fibrosis:** 350-500 mg/kg/day in divided doses every 4-6 hours

Adults:

Burn wound sepsis: I.V.: 4 g every 4 hours with vancomycin and amikacin

Cholangitis, acute: I.V.: 4 g every 6 hours

Keratitis *(Pseudomonas)*: Ophthalmic: 6-12 mg/mL every 15-60 minutes around the clock for 24-72 hours, then slow reduction

Malignant otitis externa: I.V.: 4-6 g every 4-6 hours with tobramycin
Moderate infections: I.M., I.V.: 2-3 g/dose every 6-12 hours (maximum: 2 g I.M./site)
Prosthetic joint *(Pseudomonas)*: I.V.: 3 g every 6 hours with aminoglycoside
***Pseudomonas* infections:** I.V.: 4 g every 4 hours
Severe infections: I.M., I.V.: 3-4 g/dose every 4-6 hours (maximum: 24 g/24 hours)
Urinary tract infections: I.V.: 2-3 g/dose every 6-12 hours
Uncomplicated gonorrhea: I.M.: 2 g in a single dose accompanied by 1 g probenecid 30 minutes prior to injection

Dosage Forms
Injection, powder for reconstitution: 2 g, 3 g, 4 g, 40 g

piperacillin and tazobactam sodium (pi PER a sil in & ta zoe BAK tam SOW dee um)

Sound-Alike/Look-Alike Issues
Zosyn® may be confused with Zofran®, Zyvox®

Synonyms piperacillin sodium and tazobactam sodium; tazobactam and piperacillin

U.S./Canadian Brand Names Tazocin® [Can]; Zosyn® [US]

Therapeutic Category Penicillin

Use Treatment of moderate-to-severe infections caused by susceptible organisms, including infections of the lower respiratory tract (community-acquired pneumonia, nosocomial pneumonia); urinary tract; uncomplicated and complicated skin and skin structures; gynecologic (endometritis, pelvic inflammatory disease); bone and joint infections; intraabdominal infections (appendicitis with rupture/abscess, peritonitis); and septicemia. Tazobactam expands activity of piperacillin to include beta-lactamase producing strains of *S. aureus*, *H. influenzae*, *Bacteroides*, and other gram-negative bacteria.

Usual Dosage
Usual dosage range:
Children: I.V.:
2-8 months: 80 mg of piperacillin component/kg every 8 hours
≥9 months and ≤40 kg: 100 mg of piperacillin component/kg every 8 hours
Adults: I.V.: 3.375 g every 6 hours **or** 4.5 g every 6-8 hours; maximum: 18 g/day

Indication-specific dosing: I.V.:
Children: **Note:** Dosing based on piperacillin component:
Appendicitis, peritonitis:
2-8 months: 80 mg/kg every 8 hours
≥9 months and ≤40 kg: 100 mg/kg every 8 hours
>40 kg: refer to Adult dosing
Adults:
Diverticulitis, intraabdominal abscess, peritonitis: I.V.: 3.375 g every 6 hours; **Note:** Some clinicians use 4.5 g every 8 hours for empiric coverage since the %time>MIC is similar between the regimens for most pathogens; however, this regimen is NOT recommended for nosocomial pneumonia or *Pseudomonas* coverage.
Pneumonia (nosocomial): I.V.: 4.5 g every 6 hours for 7-14 days (when used empirically, combination with an aminoglycoside or antipseudomonal fluoroquinolone is recommended; consider discontinuation of additional agent if *P. aeruginosa* is not isolated)
Severe infections: I.V.: 3.375 g every 6 hours for 7-10 days; **Note:** Some clinicians use 4.5 g every 8 hours for empiric coverage since the %time>MIC is similar between the regimens for most pathogens; however, this regimen is NOT recommended for nosocomial pneumonia or *Pseudomonas* coverage.

Dosage Forms 8:1 ratio of piperacillin sodium/tazobactam sodium
Infusion [premixed iso-osmotic solution, frozen]:
Zosyn®
2.25 g: Piperacillin 2 g and tazobactam 0.25 g (50 mL)
3.375 g: Piperacillin 3 g and tazobactam 0.375 g (50 mL)
4.5 g: Piperacillin 4 g and tazobactam 0.5 g (50 mL)
Injection, powder for reconstitution:
Zosyn®
2.25 g: Piperacillin 2 g and tazobactam 0.25 g
3.375 g: Piperacillin 3 g and tazobactam 0.375 g
4.5 g: Piperacillin 4 g and tazobactam 0.5 g
40.5 g: Piperacillin 36 g and tazobactam 4.5 g

Piperacillin for Injection, USP [Can] *see* piperacillin *on page* 786

piperacillin sodium *see* piperacillin *on page* 786

piperacillin sodium and tazobactam sodium *see* piperacillin and tazobactam sodium *on page 787*
piperazine estrone sulfate *see* estropipate *on page 381*
piperonyl butoxide and pyrethrins *see* pyrethrins and piperonyl butoxide *on page 839*
Pipracil® *(Discontinued)* *see* piperacillin *on page 786*

pirbuterol (peer BYOO ter ole)

Synonyms pirbuterol acetate

U.S./Canadian Brand Names Maxair™ Autohaler™ [US]

Therapeutic Category Adrenergic Agonist Agent

Use Prevention and treatment of reversible bronchospasm including asthma

Usual Dosage Children ≥12 years and Adults: 2 inhalations every 4-6 hours for prevention; two inhalations at an interval of at least 1-3 minutes, followed by a third inhalation in treatment of bronchospasm, not to exceed 12 inhalations/day

Dosage Forms

Aerosol for oral inhalation:
Maxair™ Autohaler™: 200 mcg/actuation (14 g)

pirbuterol acetate *see* pirbuterol *on page 788*

piroxicam (peer OKS i kam)

Sound-Alike/Look-Alike Issues
Feldene® may be confused with FLUoxetine

U.S./Canadian Brand Names Apo-Piroxicam® [Can]; Dom-Piroxicam [Can]; Feldene® [US]; Gen-Piroxicam [Can]; Novo-Pirocam [Can]; Nu-Pirox [Can]; PMS-Piroxicam [Can]; Pro-Piroxicam [Can]

Therapeutic Category Analgesic, Nonnarcotic; Nonsteroidal Antiinflammatory Drug (NSAID)

Use Symptomatic treatment of acute and chronic rheumatoid arthritis and osteoarthritis

Usual Dosage Oral: Adults: 10-20 mg/day once daily; although associated with increase in GI adverse effects, doses >20 mg/day have been used (ie, 30-40 mg/day)

Dosage Forms

Capsule: 10 mg, 20 mg
Feldene®: 10 mg, 20 mg

***p*-isobutylhydratropic acid** *see* ibuprofen *on page 515*
pit *see* oxytocin *on page 742*
Pitocin® [US/Can] *see* oxytocin *on page 742*
Pitrex [Can] *see* tolnaftate *on page 968*
pivampicillin *see* pivampicillin *(Canada only) on page 788*

pivampicillin *(Canada only)* (piv am pi SIL in)

Synonyms MK-191; pivampicilin

U.S./Canadian Brand Names Pondocillin® [Can]

Therapeutic Category Penicillin

Use Treatment of susceptible bacterial infections (nonbeta-lactamase-producing organisms); susceptible bacterial infections caused by streptococci, pneumococci, nonpenicillinase-producing staphylococci, *H. influenzae*, *N. gonorrhoeae*, *E. coli*, *P. mirabilis*, *Listeria*, *Salmonella*, *Shigella*, *Enterobacter*, and *Klebsiella*

Usual Dosage Oral:

Infants and Children: Bacterial infections: Oral suspension:
- Infants <3 months: Use of pivampicillin in this age group should be avoided
- Infants 3-12 months: Dosage range: 40-60 mg/kg/day in 2 divided doses
- Children ≤10 years: Dosage range: 25-35 mg/kg/day, not to exceed recommended daily adult dose of 500 mg twice daily
- Alternatively: Children:
  - 1-3 years: 175 mg twice daily
  - 4-6 years: 262.5 mg twice daily
  - 7-10 years: 350 mg twice daily

Children >10 years and Adults: Usual dose: 500 mg (tablet) or 525 mg (suspension) twice daily; dosage may be doubled in severe infections
- Gonococcal urethritis: 1.5 g as a single dose with 1 g probenecid concurrently

Dosage Forms [CAN] = Canadian brand name

Powder for oral suspension:

Pondocillin® [CAN]: 175 mg/5 mL (100 mL, 150 mL, 200 mL) [not available in the U.S.]

Tablet:

Pondocillin® [CAN]: 500 mg [equivalent to 377 mg ampicillin; not available in the U.S.]

pix carbonis *see* coal tar *on page 250*

pizotifen *(Canada only)* (pi ZOE ti fen)

Synonyms pizotifen malate

U.S./Canadian Brand Names Sandomigran DS® [Can]; Sandomigran® [Can]

Therapeutic Category Antimigraine Agent

Use Migraine prophylaxis

Usual Dosage Oral: Children ≥12 years and Adults: Migraine prophylaxis: Initial: 0.5 mg at bedtime; increase gradually to 0.5 mg 3 times/day; usual dosage range: 1-6 mg/day

Note: Therapeutic response may require several weeks of therapy. Do not discontinue abruptly (reduce gradually over 2-week period).

Dosage Forms [CAN] = Canadian brand name

Tablet:

Sandomigran® [CAN]: 0.5 mg [not available in the U.S.]

Tablet, double strength:

Sandomigran® DS [CAN]: 1 mg [not available in the U.S.]

pizotifen malate *see* pizotifen *(Canada only) on page 789*

Plan B® [US-RX/OTC/Can] *see* levonorgestrel *on page 582*

Plan B® One-Step [US-RX/OTC] *see* levonorgestrel *on page 582*

plantago seed *see* psyllium *on page 837*

plantain seed *see* psyllium *on page 837*

Plaquase® ***(Discontinued)*** *see* collagenase *on page 255*

Plaquenil® [US/Can] *see* hydroxychloroquine *on page 509*

Plaretase® 8000 ***(Discontinued)*** *see* pancrelipase *on page 746*

Plasbumin® [US] *see* albumin *on page 40*

Plasbumin®-5 [Can] *see* albumin *on page 40*

Plasbumin®-25 [Can] *see* albumin *on page 40*

Plasmanate® [US] *see* plasma protein fraction *on page 789*

Plasma-Plex® ***(Discontinued)*** *see* plasma protein fraction *on page 789*

plasma protein fraction (PLAS mah PROE teen FRAK shun)

U.S./Canadian Brand Names Plasmanate® [US]

Therapeutic Category Blood Product Derivative

Use Plasma volume expansion and maintenance of cardiac output in the treatment of certain types of shock or impending shock

Usual Dosage I.V.: Adults: Usual minimum dose: 250-500 mL; adjust dose based on response

Dosage Forms

Injection, solution [human, preservative free]:

Plasmanate®: 5% (50 mL, 250 mL)

Plasmatein® ***(Discontinued)*** *see* plasma protein fraction *on page 789*

Platinol®-AQ ***(Discontinued)*** *see* cisplatin *on page 233*

Plavix® [US/Can] *see* clopidogrel *on page 247*

Plegine® [Can] *see* phendimetrazine *on page 770*

Plegine® ***(Discontinued)*** *see* phendimetrazine *on page 770*

Plenaxis™ ***(Discontinued)***

Plendil® [Can] *see* felodipine *on page 408*

Plendil® ***(Discontinued)*** *see* felodipine *on page 408*

plerixafor (pler IX a fore)

Synonyms AMD3100; LM3100

U.S./Canadian Brand Names Mozobil™ [US]

Therapeutic Category Hematopoietic Stem Cell Mobilizer

Use Mobilization of hematopoietic stem cells (HSC) for collection and subsequent autologous transplantation (in combination with filgrastim) in patients with non-Hodgkin lymphoma (NHL) and multiple myeloma (MM)

Usual Dosage Note: Dosing is based on actual body weight. Begin plerixafor after patient has received filgrastim 10 mcg/kg once daily for 4 days; plerixafor, filgrastim and apheresis should be continued daily until sufficient cell collection up to a maximum of 4 days.

SubQ: Adults: HSC mobilization: 0.24 mg/kg once daily ~11 hours prior to apheresis for up to 4 consecutive days; maximum dose: 40 mg/day

Dosage Forms

Injection, solution [preservative free]:

Mozobil™: 20 mg/mL (1.2 mL)

Pletal® [US/Can] *see* cilostazol *on page* *228*
Plexion® [US] *see* sulfur and sulfacetamide *on page* *931*
Plexion SCT® [US] *see* sulfur and sulfacetamide *on page* *931*
Plexion TS® ***(Discontinued)*** *see* sulfur and sulfacetamide *on page* *931*
Pliaglis™ [US] *see* lidocaine and tetracaine *on page* *589*
PMPA *see* tenofovir *on page* *944*
PMS-Alendronate [Can] *see* alendronate *on page* *44*
PMS-Alendronate-FC [Can] *see* alendronate *on page* *44*
PMS-Amantadine [Can] *see* amantadine *on page* *57*
PMS-Amiodarone [Can] *see* amiodarone *on page* *64*
PMS-Amitriptyline [Can] *see* amitriptyline *on page* *65*
PMS-Amlodipine [Can] *see* amlodipine *on page* *66*
PMS-Amoxicillin [Can] *see* amoxicillin *on page* *70*
PMS-Anagrelide [Can] *see* anagrelide *on page* *78*
PMS-Atenolol [Can] *see* atenolol *on page* *107*
PMS-Azithromycin [Can] *see* azithromycin *on page* *116*
PMS-Baclofen [Can] *see* baclofen *on page* *120*
PMS-Benzydamine [Can] *see* benzydamine *(Canada only) on page* *135*
PMS-Bethanechol [Can] *see* bethanechol *on page* *139*
PMS-Bezafibrate [Can] *see* bezafibrate *(Canada only) on page* *140*
PMS-Bicalutamide [Can] *see* bicalutamide *on page* *141*
PMS-Bisoprolol [Can] *see* bisoprolol *on page* *144*
PMS-Brimonidine Tartrate [Can] *see* brimonidine *on page* *147*
PMS-Bromocriptine [Can] *see* bromocriptine *on page* *148*
PMS-Bupropion SR [Can] *see* bupropion *on page* *158*
PMS-Buspirone [Can] *see* buspirone *on page* *160*
PMS-Butorphanol [Can] *see* butorphanol *on page* *164*
PMS-Captopril [Can] *see* captopril *on page* *178*
PMS-Carbamazepine [Can] *see* carbamazepine *on page* *180*
PMS-Carvedilol [Can] *see* carvedilol *on page* *188*
PMS-Cefaclor [Can] *see* cefaclor *on page* *191*
PMS-Cetirizine [Can] *see* cetirizine *on page* *204*
PMS-Chloral Hydrate [Can] *see* chloral hydrate *on page* *208*
PMS-Cholestyramine [Can] *see* cholestyramine resin *on page* *224*
PMS-Cilazapril [Can] *see* cilazapril *(Canada only) on page* *228*
PMS-Cimetidine [Can] *see* cimetidine *on page* *228*
PMS-Ciprofloxacin [Can] *see* ciprofloxacin *on page* *229*
PMS-Citalopram [Can] *see* citalopram *on page* *234*
PMS-Clarithromycin [Can] *see* clarithromycin *on page* *236*
PMS-Clindamycin [Can] *see* clindamycin *on page* *239*
PMS-Clobazam [Can] *see* clobazam *(Canada only) on page* *241*

PMS-Sertraline [Can] *see* sertraline *on page 898*
PMS-Simvastatin [Can] *see* simvastatin *on page 902*
PMS-Sodium Polystyrene Sulfonate [Can] *see* sodium polystyrene sulfonate *on page 914*
PMS-Sotalol [Can] *see* sotalol *on page 919*
PMS-Sucralate [Can] *see* sucralfate *on page 925*
PMS-Sumatriptan [Can] *see* sumatriptan *on page 932*
PMS-Tamoxifen [Can] *see* tamoxifen *on page 937*
PMS-Temazepam [Can] *see* temazepam *on page 942*
PMS-Terazosin [Can] *see* terazosin *on page 945*
PMS-Testosterone [Can] *see* testosterone *on page 947*
PMS-Theophylline [Can] *see* theophylline *on page 953*
PMS-Tiaprofenic [Can] *see* tiaprofenic acid *(Canada only) on page 959*
PMS-Timolol [Can] *see* timolol *on page 961*
PMS-Tobramycin [Can] *see* tobramycin *on page 965*
PMS-Topiramate [Can] *see* topiramate *on page 969*
PMS-Trazodone [Can] *see* trazodone *on page 979*
PMS-Trifluoperazine [Can] *see* trifluoperazine *on page 986*
PMS-Ursodiol C [Can] *see* ursodiol *on page 1000*
PMS-Valacyclovir [Can] *see* valacyclovir *on page 1001*
PMS-Valproic Acid [Can] *see* valproic acid and derivatives *on page 1002*
PMS-Valproic Acid E.C. [Can] *see* valproic acid and derivatives *on page 1002*
PMS-Venlafaxine XR [Can] *see* venlafaxine *on page 1009*
PMS-Verapamil SR [Can] *see* verapamil *on page 1010*
PMS-Yohimbine [Can] *see* yohimbine *on page 1025*
PMS-Zopiclone [Can] *see* zopiclone *(Canada only) on page 1034*
PN *see* total parenteral nutrition *on page 972*
Pneumo 23™ [Can] *see* pneumococcal polysaccharide vaccine (polyvalent) *on page 794*
pneumococcal 7-valent conjugate vaccine *see* pneumococcal conjugate vaccine (7-valent) *on page 793*

pneumococcal conjugate vaccine (7-valent)

(noo moe KOK al KON ju gate vak SEEN, seven vay lent)

Sound-Alike/Look-Alike Issues

pneumococcal conjugate vaccine (7-valent) may be confused with pneumococcal polysaccharide vaccine (polyvalent)

Prevnar® may be confused with PREVEN®

Synonyms diphtheria CRM_{197} protein; PCV7; pneumococcal 7-valent conjugate vaccine

U.S./Canadian Brand Names Prevnar® [US/Can]

Therapeutic Category Vaccine

Use

Immunization of infants and toddlers against *Streptococcus pneumoniae* infection caused by serotypes included in the vaccine

Immunization of infant and toddlers against otitis media caused by serotypes included in the vaccine

Advisory Committee on Immunization Practices (ACIP) recommends routine vaccination for the following:

- All children 2-23 months
- Children ≥2-59 months with cochlear implants
- Children ages 24-59 months with: Sickle cell disease (including other sickle cell hemoglobinopathies, asplenia, splenic dysfunction), HIV infection, immunocompromising conditions (congenital immunodeficiencies excluding chronic granulomatous disease, renal failure, nephrotic syndrome, diseases associated with immunosuppressive or radiation therapy, solid organ transplant), chronic illnesses (cardiac disease, cerebrospinal fluid leaks, diabetes mellitus, pulmonary disease excluding asthma unless on high dose corticosteroids)
- Consider use in all children 24-59 months with priority given to:
  - Children 24-35 months
  - Children 24-59 months who are of Alaska native, American Indian, or African-American descent
  - Children 24-59 months who attend group day care centers

Usual Dosage I.M.:

Infants: 2-6 months: 0.5 mL at approximately 2-month intervals for 3 consecutive doses, followed by a fourth dose of 0.5 mL at 12-15 months of age; first dose may be given as young as 6 weeks of age, but is typically given at 2 months of age. In case of a moderate shortage of vaccine, defer the fourth dose until shortage is resolved; in case of a severe shortage of vaccine, defer third and fourth doses until shortage is resolved.

Previously Unvaccinated Older Infants and Children:

7-11 months: 0.5 mL for a total of 3 doses; 2 doses at least 4 weeks apart, followed by a third dose after the 1-year birthday (12-15 months), separated from the second dose by at least 2 months. In case of a severe shortage of vaccine, defer the third dose until shortage is resolved.

12-23 months: 0.5 mL for a total of 2 doses, separated by at least 2 months. In case of a severe shortage of vaccine, defer the second dose until shortage is resolved.

24-59 months:

Healthy Children: 0.5 mL as a single dose. In case of a severe shortage of vaccine, defer dosing until shortage is resolved.

Children with sickle cell disease, asplenia, HIV infection, chronic illness or immunocompromising conditions: 0.5 mL for a total of 2 doses, separated by 2 months

Previously Vaccinated with PPSV23 (ACIP recommendations): Children 24-59 months of age at high risk for pneumococcal disease but have already received the PPSV23 may benefit from the immunologic response induced by PCV7. Suggested dosing: Starting ≥2 months after last PPSV23 dose: One dose of PCV7, followed by a second dose ≥2 months later.

Previously Vaccinated with PCV7 and with a lapse in vaccine administration (ACIP recommendations):

7-11 months: Previously received 1 or 2 doses PCV7: 0.5 mL dose at 7-11 months of age, followed by a second dose ≥2 months later at 12-15 months of age

12-23 months:

Previously received 1 dose before 12 months of age: 0.5 mL dose, followed by a second dose ≥2 months later

Previously received 2 doses before age 12 months: 0.5 mL dose ≥2 months after the most recent dose

24-59 months: Any incomplete schedule: 0.5 mL as a single dose; **Note:** Patients with chronic diseases or immunosuppressing conditions should receive 2 doses ≥2 months apart

Dosage Forms

Injection, suspension:

Prevnar®: 2 mcg of each capsular saccharide for serotypes 4, 9V, 14, 18C, 19F, and 23F, and 4 mcg of serotype 6B per 0.5 mL (0.5 mL)

pneumococcal polysaccharide vaccine (polyvalent)

(noo moe KOK al pol i SAK a ride vak SEEN, pol i VAY lent)

Sound-Alike/Look-Alike Issues

pneumococcal polysaccharide vaccine (polyvalent) may be confused with pneumococcal conjugate vaccine (7-valent)

Synonyms 23-valent pneumococcal polysaccharide vaccine; 23PS; PPSV; PPSV23; PPV23

U.S./Canadian Brand Names Pneumo 23™ [Can]; Pneumovax® 23 [US/Can]

Therapeutic Category Vaccine, Inactivated Bacteria

Use Immunization against pneumococcal disease caused by serotypes included in the vaccine. Use is recommended for the following:

Immunocompetent individuals:

Routine vaccination for persons ≥50 years of age

Persons ≥2 years with the following chronic conditions: cardiovascular disease, pulmonary disease, diabetes mellitus, liver disease

Persons ≥2 years with alcoholism, cerebrospinal fluid leaks, functional or anatomic asplenia

Persons ≥2 years in special living environments or social settings

Adults 19-64 years who smoke cigarettes

Immunocompromised individuals: Persons ≥2 years with HIV infection, leukemia, lymphoma, Hodgkin disease, multiple myeloma, generalized malignancy, chronic renal failure, nephritic syndrome, chronic immunosuppressive therapy (including corticosteroids), persons who received an organ or bone marrow transplant

In addition, the Advisory Committee on Immunization Practices (ACIP) recommends routine vaccination for all immunocompetent persons ≥65 years of age and persons aged 2-64 years with cochlear implants. Routine vaccination is not recommended for Alaska Natives or American Indian persons unless they have underlying conditions which are indications for vaccination; in special situations, vaccination may be recommended when living in an area at increased risk of invasive pneumococcal disease.

Usual Dosage I.M., SubQ: Children >2 years and Adults: 0.5 mL

Revaccination:

Immunocompetent individuals: Revaccination generally not recommended

Children ≥2 years and Adults at highest risk for infection: One revaccination ≥5 years after first dose of PPSV23. May consider giving the revaccination dose ≥3 years after first dose of PPSV23 in children who will be ≤10 years of age at the time of revaccination. Patients at highest risk for infection include those with asplenia, sickle cell anemia, HIV infection, leukemia, lymphoma, Hodgkin disease, multiple myeloma, generalized malignancy, chronic renal failure, nephrotic syndrome, conditions associated with immunosuppression, and patients on immunosuppressive therapy (including corticosteroids)

Adults ≥65 years: One revaccination if ≥5 years after first dose of PPSV23 and if <65 years of age of initial vaccination.

Previously vaccinated with PCV7 vaccine: Children ≥2 years and Adults:

With sickle cell disease, asplenia, immunocompromised or HIV infection: 0.5 mL at ≥2 years of age and ≥2 months after last dose of PCV7; one revaccination with PPSV23 should be given ≥5 years for children >10 years of age and after 3-5 years for children ≤10 years of age; revaccination should not be administered <3 years after the previous PPSV23 dose

With chronic illness: 0.5 mL at ≥2 years of age and ≥2 months after last dose of PCV7; revaccination with PPSV23 is not recommended

Dosage Forms

Injection, solution:

Pneumovax® 23: 25 mcg each of 23 capsular polysaccharide isolates/0.5 mL (0.5 mL, 2.5 mL)

Pneumomist® ***(Discontinued)*** *see* guaifenesin *on page* 473

Pneumotussin® ***(Discontinued)***

Pneumovax® 23 [US/Can] *see* pneumococcal polysaccharide vaccine (polyvalent) *on page* 794

PNU-140690E *see* tipranavir *on page* 963

Pnu-Imune® 23 ***(Discontinued)***

Podactin Cream [US-OTC] *see* miconazole *on page* 654

Podactin Powder [US-OTC] *see* tolnaftate *on page* 968

Pod-Ben-25® ***(Discontinued)*** *see* podophyllum resin *on page* 795

Podocon-25® [US] *see* podophyllum resin *on page* 795

Podofilm® [Can] *see* podophyllum resin *on page* 795

podofilox (poe DOF il oks)

U.S./Canadian Brand Names Condyline™ [Can]; Condylox® [US]; Wartec® [Can]

Therapeutic Category Keratolytic Agent

Use Treatment of external genital warts

Usual Dosage Topical: Adults: Apply twice daily (morning and evening) for 3 consecutive days, then withhold use for 4 consecutive days; this cycle may be repeated up to 4 times until there is no visible wart tissue

Dosage Forms

Gel:

Condylox®: 0.5% (3.5 g)

Solution, topical: 0.5% (3.5 mL)

Condylox®: 0.5% (3.5 mL)

Podofin® ***(Discontinued)*** *see* podophyllum resin *on page* 795

podophyllin *see* podophyllum resin *on page* 795

podophyllum resin (po DOF fil um REZ in)

Synonyms mandrake; may apple; podophyllin

U.S./Canadian Brand Names Podocon-25® [US]; Podofilm® [Can]

Therapeutic Category Keratolytic Agent

Use Topical treatment of benign growths including external genital and perianal warts, papillomas, fibroids; compound benzoin tincture generally is used as the medium for topical application

Usual Dosage Topical:

Children and Adults: 10% to 25% solution in compound benzoin tincture; apply drug to dry surface, use 1 drop at a time allowing drying between drops until area is covered; total volume should be limited to <0.5 mL per treatment session

Condylomata acuminatum: 25% solution is applied daily; use a 10% solution when applied to or near mucous membranes

Verrucae: 25% solution is applied 3-5 times/day directly to the wart

Dosage Forms

Liquid, topical:

Podocon-25®: 25% (15 mL)

Point-Two® ***(Discontinued)*** *see* fluoride *on page 430*

Poladex® ***(Discontinued)*** *see* dexchlorpheniramine *on page 290*

Polaramine® ***(Discontinued)*** *see* dexchlorpheniramine *on page 290*

poliovirus vaccine (inactivated) (POE lee oh VYE rus vak SEEN, in ak ti VAY ted)

Synonyms enhanced-potency inactivated poliovirus vaccine; IPV; salk vaccine

U.S./Canadian Brand Names IPOL® [US/Can]

Therapeutic Category Vaccine, Live Virus and Inactivated Virus

Use Active immunization against poliomyelitis caused by poliovirus types 1, 2 and 3. **Note:** Combination products containing polio vaccine are also available and may be preferred in certain age groups if recipients are likely to be susceptible to the agents contained within each vaccine.

The Advisory Committee on Immunization Practices (ACIP) recommends routine vaccination for the following:

- All children (first dose given at 2 months of age). Routine immunization of adults in the United States is generally not recommended. Adults with previous wild poliovirus disease, who have never been immunized, or those who are incompletely immunized may receive inactivated poliovirus vaccine if they fall into one of the following categories:
- Travelers to regions or countries where poliomyelitis is endemic or epidemic
- Healthcare workers in close contact with patients who may be excreting poliovirus
- Laboratory workers handling specimens that may contain poliovirus
- Members of communities or specific population groups with diseases caused by wild poliovirus
- Incompletely vaccinated or unvaccinated adults in a household or with other close contact with children receiving oral poliovirus (may be at increased risk of vaccine associated paralytic poliomyelitis)

Usual Dosage I.M., SubQ:

Children:

Primary immunization: Administer three 0.5 mL doses, preferably 8 or more weeks apart, at 2, 4, and 6-18 months of age. First dose may be given as early as 6 weeks of age. Do not administer more frequently than 4 weeks apart.

Booster dose: 0.5 mL at 4-6 years of age

Adults:

Previously unvaccinated: Two 0.5 mL doses administered at 1- to 2-month intervals, followed by a third dose 6-12 months later. If <3 months, but at least 2 months are available before protection is needed, 3 doses may be administered at least 1 month apart. If administration must be completed within 1-2 months, give 2 doses at least 1 month apart. If <1 month is available, give 1 dose.

Incompletely vaccinated: Adults with at least 1 previous dose of OPV, <3 doses of IPV, or a combination of OPV and IPV equaling <3 doses, administer at least one 0.5 mL dose of IPV. Additional doses to complete the series may be given if time permits.

Completely vaccinated and at increased risk of exposure: One 0.5 mL dose

Dosage Forms

Injection, suspension:

IPOL®: Type 1 poliovirus 40 D-antigen units, type 2 poliovirus 8 D-antigen units, and type 3 poliovirus 32 D-antigen units per 0.5 mL (0.5 mL, 5 mL)

Polocaine® [US/Can] *see* mepivacaine *on page 628*

Polocaine® 2% and Levonordefrin 1:20,000 [Can] *see* mepivacaine and levonordefrin *on page 628*

Polocaine® Dental [US] *see* mepivacaine *on page 628*

Polocaine® Dental with Levonordefrin [US] *see* mepivacaine and levonordefrin *on page 628*

Polocaine® MPF [US] *see* mepivacaine *on page 628*

polycarbophil (pol i KAR boe fil)

U.S./Canadian Brand Names Equalactin® [US-OTC]; Fiber-Lax® [US-OTC]; Fiber-Tabs™ [US-OTC]; FiberCon® [US-OTC]; Konsyl® Fiber Caplets [US-OTC]

Therapeutic Category Gastrointestinal Agent, Miscellaneous; Laxative

Use Treatment of constipation or diarrhea

Usual Dosage Oral: General dosing guidelines (OTC labeling):

Children 6-12 years: 625 mg calcium polycarbophil 1-4 times/day

Children ≥12 years and Adults: 1250 mg calcium polycarbophil 1-4 times/day

Dosage Forms

Caplet: Calcium polycarbophil 625 mg [equivalent to polycarbophil 500 mg]

FiberCon® [OTC], Konsyl® Fiber [OTC]: Calcium polycarbophil 625 mg

Captab:

Fiber-Lax® [OTC]: Calcium polycarbophil 625 mg

Tablet: Calcium polycarbophil 625 mg

Fiber-Tabs™ [OTC]: Calcium polycarbophil 625 mg

Tablet, chewable:

Equalactin® [OTC]: Calcium polycarbophil 625 mg

Polycitra® [US] *see* citric acid, sodium citrate, and potassium citrate *on page* 235

Polycitra®-K [US] *see* potassium citrate and citric acid *on page* 804

Polycitra®-LC [US] *see* citric acid, sodium citrate, and potassium citrate *on page* 235

Polycose® [US-OTC] *see* glucose polymers *on page* 466

Poly-Dex™ [US] *see* neomycin, polymyxin B, and dexamethasone *on page* 687

polyethylene glycol-L-asparaginase *see* pegaspargase *on page* 755

polyethylene glycol 3350 (pol i ETH i leen GLY kol 3350)

Sound-Alike/Look-Alike Issues

polyethylene glycol 3350 may be confused with polyethylene glycol electrolyte solution

MiraLax® may be confused with Mirapex®

Synonyms PEG

U.S./Canadian Brand Names GlycoLax® [US]; MiraLax® [US-OTC]

Therapeutic Category Laxative, Osmotic

Use Treatment of occasional constipation in adults

Usual Dosage Oral: Adults: Occasional constipation: 17 g of powder (~1 heaping tablespoon) dissolved in 4-8 ounces of beverage, once daily; do not use for >2 weeks

Dosage Forms

Powder, for oral solution: PEG 3350 17 g/packet (14s); PEG 3350 255 g (16 oz); PEG 3350 527 g (32 oz)

GlycoLax®: PEG 3350 527 g (24 oz)

MiraLax® [OTC]: PEG 3350 255 g (14 oz)

polyethylene glycol-electrolyte solution
(pol i ETH i leen GLY kol ee LEK troe lite soe LOO shun)

Sound-Alike/Look-Alike Issues

GoLYTELY® may be confused with NuLYTELY®

NuLYTELY® may be confused with GoLYTELY®

TriLyte® may be confused with TriLipix™

Synonyms electrolyte lavage solution

U.S./Canadian Brand Names Colyte® [US/Can]; GoLYTELY® [US]; Klean-Prep® [Can]; MoviPrep® [US]; NuLYTELY® [US]; PegLyte® [Can]; TriLyte® [US]

Therapeutic Category Laxative

Use Bowel cleansing prior to GI examination

Usual Dosage

Oral:

Children ≥6 months: Bowel cleansing prior to GI exam (CoLyte®, GoLYTELY®, NuLYTELY®, TriLyte®): 25 mL/kg/hour (some studies have used up to 40 mL/kg/hour) for 4-10 hours (until rectal effluent is clear). Maximum total dose: 4 L. **Note:** The solution may be given via nasogastric tube to patients who are unwilling or unable to drink the solution. Patients <2 years should be monitored closely.

Adults: Bowel cleansing prior to GI exam:
CoLyte®, GoLYTELY®, NuLYTELY®, TriLyte®: 240 mL (8 oz) every 10 minutes, until 4 L are consumed or the rectal effluent is clear; rapid drinking of each portion is preferred to drinking small amounts continuously. Ideally, patients should fast for ~3-4 hours prior to administration; absolutely no solid food for at least 2 hours before the solution is given. **Note:** The solution may be given via nasogastric tube to patients who are unwilling or unable to drink the solution.
MoviPrep®: Administer 2 L total with an additional 1 L of clear fluid prior to colonoscopy as follows:
Split dose: Evening before colonoscopy: 240 mL (8 oz) every 15 minutes until 1 L is consumed. Then drink 16 oz of clear liquid. On the morning of the colonoscopy, repeat process with second liter over 1 hour and then drink 16 oz of clear liquid at least 1 hour before the procedure.
Full dose: Evening before colonoscopy (~6 PM): 240 mL (8 oz every 15 minutes) until 1 L is consumed; 90 minutes later (~7:30 PM), repeat dose. Then drink 32 oz of clear liquid.
Nasogastric tube (CoLyte®, GoLYTELY®, NuLYTELY®, TriLyte®):
Bowel cleansing prior to GI exam:
Children ≥6 months: 25 mL/kg/hour until rectal effluent is clear.
Adults: Bowel cleansing prior to GI exam: 20-30 mL/minute (1.2-1.8 L/hour); the first bowel movement should occur ~1 hour after the start of administration.

Dosage Forms

Powder, for oral solution: PEG 3350 240 g, sodium sulfate 22.72 g, sodium bicarbonate 6.72 g, sodium chloride 5.84 g, and potassium 2.98 g
Colyte®: PEG 3350 240 g, sodium sulfate 22.72 g, sodium bicarbonate 6.72 g, sodium chloride 5.84 g, and potassium 2.98 g
GoLYTELY®:
PEG 3350 236 g, sodium sulfate 22.74 g, sodium bicarbonate 6.74 g, sodium chloride 5.86 g, and potassium2.97 g
PEG 3350 227.1 g, sodium sulfate 21.5 g, sodium bicarbonate 6.36 g, sodium chloride 5.53 g, and potassium 2.82 g per packet (1s)
MoviPrep®: Pouch A: PEG 3350 100g, sodium sulfate 7.5 g, sodium chloride 2.69 g, potassium chloride 1.015 g; Pouch B: Ascorbic acid 4.7 g, sodium ascorbate 5.9 g
NuLYTELY®: PEG 3350 420 g, sodium bicarbonate 5.72 g, sodium chloride 11.2 g, and potassium 1.48
TriLyte®: PEG 3350 420 g, sodium bicarbonate 5.72 g, sodium chloride 11.2 g, and potassium 1.48

polyethylene glycol-electrolyte solution and bisacodyl

(pol i ETH i leen GLY kol ee LEK troe lite soe LOO shun & bis a KOE dil)

Synonyms electrolyte lavage solution

U.S./Canadian Brand Names HalfLytely® and Bisacodyl [US]

Therapeutic Category Laxative, Bowel Evacuant; Laxative, Stimulant

Use Bowel cleansing prior to colonoscopy

Usual Dosage Oral: Adults: Bowel cleansing:
Bisacodyl: 2 tablets as a single dose. After bowel movement or 6 hours (whichever occurs first), initiate polyethylene glycol-electrolyte solution
Polyethylene glycol-electrolyte solution: 8 ounces every 10 minutes until 2 L are consumed

Dosage Forms

Kit [each kit contains]:
HalfLytely® and Bisacodyl:
Powder for oral solution (HalfLytely®): PEG 3350 210 g, sodium bicarbonate 2.86 g, sodium chloride 5.6 g, potassium 0.74 g
Tablet, delayed release (Bisacodyl): 5 mg (2s)

Polygam® S/D *(Discontinued)* *see* immune globulin (intravenous) *on page* 523
Poly-Hist DM [US] *see* phenylephrine, pyrilamine, and dextromethorphan *on page* 778
Poly Hist Forte® [US] *see* chlorpheniramine, pyrilamine, and phenylephrine *on page* 221
Poly-Histine-D® Capsule *(Discontinued)*
Poly Hist PD [US] *see* chlorpheniramine, pyrilamine, and phenylephrine *on page* 221
Poly-Iron 150 [US-OTC] *see* polysaccharide-iron complex *on page* 799

polymyxin B (pol i MIKS in bee)

Synonyms polymyxin B sulfate

U.S./Canadian Brand Names Poly-Rx [US]

Therapeutic Category Antibiotic, Irrigation; Antibiotic, Miscellaneous

Use Treatment of acute infections caused by susceptible strains of *Pseudomonas aeruginosa*; used occasionally for gut decontamination; parenteral use of polymyxin B has mainly been replaced by less toxic antibiotics, reserved for life-threatening infections caused by organisms resistant to the preferred drugs (eg, pseudomonal meningitis - intrathecal administration)

Usual Dosage

Otic (in combination with other drugs): 1-2 drops, 3-4 times/day; should be used sparingly to avoid accumulation of excess debris

Infants <2 years:

I.M.: Up to 40,000 units/kg/day divided every 6 hours (not routinely recommended due to pain at injection sites)

I.V.: Up to 40,000 units/kg/day divided every 12 hours

Intrathecal: 20,000 units/day for 3-4 days, then 25,000 units every other day for at least 2 weeks after CSF cultures are negative and CSF (glucose) has returned to within normal limits

Children ≥2 years and Adults:

I.M.: 25,000-30,000 units/kg/day divided every 4-6 hours (not routinely recommended due to pain at injection sites)

I.V.: 15,000-25,000 units/kg/day divided every 12 hours

Intrathecal: 50,000 units/day for 3-4 days, then every other day for at least 2 weeks after CSF cultures are negative and CSF (glucose) has returned to within normal limits

Total daily dose should not exceed 2,000,000 units/day

Bladder irrigation: Continuous irrigant or rinse in the urinary bladder for up to 10 days using 20 mg (equal to 200,000 units) added to 1 L of normal saline; usually no more than 1 L of irrigant is used per day unless urine flow rate is high; administration rate is adjusted to patient's urine output

Topical irrigation or topical solution: 500,000 units/L of normal saline; topical irrigation should not exceed 2 million units/day in adults

Gut sterilization: Oral: 15,000-25,000 units/kg/day in divided doses every 6 hours

Clostridium difficile enteritis: Oral: 25,000 units every 6 hours for 10 days

Ophthalmic: A concentration of 0.1% to 0.25% is administered as 1-3 drops every hour, then increasing the interval as response indicates to 1-2 drops 4-6 times/day

Dosage Forms

Injection, powder for reconstitution: 500,000 units

Powder [for prescription compounding]:

Poly-Rx: 100 million units (13 g)

polymyxin B and bacitracin *see* bacitracin and polymyxin B *on page 119*

polymyxin B and neomycin *see* neomycin and polymyxin B *on page 687*

polymyxin B and trimethoprim *see* trimethoprim and polymyxin B *on page 988*

polymyxin B, bacitracin, and neomycin *see* bacitracin, neomycin, and polymyxin B *on page 119*

polymyxin B, bacitracin, neomycin, and hydrocortisone *see* bacitracin, neomycin, polymyxin B, and hydrocortisone *on page 120*

polymyxin B, neomycin, and dexamethasone *see* neomycin, polymyxin B, and dexamethasone *on page 687*

polymyxin B, neomycin, and gramicidin *see* neomycin, polymyxin B, and gramicidin *on page 688*

polymyxin B, neomycin, and hydrocortisone *see* neomycin, polymyxin B, and hydrocortisone *on page 688*

polymyxin B, neomycin, and prednisolone *see* neomycin, polymyxin B, and prednisolone *on page 689*

polymyxin B, neomycin, bacitracin, and pramoxine *see* bacitracin, neomycin, polymyxin B, and pramoxine *on page 120*

polymyxin B sulfate *see* polymyxin B *on page 798*

polyphenols *see* sinecatechins *on page 903*

polyphenon E *see* sinecatechins *on page 903*

Poly-Pred® [US] *see* neomycin, polymyxin B, and prednisolone *on page 689*

Poly-Rx [US] *see* polymyxin B *on page 798*

polysaccharide-iron complex (pol i SAK a ride-EYE ern KOM pleks)

Sound-Alike/Look-Alike Issues

Niferex® may be confused with Nephrox®

Synonyms iron-polysaccharide complex

U.S./Canadian Brand Names Ferrex 150 [US-OTC]; Niferex® [US-OTC]; Nu-Iron® 150 [US-OTC]; Poly-Iron 150 [US-OTC]; ProFe [US-OTC]

Therapeutic Category Electrolyte Supplement, Oral

Use Prevention and treatment of iron-deficiency anemias

Usual Dosage

Dietary Reference Intake: Dose is RDA presented as elemental iron unless otherwise noted:

0-6 months: 0.27 mg/day (adequate intake)
7-12 months: 11 mg/day
1-3 years: 7 mg/day
4-8 years: 10 mg/day
9-13 years: 8 mg/day
14-18 years: Male: 11 mg/day; Female: 15 mg/day; Pregnant female: 27 mg/day; Lactating female: 10 mg/day
19-50 years: Male: 8 mg/day; Female: 18 mg/day; Pregnant female: 27 mg/day; Lactating female: 9 mg/day
≥50 years: 8 mg/day

Iron deficiency: Oral:

Children ≥6 years: Tablets/elixir: 50-100 mg/day; may be given in divided doses
Adults:
Elixir: 50-100 mg twice daily
Capsules: 150-300 mg/day

Dosage Forms

Capsule: Elemental iron 150 mg
Ferrex 150 [OTC], Nu-Iron® 150 [OTC], Poly-Iron 150 [OTC]: Elemental iron 150 mg
Niferex® [OTC]: Elemental iron 60 mg
ProFe [OTC]: Elemental iron 180 mg

Elixir:
Niferex® [OTC]: Elemental iron 100 mg/5 mL

Polysporin® [US-OTC] *see* bacitracin and polymyxin B *on page* 119

Polytar® ***(Discontinued)*** *see* coal tar *on page* 250

Polytrim® [US/Can] *see* trimethoprim and polymyxin B *on page* 988

Poly Tussin DM [US] *see* chlorpheniramine, phenylephrine, and dextromethorphan *on page* 217

PolyTussin HD [US] *see* phenylephrine, hydrocodone, and chlorpheniramine *on page* 778

Poly-Vi-Flor® ***(Discontinued)*** *see* vitamins (multiple/pediatric) *on page* 1020

polyvinyl alcohol *see* artificial tears *on page* 100

polyvinylpyrrolidone with iodine *see* povidone-iodine *on page* 807

Poly-Vi-Sol® [US-OTC] *see* vitamins (multiple/pediatric) *on page* 1020

Poly-Vi-Sol® with Iron [US-OTC] *see* vitamins (multiple/pediatric) *on page* 1020

Pondocillin® [Can] *see* pivampicillin *(Canada only) on page* 788

Ponstan® [Can] *see* mefenamic acid *on page* 621

Ponstel® [US] *see* mefenamic acid *on page* 621

Pontocaine® [US/Can] *see* tetracaine *on page* 950

Pontocaine® Niphanoid® [US] *see* tetracaine *on page* 950

poractant alfa (por AKT ant AL fa)

U.S./Canadian Brand Names Curosurf® [US/Can]

Therapeutic Category Lung Surfactant

Use Treatment of respiratory distress syndrome (RDS) in premature infants

Usual Dosage Intratracheal use **only**: Premature infant with RDS: Initial dose is 2.5 mL/kg of birth weight. Up to 2 subsequent doses of 1.25 mL/kg birth weight can be administered at 12-hour intervals if needed in infants who continue to require mechanical ventilation and supplemental oxygen. Maximum total dose: 5 mL/kg (sum of the initial dose and 2 repeat doses)

Dosage Forms

Suspension, intratracheal [preservative free; porcine derived]:
Curosurf®: 80 mg/mL

Porcelana® Sunscreen ***(Discontinued)*** *see* hydroquinone *on page* 508

porfimer (POR fi mer)

Synonyms CL-184116; dihematoporphyrin ether; porfimer sodium

U.S./Canadian Brand Names Photofrin® [US/Can]

Therapeutic Category Antineoplastic Agent

Use Palliation in patients with obstructing (partial or complete) esophageal cancer; treatment of microinvasive endobronchial nonsmall cell lung cancer (NSCLC); reduction of obstruction and palliation in patients with obstructing (partial or complete) NSCLC; ablation of high-grade dysplasia in Barrett esophagus

Usual Dosage I.V.: Adults: 2 mg/kg, followed by exposure to the appropriate laser light; repeat courses must be separated by at least 30 days (esophageal or endobronchial cancer) or 90 days (Barrett esophagus; delay subsequent treatment for insufficient healing) for a maximum of 3 courses

Dosage Forms

Injection, powder for reconstitution:

Photofrin®: 75 mg

porfimer sodium *see* porfimer *on page 801*

Portagen® [US-OTC] *see* nutritional formula, enteral/oral *on page 715*

Portia™ [US] *see* ethinyl estradiol and levonorgestrel *on page 387*

posaconazole (poe sa KON a zole)

Sound-Alike/Look-Alike Issues

Noxafil® may be confused with minoxidil

Synonyms SCH 56592

U.S./Canadian Brand Names Noxafil® [US]; Posanol™ [Can]

Therapeutic Category Antifungal Agent, Oral

Use Prophylaxis of invasive *Aspergillus* and *Candida* infections in severely-immunocompromised patients [eg, hematopoietic stem cell transplant (HSCT) recipients with graft-versus-host disease (GVHD) or those with prolonged neutropenia secondary to chemotherapy for hematologic malignancies]; treatment of oropharyngeal candidiasis (including patients refractory to itraconazole and/or fluconazole)

Usual Dosage Oral: Children ≥13 years and Adults:

Aspergillosis, invasive: *Prophylaxis:* 200 mg 3 times/day

Candidal infections:

Prophylaxis: 200 mg 3 times/day

Treatment of oropharyngeal infection: Initial: 100 mg twice daily for 1 day; maintenance: 100 mg once daily for 13 days

Treatment of refractory oropharyngeal infection: 400 mg twice daily

Dosage Forms

Suspension, oral:

Noxafil®: 40 mg/mL

Posanol™ [Can] *see* posaconazole *on page 801*

Post Peel Healing Balm [US-OTC] *see* hydrocortisone (topical) *on page 505*

Posture® [US-OTC] *see* calcium phosphate (tribasic) *on page 175*

Potasalan® *(Discontinued)* *see* potassium chloride *on page 803*

potassium acetate (poe TASS ee um AS e tate)

Therapeutic Category Electrolyte Supplement, Oral

Use Potassium deficiency; to avoid chloride when high concentration of potassium is needed, source of bicarbonate

Usual Dosage I.V. doses should be incorporated into the patient's maintenance I.V. fluids, intermittent I.V. potassium administration should be reserved for severe depletion situations and requires ECG monitoring; doses listed as mEq of potassium

Children:

Treatment of hypokalemia: I.V.: 2-5 mEq/kg/day

I.V. intermittent infusion (must be diluted prior to administration): 0.5-1 mEq/kg/dose (maximum: 30 mEq/dose) to infuse at 0.3-0.5 mEq/kg/hour (maximum: 1 mEq/kg/hour)

Note: Use caution in premature neonates; potassium acetate for injection contains aluminum.

Adults:

Treatment of hypokalemia: I.V.: 40-100 mEq/day

I.V. intermittent infusion (must be diluted prior to administration): 5-10 mEq/dose (maximum: 40 mEq/dose) to infuse over 2-3 hours (maximum: 40 mEq over 1 hour)

Note: Continuous cardiac monitor recommended for rates >0.5 mEq/hour

Potassium dosage/rate of infusion guidelines:

Serum potassium >2.5 mEq/L: Maximum infusion rate: 10 mEq/hour; maximum concentration: 40 mEq/L; maximum 24-hour dose: 200 mEq

Serum potassium <2.5 mEq/L: Maximum infusion rate: 40 mEq/hour; maximum concentration: 80 mEq/L; maximum 24-hour dose: 400 mEq

Dosage Forms

Injection, solution: 2 mEq/mL (20 mL, 50 mL, 100 mL) [contains aluminum]

Injection, solution [concentrate]: 4 mEq/mL (50 mL) [contains aluminum]

potassium acid phosphate (poe TASS ee um AS id FOS fate)

U.S./Canadian Brand Names K-Phos® Original [US]

Therapeutic Category Urinary Acidifying Agent

Use Acidifies urine and lowers urinary calcium concentration; reduces odor and rash caused by ammoniacal urine; increases the antibacterial activity of methenamine

Usual Dosage Oral: Adults: 1000 mg dissolved in 6-8 oz of water 4 times/day with meals and at bedtime; for best results, soak tablets in water for 2-5 minutes, then stir and swallow

Dosage Forms

Tablet [scored]:

K-Phos® Original: 500 mg

potassium bicarbonate (poe TASS ee um bye KAR bun ate)

Therapeutic Category Electrolyte Supplement, Oral

Use Potassium deficiency, hypokalemia

Usual Dosage Oral:

Children: 1-4 mEq/kg/day

Adults: 25 mEq 2-4 times/day

Dosage Forms

Tablet for oral solution, effervescent: Potassium 25 mEq

potassium bicarbonate and potassium chloride
(poe TASS ee um bye KAR bun ate & poe TASS ee um KLOR ide)

Synonyms potassium bicarbonate and potassium chloride (effervescent)

Therapeutic Category Electrolyte Supplement, Oral

Use Treatment or prevention of hypokalemia

Usual Dosage Oral:

Children: 1-4 mEq/kg/24 hours in divided doses as required to maintain normal serum potassium

Adults:

Prevention: 16-24 mEq/day in 2-4 divided doses

Treatment: 40-100 mEq/day in 2-4 divided doses

Dosage Forms

Tablet for solution, oral [effervescent]: Potassium chloride 25 mEq

potassium bicarbonate and potassium chloride (effervescent) *see* potassium bicarbonate and potassium chloride *on page 802*

potassium bicarbonate and potassium citrate
(poe TASS ee um bye KAR bun ate & poe TASS ee um SIT rate)

Sound-Alike/Look-Alike Issues

Klor-Con® may be confused with Klaron®, K-Lor®

Synonyms potassium bicarbonate and potassium citrate (effervescent)

U.S./Canadian Brand Names Effer-K™ [US]; K-Lyte® DS [US]; K-Lyte® [US]; Klor-Con®/EF [US]

Therapeutic Category Electrolyte Supplement, Oral

Use Treatment or prevention of hypokalemia

Usual Dosage Oral:

Children: 1-4 mEq/kg/24 hours in divided doses as required to maintain normal serum potassium

Adults:

Prevention: 16-24 mEq/day in 2-4 divided doses

Treatment: 40-100 mEq/day in 2-4 divided doses

Dosage Forms

Tablet, effervescent:

Effer-K™, Klor-Con®/EF, K-Lyte®: Potassium 25 mEq

K-Lyte® DS: Potassium 50 mEq

potassium bicarbonate and potassium citrate (effervescent) *see* potassium bicarbonate and potassium citrate *on page 802*

potassium chloride (poe TASS ee um KLOR ide)

Sound-Alike/Look-Alike Issues

Kaon-Cl-10® may be confused with kaolin

KCl may be confused with HCl

K-Lor® may be confused with Klor-Con®

Klor-Con® may be confused with Klaron®, K-Lor®

microK® may be confused with Macrobid®, Micronase®

Synonyms KCl; kdur

U.S./Canadian Brand Names Apo-K® [Can]; K-10® [Can]; K-Dur® [Can]; K-Lor® [US/Can]; K-Lyte®/Cl [Can]; K-Tab® [US]; Kaon-Cl-10® [US]; Klor-Con® 10 [US]; Klor-Con® 8 [US]; Klor-Con® M [US]; Klor-Con® [US]; Klor-Con®/25 [US]; Micro-K Extencaps® [Can]; microK® 10 [US]; microK® [US]; Roychlor® [Can]; Slo-Pot [Can]; Slow-K® [Can]

Therapeutic Category Electrolyte Supplement, Oral

Use Treatment or prevention of hypokalemia

Usual Dosage I.V. doses should be incorporated into the patient's maintenance I.V. fluids; intermittent I.V. potassium administration should be reserved for severe depletion situations in patients undergoing ECG monitoring. Doses expressed as mEq of potassium.

Normal daily requirements: Oral, I.V.:
- Children: 1-2 mEq/kg/day
- Adults: 40-80 mEq/day

Prevention of hypokalemia: Oral:
- Children: 1-2 mEq/kg/day in 1-2 divided doses
- Adults: 20-40 mEq/day in 1-2 divided doses

Treatment of hypokalemia: Children:
- Oral: 1-2 mEq/kg initially, then as needed based on frequently obtained lab values. If deficits are severe or ongoing losses are great, I.V. route should be considered.
- I.V. intermittent infusion: 0.5-1 mEq/kg/dose (maximum dose: 40 mEq). If infusion exceeds 0.5 mEq/kg/hour, physician should be at bedside and patient should have continuous ECG monitoring; repeat as needed based on frequently obtained lab values.

Treatment of hypokalemia: Adults:
- Oral:
  - Asymptomatic, mild hypokalemia: Usual dosage range: 40-100 mEq/day divided in 2-5 doses; generally recommended to limit doses to 20-25 mEq/dose to avoid GI discomfort.
  - Mild-to-moderate hypokalemia: Some clinicians may administer up to 120-240 mEq/day divided in 3-4 doses; limit doses to 40-60 mEq/dose. If deficits are severe or ongoing losses are great, I.V. route should be considered.
- I.V. intermittent infusion: Peripheral or central line: ≤10 mEq/hour; repeat as needed based on frequently obtained lab values; central line infusion and continuous ECG monitoring highly recommended for infusions >10 mEq/hour.
  - Potassium dosage/rate of infusion general guidelines (per product labeling): **Note:** High variability exists in dosing/infusion rate recommendations; therapy guided by patient condition and specific institutional guidelines.
    - Serum potassium >2.5 mEq/L: Maximum infusion rate: 10 mEq/hour; maximum concentration: 40 mEq/L; maximum 24-hour dose: 200 mEq
    - Serum potassium <2 mEq/L and symptomatic (excluding emergency treatment of cardiac arrest): Maximum infusion rate (central line only): 40 mEq/hour in presence of continuous ECG monitoring and frequent lab monitoring; In selected situations, patients may require up to 400 mEq/24 hours.

Dosage Forms

Capsule, extended release, microencapsulated: 8 mEq [600 mg]; 10 mEq [750 mg]

microK®: 8 mEq [600 mg]

microK® 10: 10 mEq [750 mg]

Infusion [premixed in D_5W]: 20 mEq (1000 mL); 30 mEq (1000 mL); 40 mEq (1000 mL)

Infusion [premixed in D_5W and LR]: 20 mEq (1000 mL); 30 mEq (1000 mL); 40 mEq (1000 mL)
Infusion [premixed in D_5W and sodium chloride 0.2%]: 5 mEq (250 mL); 10 mEq (500 mL, 1000 mL); 20 mEq (1000 mL); 30 mEq (1000 mL); 40 mEq (1000 mL)
Infusion [premixed in D_5W and sodium chloride 0.225%]: 10 mEq (500 mL, 1000 mL); 20 mEq (1000 mL); 30 mEq (1000 mL); 40 mEq (1000 mL)
Infusion [premixed in D_5W and sodium chloride 0.3%]: 10 mEq (500 mL); 20 mEq (1000 mL)
Infusion [premixed in D_5W and sodium chloride 0.33%]: 10 mEq (500 mL); 20 mEq (1000 mL)
Infusion [premixed in D_5W and sodium chloride 0.45%]: 10 mEq (500 mL, 1000 mL); 20 mEq (1000 mL); 30 mEq (1000 mL); 40 mEq (1000 mL)
Infusion [premixed in D_5W and NS]: 20 mEq (1000 mL); 40 mEq (1000 mL)
Infusion [premixed in $D_{10}W$ and sodium chloride 0.2%]: 5 mEq (250 mL)
Infusion [premixed in sodium chloride 0.45%]: 20 mEq (1000 mL); 40 mEq (1000 mL)
Infusion [premixed in NS]: 20 mEq (1000 mL); 40 mEq (1000 mL)
Infusion [premixed in SWFI; highly concentrated]: 10 mEq (50 mL, 100 mL); 20 mEq (50 mL, 100 mL); 30 mEq (100 mL); 40 mEq (100 mL)
Injection, solution [concentrate]: 2 mEq/mL (5 mL, 10 mL, 15 mL, 20 mL, 30 mL, 250 mL, 500 mL)
Powder, for oral solution: 20 mEq/packet
K-Lor®, Klor-Con®: 20 mEq/packet
Klor-Con®/25: 25 mEq/packet
Solution, oral: 20 mEq/15 mL, 40 mEq/15 mL
Tablet, extended release: 8 mEq [600 mg]; 10 mEq [750 mg]; 20 mEq [1500 mg]
K-Tab®, Kaon-Cl®: 10 mEq
Tablet, extended release, microencapsulated: 10 mEq, 20 mEq
Klor-Con® M10: 10 mEq
Klor-Con® M15: 15 mEq
Klor-Con® M20: 20 mEq
Tablet, extended release, wax matrix: 8 mEq, 10 mEq
Klor-Con® 8: 8 mEq [600 mg]
Klor-Con® 10: 10 mEq)750 mg]

potassium citrate (poe TASS ee um SIT rate)

Sound-Alike/Look-Alike Issues
Urocit®-K may be confused with Urised®

U.S./Canadian Brand Names K-Citra® [Can]; K-Lyte® [Can]; Urocit®-K [US]

Therapeutic Category Alkalinizing Agent

Use Prevention of uric acid nephrolithiasis; prevention of calcium renal stones in patients with hypocitraturia; urinary alkalinizer when sodium citrate is contraindicated

Usual Dosage Oral: Adults: 10-20 mEq 3 times/day with meals up to 100 mEq/day

Dosage Forms
Tablet: 540 mg [5 mEq]; 1080 mg [10 mEq]
Urocit®-K: 540 mg [5 mEq]; 1080 mg [10 mEq]
Tablet, extended release: 540 mg [5 mEq]; 1080 mg [10 mEq]

potassium citrate and citric acid (poe TASS ee um SIT rate & SI trik AS id)

Synonyms citric acid and potassium citrate

U.S./Canadian Brand Names Cytra-K [US]; Polycitra®-K [US]

Therapeutic Category Alkalinizing Agent

Use Treatment of metabolic acidosis; alkalinizing agent in conditions where long-term maintenance of an alkaline urine is desirable

Usual Dosage Urine alkalizing agent:
Children: Solution: 5-15 mL after meals and at bedtime; adjust dose based on urinary pH
Adults:
Powder: One packet dissolved in water after meals and at bedtime; adjust dose to urinary pH
Solution: 15-30 mL after meals and at bedtime; adjust dose based on urinary pH

Dosage Forms Equivalent to potassium 2 mEq/mL and bicarbonate 2 mEq/mL
Powder for solution, oral:
Cytra-K: Potassium citrate 3300 mg and citric acid 1002 mg per packet (100s)
Polycitra®-K: Potassium citrate 3300 mg and citric acid 1002 mg per packet (100s)
Solution:
Cytra-K: Potassium citrate 1100 mg and citric acid 334 mg per 5 mL
Polycitra®-K: Potassium citrate 1100 mg and citric acid 334 mg per 5 mL

potassium citrate, citric acid, and sodium citrate *see* citric acid, sodium citrate, and potassium citrate *on page 235*

potassium gluconate (poe TASS ee um GLOO coe nate)

Therapeutic Category Electrolyte Supplement, Oral

Use Treatment or prevention of hypokalemia

Usual Dosage Oral (doses listed as mEq of potassium):

Normal daily requirement:
- Children: 2-3 mEq/kg/day
- Adults: 40-80 mEq/day

Prevention of hypokalemia during diuretic therapy:
- Children: 1-2 mEq/kg/day in 1-2 divided doses
- Adults: 16-24 mEq/day in 1-2 divided doses

Treatment of hypokalemia:
- Children: 2-5 mEq/kg/day in 2-4 divided doses
- Adults: 40-100 mEq/day in 2-4 divided doses

Dosage Forms

Caplet: 595 mg

Capsule: 99 mg

Tablet: 99 mg, 550 mg, 595 mg

Tablet, timed release: 95 mg

potassium iodide (poe TASS ee um EYE oh dide)

Sound-Alike/Look-Alike Issues

potassium iodide products, including saturated solution of potassium iodide (SSKI®) may be confused with potassium iodide and iodine (Strong Iodide Solution or Lugol's solution)

Synonyms KI

U.S./Canadian Brand Names Iosat™ [US-OTC]; SSKI® [US]; ThyroSafe™ [US-OTC]; ThyroShield™ [US-OTC]

Therapeutic Category Antithyroid Agent; Expectorant

Use Expectorant for the symptomatic treatment of chronic pulmonary diseases complicated by mucus; reduce thyroid vascularity prior to thyroidectomy and management of thyrotoxic crisis; block thyroidal uptake of radioactive isotopes of iodine in a radiation emergency or other exposure to radioactive iodine

Usual Dosage Oral:

Adults: RDA: 150 mcg (iodine)

Expectorant: Adults: SSKI®: 300-600 mg 3-4 times/day

Preoperative thyroidectomy: Children and Adults: 50-250 mg (1-5 drops SSKI®) 3 times/day; administer for 10 days before surgery

To reduce risk of thyroid cancer following nuclear accident (Iosat™, ThyroSafe™, ThyroShield™): Dosing should continue until risk of exposure has passed or other measures are implemented:
- Children (see adult dose for children >68 kg):
  - Infants <1 month: 16.25 mg once daily
  - 1 month to 3 years: 32.5 mg once daily
  - 3-18 years: 65 mg once daily
- Children >68 kg and Adults (including pregnant/lactating women): 130 mg once daily

Thyrotoxic crisis:
- Infants <1 year: 150-250 mg (3-5 drops SSKI®) 3 times/day
- Children and Adults: 300-500 mg (6-10 drops SSKI®) 3 times/day

Dosage Forms

Solution, oral:
- SSKI®: 1 g/mL
- ThyroShield™ [OTC]: 65 mg/mL

Tablet:
- Iosat™ [OTC]: 130 mg
- ThyroSafe™ [OTC]: 65 mg

potassium iodide, chlorpheniramine, phenylephrine, and codeine *see* chlorpheniramine, phenylephrine, codeine, and potassium iodide *on page 220*

potassium phosphate (poe TASS ee um FOS fate)

Sound-Alike/Look-Alike Issues

Neutra-Phos®-K may be confused with K-Phos Neutral®

Synonyms phosphate, potassium

Therapeutic Category Electrolyte Supplement, Oral

Use Treatment and prevention of hypophosphatemia; **Note:** The concomitant amount of potassium must be calculated into the total electrolyte content. For each 1 mmol of phosphate, ~1.5 mEq of potassium will be administered. Therefore, if ordering 30 mmol of potassium phosphate, the patient will receive ~45 mEq of potassium.

Usual Dosage

Oral:

Normal Requirements Elemental Phosphorus:

0-6 months: 100 mg
7-12 months: 275 mg
1-3 years: 460 mg
4-8 years: 500 mg
9-18 years: 1250 mg

Adults: 700 mg

Oral maintenance:

Children <4 years: 250 mg phosphorus/8 mmol 4 times/day; dilute as instructed

Children >4 years and Adults: 250-500 mg phosphorus/8-16 mmol 4 times/day; dilute as instructed

I.V.: **Caution: The concomitant amount of potassium must be calculated into the total electrolyte content. For each 1 mmol of phosphate, ~1.5 mEq of potassium will be administered. Therefore, if ordering 30 mmol of potassium phosphate, the patient will receive ~45 mEq of potassium. With orders for I.V. phosphate, there is considerable confusion associated with the use of millimoles (mmol) versus milliequivalents (mEq) to express the phosphate requirement.** The most reliable method of ordering I.V. phosphate is by millimoles, then specifying the potassium or sodium salt. Doses listed as mmol of phosphate.

Acute treatment of hypophosphatemia: It is recommended that repletion of severe hypophosphatemia be done I.V. because large doses of oral phosphate may cause diarrhea and intestinal absorption may be unreliable. Intermittent I.V. infusion should be reserved for severe depletion situations; requires continuous cardiac monitoring. Guidelines differ based on degree of illness, need/use of TPN, and severity of hypophosphatemia. If potassium >4.0 mEq/L consider phosphate replacement strategy without potassium (eg, sodium phosphates). Obese patients and/or severe renal impairment were excluded from phosphate supplement trials. **Note:** 1 mmol phosphate = 31 mg phosphorus; 1 mg phosphorus = 0.032 mmol phosphate.

Children and Adults: **Note:** There are no prospective studies of parenteral phosphate replacement in children. The following weight-based guidelines for adult dosing may be cautiously employed in pediatric patients.

General replacement guidelines:

Low dose: 0.08 mmol/kg over 6 hours; use if losses are recent and uncomplicated

Intermediate dose: 0.16-0.24 mmol/kg over 4-6 hours; use if serum phosphorus level 0.5-1 mg/dL (0.16-0.32 mmol/L)

Note: The initial dose may be increased by 25% to 50% if the patient is symptomatic secondary to hypophosphatemia and lowered by 25% to 50% if the patient is hypercalcemic.

Critically-ill adult trauma patients receiving concurrent TPN:

Low dose: 0.32 mmol/kg over 4-6 hours; use if serum phosphorus level 2.3-3 mg/dL (0.73-0.96 mmol/L)

Intermediate dose: 0.64 mmol/kg over 4-6 hours; use if serum phosphorus level 1.6-2.2 mg/dL (0.51-0.72 mmol/L)

High dose: 1 mmol/kg over 8-12 hours; use if serum phosphorus <1.5 mg/dL (<0.5 mmol/L)

Parenteral nutrition: Adults: 10-15 mmol/1000 kcal **or** 20-40 mmol/24 hours

Dosage Forms

Injection, solution: Potassium 4.4 mEq and phosphorus 3 mmol per mL (5 mL, 15 mL, 50 mL)

potassium phosphate and sodium phosphate

(poe TASS ee um FOS fate & SOW dee um FOS fate)

Sound-Alike/Look-Alike Issues

K-Phos® Neutral may be confused with Neutra-Phos-K®

Synonyms sodium phosphate and potassium phosphate

U.S./Canadian Brand Names K-Phos® MF [US]; K-Phos® Neutral [US]; K-Phos® No. 2 [US]; Phos-NaK [US]; Phospha 250™ Neutral [US]; Uro-KP-Neutral® [US]

Therapeutic Category Electrolyte Supplement, Oral

Use Treatment of conditions associated with excessive renal phosphate loss or inadequate GI absorption of phosphate; to acidify the urine to lower calcium concentrations; to increase the antibacterial activity of methenamine; reduce odor and rash caused by ammonia in urine

Usual Dosage Oral:

Children ≥4 years: Elemental phosphorus 250 mg 4 times/day after meals and at bedtime

Adults: Elemental phosphorus 250-500 mg 4 times/day after meals and at bedtime

Dosage Forms

Caplet:

Uro-KP-Neutral®: Dipotassium phosphate, disodium phosphate, and monobasic sodium phosphate

Powder, for oral solution:

Phos-NaK: Dibasic potassium phosphate, monobasic potassium phosphate, dibasic sodium phosphate, and monosodium phosphate per packet (100s)

Tablet:

K-Phos® MF: Potassium phosphate 155 mg and sodium phosphate 350 mg

K-Phos® Neutral: Monobasic potassium phosphate 155 mg, dibasic sodium phosphate 852 mg, and monobasic sodium phosphate 130 mg

K-Phos® No. 2: Potassium phosphate 305 mg and sodium phosphate 700 mg

Phospha 250™ Neutral: Monobasic potassium phosphate 155 mg, dibasic sodium phosphate 852 mg, and monobasic sodium phosphate 130 mg

Povidine™ [US-OTC] *see* povidone-iodine *on page 807*

povidone-iodine (POE vi done EYE oh dyne)

Sound-Alike/Look-Alike Issues

Betadine® may be confused with Betagan®, betaine

Synonyms polyvinylpyrrolidone with iodine; PVP-I

U.S./Canadian Brand Names Betadine® [US/Can]; Operand® [US-OTC]; Povidine™ [US-OTC]; Proviodine [Can]; Summer's Eve® Medicated Douche [US-OTC]; Vagi-Gard® [US-OTC]

Therapeutic Category Antibacterial, Topical

Use External antiseptic with broad microbicidal spectrum for the prevention or treatment of topical infections associated with surgery, burns, minor cuts/scrapes; relief of minor vaginal irritation

Usual Dosage

Antiseptic: Apply topically to affected area as needed. Ophthalmic solution may be used to irrigate the eye or applied to area around the eye such as skin, eyelashes, or lid margins.

Surgical scrub: Topical: Apply solution to wet skin or hands, scrub for ~5 minutes, rinse; refer to product labeling for specific procedure-related instructions.

Vaginal irritation: Douche: Insert 0.3% solution vaginally once daily for 5-7 days

Dosage Forms

Gel, topical: 10% (120 g)

Operand® [OTC]: 10% (120 g)

Liquid, topical [prep-swab ampule]: 10% (0.65 mL)

Ointment, topical: 10% (1 g)

Povidine™ [OTC]: 10% (30 g)

Pad [prep pads]: 10% (200s)

Betadine® SwabAids [OTC]: 10% (100s)

Solution, ophthalmic: 5% (30 mL)

Betadine® [OTC]: 5% (30 mL)

Solution, perineal [concentrate]:

Operand® [OTC]: 10% (240 mL)

Solution, topical: 10% (22 mL, 60 mL, 90 mL, 240 mL, 480 mL, 3840 mL)

Betadine® [OTC]: 10% (15 mL, 120 mL, 240 mL, 480 mL, 960 mL, 3840 mL)

Operand® [OTC]: 10% (60 mL, 120 mL, 240 mL, 480 mL, 960 mL, 3840 mL)

Povidine™ [OTC}: 10% (240 mL)

Solution, topical [cleanser]:

Betadine® Skin Cleanser [OTC]: 7.5% (120 mL)

Solution, topical [paint sponge]: 10% (50s)

Solution, topical [paint]: 10% (60 mL, 90 mL, 120 mL)

Solution, topical [surgical scrub]: 7.5% (60 mL, 120 mL)
Betadine® Surgical Scrub [OTC]: 7.5% (120 mL, 480 mL, 960 mL, 3840 mL)
Operand® [OTC]: 7.5% (60 mL, 120 mL, 240 mL, 480 mL, 960 mL, 3840 mL)
Solution, topical [spray]: 10% (60 mL)
Betadine® [OTC]: 5% (90 mL)
Operand® [OTC]: 10% (59 mL)
Solution, topical [surgical scrub sponge]: 10% (50s)
Solution, vaginal [concentrate, douche]:
Operand® [OTC]: 10% (240 mL)
Vagi-Gard® [OTC]: 10% (180 mL, 240 mL)
Solution, vaginal [douche]:
Summer's Eve® Medicated Douche [OTC]: 0.3% (135 mL) [contains sodium benzoate]
Solution [concentrate, whirlpool]:
Operand® [OTC]: 10% (3840 mL)
Swabsticks: 10% (25s, 50s, 1000s)
Betadine® [OTC]: 10% (50s, 200s)
Swabsticks [gel saturated]: 10% (50s)
Swabsticks, topical [surgical scrub]: 7.5% (25s, 50s, 1000s)

PPD *see* tuberculin tests *on page 993*
PPS *see* pentosan polysulfate sodium *on page 766*
PPSV *see* pneumococcal polysaccharide vaccine (polyvalent) *on page 794*
PPSV23 *see* pneumococcal polysaccharide vaccine (polyvalent) *on page 794*
PPV23 *see* pneumococcal polysaccharide vaccine (polyvalent) *on page 794*
Pradax™ [Can] *see* dabigatran etexilate *(Canada only) on page 272*

pralidoxime (pra li DOKS eem)

Sound-Alike/Look-Alike Issues
pralidoxime may be confused with pramoxine, pyridoxine
Protopam® may be confused with Proloprim®, protamine, Protropin®

Synonyms 2-PAM; 2-pyridine aldoxime methochloride; pralidoxime chloride

U.S./Canadian Brand Names Protopam® [US/Can]

Therapeutic Category Antidote

Use Reverse muscle paralysis caused by toxic exposure to organophosphate acetylcholinesterase-inhibiting pesticides and chemicals; control of overdose of acetylcholinesterase medications used to treat myasthenia gravis (ambenonium, neostigmine, pyridostigmine)

Usual Dosage
Organic phosphorus poisoning (use in conjunction with atropine; atropine effects should be established before pralidoxime is administered): I.V. (may be given I.M. or SubQ if I.V. is not feasible):
Children: 20-50 mg/kg/dose; repeat in 1-2 hours if muscle weakness has not been relieved, then at 8- to 12-hour intervals if cholinergic signs recur
Adults: Initial: 30 mg/kg over 20 minutes, maintenance: I.V. infusion: 4-8 mg/kg/hour
Treatment of acetylcholinesterase inhibitor toxicity: Adults: I.V.: Initial: 1-2 g followed by increments of 250 mg every 5 minutes until response is observed

Dosage Forms
Injection, powder for reconstitution:
Protopam®: 1 g
Injection, solution: 300 mg/mL (2 mL)

pralidoxime and atropine *see* atropine and pralidoxime *on page 112*
pralidoxime chloride *see* pralidoxime *on page 808*
Pramet® FA *(Discontinued)*
Pramilet® FA *(Discontinued)*

pramipexole (pra mi PEKS ole)

Sound-Alike/Look-Alike Issues
Mirapex® may be confused with Mifeprex®, MiraLax™

U.S./Canadian Brand Names Apo-Pramipexole [Can]; Mirapex® [US/Can]; Novo-Pramipexole [Can]; PMS-Pramipexole [Can]; SANDOZ-Pramipexole [Can]

Therapeutic Category Anti-Parkinson Agent (Dopamine Agonist)

Use Treatment of the signs and symptoms of idiopathic Parkinson disease; treatment of moderate-to-severe primary Restless Legs Syndrome (RLS)

Usual Dosage Oral: Adults:

Parkinson disease: Initial: 0.375 mg/day given in 3 divided doses, increase gradually by 0.125 mg/dose every 5-7 days; range: 1.5-4.5 mg/day

Restless legs syndrome: Initial: 0.125 mg once daily 2-3 hours before bedtime. Dose may be doubled every 4-7 days up to 0.5 mg/day. Maximum dose: 0.5 mg/day (manufacturer's recommendation).

Note: Most patients require <0.5 mg/day, but higher doses have been used (2 mg/day). If augmentation occurs, dose earlier in the day.

Dosage Forms [CAN] = Canadian product

Tablet: 0.25 mg [CAN; generic not available in U.S.], 0.5 mg [CAN; generic not available in U.S.], 1 mg [CAN; generic not available in U.S.], 1.5 mg [CAN; generic not available in U.S.]

Mirapex®: 0.125 mg, 0.25 mg, 0.5 mg, 0.75 mg, 1 mg, 1.5 mg

pramlintide (PRAM lin tide)

Synonyms pramlintide acetate

U.S./Canadian Brand Names Symlin® [US]

Therapeutic Category Antidiabetic Agent

Use

Adjunctive treatment with mealtime insulin in type 1 diabetes mellitus (insulin-dependent, IDDM) patients who have failed to achieve desired glucose control despite optimal insulin therapy

Adjunctive treatment with mealtime insulin in type 2 diabetes mellitus (noninsulin-dependent, NIDDM) patients who have failed to achieve desired glucose control despite optimal insulin therapy, with or without concurrent sulfonylurea and/or metformin

Usual Dosage SubQ: Adults: **Note:** When initiating pramlintide, reduce current insulin dose (including rapidly- and mixed-acting preparations) by 50% to avoid hypoglycemia.

Type 1 diabetes mellitus (insulin-dependent, IDDM): Initial: 15 mcg immediately prior to meals; titrate in 15 mcg increments every 3 days (if no significant nausea occurs) to target dose of 30-60 mcg (consider discontinuation if intolerant of 30 mcg dose)

Type 2 diabetes mellitus (noninsulin-dependent, NIDDM): Initial: 60 mcg immediately prior to meals; after 3-7 days, increase to 120 mcg prior to meals if no significant nausea occurs (if nausea occurs at 120 mcg dose, reduce to 60 mcg)

If pramlintide is discontinued for any reason, restart therapy with same initial titration protocol.

Dosage Forms

Injection, solution:

Symlin®: 600 mcg/mL (5 mL); 1000 mcg/mL (1.5 mL); 1000 mcg/mL (2.7 mL)

pramlintide acetate *see* pramlintide *on page 809*

Pramosone® [US] *see* pramoxine and hydrocortisone *on page 810*

Pramox® HC [Can] *see* pramoxine and hydrocortisone *on page 810*

pramoxine (pra MOKS een)

Sound-Alike/Look-Alike Issues

pramoxine may be confused with pralidoxime

Anusol® may be confused with Anusol-HC®, Aplisol®, Aquasol®

Synonyms pramoxine hydrochloride

U.S./Canadian Brand Names Anusol® Ointment [US-OTC]; Caladryl® Clear [US-OTC]; CalaMycin® Cool and Clear [US-OTC]; Callergy Clear [US-OTC]; Curasore® [US-OTC]; Itch-X® [US-OTC]; Prax® [US-OTC]; ProctoFoam® NS [US-OTC]; Sarna® Sensitive [US-OTC]; Soothing Care™ Itch Relief [US-OTC]; Summer's Eve® Anti-Itch Maximum Strength [US-OTC]; Tronolane® Cream [US-OTC]; Tucks® Hemorrhoidal [US-OTC]

Therapeutic Category Local Anesthetic

Use Temporary relief of pain and itching associated with anogenital pruritus or irritation; dermatosis, minor burns, or hemorrhoids

Usual Dosage Topical: Adults: Apply as directed, usually 3-5 times daily to affected area

Dosage Forms

Aerosol, topical [foam]:

ProctoFoam® NS [OTC]: 1% (15 g)

Cloth:

Summer's Eve® Anti-Itch Maximum Strength [OTC]: 1% (12s)

Cream, topical:
Tronolane® [OTC]: 1% (30 g, 60 g)
Gel, topical:
Itch-X® [OTC]: 1% (35.4 g)
Summer's Eve® Anti-Itch Maximum Strength [OTC]: 1% (30 mL)
Liquid, topical:
Curasore® [OTC]: 1% (15 mL)
Lotion, topical:
Caladryl® Clear [OTC]: 1% (177 mL)
Callergy Clear [OTC]: 1% (180 mL)
Prax® [OTC]: 1% (15 mL, 120 mL, 240 mL)
Sarna® Sensitive: 1% (222 mL)
Ointment, rectal:
Anusol® [OTC], Tucks® Hemorrhoidal [OTC]: 1% (30 g)
Solution, topical [spray]:
CalaMycin® Cool and Clear [OTC], Itch-X® [OTC]: 1% (60 mL)
Soothing Care™ Itch Relief [OTC]: 1% (74 mL)

pramoxine and hydrocortisone (pra MOKS een & hye droe KOR ti sone)

Sound-Alike/Look-Alike Issues
Pramosone® may be confused with predniSONE

Synonyms hydrocortisone and pramoxine; pramoxine hydrochloride and hydrocortisone acetate

U.S./Canadian Brand Names Analpram-HC® [US]; Epifoam® [US]; Pramosone® [US]; Pramox® HC [Can]; ProctoFoam®-HC [US/Can]

Therapeutic Category Anesthetic/Corticosteroid

Use Relief of inflammatory and pruritic manifestations of corticosteroid-responsive dermatoses

Usual Dosage Topical/rectal: Apply to affected areas 3-4 times/day

Dosage Forms
Cream, topical:
Analpram-HC®: Pramoxine 1% and hydrocortisone 1% (4 g, 30 g); pramoxine 1% and hydrocortisone 2.5% (4 g, 30 g)
Pramosone®: Pramoxine 1% and hydrocortisone 1% (30 g, 60 g); pramoxine 1% and hydrocortisone 2.5% (30 g, 60 g)
Foam, rectal:
ProctoFoam®-HC: Pramoxine 1% and hydrocortisone 1% (10 g)
Foam, topical:
Epifoam®: Pramoxine 1% and hydrocortisone 1% (10 g)
Lotion, topical:
Analpram-HC®: Pramoxine 1% and hydrocortisone 2.5% (60 mL)
Pramosone®: Pramoxine 1% and hydrocortisone 1% (60 mL, 120 mL, 240 mL); pramoxine 1% and hydrocortisone 2.5% (60 mL, 120 mL)
Ointment, topical:
Pramosone®: Pramoxine 1% and hydrocortisone 1% (30 g); pramoxine 1% and hydrocortisone 2.5% (30 g)

pramoxine hydrochloride *see* pramoxine *on page 809*

pramoxine hydrochloride and hydrocortisone acetate *see* pramoxine and hydrocortisone *on page 810*

pramoxine, neomycin, bacitracin, and polymyxin B *see* bacitracin, neomycin, polymyxin B, and pramoxine *on page 120*

PrandiMet® [US] *see* repaglinide and metformin *on page 859*

Prandin® [US/Can] *see* repaglinide *on page 858*

Prascion® [US] *see* sulfur and sulfacetamide *on page 931*

Prascion® AV *(Discontinued)* *see* sulfur and sulfacetamide *on page 931*

Prascion® FC [US] *see* sulfur and sulfacetamide *on page 931*

Prascion® RA [US] *see* sulfur and sulfacetamide *on page 931*

Prascion® TS *(Discontinued)* *see* sulfur and sulfacetamide *on page 931*

prasugrel (PRA soo grel)

Synonyms CS-747; LY-640315; prasugrel hydrochloride

U.S./Canadian Brand Names Effient™ [US]

Therapeutic Category Antiplatelet Agent

Use Reduces rate of thrombotic cardiovascular (eg, stent thrombosis) events in patients with unstable angina, non-ST-segment elevation MI, or ST-elevation MI (STEMI) managed with percutaneous coronary intervention (PCI)

Usual Dosage Oral: Adults: ≥60 kg: Loading dose: 60 mg; Maintenance dose: 10 mg once daily (in combination with aspirin 75-325 mg/day)

Note: In patients weighing <60 kg, consider decreasing maintenance dose to 5 mg once daily.

Dosage Forms

Tablet:

Effient™: 5 mg, 10 mg

prasugrel hydrochloride *see* prasugrel *on page 810*

Pravachol® [US/Can] *see* pravastatin *on page 811*

pravastatin (prav a STAT in)

Sound-Alike/Look-Alike Issues

pravastatin may be confused with nystatin

Pravachol® may be confused with atorvastatin, Prevacid®, Prinivil®, propranolol

Synonyms pravastatin sodium

U.S./Canadian Brand Names Apo-Pravastatin® [Can]; CO Pravastatin [Can]; DOM-Pravastatin [Can]; GEN-Pravastatin [Can]; Novo-Pravastatin [Can]; NU-Pravastatin [Can]; PHL-Pravastatin [Can]; PMS-Pravastatin [Can]; Pravachol® [US/Can]; RAN-Pravastatin [Can]; ratio-Pravastatin [Can]; Riva-Pravastatin [Can]; Sandoz-Pravastatin [Can]

Therapeutic Category HMG-CoA Reductase Inhibitor

Use Use with dietary therapy for the following:

Primary prevention of coronary events: In hypercholesterolemic patients without established coronary heart disease to reduce cardiovascular morbidity (myocardial infarction, coronary revascularization procedures) and mortality.

Secondary prevention of cardiovascular events in patients with established coronary heart disease: To slow the progression of coronary atherosclerosis; to reduce cardiovascular morbidity (myocardial infarction, coronary vascular procedures) and to reduce mortality; to reduce the risk of stroke and transient ischemic attacks

Hyperlipidemias: Reduce elevations in total cholesterol, LDL-C, apolipoprotein B, and triglycerides (elevations of 1 or more components are present in Fredrickson type IIa, IIb, III, and IV hyperlipidemias)

Heterozygous familial hypercholesterolemia (HeFH): In pediatric patients, 8-18 years of age, with HeFH having LDL-C ≥190 mg/dL **or** LDL ≥160 mg/dL with positive family history of premature cardiovascular disease (CVD) or 2 or more CVD risk factors in the pediatric patient

Usual Dosage Oral: **Note:** Doses should be individualized according to the baseline LDL-cholesterol levels, the recommended goal of therapy, and patient response; adjustments should be made at intervals of 4 weeks or more; doses may need adjusted based on concomitant medications

Children: HeFH:

8-13 years: 20 mg/day

14-18 years: 40 mg/day

Dosage Forms

Tablet: 10 mg, 20 mg, 40 mg, 80 mg

Pravachol®: 10 mg, 40 mg, 80 mg

pravastatin sodium *see* pravastatin *on page 811*

Pravigard™ PAC *(Discontinued)*

Prax® [US-OTC] *see* pramoxine *on page 809*

praziquantel (pray zi KWON tel)

U.S./Canadian Brand Names Biltricide® [US/Can]

Therapeutic Category Anthelmintic

Use All stages of schistosomiasis caused by all *Schistosoma* species pathogenic to humans; clonorchiasis and opisthorchiasis

Usual Dosage Oral: Children >4 years and Adults:

Schistosomiasis: 20 mg/kg/dose 2-3 times/day for 1 day at 4- to 6-hour intervals

Clonorchiasis/opisthorchiasis: 3 doses of 25 mg/kg as a 1-day treatment

Dosage Forms

Tablet [tri-scored]:

Biltricide®: 600 mg

prazosin (PRAZ oh sin)

Sound-Alike/Look-Alike Issues

prazosin may be confused with predniSONE

Synonyms furazosin; prazosin hydrochloride

U.S./Canadian Brand Names Apo-Prazo® [Can]; Minipress® [US/Can]; Novo-Prazin [Can]; Nu-Prazo [Can]

Therapeutic Category Alpha-Adrenergic Blocking Agent

Use Treatment of hypertension

Usual Dosage Oral: Adults:

Hypertension: Initial: 1 mg/dose 2-3 times/day; usual maintenance dose: 3-15 mg/day in divided doses 2-4 times/day; maximum daily dose: 20 mg

Hypertensive urgency: 10-20 mg once, may repeat in 30 minutes

Dosage Forms

Capsule: 1 mg, 2 mg, 5 mg

Minipress®: 1 mg, 2 mg, 5 mg

prazosin and polythiazide ***(Discontinued)***

prazosin hydrochloride *see* prazosin *on page 812*

PreCare® [US] *see* vitamins (multiple/prenatal) *on page 1020*

PreCare Conceive® [US] *see* vitamins (multiple/prenatal) *on page 1020*

PreCare Premier® [US] *see* vitamins (multiple/prenatal) *on page 1020*

Precedex® [US/Can] *see* dexmedetomidine *on page 291*

Precose® [US] *see* acarbose *on page 18*

Pred Forte® [US/Can] *see* prednisolone (ophthalmic) *on page 813*

Pred-G® [US] *see* prednisolone and gentamicin *on page 812*

Pred Mild® [US/Can] *see* prednisolone (ophthalmic) *on page 813*

prednicarbate (pred ni KAR bate)

Sound-Alike/Look-Alike Issues

Dermatop® may be confused with Dimetapp®

U.S./Canadian Brand Names Dermatop® [US/Can]

Therapeutic Category Corticosteroid, Topical

Use Relief of the inflammatory and pruritic manifestations of corticosteroid-responsive dermatoses (medium potency topical corticosteroid)

Usual Dosage Topical: Adults: Apply a thin film to affected area twice daily. Therapy should be discontinued when control is achieved; if no improvement is seen, reassessment of diagnosis may be necessary.

Dosage Forms

Cream: 0.1% (15 g, 60 g)

Dermatop®: 0.1% (60 g)

Ointment: 0.1% (15 g, 60 g)

Dermatop®: 0.1% (60 g)

Prednicen-M® ***(Discontinued)*** *see* prednisone *on page 814*

prednisolone acetate *see* prednisolone (systemic) *on page 813*

prednisolone acetate, ophthalmic *see* prednisolone (ophthalmic) *on page 813*

prednisolone and gentamicin (pred NIS oh lone & jen ta MYE sin)

Synonyms gentamicin and prednisolone

U.S./Canadian Brand Names Pred-G® [US]

Therapeutic Category Antibiotic/Corticosteroid, Ophthalmic

Use Treatment of steroid responsive inflammatory conditions and superficial ocular infections due to microorganisms susceptible to gentamicin

Usual Dosage Ophthalmic: Children and Adults:

Ointment: Apply 1/2 inch ribbon in the conjunctival sac 1-3 times/day

Suspension: 1 drop 2-4 times/day; during the initial 24-48 hours, the dosing frequency may be increased if necessary up to 1 drop every hour

Dosage Forms

Ointment, ophthalmic:

Pred-G®: Prednisolone 0.6% and gentamicin 0.3% (3.5 g)

prednisolone and sulfacetamide *see* sulfacetamide and prednisolone *on page 927*

prednisolone, neomycin, and polymyxin B *see* neomycin, polymyxin B, and prednisolone *on page 689*

prednisolone (ophthalmic) (pred NISS oh lone op THAL mik)

Sound-Alike/Look-Alike Issues

prednisoLONE may be confused with predniSONE

Synonyms prednisolone acetate, ophthalmic; prednisolone sodium phosphate, ophthalmic

Tall-Man predniso**LONE** (ophthalmic)

U.S./Canadian Brand Names AK-Pred® [US]; Econopred® Plus [US]; Inflamase® Mild [Can]; Ophtho-Tate® [Can]; Pred Forte® [US/Can]; Pred Mild® [US/Can]

Therapeutic Category Adrenal Corticosteroid

Use Treatment of palpebral and bulbar conjunctivitis; corneal injury from chemical, radiation, thermal burns, or foreign body penetration

Usual Dosage Ophthalmic suspension/solution: Children and Adults: Conjunctivitis, corneal injury: Instill 1-2 drops into conjunctival sac every hour during day, every 2 hours at night until favorable response is obtained, then use 1 drop every 4 hours.

Dosage Forms

Solution, ophthalmic: 1% (5 mL, 10 mL, 15 mL)

Suspension, ophthalmic: 1% (5 mL, 10 mL, 15 mL)

Econopred® Plus: 1% (5 mL, 10 mL)

Pred Forte®: 1% (1 mL, 5 mL, 10 mL, 15 mL)

Pred Mild®: 0.12% (5 mL, 10 mL)

prednisolone sodium phosphate *see* prednisolone (systemic) *on page 813*

prednisolone sodium phosphate, ophthalmic *see* prednisolone (ophthalmic) *on page 813*

prednisolone (systemic) (pred NISS oh lone sis TEM ik)

Sound-Alike/Look-Alike Issues

prednisoLONE may be confused with predniSONE

Pediapred® may be confused with Pediazole®

Synonyms deltahydrocortisone; metacortandralone; prednisolone acetate; prednisolone sodium phosphate

Tall-Man predniso**LONE** (systemic)

U.S./Canadian Brand Names Bubbli-Pred™ [US]; Diopred® [Can]; Hydeltra T.B.A.® [Can]; Novo-Prednisolone [Can]; Orapred® [US]; Pediapred® [US/Can]; Prelone® [US]; Sab-Prenase [Can]

Therapeutic Category Adrenal Corticosteroid

Use Treatment of endocrine disorders, rheumatic disorders, collagen diseases, dermatologic diseases, allergic states, ophthalmic diseases, respiratory diseases, hematologic disorders, neoplastic diseases, edematous states, and gastrointestinal diseases; resolution of acute exacerbations of multiple sclerosis

Usual Dosage Dose depends upon condition being treated and response of patient; dosage for infants and children should be based on severity of the disease and response of the patient rather than on strict adherence to dosage indicated by age, weight, or body surface area. Consider alternate day therapy for long-term therapy. Discontinuation of long-term therapy requires gradual withdrawal by tapering the dose. Patients undergoing unusual stress while receiving corticosteroids, should receive increased doses prior to, during, and after the stressful situation.

Children: Oral:

Acute asthma: 1-2 mg/kg/day in divided doses 1-2 times/day for 3-5 days

Antiinflammatory or immunosuppressive dose: 0.1-2 mg/kg/day in divided doses 1-4 times/day

Nephrotic syndrome:
Initial (first 3 episodes): 2 mg/kg/day **or** 60 mg/m^2/day (maximum: 80 mg/day) in divided doses 3-4 times/day until urine is protein free for 3 consecutive days (maximum: 28 days); followed by 1-1.5 mg/kg/dose **or** 40 mg/m^2/dose given every other day for 4 weeks
Maintenance (long-term maintenance dose for frequent relapses): 0.5-1 mg/kg/dose given every other day for 3-6 months
Adults: Oral:
Usual range: 5-60 mg/day
Multiple sclerosis: 200 mg/day for 1 week followed by 80 mg every other day for 1 month
Rheumatoid arthritis: Initial: 5-7.5 mg/day; adjust dose as necessary

Dosage Forms
Solution, oral: Prednisolone 15 mg/5 mL
Solution, oral: Prednisolone 5 mg/5 mL
Orapred®: 20 mg/5 mL
Pediapred®: 6.7 mg/5 mL
Syrup: 5 mg/5 m, 15 mg/5 mL
Prelone®: 15 mg/5 mL
Tablet: 5 mg
Tablet, orally disintegrating:
Orapred ODT™: 10 mg, 15 mg, 30 mg [grape flavor]

prednisone (PRED ni sone)

Sound-Alike/Look-Alike Issues
predniSONE may be confused with methylPREDNISolone, Pramosone®, prazosin, prednisoLONE, Prilosec®, primidone, promethazine

Synonyms deltacortisone; deltadehydrocortisone

Tall-Man predni**SONE**

U.S./Canadian Brand Names Apo-Prednisone® [Can]; Novo-Prednisone [Can]; PredniSONE Intensol™ [US]; Sterapred® DS [US]; Sterapred® [US]; Winpred™ [Can]

Therapeutic Category Adrenal Corticosteroid

Use Treatment of a variety of diseases, including:
Allergic states (including adjunctive treatment of anaphylaxis)
Autoimmune disorders (including systemic lupus erythematosus [SLE])
Collagen diseases
Dermatologic conditions/diseases
Edematous states (including nephrotic syndrome)
Endocrine disorders
Gastrointestinal diseases
Hematologic disorders (including idiopathic thrombocytopenia purpura [ITP])
Multiple sclerosis exacerbations
Neoplastic diseases
Ophthalmic diseases
Respiratory diseases (including acute asthma exacerbation)
Rheumatic disorders (including rheumatoid arthritis)
Trichinosis with neurologic or myocardial involvement
Tuberculous meningitis

Usual Dosage Oral:
General dosing range: Children and Adults: Initial: 5-60 mg/day: **Note:** Dose depends upon condition being treated and response of patient; dosage for infants and children should be based on severity of the disease and response of the patient rather than on strict adherence to dosage indicated by age, weight, or body surface area. Consider alternate day therapy for long-term therapy. Discontinuation of long-term therapy requires gradual withdrawal by tapering the dose.
Prednisone taper (other regimens also available):
Day 1: 30 mg divided as 10 mg before breakfast, 5 mg at lunch, 5 mg at dinner, 10 mg at bedtime
Day 2: 5 mg at breakfast, 5 mg at lunch, 5 mg at dinner, 10 mg at bedtime
Day 3: 5 mg 4 times/day (with meals and at bedtime)
Day 4: 5 mg 3 times/day (breakfast, lunch, bedtime)
Day 5: 5 mg 2 times/day (breakfast, bedtime)
Day 6: 5 mg before breakfast

Indication-specific dosing:

Children:

Acute asthma:

0-11 years 1-2 mg/kg/day for 3-10 days (maximum: 60 mg/day)

≥12 years: Refer to adult dosing

Nephrotic syndrome: Initial: 2 mg/kg/day or 60 mg/m^2/day given every day in 1-3 divided doses (maximum: 80 mg/day) until urine is protein free or for 4-6 weeks; followed by maintenance dose: 2 mg/kg/dose or 40 mg/m^2/dose given every other day in the morning; gradually taper and discontinue after 4-6 weeks. **Note:** No definitive treatment guidelines exist. Dosing is dependant on institution protocols and individual response.

PCP pneumonia: 1 mg/kg twice daily for 5 days, *followed by* 0.5-1 mg/kg twice daily for 5 days, *followed by* 0.5 mg/kg once daily for 11-21 days

Adolescents and Adults:

PCP pneumonia: Note: Begin within 72 hours of PCP therapy: 40 mg twice daily for 5 days, *followed by* 40 mg once daily for 5 days, *followed by* 20 mg once daily for 11 days or until antimicrobial regimen is completed

Adults:

Acute asthma: 40-60 mg per day for 3-10 days; administer as single or 2 divided doses

Anaphylaxis, adjunctive treatment: 0.5 mg/kg

Antineoplastic: Usual range: 10 mg/day to 100 mg/m^2/day (depending on indication). **Note:** Details concerning dosing in combination regimens should also be consulted.

Idiopathic thrombocytopenia purpura: 1-2 mg/kg/day

Rheumatoid arthritis: ≤10 mg/day

Systemic lupus erythematosus:

Mild SLE: ≤10 mg/day

Refractory or severe organ-threatening disease: 20-60 mg/day

Dosage Forms

Solution, oral: 1 mg/mL

Solution, oral [concentrate]:

PredniSONE Intensol™: 5 mg/mL

Tablet: 1 mg, 2.5 mg, 5 mg, 10 mg, 20 mg, 50 mg

Sterapred®: 5 mg

Sterapred® DS: 10 mg

PredniSONE Intensol™ [US] *see* prednisone *on page 814*

Prefest™ [US] *see* estradiol and norgestimate *on page 377*

Prefrin™ *(Discontinued)* *see* phenylephrine *on page 774*

pregabalin (pre GAB a lin)

Sound-Alike/Look-Alike Issues

Lyrica® may be confused with Lopressor®

Synonyms CI-1008; S-(+)-3-isobutylgaba

U.S./Canadian Brand Names Lyrica® [US/Can]

Therapeutic Category Analgesic, Miscellaneous; Anticonvulsant, Miscellaneous

Controlled Substance C-V

Use Management of pain associated with diabetic peripheral neuropathy; management of postherpetic neuralgia; adjunctive therapy for partial-onset seizure disorder in adults; management of fibromyalgia

Usual Dosage Oral: Adults:

Fibromyalgia: Initial: 150 mg/day in divided doses (75 mg 2 times/day); may be increased to 300 mg/day (150 mg 2 times/day) within 1 week based on tolerability and effect; may be further increased to 450 mg/day (225 mg 2 times/day). Maximum dose: 450 mg/day (dosages up to 600 mg/day were evaluated with no significant additional benefit and an increase in adverse effects)

Neuropathic pain (diabetes-associated): Initial: 150 mg/day in divided doses (50 mg 3 times/day); may be increased within 1 week based on tolerability and effect; maximum dose: 300 mg/day (dosages up to 600 mg/day were evaluated with no significant additional benefit and an increase in adverse effects)

Postherpetic neuralgia: Initial: 150 mg/day in divided doses (75 mg 2 times/day or 50 mg 3 times/day); may be increased to 300 mg/day within 1 week based on tolerability and effect; further titration (to 600 mg/day) after 2-4 weeks may be considered in patients who do not experience sufficient relief of pain provided they are able to tolerate pregabalin. Maximum dose: 600 mg/day

Partial-onset seizures (adjunctive therapy): Initial: 150 mg per day in divided doses (75 mg 2 times/day or 50 mg 3 times/day); may be increased based on tolerability and effect (optimal titration schedule has not been defined). Maximum dose: 600 mg/day

Discontinuing therapy: Pregabalin should not be abruptly discontinued; taper dosage over at least 1 week

Dosage Forms

Capsule:

Lyrica®: 25 mg, 50 mg, 75 mg, 100 mg, 150 mg, 200 mg, 225 mg, 300 mg

Previfem® [US] *see* ethinyl estradiol and norgestimate *on page 393*
Prevnar® [US/Can] *see* pneumococcal conjugate vaccine (7-valent) *on page 793*
Prevpac® [US] *see* lansoprazole, amoxicillin, and clarithromycin *on page 571*
Prezista® [US/Can] *see* darunavir *on page 277*
Prialt® [US] *see* ziconotide *on page 1028*
Priftin® [US/Can] *see* rifapentine *on page 867*

prilocaine (PRIL oh kane)

Sound-Alike/Look-Alike Issues
prilocaine may be confused with Polocaine®, Prilosec®

U.S./Canadian Brand Names Citanest® Plain Dental [US]; Citanest® Plain [Can]

Therapeutic Category Local Anesthetic

Use Amide-type anesthetic used for local infiltration anesthesia; injection near nerve trunks to produce nerve block

Usual Dosage
Children <10 years: Doses >40 mg (1 mL) as a 4% solution per procedure rarely needed
Children >10 years and Adults: Dental anesthesia, infiltration, or conduction block: Initial: 40-80 mg (1-2 mL) as a 4% solution; up to a maximum of 400 mg (10 mL) as a 4% solution within a 2-hour period. Manufacturer's maximum recommended dose is not more than 600 mg to normal healthy adults. The effective anesthetic dose varies with procedure, intensity of anesthesia needed, duration of anesthesia required and physical condition of the patient. Always use the lowest effective dose along with careful aspiration.
Note: Adult and children doses of prilocaine hydrochloride cited from USP Dispensing Information (USP DI), 17th ed, The United States Pharmacopeial Convention, Inc, Rockville, MD, 1997, 139.

Dosage Forms
Injection, solution [for dental use]:
Citanest® Plain Dental: 4% (1.8 mL)

prilocaine and lidocaine *see* lidocaine and prilocaine *on page 588*
Prilosec® [US] *see* omeprazole *on page 723*
Prilosec OTC™ [US-OTC] *see* omeprazole *on page 723*
PrimaCare® [US] *see* vitamins (multiple/prenatal) *on page 1020*
PrimaCare® One [US] *see* vitamins (multiple/prenatal) *on page 1020*
primaclone *see* primidone *on page 818*
Primacor® [Can] *see* milrinone *on page 659*
Primacor® *(Discontinued)* *see* milrinone *on page 659*
Primalev™ [US] *see* oxycodone and acetaminophen *on page 738*

primaquine (PRIM a kween)

Sound-Alike/Look-Alike Issues
primaquine may be confused with primidone

Synonyms primaquine phosphate; prymaccone

Therapeutic Category Aminoquinoline (Antimalarial)

Use Prevention of relapse of *P. vivax* malaria

Usual Dosage Oral: Dosage expressed as mg of base (15 mg base = 26.3 mg primaquine phosphate).
Note: The CDC recommends screening for G6PD deficiency prior to initiating treatment with primaquine.
Relapse prevention of *P. vivax* malaria: CDC recommendations: Uncomplicated malaria (*P. vivax* and *P. ovale*):
Children: 0.5 mg/kg once daily for 14 days (maximum dose: 30 mg/day); alternative regimen (recommended for mild G6PD deficiency): 45 mg once weekly for 8 weeks
Adults: 30 mg once daily for 14 days; alternative regimen (recommended for mild G6PD deficiency): 45 mg once weekly for 8 weeks

Dosage Forms
Tablet: 26.3 mg

primaquine phosphate *see* primaquine *on page 817*
Primatene® Mist [US-OTC] *see* epinephrine *on page 358*
Primaxin® [US/Can] *see* imipenem and cilastatin *on page 520*
Primaxin® I.V. [Can] *see* imipenem and cilastatin *on page 520*

Primene® [Can] *see* amino acid injection *on page 62*

primidone (PRI mi done)

Sound-Alike/Look-Alike Issues

primidone may be confused with predniSONE, primaquine, pyridoxine

Synonyms desoxyphenobarbital; primaclone

U.S./Canadian Brand Names Apo-Primidone® [Can]; Mysoline® [US]

Therapeutic Category Anticonvulsant; Barbiturate

Use Management of grand mal, psychomotor, and focal seizures

Usual Dosage Oral: Seizure disorders:

Children <8 years: Initial: Days 1-3: 50 mg/day given at bedtime; days 4-6: 50 mg twice daily; days 7-9: 100 mg twice daily; usual dose: 375-750 mg/day in 3-4 divided doses (10-25 mg/kg/day)

Children ≥8 years and Adults: Days 1-3: 100-125 mg/day at bedtime; days 4-6: 100-125 twice daily; days 7-9: 100-125 mg 3 times daily; usual dose: 750-1500 mg/day in divided doses 3-4 times/day with maximum dosage of 2 g/day

Patients already receiving other anticonvulsants: Initial: 100-125 mg at bedtime; gradually increase to maintenance dose as other drug is gradually decreased, continue until desired level obtained or other drug completely withdrawn. If goal is monotherapy, conversion should be completed over ≥2 weeks.

Dosage Forms [CAN] = Canadian brand name

Tablet: 50 mg [U.S. only], 125 [CAN only], 250 mg

Mysoline®: 50 mg, 250 mg

Primsol® [US] *see* trimethoprim *on page 988*
Prinivil® [US/Can] *see* lisinopril *on page 593*
Prinzide® [US/Can] *see* lisinopril and hydrochlorothiazide *on page 594*
Priorix™ [Can] *see* measles, mumps, and rubella virus vaccine *on page 615*
Priscoline® *(Discontinued)*
PrismaSol [US] *see* electrolyte solution, renal replacement *on page 350*
pristinamycin *see* quinupristin and dalfopristin *on page 846*
Pristiq™ [US] *see* desvenlafaxine *on page 287*
Privigen™ [US] *see* immune globulin (intravenous) *on page 523*
Privine® [US-OTC] *see* naphazoline *on page 680*
ProAir® HFA [US] *see* albuterol *on page 41*
ProAmatine® [US] *see* midodrine *on page 657*
PRO-Amiodarone [Can] *see* amiodarone *on page 64*
PRO-Azithromycin [Can] *see* azithromycin *on page 116*
Pro-Banthine® *(Discontinued)* *see* propantheline *on page 826*

probenecid (proe BEN e sid)

Sound-Alike/Look-Alike Issues

probenecid may be confused with Procanbid®

U.S./Canadian Brand Names Benuryl™ [Can]

Therapeutic Category Uricosuric Agent

Use Prevention of hyperuricemia associated with gout or gouty arthritis; prolongation and elevation of beta-lactam plasma levels

Usual Dosage Oral:

Children:

2-14 years: Prolong penicillin serum levels: Initial: 25 mg/kg, then 40 mg/kg/day given 4 times/day (maximum: 500 mg/dose)

Gonorrhea: >45 kg: Refer to adult guidelines

Adults:

Hyperuricemia with gout: 250 mg twice daily for one week; increase to 250-500 mg/day; may increase by 500 mg/month, if needed, to maximum of 2-3 g/day (dosages may be increased by 500 mg every 6 months if serum urate concentrations are controlled)

Prolong penicillin serum levels: 500 mg 4 times/day

Gonorrhea: CDC guidelines (alternative regimen): Probenecid 1 g orally with cefoxitin 2 g I.M.

Pelvic inflammatory disease: CDC guidelines: Cefoxitin 2 g I.M. plus probenecid 1 g orally as a single dose

Neurosyphilis: CDC guidelines (alternative regimen): Procaine penicillin 2.4 million units/day I.M. plus probenecid 500 mg 4 times/day; both administered for 10-14 days

Dosage Forms

Tablet: 500 mg

probenecid and colchicine *see* colchicine and probenecid *on page 253*

Pro-Bicalutamide [Can] *see* bicalutamide *on page 141*

Pro-Bionate® *(Discontinued)*

PRO-Bisoprolol [Can] *see* bisoprolol *on page 144*

procainamide (pro KANE a mide)

Sound-Alike/Look-Alike Issues

PCA (error-prone abbreviation)
Procanbid® may be confused with probenecid, Procan SR®
Procan SR® may be confused with procanbid
Pronestyl® may be confused with Ponstel®

Synonyms procainamide hydrochloride; procaine amide hydrochloride

U.S./Canadian Brand Names Apo-Procainamide® [Can]; Procainamide Hydrochloride Injection, USP [Can]; Procan SR® [Can]

Therapeutic Category Antiarrhythmic Agent, Class I-A

Use

Intravenous: Treatment of ventricular arrhythmias (eg, sustained ventricular tachycardia [VT]); **Note:** Due to proarrhythmic effects, use should be reserved for life-threatening arrhythmias

Oral (Canadian labeling; not available in U.S.): Treatment of supraventricular arrhythmias. **Note:** In the treatment of atrial fibrillation, use only when preferred treatment is ineffective or cannot be used. Use in paroxysmal atrial tachycardia when reflex stimulation or other measures are ineffective.

Usual Dosage Must be titrated to patient's response

Children:

I.M.: 50 mg/kg/24 hours divided into doses of $1/8$ to $1/4$ every 3-6 hours in divided doses

I.V.:

Load: 3-6 mg/kg/dose over 5 minutes not to exceed 100 mg/dose; may repeat every 5-10 minutes to maximum of 15 mg/kg/load

Maintenance as continuous I.V. infusion: 20-80 mcg/kg/minute; maximum: 2 g/24 hours

Possible VT (pulses and poor perfusion): I.V.; I.O.: 15 mg/kg over 30-60 minutes

Adults:

I.M.: 0.5-1 g every 4-8 hours

I.V.:

Loading dose: 15-18 mg/kg administered as slow infusion over 25-30 minutes **or** 100-200 mg/dose repeated every 5 minutes as needed to a total dose of 1 g. Reduce loading dose to 12 mg/kg in severe renal or cardiac impairment.

Maintenance dose: 1-4 mg/minute by continuous infusion. Maintenance infusions should be reduced by one-third in patients with moderate renal or cardiac impairment and by two-thirds in patients with severe renal or cardiac impairment.

ACLS guidelines: Infuse 20-50 mg/minute until arrhythmia is controlled, hypotension occurs, QRS complex widens by 50% of its original width, or total of 17 mg/kg is given. **Note:** Not recommended for use in ongoing ventricular fibrillation (VF) or pulseless ventricular tachycardia (VT) due to prolonged administration time and uncertain efficacy.

Oral (not available in the U.S.; Canadian labeling): Sustained release formulation (Procan SR®):

Maintenance: 50 mg/kg/24 hours given in divided doses every 6 hours

Suggested Procan SR® maintenance dose:

<55 kg: 500 mg every 6 hours
55-91 kg: 750 mg every 6 hours
>91 kg: 1000 mg every 6 hours

Dosage Forms [CAN] = Canadian brand name

Injection, solution: 100 mg/mL (10 mL); 500 mg/mL (2 mL)

Tablet, sustained release, oral:

Procan SR® [CAN]: 250 mg, 500 mg, 750 mg [not available in U.S.]

procainamide hydrochloride *see* procainamide *on page 819*

Procainamide Hydrochloride Injection, USP [Can] *see* procainamide *on page 819*

procaine (PROE kane)

Synonyms procaine hydrochloride

U.S./Canadian Brand Names Novocain® [US]

Therapeutic Category Local Anesthetic

Use Produces spinal anesthesia

Usual Dosage Dose varies with procedure, desired depth, and duration of anesthesia, desired muscle relaxation, vascularity of tissues, physical condition, and age of patient

Adults: Spinal analgesia: Extent of anesthesia:

Perineum: Total dose: 50 mg; Procaine 10%: 0.5 mL with 0.5 mL diluent

Perineum and lower extremities: Total dose: 100 mg; Procaine 10%: 1 mL with 1 mL diluent

Up to costal margin: Total dose: 200 mg; Procaine 10%: 2 mL with 1 mL diluent

Dosage Forms

Injection, solution:

Novocain®: 10% (2 mL)

procaine amide hydrochloride *see* procainamide *on page 819*

procaine benzylpenicillin *see* penicillin G procaine *on page 762*

procaine hydrochloride *see* procaine *on page 820*

procaine penicillin G *see* penicillin G procaine *on page 762*

Pro-Calcitonin [Can] *see* calcitonin *on page 167*

Pro-Cal-Sof® ***(Discontinued)*** *see* docusate *on page 326*

Procanbid® ***(Discontinued)*** *see* procainamide *on page 819*

Procan SR® [Can] *see* procainamide *on page 819*

procarbazine (proe KAR ba zeen)

Sound-Alike/Look-Alike Issues

procarbazine may be confused with dacarbazine

Matulane® may be confused with Materna®, Modane®

Synonyms benzmethyzin; N-methylhydrazine; NSC-77213; procarbazine hydrochloride

U.S./Canadian Brand Names Matulane® [US/Can]; Natulan® [Can]

Therapeutic Category Antineoplastic Agent

Use Treatment of Hodgkin disease

Usual Dosage Refer to individual protocols. Manufacturer states that the dose is based on patient's ideal weight if the patient is obese or has abnormal fluid retention. Other studies suggest that ideal body weight may not be necessary. Oral (may be given as a single daily dose or in 2-3 divided doses):

Children:

BMT aplastic anemia conditioning regimen: 12.5 mg/kg/day every other day for 4 doses

Hodgkin disease: MOPP/IC-MOPP regimens: 100 mg/m^2/day for 14 days and repeated every 4 weeks

Neuroblastoma and medulloblastoma: Doses as high as 100-200 mg/m^2/day once daily have been used

Adults: Initial: 2-4 mg/kg/day in single or divided doses for 7 days then increase dose to 4-6 mg/kg/day until response is obtained or leukocyte count decreased <4000/mm^3 or the platelet count decreased <100,000/mm^3; maintenance: 1-2 mg/kg/day

Dosage Forms

Capsule:

Matulane®: 50 mg

procarbazine hydrochloride *see* procarbazine *on page 820*

Procardia® [US] *see* nifedipine *on page 697*

Procardia XL® [US] *see* nifedipine *on page 697*

Pro-Cefadroxil [Can] *see* cefadroxil *on page 191*

Pro-Cefuroxime [Can] *see* cefuroxime *on page 199*

procetofene *see* fenofibrate *on page 408*

Prochieve® [US] *see* progesterone *on page 822*

prochlorperazine (proe klor PER a zeen)

Sound-Alike/Look-Alike Issues

prochlorperazine may be confused with chlorproMAZINE

Compazine® may be confused with Copaxone®, Coumadin®
CPZ (occasional abbreviation for Compazine®) is an error-prone abbreviation (mistaken as chlorpromazine)

Synonyms chlormeprazine; prochlorperazine edisylate; prochlorperazine maleate

U.S./Canadian Brand Names Apo-Prochlorperazine® [Can]; Compro™ [US]; Nu-Prochlor [Can]; Stemetil® [Can]

Therapeutic Category Phenothiazine Derivative

Use Management of nausea and vomiting; psychotic disorders, including schizophrenia and anxiety

Usual Dosage

Antiemetic: Children (therapy >1 day usually not required): **Note:** Not recommended for use in children <9 kg or <2 years:
Oral, rectal: >9 kg: 0.4 mg/kg/24 hours in 3-4 divided doses; **or**
9-13 kg: 2.5 mg every 12-24 hours as needed; maximum: 7.5 mg/day
13.1-17 kg: 2.5 mg every 8-12 hours as needed; maximum: 10 mg/day
17.1-37 kg: 2.5 mg every 8 hours or 5 mg every 12 hours as needed; maximum: 15 mg/day
I.M.: 0.13 mg/kg/dose; change to oral as soon as possible

Antiemetic: Adults:
Oral (tablet): 5-10 mg 3-4 times/day; usual maximum: 40 mg/day; larger doses may rarely be required
I.M. (deep): 5-10 mg every 3-4 hours; usual maximum: 40 mg/day
I.V.: 2.5-10 mg; maximum 10 mg/dose or 40 mg/day; may repeat dose every 3-4 hours as needed
Rectal: 25 mg twice daily

Surgical nausea/vomiting: Adults: **Note:** Should not exceed 40 mg/day
I.M.: 5-10 mg 1-2 hours before induction or to control symptoms during or after surgery; may repeat once if necessary
I.V. (administer slow IVP <5 mg/minute): 5-10 mg 15-30 minutes before induction or to control symptoms during or after surgery; may repeat once if necessary

Antipsychotic:
Children 2-12 years (not recommended in children <9 kg or <2 years):
Oral, rectal: 2.5 mg 2-3 times/day; do not give more than 10 mg the first day; increase dosage as needed to maximum daily dose of 20 mg for 2-5 years and 25 mg for 6-12 years
I.M.: 0.13 mg/kg/dose; change to oral as soon as possible
Adults:
Oral: 5-10 mg 3-4 times/day; titrate dose slowly every 2-3 days; doses up to 150 mg/day may be required in some patients for treatment of severe disturbances
I.M.: Initial: 10-20 mg; if necessary repeat initial dose every 1-4 hours to gain control; more than 3-4 doses are rarely needed. If parenteral administration is still required; give 10-20 mg every 4-6 hours; change to oral as soon as possible.

Nonpsychotic anxiety: Oral (tablet): Adults: Usual dose: 15-20 mg/day in divided doses; do not give doses >20 mg/day or for longer than 12 weeks

Dosage Forms

Injection, solution: 5 mg/mL (2 mL, 10 mL)
Suppository, rectal: 25 mg (12s)
Compro™: 25 mg (12s)
Tablet: 5 mg, 10 mg

prochlorperazine edisylate *see* prochlorperazine *on page 820*
prochlorperazine maleate *see* prochlorperazine *on page 820*
PRO-Ciprofloxacin [Can] *see* ciprofloxacin *on page 229*
Pro-Clonazepam [Can] *see* clonazepam *on page 245*
Procrit® [US] *see* epoetin alfa *on page 361*
Proctocort® [US] *see* hydrocortisone (rectal) *on page 503*
ProctoCream® HC [US] *see* hydrocortisone (rectal) *on page 503*
proctofene *see* fenofibrate *on page 408*
ProctoFoam®-HC [US/Can] *see* pramoxine and hydrocortisone *on page 810*
ProctoFoam® NS [US-OTC] *see* pramoxine *on page 809*
Procto-Kit™ [US] *see* hydrocortisone (rectal) *on page 503*
Procto-Pak™ [US] *see* hydrocortisone (rectal) *on page 503*
Proctosert [US] *see* hydrocortisone (rectal) *on page 503*
Proctosol-HC® [US] *see* hydrocortisone (rectal) *on page 503*
Proctozone-HC™ [US] *see* hydrocortisone (rectal) *on page 503*

procyclidine (proe SYE kli deen)

Sound-Alike/Look-Alike Issues
Kemadrin® may be confused with Coumadin®

Synonyms procyclidine hydrochloride

U.S./Canadian Brand Names PMS-Procyclidine [Can]

Therapeutic Category Anti-Parkinson Agent; Anticholinergic Agent

Use Relieves symptoms of parkinsonian syndrome and drug-induced extrapyramidal symptoms

Usual Dosage Oral: Adults: 2.5 mg 3 times/day after meals; if tolerated, gradually increase dose, maximum of 20 mg/day if necessary

procyclidine hydrochloride *see* procyclidine *on page* 822
Procytox® [Can] *see* cyclophosphamide *on page* 265
Pro-Diclo-Rapide [Can] *see* diclofenac *on page* 303
Prodium® [US-OTC] *see* phenazopyridine *on page* 770
Pro Doc Limitee Bromazepam [Can] *see* bromazepam *(Canada only) on page* 148
Pro-Enalapril [Can] *see* enalapril *on page* 352
Profasi® HP [Can] *see* chorionic gonadotropin (human) *on page* 225
ProFe [US-OTC] *see* polysaccharide-iron complex *on page* 799
Profen II® ***(Discontinued)*** *see* guaifenesin and pseudoephedrine *on page* 477
Profen II DM® [US] *see* guaifenesin, pseudoephedrine, and dextromethorphan *on page* 479
Profen Forte™ DM [US] *see* guaifenesin, pseudoephedrine, and dextromethorphan *on page* 479
Profen LA® ***(Discontinued)***
Pro-Feno-Super [Can] *see* fenofibrate *on page* 408
Profilnine® SD [US] *see* factor IX complex (human) *on page* 404
Proflavanol C™ [Can] *see* ascorbic acid *on page* 100
Pro-Fluconazole [Can] *see* fluconazole *on page* 424
PRO-Fluoxetine [Can] *see* fluoxetine *on page* 432

progesterone (proe JES ter one)

Synonyms pregnenedione; progestin

U.S./Canadian Brand Names Crinone® [US/Can]; Endometrin® [US]; First™-Progesterone VGS [US]; Prochieve® [US]; Prometrium® [US/Can]

Therapeutic Category Progestin

Use
Oral: Prevention of endometrial hyperplasia in nonhysterectomized, postmenopausal women who are receiving conjugated estrogen tablets; secondary amenorrhea
I.M.: Amenorrhea; abnormal uterine bleeding due to hormonal imbalance
Intravaginal gel: Part of assisted reproductive technology (ART) for infertile women with progesterone deficiency; secondary amenorrhea
Vaginal tablet: Part of ART for infertile women with progesterone deficiency

Usual Dosage Adults:
I.M.: Females:
Amenorrhea: 5-10 mg/day for 6-8 consecutive days
Functional uterine bleeding: 5-10 mg/day for 6 doses
Oral: Females:
Prevention of endometrial hyperplasia (in postmenopausal women with a uterus who are receiving daily conjugated estrogen tablets): 200 mg as a single daily dose every evening for 12 days sequentially per 28-day cycle
Amenorrhea: 400 mg every evening for 10 days
Intravaginal gel: Females:
ART in women who require progesterone supplementation: 90 mg (8% gel) once daily; if pregnancy occurs, may continue treatment for up to 10-12 weeks
ART in women with partial or complete ovarian failure: 90 mg (8% gel) intravaginally twice daily; if pregnancy occurs, may continue up to 10-12 weeks
Secondary amenorrhea: 45 mg (4% gel) intravaginally every other day for up to 6 doses; women who fail to respond may be increased to 90 mg (8% gel) every other day for up to 6 doses
Intravaginal tablet: Females: ART: 100 mg 2-3 times daily starting at oocyte retrieval and continuing for up to 10 weeks.

Dosage Forms

Capsule:

Prometrium®: 100 mg, 200 mg

Gel, vaginal:

Crinone®: 8% (1.45 g) [90 mg/dose; contains palm oil; 6 or 18 prefilled applicators]

Prochieve®: 4% (1.45 mg) [45 mg/dose; contains palm oil; 6 prefilled applicators]; 8% (1.45 g) [90 mg/dose; contains palm oil; 6 or 18 prefilled applicators]

Injection, oil: 50 mg/mL (10 mL)

Powder, for prescription compounding [micronized]: Progesterone USP (10 g, 25 g, 100 g, 1000 g)

Powder, for prescription compounding [wettable]: Progesterone USP (10 g, 25 g, 100 g, 1000 g)

First™-Progesterone VGS 25: Progesterone USP (0.75 g)

First™-Progesterone VGS 50: Progesterone USP (1.5 g)

First™-Progesterone VGS 100: Progesterone USP (3 g)

First™-Progesterone VGS 200: Progesterone USP (6 g)

First™-Progesterone VGS 400: Progesterone USP (12 g)

Tablet, vaginal:

Endometrin®: 100 mg (21s)

progestin *see* progesterone *on page 822*

PRO-Glyburide [Can] *see* glyburide *on page 467*

Proglycem® [US/Can] *see* diazoxide *on page 302*

Prograf® [US/Can] *see* tacrolimus *on page 935*

proguanil and atovaquone *see* atovaquone and proguanil *on page 109*

proguanil hydrochloride and atovaquone *see* atovaquone and proguanil *on page 109*

ProHance® [US] *see* gadoteridol *on page 452*

ProHIBiT® *(Discontinued)*

Pro-Hydroxyquine [Can] *see* hydroxychloroquine *on page 509*

Pro-Indapamide [Can] *see* indapamide *on page 525*

Pro-ISMN [Can] *see* isosorbide mononitrate *on page 551*

Prolastin® [US/Can] *see* alpha$_1$-proteinase inhibitor *on page 50*

Proleukin® [US/Can] *see* aldesleukin *on page 43*

Pro-Levocarb [US] *see* carbidopa and levodopa *on page 184*

Prolex®-D *(Discontinued)* *see* guaifenesin and phenylephrine *on page 475*

Prolex®-PD *(Discontinued)* *see* guaifenesin and phenylephrine *on page 475*

Pro-Lisinopril [Can] *see* lisinopril *on page 593*

Prolixin® *(Discontinued)* *see* fluphenazine *on page 434*

Prolixin Enanthate® *(Discontinued)* *see* fluphenazine *on page 434*

Prolopa® [Can] *see* benserazide and levodopa *(Canada only) on page 128*

PRO-Lovastatin [Can] *see* lovastatin *on page 602*

Promacet [US] *see* butalbital and acetaminophen *on page 162*

Promacta® [US] *see* eltrombopag *on page 351*

Prometa® *(Discontinued)*

promethazine (proe METH a zeen)

Sound-Alike/Look-Alike Issues

promethazine may be confused with chlorproMAZINE, predniSONE, promazine

Phenergan® may be confused with Phenaphen®, PHENobarbital, Phrenilin®, Theragran®

Synonyms promethazine hydrochloride

U.S./Canadian Brand Names Bioniche Promethazine [Can]; Histantil [Can]; Phenadoz™ [US]; Phenergan® [US/Can]; PMS-Promethazine [Can]; Promethegan™ [US]

Therapeutic Category Antiemetic; Phenothiazine Derivative

Use Symptomatic treatment of various allergic conditions; antiemetic; motion sickness; sedative

Usual Dosage

Children ≥2 years:

Allergic conditions: Oral, rectal: 0.1 mg/kg/dose (maximum: 12.5 mg) every 6 hours during the day and 0.5 mg/kg/dose (maximum: 25 mg) at bedtime as needed

Antiemetic: Oral, I.M., I.V., rectal: 0.25-1 mg/kg 4-6 times/day as needed (maximum: 25 mg/dose)

Motion sickness: Oral, rectal: 0.5 mg/kg/dose 30 minutes to 1 hour before departure, then every 12 hours as needed (maximum dose: 25 mg twice daily)
Sedation: Oral, I.M., I.V., rectal: 0.5-1 mg/kg/dose every 6 hours as needed (maximum: 50 mg/dose)
Adults:
Allergic conditions (including allergic reactions to blood or plasma):
Oral, rectal: 25 mg at bedtime **or** 12.5 mg before meals and at bedtime (range: 6.25-12.5 mg 3 times/day)
I.M., I.V.: 25 mg, may repeat in 2 hours when necessary; switch to oral route as soon as feasible
Antiemetic: Oral, I.M., I.V., rectal: 12.5-25 mg every 4-6 hours as needed
Motion sickness: Oral, rectal: 25 mg 30-60 minutes before departure, then every 12 hours as needed
Sedation: Oral, I.M., I.V., rectal: 12.5-50 mg/dose

Dosage Forms
Injection, solution: 25 mg/mL (1 mL); 50 mg/mL (1 mL)
Phenergan®: 25 mg/mL (1 mL); 50 mg/mL (1 mL)
Suppository, rectal: 12.5 mg, 25 mg, 50 mg
Phenadoz™: 12.5 mg, 25 mg
Promethegan™: 12.5 mg, 25 mg, 50 mg
Syrup: 6.25 mg/5 mL
Tablet: 12.5 mg, 25 mg, 50 mg

promethazine and codeine (proe METH a zeen & KOE deen)

Synonyms codeine and promethazine
Therapeutic Category Antihistamine/Antitussive
Controlled Substance C-V
Use Temporary relief of coughs and upper respiratory symptoms associated with allergy or the common cold
Usual Dosage Oral:
Children:
<6 years: **Note:** Use of promethazine/codeine combination is contraindicated in children <6 years of age
6-11 years: 2.5-5 mL every 4-6 hours (maximum: 30 mL/24 hours)
Children ≥12 years and Adults: 5 mL every 4-6 hours (maximum: 30 mL/24 hours)
Dosage Forms
Syrup: Promethazine 6.25 mg and codeine 10 mg per 5 mL

promethazine and dextromethorphan (proe METH a zeen & deks troe meth OR fan)

Synonyms dextromethorphan and promethazine
Therapeutic Category Antihistamine/Antitussive
Use Temporary relief of coughs and upper respiratory symptoms associated with allergy or the common cold
Usual Dosage Oral:
Children:
2-6 years: 1.25-2.5 mL every 4-6 hours up to 10 mL in 24 hours
6-12 years: 2.5-5 mL every 4-6 hours up to 20 mL in 24 hours
Adults: 5 mL every 4-6 hours up to 30 mL in 24 hours
Dosage Forms
Syrup: Promethazine 6.25 mg and dextromethorphan 15 mg per 5 mL

promethazine and meperidine *see* meperidine and promethazine *on page 627*

promethazine and phenylephrine (proe METH a zeen & fen il EF rin)

Synonyms phenylephrine and promethazine
Therapeutic Category Antihistamine/Decongestant Combination
Use Temporary relief of upper respiratory symptoms associated with allergy or the common cold
Usual Dosage Oral:
Children:
<2 years: Use of promethazine is contraindicated
2-6 years: 1.25-2.5 mL every 4-6 hours, not to exceed 7.5 mL in 24 hours
6-12 years: 2.5-5 mL every 4-6 hours, not to exceed 30 mL in 24 hours
Children >12 years and Adults: 5 mL every 4-6 hours, not to exceed 30 mL in 24 hours

Dosage Forms

Syrup: Promethazine 6.25 mg and phenylephrine 5 mg per 5 mL

promethazine hydrochloride *see* promethazine *on page 823*

promethazine, phenylephrine, and codeine

(proe METH a zeen, fen il EF rin, & KOE deen)

Synonyms codeine, phenylephrine, and promethazine; phenylephrine, promethazine, and codeine

Therapeutic Category Antihistamine/Decongestant/Antitussive

Controlled Substance C-V

Use Temporary relief of coughs and upper respiratory symptoms including nasal congestion associated with allergy or the common cold

Usual Dosage Oral:

Children:

<6 years: **Note:** Use of this combination is contraindicated in children <6 years of age

6-11 years: 2.5-5 mL every 4-6 hours (maximum: 30 mL/24 hours)

Children ≥12 years and Adults: 5 mL every 4-6 hours (maximum: 30 mL/24 hours)

Dosage Forms

Syrup: Promethazine 6.25 mg, phenylephrine 5 mg, and codeine 10 mg per 5 mL

Promethegan™ [US] *see* promethazine *on page 823*

Promethist® With Codeine *(Discontinued)* *see* promethazine, phenylephrine, and codeine *on page 825*

Prometh® VC Plain Liquid *(Discontinued)* *see* promethazine and phenylephrine *on page 824*

Prometh® VC With Codeine *(Discontinued)* *see* promethazine, phenylephrine, and codeine *on page 825*

Prometrium® [US/Can] *see* progesterone *on page 822*

PRO-Mirtazapine [Can] *see* mirtazapine *on page 661*

Promit® *(Discontinued)*

Pro-Naproxen EC [Can] *see* naproxen *on page 681*

Pronestyl® *(Discontinued)* *see* procainamide *on page 819*

Pronto® Complete Lice Removal System [US-OTC] *see* pyrethrins and piperonyl butoxide *on page 839*

Pronto® Lice Control [Can] *see* pyrethrins and piperonyl butoxide *on page 839*

Pronto® Plus Hair and Scalp Masque *(Discontinued)* *see* pyrethrins and piperonyl butoxide *on page 839*

Pronto® Plus Lice Egg Remover Kit [US-OTC] *see* benzalkonium chloride *on page 129*

Pronto® Plus Lice Killing Mousse Plus Vitamin E [US-OTC] *see* pyrethrins and piperonyl butoxide *on page 839*

Pronto® Plus Lice Killing Mousse Shampoo Plus Natural Extracts and Oils [US-OTC] *see* pyrethrins and piperonyl butoxide *on page 839*

Pronto® Plus Warm Oil Treatment and Conditioner [US-OTC] *see* pyrethrins and piperonyl butoxide *on page 839*

Propac™ [US-OTC] *see* nutritional formula, enteral/oral *on page 715*

Propacet® *(Discontinued)* *see* propoxyphene and acetaminophen *on page 828*

Propaderm® [Can] *see* beclomethasone *on page 125*

propafenone (pro PAF en one)

Synonyms propafenone hydrochloride

U.S./Canadian Brand Names Apo-Propafenone® [Can]; PMS-Propafenone [Can]; Rythmol® Gen-Propafenone [Can]; Rythmol® SR [US]; Rythmol® [US]

Therapeutic Category Antiarrhythmic Agent, Class I-C

Use Treatment of life-threatening ventricular arrhythmias

Rythmol® SR: Maintenance of normal sinus rhythm in patients with symptomatic atrial fibrillation

Usual Dosage Oral: Adults: **Note:** Patients who exhibit significant widening of QRS complex or second- or third-degree AV block may need dose reduction.

Ventricular arrhythmias:

Immediate release tablet: Initial: 150 mg every 8 hours, increase at 3- to 4-day intervals up to 300 mg every 8 hours.

Extended release capsule: Initial: 225 mg every 12 hours; dosage increase may be made at a minimum of 5-day intervals; may increase to 325 mg every 12 hours; if further increase is necessary, may increase to 425 mg every 12 hours

Dosage Forms

Capsule, extended release:
Rythmol® SR: 225 mg, 325 mg, 425 mg

Tablet: 150 mg, 225 mg, 300 mg
Rythmol®: 150 mg, 225 mg, 300 mg

propafenone hydrochloride *see* propafenone *on page 825*

Propagest® ***(Discontinued)***

propantheline (proe PAN the leen)

Synonyms propantheline bromide

Therapeutic Category Anticholinergic Agent

Use Adjunctive treatment of peptic ulcer, irritable bowel syndrome, pancreatitis, ureteral and urinary bladder spasm; reduce duodenal motility during diagnostic radiologic procedures

Usual Dosage Oral:
Antisecretory:
Children: 1-2 mg/kg/day in 3-4 divided doses
Adults: 15 mg 3 times/day before meals or food and 30 mg at bedtime
Antispasmodic:
Children: 2-3 mg/kg/day in divided doses every 4-6 hours and at bedtime
Adults: 15 mg 3 times/day before meals or food and 30 mg at bedtime

Dosage Forms

Tablet: 15 mg

propantheline bromide *see* propantheline *on page 826*

proparacaine (proe PAR a kane)

Sound-Alike/Look-Alike Issues
proparacaine may be confused with propoxyphene

Synonyms proparacaine hydrochloride; proxymetacaine

U.S./Canadian Brand Names Alcaine® [US/Can]; Diocaine® [Can]; Parcaine™ [US]

Therapeutic Category Local Anesthetic

Use Anesthesia for tonometry, gonioscopy; suture removal from cornea; removal of corneal foreign body; cataract extraction, glaucoma surgery; short operative procedure involving the cornea and conjunctiva

Usual Dosage Children and Adults:
Ophthalmic surgery: Instill 1 drop of 0.5% solution in eye every 5-10 minutes for 5-7 doses
Tonometry, gonioscopy, suture removal: Instill 1-2 drops of 0.5% solution in eye just prior to procedure

Dosage Forms

Solution, ophthalmic: 0.5% (15 mL)
Alcaine®, Parcaine™: 0.5% (15 mL)

proparacaine and fluorescein (proe PAR a kane & FLURE e seen)

Synonyms fluorescein and proparacaine

U.S./Canadian Brand Names Flucaine® [US]

Therapeutic Category Diagnostic Agent; Local Anesthetic

Use Anesthesia for tonometry, gonioscopy; suture removal from cornea; removal of corneal foreign body; cataract extraction, glaucoma surgery

Usual Dosage
Ophthalmic surgery: Children and Adults: Instill 1 drop in each eye every 5-10 minutes for 5-7 doses
Tonometry, gonioscopy, suture removal: Adults: Instill 1-2 drops in each eye just prior to procedure

Dosage Forms

Solution, ophthalmic: Proparacaine 0.5% and fluorescein 0.25% (5 mL)
Flucaine®: Proparacaine 0.5% and fluorescein 0.25% (5 mL)

proparacaine hydrochloride *see* proparacaine *on page 826*
Propecia® [US/Can] *see* finasteride *on page 420*
Propine® [Can] *see* dipivefrin *on page 323*

Propine® *(Discontinued)* *see* dipivefrin *on page 323*
Pro-Piroxicam [Can] *see* piroxicam *on page 788*
Proplex® T *(Discontinued)* *see* factor IX complex (human) *on page 404*

propofol (PROE po fole)

Sound-Alike/Look-Alike Issues
propofol may be confused with fospropofol
Diprivan® may be confused with Diflucan®, Ditropan®

U.S./Canadian Brand Names Diprivan® [US/Can]

Therapeutic Category General Anesthetic

Use Induction of anesthesia in patients ≥3 years of age; maintenance of anesthesia in patients >2 months of age; in adults, for monitored anesthesia care sedation during procedures; sedation in intubated, mechanically-ventilated ICU patients

Usual Dosage Dosage must be individualized based on total body weight and titrated to the desired clinical effect; wait at least 3-5 minutes between dosage adjustments to clinically assess drug effects; smaller doses are required when used with narcotics; the following are general dosing guidelines:

General anesthesia:
Induction: I.V.:
Children (healthy) 3-16 years, ASA-PS 1 or 2: 2.5-3.5 mg/kg over 20-30 seconds; use a lower dose for children ASA-PS 3 or 4
Adults (healthy), ASA-PS 1 or 2, <55 years: 2-2.5 mg/kg (~40 mg every 10 seconds until onset of induction)
Maintenance: I.V. infusion:
Children (healthy) 2 months to 16 years, ASA-PS 1 or 2: Initial: 200-300 mcg/kg/minute; after 30 minutes, if clinical signs of light anesthesia are absent, decrease the infusion rate; usual infusion rate: 125-150 mcg/kg/minute (range: 125-300 mcg/kg/minute); children ≤5 years may require larger infusion rates compared to older children
Adults (healthy), ASA-PS 1 or 2, <55 years: Initial: 100-200 mcg/kg/minute for 10-15 minutes; decrease by 30% to 50% during first 30 minutes of maintenance; usual infusion rate: 50-100 mcg/kg/minute to optimize recovery time
Maintenance: I.V. intermittent bolus: Adults (healthy), ASA-PS 1 or 2, <55 years: 25-50 mg increments as needed

Monitored anesthesia care sedation:
Initiation: Adults (healthy), ASA-PS 1 or 2, <55 years: Slow I.V. infusion: 100-150 mcg/kg/minute for 3-5 minutes **or** slow injection: 0.5 mg/kg over 3-5 minutes
Maintenance: Adults (healthy), ASA-PS 1 or 2, <55 years: I.V. infusion using variable rates (preferred over intermittent boluses): 25-75 mcg/kg/minute **or** incremental bolus doses: 10 mg or 20 mg

ICU sedation in intubated mechanically-ventilated patients: Avoid rapid bolus injection; individualize dose and titrate to response. Continuous infusion: Initial: 5 mcg/kg/minute; increase by 5-10 mcg/kg/minute every 5-10 minutes until desired sedation level is achieved; usual maintenance (Jacobi, 2002): 5-80 mcg/kg/minute; use 80% of healthy adult dose in elderly, debilitated, and ASA-PS 3 or 4 patients; reduce dose after adequate sedation established and adjust to response (eg, evaluate frequently to use minimum dose for sedation). Daily interruption with retitration is recommended to minimize prolonged sedative effects.

Dosage Forms
Injection, emulsion: 10 mg/mL (20 mL, 50 mL, 100 mL)
Diprivan®: 10 mg/mL (20 mL, 50 mL, 100 mL)

Propoxacet-N® *(Discontinued)* *see* propoxyphene and acetaminophen *on page 828*

propoxyphene (proe POKS i feen)

Sound-Alike/Look-Alike Issues
propoxyphene may be confused with proparacaine
Darvon® may be confused with Devrom®, Diovan®
Darvon-N® may be confused with Darvocet-N®

Synonyms dextropropoxyphene; propoxyphene hydrochloride; propoxyphene napsylate

U.S./Canadian Brand Names 642® Tablet [Can]; Darvon-N® [US/Can]; Darvon® [US]

Therapeutic Category Analgesic, Narcotic

Controlled Substance C-IV

Use Management of mild-to-moderate pain

Usual Dosage Oral: Adults:
Hydrochloride: 65 mg every 3-4 hours as needed for pain; maximum: 390 mg/day
Napsylate: 100 mg every 4 hours as needed for pain; maximum: 600 mg/day

Dosage Forms
Capsule: 65 mg
Darvon®: 65 mg
Tablet:
Darvon-N®: 100 mg

propoxyphene and acetaminophen (proe POKS i feen & a seet a MIN oh fen)

Sound-Alike/Look-Alike Issues
Darvocet® may be confused with Percocet®
Darvocet-N® may be confused with Darvon-N®

Synonyms acetaminophen and propoxyphene; propoxyphene hydrochloride and acetaminophen; propoxyphene napsylate and acetaminophen

U.S./Canadian Brand Names Balacet 325™ [US]; Darvocet A500® [US]; Darvocet-N® 100 [US/Can]; Darvocet-N® 50 [US/Can]

Therapeutic Category Analgesic, Narcotic

Controlled Substance C-IV

Use Management of mild-to-moderate pain

Usual Dosage Oral: Adults:
Darvocet A500®, Darvocet-N® 100: 1 tablet every 4 hours as needed; maximum: 600 mg propoxyphene napsylate/day
Darvocet-N® 50: 1-2 tablets every 4 hours as needed; maximum: 600 mg propoxyphene napsylate/day
Propoxyphene hydrochloride 65 mg and acetaminophen 650 mg: 1 tablet every 4 hours as needed; maximum: 390 mg/day propoxyphene hydrochloride, 4 g/day acetaminophen)
Note: Formulations contain significant amounts of acetaminophen; intake should be limited to <4 g acetaminophen/day (less in patients with hepatic impairment/ethanol abuse)

Dosage Forms
Tablet:
65/650: Propoxyphene 65 mg and acetaminophen 650 mg; 100/500: Propoxyphene 100 mg and acetaminophen 500 mg; 100/650: Propoxyphene 100 mg and acetaminophen 650 mg
Balacet 325™: Propoxyphene 100 mg and acetaminophen 325 mg
Darvocet A500®: Propoxyphene 100 mg and acetaminophen 500 mg
Darvocet-N® 50: Propoxyphene 50 mg and acetaminophen 325 mg
Darvocet-N® 100: Propoxyphene 100 mg and acetaminophen 650 mg

propoxyphene, aspirin, and caffeine *(Discontinued)*

propoxyphene hydrochloride *see* propoxyphene *on page 827*

propoxyphene hydrochloride and acetaminophen *see* propoxyphene and acetaminophen *on page 828*

propoxyphene napsylate *see* propoxyphene *on page 827*

propoxyphene napsylate and acetaminophen *see* propoxyphene and acetaminophen *on page 828*

propranolol (proe PRAN oh lole)

Sound-Alike/Look-Alike Issues
propranolol may be confused with Pravachol®, Propulsid®
Inderal® may be confused with Adderall®, Enduron®, Enduronyl®, Imdur®, Imuran®, Inderide®, Isordil®, Toradol®
Inderal® 40 may be confused with Enduronyl® Forte

Synonyms propranolol hydrochloride

U.S./Canadian Brand Names Apo-Propranolol® [Can]; Dom-Propranolol [Can]; Inderal® LA [US/Can]; Inderal® [Can]; InnoPran XL™ [US]; Novo-Pranol [Can]; Nu-Propranolol [Can]; PMS-Propranolol [Can]; Propranolol Hydrochloride Injection, USP [Can]

Therapeutic Category Antiarrhythmic Agent, Class II; Beta-Adrenergic Blocker

Use Management of hypertension; angina pectoris; pheochromocytoma; essential tremor; supraventricular arrhythmias (such as atrial fibrillation and flutter, AV nodal reentrant tachycardias), ventricular tachycardias (catecholamine-induced arrhythmias, digoxin toxicity); prevention of myocardial infarction; migraine headache prophylaxis; symptomatic treatment of hypertrophic subaortic stenosis (hypertrophic obstructive cardiomyopathy)

Usual Dosage

Essential tremor: Oral: Adults: 40 mg twice daily initially; maintenance doses: Usually 120-320 mg/day

Hypertension: Oral: Adults: Initial: 40 mg twice daily; increase dosage every 3-7 days; usual dose: 120-240 mg divided in 2-3 doses/day; maximum daily dose: 640 mg; usual dosage range (JNC 7): 40-160 mg/day in 2 divided doses

Extended release formulations:

Inderal® LA: Initial: 80 mg once daily; usual maintenance: 120-160 mg once daily; maximum daily dose: 640 mg; usual dosage range (JNC 7): 60-180 mg/day once daily

InnoPran XL™: Initial: 80 mg once daily at bedtime; if initial response is inadequate, may be increased at 2-3 week intervals to a maximum dose of 120 mg

Hypertrophic subaortic stenosis: Oral: Adults: 20-40 mg 3-4 times/day

Inderal® LA: 80-160 mg once daily

Migraine headache prophylaxis: Oral: Adults: Initial: 80 mg/day divided every 6-8 hours; increase by 20-40 mg/dose every 3-4 weeks to a maximum of 160-240 mg/day given in divided doses every 6-8 hours; if satisfactory response not achieved within 6 weeks of starting therapy, drug should be withdrawn gradually over several weeks

Inderal® LA: Initial: 80 mg once daily; effective dose range: 160-240 mg once daily

Post-MI mortality reduction: Oral: Adults: Initial: 40 mg 3 times/day; usual dosage range: 180-240 mg/day in 3-4 divided doses

Pheochromocytoma: Oral: Adults: 30-60 mg/day in divided doses

Stable angina: Oral: Adults: 80-320 mg/day in doses divided 2-4 times/day

Inderal® LA: Initial: 80 mg once daily; maximum dose: 320 mg once daily

Tachyarrhythmias:

Oral: Adults: 10-30 mg/dose every 6-8 hours

I.V.: Adults: 1-3 mg/dose slow IVP; repeat every 2-5 minutes up to a total of 5 mg; titrate initial dose to desired response

or

0.1 mg/kg divided into 3 equal doses given at 2-3 minute intervals. May repeat total dose in 2 minutes if necessary

Note: Once response achieved or maximum dose administered, additional doses should not be given for at least 4 hours.

Dosage Forms

Capsule, extended release: 60 mg, 80 mg, 120 mg, 160 mg

InnoPran XL®: 80 mg, 120 mg

Capsule, sustained release:

Inderal® LA: 60 mg, 80 mg, 120 mg, 160 mg

Injection, solution: 1 mg/mL (1 mL)

Solution, oral: 4 mg/mL, 8 mg/mL

Tablet: 10 mg, 20 mg, 40 mg, 60 mg, 80 mg

propranolol and hydrochlorothiazide (proe PRAN oh lole & hye droe klor oh THYE a zide)

Sound-Alike/Look-Alike Issues

Inderide® may be confused with Inderal®

Synonyms hydrochlorothiazide and propranolol

Therapeutic Category Antihypertensive Agent, Combination

Use Management of hypertension

Usual Dosage Oral: Adults: Hypertension: Dose is individualized; typical dosages of **hydrochlorothiazide**: 12.5-50 mg/day; initial dose of **propranolol**: 80 mg/day

Daily dose of tablet form should be divided into 2 daily doses; may be used to maximum dosage of up to 160 mg of propranolol; higher dosages would result in higher than optimal thiazide dosages.

Dosage Forms

Tablet: Propranolol 40 mg and hydrochlorothiazide 25 mg; propranolol 80 mg and hydrochlorothiazide 25 mg

propranolol hydrochloride *see* propranolol *on page* 828

Propranolol Hydrochloride Injection, USP [Can] *see* propranolol *on page* 828

Proprinal [US-OTC] *see* ibuprofen *on page* 515

Proprinal® Cold and Sinus [US-OTC] *see* pseudoephedrine and ibuprofen *on page* 835

Propulsid® [US] *see* cisapride *on page* 232

propylene glycol diacetate, acetic acid, and hydrocortisone *see* acetic acid, propylene glycol diacetate, and hydrocortisone *on page* 30

propylhexedrine (proe pil HEKS e dreen)

U.S./Canadian Brand Names Benzedrex® [US-OTC]

Therapeutic Category Adrenergic Agonist Agent

Use Topical nasal decongestant

Usual Dosage Nasal: Children 6-12 years and Adults: Two inhalations in each nostril, not more frequently than every 2 hours

Dosage Forms

Inhaler, nasal:

Benzedrex® [OTC]: 0.4-0.5 mg/inhalation (1s)

2-propylpentanoic acid *see* valproic acid and derivatives *on page* 1002

propylthiouracil (proe pil thye oh YOOR a sil)

Sound-Alike/Look-Alike Issues

propylthiouracil may be confused with Purinethol®

PTU is an error-prone abbreviation (mistaken as mercaptopurine [Purinethol®; 6-MP])

U.S./Canadian Brand Names Propyl-Thyracil® [Can]

Therapeutic Category Antithyroid Agent

Use Palliative treatment of hyperthyroidism as an adjunct to ameliorate hyperthyroidism in preparation for surgical treatment or radioactive iodine therapy; management of thyrotoxic crisis

Usual Dosage Oral: Administer in 3 equally divided doses at approximately 8-hour intervals. Adjust dosage to maintain T_3, T_4, and TSH levels in normal range; elevated T_3 may be sole indicator of inadequate treatment. Elevated TSH indicates excessive antithyroid treatment.

Children: Initial: 5-7 mg/kg/day **or** 150-200 mg/m^2/day in divided doses every 8 hours

or

6-10 years: 50-150 mg/day

>10 years: 150-300 mg/day

Maintenance: Determined by patient response **or** 1/3 to 2/3 of the initial dose in divided doses every 8-12 hours. This usually begins after 2 months on an effective initial dose.

Adults: Initial: 300-400 mg/day in divided doses every 6-8 hours. In patients with severe hyperthyroidism, very large goiters, or both, the initial dosage is usually 400 mg/day; an occasional patient will require 600-900 mg/day; maintenance: 100-150 mg/day in divided doses every 8-12 hours

Thyrotoxic crisis (recommendations vary widely and have not been evaluated in comparative trials): Dosages of 200-300 mg every 4-6 hours have been recommended for short-term initial therapy (until initial response), followed by gradual reduction to a maintenance dosage (100-150 mg/day in divided doses).

Dosage Forms

Tablet: 50 mg

Propyl-Thyracil® [Can] *see* propylthiouracil *on page* 830

2-propylvaleric acid *see* valproic acid and derivatives *on page* 1002

ProQuad® [US] *see* measles, mumps, rubella, and varicella virus vaccine *on page* 616

PRO-Quetiapine [Can] *see* quetiapine *on page* 844

Proquin® XR [US] *see* ciprofloxacin *on page* 229

PRO-Risperidone [Can] *see* risperidone *on page* 870

Proscar® [US/Can] *see* finasteride *on page* 420

Prosed®/DS [US] *see* methenamine, phenyl salicylate, methylene blue, benzoic acid, and hyoscyamine *on page* 637

Prosol [US] *see* amino acid injection *on page* 62

ProSom® *(Discontinued)* *see* estazolam *on page* 373

PRO-Sotalol [Can] *see* sotalol *on page* 919

prostacyclin *see* epoprostenol *on page* 363

prostacyclin PGI_2 *see* iloprost *on page* 519

prostaglandin E_1 *see* alprostadil *on page* 51

prostaglandin E_2 *see* dinoprostone *on page* 314

prostaglandin F_2 *see* carboprost tromethamine *on page 186*
ProStep® Patch *(Discontinued)* *see* nicotine *on page 695*
Prostigmin® [US/Can] *see* neostigmine *on page 689*
Prostin E_2® [US/Can] *see* dinoprostone *on page 314*
Prostin F_2 Alpha® *(Discontinued)*
Prostin® VR [Can] *see* alprostadil *on page 51*
Prostin VR Pediatric® [US] *see* alprostadil *on page 51*

protamine sulfate (PROE ta meen SUL fate)

Sound-Alike/Look-Alike Issues
protamine may be confused with ProAmatine®, Protonix®, Protopam®, Protropin®

Therapeutic Category Antidote

Use Treatment of heparin overdosage; neutralize heparin during surgery or dialysis procedures

Usual Dosage
Heparin neutralization: I.V.: Protamine dosage is determined by the dosage of heparin; 1 mg of protamine neutralizes 90 USP units of heparin (lung) and 115 USP units of heparin (intestinal); maximum dose: 50 mg

Heparin overdosage, following intravenous administration: I.V.: Since blood heparin concentrations decrease rapidly **after** administration, adjust the protamine dosage depending upon the duration of time since heparin administration.

Note: Excessive protamine doses may worsen bleeding potential.

Dosage Forms
Injection, solution [preservative free]: 10 mg/mL (5 mL, 25 mL)

Protection Plus® [US-OTC] *see* alcohol (ethyl) *on page 42*
protein C *see* protein C concentrate (human) *on page 831*
protein C (activated), human, recombinant *see* drotrecogin alfa *on page 340*
protein-bound paclitaxel *see* paclitaxel (protein bound) *on page 743*

protein C concentrate (human) (PROE teen cee KON suhn trate HYU man)

Sound-Alike/Look-Alike Issues
protein C concentrate (human) may be confused with activated protein C (human, recombinant) which refers to drotrecogin alfa
Ceprotin may be confused with aprotinin, Cipro®

Synonyms protein C

U.S./Canadian Brand Names Ceprotin [US]

Therapeutic Category Anticoagulant

Use Replacement therapy for severe congenital protein C deficiency for the prevention and/or treatment of venous thromboembolism and purpura fulminans

Usual Dosage Patient variables (including age, clinical condition, and plasma levels of protein C) will influence dosing and duration of therapy. Individualize dosing based on protein C activity and patient pharmacokinetic profile. Dosing is dependent on the severity of protein C deficiency, age of patient, clinical condition, and patient's level of protein C. The frequency, duration, and dose should be individualized.

I.V.: Children and Adults: Severe congenital protein C deficiency:
- Acute episode/short-term prophylaxis: Initial dose: 100-120 int. units/kg (for determination of recovery and half-life)
  - Subsequent 3 doses: 60-80 int. units/kg every 6 hours (adjust to maintain peak protein C activity of 100%)
  - Maintenance dose: 45-60 int. units/kg every 6 or 12 hours (adjust to maintain recommended maintenance trough protein C activity levels >25%)
- Long-term prophylaxis: Maintenance dose: 45-60 int. units/kg every 12 hours (recommended maintenance trough protein C activity levels >25%)

Note: Maintain target peak protein C activity of 100% during acute episodes and short-term prophylaxis. Maintain trough levels of protein C activity >25%. Higher peak levels of protein C may be necessary in prophylactic therapy of patients at increased risk for thrombosis (eg, infection, trauma, surgical intervention).

Dosage Forms

Injection, powder for reconstitution:

Ceprotin: ~500 int. units, ~1000 int. units

Protenate® ***(Discontinued)*** *see* plasma protein fraction *on page 789*

Prothazine-DC® ***(Discontinued)*** *see* promethazine and codeine *on page 824*

prothrombin complex concentrate *see* prothrombin complex (human) [(factors II, VII, IX, X), protein C, and protein S] *(Canada only) on page 832*

prothrombin complex (human) [(factors II, VII, IX, X), protein C, and protein S] *(Canada only)*

(PRO throm bin KOM pleks HYU man FAK ters too SEV en nyne ten PROE teen cee & PROE teen ess)

Synonyms prothrombin complex concentrate

U.S./Canadian Brand Names Octaplex® [Can]

Therapeutic Category Hemostatic Agent

Use Prophylaxis (perioperative) and treatment of bleeding due to acquired deficiency (eg, overdose of vitamin K antagonist) of one or more of the prothrombin complex coagulation factors II, VII, IX, and X, when rapid correction of factor deficiency is necessary

Usual Dosage Dosing should be individualized based on severity of disorder, extent and location of bleeding, and clinical status of patient. Maximum dose not to exceed 120 mL.

I.V. Adolescents ≥17 years and Adults: Approximate doses required for normalization of INR (≤1.2 within 1 hour):

Initial INR: 2-2.5: Administer 0.9-1.3 mL/kg

2.5-3: Administer 1.3-1.6 mL/kg

3-3.5: Administer 1.6-1.9 mL/kg

>3.5: Administer >1.9 mL/kg

With the correction of vitamin K antagonist-induced impairment of hemostasis in patients who have been treated concomitantly with an appropriate vitamin K dose, repeat dosing with PCC is usually not necessary.

Dosage Forms

Injection, powder for reconstitution:

Octaplex®: Human coagulation factor II: 11-38 int. units/mL; factor VII: 9-24 int. units/mL; factor IX: 20-31 int. units/mL; factor X: 18-30 int. units/mL: protein C: 7-31 int. units/mL; protein S: 7-32 int. units/mL (20 mL)

Protilase® ***(Discontinued)*** *see* pancrelipase *on page 746*

Protonix® [US/Can] *see* pantoprazole *on page 748*

Protopam® [US/Can] *see* pralidoxime *on page 808*

Protopic® [US/Can] *see* tacrolimus *on page 935*

PRO-Topiramate [Can] *see* topiramate *on page 969*

Protostat® Oral ***(Discontinued)*** *see* metronidazole *on page 651*

protriptyline (proe TRIP ti leen)

Sound-Alike/Look-Alike Issues

Vivactil® may be confused with Vyvanse™

Synonyms protriptyline hydrochloride

U.S./Canadian Brand Names Vivactil® [US]

Therapeutic Category Antidepressant, Tricyclic (Secondary Amine)

Use Treatment of depression

Usual Dosage Oral:

Adolescents: 15-20 mg/day

Adults: 15-60 mg/day in 3-4 divided doses

Dosage Forms

Tablet: 5 mg, 10 mg

Vivactil®: 5 mg, 10 mg

protriptyline hydrochloride *see* protriptyline *on page 832*

Protuss®-DM ***(Discontinued)*** *see* guaifenesin, pseudoephedrine, and dextromethorphan *on page 479*

Proventil® ***(Discontinued)*** *see* albuterol *on page 41*

Proventil® HFA [US] *see* albuterol *on page 41*
Proventil® Inhaler *(Discontinued)* *see* albuterol *on page 41*
Proventil® Solution *(Discontinued)* *see* albuterol *on page 41*
Proventil® Tablet *(Discontinued)* *see* albuterol *on page 41*
Provera® [US/Can] *see* medroxyprogesterone *on page 620*
Provera-Pak [Can] *see* medroxyprogesterone *on page 620*
PRO-Verapamil SR [Can] *see* verapamil *on page 1010*
Provigil® [US] *see* modafinil *on page 664*
Proviodine [Can] *see* povidone-iodine *on page 807*
Provisc® [US] *see* hyaluronate and derivatives *on page 496*
Provocholine® [US/Can] *see* methacholine *on page 634*
proxymetacaine *see* proparacaine *on page 826*
Prozac® [US/Can] *see* fluoxetine *on page 432*
Prozac® Weekly™ [US] *see* fluoxetine *on page 432*
PRP-OMP *see Haemophilus* B conjugate vaccine *on page 483*
PRP-T *see Haemophilus* B conjugate vaccine *on page 483*
Prudoxin™ [US] *see* doxepin *on page 334*
prussian blue *see* ferric hexacyanoferrate *on page 413*
prymaccone *see* primaquine *on page 817*
P&S® [US-OTC] *see* salicylic acid *on page 884*
23PS *see* pneumococcal polysaccharide vaccine (polyvalent) *on page 794*
PS-341 *see* bortezomib *on page 146*
Pseudacarb™ [US] *see* carbetapentane and pseudoephedrine *on page 182*

pseudoephedrine (soo doe e FED rin)

Sound-Alike/Look-Alike Issues
Dimetapp® may be confused with Dermatop®, Dimetabs®, Dimetane®
Sudafed® may be confused with sotalol, Sudafed PE™, Sufenta®

Synonyms *d*-isoephedrine hydrochloride; pseudoephedrine hydrochloride; pseudoephedrine sulfate

U.S./Canadian Brand Names Balminil Decongestant [Can]; Benylin® D for Infants [Can]; Contac® Cold 12 Hour Relief Non Drowsy [Can]; Drixoral® ND [Can]; Eltor® [Can]; Genaphed® [US-OTC]; Kidkare Decongestant [US-OTC]; Oranyl [US-OTC]; PMS-Pseudoephedrine [Can]; Pseudofrin [Can]; Robidrine® [Can]; Silfedrine Children's [US-OTC]; Sudafed® 12 Hour [US-OTC]; Sudafed® 24 Hour [US-OTC]; Sudafed® Children's [US-OTC]; Sudafed® Decongestant [Can]; Sudafed® Maximum Strength Nasal Decongestant [US-OTC]; Sudo-Tab® [US-OTC]; SudoGest Children's [US-OTC]; SudoGest [US-OTC]

Therapeutic Category Adrenergic Agonist Agent

Use Temporary symptomatic relief of nasal congestion due to common cold, upper respiratory allergies, and sinusitis; also promotes nasal or sinus drainage

Usual Dosage Oral:
Hydrochloride salt: General dosing guidelines:
Children:
<2 years: 4 mg/kg/day in divided doses every 6 hours
2-5 years: 15 mg every 4-6 hours; maximum: 60 mg/24 hours
6-12 years: 30 mg every 4-6 hours; maximum: 120 mg/24 hours
Adults: 30-60 mg every 4-6 hours, sustained release: 120 mg every 12 hours; maximum: 240 mg/24 hours
Tannate salt: Nasofed™ oral suspension:
Children 2-5 years: 1.25-2.5 mL (12.5-25 mg) every 12 hours
Children 6-11 years: 2.5-5 mL (25-50 mg) every 12 hours
Children ≥12 years and Adults: 5-10 mL (50-100 mg) every 12 hours

Dosage Forms
Caplet, extended release, oral:
Sudafed® 12 Hour [OTC]: 120 mg
Liquid, oral: 30 mg/5 mL
Silfedrine Children's [OTC], Sudafed® Children's [OTC]: 15 mg/5 mL
Liquid, oral [drops]:
Kidkare Decongestant [OTC]: 7.5 mg/0.8 mL

Syrup, oral: 30 mg/5 mL
SudoGest Children's [OTC]: 15 mg/5 mL (118 mL)
Tablet, oral: 30 mg, 60 mg
Genaphed® [OTC], Oranyl [OTC], Sudafed® [OTC], Sudo-Tab® [OTC]: 30 mg
SudoGest [OTC]: 30 mg, 60 mg
Tablet, chewable, oral:
Sudafed® Children's [OTC]: 15 mg
Tablet, extended release, oral:
Sudafed® 24 Hour [OTC]: 240 mg

pseudoephedrine, acetaminophen, and chlorpheniramine *see* acetaminophen, chlorpheniramine, and pseudoephedrine *on page 26*

pseudoephedrine and acetaminophen *see* acetaminophen and pseudoephedrine *on page 24*

pseudoephedrine and brompheniramine *see* brompheniramine and pseudoephedrine *on page 150*

pseudoephedrine and carbetapentane *see* carbetapentane and pseudoephedrine *on page 182*

pseudoephedrine and chlorpheniramine *see* chlorpheniramine and pseudoephedrine *on page 215*

pseudoephedrine and codeine (soo doe e FED rin & KOE deen)

Synonyms codeine and pseudoephedrine; codeine phosphate and pseudoephedrine hydrochloride; pseudoephedrine hydrochloride and codeine phosphate

U.S./Canadian Brand Names Notuss®-DC [US]

Therapeutic Category Antitussive/Decongestant

Controlled Substance Capsule: C-III; Liquid: C-V

Use Temporary symptomatic relief of congestion and cough due to upper respiratory infections including common cold, bronchitis, sinusitis, and influenza

Usual Dosage Oral: Relief of congestion and cough:
Children 6-11 years: 2.5-5 mL every 4-6 hours as needed (maximum: 20 mL/24 hours)
Children ≥12 years and Adults: One capsule every 6 hours as needed (maximum: 4 capsules/24 hours) **or** 5-10 mL every 4-6 hours as needed (maximum: 40 mL/24 hours)

Dosage Forms
Liquid, oral:
Notuss®-DC: Pseudoephedrine 30 mg and codeine 10 mg per 5 mL

pseudoephedrine and desloratadine *see* desloratadine and pseudoephedrine *on page 284*

pseudoephedrine and dexbrompheniramine *see* dexbrompheniramine and pseudoephedrine *on page 289*

pseudoephedrine and dextromethorphan (soo doe e FED rin & deks troe meth OR fan)

Synonyms dextromethorphan and pseudoephedrine

U.S./Canadian Brand Names Balminil DM D [Can]; Benylin® DM-D [Can]; Koffex DM-D [Can]; Novahistex® DM Decongestant [Can]; Novahistine® DM Decongestant [Can]; Pedia Relief Cough and Cold [US-OTC]; Pedia Relief Infants [US-OTC]; Robitussin® Childrens Cough & Cold [Can]; Sudafed® Children's Cold & Cough [US-OTC]; SudoGest Children's [US-OTC]

Therapeutic Category Antitussive/Decongestant

Use Temporary symptomatic relief of nasal congestion and cough due to common cold, hay fever, upper respiratory allergies

Usual Dosage Relief of nasal congestion and cough: Oral:
General dosing guidelines base on pseudoephedrine component:
Children 2-6 years: 15 mg every 4-6 hours (maximum: 60 mg/24 hours)
Children 6-12 years: 30 mg every 4-6 hours (maximum: 120 mg/24 hours)
Children ≥12 years and Adults: 60 mg every 4-6 hours (maximum: 240 mg/24 hours)
Product-specific dosing:
Children 2-6 years (Sudafed® Children's Cold & Cough): 5 mL every 4 hours (maximum: 20 mL/24 hours)
Children 6-12 years (Sudafed® Children's Cold & Cough): 10 mL every 4 hours (maximum: 40 mL/24 hours)
Children ≥12 years and Adults (Sudafed® Children's Cold & Cough): 20 mL every 4 hours (maximum: 80 mL/24 hours)

Dosage Forms

Liquid:

Sudafed® Children's Cold & Cough [OTC]: Pseudoephedrine 15 mg and dextromethorphan 5 mg per 5 mL

Liquid, oral [drops]:

Pedia Relief Infants [OTC]: Pseudoephedrine 7.5 mg and dextromethorphan 2.5 mg per 0.8 mL

Syrup:

Pedia Relief Cough and Cold [OTC]: Pseudoephedrine 15 mg and dextromethorphan 7.5 mg per 5 mL
SudoGest Children's [OTC]: Pseudoephedrine 15 mg and dextromethorphan 5 mg per 5 mL

pseudoephedrine and fexofenadine *see* fexofenadine and pseudoephedrine *on page 417*

pseudoephedrine and guaifenesin *see* guaifenesin and pseudoephedrine *on page 477*

pseudoephedrine and ibuprofen (soo doe e FED rin & eye byoo PROE fen)

Synonyms ibuprofen and pseudoephedrine

U.S./Canadian Brand Names Advil® Cold & Sinus [US-OTC/Can]; Children's Advil® Cold [Can]; Proprinal® Cold and Sinus [US-OTC]; Sudafed® Sinus Advance [Can]

Therapeutic Category Decongestant/Analgesic

Use For temporary relief of cold, sinus, and flu symptoms (including nasal congestion, sinus pressure, headache, minor body aches and pains, and fever)

Usual Dosage OTC labeling: Oral: Children ≥12 years and Adults: Ibuprofen 200 mg and pseudoephedrine 30 mg per dose: One dose every 4-6 hours as needed; may increase to 2 doses if necessary (maximum: 6 doses/24 hours). Contact healthcare provider if symptoms have not improved within 7 days when treating cold symptoms or within 3 days when treating fever.

Dosage Forms

Caplet:

Advil® Cold & Sinus [OTC], Proprinal® Cold and Sinus [OTC]: Pseudoephedrine 30 mg and ibuprofen 200 mg

Capsule, liquid filled:

Advil® Cold & Sinus [OTC]: Pseudoephedrine 30 mg and ibuprofen 200 mg

pseudoephedrine and loratadine *see* loratadine and pseudoephedrine *on page 599*

pseudoephedrine and methscopolamine (soo doe e FED rin & meth skoe POL a meen)

Synonyms methscopolamine and pseudoephedrine; pseudoephedrine hydrochloride and methscopolamine nitrate

U.S./Canadian Brand Names AlleRx™-D [US]; Extendryl PSE [US]

Therapeutic Category Decongestant/Anticholingeric Combination

Use Relief of symptoms of allergic rhinitis, vasomotor rhinitis, sinusitis, and the common cold

Usual Dosage Oral: Children ≥12 years and Adults (Allerx™-D): One tablet every 12 hours (maximum: 2 tablets/24 hours)

Dosage Forms

Tablet: Pseudoephedrine hydrochloride 120 mg and methscopolamine nitrate 2.5 mg
Allerx™-D: Pseudoephedrine 120 mg and methscopolamine 2.5 mg

Tablet, extended release:

Extendryl PSE: Pseudoephedrine 120 mg and methscopolamine 2.5 mg

pseudoephedrine and naproxen *see* naproxen and pseudoephedrine *on page 682*

pseudoephedrine and triprolidine *see* triprolidine and pseudoephedrine *on page 989*

pseudoephedrine, chlorpheniramine, and acetaminophen *see* acetaminophen, chlorpheniramine, and pseudoephedrine *on page 26*

pseudoephedrine, chlorpheniramine, and codeine *see* chlorpheniramine, pseudoephedrine, and codeine *on page 220*

pseudoephedrine, chlorpheniramine, and dextromethorphan *see* chlorpheniramine, pseudoephedrine, and dextromethorphan *on page 220*

pseudoephedrine, chlorpheniramine, and dihydrocodeine *see* pseudoephedrine, dihydrocodeine, and chlorpheniramine *on page 836*

pseudoephedrine, chlorpheniramine, and ibuprofen *see* ibuprofen, pseudoephedrine, and chlorpheniramine *on page 517*

pseudoephedrine, codeine, and triprolidine *see* triprolidine, pseudoephedrine, and codeine *(Canada only) on page 990*

pseudoephedrine, dextromethorphan, and guaifenesin *see* guaifenesin, pseudoephedrine, and dextromethorphan *on page 479*

pseudoephedrine, dextromethorphan, doxylamine, and acetaminophen *see* acetaminophen, dextromethorphan, doxylamine, and pseudoephedrine *on page 28*

pseudoephedrine, dihydrocodeine, and chlorpheniramine

(soo doe e FED rin, dye hye droe KOE deen, & klor fen IR a meen)

Synonyms chlorpheniramine, dihydrocodeine, and pseudoephedrine; dihydrocodeine bitartrate, pseudoephedrine hydrochloride, and chlorpheniramine maleate; pseudoephedrine, chlorpheniramine, and dihydrocodeine

U.S./Canadian Brand Names Coldcough [US]; DiHydro-CP [US]

Therapeutic Category Antihistamine/Decongestant/Antitussive

Controlled Substance C-III

Use Temporary relief of cough, congestion, and sneezing due to colds, respiratory infections, or hay fever

Usual Dosage Oral:

Children:

2-6 years: 1.25-2.5 mL every 4-6 hours; do not exceed 4 doses in 24 hours

6-12 years: 2.5-5 mL every 4-6 hours; do not exceed 4 doses in 24 hours

Children >12 years and Adults: 5-10 mL every 4-6 hours; do not exceed 4 doses in 24 hours

Dosage Forms

Syrup:

Coldcough, DiHydro-CP: Pseudoephedrine 15 mg, dihydrocodeine 7.5 mg, and chlorpheniramine 2 mg per 5 mL

pseudoephedrine, guaifenesin, and codeine *see* guaifenesin, pseudoephedrine, and codeine *on page 479*

pseudoephedrine hydrochloride *see* pseudoephedrine *on page 833*

pseudoephedrine hydrochloride and acetaminophen *see* acetaminophen and pseudoephedrine *on page 24*

pseudoephedrine hydrochloride and acrivastine *see* acrivastine and pseudoephedrine *on page 32*

pseudoephedrine hydrochloride and cetirizine hydrochloride *see* cetirizine and pseudoephedrine *on page 204*

pseudoephedrine hydrochloride and codeine phosphate *see* pseudoephedrine and codeine *on page 834*

pseudoephedrine hydrochloride and methscopolamine nitrate *see* pseudoephedrine and methscopolamine *on page 835*

pseudoephedrine hydrochloride, guaifenesin, and dihydrocodeine bitartrate *see* dihydrocodeine, pseudoephedrine, and guaifenesin *on page 310*

pseudoephedrine hydrochloride, methscopolamine nitrate, and chlorpheniramine maleate *see* chlorpheniramine, pseudoephedrine, and methscopolamine *on page 221*

pseudoephedrine, hydrocodone, and chlorpheniramine *(Discontinued)*

pseudoephedrine, methscopolamine, and chlorpheniramine *see* chlorpheniramine, pseudoephedrine, and methscopolamine *on page 221*

pseudoephedrine sulfate *see* pseudoephedrine *on page 833*

pseudoephedrine tannate and dexchlorpheniramine tannate *see* dexchlorpheniramine and pseudoephedrine *on page 290*

pseudoephedrine tannate, dextromethorphan tannate, and brompheniramine tannate *see* brompheniramine, pseudoephedrine, and dextromethorphan *on page 152*

pseudoephedrine, triprolidine, and codeine *see* triprolidine, pseudoephedrine, and codeine *(Canada only) on page 990*

Pseudofrin [Can] *see* pseudoephedrine *on page 833*

Pseudo-Gest Plus® Tablet *(Discontinued)* *see* chlorpheniramine and pseudoephedrine *on page 215*

Pseudo GG TR [US] *see* guaifenesin and pseudoephedrine *on page 477*

Pseudo Max [US] *see* guaifenesin and pseudoephedrine *on page 477*

Pseudo Max DMX [US] *see* guaifenesin, pseudoephedrine, and dextromethorphan *on page 479*

pseudomonic acid A *see* mupirocin *on page 672*

Pseudovent™ 400 ***(Discontinued)*** *see* guaifenesin and pseudoephedrine *on page* *477*
Pseudovent™ ***(Discontinued)*** *see* guaifenesin and pseudoephedrine *on page* *477*
Pseudovent™ DM ***(Discontinued)*** *see* guaifenesin, pseudoephedrine, and dextromethorphan *on page* *479*
Pseudovent™-Ped ***(Discontinued)*** *see* guaifenesin and pseudoephedrine *on page* *477*
P & S™ Liquid Phenol [Can] *see* phenol *on page* *772*
Psorcon® ***(Discontinued)*** *see* diflorasone *on page* *307*
Psorcon® e™ ***(Discontinued)*** *see* diflorasone *on page* *307*
Psoriatec™ [US] *see* anthralin *on page* *80*
PsoriGel® ***(Discontinued)*** *see* coal tar *on page* *250*
Psorion® Topical ***(Discontinued)***

psyllium (SIL i yum)

Sound-Alike/Look-Alike Issues

Fiberall® may be confused with Feverall®
Hydrocil® may be confused with Hydrocet®

Synonyms plantago seed; plantain seed; psyllium husk; psyllium hydrophilic mucilloid

U.S./Canadian Brand Names Bulk-K [US-OTC]; Fiberall® [US]; Fibro-Lax [US-OTC]; Fibro-XL [US-OTC]; Genfiber™ [US-OTC]; Hydrocil® Instant [US-OTC]; Konsyl-D™ [US-OTC]; Konsyl® Easy Mix™ [US-OTC]; Konsyl® Orange [US-OTC]; Konsyl® Original [US-OTC]; Konsyl® [US-OTC]; Metamucil® Plus Calcium [US-OTC]; Metamucil® Smooth Texture [US-OTC]; Metamucil® [US-OTC/Can]; Natural Fiber Therapy Smooth Texture [US-OTC]; Natural Fiber Therapy [US-OTC]; Reguloid [US-OTC]

Therapeutic Category Laxative

Use OTC labeling: Dietary fiber supplement; treatment of occasional constipation; reduce risk of coronary heart disease (CHD)

Usual Dosage Oral: General dosing guidelines; consult specific product labeling.

Adequate intake for total fiber: Note: The definition of "fiber" varies; however, the soluble fiber in psyllium is only one type of fiber which makes up the daily recommended intake of total fiber.

Children 1-3 years: 19 g/day
Children 4-8 years: 25 g/day
Children 9-13 years: Male: 31 g/day; Female: 26 g/day
Children 14-18 years: Male: 38 g/day; Female: 26 g/day
Adults 19-50 years: Male: 38 g/day; Female: 25 g/day
Adults ≥51 years: Male: 30 g/day; Female: 21 g/day
Pregnancy: 28 g/day
Lactation: 29 g/day

Constipation:

Children 6-11 years: Psyllium: 1.25-15 g per day in divided doses
Children ≥12 years and Adults: Psyllium: 2.5-30 g per day in divided doses

Reduce risk of CHD: Children ≥12 years and Adults: Soluble fiber ≥7 g (psyllium seed husk ≥10.2 g) per day

Dosage Forms

Capsule:

Fibro XL [OTC]: 0.675 g
Genfiber™ [OTC], Konsyl® [OTC], Metamucil® [OTC], Metamucil® Plus Calcium [OTC], Reguloid [OTC]: 0.52 g

Powder:

Bulk-K [OTC], Fibro-Lax [OTC]: 4.7 g/teaspoon
Fiberall®: 0.05 g/tablespoon
Genfiber™ [OTC], Konsyl-D™ [OTC], Konsyl® Orange [OTC], Metamucil® [OTC], Metamucil® Smooth Texture [OTC], Natural Fiber Therapy Smooth Texture [OTC], Reguloid [OTC]: 3.4 g/teaspoon
Genfiber™ [OTC], Konsyl® Orange [OTC], Metamucil® [OTC], Metamucil® Smooth Texture [OTC], Natural Fiber Therapy [OTC], Reguloid [OTC]: 3.4 g/tablespoon
Hydrocil® Instant: [OTC]: 3.5 g/packet, 3.5 g/teaspoon
Konsyl-D™ [OTC], Konsyl® Orange [OTC]: 3.4 g/packet
Konsyl® Original [OTC], Konsyl® Easy Mix™ [OTC]: 6 g/packet, 6 g/teaspoon
Metamucil® Smooth Texture [OTC]: 3.3 g/teaspoon, 3.4 g/packet

Wafers:

Metamucil® [OTC]: 3.4 g/2 wafers

psyllium husk *see* psyllium *on page* *837*
psyllium hydrophilic mucilloid *see* psyllium *on page* *837*
P-Tann [US] *see* chlorpheniramine *on page* *213*
pteroylglutamic acid *see* folic acid *on page* *439*
Pulmicort® [Can] *see* budesonide *on page* *153*
Pulmicort Flexhaler™ [US] *see* budesonide *on page* *153*
Pulmicort Respules® [US] *see* budesonide *on page* *153*
Pulmicort Turbuhaler® *(Discontinued)* *see* budesonide *on page* *153*
Pulmophylline [Can] *see* theophylline *on page* *953*
Pulmozyme® [US/Can] *see* dornase alfa *on page* *332*
Puralube® Tears [US-OTC] *see* artificial tears *on page* *100*
Puregon® [Can] *see* follitropin beta *on page* *441*
Purell® [US-OTC] *see* alcohol (ethyl) *on page* *42*
Purell® 2 in 1 [US-OTC] *see* alcohol (ethyl) *on page* *42*
Purell® with Aloe [US-OTC] *see* alcohol (ethyl) *on page* *42*
purified chick embryo cell *see* rabies vaccine *on page* *848*
Purinethol® [US/Can] *see* mercaptopurine *on page* *630*
PVP-I *see* povidone-iodine *on page* *807*
Pylera™ [US] *see* bismuth, metronidazole, and tetracycline *on page* *143*

pyrantel pamoate (pi RAN tel PAM oh ate)

U.S./Canadian Brand Names Combantrin™ [Can]; Pin-X® [US-OTC]; Reese's® Pinworm Medicine [US-OTC]

Therapeutic Category Anthelmintic

Use Treatment of pinworms (*Enterobius vermicularis*) and roundworms (*Ascaris lumbricoides*)

Usual Dosage Oral: Children and Adults (purgation is not required prior to use): **Note:** Dose is expressed as pyrantel base: Roundworm, pinworm, or trichostrongyliasis: 11 mg/kg administered as a single dose; maximum dose: 1 g. (**Note:** For pinworm infection, dosage should be repeated in 2 weeks and all family members should be treated).

Dosage Forms

Caplet:

Reese's® Pinworm Medicine [OTC]: 180 mg

Suspension, oral:

Pin-X® [OTC], Reese's® Pinworm Medicine [OTC]: 144 mg/mL

Tablet:

Pin-X® [OTC]: 720.5 mg

pyrazinamide (peer a ZIN a mide)

Synonyms pyrazinoic acid amide

U.S./Canadian Brand Names Tebrazid™ [Can]

Therapeutic Category Antitubercular Agent

Use Adjunctive treatment of tuberculosis in combination with other antituberculosis agents

Usual Dosage Oral: Treatment of tuberculosis:

Note: Used as part of a multidrug regimen. Treatment regimens consist of an initial 2-month phase, followed by a continuation phase of 4 or 7 additional months; frequency of dosing may differ depending on phase of therapy.

Children:

Daily therapy: 15-30 mg/kg/day (maximum: 2 g/day)
Twice weekly directly observed therapy (DOT): 50 mg/kg/dose (maximum: 4 g/dose)

Adults (dosing is based on lean body weight):

Daily therapy: 15-30 mg/kg/day
40-55 kg: 1000 mg
56-75 kg: 1500 mg
76-90 kg: 2000 mg (maximum dose regardless of weight)
Twice weekly directly observed therapy (DOT): 50 mg/kg
40-55 kg: 2000 mg
56-75 kg: 3000 mg

76-90 kg: 4000 mg (maximum dose regardless of weight)
Three times/week DOT: 25-30 mg/kg (maximum: 2.5 g)
40-55 kg: 1500 mg
56-75 kg: 2500 mg
76-90 kg: 3000 mg (maximum dose regardless of weight)

Dosage Forms

Tablet: 500 mg

pyrazinamide, rifampin, and isoniazid *see* rifampin, isoniazid, and pyrazinamide *on page 867*

pyrazinoic acid amide *see* pyrazinamide *on page 838*

pyrethrins and piperonyl butoxide (pye RE thrins & pi PER oh nil byo TOKS ide)

Synonyms piperonyl butoxide and pyrethrins

U.S./Canadian Brand Names A-200® Lice Treatment Kit [US-OTC]; A-200® Maximum Strength [US-OTC]; Licide® [US-OTC]; Pronto® Complete Lice Removal System [US-OTC]; Pronto® Lice Control [Can]; Pronto® Plus Lice Killing Mousse Plus Vitamin E [US-OTC]; Pronto® Plus Lice Killing Mousse Shampoo Plus Natural Extracts and Oils [US-OTC]; Pronto® Plus Warm Oil Treatment and Conditioner [US-OTC]; R & C™ II [Can]; R & C™ Shampoo/Conditioner [Can]; RID® Maximum Strength [US-OTC]; RID® Mousse [Can]

Therapeutic Category Scabicides/Pediculicides

Use Treatment of *Pediculus humanus* infestations (head lice, body lice, pubic lice, and their eggs)

Usual Dosage Application of pyrethrins: Topical products:

Apply enough solution to completely wet infested area, including hair
Allow to remain on area for 10 minutes
Wash and rinse with large amounts of warm water.
Use fine-toothed comb to remove lice and eggs from hair
Shampoo hair to restore body and luster
Treatment may be repeated if necessary once in a 24-hour period
Repeat treatment in 7-10 days to kill newly hatched lice
Note: Keep out of eyes when rinsing hair; protect eyes with a wash cloth or towel

Dosage Forms

Kit:

A-200® Lice Treatment Kit [OTC]:
Shampoo: Pyrethrins 0.33% and piperonyl butoxide 4% (120 mL)
Solution: Permethrin 0.5% (180 mL)
Pronto® Complete Lice Removal System [OTC]:
Shampoo: Pyrethrins 0.33% and piperonyl butoxide 4% (60 mL)
Solution, topical: Benzalkonium chloride 0.1% (60 mL)

Oil, topical:

Pronto® Plus Warm Oil Treatment and Conditioner [OTC]: Pyrethrins 0.33% and piperonyl butoxide 4% (36 mL)

Shampoo: Pyrethrins 0.33% and piperonyl butoxide 4% (60 mL, 120 mL)

A-200® Maximum Strength [OTC]: Pyrethrins 0.33% and piperonyl butoxide 4% (60 mL, 120 mL)
Licide® [OTC], Pronto® Plus Lice Killing Mousse Shampoo Plus Vitamin E [OTC]: Pyrethrins 0.33% and piperonyl butoxide 4% (120 mL)
Pronto® Plus Lice Killing Mousse Shampoo Plus Natural Extracts and Oils [OTC]: Pyrethrins 0.33% and piperonyl butoxide 4% (60 mL)
Pronto® Plus Lice Killing Mousse Shampoo Plus Vitamin E [OTC]: Pyrethrins 0.33% and piperonyl butoxide 4% (120 mL)
RID® Maximum Strength [OTC]: Pyrethrins 0.33% and piperonyl butoxide 4% (60 mL, 120 mL, 180 mL, 240 mL)

Pyri-500 [US-OTC] *see* pyridoxine *on page 840*

2-pyridine aldoxime methochloride *see* pralidoxime *on page 808*

Pyridium® [US] *see* phenazopyridine *on page 770*

pyridostigmine (peer id oh STIG meen)

Sound-Alike/Look-Alike Issues

pyridostigmine may be confused with physostigmine
Mestinon® may be confused with Metatensin®
Regonol® may be confused with Reglan®, Renagel®

Synonyms pyridostigmine bromide

U.S./Canadian Brand Names Mestinon® Timespan® [US]; Mestinon® [US/Can]; Mestinon®-SR [Can]; Regonol® [US]

Therapeutic Category Cholinergic Agent

Use Symptomatic treatment of myasthenia gravis; antagonism of nondepolarizing neuromuscular blockers

Military use: Pretreatment for soman nerve gas exposure

Usual Dosage

Myasthenia gravis:

Oral:

Children: 7 mg/kg/24 hours divided into 5-6 doses

Adults: Highly individualized dosing ranges: 60-1500 mg/day, usually 600 mg/day divided into 5-6 doses, spaced to provide maximum relief

Sustained release formulation: Highly individualized dosing ranges: 180-540 mg once or twice daily (doses separated by at least 6 hours); **Note:** Most clinicians reserve sustained release dosage form for bedtime dose only.

I.M., slow I.V. push:

Children: 0.05-0.15 mg/kg/dose

Adults: To supplement oral dosage pre- and postoperatively during labor and postpartum, during myasthenic crisis, or when oral therapy is impractical: ~1/30th of oral dose; observe patient closely for cholinergic reactions

or

I.V. infusion: Initial: 2 mg/hour with gradual titration in increments of 0.5-1 mg/hour, up to a maximum rate of 4 mg/hour

Reversal of nondepolarizing muscle relaxants: **Note:** Atropine sulfate (0.6-1.2 mg) I.V. immediately prior to pyridostigmine to minimize side effects: I.V.:

Children: Dosing range: 0.1-0.25 mg/kg/dose*

Adults: 0.1-0.25 mg/kg/dose; 10-20 mg is usually sufficient*

*Full recovery usually occurs ≤15 minutes, but ≥30 minutes may be required

Pretreatment for soman nerve gas exposure (military use): Oral: Adults: 30 mg every 8 hours beginning several hours prior to exposure; discontinue at first sign of nerve agent exposure, then begin atropine and pralidoxime

Dosage Forms

Injection, solution:

Regonol®: 5 mg/mL (2 mL)

Syrup:

Mestinon®: 60 mg/5 mL

Tablet: 60 mg

Mestinon®: 60 mg

Tablet, sustained release:

Mestinon® Timespan®: 180 mg

pyridostigmine bromide *see* pyridostigmine *on page 839*

pyridoxine (peer i DOKS een)

Sound-Alike/Look-Alike Issues

pyridoxine may be confused with paroxetine, pralidoxime, Pyridium®

Synonyms pyridoxine hydrochloride; vitamin B_6

U.S./Canadian Brand Names Aminoxin [US-OTC]; Pyri-500 [US-OTC]

Therapeutic Category Vitamin, Water Soluble

Use Prevention and treatment of vitamin B_6 deficiency, pyridoxine-dependent seizures in infants

Usual Dosage

Recommended daily allowance (RDA):

Children:

1-3 years: 0.9 mg

4-6 years: 1.3 mg

7-10 years: 1.6 mg

Adults:

Male: 1.7-2.0 mg

Female: 1.4-1.6 mg

Pyridoxine-dependent Infants:
Oral: 2-100 mg/day
I.M., I.V., SubQ: 10-100 mg
Dietary deficiency: Oral:
Children: 5-25 mg/24 hours for 3 weeks, then 1.5-2.5 mg/day in multiple vitamin product
Adults: 10-20 mg/day for 3 weeks
Drug-induced neuritis (eg, isoniazid, hydralazine, penicillamine, cycloserine): Oral:
Children:
Treatment: 10-50 mg/24 hours
Prophylaxis: 1-2 mg/kg/24 hours
Adults:
Treatment: 100-200 mg/24 hours
Prophylaxis: 25-100 mg/24 hours

Dosage Forms

Capsule: 50 mg, 250 mg
Aminoxin [OTC]: 20 mg
Injection, solution:100 mg/mL (1 mL)
Liquid, oral: 200 mg/5 mL (120 mL)
Tablet: 25 mg, 50 mg, 100 mg, 250 mg, 500 mg
Tablet, sustained release:
Pyri-500 [OTC]: 500 mg

pyridoxine and doxylamine *see* doxylamine and pyridoxine *(Canada only) on page 338*
pyridoxine, folic acid, and cyanocobalamin *see* folic acid, cyanocobalamin, and pyridoxine *on page 440*
pyridoxine hydrochloride *see* pyridoxine *on page 840*
Pyrilafen Tannate-12™ *(Discontinued)* *see* phenylephrine and pyrilamine *on page 776*
pyrilamine, chlorpheniramine, and phenylephrine *see* chlorpheniramine, pyrilamine, and phenylephrine *on page 221*
pyrilamine maleate, dextromethorphan hydrobromide, and phenylephrine hydrochloride *see* phenylephrine, pyrilamine, and dextromethorphan *on page 778*
pyrilamine, phenylephrine, and carbetapentane *see* carbetapentane, phenylephrine, and pyrilamine *on page 183*
pyrilamine tannate and phenylephrine tannate *see* phenylephrine and pyrilamine *on page 776*
pyrilamine tannate, guaifenesin, and phenylephrine tannate *see* phenylephrine, pyrilamine, and guaifenesin *on page 779*

pyrimethamine (peer i METH a meen)

Sound-Alike/Look-Alike Issues
Daraprim® may be confused with Dantrium®, Daranide®

U.S./Canadian Brand Names Daraprim® [US/Can]

Therapeutic Category Folic Acid Antagonist (Antimalarial)

Use Prophylaxis of malaria due to susceptible strains of plasmodia; used in conjunction with quinine and sulfadiazine for the treatment of uncomplicated attacks of chloroquine-resistant *P. falciparum* malaria; used in conjunction with fast-acting schizonticide to initiate transmission control and suppression cure; synergistic combination with sulfonamide in treatment of toxoplasmosis

Usual Dosage

Malaria chemoprophylaxis (for areas where chloroquine-resistant *P. falciparum* exists): Begin prophylaxis 2 weeks before entering endemic area:
Children: 0.5 mg/kg once weekly; not to exceed 25 mg/dose
or
Children:
<4 years: 6.25 mg once weekly
4-10 years: 12.5 mg once weekly
Children >10 years and Adults: 25 mg once weekly
Dosage should be continued for all age groups for at least 6-10 weeks after leaving endemic areas
Chloroquine-resistant *P. falciparum* malaria (when used in conjunction with quinine and sulfadiazine):
Children:
<10 kg: 6.25 mg/day once daily for 3 days
10-20 kg: 12.5 mg/day once daily for 3 days
20-40 kg: 25 mg/day once daily for 3 days

Adults: 25 mg twice daily for 3 days

Toxoplasmosis:

Infants (congenital toxoplasmosis): Oral: 1 mg/kg once daily for 6 months with sulfadiazine then every other month with sulfa, alternating with spiramycin.

Children: Loading dose: 2 mg/kg/day divided into 2 equal daily doses for 1-3 days (maximum: 100 mg/day) followed by 1 mg/kg/day divided into 2 doses for 4 weeks; maximum: 25 mg/day

With sulfadiazine or trisulfapyrimidines: 2 mg/kg/day divided every 12 hours for 3 days, followed by 1 mg/kg/day once daily or divided twice daily for 4 weeks given with trisulfapyrimidines or sulfadiazine

Adults: 50-75 mg/day together with 1-4 g of a sulfonamide for 1-3 weeks depending on patient's tolerance and response, then reduce dose by 50% and continue for 4-5 weeks **or** 25-50 mg/day for 3-4 weeks

Prophylaxis for first episode of *Toxoplasma gondii*:

Children ≥1 month of age: 1 mg/kg/day once daily with dapsone, plus oral folinic acid 5 mg every 3 days

Adolescents and Adults: 50 mg once weekly with dapsone, plus oral folinic acid 25 mg once weekly

Prophylaxis to prevent recurrence of *Toxoplasma gondii*:

Children ≥1 month of age: 1 mg/kg/day once daily given with sulfadiazine or clindamycin, plus oral folinic acid 5 mg every 3 days

Adolescents and Adults: 25-50 mg once daily in combination with sulfadiazine or clindamycin, plus oral folinic acid 10-25 mg daily; atovaquone plus oral folinic acid has also been used in combination with pyrimethamine.

Dosage Forms

Tablet:

Daraprim®: 25 mg

pyrimethamine and sulfadoxine *see* sulfadoxine and pyrimethamine *on page 928*

pyrithione zinc (peer i THYE one zingk)

Sound-Alike/Look-Alike Issues

pyrithione may be confused with Pyridium®

U.S./Canadian Brand Names BetaMed [US-OTC]; Denorex® Daily Protection [US-OTC]; DermaZinc™ [US-OTC]; DHS™ Zinc [US-OTC]; Head & Shoulders® Citrus Breeze 2-in-1 [US-OTC]; Head & Shoulders® Citrus Breeze [US-OTC]; Head & Shoulders® Classic Clean 2-In-1 [US-OTC]; Head & Shoulders® Classic Clean [US-OTC]; Head & Shoulders® Dry Scalp Care 2-in-1 [US-OTC]; Head & Shoulders® Dry Scalp Care [US-OTC]; Head & Shoulders® Extra Volume [US-OTC]; Head & Shoulders® intensive solutions 2-in-1 [US-OTC]; Head & Shoulders® intensive solutions for dry/damaged hair [US-OTC]; Head & Shoulders® intensive solutions for fine/oily hair [US-OTC]; Head & Shoulders® intensive solutions for normal hair [US-OTC]; Head & Shoulders® Ocean Lift 2-in-1 [US-OTC]; Head & Shoulders® Ocean Lift [US-OTC]; Head & Shoulders® Refresh 2-in-1 [US-OTC]; Head & Shoulders® Refresh [US-OTC]; Head & Shoulders® Restoring Shine 2-in-1 [US-OTC]; Head & Shoulders® Restoring Shine [US-OTC]; Head & Shoulders® Sensitive Care 2-in-1 [US-OTC]; Head & Shoulders® Sensitive Care [US-OTC]; Head & Shoulders® Smooth & Silky 2-In-1 [US-OTC]; Head & Shoulders® Smooth & Silky [US-OTC]; Selsun® Salon™ 2-in-1 [US-OTC]; Selsun® Salon™ Classic [US-OTC]; Selsun® Salon™ Moisturizing [US-OTC]; Selsun® Salon™ Volumizing [US-OTC]; Skin Care™ [US-OTC]; T/Gel® Daily Control 2 in 1 [US-OTC]; T/Gel® Daily Control [US-OTC]; Zincon® [US-OTC]; ZNP® Bar [US-OTC]

Therapeutic Category Antiseborrheic Agent, Topical

Use Relieves the itching, irritation, and scalp flaking associated with dandruff and/or seborrheal dermatitis

Usual Dosage Adults: Products should be used at least twice weekly for best results, but may be used with each washing.

Bar: May be used on body and or scalp; wet area, massage in, and rinse.

Shampoo: Should be applied to wet hair and massaged into scalp; rinse. May be followed with conditioner

Dosage Forms

Conditioner, topical:

Head & Shoulders® Classic Clean [OTC], Head & Shoulders® Dry Scalp Care [OTC]: 0.5% (400 mL)

Cream, topical:

DermaZinc™ [OTC]: 0.25% (120 g)

Lotion, topical:

Skin Care™ [OTC]: 0.25% (120 mL)

Shampoo, topical:

BetaMed [OTC]: 2% (480 mL)

Denorex® Daily Protection [OTC]: 2% (120 mL, 360 mL) [alcohol free]

DermaZinc™ [OTC]: 2% (240 mL)
DHS™ Zinc [OTC]: 2% (240 mL, 360 mL)
Head & Shoulders® Citrus Breeze [OTC], Head & Shoulders® Extra Volume [OTC], Head & Shoulders® Sensitive Care [OTC], Head & Shoulders® Ocean Lift [OTC], Head & Shoulders® Restoring Shine [OTC]: 1% (420 mL, 700 mL)
Head & Shoulders® Classic Clean [OTC]: 1% (50 mL, 420 mL, 700 mL, 1000 mL, 1200 mL)
Head & Shoulders® Dry Scalp Care [OTC]: 1% (340 mL, 420 mL, 700 mL, 1200 mL)
Head & Shoulders® intensive solutions for dry/damaged hair [OTC], Head & Shoulders® intensive solutions for fine/oily hair [OTC], Head & Shoulders® intensive solutions for normal hair [OTC]: 2% (251 mL)
Head & Shoulders® Refresh [OTC]: 1% (420 mL, 700 mL, 1000 mL, 1200 mL)
Head & Shoulders® Smooth & Silky [OTC]: 1% (420 mL)
Selsun® Salon™ Classic [OTC], Selsun® Salon™ Moisturizing [OTC], Selsun® Salon™ Volumizing [OTC]: 1% (384 mL)
T/Gel® Daily Control [OTC]: 1% (250 mL)
Zincon® [OTC]: 1% (120 mL, 240 mL)

Shampoo, topical [with conditioner]:
Head & Shoulders® Citrus Breeze 2-in-1 [OTC], Head & Shoulders® Refresh 2-in-1 [OTC], Head & Shoulders® Restoring Shine 2-in-1 [OTC]: 1% (420 mL)
Head & Shoulders® Classic Clean 2-in-1 [OTC], Head & Shoulders® Dry Scalp Care 2-in-1 [OTC], Head & Shoulders® Smooth and Silky 2-in-1 [OTC], Head & Shoulders® Ocean Lift 2-in-1 [OTC], Head & Shoulders® Sensitive Care 2-in-1 [OTC]: 1% (420 mL, 700 mL)
Head & Shoulders® intensive solutions 2-in-1 [OTC]: 2% (251 mL)
Selsun® Salon™ 2-in-1 [OTC]: 1% (384 mL)
T/Gel® Daily Control 2 in 1 [OTC]: 1% (250 mL)

Soap, topical:
DermaZinc™ [OTC]: 2% (112.5 g)
ZNP® [OTC] 2% (119 g) [bar]

Solution, topical [spray/drops]:
DermaZinc™ [OTC]: 0.25% (120 mL)

QDALL® ***(Discontinued)*** *see* chlorpheniramine and pseudoephedrine *on page 215*

quadrivalent human papillomavirus vaccine *see* papillomavirus (types 6, 11, 16, 18) vaccine (human, recombinant) *on page 750*

Quad Tann® [US] *see* chlorpheniramine, ephedrine, phenylephrine, and carbetapentane *on page 216*

Qualaquin™ [US] *see* quinine *on page 846*

Quartuss™ [US] *see* dextromethorphan, chlorpheniramine, phenylephrine, and guaifenesin *on page 297*

Quasense™ [US] *see* ethinyl estradiol and levonorgestrel *on page 387*

quaternium-18 bentonite *see* bentoquatam *on page 128*

quazepam (KWAZ e pam)

Sound-Alike/Look-Alike Issues
quazepam may be confused with oxazepam

U.S./Canadian Brand Names Doral® [US/Can]

Therapeutic Category Benzodiazepine

Controlled Substance C-IV

Use Treatment of insomnia

Usual Dosage Oral: Adults: Initial: 15 mg at bedtime, in some patients the dose may be reduced to 7.5 mg after a few nights

Dosage Forms

Tablet:
Doral®: 15 mg

Quelicin® [US/Can] *see* succinylcholine *on page 924*

Queltuss® ***(Discontinued)*** *see* guaifenesin and dextromethorphan *on page 474*

Questran® [US/Can] *see* cholestyramine resin *on page 224*

Questran® Light [US] *see* cholestyramine resin *on page 224*

Questran® Light Sugar Free [Can] *see* cholestyramine resin *on page 224*

quetiapine (kwe TYE a peen)

Sound-Alike/Look-Alike Issues
QUEtiapine may be confused with OLANZapine
Seroquel® may be confused with Serentil®, Serzone®, Sinequan®

Synonyms quetiapine fumarate

Tall-Man QUEtiapine

U.S./Canadian Brand Names Apo-Quetiapine® [Can]; CO Quetiapine [Can]; Gen-Quetiapine [Can]; Novo-Quetiapine [Can]; PMS-Quetiapine [Can]; PRO-Quetiapine [Can]; ratio-Quetiapine [Can]; Riva-Quetiapine [Can]; Sandoz-Quetiapine [Can]; Seroquel XR® [US/Can]; Seroquel® [US/Can]; ZYM-Quetiapine [Can]

Therapeutic Category Antipsychotic Agent

Use Treatment of schizophrenia; treatment of acute manic episodes associated with bipolar I disorder (as monotherapy or in combination with lithium or divalproex); maintenance treatment of bipolar I disorder (in combination with lithium or divalproex); treatment of depressive episodes associated with bipolar disorder

Usual Dosage Oral: Adults:

Bipolar disorder:

Depression:

Immediate release tablet: Initial: 50 mg/day the first day; increase to 100 mg/day on day 2, further increasing by 100 mg/day each day until a target dose of 300 mg/day is reached by day 4. Further increases up to 600 mg/day by day 8 have been evaluated in clinical trials, but no additional antidepressant efficacy was noted.

Extended release tablet: Initial: 50 mg/day the first day; increase to 100 mg on day 2, further increasing by 100 mg/day each day until a target dose of 300 mg/day is reached by day 4.

Mania:

Immediate release tablet: Initial: 50 mg twice daily on day 1, increase dose in increments of 100 mg/day to 200 mg twice daily on day 4; may increase to a target dose of 800 mg/day by day 6 at increments ≤200 mg/day. Usual dosage range: 400-800 mg/day.

Extended release tablet: Initial: 300 mg on day 1; increase to 600 mg on day 2 and adjust dose to 400-800 mg once daily on day 3, depending on response and tolerance.

Maintenance therapy: Immediate release tablet: 200-400 mg twice daily with lithium or divalproex; **Note:** Average time of stabilization was 15 weeks in clinical trials.

Schizophrenia/psychoses:

Immediate release tablet: Initial: 25 mg twice daily; increase in increments of 25-50 mg 2-3 times/day on the second and third day, if tolerated, to a target dose of 300-400 mg/day in 2-3 divided doses by day 4. Make further adjustments as needed at intervals of at least 2 days in adjustments of 25-50 mg twice daily. Usual maintenance range: 300-800 mg/day.

Extended release tablet: Initial: 300 mg once daily; increase in increments of up to 300 mg/day (in intervals of ≥1 day). Usual maintenance range: 400-800 mg/day.

Note: Dose reductions should be attempted periodically to establish lowest effective dose in patients with psychosis. Patients being restarted after 1 week of no drug need to be titrated as above.

Dosage Forms

Tablet:
Seroquel®: 25 mg, 50 mg, 100 mg, 200 mg, 300 mg, 400 mg

Tablet, extended release:
Seroquel XR®: 50 mg, 150 mg, 200 mg, 300 mg, 400 mg

quetiapine fumarate *see* quetiapine *on page* 844
Quibron® ***(Discontinued)***
Quibron®-T ***(Discontinued)*** *see* theophylline *on page* 953
Quibron®-T/SR ***(Discontinued)*** *see* theophylline *on page* 953
Quiess® Injection ***(Discontinued)*** *see* hydroxyzine *on page* 511
Quinaglute® Dura-Tabs® ***(Discontinued)*** *see* quinidine *on page* 845
quinagolide ***(Discontinued)***
Quinalan® ***(Discontinued)*** *see* quinidine *on page* 845
quinalbarbitone sodium *see* secobarbital *on page* 894

quinapril (KWIN a pril)

Sound-Alike/Look-Alike Issues
Accupril® may be confused with Accolate®, Accutane®, AcipHex®, Monopril®

Synonyms quinapril hydrochloride

U.S./Canadian Brand Names Accupril® [US/Can]; GD-Quinapril [Can]

Therapeutic Category Angiotensin-Converting Enzyme (ACE) Inhibitor

Use Treatment of hypertension; treatment of heart failure

Usual Dosage Oral: Adults:

Heart failure: Initial: 5 mg once or twice daily, titrated at weekly intervals to 20-40 mg daily in 2 divided doses; target dose (heart failure): 20 mg twice daily

Hypertension: Initial: 10-20 mg once daily, adjust according to blood pressure response at peak-and-trough blood levels; initial dose may be reduced to 5 mg in patients receiving diuretic therapy if the diuretic is continued; usual dose range (JNC 7): 10-40 mg once daily

Dosage Forms

Tablet: 5 mg, 10 mg, 20 mg, 40 mg

Accupril®: 5 mg, 10 mg, 20 mg, 40 mg

quinapril and hydrochlorothiazide (KWIN a pril & hye droe klor oh THYE a zide)

Synonyms hydrochlorothiazide and quinapril

U.S./Canadian Brand Names Accuretic® [US/Can]; Quinaretic [US]

Therapeutic Category Antihypertensive Agent, Combination

Use Treatment of hypertension (not for initial therapy)

Usual Dosage Oral: Adults: Initial:

Patients who have failed quinapril monotherapy:

Quinapril 10 mg/hydrochlorothiazide 12.5 mg **or**

Quinapril 20 mg/hydrochlorothiazide 12.5 mg once daily

Patients with adequate blood pressure control on hydrochlorothiazide 25 mg/day, but significant potassium loss:

Quinapril 10 mg/hydrochlorothiazide 12.5 mg **or**

Quinapril 20 mg/hydrochlorothiazide 12.5 mg once daily

Note: Clinical trials of quinapril/hydrochlorothiazide combinations used quinapril doses of 2.5-40 mg/day and hydrochlorothiazide doses of 6.25-25 mg/day.

Dosage Forms

Tablet: 10/12.5: Quinapril 10 mg and hydrochlorothiazide 12.5 mg; 20/12.5: Quinapril 20 mg and hydrochlorothiazide 12.5 mg; 20/25: Quinapril 20 mg and hydrochlorothiazide 25 mg

Accuretic®, Quinaretic: 10/12.5: Quinapril 10 mg and hydrochlorothiazide 12.5 mg; 20/12.5: Quinapril 20 mg and hydrochlorothiazide 12.5 mg; 20/25: Quinapril 20 mg and hydrochlorothiazide 25 mg

quinapril hydrochloride *see* quinapril *on page 844*

Quinaretic [US] *see* quinapril and hydrochlorothiazide *on page 845*

Quinate® [Can] *see* quinidine *on page 845*

Quin B Strong [US-OTC] *see* vitamin B complex combinations *on page 1017*

Quin B Strong with C and Zinc [US-OTC] *see* vitamin B complex combinations *on page 1017*

quinidine (KWIN i deen)

Sound-Alike/Look-Alike Issues

quiNIDine may be confused with cloNIDine, quiNINE, Quinora®

Synonyms quinidine gluconate; quinidine polygalacturonate; quinidine sulfate

Tall-Man quiNIDine

U.S./Canadian Brand Names Apo-Quinidine® [Can]; BioQuin® Durules™ [Can]; Novo-Quinidin [Can]; Quinate® [Can]

Therapeutic Category Antiarrhythmic Agent, Class I-A

Use

Quinidine gluconate and sulfate salts: Conversion and prevention of relapse into atrial fibrillation and/or flutter; suppression of ventricular arrhythmias. **Note:** Due to proarrhythmic effects, use should be reserved for life-threatening arrhythmias. Moreover, the use of quinidine has largely been replaced by more effective/safer antiarrhythmic agents and/or nonpharmacologic therapies (eg, radiofrequency ablation).

Quinidine gluconate (I.V. formulation): Conversion of atrial fibrillation/flutter and ventricular tachycardia. **Note:** The use of I.V. quinidine gluconate for these indications has been replaced by more effective/safer antiarrhythmic agents (eg, amiodarone and procainamide).

Quinidine gluconate (I.V. formulation) and quinidine sulfate: Treatment of malaria (*Plasmodium falciparum*)

Usual Dosage Dosage expressed in terms of the salt: 267 mg of quinidine gluconate = 200 mg of quinidine sulfate.

Children: Test dose for idiosyncratic reaction (sulfate, oral or gluconate, I.M.): 2 mg/kg or 60 mg/m²
Oral (quinidine sulfate): 15-60 mg/kg/day in 4-5 divided doses or 6 mg/kg every 4-6 hours; usual 30 mg/kg/day or 900 mg/m²/day given in 5 daily doses
I.V. **not** recommended (quinidine gluconate): 2-10 mg/kg/dose given at a rate ≤10 mg/minute every 3-6 hours as needed

Adults: Test dose: Oral, I.M.: 200 mg administered several hours before full dosage (to determine possibility of idiosyncratic reaction)
Oral (for malaria):
Sulfate: 100-600 mg/dose every 4-6 hours; begin at 200 mg/dose and titrate to desired effect (maximum daily dose: 3-4 g)
Gluconate: 324-972 mg every 8-12 hours
I.M.: 400 mg/dose every 2-6 hours; initial dose: 600 mg (gluconate)
I.V.: 200-400 mg/dose diluted and given at a rate ≤10 mg/minute; may require as much as 500-750 mg

Dosage Forms
Injection, solution: 80 mg/mL (10 mL)
Tablet: 200 mg, 300 mg
Tablet, extended release: 300 mg, 324 mg

quinidine gluconate *see* quinidine *on page 845*
quinidine polygalacturonate *see* quinidine *on page 845*
quinidine sulfate *see* quinidine *on page 845*

quinine (KWYE nine)

Sound-Alike/Look-Alike Issues
quiNINE may be confused with quiNIDine

Synonyms quinine sulfate

Tall-Man qui**NINE**

U.S./Canadian Brand Names Apo-Quinine® [Can]; Novo-Quinine [Can]; Qualaquin™ [US]; Quinine-Odan™ [Can]

Therapeutic Category Antimalarial Agent

Use In conjunction with other antimalarial agents, treatment of uncomplicated chloroquine-resistant *P. falciparum* malaria

Usual Dosage Note: Actual duration of treatment for malaria may be dependent upon the geographic region or pathogen. Oral:
Children: Treatment of chloroquine-resistant malaria (CDC guidelines): 30 mg/kg/day in divided doses every 8 hours for 3-7 days with tetracycline, doxycycline, or clindamycin (consider risk versus benefit of using tetracycline or doxycycline in children <8 years of age)
Adults: Treatment of chloroquine-resistant malaria: 648 mg every 8 hours for 7 days with tetracycline, doxycycline, or clindamycin

Dosage Forms
Capsule:
Qualaquin™: 324 mg

Quinine-Odan™ [Can] *see* quinine *on page 846*
quinine sulfate *see* quinine *on page 846*
quinol *see* hydroquinone *on page 508*
Quinora® *(Discontinued)* *see* quinidine *on page 845*
Quintabs [US-OTC] *see* vitamins (multiple/oral) *on page 1019*
Quintabs-M [US-OTC] *see* vitamins (multiple/oral) *on page 1019*
Quintabs-M Iron-Free [US-OTC] *see* vitamins (multiple/oral) *on page 1019*

quinupristin and dalfopristin (kwi NYOO pris tin & dal FOE pris tin)

Synonyms dalfopristin and quinupristin; pristinamycin; RP-59500

U.S./Canadian Brand Names Synercid® [US/Can]

Therapeutic Category Antibiotic, Streptogramin

Use Treatment of serious or life-threatening infections associated with vancomycin-resistant *Enterococcus faecium* bacteremia; treatment of complicated skin and skin structure infections caused by methcillin-susceptible *Staphylococcus aureus* or *Streptococcus pyogenes*

Has been studied in the treatment of a variety of infections caused by *Enterococcus faecium* (not *E. fecalis*) including vancomycin-resistant strains. May also be effective in the treatment of serious infections caused by *Staphylococcus* species including those resistant to methicillin.

Usual Dosage I.V.:

Children (limited information): Dosages similar to adult dosing have been used in the treatment of complicated skin/soft tissue infections and infections caused by vancomycin-resistant *Enterococcus faecium*

CNS shunt infection due to vancomycin-resistant *Enterococcus faecium*: 7.5 mg/kg/dose every 8 hours; concurrent intrathecal doses of 1-2 mg/day have been administered for up to 68 days

Adults:

Vancomycin-resistant *Enterococcus faecium*: 7.5 mg/kg every 8 hours

Complicated skin and skin structure infection: 7.5 mg/kg every 12 hours

Dosage Forms

Injection, powder for reconstitution:

Synercid®: 500 mg: Quinupristin 150 mg and dalfopristin 350 mg

Quixin® [US] *see* levofloxacin *on page* 580

QVAR® [US/Can] *see* beclomethasone *on page* 125

R & C™ II [Can] *see* pyrethrins and piperonyl butoxide *on page* 839

R & C® Lice *(Discontinued)* *see* permethrin *on page* 769

R & C™ Shampoo/Conditioner [Can] *see* pyrethrins and piperonyl butoxide *on page* 839

RabAvert® [US/Can] *see* rabies vaccine *on page* 848

rabeprazole (ra BEP ra zole)

Sound-Alike/Look-Alike Issues

rabeprazole may be confused with aripiprazole,donepezil, lansoprazole, omeprazole, raloxifene

AcipHex® may be confused with Acephen®, Accupril®, Aricept®, pHisoHex®

Synonyms pariprazole

U.S./Canadian Brand Names AcipHex® [US/Can]; Novo-Rabeprazole EC [Can]; Pariet® [Can]; PMS-Rabeprazole [Can]; Ran-Rabeprazole [Can]; Sandoz-Rabeprazole [Can]

Therapeutic Category Gastric Acid Secretion Inhibitor

Use Short-term (4-8 weeks) treatment and maintenance of erosive or ulcerative gastroesophageal reflux disease (GERD); symptomatic GERD; short-term (up to 4 weeks) treatment of duodenal ulcers; long-term treatment of pathological hypersecretory conditions, including Zollinger-Ellison syndrome; *H. pylori* eradication (in combination therapy)

Canadian labeling: Additional uses (not in U.S. labeling): Treatment of nonerosive reflux disease (NERD); treatment of gastric ulcers

Usual Dosage Oral:

Children ≥12 years: *U.S. labeling:* Short-term treatment of GERD: 20 mg once daily for ≤8 weeks

Adults >18 years:

Erosive/ulcerative GERD: Treatment: 20 mg once daily for 4-8 weeks; if inadequate response, may repeat up to an additional 8 weeks; maintenance: 20 mg once daily

Canadian labeling: 20 mg once daily for 4 weeks; if inadequate response, may repeat for an additional 4 weeks (lack of symptom control after 4 weeks warrants further evaluation); maintenance: 10 mg once daily (maximum: 20 mg once daily)

Symptomatic GERD: Treatment: 20 mg once daily for 4 weeks; if inadequate response, may repeat for an additional 4 weeks

Canadian labeling: 10 mg once daily (maximum: 20 mg once daily) for 4 weeks; lack of symptom control after 4 weeks warrants further evaluation

Duodenal ulcer: 20 mg/day before breakfast for 4 weeks; additional therapy may be required for some patients

Gastric ulcers (*Canadian labeling*): 20 mg once daily up to 6 weeks; additional therapy may be required for some patients

Helicobacter pylori eradication:

Manufacturer labeling: 20 mg twice daily administered with amoxicillin 1000 mg *and* clarithromycin 500 mg twice daily for 7 days

American College of Gastroenterology guidelines:
Nonpenicillin allergy: 20 mg twice daily administered with amoxicillin 1000 mg *and* clarithromycin 500 mg twice daily for 10-14 days
Penicillin allergy: 20 mg twice daily administered with clarithromycin 500 mg *and* metronidazole 500 mg twice daily for 10-14 days **or** 20 mg once or twice daily administered with bismuth subsalicylate 525 mg *and* metronidazole 250 mg *plus* tetracycline 500 mg 4 times/day for 10-14 days

Hypersecretory conditions: 60 mg once daily; dose may need to be adjusted as necessary. Doses as high as 100 mg once daily and 60 mg twice daily have been used, and continued as long as necessary (up to 1 year in some patients).

NERD (*Canadian labeling*): Treatment: 10 mg (maximum: 20 mg once daily) for 4 weeks; lack of symptom control after 4 weeks warrants further evaluation

Dosage Forms [CAN] = Canadian brand name

Tablet, delayed release, enteric coated:
AcipHex®: 20 mg
Pariet® [CAN]: 10 mg, 20 mg

rabies immune globulin (human) (RAY beez i MYUN GLOB yoo lin, HYU man)

Synonyms RIG

U.S./Canadian Brand Names HyperRAB™ S/D [US/Can]; Imogam® Rabies Pasteurized [Can]; Imogam® Rabies-HT [US]

Therapeutic Category Immune Globulin

Use Part of postexposure prophylaxis of persons with rabies exposure who lack a history of preexposure or postexposure prophylaxis with rabies vaccine or a recently documented neutralizing antibody response to previous rabies vaccination

Usual Dosage Children and Adults: Postexposure prophylaxis: Local wound infiltration: 20 units/kg in a single dose, RIG should always be administered as part of rabies vaccine regimen. If anatomically feasible, the full rabies immune globulin dose should be infiltrated around and into the wound(s); remaining volume should be administered I.M. at a site distant from the vaccine administration site. If rabies vaccine was initiated without rabies immune globulin, rabies immune globulin may be administered through the seventh day after the administration of the first dose of the vaccine. Administration of RIG is not recommended after the seventh day post vaccine since an antibody response to the vaccine is expected during this time period.

Note: Persons known to have an adequate titer or who have previously received postexposure prophylaxis with rabies vaccine should not receive RIG.

Dosage Forms

Injection, solution [preservative free]:
HyperRAB™ S/D, Imogam® Rabies-HT: 150 int. units/mL (2 mL, 10 mL)

rabies vaccine (RAY beez vak SEEN)

Synonyms HDCV; human diploid cell cultures rabies vaccine; PCEC; purified chick embryo cell

U.S./Canadian Brand Names Imovax® Rabies [US/Can]; RabAvert® [US/Can]

Therapeutic Category Vaccine, Inactivated Virus

Use Preexposure and postexposure vaccination against rabies

The Advisory Committee on Immunization Practices (ACIP) recommends a primary course of prophylactic immunization (preexposure vaccination) for the following:

- Persons with continuous risk of infection including rabies research laboratory and biologics production workers
- Persons with frequent risk of infection in areas where rabies is enzootic, including rabies diagnostic laboratory workers, cavers, veterinarians and their staff, animal control and wildlife workers; persons who frequently handle bats
- Persons with infrequent risk of infection, including veterinarians and animal control staff with terrestrial animals in areas where rabies infection is rare, veterinary students, travelers visiting areas where rabies is enzootic and immediate access to medical care and biologicals is limited

The ACIP recommends the use of postexposure vaccination for a particular person be assessed by the severity and likelihood versus the actual risk of acquiring rabies. Consideration should include the type of exposure, epidemiology of rabies in the area, species of the animal, circumstances of the incident, and the availability of the exposing animal for observation or rabies testing. Postexposure vaccination is used in both previously vaccinated and previously unvaccinated individuals.

Usual Dosage

Preexposure vaccination: 1 mL I.M. on days 0, 7, and 21 to 28. **Note:** Prolonging the interval between doses does not interfere with immunity achieved after the concluding dose of the basic series.

Postexposure vaccination: All postexposure treatment should begin with immediate cleansing of the wound with soap and water

Persons not previously immunized as above: I.M.: 5 doses (1 mL each) on days 0, 3, 7, 14, 28. In addition, patients should also receive rabies immune globulin with the first dose (day 0). **Note:** A regimen of 4 doses (1 mL each) on days 0, 3, 7, 14 may be used in persons who are not immununosuppressed.

Persons who have previously received postexposure prophylaxis with rabies vaccine, received a recommended I.M. preexposure series of rabies vaccine or have a previously documented rabies antibody titer considered adequate: I.M.: Two doses (1 mL each) on days 0 and 3; do not administer rabies immune globulin

Booster (for persons with continuous or frequent risk of infection): 1 mL I.M. based on antibody titers

Dosage Forms

Injection, powder for reconstitution [preservative free]:

Imovax® Rabies: ≥2.5 int. units [HDCV]

RabAvert®: ≥2.5 int. units [PCEC]

racemic epinephrine *see* epinephrine *on page 358*

racepinephrine *see* epinephrine *on page 358*

RAD001 *see* everolimus *on page 400*

Radiogardase® [US] *see* ferric hexacyanoferrate *on page 413*

rAHF *see* antihemophilic factor (recombinant) *on page 82*

R-albuterol *see* levalbuterol *on page 576*

Ralivia™ ER [Can] *see* tramadol *on page 975*

Ralix [US] *see* chlorpheniramine, phenylephrine, and methscopolamine *on page 218*

raloxifene (ral OKS i feen)

Sound-Alike/Look-Alike Issues

Evista® may be confused with Avinza™, Eovist®

Synonyms keoxifene hydrochloride; NSC-706725; raloxifene hydrochloride

U.S./Canadian Brand Names Apo-Raloxifene [Can]; Evista® [US/Can]; Novo-Raloxifene [Can]

Therapeutic Category Selective Estrogen Receptor Modulator (SERM)

Use Prevention and treatment of osteoporosis in postmenopausal women; risk reduction for invasive breast cancer in postmenopausal women with osteoporosis and in postmenopausal women with high risk for invasive breast cancer

Usual Dosage Oral: Adults: Females:

Osteoporosis: 60 mg/day

Invasive breast cancer risk reduction: 60 mg/day

Dosage Forms

Tablet:

Evista®: 60 mg

raloxifene hydrochloride *see* raloxifene *on page 849*

raltegravir (ral TEG ra vir)

Synonyms MK-0518

U.S./Canadian Brand Names Isentress® [US/Can]

Therapeutic Category Antiretroviral Agent, Integrase Inhibitor

Use Treatment of HIV-1 infection in combination with other antiretroviral agents

Usual Dosage Oral: Adolescents ≥16 years and Adults: 400 mg twice daily

Dosage Forms

Tablet:

Isentress®: 400 mg

raltitrexed *(Canada only)* (ral ti TREX ed)

Synonyms ICI-D1694; NSC-639186; raltitrexed disodium; ZD1694

U.S./Canadian Brand Names Tomudex® [Can]

Therapeutic Category Antineoplastic Agent

Use Treatment of advanced colorectal neoplasms

Usual Dosage I.V. (refer to individual protocols): 3 mg/m^2 every 3 weeks

Dosage Forms

Injection, powder for reconstitution:
2 mg [not available in the U.S.; investigational]

raltitrexed disodium *see* raltitrexed *(Canada only) on page 849*

ramelteon (ra MEL tee on)

Sound-Alike/Look-Alike Issues

ramelteon may be confused with Remeron®
Rozerem® may be confused with Razadyne™, Remeron®

Synonyms TAK-375

U.S./Canadian Brand Names Rozerem® [US]

Therapeutic Category Hypnotic, Nonbenzodiazepine

Use Treatment of insomnia characterized by difficulty with sleep onset

Usual Dosage Oral: Adults: One 8 mg tablet within 30 minutes of bedtime

Dosage Forms

Tablet:
Rozerem®: 8 mg

ramipril (RA mi pril)

Sound-Alike/Look-Alike Issues

ramipril may be confused with enalapril, Monopril®
Altace® may be confused with alteplase, Amaryl®, Amerge®, Artane®

U.S./Canadian Brand Names Altace® [US/Can]; Apo-Ramipril® [Can]; CO Ramipril [Can]; GEN-Ramipril [Can]; Novo-Ramipril [Can]; RAN-Ramipril [Can]; ratio-Ramipril [Can]; Sandoz-Ramipril [Can]

Therapeutic Category Angiotensin-Converting Enzyme (ACE) Inhibitor

Use Treatment of hypertension, alone or in combination with thiazide diuretics; treatment of left ventricular dysfunction after MI; to reduce risk of MI, stroke, and death in patients at increased risk for these events

Usual Dosage Oral: Adults:

Hypertension: 2.5-5 mg once daily, maximum: 20 mg/day

LV dysfunction postmyocardial infarction: Initial: 2.5 mg twice daily titrated upward, if possible, to 5 mg twice daily

Reduction in risk of MI, stroke, and death from cardiovascular causes: Initial: 2.5 mg once daily for 1 week, then 5 mg once daily for the next 3 weeks, then increase as tolerated to 10 mg once daily (may be given as divided dose)

Note: The dose of any concomitant diuretic should be reduced. If the diuretic cannot be discontinued, initiate therapy with 1.25 mg. After the initial dose, the patient should be monitored carefully until blood pressure has stabilized.

Dosage Forms

Capsule: 1.25 mg, 2.5 mg, 5 mg, 10 mg
Altace®: 1.25 mg, 2.5 mg, 5 mg, 10 mg

Tablet:
Altace®: 1.25 mg, 2.5 mg, 5 mg, 10 mg

ramipril and felodipine *(Canada only)* (RA mi pril & fe LOE di peen)

Synonyms felodipine and ramipril; ramipril and felodipine ER

U.S./Canadian Brand Names Altace® Plus Felodipine [Can]

Therapeutic Category Antihypertensive Agent, Combination

Use Treatment of hypertension when combination therapy is appropriate (not for initial therapy)

Usual Dosage Oral: **Note:** Not for initial therapy; titration of individual agents to an appropriate clinical response is required before patient is converted over to an equivalent dose of the combination product.

Adults (dose is individualized): Ramipril 2.5-10 mg and felodipine ER 2.5-10 mg once daily; adjust dose no more frequently than every 2 weeks

Dosage Forms [CAN] = Canadian brand name

Tablet, variable release:

Altace® Plus Felodipine 2.5/2.5 [CAN]: Ramipril 2.5 mg [immediate release] and felodipine 2.5 mg [extended release] [not available in the U.S.]

Altace® Plus Felodipine 5/5 [CAN]: Ramipril 5 mg [immediate release] and felodipine 5 mg [extended release] [not available in the U.S.]

ramipril and felodipine ER *see* ramipril and felodipine *(Canada only) on page 850*

ramipril and hydrochlorothiazide *(Canada only)*

(RA mi pril & hye droe klor oh THYE a zide)

Sound-Alike/Look-Alike Issues

Altace® HCT may be confused with alteplase, Artane®, Altace®

Synonyms hydrochlorothiazide and ramipril

U.S./Canadian Brand Names Altace® HCT [Can]

Therapeutic Category Angiotensin-Converting Enzyme (ACE) Inhibitor; Antihypertensive Agent, Combination; Diuretic, Thiazide

Use Treatment of essential hypertension (not for initial therapy)

Usual Dosage Oral: Adults: **Note:** Not for initial therapy; titration of individual agents to an appropriate clinical response is required before patient is converted over to an equivalent dose of the combination product.

Usual dosage: Ramipril 2.5 mg/hydrochlorothiazide 12.5 mg once daily; titrate to maximum ramipril 10 mg/hydrochlorothiazide 50 mg once daily

Dosage Forms

Tablet:

Altace® HCT 2.5/12.5 [CAN]: Ramipril 2.5 mg and hydrochlorothiazide 12.5 mg [not available in the U.S.]

Altace® HCT 5/12.5 [CAN]: Ramipril 5 mg and hydrochlorothiazide 12.5 mg [not available in the U.S.]

Altace® HCT 5/25 [CAN]: Ramipril 5 mg and hydrochlorothiazide 25 mg [not available in the U.S.]

Altace® HCT 10/12.5 [CAN]: Ramipril 10 mg and hydrochlorothiazide 12.5 mg [not available in the U.S.]

Altace® HCT 10/25 [CAN]: Ramipril 10 mg and hydrochlorothiazide 25 mg [not available in the U.S.]

RAN™-Atenolol [Can] *see* atenolol *on page 107*

RAN™-Carvedilol [Can] *see* carvedilol *on page 188*

Ran-Cefprozil [Can] *see* cefprozil *on page 196*

RAN-Ciprofloxacin [Can] *see* ciprofloxacin *on page 229*

RAN™-Citalopram [Can] *see* citalopram *on page 234*

RAN™-Domperidone [Can] *see* domperidone *(Canada only) on page 330*

Ranexa® [US] *see* ranolazine *on page 853*

RAN™-Fentanyl Transdermal System [Can] *see* fentanyl *on page 410*

RAN-Fosinopril [Can] *see* fosinopril *on page 446*

ranibizumab (ra ni BIZ oo mab)

Synonyms rhuFabV2

U.S./Canadian Brand Names Lucentis® [US/Can]

Therapeutic Category Monoclonal Antibody; Ophthalmic Agent; Vascular Endothelial Growth Factor (VEGF) Inhibitor

Use Treatment of neovascular (wet) age-related macular degeneration (AMD)

Usual Dosage Intravitreal: Adults:

Age-related macular degeneration (AMD): 0.5 mg (0.05 mL) once a month. **Note:** Frequency may be reduced after the first 4 injections to once every 3 months if monthly injections are not feasible; however, this regimen has reportedly resulted in a ~5 letter (1 line) loss of visual acuity over 9 months, as compared to monthly dosing.

Canadian labeling: AMD: 0.5 mg (0.05 mL) once a month. Frequency may be reduced after the first 3 injections to once every 3 months if monthly injections are not feasible.

Dosage Forms [CAN] = Canadian product availability

Injection, solution [preservative free]:

Lucentis®: 10 mg/mL (0.2 mL)

Lucentis® [CAN]: 10 mg/mL (0.3 mL)

Raniclor™ [US] *see* cefaclor *on page* 191

ranitidine (ra NI ti deen)

Sound-Alike/Look-Alike Issues
ranitidine may be confused with amantadine, rimantadine
Zantac® may be confused with Xanax®, Zarontin®, Zofran®, Zyrtec®

Synonyms ranitidine hydrochloride

U.S./Canadian Brand Names Acid Reducer Maximum Strength Non Prescription [Can]; Acid Reducer [Can]; Apo-Ranitidine® [Can]; CO Ranitidine [Can]; Dom-Ranitidine [Can]; Gen-Ranidine [Can]; Novo-Ranidine [Can]; Nu-Ranit [Can]; PMS-Ranitidine [Can]; Ranitidine Injection, USP [Can]; ratio-Ranitidine [Can]; Riva-Ranitidine [Can]; Sandoz-Ranitidine [Can]; ScheinPharm Ranitidine [Can]; Zantac 150® [US-OTC]; Zantac 75® [US-OTC/Can]; Zantac Maximum Strength Non-Prescription [Can]; Zantac® EFFERdose® [US]; Zantac® [US/Can]

Therapeutic Category Histamine H_2 Antagonist

Use
Zantac®: Short-term and maintenance therapy of duodenal ulcer, gastric ulcer, gastroesophageal reflux disease (GERD), active benign ulcer, erosive esophagitis, and pathological hypersecretory conditions; as part of a multidrug regimen for *H. pylori* eradication to reduce the risk of duodenal ulcer recurrence
Zantac 75® [OTC]: Relief of heartburn, acid indigestion, and sour stomach

Usual Dosage
Children 1 month to 16 years:
Duodenal and gastric ulcer:
Oral:
Treatment: 4-8 mg/kg/day divided twice daily; maximum: 300 mg/day
Maintenance: 2-4 mg/kg/day once daily; maximum: 150 mg/day
I.V.: 2-4 mg/kg/day divided every 6-8 hours; maximum: 200 mg/day
GERD and erosive esophagitis: Oral: 5-10 mg/kg/day divided twice daily; maximum: GERD: 300 mg/day, erosive esophagitis: 600 mg/day
Children ≥12 years: Prevention of heartburn: Oral: Zantac 75® [OTC]: 75 mg 30-60 minutes before eating food or drinking beverages which cause heartburn; maximum: 150 mg/24 hours; do not use for more than 14 days
Adults:
Duodenal ulcer: Oral: Treatment: 150 mg twice daily, or 300 mg once daily after the evening meal or at bedtime; maintenance: 150 mg once daily at bedtime
Helicobacter pylori eradication: 150 mg twice daily; requires combination therapy
Pathological hypersecretory conditions:
Oral: 150 mg twice daily; adjust dose or frequency as clinically indicated; doses of up to 6 g/day have been used
I.V.: Continuous infusion for Zollinger-Ellison: Initial: 1 mg/kg/hour; measure gastric acid output at 4 hours, if >10 mEq or if patient is symptomatic, increase dose in increments of 0.5 mg/kg/hour; doses of up to 2.5 mg/kg/hour (or 220 mg/hour) have been used
Gastric ulcer, benign: Oral: 150 mg twice daily; maintenance: 150 mg once daily at bedtime
GERD: Oral: 150 mg twice daily
Erosive esophagitis: Oral: Treatment: 150 mg 4 times/day; maintenance: 150 mg twice daily
Prevention of heartburn: Oral: Zantac 75® [OTC]: 75 mg 30-60 minutes before eating food or drinking beverages which cause heartburn; maximum: 150 mg in 24 hours; do not use for more than 14 days
Patients not able to take oral medication:
I.M.: 50 mg every 6-8 hours
I.V.: Intermittent bolus or infusion: 50 mg every 6-8 hours
Continuous I.V. infusion: 6.25 mg/hour

Dosage Forms
Capsule: 150 mg, 300 mg
Infusion, premixed in ½NS [preservative free]:
Zantac®: 50 mg (50 mL)
Injection, solution: 25 mg/mL (2 mL, 6 mL, 40 mL)
Zantac®: 25 mg/mL (2 mL, 6 mL, 40 mL)
Syrup: 15 mg/mL
Zantac®: 15 mg/mL

Tablet: 75 mg [OTC], 150 mg, 300 mg
Zantac®: 150 mg, 300 mg
Zantac 75® [OTC]: 75 mg
Zantac 150® [OTC]: 150 mg
Tablet, effervescent:
Zantac® EFFERdose®: 25 mg

ranitidine hydrochloride *see* ranitidine *on page* *852*
Ranitidine Injection, USP [Can] *see* ranitidine *on page* *852*
Ran-Lisinopril [Can] *see* lisinopril *on page* *593*
RAN™-Lovastatin [Can] *see* lovastatin *on page* *602*
RAN™-Metformin [Can] *see* metformin *on page* *633*

ranolazine (ra NOE la zeen)

Sound-Alike/Look-Alike Issues
Ranexa® may be confused with Celexa®
U.S./Canadian Brand Names Ranexa® [US]
Therapeutic Category Cardiovascular Agent, Miscellaneous
Use Treatment of chronic angina
Usual Dosage Oral: Adults: Chronic angina: Initial: 500 mg twice daily; maximum recommended dose: 1000 mg twice daily
Dosage Forms
Tablet, extended release:
Ranexa®: 500 mg, 1000 mg

RAN-Ondansetron [Can] *see* ondansetron *on page* *726*
Ran-Pantoprazole [Can] *see* pantoprazole *on page* *748*
RAN-Pravastatin [Can] *see* pravastatin *on page* *811*
Ran-Rabeprazole [Can] *see* rabeprazole *on page* *847*
RAN-Ramipril [Can] *see* ramipril *on page* *850*
Ran-Risperidone [Can] *see* risperidone *on page* *870*
RAN-Ropinirole [Can] *see* ropinirole *on page* *877*
Ran-Tamsulosin [Can] *see* tamsulosin *on page* *938*
RAN™-Zopiclone [Can] *see* zopiclone *(Canada only) on page* *1034*
Rapaflo™ [US] *see* silodosin *on page* *900*
Rapamune® [US/Can] *see* sirolimus *on page* *904*
Raphon *(Discontinued)* *see* epinephrine *on page* *358*
Raplon® *(Discontinued)*
Raptiva® *(Discontinued)* *see* efalizumab *on page* *348*

rasagiline (ra SA ji leen)

Sound-Alike/Look-Alike Issues
Azilect® may be confused with Aricept®
Synonyms AGN 1135; rasagiline mesylate; TVP-1012
U.S./Canadian Brand Names Azilect® [US]
Therapeutic Category Anti-Parkinson Agent, MAO Type B Inhibitor
Use Initial monotherapy or as adjunct to levodopa in the treatment of idiopathic Parkinson disease
Usual Dosage Oral: Adults: Parkinson disease:
Monotherapy: 1 mg once daily
Adjunctive therapy with levodopa: Initial: 0.5 mg once daily; may increase to 1 mg once daily based on response and tolerability
Note: When added to existing levodopa therapy, a dose reduction of levodopa may be required to avoid exacerbation of dyskinesias; typical dose reductions of ~9% to 13% were employed in clinical trials
Dosage Forms
Tablet:
Azilect®: 0.5 mg, 1 mg

rasagiline mesylate *see* rasagiline *on page* *853*

rasburicase (ras BYOOR i kayse)

Synonyms NSC-721631; recombinant urate oxidase

U.S./Canadian Brand Names Elitek™ [US]; Fasturtec® [Can]

Therapeutic Category Enzyme

Use Initial management of uric acid levels in pediatric patients with leukemia, lymphoma, and solid tumor malignancies receiving chemotherapy expected to result in tumor lysis and elevation of plasma uric acid

Usual Dosage I.V.: Children: Management of uric acid levels: 0.15 mg/kg or 0.2 mg/kg once daily for 5 days (manufacturer-recommended duration); begin chemotherapy 4-24 hours after the first dose

Limited data suggest that a single prechemotherapy dose (versus multiple-day administration) may be sufficiently efficacious. Monitoring electrolytes, hydration status, and uric acid concentrations are necessary to identify the need for additional doses. Other clinical manifestations of tumor lysis syndrome (eg, hyperphosphatemia, hypocalcemia, and hyperkalemia) may occur.

Dosage Forms

Injection, powder for reconstitution:

Elitek®: 1.5 mg, 7.5 mg

Rasilez® [Can] *see* aliskiren *on page* *47*
rATG *see* antithymocyte globulin (rabbit) *on page* *86*
ratio-Aclavulanate [Can] *see* amoxicillin and clavulanate potassium *on page* *71*
ratio-Acyclovir [Can] *see* acyclovir *on page* *33*
ratio-Alendronate [Can] *see* alendronate *on page* *44*
ratio-Amcinonide [Can] *see* amcinonide *on page* *59*
ratio-Amiodarone [Can] *see* amiodarone *on page* *64*
ratio-Amiodarone I.V. [Can] *see* amiodarone *on page* *64*
ratio-Amlodipine [Can] *see* amlodipine *on page* *66*
ratio-Azithromycin [Can] *see* azithromycin *on page* *116*
ratio-Benzydamine [Can] *see* benzydamine *(Canada only) on page* *135*
ratio-Bicalutamide [Can] *see* bicalutamide *on page* *141*
ratio-Brimonidine [Can] *see* brimonidine *on page* *147*
ratio-Bupropion SR [Can] *see* bupropion *on page* *158*
ratio-Buspirone [Can] *see* buspirone *on page* *160*
ratio-Carvedilol [Can] *see* carvedilol *on page* *188*
ratio-Cefuroxime [Can] *see* cefuroxime *on page* *199*
ratio-Ciprofloxacin [Can] *see* ciprofloxacin *on page* *229*
ratio-Citalopram [Can] *see* citalopram *on page* *234*
ratio-Clarithromycin [Can] *see* clarithromycin *on page* *236*
ratio-Clindamycin [Can] *see* clindamycin *on page* *239*
ratio-Clobazam [Can] *see* clobazam *(Canada only) on page* *241*
ratio-Clobetasol [Can] *see* clobetasol *on page* *242*
ratio-Cotridin [Can] *see* triprolidine, pseudoephedrine, and codeine *(Canada only) on page* *990*
ratio-Diltiazem CD [Can] *see* diltiazem *on page* *311*
ratio-Domperidone [Can] *see* domperidone *(Canada only) on page* *330*
ratio-Emtec [Can] *see* acetaminophen and codeine *on page* *20*
ratio-Enalapril [Can] *see* enalapril *on page* *352*
ratio-Famotidine [Can] *see* famotidine *on page* *405*
ratio-Fenofibrate MC [Can] *see* fenofibrate *on page* *408*
ratio-Fentanyl [Can] *see* fentanyl *on page* *410*
ratio-Fluoxetine [Can] *see* fluoxetine *on page* *432*
ratio-Gabapentin [Can] *see* gabapentin *on page* *450*
ratio-Glimepiride [Can] *see* glimepiride *on page* *464*
ratio-Glyburide [Can] *see* glyburide *on page* *467*
ratio-Inspra-Sal [Can] *see* albuterol *on page* *41*
ratio-Ipra Sal UDV [Can] *see* ipratropium and albuterol *on page* *545*
ratio-Ketorolac [Can] *see* ketorolac *on page* *558*
ratio-Lamotrigine [Can] *see* lamotrigine *on page* *567*

recombinant α-L-iduronidase (glycosaminoglycan α-L-iduronohydrolase) *see* laronidase *on page 573*
recombinant hirudin *see* lepirudin *on page 574*
recombinant human deoxyribonuclease *see* dornase alfa *on page 332*
recombinant human insulin-like growth factor-1 *see* mecasermin *on page 618*
recombinant human interleukin-11 *see* oprelvekin *on page 728*
recombinant human luteinizing hormone *see* lutropin alfa *on page 604*
recombinant human parathyroid hormone (1-34) *see* teriparatide *on page 946*
recombinant human platelet-derived growth factor B *see* becaplermin *on page 124*
recombinant human thyrotropin *see* thyrotropin alpha *on page 958*
recombinant interleukin-11 *see* oprelvekin *on page 728*
recombinant N-acetylgalactosamine 4-sulfatase *see* galsulfase *on page 454*
recombinant plasminogen activator *see* reteplase *on page 860*
recombinant urate oxidase *see* rasburicase *on page 854*
Recombinate [US/Can] *see* antihemophilic factor (recombinant) *on page 82*
Recombivax HB® [US/Can] *see* hepatitis B vaccine (recombinant) *on page 490*
Recothrom™ [US] *see* thrombin (topical) *on page 957*
Rectacaine [US-OTC] *see* phenylephrine *on page 774*
RectaGel™ HC [US] *see* lidocaine and hydrocortisone *on page 587*
Red Cross™ Canker Sore [US-OTC] *see* benzocaine *on page 129*
Redisol® *(Discontinued)* *see* cyanocobalamin *on page 263*
Reese's® Pinworm Medicine [US-OTC] *see* pyrantel pamoate *on page 838*
ReFacto® [Can] *see* antihemophilic factor (recombinant) *on page 82*
ReFacto® *(Discontinued)* *see* antihemophilic factor (recombinant) *on page 82*
Refenesen™ [US-OTC] *see* guaifenesin *on page 473*
Refenesen™ 400 [US-OTC] *see* guaifenesin *on page 473*
Refenesen™ DM [US-OTC] *see* guaifenesin and dextromethorphan *on page 474*
Refenesen™ PE [US-OTC] *see* guaifenesin and phenylephrine *on page 475*
Refenesen Plus [US-OTC] *see* guaifenesin and pseudoephedrine *on page 477*
Refissa™ [US] *see* tretinoin (topical) *on page 981*
Refludan® [US/Can] *see* lepirudin *on page 574*
Refresh® [US-OTC] *see* artificial tears *on page 100*
Refresh Liquigel® [US-OTC] *see* carboxymethylcellulose *on page 186*
Refresh Plus® [US-OTC] *see* artificial tears *on page 100*
Refresh Plus® [US-OTC/Can] *see* carboxymethylcellulose *on page 186*
Refresh Tears® [US-OTC] *see* artificial tears *on page 100*
Refresh Tears® [US-OTC/Can] *see* carboxymethylcellulose *on page 186*

regadenoson (re ga DEN of son)

Synonyms CVT-3146

U.S./Canadian Brand Names Lexiscan™ [US]

Therapeutic Category Diagnostic Agent

Use Radionuclide myocardial perfusion imaging (MPI) in patients unable to undergo adequate exercise stress testing

Usual Dosage I.V.: Adults: 0.4 mg (5 mL) over ~10 seconds, followed immediately by a 5 mL saline flush. Wait 10-20 seconds, then administer the radionuclide myocardial perfusion imaging agent.

Dosage Forms

Injection, solution [preservative free]:
Lexiscan™ 0.08 mg/mL (5 mL)

Regitine® [Can] *see* phentolamine *on page 774*
Regitine *(Discontinued)* *see* phentolamine *on page 774*
Reglan® [US] *see* metoclopramide *on page 649*
Reglan® Syrup *(Discontinued)* *see* metoclopramide *on page 649*
Regonol® [US] *see* pyridostigmine *on page 839*

Regranex® [US/Can] *see* becaplermin *on page 124*
Regular Iletin® II *(Discontinued)*
regular insulin *see* insulin regular *on page 533*
Regulax SS® *(Discontinued)* *see* docusate *on page 326*
Regulex® [Can] *see* docusate *on page 326*
Reguloid [US-OTC] *see* psyllium *on page 837*
Rejuva-A® [Can] *see* tretinoin (topical) *on page 981*
Relacon-DM NR [US] *see* guaifenesin, pseudoephedrine, and dextromethorphan *on page 479*
Relafen® [Can] *see* nabumetone *on page 675*
Relafen® *(Discontinued)* *see* nabumetone *on page 675*
Relenza® [US/Can] *see* zanamivir *on page 1026*
Relief® *(Discontinued)* *see* phenylephrine *on page 774*
Relief® Ophthalmic Solution *(Discontinued)* *see* phenylephrine *on page 774*
Relief-SF® [US] *see* acetaminophen, chlorpheniramine, and pseudoephedrine *on page 26*
Relistor™ [US/Can] *see* methylnaltrexone *on page 645*
Relpax® [US/Can] *see* eletriptan *on page 350*
Remeron® [US/Can] *see* mirtazapine *on page 661*
Remeron® RD [Can] *see* mirtazapine *on page 661*
Remeron SolTab® [US] *see* mirtazapine *on page 661*
Reme-T™ [US-OTC] *see* coal tar *on page 250*
Remicade® [US/Can] *see* infliximab *on page 527*

remifentanil (rem i FEN ta nil)

Sound-Alike/Look-Alike Issues
remifentanil may be confused with alfentanil

Synonyms GI87084B

U.S./Canadian Brand Names Ultiva® [US/Can]

Therapeutic Category Analgesic, Narcotic

Controlled Substance C-II

Use Analgesic for use during the induction and maintenance of general anesthesia; for continued analgesia into the immediate postoperative period; analgesic component of monitored anesthesia

Usual Dosage I.V. continuous infusion: Dose should be based on ideal body weight (IBW) in obese patients (>30% over IBW).

Children birth to 2 months: Maintenance of anesthesia with nitrous oxide (70%): 0.4 mcg/kg/minute (range: 0.4-1 mcg/kg/minute); supplemental bolus dose of 1 mcg/kg may be administered, smaller bolus dose may be required with potent inhalation agents, potent neuraxial anesthesia, significant comorbidities, significant fluid shifts, or without atropine pretreatment. Clearance in neonates is highly variable; dose should be carefully titrated.

Children 1-12 years: Maintenance of anesthesia with halothane, sevoflurane, or isoflurane: 0.25 mcg/kg/minute (range: 0.05-1.3 mcg/kg/minute); supplemental bolus dose of 1 mcg/kg may be administered every 2-5 minutes. Consider increasing concomitant anesthetics with infusion rate >1 mcg/kg/minute. Infusion rate can be titrated upward in increments up to 50% or titrated downward in decrements of 25% to 50%. May titrate every 2-5 minutes.

Adults:

Induction of anesthesia: 0.5-1 mcg/kg/minute; if endotracheal intubation is to occur in <8 minutes, an initial dose of 1 mcg/kg may be given over 30-60 seconds

Coronary bypass surgery: 1 mcg/kg/minute

Maintenance of anesthesia: **Note:** Supplemental bolus dose of 1 mcg/kg may be administered every 2-5 minutes. Consider increasing concomitant anesthetics with infusion rate >1 mcg/kg/minute. Infusion rate can be titrated upward in increments of 25% to 100% or downward in decrements of 25% to 50%. May titrate every 2-5 minutes.

With nitrous oxide (66%): 0.4 mcg/kg/minute (range: 0.1-2 mcg/kg/minute)

With isoflurane: 0.25 mcg/kg/minute (range: 0.05-2 mcg/kg/minute)

With propofol: 0.25 mcg/kg/minute (range: 0.05-2 mcg/kg/minute)

Coronary bypass surgery: 1 mcg/kg/minute (range: 0.125-4 mcg/kg/minute); supplemental dose: 0.5-1 mcg/kg

Continuation as an analgesic in immediate postoperative period: 0.1 mcg/kg/minute (range: 0.025-0.2 mcg/kg/minute). Infusion rate may be adjusted every 5 minutes in increments of 0.025 mcg/kg/minute.

Bolus doses are not recommended. Infusion rates >0.2 mcg/kg/minute are associated with respiratory depression.

Coronary bypass surgery, continuation as an analgesic into the ICU: 1 mcg/kg/minute (range: 0.05-1 mcg/kg/minute)

Analgesic component of monitored anesthesia care: **Note:** Supplemental oxygen is recommended:

Single I.V. dose given 90 seconds prior to local anesthetic:

Remifentanil alone: 1 mcg/kg over 30-60 seconds

With midazolam: 0.5 mcg/kg over 30-60 seconds

Continuous infusion beginning 5 minutes prior to local anesthetic:

Remifentanil alone: 0.1 mcg/kg minute

With midazolam: 0.05 mcg/kg/minute

Continuous infusion given after local anesthetic:

Remifentanil alone: 0.05 mcg/kg/minute (range: 0.025-0.2 mcg/kg/minute)

With midazolam: 0.025 mcg/kg/minute (range: 0.025-0.2 mcg/kg/minute)

Note: Following local or anesthetic block, infusion rate should be decreased to 0.05 mcg/kg/minute; rate adjustments of 0.025 mcg/kg/minute may be done at 5-minute intervals

Dosage Forms

Injection, powder for reconstitution:

Ultiva®: 1 mg, 2 mg, 5 mg

Reminyl® [Can] *see* galantamine *on page 453*

Reminyl® *(Discontinued)* *see* galantamine *on page 453*

Reminyl® ER [Can] *see* galantamine *on page 453*

Remodulin® [US/Can] *see* treprostinil *on page 980*

Renacidin® [US] *see* citric acid, magnesium carbonate, and glucono-delta-lactone *on page 234*

Renagel® [US/Can] *see* sevelamer *on page 898*

Renal Caps [US] *see* vitamin B complex combinations *on page 1017*

renal replacement solution *see* electrolyte solution, renal replacement *on page 350*

Renamin® [US] *see* amino acid injection *on page 62*

Rena-Vite [US-OTC] *see* vitamin B complex combinations *on page 1017*

Rena-Vite RX [US] *see* vitamin B complex combinations *on page 1017*

Renax® [US] *see* vitamins (multiple/oral) *on page 1019*

Renax® 5.5 [US] *see* vitamins (multiple/oral) *on page 1019*

Renedil® [Can] *see* felodipine *on page 408*

Reno-30® *(Discontinued)* *see* diatrizoate meglumine *on page 300*

Reno-60® *(Discontinued)* *see* diatrizoate meglumine *on page 300*

RenoCal-76® *(Discontinued)* *see* diatrizoate meglumine and diatrizoate sodium *on page 300*

Reno-Dip® *(Discontinued)* *see* diatrizoate meglumine *on page 300*

Renografin®-60 *(Discontinued)* *see* diatrizoate meglumine and diatrizoate sodium *on page 300*

Renoquid® *(Discontinued)*

Renova® [US/Can] *see* tretinoin (topical) *on page 981*

Renvela® [US] *see* sevelamer *on page 898*

ReoPro® [US/Can] *see* abciximab *on page 17*

repaglinide (re PAG li nide)

Sound-Alike/Look-Alike Issues

Prandin® may be confused with Avandia®

U.S./Canadian Brand Names GlucoNorm® [Can]; Prandin® [US/Can]

Therapeutic Category Hypoglycemic Agent, Oral

Use Management of type 2 diabetes mellitus (noninsulin-dependent, NIDDM) as an adjunct to diet and exercise; may be used in combination with metformin or thiazolidinediones

Usual Dosage Oral: Adults: Should be taken within 15 minutes of the meal, but time may vary from immediately preceding the meal to as long as 30 minutes before the meal

Initial: For patients not previously treated or whose Hb A_{1c} is <8%, the starting dose is 0.5 mg before each meal. For patients previously treated with blood glucose-lowering agents whose Hb A_{1c} is ≥8%, the initial dose is 1 or 2 mg before each meal.

Dose adjustment: Determine dosing adjustments by blood glucose response, usually fasting blood glucose. Double the preprandial dose up to 4 mg until satisfactory blood glucose response is achieved. At least 1 week should elapse to assess response after each dose adjustment.

Dose range: 0.5-4 mg taken with meals. Repaglinide may be dosed preprandial 2, 3, or 4 times/day in response to changes in the patient's meal pattern. Maximum recommended daily dose: 16 mg.

Dosage Forms

Tablet:

Prandin®: 0.5 mg, 1 mg, 2 mg

repaglinide and metformin (re PAG li nide & met FOR min)

Sound-Alike/Look-Alike Issues

PrandiMet® may be confused with Avandamet®, Prandin®

Synonyms metformin and repaglinide; repaglinide and metformin hydrochloride

U.S./Canadian Brand Names PrandiMet® [US]

Therapeutic Category Antidiabetic Agent, Biguanide; Antidiabetic Agent, Meglitinide Derivative; Hypoglycemic Agent, Oral

Use Management of type 2 diabetes mellitus (noninsulin-dependent, NIDDM), as an adjunct to diet and exercise, in patients currently receiving or not adequately controlled on metformin and/or a meglitinide

Usual Dosage Oral: Adults: Type 2 diabetes mellitus:

Patients currently taking repaglinide and metformin: Initial doses should be based on (but not exceeding) the patient's current doses of repaglinide and metformin; daily doses should be divided and given 2-3 times daily with meals (maximum single dose: 4 mg/dose [repaglinide], 1000 mg/dose [metformin]; maximum daily dose: 10 mg/day [repaglinide], 2500 mg/day [metformin])

Patients inadequately controlled on metformin alone: Initial dose: repaglinide 1 mg/metformin 500 mg twice daily with meals. Titrate slowly to reduce the risk of repaglinide-induced hypoglycemia.

Patients inadequately controlled on a meglitinide alone: Initial dose: metformin 500 mg twice daily plus repaglinide at a dose similar to (but not exceeding) the patient's current dose. Titrate slowly to reduce the risk of metformin-induced gastrointestinal adverse effects.

Dosage Forms

Tablet:

PrandiMet®: 1/500: Repaglinide 1 mg and metformin hydrochloride 500 mg; 2/500: Repaglinide 2 mg and metformin hydrochloride 500 mg

repaglinide and metformin hydrochloride *see* repaglinide and metformin *on page* 859

Repan® [US] *see* butalbital, acetaminophen, and caffeine *on page* 161

Replace [US-OTC] *see* vitamins (multiple/oral) *on page* 1019

Replace Without Iron [US-OTC] *see* vitamins (multiple/oral) *on page* 1019

Replagal™ [Can] *see* agalsidase alfa *(Canada only) on page* 38

Repliva 21/7® [US] *see* vitamins (multiple/oral) *on page* 1019

Reposans-10® Oral *(Discontinued)* *see* chlordiazepoxide *on page* 209

Reprexain® [US] *see* hydrocodone and ibuprofen *on page* 503

Repronex® [US/Can] *see* menotropins *on page* 625

Requa® Activated Charcoal [US-OTC] *see* charcoal *on page* 206

Requip® [US/Can] *see* ropinirole *on page* 877

Requip® XL™ [US] *see* ropinirole *on page* 877

Resa® *(Discontinued)* *see* reserpine *on page* 859

Rescon® [US] *see* chlorpheniramine, phenylephrine, and methscopolamine *on page* 218

Rescon® MX [US] *see* chlorpheniramine, phenylephrine, and methscopolamine *on page* 218

Rescon DM [US-OTC] *see* chlorpheniramine, pseudoephedrine, and dextromethorphan *on page* 220

Rescon GG [US-OTC] *see* guaifenesin and phenylephrine *on page* 475

Rescon-Jr® [US] *see* chlorpheniramine and phenylephrine *on page* 214

Rescriptor® [US/Can] *see* delavirdine *on page* 281

Rescula® *(Discontinued)*

Resectisol® [US] *see* mannitol *on page* 613

reserpine (re SER peen)

Sound-Alike/Look-Alike Issues

reserpine may be confused with Risperdal®, risperidone

Therapeutic Category Rauwolfia Alkaloid

Use Management of mild-to-moderate hypertension; treatment of agitated psychotic states (schizophrenia)

Usual Dosage Note: When used for management of hypertension, full antihypertensive effects may take as long as 3 weeks.

Oral:

Children: Hypertension: 0.01-0.02 mg/kg/24 hours divided every 12 hours; maximum dose: 0.25 mg/day (not recommended in children)

Adults: Hypertension:

Manufacturer's labeling: Initial: 0.5 mg/day for 1-2 weeks; maintenance: 0.1-0.25 mg/day

Note: Clinically, the need for a "loading" period (as recommended by the manufacturer) is not well supported, and alternative dosing is preferred.

Usual dose range (JNC 7): 0.05-0.25 mg once daily; 0.1 mg every other day may be given to achieve 0.05 mg once daily

Dosage Forms

Tablet: 0.1 mg, 0.25 mg

Respa®-1st [US] *see* guaifenesin and pseudoephedrine *on page* *477*

Respa-DM® [US] *see* guaifenesin and dextromethorphan *on page* *474*

Respa-GF® ***(Discontinued)*** *see* guaifenesin *on page* *473*

Respahist® [US] *see* brompheniramine and pseudoephedrine *on page* *150*

Respaire®-60 SR ***(Discontinued)*** *see* guaifenesin and pseudoephedrine *on page* *477*

Respaire®-120 SR ***(Discontinued)*** *see* guaifenesin and pseudoephedrine *on page* *477*

Respa® PE ***(Discontinued)*** *see* guaifenesin and phenylephrine *on page* *475*

Respbid® ***(Discontinued)*** *see* theophylline *on page* *953*

Respi-Tann™ ***(Discontinued)*** *see* carbetapentane and pseudoephedrine *on page* *182*

Resporal® ***(Discontinued)*** *see* dexbrompheniramine and pseudoephedrine *on page* *289*

Restall® ***(Discontinued)*** *see* hydroxyzine *on page* *511*

Restasis® [US] *see* cyclosporine *on page* *266*

Restoril™ [US/Can] *see* temazepam *on page* *942*

Restylane® [US] *see* hyaluronate and derivatives *on page* *496*

retapamulin (re te PAM ue lin)

U.S./Canadian Brand Names Altabax™ [US]

Therapeutic Category Antibiotic, Pleuromutilin; Antibiotic, Topical

Use Treatment of impetigo caused by susceptible strains of *S. pyogenes* or methicillin-susceptible *S. aureus*

Usual Dosage Topical: Impetigo:

Children ≥9 months: Apply to affected area twice daily for 5 days. Total treatment area should not exceed 2% of total body surface area.

Adults: Apply to affected area twice daily for 5 days. Total treatment area should not exceed 100 cm^2 total body surface area.

Dosage Forms

Ointment, topical:

Altabax™: 1% (5 g, 10 g, 15 g)

Retavase® [US/Can] *see* reteplase *on page* *860*

reteplase (RE ta plase)

Synonyms r-PA; recombinant plasminogen activator

U.S./Canadian Brand Names Retavase® [US/Can]

Therapeutic Category Fibrinolytic Agent

Use Management of ST-elevation myocardial infarction (STEMI); improvement of ventricular function; reduction of the incidence of CHF and the reduction of mortality following AMI

Recommended criteria for treatment: STEMI: Chest pain ≥20 minutes duration, onset of chest pain within 12 hours of treatment (or within prior 12-24 hours in patients with continuing ischemic symptoms), and ST-segment elevation >0.1 mV in at least two contiguous precordial leads or two adjacent limb leads on ECG or new or presumably new left bundle branch block (LBBB)

Usual Dosage Adults: 10 units I.V. over 2 minutes, followed by a second dose 30 minutes later of 10 units I.V. over 2 minutes; withhold second dose if serious bleeding or anaphylaxis occurs

Note: All patients should receive 162-325 mg of chewable nonenteric coated aspirin as soon as possible and then daily. Administer concurrently with heparin 60 units/kg bolus (maximum: 4000 units) followed by continuous infusion of 12 units/kg/hour (maximum: 1000 units/hour) and adjust to aPTT target of 50-70 seconds (or 1.5-2 times the upper limit of control).

Dosage Forms

Injection, powder for reconstitution [preservative free]:
Retavase®: 10.4 units

Retin-A® [US/Can] *see* tretinoin (topical) *on page 981*
Retin-A® Micro [US/Can] *see* tretinoin (topical) *on page 981*
retinoic acid *see* tretinoin (topical) *on page 981*
Retinova® [Can] *see* tretinoin (topical) *on page 981*
Retisert® [US] *see* fluocinolone *on page 428*
Retrovir® [US/Can] *see* zidovudine *on page 1028*
Revatio® [US] *see* sildenafil *on page 900*
Revex® *(Discontinued)*
ReVia® [US/Can] *see* naltrexone *on page 679*
Revitalose C-1000® [Can] *see* ascorbic acid *on page 100*
Revlimid® [US/Can] *see* lenalidomide *on page 574*
Revolade® *see* eltrombopag *on page 351*
Rexigen Forte® *(Discontinued)* *see* phendimetrazine *on page 770*
Reyataz® [US/Can] *see* atazanavir *on page 106*
Rezulin® *(Discontinued)*
rFSH-alpha *see* follitropin alfa *on page 440*
rFSH-beta *see* follitropin beta *on page 441*
rFVIIa *see* factor VIIa (recombinant) *on page 402*
R-Gel® *(Discontinued)* *see* capsaicin *on page 178*
R-Gene® 10 [US] *see* arginine *on page 97*
rGM-CSF *see* sargramostim *on page 891*
rhASB *see* galsulfase *on page 454*
r-hCG *see* chorionic gonadotropin (recombinant) *on page 225*
rhDNase *see* dornase alfa *on page 332*
Rheaban® *(Discontinued)*
Rheomacrodex® *(Discontinued)* *see* dextran *on page 292*
Rheumatrex® [US] *see* methotrexate *on page 639*
rhFSH-alpha *see* follitropin alfa *on page 440*
rhFSH-beta *see* follitropin beta *on page 441*
rhGAA *see* alglucosidase alfa *on page 46*
r-h α-GAL *see* agalsidase beta *on page 38*
RhIG *see* Rh_o(D) immune globulin *on page 862*
rhIGF-1 (mecasermin [Increlex™]) *see* mecasermin *on page 618*
rhIGF-1/rhIGFBP-3 (mecasermin rinfabate [Iplex™]) *see* mecasermin *on page 618*
rhIL-11 *see* oprelvekin *on page 728*
Rhinacon A [US] *see* chlorpheniramine, phenylephrine, and phenyltoloxamine *on page 219*
Rhinalar® [Can] *see* flunisolide *on page 427*
Rhinall [US-OTC] *see* phenylephrine *on page 774*
Rhinaris-CS Anti-Allergic Nasal Mist [Can] *see* cromolyn sodium *on page 261*
Rhinocort® Aqua® [US/Can] *see* budesonide *on page 153*
Rhinocort® Nasal Inhaler *(Discontinued)* *see* budesonide *on page 153*
Rhinocort® Turbuhaler® [Can] *see* budesonide *on page 153*
RhinoFlex™ [US] *see* acetaminophen and phenyltoloxamine *on page 23*
RhinoFlex™-650 [US] *see* acetaminophen and phenyltoloxamine *on page 23*
rhKGF *see* palifermin *on page 743*
r-hLH *see* lutropin alfa *on page 604*
Rho(D) immune globulin (human) *see* Rh_o(D) immune globulin *on page 862*

Rho®-Clonazepam [Can] *see* clonazepam *on page* 245
Rhodacine® [Can] *see* indomethacin *on page* 526

Rh_o(D) immune globulin (ar aych oh (dee) i MYUN GLOB yoo lin)

Synonyms RhIG; Rho(D) immune globulin (human); RhoIGIV; RhoIVIM

U.S./Canadian Brand Names HyperRHO™ S/D Full Dose [US]; HyperRHO™ S/D Mini Dose [US]; MICRhoGAM® [US]; RhoGAM® [US]; Rhophylac® [US]; WinRho® SDF [US/Can]

Therapeutic Category Immune Globulin

Use

Suppression of Rh isoimmunization: Use in the following situations when an Rh_o(D)-negative individual is exposed to Rh_o(D)-positive blood: During delivery of an Rh_o(D)-positive infant; abortion; amniocentesis; chorionic villus sampling; ruptured tubal pregnancy; abdominal trauma; hydatidiform mole; transplacental hemorrhage. Used when the mother is Rh_o(D) negative, the father of the child is either Rh_o(D) positive or Rh_o(D) unknown, the baby is either Rh_o(D) positive or Rh_o(D) unknown.

Transfusion: Suppression of Rh isoimmunization in Rh_o(D)-negative individuals transfused with Rh_o(D) antigen-positive RBCs or blood components containing Rh_o(D) antigen-positive RBCs

Treatment of idiopathic thrombocytopenic purpura (ITP): Used in the following nonsplenectomized Rh_o(D) positive individuals: Children with acute or chronic ITP, adults with chronic ITP, children and adults with ITP secondary to HIV infection

Usual Dosage

ITP: Children and Adults:
- Rhophylac®: I.V.: 50 mcg/kg
- WinRho® SDF: I.V.:
  - Initial: 50 mcg/kg as a single injection, or can be given as a divided dose on separate days. If hemoglobin is <10 g/dL: Dose should be reduced to 25-40 mcg/kg.
  - Subsequent dosing: 25-60 mcg/kg can be used if required to elevate platelet count
  - Maintenance dosing if patient **did respond** to initial dosing: 25-60 mcg/kg based on platelet and hemoglobin levels
  - Maintenance dosing if patient **did not respond** to initial dosing:
    - Hemoglobin 8-10 g/dL: Redose between 25-40 mcg/kg
    - Hemoglobin >10 g/dL: Redose between 50-60 mcg/kg
    - Hemoglobin <8 g/dL: Use with caution

Rh_o(D) suppression: Adults: **Note:** One "full dose" (300 mcg) provides enough antibody to prevent Rh sensitization if the volume of RBC entering the circulation is ≤15 mL. When >15 mL is suspected, a fetal red cell count should be performed to determine the appropriate dose.

Pregnancy:
- Antepartum prophylaxis: In general, dose is given at 28 weeks. If given early in pregnancy, administer every 12 weeks to ensure adequate levels of passively acquired anti-Rh
  - HyperRHO™ S/D Full Dose, RhoGAM®: I.M.: 300 mcg
  - Rhophylac®, WinRho® SDF: I.M., I.V.: 300 mcg
- Postpartum prophylaxis: In general, dose is administered as soon as possible after delivery, preferably within 72 hours. Can be given up to 28 days following delivery
  - HyperRHO™ S/D Full Dose, RhoGAM®: I.M.: 300 mcg
  - Rhophylac®: I.M., I.V.: 300 mcg
  - WinRho® SDF: I.M., I.V.: 120 mcg

Threatened abortion, any time during pregnancy (with continuation of pregnancy):
- HyperRHO™ S/D Full Dose, RhoGAM®: I.M.: 300 mcg; administer as soon as possible
- Rhophylac®, WinRho® SDF: I.M., I.V.: 300 mcg; administer as soon as possible

Abortion, miscarriage, termination of ectopic pregnancy:
- RhoGAM®: I.M.: ≥13 weeks gestation: 300 mcg.
- HyperRHO™ S/D Mini Dose, MICRhoGAM®: <13 weeks gestation: I.M.: 50 mcg
- Rhophylac®: I.M., I.V.: 300 mcg
- WinRho® SDF: I.M., I.V.: After 34 weeks gestation: 120 mcg; administer immediately or within 72 hours

Amniocentesis, chorionic villus sampling:
- HyperRHO™ S/D Full Dose, RhoGAM®: I.M.: At 15-18 weeks gestation or during the 3rd trimester: 300 mcg. If dose is given between 13-18 weeks, repeat at 26-28 weeks and within 72 hours of delivery.
- Rhophylac®: I.M., I.V.: 300 mcg
- WinRho® SDF: I.M., I.V.: Before 34 weeks gestation: 300 mcg; administer immediately, repeat dose every 12 weeks during pregnancy; After 34 weeks gestation: 120 mcg, administered immediately or within 72 hours

Excessive fetomaternal hemorrhage (>15 mL): Rhophylac®: I.M., I.V.: 300 mcg within 72 hours plus 20 mcg/mL fetal RBCs in excess of 15 mL if excess transplacental bleeding is quantified **or** 300 mcg/dose if bleeding cannot be quantified

Abdominal trauma, manipulation:

HyperRHO™ S/D Full Dose, RhoGAM®: I.M.: 2nd or 3rd trimester: 300 mcg. If dose is given between 13-18 weeks, repeat at 26-28 weeks and within 72 hours of delivery

Rhophylac®: I.M., I.V.: 300 mcg within 72 hours

WinRho® SDF: I.M./I.V.: After 34 weeks gestation: 120 mcg; administer immediately or within 72 hours

Transfusion:

Children and Adults: WinRho® SDF: Administer within 72 hours after exposure of incompatible blood transfusions or massive fetal hemorrhage.

I.V.: Calculate dose as follows; administer 600 mcg every 8 hours until the total dose is administered:

Exposure to Rh$_o$(D) positive whole blood: 9 mcg/mL blood

Exposure to Rh$_o$(D) positive red blood cells: 18 mcg/mL cells

I.M.: Calculate dose as follows; administer 1200 mcg every 12 hours until the total dose is administered:

Exposure to Rh$_o$(D) positive whole blood: 12 mcg/mL blood

Exposure to Rh$_o$(D) positive red blood cells: 24 mcg/mL cells

Adults:

HyperRHO™ S/D Full Dose, RhoGAM®: I.M.: Multiply the volume of Rh positive whole blood administered by the hematocrit of the donor unit to equal the volume of RBCs transfused. The volume of RBCs is then divided by 15 mL, providing the number of 300 mcg doses (vials/syringes) to administer. If the dose calculated results in a fraction, round up to the next higher whole 300 mcg dose (vial/syringe).

Rhophylac®: I.M., I.V.: 20 mcg/2 mL transfused blood or 20 mcg/mL erythrocyte concentrate

Dosage Forms

Injection, solution [preservative free]:

HyperRHO™ S/D Full Dose, RhoGAM®: 300 mcg [I.M. use only]

HyperRHO™ S/D Mini Dose, MICRhoGAM®: 50 mcg [I.M. use only]

WinRho® SDF:

300 mcg/~1.3 mL (~1.3 mL)

500 mcg/~2.2 mL (~2.2 mL)

1000 mcg/~4.4 mL (~4.4 mL)

3000 mcg/~13 mL (~13 mL)

Rhodis™ [Can] *see* ketoprofen *on page 558*

Rhodis-EC™ [Can] *see* ketoprofen *on page 558*

Rhodis SR™ [Can] *see* ketoprofen *on page 558*

RhoGAM® [US] *see* Rh$_o$(D) immune globulin *on page 862*

RhoIGIV *see* Rh$_o$(D) immune globulin *on page 862*

RhoIVIM *see* Rh$_o$(D) immune globulin *on page 862*

Rho®-Loperamine [Can] *see* loperamide *on page 597*

Rho®-Nitro [Can] *see* nitroglycerin *on page 700*

Rhophylac® [US] *see* Rh$_o$(D) immune globulin *on page 862*

Rhotral [Can] *see* acebutolol *on page 19*

Rhotrimine® [Can] *see* trimipramine *on page 988*

Rhovane® [Can] *see* zopiclone *(Canada only) on page 1034*

Rhoxal-acebutolol [Can] *see* acebutolol *on page 19*

Rhoxal-atenolol [Can] *see* atenolol *on page 107*

Rhoxal-cyclosporine [Can] *see* cyclosporine *on page 266*

Rhoxal-fluvoxamine [Can] *see* fluvoxamine *on page 439*

Rhoxal-glimepiride [Can] *see* glimepiride *on page 464*

Rhoxal-loperamide [Can] *see* loperamide *on page 597*

Rhoxal-metformin [Can] *see* metformin *on page 633*

Rhoxal-minocycline [Can] *see* minocycline *on page 659*

Rhoxal-nabumetone [Can] *see* nabumetone *on page 675*

Rhoxal-orphendrine [Can] *see* orphenadrine *on page 730*

Rhoxal-pamidronate [Can] *see* pamidronate *on page 745*

Rhoxal-paroxetine [Can] *see* paroxetine *on page 752*

Rhoxal-salbutamol [Can] *see* albuterol *on page 41*
Rhoxal-Sertraline [Can] *see* sertraline *on page 898*
Rhoxal-sotalol [Can] *see* sotalol *on page 919*
Rhoxal-sumatriptan [Can] *see* sumatriptan *on page 932*
Rhoxal-ticlopidine [Can] *see* ticlopidine *on page 960*
Rhoxal-valproic [Can] *see* valproic acid and derivatives *on page 1002*
Rhoxal-zopiclone [Can] *see* zopiclone *(Canada only) on page 1034*
rhPTH(1-34) *see* teriparatide *on page 946*
Rh-TSH *see* thyrotropin alpha *on page 958*
***r*HuEPO-α** *see* epoetin alfa *on page 361*
rhuFabV2 *see* ranibizumab *on page 851*
rhu keratinocyte growth factor *see* palifermin *on page 743*
rHu-KGF *see* palifermin *on page 743*
Rhulicaine® *(Discontinued)* *see* benzocaine *on page 129*
rhuMAb-E25 *see* omalizumab *on page 722*
rHuMAb-EGFr *see* panitumumab *on page 748*
rhuMAb-VEGF *see* bevacizumab *on page 140*
RiaSTAP™ [US] *see* fibrinogen concentrate (human) *on page 417*
RibaPak™ [US] *see* ribavirin *on page 864*
Ribasphere® [US] *see* ribavirin *on page 864*

ribavirin (rye ba VYE rin)

Sound-Alike/Look-Alike Issues

ribavirin may be confused with riboflavin, rifampin, Robaxin®

Synonyms RTCA; tribavirin

U.S./Canadian Brand Names Copegus® [US]; Rebetol® [US]; RibaPak™ [US]; Ribasphere® [US]; Virazole® [US/Can]

Therapeutic Category Antiviral Agent

Use

Inhalation: Treatment of patients with respiratory syncytial virus (RSV) infections; specially indicated for treatment of severe lower respiratory tract RSV infections in patients with an underlying compromising condition (prematurity, bronchopulmonary dysplasia and other chronic lung conditions, congenital heart disease, immunodeficiency, immunosuppression), and recent transplant recipients

Oral capsule:

In combination with interferon alfa-2b (Intron® A) injection for the treatment of chronic hepatitis C in patients with compensated liver disease who have relapsed after alpha interferon therapy or were previously untreated with alpha interferons

In combination with peginterferon alfa-2b (PEG-Intron®) injection for the treatment of chronic hepatitis C in patients with compensated liver disease who were previously untreated with alpha interferons

Oral solution: In combination with interferon alfa 2b (Intron® A) injection for the treatment of chronic hepatitis C in patients with compensated liver disease who were previously untreated with alpha interferons or patients who have relapsed after alpha interferon therapy

Oral tablet: In combination with peginterferon alfa-2a (Pegasys®) injection for the treatment of chronic hepatitis C in patients with compensated liver disease who were previously untreated with alpha interferons (includes patients with histological evidence of cirrhosis [Child-Pugh class A] and patients with clinically-stable HIV disease)

Usual Dosage

Infants and Children: Aerosol inhalation: RSV infection: Use with Viratek® small particle aerosol generator (SPAG-2) at a concentration of 20 mg/mL (6 g reconstituted with 300 mL of sterile water without preservatives). Continuous aerosol administration: 12-18 hours/day for 3 days, up to 7 days in length

Children ≥3 years: Oral capsule or solution (Rebetol®): Chronic hepatitis C (in combination with interferon alfa-2b): **Note:** Oral solution should be used in children 3-5 years of age, children ≤25 kg, or those unable to swallow capsules. Recommended therapy duration (manufacturer labeling): Genotype 1: 48 weeks; genotypes 2,3: 24 weeks

Capsule/solution: 15 mg/kg/day in 2 divided doses (morning and evening)

Capsule dosing recommendations:
25-36 kg: 400 mg/day (200 mg morning and evening)
37-49 kg: 600 mg/day (200 mg in the morning and 400 mg in the evening)
50-61 kg: 800 mg/day (400 mg in the morning and evening)
>61 kg: Refer to adult dosing
Note: *American Association for the Study of Liver Diseases (AASLD) guidelines recommendation:* Children 2-17 years with chronic HCV infection: Treatment of choice: Ribavirin 15 mg/kg daily in combination with SubQ peginterferon alfa-2b 60 mcg/m^2 once weekly for 48 weeks
Adults:
Oral capsule (Rebetol®, Ribasphere®):
Chronic hepatitis C (in combination with interferon alfa-2b):
≤75 kg: 400 mg in the morning, then 600 mg in the evening
>75 kg: 600 mg in the morning, then 600 mg in the evening
Chronic hepatitis C (in combination with peginterferon alfa-2b): 400 mg twice daily
Tablet (Copegus®): Chronic hepatitis C (in combination with peginterferon alfa-2a):
Monoinfection, genotype 1,4:
<75 kg: 1000 mg/day in 2 divided doses for 48 weeks
≥75 kg: 1200 mg/day in 2 divided doses for 48 weeks
Monoinfection, genotype 2,3: 800 mg/day in 2 divided doses for 24 weeks
Coinfection with HIV: 800 mg/day in 2 divided doses for 48 weeks (regardless of genotype)
Note: *American Association for the Study of Liver Diseases (AASLD) guidelines recommendation:* Adults with chronic HCV infection (Ghany, 2009): Treatment of choice: Ribavirin plus **peginterferon**; clinical condition and ability of patient to tolerate therapy should be evaluated to determine length and/or likely benefit of therapy. Recommended treatment duration (AASLD guidelines): Genotypes 1,4: 48 weeks; Genotypes 2,3: 24 weeks; Coinfection with HIV: 48 weeks.

Dosage Forms
Capsule: 200 mg
Rebetol®, Ribasphere®: 200 mg
Combination package [dose pack]:
RibaPak™ 400/600 [each package contains]:
Tablet: 400 mg (7s)
Tablet: 600 mg (7s)
Powder for solution, for nebulization:
Virazole®: 6 g (1s)
Solution, oral:
Rebetol®: 40 mg/mL
Tablet: 200 mg
Copegus®: 200 mg
Ribasphere®: 200 mg, 400 mg, 600 mg
Tablet [dose pack]:
RibaPak™: 400 mg (14s), 600 mg (14s)

ribavirin and peginterferon alfa-2b *see* peginterferon alfa-2b and ribavirin *(Canada only) on page 757*

Ribo-100 [US] *see* riboflavin *on page 865*

riboflavin (RYE boe flay vin)

Sound-Alike/Look-Alike Issues
riboflavin may be confused with ribavirin

Synonyms lactoflavin; vitamin B_2; vitamin G

U.S./Canadian Brand Names Ribo-100 [US]

Therapeutic Category Vitamin, Water Soluble

Use Prevention of riboflavin deficiency and treatment of ariboflavinosis

Usual Dosage Oral:
Riboflavin deficiency:
Children: 2.5-10 mg/day in divided doses
Adults: 5-30 mg/day in divided doses
Recommended daily allowance:
Children: 0.4-1.8 mg
Adults: 1.2-1.7 mg

Dosage Forms
Tablet: 25 mg, 50 mg, 100 mg
Ribo-100: 100 mg

Rid-A-Pain Dental [US-OTC] *see* benzocaine *on page 129*
Ridaura® [US/Can] *see* auranofin *on page 113*
RID® *(Discontinued)* *see* pyrethrins and piperonyl butoxide *on page 839*
RID® Maximum Strength [US-OTC] *see* pyrethrins and piperonyl butoxide *on page 839*
RID® Mousse [Can] *see* pyrethrins and piperonyl butoxide *on page 839*
Rid® Spray [US-OTC] *see* permethrin *on page 769*

rifabutin (rif a BYOO tin)

Sound-Alike/Look-Alike Issues
rifabutin may be confused with rifampin

Synonyms ansamycin

U.S./Canadian Brand Names Mycobutin® [US/Can]

Therapeutic Category Antibiotic, Miscellaneous

Use Prevention of disseminated *Mycobacterium avium* complex (MAC) in patients with advanced HIV infection

Usual Dosage Oral: Prophylaxis:
Children >1 year: 5 mg/kg daily; higher dosages have been used in limited trials
Adults: 300 mg once daily (alone or in combination with azithromycin)

Dosage Forms
Capsule:
Mycobutin®: 150 mg

Rifadin® [US/Can] *see* rifampin *on page 866*
Rifamate® [US/Can] *see* rifampin and isoniazid *on page 867*
rifampicin *see* rifampin *on page 866*

rifampin (rif AM pin)

Sound-Alike/Look-Alike Issues
rifampin may be confused with ribavirin, rifabutin, Rifamate®, rifapentine, rifaximin
Rifadin® may be confused with Rifater®, Ritalin®

Synonyms rifampicin

U.S./Canadian Brand Names Rifadin® [US/Can]; Rofact™ [Can]

Therapeutic Category Antibiotic, Miscellaneous

Use Management of active tuberculosis in combination with other agents; elimination of meningococci from the nasopharynx in asymptomatic carriers

Usual Dosage
Usual dosage ranges: Oral, I.V.:
Infants and Children: 10-20 mg/kg/day as a single dose or in 2 divided doses; maximum: 600 mg/day
Adults: 600 mg once or twice daily
Indication-specific dosing: Oral, I.V.:
Tuberculosis, active: Note: A four-drug regimen (isoniazid, rifampin, pyrazinamide, and ethambutol) is preferred for the initial, empiric treatment of TB. When the drug susceptibility results are available, the regimen should be altered as appropriate.
Infants and Children <12 years:
Daily therapy: 10-20 mg/kg/day usually as a single dose (maximum: 600 mg/day)
Twice weekly directly observed therapy (DOT): 10-20 mg/kg (maximum: 600 mg)
Adults:
Daily therapy: 10 mg/kg/day (maximum: 600 mg/day)
Twice weekly directly observed therapy (DOT): 10 mg/kg (maximum: 600 mg); 3 times/week: 10 mg/kg (maximum: 600 mg)
Tuberculosis, latent infection (LTBI): As an alternative to isoniazid:
Children: 10-20 mg/kg/day (maximum: 600 mg/day) for 6 months
Adults: 10 mg/kg/day (maximum: 600 mg/day) for 4 months. **Note:** Combination with pyrazinamide should not generally be offered.

Dosage Forms
Capsule: 150 mg, 300 mg
Rifadin®: 150 mg, 300 mg
Injection, powder for reconstitution: 600 mg
Rifadin®: 600 mg

rifampin and isoniazid (rif AM pin & eye soe NYE a zid)

Sound-Alike/Look-Alike Issues
Rifamate® may be confused with rifampin
Synonyms isoniazid and rifampin
U.S./Canadian Brand Names IsonaRif™ [US]; Rifamate® [US/Can]
Therapeutic Category Antibiotic, Miscellaneous
Use Management of active tuberculosis; see individual agents for additional information
Usual Dosage Oral: 2 capsules/day
Dosage Forms
Capsule:
IsonaRif™, Rifamate®: 300/150: Rifampin 300 mg and isoniazid 150 mg

rifampin, isoniazid, and pyrazinamide
(rif AM pin, eye soe NYE a zid, & peer a ZIN a mide)

Sound-Alike/Look-Alike Issues
Rifater® may be confused with Rifadin®
Synonyms isoniazid, pyrazinamide, and rifampin; pyrazinamide, rifampin, and isoniazid
U.S./Canadian Brand Names Rifater® [US/Can]
Therapeutic Category Antibiotic, Miscellaneous
Use Initial phase, short-course treatment of pulmonary tuberculosis; see individual agents for additional information
Usual Dosage Oral: Children ≥15 years and Adults: Tuberculosis: Patients weighing:
≤44 kg: 4 tablets once daily
45-54 kg: 5 tablets once daily
≥55 kg: 6 tablets once daily
Dosage Forms
Tablet:
Rifater®: Rifampin 120 mg, isoniazid 50 mg, and pyrazinamide 300 mg

rifapentine (rif a PEN teen)

Sound-Alike/Look-Alike Issues
rifapentine may be confused with rifampin
U.S./Canadian Brand Names Priftin® [US/Can]
Therapeutic Category Antitubercular Agent
Use Treatment of pulmonary tuberculosis; rifapentine must always be used in conjunction with at least one other antituberculosis drug to which the isolate is susceptible; it may also be necessary to add a third agent (either streptomycin or ethambutol) until susceptibility is known.
Usual Dosage
Children: No dosing information available
Adults: **Rifapentine should not be used alone**; initial phase should include a 3- to 4-drug regimen
Intensive phase (initial 2 months) of short-term therapy: 600 mg (four 150 mg tablets) given twice weekly (with an interval of not less than 72 hours between doses); following the intensive phase, treatment should continue with rifapentine 600 mg once weekly for 4 months in combination with INH or appropriate agent for susceptible organisms
Dosage Forms
Tablet:
Priftin®: 150 mg

Rifater® [US/Can] *see* rifampin, isoniazid, and pyrazinamide *on page* 867

rifaximin (rif AX i min)

Sound-Alike/Look-Alike Issues
rifaximin may be confused with rifampin

U.S./Canadian Brand Names Xifaxan™ [US]
Therapeutic Category Antibiotic, Miscellaneous
Use Treatment of traveler's diarrhea caused by noninvasive strains of *E. coli*
Usual Dosage Oral: Children ≥12 years and Adults: Traveler's diarrhea: 200 mg 3 times/day for 3 days
Dosage Forms
Tablet:
Xifaxan™: 200 mg

rIFN beta-1a *see* interferon beta-1a *on page 535*
rIFN beta-1b *see* interferon beta-1b *on page 536*
RIG *see* rabies immune globulin (human) *on page 848*
rIL-11 *see* oprelvekin *on page 728*

rilonacept (ri LON a sept)

U.S./Canadian Brand Names Arcalyst™ [US]
Therapeutic Category Interleukin-1 Inhibitor
Use Orphan drug: Treatment of cryopyrin-associated periodic syndromes (CAPS) including familial cold autoinflammatory syndrome (FCAS) and Muckle-Wells syndrome (MWS)
Usual Dosage SubQ: Cryopyrin-associated periodic syndromes:
Children ≥12 years: Loading dose 4.4 mg/kg (maximum dose: 320 mg) given as 1-2 separate injections (maximum: 2 mL/injection) on the same day, followed by 2.2 mg/kg (maximum dose: 160 mg) once weekly. **Note:** Do not administer more frequently than once weekly.
Adults: Loading dose 320 mg given as 2 separate injections (160 mg each) on the same day at 2 different sites, followed a week later by 160 mg, then once weekly. **Note:** Do not administer more frequently than once weekly.
Dosage Forms
Injection, powder for reconstitution:
Arcalyst™: 220 mg

Rilutek® [US/Can] *see* riluzole *on page 868*

riluzole (RIL yoo zole)

Synonyms 2-amino-6-trifluoromethoxy-benzothiazole; RP-54274
U.S./Canadian Brand Names Rilutek® [US/Can]
Therapeutic Category Miscellaneous Product
Use Treatment of amyotrophic lateral sclerosis (ALS); riluzole can extend survival or time to tracheostomy
Usual Dosage Oral: Adults: 50 mg every 12 hours; no increased benefit can be expected from higher daily doses, but adverse events are increased
Dosage Forms
Tablet:
Rilutek®: 50 mg

rimabotulinumtoxinB (rime uh BOT yoo lin num TOKS in bee)

Synonyms botulinum toxin type B
U.S./Canadian Brand Names Myobloc® [US]
Therapeutic Category Neuromuscular Blocker Agent, Toxin
Use Treatment of cervical dystonia (spasmodic torticollis)
Usual Dosage I.M.: Adults: Cervical dystonia: Initial: 2500-5000 units divided among the affected muscles in patients **previously treated** with botulinum toxin; initial dose in **previously untreated** patients should be lower. Subsequent dosing should be optimized according to patient's response.
Dosage Forms
Injection, solution [preservative free]:
Myobloc®: 5000 units/mL (0.5 mL, 1 mL, 2 mL)

rimantadine (ri MAN ta deen)

Sound-Alike/Look-Alike Issues
rimantadine may be confused with amantadine, ranitidine, Rimactane®
Flumadine® may be confused with fludarabine, flunisolide, flutamide
Synonyms rimantadine hydrochloride

U.S./Canadian Brand Names Flumadine® [US/Can]

Therapeutic Category Antiviral Agent

Use Prophylaxis (adults and children >1 year of age) and treatment (adults) of influenza A viral infection (per manufacturer labeling; also refer to current ACIP guidelines for recommendations during current flu season)

Note: In certain circumstances, the ACIP recommends use of rimantadine in combination with oseltamivir for the treatment or prophylaxis of influenza A infection when resistance to oseltamivir is suspected.

Usual Dosage Oral:

Prophylaxis:

Children 1-10 years: CDC recommendation: 5 mg/kg/day in 2 divided doses; maximum: 150 mg/day

Children >10 years and Adults: 100 mg twice daily

Treatment: Adults: 100 mg twice daily

Dosage Forms

Tablet: 100 mg

Flumadine®: 100 mg

rimantadine hydrochloride *see* rimantadine *on page 868*

rimexolone (ri MEKS oh lone)

Sound-Alike/Look-Alike Issues

Vexol® may be confused with VoSol®

U.S./Canadian Brand Names Vexol® [US/Can]

Therapeutic Category Adrenal Corticosteroid

Use Treatment of inflammation after ocular surgery and the treatment of anterior uveitis

Usual Dosage Ophthalmic: Adults: Instill 1 drop in conjunctival sac 2-4 times/day up to every 4 hours; may use every 1-2 hours during first 1-2 days

Dosage Forms

Suspension, ophthalmic:

Vexol®: 1% (5 mL, 10 mL)

Rimso®-50 [US/Can] *see* dimethyl sulfoxide *on page 314*

Rinate™ Pediatric [US] *see* chlorpheniramine and phenylephrine *on page 214*

Rindal HD Plus [US] *see* phenylephrine, hydrocodone, and chlorpheniramine *on page 778*

Rindal HPD *(Discontinued)*

Riobin® *(Discontinued)* *see* riboflavin *on page 865*

Riomet® [US] *see* metformin *on page 633*

Riopan® Plus *(Discontinued)* *see* magaldrate and simethicone *on page 606*

Riopan® Plus Double Strength *(Discontinued)* *see* magaldrate and simethicone *on page 606*

risedronate (ris ED roe nate)

Sound-Alike/Look-Alike Issues

risedronate may be confused with alendronate

Actonel® may be confused with Actos®

Synonyms risedronate sodium

U.S./Canadian Brand Names Actonel® [US/Can]

Therapeutic Category Bisphosphonate Derivative

Use Treatment of Paget disease of the bone; treatment and prevention of glucocorticoid-induced osteoporosis; treatment and prevention of osteoporosis in postmenopausal women; treatment of osteoporosis in men

Usual Dosage Oral: Adults:

Paget disease of bone: 30 mg once daily for 2 months

Retreatment may be considered (following post-treatment observation of at least 2 months) if relapse occurs, or if treatment fails to normalize serum alkaline phosphatase. For retreatment, the dose and duration of therapy are the same as for initial treatment. No data are available on more than one course of retreatment.

Osteoporosis (postmenopausal) prevention and treatment: 5 mg once daily **or** 35 mg once weekly **or** one 75 mg tablet taken on 2 consecutive days once a month (total of 2 tablets/month) **or** 150 mg once a month

Osteoporosis (male) treatment: 35 mg once weekly

Osteoporosis (glucocorticoid-induced) prevention and treatment: 5 mg once daily

Dosage Forms

Tablet:

Actonel®: 5 mg, 30 mg, 35 mg, 150 mg

risedronate and calcium (ris ED roe nate & KAL see um)

Sound-Alike/Look-Alike Issues

Actonel® may be confused with Actos®

Synonyms calcium and risedronate; risedronate sodium and calcium carbonate

U.S./Canadian Brand Names Actonel® and Calcium [US]

Therapeutic Category Bisphosphonate Derivative; Calcium Salt

Use Treatment and prevention of osteoporosis in postmenopausal women

Usual Dosage Oral: Adults: Osteoporosis in postmenopausal females:

Risedronate: 35 mg once weekly on day 1 of 7-day treatment cycle

Calcium carbonate: 1250 mg (elemental calcium 500 mg) once daily on days 2 through 7 of 7-day treatment cycle

Dosage Forms

Combination package [each package contains]:

Actonel® and Calcium:

Tablet (Actonel®): Risedronate 35 mg (4s)

Tablet: Calcium 1250 mg (24s)

risedronate sodium *see* risedronate *on page 869*

risedronate sodium and calcium carbonate *see* risedronate and calcium *on page 870*

Risperdal® [US/Can] *see* risperidone *on page 870*

Risperdal® M-Tab® [US/Can] *see* risperidone *on page 870*

Risperdal® Consta® [US/Can] *see* risperidone *on page 870*

risperidone (ris PER i done)

Sound-Alike/Look-Alike Issues

risperidone may be confused with reserpine, ropinirole

Risperdal® may be confused with lisinopril, reserpine, Restoril™

U.S./Canadian Brand Names Apo-Risperidone® [Can]; CO Risperidone [Can]; Dom-Risperidone [Can]; Gen-Risperidone [Can]; Novo-Risperidone [Can]; PHL-Risperidone [Can]; PMS-Risperidone ODT [Can]; PRO-Risperidone [Can]; Ran-Risperidone [Can]; Ratio-Risperidone [Can]; Risperdal® Consta® [US/Can]; Risperdal® M-Tab® [US/Can]; Risperdal® [US/Can]; Riva-Risperidone [Can]; Sandoz Risperidone [Can]; ZYM-Risperidone [Can]

Therapeutic Category Antipsychotic Agent, Benzisoxazole

Use

Oral: Treatment of schizophrenia; treatment of acute mania or mixed episodes associated with bipolar I disorder (as monotherapy in children or adults, or in combination with lithium or valproate in adults); treatment of irritability/aggression associated with autistic disorder

Injection: Treatment of schizophrenia; maintenance treatment of bipolar I disorder in adults as monotherapy or in combination with lithium or valproate

Usual Dosage

Oral:

Children ≥5 years and Adolescents: Autism:

<15 kg: Use with caution; specific dosing recommendations not available

<20 kg: Initial: 0.25 mg/day; may increase dose to 0.5 mg/day after ≥4 days, maintain dose for ≥14 days. In patients not achieving sufficient clinical response, may increase dose by 0.25 mg/day in ≥2-week intervals. Therapeutic effect reached plateau at 1 mg/day in clinical trials. Following clinical response, consider gradually lowering dose. May be administered once daily or in divided doses twice daily.

≥20 kg: Initial: 0.5 mg/day; may increase dose to 1 mg/day after ≥4 days, maintain dose for ≥14 days. In patients not achieving sufficient clinical response, may increase dose by 0.5 mg/day in ≥2-week intervals. Therapeutic effect reached plateau at 2.5 mg/day (3 mg/day in children >45 kg) in clinical trials. Following clinical response, consider gradually lowering dose. May be administered once daily or in divided doses twice daily.

Children and Adolescents:

Schizophrenia: Adolescents 13-17 years: Initial: 0.5 mg once daily; dose may be adjusted in increments of 0.5-1 mg/day at intervals ≥24 hours to a dose of 3 mg/day. Doses ranging from 1-6 mg/day have been evaluated, however, doses >3 mg/day do not confer additional benefit and are associated with increased adverse events.

Bipolar disorder: Children and Adolescents 10-17 years: Initial: 0.5 mg once daily; dose may be adjusted in increments of 0.5-1 mg/day at intervals ≥24 hours to a dose of 2.5 mg/day. Doses ranging from 0.5-6 mg/day have been evaluated, however doses >2.5 mg/day do not confer additional benefit and are associated with increased adverse events.

Adults:

Schizophrenia:

Initial: 1 mg twice daily; may be increased by 1-2 mg/day at intervals ≥24 hours to a recommended dosage range of 4-8 mg/day; may be given as a single daily dose once maintenance dose is achieved; daily dosages >6 mg do not appear to confer any additional benefit, and the incidence of extrapyramidal symptoms is higher than with lower doses. Further dose adjustments should be made in increments/decrements of 1-2 mg/day on a weekly basis. Dose range studied in clinical trials: 4-16 mg/day.

Maintenance: Recommended dosage range: 2-8 mg/day

Bipolar mania:

Initial: 2-3 mg once daily; if needed, adjust dose by 1 mg/day in intervals ≥24 hours; dosing range: 1-6 mg/day

Maintenance: No dosing recommendation available for treatment >3 weeks duration.

I.M.: Adults: Schizophrenia, bipolar I maintenance (Risperdal® Consta®): 25 mg every 2 weeks; some patients may benefit from larger doses; maximum dose not to exceed 50 mg every 2 weeks. Dosage adjustments should not be made more frequently than every 4 weeks. A lower initial dose of 12.5 mg may be appropriate in some patients.

Note: Oral risperidone (or other antipsychotic) should be administered with the initial injection of Risperdal® Consta® and continued for 3 weeks (then discontinued) to maintain adequate therapeutic plasma concentrations prior to main release phase of risperidone from injection site. When switching from depot administration to a short-acting formulation, administer short-acting agent in place of the next regularly-scheduled depot injection.

Dosage Forms

Injection, microspheres for reconstitution, extended release:

Risperdal® Consta®: 12.5 mg, 25 mg, 37.5 mg, 50 mg

Solution, oral: 1 mg/mL (30 mL)

Risperdal®: 1 mg/mL

Tablet: 0.25 mg, 0.5 mg, 1 mg, 2 mg, 3 mg, 4 mg

Risperdal®: 0.25 mg, 0.5 mg, 1 mg, 2 mg, 3 mg, 4 mg

Tablet, orally disintegrating: 0.25 mg, 0.5 mg, 1 mg, 2 mg, 3 mg, 4 mg

Risperdal® M-Tab®: 0.5 mg, 1 mg, 2 mg, 3 mg, 4 mg

Ritalin® [US/Can] *see* methylphenidate *on page* 645

Ritalin LA® [US] *see* methylphenidate *on page* 645

Ritalin-SR® [US/Can] *see* methylphenidate *on page* 645

ritonavir (ri TOE na veer)

Sound-Alike/Look-Alike Issues

ritonavir may be confused with Retrovir®

Norvir® may be confused with Norvasc®

U.S./Canadian Brand Names Norvir® SEC [Can]; Norvir® [US/Can]

Therapeutic Category Antiviral Agent

Use Treatment of HIV infection; should always be used as part of a multidrug regimen (at least three antiretroviral agents); may be used as a pharmacokinetic "booster" for other protease inhibitors

Usual Dosage Oral: Treatment of HIV infection:

Children >1 month: 350-400 mg/m^2 twice daily (maximum dose: 600 mg twice daily). Initiate dose at 250 mg/m^2 twice daily; titrate dose upward every 2-3 days by 50 mg/m^2 twice daily.

Adults: 600 mg twice daily; dose escalation tends to avoid nausea that many patients experience upon initiation of full dosing. Escalate the dose as follows: 300 mg twice daily for 1 day, 400 mg twice daily for 2 days, 500 mg twice daily for 1 day, then 600 mg twice daily. Ritonavir may be better tolerated when used in combination with other antiretrovirals by initiating the drug alone and subsequently adding the second agent within 2 weeks.

Dosage Forms

Capsule, soft gelatin:

Norvir®: 100 mg

Solution:

Norvir®: 80 mg/mL

ritonavir and lopinavir *see* lopinavir and ritonavir *on page* 598

Rituxan® [US/Can] *see* rituximab *on page* 872

rituximab (ri TUK si mab)

Sound-Alike/Look-Alike Issues

riTUXimab may be confused with inFLIXimab

Rituxan® may be confused with Remicade®

Synonyms anti-CD20 monoclonal antibody; C2B8 monoclonal antibody; IDEC-C2B8; NSC-687451

Tall-Man riTUXimab

U.S./Canadian Brand Names Rituxan® [US/Can]

Therapeutic Category Antineoplastic Agent

Use Treatment of low-grade or follicular CD20-positive, B-cell non-Hodgkin lymphoma (NHL); treatment of diffuse large B-cell CD20-positive NHL; treatment of moderately- to severely-active rheumatoid arthritis (RA) in combination with methotrexate

Usual Dosage Note: Pretreatment with acetaminophen and an antihistamine is recommended.

Adults: I.V. infusion (refer to individual protocols):

NHL (relapsed/refractory, low-grade or follicular CD20-positive, B-cell): 375 mg/m^2 once weekly for 4 or 8 doses

Retreatment following disease progression: 375 mg/m^2 once weekly for 4 doses

NHL (diffuse large B-cell): 375 mg/m^2 given on day 1 of each chemotherapy cycle for up to 8 doses

NHL (follicular, CD20-positive, B-cell, previously untreated): 375 mg/m^2 given on day 1 of each chemotherapy cycle for up to 8 doses

NHL (nonprogressing, low-grade, CD20-positive, B-cell, after first line CVP): 375 mg/m^2 once weekly for 4 doses every 6 months for up to 4 cycles (initiate after 6-8 cycles of chemotherapy are completed)

Rheumatoid arthritis: 1000 mg on days 1 and 15 in combination with methotrexate

Note: Premedication with a corticosteroid (eg, methylprednisolone 100 mg I.V.) 30 minutes prior to each rituximab dose is recommended. In clinical trials, patients received oral corticosteroids on a tapering schedule from baseline through day 16.

Combination therapy with ibritumomab: 250 mg/m^2 I.V. day 1; repeat in 7-9 days with ibritumomab (also see Ibritumomab monograph):

Dosage Forms

Injection, solution [preservative free]:

Rituxan®: 10 mg/mL (10 mL, 50 mL)

Riva-Alendronate [Can] *see* alendronate *on page* 44

Riva-Amiodarone [Can] *see* amiodarone *on page* 64

Riva-Atenolol [Can] *see* atenolol *on page* 107

Riva-Azithromycin [Can] *see* azithromycin *on page* 116

Riva-Buspirone [Can] *see* buspirone *on page* 160

Riva-Ciprofloxacin [Can] *see* ciprofloxacin *on page* 229

Riva-Citalopram [Can] *see* citalopram *on page* 234

Riva-Clindamycin [Can] *see* clindamycin *on page* 239

Riva-Diclofenac [Can] *see* diclofenac *on page* 303

Riva-Diclofenac-K [Can] *see* diclofenac *on page* 303

Riva-Dicyclomine [Can] *see* dicyclomine *on page* 305

Riva-Enalapril [Can] *see* enalapril *on page* 352

Riva-Famotidine [Can] *see* famotidine *on page* 405

Riva-Fenofibrate Micro [Can] *see* fenofibrate *on page* 408

Riva-Fluconazole [Can] *see* fluconazole *on page* 424

Riva-Fluoxetine [Can] *see* fluoxetine *on page* 432

Riva-Fluvox [Can] *see* fluvoxamine *on page* 439

Riva-Fosinopril [Can] *see* fosinopril *on page* 446

Riva-Gabapentin [Can] *see* gabapentin *on page* 450

Riva-Indapamide [Can] *see* indapamide *on page 525*
Riva-Lisinopril [Can] *see* lisinopril *on page 593*
Riva-Loperamine [Can] *see* loperamide *on page 597*
Riva-Lorazepam [Can] *see* lorazepam *on page 599*
Riva-Lovastatin [Can] *see* lovastatin *on page 602*
Riva-Metformin [Can] *see* metformin *on page 633*
Riva-Metoprolol [Can] *see* metoprolol *on page 650*
Riva-Mirtazapine [Can] *see* mirtazapine *on page 661*
Riva-Naproxen [Can] *see* naproxen *on page 681*
Rivanase AQ [Can] *see* beclomethasone *on page 125*
Riva-Norfloxacin [Can] *see* norfloxacin *on page 705*
Riva-Oxazepam [Can] *see* oxazepam *on page 734*
Riva-Oxybutynin [Can] *see* oxybutynin *on page 736*
Riva-Pantoprazole [Can] *see* pantoprazole *on page 748*
Riva-Pravastatin [Can] *see* pravastatin *on page 811*
Riva-Quetiapine [Can] *see* quetiapine *on page 844*
Riva-Ranitidine [Can] *see* ranitidine *on page 852*
Riva-Risperidone [Can] *see* risperidone *on page 870*

rivaroxaban *(Canada only)* (riv a ROX a ban)

Synonyms BAY 59-7939

U.S./Canadian Brand Names Xarelto® [Can]

Therapeutic Category Factor Xa Inhibitor

Use Postoperative thromboprophylaxis in patients who have undergone elective total hip or knee replacement procedures

Usual Dosage Oral: **Note:** Therapy should not be initiated until hemostasis has been established.

Adults: Postoperative thromboprophylaxis:

Knee replacement: 10 mg once daily; initial dose should be administered within 6-10 hours after completion of surgery and establishment of hemostasis (total duration of therapy: 14 days)

Hip replacement: 10 mg once daily; initial dose should be administered within 6-10 hours after completion of surgery and establishment of hemostasis (total duration of therapy: 35 days)

Dosage Forms [CAN] = Canadian brand name

Tablet:

Xarelto® [CAN]: 10 mg [not available in U.S.]

Riva-Sertraline [Can] *see* sertraline *on page 898*
Riva-Simvastatin [Can] *see* simvastatin *on page 902*
Rivasol [Can] *see* zinc sulfate *on page 1031*
Riva-Sotalol [Can] *see* sotalol *on page 919*

rivastigmine (ri va STIG meen)

Synonyms ENA 713; rivastigmine tartrate; SDZ ENA 713

U.S./Canadian Brand Names Exelon® [US/Can]; PMS-Rivastigmine [Can]; Sandoz-Rivastigmine [Can]

Therapeutic Category Acetylcholinesterase Inhibitor; Cholinergic Agent

Use Treatment of mild-to-moderate dementia associated with Alzheimer disease or Parkinson disease

Usual Dosage Adults:

Oral: **Note:** Exelon® oral solution and capsules are bioequivalent.

Mild-to-moderate Alzheimer dementia: Initial: 1.5 mg twice daily; may increase by 3 mg/day (1.5 mg/dose) every 2 weeks based on tolerability (maximum recommended dose: 6 mg twice daily)

Note: If GI adverse events occur, discontinue treatment for several doses then restart at the same or next lower dosage level; antiemetics have been used to control GI symptoms. If treatment is interrupted for longer than several days, restart the treatment at the lowest dose and titrate as previously described.

Mild-to-moderate Parkinson-related dementia: Initial: 1.5 mg twice daily; may increase by 3 mg/day (1.5 mg/dose) every 4 weeks based on tolerability (maximum recommended dose: 6 mg twice daily) ▶

Transdermal patch: Mild-to-moderate Alzheimer- or Parkinson-related dementia:
Initial: 4.6 mg/24 hours; if well tolerated, may be increased (after at least 4 weeks) to 9.5 mg/24 hours (recommended effective dose)
Maintenance: 9.5 mg/24 hours (maximum dose: 9.5 mg/24 hours)
Note: If intolerance is noted (nausea, vomiting), patch should be removed and treatment interrupted for several days and restarted at the same or lower dosage. If interrupted for more than several days, reinitiate at lowest dosage and increase to maintenance dose after 4 weeks.
Conversion from oral therapy: If oral daily dose <6 mg, switch to 4.6 mg/24 hours patch; if oral daily dose 6-12 mg, switch to 9.5 mg/24 hours patch. Apply patch on the next day following last oral dose.

Dosage Forms
Capsule:
Exelon®: 1.5 mg, 3 mg, 4.5 mg, 6 mg
Solution, oral:
Exelon®: 2 mg/mL
Transdermal system [once-daily patch]:
Exelon®: 4.6 mg/24hours (30s); 9.5 mg/24hours (30s)

rivastigmine tartrate *see* rivastigmine *on page 873*
Riva-Sumatriptan [Can] *see* sumatriptan *on page 932*
Riva-Valacyclovir [Can] *see* valacyclovir *on page 1001*
Riva-Venlafaxine XR [Can] *see* venlafaxine *on page 1009*
Riva-Verapamil SR [Can] *see* verapamil *on page 1010*
Riva-Zide [Can] *see* hydrochlorothiazide and triamterene *on page 500*
Riva-Zopiclone [Can] *see* zopiclone *(Canada only) on page 1034*
Rivotril® [Can] *see* clonazepam *on page 245*

rizatriptan (rye za TRIP tan)

Synonyms MK462
U.S./Canadian Brand Names Maxalt RPD™ [Can]; Maxalt-MLT® [US]; Maxalt® [US/Can]
Therapeutic Category Antimigraine Agent; Serotonin Agonist
Use Acute treatment of migraine with or without aura
Usual Dosage Note: In patients with risk factors for coronary artery disease, following adequate evaluation to establish the absence of coronary artery disease, the initial dose should be administered in a setting where response may be evaluated (physician's office or similarly staffed setting). ECG monitoring may be considered.
Oral: 5-10 mg, repeat after 2 hours if significant relief is not attained; maximum: 30 mg in a 24-hour period (use 5 mg dose in patients receiving propranolol with a maximum of 15 mg in 24 hours)
Note: For orally-disintegrating tablets (Maxalt-MLT®): Patient should be instructed to place tablet on tongue and allow to dissolve. Dissolved tablet will be swallowed with saliva.

Dosage Forms
Tablet:
Maxalt®: 5 mg, 10 mg
Tablet, orally disintegrating:
Maxalt-MLT®: 5 mg, 10 mg

rLFN-α2 *see* interferon alfa-2b *on page 534*
R-modafinil *see* armodafinil *on page 98*
RMS® *(Discontinued)* *see* morphine sulfate *on page 667*
Ro 5488 *see* tretinoin (systemic) *on page 980*
Robafen® AC [US] *see* guaifenesin and codeine *on page 473*
Robafen® CF *(Discontinued)*
Robafen Cough [US-OTC] *see* dextromethorphan *on page 295*
Robafen DM [US-OTC] *see* guaifenesin and dextromethorphan *on page 474*
Robafen DM Clear [US-OTC] *see* guaifenesin and dextromethorphan *on page 474*
Robaxin® [US/Can] *see* methocarbamol *on page 638*
Robidrine® [Can] *see* pseudoephedrine *on page 833*
Robinul® [US] *see* glycopyrrolate *on page 469*
Robinul® Forte [US] *see* glycopyrrolate *on page 469*
Robitussin® [US-OTC/Can] *see* guaifenesin *on page 473*

Robitussin® A-C ***(Discontinued)*** *see* guaifenesin and codeine *on page* *473*
Robitussin® Childrens Cough & Cold [Can] *see* pseudoephedrine and dextromethorphan *on page* *834*
Robitussin® Children's Cough Long Acting [US-OTC] *see* dextromethorphan *on page* *295*
Robitussin® Children's Cough & Cold Long-Acting [US-OTC] *see* dextromethorphan and chlorpheniramine *on page* *296*
Robitussin® Cold and Cough CF [US-OTC] *see* guaifenesin, dextromethorphan, and phenylephrine *on page* *478*
Robitussin® Cough and Allergy ***(Discontinued)*** *see* chlorpheniramine, phenylephrine, and dextromethorphan *on page* *217*
Robitussin® Cough and Cold [US-OTC/Can] *see* guaifenesin, pseudoephedrine, and dextromethorphan *on page* *479*
Robitussin® Cough and Cold CF [US-OTC] *see* guaifenesin, pseudoephedrine, and dextromethorphan *on page* *479*
Robitussin® Cough and Cold Infant CF [US-OTC] *see* guaifenesin, pseudoephedrine, and dextromethorphan *on page* *479*
Robitussin® Cough and Cold Nighttime [US-OTC] *see* chlorpheniramine, phenylephrine, and dextromethorphan *on page* *217*
Robitussin® Cough and Congestion [US-OTC] *see* guaifenesin and dextromethorphan *on page* *474*
Robitussin® Cough & Cold Long-Acting [US-OTC] *see* dextromethorphan and chlorpheniramine *on page* *296*
Robitussin® CoughGels™ [US-OTC] *see* dextromethorphan *on page* *295*
Robitussin® Cough Long-Acting [US-OTC] *see* dextromethorphan *on page* *295*
Robitussin®-DAC ***(Discontinued)*** *see* guaifenesin, pseudoephedrine, and codeine *on page* *479*
Robitussin® DM [US-OTC/Can] *see* guaifenesin and dextromethorphan *on page* *474*
Robitussin® DM Infant ***(Discontinued)*** *see* guaifenesin and dextromethorphan *on page* *474*
Robitussin® Maximum Strength Cough & Cold ***(Discontinued)*** *see* pseudoephedrine and dextromethorphan *on page* *834*
Robitussin® Night Time Cough & Cold [US-OTC] *see* diphenhydramine and phenylephrine *on page* *317*
Robitussin® Pediatric Cold and Cough CF [US-OTC] *see* guaifenesin, dextromethorphan, and phenylephrine *on page* *478*
Robitussin® Pediatric Cough and Cold Nighttime [US-OTC] *see* chlorpheniramine, phenylephrine, and dextromethorphan *on page* *217*
Robitussin® Pediatric Cough & Cold ***(Discontinued)*** *see* pseudoephedrine and dextromethorphan *on page* *834*
Robitussin® Pediatric Cough ***(Discontinued)*** *see* dextromethorphan *on page* *295*
Robitussin® Pediatric Night Relief ***(Discontinued)*** *see* chlorpheniramine, pseudoephedrine, and dextromethorphan *on page* *220*
Robitussin-PE® ***(Discontinued)*** *see* guaifenesin and pseudoephedrine *on page* *477*
Robitussin® Severe Congestion ***(Discontinued)*** *see* guaifenesin and pseudoephedrine *on page* *477*
Robitussin® Sugar Free Cough [US-OTC] *see* guaifenesin and dextromethorphan *on page* *474*
Rocaltrol® [US/Can] *see* calcitriol *on page* *168*
Rocephin® [US/Can] *see* ceftriaxone *on page* *198*

rocuronium (roe kyoor OH nee um)

Sound-Alike/Look-Alike Issues

Zemuron® may be confused with Remeron®

Synonyms ORG 946; rocuronium bromide

U.S./Canadian Brand Names Zemuron® [US/Can]

Therapeutic Category Skeletal Muscle Relaxant

Use Facilitate both rapid sequence and routine endotracheal intubation and to relax skeletal muscles during surgery; to facilitate mechanical ventilation in ICU patients

Usual Dosage Administer I.V.; dose to effect; doses will vary due to interpatient variability; use ideal body weight for obese patients

Children ≥3 months:

Initial: 0.6 mg/kg under halothane anesthesia produce excellent to good intubating conditions within 1 minute and will provide a median time of 41 minutes of clinical relaxation in children 3 months to 1 year of age, and 27 minutes in children 1-12 years

Maintenance: 0.075-0.125 mg/kg administered upon return of T_1 to 25% of control provides clinical relaxation for 7-10 minutes

Adults:

Tracheal intubation: I.V.:

Initial: 0.6 mg/kg is expected to provide approximately 31 minutes of clinical relaxation under opioid/nitrous oxide/oxygen anesthesia with neuromuscular block sufficient for intubation attained in 1-2 minutes; lower doses (0.45 mg/kg) may be used to provide 22 minutes of clinical relaxation with median time to neuromuscular block of 1-3 minutes; maximum blockade is achieved in <4 minutes

Maximum: 0.9-1.2 mg/kg may be given during surgery under opioid/nitrous oxide/oxygen anesthesia without adverse cardiovascular effects and is expected to provide 58-67 minutes of clinical relaxation; neuromuscular blockade sufficient for intubation is achieved in <2 minutes with maximum blockade in <3 minutes

Maintenance: 0.1, 0.15, and 0.2 mg/kg administered at 25% recovery of control T_1 (defined as 3 twitches of train-of-four) provides a median of 12, 17, and 24 minutes of clinical duration under anesthesia

Rapid sequence intubation: 0.6-1.2 mg/kg in appropriately premedicated and anesthetized patients with excellent or good intubating conditions within 2 minutes

Continuous infusion: Initial: 0.01-0.012 mg/kg/minute only after early evidence of spontaneous recovery of neuromuscular function is evident; infusion rates have ranged from 4-16 mcg/kg/minute

ICU: 10 mcg/kg/minute; adjust dose to maintain appropriate degree of neuromuscular blockade (eg, 1 or 2 twitches on train-of-four)

Dosage Forms

Injection, solution: 10 mg/mL (5 mL, 10 mL)

Zemuron®: 10 mg/mL (5 mL, 10 mL)

rocuronium bromide *see* rocuronium *on page 875*

Rofact™ [Can] *see* rifampin *on page 866*

Roferon®-A *(Discontinued)*

Rogaine® [Can] *see* minoxidil *on page 660*

Rogaine® Extra Strength for Men [US-OTC] *see* minoxidil *on page 660*

Rogaine® for Men [US-OTC] *see* minoxidil *on page 660*

Rogaine® for Women [US-OTC] *see* minoxidil *on page 660*

Rogitine® [Can] *see* phentolamine *on page 774*

Rolaids® [US-OTC] *see* calcium carbonate and magnesium hydroxide *on page 171*

Rolaids® Extra Strength [US-OTC] *see* calcium carbonate and magnesium hydroxide *on page 171*

Rolaids® Softchews [US-OTC] *see* calcium carbonate *on page 170*

Rolatuss® Plain Liquid *(Discontinued)* *see* chlorpheniramine and phenylephrine *on page 214*

Romazicon® [US/Can] *see* flumazenil *on page 426*

Romilar® AC [US] *see* guaifenesin and codeine *on page 473*

romiplostim (roe mi PLOE stim)

Synonyms AMG 531

U.S./Canadian Brand Names Nplate™ [US/Can]

Therapeutic Category Colony-Stimulating Factor; Thrombopoietic Agent

Use Treatment of thrombocytopenia in patients with chronic immune (idiopathic) thrombocytopenia purpura (ITP) who have had insufficient response to corticosteroids, immune globulin, or splenectomy

Usual Dosage Note: Initial dose is based on actual body weight. Discontinue if platelet count does not respond to a level that avoids clinically important bleeding after 4 weeks at the maximum recommended dose.

SubQ: Adults: ITP: Initial: 1 mcg/kg once weekly; adjust dose by 1 mcg/kg/week to achieve platelet count ≥50,000/mm^3 and to reduce the risk of bleeding; Maximum: 10 mcg/kg (median dose needed to achieve response in clinical trials: 2 mcg/kg)

Dosage Forms

Injection, powder for reconstitution:

Nplate™: 250 mcg, 500 mcg

Romycin® [US] *see* erythromycin *on page 368*

Rondec® [US] *see* chlorpheniramine and phenylephrine *on page 214*

Rondec®-DM [US] *see* chlorpheniramine, phenylephrine, and dextromethorphan *on page 217*

Rondec®-DM Drops *(Discontinued)*

Rondec®-DM Syrup *(Discontinued)* *see* brompheniramine, pseudoephedrine, and dextromethorphan *on page 152*

Rondec® Drops *(Discontinued)*

Rondec® Syrup *(Discontinued)* *see* brompheniramine and pseudoephedrine *on page 150*

Rondomycin® Capsule *(Discontinued)*

ropinirole (roe PIN i role)

Sound-Alike/Look-Alike Issues

ropinirole may be confused with ropivacaine

Requip® may be confused with Reglan®

Synonyms ropinirole hydrochloride

U.S./Canadian Brand Names CO Ropinirole [Can]; PMS-Ropinirole [Can]; RAN-Ropinirole [Can]; Requip® XL™ [US]; Requip® [US/Can]

Therapeutic Category Anti-Parkinson Agent (Dopamine Agonist)

Use Treatment of idiopathic Parkinson disease; in patients with early Parkinson disease who were not receiving concomitant levodopa therapy as well as in patients with advanced disease on concomitant levodopa; treatment of moderate-to-severe primary restless legs syndrome (RLS)

Usual Dosage Oral: Adults:

Parkinson disease:

Immediate release tablet: The dosage should be increased to achieve a maximum therapeutic effect, balanced against the principal side effects of nausea, dizziness, somnolence and dyskinesia. Recommended starting dose is 0.25 mg 3 times/day; based on individual patient response, the dosage should be titrated with weekly increments as described below:

- Week 1: 0.25 mg 3 times/day; total daily dose: 0.75 mg
- Week 2: 0.5 mg 3 times/day; total daily dose: 1.5 mg
- Week 3: 0.75 mg 3 times/day; total daily dose: 2.25 mg
- Week 4: 1 mg 3 times/day; total daily dose: 3 mg

Note: After week 4, if necessary, daily dosage may be increased by 1.5 mg/day on a weekly basis up to a dose of 9 mg/day, and then by up to 3 mg/day weekly to a total of 24 mg/day

Parkinson disease discontinuation taper: Ropinirole should be gradually tapered over 7 days as follows: reduce frequency of administration from 3 times daily to twice daily for 4 days, then reduce to once daily for remaining 3 days.

Extended release tablet: Initial: 2 mg once daily for 1-2 weeks, followed by increases of 2 mg/day at weekly or longer intervals based on therapeutic response and tolerability (maximum: 24 mg/day); **Note:** When discontinuing gradually taper over 7 days.

Restless legs syndrome: Immediate release tablets: Initial: 0.25 mg once daily 1-3 hours before bedtime. Dose may be increased after 2 days to 0.5 mg daily, and after 7 days to 1 mg daily. Dose may be further titrated upward in 0.5 mg increments every week until reaching a daily dose of 3 mg during week 6. If symptoms persist or reappear, the daily dose may be increased to a maximum of 4 mg beginning week 7.

Note: Doses up to 4 mg per day may be discontinued without tapering.

Converting from ropinirole immediate release tablets to ropinirole extended release tablets: Choose a once daily extended release dose that most closely matches current immediate release daily dose.

Dosage Forms

Tablet: 0.25 mg, 0.5 mg, 1 mg, 2 mg, 3 mg, 4 mg, 5 mg

Requip®: 0.25 mg, 0.5 mg, 1 mg, 2 mg, 3 mg, 4 mg, 5 mg

Tablet, extended-release:

Requip® XL™: 2 mg, 4 mg, 6 mg, 8 mg, 12 mg

ropinirole hydrochloride *see* ropinirole *on page 877*

ropivacaine (roe PIV a kane)

Sound-Alike/Look-Alike Issues

ropivacaine may be confused with bupivacaine, ropinirole

Synonyms ropivacaine hydrochloride

U.S./Canadian Brand Names Naropin® [US/Can]

Therapeutic Category Local Anesthetic

Use Local anesthetic for use in surgery, postoperative pain management, and obstetrical procedures when local or regional anesthesia is needed

Usual Dosage Dose varies with procedure, onset and depth of anesthesia desired, vascularity of tissues, duration of anesthesia, and condition of patient: Adults:

Surgical anesthesia:

Lumbar epidural: 15-30 mL of 0.5% to 1% solution

Lumbar epidural block for cesarean section:

20-30 mL dose of 0.5% solution

15-20 mL dose of 0.75% solution

Thoracic epidural block: 5-15 mL dose of 0.5% to 0.75% solution

Major nerve block:

35-50 mL dose of 0.5% solution (175-250 mg)

10-40 mL dose of 0.75% solution (75-300 mg)

Field block: 1-40 mL dose of 0.5% solution (5-200 mg)

Labor pain management: Lumbar epidural: Initial: 10-20 mL 0.2% solution; continuous infusion dose: 6-14 mL/hour of 0.2% solution with incremental injections of 10-15 mL/hour of 0.2% solution

Postoperative pain management:

Lumbar or thoracic epidural: Continuous infusion dose: 6-14 mL/hour of 0.2% solution

Infiltration/minor nerve block:

1-100 mL dose of 0.2% solution

1-40 mL dose of 0.5% solution

Dosage Forms

Infusion:

Naropin®: 2 mg/mL (100 mL, 200 mL)

Injection, solution [preservative free]:

Naropin®: 2 mg/mL (10 mL, 20 mL); 5 mg/mL (20 mL, 30 mL); 7.5 mg/mL (20 mL); 10 mg/mL (10 mL, 20 mL)

ropivacaine hydrochloride *see* ropivacaine *on page* 877

Rosac® [US] *see* sulfur and sulfacetamide *on page* 931

Rosanil® [US] *see* sulfur and sulfacetamide *on page* 931

rosiglitazone (roh si GLI ta zone)

Sound-Alike/Look-Alike Issues

Avandia® may be confused with Avalide®, Coumadin®, Prandin®

U.S./Canadian Brand Names Avandia® [US/Can]

Therapeutic Category Hypoglycemic Agent, Oral; Thiazolidinedione Derivative

Use Type 2 diabetes mellitus (noninsulin-dependent, NIDDM):

Monotherapy: Improve glycemic control as an adjunct to diet and exercise

Note: Canadian labeling approves use as monotherapy only when metformin is contraindicated or not tolerated.

Combination therapy: **Note:** Use when diet, exercise, and a single agent do not result in adequate glycemic control.

U.S. labeling: In combination with a sulfonylurea, metformin, or sulfonylurea plus metformin

Canadian labeling: In combination with metformin; in combination with a sulfonylurea only when metformin use is contraindicated or not tolerated

Usual Dosage Oral: Adults: **Note:** All patients should be initiated at the lowest recommended dose.

Monotherapy: Initial: 4 mg daily as a single daily dose or in divided doses twice daily. If response is inadequate after 8-12 weeks of treatment, the dosage may be increased to 8 mg daily as a single daily dose or in divided doses twice daily. In clinical trials, the 4 mg twice-daily regimen resulted in the greatest reduction in fasting plasma glucose and Hb A_{1c}.

Combination therapy: When adding rosiglitazone to existing therapy, continue current dose(s) of previous agents:

U.S. labeling: With sulfonylureas or metformin (or sulfonylurea plus metformin): Initial: 4 mg daily as a single daily dose or in divided doses twice daily. If response is inadequate after 8-12 weeks of treatment, the dosage may be increased to 8 mg daily as a single daily dose or in divided doses twice daily. Reduce dose of sulfonylurea if hypoglycemia occurs. It is unlikely that the dose of metformin will need to be reduced due to hypoglycemia.

Canadian labeling:
With metformin: Initial: 4 mg daily as a single daily dose or in divided doses twice daily. If response is inadequate after 8-12 weeks of treatment, the dosage may be increased to 8 mg daily as a single daily dose or in divided doses twice daily.
With a sulfonylurea: 4 mg daily as a single daily dose or in divided doses twice daily. Dose should not exceed 4 mg daily when using in combination with a sulfonylurea. Reduce dose of sulfonylurea if hypoglycemia occurs.

Dosage Forms

Tablet:
Avandia®: 2 mg, 4 mg, 8 mg

rosiglitazone and glimepiride (roh si GLI ta zone & GLYE me pye ride)

Synonyms glimepiride and rosiglitazone maleate

U.S./Canadian Brand Names Avandaryl® [US]

Therapeutic Category Antidiabetic Agent, Sulfonylurea; Antidiabetic Agent, Thiazolidinedione

Use Management of type 2 diabetes mellitus (noninsulin-dependent, NIDDM) as an adjunct to diet and exercise

Usual Dosage Oral: Adults: Type 2 diabetes mellitus:
Initial: Rosiglitazone 4 mg and glimepiride 1 mg once daily **or** rosiglitazone 4 mg and glimepiride 2 mg once daily (for patients previously treated with sulfonylurea or thiazolidinedione monotherapy)
Patients switching from combination rosiglitazone and glimepiride as separate tablets: Use current dose
Titration:
Dose adjustment in patients previously on sulfonylurea monotherapy: May take 2 weeks to observe decreased blood glucose and 2-3 months to see full effects of rosiglitazone component. If not adequately controlled after 8-12 weeks, increase daily dose of rosiglitazone component.
Dose adjustment in patients previously on thiazolidinedione monotherapy: If not adequately controlled after 1-2 weeks, increase daily dose of glimepiride component in ≤2 mg increments in 1-2 week intervals.
Maximum dose:
U.S. labeling: Rosiglitazone 8 mg and glimepiride 4 mg once daily
Canadian labeling: Rosiglitazone 4 mg and glimepiride 4 mg once daily

Dosage Forms

Tablet:
Avandaryl®: 4 mg/1 mg: Rosiglitazone 4 mg and glimepiride 1 mg; 4 mg/2 mg: Rosiglitazone 4 mg and glimepiride 2 mg; 4 mg/4 mg: Rosiglitazone 4 mg and glimepiride 4 mg; 8 mg/2 mg: Rosiglitazone 8 mg and glimepiride 2 mg; 8 mg/4 mg: Rosiglitazone 8 mg and glimepiride 4 mg

rosiglitazone and metformin (roh si GLI ta zone & met FOR min)

Sound-Alike/Look-Alike Issues
Avandamet® may be confused with Anzemet®

Synonyms metformin and rosiglitazone; metformin hydrochloride and rosiglitazone maleate; rosiglitazone maleate and metformin hydrochloride

U.S./Canadian Brand Names Avandamet® [US/Can]

Therapeutic Category Antidiabetic Agent (Biguanide); Antidiabetic Agent (Thiazolidinedione)

Use Management of type 2 diabetes mellitus (noninsulin-dependent, NIDDM) as an adjunct to diet and exercise in patients where dual rosiglitazone and metformin therapy is appropriate

Usual Dosage Oral: Adults: Type 2 diabetes mellitus: Daily dose should be divided and given with meals:
First-line therapy (drug-naive patients): Initial: Rosiglitazone 2 mg and metformin 500 mg once or twice daily; may increase by 2 mg/500 mg per day after 4 weeks to a maximum of 8 mg/2000 mg per day.
Second-line therapy:
Patients inadequately controlled on **metformin alone**: Initial dose: Rosiglitazone 4 mg/day plus current dose of metformin
Patients inadequately controlled on **rosiglitazone alone**: Initial dose: Metformin 1000 mg/day plus current dose of rosiglitazone
Note: When switching from combination rosiglitazone and metformin as separate tablets: Use current dose
Dose adjustment: Doses may be increased as increments of rosiglitazone 4 mg and/or metformin 500 mg, up to the maximum dose; doses should be titrated gradually.
After a change in the metformin dosage, titration can be done after 1-2 weeks
After a change in the rosiglitazone dosage, titration can be done after 8-12 weeks
Maximum dose: Rosiglitazone 8 mg/metformin 2000 mg daily

Dosage Forms

Tablet:

Avandamet®: 2/500: Rosiglitazone 2 mg and metformin 500 mg
Avandamet®: 4/500: Rosiglitazone 4 mg and metformin 500 mg
Avandamet®: 2/1000: Rosiglitazone 2 mg and metformin 1000 mg
Avandamet®: 4/1000: Rosiglitazone 4 mg and metformin 1000 mg

rosiglitazone maleate and metformin hydrochloride *see* rosiglitazone and metformin *on page 879*

Rosula® [US] *see* sulfur and sulfacetamide *on page 931*

Rosula® Clarifying [US] *see* sulfur and sulfacetamide *on page 931*

Rosula® NS [US] *see* sulfacetamide *on page 927*

rosuvastatin (roe soo va STAT in)

Sound-Alike/Look-Alike Issues

rosuvastatin may be confused with atorvastatin, nystatin

Synonyms rosuvastatin calcium

U.S./Canadian Brand Names Crestor® [US/Can]

Therapeutic Category Antilipemic Agent, HMG-CoA Reductase Inhibitor

Use Used with dietary therapy for hyperlipidemias to reduce elevations in total cholesterol (TC), LDL-C, apolipoprotein B, nonHDL-C, and triglycerides (TG) in patients with primary hypercholesterolemia (elevations of 1 or more components are present in Fredrickson type IIa, IIb, and IV hyperlipidemias); treatment of primary dysbetalipoproteinemia (Fredrickson type III hyperlipidemia); treatment of homozygous familial hypercholesterolemia (FH); to slow progression of atherosclerosis as an adjunct to diet to lower TC and LDL-C

Usual Dosage Oral: Adults:

Hyperlipidemia, mixed dyslipidemia, hypertriglyceridemia, slowing progression of atherosclerosis:

Initial dose:

General dosing: 10 mg once daily; 20 mg once daily may be used in patients with severe hyperlipidemia (LDL >190 mg/dL) and aggressive lipid targets

Conservative dosing: Patients requiring less aggressive treatment or predisposed to myopathy (including patients of Asian descent): 5 mg once daily

Titration: After 2 weeks, may be increased by 5-10 mg once daily; dosing range: 5-40 mg/day (maximum dose: 40 mg once daily)

Note: The 40 mg dose should be reserved for patients who have not achieved goal cholesterol levels on a dose of 20 mg/day, including patients switched from another HMG-CoA reductase inhibitor.

Homozygous familial hypercholesterolemia (FH): Initial: 20 mg once daily (maximum dose: 40 mg/day)

Dosage Forms

Tablet:

Crestor®: 5 mg, 10 mg, 20 mg, 40 mg

rosuvastatin calcium *see* rosuvastatin *on page 880*

Rotarix® [US/Can] *see* rotavirus vaccine *on page 880*

RotaShield® *(Discontinued)*

RotaTeq® [US] *see* rotavirus vaccine *on page 880*

rotavirus vaccine (ROE ta vye rus vak SEEN)

Synonyms human rotavirus vaccine, attenuated (HRV); pentavalent human-bovine reassortant rotavirus vaccine (PRV); rotavirus vaccine, pentavalent; RV1 (RotaTeq®); RV5 (Rotarix®)

U.S./Canadian Brand Names Rotarix® [US/Can]; RotaTeq® [US]

Therapeutic Category Vaccine

Use Prevention of rotavirus gastroenteritis in infants and children

The Advisory Committee on Immunization Practices (ACIP) recommends routine vaccination of all infants.

Usual Dosage Oral:

Manufacturer's labeling:

Infants 6-24 weeks of age: Rotarix®: A total of two 1mL doses, the first dose given at 6-14 weeks of age. The first and second dose should be separated by ≥4 weeks. The 2-dose series should be completed by 24 weeks of age.

Infants 6-32 weeks: RotaTeq®: A total of three 2 mL doses given at 2-, 4-, and 6 months of age; the first given at 6-12 weeks of age, followed by subsequent doses at 4- to 10-week intervals. Routine administration of the first dose at >12 weeks of age is not recommended (insufficient data). Administer all doses by 32 weeks of age. Infants who have had rotavirus gastroenteritis before getting the full course of vaccine should still initiate or complete the 3-dose schedule; initial infection provides only partial immunity.

ACIP recommendations: The first dose can be given at 6-14 weeks of age. The series should not be started in infants ≥15 weeks. The final dose in the series should be administered by 8 months 0 days of age. The minimum interval between doses is 4 weeks. A total of three doses (administered at 2-, 4-, and 6 months of age) is recommended; however, if Rotarix® is used at ages 2- and 4 months, a dose at 6 months is not indicated. For infants inadvertently administered rotavirus vaccine at ≥15 weeks of age, the vaccine series may be completed according to schedule and prior to 8 months and 0 days of age. The ACIP recommendations for vaccination recommend completing the vaccine series with the same product whenever possible. If continuing with same product will cause vaccination to be deferred, or if product used previously is unknown, vaccination should be completed with the product available. If RotaTeq® was used in any previous doses, or if the specific product used was unknown, a total of three doses should be given

Dosage Forms

Powder, for suspension, oral [preservative free; human derived]:

Rotarix®: G1P[8] ≥10^6 infectious units per 1 mL [oral applicator contains natural latex/natural rubber]

Suspension, oral [preservative free]:

RotaTeq®: G1 ≥2.2 10^6 infectious units, G2 ≥2.8 10^6 infectious units, G3 ≥2.2 10^6 infectious units, G4 ≥2 10^6 infectious units, and P1 [8] ≥2.3 10^6 infectious units per 2 mL (2 mL)

rotavirus vaccine, pentavalent *see* rotavirus vaccine *on page* *880*

rotigotine *(Discontinued)*

Rowasa® [US] *see* mesalamine *on page* *631*

Roxanol™ [US] *see* morphine sulfate *on page* *667*

Roxanol SR™ Oral *(Discontinued)* *see* morphine sulfate *on page* *667*

Roxanol™-T *(Discontinued)* *see* morphine sulfate *on page* *667*

Roxicet™ [US] *see* oxycodone and acetaminophen *on page* *738*

Roxicet™ 5/500 [US] *see* oxycodone and acetaminophen *on page* *738*

Roxicodone® [US] *see* oxycodone *on page* *737*

Roxiprin® *(Discontinued)* *see* oxycodone and aspirin *on page* *739*

Roychlor® [Can] *see* potassium chloride *on page* *803*

Rozerem® [US] *see* ramelteon *on page* *850*

RP-6976 *see* docetaxel *on page* *326*

RP-54274 *see* riluzole *on page* *868*

RP-59500 *see* quinupristin and dalfopristin *on page* *846*

r-PA *see* reteplase *on page* *860*

rPDGF-BB *see* becaplermin *on page* *124*

(R,R)-formoterol L-tartrate *see* arformoterol *on page* *95*

RS-25259 *see* palonosetron *on page* *744*

RS-25259-197 *see* palonosetron *on page* *744*

R-Tanna [US] *see* chlorpheniramine and phenylephrine *on page* *214*

R-Tanna Pediatric [US] *see* chlorpheniramine and phenylephrine *on page* *214*

RTCA *see* ribavirin *on page* *864*

RU 0211 *see* lubiprostone *on page* *603*

RU-486 *see* mifepristone *on page* *657*

RU-23908 *see* nilutamide *on page* *697*

RU-38486 *see* mifepristone *on page* *657*

rubella, measles, and mumps vaccines *see* measles, mumps, and rubella virus vaccine *on page* *615*

rubella, varicella, measles, and mumps vaccine *see* measles, mumps, rubella, and varicella virus vaccine *on page* *616*

rubella virus vaccine (live) (rue BEL a VYE rus vak SEEN, live)

Sound-Alike/Look-Alike Issues
Meruvax® II may be confused with Attenuvax®

Synonyms German measles vaccine

U.S./Canadian Brand Names Meruvax® II [US]

Therapeutic Category Vaccine, Live Virus

Use Active immunization against rubella

Note: Unless otherwise contraindicated, trivalent measles - mumps - rubella (MMR) is the vaccine of choice if recipients are likely to be susceptible to mumps and/or measles as well as to rubella.

The Advisory Committee on Immunization Practices (ACIP) recommends routine vaccination for the following:

- All children (first dose given at 12-15 months of age)
- Adults born 1957 or later (without evidence of immunity or documentation of vaccination)
- Adults at higher risk for exposure to and transmission of rubella should receive special consideration for vaccination, unless an acceptable evidence of immunity exists. This includes international travelers, persons attending colleges and other post-high school education, persons working in healthcare facilities.

Usual Dosage Note: Trivalent measles - mumps - rubella (MMR) vaccine should be used unless contraindicated in adults and children ≥12 months of age.

Children ≥12 months and Adults: SubQ: 0.5 mL. Primary vaccination recommended at 12-15 months of age and repeated at 4-6 years of age. For older children and adults not previously vaccinated, at least 28 days should elapse between doses.

Adults born in or after 1957 without documentation of immunity: A single dose is recommended for students entering colleges and other institutions of higher education, for military personal, for healthcare workers, for international travelers who visit endemic areas.

Women of childbearing potential, without documentation of immunity, regardless of birth year, should also receive one dose of the vaccine. Do not administer to women who are or who may become pregnant within 1 month of receiving vaccine; administer following completion or termination of pregnancy

Dosage Forms

Injection, powder for reconstitution [preservative free]:
Meruvax® II: ≥1000 $TCID_{50}$ (Wistar RA 27/3 Strain)

rubeola vaccine *see* measles virus vaccine (live) *on page 616*

Rubex® ***(Discontinued)*** *see* doxorubicin *on page 335*

rubidomycin hydrochloride *see* daunorubicin hydrochloride *on page 278*

Rubramin-PC® ***(Discontinued)*** *see* cyanocobalamin *on page 263*

RUF 331 *see* rufinamide *on page 882*

rufinamide (roo FIN a mide)

Synonyms CGP 33101; E 2080; RUF 331; xilep

U.S./Canadian Brand Names Banzel™ [US]

Therapeutic Category Anticonvulsant, Triazole Derivative

Use Adjunctive therapy in the treatment of generalized seizures of Lennox-Gastaut syndrome

Usual Dosage Oral: Lennox-Gastaut (adjunctive):

Children ≥4 years: Initial: 10 mg/kg/day in 2 equally divided doses; increase dose by ~10 mg/kg/day every other day to a target dose of 45 mg/kg/day or 3200 mg/day (whichever is lower) in 2 equally divided doses

Adults: Initial: 400-800 mg/day in 2 equally divided doses; increase dose by 400-800 mg/day every 2 days until maximum daily dose: 3200 mg/day in 2 equally divided doses

Dosage Forms

Tablet:
Banzel™: 200 mg, 400 mg

Ru-Hist Forte [US] *see* chlorpheniramine, pyrilamine, and phenylephrine *on page 221*

Rulox [US-OTC] *see* aluminum hydroxide and magnesium hydroxide *on page 55*

Rulox No. 1 ***(Discontinued)*** *see* aluminum hydroxide and magnesium hydroxide *on page 55*

Ru-Tuss DM [US] *see* guaifenesin, pseudoephedrine, and dextromethorphan *on page 479*

Rutuss Jr [US] *see* guaifenesin and pseudoephedrine *on page 477*

Ru-Tuss® Liquid ***(Discontinued)*** *see* chlorpheniramine and phenylephrine *on page* *214*
Ru-Vert-M® ***(Discontinued)*** *see* meclizine *on page* *619*
RV1 (RotaTeq®) *see* rotavirus vaccine *on page* *880*
RV5 (Rotarix®) *see* rotavirus vaccine *on page* *880*
Rylosol [Can] *see* sotalol *on page* *919*
Rymed® ***(Discontinued)*** *see* guaifenesin and pseudoephedrine *on page* *477*
Rymed-TR® ***(Discontinued)***
Ryna®-12 [US] *see* phenylephrine and pyrilamine *on page* *776*
Ryna-12 S® [US] *see* phenylephrine and pyrilamine *on page* *776*
Ryna-12X® [US] *see* phenylephrine, pyrilamine, and guaifenesin *on page* *779*
Ryna-C® ***(Discontinued)*** *see* chlorpheniramine, pseudoephedrine, and codeine *on page* *220*
Ryna® ***(Discontinued)*** *see* chlorpheniramine, pseudoephedrine, and codeine *on page* *220*
Rynatan® [US] *see* chlorpheniramine and phenylephrine *on page* *214*
Rynatan® Pediatric [US] *see* chlorpheniramine and phenylephrine *on page* *214*
Rynatuss® [US] *see* chlorpheniramine, ephedrine, phenylephrine, and carbetapentane *on page* *216*
Rynatuss® Pediatric ***(Discontinued)*** *see* chlorpheniramine, ephedrine, phenylephrine, and carbetapentane *on page* *216*
Rynesa 12S ***(Discontinued)*** *see* phenylephrine and pyrilamine *on page* *776*
Ry-T-12 ***(Discontinued)*** *see* phenylephrine and pyrilamine *on page* *776*
Rythmodan® [Can] *see* disopyramide *on page* *324*
Rythmodan®-LA [Can] *see* disopyramide *on page* *324*
Rythmol® [US] *see* propafenone *on page* *825*
Rythmol® Gen-Propafenone [Can] *see* propafenone *on page* *825*
Rythmol® SR [US] *see* propafenone *on page* *825*
Ryzolt™ [US] *see* tramadol *on page* *975*
Rēv-Eyes™ ***(Discontinued)***
S2® [US-OTC] *see* epinephrine *on page* *358*
S-(+)-3-isobutylgaba *see* pregabalin *on page* *815*
6(S)-5-methyltetrahydrofolate *see* methylfolate *on page* *644*
6(S)-5-MTHF *see* methylfolate *on page* *644*
S-4661 *see* doripenem *on page* *331*
Sab-Diclofenac [Can] *see* diclofenac *on page* *303*
SAB-Gentamicin [Can] *see* gentamicin *on page* *461*
Sab-Naproxen [Can] *see* naproxen *on page* *681*
Sab-Prenase [Can] *see* prednisolone (systemic) *on page* *813*
Sabril® [Can] *see* vigabatrin *(Canada only) on page* *1013*
SAB-Trifluridine [Can] *see* trifluridine *on page* *986*

Saccharomyces boulardii (sak roe MYE sees boo LAR dee)

Synonyms *S. boulardii*; *Saccharomyces boulardii lyo*

U.S./Canadian Brand Names Florastor® Kids [US-OTC]; Florastor® [US-OTC]

Therapeutic Category Dietary Supplement; Probiotic

Use Promote maintenance of normal microflora in the gastrointestinal tract; used in management of bloating, gas, and diarrhea, particularly to decrease the incidence of diarrhea associated with antibiotic use

Usual Dosage Oral: Dietary supplement: Dosing varies by manufacturer; consult product labeling.
Children (Florastor® Kids): 250 mg twice daily
Adults (Florastor®): 250 mg twice daily

Dosage Forms
Capsule, oral:
Florastor® [OTC]: *S. boulardii lyo* 250 mg
Powder, oral:
Florastor® Kids [OTC]: *S. boulardii lyo* 250 mg/packet (10s)

Saccharomyces boulardii lyo *see Saccharomyces boulardii on page* *883*

sacrosidase (sak ROE si dase)

U.S./Canadian Brand Names Sucraid® [US/Can]

Therapeutic Category Enzyme

Use **Orphan drug:** Oral replacement therapy in sucrase deficiency, as seen in congenital sucrase-isomaltase deficiency (CSID)

Usual Dosage Oral:

Infants ≥5 months and Children <15 kg: 8500 int. units (1 mL) per meal or snack

Children >15 kg and Adults: 17,000 int. units (2 mL) per meal or snack

Doses should be diluted with 2-4 oz of water, milk, or formula with each meal or snack. Approximately one-half of the dose may be taken before, and the remainder of a dose taken at the completion of each meal or snack.

Dosage Forms

Solution, oral:

Sucraid®: 8500 int. units per mL

Safetussin® CD [US-OTC] *see* dextromethorphan and phenylephrine *on page* 296
Safe Tussin® DM [US-OTC] *see* guaifenesin and dextromethorphan *on page* 474
SAHA *see* vorinostat *on page* 1022
Saizen® [US/Can] *see* somatropin *on page* 916
SalAc® ***(Discontinued)*** *see* salicylic acid *on page* 884
Sal-Acid® [US-OTC] *see* salicylic acid *on page* 884
Salacid® Ointment ***(Discontinued)*** *see* salicylic acid *on page* 884
Salactic® [US-OTC] *see* salicylic acid *on page* 884
Salagen® [US/Can] *see* pilocarpine *on page* 783
Salazopyrin® [Can] *see* sulfasalazine *on page* 930
Salazopyrin En-Tabs® [Can] *see* sulfasalazine *on page* 930
Salbu-2 [Can] *see* albuterol *on page* 41
Salbu-4 [Can] *see* albuterol *on page* 41
salbutamol *see* albuterol *on page* 41
salbutamol and ipratropium *see* ipratropium and albuterol *on page* 545
salbutamol sulphate *see* albuterol *on page* 41
Saleto-200® ***(Discontinued)*** *see* ibuprofen *on page* 515
Saleto-400® ***(Discontinued)*** *see* ibuprofen *on page* 515
Salex™ ***(Discontinued)*** *see* salicylic acid *on page* 884
Salflex® [Can] *see* salsalate *on page* 888
Salgesic® ***(Discontinued)*** *see* salsalate *on page* 888
salicylazosulfapyridine *see* sulfasalazine *on page* 930

salicylic acid (sal i SIL ik AS id)

Sound-Alike/Look-Alike Issues

Occlusal®-HP may be confused with Ocuflox®

U.S./Canadian Brand Names Aliclen™ [US]; Beta Sal® [US-OTC]; Compound W® One-Step Wart Remover for Feet [US-OTC]; Compound W® One-Step Wart Remover for Kids [US-OTC]; Compound W® One-Step Wart Remover [US-OTC]; Compound W® [US-OTC]; Dermarest® Psoriasis Medicated Moisturizer [US-OTC]; Dermarest® Psoriasis Medicated Scalp Treatment [US-OTC]; Dermarest® Psoriasis Medicated Shampoo/Conditioner [US-OTC]; Dermarest® Psoriasis Medicated Skin Treatment [US-OTC]; Dermarest® Psoriasis Overnight Treatment [US-OTC]; DHS™ Sal [US-OTC]; Duofilm® [Can]; Duoforte® 27 [Can]; Freezone® [US-OTC]; Fung-O® [US-OTC]; Gordofilm® [US-OTC]; Hydrisalic™ [US-OTC]; Ionil Plus® [US-OTC]; Ionil® [US-OTC]; Keralyt® [US-OTC]; LupiCare® Dandruff [US-OTC]; LupiCare® Psoriasis [US-OTC]; Mosco® Callus & Corn Remover [US-OTC]; Neutrogena® Advanced Solutions™ [US-OTC]; Neutrogena® Blackhead Eliminating™ 2-in-1 Foaming Pads [US-OTC]; Neutrogena® Blackhead Eliminating™ Daily Scrub [US-OTC]; Neutrogena® Body Clear® [US-OTC]; Neutrogena® Clear Pore™ Oil-Controlling Astringent [US-OTC]; Neutrogena® Oil-Free Acne Wash 60 Second Mask Scrub [US-OTC]; Neutrogena® Oil-Free Acne Wash Cream Cleanser [US-OTC]; Neutrogena® Oil-Free Acne Wash Foam Cleanser [US-OTC]; Neutrogena® Oil-Free Acne Wash [US-OTC]; Neutrogena® Rapid Clear® Acne Defense [US-OTC]; Neutrogena® Rapid Clear® Acne Eliminating [US-OTC]; Occlusal®-HP [US-OTC/Can]; P&S® [US-OTC]; Palmer's® Skin Success Acne Cleanser [US-OTC]; Sal-Acid® [US-OTC]; Sal-Plant® [US-OTC]; Salactic® [US-OTC]; Salitop™ [US];

Salvax [US]; Sebcur® [Can]; Soluver® Plus [Can]; Soluver® [Can]; Stridex® Essential Care® [US-OTC]; Stridex® Facewipes To Go® [US-OTC]; Stridex® Maximum Strength [US-OTC]; Stridex® Sensitive Skin [US-OTC]; Tinamed® Corn and Callus Remover [US-OTC]; Tinamed® Wart Remover [US-OTC]; Trans-Plantar® [Can]; Trans-Ver-Sal® [US-OTC/Can]; Wart-Off® Maximum Strength [US-OTC]

Therapeutic Category Keratolytic Agent

Use Topically for its keratolytic effect in controlling seborrheic dermatitis or psoriasis of body and scalp, dandruff, and other scaling dermatoses; also used to remove warts, corns, and calluses; acne

Usual Dosage Topical: Children and Adults (consult specific product labeling for use in children <12 years):

Acne:

Cream, cloth, foam, or liquid cleansers (2%): Use to cleanse skin once or twice daily. Massage gently into skin, work into lather and rinse thoroughly. Cloths should be wet with water prior to using and disposed of (not flushed) after use.

Gel (0.5% or 2%): Apply small amount to face in the morning or evening; if peeling occurs, may be used every other day. Some products may be labeled for OTC use up to 3 or 4 times per day. Apply to clean, dry skin

Pads (0.5% or 2%): Use pad to cover affected area with thin layer of salicylic acid one to three times a day. Apply to clean, dry skin. Do not leave pad on skin.

Patch (2%): At bedtime, after washing face, allow skin to dry at least 5 minutes. Apply patch directly over pimple being treated. Remove in the morning.

Shower/bath gels or soap (2%): Use once daily in shower or bath to massage over skin prone to acne. Rinse well.

Callus, corns, or warts:

Foam: Apply to affected area twice daily; rub into skin until completely absorbed

Gel or liquid (17%): Apply to each wart and allow to dry. May repeat once or twice daily, up to 12 weeks. Apply to clean dry area.

Gel (6%): Apply to affected area once daily, generally used at night and rinsed off in the morning.

Plaster or transdermal patch (40%): Apply directly over affected area, leave in place for 48 hours. Some products may be cut to fit area or secured with adhesive strips. May repeat procedure for up to 12 weeks. Apply to clean, dry skin

Transdermal patch (15%): Apply directly over affected area at bedtime, leave in place overnight and remove in the morning. Patch should be trimmed to cover affected area. May repeat daily for up to 12 weeks.

Dandruff, psoriasis, or seborrheic dermatitis:

Cream (2.5%): Apply to affected area 3-4 times daily. Apply to clean, dry skin. Some products may be left in place overnight.

Foam: Apply to affected area twice daily; rub into skin until completely absorbed

Ointment (3%): Apply to scales or plaques on skin up to 4 times per day (not for scalp or face)

Shampoo (1.8% to 3%): Massage into wet hair or affected area; leave in place for several minutes; rinse thoroughly. Labeled for OTC use 2-3 times a week, or as directed by healthcare provider. Some products may be left in place overnight.

Dosage Forms

Aerosol, topical [foam]:

Salvax: 6% (70 g)

Bar, topical [soap]: 2%

Cloth, topical:

Neutrogena® Oil-Free Acne Wash [OTC]: 2% (30s)

Cream, topical: 6% (400 g)

LupiCare™ Psoriasis [OTC]: 2% (227 g)

Neutrogena® Oil-Free Acne Wash Cream Cleanser [OTC]: 2% (200 mL)

Salex®: 6% (454 g)

Salitop™: 6% (400 g)

Gel, topical:

Compound W® [OTC]: 17.6% (7 g)

Dermarest® Psoriasis Medicated Scalp Treatment [OTC], Dermarest® Psoriasis Medicated Skin Treatment [OTC]: 3% (118 mL)

Dermarest® Psoriasis Overnight Treatment [OTC]: 3% (56.7 g)

Hydrisalic™ [OTC]: 6% (28 g)

Keralyt® [OTC]: 3% (30 g); 6% (40 g, 100 g)

Neutrogena® Oil-Free Acne Wash [OTC]: 2% (177 mL)

Neutrogena® Rapid Clear® Acne Eliminating [OTC]: 2% (15 mL)

Sal-Plant® [OTC]: 17% (14 g)

Gel, topical [peel]:
Neutrogena® Advanced Solutions™ [OTC]: 2% (40 g)
Liquid, topical: 17% (14.8 mL)
Compound W® [OTC], Mosco® Callus & Corn Remover [OTC]: 17.6% (9 mL)
Freezone® [OTC]: 17.6% (9.3 mL)
Fung-O® [OTC], Salactic® [OTC], Tinamed® Corn and Callus Remover [OTC], Tinamed® Wart Remover [OTC]: 17% (15 mL)
Gordofilm® [OTC]: 16.7% (15 mL)
Neutrogena® Blackhead Eliminating™ Daily Scrub [OTC]: 2% (125 mL)
Neutrogena® Clear Pore™ Oil-Controlling Astringent [OTC]: 2% (236 mL)
Occlusal®-HP [OTC]: 17% (10 mL)
Palmer's® Skin Success Acne Cleanser [OTC]: 0.5% (240 mL)
Wart-Off® Maximum Strength [OTC]: 17.5% (14.8 mL)
Liquid, topical [body scrub with microbeads]:
Neutrogena® Body Clear® [OTC]: 2% (250 mL)
Liquid, topical [body wash]:
Neutrogena® Body Clear® [OTC]: 2% (250 mL)
Liquid, topical [foam]:
Neutrogena® Oil-Free Acne Wash Foam Cleanser [OTC]: 2% (150 mL)
Liquid, topical [mask/wash]:
Neutrogena® Oil-Free Acne Wash 60 Second Mask Scrub [OTC]: 1% (170 g)
Lotion, topical: 6% (414 mL, 420 mL)
Dermarest® Psoriasis Medicated Moisturizer [OTC]: 2% (118 mL)
Neutrogena® Rapid Clear® Acne Defense [OTC]: 2% (50 mL)
Salex®: 6% (237 mL)
Salitop™: 6% (414 mL)
Pad, topical:
Neutrogena® Blackhead Eliminating™ 2-in-1 Foaming Pads [OTC]: 0.5% (28s)
Stridex® Essential Care® [OTC]: 1% (55s)
Stridex® Facewipes To Go® [OTC]: 0.5% (32s)
Stridex® Maximum Strength [OTC]: 2% (55s, 90s)
Stridex® Sensitive Skin [OTC]: 0.5% (55s, 90s)
Patch, topical:
Compound W® One-Step Wart Remover for Feet [OTC]: 40% (20s)
Compound W® One-Step Wart Remover [OTC]: 40% (14s)
Compound W® One-Step Wart Remover for Kids [OTC]: 40% (12s)
Trans-Ver-Sal® [OTC]: 15% (10s, 25s)
Trans-Ver-Sal® [OTC]: 15% (15s, 40s)
Trans-Ver-Sal® [OTC]: 15% (12s, 40s)
Plaster, topical:
Sal-Acid® [OTC]: 40% (14s)
Shampoo, topical: 6% (177 mL)
Aliclen™, Salex®: 6% (177 mL)
Beta Sal® [OTC]: 3% (480 mL)
DHS™ Sal [OTC]: 3% (120 mL)
Ionil Plus® [OTC]: 2% (240 mL)
Ionil® [OTC]: 2% (120 mL)
LupiCare® Dandruff [OTC], LupiCare® Psoriasis [OTC]: 2% (237 mL)
P&S® [OTC]: 2% (118 mL, 236 mL)
Shampoo/conditioner, topical:
Dermarest® Psoriasis Medicated Shampoo/Conditioner [OTC]: 3% (236 mL)

salicylic acid and coal tar *see* coal tar and salicylic acid *on page* *251*
salicylsalicylic acid *see* salsalate *on page* *888*
Saline Mist [US-OTC] *see* sodium chloride *on page* *908*
SalineX® *(Discontinued)* *see* sodium chloride *on page* *908*
Salitop™ [US] *see* salicylic acid *on page* *884*
Salivart® [US-OTC] *see* saliva substitute *on page* *887*

saliva substitute (sa LYE va SUB stee tute)

Synonyms artificial saliva

U.S./Canadian Brand Names Aquoral™ [US]; Caphosol® [US]; Entertainer's Secret® [US-OTC]; Moi-Stir® [US-OTC]; Mouthkote® [US-OTC]; Numoisyn™ [US]; Oasis® [US]; Oral Balance® [US-OTC]; Salivart® [US-OTC]; SalivaSure™ [US-OTC]

Therapeutic Category Gastrointestinal Agent, Miscellaneous

Use Relief of dry mouth and throat in xerostomia or hyposalivation; adjunct to standard oral care in relief of symptoms associated with chemotherapy or radiation therapy-induced mucositis

Usual Dosage Adults: Use as needed or product-specific dosing:

Caphosol®:

Mucositis symptoms: Swish and spit 4-10 doses per day (begin at onset of chemo-or radiation therapy)

Xerostomia: Swish and spit 2-10 doses per day

Numoisyn™ liquid: Use 2 mL as needed

Numoisyn™ lozenges: Dissolve 1 slowly; maximum 16 lozenges/day

Oasis® mouthwash: Rinse mouth with ~30 mL twice daily or as needed; do not swallow

Oasis® spray: 1-2 sprays as needed; maximum 60 sprays/day

Oral Balance®: Use after meals, at bedtime and as needed

Dosage Forms

Liquid:

Numoisyn™: Water, sorbitol, linseed extract, *Chondrus crispus*, methylparaben, sodium benzoate, potassium sorbate, dipotassium phosphate, propylparaben

Oral Balance® [OTC]: Water, starch, sunflower oil, propylene glycol, xylitol, glycerine, purified milk extract

Lozenge:

Numoisyn™: Sorbitol 0.3 g/lozenge, polyethylene glycol, malic acid, sodium citrate, calcium phosphate dibasic, hydrogenated cottonseed oil, citric acid, magnesium stearate, silicon dioxide

SalivaSure™ [OTC]: Xylitol, citric acid, apple acid, sodium citrate dihydrate, sodium carboxymethylcellulose, dibasic calcium phosphate, silica colloidal, magnesium stearate, stearic acid

Solution, oral:

Caphosol: Dibasic sodium phosphate 0.032%, monobasic sodium phosphate 0.009%, calcium chloride 0.052%, sodium chloride 0.569%, purified water

Entertainer's Secret® [OTC]: Sodium carboxymethylcellulose, aloe vera gel, glycerin (60 mL)

Solution, oral [mouthwash/gargle]:

Oasis®: Water, glycerin, sorbitol, poloxamer 338, PEG-60, hydrogenated castor oil, copovidone, sodium benzoate, carboxymethycellulose

Solution, oral [preservative free; spray]:

Salivart® [OTC]: Water, sodium carboxymethylcellulose, sorbitol, sodium chloride, potassium chloride, calcium chloride, magnesium chloride, potassium phosphate

Solution, oral [spray]:

Aquoral™: Oxidized glycerol triesters and silicon dioxide

Moi-Stir® [OTC]: Water, sorbitol, sodium carboxymethylcellulose, methylparaben, propylparaben, potassium chloride, dibasic sodium phosphate, calcium chloride, magnesium chloride, sodium chloride

Mouthkote® [OTC]: Water, xylitol, sorbitol, yerba santa, citric acid, ascorbic acid, sodium saccharin, sodium benzoate

Oasis®: Glycerin, cetylpyridinium, copovidone

Saliva Substitute® *(Discontinued)* *see* saliva substitute *on page 887*

SalivaSure™ [US-OTC] *see* saliva substitute *on page 887*

salk vaccine *see* poliovirus vaccine (inactivated) *on page 796*

salmeterol (sal ME te role)

Sound-Alike/Look-Alike Issues

salmeterol may be confused with Salbutamol, Solu-Medrol®

Serevent® may be confused with Atrovent®, Combivent®, Serentil®, sertraline, Sinemet®, Spiriva®, Zoloft®

Synonyms salmeterol xinafoate

U.S./Canadian Brand Names Serevent® Diskhaler® Disk [Can]; Serevent® Diskus® [US/Can]

Therapeutic Category Adrenergic Agonist Agent

Use Maintenance treatment of asthma; prevention of bronchospasm with reversible obstructive airway disease, including patients with symptoms of nocturnal asthma; prevention of exercise-induced bronchospasm; maintenance treatment of bronchospasm associated with COPD

Usual Dosage Inhalation, powder (50 mcg/inhalation):

Asthma, maintenance and prevention: Children ≥4 years and Adults: One inhalation twice daily (~12 hours apart); maximum: 1 inhalation twice daily. **Note:** For long-term asthma control, long acting $beta_2$-agonists (LABAs) should be used in combination with inhaled corticosteroids and not as monotherapy.

Exercise-induced asthma, prevention: Children ≥4 years and Adults: One inhalation at least 30 minutes prior to exercise; additional doses should not be used for 12 hours; should not be used in individuals already receiving salmeterol twice daily. **Note:** Because LABAs may disguise poorly controlled persistent asthma, frequent or chronic use of LABAs for exercise-induced bronchospasm is discouraged by the NIH Asthma Guidelines.

COPD maintenance: Adults: One inhalation twice daily (~12 hours apart); maximum: 1 inhalation twice daily

Dosage Forms [CAN] = Canadian brand name

Powder for oral inhalation:

Serevent® Diskus®: 50 mcg (28s, 60s)

Serevent® Diskhaler® Disk [CAN]: 50 mcg (60s)

salmeterol and fluticasone *see* fluticasone and salmeterol *on page* 436

salmeterol xinafoate *see* salmeterol *on page* 887

Salmonine® ***(Discontinued)*** *see* calcitonin *on page* 167

Salofalk® [Can] *see* mesalamine *on page* 631

Sal-Plant® [US-OTC] *see* salicylic acid *on page* 884

salsalate (SAL sa late)

Sound-Alike/Look-Alike Issues

salsalate may be confused with sucralfate, sulfasalazine

Synonyms disalicylic acid; salicylsalicylic acid

U.S./Canadian Brand Names Amigesic® [Can]; Salflex® [Can]

Therapeutic Category Analgesic, Nonnarcotic; Antipyretic; Nonsteroidal Antiinflammatory Drug (NSAID)

Use Treatment of minor pain or fever; arthritis

Usual Dosage Oral: Adults: 3 g/day in 2-3 divided doses

Dosage Forms

Tablet: 500 mg, 750 mg

Salsitab® ***(Discontinued)*** *see* salsalate *on page* 888

salt *see* sodium chloride *on page* 908

salt-poor albumin *see* albumin *on page* 40

Sal-Tropine™ [US] *see* atropine *on page* 110

Salvax [US] *see* salicylic acid *on page* 884

Samsca™ [US] *see* tolvaptan *on page* 969

Sanctura® [US] *see* trospium *on page* 992

Sanctura® XR [US] *see* trospium *on page* 992

Sancuso® [US] *see* granisetron *on page* 471

Sandimmune® [US] *see* cyclosporine *on page* 266

Sandimmune® I.V. [Can] *see* cyclosporine *on page* 266

Sandomigran® [Can] *see* pizotifen *(Canada only) on page* 789

Sandomigran DS® [Can] *see* pizotifen *(Canada only) on page* 789

Sandostatin® [US/Can] *see* octreotide *on page* 717

Sandostatin LAR® [US/Can] *see* octreotide *on page* 717

Sandoz-Acebutolol [Can] *see* acebutolol *on page* 19

Sandoz Alendronate [Can] *see* alendronate *on page* 44

Sandoz-Alfuzosin [Can] *see* alfuzosin *on page* 46

Sandoz-Amiodarone [Can] *see* amiodarone *on page* 64

Sandoz-Anagrelide [Can] *see* anagrelide *on page* 78

Sandoz-Atenolol [Can] *see* atenolol *on page* 107

sapropterin (sap roe TER in)

Sound-Alike/Look-Alike Issues

sapropterin may be confused with cyproterone

Synonyms 6R-BH4; phenoptin; sapropterin dihydrochloride

U.S./Canadian Brand Names Kuvan™ [US]

Therapeutic Category Enzyme Cofactor

Use Adjunct to dietary management in the treatment of tetrahydrobiopterin (BH4) responsive phenylketonuria (PKU)

Usual Dosage Oral: Children ≥4 years and Adults: PKU: Initial: 10 mg/kg once daily; adjust after 1 month based on blood phenylalanine levels (if phenylalanine levels do not decrease from baseline, increase dose to 20 mg/kg once daily); discontinue if phenylalanine levels do not decrease after 1 month of treatment at 20 mg/kg/day (nonresponder). Maintenance range: 5-20 mg/kg once daily

Dosage Forms

Tablet:

Kuvan™: 100 mg

saquinavir (sa KWIN a veer)

Sound-Alike/Look-Alike Issues

saquinavir may be confused with Sinequan®

Synonyms saquinavir mesylate

U.S./Canadian Brand Names Invirase® [US/Can]

Therapeutic Category Antiviral Agent

Use Treatment of HIV infection; used in combination with at least two other antiretroviral agents

Usual Dosage Oral:

Children >16 years and Adults (Invirase®): 1000 mg (five 200 mg capsules or two 500 mg tablets) twice daily given in combination with ritonavir 100 mg twice daily. This combination should be given together and within 2 hours after a full meal in combination with a nucleoside analog. **Note:** Saquinavir (Invirase®) should not be used in "unboosted regimens."

Dosage adjustments when administered in combination therapy: Lopinavir and ritonavir (Kaletra™): Invirase® 1000 mg twice daily

Dosage Forms

Capsule:

Invirase®: 200 mg

Tablet:

Invirase®: 500 mg

saquinavir mesylate *see* saquinavir *on page 890*
Sarafem® [US] *see* fluoxetine *on page 432*

sargramostim (sar GRAM oh stim)

Sound-Alike/Look-Alike Issues

Leukine® may be confused with Leukeran®, leucovorin

Synonyms GM-CSF; granulocyte-macrophage colony-stimulating factor; NSC-613795; rGM-CSF

U.S./Canadian Brand Names Leukine® [US/Can]

Therapeutic Category Colony-Stimulating Factor

Use

Acute myelogenous leukemia (AML) following induction chemotherapy in older adults (≥55 years of age) to shorten time to neutrophil recovery and to reduce the incidence of severe and life-threatening infections and infections resulting in death

Bone marrow transplant (allogeneic or autologous) failure or engraftment delay

Myeloid reconstitution after allogeneic bone marrow transplantation

Myeloid reconstitution after autologous bone marrow transplantation: Non-Hodgkin lymphoma (NHL), acute lymphoblastic leukemia (ALL), Hodgkin lymphoma

Peripheral stem cell transplantation: Mobilization and myeloid reconstitution following autologous peripheral stem cell transplantation

Usual Dosage Adults: I.V. infusion over ≥2 hours or SubQ: **Rounding the dose to the nearest vial size enhances patient convenience and reduces costs without clinical detriment**

Myeloid reconstitution after allogeneic or autologous bone marrow transplant: I.V.: 250 mcg/m^2/day (over 2 hours), begin 2-4 hours after the marrow infusion and ≥24 hours after chemotherapy or radiotherapy, when the post marrow infusion ANC is <500 cells/mm^3, and continue until ANC >1500 cells/mm^3 for 3 consecutive days

If a severe adverse reaction occurs, reduce dose by 50% or temporarily discontinue the dose until the reaction abates

If blast cells appear or progression of the underlying disease occurs, discontinue treatment

If ANC >20,000 cells/mm^3, interrupt treatment or reduce the dose by 50%

Neutrophil recovery following chemotherapy in AML: I.V.: 250 mcg/m^2/day (over 4 hours) starting approximately on day 11 or 4 days following the completion of induction chemotherapy, if day 10 bone marrow is hypoplastic with <5% blasts

If a second cycle of chemotherapy is necessary, administer ~4 days after the completion of chemotherapy if the bone marrow is hypoplastic with <5% blasts

Continue sargramostim until ANC is >1500 cells/mm^3 for 3 consecutive days or a maximum of 42 days

Discontinue sargramostim immediately if leukemic regrowth occurs

If a severe adverse reaction occurs, reduce the dose by 50% or temporarily discontinue the dose until the reaction abates

If ANC >20,000 cells/mm^3, interrupt treatment or reduce the dose by 50%

Mobilization of peripheral blood progenitor cells: I.V., SubQ: 250 mcg/m^2/day I.V. over 24 hours or SubQ once daily

Continue the same dose through the period of PBPC collection

The optimal schedule for PBPC collection has not been established (usually begun by day 5 and performed daily until protocol specified targets are achieved)

If WBC >50,000 cells/mm^3, reduce the dose by 50%

If adequate numbers of progenitor cells are not collected, consider other mobilization therapy

Postperipheral blood progenitor cell transplantation: I.V., SubQ: 250 mcg/m^2/day I.V. over 24 hours or SubQ once daily beginning immediately following infusion of progenitor cells and continuing until ANC is >1500 cells/mm^3 for 3 consecutive days is attained

BMT failure or engraftment delay: I.V.: 250 mcg/m^2/day over 2 hours for 14 days

May be repeated after 7 days off therapy if engraftment has not occurred

If engraftment still has not occurred, a third course of 500 mcg/m^2/day for 14 days may be tried after another 7 days off therapy; if there is still no improvement, it is unlikely that further dose escalation will be beneficial

If a severe adverse reaction occurs, reduce the dose by 50% or temporarily discontinue the dose until the reaction abates

If blast cells appear or disease progression occurs, discontinue treatment

If ANC >20,000 cells/mm^3, interrupt treatment or reduce the dose by 50%

Dosage Forms

Injection, powder for reconstitution:

Leukine®: 250 mcg

Injection, solution:

Leukine®: 500 mcg/mL (1 mL)

Sarna® HC [Can] *see* hydrocortisone (topical) *on page* 505
Sarna® Sensitive [US-OTC] *see* pramoxine *on page* 809
Sarnol®-HC [US-OTC] *see* hydrocortisone (topical) *on page* 505
Sativex® [Can] *see* tetrahydrocannabinol and cannabidiol *(Canada only) on page* 951
Savella™ [US] *see* milnacipran *on page* 659

saxagliptin (sax a GLIP tin)

Sound-Alike/Look-Alike Issues

saxagliptin may be confused with sitaGLIPtin, SUMAtriptan

Synonyms BMS-477118

U.S./Canadian Brand Names Onglyza™ [US]

Therapeutic Category Antidiabetic Agent, Dipeptidyl Peptidase IV (DPP-IV) Inhibitor

Use Treatment of type 2 diabetes mellitus (noninsulin-dependent, NIDDM) as an adjunct to diet and exercise as monotherapy or in combination therapy with other antidiabetic agents to improve glycemic control

Usual Dosage Oral: Adults: Type 2 diabetes: 2.5-5 mg once daily

Dosage Forms

Tablet, oral:

Onglyza™: 2.5 mg, 5 mg

SB-265805 *see* gemifloxacin *on page* 458
SB-497115 *see* eltrombopag *on page* 351
SB-497115-GR *see* eltrombopag *on page* 351
S. boulardii *see Saccharomyces boulardii on page* 883
SC 33428 *see* idarubicin *on page* 518
Scandonest® 2% L [US] *see* mepivacaine and levonordefrin *on page* 628
Scandonest® 3% Plain [US] *see* mepivacaine *on page* 628
SCH 13521 *see* flutamide *on page* 436
SCH 56592 *see* posaconazole *on page* 801
ScheinPharm Ranitidine [Can] *see* ranitidine *on page* 852
SCIG *see* immune globulin (subcutaneous) *on page* 524
S-citalopram *see* escitalopram *on page* 370
Scleromate® [US] *see* morrhuate sodium *on page* 669
Sclerosol® [US] *see* talc (sterile) *on page* 937
Scopace™ [US] *see* scopolamine derivatives *on page* 892
scopolamine and phenylephrine *see* phenylephrine and scopolamine *on page* 777
scopolamine base *see* scopolamine derivatives *on page* 892
scopolamine butylbromide *see* scopolamine derivatives *on page* 892

scopolamine derivatives (skoe POL a meen dah RIV ah tives)

Synonyms hyoscine butylbromide; hyoscine hydrobromide; scopolamine base; scopolamine butylbromide; scopolamine hydrobromide

U.S./Canadian Brand Names Buscopan® [Can]; Isopto® Hyoscine [US]; Scopace™ [US]; Transderm Scōp® [US]; Transderm-V® [Can]

Therapeutic Category Anticholinergic Agent

Use

Scopolamine base:

Transdermal: Prevention of nausea/vomiting associated with motion sickness and recovery from anesthesia and surgery

Scopolamine hydrobromide:

Injection: Preoperative medication to produce amnesia, sedation, tranquilization, antiemetic effects, and decrease salivary and respiratory secretions

Ophthalmic: Produce cycloplegia and mydriasis; treatment of iridocyclitis

Oral: Symptomatic treatment of postencephalitic parkinsonism and paralysis agitans; in spastic states; inhibits excessive motility and hypertonus of the gastrointestinal tract in such conditions as the irritable colon syndrome, mild dysentery, diverticulitis, pylorospasm, and cardiospasm

Scopolamine butylbromide [not available in the U.S.]:

Oral/injection: Treatment of smooth muscle spasm of the genitourinary or gastrointestinal tract; injection may also be used to prior to radiological/diagnostic procedures to prevent spasm

Usual Dosage Note: Scopolamine (hyoscine) hydrobromide should not be interchanged with scopolamine butylbromide formulations. Dosages are not equivalent.

Scopolamine base: Transdermal patch: Adults:

Preoperative: Apply 1 patch to hairless area behind ear the night before surgery or 1 hour prior to cesarean section (apply no sooner than 1 hour before surgery to minimize newborn exposure); remove 24 hours after surgery

Motion sickness: Apply 1 patch behind the ear at least 4 hours prior to exposure and every 3 days as needed; effective if applied as soon as 2-3 hours before anticipated need, best if 12 hours before

Scopolamine hydrobromide:

Antiemetic: SubQ:
- Children: 0.006 mg/kg
- Adults: 0.6-1 mg

Preoperative: I.M., I.V., SubQ:
- Children 6 months to 3 years: 0.1-0.15 mg
- Children 3-6 years: 0.2-0.3 mg
- Adults: 0.3-0.65 mg

Sedation, tranquilization: I.M., I.V., SubQ: Adults: 0.6 mg 3-4 times/day

Refraction: Ophthalmic:
- Children: Instill 1 drop of 0.25% to eye(s) twice daily for 2 days before procedure
- Adults: Instill 1-2 drops of 0.25% to eye(s) 1 hour before procedure

Iridocyclitis: Ophthalmic:
- Children: Instill 1 drop of 0.25% to eye(s) up to 3 times/day
- Adults: Instill 1-2 drops of 0.25% to eye(s) up to 4 times/day

Parkinsonism, spasticity, motion sickness: Adults: Oral: 0.4-0.8 mg. May repeat every 8-12 hours as needed; the dosage may be cautiously increased in parkinsonism and spastic states. For motion sickness, administration at least 1 hour before exposure is recommended.

Scopolamine butylbromide:

Gastrointestinal/genitourinary spasm (Buscopan® [CAN]; not available in the U.S.): Adults:
- Oral: 10-20 mg daily (1-2 tablets); maximum: 6 tablets/day
- I.M., I.V., SubQ: 10-20 mg; maximum: 100 mg/day. Intramuscular injections should be administered 10-15 minutes prior to radiological/diagnostic procedures

Dosage Forms [CAN] = Canadian brand name

Injection, solution: 0.4 mg/mL (1 mL)

Buscopan® [CAN]: 20 mg/mL [not available in the U.S.]

Solution, ophthalmic:

Isopto® Hyoscine: 0.25% (5 mL)

Tablet:

Buscopan® [CAN]: 10 mg [not available in the U.S.]

Tablet, soluble:

Scopace™: 0.4 mg

Transdermal system:

Transderm Scōp®: 1.5 mg (4s, 10s, 24s)

scopolamine hydrobromide *see* scopolamine derivatives *on page 892*

scopolamine, hyoscyamine, atropine, and phenobarbital *see* hyoscyamine, atropine, scopolamine, and phenobarbital *on page 513*

Scot-Tussin® Diabetes [US-OTC] *see* dextromethorphan *on page 295*

Scot-Tussin DM® Cough Chasers *(Discontinued)* *see* dextromethorphan *on page 295*

Scot-Tussin® DM Maximum Strength [US-OTC] *see* dextromethorphan and chlorpheniramine *on page 296*

Scot-Tussin® Expectorant [US-OTC] *see* guaifenesin *on page 473*
Scot-Tussin® Senior [US-OTC] *see* guaifenesin and dextromethorphan *on page 474*
Scytera™ [US-OTC] *see* coal tar *on page 250*
SD/01 *see* pegfilgrastim *on page 755*
SDX-105 *see* bendamustine *on page 127*
SDZ ENA 713 *see* rivastigmine *on page 873*
Seasonale® [US/Can] *see* ethinyl estradiol and levonorgestrel *on page 387*
Seasonique™ [US] *see* ethinyl estradiol and levonorgestrel *on page 387*
Sebcur® [Can] *see* salicylic acid *on page 884*
Sebcur/T® [Can] *see* coal tar and salicylic acid *on page 251*
Sebivo® [Can] *see* telbivudine *on page 941*
Sebizon® *(Discontinued)* *see* sulfacetamide *on page 927*
Seb-Prev™ [US] *see* sulfacetamide *on page 927*

secobarbital (see koe BAR bi tal)

Sound-Alike/Look-Alike Issues
Seconal® may be confused with Sectral®

Synonyms quinalbarbitone sodium; secobarbital sodium

U.S./Canadian Brand Names Seconal® [US]

Therapeutic Category Barbiturate

Controlled Substance C-II

Use Preanesthetic agent; short-term treatment of insomnia

Usual Dosage Oral:
Children:
Preoperative sedation: 2-6 mg/kg (maximum dose: 100 mg/dose) 1-2 hours before procedure
Sedation: 6 mg/kg/day divided every 8 hours
Adults:
Hypnotic: Usual: 100 mg/dose at bedtime; range 100-200 mg/dose
Preoperative sedation: 100-300 mg 1-2 hours before procedure

Dosage Forms
Capsule:
Seconal®: 100 mg

secobarbital sodium *see* secobarbital *on page 894*
Seconal® [US] *see* secobarbital *on page 894*
Secran® *(Discontinued)*
SecreFlo™ *(Discontinued)* *see* secretin *on page 894*

secretin (SEE kr tin)

Synonyms secretin, human; secretin, porcine

U.S./Canadian Brand Names ChiRhoStim® [US]

Therapeutic Category Diagnostic Agent

Use Secretin-stimulation testing to aid in diagnosis of pancreatic exocrine dysfunction; diagnosis of gastrinoma (Zollinger-Ellison syndrome); facilitation of endoscopic retrograde cholangiopancreatography (ERCP) visualization

Usual Dosage I.V.: Adults: **Note:** A test dose of 0.1 mL (0.2-0.4 mcg) is injected to test for possible allergy. Dosing may be completed if no reaction occurs after 1 minute.
Diagnosis of pancreatic dysfunction, facilitation of ERCP: 0.2 mcg/kg over 1 minute
Diagnosis of gastrinoma: 0.4 mcg/kg over 1 minute

Dosage Forms
Injection, powder for reconstitution [human derived]:
ChiRhoStim®: 16 mcg

secretin, human *see* secretin *on page 894*
secretin, porcine *see* secretin *on page 894*
Sectral® [US/Can] *see* acebutolol *on page 19*
Secura® Antifungal Extra Thick [US-OTC] *see* miconazole *on page 654*
Secura® Antifungal Greaseless [US-OTC] *see* miconazole *on page 654*

Sedapap® [US] *see* butalbital and acetaminophen *on page 162*
Selax® [Can] *see* docusate *on page 326*
Select™ 1/35 [Can] *see* ethinyl estradiol and norethindrone *on page 390*
Select-OB™ [US-OTC] *see* vitamins (multiple/prenatal) *on page 1020*

selegiline (se LE ji leen)

Sound-Alike/Look-Alike Issues
selegiline may be confused with Salagen®, Serentil®, sertraline, Serzone®, Stelazine®
Eldepryl® may be confused with Elavil®, enalapril
Zelapar™ may be confused with zaleplon, Zemplar®, Zyprexa® Zydis®

Synonyms deprenyl; L-deprenyl; selegiline hydrochloride

U.S./Canadian Brand Names Apo-Selegiline® [Can]; Eldepryl® [US]; Emsam® [US]; Gen-Selegiline [Can]; Novo-Selegiline [Can]; Nu-Selegiline [Can]; Zelapar™ [US]

Therapeutic Category Anti-Parkinson Agent; Dopaminergic Agent (Anti-Parkinson)

Use Adjunct in the management of parkinsonian patients in which levodopa/carbidopa therapy is deteriorating (oral products); treatment of major depressive disorder (transdermal product)

Usual Dosage Adults:
Capsule/tablet: Parkinson disease: 5 mg twice daily with breakfast and lunch or 10 mg in the morning
Orally disintegrating tablet (Zelapar™): Parkinson disease: Initial 1.25 mg daily for at least 6 weeks; may increase to 2.5 mg daily based on clinical response (maximum: 2.5 mg daily)
Transdermal (Emsam®): Depression: Initial: 6 mg/24 hours once daily; may titrate based on clinical response in increments of 3 mg/day every 2 weeks up to a maximum of 12 mg/24 hours

Dosage Forms
Capsule, oral: 5 mg
Eldepryl®: 5 mg
Tablet, oral: 5 mg
Tablet, orally-disintegrating:
Zelapar™: 1.25 mg
Transdermal system, topical [once-daily patch]:
Emsam®: 6 mg/24 hours (30s) [20 cm^2, total selegiline 20 mg]; 9 mg/24 hours (30s) [30 cm^2, total selegiline 30 mg]; 12 mg/24 hours (30s) [40 cm^2, total selegiline 40 mg]

selegiline hydrochloride *see* selegiline *on page 895*
selenium *see* trace metals *on page 974*

selenium sulfide (se LEE nee um SUL fide)

U.S./Canadian Brand Names Dandrex [US-OTC]; Head & Shoulders® Intensive Treatment [US-OTC]; Selseb® [US]; Selsun blue® 2-in-1 Treatment [US-OTC]; Selsun blue® Daily Treatment [US-OTC]; Selsun blue® Medicated Treatment [US-OTC]; Selsun blue® Moisturizing Treatment [US-OTC]; Tersi [US]; Versel® [Can]

Therapeutic Category Antiseborrheic Agent, Topical

Use Treatment of itching and flaking of the scalp associated with dandruff, to control scalp seborrheic dermatitis; treatment of tinea versicolor

Usual Dosage Topical: Adults:
Dandruff, seborrhea: Massage 5-10 mL of shampoo into wet scalp, leave on scalp 2-3 minutes, rinse thoroughly; rub foam into affected skin twice daily
Tinea versicolor: Apply the 2.5% lotion to affected area and lather with small amounts of water; leave on skin for 10 minutes, then rinse thoroughly; apply every day for 7 days; rub foam into affected skin twice daily

Dosage Forms
Aerosol, topical [foam]:
Tersi: 2.25% (70 g)
Lotion, topical: 2.5% (120 mL)
Shampoo, topical: 1% (210 mL)
Dandrex [OTC]: 1% (240 mL)
Head & Shoulders® Intensive Treatment [OTC]: 1% (420 mL)
Selseb®: 2.5% (180 mL)
Selsun blue® Daily Treatment [OTC], Selsun blue® Moisturizing Treatment [OTC], Selsun blue® 2-in-1 Treatment [OTC]: 1% (207 mL, 325 mL)
Selsun blue® Medicated Treatment [OTC]: 1% (120 mL, 207 mL, 325 mL)

senna (SEN na)

Sound-Alike/Look-Alike Issues
Perdiem® may be confused with Pyridium®
Senexon® may be confused with Cenestin®
Senokot® may be confused with Depakote®

Synonyms sennosides

U.S./Canadian Brand Names Black-Draught™ Tablets [US-OTC]; Evac-U-Gen [US-OTC]; ex-lax® Maximum Strength [US-OTC]; ex-lax® [US-OTC]; Fleet® Pedia-Lax™ Quick Dissolve [US-OTC]; Fletcher's® [US-OTC]; Little Tummys® Laxative [US-OTC]; Perdiem® Overnight Relief [US-OTC]; Senexon® [US-OTC]; Senna-Gen® [US-OTC]; SenokotXTRA® [US-OTC]; Senokot® [US-OTC]

Therapeutic Category Laxative

Use Short-term treatment of constipation; evacuate the colon for bowel or rectal examinations

Usual Dosage Oral:
Bowel evacuation: OTC labeling: Children ≥12 years and Adults: Usual dose: Sennosides 130 mg between 2-4 PM the afternoon of the day prior to procedure
Constipation: OTC ranges:
Children:
2-6 years:
Sennosides: Initial: 3.75 mg once daily (maximum: 15 mg/day, divided twice daily)
Senna concentrate: 33.3 mg/mL: 5-10 mL up to twice daily
6-12 years:
Sennosides: Initial: 8.6 mg once daily (maximum: 50 mg/day, divided twice daily)
Senna concentrate: 33.3 mg/mL: 10-30 mL up to twice daily
Children ≥12 years and Adults: Sennosides 15 mg once daily (maximum: 70-100 mg/day, divided twice daily)

Dosage Forms
Liquid:
Senexon® [OTC]: Sennosides 8.8 mg/5 mL
Liquid [concentrate]:
Fletcher's® [OTC]: Senna concentrate 33.3 mg/mL
Liquid [concentrate; drops]:
Little Tummys® Laxative [OTC]: Sennosides 8.8 mg/1 mL
Strip, orally disintegrating:
Fleet® Pedia-Lax™ Quick Dissolve [OTC]: Sennosides 8.6 mg (12s)
Syrup: Sennosides 8.8 mg/5 mL
Tablet: Sennosides 8.6 mg
ex-lax® [OTC], Perdiem® Overnight Relief [OTC]: Sennosides USP 15 mg
ex-lax® Maximum Strength [OTC]: Sennosides USP 25 mg
Senokot® [OTC], Senexon® [OTC], Senna-Gen® [OTC]: Sennosides 8.6 mg
SenokotXTRA® [OTC]: Sennosides 17 mg

Tablet, chewable:
Black-Draught™ [OTC]: Sennosides 10 mg
Evac-U-Gen [OTC]: Sennosides 10 mg
ex-lax® [OTC]: Sennosides USP 15 mg

senna and docusate *see* docusate and senna *on page 327*
Senna-Gen® [US-OTC] *see* senna *on page 896*
senna-S *see* docusate and senna *on page 327*
sennosides *see* senna *on page 896*
Senokot® [US-OTC] *see* senna *on page 896*
Senokot-S® [US-OTC] *see* docusate and senna *on page 327*
SenokotXTRA® [US-OTC] *see* senna *on page 896*
SenoSol™-X ***(Discontinued)*** *see* senna *on page 896*
SenoSol™ ***(Discontinued)*** *see* senna *on page 896*
SenoSol™-SS [US-OTC] *see* docusate and senna *on page 327*
Sensipar® [US/Can] *see* cinacalcet *on page 229*
Sensorcaine® [US/Can] *see* bupivacaine *on page 156*
Sensorcaine®-MPF [US] *see* bupivacaine *on page 156*
Sensorcaine®-MPF Spinal [US] *see* bupivacaine *on page 156*
Sensorcaine®-MPF with Epinephrine [US] *see* bupivacaine and epinephrine *on page 157*
Sensorcaine® with Epinephrine [US/Can] *see* bupivacaine and epinephrine *on page 157*
Sepasoothe® [US] *see* benzocaine *on page 129*
Septanest® N [Can] *see* articaine and epinephrine *on page 99*
Septanest® SP [Can] *see* articaine and epinephrine *on page 99*
Septa® Topical Ointment ***(Discontinued)*** *see* bacitracin, neomycin, and polymyxin B *on page 119*
Septisol® ***(Discontinued)*** *see* hexachlorophene *on page 493*
Septocaine® with epinephrine 1:100,000 [US] *see* articaine and epinephrine *on page 99*
Septocaine® with epinephrine 1:200,000 [US] *see* articaine and epinephrine *on page 99*
Septra® [US] *see* sulfamethoxazole and trimethoprim *on page 929*
Septra® DS [US] *see* sulfamethoxazole and trimethoprim *on page 929*
Septra® Injection [Can] *see* sulfamethoxazole and trimethoprim *on page 929*
Serax® [US] *see* oxazepam *on page 734*
Serc® [Can] *see* betahistine *(Canada only) on page 136*
Serevent® ***(Discontinued)*** *see* salmeterol *on page 887*
Serevent® Diskhaler® Disk [Can] *see* salmeterol *on page 887*
Serevent® Diskus® [US/Can] *see* salmeterol *on page 887*

sermorelin acetate (ser moe REL in AS e tate)

Therapeutic Category Diagnostic Agent

Use Geref® Diagnostic: For evaluation of the ability of the pituitary gland to secrete growth hormone (GH)

Usual Dosage I.V.: Children and Adults: Diagnostic: 1 mcg/kg as a single dose in the morning following an overnight fast

Note: Response to diagnostic test may be decreased in patients >40 years

Seromycin® [US] *see* cycloserine *on page 266*
Serophene® [US/Can] *see* clomiphene *on page 244*
Seroquel® [US/Can] *see* quetiapine *on page 844*
Seroquel XR® [US/Can] *see* quetiapine *on page 844*
Serostim® [US/Can] *see* somatropin *on page 916*
Serpalan® ***(Discontinued)*** *see* reserpine *on page 859*
Serpatabs® ***(Discontinued)*** *see* reserpine *on page 859*

sertaconazole (ser ta KOE na zole)

Synonyms sertaconazole nitrate

U.S./Canadian Brand Names Ertaczo® [US]

Therapeutic Category Antifungal Agent, Topical

Use Topical treatment of tinea pedis (athlete's foot)

Usual Dosage Topical: Children ≥12 years and Adults: Apply between toes and to surrounding healthy skin twice daily for 4 weeks

Dosage Forms

Cream, topical:

Ertaczo®: 2% (30 g, 60 g)

sertaconazole nitrate *see* sertaconazole *on page 897*

sertraline (SER tra leen)

Sound-Alike/Look-Alike Issues

sertraline may be confused with selegiline, Serentil®, Serevent®, Soriatane®

Zoloft® may be confused with Zocor®

Synonyms sertraline hydrochloride

U.S./Canadian Brand Names Apo-Sertraline® [Can]; CO Sertraline [Can]; Dom-Sertraline [Can]; Gen-Sertraline [Can]; GMD-Sertraline [Can]; Novo-Sertraline [Can]; Nu-Sertraline [Can]; PHL-Sertraline [Can]; PMS-Sertraline [Can]; ratio-Sertraline [Can]; Rhoxal-Sertraline [Can]; Riva-Sertraline [Can]; Sandoz-Sertraline [Can]; Zoloft® [US/Can]

Therapeutic Category Antidepressant, Selective Serotonin Reuptake Inhibitor

Use Treatment of major depression; obsessive-compulsive disorder (OCD); panic disorder; posttraumatic stress disorder (PTSD); premenstrual dysphoric disorder (PMDD); social anxiety disorder

Usual Dosage Oral:

Children and Adolescents: Obsessive-compulsive disorder:

6-12 years: Initial: 25 mg once daily

13-17 years: Initial: 50 mg once daily

Note: May increase daily dose, at intervals of not less than 1 week, to a maximum of 200 mg/day. If somnolence is noted, give at bedtime.

Adults:

Depression/obsessive-compulsive disorder: Oral: Initial: 50 mg/day (see **"Note"** above)

Panic disorder, posttraumatic stress disorder, social anxiety disorder: Initial: 25 mg once daily; increase to 50 mg once daily after 1 week (see **"Note"** above)

Premenstrual dysphoric disorder: 50 mg/day either daily throughout menstrual cycle **or** limited to the luteal phase of menstrual cycle, depending on physician assessment. Patients not responding to 50 mg/day may benefit from dose increases (50 mg increments per menstrual cycle) up to 150 mg/day when dosing throughout menstrual cycle **or** up to 100 mg day when dosing during luteal phase only. If a 100 mg/day dose has been established with luteal phase dosing, a 50 mg/day titration step for 3 days should be utilized at the beginning of each luteal phase dosing period.

Dosage Forms

Solution, oral [concentrate]: 20 mg/mL (60 mL)

Zoloft®: 20 mg/mL

Tablet: 25 mg, 50 mg, 100 mg

Zoloft®: 25 mg, 50 mg, 100 mg

sertraline hydrochloride *see* sertraline *on page 898*

Serzone® *(Discontinued)* *see* nefazodone *on page 685*

sevelamer (se VEL a mer)

Sound-Alike/Look-Alike Issues

sevelamer may be confused with Savella™

Renagel® may be confused with Reglan®, Regonol®, Renal Caps, Renvela®

Renvela® may be confused with Reglan®, Regonol®, Renagel®, Renal Caps

Synonyms sevelamer carbonate; sevelamer hydrochloride

U.S./Canadian Brand Names Renagel® [US/Can]; Renvela® [US]

Therapeutic Category Phosphate Binder

Use Reduction or control of serum phosphorous in patients with chronic kidney disease on hemodialysis

Usual Dosage Oral: **Note:** The dosing of sevelamer carbonate and sevelamer hydrochloride are expected to be similar, when switching from one product to another, the same dose (on a mg per mg basis) should be utilized.

Adults: Patients not taking a phosphate binder: 800-1600 mg 3 times/day with meals; the initial dose may be based on serum phosphorous levels:

>5.5 mg/dL to <7.5 mg/dL: 800 mg 3 times/day

≥7.5 mg/dL to <9.0 mg/dL: 1200-1600 mg 3 times/day
≥9.0 mg/dL: 1600 mg 3 times/day

Maintenance dose adjustment based on serum phosphorous concentration (goal range of 3.5-5.5 mg/dL; maximum dose studied was equivalent to 13 g/day [sevelamer hydrochloride] or 14 g/day [sevelamer carbonate]):
>5.5 mg/dL: Increase by 1 tablet per meal at 2-week intervals
3.5-5.5 mg/dL: Maintain current dose
<3.5 mg/dL: Decrease by 1 tablet per meal

Dosage adjustment when switching between phosphate binder products: 667 mg of calcium acetate is equivalent to 800 mg sevelamer (carbonate or hydrochloride)

Dosage Forms

Tablet:
Renagel®: 400 mg, 800 mg
Renvela®: 800 mg

sevelamer carbonate *see* sevelamer *on page 898*
sevelamer hydrochloride *see* sevelamer *on page 898*

sevoflurane (see voe FLOO rane)

Sound-Alike/Look-Alike Issues
Ultane® may be confused with Ultram®

U.S./Canadian Brand Names Sevorane® AF [Can]; Sojourn™ [US]; Ultane® [US]

Therapeutic Category General Anesthetic

Use Induction and maintenance of general anesthesia

Usual Dosage Minimum alveolar concentration (MAC), the concentration that abolishes movement in response to a noxious stimulus (surgical incision) in 50% of patients, is 2.6% (25 years of age) for sevoflurane. Surgical levels of anesthesia are generally achieved with concentrations from 0.5% to 3%; the concentration at which amnesia and loss of awareness occur is 0.6%.

Minimum alveolar concentrations (MAC) values for surgical levels of anesthesia:
0 to 1 month old full-term neonates: Sevoflurane in oxygen: 3.3%
1 to <6 months: Sevoflurane in oxygen: 3%
6 months to <3 years:
Sevoflurane in oxygen: 2.8%
Sevoflurane in 60% N_2O/40% oxygen: 2%
3-12 years: Sevoflurane in oxygen: 2.5%
25 years:
Sevoflurane in oxygen: 2.6%
Sevoflurane in 65% N_2O/35% oxygen: 1.4%
40 years:
Sevoflurane in oxygen: 2.1%
Sevoflurane in 65% N_2O/35% oxygen: 1.1%
60 years:
Sevoflurane in oxygen: 1.7%
Sevoflurane in 65% N_2O/35% oxygen: 0.9%
80 years:
Sevoflurane in oxygen: 1.4%
Sevoflurane in 65% N_2O/35% oxygen: 0.7%

Dosage Forms

Liquid for inhalation: 100% (250 mL)
Sojourn™, Ultane®: 100% (250 mL)

Sevorane® AF [Can] *see* sevoflurane *on page 899*
shingles vaccine *see* zoster vaccine *on page 1035*
Shur-Seal® *(Discontinued)* *see* nonoxynol 9 *on page 703*
Sibelium® [Can] *see* flunarizine *(Canada only) on page 427*

sibutramine (si BYOO tra meen)

Sound-Alike/Look-Alike Issues
Meridia® may be confused with Aredia®

Synonyms sibutramine hydrochloride monohydrate

U.S./Canadian Brand Names Meridia® [US/Can]

Therapeutic Category Anorexiant
Controlled Substance C-IV
Use Management of obesity
Usual Dosage Children ≥16 years and Adults:
Initial: 10 mg once daily; after 4 weeks may titrate up to 15 mg once daily as needed and tolerated (may be used for up to 2 years, per manufacturer labeling)
Maintenance: 5-15 mg once daily
Dosage Forms
Capsule:
Meridia®: 5 mg, 10 mg, 15 mg

sibutramine hydrochloride monohydrate *see* sibutramine *on page 899*
Silace [US-OTC] *see* docusate *on page 326*
Siladryl Allergy [US-OTC] *see* diphenhydramine *on page 315*
Silafed [US-OTC] *see* triprolidine and pseudoephedrine *on page 989*
Silain® ***(Discontinued)*** *see* simethicone *on page 901*
Silaminic® Expectorant ***(Discontinued)***
Silapap Children's [US-OTC] *see* acetaminophen *on page 19*
Silapap Infants [US-OTC] *see* acetaminophen *on page 19*
Sildec ***(Discontinued)***
Sildec-DM ***(Discontinued)***
Sildec PE ***(Discontinued)*** *see* chlorpheniramine and phenylephrine *on page 214*
Sildec PE-DM ***(Discontinued)*** *see* chlorpheniramine, phenylephrine, and dextromethorphan *on page 217*
Sildec Syrup [US] *see* brompheniramine and pseudoephedrine *on page 150*

sildenafil (sil DEN a fil)

Sound-Alike/Look-Alike Issues
sildenafil may be confused with silodosin, tadalafil, vardenafil
Revatio® may be confused with ReVia®
Viagra® may be confused with Allegra®, Vaniqa™
Synonyms UK92480
U.S./Canadian Brand Names Revatio® [US]; Viagra® [US/Can]
Therapeutic Category Phosphodiesterase (Type 5) Enzyme Inhibitor
Use
Revatio®: Treatment of pulmonary arterial hypertension (WHO Group I) to improve exercise ability and delay clinical worsening
Viagra®: Treatment of erectile dysfunction (ED)
Usual Dosage Oral: Adults:
Erectile dysfunction (Viagra®): Usual dose: 50 mg once daily 1 hour (range: 30 minutes to 4 hours) before sexual activity; dosing range: 25-100 mg once daily
Pulmonary arterial hypertension (Revatio®): Pulmonary arterial hypertension (Revatio®): 20 mg 3 times/day, taken 4-6 hours apart
Dosage Forms
Tablet:
Revatio®: 20 mg
Viagra®: 25 mg, 50 mg, 100 mg

Sildicon-E® ***(Discontinued)***
Silexin [US-OTC] *see* guaifenesin and dextromethorphan *on page 474*
Silfedrine Children's [US-OTC] *see* pseudoephedrine *on page 833*

silodosin (SI lo doe sin)

Sound-Alike/Look-Alike Issues
silodosin may be confused with sildenafil
Rapaflo™ may be confused with Rapamune®, Raptiva®
Synonyms KMD 3213
U.S./Canadian Brand Names Rapaflo™ [US]

Therapeutic Category Alpha$_1$ Blocker

Use Treatment of signs and symptoms of benign prostatic hyperplasia (BPH)

Usual Dosage Oral: Adults: BPH: 8 mg once daily with a meal

Dosage Forms

Capsule:

Rapaflo™: 4 mg, 8 mg

Silphen Cough [US-OTC] *see* diphenhydramine *on page 315*

Silphen DM® [US-OTC] *see* dextromethorphan *on page 295*

Sil-Tex [US] *see* guaifenesin and phenylephrine *on page 475*

Siltussin-CF® ***(Discontinued)***

Siltussin DAS [US-OTC] *see* guaifenesin *on page 473*

Siltussin DM [US-OTC] *see* guaifenesin and dextromethorphan *on page 474*

Siltussin DM DAS [US-OTC] *see* guaifenesin and dextromethorphan *on page 474*

Siltussin SA [US-OTC] *see* guaifenesin *on page 473*

Silvadene® [US] *see* silver sulfadiazine *on page 901*

silver nitrate (SIL ver NYE trate)

Synonyms $AgNO_3$

Therapeutic Category Topical Skin Product

Use Cauterization of wounds and sluggish ulcers, removal of granulation tissue and warts; aseptic prophylaxis of burns

Usual Dosage Children and Adults:

Sticks: Apply to mucous membranes and other moist skin surfaces only on area to be treated 2-3 times/week for 2-3 weeks

Topical solution: Apply a cotton applicator dipped in solution on the affected area 2-3 times/week for 2-3 weeks

Dosage Forms

Applicator sticks, topical: Silver nitrate 75% and potassium 25% (6", 12", 18")

Solution, topical: 0.5% (960 mL); 10% (30 mL); 25% (30 mL); 50% (30 mL)

silver sulfadiazine (SIL ver sul fa DYE a zeen)

U.S./Canadian Brand Names Flamazine® [Can]; Silvadene® [US]; SSD® AF [US]; SSD® [US]; Thermazene® [US]

Therapeutic Category Antibacterial, Topical

Use Prevention and treatment of infection in second and third degree burns

Usual Dosage Topical: Children and Adults: Apply once or twice daily with a sterile-gloved hand; apply to a thickness of 1/16"; burned area should be covered with cream at all times

Dosage Forms

Cream, topical: 1% (25 g, 50 g, 85 g, 400 g)

Silvadene®, Thermazene®: 1% (20 g, 50 g, 85 g, 400 g, 1000 g)

SSD®: 1% (25 g, 50 g, 85 g, 400 g)

SSD® AF: 1% (50 g, 400 g)

Simcor® [US] *see* niacin and simvastatin *on page 694*

simethicone (sye METH i kone)

Sound-Alike/Look-Alike Issues

simethicone may be confused with cimetidine

Mylanta® may be confused with Mynatal®

Mylicon® may be confused with Modicon®, Myleran®

Phazyme® may be confused with Pherazine®

Synonyms activated dimethicone; activated methylpolysiloxane

U.S./Canadian Brand Names Equalizer Gas Relief [US-OTC]; Gas-X® Extra Strength [US-OTC]; Gas-X® Infant [US-OTC]; Gas-X® Maximum Strength [US-OTC]; Gas-X® Thin Strips™ [US-OTC]; Gas-X® [US-OTC]; Gas-X®, Children's Tongue Twisters™ [US-OTC]; Genasyme® [US-OTC]; Infantaire Gas Drops [US-OTC]; Little Tummys® Gas Relief [US-OTC]; Mylanta® Gas Maximum Strength [US-OTC]; Mylicon® Infants [US-OTC]; Ovol® [Can]; Phazyme® Ultra Strength [US-OTC]; Phazyme™ [Can]

Therapeutic Category Antiflatulent

Use Postoperative gas pain or for use in endoscopic examination; relief of bloating, pressure, and discomfort of gas

Usual Dosage Oral:

Infants and Children <2 years or <11 kg: 20 mg 4 times/day, as needed

Children >2 years or >11 kg: 40 mg 4 times/day, as needed

Children >12 years and Adults: 40-360 mg after meals and at bedtime, as needed

Dosage Forms

Softgels: 125 mg

Gas-X® Extra Strength [OTC], Mylanta® Gas Maximum Strength [OTC]: 125 mg

Gas-X® Maximum Strength [OTC]: 166 mg

Phazyme® Ultra Strength [OTC]: 180 mg

Strips, oral:

Gas-X®, Children's Tongue Twisters™ [OTC]: 40 mg (16s)

Gas-X® Thin Strips™ [OTC]: 62.5 mg (18s, 32s)

Suspension, oral [drops]: 40 mg/0.6 mL

Equalizer Gas Relief [OTC], Gas-X® Infant [OTC], Genasyme® [OTC], Infantaire Gas [OTC], Little Tummys® Gas Relief [OTC], Mylicon® Infants [OTC]: 40 mg/0.6 mL

Tablet, chewable: 80 mg, 125 mg

Gas-X® [OTC], Genasyme® [OTC]: 80 mg

Gas-X® Extra Strength [OTC], Mylanta® Gas Maximum Strength [OTC]: 125 mg

simethicone, aluminum hydroxide, and magnesium hydroxide *see* aluminum hydroxide, magnesium hydroxide, and simethicone *on page 56*

simethicone and calcium carbonate *see* calcium carbonate and simethicone *on page 171*

simethicone and loperamide hydrochloride *see* loperamide and simethicone *on page 598*

simethicone and magaldrate *see* magaldrate and simethicone *on page 606*

Similac® Glucose [US] *see* dextrose *on page 298*

Simply Cough® ***(Discontinued)*** *see* dextromethorphan *on page 295*

Simply Saline® [US-OTC] *see* sodium chloride *on page 908*

Simply Saline® Baby [US-OTC] *see* sodium chloride *on page 908*

Simply Saline® Nasal Moist® [US-OTC] *see* sodium chloride *on page 908*

Simply Sleep™ [US-OTC/Can] *see* diphenhydramine *on page 315*

Simply Stuffy™ ***(Discontinued)*** *see* pseudoephedrine *on page 833*

Simponi™ [US] *see* golimumab *on page 470*

Simuc ***(Discontinued)*** *see* guaifenesin and phenylephrine *on page 475*

Simuc-DM [US] *see* guaifenesin and dextromethorphan *on page 474*

Simulect® [US/Can] *see* basiliximab *on page 123*

simvastatin (sim va STAT in)

Sound-Alike/Look-Alike Issues

simvastatin may be confused with atorvastatin, nystatin

Zocor® may be confused with Cozaar®, Lipitor®, Yocon®, Zoloft®, Zyrtec®

U.S./Canadian Brand Names Apo-Simvastatin® [Can]; CO Simvastatin [Can]; Dom-Simvastatin [Can]; Gen-Simvastatin [Can]; Novo-Simvastatin [Can]; Nu-Simvastatin [Can]; PHL-Simvastatin [Can]; PMS-Simvastatin [Can]; ratio-Simvastatin [Can]; Riva-Simvastatin [Can]; Sandoz-Simvastatin [Can]; Taro-Simvastatin [Can]; Zocor® [US/Can]; ZYM-Simvastatin [Can]

Therapeutic Category HMG-CoA Reductase Inhibitor

Use Used with dietary therapy for the following:

Secondary prevention of cardiovascular events in hypercholesterolemic patients with established coronary heart disease (CHD) or at high risk for CHD: To reduce cardiovascular morbidity (myocardial infarction, coronary revascularization procedures) and mortality; to reduce the risk of stroke and transient ischemic attacks

Hyperlipidemias: To reduce elevations in total cholesterol, LDL-C, apolipoprotein B, and triglycerides, and increase HDL-C in patients with primary hypercholesterolemia (elevations of 1 or more components are present in Fredrickson type IIa, IIb, III, and IV hyperlipidemias); treatment of homozygous familial hypercholesterolemia

Heterozygous familial hypercholesterolemia (HeFH): In adolescent patients (10-17 years of age, females >1 year postmenarche) with HeFH having LDL-C ≥190 mg/dL **or** LDL ≥160 mg/dL with positive family history of premature cardiovascular disease (CVD), or 2 or more CVD risk factors in the adolescent patient

Usual Dosage Oral: **Note:** Doses should be individualized according to the baseline LDL-cholesterol levels, the recommended goal of therapy, and the patient's response; adjustments should be made at intervals of 4 weeks or more; doses may need adjusted based on concomitant medications

Children 10-17 years (females >1 year postmenarche): HeFH: 10 mg once daily in the evening; range: 10-40 mg/day (maximum: 40 mg/day)

Adults:

Homozygous familial hypercholesterolemia: 40 mg once daily in the evening **or** 80 mg/day (given as 20 mg, 20 mg, and 40 mg evening dose)

Prevention of cardiovascular events, hyperlipidemias: 20-40 mg once daily in the evening; range: 5-80 mg/day

Patients requiring only moderate reduction of LDL-cholesterol may be started at 10 mg once daily

Patients requiring reduction of >45% in low-density lipoprotein (LDL) cholesterol may be started at 40 mg once daily in the evening

Patients with CHD or at high risk for CHD: Dosing should be started at 40 mg once daily in the evening; simvastatin should be started simultaneously with diet therapy.

Dosage Forms

Tablet: 5 mg, 10 mg, 20 mg, 40 mg, 80 mg

Zocor®: 5 mg, 10 mg, 20 mg, 40 mg, 80 mg

simvastatin and ezetimibe *see* ezetimibe and simvastatin *on page 402*

simvastatin and niacin *see* niacin and simvastatin *on page 694*

Sina-12X [US] *see* guaifenesin and phenylephrine *on page 475*

sincalide (SIN ka lide)

Synonyms C8-CCK; OP-CCK

U.S./Canadian Brand Names Kinevac® [US]

Therapeutic Category Diagnostic Agent

Use Postevacuation cholecystography; gallbladder bile sampling; stimulate pancreatic secretion for analysis; accelerate the transit of barium through the small bowel

Usual Dosage Adults:

Contraction of gallbladder:

I.V.: 0.02 mcg/kg over 30-60 seconds; may repeat in 15 minutes with a 0.04 mcg/kg dose

Infusion: 0.12 mcg/kg in 100 mL of NS; administer over 50 minutes

I.M.: 0.1 mcg/kg

Pancreatic function: I.V.: 0.02 mcg/kg over 30 minutes

Accelerate barium transit through small bowel:

I.V.: 0.04 mcg/kg over 30-60 seconds; if movement of barium has not occurred in 30 minutes, may repeat dose

Infusion: 0.12 mcg/kg in 30 mL of NS; administer over 30 minutes

Dosage Forms

Injection, powder for reconstitution:

Kinevac®: 5 mcg

Sine-Aid® IB *(Discontinued)* *see* pseudoephedrine and ibuprofen *on page 835*

sinecatechins (sin e KAT e kins)

Synonyms catechins; green tea extract; kunecatechins; polyphenols; polyphenon E

U.S./Canadian Brand Names Veregen® [US]

Therapeutic Category Immunomodulator, Topical; Topical Skin Product

Use Treatment of external genital and perianal warts secondary to *Condylomata acuminata*

Usual Dosage Topical: Adults: Apply a thin layer (~0.5 cm strand) 3 times/day to all external genital and perianal warts until all warts have been cleared (maximum duration: 16 weeks)

Dosage Forms

Ointment, topical:

Veregen®: 15% (15 g)

Sinemet® [US/Can] *see* carbidopa and levodopa *on page 184*

Sinemet® CR [US/Can] *see* carbidopa and levodopa *on page* 184
Sinequan® [Can] *see* doxepin *on page* 334
Sinequan® *(Discontinued)* *see* doxepin *on page* 334
Singulair® [US/Can] *see* montelukast *on page* 667
Sinografin® [US] *see* diatrizoate meglumine and iodipamide meglumine *on page* 300
Sinubid® *(Discontinued)*
Sinufed® Timecelles® *(Discontinued)* *see* guaifenesin and pseudoephedrine *on page* 477
Sinumed® *(Discontinued)* *see* acetaminophen, chlorpheniramine, and pseudoephedrine *on page* 26
Sinumist®-SR Capsulets® *(Discontinued)* *see* guaifenesin *on page* 473
Sinus Pain & Pressure [US-OTC] *see* acetaminophen and phenylephrine *on page* 22
Sinus-Relief *(Discontinued)* *see* acetaminophen and pseudoephedrine *on page* 24
Sinutab® Non Drowsy [Can] *see* acetaminophen and pseudoephedrine *on page* 24
Sinutab® Non-Drying [US-OTC] *see* guaifenesin and pseudoephedrine *on page* 477
Sinutab® Sinus [US-OTC] *see* acetaminophen and phenylephrine *on page* 22
SINUtuss® DM [US] *see* guaifenesin, dextromethorphan, and phenylephrine *on page* 478
SINUvent® PE [US] *see* guaifenesin and phenylephrine *on page* 475
Sirdalud® *(Discontinued)* *see* tizanidine *on page* 964

sirolimus (sir OH li mus)

Sound-Alike/Look-Alike Issues
sirolimus may be confused with everolimus, tacrolimus, temsirolimus
Rapamune® may be confused with Rapaflo™

U.S./Canadian Brand Names Rapamune® [US/Can]

Therapeutic Category Immunosuppressant Agent

Use Prophylaxis of organ rejection in patients receiving renal transplants

Usual Dosage Oral:
Combination therapy with cyclosporine: Doses should be taken 4 hours after cyclosporine, and should be taken consistently either with or without food.
Low-to-moderate immunologic risk renal transplant patients: Children ≥13 years and Adults: Dosing by body weight:
<40 kg: Loading dose: 3 mg/m^2 on day 1, followed by maintenance dosing of 1 mg/m^2 once daily
≥40 kg: Loading dose: 6 mg on day 1; maintenance: 2 mg once daily
High immunologic risk renal transplant patients: Adults: Loading dose: Up to 15 mg on day 1; maintenance: 5 mg/day; obtain trough concentration between days 5-7 and adjust accordingly. Continue concurrent cyclosporine/sirolimus therapy for 1 year following transplantation. Further adjustment of the regimen must be based on clinical status.

Dosage Forms
Solution, oral:
Rapamune®: 1 mg/mL
Tablet:
Rapamune®: 1 mg, 2 mg

sitagliptin (sit a GLIP tin)

Sound-Alike/Look-Alike Issues
sitaGLIPtin may be confused with saxagliptin, SUMAtriptan
Januvia™ may be confused with Enjuvia™, Janumet™, Jantoven™

Synonyms MK-0431; sitagliptin phosphate

Tall-Man sita**GLIP**tin

U.S./Canadian Brand Names Januvia™ [US]

Therapeutic Category Antidiabetic Agent, Dipeptidyl Peptidase IV (DPP-IV) Inhibitor

Use
U.S. labeling: Management of type 2 diabetes mellitus (noninsulin-dependent, NIDDM) as an adjunct to diet and exercise as monotherapy or in combination therapy with other antidiabetic agents
Canadian labeling: Management of NIDDM in combination with metformin therapy, diet, and exercise. **Note:** Use as monotherapy is not approved in Canadian labeling.

Usual Dosage Oral: Adults: Type 2 diabetes: 100 mg once daily

Dosage Forms

Tablet:

Januvia™: 25 mg, 50 mg, 100 mg

sitagliptin and metformin (sit a GLIP tin & met FOR min)

Sound-Alike/Look-Alike Issues

Janumet™ may be confused with Jantoven™, Januvia™

Synonyms metformin and sitagliptin; sitagliptin phosphate and metformin hydrochloride

U.S./Canadian Brand Names Janumet™ [US]

Therapeutic Category Antidiabetic Agent, Biguanide; Antidiabetic Agent, Dipeptidyl Peptidase IV (DPP-IV) Inhibitor; Hypoglycemic Agent, Oral

Use Management of type 2 diabetes mellitus (noninsulin-dependent, NIDDM) in patients not adequately controlled on metformin or sitagliptin monotherapy and as an adjunct to diet and exercise

Usual Dosage Oral: Type 2 diabetes mellitus: Adults: Initial doses should be based on current dose of sitagliptin and metformin; daily doses should be divided and given twice daily with meals. Maximum: Sitagliptin 100 mg/metformin 2000 mg daily

Patients inadequately controlled on metformin alone: Initial dose: Sitagliptin 100 mg/day plus current dose of metformin. **Note:** Per manufacturer labeling, patients currently receiving metformin 850 mg twice daily should receive an initial dose of sitagliptin 50 mg and metformin 1000 mg twice daily

Patients inadequately controlled on sitagliptin alone: Initial dose: Metformin 1000 mg/day plus sitagliptin 100 mg/day. **Note:** Patients currently receiving a renally adjusted dose of sitagliptin should not be switched to combination product.

Dosage Forms

Tablet:

Janumet™:

50/500: Sitagliptin 50 mg and metformin 500 mg

50/1000: Sitagliptin 50 mg and metformin 1000 mg

sitagliptin phosphate *see* sitagliptin *on page* *904*

sitagliptin phosphate and metformin hydrochloride *see* sitagliptin and metformin *on page* *905*

sitaxsentan *(Canada only)* (sye TACKS en tan)

Synonyms sitaxsentan sodium

U.S./Canadian Brand Names Thelin™ [Can]

Therapeutic Category Endothelin Antagonist

Use Treatment of primary pulmonary arterial hypertension (PAH) or pulmonary hypertension secondary to connective tissue disease, in World Health Organization (WHO) class III patients unresponsive to conventional therapy; treatment of PAH in WHO class II patients who are unresponsive to conventional therapy and have no alternative treatment options

Usual Dosage Oral: Adults: 100 mg once daily. (**Note:** Doses above 100 mg/day are not recommended; higher doses have not been shown to provide additional benefit and may increase risk of hepatic toxicity).

Dosage Forms CAN = Canadian brand name

Tablet:

Thelin™ [CAN]: 100 mg [not available in U.S.]

sitaxsentan sodium *see* sitaxsentan *(Canada only)* *on page* *905*

Skeeter Stik [US-OTC] *see* benzocaine *on page* *129*

Skelaxin® [US/Can] *see* metaxalone *on page* *633*

Skelid® [US] *see* tiludronate *on page* *961*

SKF 104864 *see* topotecan *on page* *970*

SKF 104864-A *see* topotecan *on page* *970*

Skin Care™ [US-OTC] *see* pyrithione zinc *on page* *842*

Sleep-ettes D [US-OTC] *see* diphenhydramine *on page* *315*

Sleep-eze 3® Oral *(Discontinued)* *see* diphenhydramine *on page* *315*

Sleepinal® [US-OTC] *see* diphenhydramine *on page* *315*

Sleep-Tabs [US-OTC] *see* diphenhydramine *on page* *315*

Sleepwell 2-nite® *(Discontinued)* *see* diphenhydramine *on page* *315*

S-leucovorin *see* LEVOleucovorin *on page* *581*

6S-leucovorin *see* LEVOleucovorin *on page* 581
Slim-Mint® ***(Discontinued)*** *see* benzocaine *on page* 129
Slo-bid™ ***(Discontinued)*** *see* theophylline *on page* 953
Slo-Niacin® [US-OTC] *see* niacin *on page* 692
Slo-Phyllin® (all products) ***(Discontinued)*** *see* theophylline *on page* 953
Slo-Phyllin® GG ***(Discontinued)***
Slo-Pot [Can] *see* potassium chloride *on page* 803
Slow FE® [US-OTC] *see* ferrous sulfate *on page* 414
Slow-K® [Can] *see* potassium chloride *on page* 803
Slow-K® ***(Discontinued)*** *see* potassium chloride *on page* 803
Slow-Mag® [US-OTC] *see* magnesium chloride *on page* 606

smallpox vaccine (SMAL poks vak SEEN)

Synonyms live smallpox vaccine; vaccinia vaccine

U.S./Canadian Brand Names ACAM2000™ [US]

Therapeutic Category Vaccine

Use Active immunization against vaccinia virus, the causative agent of smallpox in persons determined to be at risk for smallpox infection.

The Advisory Committee on Immunization Practices (ACIP) recommends routine vaccination for the following:

- Laboratory workers at risk of exposure from cultures or contaminated animals which may be a source of vaccinia or related Orthopoxviruses capable of causing infections in humans (monkeypox, cowpox, or variola).
- Consideration may also be given for vaccination of healthcare workers having contact with clinical specimens, contaminated material, or patients receiving vaccinia or recombinant vaccinia viruses.

In a Pre-Event Vaccination Program, the ACIP recommends vaccination for the following:

- Persons designated by authorities to investigate smallpox cases with the likelihood of direct patient contact
- Persons responsible for administering smallpox vaccine

In the event of an intentional release of smallpox virus, the ACIP recommends vaccination for the following:

- Persons exposed to the initial release of the virus
- Persons who had close contact with a confirmed or suspected smallpox patient at any time from the onset of the patient's fever until all scabs have separated
- Healthcare providers involved in evaluation, care, or transport of confirmed or suspected smallpox patients
- Laboratory personnel involved in processing specimens of confirmed or suspected smallpox patients
- Persons likely to have increased contact with infectious materials from smallpox patients

Usual Dosage Percutaneous: Not for I.M., I.V., or SubQ injection: Vaccination by scarification (multiple-puncture technique) only: **Note:** A trace of blood should appear at vaccination site after 15-20 seconds; if no trace of blood is visible, an additional 3 insertions should be made using the same needle, without reinserting the needle into the vaccine bottle.

Children ≥12 months (in emergency conditions only) and Adults (ACAM2000™):

Primary vaccination and revaccination: Use a single drop of vaccine suspension and 15 needle punctures (using the same bifurcated needle) into the superficial skin

Note: According to the manufacturer, revaccination is recommended every 3 years for patients at a continued high risk for smallpox infection. The ACIP recommends routine nonemergency revaccination every 3-10 years, depending on type of exposure. Additional information can be obtained from the Department of Defense and the CDC.

Dosage Forms

Injection, powder for reconstitution [purified monkey cell source]:
ACAM2000™: 1-5 x 10^8 plaque-forming units per mL

smelling salts *see* ammonia spirit (aromatic) *on page* 69
SMZ-TMP *see* sulfamethoxazole and trimethoprim *on page* 929
snake antivenin *see* crotalidae polyvalent immune FAB (ovine) *on page* 262
Snaplets-EX® ***(Discontinued)***
(+)-(*S*)-*N*-methyl-γ-(1-naphthyloxy)-2-thiophenepropylamine hydrochloride *see* duloxetine *on page* 341

sodium 2-mercaptoethane sulfonate *see* mesna *on page 631*
sodium 4-hydroxybutyrate *see* sodium oxybate *on page 911*
sodium *L*-triiodothyronine *see* liothyronine *on page 591*

sodium acetate (SOW dee um AS e tate)

Therapeutic Category Alkalinizing Agent; Electrolyte Supplement, Oral

Use Sodium source in large volume I.V. fluids to prevent or correct hyponatremia in patients with restricted intake; used to counter acidosis through conversion to bicarbonate

Usual Dosage Sodium acetate is metabolized to bicarbonate on an equimolar basis outside the liver; administer in large volume I.V. fluids as a sodium source. Refer to sodium bicarbonate monograph.

Maintenance electrolyte requirements of sodium in parenteral nutrition solutions:

Daily requirements: 3-4 mEq/kg/24 hours or 25-40 mEq/1000 kcal/24 hours

Maximum: 100-150 mEq/24 hours

Dosage Forms

Injection, solution [concentrate]: 2 mEq/mL (20 mL, 50 mL, 100 mL); 4 mEq/mL (50 mL, 100 mL)

sodium acid carbonate *see* sodium bicarbonate *on page 907*
sodium aurothiomalate *see* gold sodium thiomalate *on page 470*
sodium benzoate and caffeine *see* caffeine *on page 165*
sodium benzoate and sodium phenylacetate *see* sodium phenylacetate and sodium benzoate *on page 912*

sodium bicarbonate (SOW dee um bye KAR bun ate)

Synonyms baking soda; $NaHCO_3$; sodium acid carbonate; sodium hydrogen carbonate

U.S./Canadian Brand Names Brioschi® [US-OTC]; Neut® [US]

Therapeutic Category Alkalinizing Agent; Antacid; Electrolyte Supplement, Oral

Use Management of metabolic acidosis; gastric hyperacidity; as an alkalinization agent for the urine; treatment of hyperkalemia; management of overdose of certain drugs, including tricyclic antidepressants and aspirin

Usual Dosage

Cardiac arrest: **Routine use of $NaHCO_3$ is not recommended.** May be considered in the setting of prolonged cardiac arrest only after adequate alveolar ventilation has been established and effective cardiac compressions. **Note:** In some cardiac arrest situations (eg, metabolic acidosis, hyperkalemia, or tricyclic antidepressant overdose), sodium bicarbonate may be beneficial.

Infants and Children: I.V.: 0.5-1 mEq/kg/dose repeated every 10 minutes or as indicated by arterial blood gases; rate of infusion should not exceed 10 mEq/minute; neonates and children <2 years of age should receive 4.2% (0.5 mEq/mL) solution

Adults: I.V.: Initial: 1 mEq/kg/dose one time; maintenance: 0.5 mEq/kg/dose every 10 minutes or as indicated by arterial blood gases

Metabolic acidosis: Infants, Children, and Adults: Dosage should be based on the following formula if blood gases and pH measurements are available:

HCO_3^- (mEq) = 0.3 x weight (kg) x base deficit (mEq/L)

Administer 1/2 dose initially, then remaining 1/2 dose over the next 24 hours; monitor pH, serum HCO_3^-, and clinical status

Note: If acid-base status is not available: Dose for older Children and Adults: 2-5 mEq/kg I.V. infusion over 4-8 hours; subsequent doses should be based on patient's acid-base status

Chronic renal failure: Oral: Initiate when plasma HCO_3^- <15 mEq/L

Children: 1-3 mEq/kg/day

Adults: Start with 20-36 mEq/day in divided doses, titrate to bicarbonate level of 18-20 mEq/L

Hyperkalemia: Adults: I.V.: 50 mEq over 5 minutes (as appropriate, consider methods of enhancing potassium removal/excretion)

Renal tubular acidosis: Oral:

Distal:

Children: 2-3 mEq/kg/day

Adults: 0.5-2 mEq/kg/day in 4-5 divided doses

Proximal: Children and Adults: Initial: 5-10 mEq/kg/day; maintenance: Increase as required to maintain serum bicarbonate in the normal range

Urine alkalinization: Oral:

Children: 1-10 mEq (84-840 mg)/kg/day in divided doses every 4-6 hours; dose should be titrated to desired urinary pH

Adults: Initial: 48 mEq (4 g), then 12-24 mEq (1-2 g) every 4 hours; dose should be titrated to desired urinary pH; doses up to 16 g/day (200 mEq) in patients <60 years and 8 g (100 mEq) in patients >60 years

Antacid: Adults: Oral: 325 mg to 2 g 1-4 times/day

Dosage Forms

Granules, for solution, oral [effervescent]:

Brioschi® [OTC]: 2.69 g/packet, 2.69 g/capful

Infusion [premixed in water for injection]: 5% (500 mL)

Injection, solution:

4.2% (10 mL) [5 mEq/10 mL]

7.5% (50 mL) [8.92 mEq/10 mL]

8.4% (10 mL, 50 mL, 250 mL, 500 mL) [10 mEq/10 mL]

Neut®: 4% (5 mL) [2.4 mEq/5 mL]

Powder: Sodium bicarbonate USP (120 g, 480 g)

Tablet: 325 mg [3.8 mEq]; 650 mg [7.6 mEq]

sodium bicarbonate and omeprazole *see* omeprazole and sodium bicarbonate *on page 724*

sodium chloride (SOW dee um KLOR ide)

Synonyms NaCl; normal saline; salt

U.S./Canadian Brand Names 4-Way® Saline Moisturizing Mist [US-OTC]; Altachlore [US-OTC]; Altamist [US-OTC]; Ayr® Allergy Sinus [US-OTC]; Ayr® Baby Saline [US-OTC]; Ayr® Saline No-Drip [US-OTC]; Ayr® Saline [US-OTC]; Breathe Free® [US-OTC]; Deep Sea [US-OTC]; Entsol® [US-OTC]; Humist® for Kids [US-OTC]; Humist® [US-OTC]; Hyper-Sal™ [US]; Little Noses® Saline [US-OTC]; Little Noses® Stuffy Nose Kit [US-OTC]; Muro 128® [US-OTC]; Na-Zone® [US-OTC]; Nasal Moist® Saline [US-OTC]; Nasal Spray [US-OTC]; NāSal™ [US-OTC]; Ocean® for Kids [US-OTC]; Ocean® [US-OTC]; Pretz® [US-OTC]; Saline Mist [US-OTC]; Simply Saline® Baby [US-OTC]; Simply Saline® Nasal Moist® [US-OTC]; Simply Saline® [US-OTC]; Syrex [US]; Wound Wash Saline™ [US-OTC]

Therapeutic Category Electrolyte Supplement, Oral; Lubricant, Ocular

Use

Parenteral: Restores sodium ion in patients with restricted oral intake (especially hyponatremia states or low salt syndrome). In general, parenteral saline uses:

Bacteriostatic sodium chloride: Dilution or dissolving drugs for I.M., I.V., or SubQ injections

Concentrated sodium chloride: Additive for parenteral fluid therapy

Hypertonic sodium chloride: For severe hyponatremia and hypochloremia

Hypotonic sodium chloride: Hydrating solution

Normal saline: Restores water/sodium losses

Pharmaceutical aid/diluent for infusion of compatible drug additives

Ophthalmic: Reduces corneal edema

Inhalation: Restores moisture to pulmonary system; loosens and thins congestion caused by colds or allergies; diluent for bronchodilator solutions that require dilution before inhalation

Intranasal: Restores moisture to nasal membranes

Irrigation: Wound cleansing, irrigation, and flushing

Usual Dosage

Children: I.V.: Hypertonic solutions (>0.9%) should only be used for the initial treatment of acute serious symptomatic hyponatremia; maintenance: 3-4 mEq/kg/day; maximum: 100-150 mEq/day; dosage varies widely depending on clinical condition

Replacement: Determined by laboratory determinations mEq

Sodium deficiency (mEq/kg) = [% dehydration (L/kg)/100 x 70 (mEq/L)] + [0.6 (L/kg) x (140 - serum sodium) (mEq/L)]

Children ≥2 years and Adults:

Intranasal: 2-3 sprays in each nostril as needed

Irrigation: Spray affected area

Children and Adults: Inhalation: Bronchodilator diluent: 1-3 sprays (1-3 mL) to dilute bronchodilator solution in nebulizer prior to administration

Adults:

GU irrigant: 1-3 L/day by intermittent irrigation

Replacement I.V.: Determined by laboratory determinations mEq

Sodium deficiency (mEq/kg) = [% dehydration (L/kg)/100 x 70 (mEq/L)] + [0.6 (L/kg) x (140 - serum sodium) (mEq/L)]

To correct acute, serious hyponatremia: mEq sodium = [desired sodium (mEq/L) - actual sodium (mEq/L)] x [0.6 x wt (kg)]; for acute correction use 125 mEq/L as the desired serum sodium; acutely correct serum sodium in 5 mEq/L/dose increments; more gradual correction in increments of 10 mEq/L/day is indicated in the asymptomatic patient

Chloride maintenance electrolyte requirement in parenteral nutrition: 2-4 mEq/kg/24 hours or 25-40 mEq/1000 kcals/24 hours; maximum: 100-150 mEq/24 hours

Sodium maintenance electrolyte requirement in parenteral nutrition: 3-4 mEq/kg/24 hours or 25-40 mEq/1000 kcals/24 hours; maximum: 100-150 mEq/24 hours.

Ophthalmic:

Ointment: Apply once daily or more often

Solution: Instill 1-2 drops into affected eye(s) every 3-4 hours

Dosage Forms

Aerosol, intranasal [spray; preservative free]:

Entsol® [OTC]: 3% (100 mL)

Gel, intranasal:

Ayr® Saline [OTC]: <0.5% (14 g)

Entsol® [OTC]: 3% (20 g)

Simply Saline® Nasal Moist® [OTC]: 0.65% (30 g) [contains aloe]

Gel, intranasal [spray]:

Ayr® Saline No-Drip [OTC]: <0.5% (22 mL)

Injection, solution: 0.45% (25 mL, 50 mL, 100 mL, 250 mL, 500 mL, 1000 mL); 0.9% (25 mL, 50 mL, 100 mL, 150 mL, 250 mL, 500 mL, 1000 mL, 1 g); 3% (500 mL); 5% (500 mL)

Injection, solution [preservative free]: 0.9% (2 mL, 3 mL, 5 mL, 10 mL, 20 mL, 50 mL, 100 mL)

Injection, solution [I.V. flush]: 0.9% (10 mL)

Injection, solution [I.V. flush; preservative free]: 0.9% (1 mL, 2 mL, 2.5 mL, 3 mL, 5 mL, 10 mL)

Syrex: 0.9% (2.5 mL, 3 mL, 5 mL, 10 mL)

Injection, solution [bacteriostatic]: 0.9% (10 mL, 20 mL, 30 mL)

Injection, solution [concentrate]: 14.6% (40 mL); 23.4% (100 mL, 250 mL)

Injection, solution [concentrate; preservative free]: 14.6% (20 mL, 40 mL); 23.4% (30 mL, 100 mL, 200 mL)

Ointment, ophthalmic: 5% (3.5 g)

Altachlore [OTC]: 5% (3.5 g)

Ointment, ophthalmic [preservative free]:

Muro 128® [OTC]: 5% (3.5 g)

Powder for solution, intranasal [preservative free]:

Entsol® [OTC]: 3% (10.5 g)

Solution for blood processing [not for injection]: 0.9% (3000 mL)

Solution for inhalation [preservative free]: 0.9% (3 mL, 5 mL, 15 mL); 3% (15 mL)

Solution for inhalation [hypertonic; preservative free]: 10% (15 mL)

Solution for inhalation [hypotonic; preservative free]: 0.45% (5 mL)

Solution for injection [I.V. flush; preservative free]: 0.9% (2.5 mL, 5 mL, 10 mL)

Solution for irrigation: 0.45% (2000 mL); 0.9% (250 mL, 500 mL, 1000 mL, 1500 mL, 2000 mL, 3000 mL, 4000 mL, 5000 mL)

Solution for irrigation [preservative free]: 0.45% (2000 mL); 0.9% (250 mL, 500 mL, 1000 mL, 1500 mL, 2000 mL, 3000 mL)

Solution for irrigation [slush solution]: 0.9% (1000 mL)

Solution for nebulization [preservative free]:

Hyper-Sal™: 7% (4 mL)

Solution, intranasal [preservative free]:

Simply Saline® [OTC]: 3% (44 mL)

Solution, intranasal [drops]:

Humist® [OTC]: 0.65% (45 mL)

Humist® for Kids [OTC]: 0.65% (30 mL)

Ayr® Saline [OTC]: 0.65% (50 mL)

NāSal™ [OTC]: 0.65% (15 mL)

Solution, intranasal [drops, mist, spray]

Ocean® [OTC]: 0.65% (45 mL, 473 mL)

Ocean® for Kids [OTC]: 0.65% (37.5 mL)

Solution, intranasal [drops, spray]:

Ayr® Baby Saline [OTC]: 0.65% (30 mL)

Little Noses® Saline [OTC]: 0.65% (30 mL)

Little Noses® Stuffy Nose Kit [OTC]: 0.65% (15 mL)

Solution, intranasal [irrigation]:
Pretz® [OTC]: 0.75% (237 mL, 960 mL)
Solution, intranasal [mist]:
Ayr® Allergy Sinus [OTC]: 2.65% (50 mL)
Ayr® Saline [OTC]: 0.65% (50 mL)
Entsol® [OTC]: 3% (30 mL)
Saline Mist [OTC]: 0.65% (45 mL)
4-Way® Moisturizing Mist [OTC]: 0.74% (29.6 mL)
Solution, intranasal [mist, preservative free]:
Simply Saline® [OTC]: 0.9% (44 mL, 90 mL)
Simply Saline® Baby [OTC]: 0.9% (45 mL)
Solution, intranasal [nasal wash; preservative free]:
Entsol® [OTC]: 3% (240 mL)
Solution, intranasal [spray]:
Altamist [OTC], Na-Zone® [OTC]: 0.65% (60 mL)
Breathe Free® [OTC]: 0.65% (44.3 mL)
Deep Sea [OTC], Nasal Moist® Saline [OTC], Nasal Spray [OTC]: 0.65% (45 mL)
NāSal™ [OTC]: 0.65% (30 mL)
Solution, intranasal [spray, isotonic, buffered]:
Pretz® [OTC]: 0.75% (50 mL)
Solution, ophthalmic: 5% (15 mL)
Solution, ophthalmic [drops]: 5% (15 mL)
Altachlore [OTC]: 5% (15 mL, 30 mL)
Muro 128® [OTC]: 2% (15 mL); 5% (15 mL, 30 mL)
Solution, topical [preservative free]:
Wound Wash Saline™ [OTC]: 0.9% (90 mL, 210 mL)
Swab, intranasal:
Ayr® Saline [OTC]: <0.5% (20)
Tablet for solution, topical: 1000 mg

sodium chondroitin sulfate and sodium hyaluronate

(SOW de um kon DROY tin SUL fate & SOW de um hye al yoor ON ate)

Synonyms chondroitin sulfate and sodium hyaluronate; sodium hyaluronate and chondroitin sulfate

U.S./Canadian Brand Names DisCoVisc® [US]; Viscoat® [US]

Therapeutic Category Ophthalmic Agent, Viscoelastic

Use Ophthalmic surgical aid in the anterior segment during cataract extraction and intraocular lens implantation

Usual Dosage Ophthalmic: Adults: Carefully introduce (using a 27-gauge cannula) into anterior chamber during surgery

Dosage Forms

Injection, solution, intraocular:
DisCoVisc®: Sodium chondroitin sulfate ≤4% and sodium hyaluronate ≤1.7% (0.5 mL, 1 mL)
Viscoat®: Sodium chondroitin sulfate ≤4% and sodium hyaluronate ≤3% (0.5 mL, 0.75 mL)

sodium citrate, citric acid, and potassium citrate *see* citric acid, sodium citrate, and potassium citrate *on page* 235
Sodium Diuril® [US] *see* chlorothiazide *on page* 213
Sodium Edecrin® [US] *see* ethacrynic acid *on page* 382
sodium edetate *see* edetate disodium *on page* 347
sodium etidronate *see* etidronate disodium *on page* 397
sodium ferric gluconate *see* ferric gluconate *on page* 413
sodium fluorescein *see* fluorescein *on page* 429
sodium fluoride *see* fluoride *on page* 430
sodium fusidate *see* fusidic acid *(Canada only) on page* 450
sodium hyaluronate *see* hyaluronate and derivatives *on page* 496
sodium hyaluronate and chondroitin sulfate *see* sodium chondroitin sulfate and sodium hyaluronate *on page* 910
sodium hydrogen carbonate *see* sodium bicarbonate *on page* 907

sodium hypochlorite solution (SOW dee um hye poe KLOR ite soe LOO shun)

Synonyms modified Dakin's solution

U.S./Canadian Brand Names Dakin's Solution [US]; Di-Dak-Sol [US]

Therapeutic Category Disinfectant

Use Treatment of athlete's foot (0.5%); wound irrigation (0.5%); disinfection of utensils and equipment (5%)

Usual Dosage Topical irrigation

Dosage Forms

Solution, topical:

Dakin's: 0.125% (480 mL); 0.25% (480 mL); 0.5% (480 mL, 3840 mL)

Di-Dak-Sol: 0.0125% (480 mL)

sodium hyposulfate *see* sodium thiosulfate *on page 915*

sodium lactate (SOW dee um LAK tate)

Therapeutic Category Alkalinizing Agent

Use Source of bicarbonate for prevention and treatment of mild-to-moderate metabolic acidosis

Usual Dosage Dosage depends on degree of acidosis

Dosage Forms

Infusion: 18.7 g (1000 mL)

Injection, solution [concentrate; preservative free]: 560 mg/mL (10 mL)

sodium nafcillin *see* nafcillin *on page 677*

sodium nitrite, sodium thiosulfate, and amyl nitrite

(SOW dee um NYE trite, SOW dee um thye oh SUL fate, & AM il NYE trite)

Synonyms amyl nitrite, sodium nitrite, and sodium thiosulfate; cyanide antidote kit; sodium thiosulfate, sodium nitrite, and amyl nitrite

U.S./Canadian Brand Names Cyanide Antidote Package [US]

Therapeutic Category Antidote

Use Treatment of cyanide poisoning

Usual Dosage Cyanide poisoning:

Children: 0.3 mL ampul of amyl nitrite is crushed every minute and vapor is inhaled for 15-30 seconds until an I.V. sodium nitrite infusion is available. Following administration of sodium nitrite I.V. 10 mg/kg (0.33 mL/kg or 6-8 mL/m^2 of a 3% solution; maximum: 10 mL), inject sodium thiosulfate I.V. 7 g/m^2 (maximum: 12.5 g) over ~10 minutes, if needed; injection of both may be repeated at 1/2 the original dose.

Adults: 0.3 mL ampul of amyl nitrite is crushed every minute and vapor is inhaled for 15-30 seconds until an I.V. sodium nitrite infusion is available. Following administration of 300 mg or 10 mg/kg I.V. sodium nitrite, inject 12.5 g sodium thiosulfate I.V. (over ~10 minutes), if needed; injection of both may be repeated at 1/2 the original dose.

Dosage Forms Kit [each kit contains]:

Cyanide Antidote Package:

Injection, solution:

Sodium nitrite 300 mg/10 mL (2)

Sodium thiosulfate 12.5 g/50 mL (2)

Inhalant: Amyl nitrite 0.3 mL (12)

sodium nitroferricyanide *see* nitroprusside *on page 701*

sodium nitroprusside *see* nitroprusside *on page 701*

sodium oxybate (SOW dee um ox i BATE)

Synonyms 4-hydroxybutyrate; gamma hydroxybutyric acid; GHB; sodium 4-hydroxybutyrate

U.S./Canadian Brand Names Xyrem® [US/Can]

Therapeutic Category Central Nervous System Depressant

Controlled Substance C-I (illicit use); C-III (medical use)

Use Treatment of cataplexy and daytime sleepiness in patients with narcolepsy

Usual Dosage Oral: Children ≥16 years and Adults: Narcolepsy: Initial: 4.5 g/day, in 2 equal doses; first dose to be given at bedtime after the patient is in bed, and second dose to be given 2.5-4 hours later. Dose may be increased or adjusted in 2-week intervals; average dose: 6-9 g/day (maximum: 9 g/day)

Dosage Forms

Solution, oral:

Xyrem®: 500 mg/mL

sodium PAS *see* aminosalicylic acid *on page 64*

sodium-PCA and lactic acid *see* lactic acid *on page 563*

sodium phenylacetate and sodium benzoate

(SOW dee um fen il AS e tate & SOW dee um BENZ oh ate)

Synonyms NAPA and NABZ; sodium benzoate and sodium phenylacetate

U.S./Canadian Brand Names Ammonul® [US]

Therapeutic Category Ammonium Detoxicant

Use Adjunct to treatment of acute hyperammonemia and encephalopathy in patients with urea cycle disorders involving partial or complete deficiencies of carbamyl-phosphate synthetase (CPS), ornithine transcarbamoylase (OTC), argininosuccinate lysase (ASL), or argininosuccinate synthetase (ASS); for use with hemodialysis in acute neonatal hyperammonemic coma, moderate-to-severe hyperammonemic encephalopathy and hyperammonemia which fails to respond to initial therapy

Usual Dosage Administer as a loading dose over 90-120 minutes, followed by an equivalent maintenance infusion given over 24 hours. Dosage based on weight and specific enzyme deficiency; therapy should continue until ammonia levels are in normal range. Repeat loading doses are not recommended due to the prolonged plasma levels.

Children ≤20 kg:

CPS and OTC deficiency: Ammonul® 2.5 mL/kg and arginine 10% 2 mL/kg (provides sodium phenylacetate 250 mg/kg, sodium benzoate 250 mg/kg, and arginine hydrochloride 200 mg/kg).

ASS and ASL deficiency: Ammonul® 2.5 mL/kg and arginine 10% 6 mL/kg (provides sodium phenylacetate 250 mg/kg, sodium benzoate 250 mg/kg, and arginine hydrochloride 600 mg/kg)

Note: Pending a specific diagnosis in infants, the bolus and maintenance dose of arginine should be 6 mL/kg. If ASS or ASL are excluded as diagnostic possibilities, reduce dose of arginine to 2 mL/kg/day.

Children >20 kg and Adults:

CPS and OTC deficiency: Ammonul® 55 mL/m^2 and arginine 10% 2 mL/kg (provides sodium phenylacetate 5.5 g/m^2, sodium benzoate 5.5 g/m^2, and arginine hydrochloride 200 mg/kg)

ASS and ASL deficiency: Ammonul® 55 mL/m^2 and arginine 10% 6 mL/kg (provides sodium phenylacetate 5.5 g/m^2, sodium benzoate 5.5 g/m^2, and arginine hydrochloride 600 mg/kg)

Dosage Forms

Injection, solution [concentrate]:

Ammonul®: Sodium phenylacetate 100 mg and sodium benzoate 100 mg per 1 mL (50 mL)

sodium phenylbutyrate (SOW dee um fen il BYOO ti rate)

Synonyms ammonapse

U.S./Canadian Brand Names Buphenyl® [US]

Therapeutic Category Miscellaneous Product

Use Adjunctive therapy in the chronic management of patients with urea cycle disorder involving deficiencies of carbamoylphosphate synthetase, ornithine transcarbamylase, or argininosuccinic acid synthetase

Usual Dosage Oral: Management of urea cycle disorders:

Children <20 kg: Powder: 450-600 mg/kg/day, administered in equally divided amounts with each meal or feeding, 3-6 times daily (maximum dose: 20 g/day)

Children ≥20 kg and Adults: Powder or tablet: 9.9-13 g/m^2/day, administered in equally divided amounts with each meal or feeding, 3-6 times daily (maximum dose: 20 g/day)

Dosage Forms

Powder, for oral solution:

Buphenyl®: 3 g/level teaspoon

Tablet:

Buphenyl®: 500 mg

sodium phosphate and potassium phosphate *see* potassium phosphate and sodium phosphate *on page 806*

sodium phosphates (SOW dee um FOS fates)

Sound-Alike/Look-Alike Issues

Visicol® may be confused with Asacol®, VESIcare®

Synonyms phosphates, sodium

U.S./Canadian Brand Names Fleet® Enema Extra® [US-OTC]; Fleet® Enema [US-OTC/Can]; Fleet® Pedia-Lax™ Enema [US-OTC]; LaCrosse Complete [US-OTC]; OsmoPrep® [US]; Visicol® [US]

Therapeutic Category Electrolyte Supplement, Oral; Laxative

Use

Oral, rectal: Short-term treatment of constipation and to evacuate the colon for rectal and bowel exams

I.V.: Source of phosphate in large volume I.V. fluids and parenteral nutrition; treatment and prevention of hypophosphatemia

Usual Dosage **Caution: With orders for I.V. phosphate, there is considerable confusion associated with the use of millimoles (mmol) versus milliequivalents (mEq) to express the phosphate requirement.** The most reliable method of ordering I.V. phosphate is by millimoles, then specifying the potassium or sodium salt. Intravenous doses listed as mmol of phosphate.

Acute treatment of hypophosphatemia: I.V.: It is difficult to provide concrete guidelines for the treatment of severe hypophosphatemia because the extent of total body deficits and response to therapy are difficult to predict. Aggressive doses of phosphate may result in a transient serum elevation followed by redistribution into intracellular compartments or bone tissue. It is recommended that repletion of severe hypophosphatemia be done I.V. because large doses of oral phosphate may cause diarrhea and intestinal absorption may be unreliable. Intermittent I.V. infusion should be reserved for severe depletion situations; requires continuous cardiac monitoring. Guidelines differ based on degree of illness, need/use of TPN, and severity of hypophosphatemia. If hypokalemia exists (some clinicians recommend threshold of <4 mmol/L), consider phosphate replacement strategy with potassium (eg, potassium phosphates). Obese patients and/or severe renal impairment were excluded from phosphate supplement trials.

Children and Adults: There are no prospective studies of parenteral phosphate replacement in children. The following weight-based guidelines for adult dosing may be cautiously employed in pediatric patients. **Note:** 1 mmol phosphate = 31 mg phosphorus; 1 mg phosphorus = 0.032 mmol phosphate

General replacement guidelines:

Low dose: 0.08 mmol/kg over 6 hours; use if losses are recent and uncomplicated

Intermediate dose: 0.16-0.24 mmol/kg over 4-6 hours; use if serum phosphorus level 0.5-1 mg/dL (0.16-0.32 mmol/L)

Note: The initial dose may be increased by 25% to 50% if the patient is symptomatic secondary to hypophosphatemia and lowered by 25% to 50% if the patient is hypercalcemic.

Critically-ill adult trauma patients receiving concurrent TPN:

Low dose: 0.32 mmol/kg over 4-6 hours; use if serum phosphorus level 2.3-3 mg/dL (0.73-0.96 mmol/L)

Intermediate dose: 0.64 mmol/kg over 4-6 hours; use if serum phosphorus level 1.6-2.2 mg/dL (0.51-0.72 mmol/L)

High dose: 1 mmol/kg over 8-12 hours; use if serum phosphorus <1.5 mg/dL (<0.5 mmol/L)

Parenteral nutrition: I.V.:

Infants and Children: 0.5-2 mmol/kg/24 hours (Mirtallo, 2004 [ASPEN guidelines])

Children >50 kg and Adolescents: 10-40 mmol/24 hours

Adults: 10-15 mmol/1000 kcal **or** 20-40 mmol/24 hours

Laxative (Fleet®): Rectal:

Children 2-<5 years: One-half contents of one 2.25 oz pediatric enema

Children 5-12 years: Contents of one 2.25 oz pediatric enema, may repeat

Children ≥12 years and Adults: Contents of one 4.5 oz enema as a single dose, may repeat

Laxative (Fleet® Phospho-soda®): Oral: Take on an empty stomach; dilute dose with 8 ounces cool water, then follow dose with 8 ounces water; **do not repeat dose within 24 hours**

Children 5-9 years: 7.5 mL as a single dose; maximum daily dose: 7.5 mL

Children 10-12 years: 15 mL as a single dose; maximum daily dose: 15 mL

Children ≥12 years and Adults: 15 mL as a single dose; maximum daily dose: 45 mL

Bowel cleansing prior to colonoscopy: Adults: Oral: **Note:** Each dose should be taken with a minimum of 8 ounces of clear liquids. Do not repeat treatment within 7 days. Do not use additional agents, especially sodium phosphate products.

Fleet® Phospho-Soda® (as component of Fleet® Prep Kit 3): Prior to procedure (timing of doses determined by prescriber): Mix 15 mL with 240 mL clear liquid; drink, then follow with 240 mL clear liquid; repeat every 10 minutes for a total of 45 mL

Visicol®: A total of 40 tablets divided as follows:

Evening before colonoscopy: 3 tablets every 15 minutes for 6 doses, then 2 additional tablets in 15 minutes (total of 20 tablets)

3-5 hours prior to colonoscopy: 3 tablets every 15 minutes for 6 doses, then 2 additional tablets in 15 minutes (total of 20 tablets)

OsmoPrep®: A total of 32 tablets divided as follows:

Evening before colonoscopy: 4 tablets every 15 minutes for 5 doses (total of 20 tablets)

3-5 hours prior to colonoscopy: 4 tablets every 15 minutes for 3 doses (total of 12 tablets)

Dosage Forms

Injection, solution [concentrate; preservative free]: Phosphorus 3 mmol and sodium 4 mEq per 1 mL (5 mL, 15 mL, 50 mL)

Solution, oral: Monobasic sodium phosphate 2.4 g and dibasic sodium phosphate 0.9 g per 5 mL (45 mL)

Solution, rectal [enema]: Monobasic sodium phosphate 19 g and dibasic sodium phosphate 7 g per 118 mL delivered dose (133 mL)

Fleet® Enema [OTC], LaCrosse Complete [OTC]: Monobasic sodium phosphate 19 g and dibasic sodium phosphate 7 g per 118 mL delivered dose (133 mL)

Fleet® Enema Extra® [OTC]: Monobasic sodium phosphate 19 g and dibasic sodium phosphate 7 g per 197 mL delivered dose (230 mL)

Fleet® Pedia-Lax™ Enema [OTC]: Monobasic sodium phosphate 9.5 g and dibasic sodium phosphate 3.5 g per 59 mL delivered dose (66 mL)

Tablet, oral [scored]:

OsmoPrep®, Visicol®: Monobasic sodium phosphate 1.102 g and dibasic sodium phosphate 0.398 g

sodium polystyrene sulfonate (SOW dee um pol ee STYE reen SUL fon ate)

Sound-Alike/Look-Alike Issues

Kayexalate® may be confused with Kaopectate®

U.S./Canadian Brand Names Kalexate [US]; Kayexalate® [US/Can]; Kionex® [US]; PMS-Sodium Polystyrene Sulfonate [Can]; SPS® [US]

Therapeutic Category Antidote

Use Treatment of hyperkalemia

Usual Dosage

Children:

Oral: 1 g/kg/dose every 6 hours

Rectal: 1 g/kg/dose every 2-6 hours (In small children and infants, employ lower doses by using the practical exchange ratio of 1 mEq K^+/g of resin as the basis for calculation)

Adults: Hyperkalemia:

Oral: 15 g 1-4 times/day

Rectal: 30-50 g every 6 hours

Dosage Forms

Powder for suspension, oral/rectal: 15 g/4 level teaspoons

Kalexate, Kayexalate®, Kionex®: 15 g/4 level teaspoons

Suspension, oral/rectal:

SPS®: 15 g/60 mL

sodium sulfacetamide *see* sulfacetamide *on page* *927*

sodium sulfacetamide and sulfur *see* sulfur and sulfacetamide *on page* *931*

sodium tetradecyl (SOW dee um tetra DEK il)

Synonyms sodium tetradecyl sulfate

U.S./Canadian Brand Names Sotradecol® [US]; Trombovar® [Can]

Therapeutic Category Sclerosing Agent

Use Treatment of small, uncomplicated varicose veins of the lower extremities

Usual Dosage I.V.: Test dose: 0.5 mL given several hours prior to administration of larger dose; 0.5-2 mL (preferred maximum: 1 mL) in each vein, maximum: 10 mL per treatment session; 3% solution reserved for large varices

Dosage Forms

Injection:

Sotradecol®: 1% (2 mL); 3% (2 mL)

sodium tetradecyl sulfate *see* sodium tetradecyl *on page* *914*

sodium thiosulfate (SOW dee um thye oh SUL fate)

Synonyms disodium thiosulfate pentahydrate; pentahydrate; sodium hyposulfate; sodium thiosulphate; thiosulfuric acid disodium salt

U.S./Canadian Brand Names Versiclear™ [US]

Therapeutic Category Antidote; Antifungal Agent

Use

Parenteral: Used alone or with sodium nitrite or amyl nitrite in cyanide poisoning; reduce the risk of nephrotoxicity associated with cisplatin therapy; treatment of cyanide poisoning due to nitroprusside

Topical: Treatment of tinea versicolor

Usual Dosage

Cyanide poisoning: I.V.: **Note:** Death from cyanide poisoning may occur rapidly, do not delay antidote administration in the event of highly suspected or confirmed cyanide poisoning; usually given in conjunction with amyl nitrite and sodium nitrite

Children: 7 g/m^2 (maximum dose: 12.5 g) given over 10 minutes; may repeat at 1/2 the original dose if symptoms return

Adults: 12.5 g given over 10 minutes; may repeat at 1/2 the original dose if symptoms return

Cisplatin rescue should be given before or during cisplatin administration: I.V. infusion (in sterile water): 12 g/m^2 over 6 hours or 9 g/m^2 I.V. push followed by 1.2 g/m^2 continuous infusion for 6 hours

Tinea versicolor: Children and Adults: Topical: 20% to 25% solution: Apply a thin layer to affected areas twice daily

Dosage Forms

Injection, solution [preservative free]: 100 mg/mL (10 mL); 250 mg/mL (50 mL)

Versiclear™: 100 mg/mL (10 mL); 250 mg/mL (50 mL)

Lotion:

Versiclear™: Sodium thiosulfate 25% and salicylic acid 1% (120 mL)

sodium thiosulfate, sodium nitrite, and amyl nitrite *see* sodium nitrite, sodium thiosulfate, and amyl nitrite *on page 911*

sodium thiosulphate *see* sodium thiosulfate *on page 915*

Soflax™ [Can] *see* docusate *on page 326*

Sojourn™ [US] *see* sevoflurane *on page 899*

Solagé® [US/Can] *see* mequinol and tretinoin *on page 629*

Solaquin® [Can] *see* hydroquinone *on page 508*

Solaquin® *(Discontinued)* *see* hydroquinone *on page 508*

Solaquin Forte® [Can] *see* hydroquinone *on page 508*

Solaquin Forte® *(Discontinued)* *see* hydroquinone *on page 508*

Solaraze® [US] *see* diclofenac *on page 303*

Solarcaine® Aloe Extra Burn Relief [US-OTC] *see* lidocaine *on page 584*

Solfoton® *(Discontinued)* *see* phenobarbital *on page 771*

Solia™ [US] *see* ethinyl estradiol and desogestrel *on page 383*

solifenacin (sol i FEN a sin)

Sound-Alike/Look-Alike Issues

VESIcare® may be confused with Visicol®

Synonyms solifenacin succinate; YM905

U.S./Canadian Brand Names VESIcare® [US]

Therapeutic Category Anticholinergic Agent

Use Treatment of overactive bladder with symptoms of urinary frequency, urgency, or urge incontinence

Usual Dosage Oral: Adults: 5 mg/day; if tolerated, may increase to 10 mg/day

Dosage Forms

Tablet:

VESIcare®: 5 mg, 10 mg

solifenacin succinate *see* solifenacin *on page 915*

Soliris™ [US] *see* eculizumab *on page 345*

Solodyn® [US] *see* minocycline *on page 659*

Soltamox™ *(Discontinued)* *see* tamoxifen *on page 937*

Soluble Fiber Therapy [US-OTC] *see* methylcellulose *on page 642*

soluble fluorescein *see* fluorescein *on page* 429
Solu-Cortef® [US/Can] *see* hydrocortisone (systemic) *on page* 504
Solugel® [Can] *see* benzoyl peroxide *on page* 132
Solu-Medrol® [US/Can] *see* methylprednisolone *on page* 647
solumedrol *see* methylprednisolone *on page* 647
Soluver® [Can] *see* salicylic acid *on page* 884
Soluver® Plus [Can] *see* salicylic acid *on page* 884
Soma® [US/Can] *see* carisoprodol *on page* 187
Soma® Compound [US] *see* carisoprodol and aspirin *on page* 187
Soma® Compound w/Codeine *(Discontinued)* *see* carisoprodol, aspirin, and codeine *on page* 187
somatrem *see* somatropin *on page* 916

somatropin (soe ma TROE pin)

Sound-Alike/Look-Alike Issues

somatropin may be confused with homatropine, somatrem, sumatriptan
Humatrope® may be confused with homatropine
somatrem may be confused with somatropin

Synonyms growth hormone, human; hGH; human growth hormone; somatrem

U.S./Canadian Brand Names Genotropin Miniquick® [US]; Genotropin® [US]; Humatrope® [US/Can]; Norditropin® NordiFlex® [US]; Norditropin® [US]; Nutropin AQ® [US/Can]; Nutropin® [US/Can]; Omnitrope® [US]; Saizen® [US/Can]; Serostim® [US/Can]; Tev-Tropin® [US]; Zorbtive® [US]

Therapeutic Category Growth Hormone

Use

Children:

- Treatment of growth failure due to inadequate endogenous growth hormone secretion (Genotropin®, Humatrope®, Norditropin®, Nutropin®, Nutropin AQ®, Omnitrope®, Saizen®, Tev-Tropin®)
- Treatment of short stature associated with Turner syndrome (Genotropin®, Humatrope®, Norditropin®, Nutropin®, Nutropin AQ®)
- Treatment of Prader-Willi syndrome (Genotropin®)
- Treatment of growth failure associated with chronic renal insufficiency (CRI) up until the time of renal transplantation (Nutropin®, Nutropin AQ®)
- Treatment of growth failure in children born small for gestational age who fail to manifest catch-up growth by 2 years of age (Genotropin®) or by 2-4 years of age (Humatrope®, Norditropin®)
- Treatment of idiopathic short stature (nongrowth hormone-deficient short stature) defined by height standard deviation score (SDS) ≤ -2.25 and growth rate not likely to attain normal adult height (Genotropin®, Humatrope®, Nutropin®, Nutropin AQ®)
- Treatment of short stature or growth failure associated with short stature homeobox gene (SHOX) deficiency (Humatrope®)
- Treatment of short stature associated with Noonan syndrome (Norditropin®)

Adults:

- HIV patients with wasting or cachexia with concomitant antiviral therapy (Serostim®)
- Replacement of endogenous growth hormone in patients with adult growth hormone deficiency who meet both of the following criteria (Genotropin®, Humatrope®, Norditropin®, Nutropin®, Nutropin AQ®, Omnitrope®, Saizen®):
  - Biochemical diagnosis of adult growth hormone deficiency by means of a subnormal response to a standard growth hormone stimulation test (peak growth hormone ≤5 mcg/L). Confirmatory testing may not be required in patients with congenital/genetic growth hormone deficiency or multiple pituitary hormone deficiencies due to organic diseases.

    and

  - Adult-onset: Patients who have adult growth hormone deficiency whether alone or with multiple hormone deficiencies (hypopituitarism) as a result of pituitary disease, hypothalamic disease, surgery, radiation therapy, or trauma

    or

  - Childhood-onset: Patients who were growth hormone deficient during childhood, confirmed as an adult before replacement therapy is initiated
- Treatment of short-bowel syndrome (Zorbtive®)

Usual Dosage

Children (individualize dose):

Chronic renal insufficiency (CRI): Nutropin®, Nutropin® AQ: SubQ: Weekly dosage: 0.35 mg/kg divided into daily injections; continue until the time of renal transplantation

Dosage recommendations in patients treated for CRI who require dialysis:

Hemodialysis: Administer dose at night prior to bedtime or at least 3-4 hours after hemodialysis to prevent hematoma formation from heparin

CCPD: Administer dose in the morning following dialysis

CAPD: Administer dose in the evening at the time of overnight exchange

Growth hormone deficiency:

Genotropin®, Omnitrope®: SubQ: Weekly dosage: 0.16-0.24 mg/kg divided into equal doses 6-7 days per week

Humatrope®: SubQ: Weekly dosage: 0.18-0.3 mg/kg divided into equal doses 6-7 days per week

Norditropin®: SubQ: 0.024-0.034 mg/kg/day, 6-7 days per week

Nutropin®, Nutropin® AQ: SubQ: Weekly dosage: 0.3 mg/kg divided into equal daily doses; pubertal patients: ≤0.7 mg/kg divided into equal daily doses

Tev-Tropin®: SubQ: Up to 0.1 mg/kg administered 3 days per week

Saizen®: I.M., SubQ: Weekly dosage: 0.18 mg/kg divided into equal daily doses **or** as 0.06 mg/kg/dose administered 3 days per week **or** as 0.03 mg/kg/dose administered 6 days per week

Note: Therapy should be discontinued when patient has reached satisfactory adult height, when epiphyses have fused, or when the patient ceases to respond. Growth of 5 cm/year or more is expected, if growth rate does not exceed 2.5 cm in a 6-month period, double the dose for the next 6 months; if there is still no satisfactory response, discontinue therapy

Idiopathic short stature:

Genotropin®: SubQ: Weekly dosage: 0.47 mg/kg divided into equal doses 6-7 days per week

Humatrope®: SubQ: Weekly dosage: 0.37 mg/kg divided into equal doses 6-7 days per week

Nutropin®, Nutropin AQ®: SubQ: Weekly dosage: Up to 0.3 mg/kg divided into equal daily doses

Noonan syndrome: Norditropin®: SubQ: Up to 0.066 mg/kg/day

Prader-Willi syndrome: Genotropin®: SubQ: Weekly dosage: 0.24 mg/kg divided into equal doses 6-7 days per week

SHOX deficiency: Humatrope®: SubQ: Weekly dosage: 0.35 mg/kg divided into equal doses 6-7 days per week

Small for gestational age:

Genotropin®: SubQ: Weekly dosage: 0.48 mg/kg divided into equal doses 6-7 days per week

Humatrope®: SubQ: Weekly dosage: 0.47 mg/kg divided into equal doses 6-7 days per week

Norditropin®: SubQ: Up to 0.067 mg/kg/day

Alternate dosing (small for gestational age): In older/early pubertal children or children with very short stature, consider initiating therapy at higher doses (0.067 mg/kg/day) and then consider reducing the dose (0.033 mg/kg/day) if substantial catch-up growth observed. In younger children (<4 years) with less severe short stature, consider initiating therapy with lower doses (0.033 mg/kg/day) and then titrating the dose upwards as needed.

Turner syndrome:

Genotropin®: SubQ: Weekly dosage: 0.33 mg/kg divided into equal doses 6-7 days per week

Humatrope®: SubQ: Weekly dosage: 0.375 mg/kg divided into equal doses 6-7 days per week

Norditropin®: SubQ: Up to 0.067 mg/kg/day

Nutropin®, Nutropin® AQ: SubQ: Weekly dosage: ≤0.375 mg/kg divided into equal doses 3-7 days per week

Adults:

Growth hormone deficiency: Adjust dose based on individual requirements: To minimize adverse events in older or overweight patients, reduced dosages may be necessary. During therapy, dosage should be decreased if required by the occurrence of side effects or excessive IGF-I levels.

Weight-based dosing:

Norditropin®: SubQ: Initial dose ≤0.004 mg/kg/day; after 6 weeks of therapy, may increase dose up to 0.016 mg/kg/day

Nutropin®, Nutropin® AQ: SubQ: ≤0.006 mg/kg/day; dose may be increased up to a maximum of 0.025 mg/kg/day in patients <35 years of age, or up to a maximum of 0.0125 mg/kg/day in patients ≥35 years of age

Humatrope®: SubQ: ≤0.006 mg/kg/day; dose may be increased up to a maximum of 0.0125 mg/kg/day

Genotropin®, Omnitrope®: SubQ: Weekly dosage: ≤0.04 mg/kg divided into equal doses 6-7 days per week; dose may be increased at 4- to 8-week intervals to a maximum of 0.08 mg/kg/week

Saizen®: SubQ: ≤0.005 mg/kg/day; dose may be increased to not more than 0.01 mg/kg/day after 4 weeks

Nonweight-based dosing: SubQ: Initial: 0.2 mg/day (range: 0.15-0.3 mg/day); may increase every 1-2 months by 0.1-0.2 mg/day based on response and/or serum IGF-I levels

Dosage adjustment with estrogen supplementation (growth hormone deficiency): Larger doses of somatropin may be needed for women taking oral estrogen replacement products; dosing not affected by topical products

HIV patients with wasting or cachexia: Serostim®: SubQ: 0.1 mg/kg once daily at bedtime (maximum: 6 mg/day). Alternately, patients at risk for side effects may be started at 0.1 mg/kg every other day. Patients who continue to lose weight after 12 weeks should be re-evaluated for opportunistic infections or other clinical events; rotate injection sites to avoid lipodystrophy Adjust dose if needed to manage side effects.

Daily dose based on body weight:

<35 kg: 0.1 mg/kg
35-45 kg: 4 mg
45-55 kg: 5 mg
>55 kg: 6 mg

Short-bowel syndrome (Zorbtive®): SubQ: 0.1 mg/kg once daily for 4 weeks (maximum: 8 mg/day)

Fluid retention (moderate) or arthralgias: Treat symptomatically or reduce dose by 50%

Severe toxicity: Discontinue therapy for up to 5 days; when symptoms resolve, restart at 50% of dose. If severe toxicity recurs or does not disappear within 5 days after discontinuation, permanently discontinue treatment.

Dosage Forms

Injection, powder for reconstitution [rDNA origin]:

Genotropin®: 5.8 mg [~15 int. units/mL]; 13.8 mg [~36 int. units/mL]
Genotropin Miniquick® [preservative free]: 0.2 mg, 0.4 mg, 0.6 mg, 0.8 mg, 1 mg, 1.2 mg, 1.4 mg, 1.6 mg, 1.8 mg, 2 mg
Humatrope®: 5 mg [15 int. units], 6 mg [18 int. units], 12 mg [36 int. units], 24 mg [72 int. units]
Nutropin®: 5 mg [~15 int. units]; 10 mg [~30 int. units]
Omnitrope®: 5.8 mg [~17.4 int. units]
Saizen®: 5 mg [~15 int. units]; 8.8 mg [~26.4 int. units]
Serostim®: 4 mg [~12 int. units]; 5 mg [~15 int. units]; 6 mg [~18 int. units]
Tev-Tropin®: 5 mg [15 int. units/mL]
Zorbtive®: 8.8 mg [~26.4 int. units]

Injection, solution [rDNA origin]:

Norditropin®: 5 mg/1.5 mL (1.5 mL); 15 mg/1.5 mL (1.5 mL)
Norditropin® NordiFlex®: 5 mg/1.5 mL (1.5 mL); 10 mg/1.5 mL (1.5 mL); 15 mg/1.5 mL (1.5 mL)
Nutropin AQ®: 5 mg/mL [~15 int. units/mL] (2 mL)
Omnitrope®: 5 mg/1.5 mL (1.5 mL); 10 mg/1.5 mL (1.5 mL)

Somatuline® Autogel® [Can] *see* lanreotide *on page* *570*

Somatuline® Depot [US] *see* lanreotide *on page* *570*

Somavert® [US/Can] *see* pegvisomant *on page* *758*

Sominex® [US-OTC] *see* diphenhydramine *on page* *315*

Sominex® Maximum Strength [US-OTC] *see* diphenhydramine *on page* *315*

Somnote® [US] *see* chloral hydrate *on page* *208*

Som Pam [Can] *see* flurazepam *on page* *435*

Sonata® [US] *see* zaleplon *on page* *1026*

Soothe® [US-OTC] *see* artificial tears *on page* *100*

Soothing Care™ Itch Relief [US-OTC] *see* pramoxine *on page* *809*

sorafenib (sor AF e nib)

Sound-Alike/Look-Alike Issues

sorafenib may be confused with imatinib, sunitinib
Nexavar® may be confused with Nexium®

Synonyms BAY 43-9006; NSC-724772; sorafenib tosylate

U.S./Canadian Brand Names Nexavar® [US/Can]

Therapeutic Category Antineoplastic Agent, Tyrosine Kinase Inhibitor; Vascular Endothelial Growth Factor (VEGF) Inhibitor

Use Treatment of advanced renal cell cancer (RCC), unresectable hepatocellular cancer (HCC)

Usual Dosage Oral: Adults:
Advanced renal cell carcinoma: 400 mg twice daily
Hepatocellular cancer: 400 mg twice daily

Dosage Forms
Tablet:
Nexavar®: 200 mg

sorafenib tosylate *see* sorafenib *on page 918*

sorbitol (SOR bi tole)

Therapeutic Category Genitourinary Irrigant; Laxative

Use Genitourinary irrigant in transurethral prostatic resection or other transurethral resection or other transurethral surgical procedures; diuretic; humectant; sweetening agent; hyperosmotic laxative; facilitate the passage of sodium polystyrene sulfonate through the intestinal tract

Usual Dosage Hyperosmotic laxative (as single dose, at infrequent intervals):
Children 2-11 years:
Oral: 2 mL/kg (as 70% solution)
Rectal enema: 30-60 mL as 25% to 30% solution
Children >12 years and Adults:
Oral: 30-150 mL (as 70% solution)
Rectal enema: 120 mL as 25% to 30% solution
Adjunct to sodium polystyrene sulfonate: 15 mL as 70% solution orally until diarrhea occurs (10-20 mL/2 hours) or 20-100 mL as an oral vehicle for the sodium polystyrene sulfonate resin
When administered with charcoal:
Oral:
Children: 4.3 mL/kg of 35% sorbitol with 1 g/kg of activated charcoal
Adults: 4.3 mL/kg of 70% sorbitol with 1 g/kg of activated charcoal every 4 hours until first stool containing charcoal is passed
Topical: 3% to 3.3% as transurethral surgical procedure irrigation

Dosage Forms
Solution, genitourinary irrigation: 3% (3000 mL, 5000 mL); 3.3% (2000 mL, 4000 mL)
Solution, oral: 70%

Sorbitrate® *(Discontinued)* *see* isosorbide dinitrate *on page 550*
Soriatane® [Can] *see* acitretin *on page 32*
Soriatane® CK Convenience Kit™ [US] *see* acitretin *on page 32*
Soriatane® *(Discontinued)* *see* acitretin *on page 32*
Sorine® [US] *see* sotalol *on page 919*

sotalol (SOE ta lole)

Sound-Alike/Look-Alike Issues
sotalol may be confused with Stadol®, Sudafed®
Betapace® may be confused with Betapace AF®
Betapace AF® may be confused with Betapace®

Synonyms sotalol hydrochloride

U.S./Canadian Brand Names Apo-Sotalol® [Can]; Betapace AF® [US/Can]; Betapace® [US]; CO Sotalol [Can]; DOM-Sotalol [Can]; Gen-Sotalol [Can]; Lin-Sotalol [Can]; MED-Sotalol [Can]; Novo-Sotalol [Can]; Nu-Sotalol [Can]; PHL-Sotalol [Can]; PMS-Sotalol [Can]; PRO-Sotalol [Can]; ratio-Sotalol [Can]; Rhoxal-sotalol [Can]; Riva-Sotalol [Can]; Rylosol [Can]; Sandoz-Sotalol [Can]; Sorine® [US]; ZYM-Sotalol [Can]

Therapeutic Category Antiarrhythmic Agent, Class II; Antiarrhythmic Agent, Class III; Beta-Adrenergic Blocker, Nonselective

Use Treatment of documented ventricular arrhythmias (ie, sustained ventricular tachycardia), that in the judgment of the physician are life-threatening; maintenance of normal sinus rhythm in patients with symptomatic atrial fibrillation and atrial flutter who are currently in sinus rhythm. Manufacturer states substitutions should not be made for Betapace AF® since Betapace AF® is distributed with a patient package insert specific for atrial fibrillation/flutter.

Usual Dosage Sotalol should be initiated and doses increased in a hospital with facilities for cardiac rhythm monitoring and assessment. Proarrhythmic events can occur after initiation of therapy and with each upward dosage adjustment.

Children: Oral: The safety and efficacy of sotalol in children have not been established

Note: Dosing per manufacturer, based on pediatric pharmacokinetic data; wait at least 36 hours between dosage adjustments to allow monitoring of QT intervals

≤2 years: Dosage should be adjusted (decreased) by plotting of the child's age on a logarithmic scale; refer to manufacturer's package labeling.

>2 years: Initial: 90 mg/m^2/day in 3 divided doses; may be incrementally increased to a maximum of 180 mg/m^2/day

Adults: Oral:

Ventricular arrhythmias (Betapace®, Sorine®):

Initial: 80 mg twice daily

Dose may be increased gradually to 240-320 mg/day; allow 3 days between dosing increments in order to attain steady-state plasma concentrations and to allow monitoring of QT intervals

Most patients respond to a total daily dose of 160-320 mg/day in 2-3 divided doses.

Some patients, with life-threatening refractory ventricular arrhythmias, may require doses as high as 480-640 mg/day; however, these doses should only be prescribed when the potential benefit outweighs the increased of adverse events.

Atrial fibrillation or atrial flutter (Betapace AF®): Initial: 80 mg twice daily

If the initial dose does not reduce the frequency of relapses of atrial fibrillation/flutter and is tolerated without excessive QT prolongation (not >520 msec) after 3 days, the dose may be increased to 120 mg twice daily. This may be further increased to 160 mg twice daily if response is inadequate and QT prolongation is not excessive.

Dosage Forms

Tablet: 80 mg, 80 mg [atrial fibrillation], 120 mg, 120 mg [atrial fibrillation], 160 mg, 160 mg [atrial fibrillation], 240 mg

Betapace®: 80 mg, 120 mg, 160 mg, 240 mg

Betapace AF®: 80 mg, 120 mg, 160 mg [atrial fibrillation]

Sorine®: 80 mg, 120 mg, 160 mg, 240 mg

sotalol hydrochloride *see* sotalol *on page* *919*

Sotradecol® [US] *see* sodium tetradecyl *on page* *914*

Sotret® [US] *see* isotretinoin *on page* *551*

SourceCF® [US] *see* vitamins (multiple/oral) *on page* *1019*

Soyacal® *(Discontinued)* *see* fat emulsion *on page* *406*

Soyalac® [US-OTC] *see* nutritional formula, enteral/oral *on page* *715*

SPA *see* albumin *on page* *40*

Spacol *(Discontinued)* *see* hyoscyamine *on page* *512*

Spacol T/S *(Discontinued)* *see* hyoscyamine *on page* *512*

Span-FF® *(Discontinued)* *see* ferrous fumarate *on page* *413*

Spasmolin® *(Discontinued)* *see* hyoscyamine, atropine, scopolamine, and phenobarbital *on page* *513*

Spastrin® *(Discontinued)*

SPD417 *see* carbamazepine *on page* *180*

Spectazole® *(Discontinued)* *see* econazole *on page* *345*

Spec-T® *(Discontinued)* *see* benzocaine *on page* *129*

spectinomycin *(Discontinued)*

Spectracef® [US] *see* cefditoren *on page* *192*

Spectrocin Plus™ *(Discontinued)* *see* bacitracin, neomycin, polymyxin B, and pramoxine *on page* *120*

SPEF-Pioglitazone [Can] *see* pioglitazone *on page* *785*

SPI 0211 *see* lubiprostone *on page* *603*

Spiriva® [Can] *see* tiotropium *on page* *963*

Spiriva® HandiHaler® [US] *see* tiotropium *on page* *963*

Spironazide® *(Discontinued)* *see* hydrochlorothiazide and spironolactone *on page* *500*

spironolactone (speer on oh LAK tone)

Sound-Alike/Look-Alike Issues

Aldactone® may be confused with Aldactazide®

U.S./Canadian Brand Names Aldactone® [US/Can]; Novo-Spiroton [Can]

Therapeutic Category Diuretic, Potassium Sparing

Use Management of edema associated with excessive aldosterone excretion; hypertension; primary hyperaldosteronism; hypokalemia; cirrhosis of liver accompanied by edema or ascites; nephritic syndrome; severe heart failure (NYHA class III-IV) to increase survival and reduce hospitalization when added to standard therapy

Usual Dosage Oral: Adults:

Edema: 25-200 mg/day in 1-2 divided doses

Hypokalemia: 25-100 mg daily

Hypertension (JNC 7): 25-50 mg/day in 1-2 divided doses

Diagnosis of primary aldosteronism: Long test: 400 mg daily for 3-4 weeks; short test: 400 mg daily for 4 days; maintenance until surgical correction: 100-400 mg/day in 1-2 divided doses

Heart failure, severe (NYHA class III-IV; with ACE inhibitor and a loop diuretic ± digoxin): 12.5-25 mg/day; maximum daily dose: 50 mg. If 25 mg once daily not tolerated, reduce to 25 mg every other day was the lowest maintenance dose possible.

Note: If potassium >5 mEq/L or serum creatinine >4 mg/dL, discontinue or interrupt therapy.

Dosage Forms

Tablet: 25 mg, 50 mg, 100 mg

Aldactone®: 25 mg

Aldactone®: 50 mg, 100 mg [scored]

spironolactone and hydrochlorothiazide *see* hydrochlorothiazide and spironolactone *on page 500*

Spirozide® *(Discontinued)* *see* hydrochlorothiazide and spironolactone *on page 500*

SPM 927 *see* lacosamide *on page 563*

Sporanox® [US/Can] *see* itraconazole *on page 552*

Sportscreme® [US-OTC] *see* trolamine *on page 991*

SPP100 *see* aliskiren *on page 47*

Sprayzoin™ [US-OTC] *see* benzoin *on page 132*

Sprintec® [US] *see* ethinyl estradiol and norgestimate *on page 393*

Sprycel® [US/Can] *see* dasatinib *on page 278*

SPS® [US] *see* sodium polystyrene sulfonate *on page 914*

SR33589 *see* dronedarone *on page 339*

SRC® Expectorant *(Discontinued)*

Sronyx™ [US] *see* ethinyl estradiol and levonorgestrel *on page 387*

SS734 *see* besifloxacin *on page 136*

SSD® [US] *see* silver sulfadiazine *on page 901*

SSD® AF [US] *see* silver sulfadiazine *on page 901*

SSKI® [US] *see* potassium iodide *on page 805*

S.T. 37® [US-OTC] *see* hexylresorcinol *on page 493*

Stadol® *(Discontinued)* *see* butorphanol *on page 164*

Stadol® NS *(Discontinued)* *see* butorphanol *on page 164*

Staflex [US] *see* acetaminophen and phenyltoloxamine *on page 23*

Stagesic™ [US] *see* hydrocodone and acetaminophen *on page 501*

Stalevo® [US/Can] *see* levodopa, carbidopa, and entacapone *on page 579*

StanGard® [US] *see* fluoride *on page 430*

StanGard® Perio [US] *see* fluoride *on page 430*

stannous fluoride *see* fluoride *on page 430*

stanozolol *(Discontinued)*

Starlix® [US/Can] *see* nateglinide *on page 684*

Statex® [Can] *see* morphine sulfate *on page 667*

Staticin® *(Discontinued)* *see* erythromycin *on page 368*

Statobex® [Can] *see* phendimetrazine *on page 770*

Statuss™ DM [US] *see* chlorpheniramine, phenylephrine, and dextromethorphan *on page 217*

stavudine (STAV yoo deen)

Sound-Alike/Look-Alike Issues

Zerit® may be confused with Zestril®, Ziac®, Zyrtec®

Synonyms d4T

U.S./Canadian Brand Names Zerit® [US/Can]

Therapeutic Category Antiviral Agent
Use Treatment of HIV infection in combination with other antiretroviral agents
Usual Dosage Oral:
Newborns (Birth to 13 days): 0.5 mg/kg every 12 hours
Children:
>14 days and <30 kg: 1 mg/kg every 12 hours
≥30 kg: Refer to adult dosing
Adults:
<60 kg: 30 mg every 12 hours
≥60 kg: 40 mg every 12 hours
Dosage Forms
Capsule: 15 mg, 20 mg, 30 mg, 40 mg
Zerit®: 15 mg, 20 mg, 30 mg, 40 mg
Powder for solution, oral:
Zerit®: 1 mg/mL

Stavzor™ [US] *see* valproic acid and derivatives *on page* 1002
Stelara® [Can] *see* ustekinumab *(Canada only) on page* 1000
Stelazine® *(Discontinued)* *see* trifluoperazine *on page* 986
Stemetil® [Can] *see* prochlorperazine *on page* 820
Sterapred® [US] *see* prednisone *on page* 814
Sterapred® DS [US] *see* prednisone *on page* 814
sterile talc *see* talc (sterile) *on page* 937
Sterile Talc Powder™ [US] *see* talc (sterile) *on page* 937
STI-571 *see* imatinib *on page* 519
Stieprox® [Can] *see* ciclopirox *on page* 227
Stimate® [US] *see* desmopressin acetate *on page* 285
Sting-Kill [US-OTC] *see* benzocaine *on page* 129
St. Joseph® Adult Aspirin [US-OTC] *see* aspirin *on page* 103
St. Joseph® Cough Suppressant *(Discontinued)* *see* dextromethorphan *on page* 295
St. Joseph® Measured Dose Nasal Solution *(Discontinued)* *see* phenylephrine *on page* 774
Stop® [US] *see* fluoride *on page* 430
Strattera® [US/Can] *see* atomoxetine *on page* 108
Streptase® *(Discontinued)*
streptokinase *(Discontinued)*

streptomycin (strep toe MYE sin)

Sound-Alike/Look-Alike Issues
streptomycin may be confused with streptozocin
Synonyms streptomycin sulfate
Therapeutic Category Antibiotic, Aminoglycoside; Antitubercular Agent
Use Part of combination therapy of active tuberculosis; used in combination with other agents for treatment of streptococcal or enterococcal endocarditis, mycobacterial infections, plague, tularemia, and brucellosis
Usual Dosage Note: For I.M. administration; I.V. use is not recommended
Usual dosage range:
Children: 20-40 mg/kg/day (maximum: 1 g)
Adults: 15-30 mg/kg/day or 1-2 g/day
Indication-specific dosing:
Children: **Tuberculosis:** I.M.:
Daily therapy: 20-40 mg/kg/day (maximum: 1 g/day)
Directly observed therapy (DOT): Twice weekly: 25-30 mg/kg (maximum: 1.5 g)
Directly observed therapy (DOT): 3 times/week: 25-30 mg/kg (maximum: 1.5 g)
Adults: I.M.:
Brucellosis: 1 g/day for 14-21 days (with doxycycline, 100 mg twice daily for 6 weeks)
Endocarditis:
Enterococcal: 1 g every 12 hours for 2 weeks, 500 mg every 12 hours for 4 weeks in combination with penicillin
Streptococcal: 1 g every 12 hours for 1 week, 500 mg every 12 hours for 1 week

***Mycobacterium avium* complex:** Adjunct therapy (with macrolide, rifamycin, and ethambutol): 15 mg/kg 3 times/week for first 2-3 months for severe disease

Plague: 15 mg/kg (or 1 g) every 12 hours until the patient is afebrile for at least 3 days

Tuberculosis:

Daily therapy: 15 mg/kg/day (maximum: 1 g)

Directly observed therapy (DOT): Twice weekly: 25-30 mg/kg (maximum: 1.5 g)

Directly observed therapy (DOT): 3 times/week: 25-30 mg/kg (maximum: 1.5 g)

Tularemia: 10-15 mg/kg every 12 hours (maximum: 2 g/day) for 7-10 days or until patient is afebrile for 5-7 days

Dosage Forms

Injection, powder for reconstitution: 1 g

streptomycin sulfate *see* streptomycin *on page* 922

streptozocin (strep toe ZOE sin)

Sound-Alike/Look-Alike Issues

streptozocin may be confused with streptomycin

Synonyms NSC-85998

U.S./Canadian Brand Names Zanosar® [US/Can]

Therapeutic Category Antineoplastic Agent

Use Treatment of metastatic islet cell carcinoma of the pancreas, carcinoid tumor and syndrome, Hodgkin disease, palliative treatment of colorectal cancer

Usual Dosage I.V. (refer to individual protocols): Children and Adults:

Single agent therapy: 1-1.5 g/m^2 weekly for 6 weeks followed by a 4-week rest period

Combination therapy: 0.5-1 g/m^2 for 5 consecutive days followed by a 4- to 6-week rest period

Dosage Forms

Injection, powder for reconstitution:

Zanosar®: 1 g

Stresstabs® High Potency Advanced [US-OTC] *see* vitamin B complex combinations *on page* 1017

Stresstabs® High Potency Energy [US-OTC] *see* vitamin B complex combinations *on page* 1017

Stresstabs® High Potency Weight [US-OTC] *see* vitamin B complex combinations *on page* 1017

Striant® [US] *see* testosterone *on page* 947

Stridex® Essential Care® [US-OTC] *see* salicylic acid *on page* 884

Stridex® Facewipes To Go® [US-OTC] *see* salicylic acid *on page* 884

Stridex® Maximum Strength [US-OTC] *see* salicylic acid *on page* 884

Stridex® Sensitive Skin [US-OTC] *see* salicylic acid *on page* 884

Strifon Forte® [Can] *see* chlorzoxazone *on page* 223

Stromectol® [US] *see* ivermectin *on page* 553

strontium-89 chloride *see* strontium-89 *on page* 923

strontium-89 (STRON shee um atey nine)

Synonyms strontium-89 chloride

U.S./Canadian Brand Names Metastron® [US/Can]

Therapeutic Category Radiopharmaceutical

Use Relief of bone pain in patients with skeletal metastases

Usual Dosage I.V.: Adults: 148 megabecquerel (4 millicurie) administered by slow I.V. injection over 1-2 minutes or 1.5-2.2 megabecquerel (40-60 microcurie)/kg; repeated doses are generally not recommended at intervals <90 days; measure the patient dose by a suitable radioactivity calibration system immediately prior to administration

Dosage Forms

Injection, solution [preservative free]:

Metastron®: 1 mCi/mL (4 mL) [37 megabecquerel per mL]

Strovite® [US] *see* vitamins (multiple/oral) *on page* 1019

Strovite® Advance [US] *see* vitamins (multiple/oral) *on page* 1019

Strovite® Forte [US] *see* vitamins (multiple/oral) *on page* 1019

Strovite® Plus [US] *see* vitamins (multiple/oral) *on page* 1019

Stuartnatal® Plus 3™ ***(Discontinued)*** *see* vitamins (multiple/prenatal) *on page 1020*
Stuart Prenatal® [US-OTC] *see* vitamins (multiple/prenatal) *on page 1020*
SU011248 *see* sunitinib *on page 933*
suberoylanilide hydroxamic acid *see* vorinostat *on page 1022*
Sublimaze® [US] *see* fentanyl *on page 410*
Suboxone® [US] *see* buprenorphine and naloxone *on page 158*
Subutex® [US/Can] *see* buprenorphine *on page 157*

succimer (SUKS si mer)

Synonyms DMSA

U.S./Canadian Brand Names Chemet® [US/Can]

Therapeutic Category Chelating Agent

Use Treatment of lead poisoning in children with serum lead levels >45 mcg/dL

Usual Dosage Note: For the treatment of high blood lead levels in children, the CDC recommends chelation treatment when blood lead levels are >45 mcg/dL. Children with blood lead levels >70 mcg/dL or symptomatic lead poisoning should be treated with parenteral agents. In adults, available guidelines recommend chelation therapy with blood lead levels >50 mcg/dL and significant symptoms; chelation therapy may also be indicated with blood lead levels ≥100 mcg/dL and/or symptoms.

Children: Oral: 10 mg/kg/dose (or 350 mg/m^2/dose) every 8 hours for 5 days followed by 10 mg/kg/dose (or 350 mg/m^2/dose) every 12 hours for 14 days. Maximum: 500 mg/dose. For children <5 years of age, dose should be based on mg/m^2; dosing by mg/kg may be suboptimal.

Note: Treatment courses may be repeated, but 2-week intervals between courses is generally recommended.

Dosage Forms

Capsule:

Chemet®: 100 mg

succinylcholine (suks in il KOE leen)

Synonyms succinylcholine chloride; suxamethonium chloride

U.S./Canadian Brand Names Anectine® [US]; Quelicin® [US/Can]

Therapeutic Category Skeletal Muscle Relaxant

Use To facilitate both rapid sequence and routine endotracheal intubation and to relax skeletal muscles during surgery; to reduce the intensity of muscle contractions of pharmacologically- or electrically-induced convulsions; does not relieve pain or produce sedation

Usual Dosage I.M., I.V.: Dose to effect; doses will vary due to interpatient variability; use ideal body weight for obese patients

I.M.: Children and Adults: Up to 3-4 mg/kg, total dose should not exceed 150 mg

I.V.:

Children: **Note:** Because of the risk of malignant hyperthermia, use of continuous infusions is not recommended in infants and children

Smaller Children: Intermittent: Initial: 2 mg/kg/dose one time; maintenance: 0.3-0.6 mg/kg/dose every 5-10 minutes as needed

Older Children and Adolescents: Intermittent: Initial: 1 mg/kg/dose one time; maintenance: 0.3-0.6 mg/kg every 5-10 minutes as needed

Adults: Initial:

Short surgical procedures: 0.6 mg/kg (range 0.3-1.1 mg/kg)

Long surgical procedures:

Continuous infusion: 2.5-4.3 mg/minute; adjust dose based on response

Intermittent: Initial: 0.3-1.1 mg/kg; maintenance: 0.04-0.07 mg/kg/dose as required

Note: Initial dose of succinylcholine must be increased when nondepolarizing agent pretreatment used because of the antagonism between succinylcholine and nondepolarizing neuromuscular-blocking agents.

Dosage Forms

Injection, solution:

Anectine®: 20 mg/mL (10 mL)

Quelicin®: 20 mg/mL (10 mL)

Injection, solution [preservative free]:

Quelicin®: 100 mg/mL (10 mL)

succinylcholine chloride *see* succinylcholine *on page 924*

Suclor™ [US] *see* chlorpheniramine and pseudoephedrine *on page* 215
Sucraid® [US/Can] *see* sacrosidase *on page* 884

sucralfate (soo KRAL fate)

Sound-Alike/Look-Alike Issues
sucralfate may be confused with salsalate
Carafate® may be confused with Cafergot®

Synonyms aluminum sucrose sulfate, basic

U.S./Canadian Brand Names Carafate® [US]; Novo-Sucralate [Can]; Nu-Sucralate [Can]; PMS-Sucralate [Can]; Sulcrate® Suspension Plus [Can]; Sulcrate® [Can]

Therapeutic Category Gastrointestinal Agent, Gastric or Duodenal Ulcer Treatment

Use Short-term (≤8 weeks) management of duodenal ulcers; maintenance therapy for duodenal ulcers

Usual Dosage Oral: Adults: Duodenal ulcer:
Treatment: 1 g 4 times/day on an empty stomach and at bedtime for 4-8 weeks, or alternatively 2 g twice daily; treatment is recommended for 4-8 weeks in adults
Maintenance: Prophylaxis: 1 g twice daily

Dosage Forms
Suspension, oral: 1 g/10 mL (10 mL)
Carafate®: 1 g/10 mL
Tablet: 1 g
Carafate®: 1 g

Sucrets® [US-OTC] *see* dyclonine *on page* 343
Sucrets® Cough Calmers ***(Discontinued)*** *see* dextromethorphan *on page* 295
Sucrets® Original [US-OTC] *see* hexylresorcinol *on page* 493
Sudafed® 12 Hour [US-OTC] *see* pseudoephedrine *on page* 833
Sudafed® 24 Hour [US-OTC] *see* pseudoephedrine *on page* 833
Sudafed® Children's [US-OTC] *see* pseudoephedrine *on page* 833
Sudafed® Children's Cold & Cough [US-OTC] *see* pseudoephedrine and dextromethorphan *on page* 834
Sudafed® Decongestant [Can] *see* pseudoephedrine *on page* 833
Sudafed® Head Cold and Sinus Extra Strength [Can] *see* acetaminophen and pseudoephedrine *on page* 24
Sudafed® Maximum Strength Nasal Decongestant [US-OTC] *see* pseudoephedrine *on page* 833
Sudafed® Maximum Strength Sinus Nighttime ***(Discontinued)*** *see* triprolidine and pseudoephedrine *on page* 989
Sudafed® Non-Drying Sinus ***(Discontinued)*** *see* guaifenesin and pseudoephedrine *on page* 477
Sudafed PE™ [US-OTC] *see* phenylephrine *on page* 774
Sudafed PE® Nighttime Cold [US-OTC] *see* acetaminophen, diphenhydramine, and phenylephrine *on page* 28
Sudafed PE® Severe Cold [US-OTC] *see* acetaminophen, diphenhydramine, and phenylephrine *on page* 28
Sudafed PE® Sinus & Allergy [US-OTC] *see* chlorpheniramine and phenylephrine *on page* 214
Sudafed PE® Sinus Headache [US-OTC] *see* acetaminophen and phenylephrine *on page* 22
Sudafed® Sinus Advance [Can] *see* pseudoephedrine and ibuprofen *on page* 835
Sudafed® Sinus & Allergy [US-OTC] *see* chlorpheniramine and pseudoephedrine *on page* 215
SudaHist® [US] *see* chlorpheniramine and pseudoephedrine *on page* 215
Sudal® 12 [US] *see* chlorpheniramine and pseudoephedrine *on page* 215
SudaTex-DM [US] *see* guaifenesin, pseudoephedrine, and dextromethorphan *on page* 479
SudaTex-G [US] *see* guaifenesin and pseudoephedrine *on page* 477
Sudex® ***(Discontinued)*** *see* guaifenesin and pseudoephedrine *on page* 477
SudoGest [US-OTC] *see* pseudoephedrine *on page* 833
SudoGest Children's [US-OTC] *see* pseudoephedrine *on page* 833
SudoGest Children's [US-OTC] *see* pseudoephedrine and dextromethorphan *on page* 834
Sudo-Tab® [US-OTC] *see* pseudoephedrine *on page* 833
Sufedrin® ***(Discontinued)*** *see* pseudoephedrine *on page* 833

Sufenta® [US/Can] *see* sufentanil *on page 926*

sufentanil (soo FEN ta nil)

Sound-Alike/Look-Alike Issues

SUFentanil may be confused with alfentanil, fentaNYL

Sufenta® may be confused with Alfenta®, Sudafed®, Survanta®

Synonyms sufentanil citrate

Tall-Man SUFentanil

U.S./Canadian Brand Names Sufentanil Citrate Injection, USP [Can]; Sufenta® [US/Can]

Therapeutic Category Analgesic, Narcotic; General Anesthetic

Controlled Substance C-II

Use Analgesic supplement in maintenance of general anesthesia; epidural analgesic in conjunction with a local anesthetic

Usual Dosage

I.V.:

Children 2-12 years: Induction: 10-25 mcg/kg (10-15 mcg/kg most common dose) with 100% O_2; Maintenance: Up to 1-2 mcg/kg total dose

Adults: Dose should be based on body weight. **Note:** In obese patients (eg, >20% above ideal body weight), use lean body weight to determine dosage.

Surgical analgesia (surgery 1-2 hours long): Total dose: 1-2 mcg/kg; ≥75% of dose administered prior to intubation; administered with N_2O/O_2; Maintenance: 5-20 mcg as needed. Total dose should not exceed 1 mcg/kg/hour of expected surgical time.

Epidural: Adults: Analgesia: Labor and delivery: 10-15 mcg with 10 mL bupivacaine 0.125% with/without epinephrine. May repeat at ≥1-hour interval for 2 additional doses.

Dosage Forms

Injection, solution [preservative free]: 50 mcg/mL (1 mL, 2 mL, 5 mL)

Sufenta®: 50 mcg/mL (1 mL, 2 mL, 5 mL)

sufentanil citrate *see* sufentanil *on page 926*

Sufentanil Citrate Injection, USP [Can] *see* sufentanil *on page 926*

sulamyd *see* sulfacetamide *on page 927*

Sular® [US] *see* nisoldipine *on page 698*

sulbactam and ampicillin *see* ampicillin and sulbactam *on page 77*

sulconazole (sul KON a zole)

Synonyms sulconazole nitrate

U.S./Canadian Brand Names Exelderm® [US/Can]

Therapeutic Category Antifungal Agent

Use Treatment of superficial fungal infections of the skin, including tinea cruris (jock itch), tinea corporis (ringworm), tinea versicolor, and possibly tinea pedis (athlete's foot, cream only)

Usual Dosage Topical: Adults: Apply a small amount to the affected area and gently massage once or twice daily for 3 weeks (tinea cruris, tinea corporis, tinea versicolor) to 4 weeks (tinea pedis).

Dosage Forms

Cream:

Exelderm®: 1% (15 g, 30 g, 60 g)

Solution, topical:

Exelderm®: 1% (30 mL)

sulconazole nitrate *see* sulconazole *on page 926*

Sulcrate® [Can] *see* sucralfate *on page 925*

Sulcrate® Suspension Plus [Can] *see* sucralfate *on page 925*

sulfabenzamide, sulfacetamide, and sulfathiazole

(sul fa BENZ a mide, sul fa SEE ta mide, & sul fa THYE a zole)

Synonyms triple sulfa

U.S./Canadian Brand Names V.V.S.® [US]

Therapeutic Category Antibiotic, Vaginal

Use Treatment of *Haemophilus vaginalis* vaginitis

Usual Dosage Intravaginal: Adults: Female: Cream: Insert one applicatorful into vagina twice daily for 4-6 days; dosage may then be decreased to 1/2 to 1/4 of an applicatorful twice daily

Dosage Forms

Cream, vaginal: Sulfabenzamide 3.7%, sulfacetamide 2.86%, and sulfathiazole 3.42% (78 g with applicator)

V.V.S.®: Sulfabenzamide 3.7%, sulfacetamide 2.86%, and sulfathiazole 3.42% (78 g with applicator)

sulfacetamide (sul fa SEE ta mide)

Sound-Alike/Look-Alike Issues

Bleph®-10 may be confused with Blephamide®

Klaron® may be confused with Klor-Con®

Synonyms sodium sulfacetamide; sulamyd; sulfacetamide sodium

U.S./Canadian Brand Names Bleph®-10 [US]; Carmol® Scalp Treatment [US]; Cetamide™ [Can]; Diosulf™ [Can]; Klaron® [US]; Ovace® Plus [US]; Ovace® [US]; Rosula® NS [US]; Seb-Prev™ [US]

Therapeutic Category Antibiotic, Ophthalmic

Use

Ophthalmic: Treatment and prophylaxis of conjunctivitis due to susceptible organisms; corneal ulcers; adjunctive treatment with systemic sulfonamides for therapy of trachoma

Dermatologic: Scaling dermatosis (seborrheic); bacterial infections of the skin; acne vulgaris

Usual Dosage

Children >2 months and Adults: Ophthalmic: Solution: Instill 1-2 drops several times daily up to every 2-3 hours in lower conjunctival sac during waking hours and less frequently at night; increase dosing interval as condition responds. Usual duration of treatment: 7-10 days

Trachoma: Instill 2 drops into the conjunctival sac every 2 hours; must be used in conjunction with systemic therapy

Children >12 years and Adults: Topical:

Acne: Apply thin film to affected area twice daily

Seborrheic dermatitis: Apply at bedtime and allow to remain overnight; in severe cases, may apply twice daily. Duration of therapy is usually 8-10 applications; dosing interval may be increased as eruption subsides. Applications once or twice weekly, or every other week may be used to prevent eruptions.

Secondary cutaneous bacterial infections: Apply 2-4 times/day until infection clears

Dosage Forms

Aerosol, topical:

Ovace®: 10% (100 g)

Cream, topical:

Seb-Prev™: 10% (30 g, 60 g)

Gel, topical:

Seb-Prev™: 10% (30 g, 60 g)

Lotion, topical: 10% (120 mL)

Carmol® Scalp Treatment: 10% (85 g)

Klaron®: 10% (120 mL)

Lotion, topical [wash]:

Ovace®: 10% (180 mL, 360 mL)

Lotion, topical [emulsion-based wash]:

Ovace® Plus: 10% (480 mL)

Pad, topical:

Rosula® NS: 10% (30s)

Soap, topical [wash]:

Seb-Prev™: 10% (170 mL, 340 mL)

Solution, ophthalmic [drops]: 10% (15 mL)

Bleph®-10: 10% (5 mL)

Suspension, topical: 10% (118 mL)

sulfacetamide and prednisolone (sul fa SEE ta mide & pred NIS oh lone)

Sound-Alike/Look-Alike Issues

Blephamide® may be confused with Bleph®-10

Synonyms prednisolone and sulfacetamide

U.S./Canadian Brand Names Blephamide® [US/Can]; Dioptimyd® [Can]

Therapeutic Category Antibiotic/Corticosteroid, Ophthalmic

Use Steroid-responsive inflammatory ocular conditions in which a corticosteroid is indicated and where infection is present or there is a risk of infection

Usual Dosage Ophthalmic: Children ≥6 years and Adults:

Ointment: Apply ~1/2 inch ribbon to lower conjunctival sac 3-4 times/day and 1-2 times at night

Solution: Instill 2 drops every 4 hours

Suspension: Instill 2 drops every 4 hours during the day and at bedtime

Dosage Forms

Ointment, ophthalmic:

Blephamide®: Sulfacetamide 10% and prednisolone 0.2% (3.5 g)

Solution, ophthalmic: Sulfacetamide 10% and prednisolone 0.25% (5 mL, 10 mL)

Suspension, ophthalmic:

Blephamide®: Sulfacetamide 10% and prednisolone 0.2% (5 mL, 10 mL)

sulfacetamide and sulfur *see* sulfur and sulfacetamide *on page* 931

sulfacetamide sodium *see* sulfacetamide *on page* 927

sulfacetamide sodium and fluorometholone *(Discontinued)*

Sulfacet-R® [US/Can] *see* sulfur and sulfacetamide *on page* 931

sulfadiazine (sul fa DYE a zeen)

Sound-Alike/Look-Alike Issues

sulfaDIAZINE may be confused with sulfasalazine, sulfiSOXAZOLE

Tall-Man sulf**ADIAZINE**

Therapeutic Category Sulfonamide

Use Treatment of urinary tract infections and nocardiosis; adjunctive treatment in toxoplasmosis; uncomplicated attack of malaria

Usual Dosage Oral:

Asymptomatic meningococcal carriers:

Infants 1-12 months: 500 mg once daily for 2 days

Children 1-12 years: 500 mg twice daily for 2 days

Adults: 1 g twice daily for 2 days

Congenital toxoplasmosis:

Newborns and Children <2 months: 100 mg/kg/day divided every 6 hours in conjunction with pyrimethamine 1 mg/kg/day once daily and supplemental folinic acid 5 mg every 3 days for 6 months

Children >2 months: 25-50 mg/kg/dose 4 times/day

Nocardiosis: 4-8 g/day for a minimum of 6 weeks

Toxoplasmosis:

Children >2 months: Loading dose: 75 mg/kg; maintenance dose: 120-150 mg/kg/day, maximum dose: 6 g/day; divided every 4-6 hours in conjunction with pyrimethamine 2 mg/kg/day divided every 12 hours for 3 days followed by 1 mg/kg/day once daily with supplemental folinic acid

Adults: 2-6 g/day in divided doses every 6 hours in conjunction with pyrimethamine 50-75 mg/day and with supplemental folinic acid

Dosage Forms

Tablet: 500 mg

sulfadoxine and pyrimethamine (sul fa DOKS een & peer i METH a meen)

Synonyms pyrimethamine and sulfadoxine

U.S./Canadian Brand Names Fansidar® [US]

Therapeutic Category Antimalarial Agent

Use Treatment of *Plasmodium falciparum* malaria in patients in whom chloroquine resistance is suspected; malaria prophylaxis for travelers to areas where chloroquine-resistant malaria is endemic

Usual Dosage Oral: Children and Adults:

Treatment of acute attack of malaria: A single dose of the following number of Fansidar® tablets is used in sequence with quinine or alone:

2-11 months: 1/4 tablet

1-3 years: 1/2 tablet

4-8 years: 1 tablet

9-14 years: 2 tablets

>14 years: 3 tablets

Malaria prophylaxis: A single dose should be carried for self-treatment in the event of febrile illness when medical attention is not immediately available:
2-11 months: 1/4 tablet
1-3 years: 1/2 tablet
4-8 years: 1 tablet
9-14 years: 2 tablets
>14 years and Adults: 3 tablets

Dosage Forms

Tablet:
Fansidar®: Sulfadoxine 500 mg and pyrimethamine 25 mg

Sulfa-Gyn® ***(Discontinued)*** *see* sulfabenzamide, sulfacetamide, and sulfathiazole *on page 926*

Sulfamethoprim® ***(Discontinued)***

sulfamethoxazole and trimethoprim (sul fa meth OKS a zole & trye METH oh prim)

Sound-Alike/Look-Alike Issues
Bactrim™ may be confused with bacitracin, Bactine®, Bactroban®
co-trimoxazole may be confused with clotrimazole
Septra® may be confused with Ceptaz®, Sectral®
Septra® DS may be confused with Semprex®-D

Synonyms co-trimoxazole; SMZ-TMP; TMP-SMZ; trimethoprim and sulfamethoxazole

U.S./Canadian Brand Names Apo-Sulfatrim® DS [Can]; Apo-Sulfatrim® Pediatric [Can]; Apo-Sulfatrim® [Can]; Bactrim™ DS [US]; Bactrim™ [US]; Novo-Trimel D.S. [Can]; Novo-Trimel [Can]; Nu-Cotrimox [Can]; Septra® DS [US]; Septra® Injection [Can]; Septra® [US]; Sulfatrim® [US]

Therapeutic Category Sulfonamide

Use

Oral treatment of urinary tract infections due to *E. coli*, *Klebsiella* and *Enterobacter* sp, *M. morganii*, *P. mirabilis* and *P. vulgaris*; acute otitis media in children; acute exacerbations of chronic bronchitis in adults due to susceptible strains of *H. influenzae* or *S. pneumoniae*; treatment and prophylaxis of *Pneumocystis jiroveci* pneumonitis (PCP); traveler's diarrhea due to enterotoxigenic *E. coli*; treatment of enteritis caused by *Shigella flexneri* or *Shigella sonnei*

I.V. treatment or severe or complicated infections when oral therapy is not feasible, for documented PCP, empiric treatment of PCP in immune compromised patients; treatment of documented or suspected shigellosis, typhoid fever, *Nocardia asteroides* infection, or other infections caused by susceptible bacteria

Usual Dosage Dosage recommendations are based on the trimethoprim component. double strength tablets are equivalent to sulfamethoxazole 800 mg and trimethoprim 160 mg.

Usual dosage range:

Children >2 months:
Mild-to-moderate infections: Oral: 8-12 mg TMP/kg/day in divided doses every 12 hours
Serious infection:
Oral: 20 mg TMP/kg/day in divided doses every 6 hours
I.V.: 8-12 mg TMP/kg/day in divided doses every 6 hours

Adults:
Oral: One double strength tablet (sulfamethoxazole 800 mg; trimethoprim 160 mg) every 12-24 hours
I.V.: 8-20 mg TMP/kg/day divided every 6-12 hours

Indication-specific dosing:

Children >2 months:

Acute otitis media: Oral: 8 mg TMP/kg/day in divided doses every 12 hours for 10 days. **Note:** Recommended by the American Academy of Pediatrics as an alternative agent in penicillin-allergic patients at a dose of 6-10 mg TMP/kg/day.

Pneumocystis jiroveci:
Treatment: Oral, I.V.: 15-20 mg TMP/kg/day in divided doses every 6-8 hours
Prophylaxis: Oral, 150 mg TMP/m^2/day in divided doses every 12 hours for 3 days/week; dose should not exceed trimethoprim 320 mg and sulfamethoxazole 1600 mg daily
Alternative prophylaxis dosing schedules include:
150 mg TMP/m^2/day as a single daily dose 3 times/week on consecutive days
or
150 mg TMP/m^2/day in divided doses every 12 hours administered 7 days/week
or
150 mg TMP/m^2/day in divided doses every 12 hours administered 3 times/week on alternate days ▶

Shigellosis:
Oral: 8 mg TMP/kg/day in divided doses every 12 hours for 5 days
I.V.: 8-10 mg TMP/kg/day in divided doses every 6, 8, or 12 hours for up to 5 days
Urinary tract infection:
Treatment:
Oral: 6-12 mg TMP/kg/day in divided doses every 12 hours
I.V.: 8-10 mg TMP/kg/day in divided doses every 6, 8, or 12 hours for up to 14 days with serious infections
Prophylaxis: Oral: 2 mg TMP/kg/dose daily or 5 mg TMP/kg/dose twice weekly
Adults:
Chronic bronchitis (acute): Oral: One double strength tablet every 12 hours for 10-14 days
Meningitis (bacterial): I.V.: 10-20 mg TMP/kg/day in divided doses every 6-12 hours
***Pneumocystis jiroveci*:**
Prophylaxis: Oral: One double strength tablet daily or 3 times/week
Treatment: Oral, I.V.: 15-20 mg TMP/kg/day in 3-4 divided doses
Sepsis: I.V.: 20 TMP/kg/day divided every 6 hours
Shigellosis:
Oral: One double strength tablet every 12 hours for 5 days
I.V.: 8-10 mg TMP/kg/day in divided doses every 6, 8, or 12 hours for up to 5 days
Traveler's diarrhea: Oral: One double strength tablet every 12 hours for 5 days
Urinary tract infection:
Oral: One double strength tablet every 12 hours
Duration of therapy: Uncomplicated: 3-5 days; Complicated: 7-10 days
Pyelonephritis: 14 days
Prostatitis: Acute: 2 weeks; Chronic: 2-3 months
I.V.: 8-10 mg TMP/kg/day in divided doses every 6, 8, or 12 hours for up to 14 days with severe infections

Dosage Forms The 5:1 ratio (SMX:TMP) remains constant in all dosage forms.
Injection, solution: Sulfamethoxazole 80 mg and trimethoprim 16 mg per mL (5 mL, 10 mL, 30 mL)
Suspension, oral: Sulfamethoxazole 200 mg and trimethoprim 40 mg per 5 mL
Sulfatrim®: Sulfamethoxazole 200 mg and trimethoprim 40 mg per 5 mL
Tablet: Sulfamethoxazole 400 mg and trimethoprim 80 mg
Bactrim™, Septra®: Sulfamethoxazole 400 mg and trimethoprim 80 mg
Tablet, double strength: Sulfamethoxazole 800 mg and trimethoprim 160 mg
Bactrim™ DS, Septra® DS: Sulfamethoxazole 800 mg and trimethoprim 160 mg

Sulfamylon® [US] *see* mafenide *on page* 605

sulfasalazine (sul fa SAL a zeen)

Sound-Alike/Look-Alike Issues
sulfasalazine may be confused with salsalate, sulfaDIAZINE, sulfiSOXAZOLE
Azulfidine® may be confused with Augmentin®, azaTHIOprine

Synonyms salicylazosulfapyridine

U.S./Canadian Brand Names Alti-Sulfasalazine [Can]; Azulfidine® EN-tabs® [US]; Azulfidine® [US]; Salazopyrin En-Tabs® [Can]; Salazopyrin® [Can]; Sulfazine EC [US]; Sulfazine [US]

Therapeutic Category 5-Aminosalicylic Acid Derivative

Use Management of ulcerative colitis; enteric coated tablets are also used for rheumatoid arthritis (including juvenile rheumatoid arthritis) in patients who inadequately respond to analgesics and NSAIDs

Usual Dosage Oral:
Children ≥2 years: Ulcerative colitis: Initial: 40-60 mg/kg/day in 3-6 divided doses; maintenance dose: 20-30 mg/kg/day in 4 divided doses
Children ≥6 years: Juvenile rheumatoid arthritis: Enteric coated tablet: 30-50 mg/kg/day in 2 divided doses; Initial: Begin with 1/4 to 1/3 of expected maintenance dose; increase weekly; maximum: 2 g/day typically
Adults:
Ulcerative colitis: Initial: 1 g 3-4 times/day, 2 g/day maintenance in divided doses; may initiate therapy with 0.5-1 g/day
Rheumatoid arthritis: Enteric coated tablet: Initial: 0.5-1 g/day; increase weekly to maintenance dose of 2 g/day in 2 divided doses; maximum: 3 g/day (if response to 2 g/day is inadequate after 12 weeks of treatment)

Dosage Forms

Tablet: 500 mg

Azulfidine®, Sulfazine: 500 mg

Tablet, delayed release, enteric coated: 500 mg

Azulfidine® EN-tabs®, Sulfazine EC: 500 mg

Sulfatol® [US] *see* sulfur and sulfacetamide *on page 931*

Sulfatol®-M [US] *see* sulfur and sulfacetamide *on page 931*

Sulfatrim® [US] *see* sulfamethoxazole and trimethoprim *on page 929*

Sulfa-Trip® *(Discontinued)* *see* sulfabenzamide, sulfacetamide, and sulfathiazole *on page 926*

Sulfazine [US] *see* sulfasalazine *on page 930*

Sulfazine EC [US] *see* sulfasalazine *on page 930*

sulfinpyrazone *(Discontinued)*

sulfisoxazole (sul fi SOKS a zole)

Sound-Alike/Look-Alike Issues

sulfiSOXAZOLE may be confused with sulfaDIAZINE, sulfamethoxazole, sulfasalazine

Gantrisin® may be confused with Gastrosed™

Synonyms sulfisoxazole acetyl; sulphafurazole

Tall-Man sulfi**SOXAZOLE**

U.S./Canadian Brand Names Gantrisin® [US]; Novo-Soxazole [Can]; Sulfizole® [Can]

Therapeutic Category Sulfonamide

Use Treatment of urinary tract infections, otitis media, *Chlamydia*; nocardiosis

Usual Dosage Oral: Not for use in patients <2 months of age:

Children >2 months: Initial: 75 mg/kg, followed by 120-150 mg/kg/day in divided doses every 4-6 hours; not to exceed 6 g/day

Adults: Initial: 2-4 g, then 4-8 g/day in divided doses every 4-6 hours

Dosage Forms

Suspension, oral [pediatric]:

Gantrisin®: 500 mg/5 mL

sulfisoxazole acetyl *see* sulfisoxazole *on page 931*

sulfisoxazole and erythromycin *see* erythromycin and sulfisoxazole *on page 370*

Sulfizole® [Can] *see* sulfisoxazole *on page 931*

sulfur and sulfacetamide (SUL fur & sul fa SEE ta mide)

Synonyms sodium sulfacetamide and sulfur; sulfacetamide and sulfur; sulfur and sulfacetamide sodium

U.S./Canadian Brand Names AVAR™-e [US]; Clarifoam™ EF [US]; Clenia™ [US]; Plexion SCT® [US]; Plexion® [US]; Prascion® FC [US]; Prascion® RA [US]; Prascion® [US]; Rosac® [US]; Rosanil® [US]; Rosula® Clarifying [US]; Rosula® [US]; Sulfacet-R® [US/Can]; Sulfatol® [US]; Sulfatol®-M [US]; Sumaxin™ [US]; Suphera™ [US]

Therapeutic Category Antiseborrheic Agent, Topical

Use Aid in the treatment of acne vulgaris, acne rosacea, and seborrheic dermatitis

Usual Dosage Topical: Children ≥12 years and Adults: Apply in a thin film 1-3 times/day. Cleansing products should be used 1-2 times/day.

Dosage Forms

Aerosol, topical [foam]:

Clarifoam™ EF: Sulfur 5% and sulfacetamide 10% (60 g)

Cleanser, topical:

Plexion®, Prascion®: Sulfur 5% and sulfacetamide 10% (170 g, 340 g)

Rosanil®: Sulfur 5% and sulfacetamide 10% (170 g, 390 g)

Rosula®: Sulfur 5% and sulfacetamide 10% (355 mL)

Cleanser, topical [emulsion-based]:

Sulfatol®: Sulfur 5% and sulfacetamide 10% (355 mL)

Cream, topical:

AVAR™-e, Prascion® RA, Rosac®: Sulfur 5% and sulfacetamide 10% (45 g)

Clenia™: Sulfur 5% and sulfacetamide sodium 10% (28 g)

Plexion SCT®: Sulfur 5% and sulfacetamide sodium 10% (120 g)

Suphera™: Sulfur 5% and sulfacetamide sodium 10% (113 g)

Gel, topical:
Rosula®: Sulfur 5% and sulfacetamide 10% (45 g)
Gel, topical [emulsion-based]:
Sulfatol®: Sulfur 5% and sulfacetamide 10% (45 mL)
Lotion, topical: Sulfur 5% and sulfacetamide 10% (25 g, 30 g, 45 g, 60 g)
Sulfacaet-R®, Sulfatol®-M: Sulfur 5% and sulfacetamide 10% (25 g)
Pad, topical [cleansing cloth]:
Plexion®, Prascion®: Sulfur 5% and sulfacetamide 10% (30s, 60s)
Sumaxin™: Sulfur 4% and sulfacetamide 10% (60s)
Suspension, topical: Sulfur 5% and sulfacetamide 10% (30 g)
Wash, topical: Sulfur 5% and sulfacetamide 10% (170 g, 340 g)
Rosac®: Sulfur 1% and sulfacetamide sodium 10% (170 g)
Clenia™: Sulfur 5% and sulfacetamide 10% (170 g, 340 g)
Wash, topical [emulsion-based]:
Rosula® Clarifying: Sulfur 4% and sulfacetamide 10% (473 mL)

sulfur and sulfacetamide sodium *see* sulfur and sulfacetamide *on page 931*

sulindac (SUL in dak)

Sound-Alike/Look-Alike Issues
Clinoril® may be confused with Cleocin®, Clozaril®, Oruvail®

U.S./Canadian Brand Names Apo-Sulin® [Can]; Clinoril® [US]; Novo-Sundac [Can]; Nu-Sundac [Can]

Therapeutic Category Analgesic, Nonnarcotic; Nonsteroidal Antiinflammatory Drug (NSAID)

Use Management of inflammatory diseases including osteoarthritis, rheumatoid arthritis, acute gouty arthritis, ankylosing spondylitis, acute painful shoulder (bursitis/tendonitis)

Usual Dosage Oral: Adults: **Note:** Maximum daily dose: 400 mg
Osteoarthritis, rheumatoid arthritis, ankylosing spondylitis: 150 mg twice daily
Acute painful shoulder (bursitis/tendonitis): 200 mg twice daily; usual treatment: 7-14 days
Acute gouty arthritis: 200 mg twice daily; usual treatment: 7 days

Dosage Forms
Tablet: 150 mg, 200 mg
Clinoril®: 200 mg

sulphafurazole *see* sulfisoxazole *on page 931*
Sultrin™ ***(Discontinued)*** *see* sulfabenzamide, sulfacetamide, and sulfathiazole *on page 926*

sumatriptan (soo ma TRIP tan)

Sound-Alike/Look-Alike Issues
SUMAtriptan may be confused with saxagliptin, sitaGLIPtin, somatropin, zolmitriptan

Synonyms sumatriptan succinate

Tall-Man **SUMA**triptan

U.S./Canadian Brand Names Apo-Sumatriptan® [Can]; CO Sumatriptan [Can]; Dom-Sumatriptan [Can]; Gen-Sumatriptan [Can]; Imitrex® DF [Can]; Imitrex® Nasal Spray [Can]; Imitrex® [US/Can]; Novo-Sumatriptan [Can]; PHL-Sumatriptan [Can]; PMS-Sumatriptan [Can]; ratio-Sumatriptan [Can]; Rhoxal-sumatriptan [Can]; Riva-Sumatriptan [Can]; Sandoz-Sumatriptan [Can]; Sumatryx [Can]

Therapeutic Category Antimigraine Agent

Use
Oral, SubQ: Acute treatment of migraine with or without aura
SubQ: Acute treatment of cluster headache episodes

Usual Dosage Adults:
Oral: A single dose of 25 mg, 50 mg, or 100 mg (taken with fluids). If a satisfactory response has not been obtained at 2 hours, a second dose may be administered. Results from clinical trials show that initial doses of 50 mg and 100 mg are more effective than doses of 25 mg, and that 100 mg doses do not provide a greater effect than 50 mg and may have increased incidence of side effects. Although doses of up to 300 mg/day have been studied, the total daily dose should not exceed 200 mg. The safety of treating an average of >4 headaches in a 30-day period have not been established.
Intranasal: A single dose of 5 mg, 10 mg, or 20 mg administered in one nostril. A 10 mg dose may be achieved by administering a single 5 mg dose in each nostril. If headache returns, the dose may be repeated once after 2 hours, not to exceed a total daily dose of 40 mg. The safety of treating an average of >4 headaches in a 30-day period has not been established.

SubQ: Up to 6 mg; if side effects are dose-limiting, lower doses may be used. A second injection may be administered at least 1 hour after the initial dose, but not more than 2 injections in a 24-hour period.

Dosage Forms

Injection, solution: 8 mg/mL (0.5 mL); 12 mg/mL (0.5 mL)
Imitrex®: 8 mg/mL (0.5 mL); 12 mg/mL (0.5 mL)
Solution, intranasal [spray]: 5 mg/0.1 mL (6s); 20 mg/0.1 mL (6s)
Imitrex®: 5 mg/0.1 mL (6s); 20 mg/0.1 mL (6s)
Tablet: 25 mg, 50 mg, 100 mg
Imitrex®: 25 mg, 50 mg, 100 mg

sumatriptan and naproxen (soo ma TRIP tan & na PROKS en)

Sound-Alike/Look-Alike Issues

naproxen may be confused with Natacyn®, Nebcin®, neomycin, niacin
SUMAtriptan may be confused with somatropin, zolmitriptan
Treximet™ may be confused with Trexall™

Synonyms naproxen and sumatriptan; naproxen sodium and sumatriptan; naproxen sodium and sumatriptan succinate; sumatriptan succinate and naproxen; sumatriptan succinate and naproxen sodium

U.S./Canadian Brand Names Treximet™ [US]

Therapeutic Category Antimigraine Agent; Nonsteroidal Antiinflammatory Drug (NSAID); Serotonin 5-$HT_{1B,\ 1D}$ Receptor Agonist

Use Acute treatment of migraine with or without aura

Usual Dosage Oral: Adults: 1 tablet (sumatriptan 85 mg and naproxen 500 mg). If a satisfactory response has not been obtained at 2 hours, a second dose may be administered (maximum: 2 tablets/24 hours). **Note:** The safety of treating an average of >5 migraine headaches in a 30-day period has not been established.

Dosage Forms

Tablet:
Treximet™ 85/500: Sumatriptan 85 mg and naproxen sodium 500 mg

sumatriptan succinate *see* sumatriptan *on page* 932
sumatriptan succinate and naproxen *see* sumatriptan and naproxen *on page* 933
sumatriptan succinate and naproxen sodium *see* sumatriptan and naproxen *on page* 933
Sumatryx [Can] *see* sumatriptan *on page* 932
Sumaxin™ [US] *see* sulfur and sulfacetamide *on page* 931
Summer's Eve® Anti-Itch Maximum Strength [US-OTC] *see* pramoxine *on page* 809
Summer's Eve® Medicated Douche [US-OTC] *see* povidone-iodine *on page* 807
Summer's Eve® SpecialCare™ Medicated Anti-Itch Cream *(Discontinued)* *see* hydrocortisone (topical) *on page* 505
Sumycin® *(Discontinued)* *see* tetracycline *on page* 950
Sun-Benz® [Can] *see* benzydamine *(Canada only) on page* 135

sunitinib (su NIT e nib)

Sound-Alike/Look-Alike Issues

sunitinib may be confused with imatinib, sorafenib

Synonyms SU011248; SU11248; sunitinib malate

U.S./Canadian Brand Names Sutent® [US/Can]

Therapeutic Category Antineoplastic Agent, Tyrosine Kinase Inhibitor; Vascular Endothelial Growth Factor (VEGF) Inhibitor

Use Treatment of gastrointestinal stromal tumor (GIST) intolerance to or disease progression on imatinib; treatment of advanced renal cell cancer (RCC)

Usual Dosage Oral: Adults: Gastrointestinal stromal tumor, renal cell cancer: 50 mg once daily for 4 weeks of a 6-week treatment cycle (4 weeks on, 2 weeks off). **Note:** Dosage modifications should be done in increments of 12.5 mg; individualize based on safety and tolerability.

Dosage Forms

Capsule:
Sutent®: 12.5 mg, 25 mg, 50 mg

sunitinib malate *see* sunitinib *on page* 933

Syntocinon® [Can] *see* oxytocin *on page 742*
Synvisc® [US] *see* hyaluronate and derivatives *on page 496*
Syprine® [US/Can] *see* trientine *on page 985*
Syrex [US] *see* sodium chloride *on page 908*
SyringeAvitene™ [US] *see* collagen hemostat *on page 255*
syrup of ipecac *see* ipecac syrup *on page 543*
Systane® [US-OTC] *see* artificial tears *on page 100*
Systane® Free [US-OTC] *see* artificial tears *on page 100*
Sytobex® ***(Discontinued)*** *see* cyanocobalamin *on page 263*
T_3/T_4 liotrix *see* liotrix *on page 592*
T_4 *see* levothyroxine *on page 583*
T-20 *see* enfuvirtide *on page 354*
642® Tablet [Can] *see* propoxyphene *on page 827*
Tabloid® [US] *see* thioguanine *on page 955*
Tac™-40 Injection ***(Discontinued)***
Taclonex® [US] *see* calcipotriene and betamethasone *on page 167*
Taclonex Scalp® [US] *see* calcipotriene and betamethasone *on page 167*

tacrine (TAK reen)

Sound-Alike/Look-Alike Issues

Cognex® may be confused with Corgard®

Synonyms tacrine hydrochloride; tetrahydroaminoacrine; THA

U.S./Canadian Brand Names Cognex® [US]

Therapeutic Category Acetylcholinesterase Inhibitor; Cholinergic Agent

Use Treatment of mild-to-moderate dementia of the Alzheimer type

Usual Dosage Adults: Initial: 10 mg 4 times/day; may increase by 40 mg/day adjusted every 6 weeks; maximum: 160 mg/day; best administered separate from meal times.

Dose adjustment based upon transaminase elevations:

ALT ≤3 times ULN*: Continue titration

ALT >3 to ≤5 times ULN*: Decrease dose by 40 mg/day, resume when ALT returns to normal

ALT >5 times ULN*: Stop treatment, may rechallenge upon return of ALT to normal

*ULN = upper limit of normal

Patients with clinical jaundice confirmed by elevated total bilirubin (>3 mg/dL) should not be rechallenged with tacrine

Dosage Forms

Capsule:

Cognex®: 10 mg, 20 mg, 30 mg, 40 mg

tacrine hydrochloride *see* tacrine *on page 935*

tacrolimus (ta KROE li mus)

Sound-Alike/Look-Alike Issues

tacrolimus may be confused with everolimus, pimecrolimus, sirolimus, temsirolimus

Prograf® may be confused with Gengraf®, Prozac®

Synonyms FK506

U.S./Canadian Brand Names Advagraf™ [Can]; Prograf® [US/Can]; Protopic® [US/Can]

Therapeutic Category Immunosuppressant Agent

Use

Oral/injection: Prevention of organ rejection in heart, kidney, or liver transplant recipients

Topical: Moderate-to-severe atopic dermatitis in patients not responsive to conventional therapy or when conventional therapy is not appropriate

Usual Dosage

Oral:

Prevention of organ rejection in transplant recipients: The initial dose of tacrolimus should begin no sooner than 6 hours post-transplant; adjunctive therapy with corticosteroids is recommended early post-transplant. I.V. route should only be used in patients not able to take oral medications and continued only until oral medication can be tolerated; anaphylaxis has been reported with I.V. administration. If switching from I.V. to oral, the oral dose should be started 8-12 hours after stopping the infusion.

Children: Patients without preexisting renal or hepatic dysfunction have required (and tolerated) higher doses than adults to achieve similar blood concentrations. It is recommended that therapy be initiated at ***high end*** of the recommended adult I.V. and oral dosing ranges; dosage adjustments may be required.

Liver transplant: Initial dose: 0.15-0.20 mg/kg/day in 2 divided doses, given every 12 hours

Adults:

Heart transplant: Initial dose: 0.075 mg/kg/day in 2 divided doses, given every 12 hours. Use in combination with azathioprine or mycophenolate mofetil is recommended.

Kidney transplant: Initial dose: 0.2 mg/kg/day in combination with azathioprine **or** 0.1 mg/kg/day in combination with mycophenolate mofetil. Administer in 2 divided doses, given every 12 hours; initial dose may be given within 24 hours of transplant, but should be delayed until renal function has recovered; African-American patients may require larger doses to maintain trough concentration.

Liver transplant: Initial dose: 0.1-0.15 mg/kg/day in 2 divided doses, given every 12 hours

I.V.:

Prevention of organ rejection in transplant recipients: The initial dose of tacrolimus should begin no sooner than 6 hours post-transplant; adjunctive therapy with corticosteroids is recommended early post-transplant. I.V. route should only be used in patients not able to take oral medications and continued only until oral medication can be tolerated; anaphylaxis has been reported with I.V. administration. If switching from I.V. to oral, the oral dose should be started 8-12 hours after stopping the infusion.

Children: It is recommended that therapy be initiated at the ***high end*** of the dosing range.

Liver transplant: Initial dose: 0.03-0.05 mg/kg/day as a continuous infusion

Adults: It is recommended that therapy be initiated at the ***lower end*** of the dosing range.

Heart transplant: Initial dose: 0.01 mg/kg/day as a continuous infusion. Use in combination with azathioprine or mycophenolate mofetil is recommended.

Kidney transplant: Initial dose: 0.03-0.05 mg/kg/day as a continuous infusion. Use in combination with azathioprine or mycophenolate mofetil is recommended.

Liver transplant: Initial dose: 0.03-0.05 mg/kg/day as a continuous infusion.

Topical:

Atopic dermatitis (moderate-to-severe):

Children ≥2 years: Apply minimum amount of 0.03% ointment to affected area twice daily; rub in gently and completely. Discontinue use when symptoms have cleared. If no improvement within 6 weeks, patients should be re-examined to confirm diagnosis.

Adults: Apply minimum amount of 0.03% or 0.1% ointment to affected area twice daily; rub in gently and completely. Discontinue use when symptoms have cleared. If no improvement within 6 weeks, patients should be reexamined to confirm diagnosis.

Dosage Forms

Capsule: 0.5 mg, 1 mg, 5 mg

Prograf®: 0.5 mg, 1 mg, 5 mg

Injection, solution:

Prograf®: 5 mg/mL (1 mL)

Ointment, topical:

Protopic®: 0.03% (30 g, 60 g, 100 g); 0.1% (30 g, 60 g, 100 g)

tadalafil (tah DA la fil)

Sound-Alike/Look-Alike Issues

tadalafil may be confused with sildenafil, vardenafil

Adcirca™ may be confused with Advair® Diskus®, Advair® HFA, Advicor®

Synonyms GF196960

U.S./Canadian Brand Names Adcirca™ [US]; Cialis® [US/Can]

Therapeutic Category Phosphodiesterase (Type 5) Enzyme Inhibitor

Use

Adcirca™: Treatment of pulmonary arterial hypertension (PAH) (WHO Group I) to improve exercise ability

Cialis®: Treatment of erectile dysfunction (ED)

Usual Dosage Oral: Adults:

Erectile dysfunction (Cialis®):

As-needed dosing: 10 mg at least 30 minutes prior to anticipated sexual activity (dosing range: 5-20 mg); to be given as one single dose and not given more than once daily. **Note:** Erectile function may be improved for up to 36 hours following a single dose; adjust dose.

Once-daily dosing: 2.5 mg once daily (dosing range: 2.5-5 mg/day) to be given at approximately the same time daily without regard to timing of sexual activity

Pulmonary arterial hypertension (Adcirca™): 40 mg once daily

Dosage Forms

Tablet:

Adcirca™: 20 mg

Cialis®: 2.5 mg, 5 mg, 10 mg, 20 mg

Tagamet® *(Discontinued)* *see* cimetidine *on page 228*

Tagamet® HB [Can] *see* cimetidine *on page 228*

Tagamet® HB 200 [US-OTC] *see* cimetidine *on page 228*

TAK-375 *see* ramelteon *on page 850*

TAK-390MR *see* dexlansoprazole *on page 290*

Talacen® [US] *see* pentazocine and acetaminophen *on page 765*

talc *see* talc (sterile) *on page 937*

talc for pleurodesis *see* talc (sterile) *on page 937*

talc (sterile) (talk STARE il)

Synonyms intrapleural talc; sterile talc; talc; talc for pleurodesis

U.S./Canadian Brand Names Sclerosol® [US]; Sterile Talc Powder™ [US]

Therapeutic Category Sclerosing Agent

Use Prevention of recurrence of malignant pleural effusion in symptomatic patients

Usual Dosage Adults: Pleural effusion:

Intrapleural aerosol: 4-8 g (1-2 cans) as a single dose

Intrapleural instillation: 5 g

Dosage Forms

Aerosol, intrapleural [powder]:

Sclerosol®: 4 g

Powder, intrapleural:

Sterile Talc Powder™: Talc USP 5 g

Talwin® [US/Can] *see* pentazocine *on page 764*

Talwin® Nx [US] *see* pentazocine *on page 764*

Tambocor™ [US/Can] *see* flecainide *on page 422*

Tamiflu® [US/Can] *see* oseltamivir *on page 731*

Tamofen® [Can] *see* tamoxifen *on page 937*

tamoxifen (ta MOKS i fen)

Sound-Alike/Look-Alike Issues

tamoxifen may be confused with pentoxifylline, Tambocor™, tamsulosin, temazepam

Synonyms ICI-46474; tamoxifen citras; tamoxifen citrate

U.S./Canadian Brand Names Apo-Tamox® [Can]; Mylan-Tamoxifen [Can]; Nolvadex®-D [Can]; Novo-Tamoxifen [Can]; PMS-Tamoxifen [Can]; Tamofen® [Can]

Therapeutic Category Antineoplastic Agent

Use Treatment of metastatic (female and male) breast cancer; adjuvant treatment of breast cancer; reduce risk of invasive breast cancer in women with ductal carcinoma *in situ* (DCIS); reduce the incidence of breast cancer in women at high risk

Usual Dosage Oral: Adults: **Note:** For the treatment of breast cancer, patients receiving both tamoxifen and chemotherapy, should receive treatment sequentially, with tamoxifen following completion of chemotherapy.

Breast cancer treatment:

Adjuvant therapy (females): 20 mg once daily for 5 years

Metastatic (males and females): 20-40 mg/day; daily doses >20 mg should be given in 2 divided doses (morning and evening)

DCIS (females): 20 mg once daily for 5 years

Breast cancer risk reduction (pre- and postmenopausal high-risk females): 20 mg once daily for 5 years

Paget disease of the breast (risk reduction; with DCIS or without associated cancer): 20 mg once daily for 5 years

Dosage adjustment for DVT, pulmonary embolism, cerebrovascular accident, or prolonged immobilization: Discontinue tamoxifen

Dosage Forms

Tablet: 10 mg, 20 mg

tamoxifen citras *see* tamoxifen *on page* *937*
tamoxifen citrate *see* tamoxifen *on page* *937*

tamsulosin (tam SOO loe sin)

Sound-Alike/Look-Alike Issues
tamsulosin may be confused with tacrolimus, tamoxifen, terazosin
Flomax® may be confused with Flonase®, Flovent®, Foltx®, Fosamax®, Volmax®

Synonyms tamsulosin hydrochloride

U.S./Canadian Brand Names Flomax® CR [Can]; Flomax® [US/Can]; Gen-Tamsulosin [Can]; Mylan-Tamsulosin [Can]; Novo-Tamsulosin [Can]; Ran-Tamsulosin [Can]; ratio-Tamsulosin [Can]; Sandoz-Tamsulosin [Can]

Therapeutic Category Alpha-Adrenergic Blocking Agent

Use Treatment of signs and symptoms of benign prostatic hyperplasia (BPH)

Usual Dosage Oral: Adults: BPH: 0.4 mg once daily ~30 minutes after the same meal each day; dose may be increased after 2-4 weeks to 0.8 mg once daily in patients who fail to respond. If therapy is interrupted for several days, restart with 0.4 mg once daily.

Dosage Forms
Capsule:
Flomax®: 0.4 mg

tamsulosin hydrochloride *see* tamsulosin *on page* *938*
Tanac® [US-OTC] *see* benzocaine *on page* *129*
TanaCof-XR [US] *see* brompheniramine *on page* *149*
Tanafed® *(Discontinued)* *see* chlorpheniramine and pseudoephedrine *on page* *215*
Tanafed DMX™ [US] *see* chlorpheniramine, pseudoephedrine, and dextromethorphan *on page* *220*
Tandem® DHA [US] *see* vitamins (multiple/prenatal) *on page* *1020*
Tandem® OB [US] *see* vitamins (multiple/prenatal) *on page* *1020*
Tannate-V-DM *(Discontinued)* *see* phenylephrine, pyrilamine, and dextromethorphan *on page* *778*
Tannate 12 S *(Discontinued)* *see* carbetapentane and chlorpheniramine *on page* *182*
Tannate PD-DM [US] *see* chlorpheniramine, pseudoephedrine, and dextromethorphan *on page* *220*
Tannate Pediatric [US] *see* chlorpheniramine and phenylephrine *on page* *214*
Tannic-12 *(Discontinued)* *see* carbetapentane and chlorpheniramine *on page* *182*
Tannic-12 S [US] *see* carbetapentane and chlorpheniramine *on page* *182*
Tannihist-12 D *(Discontinued)* *see* carbetapentane, phenylephrine, and pyrilamine *on page* *183*
Tannihist-12 RF *(Discontinued)* *see* carbetapentane and chlorpheniramine *on page* *182*
Tanta-Orciprenaline® [Can] *see* metaproterenol *on page* *632*
Tantum® [Can] *see* benzydamine *(Canada only) on page* *135*
TAP-144 *see* leuprolide *on page* *575*
Tapazole® [US/Can] *see* methimazole *on page* *637*

tapentadol (ta PEN ta dol)

Sound-Alike/Look-Alike Issues
tapentadol may be confused with traMADol

Synonyms CG5503; tapentadol hydrochloride

U.S./Canadian Brand Names Nucynta™ [US]

Therapeutic Category Analgesic, Opioid

Controlled Substance C-II

Use Relief of moderate-to-severe acute pain

Usual Dosage Oral: **Note:** Dose and dosage intervals should be individualized according to pain severity with respect to patient's previous experience with similar opioid analgesics.
Adults: Acute moderate-to-severe pain: Day 1: 50-100 mg every 4-6 hours as needed; may administer a second dose ≥1 hour after the initial dose (maximum dose on first day: 700 mg/day); Day 2 and subsequent dosing: 50-100 mg every 4-6 hours as needed (maximum: 600 mg/day)

Dosage Forms
Tablet, oral:
Nucynta™: 50 mg, 75 mg, 100 mg

tapentadol hydrochloride *see* tapentadol *on page* *938*

Tarabine® PFS *(Discontinued)* *see* cytarabine *on page 270*
Tarceva® [US/Can] *see* erlotinib *on page 367*
Targel® [Can] *see* coal tar *on page 250*
Targretin® [US/Can] *see* bexarotene *on page 140*
Tarka® [US/Can] *see* trandolapril and verapamil *on page 976*
Taro-Amcinonide [Can] *see* amcinonide *on page 59*
Taro-Carbamazepine Chewable [Can] *see* carbamazepine *on page 180*
Taro-Ciprofloxacin [Can] *see* ciprofloxacin *on page 229*
Taro-Clindamycin [Can] *see* clindamycin *on page 239*
Taro-Clobetasol [Can] *see* clobetasol *on page 242*
Taro-Desoximetasone [Can] *see* desoximetasone *on page 287*
Taro-Enalapril [Can] *see* enalapril *on page 352*
Taro-Fluconazole [Can] *see* fluconazole *on page 424*
Taro-Mometasone [Can] *see* mometasone *on page 665*
Taro-Simvastatin [Can] *see* simvastatin *on page 902*
Taro-Sone® [Can] *see* betamethasone (topical) *on page 138*
Taro-Warfarin [Can] *see* warfarin *on page 1022*
Tarsum® [US-OTC] *see* coal tar and salicylic acid *on page 251*
Tasigna® [US/Can] *see* nilotinib *on page 697*
Tasmar® [US] *see* tolcapone *on page 967*
Tavist® Allergy [US-OTC] *see* clemastine *on page 237*
Tavist® ND Allergy [US-OTC] *see* loratadine *on page 599*
Taxol® [Can] *see* paclitaxel *on page 742*
Taxol® *(Discontinued)* *see* paclitaxel *on page 742*
Taxotere® [US/Can] *see* docetaxel *on page 326*

tazarotene (taz AR oh teen)

U.S./Canadian Brand Names Avage™ [US]; Tazorac® [US/Can]

Therapeutic Category Keratolytic Agent

Use Topical treatment of facial acne vulgaris; topical treatment of stable plaque psoriasis of up to 20% body surface area involvement; mitigation (palliation) of facial skin wrinkling, facial mottled hyper-/hypopigmentation, and benign facial lentigines

Usual Dosage Topical: **Note:** In patients experiencing excessive pruritus, burning, skin redness, or peeling, discontinue until integrity of the skin is restored, or reduce dosing to an interval the patient is able to tolerate.

Children ≥12 years and Adults:

Acne: Tazorac® cream/gel 0.1%: Cleanse the face gently. After the skin is dry, apply a thin film of tazarotene (2 mg/cm^2) once daily, in the evening, to the skin where the acne lesions appear; use enough to cover the entire affected area

Psoriasis: Tazorac® gel 0.05% or 0.1%: Apply once daily, in the evening, to psoriatic lesions using enough (2 mg/cm^2) to cover only the lesion with a thin film to no more than 20% of body surface area. If a bath or shower is taken prior to application, dry the skin before applying. Unaffected skin may be more susceptible to irritation, avoid application to these areas.

Children ≥17 years and Adults: Palliation of fine facial wrinkles, facial mottled hyper/hypopigmentation, benign facial lentigines: Avage™: Apply a pea-sized amount once daily to clean dry face at bedtime; lightly cover entire face including eyelids if desired. Emollients or moisturizers may be applied before or after; if applied before tazarotene, ensure cream or lotion has absorbed into the skin and has dried completely.

Adults: Psoriasis: Tazorac® cream 0.05% or 0.1%: Apply once daily, in the evening, to psoriatic lesions using enough (2 mg/cm^2) to cover only the lesion with a thin film to no more than 20% of body surface area. If a bath or shower is taken prior to application, dry the skin before applying. Unaffected skin may be more susceptible to irritation, avoid application to these areas.

Dosage Forms

Cream:

Avage™: 0.1% (30 g)

Tazorac®: 0.05% (30 g, 60 g); 0.1% (30 g, 60 g)

Gel:

Tazorac®: 0.05% (30 g, 100 g); 0.1% (30 g, 100 g)

tegaserod (teg a SER od)

Synonyms HTF919; tegaserod maleate

U.S./Canadian Brand Names Zelnorm® [US]

Therapeutic Category Serotonin 5-HT_4 Receptor Agonist

Use Emergency treatment of irritable bowel syndrome with constipation (IBS-C) and chronic idiopathic constipation (CIC) in women (<55 years of age) in which no alternative therapy exists

Usual Dosage Oral: Adults (<55 years of age): Females:

IBS with constipation: 6 mg twice daily, before meals, for 4-6 weeks; may consider continuing treatment for an additional 4-6 weeks in patients who respond initially

Chronic idiopathic constipation: 6 mg twice daily, before meals; the need for continued therapy should be reassessed periodically

Dosage Forms

Tablet:

Zelnorm®: 2 mg, 6 mg

tegaserod maleate *see* tegaserod *on page* *940*

Tega-Vert® Oral *(Discontinued)* *see* dimenhydrinate *on page* *312*

Tegretol® [US/Can] *see* carbamazepine *on page* *180*

Tegretol®-XR [US] *see* carbamazepine *on page* *180*

TEI-6720 *see* febuxostat *on page* *407*

Tekturna® [US] *see* aliskiren *on page* *47*

Tekturna HCT® [US] *see* aliskiren and hydrochlorothiazide *on page* *47*

Telachlor® Oral *(Discontinued)* *see* chlorpheniramine *on page* *213*

Teladar® Topical *(Discontinued)*

telbivudine (tel BI vyoo deen)

Synonyms L-deoxythymidine

U.S./Canadian Brand Names Sebivo® [Can]; Tyzeka® [US]

Therapeutic Category Antiretroviral Agent, Reverse Transcriptase Inhibitor (Nucleoside)

Use Treatment of chronic hepatitis B with evidence of viral replication and either persistent transaminase elevations or histologically-active disease

Usual Dosage Oral: Adolescents ≥16 years and Adults: Chronic hepatitis B: 600 mg once daily. **Note:** Usual treatment duration is at least 1 year and varies with HBeAg status, consult current guidelines and literature.

Product Availability Oral solution: FDA approved April 2009; anticipated availability is currently undetermined

Dosage Forms

Tablet:

Tyzeka®: 600 mg

Teldrin® HBP [US-OTC] *see* chlorpheniramine *on page* *213*

Teldrin® Oral *(Discontinued)* *see* chlorpheniramine *on page* *213*

telithromycin (tel ith roe MYE sin)

Sound-Alike/Look-Alike Issues

Sound-alike/look-alike issues:

Telithromycin may be confused with telavancin

Synonyms HMR 3647

U.S./Canadian Brand Names Ketek® [US/Can]

Therapeutic Category Antibiotic, Ketolide

Use Treatment of community-acquired pneumonia (mild-to-moderate) caused by susceptible strains of *Streptococcus pneumoniae* (including multidrug-resistant isolates), *Haemophilus influenzae*, *Chlamydophila pneumoniae*, *Moraxella catarrhalis*, and *Mycoplasma pneumoniae*

Usual Dosage Oral: Adults: Community-acquired pneumonia: 800 mg once daily for 7-10 days

Dosage Forms

Tablet:

Ketek®: 300 mg [not available in Canada], 400 mg

telmisartan (tel mi SAR tan)

U.S./Canadian Brand Names Micardis® [US/Can]

Therapeutic Category Angiotensin II Receptor Antagonist

Use Treatment of hypertension; may be used alone or in combination with other antihypertensive agents

Usual Dosage Oral: Adults: Initial: 40 mg once daily; usual maintenance dose range: 20-80 mg/day. Patients with volume depletion should be initiated on the lower dosage with close supervision.

Dosage Forms

Tablet:

Micardis®: 20 mg, 40 mg, 80 mg

telmisartan and hydrochlorothiazide (tel mi SAR tan & hye droe klor oh THYE a zide)

Synonyms hydrochlorothiazide and telmisartan

U.S./Canadian Brand Names Micardis® HCT [US]; Micardis® Plus [Can]

Therapeutic Category Antihypertensive Agent, Combination

Use Treatment of hypertension; combination product should not be used for initial therapy

Usual Dosage Oral: Adults: Replacement therapy: Combination product can be substituted for individual titrated agents. Initiation of combination therapy when monotherapy has failed to achieve desired effects:

Patients currently on telmisartan: Initial dose if blood pressure is not currently controlled on monotherapy of 80 mg telmisartan: Telmisartan 80 mg/hydrochlorothiazide 12.5 mg once daily; may titrate up to telmisartan 160 mg/hydrochlorothiazide 25 mg if needed

Patients currently on hydrochlorothiazide: Initial dose if blood pressure is not currently controlled on monotherapy of 25 mg once daily: Telmisartan 80 mg/hydrochlorothiazide 12.5 mg once daily or telmisartan 80 mg/hydrochlorothiazide 25 mg once daily; may titrate up to telmisartan 160 mg/hydrochlorothiazide 25 mg if blood pressure remains uncontrolled after 2-4 weeks of therapy. Patients who develop hypokalemia may be switched to telmisartan 80 mg/hydrochlorothiazide 12.5 mg.

Dosage Forms [CAN]: Canadian brand name

Tablet:

Micardis® HCT: 40/12.5: Telmisartan 40 mg and hydrochlorothiazide 12.5 mg; 80/12.5: Telmisartan 80 mg and hydrochlorothiazide 12.5 mg; 80/25: Telmisartan 80 mg and hydrochlorothiazide 25 mg

Micardis® Plus [CAN]: 80/25: Telmisartan 80 mg and hydrochlorothiazide 25 mg [not available in the U.S.]

Telzir® [Can] *see* fosamprenavir *on page 444*

temazepam (te MAZ e pam)

Sound-Alike/Look-Alike Issues

temazepam may be confused with flurazepam, LORazepam, tamoxifen

Restoril™ may be confused with, Risperdal®, Vistaril®, Zestril®

U.S./Canadian Brand Names Apo-Temazepam® [Can]; CO Temazepam [Can]; Dom-Temazepam [Can]; Gen-Temazepam [Can]; Novo-Temazepam [Can]; Nu-Temazepam [Can]; PHL-Temazepam [Can]; PMS-Temazepam [Can]; ratio-Temazepam [Can]; Restoril™ [US/Can]

Therapeutic Category Benzodiazepine

Controlled Substance C-IV

Use Short-term treatment of insomnia

Usual Dosage Oral: Adults: 15-30 mg at bedtime

Dosage Forms

Capsule: 7.5 mg, 15 mg, 22.5 mg, 30 mg

Restoril™: 7.5 mg, 15 mg, 22.5 mg, 30 mg

Temodal® [Can] *see* temozolomide *on page 942*

Temodar® [US] *see* temozolomide *on page 942*

Temovate® [US] *see* clobetasol *on page 242*

Temovate E® [US] *see* clobetasol *on page 242*

temozolomide (te moe ZOE loe mide)

Sound-Alike/Look-Alike Issues

Temodar® may be confused with Tambocor®

Synonyms TMZ

U.S./Canadian Brand Names Temodal® [Can]; Temodar® [US]

Therapeutic Category Antineoplastic Agent, Alkylating Agent

Use Treatment of newly-diagnosed glioblastoma multiforme (initially in combination with radiotherapy, then as maintenance treatment); treatment of refractory anaplastic astrocytoma

Note: The following use is approved in Canada (not an approved indication in the U.S.): Treatment of recurrent glioblastoma multiforme

Usual Dosage Oral, I.V.: Adults:

Anaplastic astrocytoma (refractory): Initial dose: 150 mg/m^2/day for 5 days; repeat every 28 days. Subsequent doses of 100-200 mg/m^2/day for 5 days per treatment cycle; based upon hematologic tolerance.

Glioblastoma multiforme (newly diagnosed, high-grade glioma):

Concomitant phase: 75 mg/m²/day for 42 days with focal radiotherapy (60Gy administered in 30 fractions). **Note:** PCP prophylaxis is required during concomitant phase and should continue in patients who develop lymphocytopenia until lymphocyte recovery to ≤ grade 1. Obtain weekly CBC.

ANC ≥1500/mm³, platelet count ≥100,000/mm³, and nonhematologic toxicity ≤ grade 1 (excludes alopecia, nausea/vomiting): Temodar® 75 mg/m²/day may be continued throughout the 42-day concomitant period up to 49 days

Maintenance phase (consists of 6 treatment cycles): Begin 4 weeks after concomitant phase completion. **Note:** Each subsequent cycle is 28 days (consisting of 5 days of drug treatment followed by 23 days without treatment). Draw CBC within 48 hours of day 22; hold next cycle and do weekly CBC until ANC >1500/mm³ and platelet count >100,000/mm³; dosing modification should be based on lowest blood counts and worst nonhematologic toxicity during the previous cycle.

Cycle 1: 150 mg/m²/day for 5 days; repeat every 28 days

Cycles 2-6: May increase to 200 mg/m²/day for 5 days every 28 days (if ANC >1500/mm³, platelets >100,000/mm³ and nonhematologic toxicities for cycle 1 are ≤ grade 2; if dose was not escalated at the onset of cycle 2, do not increase for cycles 3-6)

Glioblastoma multiforme (recurrent glioma): *Canadian labeling (not an approved use in the U.S.):* 200 mg/m²/day for 5 days every 28 days; if previously treated with chemotherapy, initiate at 150 mg/m²/day for 5 days every 28 days and increase to 200 mg/m²/day for 5 days every 28 days with cycle 2 if no hematologic toxicity

Dosage Forms

Capsule:

Temodar®: 5 mg, 20 mg, 100 mg, 140 mg, 180 mg, 250 mg

Injection, powder for reconstitution:

Temodar®: 100 mg

Tempra® [Can] *see* acetaminophen *on page 19*

Tempra® *(Discontinued)* *see* acetaminophen *on page 19*

temsirolimus (tem sir OH li mus)

Sound-Alike/Look-Alike Issues

temsirolimus may be confused with everolimus, sirolimus, tacrolimus

Synonyms CCI-779; NSC-683864

U.S./Canadian Brand Names Torisel [US/Can]

Therapeutic Category Antineoplastic Agent, mTOR Kinase Inhibitor

Use Treatment of advanced renal cell cancer (RCC)

Usual Dosage **Note:** For infusion reaction prophylaxis, premedicate with an H_1 antagonist (eg, diphenhydramine 25-50 mg I.V.) 30 minutes prior to infusion. I.V.: Adults: RCC: 25 mg weekly

Dosage Forms

Injection, solution [concentrate]:

Torisel®: 25 mg/mL

tenecteplase (ten EK te plase)

Sound-Alike/Look-Alike Issues

TNKase® may be confused with Activase®, t-PA

TNK (occasional abbreviation for TNKase®) is an error-prone abbreviation (mistaken as TPA)

U.S./Canadian Brand Names TNKase® [US/Can]

Therapeutic Category Thrombolytic Agent

Use Thrombolytic agent used in the management of ST-elevation myocardial infarction (STEMI) for the lysis of thrombi in the coronary vasculature to restore perfusion and reduce mortality.

Recommended criteria for treatment: STEMI: Chest pain ≥20 minutes duration, onset of chest pain within 12 hours of treatment (or within prior 12-24 hours in patients with continuing ischemic symptoms), and S-T segment elevation >0.1 mV in at least two contiguous precordial leads or two adjacent limb leads on ECG or new or presumably new left bundle branch block (LBBB)

Usual Dosage I.V.: Adults: Recommended total dose should not exceed 50 mg and is based on patient's weight; administer as a bolus over 5 seconds

If patient's weight:

<60 kg, dose: 30 mg

≥60 to <70 kg, dose: 35 mg

≥70 to <80 kg, dose: 40 mg

≥80 to <90 kg, dose: 45 mg

≥90 kg, dose: 50 mg

Note: All patients should receive 162-325 mg of chewable nonenteric coated aspirin as soon as possible and then daily. Administer concurrently with heparin 60 units/kg bolus (maximum: 4000 units) followed by continuous infusion of 12 units/kg/hour (maximum: 1000 units/hour) and adjust to aPTT target of 50-70 seconds (or 1.5-2 times the upper limit of control).

Dosage Forms

Injection, powder for reconstitution, recombinant:

TNKase®: 50 mg

Tenex® [US/Can] *see* guanfacine *on page* 481

teniposide (ten i POE side)

Sound-Alike/Look-Alike Issues

teniposide may be confused with etoposide

Synonyms EPT; VM-26

U.S./Canadian Brand Names Vumon® [US/Can]

Therapeutic Category Antineoplastic Agent

Use Treatment of acute lymphocytic leukemia, small cell lung cancer

Usual Dosage I.V.:

Children: 130 mg/m^2/week, increasing to 150 mg/m^2 after 3 weeks and up to 180 mg/m^2 after 6 weeks

Acute lymphoblastic leukemia (ALL): 165 mg/m^2 twice weekly for 8-9 doses **or** 250 mg/m^2 weekly for 4-8 weeks

Adults: 50-180 mg/m^2 once or twice weekly for 4-6 weeks or 20-60 mg/m^2/day for 5 days

Small cell lung cancer: 80-90 mg/m^2/day for 5 days every 4-6 weeks

Dosage Forms

Injection, solution:

Vumon®: 10 mg/mL (5 mL)

Ten-K® *(Discontinued)* *see* potassium chloride *on page* 803

tenofovir (te NOE fo veer)

Synonyms PMPA; TDF; tenofovir disoproxil fumarate

U.S./Canadian Brand Names Viread® [US/Can]

Therapeutic Category Antiretroviral Agent, Reverse Transcriptase Inhibitor (Nucleotide)

Use Management of HIV infections in combination with at least two other antiretroviral agents; treatment of chronic hepatitis B virus (HBV)

Usual Dosage Oral: Adults: HIV infection, hepatitis B infection: 300 mg once daily

Note: Concurrent use with adefovir and/or tenofovir combination products should be avoided.

Dosage Forms

Tablet:

Viread®: 300 mg

tenofovir and emtricitabine *see* emtricitabine and tenofovir *on page* 352
tenofovir disoproxil fumarate *see* tenofovir *on page* 944
tenofovir disoproxil fumarate, efavirenz, and emtricitabine *see* efavirenz, emtricitabine, and tenofovir *on page* 349
Tenolin [Can] *see* atenolol *on page* 107
Tenoretic® [US/Can] *see* atenolol and chlorthalidone *on page* 107
Tenormin® [US/Can] *see* atenolol *on page* 107
Tensilon® [Can] *see* edrophonium *on page* 347
Tenuate® [Can] *see* diethylpropion *on page* 306
Tenuate® *(Discontinued)* *see* diethylpropion *on page* 306
Tenuate® Dospan® [Can] *see* diethylpropion *on page* 306
Tenuate® Dospan® *(Discontinued)* *see* diethylpropion *on page* 306
Tequin® *(Discontinued)* *see* gatifloxacin *on page* 456
Tera-Gel™ [US-OTC] *see* coal tar *on page* 250
Terazol® [Can] *see* terconazole *on page* 946
Terazol® 3 [US] *see* terconazole *on page* 946
Terazol® 7 [US] *see* terconazole *on page* 946

terazosin (ter AY zoe sin)

U.S./Canadian Brand Names Alti-Terazosin [Can]; Apo-Terazosin® [Can]; Hytrin® [Can]; Novo-Terazosin [Can]; Nu-Terazosin [Can]; PMS-Terazosin [Can]

Therapeutic Category Alpha-Adrenergic Blocking Agent

Use Management of mild-to-moderate hypertension; alone or in combination with other agents such as diuretics or beta-blockers; benign prostate hyperplasia (BPH)

Usual Dosage Oral: Adults:

Hypertension: Initial: 1 mg at bedtime; slowly increase dose to achieve desired blood pressure, up to 20 mg/day; usual dose range (JNC 7): 1-20 mg once daily

Dosage reduction may be needed when adding a diuretic or other antihypertensive agent; if drug is discontinued for greater than several days, consider beginning with initial dose and retitrate as needed; dosage may be given on a twice daily regimen if response is diminished at 24 hours and hypotensive is observed at 2-4 hours following a dose

Benign prostatic hyperplasia: Initial: 1 mg at bedtime, increasing as needed; most patients require 10 mg/day; if no response after 4-6 weeks of 10 mg/day, may increase to 20 mg/day

Dosage Forms

Capsule: 1 mg, 2 mg, 5 mg, 10 mg

terbinafine (oral) (TER bin a feen OR al)

Sound-Alike/Look-Alike Issues

terbinafine may be confused with terbutaline

Lamisil® may be confused with Lamictal®, Lomotil®

U.S./Canadian Brand Names Lamisil® Oral [US/Can]

Therapeutic Category Antifungal Agent

Use Treatment of onychomycosis infections of the toenail or fingernail

Usual Dosage Oral: Adults:

Fingernail onychomycosis: 250 mg once daily for 6 weeks

Toenail onychomycosis: 250 mg once daily for 12 weeks

Dosage Forms

Tablet: 250 mg

Lamisil®: 250 mg

terbinafine (topical) (TER bin a feen TOP i kal)

Sound-Alike/Look-Alike Issues

terbinafine may be confused with terbutaline

Lamisil® may be confused with Lamictal®, Lomotil®

U.S./Canadian Brand Names Lamisil® Topical [US/Can]

Therapeutic Category Antifungal Agent

Use Topical antifungal for the treatment of tinea pedis (athlete's foot), tinea cruris (jock itch), and tinea corporis (ring worm); tinea versicolor (lotion)

Usual Dosage Topical: Adults:

Athlete's foot: Apply to affected area twice daily for at least 1 week, not to exceed 4 weeks

Ringworm and jock itch: Apply to affected area once or twice daily for at least 1 week, not to exceed 4 weeks

Dosage Forms

Cream: 1% (12 g, 24 g)

Lamisil® AT™: 1% (12 g)

Solution [topical spray]:

Lamisil® AT™ [OTC]: 1% (30 mL)

terbutaline (ter BYOO ta leen)

Sound-Alike/Look-Alike Issues

terbutaline may be confused with terbinafine, TOLBUTamide

brethine may be confused with Methergine®

Synonyms brethine

U.S./Canadian Brand Names Bricanyl® [Can]

Therapeutic Category Adrenergic Agonist Agent

Use Bronchodilator in reversible airway obstruction and bronchial asthma

Usual Dosage

Children <12 years: Bronchoconstriction:

Oral: Initial: 0.05 mg/kg/dose 3 times/day, increased gradually as required; maximum: 0.15 mg/kg/dose 3-4 times/day or a total of 5 mg/24 hours

SubQ: 0.005-0.01 mg/kg/dose to a maximum of 0.3 mg/dose; may repeat in 15-20 minutes

Children ≥6 years and Adults: Bronchospasm (acute): Inhalation (Bricanyl® [CAN] MDI: 500 mcg/puff, *not labeled for use in the U.S.*): One puff as needed; may repeat with 1 inhalation (after 5 minutes); more than 6 inhalations should not be necessary in any 24 hour period. **Note:** If a previously effective dosage regimen fails to provide the usual relief, or the effects of a dose last for >3 hours, medical advice should be sought immediately; this is a sign of seriously worsening asthma that requires reassessment of therapy.

Children >12 years and Adults: Bronchoconstriction:

Oral:

12-15 years: 2.5 mg every 6 hours 3 times/day; not to exceed 7.5 mg in 24 hours

>15 years: 5 mg/dose every 6 hours 3 times/day; if side effects occur, reduce dose to 2.5 mg every 6 hours; not to exceed 15 mg in 24 hours

SubQ: 0.25 mg/dose; may repeat in 15-30 minutes (maximum: 0.5 mg/4-hour period)

Dosage Forms [CAN] = Canadian brand name

Injection, solution: 1 mg/mL (1 mL)

Powder for oral inhalation:

Bricanyl® Turbuhaler [CAN]: 500 mcg/actuation [50 or 200 metered actuations] [not available in the U.S.]

Tablet: 2.5 mg, 5 mg

terconazole (ter KONE a zole)

Sound-Alike/Look-Alike Issues

terconazole may be confused with tioconazole

Synonyms triaconazole

U.S./Canadian Brand Names Terazol® 3 [US]; Terazol® 7 [US]; Terazol® [Can]; Zazole™ [US]

Therapeutic Category Antifungal Agent

Use Local treatment of vulvovaginal candidiasis

Usual Dosage Adults: Female:

Terazol® 3, Zazole™ 0.8% vaginal cream: Insert 1 applicatorful intravaginally at bedtime for 3 consecutive days

Terazol® 7, Zazole™ 0.4% vaginal cream: Insert 1 applicatorful intravaginally at bedtime for 7 consecutive days

Terazol® 3 vaginal suppository: Insert 1 suppository intravaginally at bedtime for 3 consecutive days

Dosage Forms

Cream, vaginal: 0.4% (45 g); 0.8% (20 g)

Terazol® 7, Zazole™: 0.4% (45 g)

Terazol® 3, Zazole™: 0.8% (20 g)

Suppository, vaginal:

Terazol® 3: 80 mg (3s)

Terfluzine [Can] *see* trifluoperazine *on page 986*

teriparatide (ter i PAR a tide)

Synonyms parathyroid hormone (1-34); recombinant human parathyroid hormone (1-34); rhPTH(1-34)

U.S./Canadian Brand Names Forteo® [US/Can]

Therapeutic Category Diagnostic Agent

Use Treatment of osteoporosis in postmenopausal women at high risk of fracture; treatment of primary or hypogonadal osteoporosis in men at high risk of fracture; treatment of glucocorticoid-induced osteoporosis in men and women at high risk for fracture

Usual Dosage SubQ: Adults: 20 mcg once daily; **Note:** Initial administration should occur under circumstances in which the patient may sit or lie down, in the event of orthostasis.

Dosage Forms

Injection, solution:

Forteo®: 250 mcg/mL (2.4 mL)

terpin hydrate *(Discontinued)*

Terra-Cortril® Ophthalmic Suspension *(Discontinued)*

Terramycin® I.M. ***(Discontinued)***
Terramycin® Oral ***(Discontinued)***
Terrell™ [US] *see* isoflurane *on page 548*
Tersi [US] *see* selenium sulfide *on page 895*
Tesamone® Injection ***(Discontinued)*** *see* testosterone *on page 947*
Teslac® ***(Discontinued)***
TESPA *see* thiotepa *on page 956*
Tessalon® [US/Can] *see* benzonatate *on page 132*
Tessalon Perles *see* benzonatate *on page 132*
Testim® [US/Can] *see* testosterone *on page 947*
Testoderm® ***(Discontinued)*** *see* testosterone *on page 947*
Testoderm® TTS ***(Discontinued)*** *see* testosterone *on page 947*
Testoderm® With Adhesive ***(Discontinued)*** *see* testosterone *on page 947*
testolactone ***(Discontinued)***
Testomar® ***(Discontinued)*** *see* yohimbine *on page 1025*
Testopel® [US] *see* testosterone *on page 947*
Testopel® Pellet ***(Discontinued)*** *see* testosterone *on page 947*

testosterone (tes TOS ter one)

Sound-Alike/Look-Alike Issues
testosterone may be confused with testolactone
Testoderm® may be confused with Estraderm®

Synonyms testosterone cypionate; testosterone enanthate

U.S./Canadian Brand Names Andriol® [Can]; Androderm® [US/Can]; AndroGel® [US/Can]; Andropository [Can]; Delatestryl® [US/Can]; Depotest® 100 [Can]; Depo®-Testosterone [US]; Everone® 200 [Can]; First® Testosterone MC [US]; First® Testosterone [US]; PMS-Testosterone [Can]; Striant® [US]; Testim® [US/Can]; Testopel® [US]

Therapeutic Category Androgen

Controlled Substance C-III

Use

Injection: Androgen replacement therapy in the treatment of delayed male puberty; male hypogonadism (primary or hypogonadotropic); inoperable metastatic female breast cancer (enanthate only)

Pellet: Androgen replacement therapy in the treatment of delayed male puberty; male hypogonadism (primary or hypogonadotropic)

Topical (buccal system, gel, transdermal system): Male hypogonadism (primary or hypogonadotropic)

Capsule (not available in U.S.): Androgen replacement therapy in the treatment of delayed male puberty; male hypogonadism (primary or hypogonadotropic); replacement therapy in impotence or for male climacteric symptoms due to androgen deficiency

Usual Dosage

Adolescents and Adults: Male:

I.M.:

Hypogonadism: Testosterone enanthate or testosterone cypionate: 50-400 mg every 2-4 weeks (FDA-approved dosing range); 75-100 mg/week or 150-200 mg every 2 weeks (per practice guidelines)

Delayed puberty: Testosterone enanthate: 50-200 mg every 2-4 weeks for a limited duration

Pellet (for subcutaneous implantation): Delayed male puberty, male hypogonadism: 150-450 mg every 3-6 months

Oral: Delayed puberty, hypogonadism, or hypogonadotropic hypogonadism: Capsule (Andriol®; not available in U.S.): Initial: 120-160 mg/day in 2 divided doses for 2-3 weeks; adjust according to individual response; usual maintenance dose: 40-120 mg/day (in divided doses)

Adults:

I.M.: Females: Inoperable metastatic breast cancer: Testosterone enanthate: 200-400 mg every 2-4 weeks

Topical: Primary male hypogonadism **or** hypogonadotropic hypogonadism:

Buccal: 30 mg twice daily (every 12 hours) applied to the gum region above the incisor tooth

Transdermal system: Androderm®: Initial: Apply 5 mg/day once nightly to clean, dry area on the back, abdomen, upper arms, or thighs (do **not** apply to scrotum); dosing range: 2.5-7.5 mg/day; in nonvirilized patients, dose may be initiated at 2.5 mg/day

Gel: AndroGel®, Testim®: 5 g (to deliver 50 mg of testosterone with 5 mg systemically absorbed) applied once daily (preferably in the morning) to clean, dry, intact skin of the shoulder and upper arms. AndroGel® may also be applied to the abdomen. Dosage may be increased to a maximum of 10 g (100 mg). **Do not apply testosterone gel to the genitals.**

Dose adjustment based on testosterone levels:

Less than normal range: Increase dose from 5 g to 7.5 g to 10 g

Greater than normal range: Decrease dose. Discontinue if consistently above normal at 5 g/day

Dosage Forms [CAN] = Canadian brand name

Capsule, gelatin:

Andriol™ [CAN]: 40 mg (10s) [not available in the U.S.]

Gel, topical:

AndroGel®: 1.25 g/actuation (75 g); 2.5 g (30s); 5 g (30s)

Testim®: 5 g (30s)

Implant, subcutaneous:

Testopel®: 75 mg (10s, 100s)

Injection, in oil: 100 mg/mL (10 mL); 200 mg/mL (1 mL, 5 mL, 10 mL)

Depo®-Testosterone: 100 mg/mL (10 mL); 200 mg/mL (1 mL, 10 mL)

Delatestryl®: 200 mg/mL (1 mL, 5 mL)

Kit [for prescription compounding; testosterone 2%]:

First®-Testosterone:

Injection, in oil: Testosterone 100 mg/mL (12 mL)

Ointment: White petrolatum (48 g)

First®-Testosterone MC:

Injection, in oil: Testosterone 100 mg/mL (12 mL)

Cream: Moisturizing cream (48 g)

Mucoadhesive, for buccal application [buccal system]:

Striant®: 30 mg (10s)

Transdermal system:

Androderm®: 2.5 mg/day (60s); 5 mg/day (30s)

testosterone cypionate *see* testosterone *on page* 947

testosterone enanthate *see* testosterone *on page* 947

Testred® [US] *see* methyltestosterone *on page* 648

tetanus and diphtheria toxoid *see* diphtheria and tetanus toxoid *on page* 318

tetanus immune globulin (human) (TET a nus i MYUN GLOB yoo lin HYU man)

Synonyms TIG

U.S./Canadian Brand Names HyperTET™ S/D [US/Can]

Therapeutic Category Immune Globulin

Use Prophylaxis against tetanus following injury in patients where immunization status is not known or uncertain

The Advisory Committee on Immunization Practices (ACIP) recommends passive immunization with TIG for the following:

- Persons with a wound that is not clean or minor and in whom contraindications to a tetanus-toxoid containing vaccine exist and they have not completed a primary series of tetanus toxoid immunization.
- Persons who are wounded in bombings or similar mass casualty events who have penetrating injuries or nonintact skin exposure and who cannot confirm receipt of a tetanus booster within the previous 5 years. In case of shortage, use should be reserved for persons ≥60 years of age.

Usual Dosage I.M.:

Prophylaxis of tetanus:

Children: 4 units/kg; some recommend administering 250 units to small children

Adults: 250 units

Treatment of tetanus:

Children: 500-3000 units; some should infiltrate locally around the wound

Adults: 3000-6000 units

Dosage Forms

Injection, solution [preservative free]:

HyperTET™ S/D: 250 units/mL (1 mL)

tetanus toxoid *see* diphtheria and tetanus toxoids, acellular pertussis, poliovirus and *Haemophilus* b conjugate vaccine *on page* 320

tetanus toxoid (adsorbed) (TET a nus TOKS oyd, ad SORBED)

Sound-Alike/Look-Alike Issues

Tetanus toxoid products may be confused with influenza virus vaccine and tuberculin products. Medication errors have occurred when tetanus toxoid products have been inadvertently administered instead of tuberculin skin tests (PPD) and influenza virus vaccine. These products are refrigerated and often stored in close proximity to each other.

Synonyms TT

Therapeutic Category Toxoid

Use Active immunization against tetanus when combination antigen preparations are not indicated. **Note:** Tetanus and diphtheria toxoids for adult use (Td) is the preferred immunizing agent for most adults and for children after their seventh birthday. Young children should receive trivalent DTaP (diphtheria/tetanus/acellular pertussis), as part of their childhood immunization program, unless pertussis is contraindicated, then DT is warranted.

Usual Dosage I.M.: Children ≥7 years and Adults:

Primary immunization: 0.5 mL; repeat 0.5 mL at 4-8 weeks after first dose and at 6-12 months after second dose

Routine booster dose: Recommended every 10 years

Note: In most patients, Td is the recommended product for primary immunization, booster doses, and tetanus immunization in wound management (refer to diphtheria and tetanus toxoid monograph)

Dosage Forms

Injection, suspension:

Tetanus 5 Lf units per 0.5 mL (0.5 mL)

tetanus toxoid (fluid) (TET a nus TOKS oyd FLOO id)

Sound-Alike/Look-Alike Issues

Tetanus toxoid products may be confused with influenza virus vaccine and tuberculin products. Medication errors have occurred when tetanus toxoid products have been inadvertently administered instead of tuberculin skin tests (PPD) and influenza virus vaccine. These products are refrigerated and often stored in close proximity to each other.

Synonyms tetanus toxoid plain

Therapeutic Category Toxoid

Use Indicated as booster dose in the active immunization against tetanus in the rare adult or child who is allergic to the aluminum adjuvant (a product containing adsorbed tetanus toxoid is preferred); not indicated for primary immunization

Usual Dosage Booster doses: I.M., SubQ: 0.5 mL every 10 years

tetanus toxoid plain *see* tetanus toxoid (fluid) *on page 949*

tetanus toxoid, reduced diphtheria toxoid, and acellular pertussis, adsorbed *see* diphtheria, tetanus toxoids, and acellular pertussis vaccine *on page 321*

tetrabenazine (tet ra BEN a zeen)

U.S./Canadian Brand Names Nitoman™ [Can]; Xenazine® [US]

Therapeutic Category Monoamine Depleting Agent

Use Treatment of chorea associated with Huntington disease

Canadian labeling: Treatment of hyperkinetic movement disorders, including Huntington chorea, hemiballismus, senile chorea, Tourette syndrome, and tardive dyskinesia

Usual Dosage Oral: Dose should be individualized; titrate slowly

Chorea associated with Huntington disease: Adults:

Initial: 12.5 mg once daily, may increase to 12.5 mg twice daily after 1 week

Maintenance: May be increased by 12.5 mg/day at weekly intervals; doses >37.5 mg/day should be divided into 3 doses (maximum single dose 25 mg)

Canadian labeling: Hyperkinetic movement disorders:

Adults: Initial: 12.5 mg twice daily (may be given 3 times/day); may be increased by 12.5 mg/day every 3-5 days; should be titrated slowly to maximal tolerated and effective dose (dose is individualized)

Usual maximum tolerated dosage: 25 mg 3 times/day; maximum recommended dose: 200 mg/day

Note: If there is no improvement at the maximum tolerated dose after 7 days, improvement is unlikely; discontinuation should be considered.

Dosage Forms [CAN] = Canadian brand name

Tablet:

Nitoman™ [CAN]: 25 mg [not available in the U.S.]

Xenazine®: 12.5 mg, 25 mg

tetracaine (TET ra kane)

Synonyms amethocaine hydrochloride; tetracaine hydrochloride

U.S./Canadian Brand Names Ametop™ [Can]; Pontocaine® Niphanoid® [US]; Pontocaine® [US/Can]

Therapeutic Category Local Anesthetic

Use Spinal anesthesia; local anesthesia in the eye for various diagnostic and examination purposes; topically applied to nose and throat for diagnostic procedures

Usual Dosage Adults:

Ophthalmic: Short-term anesthesia of the eye: 0.5% solution: Instill 1-2 drops; prolonged use (especially for at-home self-medication) is not recommended

Injection: Spinal anesthesia: **Note:** Dosage varies with the anesthetic procedure, the degree of anesthesia required, and the individual patient response; it is administered by subarachnoid injection for spinal anesthesia.

Perineal anesthesia: 5 mg

Perineal and lower extremities: 10 mg

Anesthesia extending up to costal margin: 15 mg; doses up to 20 mg may be given, but are reserved for exceptional cases

Low spinal anesthesia (saddle block): 2-5 mg

Topical mucous membranes (rhinolaryngology): Used as a 0.25% or 0.5% solution by direct application or nebulization; total dose should not exceed 20 mg

Dosage Forms

Injection, powder for reconstitution [preservative free]:

Pontocaine® Niphanoid®: 20 mg

Injection, solution: 1% [10 mg/mL] (2 mL)

Pontocaine®: 1% [10 mg/mL] (2 mL)

Solution, ophthalmic: 0.5% [5 mg/mL] (2 mL, 15 mL)

Solution, topical:

Pontocaine®: 2% [20 mg/mL] (30 mL, 118 mL)

tetracaine and lidocaine *see* lidocaine and tetracaine *on page* 589

tetracaine, benzocaine, and butamben *see* benzocaine, butamben, and tetracaine *on page* 131

tetracaine hydrochloride *see* tetracaine *on page* 950

Tetracap® ***(Discontinued)*** *see* tetracycline *on page* 950

tetracosactide *see* cosyntropin *on page* 260

tetracycline (tet ra SYE kleen)

Sound-Alike/Look-Alike Issues

tetracycline may be confused with tetradecyl sulfate

achromycin may be confused with actinomycin, Adriamycin PFS®

Synonyms achromycin; TCN; tetracycline hydrochloride

U.S./Canadian Brand Names Apo-Tetra® [Can]; Nu-Tetra [Can]

Therapeutic Category Antibiotic, Ophthalmic; Antibiotic, Topical; Tetracycline Derivative

Use Treatment of susceptible bacterial infections of both gram-positive and gram-negative organisms; also infections due to *Mycoplasma*, *Chlamydia*, and *Rickettsia*; indicated for acne, exacerbations of chronic bronchitis, and treatment of gonorrhea and syphilis in patients who are allergic to penicillin; as part of a multidrug regimen for *H. pylori* eradication to reduce the risk of duodenal ulcer recurrence

Usual Dosage

Usual dosage range:

Children >8 years: Oral: 25-50 mg/kg/day in divided doses every 6 hours

Adults: Oral: 250-500 mg/dose every 6 hours

Indication-specific dosing:

Adults: Oral:

Acne: 250-500 twice daily

Chronic bronchitis, acute exacerbation: 500 mg 4 times/day

Erlichiosis: 500 mg 4 times/day for 7-14 days

Peptic ulcer disease: Eradication of *Helicobacter pylori*: 500 mg 2-4 times/day depending on regimen; requires combination therapy with at least one other antibiotic and an acid-suppressing agent (proton pump inhibitor or H_2 blocker)

Periodontitis: 250 mg every 6 hours until improvement (usually 10 days)

Vibrio cholerae: 500 mg 4 times/day for 3 days

Dosage Forms

Capsule: 250 mg, 500 mg

tetracycline hydrochloride *see* tetracycline *on page 950*

tetracycline, metronidazole, and bismuth subcitrate potassium *see* bismuth, metronidazole, and tetracycline *on page 143*

tetracycline, metronidazole, and bismuth subsalicylate *see* bismuth, metronidazole, and tetracycline *on page 143*

tetrahydroaminoacrine *see* tacrine *on page 935*

tetrahydrocannabinol *see* dronabinol *on page 339*

tetrahydrocannabinol and cannabidiol *(Canada only)*

(TET ra hye droe can NAB e nol & can nab e DYE ol)

Synonyms cannabidiol and tetrahydrocannabinol; delta-9-tetrahydrocannabinol and cannabinol; GW-1000-02; THC and CBD

U.S./Canadian Brand Names Sativex® [Can]

Therapeutic Category Analgesic, Miscellaneous

Controlled Substance CDSA-II

Use Adjunctive treatment of neuropathic pain in multiple sclerosis; adjunctive treatment of moderate-to-severe pain in advanced cancer

Usual Dosage Buccal spray: Adults: Neuropathic pain (MS), cancer pain: Initial: One spray every 4 hours to a maximum of 4 sprays on first day

Titration and individualization: Dosage is self-titrated by the patient. In the treatment of MS, the mean daily dosage after titration in clinical trials was 5 sprays per day. The usual maximum dose is 12 sprays per day although some patients may require and tolerate a higher number of sprays per day. In the treatment of cancer pain, the mean daily dosage after titration was 8 sprays per day. Dosage should be adjusted as necessary, based on effect and tolerance. Sprays should be evenly distributed over the course of the day during initial titration. If adverse reactions, including intoxication-type symptoms, are noted the dosage should be suspended until resolution of the symptoms; a dosage reduction or extension of the interval between doses may be used to avoid a recurrence of symptoms. Retitration may be required in the event of adverse reactions and/or worsening of symptoms.

Dosage Forms [CAN] = Canadian brand name

Solution, buccal [spray]:

Sativex® [CAN]: Delta-9 tetrahydrocannabinol 27 mg/mL and cannabidiol 25 mg/mL (5.5 mL) [not available in the U.S.]

tetrahydrozoline (tet ra hye DROZ a leen)

Sound-Alike/Look-Alike Issues

Visine® may be confused with Visken®

Synonyms tetrahydrozoline hydrochloride; tetryzoline

U.S./Canadian Brand Names Geneye [US-OTC]; Murine® Tears Plus [US-OTC]; Opti-Clear [US-OTC]; Tyzine® Pediatric [US]; Tyzine® [US]; Visine® Advanced Relief [US-OTC]; Visine® Original [US-OTC]

Therapeutic Category Adrenergic Agonist Agent

Use Symptomatic relief of nasal congestion and conjunctival congestion

Usual Dosage

Nasal congestion: Intranasal:

Children 2-6 years: Instill 2-3 drops of 0.05% solution every 4-6 hours as needed, no more frequent than every 3 hours

Children >6 years and Adults: Instill 2-4 drops or 3-4 sprays of 0.1% solution every 3-4 hours as needed, no more frequent than every 3 hours

Conjunctival congestion: Ophthalmic: Adults: Instill 1-2 drops in each eye 2-4 times/day

Dosage Forms

Solution, intranasal:

Tyzine®: 0.1% (30 mL)

Tyzine® Pediatric: 0.05% (15 mL)

Solution, intranasal [spray]:
Tyzine®: 0.1% (15 mL)
Solution, ophthalmic: 0.05% (15 mL)
Geneye [OTC], Opti-Clear [OTC]: 0.05% (15 mL)
Murine® Tears Plus [OTC], Visine® Original [OTC]: 0.05% (15 mL, 30 mL)
Visine® Advanced Relief [OTC]: 0.05% (30 mL)

tetrahydrozoline hydrochloride *see* tetrahydrozoline *on page* 951
2,2,2-tetramine *see* trientine *on page* 985
Tetramune® ***(Discontinued)***
Tetrasine® Extra Ophthalmic ***(Discontinued)*** *see* tetrahydrozoline *on page* 951
Tetrasine® Ophthalmic ***(Discontinued)*** *see* tetrahydrozoline *on page* 951
Tetra Tannate Pediatric [US] *see* chlorpheniramine, ephedrine, phenylephrine, and carbetapentane *on page* 216
tetryzoline *see* tetrahydrozoline *on page* 951
Teveten® [US/Can] *see* eprosartan *on page* 363
Teveten® HCT [US/Can] *see* eprosartan and hydrochlorothiazide *on page* 364
Teveten® Plus [Can] *see* eprosartan and hydrochlorothiazide *on page* 364
Tev-Tropin® [US] *see* somatropin *on page* 916
Texacort® [US] *see* hydrocortisone (topical) *on page* 505
TG *see* thioguanine *on page* 955
T/Gel® Daily Control [US-OTC] *see* pyrithione zinc *on page* 842
T/Gel® Daily Control 2 in 1 [US-OTC] *see* pyrithione zinc *on page* 842
T-Gen® ***(Discontinued)*** *see* trimethobenzamide *on page* 987
THA *see* tacrine *on page* 935

thalidomide (tha LI doe mide)

Sound-Alike/Look-Alike Issues
thalidomide may be confused with flutamide
Thalomid® may be confused with thiamine

Synonyms NSC-66847

U.S./Canadian Brand Names Thalomid® [US/Can]

Therapeutic Category Immunosuppressant Agent

Use Treatment of multiple myeloma; treatment and maintenance of cutaneous manifestations of erythema nodosum leprosum (ENL)

Usual Dosage Oral:
Multiple myeloma: 200 mg once daily (with dexamethasone 40 mg daily on days 1-4, 9-12, and 17-20 of a 28-day treatment cycle)
Cutaneous ENL:
Initial: 100-300 mg/day taken once daily at bedtime with water (at least 1 hour after evening meal)
Patients weighing <50 kg: Initiate at lower end of the dosing range
Severe cutaneous reaction or patients previously requiring high dose may be initiated at 400 mg/day; doses may be divided, but taken 1 hour after meals
Maintenance: Dosing should continue until active reaction subsides (usually at least 2 weeks), then tapered in 50 mg decrements every 2-4 weeks
Patients who flare during tapering or with a history or requiring prolonged maintenance should be maintained on the minimum dosage necessary to control the reaction. Efforts to taper should be repeated every 3-6 months, in increments of 50 mg every 2-4 weeks.

Dosage Forms
Capsule:
Thalomid®: 50 mg, 100 mg, 150 mg, 200 mg

Thalitone® [US] *see* chlorthalidone *on page* 223
Thalomid® [US/Can] *see* thalidomide *on page* 952
THAM® [US] *see* tromethamine *on page* 991
THC *see* dronabinol *on page* 339
THC and CBD *see* tetrahydrocannabinol and cannabidiol *(Canada only) on page* 951
Thelin™ [Can] *see* sitaxsentan *(Canada only) on page* 905
Theo-X® ***(Discontinued)*** *see* theophylline *on page* 953

Theo-24® [US] *see* theophylline *on page 953*
Theobid® *(Discontinued)* *see* theophylline *on page 953*
Theochron™ [US] *see* theophylline *on page 953*
Theochron® SR [Can] *see* theophylline *on page 953*
Theoclear-80® *(Discontinued)* *see* theophylline *on page 953*
Theoclear®-L.A. *(Discontinued)* *see* theophylline *on page 953*
Theo-Dur® (all products) *(Discontinued)* *see* theophylline *on page 953*
Theolair-SR® *(Discontinued)* *see* theophylline *on page 953*
Theolate *(Discontinued)*

theophylline (thee OFF i lin)

Synonyms theophylline anhydrous

U.S./Canadian Brand Names Apo-Theo LA® [Can]; Elixophyllin® [US]; Novo-Theophyl SR [Can]; PMS-Theophylline [Can]; Pulmophylline [Can]; ratio-Theo-Bronc [Can]; Theo-24® [US]; Theochron® SR [Can]; Theochron™ [US]; Uniphyl® SRT [Can]; Uniphyl® [US]

Therapeutic Category Theophylline Derivative

Use Treatment of symptoms and reversible airway obstruction due to chronic asthma, or other chronic lung diseases; apnea of prematurity

Note: The National Heart, Lung, and Blood Institute Guidelines (2007) do not recommend oral theophylline as a long-term control medication for asthma in children ≤4 years of age; use may be considered as an alternative (but not preferred) agent in older children and adults. The guidelines do not recommend theophylline I.V. for the treatment of exacerbations of asthma.

Usual Dosage Note: Doses should be individualized based on peak serum concentrations and should be based on ideal body weight.

Dosage Forms

Capsule, extended release:
Theo-24®: 100 mg, 200 mg, 300 mg, 400 mg [24 hours]

Elixir:
Elixophyllin®: 80 mg/15 mL (473 mL)

Infusion [premixed in D_5W]: 200 mg (50 mL, 100 mL); 400 mg (250 mL, 500 mL); 800 mg (250 mL, 500 mL, 1000 mL)

Tablet, controlled release:
Uniphyl®: 400 mg, 600 mg [24 hours]

Tablet, extended release: 100 mg, 200 mg, 300 mg, 400 mg, 450 mg, 600 mg
Theochron™: 100 mg, 200 mg, 300 mg, 450 mg [12-24 hours]

theophylline and guaifenesin *(Discontinued)*
theophylline anhydrous *see* theophylline *on page 953*
theophylline ethylenediamine *see* aminophylline *on page 63*
Theo-Sav® *(Discontinued)* *see* theophylline *on page 953*
Theospan®-SR *(Discontinued)* *see* theophylline *on page 953*
Theostat-80® *(Discontinued)* *see* theophylline *on page 953*
Theovent® *(Discontinued)* *see* theophylline *on page 953*
Therabid® *(Discontinued)*
TheraCys® [US] *see* BCG vaccine *on page 124*
Theraflu® Daytime Severe Cold & Cough [US-OTC] *see* acetaminophen, dextromethorphan, and phenylephrine *on page 27*
Thera-Flur® *(Discontinued)* *see* fluoride *on page 430*
Thera-Flur-N® *(Discontinued)* *see* fluoride *on page 430*
Thera-Flu® Severe Cold Non-Drowsy *(Discontinued)*
Theraflu® Thin Strips® Multi Symptom [US-OTC] *see* diphenhydramine *on page 315*
Theraflu® Warming Relief Daytime Severe Cold & Cough [US-OTC] *see* acetaminophen, dextromethorphan, and phenylephrine *on page 27*
Theragran-M® Advanced Formula *(Discontinued)* *see* vitamins (multiple/oral) *on page 1019*
Theragran® Heart Right™ *(Discontinued)* *see* vitamins (multiple/oral) *on page 1019*
TheraPatch® Warm *(Discontinued)* *see* capsaicin *on page 178*
therapeutic multivitamins *see* vitamins (multiple/oral) *on page 1019*

Theratears® [US] *see* carboxymethylcellulose *on page 186*
Thermazene® [US] *see* silver sulfadiazine *on page 901*

thiabendazole (thye a BEN da zole)

Synonyms tiabendazole

U.S./Canadian Brand Names Mintezol® [US]

Therapeutic Category Anthelmintic

Use Treatment of strongyloidiasis, cutaneous larva migrans, visceral larva migrans, dracunculiasis, trichinosis, and mixed helminthic infections

Usual Dosage Purgation is not required prior to use; drinking of fruit juice aids in expulsion of worms by removing the mucus to which the intestinal tapeworms attach themselves.

Children and Adults:
Oral: 50 mg/kg/day divided every 12 hours (if >68 kg: 1.5 g/dose); maximum dose: 3 g/day
Treatment duration:
Strongyloidiasis, ascariasis, uncinariasis: For 2 consecutive days
Cutaneous larva migrans: For 2 consecutive days; if active lesions are still present 2 days after completion, a second course of treatment is recommended.
Visceral larva migrans: For 7 consecutive days
Trichinosis: For 2-4 consecutive days; optimal dosage not established
Dracunculosis: 50-75 mg/kg/day divided every 12 hours for 3 days

Dosage Forms
Tablet, chewable:
Mintezol®: 500 mg

thiamazole *see* methimazole *on page 637*
thiamin *see* thiamine *on page 954*

thiamine (THYE a min)

Sound-Alike/Look-Alike Issues
thiamine may be confused with Tenormin®, Thalomid®, Thorazine®

Synonyms aneurine hydrochloride; thiamin; thiamine hydrochloride; thiaminium chloride hydrochloride; vitamin B_1

U.S./Canadian Brand Names Betaxin® [Can]

Therapeutic Category Vitamin, Water Soluble

Use Treatment of thiamine deficiency including beriberi, Wernicke encephalopathy, Korsakoff syndrome, neuritis associated with pregnancy, or in alcoholic patients; dietary supplement

Usual Dosage
Adequate Intake:
0-6 months: 0.2 mg/day
7-12 months: 0.3 mg/day
Recommended daily intake:
1-3 years: 0.5 mg
4-8 years: 0.6 mg
9-13 years: 0.9 mg
14-18 years: Female: 1 mg; Male: 1.2 mg
≥19 years: Female: 1.1 mg; Male: 1.2 mg
Pregnancy, lactation: 1.4 mg
Parenteral nutrition supplementation:
Infants: 1.2 mg/day
Adults: 6 mg/day; may be increased to 25-50 mg/day with history of alcohol abuse
Thiamine deficiency (beriberi):
Children: 10-25 mg/dose I.M. or I.V. daily (if critically ill), or 10-50 mg/dose orally every day for 2 weeks, then 5-10 mg/dose orally daily for 1 month
Adults: 5-30 mg/dose I.M. or I.V. 3 times/day (if critically ill); then orally 5-30 mg/day in single or divided doses 3 times/day for 1 month
Alcohol withdrawal syndrome: Adults: 100 mg/day I.M. or I.V. for several days, followed by 50-100 mg/day orally
Wernicke encephalopathy: Adults: Treatment: Initial: 100 mg I.V., then 50-100 mg/day I.M. or I.V. until consuming a regular, balanced diet. Larger doses may be needed in patients with alcohol abuse.

Dosage Forms
Injection, solution: 100 mg/mL (2 mL)
Tablet: 50 mg, 100 mg, 250 mg, 500 mg

thiamine hydrochloride *see* thiamine *on page 954*
thiaminium chloride hydrochloride *see* thiamine *on page 954*

thioguanine (thye oh GWAH neen)

Sound-Alike/Look-Alike Issues
6-thioguanine and 6-TG are error-prone abbreviations (associated with six-fold overdoses of thioguanine)

Synonyms 2-amino-6-mercaptopurine; NSC-752; TG; tioguanine

U.S./Canadian Brand Names Lanvis® [Can]; Tabloid® [US]

Therapeutic Category Antineoplastic Agent

Use Treatment of acute myelogenous (nonlymphocytic) leukemia (AML)

Usual Dosage Total daily dose can be given at one time. Oral (refer to individual protocols):
Infants and Children <3 years: Combination drug therapy for acute nonlymphocytic leukemia: 3.3 mg/kg/day in divided doses twice daily for 4 days
Children and Adults: 2-3 mg/kg/day calculated to nearest 20 mg or 75-200 mg/m^2/day in 1-2 divided doses for 5-7 days or until remission is attained

Dosage Forms
Tablet [scored]:
Tabloid®: 40 mg

Thiola® [US/Can] *see* tiopronin *on page 963*

thiopental (thye oh PEN tal)

Synonyms thiopental sodium

U.S./Canadian Brand Names Pentothal® [US/Can]

Therapeutic Category Barbiturate

Controlled Substance C-III

Use Induction of anesthesia; control of convulsive states; treatment of elevated intracranial pressure

Usual Dosage I.V.:
Induction anesthesia:
Infants: 5-8 mg/kg
Children 1-12 years: 5-6 mg/kg
Adults: 3-5 mg/kg
Maintenance anesthesia:
Children: 1 mg/kg as needed
Adults: 25-100 mg as needed
Increased intracranial pressure: Children and Adults: 1.5-5 mg/kg/dose; repeat as needed to control intracranial pressure
Seizures:
Children: 2-3 mg/kg/dose; repeat as needed
Adults: 75-250 mg/dose; repeat as needed

Dosage Forms
Injection, powder for reconstitution:
Pentothal®: 250 mg, 400 mg, 500 mg, 1 g

thiopental sodium *see* thiopental *on page 955*
thiophosphoramide *see* thiotepa *on page 956*
Thioplex® *(Discontinued)* *see* thiotepa *on page 956*

thioridazine (thye oh RID a zeen)

Sound-Alike/Look-Alike Issues
thioridazine may be confused with thiothixene, Thorazine®
Mellaril® may be confused with Elavil®, Mebaral®

Synonyms thioridazine hydrochloride

U.S./Canadian Brand Names Mellaril® [Can]

Therapeutic Category Phenothiazine Derivative

Use Management of schizophrenic patients who fail to respond adequately to treatment with other antipsychotic drugs, either because of insufficient effectiveness or the inability to achieve an effective dose due to intolerable adverse effects from those medications

Usual Dosage Oral: Adults: Schizophrenia/psychoses: Initial: 50-100 mg 3 times/day with gradual increments as needed and tolerated; maximum: 800 mg/day in 2-4 divided doses

Dosage Forms

Tablet: 10 mg, 25 mg, 50 mg, 100 mg

thioridazine hydrochloride *see* thioridazine *on page 955*

thiosulfuric acid disodium salt *see* sodium thiosulfate *on page 915*

thiotepa (thye oh TEP a)

Synonyms TESPA; thiophosphoramide; triethylenethiophosphoramide; TSPA

Therapeutic Category Antineoplastic Agent

Use Treatment of superficial tumors of the bladder; palliative treatment of adenocarcinoma of breast or ovary; lymphomas and sarcomas; controlling intracavitary effusions caused by metastatic tumors; I.T. use: CNS leukemia/lymphoma, CNS metastases

Usual Dosage Refer to individual protocols.

Children: Sarcomas: I.V.: 25-65 mg/m^2 as a single dose every 21 days

Adults:

I.M., I.V., SubQ: 30-60 mg/m^2 once weekly

I.V.: 0.3-0.4 mg/kg by rapid I.V. administration every 1-4 weeks, **or** 0.2 mg/kg or 6-8 mg/m^2/day for 4-5 days every 2-4 weeks

High-dose therapy for bone marrow transplant: I.V.: 500 mg/m^2, up to 900 mg/m^2

I.M.: 15-30 mg in various schedules have been given

Intracavitary: 0.6-0.8 mg/kg or 30-60 mg weekly

Intrapericardial: 15-30 mg

Intrathecal: 10-15 mg or 5-11.5 mg/m^2

Dosage Forms

Injection, powder for reconstitution: 15 mg, 30 mg

thiothixene (thye oh THIKS een)

Sound-Alike/Look-Alike Issues

thiothixene may be confused with FLUoxetine, thioridazine

Navane® may be confused with Norvasc®, Nubain®

Synonyms tiotixene

U.S./Canadian Brand Names Navane® [US/Can]

Therapeutic Category Thioxanthene Derivative

Use Management of schizophrenia

Usual Dosage Oral: Adults:

Mild-to-moderate psychosis: 2 mg 3 times/day, up to 20-30 mg/day; more severe psychosis: Initial: 5 mg 2 times/day, may increase gradually, if necessary; maximum: 60 mg/day

Rapid tranquilization of the agitated patient (administered every 30-60 minutes): 5-10 mg; average total dose for tranquilization: 15-30 mg

Dosage Forms

Capsule: 1 mg, 2 mg, 5 mg, 10 mg

Navane®: 2 mg, 5 mg, 10 mg, 20 mg

thonzonium, neomycin, colistin, and hydrocortisone *see* neomycin, colistin, hydrocortisone, and thonzonium *on page 687*

Thorazine® *(Discontinued)* *see* chlorpromazine *on page 222*

Thorets [US-OTC] *see* benzocaine *on page 129*

Thrive™ [US-OTC] *see* nicotine *on page 695*

Thrombate III® [US/Can] *see* antithrombin III *on page 85*

Thrombi-Gel® [US] *see* thrombin (topical) *on page 957*

Thrombinar® *(Discontinued)* *see* thrombin (topical) *on page 957*

Thrombin-JMI® [US] *see* thrombin (topical) *on page 957*

Thrombin-JMI® Epistaxis Kit [US] *see* thrombin (topical) *on page 957*

Thrombin-JMI® Spray Kit [US] *see* thrombin (topical) *on page 957*

Thrombin-JMI® Syringe Spray Kit [US] *see* thrombin (topical) *on page 957*

thrombin (topical) (THROM bin, TOP i kal)

U.S./Canadian Brand Names Evithrom™ [US]; Recothrom™ [US]; Thrombi-Gel® [US]; Thrombi-Pad® [US]; Thrombin-JMI® Epistaxis Kit [US]; Thrombin-JMI® Spray Kit [US]; Thrombin-JMI® Syringe Spray Kit [US]; Thrombin-JMI® [US]

Therapeutic Category Hemostatic Agent

Use Hemostasis whenever minor bleeding from capillaries and small venules is accessible

Thrombi-Gel®; Thrombi-Pad®: Temporary control as trauma dressing for moderate-to-severe bleeding wounds; control of surface bleeding from vascular access sites and percutaneous catheter/tubes

Usual Dosage Topical: Hemostasis: **Note:** For topical use only; do not administer intravenously or intraarterially:

Evithrom™: Children and Adults: Dose depends on area to be treated; up to 10 mL was used with absorbable gelatin sponge in clinical studies

Recothrom™: Adults: Dose depends on area to be treated

Thrombi-Gel® 10, 40, 100: Adults: Wet product with up to 3 mL, 10 mL, or 20 mL, respectively, of 0.9% sodium chloride or SWFI; apply directly over source of the bleeding with manual pressure

Thrombi-Pad®: Adults: Apply pad directly over source of bleeding; may apply dry or wetted with up to 10 mL of 0.9% sodium chloride. If desired, product may be left in place for up to 24 hours; do not leave in the body.

Thrombin-JMI®: Adults:

Solution: Use 1000-2000 int. units/mL of solution where bleeding is profuse; use 100 int. units/mL for bleeding from skin or mucosal surfaces

Powder: May apply powder directly to the site of bleeding or on oozing surfaces

Dosage Forms

Pad, topical [preservative free]:

Thrombi-Pad® 3x3: ≥200 units

Powder for reconstitution, topical:

Thrombin-JMI®: 5000 int. units, 20,000 int. units

Thrombin-JMI® Epistaxis kit: 5000 int. units

Thrombin-JMI® Spray Kit, Thrombin-JMI® Syringe Spray Kit: 20,000 int. units

Powder for reconstitution, topical [preservative free]:

Recothrom™: 5000 int. units; 20,000 int. units

Solution, topical:

Evithrom™: 800-1200 int. units/mL (2 mL, 5 mL, 20 mL)

Sponge, topical [preservative free]:

Thrombi-Gel® 10: ≥1000 units (10s)

Thrombi-Gel® 40: ≥1000 units (5s)

Thrombi-Gel® 100: ≥2000 units (5s)

Thrombi-Pad® [US] *see* thrombin (topical) *on page 957*

Thrombostat® ***(Discontinued)*** *see* thrombin (topical) *on page 957*

thymocyte stimulating factor *see* aldesleukin *on page 43*

Thymoglobulin® [US] *see* antithymocyte globulin (rabbit) *on page 86*

Thyrar® ***(Discontinued)*** *see* thyroid, desiccated *on page 957*

Thyrel® TRH ***(Discontinued)***

Thyro-Block® ***(Discontinued)*** *see* potassium iodide *on page 805*

Thyrogen® [US/Can] *see* thyrotropin alpha *on page 958*

thyroid, desiccated (THYE roid DES i kay tid)

Synonyms desiccated thyroid; thyroid extract; thyroid USP

U.S./Canadian Brand Names Armour® Thyroid [US]; Nature-Throid™ [US]; Westhroid™ [US]

Therapeutic Category Thyroid Product

Use Replacement or supplemental therapy in hypothyroidism; pituitary TSH suppressants (thyroid nodules, thyroiditis, multinodular goiter, thyroid cancer), thyrotoxicosis, diagnostic suppression tests

Usual Dosage Oral:

Children: Recommended pediatric dosage for congenital hypothyroidism:

0-6 months: 15-30 mg/day; 4.8-6 mg/kg/day

6-12 months: 30-45 mg/day; 3.6-4.8 mg/kg/day

1-5 years: 45-60 mg/day; 3-3.6 mg/kg/day

6-12 years: 60-90 mg/day; 2.4-3 mg/kg/day
>12 years: >90 mg/day; 1.2-1.8 mg/kg/day
Adults: Initial: 15-30 mg; increase with 15 mg increments every 2-4 weeks; use 15 mg in patients with cardiovascular disease or myxedema. Maintenance dose: Usually 60-120 mg/day; monitor TSH and clinical symptoms.
Thyroid cancer: Requires larger amounts than replacement therapy

Dosage Forms

Tablet: 30 mg, 32.5 mg, 60 mg, 65 mg, 120 mg, 130 mg, 180 mg
Armour® Thyroid: 15 mg, 30 mg, 60 mg, 90 mg, 120 mg, 180 mg, 240 mg, 300 mg
Nature-Throid™: 16.25 mg, 32.5 mg, 65 mg, 130 mg, 195 mg
Westhroid™: 32.5 mg, 65 mg, 130 mg

thyroid extract *see* thyroid, desiccated *on page* 957

Thyroid Strong® ***(Discontinued)*** *see* thyroid, desiccated *on page* 957

thyroid USP *see* thyroid, desiccated *on page* 957

Thyrolar® [US/Can] *see* liotrix *on page* 592

ThyroSafe™ [US-OTC] *see* potassium iodide *on page* 805

ThyroShield™ [US-OTC] *see* potassium iodide *on page* 805

thyrotropin alpha (thye roe TROH pin AL fa)

Sound-Alike/Look-Alike Issues
Thyrogen® may be confused with Thyrolar®

Synonyms human thyroid stimulating hormone; recombinant human thyrotropin; Rh-TSH; TSH

U.S./Canadian Brand Names Thyrogen® [US/Can]

Therapeutic Category Diagnostic Agent

Use As an adjunctive diagnostic tool for serum thyroglobulin (Tg) testing; adjunctive treatment for radioiodine ablation of thyroid tissue remnants after total or near-total thyroidectomy in patients with well-differentiated thyroid cancer without evidence of metastatic disease

Potential clinical uses include: Patients with an undetectable Tg on thyroid hormone suppressive therapy to exclude the diagnosis of residual or recurrent thyroid cancer, patients requiring serum Tg testing and radioiodine imaging who are unwilling to undergo thyroid hormone withdrawal testing and whose treating physician believes that use of a less sensitive test is justified, patients who are either unable to mount an adequate endogenous TSH response to thyroid hormone withdrawal or in whom withdrawal is medically contraindicated, and patients without evidence of metastatic disease to ablate thyroid remnants (in combination with radioiodine [I^{131}]) following near-total thyroidectomy.

Usual Dosage I.M.: Children >16 years and Adults: Radioiodine imaging or ablation: 0.9 mg, followed 24 hours later by a second 0.9 mg dose

For radioiodine imaging or remnant ablation, radioiodine administration should be given 24 hours following the second thyrotropin injection. Diagnostic scanning should be performed 48 hours after radioiodine administration (72 hours after the second thyrotropin injection). Post-therapy scanning may be delayed (additional days) to allow decline of background activity.

For serum Tg testing, serum Tg should be obtained 72 hours after final injection of thyrotropin.

Dosage Forms Injection, powder for reconstitution:
Thyrogen®: 1.1 mg

tiabendazole *see* thiabendazole *on page* 954

tiagabine (tye AG a been)

Sound-Alike/Look-Alike Issues
tiaGABine may be confused with tiZANidine

Synonyms tiagabine hydrochloride

Tall-Man tia**GAB**ine

U.S./Canadian Brand Names Gabitril® [US/Can]

Therapeutic Category Anticonvulsant

Use Adjunctive therapy in adults and children ≥12 years of age in the treatment of partial seizures

Usual Dosage Oral (administer with food):
Patients receiving enzyme-inducing AED regimens:
Children 12-18 years: 4 mg once daily for 1 week; may increase to 8 mg daily in 2 divided doses for 1 week; then may increase by 4-8 mg weekly to response or up to 32 mg daily in 2-4 divided doses

Adults: 4 mg once daily for 1 week; may increase by 4-8 mg weekly to response or up to 56 mg daily in 2-4 divided doses; usual maintenance: 32-56 mg/day

Patients **not** receiving enzyme-inducing AED regimens: The estimated plasma concentrations of tiagabine in patients not taking enzyme-inducing medications is twice that of patients receiving enzyme-inducing AEDs. Lower doses are required; slower titration may be necessary.

Dosage Forms

Tablet:

Gabitril®: 2 mg, 4 mg, 12 mg, 16 mg

tiagabine hydrochloride *see* tiagabine *on page 958*

Tiamate® ***(Discontinued)*** *see* diltiazem *on page 311*

Tiamol® [Can] *see* fluocinonide *on page 429*

Tiaprofenic-200 [Can] *see* tiaprofenic acid *(Canada only) on page 959*

Tiaprofenic-300 [Can] *see* tiaprofenic acid *(Canada only) on page 959*

tiaprofenic acid *(Canada only)* (tye ah PRO fen ik AS id)

U.S./Canadian Brand Names Apo-Tiaprofenic® [Can]; Dom-Tiaprofenic [Can]; Novo-Tiaprofenic [Can]; Nu-Tiaprofenic [Can]; PMS-Tiaprofenic [Can]; Surgam® [Can]; Tiaprofenic-200 [Can]; Tiaprofenic-300 [Can]

Therapeutic Category Nonsteroidal Antiinflammatory Drug (NSAID)

Use Relief of signs and symptoms of rheumatoid arthritis and osteoarthritis (degenerative joint disease)

Usual Dosage Oral: Adults:

Rheumatoid arthritis:

Tablet: Usual initial and maintenance dose: 600 mg/day in 3 divided doses; some patients may do well on 300 mg twice daily; maximum daily dose: 600 mg

Sustained release capsule: Initial and maintenance dose: 2 sustained release capsules of 300 mg once daily

Osteoarthritis:

Tablet: Usual initial and maintenance dose: 600 mg/day in 2 or 3 divided doses; in rare instances patients may be maintained on 300 mg/day in divided doses; maximum daily dose: 600 mg

Sustained release capsule: Initial and maintenance dose: 2 sustained release capsules of 300 mg once daily

Dosage Forms [CAN] = Canadian brand name

Capsule, sustained release: 300 mg [not available in the U.S.]

Tablet: 200 mg, 300 mg

Apo-Tiaprofenic® [CAN], Novo-Tiaprofenic [CAN], Nu-Tiaprofenic [CAN], PMS-Tiaprofenic: 200 mg, 300 mg [not available in the U.S.]

Albert® Tiafen [CAN], Dom-Tiaprofenic® [CAN], Surgam® [CAN]: 300 mg [not available in the U.S.]

Tiazac® [US/Can] *see* diltiazem *on page 311*

Tiazac® XC [Can] *see* diltiazem *on page 311*

ticarcillin and clavulanate potassium (tye kar SIL in & klav yoo LAN ate poe TASS ee um)

Synonyms ticarcillin and clavulanic acid

U.S./Canadian Brand Names Timentin® [US/Can]

Therapeutic Category Penicillin

Use Treatment of lower respiratory tract, urinary tract, skin and skin structures, bone and joint, gynecologic (endometritis) and intraabdominal (peritonitis) infections, and septicemia caused by susceptible organisms. Clavulanate expands activity of ticarcillin to include beta-lactamase producing strains of *S. aureus*, *H. influenzae*, *Bacteroides* species, and some other gram-negative bacilli

Usual Dosage Note: Timentin® (ticarcillin/clavulanate) is a combination product; each 3.1 g dosage form contains 3 g ticarcillin disodium and 0.1 g clavulanic acid.

Usual dosage range:

Children and Adults <60 kg: I.V.: 200-300 mg of ticarcillin component/kg/day in divided doses every 4-6 hours

Children ≥60 kg and Adults: I.V.: 3.1 g (ticarcillin 3 g plus clavulanic acid 0.1 g) every 4-6 hours (maximum: 24 g of ticarcillin component/day)

Indication-specific dosing:

Children: I.V.:

Bite wounds (animal): 200 mg of ticarcillin component/kg/day in divided doses

Neutropenic fever: 75 mg of ticarcillin component/kg every 6 hours (maximum: 3.1 g/dose)

Pneumonia (nosocomial): 300 mg of ticarcillin component/kg/day in 4 divided doses (maximum: 18-24 g of ticarcillin component/day)

Children ≥60 kg and Adults: I.V.:

Amnionitis, cholangitis, diverticulitis, endometritis, epididymo-orchitis, mastoiditis, orbital cellulitis, peritonitis, pneumonia (aspiration): 3.1 g every 6 hours

Liver abscess, parafascial space infections, septic thrombophlebitis: 3.1 g every 4 hours

***Pseudomonas* infections:** 3.1 g every 4 hours

Urinary tract infections: 3.1 g every 6-8 hours

Dosage Forms

Infusion [premixed, frozen]:

Timentin®: Ticarcillin 3 g and clavulanic acid 0.1 g (100 mL)

Injection, powder for reconstitution:

Timentin®: Ticarcillin 3 g and clavulanic acid 0.1 g (3.1 g, 31 g)

ticarcillin and clavulanic acid *see* ticarcillin and clavulanate potassium *on page 959*

ticarcillin *(Discontinued)*

Ticar® *(Discontinued)*

TICE® BCG [US] *see* BCG vaccine *on page 124*

Ticlid® [Can] *see* ticlopidine *on page 960*

Ticlid® *(Discontinued)* *see* ticlopidine *on page 960*

ticlopidine (tye KLOE pi deen)

Synonyms ticlopidine hydrochloride

U.S./Canadian Brand Names Alti-Ticlopidine [Can]; Apo-Ticlopidine® [Can]; Gen-Ticlopidine [Can]; Novo-Ticlopidine [Can]; Nu-Ticlopidine [Can]; Rhoxal-ticlopidine [Can]; Sandoz-Ticlopidine [Can]; Ticlid® [Can]

Therapeutic Category Antiplatelet Agent

Use Platelet aggregation inhibitor that reduces the risk of thrombotic stroke in patients who have had a stroke or stroke precursors. **Note:** Due to its association with life-threatening hematologic disorders, ticlopidine should be reserved for patients who are intolerant to aspirin, or who have failed aspirin therapy. Adjunctive therapy (with aspirin) following successful coronary stent implantation to reduce the incidence of subacute stent thrombosis.

Usual Dosage Oral: Adults:

Stroke prevention: 250 mg twice daily

Coronary artery stenting (initiate after successful implantation): 250 mg twice daily (in combination with antiplatelet doses of aspirin) for up to 30 days

Dosage Forms

Tablet: 250 mg

ticlopidine hydrochloride *see* ticlopidine *on page 960*

Ticon® *(Discontinued)* *see* trimethobenzamide *on page 987*

TIG *see* tetanus immune globulin (human) *on page 948*

Tigan® [US/Can] *see* trimethobenzamide *on page 987*

tigecycline (tye ge SYE kleen)

Synonyms GAR-936

U.S./Canadian Brand Names Tygacil® [US]

Therapeutic Category Antibiotic, Glycylcycline

Use Treatment of complicated skin and skin structure infections caused by susceptible organisms, including methicillin-resistant *Staphylococcus aureus* and vancomycin-sensitive *Enterococcus faecalis*; complicated intraabdominal infections; community-acquired pneumonia

Usual Dosage I.V.: Adults: **Note:** Duration of therapy dependant on severity/site of infection and clinical status and response to therapy.

Community-acquired pneumonia: Initial: 100 mg as a single dose; Maintenance dose: 50 mg every 12 hours for 7-14 days

Complicated intraabdominal infections: Initial: 100 mg as a single dose; Maintenance dose: 50 mg every 12 hours for 5-14 days

Complicated skin/skin structure infections: Initial: 100 mg as a single dose; Maintenance dose: 50 mg every 12 hours for 5-14 days

Dosage Forms

Injection, powder for reconstitution:

Tygacil®: 50 mg

Tikosyn® [US/Can] *see* dofetilide *on page 328*

Tilade® [US/Can] *see* nedocromil (inhalation) *on page 685*

Tilia™ Fe [US] *see* ethinyl estradiol and norethindrone *on page 390*

tiludronate (tye LOO droe nate)

Synonyms tiludronate disodium

U.S./Canadian Brand Names Skelid® [US]

Therapeutic Category Bisphosphonate Derivative

Use Treatment of Paget disease of the bone (osteitis deformans) in patients who have a level of serum alkaline phosphatase (SAP) at least twice the upper limit of normal, or who are symptomatic, or who are at risk for future complications of their disease

Usual Dosage Oral: Adults: 400 mg (2 tablets of tiludronic acid) daily for a period of 3 months; allow an interval of 3 months to assess response

Dosage Forms

Tablet:

Skelid®: 200 mg

tiludronate disodium *see* tiludronate *on page 961*

Tim-AK [Can] *see* timolol *on page 961*

Time-C [US-OTC] *see* ascorbic acid *on page 100*

Time-C-Bio [US-OTC] *see* ascorbic acid *on page 100*

Timecelles® ***(Discontinued)*** *see* ascorbic acid *on page 100*

Timentin® [US/Can] *see* ticarcillin and clavulanate potassium *on page 959*

timolol (TIM oh lol)

Sound-Alike/Look-Alike Issues

timolol may be confused with atenolol, Tylenol®

Timoptic® may be confused with Betoptic® S, Talacen®, Viroptic®

Synonyms timolol hemihydrate; timolol maleate

U.S./Canadian Brand Names Alti-Timolol [Can]; Apo-Timol® [Can]; Apo-Timop® [Can]; Betimol® [US]; Gen-Timolol [Can]; Istalol® [US]; Nu-Timolol [Can]; Phoxal-timolol [Can]; PMS-Timolol [Can]; Sandoz-Timolol [Can]; Tim-AK [Can]; Timolol GFS [US]; Timoptic-XE® [US/Can]; Timoptic® in OcuDose® [US]; Timoptic® [US/Can]

Therapeutic Category Beta-Adrenergic Blocker

Use

Ophthalmic: Treatment of elevated intraocular pressure such as glaucoma or ocular hypertension

Oral: Treatment of hypertension and angina; to reduce mortality following myocardial infarction; prophylaxis of migraine

Usual Dosage

Ophthalmic:

Children and Adults:

Solution: Initial: Instill 1 drop (0.25% solution) into affected eye(s) twice daily; increase to 0.5% solution if response not adequate; decrease to 1 drop/day if controlled; do not exceed 1 drop twice daily of 0.5% solution

Gel-forming solution (Timolol GFS, Timoptic-XE®): Instill 1 drop (either 0.25% or 0.5% solution) once daily

Adults: Solution (Istalol®): Instill 1 drop (0.5% solution) once daily in the morning

Oral: Adults:

Hypertension: Initial: 10 mg twice daily, increase gradually every 7 days, usual dosage: 20-40 mg/day in 2 divided doses; maximum: 60 mg/day

Prevention of myocardial infarction: 10 mg twice daily initiated within 1-4 weeks after infarction

Migraine headache: Initial: 10 mg twice daily, increase to maximum of 30 mg/day

Dosage Forms

Gel-forming solution, ophthalmic: 0.25% (5 mL); 0.5% (2.5 mL, 5 mL)

Timolol GFS: 0.25% (2.5 mL, 5 mL); 0.5% (2.5 mL, 5 mL)

Timoptic-XE®: 0.25% (5 mL); 0.5% (5 mL)

Solution, ophthalmic: 0.25% (5 mL, 10 mL, 15 mL); 0.5% (5 mL, 10 mL, 15 mL)
Betimol®: 0.25% (5 mL); 0.5% (5 mL, 10 mL, 15 mL)
Istalol®: 0.5% (10 mL)
Timoptic®: 0.25% (5 mL); 0.5% (5 mL, 10 mL)
Solution, ophthalmic [preservative free]: 0.25% (0.2 mL); 0.5% (0.2 mL)
Timoptic® in OcuDose®: 0.25% (0.2 mL); 0.5% (0.2 mL)
Tablet: 5 mg, 10 mg, 20 mg

timolol and brimonidine *see* brimonidine and timolol *on page 147*
timolol and dorzolamide *see* dorzolamide and timolol *on page 332*
Timolol GFS [US] *see* timolol *on page 961*
timolol hemihydrate *see* timolol *on page 961*
timolol maleate *see* timolol *on page 961*
timolol maleate and travoprost *see* travoprost and timolol *(Canada only) on page 979*
Timoptic® [US/Can] *see* timolol *on page 961*
Timoptic® in OcuDose® [US] *see* timolol *on page 961*
Timoptic-XE® [US/Can] *see* timolol *on page 961*
Tinactin® Antifungal [US-OTC] *see* tolnaftate *on page 968*
Tinactin® Antifungal Deodorant [US-OTC] *see* tolnaftate *on page 968*
Tinactin® Antifungal Jock Itch [US-OTC] *see* tolnaftate *on page 968*
Tinaderm [US-OTC] *see* tolnaftate *on page 968*
Tinamed® Corn and Callus Remover [US-OTC] *see* salicylic acid *on page 884*
Tinamed® Wart Remover [US-OTC] *see* salicylic acid *on page 884*
TinBen® *(Discontinued)* *see* benzoin *on page 132*
Tindamax® [US] *see* tinidazole *on page 962*
Ting® Cream [US-OTC] *see* tolnaftate *on page 968*
Ting® Spray Liquid [US-OTC] *see* tolnaftate *on page 968*

tinidazole (tye NI da zole)

U.S./Canadian Brand Names Tindamax® [US]

Therapeutic Category Amebicide; Antibiotic, Miscellaneous; Antiprotozoal, Nitroimidazole

Use Treatment of trichomoniasis caused by *T. vaginalis*; treatment of giardiasis caused by *G. duodenalis* (*G. lamblia*); treatment of intestinal amebiasis and amebic liver abscess caused by *E. histolytica*; treatment of bacterial vaginosis caused by *Bacteroides* spp, *Gardnerella vaginalis*, and *Prevotella* spp in nonpregnant females

Usual Dosage Oral:
Children >3 years:
Amebiasis, intestinal: 50 mg/kg/day for 3 days (maximum dose: 2 g/day)
Amebiasis, liver abscess: 50 mg/kg/day for 3-5 days (maximum dose: 2 g/day)
Giardiasis: 50 mg/kg as a single dose (maximum dose: 2 g)
Adults:
Amebiasis, intestinal: 2 g/day for 3 days
Amebiasis, liver abscess: 2 g/day for 3-5 days
Bacterial vaginosis: 2 g/day for 2 days or 1 g/day for 5 days
Giardiasis: 2 g as a single dose
Trichomoniasis: 2 g as a single dose; sexual partners should be treated at the same time

Dosage Forms
Tablet [scored]:
Tindamax®: 250 mg, 500 mg

Tinver® *(Discontinued)* *see* sodium thiosulfate *on page 915*

tinzaparin (tin ZA pa rin)

Synonyms tinzaparin sodium

U.S./Canadian Brand Names Innohep® [US/Can]

Therapeutic Category Anticoagulant (Other)

Use Treatment of acute symptomatic deep vein thrombosis, with or without pulmonary embolism, in conjunction with warfarin sodium

Usual Dosage SubQ: Adults: DVT with or without pulmonary embolism (PE): 175 anti-Xa int. units/kg of body weight once daily. The 2008 *Chest* guidelines recommend starting warfarin on the first treatment day and continuing tinzaparin until INR is between 2 and 3 (usually 5-7 days). Administer tinzaparin for at least 5 days and until INR ≥2 for at least 24 hours.

Note: To calculate the volume of solution to administer per dose: Volume to be administered (mL) = patient weight (kg) x 0.00875 mL/kg (may be rounded off to the nearest 0.05 mL)

Dosage Forms

Injection, solution:,

Innohep®: 20,000 anti-Xa int. units/mL (2 mL)

tinzaparin sodium *see* tinzaparin *on page 962*

tioconazole (tye oh KONE a zole)

Sound-Alike/Look-Alike Issues

tioconazole may be confused with terconazole

U.S./Canadian Brand Names 1-Day™ [US-OTC]; Vagistat®-1 [US-OTC]

Therapeutic Category Antifungal Agent

Use Local treatment of vulvovaginal candidiasis

Usual Dosage Adults: Vaginal: Insert 1 applicatorful in vagina, just prior to bedtime, as a single dose

Dosage Forms

Ointment, vaginal:

1-Day™ [OTC], Vagistat®-1 [OTC]: 6.5% (4.6 g)

tioguanine *see* thioguanine *on page 955*

tiopronin (tye oh PROE nin)

U.S./Canadian Brand Names Thiola® [US/Can]

Therapeutic Category Urinary Tract Product

Use Prevention of kidney stone (cystine) formation in patients with severe homozygous cystinuric who have urinary cystine >500 mg/day who are resistant to treatment with high fluid intake, alkali, and diet modification, or who have had adverse reactions to penicillamine

Usual Dosage Adults: Initial dose is 800 mg/day, average dose is 1000 mg/day

Dosage Forms

Tablet:

Thiola®: 100 mg

tiotixene *see* thiothixene *on page 956*

tiotropium (ty oh TRO pee um)

Sound-Alike/Look-Alike Issues

tiotropium may be confused with ipratropium

Spiriva® may be confused with Inspra™, Serevent®

Synonyms tiotropium bromide monohydrate

U.S./Canadian Brand Names Spiriva® HandiHaler® [US]; Spiriva® [Can]

Therapeutic Category Anticholinergic Agent

Use Maintenance treatment of bronchospasm associated with COPD (including bronchitis and emphysema)

Usual Dosage Oral inhalation: Adults: Contents of 1 capsule (18 mcg) inhaled once daily using HandiHaler® device

Dosage Forms

Powder for oral inhalation [capsule]:

Spiriva® HandiHaler®: 18 mcg/capsule (5s, 30s, 90s)

tiotropium bromide monohydrate *see* tiotropium *on page 963*

tipranavir (tip RA na veer)

Synonyms PNU-140690E; TPV

U.S./Canadian Brand Names Aptivus® [US/Can]

Therapeutic Category Antiretroviral Agent, Protease Inhibitor

Use Treatment of HIV-1 infections in combination with ritonavir and other antiretroviral agents; limited to highly treatment-experienced or multiprotease inhibitor-resistant patients.

Usual Dosage Oral:

Children ≥2 years: 14 mg/kg or 375 mg/m^2 (maximum: 500 mg/dose) twice daily. **Note:** Coadministration with ritonavir (6 mg/kg or 150 mg/m^2 [maximum 200 mg/dose] twice daily) is required.

If intolerance or toxicity develops and virus is not resistant to multiple protease inhibitors: May decrease dose to 12 mg/kg or 290 mg/m^2 twice daily. **Note:** Coadministration with ritonavir (5 mg/kg or 115 mg/m^2 twice daily) is required.

Adults: 500 mg twice daily with a high-fat meal. **Note:** Coadministration with ritonavir (200 mg twice daily) is required.

Dosage Forms

Capsule, soft gelatin:

Aptivus®: 250 mg

Solution:

Aptivus®: 100 mg/mL (95 mL)

TipTapToe *(Discontinued)* *see* tolnaftate *on page 968*

tirofiban (tye roe FYE ban)

Sound-Alike/Look-Alike Issues

Aggrastat® may be confused with Aggrenox®, argatroban

Synonyms MK383; tirofiban hydrochloride

U.S./Canadian Brand Names Aggrastat® [US/Can]

Therapeutic Category Antiplatelet Agent

Use In combination with heparin, is indicated for the treatment of acute coronary syndrome, including patients who are to be managed medically and those undergoing PTCA or atherectomy. In this setting, it has been shown to decrease the rate of a combined endpoint of death, new myocardial infarction or refractory ischemia/repeat cardiac procedure.

Usual Dosage I.V.: Adults: Initial rate of 0.4 mcg/kg/minute for 30 minutes and then continued at 0.1 mcg/kg/minute; dosing should be continued through angiography and for 12-24 hours after angioplasty or atherectomy.

Dosage Forms

Infusion [premixed in sodium chloride]:

Aggrastat®: 50 mcg/mL (100 mL, 250 mL)

tirofiban hydrochloride *see* tirofiban *on page 964*
Tisseel® VH [Can] *see* fibrin sealant kit *on page 417*
Tisseel® VH S/D [US] *see* fibrin sealant kit *on page 417*
Titralac™ [US-OTC] *see* calcium carbonate *on page 170*
Titralac® Plus [US-OTC] *see* calcium carbonate and simethicone *on page 171*
Ti-U-Lac® H [Can] *see* urea and hydrocortisone *on page 999*

tizanidine (tye ZAN i deen)

Sound-Alike/Look-Alike Issues

tiZANidine may be confused with tiaGABine

Tall-Man ti**ZAN**idine

U.S./Canadian Brand Names Apo-Tizanidine® [Can]; Gen-Tizanidine [Can]; Zanaflex Capsules™ [US]; Zanaflex® [US/Can]

Therapeutic Category Alpha$_2$-Adrenergic Agonist Agent

Use Skeletal muscle relaxant used for treatment of muscle spasticity

Usual Dosage Adults: 2-4 mg 3 times/day

Usual initial dose: 4 mg, may increase by 2-4 mg as needed for satisfactory reduction of muscle tone every 6-8 hours to a maximum of 3 doses in any 24-hour period

Maximum: 36 mg/day

Dosage Forms

Capsule:

Zanaflex Capsules™: 2 mg, 4 mg, 6 mg

Tablet: 2 mg, 4 mg

Zanaflex®: 4 mg [scored]

TMC-114 *see* darunavir *on page* *277*

TMC125 *see* etravirine *on page* *399*

TMP *see* trimethoprim *on page* *988*

TMP-SMZ *see* sulfamethoxazole and trimethoprim *on page* *929*

TMX-67 *see* febuxostat *on page* *407*

TMZ *see* temozolomide *on page* *942*

T.N. Dickinson's® Hazelets [US-OTC] *see* witch hazel *on page* *1023*

TNKase® [US/Can] *see* tenecteplase *on page* *943*

TOBI® [US/Can] *see* tobramycin *on page* *965*

TobraDex® [US/Can] *see* tobramycin and dexamethasone *on page* *966*

tobramycin (toe bra MYE sin)

Sound-Alike/Look-Alike Issues

tobramycin may be confused with Trobicin®, vancomycin

AKTob® may be confused with AK-Trol®

Nebcin® may be confused with Inapsine®, Naprosyn®, Nubain®

Tobrex® may be confused with TobraDex®

Synonyms tobramycin sulfate

U.S./Canadian Brand Names AKTob® [US]; PMS-Tobramycin [Can]; Sandoz-Tobramycin [Can]; TOBI® [US/Can]; Tobramycin Injection, USP [Can]; Tobrex® [US/Can]

Therapeutic Category Aminoglycoside (Antibiotic); Antibiotic, Ophthalmic

Use Treatment of documented or suspected infections caused by susceptible gram-negative bacilli including *Pseudomonas aeruginosa*; topically used to treat superficial ophthalmic infections caused by susceptible bacteria. Tobramycin solution for inhalation is indicated for the management of cystic fibrosis patients (>6 years of age) with *Pseudomonas aeruginosa*.

Usual Dosage Note: Dosage individualization is **critical** because of the low therapeutic index.

Use of ideal body weight (IBW) for determining the mg/kg/dose appears to be more accurate than dosing on the basis of total body weight (TBW). In morbid obesity, dosage requirement may best be estimated using a dosing weight of IBW + 0.4 (TBW - IBW).

Initial and periodic plasma drug levels (eg, peak-and-trough with conventional dosing) should be determined, particularly in critically-ill patients with serious infections or in disease states known to significantly alter aminoglycoside pharmacokinetics (eg, cystic fibrosis, burns, or major surgery).

Usual dosage range:

Infants and Children <5 years: I.M., I.V.: 2.5 mg/kg/dose every 8 hours

Children ≥5 years: I.M., I.V.: 2-2.5 mg/kg/dose every 8 hours

Note: Higher individual doses and/or more frequent intervals (eg, every 6 hours) may be required in selected clinical situations (cystic fibrosis) or serum levels document the need.

Children and Adults:

Inhalation: TOBI®: Children ≥6 years and Adults: 300 mg every 12 hours (do not administer doses <6 hours apart); administer in repeated cycles of 28 days on drug followed by 28 days off drug.

Intrathecal: 4-8 mg/day

Ophthalmic: Children ≥2 months and Adults:

Ointment: Instill 1/2" (1.25 cm) 2-3 times/day every 3-4 hours

Solution: Instill 1-2 drops every 2-4 hours, up to 2 drops every hour for severe infections

Topical: Apply 3-4 times/day to affected area

Adults: I.M., I.V.:

Conventional: 1-2.5 mg/kg/dose every 8-12 hours; to ensure adequate peak concentrations early in therapy, higher initial dosage may be considered in selected patients when extracellular water is increased (edema, septic shock, postsurgical, and/or trauma)

Once-daily: 4-7 mg/kg/dose once daily; some clinicians recommend this approach for all patients with normal renal function; this dose is at least as efficacious with similar, if not less, toxicity than conventional dosing.

Indication-specific dosing:

Neonates:

Meningitis: I.M., I.V.:

0-7 days: <2000 g: 2.5 mg/kg every 18-24 hours; >2000 g: 2.5 mg/kg every 12 hours

8-28 days: <2000 g: 2.5 mg/kg every 8-12 hours; >2000 g: 2.5 mg/kg every 8 hours

Children:

Cystic fibrosis:

I.M., I.V.: 2.5-3.3 mg/kg every 6-8 hours; **Note:** Some patients may require larger or more frequent doses if serum levels document the need (eg, cystic fibrosis or febrile granulocytopenic patients).

Inhalation: See adult dosing.

Adults:

I.M., I.V.:

Brucellosis: 240 mg (I.M.) daily or 5 mg/kg (I.V.) daily for 7 days; either regimen recommended in combination with doxycycline

Cholangitis: 4-6 mg/kg once daily with ampicillin

Diverticulitis, complicated: 1.5-2 mg/kg every 8 hours (with ampicillin and metronidazole)

Infective endocarditis or synergy (for gram-positive infections): I.M., I.V.: 1 mg/kg every 8 hours (with ampicillin)

Meningitis *(Enterococcus or Pseudomonas aeruginosa)*: I.V.: Loading dose: 2 mg/kg, then 1.7 mg/kg/dose every 8 hours (administered with another bacteriocidal drug)

Pelvic inflammatory disease: Loading dose: 2 mg/kg, then 1.5 mg/kg every 8 hours **or** 4.5 mg/kg once daily

Plague *(Yersinia pestis)*: Treatment: 5 mg/kg/day, followed by postexposure prophylaxis with doxycycline

Pneumonia, hospital- or ventilator-associated: 7 mg/kg/day (with antipseudomonal beta-lactam or carbapenem)

Prophylaxis against endocarditis (dental, oral, upper respiratory procedures, GI/GU procedures): 1.5 mg/kg with ampicillin (50 mg/kg) 30 minutes prior to procedure. **Note:** AHA guidelines now recommend prophylaxis only in patients undergoing invasive procedures and in whom underlying cardiac conditions may predispose to a higher risk of adverse outcomes should infection occur. As of April 2007, routine prophylaxis no longer recommended by the AHA.

Tularemia: 5 mg/kg/day divided every 8 hours for 1-2 weeks

Urinary tract infection: 1.5 mg/kg/dose every 8 hours

Inhalation: **Cystic fibrosis:** TOBI®: 300 mg every 12 hours (do not administer doses <6 hours apart); administer in repeated cycles of 28 days on drug followed by 28 days off drug.

Dosage Forms

Infusion [premixed in NS]: 60 mg (50 mL); 80 mg (100 mL)

Injection, powder for reconstitution: 1.2 g

Injection, solution: 10 mg/mL (2 mL, 8 mL); 40 mg/mL (2 mL, 30 mL, 50 mL)

Ointment, ophthalmic:

Tobrex®: 0.3% (3.5 g)

Solution for nebulization [preservative free]:

TOBI®: 60 mg/mL (5 mL)

Solution, ophthalmic: 0.3% (5 mL)

AKTob®, Tobrex®: 0.3% (5 mL)

tobramycin and dexamethasone (toe bra MYE sin & deks a METH a sone)

Sound-Alike/Look-Alike Issues

TobraDex® may be confused with Tobrex®

Synonyms dexamethasone and tobramycin

U.S./Canadian Brand Names TobraDex® [US/Can]

Therapeutic Category Antibiotic/Corticosteroid, Ophthalmic

Use Treatment of external ocular infection caused by susceptible gram-negative bacteria and steroid responsive inflammatory conditions of the palpebral and bulbar conjunctiva, lid, cornea, and anterior segment of the globe

Usual Dosage Ophthalmic: Children and Adults: Instill 1-2 drops of solution every 4 hours; apply ointment 2-3 times/day; for severe infections apply ointment every 3-4 hours, or solution 2 drops every 30-60 minutes initially, then reduce to less frequent intervals

Dosage Forms

Ointment, ophthalmic:

TobraDex®: Tobramycin 0.3% and dexamethasone 0.1% (3.5 g)

Suspension, ophthalmic: Tobramycin 0.3% and dexamethasone 0.1% (2.5 mL, 5 mL, 10 mL)

TobraDex®: Tobramycin 0.3% and dexamethasone 0.1% (2.5 mL, 5 mL, 10 mL)

tobramycin and loteprednol etabonate *see* loteprednol and tobramycin *on page* 602

Tobramycin Injection, USP [Can] *see* tobramycin *on page* 965

tobramycin sulfate *see* tobramycin *on page 965*
Tobrex® [US/Can] *see* tobramycin *on page 965*
tocophersolan ***(Discontinued)***
Today® [US-OTC] *see* nonoxynol 9 *on page 703*
Tofranil® [US/Can] *see* imipramine *on page 521*
Tofranil-PM® [US] *see* imipramine *on page 521*

tolazamide (tole AZ a mide)

Sound-Alike/Look-Alike Issues
TOLAZamide may be confused with tolazoline, TOLBUTamide
Tolinase® may be confused with Orinase®

Tall-Man **TOLAZ**amide

U.S./Canadian Brand Names Tolinase® [Can]

Therapeutic Category Antidiabetic Agent, Oral

Use Adjunct to diet for the management of mild to moderately severe, stable, type 2 diabetes mellitus (noninsulin-dependent, NIDDM)

Usual Dosage Oral: Adults: Doses >500 mg/day should be given in 2 divided doses:
Initial: 100-250 mg/day with breakfast or the first main meal of the day
Fasting blood sugar <200 mg/dL: 100 mg/day
Fasting blood sugar >200 mg/dL: 250 mg/day
Patient is malnourished, underweight, elderly, or not eating properly: 100 mg/day
Adjust dose in increments of 100-250 mg/day at weekly intervals to response; maximum daily dose: 1 g (doses >1 g/day are not likely to improve control)

Conversion from insulin to tolazamide
<20 units day = 100 mg/day
21-<40 units/day = 250 mg/day
≥40 units/day = 250 mg/day and 50% of insulin dose

Dosage Forms
Tablet: 250 mg, 500 mg

tolazoline ***(Discontinued)***

tolbutamide (tole BYOO ta mide)

Sound-Alike/Look-Alike Issues
TOLBUTamide may be confused with terbutaline, TOLAZamide
Orinase® may be confused with Orabase®, Ornex®, Tolinase®

Synonyms tolbutamide sodium

Tall-Man **TOLBUT**amide

U.S./Canadian Brand Names Apo-Tolbutamide® [Can]

Therapeutic Category Antidiabetic Agent, Oral

Use Adjunct to diet for the management of type 2 diabetes mellitus (noninsulin-dependent, NIDDM)

Usual Dosage Note: Divided doses may improve gastrointestinal tolerance. Oral: Adults: Initial: 1-2 g/day as a single dose in the morning or in divided doses throughout the day. Maintenance dose: 0.25-3 g/day; however, a maintenance dose >2 g/day is seldom required.

Dosage Forms
Tablet: 500 mg

tolbutamide sodium *see* tolbutamide *on page 967*

tolcapone (TOLE ka pone)

U.S./Canadian Brand Names Tasmar® [US]

Therapeutic Category Anti-Parkinson Agent

Use Adjunct to levodopa and carbidopa for the treatment of signs and symptoms of idiopathic Parkinson disease in patients with motor fluctuations not responsive to other therapies

Usual Dosage Note: If clinical improvement is not observed after 3 weeks of therapy (regardless of dose), tolcapone treatment should be discontinued.

Oral: Adults: Initial: 100 mg 3 times/day; may increase as tolerated to 200 mg 3 times/day. **Note:** Levodopa dose may need to be decreased upon initiation of tolcapone (average reduction in clinical trials was 30%). As many as 70% of patients receiving levodopa doses >600 mg daily required levodopa dosage reduction in clinical trials. Patients with moderate-to-severe dyskinesia prior to initiation are also more likely to require dosage reduction.

Dosage Forms

Tablet:

Tasmar®: 100 mg, 200 mg

Tolectin® DS *(Discontinued)* *see* tolmetin *on page 968*

Tolinase® [Can] *see* tolazamide *on page 967*

Tolinase® *(Discontinued)* *see* tolazamide *on page 967*

tolmetin (TOLE met in)

Synonyms tolmetin sodium

Therapeutic Category Analgesic, Nonnarcotic; Nonsteroidal Antiinflammatory Drug (NSAID)

Use Treatment of rheumatoid arthritis and osteoarthritis, juvenile rheumatoid arthritis

Usual Dosage Oral:

Children ≥2 years: JRA: Initial: 20 mg/kg/day in 3-4 divided doses, then 15-30 mg/kg/day in 3-4 divided doses (maximum dose: 30 mg/kg/day)

Adults: RA, osteoarthritis: 400 mg 3 times/day; usual dose: 600 mg to 1.8 g/day; maximum: 1.8 g/day

Dosage Forms

Capsule: 400 mg

Tablet: 200 mg, 600 mg

tolmetin sodium *see* tolmetin *on page 968*

tolnaftate (tole NAF tate)

Sound-Alike/Look-Alike Issues

tolnaftate may be confused with Tornalate®

Tinactin® may be confused with Talacen®

U.S./Canadian Brand Names Blis-To-Sol® [US-OTC]; FungiGuard [US-OTC]; Mycocide® NS [US-OTC]; Pitrex [Can]; Podactin Powder [US-OTC]; Tinactin® Antifungal Deodorant [US-OTC]; Tinactin® Antifungal Jock Itch [US-OTC]; Tinactin® Antifungal [US-OTC]; Tinaderm [US-OTC]; Ting® Cream [US-OTC]; Ting® Spray Liquid [US-OTC]

Therapeutic Category Antifungal Agent

Use Treatment of tinea pedis, tinea cruris, tinea corporis

Usual Dosage Topical: Children ≥2 years and Adults: Wash and dry affected area; spray aerosol or apply 1-3 drops of solution or a small amount of cream, or powder and rub into the affected areas 2 times/day

Note: May use for up to 4 weeks for tinea pedis or tinea corporis, and up to 2 weeks for tinea cruris

Dosage Forms

Aerosol, topical [spray]:

Tinactin® Antifungal [OTC]: 1% (150 g)

Ting® [OTC]: 1% (128 g)

Aerosol, topical [powder, spray]:

Tinactin® Antifungal Deodorant [OTC], Tinactin® Antifungal [OTC], Tinactin® Antifungal Jock Itch [OTC]: 1% (133 g)

Cream, topical: 1% (15 g, 30 g)

FungiGuard [OTC], Tinactin® Antifungal Jock Itch [OTC], Ting® [OTC]: 1% (15 g)

Tinactin® Antifungal [OTC]: 1% (15 g, 30 g)

Liquid, topical:

Blis-To-Sol® [OTC]: 1% (30 mL, 55 mL)

FungiGuard [OTC]: 1% (30 mL)

Liquid, topical [spray]:

Tinactin® Antifungal [OTC]: 1% (59 mL)

Powder, topical: 1% (45 g)

Podactin [OTC]: 1% (45 g)

Tinactin® Antifungal [OTC]: 1% (108 g)

Solution, topical: 1% (10 mL)

Mycocide® NS [OTC]: 1% (30 mL)

Tinaderm [OTC]: 1% (10 mL)

tolterodine (tole TER oh deen)

Sound-Alike/Look-Alike Issues

tolterodine may be confused with fesoterodine
Detrol® may be confused with Ditropan®

Synonyms tolterodine tartrate

U.S./Canadian Brand Names Detrol® LA [US/Can]; Detrol® [US/Can]; Unidet® [Can]

Therapeutic Category Anticholinergic Agent

Use Treatment of patients with an overactive bladder with symptoms of urinary frequency, urgency, or urge incontinence

Usual Dosage Oral: Adults: Treatment of overactive bladder:

Immediate release tablet: 2 mg twice daily; the dose may be lowered to 1 mg twice daily based on individual response and tolerability

Extended release capsule: 4 mg once a day; dose may be lowered to 2 mg daily based on individual response and tolerability

Dosage Forms

Capsule, extended release:

Detrol® LA: 2 mg, 4 mg

Tablet:

Detrol®: 1 mg, 2 mg

tolterodine tartrate *see* tolterodine *on page* *969*

tolvaptan (tol VAP tan)

Synonyms OPC-41061

U.S./Canadian Brand Names Samsca™ [US]

Therapeutic Category Vasopressin Antagonist

Use Treatment of clinically significant hypervolemic or euvolemic hyponatremia (associated with heart failure, cirrhosis or SIADH) with either a serum sodium <125 mEq/L or less marked hyponatremia that is symptomatic and resistant to fluid restriction

Usual Dosage Oral: Adults: Hyponatremia: Initial: 15 mg once daily; after at least 24 hours, may increase to 30 mg once daily to a maximum of 60 mg once daily titrating at 24-hour intervals to desired serum sodium concentration

Dosage Forms

Tablet, oral:

Samsca™: 15 mg, 30 mg

Tomocat® [US] *see* barium *on page* *122*

Tomocat® 1000 [US] *see* barium *on page* *122*

tomoxetine *see* atomoxetine *on page* *108*

Tomudex® [Can] *see* raltitrexed *(Canada only) on page* *849*

Tomycine® ***(Discontinued)*** *see* tobramycin *on page* *965*

Tonocard® ***(Discontinued)***

Tonojug [US] *see* barium *on page* *122*

Tonopaque [US] *see* barium *on page* *122*

Topactin [Can] *see* fluocinonide *on page* *429*

Topamax® [US/Can] *see* topiramate *on page* *969*

Topamax® 200 mg Tablet ***(Discontinued)*** *see* topiramate *on page* *969*

Topicaine® [US-OTC] *see* lidocaine *on page* *584*

Topicort® [US/Can] *see* desoximetasone *on page* *287*

Topicort®-LP [US] *see* desoximetasone *on page* *287*

Topicycline® Topical ***(Discontinued)*** *see* tetracycline *on page* *950*

Topilene® [Can] *see* betamethasone (topical) *on page* *138*

topiramate (toe PYRE a mate)

Sound-Alike/Look-Alike Issues

Topamax® may be confused with Sporanox®, Tegretol®, Tegretol®-XR, Toprol-XL®

U.S./Canadian Brand Names Apo-Topiramate® [Can]; CO Topiramate [Can]; Dom-Topiramate [Can]; Mint-Topiramate [Can]; Mylan-Topiramate [Can]; Novo-Topiramate [Can]; PHL-Topiramate [Can]; PMS-Topiramate [Can]; PRO-Topiramate [Can]; ratio-Topiramate [Can]; Sandoz-Topiramate [Can]; Topamax® [US/Can]; ZYM-Topiramate [Can]

Therapeutic Category Anticonvulsant

Use Monotherapy or adjunctive therapy for partial onset seizures and primary generalized tonic-clonic seizures; adjunctive treatment of seizures associated with Lennox-Gastaut syndrome; prophylaxis of migraine headache

Usual Dosage Oral: **Note:** Do not abruptly discontinue therapy; taper dosage gradually to prevent rebound effects. (In clinical trials, adult doses were withdrawn by decreasing in weekly intervals of 50-100 mg/day gradually over 2-8 weeks for seizure treatment, and by decreasing in weekly intervals by 25-50 mg/day for migraine prophylaxis.)

Epilepsy, monotherapy: Children ≥10 years and Adults: Partial onset seizure and primary generalized tonic-clonic seizure: Initial: 25 mg twice daily; may increase weekly by 50 mg/day up to 100 mg twice daily (week 4 dose); thereafter, may further increase weekly by 100 mg/day up to the recommended maximum of 200 mg twice daily.

Epilepsy, adjunctive therapy:

Children 2-16 years:

Partial onset seizure or seizure associated with Lennox-Gastaut syndrome: Initial dose titration should begin at 25 mg (or less, based on a range of 1-3 mg/kg/day) nightly for the first week; dosage may be increased in increments of 1-3 mg/kg/day (administered in 2 divided doses) at 1- or 2-week intervals to a total daily dose of 5-9 mg/kg/day

Primary generalized tonic-clonic seizure: Use initial dose listed above, but use slower initial titration rate; titrate to recommended maintenance dose by the end of 8 weeks

Adolescents ≥17 years and Adults:

Partial onset seizures: Initial: 25-50 mg/day (given in 2 divided doses) for 1 week; increase at weekly intervals by 25-50 mg/day until response; usual maintenance dose: 100-200 mg twice daily. Doses >1600 mg/day have not been studied.

Primary generalized tonic-clonic seizures: Use initial dose as listed above for partial onset seizures, but use slower initial titration rate; titrate upwards to recommended dose by the end of 8 weeks; usual maintenance dose: 200 mg twice daily. Doses >1600 mg/day have not been studied.

Adults: Migraine prophylaxis: Initial: 25 mg/day (in the evening), titrated at weekly intervals in 25 mg increments, up to the recommended total daily dose of 100 mg/day given in 2 divided doses

Dosage Forms

Capsule, sprinkle: 15 mg, 25 mg

Topamax®: 15 mg, 25 mg

Tablet: 25 mg, 50 mg, 100 mg, 200 mg

Topamax®: 25 mg, 50 mg, 100 mg, 200 mg

Topisone® [Can] *see* betamethasone (topical) *on page 138*

Toposar™ [US] *see* etoposide *on page 398*

topotecan (toe poe TEE kan)

Sound-Alike/Look-Alike Issues

Hycamtin® may be confused with Hycomine®, Mycamine®

Synonyms hycamptamine; NSC-609699; SKF 104864; SKF 104864-A; topotecan hydrochloride

U.S./Canadian Brand Names Hycamtin® [US/Can]

Therapeutic Category Antineoplastic Agent

Use Treatment of ovarian cancer and small cell lung cancer; cervical cancer (in combination with cisplatin)

Usual Dosage Adults (refer to individual protocols): **Note:** Baseline neutrophil count should be >1500/mm^3; retreatment neutrophil count should be >1000/mm^3; baseline and retreatment platelet count should be >100,000/mm^3; (also, for oral topotecan, retreatment hemoglobin should be ≥9 g/dL):

Small cell lung cancer:

IVPB: 1.5 mg/m^2/day for 5 days; repeated every 21 days

Oral: 2.3 mg/m^2/day for 5 days; repeated every 21 days (round dose to the nearest 0.25 mg); if patient vomits after dose is administered, do not give a replacement dose.

Metastatic ovarian cancer: IVPB: 1.5 mg/m^2/day for 5 days; repeated every 21 days

Cervical cancer: IVPB: 0.75 mg/m^2/day for 3 days (followed by cisplatin 50 mg/m^2 on day 1 only, [with hydration]); repeated every 21 days

Dosage Forms
Capsule:
Hycamtin®: 0.25 mg, 1 mg
Injection, powder for reconstitution:
Hycamtin®: 4 mg

topotecan hydrochloride *see* topotecan *on page 970*
Toprol-XL® [US/Can] *see* metoprolol *on page 650*
Topsyn® [Can] *see* fluocinonide *on page 429*
Toradol® [Can] *see* ketorolac *on page 558*
Toradol® IM [Can] *see* ketorolac *on page 558*

toremifene (tore EM i feen)

Synonyms FC1157a; toremifene citrate
U.S./Canadian Brand Names Fareston® [US/Can]
Therapeutic Category Antineoplastic Agent
Use Treatment of postmenopausal metastatic breast cancer (estrogen receptor positive or estrogen receptor status unknown)
Usual Dosage Oral: Adults: 60 mg once daily, generally continued until disease progression is observed
Dosage Forms
Tablet:
Fareston®: 60 mg

toremifene citrate *see* toremifene *on page 971*
Torisel [US/Can] *see* temsirolimus *on page 943*

torsemide (TORE se mide)

Sound-Alike/Look-Alike Issues
torsemide may be confused with furosemide
Demadex® may be confused with Denorex®
U.S./Canadian Brand Names Demadex® [US]
Therapeutic Category Diuretic, Loop
Use Management of edema associated with heart failure and hepatic or renal disease; used alone or in combination with antihypertensives in treatment of hypertension; I.V. form is indicated when rapid onset is desired
Usual Dosage Oral, I.V.: Adults:
Chronic renal failure: 20 mg once daily; increase as described above
Heart failure: Initial: 10-20 mg once daily; may increase gradually for chronic treatment by doubling dose until the diuretic response is apparent (for acute treatment, I.V. dose may be repeated every 2 hours with double the dose as needed). **Note:** ACC/AHA 2009 guidelines for heart failure recommend a maximum daily oral dose of 200 mg; maximum single I.V. dose of 100-200 mg
Continuous I.V. infusion: 20 mg I.V. load then 5-20 mg/hour
Hepatic cirrhosis: 5-10 mg once daily with an aldosterone antagonist or a potassium-sparing diuretic; increase as described above
Hypertension: 2.5-5 mg once daily; increase to 10 mg after 4-6 weeks if an adequate hypotensive response is not apparent; if still not effective, an additional antihypertensive agent may be added
Dosage Forms
Injection, solution:
Demadex®: 10 mg/mL
Tablet: 5 mg, 10 mg, 20 mg, 100 mg
Demadex®: 5 mg, 10 mg, 20 mg, 100 mg [scpred]

tositumomab I-131 *see* tositumomab and iodine I 131 tositumomab *on page 971*

tositumomab and iodine I 131 tositumomab

(toe si TYOO mo mab & EYE oh dyne eye one THUR tee one toe si TYOO mo mab)
Synonyms 131 I anti-B1 antibody; 131 I-anti-B1 monoclonal antibody; anti-CD20-murine monoclonal antibody I-131; iodine I 131 tositumomab and tositumomab; tositumomab I-131
U.S./Canadian Brand Names Bexxar® [US]
Therapeutic Category Antineoplastic Agent, Monoclonal Antibody; Radiopharmaceutical

Use Treatment of relapsed or refractory CD20 positive, low-grade, follicular, or transformed non-Hodgkin lymphoma (NHL)

Usual Dosage I.V.: Adults: NHL: Dosing consists of four components administered in 2 steps. Refer to manufacturer's labeling for additional details. Thyroid protective agents (SSKI, Lugol's solution or potassium iodide) should be administered beginning at least 24 hours prior to step 1. Premedicate with acetaminophen 650 mg and diphenhydramine 50 mg orally prior to step 1 and step 2.

Step 1: Dosimetric step (Day 0):

Tositumomab 450 mg in NS 50 mL administered over 60 minutes

Iodine I 131 tositumomab (containing I-131 5 mCi and tositumomab 35 mg) in NS 30 mL administered over 20 minutes

Note: Whole body dosimetry and biodistribution should be determined on Day 0; days 2, 3, or 4; and day 6 or 7 prior to administration of Step 2. If biodistribution is not acceptable, do not administer the therapeutic step. On day 6 or 7, calculate the patient specific activity of iodine I 131 tositumomab to deliver 75 cGy TBD or 65 cGy TBD (in mCi).

Step 2: Therapeutic step (one dose administered 7-14 days after step 1):

Tositumomab 450 mg in NS 50 mL administered over 60 minutes

Iodine I 131 tositumomab:

Platelets ≥150,000/mm^3: Iodine I 131 calculated to deliver 75 cGy total body irradiation and tositumomab 35 mg over 20 minutes

Platelets ≥100,000/mm^3 and <150,000/mm^3: Iodine I 131 calculated to deliver 65 cGy total body irradiation and tositumomab 35 mg over 20 minutes

Dosage Forms

Kit [dosimetric package]:

Bexxar®: Tositumomab 225 mg/16.1 mL [2 vials], tositumomab 35 mg/2.5 mL [1 vial], and iodine I 131 tositumomab 0.1 mg/mL and 0.61mCi/mL (20 mL) [1 vial]

Kit [therapeutic package]:

Bexxar®: Tositumomab 225 mg/16.1 mL [2 vials], tositumomab 35 mg/2.5 mL [1 vial], and iodine I 131 tositumomab 1.1 mg/mL and 5.6 mCi/mL (20 mL) [1 or 2 vials]

Totacillin® ***(Discontinued)*** *see* ampicillin *on page 76*

total parenteral nutrition (TOE tal par EN ter al noo TRISH un)

Synonyms hyperal; hyperalimentation; parenteral nutrition; PN; TPN

Therapeutic Category Caloric Agent; Intravenous Nutritional Therapy

Use Infusion of nutrient solutions into the bloodstream to support nutritional needs during a time when patient is unable to absorb nutrients via the gastrointestinal tract, cannot take adequate nutrition orally or enterally, or have had (or are expected to have) inadequate oral intake for 7-14 days

Usual Dosage PN is a highly-individualized therapy. The following general guidelines may be used in the estimation of needs. Electrolytes, vitamins, and trace minerals should be added to TPN mixtures based on patients individualized needs.

Neonates: I.V.: **Note:** When indicated for premature neonates, start on day 1 of life if possible.

Total calories:

Term: 85-105 kcal/kg/day

Preterm (stable): 90-120 kcal/kg/day

Fluid:

<1.5 kg: 130-150 mL/kg/day

1.5-2 kg: 110-130 mL/kg/day

2-10 kg: 100 mL/kg/day

Carbohydrate (dextrose): 40% to 50% of caloric intake; advance as tolerated

Term: Initial: 6-8 mg/kg/minute; goal: 10-14 mg/kg/minute

Premature: Initial: 6 mg/kg/minute; goal: 10-13 mg/kg/minute

Protein (amino acids):

Term: Initial: 2.5 g/kg/day; goal: 3 g/kg/day

Extremely (<1000 g) and very (<1500 g) low-birth-weight (stable): Initial: 1-1.5 g/kg/day; goal: 3.5-3.85 g/kg/day to promote utero growth rates.

Sepsis, hypoxia: Initial: 1 g/kg/day; goal: 3-3.85 g/kg/day

Fat:

Term: Initial: 0.5-1 g/kg/day (maximum: 3 g/kg/day); administer over 24 hours

Preterm: Initial: 0.25-0.5 g/kg/day (maximum: 3 g/kg/day or 1 g/kg/day if on phototherapy); administer over 24 hours

Note: Monitor triglycerides while receiving intralipids. If triglycerides >200 mg/dL, stop infusion and restart at 0.5-1g/kg/day

Heparin: 1 unit/mL of parenteral nutrition fluids should be added to enhance clearance of lipid emulsions

Children: I.V.: **Note:** Give within 5-7 days if unable to meet needs orally or with enteral nutrition:

Total calories:
- <6 months: 85-105 kcal/kg/day
- 6-12 months: 80-100 kcal/kg/day
- 1-7 years: 75-90 kcal/kg/day
- 7-12 years: 50-75 kcal/kg/day
- 12-18 years: 30-50 kcal/kg/day

Fluid:
- 2-10 kg: 100 mL/kg
- >10-20 kg: 1000 mL for 10 kg plus 50 mL/kg for each kg >10
- >20 kg: 1500 mL for 10 kg plus 20 mL/kg for each kg >20

Carbohydrate (dextrose): 40% to 50% of caloric intake
- <1 year: Initial: 6-8 mg/kg/minute; goal: 10-14 mg/kg/minute
- 1-10 years: Initial: 10% to 12.5%; daily increase: 5% increments (maximum: 15 mg/kg/minute)
- >10 years: Initial: 10% to 15%; daily increase: 5% increments (maximum: 8.5 mg/kg/minute)

Protein (amino acids):
- 1-12 months: Initial: 2-3 g/kg/day; daily increase: 1 g/kg/day (maximum: 3 g/kg/day)
- 1-10 years: Initial: 1-2 g/kg/day; daily increase: 1 g/kg/day (maximum: 2-2.5 g/kg/day)
- >10 years: Initial: 0.8-1.5 g/kg/day; daily increase: 1 g/kg/day (maximum: 1.5-2 g/kg/day)

Fat: Initial: 1 g/kg/day; daily increase: 1 g/kg/day (maximum: 3 g/kg/day); **Note:** Monitor triglycerides while receiving intralipids.

Adults: I.V.:

Total calories: Calculate using Harris-Benedict equation or based on stress level as indicated below:

Harris-Benedict Equation (BEE):
- Females: 655.1 + [(9.56 x W) + (1.85 x H) - (4.68 x A)]
- Males: 66.47 + [(13.75 x W) + (5 x H) - (6.76 x A)]
- Then multiply BEE x (activity factor) x (stress factor)
- W = weight in kg; H = height in cm; A = age in years
- Activity factor = 1.2 sedentary, 1.3 normal activity, 1.4 active, 1.5 very active
- Stress factor = 1.5 for trauma, stressed, or surgical patients and underweight (to promote weight gain); 2.0 for severe burn patients

Stress level:
- Normal/mild stress level: 20-25 kcal/kg/day
- Moderate stress level: 25-30 kcal/kg/day
- Severe stress level: 30-40 kcal/kg/day
- Pregnant women in second or third trimester: Add an additional 300 kcal/day

Fluid: mL/day = 30-40 mL/kg

Carbohydrate (dextrose):
- 5 g/kg/day or 3.5 mg/kg/minute (maximum rate: 4-7 mg/kg/minute)
- Minimum recommended amount: 400 calories/day or 100 g/day

Protein (amino acids):
- Maintenance: 0.8-1 g/kg/day
- Normal/mild stress level: 1-1.2 g/kg/day
- Moderate stress level: 1.2-1.5 g/kg/day
- Severe stress level: 1.5-2 g/kg/day
- Burn patients (severe): Increase protein until significant wound healing achieved
- Solid organ transplant: Perioperative: 1.5-2 g/kg/day
- Renal failure:
  - Acute (severely malnourished or hypercatabolic): 1.5-1.8 g/kg/day
  - Chronic, with dialysis: 1.2-1.3 g/kg/day
  - Chronic, without dialysis: 0.6-0.8 g/kg/day
  - Continuous hemofiltration: ≥1 g/kg/day
- Hepatic failure:
  - Acute management when other treatments have failed:
    - With encephalopathy: 0.6-1 g/kg/day
    - Without encephalopathy: 1-1.5 g/kg/day

Chronic encephalopathy: Use branch chain amino acid enriched diets only if unresponsive to pharmacotherapy

Pregnant women in second or third trimester: Add an additional 10-14 g/day

Fat:

Initial: 20% to 40% of total calories (maximum: 60% of total calories or 2.5 g/kg/day); **Note:** Monitor triglycerides while receiving intralipids.

Safe for use in pregnancy

I.V. lipids are safe in adults with pancreatitis if triglyceride levels <400 mg/dL

Dosage Forms TPN is usually compounded from optimal combinations of macronutrients (water, protein, dextrose, and lipids) and micronutrients (electrolytes, trace elements, and vitamins) to meet the specific nutritional requirements of a patient. Individual hospitals may have designated standard TPN formulas. There are a few commercially-available amino acids with electrolytes solutions; however, these products may not meet an individual's specific nutrition requirements.

Totect™ [US] *see* dexrazoxane *on page 292*

Touro® CC [US] *see* guaifenesin, pseudoephedrine, and dextromethorphan *on page 479*

Touro® CC-LD [US] *see* guaifenesin, pseudoephedrine, and dextromethorphan *on page 479*

Touro® Allergy [US] *see* brompheniramine and pseudoephedrine *on page 150*

Touro® DM [US] *see* guaifenesin and dextromethorphan *on page 474*

Touro Ex® *(Discontinued)* *see* guaifenesin *on page 473*

Touro® HC *(Discontinued)*

Touro LA® [US] *see* guaifenesin and pseudoephedrine *on page 477*

Toviaz™ [US] *see* fesoterodine *on page 416*

tPA *see* alteplase *on page 53*

TPN *see* total parenteral nutrition *on page 972*

TPV *see* tipranavir *on page 963*

tRA *see* tretinoin (systemic) *on page 980*

4 Trace Elements [US] *see* trace metals *on page 974*

Trace Elements 4 Pediatric [US] *see* trace metals *on page 974*

trace metals (trase MET als)

Synonyms chromium; copper; iodine; manganese; molybdenum; neonatal trace metals; selenium; zinc

U.S./Canadian Brand Names 4 Trace Elements [US]; Multitrace®-4 Concentrate [US]; Multitrace®-4 Neonatal [US]; Multitrace®-4 Pediatric [US]; Multitrace®-4 [US]; Multitrace®-5 Concentrate [US]; Multitrace®-5 [US]; Trace Elements 4 Pediatric [US]

Therapeutic Category Trace Element

Use Prevention and correction of trace metal deficiencies

Usual Dosage Recommended daily parenteral dosage:

Chromium:[1]

Infants: 0.2 mcg/kg

Children: 0.2 mcg/kg (maximum: 5 mcg)

Adults: 10-15 mcg

Copper:[2]

Infants: 20 mcg/kg

Children: 20 mcg/kg (maximum: 300 mcg)

Adults: 0.5-1.5 mg

Manganese:[2,3]

Infants: 1 mcg/kg

Children: 1 mcg/kg (maximum: 50 mcg)

Adults: 150-800 mcg

Molybdenum:[1,4]

Infants: 0.25 mcg/kg

Children: 0.25 mcg/kg (maximum: 5 mcg)

Adults: 20-120 mcg

Selenium:[1,4]

Infants: 2 mcg/kg

Children: 2 mcg/kg (maximum: 30 mcg)

Adults: 20-40 mcg

Zinc:
Infants, preterm: 400 mcg/kg
Infants, term <3 months: 250 mcg/kg
Infants, term >3 months: 100 mcg/kg
Children: 50 mcg/kg (maximum: 5 mg)
Adults: 2.5-4 mg

[1]Omit in patients with renal dysfunction.
[2]Omit in patients with obstructive jaundice.
[3]Current available commercial products are not in appropriate ratios to maintain this recommendation; doses of up to 10 mcg/kg have been used.
[4]Indicated for use in long-term parenteral nutrition patients.

Dosage Forms

Injection, solution [combination products]:
- Multitrace®-4: Chromium 4 mcg, copper 0.4 mg, manganese 0.1 mg, and zinc 1 mg per 1 mL (10 mL)
- Multitrace®-4 Concentrate: Chromium 10 mcg, copper 1 mg, manganese 0.5 mg, and zinc 5 mg per 1 mL (1 mL, 10 mL)
- Multitrace®-4 Neonatal: Chromium 0.85 mcg, copper 0.1 mg, manganese 0.025 mg, and zinc 1.5 mg per 1 mL (2 mL)
- Multitrace®-5: Chromium 4 mcg, copper 0.4 mg, manganese 0.1 mg, selenium 20 mcg, and zinc 1 mg per 1 mL (10 mL)
- Multitrace®-5 Concentrate: Chromium 10 mcg, copper 1 mg, manganese 0.5 mg, selenium 60 mcg, and zinc 5 mg per 1 mL (1 mL, 10 mL)
- Trace Elements 4 Pediatric: Chromium 1 mcg, copper 0.1 mg, manganese 0.03 mg, and zinc 0.5 mg per 1 mL (10 mL)

Injection, solution [combination products, preservative free]:
- 4 Trace Elements: Chromium 2 mcg, copper 0.2 mg, manganese 0.16 mg, and zinc 0.8 mg per 1 mL (5 mL, 50 mL)
- Multitrace®-4 Pediatric: Chromium 1 mcg, copper 0.1 mg, manganese 0.025 mg, and zinc 1 mg per 1 mL (3 mL)

Tracleer® [US/Can] *see* bosentan *on page 146*

Tramacet [Can] *see* acetaminophen and tramadol *on page 24*

tramadol (TRA ma dole)

Sound-Alike/Look-Alike Issues
traMADol may be confused with tapentadol, Toradol®, Trandate®, traZODone, Voltaren®
Ultram® may be confused with Ultane®, Ultracet®, Voltaren®

Synonyms tramadol hydrochloride

Tall-Man tra**MAD**ol

U.S./Canadian Brand Names Ralivia™ ER [Can]; Ryzolt™ [US]; Tridural™ [Can]; Ultram® ER [US]; Ultram® [US]; Zytram® XL [Can]

Therapeutic Category Analgesic, Nonnarcotic

Use Relief of moderate to moderately-severe pain
Extended release formulations are indicated for patients requiring around-the-clock management of moderate to moderately-severe pain for an extended period of time

Usual Dosage Oral: Moderate-to-severe pain:
Children ≥17 years and Adults: Immediate release formulation: 50-100 mg every 4-6 hours (not to exceed 400 mg/day)
For patients not requiring rapid onset of effect, tolerability may be improved by starting dose at 25 mg/day and titrating dose by 25 mg every 3 days, until reaching 25 mg 4 times/day. The total daily dose may then be increased by 50 mg every 3 days as tolerated, to reach dose of 50 mg 4 times/day. After titration, 50-100 mg may be given every 4-6 hours as needed up to a maximum 400 mg/day.
Adults: Extended release formulations:
Ultram® ER:
Patients not currently on immediate-release: 100 mg once daily; titrate every 5 days (maximum: 300 mg/day)
Patients currently on immediate-release: Calculate 24-hour immediate release total dose and initiate total extended release daily dose (round dose to the next lowest 100 mg increment); titrate (maximum: 300 mg/day)
Ralivia™ ER (Canadian labeling, not available in U.S.): 100 mg once daily; titrate every 5 days as needed based on clinical response and severity of pain (maximum: 300 mg/day)

Ryzolt™:

Patients not currently on immediate-release: 100 mg once daily; titrate every 2-3 days by 100 mg/day increments; usual daily dose: 200-300 mg/day (maximum: 300 mg/day)

Patients currently on immediate-release: Calculate 24 hour immediate release total dose and initiate total extended release daily dose (round dose to the next lowest 100 mg increment); titrate (maximum: 300 mg/day)

Tridural™ (Canadian labeling, not available in U.S.): 100 mg once daily; titrate by 100 mg/day every 2 days as needed based on clinical response and severity of pain (maximum: 300 mg/day)

Zytram® XL (Canadian labeling, not available in U.S.): 150 mg once daily; if pain relief is not achieved may titrate by increasing dosage incrementally, with sufficient time to evaluate effect of increased dosage; generally not more often than every 7 days (maximum: 400 mg/day)

Dosage Forms [CAN] = Canadian brand name

Tablet: 50 mg

Ultram®: 50 mg

Tablet, extended release:

Ultram® ER: 100 mg, 200 mg, 300 mg

Ralivia™ ER [CAN]: 100 mg, 200 mg, 300 mg [not available in the U.S.]

Ryzolt™: 100 mg, 200 mg, 300 mg

Tridural™ [CAN]: 100 mg, 200 mg, 300 mg [not available in the U.S.]

Zytram® XL [CAN]: 150 mg, 200 mg, 300 mg, 400 mg

tramadol hydrochloride *see* tramadol *on page 975*

tramadol hydrochloride and acetaminophen *see* acetaminophen and tramadol *on page 24*

Trandate® [US/Can] *see* labetalol *on page 562*

trandolapril (tran DOE la pril)

U.S./Canadian Brand Names Mavik® [US/Can]

Therapeutic Category Angiotensin-Converting Enzyme (ACE) Inhibitor

Use Treatment of hypertension alone or in combination with other antihypertensive agents; treatment of heart failure or left ventricular dysfunction after myocardial infarction

Usual Dosage Oral: Adults:

Heart failure postmyocardial infarction or left ventricular dysfunction postmyocardial infarction: Initial: 1 mg/day; titrate patients (as tolerated) towards the target dose of 4 mg/day. If a 4 mg dose is not tolerated, patients can continue therapy with the greatest tolerated dose.

Hypertension: Initial dose in patients not receiving a diuretic: 1 mg/day (2 mg/day in black patients). Adjust dosage according to the blood pressure response. Make dosage adjustments at intervals of ≥1 week. Most patients have required dosages of 2-4 mg/day. There is a little experience with doses >8 mg/day. Patients inadequately treated with once daily dosing at 4 mg may be treated with twice daily dosing. If blood pressure is not adequately controlled with trandolapril monotherapy, a diuretic may be added.

Usual dose range (JNC 7): 1-4 mg once daily

Dosage Forms

Tablet: 1 mg, 2 mg, 4 mg

Mavik®: 1 mg, 2 mg, 4 mg

trandolapril and verapamil (tran DOE la pril & ver AP a mil)

Synonyms verapamil and trandolapril

U.S./Canadian Brand Names Tarka® [US/Can]

Therapeutic Category Antihypertensive Agent, Combination

Use Treatment of hypertension; however, not indicated for initial treatment of hypertension

Usual Dosage Dose is individualized.

Dosage Forms

Tablet, variable release:

Tarka®:

1/240: Trandolapril 1 mg [immediate release] and verapamil 240 mg [sustained release]

2/180: Trandolapril 2 mg [immediate release] and verapamil 180 mg [sustained release]

2/240: Trandolapril 2 mg [immediate release] and verapamil 240 mg [sustained release]

4/240: Trandolapril 4 mg [immediate release] and verapamil 240 mg [sustained release]

tranexamic acid (tran eks AM ik AS id)

Sound-Alike/Look-Alike Issues

Cyklokapron® may be confused with cycloSPORINE

U.S./Canadian Brand Names Cyklokapron® [US/Can]; Tranexamic Acid Injection BP [Can]

Therapeutic Category Antihemophilic Agent

Use Short-term use (2-8 days) in hemophilia patients to reduce or prevent hemorrhage and reduce need for replacement therapy during and following tooth extraction

Usual Dosage I.V.: Children and Adults: Tooth extraction in patients with hemophilia (in combination with replacement therapy): 10 mg/kg immediately before surgery, then 10 mg/kg/dose 3-4 times/day; may be used for 2-8 days

Dosage Forms

Injection, solution:

Cyklokapron®: 100 mg/mL (10 mL)

Tranexamic Acid Injection BP [Can] *see* tranexamic acid *on page 977*

transamine sulphate *see* tranylcypromine *on page 977*

Transderm-V® [Can] *see* scopolamine derivatives *on page 892*

Transdermal-NTG® Patch *(Discontinued)* *see* nitroglycerin *on page 700*

Transderm-Nitro® [Can] *see* nitroglycerin *on page 700*

Transderm Scōp® [US] *see* scopolamine derivatives *on page 892*

Trans-Plantar® [Can] *see* salicylic acid *on page 884*

Trans-Plantar® Transdermal Patch *(Discontinued)* *see* salicylic acid *on page 884*

***trans*-retinoic acid** *see* tretinoin (systemic) *on page 980*

***trans*-retinoic acid** *see* tretinoin (topical) *on page 981*

Trans-Ver-Sal® [US-OTC/Can] *see* salicylic acid *on page 884*

Tranxene® SD™ [US] *see* clorazepate *on page 247*

Tranxene® SD™-Half Strength [US] *see* clorazepate *on page 247*

Tranxene® T-Tab® [US] *see* clorazepate *on page 247*

tranylcypromine (tran il SIP roe meen)

Synonyms transamine sulphate; tranylcypromine sulfate

U.S./Canadian Brand Names Parnate® [US/Can]

Therapeutic Category Antidepressant, Monoamine Oxidase Inhibitor

Use Treatment of major depressive episode without melancholia

Usual Dosage Oral: Adults: 10 mg twice daily, increase by 10 mg increments at 1- to 3-week intervals; maximum: 60 mg/day; usual effective dose: 30 mg/day

Dosage Forms

Tablet:

Parnate®: 10 mg

tranylcypromine sulfate *see* tranylcypromine *on page 977*

Trasicor® [Can] *see* oxprenolol *(Canada only) on page 736*

trastuzumab (tras TU zoo mab)

Synonyms NSC-688097

U.S./Canadian Brand Names Herceptin® [US/Can]

Therapeutic Category Antineoplastic Agent

Use Adjuvant treatment of HER-2 overexpressing breast cancer; treatment of HER-2 overexpressing metastatic breast cancer

Usual Dosage Details concerning dosing in combination regimens should also be consulted. Adults: I.V. infusion:

Adjuvant treatment of breast cancer:

With concurrent paclitaxel or docetaxel:

Initial loading dose: 4 mg/kg infused over 90 minutes

Maintenance dose: 2 mg/kg infused over 30 minutes weekly for total of 12 weeks, followed 1 week later (when concurrent chemotherapy completed) by 6 mg/kg infused over 30-60 minutes every 3 weeks for total therapy duration of 52 weeks

With concurrent docetaxel/carboplatin:
Initial loading dose: 4 mg/kg infused over 90 minutes
Maintenance dose: 2 mg/kg infused over 30 minutes weekly for total of 18 weeks, followed 1 week later (when concurrent chemotherapy completed) by 6 mg/kg infused over 30-60 minutes every 3 weeks for total therapy duration of 52 weeks
Following completion of anthracycline-based chemotherapy:
Initial loading dose: 8 mg/kg infused over 90 minutes
Maintenance dose: 6 mg/kg infused over 30 minutes every 3 weeks for total therapy duration of 52 weeks

Metastatic breast cancer (either as a single agent or in combination with paclitaxel):
Initial loading dose: 4 mg/kg infused over 90 minutes
Maintenance dose: 2 mg/kg infused over 30 minutes weekly until disease progression

Dosage Forms

Injection, powder for reconstitution:
Herceptin®: 440 mg

Trasylol® [US/Can] *see* aprotinin *on page* *94*
Trav-L-Tabs® [US-OTC] *see* meclizine *on page* *619*
Travasol® [US] *see* amino acid injection *on page* *62*
Travatan® [US/Can] *see* travoprost *on page* *979*
Travatan® Z [US/Can] *see* travoprost *on page* *979*

traveler's diarrhea and cholera vaccine *(Canada only)*

(TRAV uh lerz dahy uh REE uh & KOL er uh vak SEEN)

Synonyms *Vibrio cholera* and enterotoxigenic *Escherichia coli vaccine*; cholera and traveler's diarrhea vaccine; enterotoxigenic *Escherichia coli* and *Vibrio cholera* vaccine; traveller's diarrhea vaccine and cholera

U.S./Canadian Brand Names Dukoral™ [Can]

Therapeutic Category Vaccine

Use Protection against traveler's diarrhea and/or cholera in adults and children ≥2 years of age who will be visiting areas where there is a risk of contacting traveler's diarrhea caused by enterotoxigenic *E. coli* (ETEC) or cholera caused by *V. cholerae* O1 (classical and El Tor biotypes)

Usual Dosage Oral:
Cholera:
Primary immunization:
Children 2-6 years: 3 doses given at intervals of ≥1 week and completed at least 1 week prior to trip to endemic/epidemic areas; restart treatment if interval between doses >6 weeks
Children ≥6 years and Adults: 2 doses given at intervals of ≥1 week and completed at least 1 week prior to trip to endemic/epidemic areas; restart treatment if interval between doses >6 weeks
Booster:
Children 2-6 years: 1 dose after 6 months have elapsed since vaccination
Children ≥6 years and Adults: 1 dose after 2 years have elapsed since vaccination
ETEC:
Primary immunization: Children ≥2 years and Adults: 2 doses given at intervals of ≥1 week; restart treatment if interval between doses >6 weeks
Booster: Children ≥2 years and Adults:
Continued risk: 1 dose every 3 months
Renewed protection: 1 dose may be given if last booster or original immunization was <5 years ago (if >5 years, revaccinate)

Dosage Forms [CAN] = Canadian brand name

Suspension [vial]:
Dukoral™ [CAN]: 2.5 x 10^{10} of each of the following *Vibrio cholerae* O1 strains: Inaba classic (heat inactived), Inaba El Tor (formalin inactivated), Ogawa classic (heat inactivated), Ogawa classic (formalin inactivated), and 1 mg recombinant cholera toxin B subunit (rCTB) (3 mL) [not available in the U.S.]

traveller's diarrhea vaccine and cholera *see* traveler's diarrhea and cholera vaccine *(Canada only)* *on page* *978*

travoprost (TRA voe prost)

Sound-Alike/Look-Alike Issues

Travatan® may be confused with Xalatan®

U.S./Canadian Brand Names Travatan® Z [US/Can]; Travatan® [US/Can]

Therapeutic Category Prostaglandin, Ophthalmic

Use Reduction of elevated intraocular pressure in patients with open-angle glaucoma or ocular hypertension who are intolerant of the other IOP-lowering medications or insufficiently responsive (failed to achieve target IOP determined after multiple measurements over time) to another IOP-lowering medication

Usual Dosage Ophthalmic: Adults: Glaucoma (open angle) or ocular hypertension: Instill 1 drop into affected eye(s) once daily in the evening; do not exceed once-daily dosing (may decrease IOP-lowering effect). If used with other topical ophthalmic agents, separate administration by at least 5 minutes.

Dosage Forms

Solution, ophthalmic:

Travatan®: 0.004% (2.5 mL, 5 mL)

Travatan® Z: 0.004% (2.5 mL, 5 mL)

travoprost and timolol *(Canada only)* (TRA voe prost & TIM oh lol)

Sound-Alike/Look-Alike Issues

DuoTrav™ may be confused with DuoNeb®

Synonyms timolol maleate and travoprost

U.S./Canadian Brand Names DuoTrav™ [CAN]

Therapeutic Category Beta Blocker, Nonselective; Ophthalmic Agent, Antiglaucoma; Prostaglandin, Ophthalmic

Use Reduction of intraocular pressure (IOP) in patients with open-angle glaucoma or ocular hypertension who are insufficiently responsive to topical beta-blockers, prostaglandin analogues, or other IOP-reducing agents and in whom combination therapy is appropriate

Usual Dosage Ophthalmic: Adults: Instill 1 drop into affected eye(s) once daily in the morning

Dosage Forms [CAN] = Canadian brand name

Solution, ophthalmic:

DuoTrav™ [CAN]: Travoprost 0.004% and timolol 0.5%: (2.5 mL, 5 mL) [not available in the U.S.]

trazodone (TRAZ oh done)

Sound-Alike/Look-Alike Issues

traZODone may be confused with traMADol

Desyrel® may be confused with Demerol®, Delsym®, Zestril®

Synonyms trazodone hydrochloride

Tall-Man tra**ZOD**one

U.S./Canadian Brand Names Apo-Trazodone D® [Can]; Apo-Trazodone® [Can]; Desyrel® [Can]; Dom-Trazodone [Can]; Gen-Trazodone [Can]; Novo-Trazodone [Can]; Nu-Trazodone [Can]; PHL-Trazodone [Can]; PMS-Trazodone [Can]; ratio-Trazodone [Can]; Trazorel® [Can]; ZYM-Trazodone [Can]

Therapeutic Category Antidepressant, Triazolopyridine

Use Treatment of depression

Usual Dosage Oral: Therapeutic effects may take up to 6 weeks to occur; therapy is normally maintained for 6-12 months after optimum response is reached to prevent recurrence of depression

Adults: Depression: Initial: 150 mg/day in 3 divided doses (may increase by 50 mg/day every 3-7 days); maximum: 600 mg/day

Dosage Forms

Tablet, as hydrochloride: 50 mg, 100 mg, 150 mg, 300 mg

trazodone hydrochloride *see* trazodone *on page* 979

Trazorel® [Can] *see* trazodone *on page* 979

Treanda® [US] *see* bendamustine *on page* 127

Trecator® [US/Can] *see* ethionamide *on page* 395

Trelstar® [Can] *see* triptorelin *on page* 990

Trelstar® Depot [US/Can] *see* triptorelin *on page* 990

Trelstar® LA [US/Can] *see* triptorelin *on page* 990

Trendar® ***(Discontinued)*** *see* ibuprofen *on page* 515

Trental® [US/Can] *see* pentoxifylline *on page 766*

treprostinil (tre PROST in il)

Synonyms treprostinil sodium

U.S./Canadian Brand Names Remodulin® [US/Can]; Tyvaso™ [US]

Therapeutic Category Vasodilator

Use

Injection: Treatment of pulmonary arterial hypertension (PAH) in patients with NYHA Class II-IV symptoms to decrease exercise-associated symptoms; to diminish clinical deterioration when transitioning from epoprostenol (I.V.)

Inhalation: Treatment of pulmonary arterial hypertension (PAH) in patients with NYHA Class III symptoms to increase walk distance. **Note:** Nearly all controlled clinical trial experience has been with concomitant bosentan or sildenafil.

Usual Dosage Note: Prior to initiation, patients should be carefully evaluated for ability to administer treprostinil and care for the infusion system outside of inpatient setting. Immediate access to backup pump, infusion sets, and medication is essential to prevent treatment interruptions.

Adults: PAH: SubQ (preferred) or I.V. infusion:

Initial: New to prostacyclin therapy: 1.25 ng/kg/minute continuous; if dose cannot be tolerated due to systemic effects, reduce to 0.625 ng/kg/minute. Increase at rate not >1.25 ng/kg/minute per week for first 4 weeks, and not >2.5 ng/kg/minute per week for remainder of therapy. Limited experience with doses >40 ng/kg/minute. **Note:** Dose must be carefully and individually titrated (symptom improvement with minimal adverse effects). Avoid abrupt withdrawal. If infusion is restarted within a few hours of discontinuation, the same dose rate may be used. Interruptions for longer periods may require retitration.

Transitioning from epoprostenol (see below): SubQ (preferred) or I.V. infusion: **Note:** Transition should occur in a hospital setting to follow response (eg, walking distance, sign/symptoms of disease progression). May take 24-48 hours to transition. Transition is accomplished by initiating the infusion of treprostinil, and increasing it while simultaneously reducing the dose of intravenous epoprostenol. During transition, increases in PAH symptoms should be first treated with an increase in treprostinil dose. Occurrence of prostacyclin associated side effects should be treated by decreasing the dose of epoprostenol.

Product Availability

Tyvaso™: FDA approved in July 2009; availability anticipated in early September 2009

Dosage Forms

Injection, solution:

Remodulin®: 1 mg/mL (20 mL); 2.5 mg/mL (20 mL); 5 mg/mL (20 mL); 10 mg/mL (20 mL)

Solution for oral inhalation:

Tyvaso™: 0.6 mg/mL (2.9 mL) [delivers ~6 mcg/inhalation]

treprostinil sodium *see* treprostinil *on page 980*

Tretin-X™ [US] *see* tretinoin (topical) *on page 981*

tretinoin and clindamycin *see* clindamycin and tretinoin *on page 240*

tretinoin and mequinol *see* mequinol and tretinoin *on page 629*

tretinoin, fluocinolone acetonide, and hydroquinone *see* fluocinolone, hydroquinone, and tretinoin *on page 428*

tretinoin (systemic) (TRET i noyn, sis TEM ik)

Sound-Alike/Look-Alike Issues

tretinoin may be confused with isotretinoin, trientine

Synonyms *trans*-retinoic acid; all-*trans*-retinoic acid; ATRA; NSC-122758; Ro 5488; tRA

U.S./Canadian Brand Names Vesanoid® [US/Can]

Therapeutic Category Antineoplastic Agent

Use Induction of remission in patients with acute promyelocytic leukemia (APL), French American British (FAB) classification M3 (including the M3 variant) characterized by t(15;17) translocation and/or PML/RARα gene presence

Usual Dosage Oral: Children and Adults:

Remission induction: 45 mg/m^2/day in 2-3 divided doses for up to 30 days after complete remission (maximum duration of treatment: 90 days)

Remission maintenance: 45-200 mg/m^2/day in 2-3 divided doses for up to 12 months.

Dosage Forms
Capsule: 10 mg
Vesanoid®: 10 mg

tretinoin (topical) (TRET i noyn TOP i kal)

Sound-Alike/Look-Alike Issues
tretinoin may be confused with isotretinoin, trientine

Synonyms *trans*-retinoic acid; retinoic acid; vitamin A acid

U.S./Canadian Brand Names Atralin™ [US]; Avita® [US]; Refissa™ [US]; Rejuva-A® [Can]; Renova® [US/Can]; Retin-A® Micro [US/Can]; Retin-A® [US/Can]; Retinova® [Can]; Tretin-X™ [US]

Therapeutic Category Retinoic Acid Derivative

Use Treatment of acne vulgaris; photodamaged skin; palliation of fine wrinkles, mottled hyperpigmentation, and tactile roughness of facial skin as part of a comprehensive skin care and sun avoidance program

Usual Dosage Topical:
Children >12 years and Adults: Acne vulgaris: Begin therapy with a weaker formulation of tretinoin (0.025% cream, 0.04% microsphere gel, or 0.01% gel) and increase the concentration as tolerated; apply once daily to acne lesions before retiring or on alternate days; if stinging or irritation develop, decrease frequency of application
Adults ≥18: Palliation of fine wrinkles, mottled hyperpigmentation, and tactile roughness of facial skin: Pea-sized amount of the 0.02% or 0.05% cream applied to entire face once daily in the evening

Dosage Forms
Cream, topical: 0.025% (20 g, 45 g); 0.05% (20 g, 45 g); 0.1% (20 g, 45 g)
Avita®: 0.025% (20 g, 45 g)
Refissa™: 0.05% (40 g)
Renova®: 0.02% (40 g, 44 g, 60 g)
Retin-A®: 0.025% (20 g, 45 g); 0.05% (20 g, 45 g); 0.1% (20 g, 45 g)
Tretin-X™: 0.025% (35 g); 0.05% (35 g); 0.1% (35 g)
Gel, topical: 0.01% (15 g, 45 g); 0.025% (15 g, 45 g)
Atralin™: 0.05% (45 g)
Avita®: 0.025% (20 g, 45 g)
Retin-A®: 0.01% (15 g, 45 g); 0.025% (15 g, 45 g)
Tretin-X™: 0.025% (35 g); 0.01% (35 g)
Gel, topical [microsphere gel]:
Retin-A® Micro: 0.04% (20 g, 45 g, 50 g); 0.1% (20 g, 45 g, 50 g)

Trexall™ [US] *see* methotrexate *on page 639*
Treximet™ [US] *see* sumatriptan and naproxen *on page 933*
Trezix® [US] *see* acetaminophen, caffeine, and dihydrocodeine *on page 25*

triacetin (trye a SEE tin)

Sound-Alike/Look-Alike Issues
triacetin may be confused with Triacin®

Synonyms glycerol triacetate

U.S./Canadian Brand Names Myco-Nail [US-OTC]

Therapeutic Category Antifungal Agent

Use Fungistat for athlete's foot and other superficial fungal infections

Usual Dosage Apply twice daily, cleanse areas with dilute alcohol or mild soap and water before application; continue treatment for 7 days after symptoms have disappeared

Dosage Forms
Liquid, topical:
Myco-Nail [OTC]: 25% (30 mL)

Triacin-C® ***(Discontinued)*** *see* triprolidine, pseudoephedrine, and codeine *(Canada only) on page 990*
triaconazole *see* terconazole *on page 946*
Triaderm [Can] *see* triamcinolone (topical) *on page 983*
Triafed® ***(Discontinued)*** *see* triprolidine and pseudoephedrine *on page 989*
Triall™ [US] *see* chlorpheniramine, phenylephrine, and methscopolamine *on page 218*
triamcinolone acetonide, parenteral *see* triamcinolone (systemic) *on page 982*
triamcinolone and nystatin *see* nystatin and triamcinolone *on page 716*

triamcinolone diacetate, oral *see* triamcinolone (systemic) *on page 982*
triamcinolone diacetate, parenteral *see* triamcinolone (systemic) *on page 982*
triamcinolone hexacetonide *see* triamcinolone (systemic) *on page 982*

triamcinolone (inhalation, nasal) (trye am SIN oh lone in hil LA shun, NAY sal)

Sound-Alike/Look-Alike Issues
Nasacort® may be confused with NasalCrom®

U.S./Canadian Brand Names Nasacort® AQ [US/Can]; Nasacort® HFA [US]; Tri-Nasal® [US/Can]

Therapeutic Category Adrenal Corticosteroid

Use Nasal inhalation: Management of seasonal and perennial allergic rhinitis in patients ≥6 years of age

Usual Dosage Intranasal: Perennial allergic rhinitis, seasonal allergic rhinitis:
Nasal spray:
Children 6-11 years: 110 mcg/day as 1 spray in each nostril once daily.
Children ≥12 years and Adults: 220 mcg/day as 2 sprays in each nostril once daily
Nasal inhaler:
Children 6-11 years: Initial: 220 mcg/day as 2 sprays in each nostril once daily
Children ≥12 years and Adults: Initial: 220 mcg/day as 2 sprays in each nostril once daily; may increase dose to 440 mcg/day (given once daily or divided and given 2 or 4 times/day)

Dosage Forms
Solution, intranasal:
Tri-Nasal®: 50 mcg/inhalation (15 mL)
Suspension, intranasal:
Nasacort® AQ: 55 mcg/inhalation (16.5 g)

triamcinolone (inhalation, oral) (trye am SIN oh lone in hil LA shun, OR al)

Sound-Alike/Look-Alike Issues
TAC (occasional abbreviation for triamcinolone) is an error-prone abbreviation (mistaken as tetracaine-adrenaline-cocaine)

U.S./Canadian Brand Names Azmacort® [US]

Therapeutic Category Adrenal Corticosteroid

Use Oral inhalation: Control of bronchial asthma and related bronchospastic conditions

Usual Dosage Oral inhalation: Asthma:
Children 6-12 years: 100-200 mcg 3-4 times/day **or** 200-400 mcg twice daily; maximum dose: 1200 mcg/day
Children >12 years and Adults: 200 mcg 3-4 times/day **or** 400 mcg twice daily; maximum dose: 1600 mcg/day

Dosage Forms
Aerosol for oral inhalation:
Azmacort®: 100 mcg per actuation (20 g)

triamcinolone, oral *see* triamcinolone (systemic) *on page 982*

triamcinolone (systemic) (trye am SIN oh lone sis TEM ik)

Sound-Alike/Look-Alike Issues
Kenalog® may be confused with Ketalar®

Synonyms triamcinolone acetonide, parenteral; triamcinolone diacetate, oral; triamcinolone diacetate, parenteral; triamcinolone hexacetonide; triamcinolone, oral

U.S./Canadian Brand Names Aristospan® [US/Can]; Kenalog-10® [US]; Kenalog-40® [US]; Oracort [Can]

Therapeutic Category Adrenal Corticosteroid

Use Systemic: Adrenocortical insufficiency, rheumatic disorders, allergic states, respiratory diseases, systemic lupus erythematosus (SLE), and other diseases requiring antiinflammatory or immunosuppressive effects

Usual Dosage The lowest possible dose should be used to control the condition; when dose reduction is possible, the dose should be reduced gradually. Parenteral dose is usually 1/3 to 1/2 the oral dose given every 12 hours. In life-threatening situations, parenteral doses larger than the oral dose may be needed.

Injection:
Acetonide:
Intraarticular, intrabursal, tendon sheaths: Adults: Initial: Smaller joints: 2.5-5 mg, larger joints: 5-15 mg

Intradermal: Adults: Initial: 1 mg
I.M.: Range: 2.5-60 mg/day
Children 6-12 years: Initial: 40 mg
Children >12 years and Adults: Initial: 60 mg
Hexacetonide: Adults:
Intralesional, sublesional: Up to 0.5 mg/square inch of affected skin
Intraarticular: Range: 2-20 mg

Oral: Adults:
Acute rheumatic carditis: Initial: 20-60 mg/day; reduce dose during maintenance therapy
Acute seasonal or perennial allergic rhinitis: 8-12 mg/day
Adrenocortical insufficiency: Range 4-12 mg/day
Bronchial asthma: 8-16 mg/day
Dermatological disorders, contact/atopic dermatitis: Initial: 8-16 mg/day
Ophthalmic disorders: 12-40 mg/day
Rheumatic disorders: Range: 8-16 mg/day
SLE: Initial: 20-32 mg/day, some patients may need initial doses ≥48 mg; reduce dose during maintenance therapy

Dosage Forms

Injection, suspension:
Kenalog-10®: 10 mg/mL (5 mL) [not for I.V. or I.M. use]
Kenalog-40®: 40 mg/mL (1 mL, 5 mL, 10 mL) [not for I.V. or intradermal use]

Injection, suspension:
Aristospan®: 5 mg/mL (5 mL); 20 mg/mL (1 mL, 5 mL) [not for I.V. use]

triamcinolone (topical) (trye am SIN oh lone TOP i kal)

Sound-Alike/Look-Alike Issues
Kenalog® may be confused with Ketalar®

U.S./Canadian Brand Names Aristocort® A [US]; Kenalog® in Orabase [Can]; Kenalog® [US/Can]; Triaderm [Can]; Triderm® [US]

Therapeutic Category Corticosteroid, Topical

Use
Oral topical: Adjunctive treatment and temporary relief of symptoms associated with oral inflammatory lesions and ulcerative lesions resulting from trauma
Topical: Inflammatory dermatoses responsive to steroids

Usual Dosage

Oral topical: Oral inflammatory lesions/ulcers: Press a small dab (about 1/4 inch) to the lesion until a thin film develops. A larger quantity may be required for coverage of some lesions. For optimal results use only enough to coat the lesion with a thin film; do not rub in.

Topical:
Cream, Ointment: Apply thin film to affected areas 2-4 times/day
Spray: Apply to affected area 3-4 times/day

Product Availability Trivaris™: FDA approved June 2008; availability currently undetermined

Dosage Forms

Aerosol, topical:
Kenalog®: 0.2 mg/2-second spray (63 g)
Cream: 0.025% (15 g, 80 g, 454 g); 0.1% (15 g, 80 g, 454 g, 2270 g); 0.5% (15 g)
Triderm®: 0.1% (30 g, 85 g)
Lotion: 0.025% (60 mL); 0.1% (60 mL)
Ointment, topical: 0.025% (15 g, 80 g, 454 g); 0.1% (15 g, 80 g, 454 g); 0.5% (15 g)
Paste, oral, topical: 0.1% (5 g)

Triaminic® Children's Cough Long Acting [US-OTC] *see* dextromethorphan *on page 295*

Triaminic® Children's Softchews® Cough & Runny Nose [US-OTC] *see* dextromethorphan and chlorpheniramine *on page 296*

Triaminic® Cold & Allergy [Can] *see* chlorpheniramine and pseudoephedrine *on page 215*

Triaminic® Cold and Allergy [US-OTC] *see* chlorpheniramine and phenylephrine *on page 214*

Triaminic® Cold and Cough *(Discontinued)* *see* chlorpheniramine, pseudoephedrine, and dextromethorphan *on page 220*

Triaminic® Cough and Sore Throat Formula *(Discontinued)*

Triaminic® Cough *(Discontinued)* *see* pseudoephedrine and dextromethorphan *on page 834*

Triaminic® Cough & Nasal Congestion *(Discontinued)* *see* pseudoephedrine and dextromethorphan *on page 834*
Triaminic® Day Time Cold & Cough [US-OTC] *see* dextromethorphan and phenylephrine *on page 296*
Triaminic® Expectorant *(Discontinued)*
Triaminic® Infant Thin Strips® Decongestant *(Discontinued)* *see* phenylephrine *on page 774*
Triaminic® Night Time Cough and Cold *(Discontinued)* *see* chlorpheniramine, pseudoephedrine, and dextromethorphan *on page 220*
Triaminic Thin Strips® Children's Cough and Runny Nose [US-OTC] *see* diphenhydramine *on page 315*
Triaminic® Thin Strips® Children's Long Acting Cough [US-OTC] *see* dextromethorphan *on page 295*
Triaminic Thin Strips® Children's Day Time Cold & Cough [US-OTC] *see* dextromethorphan and phenylephrine *on page 296*
Triaminic® Thin Strips® Cold [US-OTC] *see* phenylephrine *on page 774*
Triamonide® Injection *(Discontinued)*

triamterene (trye AM ter een)

Sound-Alike/Look-Alike Issues
triamterene may be confused with trimipramine
Dyrenium® may be confused with Pyridium®

U.S./Canadian Brand Names Dyrenium® [US]

Therapeutic Category Diuretic, Potassium Sparing

Use Alone or in combination with other diuretics in treatment of edema and hypertension; decreases potassium excretion caused by kaliuretic diuretics

Usual Dosage Oral: Adults: Hypertension, edema: 100-300 mg/day in 1-2 divided doses; maximum dose: 300 mg/day; usual dosage range (JNC 7): 50-100 mg/day

Dosage Forms
Capsule:
Dyrenium®: 50 mg, 100 mg

triamterene and hydrochlorothiazide *see* hydrochlorothiazide and triamterene *on page 500*
Triant-HC™ [US] *see* phenylephrine, hydrocodone, and chlorpheniramine *on page 778*
Triapin® *(Discontinued)*
Triatec-8 [Can] *see* acetaminophen and codeine *on page 20*
Triatec-8 Strong [Can] *see* acetaminophen and codeine *on page 20*
Triatec-30 [Can] *see* acetaminophen and codeine *on page 20*
Triavil® *(Discontinued)* *see* amitriptyline and perphenazine *on page 66*
Triaz® [US] *see* benzoyl peroxide *on page 132*

triazolam (trye AY zoe lam)

Sound-Alike/Look-Alike Issues
triazolam may be confused with alPRAZolam
Halcion® may be confused with halcinonide, Haldol®

U.S./Canadian Brand Names Apo-Triazo® [Can]; Gen-Triazolam [Can]; Halcion® [US/Can]

Therapeutic Category Benzodiazepine

Controlled Substance C-IV

Use Short-term treatment of insomnia

Usual Dosage Oral (onset of action is rapid, patient should be in bed when taking medication): Adults:
Insomnia (short-term): 0.125-0.25 mg at bedtime (maximum dose: 0.5 mg/day)
Preprocedure sedation (dental): 0.25 mg taken the evening before oral surgery; or 0.25 mg 1 hour before procedure

Dosage Forms
Tablet: 0.125 mg, 0.25 mg
Halcion®: 0.25 mg

tribavirin *see* ribavirin *on page 864*
Tri Biozene [US-OTC] *see* bacitracin, neomycin, polymyxin B, and pramoxine *on page 120*

tricalcium phosphate *see* calcium phosphate (tribasic) *on page 175*

Tricardio B [US] *see* folic acid, cyanocobalamin, and pyridoxine *on page 440*

Tri-Chlor® [US] *see* trichloroacetic acid *on page 985*

Trichlor Fresh Pac™ [US] *see* trichloroacetic acid *on page 985*

trichloroacetaldehyde monohydrate *see* chloral hydrate *on page 208*

trichloroacetic acid (trye klor oh a SEE tik AS id)

U.S./Canadian Brand Names Tri-Chlor® [US]; Trichlor Fresh Pac™ [US]

Therapeutic Category Keratolytic Agent

Use Chemical used in compounding agents for the treatment of warts, skin resurfacing (chemical peels)

Usual Dosage Topical: Apply to verruca, cover with bandage for 5-6 days, remove verruca, reapply as needed

Dosage Forms

Liquid: 80%

Tri-Chlor®: 80%

Powder for reconstitution, topical: 10% (28 mL); 15% (28 mL); 20% (28 mL); 25% (28 mL); 30% (28 mL); 35% (28 mL); 40% (28 mL); 50% (28 mL)

Trichlor Fresh Pac™: 10% (28 mL); 15% (28 mL); 20% (28 mL); 25% (28 mL); 30% (28 mL); 35% (28 mL); 40% (28 mL); 50% (28 mL)

trichloromonofluoromethane and dichlorodifluoromethane *see* dichlorodifluoromethane and trichloromonofluoromethane *on page 303*

Trichophyton skin test (trye koe FYE ton skin test)

Therapeutic Category Diagnostic Agent

Use Assess cell-mediated immunity

Usual Dosage 0.1 mL intradermally, examine reaction site in 24-48 hours; induration of ≥5 mm in diameter is a positive reaction

Dosage Forms

Injection, solution: 1:200 (2 mL)

Tricitrates [US] *see* citric acid, sodium citrate, and potassium citrate *on page 235*

Tri-Clear® Expectorant *(Discontinued)*

TriCor® [US] *see* fenofibrate *on page 408*

tricosal *see* choline magnesium trisalicylate *on page 224*

Tri-Cyclen® [Can] *see* ethinyl estradiol and norgestimate *on page 393*

Tri-Cyclen® Lo [Can] *see* ethinyl estradiol and norgestimate *on page 393*

Triderm® [US] *see* triamcinolone (topical) *on page 983*

Tridil® Injection *(Discontinued)* *see* nitroglycerin *on page 700*

Tridione® *(Discontinued)*

Tridural™ [Can] *see* tramadol *on page 975*

trien *see* trientine *on page 985*

trientine (TRYE en teen)

Sound-Alike/Look-Alike Issues

trientine may be confused with Trental®, tretinoin

Synonyms 2,2,2-tetramine; trien; trientine hydrochloride; triethylene tetramine dihydrochloride

U.S./Canadian Brand Names Syprine® [US/Can]

Therapeutic Category Chelating Agent

Use Treatment of Wilson disease in patients intolerant to penicillamine

Usual Dosage Oral (administer on an empty stomach):

Children <12 years: 500-750 mg/day in divided doses 2-4 times/day; maximum: 1.5 g/day. The practice guideline suggests 20 mg/kg/day rounded off to the nearest 250 mg, given in 2-3 divided doses.

Children ≥12 years and Adults: 750-1250 mg/day in divided doses 2-4 times/day; maximum dose: 2 g/day. The practice guideline suggests typical doses of 750-1500 mg/day in 2-3 divided doses with maintenance therapy of 750-1000 mg/day

Dosage Forms

Capsule:

Syprine®: 250 mg

trientine hydrochloride *see* trientine *on page 985*

triethanolamine salicylate *see* trolamine *on page 991*

triethylene tetramine dihydrochloride *see* trientine *on page 985*

triethylenethiophosphoramide *see* thiotepa *on page 956*

Trifed-C® ***(Discontinued)*** *see* triprolidine, pseudoephedrine, and codeine *(Canada only) on page 990*

trifluoperazine (trye floo oh PER a zeen)

Sound-Alike/Look-Alike Issues

trifluoperazine may be confused with triflupromazine, trihexyphenidyl

Stelazine® may be confused with selegiline

Synonyms trifluoperazine hydrochloride

U.S./Canadian Brand Names Apo-Trifluoperazine® [Can]; Novo-Trifluzine [Can]; PMS-Trifluoperazine [Can]; Terfluzine [Can]

Therapeutic Category Phenothiazine Derivative

Use Treatment of schizophrenia

Usual Dosage Oral:

Children 6-12 years: Schizophrenia/psychoses: Hospitalized or well-supervised patients: Initial: 1 mg 1-2 times/day, gradually increase until symptoms are controlled or adverse effects become troublesome; maximum: 15 mg/day

Adults:

Schizophrenia/psychoses:

Outpatients: 1-2 mg twice daily

Hospitalized or well-supervised patients: Initial: 2-5 mg twice daily with optimum response in the 15-20 mg/day range; do not exceed 40 mg/day

Nonpsychotic anxiety: 1-2 mg twice daily; maximum: 6 mg/day; therapy for anxiety should not exceed 12 weeks; do not exceed 6 mg/day for longer than 12 weeks when treating anxiety; agitation, jitteriness, or insomnia may be confused with original neurotic or psychotic symptoms

Dosage Forms

Tablet: 1 mg, 2 mg, 5 mg, 10 mg

trifluoperazine hydrochloride *see* trifluoperazine *on page 986*

trifluorothymidine *see* trifluridine *on page 986*

trifluridine (trye FLURE i deen)

Sound-Alike/Look-Alike Issues

Viroptic® may be confused with Timoptic®

Synonyms F_3T; trifluorothymidine

U.S./Canadian Brand Names SAB-Trifluridine [Can]; Sandoz-Trifluridine [Can]; Viroptic® [US/Can]

Therapeutic Category Antiviral Agent

Use Treatment of primary keratoconjunctivitis and recurrent epithelial keratitis caused by herpes simplex virus types I and II

Usual Dosage Adults: Instill 1 drop into affected eye every 2 hours while awake, to a maximum of 9 drops/day, until reepithelialization of corneal ulcer occurs; then use 1 drop every 4 hours for another 7 days; do **not** exceed 21 days of treatment; if improvement has not taken place in 7-14 days, consider another form of therapy

Dosage Forms

Solution, ophthalmic: 1% (7.5 mL)

Viroptic®: 1% (7.5 mL)

Triglide™ [US] *see* fenofibrate *on page 408*

triglycerides, medium chain *see* medium chain triglycerides *on page 620*

trihexyphenidyl (trye heks ee FEN i dil)

Sound-Alike/Look-Alike Issues

trihexyphenidyl may be confused with trifluoperazine

Artane® may be confused with Altace®, Anturane®, Aramine®

Synonyms benzhexol hydrochloride; trihexyphenidyl hydrochloride

U.S./Canadian Brand Names Apo-Trihex® [Can]

Therapeutic Category Anti-Parkinson Agent; Anticholinergic Agent

Use Adjunctive treatment of Parkinson disease; treatment of drug-induced extrapyramidal symptoms

Usual Dosage Oral: Adults: Initial: 1-2 mg/day, increase by 2 mg increments at intervals of 3-5 days; usual dose: 5-15 mg/day in 3-4 divided doses

Dosage Forms

Elixir: 2 mg/5 mL

Tablet: 2 mg, 5 mg

trihexyphenidyl hydrochloride *see* trihexyphenidyl *on page 986*

TriHIBit® [US] *see* diphtheria, tetanus toxoids, and acellular pertussis vaccine and *Haemophilus influenzae* b conjugate vaccine *on page 323*

Tri-Hist *(Discontinued)* *see* chlorpheniramine, pyrilamine, and phenylephrine *on page 221*

Trikacide [Can] *see* metronidazole *on page 651*

Trikof-D® *(Discontinued)* *see* guaifenesin, pseudoephedrine, and dextromethorphan *on page 479*

Tri-Kort® Injection *(Discontinued)*

Trilafon® *(Discontinued)* *see* perphenazine *on page 769*

Tri-Legest™ Fe [US] *see* ethinyl estradiol and norethindrone *on page 390*

Trileptal® [US/Can] *see* oxcarbazepine *on page 734*

Tri-Levlen® *(Discontinued)* *see* ethinyl estradiol and levonorgestrel *on page 387*

TriLipix™ [US] *see* fenofibric acid *on page 409*

Trilisate® *(Discontinued)* *see* choline magnesium trisalicylate *on page 224*

Trilog® Injection *(Discontinued)*

Trilone® Injection *(Discontinued)*

Tri-Lo-Sprintec™ [US] *see* ethinyl estradiol and norgestimate *on page 393*

Tri-Luma™ [US] *see* fluocinolone, hydroquinone, and tretinoin *on page 428*

TriLyte® [US] *see* polyethylene glycol-electrolyte solution *on page 797*

Trimazide® *(Discontinued)* *see* trimethobenzamide *on page 987*

trimebutine *(Canada only)* (trye me BYOO teen)

Synonyms trimebutine maleate

U.S./Canadian Brand Names Apo-Trimebutine® [Can]; Modulon® [Can]

Therapeutic Category Antispasmodic Agent, Gastrointestinal

Use Treatment and relief of symptoms associated with irritable bowel syndrome (IBS) (spastic colon). In postoperative paralytic ileus in order to accelerate the resumption of the intestinal transit following abdominal surgery.

Usual Dosage Oral: Children ≥12 years and Adults: 200 mg 3 times/day before meals

Dosage Forms [CAN] = Canadian brand name

Tablet:

Apo-Trimebutine® [CAN], Modulon® [CAN]: 100 mg, 200 mg [not available in the U.S.]

trimebutine maleate *see* trimebutine *(Canada only) on page 987*

trimethadione *(Discontinued)*

trimethobenzamide (trye meth oh BEN za mide)

Sound-Alike/Look-Alike Issues

trimethobenzamide may be confused with metoclopramide, trimethoprim

Tigan® may be confused with Tiazac®, Ticar®, Ticlid®

Synonyms trimethobenzamide hydrochloride

U.S./Canadian Brand Names Tigan® [US/Can]

Therapeutic Category Anticholinergic Agent; Antiemetic

Use Treatment of postoperative nausea and vomiting; treatment of nausea associated with gastroenteritis ▶

Usual Dosage
Children >40 kg: Oral: 300 mg 3-4 times/day
Adults:
Oral: 300 mg 3-4 times/day
I.M.: 200 mg 3-4 times/day
Postoperative nausea and vomiting (PONV): I.M.: 200 mg, followed 1 hour later by a second 200 mg dose

Dosage Forms
Capsule: 300 mg
Tigan®: 300 mg
Injection, solution: 100 mg/mL (2 mL)
Tigan®: 100 mg/mL (20 mL)
Injection, solution [preservative free]:
Tigan®: 100 mg/mL (2 mL)

trimethobenzamide hydrochloride *see* trimethobenzamide *on page 987*

trimethoprim (trye METH oh prim)

Sound-Alike/Look-Alike Issues
trimethoprim may be confused with trimethaphan
Synonyms TMP
U.S./Canadian Brand Names Apo-Trimethoprim® [Can]; Primsol® [US]
Therapeutic Category Antibiotic, Miscellaneous
Use Treatment of urinary tract infections due to susceptible strains of *E. coli*, *P. mirabilis*, *K. pneumoniae*, *Enterobacter* sp and coagulase-negative *Staphylococcus* including *S. saprophyticus*; acute otitis media in children; acute exacerbations of chronic bronchitis in adults; in combination with other agents for treatment of toxoplasmosis, *Pneumocystis carinii*; treatment of superficial ocular infections involving the conjunctiva and cornea
Usual Dosage Oral:
Children: 4 mg/kg/day in divided doses every 12 hours
Adults: 100 mg every 12 hours or 200 mg every 24 hours for 10 days; longer treatment periods may be necessary for prostatitis (ie, 4-16 weeks); in the treatment of *Pneumocystis carinii* pneumonia; dose may be as high as 15-20 mg/kg/day in 3-4 divided doses

Dosage Forms
Solution, oral:
Primsol®: 50 mg/5 mL
Tablet: 100 mg

trimethoprim and polymyxin B (trye METH oh prim & pol i MIKS in bee)

Synonyms polymyxin B and trimethoprim
U.S./Canadian Brand Names PMS-Polytrimethoprim [Can]; Polytrim® [US/Can]
Therapeutic Category Antibiotic, Ophthalmic
Use Treatment of surface ocular bacterial conjunctivitis and blepharoconjunctivitis
Usual Dosage Instill 1-2 drops in eye(s) every 4-6 hours
Dosage Forms
Solution, ophthalmic: Trimethoprim 1 mg and polymyxin B 10,000 units per mL (10 mL)
Polytrim®: Trimethoprim 1 mg and polymyxin B 10,000 units per mL (10 mL)

trimethoprim and sulfamethoxazole *see* sulfamethoxazole and trimethoprim *on page 929*

trimetrexate *(Discontinued)*

trimipramine (trye MI pra meen)

Sound-Alike/Look-Alike Issues
trimipramine may be confused with triamterene, trimeprazine
Synonyms trimipramine maleate
U.S./Canadian Brand Names Apo-Trimip® [Can]; Nu-Trimipramine [Can]; Rhotrimine® [Can]; Surmontil® [US/Can]
Therapeutic Category Antidepressant, Tricyclic (Tertiary Amine)
Use Treatment of depression

Usual Dosage Oral: Adults: 50-150 mg/day as a single bedtime dose up to a maximum of 200 mg/day outpatient and 300 mg/day inpatient

Dosage Forms

Capsule:

Surmontil®: 25 mg, 50 mg, 100 mg

trimipramine maleate *see* trimipramine *on page* 988

Trimox® ***(Discontinued)*** *see* amoxicillin *on page* 70

Trimpex® ***(Discontinued)*** *see* trimethoprim *on page* 988

Tri-Nasal® [US/Can] *see* triamcinolone (inhalation, nasal) *on page* 982

Trinate [US-OTC] *see* vitamins (multiple/prenatal) *on page* 1020

TriNessa® [US] *see* ethinyl estradiol and norgestimate *on page* 393

Trinipatch® 0.2 [Can] *see* nitroglycerin *on page* 700

Trinipatch® 0.4 [Can] *see* nitroglycerin *on page* 700

Trinipatch® 0.6 [Can] *see* nitroglycerin *on page* 700

Tri-Norinyl® [US] *see* ethinyl estradiol and norethindrone *on page* 390

Trinsicon® ***(Discontinued)*** *see* vitamin B complex combinations *on page* 1017

Triofed® Syrup ***(Discontinued)*** *see* triprolidine and pseudoephedrine *on page* 989

Trionate® ***(Discontinued)*** *see* carbetapentane and chlorpheniramine *on page* 182

Triostat® [US] *see* liothyronine *on page* 591

Tripedia® [US] *see* diphtheria, tetanus toxoids, and acellular pertussis vaccine *on page* 321

Triphasil® [US/Can] *see* ethinyl estradiol and levonorgestrel *on page* 387

Triphenyl® Expectorant ***(Discontinued)***

triple antibiotic *see* bacitracin, neomycin, and polymyxin B *on page* 119

triple sulfa *see* sulfabenzamide, sulfacetamide, and sulfathiazole *on page* 926

Triplex™ AD [US] *see* chlorpheniramine, pyrilamine, and phenylephrine *on page* 221

Tripohist™ D [US] *see* triprolidine and pseudoephedrine *on page* 989

Triposed® Syrup ***(Discontinued)*** *see* triprolidine and pseudoephedrine *on page* 989

Tri-Previfem® [US] *see* ethinyl estradiol and norgestimate *on page* 393

triprolidine and pseudoephedrine (trye PROE li deen & soo doe e FED rin)

Sound-Alike/Look-Alike Issues

Aprodine may be confused with Aphrodyne®

Synonyms pseudoephedrine and triprolidine

U.S./Canadian Brand Names Actifed® [Can]; Allerfrim [US-OTC]; Aprodine [US-OTC]; Genac™ [US-OTC]; Pediatex® TD [US]; Silafed [US-OTC]; Tripohist™ D [US]

Therapeutic Category Antihistamine/Decongestant Combination

Use Temporary relief of nasal congestion, decongest sinus openings, running nose, sneezing, itching of nose or throat and itchy, watery eyes due to common cold, hay fever, or other upper respiratory allergies

Usual Dosage Oral:

Liquid:

Children:

2-4 years: 1.25 mL every 4-6 hours (maximum pseudoephedrine: 60 mg/24 hours)

4-6 years: 2.5 mL every 4-6 hours (maximum pseudoephedrine: 60 mg/24 hours)

6-12 years: 2.5-5 mL every 4-6 hours (maximum pseudoephedrine: 120 mg/24 hours)

Children ≥12 years and Adults: 5-10 mL every 4-6 hours (maximum pseudoephedrine: 240 mg/24 hours)

Syrup (Allerfrim, Aprodine):

Children 6-12 years: 5 mL every 4-6 hours; do not exceed 4 doses in 24 hours

Children >12 years and Adults: 10 mL every 4-6 hours; do not exceed 4 doses in 24 hours

Tablet (Aprodine):

Children 6-12 years: 1/2 tablet every 4-6 hours; do not exceed 4 doses in 24 hours

Children >12 years and Adults: One tablet every 4-6 hours; do not exceed 4 doses in 24 hours

Dosage Forms

Liquid, oral:

Pediatex® TD: Triprolidine 0.938 mg and pseudoephedrine 10 mg per 1 mL

Tripohist™ D: Triprolidine 1.25 mg and pseudoephedrine 45 mg per 5 mL

Syrup, oral:
Allerfrim [OTC], Aprodine [OTC], Silafed [OTC]: Triprolidine 1.25 mg and pseudoephedrine 30 mg per 5 mL
Tablet, oral:
Allerfrim [OTC], Aprodine [OTC], Genac™ [OTC]: Triprolidine 2.5 mg and pseudoephedrine 60 mg

triprolidine, codeine, and pseudoephedrine *see* triprolidine, pseudoephedrine, and codeine *(Canada only) on page 990*

triprolidine, pseudoephedrine, and codeine *(Canada only)*

(trye PROE li deen, soo doe e FED rin, & KOE deen)

Sound-Alike/Look-Alike Issues
Triacin-C® may be confused with triacetin

Synonyms codeine, pseudoephedrine, and triprolidine; codeine, triprolidine, and pseudoephedrine; pseudoephedrine, codeine, and triprolidine; pseudoephedrine, triprolidine, and codeine; triprolidine, codeine, and pseudoephedrine

U.S./Canadian Brand Names CoActifed® [Can]; Covan® [Can]; ratio-Cotridin [Can]

Therapeutic Category Antihistamine/Decongestant/Antitussive

Controlled Substance C-V (CDSA-I)

Use Symptomatic relief of upper respiratory symptoms and cough

Usual Dosage Oral:
Children:
2-6 years: 2.5 mL 4 times/day
7-12 years: 5 mL 4 times/day **or** 1/2 tablet 4 times/day
Children >12 years and Adults: 10 mL 4 times/day **or** 1 tablet 4 times/day

Dosage Forms [CAN] = Canadian brand name
Syrup:
CoActifed® [CAN], ratio-Cotridin [CAN]: Triprolidine 2 mg, pseudoephedrine 30 mg, and codeine 10 mg per 5 mL (100 mL, 2000 mL) [not available in the U.S.]
CoVan® [CAN]: Triprolidine 2 mg, pseudoephedrine 30 mg, and codeine 10 mg per 5 mL (500 mL) [not available in the U.S.]
Tablet:
CoActifed® [CAN]: Triprolidine 4 mg, pseudoephedrine 60 mg, and codeine 20 mg (50s) [not available in the U.S.]

Tri-Pseudo® ***(Discontinued)*** *see* triprolidine and pseudoephedrine *on page 989*

TripTone® [US-OTC] *see* dimenhydrinate *on page 312*

triptoraline *see* triptorelin *on page 990*

triptorelin (trip toe REL in)

Synonyms AY-25650; CL-118,532; D-Trp(6)-LHRH; triptoraline; triptorelin pamoate; tryptoreline

U.S./Canadian Brand Names Trelstar® Depot [US/Can]; Trelstar® LA [US/Can]; Trelstar® [Can]

Therapeutic Category Luteinizing Hormone-Releasing Hormone Analog

Use Palliative treatment of advanced prostate cancer as an alternative to orchiectomy or estrogen administration

Usual Dosage I.M.: Adults: Prostate cancer:
Trelstar® Depot: 3.75 mg once every 28 days
Trelstar® LA: 11.25 mg once every 84 days

Dosage Forms
Injection, powder for reconstitution:
Trelstar® Depot: 3.75 mg
Trelstar® LA: 11.25 mg

triptorelin pamoate *see* triptorelin *on page 990*

Triquilar® [Can] *see* ethinyl estradiol and levonorgestrel *on page 387*

tris buffer *see* tromethamine *on page 991*

Trisenox® [US] *see* arsenic trioxide *on page 98*

tris(hydroxymethyl)aminomethane *see* tromethamine *on page 991*

trisodium calcium diethylenetriaminepentaacetate (Ca-DTPA) *see* diethylene triamine pentaacetic acid *on page 306*

Tri-Sprintec® [US] *see* ethinyl estradiol and norgestimate *on page 393*
Tri-Statin® II Topical ***(Discontinued)*** *see* nystatin and triamcinolone *on page 716*
Tristoject® Injection ***(Discontinued)***
Trisudex® ***(Discontinued)*** *see* triprolidine and pseudoephedrine *on page 989*
Tri-Sudo® ***(Discontinued)*** *see* triprolidine and pseudoephedrine *on page 989*
Trital DM [US] *see* chlorpheniramine, phenylephrine, and dextromethorphan *on page 217*
Tri-Tannate Plus® ***(Discontinued)*** *see* chlorpheniramine, ephedrine, phenylephrine, and carbetapentane *on page 216*
TriTuss® [US] *see* guaifenesin, dextromethorphan, and phenylephrine *on page 478*
TriTuss® ER [US] *see* guaifenesin, dextromethorphan, and phenylephrine *on page 478*
Trivagizole-3® [Can] *see* clotrimazole *on page 248*
Trivagizole-3® ***(Discontinued)*** *see* clotrimazole *on page 248*
trivalent inactivated influenza vaccine (TIV) *see* influenza virus vaccine *on page 528*
Tri-Vent™ DM ***(Discontinued)*** *see* guaifenesin, pseudoephedrine, and dextromethorphan *on page 479*
Tri-Vent™ DPC ***(Discontinued)*** *see* chlorpheniramine, phenylephrine, and dextromethorphan *on page 217*
Tri-Vent™ HC ***(Discontinued)***
Tri-Vi-Sol® [US-OTC] *see* vitamins (multiple/pediatric) *on page 1020*
Tri-Vi-Sol® With Iron [US-OTC] *see* vitamins (multiple/pediatric) *on page 1020*
Trivora® [US] *see* ethinyl estradiol and levonorgestrel *on page 387*
Trizivir® [US/Can] *see* abacavir, lamivudine, and zidovudine *on page 16*
Trobicin® ***(Discontinued)***
Trocaine® [US-OTC] *see* benzocaine *on page 129*
Trocal® [US-OTC] *see* dextromethorphan *on page 295*

trolamine (TROLE a meen)

Sound-Alike/Look-Alike Issues
Myoflex® may be confused with Mycelex®

Synonyms TEAS; triethanolamine salicylate; trolamine salicylate

U.S./Canadian Brand Names Antiphlogistine Rub A-535 No Odour [Can]; Aspercreme® [US-OTC]; Flex-Power [US-OTC]; Mobisyl® [US-OTC]; Myoflex® [US-OTC/Can]; Sportscreme® [US-OTC]

Therapeutic Category Analgesic, Topical

Use Relief of pain of muscular aches, rheumatism, neuralgia, sprains, arthritis on intact skin

Usual Dosage Topical: Apply to area as needed

Dosage Forms

Cream, topical: 10% (90 g)
Aspercreme® [OTC]: 10% (35 g, 85 g, 142 g)
Flex-Power [OTC]: 10% (57 g, 113 g)
Mobisyl® [OTC]: 10% (100 g, 227 g)
Myoflex® [OTC]: 10% (57 g, 113 g)
Sportscreme® [OTC]: 10% (35 g, 85 g)

Lotion, topical: 10% (180 mL)
Aspercreme® [OTC]: 10% (180 mL)

trolamine salicylate *see* trolamine *on page 991*
Trombovar® [Can] *see* sodium tetradecyl *on page 914*

tromethamine (troe METH a meen)

Sound-Alike/Look-Alike Issues
tromethamine may be confused with TrophAmine®

Synonyms tris buffer; tris(hydroxymethyl)aminomethane

U.S./Canadian Brand Names THAM® [US]

Therapeutic Category Alkalinizing Agent

Use Correction of metabolic acidosis associated with cardiac bypass surgery or cardiac arrest; to correct excess acidity of stored blood that is preserved with acid citrate dextrose (ACD); indicated in infants needing alkalinization after receiving maximum sodium bicarbonate (8-10 mEq/kg/24 hours)

Usual Dosage

Neonates and Infants: Metabolic acidosis associated with RDS: Initial: Approximately 1 mL/kg for each pH unit below 7.4; additional doses determined by changes in PaO_2, pH, and pCO_2; **Note:** Although THAM® solution does not raise pCO_2 when treating metabolic acidosis with concurrent respiratory acidosis, bicarbonate may be preferred because the osmotic effects of THAM® are greater.

Adults: Dose depends on buffer base deficit; when deficit is known: tromethamine (mL of 0.3 M solution) = body weight (kg) x base deficit (mEq/L) x 1.1

Metabolic acidosis with cardiac arrest:

I.V.: 3.6-10.8 g (111-333 mL); additional amounts may be required to control acidosis after arrest reversed

Open chest: Intraventricular: 2-6 g (62-185 mL). **Note:** Do not inject into cardiac muscle

Acidosis associated with cardiac bypass surgery: Average dose: 9 mL/kg (2.7 mEq/kg); 500 mL is adequate for most adults; maximum dose: 500 mg/kg in ≤1 hour

Excess acidity of acid citrate dextrose (ACD) blood in coronary artery surgery: 15-77 mL of 0.3 molar solution added to each 500 mL of blood

Dosage Forms

Injection, solution:

THAM®: 18 g [0.3 molar] (500 mL)

Tronolane® Cream [US-OTC] *see* pramoxine *on page 809*

Tronolane® Suppository [US-OTC] *see* phenylephrine *on page 774*

TrophAmine® [US] *see* amino acid injection *on page 62*

Tropicacyl® [US] *see* tropicamide *on page 992*

tropicamide (troe PIK a mide)

Synonyms bistropamide

U.S./Canadian Brand Names Diotrope® [Can]; Mydral™ [US]; Mydriacyl® [US/Can]; Tropicacyl® [US]

Therapeutic Category Anticholinergic Agent

Use Short-acting mydriatic used in diagnostic procedures; as well as preoperatively and postoperatively; treatment of some cases of acute iritis, iridocyclitis, and keratitis

Usual Dosage Ophthalmic: Children and Adults (individuals with heavily pigmented eyes may require larger doses):

Cycloplegia: Instill 1-2 drops (1%); may repeat in 5 minutes

Exam must be performed within 30 minutes after the repeat dose; if the patient is not examined within 20-30 minutes, instill an additional drop

Mydriasis: Instill 1-2 drops (0.5%) 15-20 minutes before exam; may repeat every 30 minutes as needed

Dosage Forms

Solution, ophthalmic [drops]: 0.5% (15 mL); 1% (2 mL, 3 mL, 15 mL)

Mydriacyl®: 1% (3 mL, 15 mL)

Mydral™, Tropicacyl®: 0.5% (15 mL); 1% (15 mL)

tropicamide and hydroxyamphetamine *see* hydroxyamphetamine and tropicamide *on page 509*

Trosec [Can] *see* trospium *on page 992*

trospium (TROSE pee um)

Synonyms trospium chloride

U.S./Canadian Brand Names Sanctura® XR [US]; Sanctura® [US]; Trosec [Can]

Therapeutic Category Anticholinergic Agent

Use Treatment of overactive bladder with symptoms of urgency, incontinence, and urinary frequency

Usual Dosage Oral: Adults: Immediate release formulation: 20 mg twice daily; extended release formulation: 60 mg once daily

Dosage Forms

Capsule, extended release:

Sanctura® XR: 60 mg

Tablet:

Sanctura®: 20 mg

trospium chloride *see* trospium *on page 992*

Trovan® ***(Discontinued)***

Truphylline® ***(Discontinued)*** *see* aminophylline *on page 63*

Trusopt® [US/Can] *see* dorzolamide *on page* 332
Truvada® [US/Can] *see* emtricitabine and tenofovir *on page* 352

trypsin, balsam Peru, and castor oil (TRIP sin, BAL sam pe RUE, & KAS tor oyl)

Sound-Alike/Look-Alike Issues
Granulex® may be confused with Regranex®

Synonyms balsam Peru, castor oil, and trypsin; castor oil, trypsin, and balsam Peru

U.S./Canadian Brand Names Granulex® [US]; Optase™ [US]; Xenaderm™ [US]

Therapeutic Category Protectant, Topical

Use Treatment of decubitus ulcers, varicose ulcers, debridement of eschar, dehiscent wounds and sunburn; promote wound healing; reduce odor from necrotic wounds

Usual Dosage Topical: Apply a minimum of twice daily or as often as necessary

Dosage Forms

Aerosol, topical: Trypsin 0.12 mg, balsam Peru 87 mg, and castor oil 788 mg per gram (120 g)
Granulex®: Trypsin 0.12 mg, balsam Peru 87 mg, and castor oil 788 mg per gram (60 g, 120 g)

Gel, topical:
Optase™: Trypsin 0.12 mg, balsam Peru 87 mg, and castor oil 788 mg per gram (95 g)

Ointment, topical:
Xenaderm™: Trypsin 90 USP units, balsam Peru 87 mg, and castor oil 788 mg per gram (30 g, 60 g)

tryptoreline *see* triptorelin *on page* 990
Trysul® ***(Discontinued)*** *see* sulfabenzamide, sulfacetamide, and sulfathiazole *on page* 926
TSH *see* thyrotropin alpha *on page* 958
TSPA *see* thiotepa *on page* 956
TST *see* tuberculin tests *on page* 993
T-Stat® ***(Discontinued)*** *see* erythromycin *on page* 368
TT *see* tetanus toxoid (adsorbed) *on page* 949
tuberculin purified protein derivative *see* tuberculin tests *on page* 993
tuberculin skin test *see* tuberculin tests *on page* 993

tuberculin tests (too BER kyoo lin tests)

Sound-Alike/Look-Alike Issues
Aplisol® may be confused with Anusol®, A.P.L.®, Aplitest®, Atropisol®
Tuberculin products may be confused with tetanus toxoid products and influenza virus vaccine. Medication errors have occurred when tuberculin skin tests (PPD) have been inadvertently administered instead of tetanus toxoid products and influenza virus vaccine. These products are refrigerated and often stored in close proximity to each other.

Synonyms mantoux; PPD; TB skin test; TST; tuberculin purified protein derivative; tuberculin skin test

U.S./Canadian Brand Names Aplisol® [US]; Tubersol® [US]

Therapeutic Category Diagnostic Agent

Use Skin test in diagnosis of tuberculosis

Usual Dosage Children and Adults: Intradermal: 0.1 mL

TST interpretation: Criteria for positive TST read at 48-72 hours (see Note for healthcare workers):
Induration ≥5 mm: Persons with HIV infection (or risk factors for HIV infection, but unknown status), recent close contact to person with known active TB, persons with chest x-ray consistent with healed TB, persons who are immunosuppressed
Induration ≥10 mm: Persons with clinical conditions which increase risk of TB infection, recent immigrants, I.V. drug users, residents and employees of high-risk settings, children <4 years of age
Induration ≥15 mm: Persons who do not meet any of the above criteria (no risk factors for TB)
Note: A two-step test is recommended when testing will be performed at regular intervals (eg, for healthcare workers). If the first test is negative, a second TST should be administered 1-3 weeks after the first test was read.

TST interpretation (CDC guidelines) in a healthcare setting:
Baseline test: ≥10 mm is positive (either first or second step)
Serial testing without known exposure: Increase of ≥10 mm is positive
Known exposure:
≥5 mm is positive in patients with baseline of 0 mm
≥10 mm is positive in patients with negative baseline or previous screening result of ≥0 mm

Read test at 48-72 hours following placement. Test results with 0 mm induration or measured induration less than the defined cutoff point are considered to signify absence of infection with *M. tuberculosis*. Test results should be documented in millimeters even if classified as negative. Erythema and redness of skin are not indicative of a positive test result.

Dosage Forms

Injection, solution:

Aplisol®, Tubersol®: 5 TU/0.1 mL (1 mL, 5 mL)

Tubersol® [US] *see* tuberculin tests *on page 993*

Tucks® [US-OTC] *see* witch hazel *on page 1023*

Tucks® Anti-Itch [US-OTC] *see* hydrocortisone (rectal) *on page 503*

Tucks® Hemorrhoidal [US-OTC] *see* pramoxine *on page 809*

Tucks® Take Alongs® [US-OTC] *see* witch hazel *on page 1023*

Tuinal® *(Discontinued)*

Tums® [US-OTC] *see* calcium carbonate *on page 170*

Tums® E-X [US-OTC] *see* calcium carbonate *on page 170*

Tums® Extra Strength Sugar Free [US-OTC] *see* calcium carbonate *on page 170*

Tums® Smoothies™ [US-OTC] *see* calcium carbonate *on page 170*

Tums® Ultra [US-OTC] *see* calcium carbonate *on page 170*

Tusal® *(Discontinued)*

Tusibron® *(Discontinued)* *see* guaifenesin *on page 473*

Tusibron-DM® *(Discontinued)* *see* guaifenesin and dextromethorphan *on page 474*

Tusnel-DM Pediatric® [US] *see* guaifenesin, pseudoephedrine, and dextromethorphan *on page 479*

Tusnel Liquid® [US] *see* guaifenesin, pseudoephedrine, and dextromethorphan *on page 479*

Tusnel Pediatric® [US] *see* guaifenesin, pseudoephedrine, and dextromethorphan *on page 479*

Tussafed® *(Discontinued)*

Tussafed® HC *(Discontinued)*

Tussafed® HCG *(Discontinued)*

Tussafin® Expectorant *(Discontinued)*

Tussend® Expectorant *(Discontinued)*

Tussend® Syrup *(Discontinued)*

Tussend® Tablet *(Discontinued)*

Tussi-12® [US] *see* carbetapentane and chlorpheniramine *on page 182*

Tussi-12® D [US] *see* carbetapentane, phenylephrine, and pyrilamine *on page 183*

Tussi-12® DS [US] *see* carbetapentane, phenylephrine, and pyrilamine *on page 183*

Tussi-12 S™ [US] *see* carbetapentane and chlorpheniramine *on page 182*

Tussi-Bid® [US] *see* guaifenesin and dextromethorphan *on page 474*

TussiCaps® [US] *see* hydrocodone and chlorpheniramine *on page 502*

Tussigon® [US] *see* hydrocodone and homatropine *on page 502*

TussiNate™ *(Discontinued)*

Tussionex® [US] *see* hydrocodone and chlorpheniramine *on page 502*

Tussi-Organidin® DM NR [US] *see* guaifenesin and dextromethorphan *on page 474*

Tussi-Organidin® DM-S NR [US] *see* guaifenesin and dextromethorphan *on page 474*

Tussi-Organidin® NR [US] *see* guaifenesin and codeine *on page 473*

Tussi-Organidin® S-NR [US] *see* guaifenesin and codeine *on page 473*

Tussizone-12 RF™ [US] *see* carbetapentane and chlorpheniramine *on page 182*

Tuss-LA® *(Discontinued)* *see* guaifenesin and pseudoephedrine *on page 477*

Tusso-C™ [US] *see* guaifenesin and codeine *on page 473*

Tusso-DF® *(Discontinued)*

Tusso™-DMR [US] *see* guaifenesin, dextromethorphan, and phenylephrine *on page 478*

Tussplex™ DM [US] *see* chlorpheniramine, phenylephrine, and dextromethorphan *on page 217*

Tustan 12S™ [US] *see* carbetapentane and chlorpheniramine *on page 182*

T-Vites [US-OTC] *see* vitamins (multiple/oral) *on page 1019*

TVP-1012 *see* rasagiline *on page 853*

Twelve Resin-K [US-OTC] *see* cyanocobalamin *on page 263*

Typherix® [Can] *see* typhoid vaccine *on page* 996
Typhim Vi® [US/Can] *see* typhoid vaccine *on page* 996

typhoid vaccine (TYE foid vak SEEN)

Synonyms Ty21a vaccine; typhoid vaccine live oral Ty21a; Vi vaccine

U.S./Canadian Brand Names Typherix® [Can]; Typhim Vi® [US/Can]; Vivotif® [US/Can]

Therapeutic Category Vaccine, Inactivated Bacteria

Use Active immunization against typhoid fever caused by *Salmonella typhi*

Not for routine vaccination. In the United States and Canada, use should be limited to:
- Travelers to areas with a prolonged risk of exposure to *S. typhi*
- Persons with intimate exposure to a *S. typhi* carrier
- Laboratory technicians with exposure to *S. typhi*
- Travelers with achlorhydria or hypochlorhydria (Canadian recommendation)

Usual Dosage Immunization:

Oral: Children ≥6 years and Adults:

Primary immunization: One capsule on alternate days (day 1, 3, 5, and 7) for a total of 4 doses; all doses should be complete at least 1 week prior to potential exposure

Booster immunization: Repeat full course of primary immunization every 5 years

I.M.: Children ≥2 years and Adults: 0.5 mL given at least 2 weeks prior to expected exposure

Reimmunization:

Typhim Vi®: 0.5 mL; optimal schedule has not been established; a single dose every 2 years is currently recommended for repeated or continued exposure

Typherix®: 0.5 mL every 3 years

Dosage Forms [CAN] = Canadian brand name

Capsule, enteric coated:

Vivotif®: Viable *S. typhi* Ty21a 2-6.8 x 10^9 colony-forming units and nonviable *S. typhi* Ty21a 5-50 x 10^9 bacterial cells [contains lactose 100-180 mg/capsule and sucrose 26-130 mg/capsule]

Injection, solution:

Typherix® [CAN]: Vi capsular polysaccharide 25 mcg/0.5 mL (0.5 mL) [derived from *S. typhi* Ty2 strain] [not available in U.S.]

Typhim Vi®: Purified Vi capsular polysaccharide 25 mcg/0.5 mL (0.5 mL, 10 mL) [derived from *S. typhi* Ty2 strain]

typhoid vaccine live oral Ty21a *see* typhoid vaccine *on page* 996
Tyrodone® Liquid *(Discontinued)*
Tysabri® [US/Can] *see* natalizumab *on page* 683
Tyvaso™ [US] *see* treprostinil *on page* 980
Tyzeka® [US] *see* telbivudine *on page* 941
Tyzine® [US] *see* tetrahydrozoline *on page* 951
Tyzine® Pediatric [US] *see* tetrahydrozoline *on page* 951
506U78 *see* nelarabine *on page* 685
U-90152S *see* delavirdine *on page* 281
UAD Otic® *(Discontinued)* *see* neomycin, polymyxin B, and hydrocortisone *on page* 688
UCB-P071 *see* cetirizine *on page* 204
UK *see* urokinase *on page* 999
UK-88,525 *see* darifenacin *on page* 277
UK-427,857 *see* maraviroc *on page* 614
UK92480 *see* sildenafil *on page* 900
UK109496 *see* voriconazole *on page* 1021
Ulcerease® [US-OTC] *see* phenol *on page* 772
Ulcidine [Can] *see* famotidine *on page* 405
Uloric® [US] *see* febuxostat *on page* 407
ULR-LA® *(Discontinued)*
Ultane® [US] *see* sevoflurane *on page* 899
Ultiva® [US/Can] *see* remifentanil *on page* 857
Ultracaine® DS [Can] *see* articaine and epinephrine *on page* 99
Ultracaine® DS Forte [Can] *see* articaine and epinephrine *on page* 99

Ultracaps MT *(Discontinued)* *see* pancrelipase *on page 746*
Ultracet® [US] *see* acetaminophen and tramadol *on page 24*
Ultra Freeda A-Free [US-OTC] *see* vitamins (multiple/oral) *on page 1019*
Ultra Freeda Iron-Free [US-OTC] *see* vitamins (multiple/oral) *on page 1019*
Ultra Freeda With Iron [US-OTC] *see* vitamins (multiple/oral) *on page 1019*
Ultram® [US] *see* tramadol *on page 975*
Ultram® ER [US] *see* tramadol *on page 975*
Ultra Mide® [US-OTC] *see* urea *on page 998*
UltraMide 25™ [Can] *see* urea *on page 998*
Ultramop™ [Can] *see* methoxsalen *on page 641*
Ultra NatalCare® [US] *see* vitamins (multiple/prenatal) *on page 1020*
Ultraprin [US-OTC] *see* ibuprofen *on page 515*
Ultraquin™ [Can] *see* hydroquinone *on page 508*
Ultrase® [US/Can] *see* pancrelipase *on page 746*
Ultrase® MT [US/Can] *see* pancrelipase *on page 746*
Ultra Tears® [US-OTC] *see* artificial tears *on page 100*
Ultravate® [US/Can] *see* halobetasol *on page 484*
Ultravist® [US] *see* iopromide *on page 540*
Umecta® [US] *see* urea *on page 998*
Unasyn® [US/Can] *see* ampicillin and sulbactam *on page 77*
Unburn® [US] *see* lidocaine *on page 584*

undecylenic acid and derivatives (un de sil EN ik AS id & dah RIV ah tivs)

Synonyms zinc undecylenate
U.S./Canadian Brand Names Fungi-Nail® [US-OTC]
Therapeutic Category Antifungal Agent
Use Treatment of athlete's foot (tinea pedis); ringworm (except nails and scalp)
Usual Dosage Topical: Children ≥2 years and Adults: Apply twice daily to affected area for 4 weeks; apply to clean, dry area
Dosage Forms
Solution, topical:
Fungi-Nail® [OTC]: Undecylenic acid 25% (29.57 mL)

Unguentine® *(Discontinued)* *see* benzocaine *on page 129*
Uni-Bent® Cough Syrup *(Discontinued)* *see* diphenhydramine *on page 315*
Uni-Cenna *(Discontinued)* *see* senna *on page 896*
Uni-Cof *(Discontinued)* *see* pseudoephedrine, dihydrocodeine, and chlorpheniramine *on page 836*
Unidet® [Can] *see* tolterodine *on page 969*
Uni-Dur® *(Discontinued)* *see* theophylline *on page 953*
Unipen® [Can] *see* nafcillin *on page 677*
Uniphyl® [US] *see* theophylline *on page 953*
Uniphyl® SRT [Can] *see* theophylline *on page 953*
Uni-Pro® *(Discontinued)* *see* ibuprofen *on page 515*
Uniretic® [US/Can] *see* moexipril and hydrochlorothiazide *on page 664*
Unisom®-2 [Can] *see* doxylamine *on page 338*
Unisom® SleepGels® Maximum Strength [US-OTC] *see* diphenhydramine *on page 315*
Unisom® SleepMelts™ [US-OTC] *see* diphenhydramine *on page 315*
Unisom® SleepTabs® [US-OTC] *see* doxylamine *on page 338*
Unithroid® [US] *see* levothyroxine *on page 583*
Unitrol® *(Discontinued)*
Uni-tussin® *(Discontinued)* *see* guaifenesin *on page 473*
Uni-tussin® DM *(Discontinued)* *see* guaifenesin and dextromethorphan *on page 474*
Univasc® [US] *see* moexipril *on page 664*
unna's boot *see* zinc gelatin *on page 1030*
unna's paste *see* zinc gelatin *on page 1030*

Urabeth® ***(Discontinued)*** *see* bethanechol *on page* *139*
Uramaxin™ [US] *see* urea *on page* *998*
Urasal® [Can] *see* methenamine *on page* *637*

urea (yoor EE a)

Synonyms carbamide

U.S./Canadian Brand Names Aquacare® [US-OTC]; Aquaphilic® With Carbamide [US-OTC]; Carmol® 10 [US-OTC]; Carmol® 20 [US-OTC]; Carmol® 40 [US]; Carmol® Deep Cleaning [US]; Cerovel™ [US]; DPM™ [US-OTC]; Gormel® [US-OTC]; Hydro 40™ [US]; Kerafoam™ [US]; Keralac™ Nailstik [US]; Keralac™ [US]; Kerol™ Redi-Cloths [US]; Kerol™ ZX [US]; Kerol™ [US]; Lanaphilic® [US-OTC]; Nutraplus® [US-OTC]; Rea-Lo® [US-OTC]; Ultra Mide® [US-OTC]; UltraMide 25™ [Can]; Umecta® [US]; Uramaxin™ [US]; Ureacin® [US-OTC]; Uremol® [Can]; Urisec® [Can]; Vanamide™ [US]

Therapeutic Category Diuretic, Osmotic; Topical Skin Product

Use Keratolytic agent to soften nails or skin; OTC: Moisturizer for dry, rough skin

Usual Dosage Topical: Adults: Hyperkeratotic conditions, dry skin: Apply 1-3 times/day

Dosage Forms

Aerosol, topical [foam]:
Hydro 40™: 40% (70 g, 150 g)
Kerafoam™: 30% (60 g)

Cloth, topical:
Kerol™ Redi-Cloths: 42% (30s)

Cream, topical: 40% (30 g, 85 g, 199 g)
Aquacare® [OTC]: 10% (75 g)
Carmol® 20 [OTC]: 20% (90 g)
Carmol® 40: 40% (30 g, 90 g, 210 g)
DPM™ [OTC]: 20% (118 g)
Gormel® [OTC]: 20% (75 g, 120 g, 454 g, 2270 g)
Keralac™: 50% (142 g, 255 g)
Nutraplus® [OTC]: 10% (90 g, 454 g)
Rea-Lo® [OTC]: 30% (60 g, 240 g)
Uramaxin™: 45% (225 g)
Ureacin®-20 [OTC]: 20% (120 g)
Vanamide™: 40% (85 g, 199 g)

Emulsion, topical:
Kerol™: 50% (283.5 g)
Umecta®: 40% (120 mL, 480 mL)

Gel, topical: 40% (15 mL)
Carmol® 40: 40% (15 mL)
Cerovel™: 40% (25 mL)
Keralac™: 50% (18 mL)
Uramaxin™: 45% (28 mL)

Lotion, topical: 40% (240 mL)
Aquacare® [OTC]: 10% (240 mL)
Carmol® 10 [OTC]: 10% (180 mL)
Carmol® 40: 40% (240 mL)
Cerovel™: 40% (325 mL)
Keralac™: 35% (207 mL, 325 mL)
Nutraplus® [OTC]: 10% (240 mL, 480 mL)
Ultra Mide® [OTC]: 25% (120 mL, 240 mL)
Ureacin®-10 [OTC]: 10% (240 mL)

Ointment, topical:
Aquaphilic® with Carbamide [OTC]: 10% (180 g, 480 g); 20% (480 g)
Keralac™: 50% (90 g)
Lanaphilic® [OTC]: 10% (454 g); 20% (454 g)

Shampoo, topical:
Carmol® Deep Cleaning: 10% (240 mL)

Solution, topical:
Keralac™ Nailstick: 50% (2.4 mL)
Kerol™ ZX: 50% (12 mL)

Suspension, topical: 50% (284 g)
Kerol™: 50% (284 g)
Umecta®: 40% (18 mL, 300 mL)

urea and hydrocortisone (yoor EE a & hye droe KOR ti sone)

Synonyms hydrocortisone and urea

U.S./Canadian Brand Names Carmol-HC® [US]; Ti-U-Lac® H [Can]; Uremol® HC [Can]

Therapeutic Category Corticosteroid, Topical

Use Inflammation of corticosteroid-responsive dermatoses

Usual Dosage Apply thin film and rub in well 1-4 times/day. Therapy should be discontinued when control is achieved; if no improvement is seen, reassessment of diagnosis may be necessary.

Dosage Forms

Cream:

Carmol-HC®: Urea 10% and hydrocortisone 1% (30 g)

urea and papain *see* papain and urea *on page* 749
urea, chlorophyllin, and papain *see* chlorophyllin, papain, and urea *on page* 211
Ureacin® [US-OTC] *see* urea *on page* 998
urea peroxide *see* carbamide peroxide *on page* 181
Urecholine® [US] *see* bethanechol *on page* 139
Uremol® [Can] *see* urea *on page* 998
Uremol® HC [Can] *see* urea and hydrocortisone *on page* 999
Urex™ [US/Can] *see* methenamine *on page* 637
Urisec® [Can] *see* urea *on page* 998
Urispas® [US/Can] *see* flavoxate *on page* 421
Uristat® *(Discontinued)* *see* phenazopyridine *on page* 770
Urocit®-K [US] *see* potassium citrate *on page* 804
Urodine® *(Discontinued)* *see* phenazopyridine *on page* 770

urofollitropin (yoor oh fol li TROE pin)

Synonyms follicle-stimulating hormone, human; FSH; hFSH

U.S./Canadian Brand Names Bravelle® [US/Can]; Fertinorm® H.P. [Can]

Therapeutic Category Gonadotropin; Ovulation Stimulator

Use Ovulation induction in patients who previously received pituitary suppression; development of multiple follicles with Assisted Reproductive Technologies (ART)

Usual Dosage Note: Dose should be individualized. Use the lowest dose consistent with the expectation of good results. Over the course of treatment, doses may vary depending on individual patient response.

Adults: Female:

Ovulation induction: I.M., SubQ: Initial: 150 int. units daily for the first 5 days of treatment. Dose adjustments ≤75-150 int. units can be made every ≥2 days; maximum daily dose: 450 int. units; treatment >12 days is not recommended. If response to follitropin is appropriate, hCG is given 1 day following the last dose. Withhold hCG if serum estradiol is >2000 pg/mL, if the ovaries are abnormally enlarged, or if abdominal pain occurs.

ART: SubQ: 225 int. units daily for the first 5 days; dose may be adjusted based on patient response, but adjustments should not be made more frequently than once every 2 days; maximum adjustment: 75-150 int. units; maximum daily dose: 450 int. units; maximum duration of treatment: 12 days. When a sufficient number of follicles of adequate size are present, the final maturation of the follicles is induced by administering hCG. Withhold hCG in cases where the ovaries are abnormally enlarged on the last day of therapy.

Dosage Forms

Injection, powder for reconstitution [human origin]:

Bravelle®: 75 int. units

urokinase (ur oh KYE nase)

Synonyms UK

U.S./Canadian Brand Names Kinlytic™ [US]

Therapeutic Category Thrombolytic Agent

Use Thrombolytic agent for the lysis of acute massive pulmonary emboli or pulmonary emboli with unstable hemodynamics

Usual Dosage I.V.: Adults: Acute pulmonary embolism: Loading: 4400 int. units/kg over 10 minutes; maintenance: 4400 int. units/kg/hour for 12 hours. To prevent recurrent thrombosis, anticoagulation treatment is recommended after the completion of urokinase infusion; if heparin is used, do not administer heparin loading dose. Do not start anticoagulation until aPTT has decreased to less than twice the normal control value.

Product Availability

Kinlytic™: ImaRx Therapeutics retired the trade name Abbokinase® for urokinase and had intended to market urokinase under the trade name Kinlytic™. As of September, 2009, Microbix Biosystems, Inc. has acquired all rights to Kinlytic™, but have not yet gained FDA approval so no product is available.

Uro-KP-Neutral® [US] *see* potassium phosphate and sodium phosphate *on page 806*

Urolene Blue® *(Discontinued)* *see* methylene blue *on page 644*

Uro-Mag® [US-OTC] *see* magnesium oxide *on page 610*

Uromax® [Can] *see* oxybutynin *on page 736*

Uromitexan [Can] *see* mesna *on page 631*

Uroplus® DS *(Discontinued)*

Uroplus® SS *(Discontinued)*

Uroxatral® [US] *see* alfuzosin *on page 46*

Urso® [Can] *see* ursodiol *on page 1000*

Urso 250® [US] *see* ursodiol *on page 1000*

ursodeoxycholic acid *see* ursodiol *on page 1000*

ursodiol (ur soe DYE ol)

Synonyms ursodeoxycholic acid

U.S./Canadian Brand Names Actigall® [US]; DOM-Ursodiol C [Can]; PHL-Ursodiol C [Can]; PMS-Ursodiol C [Can]; Urso 250® [US]; Urso Forte® [US]; Urso® DS [Can]; Urso® [Can]

Therapeutic Category Gallstone Dissolution Agent

Use Actigall®: Gallbladder stone dissolution; prevention of gallstones in obese patients experiencing rapid weight loss; Urso®: Primary biliary cirrhosis

Usual Dosage Oral: Adults:

Gallstone dissolution: 8-10 mg/kg/day in 2-3 divided doses; use beyond 24 months is not established; obtain ultrasound images at 6-month intervals for the first year of therapy; 30% of patients have stone recurrence after dissolution

Gallstone prevention: 300 mg twice daily

Primary biliary cirrhosis: 13-15 mg/kg/day in 2-4 divided doses (with food)

Dosage Forms

Capsule: 300 mg
  Actigall®: 300 mg

Tablet: 250 mg, 500 mg
  Urso 250®: 250 mg
  Urso Forte®: 500 mg

Urso® DS [Can] *see* ursodiol *on page 1000*

Urso Forte® [US] *see* ursodiol *on page 1000*

ustekinumab *(Canada only)* (yoo stek in YOO mab)

Sound-Alike/Look-Alike Issues

ustekinumab may be confused with infliximab, rituximab
Stelara® may be confused with Aldara®

Synonyms CNTO 1275

U.S./Canadian Brand Names Stelara® [Can]

Therapeutic Category Antipsoriatic Agent; Interleukin-12 Inhibitor; Interleukin-23 Inhibitor; Monoclonal Antibody

Use Treatment of moderate-to-severe chronic plaque psoriasis

Usual Dosage SubQ: Adults: Plaque psoriasis:

Initial and maintenance: **Note:** Following an interruption in therapy, retreatment may be initiated at the initial dosing interval. Consider therapy discontinuation in any patient failing to demonstrate a response after 12 weeks of therapy.

≤100 kg: 45 mg at 0- and 4 weeks, and then every 12 weeks thereafter (if inadequate response, may change to every 8 weeks)
>100 kg: 45 mg or 90 mg at 0- and 4 weeks, and then every 12 weeks thereafter (if inadequate response, may change to every 8 weeks)

Dosage Forms [CAN] = Canadian product availability
Injection, solution [preservative free]:
Stelara® [CAN]: 45 mg/0.5 mL (0.5 mL); 90 mg/1 mL (1 mL) [not available in the U.S.]

UTI Relief® [US-OTC] *see* phenazopyridine *on page 770*
Utradol™ [Can] *see* etodolac *on page 397*
Uvadex® [US/Can] *see* methoxsalen *on page 641*

vaccinia immune globulin (intravenous)
(vax IN ee a i MYUN GLOB yoo lin IN tra VEE nus)

Synonyms VIGIV
U.S./Canadian Brand Names CNJ-016™ [US]
Therapeutic Category Immune Globulin
Use Treatment of infectious complications of smallpox (vaccinia virus) vaccination, such as eczema vaccinatum, progressive vaccinia, and severe generalized vaccinia; treatment of vaccinia infections in individuals with concurrent skin conditions or accidental virus exposure to eyes (except vaccinia keratitis), mouth, or other areas where viral infection would pose significant risk
Usual Dosage I.V.: Adults:
CNJ-016™ (Cangene product): 6000 units/kg; 9000 units/kg may be considered if patient does not respond to initial dose.
DynPort product: Total dose: 2 mL/kg (100 mg/kg); higher doses (200-500 mg/kg) may be considered if patient does not respond to initial recommended dose (sucrose-related renal impairment is worsened at doses ≥400 mg/kg)
Dosage Forms Injection, solution [preservative free; solvent-detergent treated]:
CNJ-016™: Cangene product: ≥50,000 units/15 mL (15 mL)
DynPort product: 50 mg/mL (50 mL)

vaccinia vaccine *see* smallpox vaccine *on page 906*
Vagifem® [US/Can] *see* estradiol *on page 373*
Vagi-Gard® [US-OTC] *see* povidone-iodine *on page 807*
Vagistat®-1 [US-OTC] *see* tioconazole *on page 963*
Vagitrol® *(Discontinued)*

valacyclovir (val ay SYE kloe veer)

Sound-Alike/Look-Alike Issues
valacyclovir may be confused with acyclovir, valganciclovir, vancomycin
Valtrex® may be confused with Valcyte™, Zovirax®
Synonyms valacyclovir hydrochloride
Tall-Man val**ACY**clovir
U.S./Canadian Brand Names Apo-Valacyclovir® [Can]; PMS-Valacyclovir [Can]; Riva-Valacyclovir [Can]; Valtrex® [US/Can]
Therapeutic Category Antiviral Agent
Use Treatment of herpes zoster (shingles) in immunocompetent patients; treatment of first-episode and recurrent genital herpes; suppression of recurrent genital herpes and reduction of heterosexual transmission of genital herpes in immunocompetent patients; suppression of genital herpes in HIV-infected individuals; treatment of herpes labialis (cold sores); chickenpox in immunocompetent children
Usual Dosage Oral:
Children 2 to <18 years: Chickenpox: 20 mg/kg/dose 3 times/day for 5 days (maximum: 1 g 3 times/day)
Children ≥12 and Adults: Herpes labialis (cold sores): 2 g twice daily for 1 day (separate doses by ~12 hours)
Adults:
Herpes zoster (shingles): 1 g 3 times/day for 7 days
Genital herpes:
Initial episode: 1 g twice daily for 10 days
Recurrent episode: 500 mg twice daily for 3 days
Reduction of transmission: 500 mg once daily (source partner)

Suppressive therapy:
Immunocompetent patients: 1000 mg once daily (500 mg once daily in patients with <9 recurrences per year)
HIV-infected patients (CD4 ≥100 cells/mm^3): 500 mg twice daily

Dosage Forms

Caplet:
Valtrex®: 500 mg, 1000 mg

valacyclovir hydrochloride *see* valacyclovir *on page 1001*

Valcyte® [US/Can] *see* valganciclovir *on page 1002*

23-valent pneumococcal polysaccharide vaccine *see* pneumococcal polysaccharide vaccine (polyvalent) *on page 794*

valganciclovir (val gan SYE kloh veer)

Sound-Alike/Look-Alike Issues
valganciclovir may be confused with valacyclovir
Valcyte® may be confused with Valium®, Valtrex®

Synonyms valganciclovir hydrochloride

Tall-Man val**GANCI**clovir

U.S./Canadian Brand Names Valcyte® [US/Can]

Therapeutic Category Antiviral Agent

Use Treatment of cytomegalovirus (CMV) retinitis in patients with acquired immunodeficiency syndrome (AIDS); prevention of CMV disease in high-risk patients (donor CMV positive/recipient CMV negative) undergoing kidney, heart, or kidney/pancreas transplantation

Usual Dosage Oral: Adults:
CMV retinitis:
Induction: 900 mg twice daily for 21 days (with food)
Maintenance: Following induction treatment, or for patients with inactive CMV retinitis who require maintenance therapy: Recommended dose: 900 mg once daily (with food)
Prevention of CMV disease following transplantation: 900 mg once daily (with food) beginning within 10 days of transplantation; continue therapy until 100 days posttransplantation

Product Availability
Valcyte® oral solution: FDA approved August 2009; availability expected January 2010

Dosage Forms

Tablet, oral: 450 mg

valganciclovir hydrochloride *see* valganciclovir *on page 1002*

Valisone® Scalp Lotion [Can] *see* betamethasone (topical) *on page 138*

Valisone® Topical *(Discontinued)*

Valium® [US/Can] *see* diazepam *on page 301*

Valorin [US-OTC] *see* acetaminophen *on page 19*

Valorin Extra [US-OTC] *see* acetaminophen *on page 19*

valproate semisodium *see* valproic acid and derivatives *on page 1002*

valproate sodium *see* valproic acid and derivatives *on page 1002*

valproic acid *see* valproic acid and derivatives *on page 1002*

valproic acid and derivatives (val PROE ik AS id & dah RIV ah tives)

Sound-Alike/Look-Alike Issues
Depakene® may be confused with Depakote®
Depakote® may be confused with Depakene®, Depakote® ER, Senokot®
Depakote® ER may be confused with Depakote®, divalproex enteric coated

Synonyms 2-propylpentanoic acid; 2-propylvaleric acid; dipropylacetic acid; divalproex sodium; DPA; valproate semisodium; valproate sodium; valproic acid

U.S./Canadian Brand Names Alti-Divalproex [Can]; Apo-Divalproex® [Can]; Apo-Valproic® [Can]; Depacon® [US]; Depakene® [US/Can]; Depakote® ER [US]; Depakote® Sprinkle [US]; Depakote® [US]; Dom-Divalproex [Can]; Epival® I.V. [Can]; Gen-Divalproex [Can]; Novo-Divalproex [Can]; Nu-Divalproex [Can]; PHL-Divalproex [Can]; PHL-Valproic Acid E.C. [Can]; PHL-Valproic Acid [Can]; PMS-Valproic Acid E.C. [Can]; PMS-Valproic Acid [Can]; ratio-Valproic ECC [Can]; ratio-Valproic [Can]; Rhoxal-valproic [Can]; Sandoz-Valporic [Can]; Stavzor™ [US]

Therapeutic Category Anticonvulsant

Use

Depacon®, Depakene®, Depakote®, Depakote® ER, Depakote® Sprinkle, Stavzor™: Monotherapy and adjunctive therapy in the treatment of patients with complex partial seizures; monotherapy and adjunctive therapy of simple and complex absence seizures; adjunctive therapy in patients with multiple seizure types that include absence seizures

Depakote®, Depakote® ER, Stavzor™: Mania associated with bipolar disorder; migraine prophylaxis

Usual Dosage

Seizure disorders: **Note:** Administer doses >250 mg/day in divided doses.

Oral:

Simple and complex absence seizures: Children and Adults: Initial: 15 mg/kg/day; increase by 5-10 mg/kg/day at weekly intervals until therapeutic levels are achieved; maximum: 60 mg/kg/day. Larger maintenance doses may be required in younger children.

Complex partial seizures: Children ≥10 years and Adults: Initial: 10-15 mg/kg/day; increase by 5-10 mg/kg/day at weekly intervals until therapeutic levels are achieved; maximum: 60 mg/kg/day. Larger maintenance doses may be required in younger children.

Note: Regular release and delayed release formulations are usually given in 2-4 divided doses/day; extended release formulation (Depakote® ER) is usually given once daily. Conversion to Depakote® ER from a stable dose of Depakote® may require an increase in the total daily dose between 8% and 20% to maintain similar serum concentrations. Depakote® ER is not recommended for use in children <10 years of age.

I.V.: Administer as a 60-minute infusion (≤20 mg/minute) with the same frequency as oral products; switch patient to oral products as soon as possible. Rapid infusions ≤45 mg/kg over 5-10 minutes (1.5-6 mg/kg/minute) were generally well tolerated in a clinical trial.

Mania: Adults: Oral:

Depakote® tablet, Stavzor™: Initial: 750 mg/day in divided doses; dose should be adjusted as rapidly as possible to desired clinical effect; maximum recommended dosage: 60 mg/kg/day

Depakote® ER: Initial: 25 mg/kg/day given once daily; dose should be adjusted as rapidly as possible to desired clinical effect; maximum recommended dose: 60 mg/kg/day.

Migraine prophylaxis:

Children ≥12 years (Stavzor™): 250 mg twice daily; adjust dose based on patient response, up to 1000 mg/day

Children ≥16 years and Adults: Oral:

Depakote® tablet: 250 mg twice daily; adjust dose based on patient response, up to 1000 mg/day

Depakote® ER: 500 mg once daily for 7 days, then increase to 1000 mg once daily; adjust dose based on patient response; usual dosage range 500-1000 mg/day

Dosage Forms Strength expressed as valproic acid.

Capsule, softgel: 250 mg

Depakene®: 250 mg

Capsule, softgel, delayed release:

Stavzor™: 125 mg, 250 mg, 500 mg

Capsule, sprinkles: 125 mg

Depakote® Sprinkle: 125 mg

Injection, solution: 100 mg/mL (5 mL)

Depacon®: 100 mg/mL (5 mL)

Syrup: 250 mg/5 mL

Depakene®: 250 mg/5 mL

Tablet, delayed release: 125 mg, 250 mg, 500 mg

Depakote®: 125 mg, 250 mg, 500 mg

Tablet, extended release: 250 mg, 500 mg

Depakote® ER: 250 mg, 500 mg

valrubicin (val ROO bi sin)

Sound-Alike/Look-Alike Issues

valrubicin may be confused with DAUNOrubicin, DOXOrubicin, epirubicin, IDArubicin

Valstar® may be confused with valsartan

Synonyms *N*-trifluoroacetyladriamycin-14-valerate; AD32

U.S./Canadian Brand Names Valstar® [US]; Valtaxin® [Can]

Therapeutic Category Antineoplastic Agent, Anthracycline

Use Intravesical therapy of BCG-refractory bladder carcinoma *in situ*

Usual Dosage Intravesical: Adults: Bladder cancer: 800 mg once weekly (retain for 2 hours) for 6 weeks

Dosage Forms

Injection, solution [preservative free]:

Valstar®: 40 mg/mL (5 mL)

valsartan (val SAR tan)

Sound-Alike/Look-Alike Issues

valsartan may be confused with losartan, Valstar™

Diovan® may be confused with Darvon®, Dioval®, Zyban®

U.S./Canadian Brand Names Diovan® [US/Can]

Therapeutic Category Angiotensin II Receptor Antagonist

Use Alone or in combination with other antihypertensive agents in the treatment of essential hypertension; reduction of cardiovascular mortality in patients with left ventricular dysfunction postmyocardial infarction; treatment of heart failure (NYHA Class II-IV)

Usual Dosage Oral:

Hypertension:

Children 6-16 years: Initial: 1.3 mg/kg once daily (maximum: 40 mg/day); dose may be increased to achieve desired effect; doses >2.7 mg/kg (maximum: 160 mg) have not been studied

Adults: Initial: 80 mg or 160 mg once daily (in patients who are not volume depleted); dose may be increased to achieve desired effect; maximum recommended dose: 320 mg/day

Heart failure: Adults: Initial: 40 mg twice daily; titrate dose to 80-160 mg twice daily, as tolerated; maximum daily dose: 320 mg

Left ventricular dysfunction after MI: Adults: Initial: 20 mg twice daily; titrate dose to target of 160 mg twice daily as tolerated; may initiate ≥12 hours following MI

Dosage Forms

Tablet:

Diovan®: 40 mg [scored]

Diovan®: 80 mg, 160 mg, 320 mg

valsartan and amlodipine *see* amlodipine and valsartan *on page 68*

valsartan and hydrochlorothiazide (val SAR tan & hye droe klor oh THYE a zide)

Sound-Alike/Look-Alike Issues

Diovan® may be confused with Darvon®, Dioval®, Zyban®

Synonyms hydrochlorothiazide and valsartan

U.S./Canadian Brand Names Diovan HCT® [US/Can]

Therapeutic Category Antihypertensive Agent, Combination

Use Treatment of hypertension

Usual Dosage Oral: Dose is individualized; combination product may be used as initial therapy or substituted for individual components in patients currently maintained on both agents separately or in patients not adequately controlled with monotherapy (using one of the agents or an agent within same antihypertensive class).

Adults: Hypertension:

Initial therapy: Valsartan 160 mg and hydrochlorothiazide 12.5 mg once daily; dose may be titrated after 1-2 weeks of therapy. Maximum recommended daily doses: Valsartan 320 mg; hydrochlorothiazide 25 mg.

Add-on/replacement therapy: Valsartan 80-160 mg and hydrochlorthiazide 12.5-25 mg once daily; dose may be titrated after 3-4 weeks of therapy. Maximum recommended daily dose: Valsartan 320 mg; hydrochlorothiazide 25 mg.

Dosage Forms

Tablet:

Diovan HCT®: 80 mg/12.5 mg: Valsartan 80 mg and hydrochlorothiazide 12.5 mg; 160 mg/12.5 mg: Valsartan 160 mg and hydrochlorothiazide 12.5 mg; 160 mg/25 mg: Valsartan 160 mg and hydrochlorothiazide 25 mg; 320 mg/12.5 mg: Valsartan 320 mg and hydrochlorothiazide 12.5 mg; 320 mg/25 mg: Valsartan 320 mg and hydrochlorothiazide 25 mg

valsartan, hydrochlorothiazide, and amlodipine *see* amlodipine, valsartan, and hydrochlorothiazide *on page 69*

Valstar® [US] *see* valrubicin *on page 1003*

Valtaxin® [Can] *see* valrubicin *on page 1003*

Valtrex® [US/Can] *see* valacyclovir *on page 1001*

Vamate® Oral ***(Discontinued)*** *see* hydroxyzine *on page 511*
Vanamide™ [US] *see* urea *on page 998*
Vanatrip® ***(Discontinued)*** *see* amitriptyline *on page 65*
Vancenase® AQ 84 mcg ***(Discontinued)*** *see* beclomethasone *on page 125*
Vancenase® Pockethaler® ***(Discontinued)*** *see* beclomethasone *on page 125*
Vanceril® AEM [Can] *see* beclomethasone *on page 125*
Vanceril® ***(Discontinued)*** *see* beclomethasone *on page 125*
Vancocin® [US/Can] *see* vancomycin *on page 1005*

vancomycin (van koe MYE sin)

Sound-Alike/Look-Alike Issues

vancomycin may be confused with clindamycin, gentamicin, tobramycin, valacyclovir, vecuronium, Vibramycin®

I.V. vancomycin may be confused with Invanz®

Synonyms vancomycin hydrochloride

U.S./Canadian Brand Names Vancocin® [US/Can]

Therapeutic Category Antibiotic, Miscellaneous

Use Treatment of patients with infections caused by staphylococcal species and streptococcal species; used orally for staphylococcal enterocolitis or for antibiotic-associated pseudomembranous colitis produced by *C. difficile*

Usual Dosage

Usual dosage range:

Infants >1 month and Children: I.V.: 10-15 mg/kg every 6 hours

Adults:

I.V.: 2-3 g/day (or 30-60 mg/kg/day) in divided doses every 8-12 hours; **Note:** Dose requires adjustment in renal impairment

Oral: 500-1000 mg/day in divided doses every 6 hours

Indication-specific dosing:

Infants >1 month and Children:

Colitis *(C. difficile)*, enterocolitis *(S. aureus)*: Oral: 40 mg/kg/day in 3-4 divided doses added to fluids for 7-10 days (maximum: 2000 mg/day)

Meningitis/CNS infection:

I.V.: 15 mg/kg every 6 hours

Intrathecal: 5-20 mg/day

Prophylaxis against infective endocarditis: I.V.:

Dental, oral, or upper respiratory tract surgery: 20 mg/kg 1 hour prior to the procedure. **Note:** American Heart Association (AHA) guidelines now recommend prophylaxis only in patients undergoing invasive procedures and in whom underlying cardiac conditions may predispose to a higher risk of adverse outcomes should infection occur.

GI/GU procedure: 20 mg/kg plus gentamicin 2 mg/kg 1 hour prior to surgery. **Note:** As of April 2007, routine prophylaxis no longer recommended by the AHA.

Susceptible gram-positive infections: I.V.: 10 mg/kg every 6 hours

Adults: Initial intravenous dosing should be based on actual body weight; subsequent dosing adjusted based on serum trough vancomycin concentrations.

Complicated infections in seriously-ill patients: I.V.: Loading dose: 25-30 mg/kg (based on actual body weight) may be used to rapidly achieve target concentration; then 15-20 mg/kg/dose every 8-12 hours.

Catheter-related infections: Antibiotic lock technique: 2 mg/mL ± 10 units heparin/mL **or** 2.5 mg/mL ± 2500 **or** 5000 units heparin/mL **or** 5 mg/mL ± 5000 units heparin/mL (preferred regimen); instill into catheter port with a volume sufficient to fill the catheter (2-5 mL). **Note:** May use SWFI/NS or D_5W as diluents. Do not mix with any other solutions. Dwell times generally should not exceed 48 hours before renewal of lock solution. Remove lock solution prior to catheter use then replace.

Colitis *(C. difficile)*, enterocolitis *(S. aureus)*: Oral: 500-2000 mg/day in 3-4 divided doses for 7-10 days (usual dose: 125-250 mg every 6 hours)

Hospital-acquired pneumonia (HAP): I.V.: 15 mg/kg/dose every 12 hours

Meningitis *(Pneumococcus* or *Staphylococcus)*:

I.V.: 30-60 mg/kg/day in divided doses every 8-12 hours **or** 500-750 mg every 6 hours (with third-generation cephalosporin for PCN-resistant *Streptococcus pneumoniae*)

Intrathecal: 5-20 mg/day

Prophylaxis against infective endocarditis: I.V.:

Dental, oral, or upper respiratory tract surgery: 1 g 1 hour before surgery. **Note:** AHA guidelines now recommend prophylaxis only in patients undergoing invasive procedures and in whom underlying cardiac conditions may predispose to a higher risk of adverse outcomes should infection occur

GI/GU procedure: 1 g plus 1.5 mg/kg gentamicin 1 hour prior to surgery. **Note:** As of April 2007, routine prophylaxis no longer recommended by the AHA.

Susceptible (MIC ≤1 mcg/mL) gram-positive infections: I.V.: 15-20 mg/kg/dose (usual: 750-1500 mg) every 8-12 hours

Note: If MIC ≥2 mcg/mL, the targeted AUC:MIC >400 is not achievable with conventional dosing methods in patients with normal renal function and alternative therapies are recommended.

Dosage Forms

Capsule:

Vancocin®: 125 mg, 250 mg

Infusion [premixed in iso-osmotic dextrose]:

Vancocin®: 500 mg (100 mL); 1 g (200 mL)

Injection, powder for reconstitution: 500 mg, 1 g, 5 g, 10 g

vancomycin hydrochloride *see* vancomycin *on page 1005*

Vandazole® [US] *see* metronidazole *on page 651*

Vanex Forte™-D *(Discontinued)* *see* chlorpheniramine, phenylephrine, and methscopolamine *on page 218*

Vanex-HD® *(Discontinued)* *see* phenylephrine, hydrocodone, and chlorpheniramine *on page 778*

Vaniqa™ [US/Can] *see* eflornithine *on page 349*

Vanos™ [US] *see* fluocinonide *on page 429*

Vanoxide® *(Discontinued)* *see* benzoyl peroxide *on page 132*

Vanoxide-HC® [US/Can] *see* benzoyl peroxide and hydrocortisone *on page 134*

Vanquish® Extra Strength Pain Reliever [US-OTC] *see* acetaminophen, aspirin, and caffeine *on page 24*

Vansil™ *(Discontinued)*

Vantin® [US/Can] *see* cefpodoxime *on page 195*

Vaponefrin® *(Discontinued)* *see* epinephrine *on page 358*

Vaprisol® [US] *see* conivaptan *on page 256*

VAQTA® [US/Can] *see* hepatitis A vaccine *on page 489*

VAR *see* varicella virus vaccine *on page 1007*

vardenafil (var DEN a fil)

Sound-Alike/Look-Alike Issues

vardenafil may be confused with sildenafil, tadalafil

Levitra® may be confused with Kaletra®, Lexiva®

Synonyms vardenafil hydrochloride

U.S./Canadian Brand Names Levitra® [US/Can]

Therapeutic Category Phosphodiesterase (Type 5) Enzyme Inhibitor

Use Treatment of erectile dysfunction (ED)

Usual Dosage Oral: Adults: Erectile dysfunction: 10 mg 60 minutes prior to sexual activity; dosing range: 5-20 mg; to be given as one single dose and not given more than once daily

Dosage Forms

Tablet:

Levitra®: 2.5 mg, 5 mg, 10 mg, 20 mg

vardenafil hydrochloride *see* vardenafil *on page 1006*

varenicline (var e NI kleen)

Synonyms varenicline tartrate

U.S./Canadian Brand Names Champix® [Can]; Chantix® [US]

Therapeutic Category Partial Nicotine Agonist

Use Treatment to aid in smoking cessation

Usual Dosage Oral: Adults:

Initial:

Days 1-3: 0.5 mg once daily

Days 4-7: 0.5 mg twice daily

Maintenance (≥ Day 8): 1 mg twice daily

Note: Start 1 week before target quit date. Patients who cannot tolerate adverse events may require temporary reduction in dose. If patient successfully quits smoking during the 12 weeks, may continue for another 12 weeks to help maintain success. If not successful in first 12 weeks, then stop medication and reassess factors contributing to failure.

Dosage Forms

Tablet:

Chantix®: 0.5 mg, 1 mg

Combination package, oral [dose-pack]:

Chantix®:

Tablet, oral: 0.5 mg (11)

Tablet, oral: 1 mg (42)

varenicline tartrate *see* varenicline *on page 1006*

Varibar® Honey [US] *see* barium *on page 122*

Varibar® Nectar [US] *see* barium *on page 122*

Varibar® Pudding [US] *see* barium *on page 122*

Varibar® Thin Honey [US] *see* barium *on page 122*

Varibar® Thin Liquid [US] *see* barium *on page 122*

varicella, measles, mumps, and rubella vaccine *see* measles, mumps, rubella, and varicella virus vaccine *on page 616*

varicella virus vaccine (var i SEL a VYE rus vak SEEN)

Sound-Alike/Look-Alike Issues

varicella virus vaccine has been given in error (instead of the indicated varicella immune globulin) to pregnant women exposed to varicella

Synonyms chickenpox vaccine; VAR; varicella-zoster virus (VZV) vaccine (varicella); VZV vaccine (varicella)

U.S./Canadian Brand Names Varilrix® [Can]; Varivax® III [Can]; Varivax® [US]

Therapeutic Category Vaccine, Live Virus

Use Immunization against varicella in children ≥12 months of age and adults

The ACIP recommends vaccination for all children, adolescents, and adults who do not have evidence of immunity. Vaccination is especially important for:

- Persons with close contact to those at high risk for severe disease
- Persons living or working in environments where transmission is likely (teachers, child-care workers, residents and staff of institutional settings)
- Persons in environments where transmission has been reported
- Nonpregnant women of childbearing age
- Adolescents and adults in households with children
- International travelers

Postexposure prophylaxis: Vaccination within 3 days (possibly 5 days) after exposure to rash is effective in preventing illness or modifying severity of disease

Usual Dosage SubQ:

Children 12 months to 12 years: 0.5 mL; a second dose may be administered ≥3 months later

Note: The ACIP recommends the routine childhood vaccination be 2 doses, with the first dose administered at 12-15 months of age. School age children should receive the second dose at 4-6 years of age, but it may be administered earlier provided ≥3 months have elapsed after the first dose. All children and adolescents who received only 1 dose of vaccine should receive a second dose.

Children ≥13 years to Adults: 2 doses of 0.5 mL separated by 4-8 weeks

Dosage Forms [CAN] = Canadian brand name

Injection, powder for reconstitution [preservative free]:

Varivax®: 1350 plaque-forming units (PFU)

Varivax® III [CAN]: 1350 plaque-forming units (PFU) [not available in the U.S.]

Injection, powder for reconstitution:

Valrilix® [CAN]: $10^{3.3}$ plaque-forming units (PFU) [not available in the U.S.]

varicella-zoster immune globulin (human)

(var i SEL a- ZOS ter i MYUN GLOB yoo lin HYU man)

Sound-Alike/Look-Alike Issues

varicella virus vaccine has been given in error (instead of the indicated varicella immune globulin) to pregnant women exposed to varicella.

Synonyms VZIG

U.S./Canadian Brand Names VariZIG™ [Can]

Therapeutic Category Immune Globulin

Use In pregnant women, for the prevention or reduction in severity of maternal infection within 4 days of exposure to the varicella zoster virus.

Usual Dosage I.M., I.V.: Adults: Prevention or reduction of maternal infection: 125 int. units/10 kg (minimum dose: 125 int. units; maximum dose: 625 int. units). Administer within 96 hours of exposure.

Dosage Forms [CAN = Canadian brand name]

Injection, powder for reconstitution [preservative free]:

VariZIG™ [CAN]: 125 int. units [package with diluent] [available in the U.S under expanded access protocol]

varicella-zoster virus (VZV) vaccine (varicella) *see* varicella virus vaccine *on page* 1007
varicella-zoster (VZV) vaccine (zoster) *see* zoster vaccine *on page* 1035
Varilrix® [Can] *see* varicella virus vaccine *on page* 1007
Varivax® [US] *see* varicella virus vaccine *on page* 1007
Varivax® III [Can] *see* varicella virus vaccine *on page* 1007
VariZIG™ [Can] *see* varicella-zoster immune globulin (human) *on page* 1008
Vaseretic® [US/Can] *see* enalapril and hydrochlorothiazide *on page* 353
VasoClear® *(Discontinued)* *see* naphazoline *on page* 680
Vasocon® [Can] *see* naphazoline *on page* 680
Vasocon®-A *(Discontinued)*
Vasocon Regular® Ophthalmic *(Discontinued)* *see* naphazoline *on page* 680
Vasodilan® *(Discontinued)* *see* isoxsuprine *on page* 552

vasopressin (vay soe PRES in)

Synonyms 8-arginine vasopressin; ADH; antidiuretic hormone

U.S./Canadian Brand Names Pressyn® AR [Can]; Pressyn® [Can]

Therapeutic Category Hormone, Posterior Pituitary

Use Treatment of diabetes insipidus; differential diagnosis of diabetes insipidus

Usual Dosage I.M., SubQ: Diabetes insipidus: **Note:** Highly variable dosage; titrated based on serum and urine sodium and osmolality in addition to fluid balance and urine output; vasopressin rarely used for this indication; other therapies are available.

Children: 2.5-10 units 2-4 times/day as needed

Adults: 5-10 units 2-3 times/day as needed

Dosage Forms

Injection, solution: 20 units/mL (0.5 mL, 1 mL, 10 mL)

Vasotec® [US/Can] *see* enalapril *on page* 352
Vasotec® I.V. [Can] *see* enalapril *on page* 352
Vasovist® [Can] *see* gadofosveset *(Canada only) on page* 452
Vaxigrip® [Can] *see* influenza virus vaccine *on page* 528
VaZol™ [US] *see* brompheniramine *on page* 149
VCF™ [US-OTC] *see* nonoxynol 9 *on page* 703
Vectibix® [US/Can] *see* panitumumab *on page* 748
Vectical™ [US] *see* calcitriol *on page* 168
Vectrin® *(Discontinued)* *see* minocycline *on page* 659

vecuronium (vek ue ROE nee um)

Sound-Alike/Look-Alike Issues

vecuronium may be confused with vancomycin

Norcuron® may be confused with Narcan®

Synonyms ORG NC 45

U.S./Canadian Brand Names Norcuron® [Can]

Therapeutic Category Skeletal Muscle Relaxant

Use To facilitate endotracheal intubation and to relax skeletal muscles during surgery; to facilitate mechanical ventilation in ICU patients; does not relieve pain or produce sedation

Usual Dosage Administer I.V.; dose to effect; doses will vary due to interpatient variability:

Children ≥1 year and Adults: Surgical relaxation: **Note:** Children 1-10 years may require slightly higher initial doses and more frequent supplementation. For obese (≥130% of IBW) adult patients, may use ideal body weight (IBW); onset time may be slightly delayed using IBW.

Tracheal intubation: I.V.: Initial: 0.08-0.1 mg/kg. **Note:** If intubation is performed using succinylcholine (not preferred agent in pediatric patients), the initial dose of vecuronium may be reduced to 0.04-0.06 mg/kg with inhalation anesthesia and 0.05-0.06 mg/kg with balanced anesthesia. Inhaled anesthetic agents prolong the duration of action of vecuronium.

Pretreatment/priming: Adults: 10% of intubating dose given 3-5 minutes before intubating dose

Maintenance for continued surgical relaxation: Intermittent dosing (see "Note"): 0.01-0.015 mg/kg administered at 25% recovery of control T_1 or continuous infusion: Initial: 1 mcg/kg/minute only after early evidence of spontaneous recovery of neuromuscular function. Infusion rates range: 0.8-1.2 mcg/kg/minute.

Note: Use lower end of the dosing range when anesthesia is maintained with an inhaled anesthetic agent, with the redosing interval guided by monitoring with a peripheral nerve stimulator.

Adults:

ICU paralysis (eg, facilitate mechanical ventilation) in selected adequately sedated patients: Initial bolus dose: 0.08-0.1 mg/kg, then a continuous I.V. infusion of 0.8-1.7 mcg/kg/minute; monitor depth of blockade every 1-2 hours initially until stable dose, then every 8-12 hours

Dosage adjustment: Adjust rate of administration in increments of 0.3 mcg/kg/minute or by 50% reductions of previous dose according to peripheral nerve stimulation response (eg, train-of-four [TOF] count) or desired clinical response as long as TOF count >1/4 is present. If no response on TOF, discontinue infusion and reinitiate when TOF count ≥1/4 occurs.

Note: When possible, minimize depth and duration of paralysis. Stopping the infusion daily for some time until forced to restart based on patient condition is recommended to reduce post-paralytic complications (eg, acute quadriplegic myopathy syndrome [AQMS]).

Intermittent bolus dosing: 0.1-0.2 mg/kg/dose; may be repeated when TOF count >1/4

Dosage Forms

Injection, powder for reconstitution: 10 mg, 20 mg

Veg-Pancreatin 4X [US-OTC] *see* pancreatin *on page 746*

Velban® *(Discontinued)* *see* vinblastine *on page 1013*

Velcade® [US/Can] *see* bortezomib *on page 146*

Velivet™ [US] *see* ethinyl estradiol and desogestrel *on page 383*

Velosulin® BR (Buffered) *(Discontinued)*

venlafaxine (ven la FAX een)

Sound-Alike/Look-Alike Issues

Effexor® may be confused with Effexor XR®

Effexor XR® may be confused with Effexor®

U.S./Canadian Brand Names CO Venlafaxine XR [Can]; Effexor XR® [US/Can]; Effexor® [US]; GEN-Venlafaxine XR [Can]; Mylan-Venlafaxine XR [Can]; Novo-Venlafaxine XR [Can]; PMS-Venlafaxine XR [Can]; ratio-Venlafaxine XR [Can]; Riva-Venlafaxine XR [Can]; Sandoz-Venlafaxine XR [Can]

Therapeutic Category Antidepressant, Phenethylamine

Use Treatment of major depressive disorder, generalized anxiety disorder (GAD), social anxiety disorder (social phobia), panic disorder

Usual Dosage Oral: Adults:

Depression:

Immediate-release tablets: 75 mg/day, administered in 2 or 3 divided doses, taken with food; dose may be increased in 75 mg/day increments at intervals of at least 4 days, up to 225-375 mg/day

Extended-release capsules or tablets: 75 mg once daily taken with food; for some new patients, it may be desirable to start at 37.5 mg/day for 4-7 days before increasing to 75 mg once daily; dose may be increased by up to 75 mg/day increments every 4 days as tolerated, up to a recommended maximum of 225 mg/day

Generalized anxiety disorder: Extended-release capsules: 75 mg once daily taken with food; for some new patients, it may be desirable to start at 37.5 mg/day for 4-7 days before increasing to 75 mg once daily; dose may be increased by up to 75 mg/day increments every 4 days as tolerated, up to a maximum of 225 mg/day

Panic disorder: Extended-release capsules: 37.5 mg once daily for 1 week; may increase to 75 mg daily, with subsequent weekly increases of 75 mg/day up to a maximum of 225 mg/day.

Social anxiety disorder:

Extended-release capsules: 75 mg once daily taken with food; for some new patients, it may be desirable to start at 37.5 mg/day for 4-7 days before increasing to 75 mg once daily; dose may be increased by up to 75 mg/day increments every 4 days as tolerated, up to a maximum of 225 mg/day

Extended release tablets: 75 mg once daily taken with food (maximum: 75 mg/day); no evidence that doses >75 mg/day offer any additional benefit

Note: When discontinuing this medication after more than 1 week of treatment, it is generally recommended that the dose be tapered. If venlafaxine is used for 6 weeks or longer, the dose should be tapered over 2 weeks when discontinuing its use.

Dosage Forms

Capsule, extended release:

Effexor XR®: 37.5 mg, 75 mg, 150 mg

Tablet: 25 mg, 37.5 mg, 50 mg, 75 mg, 100 mg

Effexor®: 25 mg, 37.5 mg, 50 mg

Tablet, extended release: 37.5 mg, 75 mg, 150 mg, 225 mg

Venofer® [US/Can] *see* iron sucrose *on page 547*

Venoglobulin®-I *(Discontinued)* *see* immune globulin (intravenous) *on page 523*

Venoglobulin®-S *(Discontinued)* *see* immune globulin (intravenous) *on page 523*

Ventavis® [US] *see* iloprost *on page 519*

Ventolin® [Can] *see* albuterol *on page 41*

Ventolin® *(Discontinued)* *see* albuterol *on page 41*

Ventolin® Diskus [Can] *see* albuterol *on page 41*

Ventolin® HFA [US/Can] *see* albuterol *on page 41*

Ventolin® Inhaler Aerosol *(Discontinued)* *see* albuterol *on page 41*

Ventolin® I.V. Infusion [Can] *see* albuterol *on page 41*

Ventrodisk [Can] *see* albuterol *on page 41*

VePesid® *(Discontinued)* *see* etoposide *on page 398*

Veracolate [US-OTC] *see* bisacodyl *on page 142*

verapamil (ver AP a mil)

Sound-Alike/Look-Alike Issues

Calan® may be confused with Colace®, diltiazem

Covera-HS® may be confused with Provera®

Isoptin® may be confused with Isopto® Tears

Verelan® may be confused with Virilon®, Voltaren®

Synonyms iproveratril hydrochloride; verapamil hydrochloride

U.S./Canadian Brand Names Apo-Verap® SR [Can]; Apo-Verap® [Can]; Calan® SR [US]; Calan® [US/Can]; Chronovera® [Can]; Covera-HS® [US/Can]; Covera® [Can]; Dom-Verapamil SR [Can]; Gen-Verapamil SR [Can]; Gen-Verapamil [Can]; Isoptin® SR [US/Can]; Med-Verapamil [Can]; Mylan-Verapamil SR [Can]; Mylan-Verapamil [Can]; Novo-Veramil SR [Can]; Novo-Veramil [Can]; Nu-Verap SR [Can]; Nu-Verap [Can]; PHL-Verapamil [Can]; PMS-Verapamil SR [Can]; PRO-Verapamil SR [Can]; Riva-Verapamil SR [Can]; Verapamil Hydrochloride Injection, USP [Can]; Verelan SRC [Can]; Verelan® PM [US]; Verelan® [US]; ZYM-Verapamil SR [Can]

Therapeutic Category Antiarrhythmic Agent, Class IV; Calcium Channel Blocker

Use Orally for treatment of angina pectoris (vasospastic, chronic stable, unstable) and hypertension; I.V. for supraventricular tachyarrhythmias (PSVT, atrial fibrillation, atrial flutter)

Usual Dosage

Children: SVT: I.V.:

<1 year: 0.1-0.2 mg/kg over 2 minutes; repeat every 30 minutes as needed

1-15 years: 0.1-0.3 mg/kg over 2 minutes; maximum: 5 mg/dose, may repeat dose in 15 minutes if adequate response not achieved; maximum for second dose: 10 mg/dose

Adults:

SVT: I.V.: 2.5-5 mg (over 2 minutes); second dose of 5-10 mg (~0.15 mg/kg) may be given 15-30 minutes after the initial dose if patient tolerates, but does not respond to initial dose; maximum total dose: 20 mg

Angina: Oral: Initial dose: 80-120 mg 3 times/day (elderly or small stature: 40 mg 3 times/day); range: 240-480 mg/day in 3-4 divided doses

Hypertension: Oral:

Immediate release: 80 mg 3 times/day; usual dose range (JNC 7): 80-320 mg/day in 2 divided doses

Sustained release: 240 mg/day; usual dose range (JNC 7): 120-360 mg/day in 1-2 divided doses; 120 mg/day in the elderly or small patients (no evidence of additional benefit in doses >360 mg/day).

Extended release:

Covera-HS®: Usual dose range (JNC 7): 120-360 mg once daily (once-daily dosing is recommended at bedtime)

Verelan® PM: Usual dose range: 200-400 mg once daily at bedtime

Dosage Forms

Caplet, sustained release: 120 mg, 180 mg, 240 mg

Calan® SR: 120 mg, 180 mg, 240 mg

Capsule, extended release: 120 mg, 180 mg, 240 mg

Capsule, extended release, controlled onset: 100 mg, 200 mg, 300 mg

Verelan® PM: 100 mg, 200 mg, 300 mg

Capsule, sustained release: 120 mg, 180 mg, 240 mg, 360 mg

Verelan®: 120 mg, 180 mg, 240 mg, 360 mg

Injection, solution: 2.5 mg/mL (2 mL, 4 mL)

Tablet: 40 mg, 80 mg, 120 mg

Calan®: 80 mg, 120 mg

Tablet, extended release: 120 mg, 180 mg, 240 mg

Tablet, extended release, controlled onset:

Covera-HS®: 180 mg, 240 mg

Tablet, sustained release: 120 mg, 180 mg, 240 mg

Isoptin® SR: 120 mg, 180 mg, 240 mg

verapamil and trandolapril *see* trandolapril and verapamil *on page 976*

verapamil hydrochloride *see* verapamil *on page 1010*

Verapamil Hydrochloride Injection, USP [Can] *see* verapamil *on page 1010*

Verazinc® Oral *(Discontinued)* *see* zinc sulfate *on page 1031*

Verdeso™ [US] *see* desonide *on page 286*

Veregen® [US] *see* sinecatechins *on page 903*

Verelan® [US] *see* verapamil *on page 1010*

Verelan® PM [US] *see* verapamil *on page 1010*

Verelan SRC [Can] *see* verapamil *on page 1010*

Vergogel® Gel *(Discontinued)* *see* salicylic acid *on page 884*

Vergon® *(Discontinued)* *see* meclizine *on page 619*

Vermox® [Can] *see* mebendazole *on page 617*

Vermox® *(Discontinued)* *see* mebendazole *on page 617*

Versed® *(Discontinued)* *see* midazolam *on page 656*

Versel® [Can] *see* selenium sulfide *on page 895*

Versiclear™ [US] *see* sodium thiosulfate *on page 915*

verteporfin (ver te POR fin)

U.S./Canadian Brand Names Visudyne® [US/Can]

Therapeutic Category Ophthalmic Agent

Use Treatment of predominantly classic subfoveal choroidal neovascularization due to macular degeneration, presumed ocular histoplasmosis, or pathologic myopia

Usual Dosage Therapy is a two-step process; first the infusion of verteporfin, then the activation of verteporfin with a nonthermal diode laser. Adults: I.V.: 6 mg/m^2 body surface area

Note: Treatment in more than one eye: Patients who have lesions in both eyes should be evaluated and treatment should first be done to the more aggressive lesion. Following safe and acceptable treatment, the second eye can be treated one week later. Patients who have had previous verteporfin therapy, with an acceptable safety profile, may then have both eyes treated concurrently. Treat the more aggressive lesion followed immediately with the second eye. The light treatment to the second eye should begin no later than 20 minutes from the start of the infusion.

Dosage Forms

Injection, powder for reconstitution:
Visudyne®: 15 mg

Vicks® Sinex® Nasal Spray [US-OTC] *see* phenylephrine *on page 774*
Vicks® Sinex® UltraFine Mist [US-OTC] *see* phenylephrine *on page 774*
Vicks® Vitamin C [US-OTC] *see* ascorbic acid *on page 100*
Vicodin® [US] *see* hydrocodone and acetaminophen *on page 501*
Vicodin® ES [US] *see* hydrocodone and acetaminophen *on page 501*
Vicodin® HP [US] *see* hydrocodone and acetaminophen *on page 501*
Vicoprofen® [US/Can] *see* hydrocodone and ibuprofen *on page 503*
Vi-Daylin® ADC *(Discontinued)* *see* vitamins (multiple/pediatric) *on page 1020*
Vi-Daylin® ADC + Iron *(Discontinued)* *see* vitamins (multiple/pediatric) *on page 1020*
Vi-Daylin® Drops *(Discontinued)* *see* vitamins (multiple/pediatric) *on page 1020*
Vi-Daylin®/F ADC *(Discontinued)* *see* vitamins (multiple/pediatric) *on page 1020*
Vi-Daylin®/F ADC + Iron *(Discontinued)* *see* vitamins (multiple/pediatric) *on page 1020*
Vi-Daylin®/F *(Discontinued)* *see* vitamins (multiple/pediatric) *on page 1020*
Vi-Daylin®/F + Iron *(Discontinued)* *see* vitamins (multiple/pediatric) *on page 1020*
Vi-Daylin® + Iron Drops *(Discontinued)* *see* vitamins (multiple/pediatric) *on page 1020*
Vi-Daylin® + Iron Liquid *(Discontinued)* *see* vitamins (multiple/oral) *on page 1019*
Vi-Daylin® Liquid *(Discontinued)* *see* vitamins (multiple/oral) *on page 1019*
Vidaza® [US] *see* azacitidine *on page 114*
Videx® [US/Can] *see* didanosine *on page 305*
Videx® EC [US/Can] *see* didanosine *on page 305*

vigabatrin *(Canada only)* (vye GA ba trin)

Sound-Alike/Look-Alike Issues
vigabatrin may be confused with Vibativ™
U.S./Canadian Brand Names Sabril® [Can]
Therapeutic Category Anticonvulsant
Use Treatment of infantile spasms; refractory complex partial seizures not controlled by usual treatments

Additional uses in Canadian labeling (not in U.S. labeling): Active management of partial or secondary generalized seizures not controlled by usual treatments

Usual Dosage Oral:
Children: **Note:** Administer daily dose in 2 divided doses, especially in the higher dosage ranges:
Adjunctive treatment of seizures: Initial: 40 mg/kg/day; maintenance dosages based on patient weight:
10-15 kg: 0.5-1 g/day
16-30 kg: 1-1.5 g/day
31-50 kg: 1.5-3 g/day
>50 kg: 2-3 g/day
Infantile spasms: 50-100 mg/kg/day, depending on severity of symptoms; higher doses (up to 150 mg/kg/day) have been used in some cases.
Adults: Adjunctive treatment of seizures: Initial: 1 g/day (severe manifestations may require 2 g/day); dose may be given as a single daily dose or divided into 2 equal doses. Increase daily dose by 0.5 g based on response and tolerability. Optimal dose range: 2-3 g/day (maximum dose: 3 g/day)

Dosage Forms [CAN] = Canadian product
Powder for solution, oral:
Sabril®: 500 mg/packet (50s)
Powder for suspension, oral [sachets]:
Sabril® [CAN]: 0.5 g
Tablet, oral:
Sabril®: 500 mg

Vigamox® [US/Can] *see* moxifloxacin *on page 670*
VIGIV *see* vaccinia immune globulin (intravenous) *on page 1001*
Vimpat® [US] *see* lacosamide *on page 563*

vinblastine (vin BLAS teen)

Sound-Alike/Look-Alike Issues
vinBLAStine may be confused with vinCRIStine, vinorelbine

Synonyms NSC-49842; vinblastine sulfate; vincaleukoblastine; VLB

Tall-Man vin**BLAS**tine

Therapeutic Category Antineoplastic Agent

Use Treatment of Hodgkin and non-Hodgkin lymphoma; testicular cancer; breast cancer; mycosis fungoides; Kaposi sarcoma; histiocytosis (Letterer-Siwe disease); choriocarcinoma

Usual Dosage Details concerning dosing in combination regimens should also be consulted. **Note:** Frequency and duration of therapy may vary by indication, concomitant combination chemotherapy and hematologic response. **For I.V. use only.**

Children: I.V.:

Hodgkin disease: Initial dose: 6 mg/m^2; do not administer more frequently than every 7 days

Letterer-Siwe disease: Initial dose: 6.5 mg/m^2; do not administer more frequently than every 7 days

Testicular cancer: Initial dose: 3 mg/m^2; do not administer more frequently than every 7 days

Adults: I.V.: Initial: 3.7 mg/m^2; adjust dose every 7 days (based on white blood cell response) up to 5.5 mg/m^2 (second dose); 7.4 mg/m^2 (third dose); 9.25 mg/m^2 (fourth dose); and 11.1 mg/m^2 (fifth dose); do not administer more frequently than every 7 days.

Usual range: 5.5-7.4 mg/m^2 every 7 days; Maximum dose: 18.5 mg/m^2; dosage adjustment goal is to reduce white blood cell count to ~3000/mm^3

Indication-specific dosing:

Hodgkin disease: Usual dose: 6 mg/m^2 every 2 weeks (as part of a combination chemotherapy regimen)

Testicular cancer: Usual dose: 0.11 mg/kg daily for 2 days every 3 weeks (as part of a combination chemotherapy regimen) **or** 6 mg/m^2/day for 2 days every 3-4 weeks (as part of a combination chemotherapy regimen)

Dosage Forms

Injection, powder for reconstitution: 10 mg

Injection, solution: 1 mg/mL (10 mL)

vinblastine sulfate *see* vinblastine *on page 1013*

vincaleukoblastine *see* vinblastine *on page 1013*

Vincasar PFS® [US/Can] *see* vincristine *on page 1014*

vincristine (vin KRIS teen)

Sound-Alike/Look-Alike Issues

vinCRIStine may be confused with vinBLAStine

Oncovin® may be confused with Ancobon®

Synonyms leurocristine sulfate; NSC-67574; vincristine sulfate

Tall-Man vin**CRIS**tine

U.S./Canadian Brand Names Vincasar PFS® [US/Can]

Therapeutic Category Antineoplastic Agent

Use Treatment of leukemias, Hodgkin disease, non-Hodgkin lymphomas, Wilms tumor, neuroblastoma, rhabdomyosarcoma

Usual Dosage Note: Doses are often capped at 2 mg; however, this may reduce the efficacy of the therapy and may not be advisable. Refer to individual protocols; orders for single doses >2.5 mg or >5 mg/treatment cycle should be verified with the specific treatment regimen and/or an experienced oncologist prior to dispensing. I.V.:

Children ≤10 kg or BSA <1 m^2: Initial therapy: 0.05 mg/kg once weekly then titrate dose

Children >10 kg or BSA ≥1 m^2: 1-2 mg/m^2, may repeat once weekly for 3-6 weeks; maximum single dose: 2 mg

Neuroblastoma: I.V. continuous infusion with doxorubicin: 1 mg/m^2/day for 72 hours

Adults: 0.4-1.4 mg/m^2, may repeat every week **or**

0.4-0.5 mg/day continuous infusion for 4 days every 4 weeks **or**

0.25-0.5 mg/m^2/day for 5 days every 4 weeks

Dosage Forms

Injection, solution [preservative free]:

Vincasar PFS®: 1 mg/mL (1 mL, 2 mL)

vincristine sulfate *see* vincristine *on page 1014*

vinorelbine (vi NOR el been)

Sound-Alike/Look-Alike Issues

vinorelbine may be confused with vinBLAStine

Synonyms dihydroxydeoxynorvinkaleukoblastine; vinorelbine tartrate

U.S./Canadian Brand Names Navelbine® [US/Can]; Vinorelbine Injection, USP [Can]; Vinorelbine Tartrate for Injection [Can]

Therapeutic Category Antineoplastic Agent

Use Treatment of nonsmall cell lung cancer (NSCLC)

Usual Dosage Details concerning dosing in combination regimens should also be consulted. I.V.: Adults: NSCLC:

Single-agent therapy: 30 mg/m^2/dose every 7 days

Combination therapy with cisplatin: 25-30 mg/m^2/dose every 7 days (in combination with cisplatin)

Dosage Forms

Injection, solution [preservative free]: 10 mg/mL (1 mL, 5 mL)

Navelbine®: 10 mg/mL (1 mL, 5 mL)

Vinorelbine Injection, USP [Can] *see* vinorelbine *on page* *1014*
vinorelbine tartrate *see* vinorelbine *on page* *1014*
Vinorelbine Tartrate for Injection [Can] *see* vinorelbine *on page* *1014*
Viokase® [US/Can] *see* pancrelipase *on page* *746*
viosterol *see* ergocalciferol *on page* *364*
Vioxx® ***(Discontinued)***
Viracept® [US/Can] *see* nelfinavir *on page* *685*
Viramune® [US/Can] *see* nevirapine *on page* *692*
Viravan® ***(Discontinued)*** *see* phenylephrine and pyrilamine *on page* *776*
Viravan®-DM [US] *see* phenylephrine, pyrilamine, and dextromethorphan *on page* *778*
Virazole® [US/Can] *see* ribavirin *on page* *864*
Viread® [US/Can] *see* tenofovir *on page* *944*
Virilon® [US] *see* methyltestosterone *on page* *648*
Viroptic® [US/Can] *see* trifluridine *on page* *986*
Viscoat® [US] *see* sodium chondroitin sulfate and sodium hyaluronate *on page* *910*
Visicol® [US] *see* sodium phosphates *on page* *912*
Visine-A® [US-OTC] *see* naphazoline and pheniramine *on page* *681*
Visine® Advanced Allergy [Can] *see* naphazoline and pheniramine *on page* *681*
Visine® Advanced Relief [US-OTC] *see* tetrahydrozoline *on page* *951*
Visine® L.R. [US-OTC] *see* oxymetazoline *on page* *740*
Visine® Original [US-OTC] *see* tetrahydrozoline *on page* *951*
Visipaque™ [US] *see* iodixanol *on page* *539*
Visken® [Can] *see* pindolol *on page* *785*
Visken® ***(Discontinued)*** *see* pindolol *on page* *785*
Vistacon-50® Injection ***(Discontinued)*** *see* hydroxyzine *on page* *511*
Vistaquel® Injection ***(Discontinued)*** *see* hydroxyzine *on page* *511*
Vistaril® [US/Can] *see* hydroxyzine *on page* *511*
Vistazine® Injection ***(Discontinued)*** *see* hydroxyzine *on page* *511*
Vistide® [US] *see* cidofovir *on page* *227*
Vistra 650 ***(Discontinued)*** *see* acetaminophen and phenyltoloxamine *on page* *23*
Visudyne® [US/Can] *see* verteporfin *on page* *1011*
Vita-C® [US-OTC] *see* ascorbic acid *on page* *100*
Vitaball® [US-OTC] *see* vitamins (multiple/pediatric) *on page* *1020*
Vitaball® Minis [US-OTC] *see* vitamins (multiple/pediatric) *on page* *1020*
Vitaball® Wild 'N Fruity [US-OTC] *see* vitamins (multiple/pediatric) *on page* *1020*
VitaCarn® Oral ***(Discontinued)*** *see* levocarnitine *on page* *578*
Vitafol [US] *see* vitamin B complex combinations *on page* *1017*
Vitafol® [US] *see* vitamins (multiple/oral) *on page* *1019*
Vitafol®-OB [US-OTC] *see* vitamins (multiple/prenatal) *on page* *1020*
Vitafol®-OB+DHA [US-OTC] *see* vitamins (multiple/prenatal) *on page* *1020*
Vitafol®-PN [US] *see* vitamins (multiple/prenatal) *on page* *1020*
Vitalets [US-OTC] *see* vitamins (multiple/pediatric) *on page* *1020*

Vital HN® [US-OTC] *see* nutritional formula, enteral/oral *on page 715*
vitamin C *see* ascorbic acid *on page 100*
vitamin D_2 *see* ergocalciferol *on page 364*
vitamin D_3 and alendronate *see* alendronate and cholecalciferol *on page 45*
vitamin D and calcium carbonate *see* calcium and vitamin D *on page 169*

vitamin A (VYE ta min aye)

Sound-Alike/Look-Alike Issues
Aquasol® may be confused with Anusol®

Synonyms oleovitamin A

U.S./Canadian Brand Names Aquasol A® [US]; Palmitate-A® [US-OTC]

Therapeutic Category Vitamin, Fat Soluble

Use Treatment and prevention of vitamin A deficiency; parenteral (I.M.) route is indicated when oral administration is not feasible or when absorption is insufficient (malabsorption syndrome)

Usual Dosage

RDA:
- <1 year: 375 mcg
- 1-3 years: 400 mcg
- 4-6 years: 500 mcg*
- 7-10 years: 700 mcg*
- >10 years: 800-1000 mcg*
- Male: 1000 mcg
- Female: 800 mcg
- *mcg retinol equivalent (0.3 mcg retinol = 1 unit vitamin A)

Vitamin A supplementation in measles (recommendation of the World Health Organization): Children: Oral: Administer as a single dose; repeat the next day and at 4 weeks for children with ophthalmologic evidence of vitamin A deficiency:
- 6 months to 1 year: 100,000 units
- >1 year: 200,000 units

Note: Use of vitamin A in measles is recommended only for patients 6 months to 2 years of age hospitalized with measles and its complications **or** patients >6 months of age who have any of the following risk factors and who are not already receiving vitamin A: immunodeficiency, ophthalmologic evidence of vitamin A deficiency including night blindness, Bitot spots or evidence of xerophthalmia, impaired intestinal absorption, moderate-to-severe malnutrition including that associated with eating disorders, or recent immigration from areas where high mortality rates from measles have been observed

Note: Monitor patients closely; dosages >25,000 units/kg have been associated with toxicity

Severe deficiency with xerophthalmia: Oral:
- Children 1-8 years: 5000-10,000 units/kg/day for 5 days or until recovery occurs
- Children >8 years and Adults: 500,000 units/day for 3 days, then 50,000 units/day for 14 days, then 10,000-20,000 units/day for 2 months

Deficiency (without corneal changes): Oral:
- Infants <1 year: 100,000 units every 4-6 months
- Children 1-8 years: 200,000 units every 4-6 months
- Children >8 years and Adults: 100,000 units/day for 3 days then 50,000 units/day for 14 days

Deficiency: I.M.: **Note:** I.M. route is indicated when oral administration is not feasible or when absorption is insufficient (malabsorption syndrome):
- Infants: 7500-15,000 units/day for 10 days
- Children 1-8 years: 17,500-35,000 units/day for 10 days
- Children >8 years and Adults: 100,000 units/day for 3 days, followed by 50,000 units/day for 2 weeks

Note: Follow-up therapy with an oral therapeutic multivitamin (containing additional vitamin A) is recommended:
- Low Birth Weight Infants: Additional vitamin A is recommended, however, no dosage amount has been established
- Children ≤8 years: 5000-10,000 units/day
- Children >8 years and Adults: 10,000-20,000 units/day

Malabsorption syndrome (prophylaxis): Children >8 years and Adults: Oral: 10,000-50,000 units/day of water miscible product

Dietary supplement: Oral:
Infants up to 6 months: 1500 units/day
Children:
6 months to 3 years: 1500-2000 units/day
4-6 years: 2500 units/day
7-10 years: 3300-3500 units/day
Children >10 years and Adults: 4000-5000 units/day

Dosage Forms

Capsule [softgel]: 10,000 units; 25,000 units
Injection, solution:
Aquasol A®: 50,000 units/mL (2 mL)
Tablet:
Palmitate-A® [OTC]: 5000 units, 15,000 units

vitamin A acid *see* tretinoin (topical) *on page* 981

vitamin A and vitamin D (VYE ta min aye & VYE ta min dee)

Synonyms cod liver oil

U.S./Canadian Brand Names A and D® Original [US-OTC]; Baza® Clear [US-OTC]; Sween Cream® [US-OTC]

Therapeutic Category Protectant, Topical

Use Temporary relief of discomfort due to chapped skin, diaper rash, minor burns, abrasions, as well as irritations associated with ostomy skin care

Usual Dosage Topical: Apply locally with gentle massage as needed

Dosage Forms

Capsule, softgel: Vitamin A 1250 int. units and vitamin D 135 int. units; vitamin A 1250 int. units and vitamin D 130 int. units; vitamin A 5,000 int. units and vitamin D 400 int. units; vitamin A 10,000 int. units and vitamin D 400 int. units; vitamin A 10,000 int. units and vitamin D 5000 int. units; vitamin A 25,000 int. units and vitamin D 1000 int. units
Cream:
Sween Cream® [OTC]: 2 g, 57 g, 85 g, 142 g, 184 g, 339 g
Ointment: 0.9 g, 5 g, 60 g, 120 g, 454 g
A and D® Original [OTC]: 45 g, 120 g, 454 g
Baza® Clear [OTC]: 50 g, 150 g, 240 g
Tablet: Vitamin A 10,000 int. units and vitamin D 400 int. units

vitamin B_1 *see* thiamine *on page* 954
vitamin B_2 *see* riboflavin *on page* 865
vitamin B_3 *see* niacin *on page* 692
vitamin B_3 *see* niacinamide *on page* 693
vitamin B_5 *see* pantothenic acid *on page* 749
vitamin B_6 *see* pyridoxine *on page* 840
vitamin B_{12} *see* cyanocobalamin *on page* 263

vitamin B complex combinations (VYE ta min bee KOM pleks kom bi NAY shuns)

Sound-Alike/Look-Alike Issues
Nephrocaps® may be confused with Nephro-Calci®
Renal Caps may be confused with Renagel®, Renvela®
Surbex® may be confused with Sebex®, Suprax®, Surfak®

Synonyms B complex combinations; B vitamin combinations

U.S./Canadian Brand Names Allbee® C-800 + Iron [US-OTC]; Allbee® C-800 [US-OTC]; Allbee® with C [US-OTC]; Apatate® [US-OTC]; DexFol™ [US]; Gevrabon® [US-OTC]; Kobee [US-OTC]; Metanx™ [US]; NephPlex® Rx [US]; Nephro-Vite® Rx [US]; Nephro-Vite® [US-OTC]; Nephrocaps® [US]; Nephron FA® [US]; Nephronex® [US]; Quin B Strong with C and Zinc [US-OTC]; Quin B Strong [US-OTC]; Rena-Vite RX [US]; Rena-Vite [US-OTC]; Renal Caps [US]; Senilezol [US]; Stresstabs® High Potency Advanced [US-OTC]; Stresstabs® High Potency Energy [US-OTC]; Stresstabs® High Potency Weight [US-OTC]; Super Dec B 100 [US-OTC]; Super Quints 50 [US-OTC]; Superplex-T™ [US-OTC]; Surbex-T® [US-OTC]; Vitafol [US]; Z-Bec® [US-OTC]

Therapeutic Category Vitamin, Water Soluble

Use Supplement for use in the wasting syndrome in chronic renal failure, uremia, impaired metabolic functions of the kidney, dialysis; labeled for OTC use as a dietary supplement

Usual Dosage Oral: Adults:
Dietary supplement: One tablet daily
Apatate® liquid: One teaspoonful daily, 1 hour prior to mid-day meal
Gevrabon® liquid: Two tablespoonsful (30 mL) once daily; shake well before use
Renal patients: One tablet or capsule daily between meals; take after treatment if on dialysis
Nephron FA®: Two tablets once daily, between meals

Dosage Forms Content varies depending on product used. For more detailed information on ingredients in these and other multivitamins, please refer to package labeling.

Vitamin D3 [US-OTC] *see* cholecalciferol *on page* 224

vitamin E (VYE ta min ee)

Sound-Alike/Look-Alike Issues
Aquasol E® may be confused with Anusol®

Synonyms *d*-alpha tocopherol; *dl*-alpha tocopherol

U.S./Canadian Brand Names Alph-E [US-OTC]; Alph-E-Mixed [US-OTC]; Aquasol E® [US-OTC]; Aquavit-E [US-OTC]; d-Alpha-Gems™ [US-OTC]; E-Gems Elite® [US-OTC]; E-Gems Plus® [US-OTC]; E-Gems® [US-OTC]; Ester-E™ [US-OTC]; Gamma E-Gems® [US-OTC]; Gamma-E Plus [US-OTC]; High Gamma Vitamin E Complete™ [US-OTC]; Key-E® Kaps [US-OTC]; Key-E® [US-OTC]

Therapeutic Category Vitamin, Fat Soluble; Vitamin, Topical

Use Dietary supplement

Usual Dosage Vitamin E may be expressed as alpha-tocopherol equivalents (ATE), which refer to the biologically active (R) stereoisomer content. Oral:
Recommended daily allowance (RDA):
Infants (adequate intake; RDA not established):
≤6 months: 4 mg
7-12 months: 6 mg
Children:
1-3 years: 6 mg; upper limit of intake should not exceed 200 mg/day
4-8 years: 7 mg; upper limit of intake should not exceed 300 mg/day
9-13 years: 11 mg; upper limit of intake should not exceed 600 mg/day
14-18 years: 15 mg; upper limit of intake should not exceed 800 mg/day
Adults: 15 mg; upper limit of intake should not exceed 1000 mg/day
Pregnant female:
≤18 years: 15 mg; upper level of intake should not exceed 800 mg/day
19-50 years: 15 mg; upper level of intake should not exceed 1000 mg/day
Lactating female:
≤18 years: 19 mg; upper level of intake should not exceed 800 mg/day
19-50 years: 19 mg; upper level of intake should not exceed 1000 mg/day
Vitamin E deficiency:
Children (with malabsorption syndrome): 1 unit/kg/day of water miscible vitamin E (to raise plasma tocopherol concentrations to the normal range within 2 months and to maintain normal plasma concentrations)
Adults: 60-75 units/day
Prevention of vitamin E deficiency: Adults: 30 units/day
Cystic fibrosis, beta-thalassemia, sickle cell anemia may require higher daily maintenance doses:
Children:
Cystic fibrosis: 100-400 units/day
Beta-thalassemia: 750 units/day
Adults: Sickle cell: 450 units/day

Dosage Forms
Capsule: 400 int. units, 1000 int. units
Key-E® Kaps [OTC]: 200 int. units, 400 int. units
Capsule, softgel: 200 int. units, 400 int. units, 600 int. units, 1000 int. units
Alph-E [OTC]: 200 int. units, 400 int. units
Alph-E-Mixed [OTC]: 200 int. units, 400 int. units, 1000 int. units
d-Alpha-Gems™ [OTC], E-Gems Elite® [OTC], Ester-E™ [OTC]: 400 int. units
E-Gems® [OTC]: 30 int. units, 100 int. units, 200 int. units, 400 int. units, 600 int. units, 800 int. units, 1000 int. units, 1200 int. units

E-Gems Plus® [OTC]: 200 int. units, 400 int. units, 800 int. units
Gamma E-Gems® [OTC]: 90 int. units
Gamma-E Plus [OTC], High Gamma Vitamin E Complete™ [OTC]: 200 int. units
Cream: 50 int. units/g (60 g), 100 int. units/g (60 g), 1000 int. units/120 g (120 g), 30,000 int. units/57 g (57g)
Key-E® [OTC]: 30 int. units/g (60 g, 120 g, 600 g)
Lip balm:
E-Gem® Lip Care: 1000 int. units/tube
Oil, oral/topical: 100 int. units/0.25 mL, 1150 units/0.25 mL, 28,000 int. units/30 mL
Alph-E [OTC]: 28,000 int. units/30 mL
E-Gems® [OTC]: 100 units/10 drops
Ointment, topical:
Key-E® [OTC]: 30 units/g (60 g, 120 g, 480 g)
Powder:
Key-E® [OTC]: 700 int. units per 1/4 teaspoon
Solution, oral drops: 15 int. units/0.3 mL
Aquasol E® [OTC], Aquavit-E [OTC]: 15 int. units/0.3 mL
Suppository, rectal/vaginal:
Key-E® [OTC]: 30 int. units (12s, 24s)
Tablet: 100 int. units, 200 int. units, 400 int. units, 500 int. units
Key-E® [OTC]: 200 int. units, 400 int. units

vitamin G *see* riboflavin *on page* 865

vitamin K_1 *see* phytonadione *on page* 782

vitamins (multiple/injectable) (VYE ta mins, MUL ti pul/in JEK ti bal)

U.S./Canadian Brand Names Infuvite® Adult [US]; Infuvite® Pediatric [US]; M.V.I. Adult™ [US]; M.V.I.®-12 [US]; M.V.I® Pediatric [US]

Therapeutic Category Vitamin

Use Nutritional supplement in patients receiving parenteral nutrition or requiring intravenous administration

Usual Dosage I.V.: Not for direct infusion
Children: ≥3 kg to 11 years: Pediatric formulation: 5 mL/day added to TPN or ≥100 mL of appropriate solution
Children >11 years and Adults: Adult formulation: 10 mL/day added to TPN or ≥500 mL of appropriate solution

Dosage Forms Content varies depending on product used. For more detailed information on ingredients in these and other multivitamins, please refer to package labeling.

vitamins (multiple/oral) (VYE ta mins, MUL ti pul/OR al)

Sound-Alike/Look-Alike Issues
Theragran® may be confused with Phenergan®

Synonyms multiple vitamins; therapeutic multivitamins; vitamins, multiple (oral); vitamins, multiple (therapeutic); vitamins, multiple with iron

U.S./Canadian Brand Names Androvite® [US-OTC]; CalciFolic-D™ [US]; Centamin [US-OTC]; Centrum Cardio® [US-OTC]; Centrum Performance® [US-OTC]; Centrum® Silver® Ultra Men's [US-OTC]; Centrum® Silver® Ultra Women's [US-OTC]; Centrum® Silver® [US-OTC]; Centrum® Ultra Men's [US-OTC]; Centrum® Ultra Women's [US-OTC]; Centrum® [US-OTC]; Diatx®Zn [US]; Drinkables® Fruits and Vegetables [US-OTC]; Drinkables® MultiVitamins [US-OTC]; Encora® [US]; Foltrin® [US]; Freedavite [US-OTC]; Geri-Freeda [US-OTC]; Geriation [US-OTC]; Geritol Complete® [US-OTC]; Geritol Extend® [US-OTC]; Geritol® Tonic [US-OTC]; Glutofac®-MX [US]; Glutofac®-ZX [US]; Gynovite® Plus [US-OTC]; Hemocyte Plus® [US]; Hi-Kovite [US-OTC]; Monocaps [US-OTC]; Myadec® [US-OTC]; Nutrimin-Plus [US-OTC]; Ocuvite® Adult 50+ [US-OTC]; Ocuvite® Extra® [US-OTC]; Ocuvite® Lutein [US-OTC]; Ocuvite® [US-OTC]; One A Day® Cholesterol Plus [US-OTC]; One A Day® Energy [US-OTC]; One A Day® Essential [US-OTC]; One A Day® Maximum [US-OTC]; One A Day® Men's 50+ Advantage [US-OTC]; One A Day® Men's Health Formula [US-OTC]; One A Day® Teen Advantage for Her [US-OTC]; One A Day® Teen Advantage for Him [US-OTC]; One A Day® Weight Smart® Advanced [US-OTC]; One A Day® Women's 50+ Advantage [US-OTC]; One A Day® Women's Active Mind & Body [US-OTC]; One A Day® Women's [US-OTC]; Optivite® P.M.T. [US-OTC]; PreserVision® AREDS [US-OTC]; PreserVision® Lutein [US-OTC]; Quintabs [US-OTC]; Quintabs-M Iron-Free [US-OTC]; Quintabs-M [US-OTC]; Renax® 5.5 [US]; Renax® [US]; Replace Without Iron [US-OTC]; Replace [US-OTC]; Repliva 21/7® [US]; SourceCF® [US]; Strovite® Advance [US]; Strovite® Forte [US]; Strovite® Plus [US];

Strovite® [US]; T-Vites [US-OTC]; Ultra Freeda A-Free [US-OTC]; Ultra Freeda Iron-Free [US-OTC]; Ultra Freeda With Iron [US-OTC]; Viactiv® Calcium Flavor Glides™ [US-OTC]; Viactiv® Flavor Glides [US-OTC]; Viactiv® for Teens [US-OTC]; Viactiv® With Calcium [US-OTC]; Viactiv® [US-OTC]; Vitafol® [US]; Xtramins [US-OTC]; Yelets [US-OTC]

Therapeutic Category Vitamin

Use Prevention/treatment of vitamin and mineral deficiencies; labeled for OTC use as a dietary supplement

Usual Dosage Oral: Adults: Daily dose of adult preparations varies by product. Generally, 1 tablet or capsule or 5-15 mL of liquid per day. Consult package labeling. Prescription doses may be higher for burn or cystic fibrosis patients.

Dosage Forms Content varies depending on product used. For more detailed information on ingredients in these and other multivitamins, please refer to package labeling.

vitamins, multiple (oral) *see* vitamins (multiple/oral) *on page* 1019

vitamins (multiple/pediatric) (VYE ta mins, MUL ti pul/pe de AT rik)

Synonyms children's vitamins; multivitamins/fluoride

U.S./Canadian Brand Names ADEKs® [US-OTC]; AquADEKs™ [US-OTC]; Centrum Kids® Complete Dora the Explorer™ [US-OTC]; Centrum Kids® Complete Rugrats™ [US-OTC]; Centrum Kids® Complete SpongeBob SquarePants™ [US-OTC]; Flintstones™ Complete [US-OTC]; Flintstones™ Gummies Vita-Packs [US-OTC]; Flintstones™ Gummies [US-OTC]; Flintstones™ Plus Bone Building Support [US-OTC]; Flintstones™ Plus Immunity Support [US-OTC]; Flintstones™ Plus Iron [US-OTC]; Flintstones™ Sour Gummies [US-OTC]; My First Flintstones™ [US-OTC]; MyKidz Iron FL™ [US]; MyKidz Iron™ [US-OTC]; One A Day® Kids Scooby-Doo!™ Gummies [US-OTC]; One-A-Day® Kids Bugs Bunny and Friends Complete [US-OTC]; One-A-Day® Kids Scooby-Doo!™ Complete [US-OTC]; One-A-Day® Kids Scooby-Doo!™ Plus Calcium [US-OTC]; Poly-Vi-Sol® with Iron [US-OTC]; Poly-Vi-Sol® [US-OTC]; Tri-Vi-Sol® With Iron [US-OTC]; Tri-Vi-Sol® [US-OTC]; Vitaball® Minis [US-OTC]; Vitaball® Wild 'N Fruity [US-OTC]; Vitaball® [US-OTC]; Vitalets [US-OTC]

Therapeutic Category Vitamin

Use Prevention/treatment of vitamin deficiency; products containing fluoride are used to prevent dental caries; labeled for OTC use as a dietary supplement

Usual Dosage Daily dose varies by product; refer to package insert for specific product labeling

Dosage Forms Content varies depending on product used. For more detailed information on ingredients in these and other multivitamins, please refer to package labeling.

vitamins (multiple/prenatal) (VYE ta mins, MUL ti pul/pree NAY tal)

Sound-Alike/Look-Alike Issues

PreCare® may be confused with Precose®

Synonyms prenatal vitamins

U.S./Canadian Brand Names A-Free Prenatal [US]; Calna [US-OTC]; CitraNatal™ 90 DHA [US]; CitraNatal™ DHA [US]; CitraNatal™ Rx [US]; Duet® DHA [US]; Duet® DHA[ec] [US]; Duet® [US]; KPN Prenatal [US-OTC]; Mini-Prenatal [US-OTC]; NataCaps™ [US]; NataChew® [US-OTC]; NataFort® [US-OTC]; NatalCare® GlossTabs™ [US]; NatalCare® PIC Forte [US]; NatalCare® PIC [US]; NatalCare® Plus [US]; NatalCare® Rx [US]; NatalCare® Three [US]; NataTab™ CFe [US]; NataTab™ FA [US]; NataTab™ Rx [US]; NutriNate® [US]; NutriSpire™ [US]; Néevo® DHA [US]; Néevo® [US]; One A Day® Women's Prenatal [US-OTC]; OptiNate® [US]; PreCare Conceive® [US]; PreCare Premier® [US]; PreCare® [US]; PremesisRx® [US]; Prenatal 19 [US-OTC]; Prenatal AD [US-OTC]; Prenatal One Daily [US-OTC]; Prenatal Rx 1 [US]; Prenatal U [US-OTC]; Prenate DHA™ [US]; Prenate Elite® [US]; PrimaCare® One [US]; PrimaCare® [US]; Select-OB™ [US-OTC]; Stuart Prenatal® [US-OTC]; Tandem® DHA [US]; Tandem® OB [US]; Trinate [US-OTC]; Ultra NatalCare® [US]; Vitafol®-OB [US-OTC]; Vitafol®-OB+DHA [US-OTC]; Vitafol®-PN [US]

Therapeutic Category Vitamin

Use Nutritional supplement for use prior to conception, during pregnancy, and postnatal (in lactating and nonlactating women)

Usual Dosage Oral: Adults:

Capsule, tablet: One daily

Powder: 4 teaspoonfuls/day; given once daily or in divided doses; mix 1 teaspoonful in 1 ounce of water

Dosage Forms Content varies depending on product used. For more detailed information on ingredients in these and other multivitamins, please refer to package labeling.

vitamins, multiple (therapeutic) *see* vitamins (multiple/oral) *on page* 1019

vitamins, multiple with iron *see* vitamins (multiple/oral) *on page 1019*
Vitaneed™ [US-OTC] *see* nutritional formula, enteral/oral *on page 715*
Vitelle™ Irospan® *(Discontinued)* *see* ferrous sulfate and ascorbic acid *on page 415*
Vitrase® [US] *see* hyaluronidase *on page 497*
Vitrasert® [US/Can] *see* ganciclovir *on page 454*
Vitrax® [US] *see* hyaluronate and derivatives *on page 496*
Vitussin *(Discontinued)*
Vivacaine™ [US] *see* bupivacaine and epinephrine *on page 157*
Vi vaccine *see* typhoid vaccine *on page 996*
Vivactil® [US] *see* protriptyline *on page 832*
Viva-Drops® [US-OTC] *see* artificial tears *on page 100*
Vivaglobin® [US] *see* immune globulin (subcutaneous) *on page 524*
Vivarin® [US-OTC] *see* caffeine *on page 165*
Vivelle® *(Discontinued)* *see* estradiol *on page 373*
Vivelle-Dot® [US] *see* estradiol *on page 373*
Vivitrol™ [US] *see* naltrexone *on page 679*
Vivonex® [US-OTC] *see* nutritional formula, enteral/oral *on page 715*
Vivonex® T.E.N. [US-OTC] *see* nutritional formula, enteral/oral *on page 715*
Vivotif® [US/Can] *see* typhoid vaccine *on page 996*
VLB *see* vinblastine *on page 1013*
VM-26 *see* teniposide *on page 944*
Volibris™ [Can] *see* ambrisentan *on page 59*
Volmax® *(Discontinued)* *see* albuterol *on page 41*
Voltaren® [US/Can] *see* diclofenac *on page 303*
Voltaren® Gel [US] *see* diclofenac *on page 303*
Voltaren Ophtha® [Can] *see* diclofenac *on page 303*
Voltaren Ophthalmic® [US] *see* diclofenac *on page 303*
Voltaren Rapide® [Can] *see* diclofenac *on page 303*
Voltaren®-XR [US] *see* diclofenac *on page 303*
VoLumen™ [US] *see* barium *on page 122*
Voluven® [US/Can] *see* hetastarch *on page 493*

voriconazole (vor i KOE na zole)

Synonyms UK109496

U.S./Canadian Brand Names VFEND® [US/Can]

Therapeutic Category Antifungal Agent

Use Treatment of invasive aspergillosis; treatment of esophageal candidiasis; treatment of candidemia (in nonneutropenic patients); treatment of disseminated *Candida* infections of the skin and viscera; treatment of serious fungal infections caused by *Scedosporium apiospermum* and *Fusarium* spp (including *Fusarium solani*) in patients intolerant of, or refractory to, other therapy

Usual Dosage

Usual dosage range:

Children ≥12 years and Adults:

Oral: 100-300 mg every 12 hours

I.V.: 6 mg/kg every 12 hours for 2 doses; followed by maintenance dose of 4 mg/kg every 12 hours

Indication-specific dosing: Children ≥12 years and Adults:

Aspergillosis, invasive, including disseminated and extrapulmonary infection: Duration of therapy should be a minimum of 6-12 weeks or throughout period of immunosuppression:

I.V.: Initial: Loading dose: 6 mg/kg every 12 hours for 2 doses; followed by maintenance dose of 4 mg/kg every 12 hours

Oral: May consider oral therapy in place of I.V. with dosing of 4 mg/kg (rounded up to convenient tablet dosage form) every 12 hours; however, I.V. administration is preferred in serious infections since comparative efficacy with the oral formulation has not been established.

Scedosporiosis, fusariosis: I.V.: Initial: Loading dose: 6 mg/kg every 12 hours for 2 doses; followed by maintenance dose of 4 mg/kg every 12 hours

Candidemia and other deep tissue *Candida* infections: I.V.: Initial: Loading dose 6 mg/kg every 12 hours for 2 doses; followed by maintenance dose of 3-4 mg/kg every 12 hours

Endophthalmitis, fungal: I.V.: 6 mg/kg every 12 hours for 2 doses, then 200 mg orally twice daily

Esophageal candidiasis: Oral:

Patients <40 kg: 100 mg every 12 hours; maximum: 300 mg/day

Patients ≥40 kg: 200 mg every 12 hours; maximum: 600 mg/day

Note: Treatment should continue for a minimum of 14 days, and for at least 7 days following resolution of symptoms.

Conversion to oral dosing:

Patients <40 kg: 100 mg every 12 hours; increase to 150 mg every 12 hours in patients who fail to respond adequately

Patients ≥40 kg: 200 mg every 12 hours; increase to 300 mg every 12 hours in patients who fail to respond adequately

Dosage Forms

Injection, powder for reconstitution:

VFEND®: 200 mg

Powder for oral suspension:

VFEND®: 200 mg/5 mL

Tablet:

VFEND®: 50 mg, 200 mg

vorinostat (vor IN oh stat)

Synonyms NSC-701852; SAHA; suberoylanilide hydroxamic acid

U.S./Canadian Brand Names Zolinza™ [US]

Therapeutic Category Antineoplastic Agent, Histone Deacetylase Inhibitor

Use Treatment of progressive, persistent, or recurrent cutaneous T-cell lymphoma (CTCL)

Usual Dosage Oral: Adults: Cutaneous T-cell lymphoma: 400 mg once daily

Dosage Forms

Capsule:

Zolinza™: 100 mg

VoSol® *(Discontinued)* *see* acetic acid *on page 30*

VoSol® HC [US] *see* acetic acid, propylene glycol diacetate, and hydrocortisone *on page 30*

VoSpire ER® [US] *see* albuterol *on page 41*

VP-16 *see* etoposide *on page 398*

VP-16-213 *see* etoposide *on page 398*

V-Tann™ *(Discontinued)* *see* phenylephrine and pyrilamine *on page 776*

Vumon® [US/Can] *see* teniposide *on page 944*

Vusion® [US] *see* miconazole and zinc oxide *on page 655*

V.V.S.® [US] *see* sulfabenzamide, sulfacetamide, and sulfathiazole *on page 926*

vWF:RCof *see* antihemophilic factor/von Willebrand factor complex (human) *on page 83*

Vytone® [US] *see* iodoquinol and hydrocortisone *on page 539*

Vytorin® [US] *see* ezetimibe and simvastatin *on page 402*

Vyvanse™ [US] *see* lisdexamfetamine *on page 593*

VZIG *see* varicella-zoster immune globulin (human) *on page 1008*

VZV vaccine (varicella) *see* varicella virus vaccine *on page 1007*

VZV vaccine (zoster) *see* zoster vaccine *on page 1035*

warfarin (WAR far in)

Sound-Alike/Look-Alike Issues

Coumadin® may be confused with Avandia®, Cardura®, Compazine®, Kemadrin®

Jantoven® may be confused with Janumet™, Januvia™

Synonyms warfarin sodium

U.S./Canadian Brand Names Apo-Warfarin® [Can]; Coumadin® [US/Can]; Gen-Warfarin [Can]; Jantoven® [US]; Novo-Warfarin [Can]; Taro-Warfarin [Can]

Therapeutic Category Anticoagulant (Other)

Use Prophylaxis and treatment of thromboembolic disorders (eg, venous, pulmonary) and embolic complications arising from atrial fibrillation or cardiac valve replacement; adjunct to reduce risk of systemic embolism (eg, recurrent MI, stroke) after myocardial infarction

Usual Dosage Note: New labeling identifies genetic factors which may increase patient sensitivity to warfarin. Specifically, genetic variations in the proteins CYP2C9 and VKORC1, responsible for warfarin's primary metabolism and pharmacodynamic activity, respectively, have been identified as predisposing factors associated with decreased dose requirement and increased bleeding risk. A genotyping test is available, and may provide important guidance on initiation of anticoagulant therapy.

Oral:

Adults: Initial dosing must be individualized. Consider the patient (hepatic function, cardiac function, age, nutritional status, concurrent therapy, risk of bleeding) in addition to prior dose response (if available) and the clinical situation. Start 2-5 mg daily for 2 days **or** 5-10 mg daily for 1-2 days. Adjust dose according to INR results; usual maintenance dose ranges from 2-10 mg daily (individual patients may require loading and maintenance doses outside these general guidelines).

Note: Lower starting doses may be required for patients with hepatic impairment, poor nutrition, CHF, elderly, high risk of bleeding, or patients who are debilitated, or those with reduced function genomic variants of the catabolic enzymes CYP2C9 (*2 or *3 alleles) or VKORC1 (-1639 polymorphism). Higher initial doses may be reasonable in selected patients (ie, receiving enzyme-inducing agents and with low risk of bleeding).

I.V.: Adults: 2-5 mg/day administered as a slow bolus injection

Dosage Forms

Injection, powder for reconstitution:

Coumadin®: 5 mg

Tablet: 1 mg, 2 mg, 2.5 mg, 3 mg, 4 mg, 5 mg, 6 mg, 7.5 mg, 10 mg

Coumadin®, Jantoven®: 1 mg, 2 mg, 2.5 mg, 3 mg, 4 mg, 5 mg, 6 mg, 7.5 mg, 10 mg

warfarin sodium *see* warfarin *on page 1022*

Wartec® [Can] *see* podofilox *on page 795*

Wart-Off® Maximum Strength [US-OTC] *see* salicylic acid *on page 884*

4-Way® 12 Hour [US-OTC] *see* oxymetazoline *on page 740*

4 Way® Fast Acting [US-OTC] *see* phenylephrine *on page 774*

4 Way® Menthol [US-OTC] *see* phenylephrine *on page 774*

4 Way® No Drip [US-OTC] *see* phenylephrine *on page 774*

4-Way® Saline Moisturizing Mist [US-OTC] *see* sodium chloride *on page 908*

WelChol® [US/Can] *see* colesevelam *on page 254*

Wellbutrin® [US/Can] *see* bupropion *on page 158*

Wellbutrin XL® [US/Can] *see* bupropion *on page 158*

Wellbutrin SR® [US] *see* bupropion *on page 158*

Wellcovorin® *(Discontinued)* *see* leucovorin calcium *on page 575*

Westcort® [US/Can] *see* hydrocortisone (topical) *on page 505*

Westhroid™ [US] *see* thyroid, desiccated *on page 957*

40 Winks® *(Discontinued)* *see* diphenhydramine *on page 315*

Winpred™ [Can] *see* prednisone *on page 814*

WinRho SD® *(Discontinued)*

WinRho® SDF [US/Can] *see* Rh_o(D) immune globulin *on page 862*

Winstrol® *(Discontinued)*

witch hazel (witch HAY zel)

Synonyms hamamelis water

U.S./Canadian Brand Names Dickinson's® Witch Hazel [US-OTC]; Preparation H® Cleansing Pads [Can]; Preparation H® Medicated Wipes [US-OTC]; T.N. Dickinson's® Hazelets [US-OTC]; Tucks® Take Alongs® [US-OTC]; Tucks® [US-OTC]

Therapeutic Category Astringent

Use After-stool wipe to remove most causes of local irritation; temporary management of vulvitis, pruritus ani and vulva; help relieve the discomfort of simple hemorrhoids, anorectal surgical wounds, and episiotomies

Usual Dosage Apply to anorectal area as needed

Dosage Forms

Liquid, topical: 100% (120 mL, 480 mL)

Dickinson's® Witch Hazel [OTC]: 100% (60 mL, 240 mL, 480 mL)

Pads, topical: 50% (100s)

Dickinson's® Witch Hazel [OTC]: 50% (20s,50s, 100s)

Preparation H® Medicated Wipes [OTC]: 50% (8s, 48s)

T.N. Dickinson's® Hazelets [OTC]: 50% (50s, 60s)

Tucks® [OTC]: 50% (40s, 100s)

Towelette, topical:

Tucks® Take Alongs® [OTC]: 50% (12s)

Xylocaine® Dental [US] *see* lidocaine *on page* *584*
Xylocaine® MPF [US] *see* lidocaine *on page* *584*
Xylocaine® MPF With Epinephrine [US] *see* lidocaine and epinephrine *on page* *586*
Xylocaine® Viscous [US] *see* lidocaine *on page* *584*
Xylocaine® With Epinephrine [US/Can] *see* lidocaine and epinephrine *on page* *586*
Xylocard® [Can] *see* lidocaine *on page* *584*
Xyntha™ [US] *see* antihemophilic factor (recombinant) *on page* *82*
Xyralid™ *(Discontinued)* *see* lidocaine and hydrocortisone *on page* *587*
Xyralid™ LP *(Discontinued)* *see* lidocaine and hydrocortisone *on page* *587*
Xyralid™ RC *(Discontinued)* *see* lidocaine and hydrocortisone *on page* *587*
Xyrem® [US/Can] *see* sodium oxybate *on page* *911*
Xyzal® [US] *see* levocetirizine *on page* *579*
Y-90 ibritumomab *see* ibritumomab *on page* *515*
Y-90 zevalin *see* ibritumomab *on page* *515*
Yasmin® [US/Can] *see* ethinyl estradiol and drospirenone *on page* *384*
Yaz® [US/Can] *see* ethinyl estradiol and drospirenone *on page* *384*
Yelets [US-OTC] *see* vitamins (multiple/oral) *on page* *1019*

yellow fever vaccine (YEL oh FEE ver vak SEEN)

U.S./Canadian Brand Names YF-VAX® [US/Can]

Therapeutic Category Vaccine, Live Virus

Use Induction of active immunity against yellow fever virus, primarily among persons traveling or living in areas where yellow fever infection exists and laboratory workers who may be exposed to the virus; vaccination may also be required for some international travelers

The Advisory Committee on Immunization Practices (ACIP) recommends vaccination for:

- Persons traveling to or living in areas where yellow fever is officially reported
- Persons traveling to countries that do not officially report yellow fever, but are in the endemic zone
- Persons traveling to countries which require vaccination for international travel
- Laboratory personnel who may be exposed to the yellow fever virus or concentrated preparations of the vaccine

Although the vaccine is approved for use in children ≥9 months of age, the CDC recommends use in children as young as 6 months under unusual circumstances (eg, travel to an area where exposure is unavoidable). Children <6 months of age should **never** receive the vaccine.

Usual Dosage SubQ: Children ≥9 months (per manufacturer) and Adults: One dose (0.5 mL) ≥10 days before travel; Booster: Every 10 years for those at continued risk of exposure

Dosage Forms

Injection, powder for reconstitution [17D-204 strain]:
YF-VAX®: ≥4.74 Log_{10} plaque-forming units (PFU) per 0.5 mL dose

YF-VAX® [US/Can] *see* yellow fever vaccine *on page* *1025*
YM087 *see* conivaptan *on page* *256*
YM905 *see* solifenacin *on page* *915*
YM-08310 *see* amifostine *on page* *60*
Yocon® [US/Can] *see* yohimbine *on page* *1025*
Yodoxin® [US] *see* iodoquinol *on page* *539*

yohimbine (yo HIM bine)

Sound-Alike/Look-Alike Issues
Aphrodyne® may be confused with Aprodine®
Yocon® may be confused with Zocor®

Synonyms yohimbine hydrochloride

U.S./Canadian Brand Names PMS-Yohimbine [Can]; Yocon® [US/Can]

Therapeutic Category Miscellaneous Product

Usual Dosage Oral: Adults:

Male erectile impotence: 5.4 mg tablet 3 times/day have been used. If side effects occur, reduce to 1/2 tablet (2.7 mg) 3 times/day followed by gradual increases to 1 tablet 3 times/day. Results of therapy >10 weeks are not known.

Orthostatic hypotension: Doses of 12.5 mg/day have been utilized; however, more research is necessary

Dosage Forms

Tablet: 5.4 mg

yohimbine hydrochloride *see* yohimbine *on page 1025*

Yohimex™ ***(Discontinued)*** *see* yohimbine *on page 1025*

Yutopar® Injection ***(Discontinued)***

Z4942 *see* ifosfamide *on page 518*

Zaditen® [Can] *see* ketotifen *on page 559*

Zaditor® [US-OTC/Can] *see* ketotifen *on page 559*

zafirlukast (za FIR loo kast)

Sound-Alike/Look-Alike Issues

Accolate® may be confused with Accupril®, Accutane®, Aclovate®

Synonyms ICI-204,219

U.S./Canadian Brand Names Accolate® [US/Can]

Therapeutic Category Leukotriene Receptor Antagonist

Use Prophylaxis and chronic treatment of asthma in adults and children ≥5 years of age

Usual Dosage Oral:

Children 5-11 years: 10 mg twice daily

Children ≥12 years and Adults: 20 mg twice daily

Dosage Forms

Tablet:

Accolate®: 10 mg, 20 mg

Zagam® ***(Discontinued)***

zalcitabine ***(Discontinued)***

zaleplon (ZAL e plon)

Sound-Alike/Look-Alike Issues

zaleplon may be confused with zolpidem

Sonata® may be confused with Soriatane®

U.S./Canadian Brand Names Sonata® [US]

Therapeutic Category Hypnotic, Nonbenzodiazepine (Pyrazolopyrimidine)

Controlled Substance C-IV

Use Short-term (7-10 days) treatment of insomnia (has been demonstrated to be effective for up to 5 weeks in controlled trial)

Usual Dosage Oral: Adults: 10 mg at bedtime (range: 5-20 mg); has been used for up to 5 weeks of treatment in controlled trial setting

Dosage Forms

Capsule: 5 mg, 10 mg

Sonata®: 5 mg, 10 mg

Zamicet™ [US] *see* hydrocodone and acetaminophen *on page 501*

Zanaflex® [US/Can] *see* tizanidine *on page 964*

Zanaflex Capsules™ [US] *see* tizanidine *on page 964*

zanamivir (za NA mi veer)

Sound-Alike/Look-Alike Issues

Relenza® may be confused with Albenza®, Aplenzin™

U.S./Canadian Brand Names Relenza® [US/Can]

Therapeutic Category Antiviral Agent, Inhalation Therapy

Use Treatment of uncomplicated acute illness due to influenza virus A and B in patients who have been symptomatic for no more than 2 days; prophylaxis against influenza virus A and B

The Advisory Committee on Immunization Practices (ACIP) recommends that **treatment** be considered for the following:

- Persons hospitalized with laboratory confirmed influenza (may also have benefit if started >48 hours after onset of illness).
- Persons with laboratory confirmed influenza pneumonia.
- Persons with laboratory confirmed influenza and bacterial infections.
- Persons with laboratory confirmed influenza and who are at higher risk for influenza complications.
- Persons presenting for care within 48 hours of laboratory confirmed influenza onset and who want to decrease duration and/or severity of their symptoms or decrease the risk of transmission to those at high risk for complications.

The ACIP recommends that **prophylaxis** be considered for the following:

- Persons at high risk for influenza infection during the first 2 weeks following vaccination (eg, children <9 years and not previously vaccinated) if the virus is circulating in the community.
- Persons at high risk for influenza infection, but the vaccination is contraindicated.
- Unvaccinated family members or healthcare providers with prolonged exposure to or close contact with high-risk persons, unvaccinated persons, or infants <6 months of age.
- Persons at high risk for influenza infection, their family members and close contacts, and healthcare workers when the circulating strain of influenza is not matched with the vaccine.
- Persons with immune deficiency or those who may not respond to vaccination.
- Unvaccinated staff and persons during response to an outbreak in a closed institutional setting that has patients at high risk for infection (eg, extended care facilities).

Usual Dosage Oral inhalation:

Children ≥5 years and Adults: Prophylaxis (household setting): Two inhalations (10 mg) once daily for 10 days. Begin within 1 1/2 days following onset of signs or symptoms of index case.

Children ≥7 years and Adults: Treatment: Two inhalations (10 mg total) twice daily for 5 days. Doses on first day should be separated by at least 2 hours; on subsequent days, doses should be spaced by ~12 hours. Begin within 2 days of signs or symptoms.

Adolescents and Adults: Prophylaxis (community outbreak): Two inhalations (10 mg) once daily for 28 days. Begin within 5 days of outbreak.

Dosage Forms

Powder for oral inhalation:

Relenza®: 5 mg/blister (20s)

Zanosar® [US/Can] *see* streptozocin *on page 923*

Zantac® [US/Can] *see* ranitidine *on page 852*

Zantac 75® [US-OTC/Can] *see* ranitidine *on page 852*

Zantac 150® [US-OTC] *see* ranitidine *on page 852*

Zantac® EFFERdose® [US] *see* ranitidine *on page 852*

Zantac Maximum Strength Non-Prescription [Can] *see* ranitidine *on page 852*

Zantryl® *(Discontinued)* *see* phentermine *on page 773*

Zapzyt® [US-OTC] *see* benzoyl peroxide *on page 132*

Zarontin® [US/Can] *see* ethosuximide *on page 395*

Zaroxolyn® [US/Can] *see* metolazone *on page 650*

Zartan® *(Discontinued)* *see* cephalexin *on page 202*

Zavesca® [US/Can] *see* miglustat *on page 658*

Zazole™ [US] *see* terconazole *on page 946*

Z-Bec® [US-OTC] *see* vitamin B complex combinations *on page 1017*

Z-chlopenthixol *see* zuclopenthixol *(Canada only) on page 1035*

Z-Cof™ 12DM [US] *see* guaifenesin, pseudoephedrine, and dextromethorphan *on page 479*

Z-Cof HC *(Discontinued)* *see* phenylephrine, hydrocodone, and chlorpheniramine *on page 778*

Z-Cof LA™ [US] *see* guaifenesin and dextromethorphan *on page 474*

ZD1033 *see* anastrozole *on page 79*

ZD1694 *see* raltitrexed *(Canada only) on page 849*

ZD1839 *see* gefitinib *on page 456*

ZDV *see* zidovudine *on page 1028*

ZDV, abacavir, and lamivudine *see* abacavir, lamivudine, and zidovudine *on page 16*

Zeasorb®-AF [US-OTC] *see* miconazole *on page 654*

Zebeta® [US/Can] *see* bisoprolol *on page 144*

Zebutal™ [US] *see* butalbital, acetaminophen, and caffeine *on page 161*
Zefazone® *(Discontinued)*
Zeftera™ [Can] *see* ceftobiprole *(Canada only) on page 198*
Zegerid® [US] *see* omeprazole and sodium bicarbonate *on page 724*
Zelapar™ [US] *see* selegiline *on page 895*
Zeldox® [Can] *see* ziprasidone *on page 1032*
Zelnorm® [US] *see* tegaserod *on page 940*
Zemaira® [US] *see* alpha$_1$-proteinase inhibitor *on page 50*
Zemplar® [US/Can] *see* paricalcitol *on page 751*
Zemuron® [US/Can] *see* rocuronium *on page 875*
Zenapax® [US/Can] *see* daclizumab *on page 272*
Zenchent™ [US] *see* ethinyl estradiol and norethindrone *on page 390*
zeneca 182,780 *see* fulvestrant *on page 448*
Zephiran® [US-OTC] *see* benzalkonium chloride *on page 129*
Zephrex LA® *(Discontinued)* *see* guaifenesin and pseudoephedrine *on page 477*
Zerit® [US/Can] *see* stavudine *on page 921*
ZerLor™ [US] *see* acetaminophen, caffeine, and dihydrocodeine *on page 25*
Zestoretic® [US/Can] *see* lisinopril and hydrochlorothiazide *on page 594*
Zestril® [US/Can] *see* lisinopril *on page 593*
Zetar® [US-OTC] *see* coal tar *on page 250*
Zetia® [US] *see* ezetimibe *on page 401*
Zevalin® [US/Can] *see* ibritumomab *on page 515*
Zgesic [US] *see* acetaminophen and phenyltoloxamine *on page 23*
Ziac® [US/Can] *see* bisoprolol and hydrochlorothiazide *on page 144*
Ziagen® [US/Can] *see* abacavir *on page 16*
Ziana™ [US] *see* clindamycin and tretinoin *on page 240*

ziconotide (zi KOE no tide)

U.S./Canadian Brand Names Prialt® [US]

Therapeutic Category Analgesic, Nonnarcotic; Calcium Channel Blocker, N-Type

Use Management of severe chronic pain in patients requiring intrathecal (I.T.) therapy and who are intolerant or refractory to other therapies

Usual Dosage I.T.: Adults: Chronic pain: Initial dose: ≤2.4 mcg/day (0.1 mcg/hour)

Dose may be titrated by ≤2.4 mcg/day (0.1 mcg/hour) at intervals ≤2-3 times/week to a maximum dose of 19.2 mcg/day (0.8 mcg/hour) by day 21; average dose at day 21: 6.9 mcg/day (0.29 mcg/hour). A faster titration should be used only if the urgent need for analgesia outweighs the possible risk to patient safety.

Dosage Forms

Injection, solution [preservative free]:

Prialt®: 25 mcg/mL (20 mL); 100 mcg/mL (1 mL, 5 mL)

zidovudine (zye DOE vyoo deen)

Sound-Alike/Look-Alike Issues

azidothymidine may be confused with azaTHIOprine, aztreonam
Retrovir® may be confused with acyclovir, ritonavir
AZT is an error-prone abbreviation (mistaken as azathioprine, aztreonam)

Synonyms azidothymidine; compound S; ZDV

U.S./Canadian Brand Names Apo-Zidovudine® [Can]; AZT™ [Can]; Retrovir® [US/Can]

Therapeutic Category Antiviral Agent

Use Treatment of HIV infection in combination with at least two other antiretroviral agents; prevention of maternal/fetal HIV transmission as monotherapy

Usual Dosage

Prevention of maternal-fetal HIV transmission: **Note:** Consider use of zidovudine in combination with nevirapine (and possibly lamivudine) in select situations (eg, infants born to mothers with suboptimal viral suppression at delivery, infants born to mothers with only intrapartum therapy or no therapy, or infants born to mothers with known antiretroviral drug-resistant virus).

Neonatal: **Note:** Dosing should begin 6-12 hours after birth and continue for the first 6 weeks of life.
Oral:
Full-term infants: 2 mg/kg/dose every 6 hours
Infants ≥30 weeks and <35 weeks gestation at birth: 2 mg/kg/dose every 12 hours; at 2 weeks of age, advance to 2 mg/kg/dose every 8 hours
Infants <30 weeks gestation at birth: 2 mg/kg/dose every 12 hours; at 4 weeks of age, advance to 2 mg/kg/dose every 8 hours
I.V.: Infants unable to receive oral dosing:
Full term: 1.5 mg/kg/dose every 6 hours
Infants ≥30 weeks and <35 weeks gestation at birth: 1.5 mg/kg/dose every 12 hours; at 2 weeks of age, advance to 1.5 mg/kg/dose every 8 hours
Infants <30 weeks gestation at birth: 1.5 mg/kg/dose every 12 hours; at 4 weeks of age, advance to 1.5 mg/kg/dose every 8 hours
Maternal: Oral (per AIDSinfo guidelines): 100 mg 5 times/day **or** 200 mg 3 times/day **or** 300 mg twice daily. Begin at 14-34 weeks gestation and continue until start of labor.
During labor and delivery, administer zidovudine I.V. at 2 mg/kg as loading dose followed by a continuous I.V. infusion of 1 mg/kg/hour until the umbilical cord is clamped
Treatment of HIV infection:
Children 6 weeks to 12 years:
Oral: Dose should be calculated by body weight (in kg) or body surface area and should not exceed the recommended adult dose. **Note:** Doses calculated by body weight may not be the same as those calculated by body surface area.
Dosing based on body surface area: 160 mg/m^2/dose every 8 hours **or** 240 mg/m^2 every 12 hours (maximum: 200 mg every 8 hours); some Working Group members use a dose of 180 mg/m^2 to 240 mg/m^2 every 12 hours when using in drug combinations with other antiretroviral compounds, but data on this dosing in children is limited.
Dosing based on weight:
4 to <9 kg: 12 mg/kg/dose twice daily **or** 8 mg/kg/dose 3 times a day
≥9 to <30 kg: 9 mg/kg/dose twice daily **or** 6 mg/kg/dose 3 times a day
≥30 kg: 300 mg twice daily **or** 200 mg 3 times a day
I.V. continuous infusion: 20 mg/m^2/hour
I.V. intermittent infusion: 120 mg/m^2/dose every 6 hours
Adults:
Oral: 300 mg twice daily or 200 mg 3 times/day
I.V.: 1 mg/kg/dose administered every 4 hours around-the-clock (5-6 doses/day)

Dosage Forms
Capsule, oral: 100 mg
Retrovir®: 100 mg
Injection, solution [preservative free]:
Retrovir®: 10 mg/mL (20 mL)
Syrup, oral: 50 mg/5 mL
Retrovir®: 50 mg/5 mL
Tablet: 300 mg
Retrovir®: 300 mg

zidovudine, abacavir, and lamivudine *see* abacavir, lamivudine, and zidovudine *on page 16*

zidovudine and lamivudine (zye DOE vyoo deen & la MI vyoo deen)

Sound-Alike/Look-Alike Issues
Combivir® may be confused with Combivent®, Epivir®
AZT is an error-prone abbreviation (mistaken as azaTHIOprine, aztreonam)

Synonyms lamivudine and zidovudine

U.S./Canadian Brand Names Combivir® [US/Can]

Therapeutic Category Antiviral Agent

Use Treatment of HIV infection when therapy is warranted based on clinical and/or immunological evidence of disease progression

Usual Dosage Oral: Adolescents ≥30 kg and Adults: One tablet twice daily. **Note:** Because this is a fixed-dose combination product, avoid use in patients requiring dosage reduction including children <30 kg, renally-impaired patients with a creatinine clearance ≤50 mL/minute, hepatic impairment, or those patients experiencing dose-limiting adverse effects.

Dosage Forms

Tablet:

Combivir®: Zidovudine 300 mg and lamivudine 150 mg

Zilactin® [Can] *see* lidocaine *on page* 584
Zilactin-L® [US-OTC] *see* lidocaine *on page* 584
Zilactin®-B [US-OTC/Can] *see* benzocaine *on page* 129
Zilactin Baby® [Can] *see* benzocaine *on page* 129
Zilactin Toothache and Gum Pain® [US-OTC] *see* benzocaine *on page* 129

zileuton (zye LOO ton)

U.S./Canadian Brand Names Zyflo CR® [US]

Therapeutic Category 5-Lipoxygenase Inhibitor

Use Prophylaxis and chronic treatment of asthma in children ≥12 years of age and adults

Usual Dosage Oral: Children ≥12 years and Adults (Zyflo CR®): 1200 mg twice daily

Dosage Forms

Tablet, extended release:

Zyflo CR®: 600 mg

Zinacef® [US/Can] *see* cefuroxime *on page* 199
zinc *see* trace metals *on page* 974
Zincate® [US] *see* zinc sulfate *on page* 1031

zinc chloride (zink KLOR ide)

Therapeutic Category Trace Element

Use Cofactor for replacement therapy to different enzymes; helps maintain normal growth rates, normal skin hydration, and senses of taste and smell

Usual Dosage Clinical response may not occur for up to 6-8 weeks

Supplemental to I.V. solutions:

Premature Infants <1500 g, up to 3 kg: 300 mcg/kg/day

Infants (full term) and Children ≤5 years: 100 mcg/kg/day

Adults:

Stable with fluid loss from small bowel: 12.2 mg zinc/L TPN or 17.1 mg zinc/kg (added to 1000 mL I.V. fluids) of stool or ileostomy output

Metabolically stable: 2.5-4 mg/day; add 2 mg/day for acute catabolic states

Dosage Forms

Injection, solution [preservative free]: 1 mg/mL (10 mL, 50 mL)

zinc diethylenetriaminepentaacetate (Zn-DTPA) *see* diethylene triamine penta-acetic acid *on page* 306
Zincfrin® [Can] *see* phenylephrine and zinc sulfate *(Canada only) on page* 777

zinc gelatin (zink JEL ah tin)

Synonyms dome paste bandage; unna's boot; unna's paste; zinc gelatin boot

U.S./Canadian Brand Names Gelucast® [US]

Therapeutic Category Protectant, Topical

Use As a protectant and to support varicosities and similar lesions of the lower limbs

Usual Dosage Topical: Apply externally as an occlusive boot

Dosage Forms

Bandage: 3" x 10 yards; 4" x 10 yards

Gelucast®: 3" x 10 yards; 4" x 10 yards

zinc gelatin boot *see* zinc gelatin *on page* 1030
Zincofax® [Can] *see* zinc oxide *on page* 1030
Zincon® [US-OTC] *see* pyrithione zinc *on page* 842

zinc oxide (zink OKS ide)

Synonyms base ointment; lassar's zinc paste

U.S./Canadian Brand Names Ammens® Medicated Deodorant [US-OTC]; Balmex® [US-OTC]; Boudreaux's® Butt Paste [US-OTC]; Critic-Aid Skin Care® [US-OTC]; Desitin® Creamy [US-OTC]; Desitin® [US-OTC]; Zincofax® [Can]

Therapeutic Category Topical Skin Product

Use Protective coating for mild skin irritations and abrasions; soothing and protective ointment to promote healing of chapped skin, diaper rash

Usual Dosage Topical: Infants, Children, and Adults: Apply as required for affected areas several times daily

Dosage Forms

Cream:

Balmex® [OTC]: 11.3% (60 g, 120 g, 480 g)

Ointment, topical: 20% (30 g, 60 g, 454 g); 40% (120 g)

Desitin® [OTC]: 40% (30 g, 60 g, 90 g, 120 g, 270 g, 480 g)

Desitin® Creamy [OTC]: 10% (60 g, 120 g)

Paste, topical:

Boudreaux's® Butt Paste [OTC]: 16% (30 g, 60 g, 120 g, 480 g)

Critic-Aid Skin Care® [OTC]: 20% (71 g, 170 g)

Powder, topical:

Ammens® Original Medicated [OTC], Ammens® Shower Fresh [OTC]: 9.1% (312 g)

zinc oxide and miconazole nitrate *see* miconazole and zinc oxide *on page 655*

zinc sulfate (zink SUL fate)

Sound-Alike/Look-Alike Issues

$ZnSO_4$ is an error-prone abbreviation (mistaken as morphine sulfate)

U.S./Canadian Brand Names Anuzinc [Can]; Orazinc® [US-OTC]; Rivasol [Can]; Zincate® [US]

Therapeutic Category Electrolyte Supplement, Oral

Use Zinc supplement (oral and parenteral); may improve wound healing in those who are deficient

Usual Dosage

RDA: Oral:

Birth to 6 months: 3 mg elemental zinc/day

6-12 months: 5 mg elemental zinc/day

1-10 years: 10 mg elemental zinc/day

≥11 years: 15 mg elemental zinc/day

Zinc deficiency: Oral:

Infants and Children: 0.5-1 mg elemental zinc/kg/day divided 1-3 times/day; somewhat larger quantities may be needed if there is impaired intestinal absorption or an excessive loss of zinc

Adults: 110-220 mg zinc sulfate (25-50 mg elemental zinc)/dose 3 times/day

Parenteral TPN: I.V.:

Infants (premature, birth weight <1500 g up to 3 kg): 300 mcg/kg/day

Infants (full-term) and Children ≤5 years: 100 mcg/kg/day

Adults:

Acute metabolic states: 4.5-6 mg/day

Metabolically stable: 2.5-4 mg/day

Stable with fluid loss from the small bowel: 12.2 mg zinc/L of TPN solution, or an additional 17.1 mg zinc (added to 1000 mL I.V. fluids) per kg of stool or ileostomy output

Dosage Forms

Capsule: 220 mg

Orazinc® [OTC], Zincate®: 220 mg

Injection, solution [preservative free]: 1 mg elemental zinc/mL (10 mL); 5 mg elemental zinc/mL (5 mL)

Tablet: 110 mg

Orazinc® [OTC]: 110 mg

zinc sulfate and phenylephrine *see* phenylephrine and zinc sulfate *(Canada only) on page 777*

zinc undecylenate *see* undecylenic acid and derivatives *on page 997*

Zinecard® [US/Can] *see* dexrazoxane *on page 292*

Zingo™ *(Discontinued)* *see* lidocaine *on page 584*

Ziox™ [US] *see* chlorophyllin, papain, and urea *on page 211*

Ziox 405™ [US] *see* chlorophyllin, papain, and urea *on page 211*

ziprasidone (zi PRAS i done)

Synonyms ziprasidone hydrochloride; ziprasidone mesylate

U.S./Canadian Brand Names Geodon® [US]; Zeldox® [Can]

Therapeutic Category Antipsychotic Agent

Use Treatment of schizophrenia; treatment of acute manic or mixed episodes associated with bipolar disorder with or without psychosis; acute agitation in patients with schizophrenia

Usual Dosage Adults:

Bipolar mania: Oral: Initial: 40 mg twice daily (with food)

Adjustment: May increase to 60 or 80 mg twice daily on second day of treatment; average dose 40-80 mg twice daily

Schizophrenia: Oral: Initial: 20 mg twice daily (with food)

Adjustment: Increases (if indicated) should be made no more frequently than every 2 days; ordinarily patients should be observed for improvement over several weeks before adjusting the dose

Maintenance: Range 20-100 mg twice daily; however, dosages >80 mg twice daily are generally not recommended

Acute agitation (schizophrenia): I.M.: 10 mg every 2 hours **or** 20 mg every 4 hours; maximum: 40 mg/day; oral therapy should replace I.M. administration as soon as possible

Dosage Forms

Capsule:

Geodon®: 20 mg, 40 mg, 60 mg, 80 mg

Injection, powder for reconstitution:

Geodon®: 20 mg

ziprasidone hydrochloride *see* ziprasidone *on page* *1032*
ziprasidone mesylate *see* ziprasidone *on page* *1032*
Zithromax® [US/Can] *see* azithromycin *on page* *116*
Zithromax® TRI-PAK™ *see* azithromycin *on page* *116*
Zithromax® Z-PAK® *see* azithromycin *on page* *116*
ZM-182,780 *see* fulvestrant *on page* *448*
Zmax® [US] *see* azithromycin *on page* *116*
Zn-DTPA *see* diethylene triamine penta-acetic acid *on page* *306*
ZNP® Bar [US-OTC] *see* pyrithione zinc *on page* *842*
Zocor® [US/Can] *see* simvastatin *on page* *902*
Zoderm® [US] *see* benzoyl peroxide *on page* *132*
Zoderm® Hydrating Wash™ [US] *see* benzoyl peroxide *on page* *132*
Zoderm® Redi-Pads™ [US] *see* benzoyl peroxide *on page* *132*
Zofran® [US/Can] *see* ondansetron *on page* *726*
Zofran® ODT [US/Can] *see* ondansetron *on page* *726*
zol 446 *see* zoledronic acid *on page* *1032*
Zoladex® [US/Can] *see* goserelin *on page* *471*
Zoladex® LA [Can] *see* goserelin *on page* *471*
zoledronate *see* zoledronic acid *on page* *1032*

zoledronic acid (zoe le DRON ik AS id)

Sound-Alike/Look-Alike Issues

Zometa® may be confused with Zofran®, Zoladex®

Synonyms CGP-42446; zol 446; zoledronate

U.S./Canadian Brand Names Aclasta® [Can]; Reclast® [US]; Zometa® [US/Can]

Therapeutic Category Bisphosphonate Derivative

Use

Oncology-related uses: Treatment of hypercalcemia of malignancy (albumin-corrected serum calcium >12 mg/dL); treatment of multiple myeloma; treatment of bone metastases of solid tumors

Nononcology uses: Treatment of Paget disease of bone; treatment of osteoporosis in postmenopausal women (to reduce the incidence of fractures or to reduce the incidence of new clinical fractures in patients with low-trauma hip fracture); prevention of osteoporosis in postmenopausal women, treatment of osteoporosis in men (to increase bone mass); treatment and prevention of glucocorticoid-induced osteoporosis (in patients initiating or continuing prednisone ≥7.5 mg/day [or equivalent] and expected to remain on glucocorticoids for at least 12 months)

Usual Dosage I.V.: Adults: **Note:** Acetaminophen administration after the infusion may reduce symptoms of acute-phase reactions. Patients treated for multiple myeloma, osteoporosis, and Paget disease should receive a daily calcium supplement and multivitamin containing vitamin D (if dietary intake is inadequate).

Hypercalcemia of malignancy (albumin-corrected serum calcium ≥12 mg/dL) (Zometa®): 4 mg (maximum) given as a single dose. Wait at least 7 days before considering retreatment. Dosage adjustment may be needed in patients with decreased renal function following treatment.

Multiple myeloma or metastatic bone lesions from solid tumors (Zometa®): 4 mg every 3-4 weeks

Osteoporosis, glucocorticoid-induced, treatment and prevention (Reclast®, Aclasta® [CAN]): 5 mg infused over at least 15 minutes once a year

Osteoporosis, prevention (Reclast®): 5 mg infused over at least 15 minutes every 2 years

Osteoporosis, treatment (Reclast®, Aclasta® [CAN]): 5 mg infused over at least 15 minutes once a year

Paget disease: 5 mg infused over at least 15 minutes. **Note:** Data concerning retreatment is not available; retreatment may be considered for relapse if appropriate, for inadequate response, or in patients who are symptomatic.

Dosage Forms [CAN] = Canadian brand name

Infusion, solution [premixed]:

Aclasta® [CAN]): 5 mg (100 mL) [not available in the U.S.]

Reclast®: 5 mg (100 mL)

Injection, solution:

Zometa®: 4 mg/5 mL (5 mL)

Zolicef® ***(Discontinued)*** *see* cefazolin *on page 191*

Zolinza™ [US] *see* vorinostat *on page 1022*

zolmitriptan (zohl mi TRIP tan)

Sound-Alike/Look-Alike Issues

zolmitriptan may be confused with SUMAtriptan

Synonyms 311C90

U.S./Canadian Brand Names Zomig-ZMT® [US]; Zomig® Nasal Spray [Can]; Zomig® Rapimelt [Can]; Zomig® [US/Can]

Therapeutic Category Antimigraine Agent; Serotonin Agonist

Use Acute treatment of migraine with or without aura

Usual Dosage Oral: Adults: Migraine:

Tablet: Initial: ≤2.5 mg at the onset of migraine headache; may break 2.5 mg tablet in half

Orally-disintegrating tablet: Initial: 2.5 mg at the onset of migraine headache

Nasal spray: Initial: 1 spray (5 mg) at the onset of migraine headache

Note: Use the lowest possible dose to minimize adverse events. If the headache returns, the dose may be repeated after 2 hours; do not exceed 10 mg within a 24-hour period. Controlled trials have not established the effectiveness of a second dose if the initial one was ineffective

Dosage Forms

Solution, intranasal [spray]:

Zomig®: 5 mg/0.1 mL (0.1 mL)

Tablet:

Zomig®: 2.5 mg, 5 mg

Tablet, orally disintegrating

Zomig-ZMT®: 2.5 mg, 5 mg

Zoloft® [US/Can] *see* sertraline *on page 898*

zolpidem (zole PI dem)

Sound-Alike/Look-Alike Issues

zolpidem may be confused with lorazepam, zaleplon

Ambien® may be confused with Abilify®, Ativan®, Ambi 10®

Synonyms zolpidem tartrate

U.S./Canadian Brand Names Ambien CR® [US]; Ambien® [US]; Edluar™ [US]; Zolpimist® [US]

Therapeutic Category Hypnotic, Nonbarbiturate

Controlled Substance C-IV

Use
Ambien®, Edluar™: Short-term treatment of insomnia (with difficulty of sleep onset)
Ambien CR®: Treatment of insomnia (with difficulty of sleep onset and/or sleep maintenance)

Usual Dosage Oral: Adults:
Immediate release, Sublingual: 10 mg immediately before bedtime; maximum dose: 10 mg
Extended release: 12.5 mg immediately before bedtime

Product Availability Zolpimist® oral spray: FDA approved December, 2008; availability currently undetermined
Zolpimist® is an oral spray of zolpidem indicated for the short-term treatment of insomnia characterized by difficulties with sleep initiation.

Dosage Forms
Tablet, oral: 5 mg, 10 mg
Ambien®: 5 mg, 10 mg
Tablet, extended release, oral:
Ambien CR®: 6.25 mg, 12.5 mg
Tablet, sublingual:
Edluar™: 5 mg, 10 mg

zolpidem tartrate *see* zolpidem *on page 1033*
Zolpimist® [US] *see* zolpidem *on page 1033*
Zometa® [US/Can] *see* zoledronic acid *on page 1032*
Zomig® [US/Can] *see* zolmitriptan *on page 1033*
Zomig® Nasal Spray [Can] *see* zolmitriptan *on page 1033*
Zomig® Rapimelt [Can] *see* zolmitriptan *on page 1033*
Zomig-ZMT® [US] *see* zolmitriptan *on page 1033*
Zomorph® [Can] *see* morphine sulfate *on page 667*
Zonalon® [US/Can] *see* doxepin *on page 334*
Zonegran® [US] *see* zonisamide *on page 1034*

zonisamide (zoe NIS a mide)

Sound-Alike/Look-Alike Issues
zonisamide may be confused with lacosamide
Zonegran® may be confused with Sinequan®

U.S./Canadian Brand Names Zonegran® [US]

Therapeutic Category Anticonvulsant, Sulfonamide

Use Adjunct treatment of partial seizures in children >16 years of age and adults with epilepsy

Usual Dosage Oral: Children >16 years and Adults: Adjunctive treatment of partial seizures: Initial: 100 mg/day; dose may be increased to 200 mg/day after 2 weeks. Further dosage increases to 300 mg/day and 400 mg/day can then be made with a minimum of 2 weeks between adjustments, in order to reach steady state at each dosage level. Doses of up to 600 mg/day have been studied, however, there is no evidence of increased response with doses above 400 mg/day.

Dosage Forms
Capsule: 25 mg, 50 mg, 100 mg
Zonegran®: 25 mg, 100 mg

zopiclone *(Canada only)* (ZOE pi clone)

U.S./Canadian Brand Names Apo-Zopiclone® [Can]; CO Zopiclone [Can]; Dom-Zopiclone [Can]; Gen-Zopiclone [Can]; Imovane® [Can]; Novo-Zopiclone [Can]; Nu-Zopiclone [Can]; PMS-Zopiclone [Can]; RAN™-Zopiclone [Can]; ratio-Zopiclone [Can]; Rhovane® [Can]; Rhoxal-zopiclone [Can]; Riva-Zopiclone [Can]; Sandoz-Zopiclone [Can]

Therapeutic Category Hypnotic

Use Symptomatic relief of transient and short-term insomnia

Usual Dosage Administer just before bedtime: Oral: Adults: 5-7.5 mg
Patients with chronic respiratory insufficiency: 3.75 mg; may increase up to 7.5 mg with caution in appropriate cases

Dosage Forms [CAN] = Canadian brand name
Tablet: 5 mg, 7.5 mg [not available in the U.S.]
Apo-Zopiclone® [CAN], Gen-Zopiclone [CAN], Imovane® [CAN], Novo-Zopiclone [CAN], Nu-Zopiclone [CAN], PMS-Zopiclone [CAN], Rhovane® [CAN], Rhoxal-zopiclone [CAN]: 5 mg, 7.5 mg

Zorbtive® [US] *see* somatropin *on page 916*
Zorcaine™ [US/Can] *see* articaine and epinephrine *on page 99*
ZORprin® [US] *see* aspirin *on page 103*
ZOS *see* zoster vaccine *on page 1035*
Zostavax® [US] *see* zoster vaccine *on page 1035*

zoster vaccine (ZOS ter vak SEEN)

Synonyms shingles vaccine; varicella-zoster (VZV) vaccine (zoster); VZV vaccine (zoster); ZOS

U.S./Canadian Brand Names Zostavax® [US]

Therapeutic Category Vaccine

Use Prevention of herpes zoster (shingles) in patients ≥60 years of age

The Advisory Committee on Immunization Practices (ACIP) recommends routine vaccination of all patients ≥60 years of age, including:

- Patients who report a previous episode of zoster.
- Patients with chronic medical conditions (eg, chronic renal failure, diabetes mellitus, rheumatoid arthritis, chronic pulmonary disease) unless those conditions are contraindications.
- Residents of nursing homes and other long-term care facilities ≥60 years of age, without contraindications.

Usual Dosage SubQ: Adults ≥60 years: 0.65 mL administered as a single dose; there is no data to support readministration of the vaccine

Dosage Forms

Injection, powder for reconstitution [preservative free]

Zostavax®: 19,400 plaque-forming units (PFU)

Zostrix® [US-OTC/Can] *see* capsaicin *on page 178*
Zostrix®-HP [US-OTC/Can] *see* capsaicin *on page 178*
Zostrix® Neuropathy [US-OTC] *see* capsaicin *on page 178*
Zosyn® [US] *see* piperacillin and tazobactam sodium *on page 787*
Zovia® [US] *see* ethinyl estradiol and ethynodiol diacetate *on page 385*
Zovirax® [US/Can] *see* acyclovir *on page 33*
Ztuss™ Tablet *(Discontinued)*
Ztuss™ ZT *(Discontinued)*
zuclopenthixol acetate *see* zuclopenthixol *(Canada only) on page 1035*

zuclopenthixol *(Canada only)* (zoo kloe pen THIX ol)

Synonyms Z-chlopenthixol; zuclopenthixol acetate; zuclopenthixol decanoate; zuclopenthixol dihydrochloride

U.S./Canadian Brand Names Clopixol-Acuphase® [Can]; Clopixol® Depot [Can]; Clopixol® [Can]

Therapeutic Category Antipsychotic Agent

Use Management of schizophrenia; acetate injection is intended for short-term acute treatment; decanoate injection is for long-term management; dihydrochloride tablets may be used in either phase

Usual Dosage Adults:

Oral: Zuclopenthixol dihydrochloride: Initial: 20-30 mg/day in 2-3 divided doses; usual maintenance dose: 20-40 mg/day; maximum daily dose: 100 mg

I.M.:

Zuclopenthixol acetate: 50-150 mg; may be repeated in 2-3 days; no more than 4 injections should be given in the course of treatment; maximum dose during course of treatment: 400 mg (maximum treatment period: 2 weeks)

Transfer of patients from I.M. acetate to oral (tablets):

50 mg = 20 mg daily
100 mg = 40 mg daily
150 mg = 60 mg daily

Zuclopenthixol decanoate: 100 mg by deep I.M. injection; additional I.M. doses of 100-200 mg may be given over the following 1-4 weeks; maximum weekly dose: 600 mg; usual maintenance dose: 150-300 mg every 2 weeks

Transfer of patients from oral (tablets) to I.M. decanoate (depot):

≤20 mg daily = 100 mg every 2 weeks
25-40 mg daily = 200 mg every 2 weeks
50-75 mg daily = 300 mg every 2 weeks
>75 mg/day = 400 mg every 2 weeks

Transfer of patients from I.M. acetate to I.M. decanoate (depot):
50 mg every 2-3 days = 100 mg every 2 weeks
100 mg every 2-3 days = 200 mg every 2 weeks
150 mg every 2-3 days = 300 mg every 2 weeks

Dosage Forms [CAN] = Canadian brand name

Injection:

Clopixol Acuphase® [CAN]: 50 mg/mL [zuclopenthixol 42.5 mg/mL] (1 mL, 2 mL) [not available in the U.S.]

Clopixol® Depot [CAN]: 200 mg/mL [zuclopenthixol 144.4 mg/mL] (10 mL) [not available in the U.S.]

Tablet:

Clopixol® [CAN]: 10 mg, 25 mg, 40 mg [not available in the U.S.]

Zyprexa Relprevv - I.M. injection form

CHEMOTHERAPY REGIMENS

5 + 2

Use Leukemia, acute myeloid (induction)

Regimen

Cytarabine: I.V.: 100-200 mg/m^2/day continuous infusion days 1 to 5
[total dose/cycle = 500-1000 mg/m^2]

with

Daunorubicin: I.V.: 45 mg/m^2/day days 1 and 2
[total dose/cycle = 90 mg/m^2]

7 + 3 (Daunorubicin)

Use Leukemia, acute myeloid (induction)

Regimen

Cytarabine: I.V.: 100 mg/m^2/day continuous infusion days 1 to 7
[total dose/cycle = 700 mg/m^2]

Daunorubicin: I.V.: 45 mg/m^2/day days 1, 2, and 3
[total dose/cycle = 135 mg/m^2]

Administer one cycle only

7 + 3 (Idarubicin)

Use Leukemia, acute myeloid (induction)

Regimen

Cytarabine: I.V.: 100-200 mg/m^2/day continuous infusion days 1 to 7
[total dose/cycle = 700-1400 mg/m^2]

Idarubicin: I.V.: 12 mg/m^2/day days 1, 2, and 3
[total dose/cycle = 36 mg/m^2]

Administer one cycle only

7 + 3 (Mitoxantrone)

Use Leukemia, acute myeloid (induction)

Regimen

Cytarabine: I.V.: 100-200 mg/m^2/day continuous infusion days 1 to 7
[total dose/cycle = 700-1400 mg/m^2]

Mitoxantrone: I.V.: 12 mg/m^2/day days 1, 2, and 3
[total dose/cycle = 36 mg/m^2]

Administer one cycle only

7 + 3 + 7

Use Leukemia, acute myeloid

Regimen

Cytarabine: I.V.: 100 mg/m^2/day continuous infusion days 1 to 7
[total dose/cycle = 700 mg/m^2]

Daunorubicin: I.V.: 50 mg/m^2/day days 1, 2, and 3
[total dose/cycle = 150 mg/m^2]

Etoposide: I.V.: 75 mg/m^2/day days 1 to 7
[total dose/cycle = 525 mg/m^2]

Repeat cycle every 21 days; up to 3 cycles may be given based on individual response

8 in 1 (Brain Tumors)

Use Brain tumors

Regimen NOTE: Multiple variations are listed below.

Variation 1:

Methylprednisolone: I.V.: 300 mg/m^2 every 6 hours day 1 (3 doses)
[total dose/cycle = 900 mg/m^2]

Vincristine: I.V.: 1.5 mg/m^2 (maximum: 2 mg) day 1

Lomustine: Oral: 75 mg/m^2 day 1

Procarbazine: Oral: 75 mg/m^2 day 1; 1 hour after methylprednisolone and vincristine

Hydroxyurea: Oral: 3000 mg/m^2 day 1; 2 hours after methylprednisolone and vincristine

Cisplatin: I.V.: 90 mg/m^2 day 1; 3 hours after methylprednisolone and vincristine

Cytarabine: I.V.: 300 mg/m^2 day 1; 9 hours after methylprednisolone and vincristine

Dacarbazine: I.V.: 150 mg/m^2 day 1; 12 hours after methylprednisolone and vincristine

Repeat cycle every 14 days

Variation 2:
Methylprednisolone: I.V.: 300 mg/m^2 every 6 hours day 1 (3 doses)
[total dose/cycle = 900 mg/m^2]
Vincristine: I.V.: 1.5 mg/m^2 (maximum: 2 mg) day 1
Lomustine: Oral: 75 mg/m^2 day 1
Procarbazine: Oral: 75 mg/m^2 day 1; 1 hour after methylprednisolone and vincristine
Hydroxyurea: Oral: 3000 mg/m^2 day 1; 2 hours after methylprednisolone and vincristine
Cisplatin: I.V.: 60 mg/m^2 day 1; 3 hours after methylprednisolone and vincristine
Cytarabine: I.V.: 300 mg/m^2 day 1; 9 hours after methylprednisolone and vincristine
Cyclophosphamide: I.V.: 300 mg/m^2 day 1; 12 hours after methylprednisolone and vincristine
Repeat cycle every 14 days

8 in 1 (Retinoblastoma)

Use Retinoblastoma

Regimen

Vincristine: I.V.: 1.5 mg/m^2 day 1
Methylprednisolone: I.V.: 300 mg/m^2 day 1
Lomustine: Oral: 75 mg/m^2 day 1
Procarbazine: Oral: 75 mg/m^2 day 1
Hydroxyurea: Oral: 1500 mg/m^2 day 1
Cisplatin: I.V.: 60 mg/m^2 day 1
Cytarabine: I.V.: 300 mg/m^2 day 1
Repeat cycle every 28 days

AAV (DD)

Use Wilms tumor

Regimen

Dactinomycin: I.V.: 15 mcg/kg/day days 1 to 5 of weeks 0, 13, 26, 39, 52, and 65
[total dose/cycle = 450 mcg/kg]
Doxorubicin: I.V.: 20 mg/m^2/day days 1, 2, and 3 of weeks 6, 19, 32, 45, and 58
[total dose/cycle = 300 mg/m^2]
Vincristine: I.V.: 1.5 mg/m^2 day 1 of weeks 0-10, 13, 14, 26, 27, 39, 40, 52, 53, 65, and 66
[total dose/cycle = 31.5 mg/m^2]

ABVD

Use Lymphoma, Hodgkin disease

Regimen

Doxorubicin: I.V.: 25 mg/m^2/day days 1 and 15
[total dose/cycle = 50 mg/m^2]
Bleomycin: I.V.: 10 units/m^2/day days 1 and 15
[total dose/cycle = 20 units/m^2]
Vinblastine: I.V.: 6 mg/m^2/day days 1 and 15
[total dose/cycle = 12 mg/m^2]
Dacarbazine: I.V.: 375 mg/m^2/day days 1 and 15
[total dose/cycle = 750 mg/m^2]
Repeat cycle every 28 days

AC

Use Breast cancer

Regimen NOTE: Multiple variations are listed below.

Variation 1: AC (conventional):
Doxorubicin: I.V.: 60 mg/m^2 day 1
[total dose/cycle = 60 mg/m^2]
Cyclophosphamide: I.V.: 600 mg/m^2 day 1
[total dose/cycle = 600 mg/m^2]
Repeat cycle every 21 days

Variation 2:
Cyclophosphamide: Oral: 200 mg/m^2/day days 3 to 6
[total dose/cycle = 800 mg/m^2]
Doxorubicin: I.V.: 40 mg/m^2 day 1
[total dose/cycle = 40 mg/m^2]
Repeat cycle every 3 weeks for 3 cycles, then every 4 weeks

ACAV (J)

Use Wilms tumor

Regimen

Dactinomycin: I.V.: 15 mcg/kg/day days 1 to 5 of weeks 0, 13, 26, 39, 52, and 65
[total dose/cycle = 450 mcg/kg]
Cyclophosphamide: I.V.: 10 mg/kg/day days 1, 2, and 3 of weeks 0, 6, 13, 19, 26, 32, 39, 45, 52, 58, and 65
[total dose/cycle = 330 mg/kg]
Doxorubicin: I.V.: 20 mg/m^2/day days 1, 2, and 3 of weeks 6, 19, 32, 45, and 58
[total dose/cycle = 300 mg/m^2]
Vincristine: I.V.: 1.5 mg/m^2 day 1 of weeks 0-10, 13, 14, 19, 20, 26, 27, 32, 33, 39, 40, 45, 52, 53, 56, 57, 65, and 66
[total dose/cycle = 42 mg/m^2]

AC/Paclitaxel (Sequential)

Use Breast cancer

Regimen

Variation 1: AC + Paclitaxel (conventional):
Doxorubicin: I.V.: 60 mg/m^2 day 1
[total dose/cycle = 60 mg/m^2]
Cyclophosphamide: I.V.: 600 mg/m^2 day 1
[total dose/cycle = 600 mg/m^2]
Repeat cycle every 21 days for 4 cycles
followed by
Paclitaxel: I.V.: 175 mg/m^2 day 1
[total dose/cycle = 175 mg/m^2]
Repeat cycle every 21 days for 4 cycles
Variation 2: AC + Paclitaxel (dose dense):
Doxorubicin: I.V.: 60 mg/m^2 day 1
[total dose/cycle = 60 mg/m^2]
Cyclophosphamide: I.V.: 600 mg/m^2 day 1
[total dose/cycle = 600 mg/m^2]
Filgrastim: SubQ: 5 mcg/kg/day days 3 to 10
[total dose/cycle = 40 mcg/kg]
Repeat cycle every 14 days for 4 cycles
followed by
Paclitaxel: I.V.: 175 mg/m^2 day 1
[total dose/cycle = 175 mg/m^2]
Filgrastim: SubQ: 5 mcg/kg/day days 3 to 10
[total dose/cycle = 40 mcg/kg]
Repeat cycle every 14 days for 4 cycles

AC-Paclitaxel-Trastuzumab

Use Breast cancer

Regimen NOTE: Multiple variations are listed below.

Variation 1:
Doxorubicin: I.V.: 60 mg/m^2 day 1
[total dose/cycle = 60 mg/m^2]
Cyclophosphamide: I.V.: 600 mg/m^2 day 1
[total dose/cycle = 600 mg/m^2]
Repeat cycle every 21 days for 4 cycles
followed by
Paclitaxel: I.V.: 175 mg/m^2 day 1
[total dose/cycle = 175 mg/m^2]

Trastuzumab: I.V.: 4 mg/kg (loading dose) day 1 (cycle 1 only)
[total dose/cycle = 4 mg/kg]
followed by I.V.: 2 mg/kg/day days 8 and 15 (cycle 1)
[total dose/cycle = 4 mg/kg]
then I.V.: 2 mg/kg/day days 1, 8, and 15 (cycles 2, 3, and 4)
[total dose/cycle = 6 mg/kg]
Repeat cycle every 21 days for 4 cycles
followed by
Trastuzumab: I.V.: 2 mg/kg weekly for 40 weeks

Variation 2:
Doxorubicin: I.V.: 60 mg/m^2 day 1
[total dose/cycle = 60 mg/m^2]
Cyclophosphamide: I.V.: 600 mg/m^2 day 1
[total dose/cycle = 600 mg/m^2]
Repeat cycle every 21 days for 4 cycles
followed by
Paclitaxel: I.V.: 80 mg/m^2day 1 week 13
[total dose/cycle = 80 mg/m^2]
Trastuzumab: I.V.: 4 mg/kg (loading dose) day 1 week 13 only
[total dose/cycle = 4 mg/kg]
followed by
Paclitaxel: I.V.: 80 mg/m^2 weekly
[total dose/cycle = 80 mg/m^2]
Trastuzumab: I.V.: 2 mg/kg /weekly
[total dose/cycle = 2 mg/kg]
Repeat cycle every week for 11 cycles
followed by
Trastuzumab: I.V.: 2 mg/kg/weekly for 40 weeks

AD

Use Soft tissue sarcoma

Regimen
Doxorubicin: I.V.: 60 mg/m^2 day 1
[total dose/cycle = 60 mg/m^2]
Dacarbazine: I.V.: 250 mg/m^2/day days 1 to 5
[total dose/cycle = 1250 mg/m^2]
Repeat cycle every 21 days

AI

Use Soft tissue sarcoma

Regimen NOTE: Multiple variations are listed below.

Variation 1:
Doxorubicin: I.V.: 25 mg/m^2/day continuous infusion days 1, 2, and 3
[total dose/cycle = 75 mg/m^2]
Ifosfamide: I.V.: 2 g/m^2/day days 1 to 5
[total dose/cycle = 10 g/m^2]
Mesna: I.V.: 400 mg/m^2 day 1
followed by I.V.: 1200 mg/m^2/day continuous infusion days 1 to 5
[total dose/cycle = 6400 mg/m^2]
Repeat cycle every 3 weeks

Variation 2:
Doxorubicin: I.V.: 30 mg/m^2/day continuous infusion days 1, 2, and 3
[total dose/cycle = 90 mg/m^2]
Ifosfamide: I.V.: 2.5 g/m^2/day days 1 to 4
[total dose/cycle = 10 g/m^2]
Mesna: I.V.: 500 mg/m^2 day 1
followed by I.V.: 1500 mg/m^2/day continuous infusion days 1 to 4
[total dose/cycle = 6500 mg/m^2]
Filgrastim: SubQ: 5 mcg/kg/day days 5 through ANC recovery
Repeat cycle every 3 weeks

AP

Use Endometrial cancer

Regimen

Doxorubicin: I.V.: 60 mg/m^2 day 1
[total dose/cycle = 60 mg/m^2]
Cisplatin: I.V.: 60 mg/m^2 day 1
[total dose/cycle = 60 mg/m^2]
Repeat cycle every 21-28 days

AT

Use Breast cancer

Regimen NOTE: Multiple variations are listed below.

Variation 1:
Doxorubicin: I.V.: 50 mg/m^2 day 1
[total dose/cycle = 50 mg/m^2]
Docetaxel: I.V.: 75 mg/m^2 day 1
[total dose/cycle = 75 mg/m^2]
Repeat cycle every 3 weeks

Variation 2:
Doxorubicin: I.V.: 60 mg/m^2 day 1
[total dose/cycle = 60 mg/m^2]
Docetaxel: I.V.: 60 mg/m^2 day 1
[total dose/cycle = 60 mg/m^2]
Repeat cycle every 3 weeks

Variation 3:
Doxorubicin: I.V.: 50 mg/m^2 day 1
[total dose/cycle = 50 mg/m^2]
Docetaxel: I.V.: 75 mg/m^2 day 1
[total dose/cycle = 75 mg/m^2]
Repeat cycle every 14 days

Variation 4:
Doxorubicin: I.V.: 50 mg/m^2 day 1
[total dose/cycle = 50 mg/m^2]
Docetaxel: I.V.: 60 mg/m^2 day 1
[total dose/cycle = 60 mg/m^2]
Repeat cycle every 3 weeks

Variation 5:
Doxorubicin: I.V.: 50 mg/m^2 day 1
[total dose/cycle = 50 mg/m^2]
Docetaxel: I.V.: 60 mg/m^2 day 1
[total dose/cycle = 60 mg/m^2]
Repeat cycle every 3-4 weeks

Variation 6:
Doxorubicin: I.V.: 56 mg/m^2 day 1
[total dose/cycle = 56 mg/m^2]
Docetaxel: I.V.: 75 mg/m^2 day 1
[total dose/cycle = 75 mg/m^2]
Repeat cycle every 3 weeks

Variation 7:
Doxorubicin: I.V.: 50 mg/m^2 day 1
[total dose/cycle = 50 mg/m^2]
Docetaxel: I.V.: 75 mg/m^2 day 2
[total dose/cycle = 75 mg/m^2]
Repeat cycle every 4 weeks

AVD

Use Wilms tumor

Regimen

Dactinomycin: I.V.: 15 mcg/kg/day days 1 to 5 of weeks 0, 13, 26, 39, 52, and 65
[total dose/cycle = 450 mcg/kg]
Doxorubicin: I.V.: 60 mg/m^2 day 1 of weeks 6, 19, 32, 45, and 58
[total dose/cycle = 300 mg/m^2]
Vincristine: I.V.: 1.5 mg/m^2 day 1 of weeks 1 to 8, 13, 14, 26, 27, 39, 40, 52, 53, 65, and 66
[total dose/cycle = 27 mg/m^2]

AV (EE)

Use Wilms tumor

Regimen

Dactinomycin: I.V.: 15 mcg/kg/day days 1 to 5 of weeks 0, 5, 13, and 26
[total dose/cycle = 300 mcg/kg]
Vincristine: I.V.: 1.5 mg/m^2/dose day 1 of weeks 1 to 10, and days 1 and 5 of weeks 13 and 26
[total dose/cycle = 21 mg/m^2]

AV (K)

Use Wilms tumor

Regimen

Dactinomycin: I.V.: 15 mcg/kg/day days 1 to 5 of weeks 0, 5, 13, 22, 31, 40, 49, and 58
[total dose/cycle = 600 mcg/kg]
Vincristine: I.V.: 1.5 mg/m^2/dose day 1 of weeks 0-10, 15-20, 24-29, 33-38, 42-47, 51-56, and 60-65
[total dose/cycle = 70.5 mg/m^2]

AV (L)

Use Wilms tumor

Regimen

Dactinomycin: I.V.: 15 mcg/kg/day days 1 to 5 of weeks 0 and 5
[total dose/cycle = 150 mcg/kg]
Vincristine: I.V.: 1.5 mg/m^2 day 1 of weeks 0-10
[total dose/cycle = 16.5 mg/m^2]

AV (Wilms Tumor)

Use Wilms tumor

Regimen

Dactinomycin: I.V.: 15 mcg/kg/day days 1 to 5 of weeks 0, 13, 26, 39, 52, and 65
[total dose/cycle = 450 mcg/kg]
Vincristine: I.V.: 1.5 mg/m^2/dose day 1 of weeks 1 to 8, 13, 14, 26, 27, 39, 40, 52, 53, 65, and 66
[total dose/cycle = 27 mg/m^2]

BEACOPP

Use Lymphoma, Hodgkin disease

Regimen

Bleomycin: I.V.: 10 units/m^2 day 8
[total dose/cycle = 10 units/m^2]
Etoposide: I.V.: 100 mg/m^2/day days 1, 2, and 3
[total dose/cycle = 300 mg/m^2]
Doxorubicin: I.V.: 25 mg/m^2 day 1
[total dose/cycle = 25 mg/m^2]
Cyclophosphamide: I.V.: 650 mg/m^2 day 1
[total dose/cycle = 650 mg/m^2]
Vincristine: I.V.: 1.4 mg/m^2 (maximum: 2 mg) day 8
[total dose/cycle = 1.4 mg/m^2; maximum: 2 mg]
Procarbazine: Oral: 100 mg/m^2/day days 1 to 7
[total dose/cycle = 700 mg/m^2]
Prednisone: Oral: 40 mg/m^2/day days 1 to 14
[total dose/cycle = 560 mg/m^2]
Repeat cycle every 21 days

Bendamustine-Rituximab

Use Lymphoma, non-Hodgkin (mantle cell or low-grade NHL)

Regimen NOTE: Multiple variations are listed below.

Variation 1:

Pretreatment:

Rituximab: I.V.: 375 mg/m^2 1 week before the start of cycle 1
[total dose/pretreatment = 375 mg/m^2]

Cycles:

Rituximab: I.V.: 375 mg/m^2 day 1
[total dose/cycle = 375 mg/m^2]

Bendamustine: I.V.: 90 mg/m^2 days 2 and 3
[total dose/cycle = 180 mg/m^2]

Repeat cycle every 4 weeks for up to 4 cycles

Post-Treatment:

Rituximab: I.V.: 375 mg/m^2 4 weeks after the last cycle
[total dose/post-treatment = 375 mg/m^2]

Variation 2:

Pretreatment:

Rituximab: I.V.: 375 mg/m^2 1 week before the start of cycle 1
[total dose/pretreatment = 375 mg/m^2]

Cycles:

Rituximab: I.V.: 375 mg/m^2 day 1
[total dose/cycle = 375 mg/m^2]

Bendamustine: I.V.: 90 mg/m^2 days 2 and 3
[total dose/cycle = 180 mg/m^2]

Repeat cycle every 4 weeks for 4-6 cycles

Post-Treatment:

Rituximab: I.V.: 375 mg/m^2 4 weeks after the last cycle
[total dose/post-treatment = 375 mg/m^2]

BEP (Ovarian Cancer)

Use Ovarian cancer

Regimen

Bleomycin: I.V.: 20 units/m^2 (maximum dose: 30 units) day 1
[total dose/cycle = 20 units/m^2]

Etoposide: I.V.: 75 mg/m^2/day days 1 to 5
[total dose/cycle = 375 mg/m^2]
or I.V.: 75 mg/m^2/day days 1 to 4 (if received prior radiation therapy)
[total dose/cycle = 300 mg/m^2]

Cisplatin: I.V.: 20 mg/m^2/day days 1 to 5
[total dose/cycle = 100 mg/m^2]

Repeat cycle every 3 weeks for 4 cycles

BEP (Ovarian Cancer, Testicular Cancer)

Use Ovarian cancer; Testicular cancer

Regimen

Bleomycin: I.V.: 30 units/day days 2, 9, and 16
[total dose/cycle = 90 units]

Etoposide: I.V.: 100 mg/m^2/day days 1 to 5
[total dose/cycle = 500 mg/m^2]
or I.V.: 120 mg/m^2/day days 1, 2, and 3
[total dose/cycle = 360 mg/m^2]

Cisplatin: I.V.: 20 mg/m^2/day days 1 to 5
[total dose/cycle = 100 mg/m^2]

Repeat cycle every 21 days

BEP (Testicular Cancer)

Use Testicular cancer

Regimen NOTE: Multiple variations are listed below.

Variation 1:

Bleomycin: I.V.: 30 units/day days 1, 8, and 15
[total dose/cycle = 90 units]

Etoposide: I.V.: 100 mg/m^2/day days 1 to 5
[total dose/cycle = 500 mg/m^2]

Cisplatin: I.V.: 20 mg/m^2/day days 1 to 5
[total dose/cycle = 100 mg/m^2]

Repeat cycle every 21 days for 3-4 cycles

Variation 2:

Bleomycin: I.V.: 30 units/day days 2, 9, and 16
[total dose/cycle = 90 units]

Etoposide: I.V.: 100 mg/m^2/day days 1 to 5
[total dose/cycle = 500 mg/m^2]

Cisplatin: I.V.: 20 mg/m^2/day days 1 to 5
[total dose/cycle = 100 mg/m^2]

Repeat cycle every 21 days

Variation 3:

Bleomycin: I.V.: 30 units once weekly
[total dose/cycle = 90 units]

Etoposide: I.V.: 120 mg/m^2/day days 1, 3, and 5
[total dose/cycle = 360 mg/m^2]

Cisplatin: I.V.: 20 mg/m^2/day days 1 to 5
[total dose/cycle = 100 mg/m^2]

Repeat cycle every 21 days

Variation 4:

Bleomycin: I.V.: 30 units/day days 1, 8, and 15
[total dose/cycle = 90 units]

Etoposide: I.V.: 165 mg/m^2/day days 1, 2, and 3
[total dose/cycle = 495 mg/m^2]

Cisplatin: I.V.: 50 mg/m^2/day days 1 and 2
[total dose/cycle = 100 mg/m^2]

Repeat cycle every 21 days

Bevacizumab-Capecitabine

Use Breast cancer

Regimen

Capecitabine: Oral: 1250 mg/m^2 twice daily days 1 to 14
[total dose/cycle = 35,000 mg/m^2]

Bevacizumab: I.V.: 15 mg/kg day 1
[total dose/cycle = 15 mg/kg]

Repeat cycle every 21 days for up to 35 cycles

Bevacizumab-Cisplatin-Gemcitabine (NSCLC)

Use Lung cancer, nonsmall cell

Regimen

Bevacizumab: I.V.: 7.5 or 15 mg/kg/dose day 1
[total dose/cycle = 7.5 or 15 mg/kg]

Cisplatin: I.V.: 80 mg/m^2/dose day 1
[total dose/cycle = 80 mg/m^2]

Gemcitabine: I.V.: 1250 mg/m^2/dose days 1 and 8
[total dose/cycle = 2500 mg/m^2]

Repeat cycle every 21 days for up to 6 cycles (bevacizumab monotherapy may be continued thereafter until disease progression)

Bevacizumab-Fluorouracil-Leucovorin

Use Colorectal cancer

Regimen

Bevacizumab: I.V.: 5 mg/kg/day days 1, 15, 29, and 43
[total dose/cycle = 20 mg/kg]
Leucovorin: I.V.: 500 mg/m^2/day days 1, 8, 15, 22, 29, and 36
[total dose/cycle = 3000 mg/m^2]
Fluorouracil: I.V.: 500 mg/m^2/day days 1, 8, 15, 22, 29, and 36
[total dose/cycle = 3000 mg/m^2]
Repeat cycle every 56 days

Bevacizumab-Interferon Alfa (RCC)

Use Renal cell cancer

Regimen NOTE: Multiple variations are listed below

Variation 1:
Interferon Alfa-2a: SubQ: 9 million units 3 times/week
[total dose/cycle = 54 million units]
Bevacizumab: I.V.: 10 mg/kg day 1
[total dose/cycle = 10 mg/kg]
Repeat cycle every 14 days for up to 1 year or until disease progression

Variation 2:
Interferon Alfa-2b: SubQ: 9 million units 3 times/week
[total dose/cycle = 108 million units]
Bevacizumab: I.V.: 10 mg/kg day 1 and 15
[total dose/cycle = 20 mg/kg]
Repeat cycle every 28 days until disease progression or unacceptable toxicity

Bevacizumab-Irinotecan-Fluorouracil-Leucovorin

Use Colorectal cancer

Regimen

Bevacizumab: I.V.: 5 mg/kg/day days 1, 15, and 29
[total dose/cycle = 15 mg/kg]
Irinotecan: I.V.: 125 mg/m^2/day days 1, 8, 15, and 22
[total dose/cycle = 500 mg/m^2]
Fluorouracil: I.V.: 500 mg/m^2/day days 1, 8, 15, and 22
[total dose/cycle = 2000 mg/m^2]
Leucovorin: I.V.: 20 mg/m^2/day days 1, 8, 15, and 22
[total dose/cycle = 80 mg/m^2]
Repeat cycle every 42 days

Bevacizumab-Irinotecan (Glioblastoma)

Use Brain tumors

Regimen Note: Patients receiving concurrent antiepileptic enzyme-inducing drugs received an increased dose of irinotecan (340 mg/m^2/dose).

Bevacizumab: I.V.: 10 mg/kg day 1
[total dose/cycle = 10 mg/kg]
Irinotecan: I.V.: 125 mg/m^2 day 1
[total dose/cycle = 125 mg/m^2]
Repeat cycle every 14 days

Bevacizumab-Oxaliplatin-Fluorouracil-Leucovorin

Use Colorectal cancer

Regimen

Bevacizumab: I.V.: 10 mg/kg day 1
[total dose/cycle = 10 mg/kg]
Oxaliplatin: I.V.: 85 mg/m^2 day 1
[total dose/cycle = 85 mg/m^2]
Leucovorin: I.V.: 200 mg/m^2/day days 1 and 2
[total dose/cycle = 400 mg/m^2]

Fluorouracil: I.V. bolus: 400 mg/m^2/day days 1 and 2
followed by I.V.: 600 mg/m^2 continuous infusion over 22 hours days 1 and 2
[total dose/cycle = 2000 mg/m^2]
Repeat cycle every 14 days

Bicalutamide-Goserelin

Use Prostate cancer

Regimen

Bicalutamide: Oral: 50 mg/day
[total dose/cycle = 1400 mg]
Goserelin acetate: SubQ: 3.6 mg day 1
[total dose/cycle = 3.6 mg]
Repeat cycle every 28 days

Bicalutamide-Leuprolide

Use Prostate cancer

Regimen

Bicalutamide: Oral: 50 mg/day
[total dose/cycle = 1400 mg]
Leuprolide depot: I.M.: 7.5 mg day 1
[total dose/cycle = 7.5 mg]
Repeat cycle every 28 days

BIP

Use Cervical cancer

Regimen

Bleomycin: I.V.: 30 units continuous infusion day 1
[total dose/cycle = 30 units]
Cisplatin: I.V.: 50 mg/m^2 day 2
[total dose/cycle = 50 mg/m^2]
Ifosfamide: I.V.: 5 g/m^2 continuous infusion day 2
[total dose/cycle = 5 g/m^2]
Mesna: I.V.: 6 g/m^2 continuous infusion over 36 hours day 2 (start with ifosfamide)
[total dose/cycle = 6 g/m^2]
Repeat cycle every 21 days

BOLD

Use Melanoma

Regimen

Dacarbazine: I.V.: 200 mg/m^2/day days 1 to 5
[total dose/cycle = 1000 mg/m^2]
Vincristine: I.V.: 1 mg/m^2/day days 1 and 4
[total dose/cycle = 2 mg/m^2]
Bleomycin: I.V.: 15 units/day days 2 and 5
[total dose/cycle = 30 units]
Lomustine: Oral: 80 mg day 1
[total dose/cycle = 80 mg]
Repeat cycle every 4 weeks

BOLD + Interferon

Use Melanoma

Regimen NOTE: Multiple variations are listed below.

Variation 1:
Bleomycin: I.V.: 15 units/day days 2 and 5
[total dose/cycle = 30 units]
Vincristine: I.V.: 1 mg/m^2/day days 1 and 4
[total dose/cycle = 2 mg/m^2]
Lomustine: Oral: 80 mg day 1
[total dose/cycle = 80 mg]
Dacarbazine: I.V.: 200 mg/m^2/day days 1 to 5
[total dose/cycle = 1000 mg/m^2]

Interferon Alfa-2b: SubQ: 3 million units/day days 8 to 49 (cycles 1 and 2)
[total dose through day 49 = 126 million units]
followed by SubQ: 6 million units 3 times/week (beginning day 50 and subsequent cycles)
[total dose/cycle = 72 million units]
Repeat cycle every 4 weeks

Variation 2:
Bleomycin: I.V.: 30 units day 1
[total dose/cycle = 30 units]
Vincristine: I.V.: 2 mg day 1
[total dose/cycle = 2 mg]
Lomustine: Oral: 80 mg day 1
[total dose/cycle = 80 mg]
Dacarbazine: I.V.: 700 mg/m^2 day 1
[total dose/cycle = 700 mg/m^2]
Interferon Alfa-2b: SubQ: 3 million units 3 times/week
[total dose/cycle = 36 million units]
Repeat cycle every 4 weeks

Variation 3:
Bleomycin: I.V.: 15 units/day days 2 and 5
[total dose/cycle = 30 units]
Vincristine: I.V.: 1-2 mg/day days 1 and 4
[total dose/cycle = 2-4 mg]
Lomustine: Oral: 80 mg day 1
[total dose/cycle = 80 mg]
Dacarbazine: I.V.: 200 mg/m^2/day days 1 to 5
[total dose/cycle = 1000 mg/m^2]
Interferon Alfa-2b: SubQ: 6 million units 3 times/week, for 6 doses, starting day 8
[total dose/cycle = 36 million units]
Repeat cycle every 4 weeks

Variation 4:
Bleomycin: I.V.: 15 units/day days 2 and 5
[total dose/cycle = 30 units]
Vincristine: I.V.: 1 mg/m^2/day (maximum: 2 mg/dose) days 1 and 4
[total dose/cycle = 2 mg/m^2]
Lomustine: Oral: 80 mg day 1
[total dose/cycle = 80 mg]
Dacarbazine: I.V.: 200 mg/m^2/day days 1 to 5
[total dose/cycle = 1000 mg/m^2]
Interferon Alfa-2b: SubQ: 3 million units/day days 8, 10, 12, 15, 17, and 19
[total dose/cycle = 18 million units]
Repeat cycle every 4 weeks

BOLD (Melanoma)

Use Melanoma

Regimen NOTE: Multiple variations are listed below.

Variation 1:
Bleomycin: SubQ: 7.5 units/day days 1 and 4 (cycle 1 only)
followed by SubQ: 15 units/day days 1 and 4 (subsequent cycles)
[total dose/cycle = 45 units; maximum total dose (all cycles): 400 units]
Vincristine: I.V.: 1 mg/m^2/day days 1 and 5
[total dose/cycle = 2 mg/m^2]
Lomustine: Oral: 80 mg/m^2 (maximum: 150 mg/dose) day 1
[total dose/cycle = 80 mg/m^2]
Dacarbazine: I.V.: 200 mg/m^2/day (maximum: 400 mg/dose) days 1 to 5
[total dose/cycle = 1000 mg/m^2; maximum: 2000 mg]
Repeat cycle every 4-6 weeks

Variation 2:
Bleomycin: I.V.: 15 units/day days 1 and 4
[total dose/cycle = 30 units]
Vincristine: I.V.: 1 mg/m^2/day days 1 and 5
[total dose/cycle = 2 mg/m^2]

Lomustine: Oral: 80 mg/m^2 (maximum: 150 mg/dose) day 1
[total dose/cycle = 80 mg/m^2]
Dacarbazine: I.V.: 200 mg/m^2/day days 1 to 5
[total dose/cycle = 1000 mg/m^2]
Repeat cycle every 4 weeks
Variation 3:
Bleomycin: I.V.: 15 units/day days 1 and 4
[total dose/cycle = 30 units]
Vincristine: I.V.: 1 mg/m^2 day 1
[total dose/cycle = 1 mg/m^2]
Lomustine: Oral: 80 mg/m^2 day 3 (odd numbered cycles)
[total dose/cycle = 80 mg/m^2; every other cycle]
Dacarbazine: I.V.: 200 mg/m^2/day days 1 to 5
[total dose/cycle = 1000 mg/m^2]
Repeat cycle every 4 weeks

Bortezomib-Dexamethasone

Use Multiple myeloma

Regimen NOTE: Multiple variations are listed below.
Variation 1:
Cycles 1 and 2:
Bortezomib: I.V.: 1.3 mg/m^2/day days 1, 4, 8, and 11
[total dose/cycle = 5.2 mg/m^2]
Dexamethasone: Oral: 40 mg/day days 1 to 4 and days 9 to 12
[total dose/cycle = 320 mg]
Treatment cycle is 21 days
Cycles 3 and 4:
Bortezomib: I.V.: 1.3 mg/m^2/day days 1, 4, 8, and 11
[total dose/cycle = 5.2 mg/m^2]
Dexamethasone: Oral: 40 mg/day days 1 to 4
[total dose/cycle = 160 mg]
Treatment cycle is 21 days
Variation 2:
Cycles 1 and 2:
Bortezomib: I.V.: 1.3 mg/m^2/day days 1, 4, 8, and 11
[total dose/cycle = 5.2 mg/m^2]
Treatment cycle is 21 days
Cycles 3 through 6 (begin dexamethasone after cycle 2 if partial response not achieved or after cycle 4 if complete response not achieved):
Bortezomib: I.V.: 1.3 mg/m^2/day days 1, 4, 8, and 11
[total dose/cycle = 5.2 mg/m^2]
Dexamethasone: Oral: 40 mg/day days 1 and 2
[total dose/cycle = 80 mg]
Treatment cycle is 21 days (for up to a total of 6 cycles)

Bortezomib-Doxorubicin-Dexamethasone

Use Multiple myeloma

Regimen NOTE: Multiple variations are listed below.
Variation 1:
Cycle 1:
Bortezomib: I.V.: 1.3 mg/m^2/day days 1, 4, 8, and 11
[total dose/cycle = 5.2 mg/m^2]
Dexamethasone: Oral: 40 mg/day days 1 to 4, 8 to 11, and 15 to 18
[total dose/cycle = 480 mg]
Doxorubicin: I.V.: 4.5 or 9 mg/m^2/day days 1 to 4
[total dose/cycle = 18 or 36 mg/m^2]
Treatment cycle is 21 days

Cycles 2-4:
Bortezomib: I.V.: 1.3 mg/m^2/day days 1, 4, 8, and 11
[total dose/cycle = 5.2 mg/m^2]
Dexamethasone: Oral: 40 mg/day days 1 to 4
[total dose/cycle = 160 mg]
Doxorubicin: I.V.: 4.5 or 9 mg/m^2/day days 1 to 4
[total dose/cycle = 18 or 36 mg/m^2]
Treatment cycle is 21 days

Variation 2:
Cycle 1:
Bortezomib: I.V.: 1 mg/m^2/day days 1, 4, 8, and 11
[total dose/cycle = 4 mg/m^2]
Dexamethasone: Oral: 40 mg/day days 1 to 4, 8 to 11, and 15 to 18
[total dose/cycle = 480 mg]
Doxorubicin: I.V.: 9 mg/m^2/day days 1 to 4
[total dose/cycle = 36 mg/m^2]
Treatment cycle is 21 days

Cycles 2-4:
Bortezomib: I.V.: 1 mg/m^2/day days 1, 4, 8, and 11
[total dose/cycle = 4 mg/m^2]
Dexamethasone: Oral: 40 mg/day days 1 to 4
[total dose/cycle = 160 mg]
Doxorubicin: I.V.: 9 mg/m^2/day days 1 to 4
[total dose/cycle = 36 mg/m^2]
Treatment cycle is 21 days

Variation 3:
Bortezomib: I.V.: 1.3 mg/m^2/day days 1, 4, 8, and 11
[total dose/cycle = 5.2 mg/m^2]
Dexamethasone: Oral: 40 mg/day days 1 to 4
[total dose/cycle = 160 mg]
Doxorubicin: I.V.: 20 mg/m^2/day days 1 and 4
[total dose/cycle = 40 mg/m^2]
Repeat cycle every 28 days for up to 6 cycles

Bortezomib-Doxorubicin (Liposomal)

Use Multiple myeloma

Regimen

Bortezomib: I.V.: 1.3 mg/m^2/day days 1, 4, 8, and 11
[total dose/cycle = 5.2 mg/m^2]
Doxorubicin (liposomal): I.V.: 30 mg/m^2 day 4
[total dose/cycle = 30 mg/m^2]
Repeat cycle every 21 days for up to 8 cycles

Bortezomib-Doxorubicin (Liposomal)-Dexamethasone

Use Multiple myeloma

Regimen

Bortezomib: I.V.: 1.3 mg/m^2/day days 1, 4, 8, and 11
[total dose/cycle = 5.2 mg/m^2]
Doxorubicin (Liposomal): I.V.: 30 mg/m^2 day 1
[total dose/cycle = 30 mg/m^2]
Dexamethasone: Oral: 40 mg/day days 1 to 4
[total dose/cycle = 160 mg]
Repeat cycle every 28 days for up to 6 cycles

Bortezomib-Melphalan-Prednisone

Use Multiple myeloma

Regimen NOTE: Multiple variations are listed below.

Variation 1:
Bortezomib: I.V.: 1.3 mg/m^2/day days 1, 4, 8, 11, 22, 25, 29, and 32
[total dose/cycle = 10.4 mg/m^2]

Melphalan: Oral: 9 mg/m^2/day days 1 to 4
[total dose/cycle = 36 mg/m^2]
Prednisone: Oral: 60 mg/m^2/day days 1 to 4
[total dose/cycle = 240 mg/m^2]
Repeat cycle every 42 days for 4 cycles
followed by
Bortezomib: I.V.: 1.3 mg/m^2/day days 1, 8, 22, and 29
[total dose/cycle = 5.2 mg/m^2]
Melphalan: Oral: 9 mg/m^2/day days 1 to 4
[total dose/cycle = 36 mg/m^2]
Prednisone: Oral: 60 mg/m^2/day days 1 to 4
[total dose/cycle = 240 mg/m^2]
Repeat cycle every 42 days for 5 cycles

Variation 2:
Bortezomib: I.V.: 1-1.3 mg/m^2/day days 1, 4, 8, 11, 22, 25, 29, and 32
[total dose/cycle = 8-10.4 mg/m^2]
Melphalan: Oral: 9 mg/m^2/day days 1 to 4
[total dose/cycle = 36 mg/m^2]
Prednisone: Oral: 60 mg/m^2/day days 1 to 4
[total dose/cycle = 240 mg/m^2]
Repeat cycle every 42 days for 4 cycles
followed by
Bortezomib: I.V.: 1-1.3 mg/m^2/day days 1, 8, 15, and 22
[total dose/cycle = 4-5.2 mg/m^2]
Melphalan: Oral: 9 mg/m^2/day days 1 to 4
[total dose/cycle = 36 mg/m^2]
Prednisone: Oral: 60 mg/m^2/day days 1 to 4
[total dose/cycle = 240 mg/m^2]
Repeat cycle every 35 days for 5 cycles

Bortezomib-Melphalan-Prednisone-Thalidomide

Use Multiple myeloma

Regimen

Bortezomib: I.V.: 1-1.3 mg/m^2/day days 1, 4, 15, and 22
[total dose/cycle = 4-5.2 mg/m^2]
Melphalan: Oral: 6 mg/m^2/day days 1 to 5
[total dose/cycle = 30 mg/m^2]
Prednisone: Oral: 60 mg/m^2/day days 1 to 5
[total dose/cycle = 300 mg/m^2]
Thalidomide: Oral: 50 mg/day days 1 to 35
[total dose/cycle = 1750 mg]
Repeat cycle every 35 days for 6 cycles

CA

Use Leukemia, acute myeloid

Regimen

Cytarabine: I.V.: 3000 mg/m^2 every 12 hours days 1 and 2 (4 doses)
[total dose/cycle = 12,000 mg/m^2]
Asparaginase: I.M.: 6000 units/m^2 at hour 42
[total dose/cycle = 6000 units/m^2]
Repeat cycle every 7 days for 2 or 3 cycles

CABO

Use Head and neck cancer

Regimen

Cisplatin: I.V.: 50 mg/m^2 day 4
[total dose/cycle = 50 mg/m^2]
Methotrexate: I.V.: 40 mg/m^2/day days 1 and 15
[total dose/cycle = 80 mg/m^2]
Bleomycin: I.V.: 10 units/day days 1, 8, and 15
[total dose/cycle = 30 units]

Vincristine: I.V.: 2 mg/day days 1, 8, and 15
[total dose/cycle = 6 mg]
Repeat cycle every 21 days

CAD/MOPP/ABV

Use Lymphoma, Hodgkin disease

Regimen

CAD:
Lomustine: Oral: 100 mg/m^2 day 1
[total dose/cycle = 100 mg/m^2]
Melphalan: Oral: 6 mg/m^2/day days 1 to 4
[total dose/cycle = 24 mg/m^2]
Vindesine: I.V.: 3 mg/m^2/day days 1 and 8
[total dose/cycle = 6 mg/m^2]

MOPP:
Mechlorethamine: I.V.: 6 mg/m^2/day days 1 and 8
[total dose/cycle = 12 mg/m^2]
Vincristine: I.V.: 1.4 mg/m^2/day days 1 and 8
[total dose/cycle = 2.8 mg/m^2]
Procarbazine: Oral: 100 mg/m^2/day days 1 to 14
[total dose/cycle = 1400 mg/m^2]
Prednisone: Oral: 40 mg/m^2/day days 1 to 14
[total dose/cycle = 560 mg/m^2]

ABV:
Doxorubicin: I.V.: 25 mg/m^2/day days 1 and 14
[total dose/cycle = 50 mg/m^2]
Bleomycin: SubQ: 6 units/m^2/day days 1 and 14
[total dose/cycle = 12 units/m^2]
Vinblastine: I.V.: 2 mg/m^2 continuous infusion days 4 to 12 and 18 to 26
[total dose/cycle = 36 mg/m^2]

CAD is administered first, then MOPP begins on day 29 or day 37 following CAD. ABV is administered on day 29 following MOPP; CAD recycles on day 29 following ABV.

CAF

Use Breast cancer

Regimen NOTE: Multiple variations are listed below.

Variation 1:
Cyclophosphamide: Oral: 100 mg/m^2/day days 1 to 14
[total dose/cycle = 1400 mg/m^2]
Doxorubicin: I.V.: 30 mg/m^2/day days 1 and 8
[total dose/cycle = 60 mg/m^2]
Fluorouracil: I.V.: 500 mg/m^2/day days 1 and 8
[total dose/cycle = 1000 mg/m^2]
Repeat cycle every 28 days

Variation 2:
Cyclophosphamide: Oral: 100 mg/m^2/day days 1 to 14
[total dose/cycle = 1400 mg/m^2]
Doxorubicin: I.V.: 25 mg/m^2/day days 1 and 8
[total dose/cycle = 50 mg/m^2]
Fluorouracil: I.V.: 500 mg/m^2/day days 1 and 8
[total dose/cycle = 1000 mg/m^2]
Repeat cycle every 28 days

CAP

Use Bladder cancer

Regimen

Cyclophosphamide: I.V.: 400 mg/m^2 day 1
[total dose = 400 mg/m^2]
Doxorubicin: I.V.: 40 mg/m^2 day 1
[total dose = 40 mg/m^2]
Cisplatin: I.V.: 60 mg/m^2 day 1
[total dose = 60 mg/m^2]
Repeat cycle every 21 days

Capecitabine + Docetaxel (Breast Cancer)

Use Breast cancer

Regimen NOTE: Multiple variations are listed below.

Variation 1:

Capecitabine: Oral: 1250 mg/m^2 twice daily days 1 to 14
[total dose/cycle = 35,000 mg/m^2]

Docetaxel: I.V.: 75 mg/m^2 day 1
[total dose/cycle = 75 mg/m^2]

Repeat cycle every 3 weeks

Variation 2:

Capecitabine: Oral: 1000 mg/m^2 twice daily days 2 to 15
[total dose/cycle = 28,000 mg/m^2]

Docetaxel: I.V.: 75 mg/m^2 day 1
[total dose/cycle = 75 mg/m^2]

Repeat cycle every 3 weeks

Variation 3:

Capecitabine: Oral: 937.5 mg/m^2 twice daily days 2 to 15
[total dose/cycle = 26,250 mg/m^2]

Docetaxel: I.V.: 60 mg/m^2 day 1
[total dose/cycle = 60 mg/m^2]

Repeat cycle every 3 weeks

Capecitabine + Docetaxel (Gastric Cancer)

Use Gastric cancer

Regimen NOTE: Multiple variations are listed below

Variation 1:

Capecitabine: Oral: 1000 mg/m^2 twice daily days 1 to 14
[total dose/cycle = 28,000 mg/m^2]

Docetaxel: I.V.: 75 mg/m^2 day 1
[total dose/cycle = 75 mg/m^2]

Repeat cycle every 3 weeks

Variation 2:

Capecitabine: Oral: 1000 mg/m^2 twice daily days 1 to 14
[total dose/cycle = 28,000 mg/m^2]

Docetaxel: I.V.: 36 mg/m^2 days 1 and 8
[total dose/cycle = 72 mg/m^2]

Repeat cycle every 3 weeks

Capecitabine-Docetaxel (NSCLC)

Use Lung cancer, nonsmall cell

Regimen NOTE: Multiple variations are listed below

Variation 1:

Capecitabine: Oral: 1000 mg/m^2 twice daily days 1 to 14
[total dose/cycle = 28,000 mg/m^2]

Docetaxel: I.V.: 36 mg/m^2 days 1 and 8
[total dose/cycle = 72 mg/m^2]

Repeat cycle every 3 weeks

Variation 2:

Capecitabine: Oral: 625 mg/m^2 twice daily days 5 to 18
[total dose/cycle = 17,500 mg/m^2]

Docetaxel: I.V.: 36 mg/m^2 days 1, 8, and 15
[total dose/cycle = 108 mg/m^2]

Repeat cycle every 4 weeks

Capecitabine + Lapatinib

Use Breast cancer

Regimen

Capecitabine: Oral: 1000 mg/m^2 twice daily days 1 to 14
[total dose/cycle = 28,000 mg/m^2]
Lapatinib: Oral: 1250 mg/day days 1 to 21
[total dose/cycle = 26,250 mg]
Repeat cycle every 3 weeks

Capecitabine-Trastuzumab

Use Breast cancer

Regimen NOTE: Multiple variations are listed below.

Variation 1:
Cycle 1:
Capecitabine: Oral: 1250 mg/m^2 twice daily days 1 to 14
[total dose/cycle 1 = 35,000 mg/m^2]
Trastuzumab: I.V.: 4 mg/kg (loading dose) day 1 cycle 1
followed by I.V.: 2 mg/kg/day days 8 and 15 cycle 1
[total dose/cycle 1 = 8 mg/kg]
Treatment cycle is 21 days
Subsequent cycles:
Capecitabine: Oral: 1250 mg/m^2 twice daily days 1 to 14
[total dose/cycle = 35,000 mg/m^2]
Trastuzumab: I.V.: 2 mg/kg/day days 1, 8, and 15
[total dose/cycle = 6 mg/kg]
Repeat cycle every 21 days

Variation 2:
Cycle 1:
Capecitabine: Oral: 1250 mg/m^2 twice daily days 1 to 14
[total dose/cycle 1 = 35,000 mg/m^2]
Trastuzumab: I.V.: 8 mg/kg (loading dose) day 1 cycle 1
[total dose/cycle 1 = 8 mg/kg]
Treatment cycle is 21 days
Subsequent cycles:
Capecitabine: Oral: 1250 mg/m^2 twice daily days 1 to 14
[total dose/cycle = 35,000 mg/m^2]
Trastuzumab: I.V.: 6 mg/kg day 1
[total dose/cycle = 6 mg/kg]
Repeat cycle every 21 days

CAPOX (Biliary Cancer)

Use Biliary adenocarcinoma

Regimen

Capecitabine: Oral: 1000 mg/m^2/dose twice daily days 1 to 14
[total dose/cycle = 28,000 mg/m^2]
Oxaliplatin: I.V.: 130 mg/m^2 over 2 hours day 1
[total dose/cycle = 130 mg/m^2]
Repeat cycle every 3 weeks

CAPOX (Colorectal Cancer)

Use Colorectal cancer

Regimen Note: Multiple variations are listed below.

Variation 1:
Oxaliplatin: I.V.: 130 mg/m^2 day 1
[total dose/cycle = 130 mg/m^2]
Capecitabine: Oral: 2500 mg/m^2/day days 1 to 14
[total dose/cycle = 35,000 mg/m^2]
Repeat cycle every 21 days

Variation 2:
Oxaliplatin: I.V.: 85 mg/m^2 day 1
[total dose/cycle = 85 mg/m^2]
Capecitabine: Oral: 3500 mg/m^2/day days 1 to 7
[total dose/cycle = 24,500 mg/m^2]
Repeat cycle every 14 days

Variation 3:
Oxaliplatin: I.V.: 50-80 mg/m^2/day days 1, 8, 22, and 29
[total dose/cycle = 200-320 mg/m^2]
Capecitabine: Oral: 1650 mg/m^2/day days 1 to 14 and 22 to 35
[total dose/cycle = 46,200 mg/m^2]

Variation 4:
Oxaliplatin: I.V.: 70 mg/m^2/day days 1 and 8
[total dose/cycle = 140 mg/m^2]
Capecitabine: Oral: 2000 mg/m^2/day days 1 to 14
[total dose/cycle = 28,000 mg/m^2]
Repeat cycle every 21 days

Variation 5:
Oxaliplatin: I.V.: 120 mg/m^2 day 1
[total dose/cycle = 120 mg/m^2]
Capecitabine: Oral: 2500 mg/m^2/day days 1 to 14
[total dose/cycle = 35,000 mg/m^2]
Repeat cycle every 21 days

Variation 6:
Oxaliplatin: I.V.: 85 mg/m^2 day 1
[total dose/cycle = 85 mg/m^2]
Capecitabine: Oral: 2500 mg/m^2/day days 1 to 7
[total dose/cycle = 17,500 mg/m^2]
or Capecitabine: Oral: 3000 mg/m^2/day days 1 to 7
[total dose/cycle = 21,000 mg/m^2]
or Capecitabine: Oral: 3500 mg/m^2/day days 1 to 7
[total dose/cycle = 24,500 mg/m^2]
or Capecitabine: Oral: 4000 mg/m^2/day days 1 to 7
[total dose/cycle = 28,000 mg/m^2]
Repeat cycle every 14 days

Variation 7:
Oxaliplatin: I.V.: 130 mg/m^2 day 1
[total dose/cycle = 130 mg/m^2]
Capecitabine: Oral: 1000 mg/m^2 twice daily days 1 (beginning with evening dose) to 15 (ending with morning dose)
[total dose/cycle = 28,000 mg/m^2]
Repeat cycle every 21 days

CAPOX (Pancreatic Cancer)

Use Pancreatic cancer

Regimen NOTE: Multiple variations are listed below.

Variation 1 (patients ≤65 years of age or ECOG PS <2):
Capecitabine: Oral: 1000 mg/m^2/dose twice daily days 1 to 14
[total dose/cycle = 28,000 mg/m^2]
Oxaliplatin: I.V.: 130 mg/m^2/dose over 2 hours day 1
[total dose/cycle = 130 mg/m^2]
Repeat cycle every 21 days until disease progression or unacceptable toxicity

Variation 2 (patients >65 years of age or ECOG PS of 2):
Capecitabine: Oral: 750 mg/m^2/dose twice daily days 1 to 14
[total dose/cycle = 21,000 mg/m^2]
Oxaliplatin: I.V.: 110 mg/m^2/dose over 2 hours day 1
[total dose/cycle = 110 mg/m^2]
Repeat cycle every 21 days until disease progression or unacceptable toxicity

Carboplatin-Cetuximab

Use Head and neck cancer

Regimen

Cycle 1:

Cetuximab: I.V.: 400 mg/m^2 (loading dose) day 1 (week 1, cycle 1 only)
[total loading dose = 400 mg/m^2]
followed by I.V.: 250 mg/m^2/day days 8 and 15
[total dose/cycle 1 = 900 mg/m^2]
Carboplatin: I.V.: AUC 5 day 1
[total dose/cycle = AUC = 5]
Treatment cycle is 3 weeks

Subsequent cycles:

Cetuximab: I.V.: 250 mg/m^2/day days 1, 8, and 15
[total dose/cycle = 750 mg/m^2]
Carboplatin: I.V.: AUC 5 day 1
[total dose/cycle = AUC = 5]
Repeat cycle every 3 weeks

Carboplatin-Paclitaxel (Ovarian Cancer)

Use Ovarian cancer

Regimen NOTE: Multiple variations are listed below.

Variation 1:

Carboplatin: I.V.: AUC 7.5 day 1
[total dose/cycle = AUC = 7.5]
Paclitaxel: I.V.: 175 mg/m^2 over 3 hours day 1
[total dose/cycle = 175 mg/m^2]
Repeat cycle every 3 weeks for a total for 6 cycles

Variation 2:

Carboplatin: I.V.: AUC 5-6 day 1
[total dose/cycle = AUC = 5-6]
Paclitaxel: I.V.: 175 mg/m^2 over 3 hours day 1
[total dose/cycle = 175 mg/m^2]
Repeat cycle every 3 weeks for a total of 6-8 cycles

Variation 3:

Carboplatin: I.V.: AUC 5 day 1
[total dose/cycle = AUC = 5]
Paclitaxel: I.V.: 175 mg/m^2 over 3 hours day 1
[total dose/cycle = 175 mg/m^2]
Repeat cycle every 3 weeks for 6 cycles

Variation 4:

Carboplatin: I.V.: AUC 6 day 1
[total dose/cycle = AUC = 6; maximum dose: 880 mg]
Paclitaxel: I.V.: 185 mg/m^2 over 3 hours day 1
[total dose/cycle = 185 mg/m^2; maximum dose: 400 mg]
Repeat cycle every 3 weeks

Variation 5:

Carboplatin: I.V.: AUC 7.5 day 1
[total dose/cycle = AUC = 7.5]
Paclitaxel: I.V.: 175 mg/m^2 over 3 hours day 1
[total dose/cycle = 175 mg/m^2]
Repeat cycle every 3 weeks for 3-6 cycles

Carbo-Tax (Adenocarcinoma)

Use Adenocarcinoma, unknown primary

Regimen

Paclitaxel: I.V.: 135 mg/m^2 infused over 24 hours day 1
[total dose = 135 mg/m^2]
followed by
Carboplatin: I.V.: Target AUC 7.5
[total dose = AUC = 7.5]
Repeat cycle every 21 days

Carbo-Tax (NSCLC)

Use Lung cancer, nonsmall cell

Regimen

Paclitaxel: I.V.: 135-215 mg/m^2 infused over 24 hours day 1
[total dose/cycle = 135-215 mg/m^2]
or I.V.: 175 mg/m^2 infused over 3 hours day 1
[total dose/cycle = 175 mg/m^2]
followed by
Carboplatin: I.V.: Target AUC 7.5
[total dose/cycle = AUC = 7.5]
Repeat cycle every 21 days

CaT (NSCLC)

Use Lung cancer, nonsmall cell

Regimen NOTE: Multiple variations are listed below.

Variation 1:
Paclitaxel: I.V.: 175 mg/m^2 day 1
[total dose/cycle = 175 mg/m^2]
or I.V.: 135 mg/m^2 continuous infusion day 1
[total dose/cycle = 135 mg/m^2]
Carboplatin: I.V.: AUC 7.5 day 1 or 2
[total dose/cycle = AUC = 7.5]
Repeat cycle every 21 days

Variation 2:
Paclitaxel: I.V.: 225 mg/m^2 day 1
[total dose/cycle = 225 mg/m^2]
Carboplatin: I.V.: AUC 6 day 1
[total dose/cycle = AUC = 6]
Repeat cycle every 21 days

CAVE

Use Lung cancer, small cell

Regimen

Cyclophosphamide: I.V.: 750 mg/m^2 day 1
[total dose/cycle = 750 mg/m^2]
Doxorubicin: I.V.: 50 mg/m^2 day 1
[total dose/cycle = 50 mg/m^2]
Vincristine: I.V.: 1.4 mg/m^2 (maximum dose: 2 mg) day 1
[total dose/cycle = 1.4 mg/m^2]
Etoposide: I.V.: 60-100 mg/m^2/day days 1, 2, and 3
[total dose/cycle = 180-300 mg/m^2]
Repeat cycle every 21 days

CAV-P/VP

Use Neuroblastoma

Regimen

Course 1, 2, 4, and 6:
Cyclophosphamide: I.V.: 70 mg/kg/day days 1 and 2
[total dose/cycle = 140 mg/kg]
Doxorubicin: I.V.: 25 mg/m^2/day continuous infusion days 1, 2, and 3
[total dose/cycle = 75 mg/m^2]
Vincristine: I.V.: 0.033 mg/kg/day continuous infusion days 1, 2, and 3
[total dose/cycle = 0.099 mg/kg]
Vincristine: I.V.: 1.5 mg/m^2 day 9
[total dose/cycle = 1.5 mg/m^2]

Course 3, 5, and 7:
Etoposide: I.V.: 200 mg/m^2/day days 1, 2, and 3 [total dose/cycle = 600 mg/m^2]
Cisplatin: I.V.: 50 mg/m^2/day days 1 to 4 [total dose/cycle = 200 mg/m^2]

CC

Use Ovarian cancer

Regimen

Carboplatin: I.V.: Target AUC 5-7.5 day 1 [total dose/cycle = AUC = 5-7.5]
Cyclophosphamide: I.V.: 600 mg/m^2 day 1 [total dose/cycle = 600 mg/m^2]
Repeat cycle every 28 days

CCCDE (Retinoblastoma)

Use Retinoblastoma

Regimen

Cyclophosphamide: I.V.: 150 mg/m^2/day days 1 to 7 [total dose/cycle = 1050 mg/m^2]
Cyclophosphamide: Oral: 150 mg/m^2/day days 22 to 28 and 43 to 49 [total dose/cycle = 2100 mg/m^2]
Doxorubicin: I.V.: 35 mg/m^2/day days 10 and 52 [total dose/cycle = 70 mg/m^2]
Cisplatin: I.V.: 90 mg/m^2/day days 8, 50, and 71 [total dose/cycle = 270 mg/m^2]
Etoposide: I.V.: 150 mg/m^2/day continuous infusion days 29, 30, and 31 and 73, 74, and 75 [total dose/cycle = 900 mg/m^2]

CCDDT (Neuroblastoma)

Use Neuroblastoma

Regimen

Cyclophosphamide: I.V.: 40 mg/kg/day days 1 and 2 [total dose/cycle = 80 mg/kg]
Cisplatin: I.V.: 20 mg/m^2/day days 1 to 5 [total dose/cycle = 100 mg/m^2]
Teniposide: I.V.: 100 mg/m^2 day 7 [total dose/cycle = 100 mg/m^2]
Doxorubicin: I.V.: 60 mg/m^2 day 1 [total dose/cycle = 60 mg/m^2]
Dacarbazine: I.V.: 250 mg/m^2/day days 1 to 5 [total dose/cycle = 1250 mg/m^2]
Repeat cycle every 21-28 days

CCDT (Melanoma)

Use Melanoma

Regimen

Dacarbazine: I.V.: 220 mg/m^2/day days 1, 2, and 3, every 21 to 28 days [total dose/cycle = 660 mg/m^2]
Carmustine: I.V.: 150 mg/m^2 day 1, every 42 to 56 days [total dose/cycle = 150 mg/m^2]
Cisplatin: I.V.: 25 mg/m^2/day days 1, 2, and 3, every 21 to 28 days [total dose/cycle = 75 mg/m^2]
Tamoxifen: Oral: 20 mg/day (use of tamoxifen is optional)

CCT (Neuroblastoma)

Use Neuroblastoma

Regimen

Cyclophosphamide: I.V.: 40 mg/kg/day days 1 and 2 [total dose/cycle = 80 mg/kg]
Cisplatin: I.V.: 20 mg/m^2/day days 22 to 26 [total dose/cycle = 100 mg/m^2]

Teniposide: I.V.: 100 mg/m^2 day 28
[total dose/cycle = 100 mg/m^2]
Repeat every 42 days for 3 cycles

CDDP/VP-16

Use Brain tumors

Regimen

Cisplatin: I.V.: 90 mg/m^2 day 1
[total dose/cycle = 90 mg/m^2]
Etoposide: I.V.: 150 mg/m^2/day days 3 and 4
[total dose/cycle = 300 mg/m^2]
Repeat cycle every 21 days

CE-CAdO

Use Neuroblastoma

Regimen

Carboplatin: I.V.: 160 mg/m^2/day days 1 to 5
[total dose/cycle = 800 mg/m^2]
Etoposide: I.V.: 100 mg/m^2/day days 1 to 5
[total dose/cycle = 500 mg/m^2]
or
Carboplatin: I.V.: 200 mg/m^2/day days 1, 2, and 3
[total dose/cycle = 600 mg/m^2]
Etoposide: I.V.: 150 mg/m^2/day days 1, 2, and 3
[total dose/cycle = 450 mg/m^2]
and
Cyclophosphamide: I.V.: 300 mg/m^2/day days 1 to 5
[total dose/cycle = 1500 mg/m^2]
Doxorubicin: I.V.: 60 mg/m^2 day 5
[total dose/cycle = 60 mg/m^2]
Vincristine: I.V.: 1.5 mg/m^2/day days 1 and 5
[total dose/cycle = 3 mg/m^2]
Repeat cycle every 21 days

CEF

Use Breast cancer

Regimen

Cyclophosphamide: Oral: 75 mg/m^2/day days 1 to 14
[total dose/cycle = 1050 mg/m^2]
Epirubicin: I.V.: 60 mg/m^2/day days 1 and 8
[total dose/cycle = 120 mg/m^2]
Fluorouracil: I.V.: 500 mg/m^2/day days 1 and 8
[total dose/cycle = 1000 mg/m^2]
Repeat cycle every 28 days

CE (Neuroblastoma)

Use Neuroblastoma

Regimen

Carboplatin: I.V.: 500 mg/m^2/day days 1 and 2
[total dose/cycle = 1000 mg/m^2]
Etoposide: I.V.: 100 mg/m^2/day days 1, 2, and 3
[total dose/cycle = 300 mg/m^2]
Repeat cycle every 21-28 days

CEPP(B)

Use Lymphoma, non-Hodgkin

Regimen

Cyclophosphamide: I.V.: 600-650 mg/m^2/day days 1 and 8
[total dose/cycle = 1200-1300 mg/m^2]
Etoposide: I.V.: 70-85 mg/m^2/day days 1, 2, and 3
[total dose/cycle = 210-255 mg/m^2]

Procarbazine: Oral: 60 mg/m^2/day days 1 to 10
[total dose/cycle = 600 mg/m^2]
Prednisone: Oral: 60 mg/m^2/day days 1 to 10
[total dose/cycle = 600 mg/m^2]
Bleomycin: I.V.: 15 units/m^2/day days 1 and 15 (Bleomycin is sometimes omitted)
[total dose/cycle = 30 units/m^2]
Repeat cycle every 28 days

CE (Retinoblastoma)

Use Retinoblastoma

Regimen

Etoposide: I.V.: 100 mg/m^2/day days 1 to 5
[total dose/cycle = 500 mg/m^2]
Carboplatin: I.V.: 160 mg/m^2/day days 1 to 5
[total dose/cycle = 800 mg/m^2]
Repeat cycle every 21 days

Cetuximab (Biweekly)-Irinotecan

Use Colorectal cancer

Regimen

Cycle 1:
Cetuximab: I.V.: 500 mg/m^2 over 120 minutes day 1 (cycle 1 only)
[total dose/cycle = 500 mg/m^2]
Irinotecan: I.V.: 180 mg/m^2 day 1
[total dose/cycle = 180 mg/m^2]
Subsequent cycles:
Cetuximab: I.V.: 500 mg/m^{2}over 60 minutes day 1
[total dose/cycle = 500 mg/m^2]
Irinotecan: I.V.: 180 mg/m^2 day 1
[total dose/cycle = 180 mg/m^2]
Repeat cycle every 14 days

Cetuximab-Carboplatin-Fluorouracil

Use Head and neck cancer

Regimen

Cycle 1:
Cetuximab: I.V.: 400 mg/m^2 (loading dose) day 1 (week 1, cycle 1 only)
[total loading dose = 400 mg/m^2]
followed by I.V.: 250 mg/m^2/day days 8 and 15
[total dose/cycle 1 = 900 mg/m^2]
Carboplatin: I.V.: AUC 5 day 1
[total dose/cycle = AUC = 5]
Fluorouracil: I.V.: 1000 mg/m^2/day continuous infusion days 1 to 4
[total dose/cycle = 4000 mg/m^2]
Treatment cycle is 3 weeks
Subsequent cycles:
Cetuximab: I.V.: 250 mg/m^2/day days 1, 8, and 15
[total dose/cycle = 750 mg/m^2]
Carboplatin: I.V.: AUC 5 day 1
[total dose/cycle = AUC = 5]
Fluorouracil: I.V.: 1000 mg/m^2/day continuous infusion days 1 to 4
[total dose/cycle = 4000 mg/m^2]
Repeat cycle every 3 weeks for a total of up to 6 cycles (cetuximab monotherapy may be continued thereafter until disease progression or unacceptable toxicity)

Cetuximab-Cisplatin-Fluorouracil

Use Head and neck cancer

Regimen

Cycle 1:

Cetuximab: I.V.: 400 mg/m^2 (loading dose) day 1 (week 1, cycle 1 only)
[total loading dose = 400 mg/m^2]
followed by I.V.: 250 mg/m^2/day days 8 and 15
[total dose/cycle 1 = 900 mg/m^2]
Cisplatin: I.V.: 100 mg/m^2 day 1
[total dose/cycle = 100 mg/m^2]
Fluorouracil: I.V.: 1000 mg/m^2/day continuous infusion days 1 to 4
[total dose/cycle = 4000 mg/m^2]
Treatment cycle is 3 weeks

Subsequent cycles:

Cetuximab: I.V.: 250 mg/m^2/day days 1, 8, and 15
[total dose/cycle = 750 mg/m^2]
Cisplatin: I.V.: 100 mg/m^2 day 1
[total dose/cycle = 100 mg/m^2]
Fluorouracil: I.V.: 1000 mg/m^2/day continuous infusion days 1 to 4
[total dose/cycle = 4000 mg/m^2]
Repeat cycle every 3 weeks for a total of up to 6 cycles (cetuximab monotherapy may be continued thereafter until disease progression or unacceptable toxicity)

Cetuximab-Cisplatin-Vinorelbine

Use Lung cancer, nonsmall cell

Regimen

Cycle 1:

Cetuximab: I.V.: 400 mg/m^2 (loading dose) day 1 (week 1, cycle 1 only)
[total loading dose = 400 mg/m^2]
followed by I.V.: 250 mg/m^2/dose days 8 and 15
[total dose/cycle 1 = 900 mg/m^2]
Cisplatin: I.V.: 80 mg/m^2/dose day 1
[total dose/cycle = 80 mg/m^2]
Vinorelbine: I.V.: 25 mg/m^2/dose days 1 and 8
[total dose/cycle = 50 mg/m^2]
Treatment cycle is 3 weeks

Subsequent cycles:

Cetuximab: I.V.: 250 mg/m^2/day days 1, 8, and 15
[total dose/cycle = 750 mg/m^2]
Cisplatin: I.V.: 80 mg/m^2 day 1
[total dose/cycle = 80 mg/m^2]
Vinorelbine: I.V.: 25 mg/m^2/dose days 1 and 8
[total dose/cycle = 50 mg/m^2]
Repeat cycle every 3 weeks

Cetuximab-FOLFOX4

Use Colorectal cancer

Regimen

Cycle 1:

Cetuximab: I.V.: 400 mg/m^2 (loading dose) day 1 (week 1, cycle 1 only)
followed by I.V.: 250 mg/m^2/day day 8
[total dose/cycle 1 = 650 mg/m^2]
Oxaliplatin: I.V.: 85 mg/m^2 (over 2 hours) day 1
[total dose/cycle = 85 mg/m^2]
Leucovorin: I.V.: 200 mg/m^2/day (over 2 hours) days 1 and 2
[total dose/cycle = 400 mg/m^2]
Fluorouracil: I.V. bolus: 400 mg/m^2/day days 1 and 2
followed by I.V.: 600 mg/m^2 continuous infusion (over 22 hours) days 1 and 2
[total dose/cycle = 2000 mg/m^2]

Note: Bolus fluorouracil and continuous infusion are both given on each day.
Treatment cycle is 14 days
Subsequent cycles:
Cetuximab: I.V.: 250 mg/m^2/day days 1 and 8
[total dose/cycle = 500 mg/m^2]
Oxaliplatin: I.V.: 85 mg/m^2 day 1
[total dose/cycle = 85 mg/m^2]
Leucovorin: I.V.: 200 mg/m^2/day (over 2 hours) days 1 and 2
[total dose/cycle = 400 mg/m^2]
Fluorouracil: I.V. bolus: 400 mg/m^2/day days 1 and 2
followed by I.V.: 600 mg/m^2 continuous infusion (over 22 hours) days 1 and 2
[total dose/cycle = 2000 mg/m^2]
Note: Bolus fluorouracil and continuous infusion are both given on each day.
Repeat cycle every 14 days

Cetuximab-Irinotecan

Use Colorectal cancer

Regimen NOTE: Multiple variations are listed below.
Variation 1:
Cycle 1:
Cetuximab: I.V.: 400 mg/m^2 (loading dose) day 1 (week 1, cycle 1 only)
[total loading dose = 400 mg/m^2]
followed by I.V.: 250 mg/m^2/day days 8, 15, 22, 29, and 36
[total dose/cycle 1 = 1650 mg/m^2]
Irinotecan: I.V.: 125 mg/m^2/day days 1, 8, 15, and 22
[total dose/cycle = 500 mg/m^2]
Subsequent cycles:
Cetuximab: I.V.: 250 mg/m^2/day days 1, 8, 15, 22, 29, and 36
[total dose/cycle = 1500 mg/m^2]
Irinotecan: I.V.: 125 mg/m^2/day days 1, 8, 15, and 22
[total dose/cycle = 500 mg/m^2]
Repeat cycle every 42 days
Variation 2:
Cycle 1:
Cetuximab: I.V.: 400 mg/m^2 (loading dose) day 1 (week 1, cycle 1 only)
[total loading dose = 400 mg/m^2]
followed by I.V.: 250 mg/m^2 day 8
[total dose/cycle 1 = 650 mg/m^2]
Irinotecan: I.V.: 180 mg/m^2 day 1
[total dose/cycle = 180 mg/m^2]
Subsequent cycles:
Cetuximab: I.V.: 250 mg/m^2/day days 1 and 8
[total dose/cycle = 500 mg/m^2]
Irinotecan: I.V.: 180 mg/m^2 day 1
[total dose/cycle = 180 mg/m^2]
Repeat cycle every 14 days
Variation 3:
Cycle 1:
Cetuximab: I.V.: 400 mg/m^2 (loading dose) day 1 (week 1, cycle 1 only)
[total loading dose = 400 mg/m^2]
followed by I.V.: 250 mg/m^2/day days 8 and 15 (cycle 1)
[total dose/cycle 1 = 900 mg/m^2]
Irinotecan: I.V.: 350 mg/m^2 day 1
[total dose/cycle = 350 mg/m^2]
Subsequent cycles:
Cetuximab: I.V.: 250 mg/m^2/day days 1, 8, and 15
[total dose/cycle = 750 mg/m^2]
Irinotecan: I.V.: 350 mg/m^2 day 1
[total dose/cycle = 350 mg/m^2]
Repeat cycle every 21 days

CEV

Use Rhabdomyosarcoma

Regimen

Carboplatin: I.V.: 500 mg/m^2 day 1
[total dose/cycle = 500 mg/m^2]
Epirubicin: I.V.: 150 mg/m^2 day 1
[total dose/cycle = 150 mg/m^2]
Vincristine: I.V.: 1.5 mg/m^2/day days 1 and 7
[total dose/cycle = 3 mg/m^2]
Repeat cycle every 21 days

CFP

Use Breast cancer

Regimen

Cyclophosphamide: I.V.: 150 mg/m^2/day days 1 to 5
[total dose/cycle = 750 mg/m^2]
Fluorouracil: I.V.: 300 mg/m^2/day days 1 to 5
[total dose/cycle = 1500 mg/m^2]
Prednisone: Oral: 30 mg/day days 1 to 14 (cycle 1 only)
followed by Oral: 20 mg/day days 15 to 21 (cycle 1 only)
followed by Oral: 10 mg daily thereafter as maintenance
[total dose/cycle = 700 mg in cycle 1; 350 mg in subsequent cycles]
Repeat cycle every 35 days

CHAMOCA (Modified Bagshawe Regimen)

Use Gestational trophoblastic tumor

Regimen NOTE: Multiple variations are listed below.

Variation 1:
Hydroxyurea: Oral: 500 mg every 6 hours, for 4 doses, day 1 (start at 6 AM)
[total dose/cycle = 2000 mg]
Dactinomycin: I.V.: 0.2 mg/day days 1, 2, and 3 (give at 7 PM)
followed by I.V.: 0.5 mg/day days 4 and 5 (give at 7 PM)
[total dose/cycle = 1.6 mg]
Cyclophosphamide: I.V.: 500 mg/m^2/day days 3 and 8 (give at 7 PM)
[total dose/cycle = 1000 mg/m^2]
Vincristine: I.V.: 1 mg/m^2 (maximum: 2 mg) day 2 (give at 7 AM)
[total dose/cycle = 1 mg/m^2; maximum: 2 mg]
Methotrexate: I.V. bolus: 100 mg/m^2 day 2 (give at 7 PM)
followed by I.V.: 200 mg/m^2 continuous infusion over 12 hours day 2
[total dose/cycle = 300 mg/m^2]
Leucovorin: I.M.: 14 mg every 6 hours, for 6 doses, days 3, 4, and 5 (begin at 7 PM on day 3; start 24 hours after the start of methotrexate)
[total dose/cycle = 84 mg]
Doxorubicin: I.V.: 30 mg/m^2 day 8 (give at 7 PM)
[total dose/cycle = 30 mg/m^2]
Repeat cycle every 18 days or as toxicity permits (cycle may be repeated 10 days after last treatment)

Variation 2:
Hydroxyurea: Oral: 500 mg every 12 hours, for 4 doses, days 1 and 2 (usually started in early morning)
[total dose/cycle = 2000 mg]
Dactinomycin: I.V.: 10 mcg/kg/day days 5, 6, and 7
[total dose/cycle = 30 mcg/kg]
Vincristine: I.V.: 1 mg/m^2 day 3
[total dose/cycle = 1 mg/m^2]
Methotrexate: I.V. bolus: 100 mg/m^2 day 3
followed by I.V.: 200 mg/m^2 continuous infusion over 12 hours day 3
[total dose/cycle = 300 mg/m^2]
Leucovorin: I.M.: 10 mg/m^2 every 12 hours, for 4 doses, days 4 and 5 (start 24 hours after the start of methotrexate)
[total dose/cycle = 40 mg/m^2]

Cyclophosphamide: I.V.: 600 mg/m^2 day 5
[total dose/cycle = 600 mg/m^2]
Doxorubicin: I.V.: 30 mg/m^2 day 10
[total dose/cycle = 30 mg/m^2]
Repeat cycle every 3 weeks

Variation 3:

Hydroxyurea: Oral: 500 mg every 12 hours, for 4 doses, days 1 and 2 (usually started in early morning)
[total dose/cycle = 2000 mg/m^2]
Vincristine: I.V.: 1 mg/m^2 day 3
[total dose/cycle = 1 mg/m^2]
Methotrexate: I.V. bolus: 100 mg/m^2 day 3
followed by I.V.: 200 mg/m^{2}continuous infusion over 12 hours day 3
[total dose/cycle = 300 mg/m^2]
Leucovorin: I.M.: 14 mg every 6 hours, for 6 doses, days 4, 5, and 6 (start 24 hours after start of methotrexate)
[total dose/cycle = 84 mg]
Dactinomycin: I.V.: 0.2 mg/day days 2, 3, and 4
followed by I.V.: 0.5 mg/day days 5 and 6
[total dose/cycle = 1.6 mg]
Cyclophosphamide: I.V.: 500 mg/m^2 day 4
[total dose/cycle = 500 mg/m^2]
Doxorubicin: I.V.: 30 mg/m^2 day 9
[total dose/cycle = 30 mg/m^2]
Melphalan: I.V.: 6 mg/m^2 day 9
[total dose/cycle = 6 mg/m^2]
Repeat cycle approximately every 3 weeks

Variation 4:

Hydroxyurea: Oral: 500 mg 4 times/day, for 4 doses, day 1
[total dose/cycle = 2000 mg/m^2]
Vincristine: I.V.: 1 mg/m^2 day 2
[total dose/cycle = 1 mg/m^2]
Methotrexate: I.V. bolus: 100 mg/m^2 day 2
followed by I.V.: 200 mg/m^2 continuous infusion over 12 hours day 2
[total dose/cycle = 300 mg/m^2]
Leucovorin: I.M.: 14 mg every 6 hours, for 6 doses, days 3, 4, and 5 (start 24 hours after the start of methotrexate)
[total dose/cycle = 84 mg]
Dactinomycin: I.V.: 0.2 mg days 1, 2, and 3
followed by I.V.: 0.5 mg days 4 and 5
[total dose/cycle = 1.6 mg]
Cyclophosphamide: I.V.: 500 mg/m^2 day 3
[total dose/cycle = 500 mg/m^2]
Cyclophosphamide: I.V.: 300 mg/m^2 on day 8
[total dose/cycle = 300 mg/m^2]
Doxorubicin: I.V.: 30 mg/m^2 day 8
[total dose/cycle = 30 mg/m^2]
Repeat cycle approximately every 3 weeks

CHAMOMA (Bagshawe Regimen)

Use Gestational trophoblastic tumor

Regimen

Hydroxyurea: Oral: 500 mg every 12 hours, for 4 doses, days 1 and 2
[total dose/cycle = 2000 mg]
Vincristine: I.V.: 1 mg/m^2 day 3
[total dose/cycle = 1 mg/m^2]
Methotrexate: I.V. bolus: 100 mg/m^2 day 3
followed by I.V.: 200 mg/m^2 continuous infusion over 12 hours day 3
[total dose/cycle = 300 mg/m^2]
Leucovorin: I.M.: 12 mg/m^2 every 12 hours, for 4 doses, days 4 and 5 (start 12 hours after the end of methotrexate infusion)
[total dose/cycle = 48 mg/m^2]

Dactinomycin: I.V.: 10 mcg/kg/day days 5, 6, and 7
[total dose/cycle = 30 mcg/kg]
Cyclophosphamide: I.V.: 600 mg/m^2 day 5
[total dose/cycle = 600 mg/m^2]
Doxorubicin: I.V.: 30 mg/m^2 day 10
[total dose/cycle = 30 mg/m^2]
Melphalan: I.V.: 6 mg/m^2 day 10
[total dose/cycle = 6 mg/m^2]
Repeat cycle approximately every 3 weeks

ChIVPP

Use Lymphoma, Hodgkin disease

Regimen

Chlorambucil: Oral: 6 mg/m^2/day (maximum: 10 mg) days 1 to 14
[total dose/cycle = 84 mg/m^2]
Vinblastine: I.V.: 6 mg/m^2/day (maximum: 10 mg) days 1 and 8
[total dose/cycle = 12 mg/m^2]
Procarbazine: Oral: 100 mg/m^2/day (maximum: 150 mg) days 1 to 14
[total dose/cycle = 1400 mg/m^2]
Prednisone: Oral: 40-50 mg/day days 1 to 14
[total dose/cycle = 560-700 mg]
Repeat cycle every 28 days

CHL + PRED

Use Leukemia, chronic lymphocytic

Regimen

Chlorambucil: Oral: 0.4 mg/kg/day for 1 day every other week; increase initial dose of 0.4 mg/kg by 0.1 mg/kg every 2 weeks until toxicity or disease control is achieved
Prednisone: Oral: 100 mg/day for 2 days every other week

CHOP

Use Lymphoma, non-Hodgkin

Regimen NOTE: Multiple variations are listed below.

Variation 1:
Cyclophosphamide: I.V.: 750 mg/m^2 day 1
[total dose/cycle = 750 mg/m^2]
Doxorubicin: I.V.: 50 mg/m^2 day 1
[total dose/cycle = 50 mg/m^2]
Vincristine: I.V.: 1.4 mg/m^2 (maximum dose: 2 mg) day 1
[total dose/cycle = 1.4 mg/m^2]
Prednisone: Oral: 100 mg/day days 1 to 5
[total dose/cycle = 500 mg]
or Oral: 50 mg/m^2/day days 1 to 5
[total dose/cycle = 250 mg/m^2]
or Oral: 100 mg/m^2/day days 1 to 5
[total dose/cycle = 500 mg/m^2]
Repeat cycle every 21 days

Variation 2:
Cyclophosphamide: I.V.: 750 mg/m^2 day 1
[total dose/cycle = 750 mg/m^2]
Doxorubicin: I.V.: 50 mg/m^2 day 1
[total dose/cycle = 50 mg/m^2]
Vincristine: I.V.: 2 mg day 1
[total dose/cycle = 2 mg]
Prednisone: Oral: 75 mg/day days 1 to 5
[total dose/cycle = 375 mg]
Repeat cycle every 21 days

Variation 3:
Cyclophosphamide: I.V.: 750 mg/m^2/day days 1 and 8
[total dose/cycle = 1500 mg/m^2]
Doxorubicin: I.V.: 25 mg/m^2/day days 1 and 8
[total dose/cycle = 50 mg/m^2]
Vincristine: I.V.: 1.4 mg/m^2/day (maximum dose: 2 mg) days 1 and 8
[total dose/cycle = 2.8 mg/m^2]
Prednisone: Oral: 50 mg/m^2/day days 1 to 8
[total dose/cycle = 400 mg/m^2]
Repeat cycle every 28 days
Variation 4 - "mini-CHOP":
Cyclophosphamide: I.V.: 250 mg/m^2/day days 1, 8, and 15
[total dose/cycle = 750 mg/m^2]
Doxorubicin: I.V.: 16.7 mg/m^2/day days 1, 8, and 15
[total dose/cycle = 50.1 mg/m^2]
Vincristine: I.V.: 0.67 mg/day days 1, 8, and 15
[total dose/cycle = 2.01 mg]
Prednisone: Oral: 75 mg/day days 1 to 5
[total dose/cycle = 375 mg]
Repeat cycle every 21 days

CI (Neuroblastoma)

Use Neuroblastoma

Regimen
Ifosfamide: I.V.: 1500 mg/m^2/day days 1, 2, and 3
[total dose/cycle = 4500 mg/m^2]
Mesna: I.V.: 500 mg/m^2 every 3 hours, for 3 doses each day, days 1, 2, and 3
[total dose/cycle = 4500 mg/m^2]
Carboplatin: I.V.: 400 mg/m^2 day 4
[total dose/cycle = 400 mg/m^2]
Repeat cycle every 21-28 days

CISCA

Use Bladder cancer

Regimen
Cyclophosphamide: I.V.: 650 mg/m^2 day 1
[total dose = 650 mg/m^2]
Doxorubicin: I.V.: 50 mg/m^2 day 1
[total dose = 50 mg/m^2]
Cisplatin: I.V.: 100 mg/m^2 day 2
[total dose = 100 mg/m^2]
Repeat cycle every 21-28 days

Cisplatin-Cetuximab

Use Head and neck cancer

Regimen NOTE: Multiple variations are listed below.
Variation 1:
Cycle 1:
Cetuximab: I.V.: 400 mg/m^2 (loading dose) day 1 (week 1, cycle 1 only)
[total loading dose = 400 mg/m^2]
followed by I.V.: 250 mg/m^2/day days 8, 15, and 22
[total dose/cycle 1 = 1150 mg/m^2]
Cisplatin: I.V.: 100 mg/m^2 day 1
[total dose/cycle = 100 mg/m^2]
Treatment cycle is 4 weeks
Subsequent cycles:
Cetuximab: I.V.: 250 mg/m^2/day days 1, 8, 15, and 22
[total dose/cycle = 1000 mg/m^2]
Cisplatin: I.V.: 100 mg/m^2 day 1
[total dose/cycle = 100 mg/m^2]
Repeat cycle every 4 weeks

Variation 2:
Cycle 1:
Cetuximab: I.V.: 400 mg/m^2 (loading dose) day 1 (week 1, cycle 1 only)
[total loading dose = 400 mg/m^2]
followed by I.V.: 250 mg/m^2/day days 8 and 15
[total dose/cycle 1 = 900 mg/m^2]
Cisplatin: I.V.: 75-100 mg/m^2 day 1
[total dose/cycle = 75-100 mg/m^2]
Treatment cycle is 3 weeks
Subsequent cycles:
Cetuximab: I.V.: 250 mg/m^2/day days 1, 8, and 15
[total dose/cycle = 750 mg/m^2]
Cisplatin: I.V.: 75-100 mg/m^2 day 1
[total dose/cycle = 75-100 mg/m^2]
Repeat cycle every 3 weeks

Cisplatin-Cytarabine-Dexamethasone (NHL Regimen)

Use Lymphoma, non-Hodgkin

Regimen NOTE: Multiple variations are listed below.
Variation 1:
Dexamethasone: I.V. or Oral: 40 mg/day days 1 to 4
[total dose/cycle = 160 mg]
Cisplatin: I.V.: 100 mg/m^2 over 24 hours day 1
[total dose/cycle = 100 mg/m^2]
Cytarabine: I.V.: 2000 mg/m^2 every 12 hours for 2 doses day 2 (begins at the end of the cisplatin infusion)
[total dose/cycle = 4000 mg/m^2]
Repeat cycle every 3-4 weeks for 6-10 cycles
Variation 2 (patients >70 years of age):
Dexamethasone: I.V. or Oral: 40 mg/day days 1 to 4
[total dose/cycle = 160 mg]
Cisplatin: I.V.: 100 mg/m^2 over 24 hours day 1
[total dose/cycle = 100 mg/m^2]
Cytarabine: I.V.: 1000 mg/m^2 every 12 hours for 2 doses day 2 (begins at the end of the cisplatin infusion)
[total dose/cycle = 2000 mg/m^2]
Repeat cycle every 3-4 weeks for 6-10 cycles

Cisplatin-Dacarbazine-Carmustine (Melanoma)

Use Melanoma

Regimen NOTE: Multiple variations are listed below.
Variation 1:
Cisplatin: I.V.: 25 mg/m^2/day days 1, 2, and 3
[total dose/cycle = 75 mg/m^2]
Dacarbazine: I.V.: 220 mg/m^2/day days 1, 2, and 3
[total dose/cycle = 660 mg/m^2]
Carmustine: I.V.: 150 mg/m^2 day 1 (every other cycle **[odd cycles]**)
[total dose/**odd** cycles = 150 mg/m^2]
Repeat cycle every 21 days
Variation 2:
Carmustine: I.V.: 150 mg/m^2 day 1
[total dose/cycle = 150 mg/m^2]
Cisplatin: I.V.: 25 mg/m^2/day days 1, 2, 3, 22, 23, and 24
[total dose/cycle = 150 mg/m^2]
Dacarbazine: I.V.: 220 mg/m^2/day days 1, 2, 3, 22, 23, and 24
[total dose/cycle = 1320 mg/m^2]
Repeat cycle every 42 days

Cisplatin-Dacarbazine-Interferon Alfa-2b-Aldesleukin

Use Melanoma

Regimen

Cisplatin: I.V.: 25 mg/m^2/day days 1, 2, and 3
[total dose/cycle = 75 mg/m^2]
Dacarbazine: 250 mg/m^2/day days 1, 2, and 3
[total dose/cycle = 750 mg/m^2]
Interferon Alfa-2b: SubQ: 5 million units/m^2/day days 6, 8, 10, 13, and 15
[total dose/cycle = 25 million units/m^2]
Aldesleukin: I.V.: 18 million units/m^2/day days 6 to 10, 13, 14, and 15
[total dose/cycle = 144 million units/m^2]
Repeat cycle every 28 days

Cisplatin-Docetaxel

Use Bladder cancer

Regimen

Cisplatin: I.V.: 30 mg/m^2 day 1
[total dose/cycle = 30 mg/m^2]
Docetaxel: I.V.: 40 mg/m^2 day 4
[total dose/cycle = 40 mg/m^2]
Repeat cycle weekly for 8 weeks

Cisplatin-Etoposide (NSCLC)

Use Lung cancer, nonsmall cell

Regimen NOTE: Multiple variations are listed below.

Variation 1:
Cisplatin: I.V.: 80 mg/m^2 day 1
[total dose/cycle = 80 mg/m^2]
Etoposide: I.V.: 100 mg/m^2/day days 1, 2, and 3
[total dose/cycle = 300 mg/m^2]
Repeat cycle every 21 days for a total of 4 cycles

Variation 2:
Cisplatin: I.V.: 100 mg/m^2 day 1
[total dose/cycle = 100 mg/m^2]
Etoposide: I.V.: 100 mg/m^2/day days 1, 2, and 3
[total dose/cycle = 300 mg/m^2]
Repeat cycle every 28 days for a total of 3 cycles

Variation 3:
Cisplatin: I.V.: 100 mg/m^2 day 1
[total dose/cycle = 100 mg/m^2]
Etoposide: I.V.: 100 mg/m^2/day days 1, 2, and 3
[total dose/cycle = 300 mg/m^2]
Repeat cycle every 28 days for a total of 4 cycles

Variation 4:
Cisplatin: I.V.: 120 mg/m^2/day days 1, 29, and 71
[total dose/treatment = 360 mg/m^2]
Etoposide: I.V.: 100 mg/m^2/day days 1, 2, 3, 29, 30, 31, 71, 72, and 73
[total dose/treatment = 900 mg/m^2]

Variation 5:
Cisplatin: I.V.: 75 mg/m^2 day 1
[total dose/cycle = 75 mg/m^2]
Etoposide: I.V.: 100 mg/m^2/day days 1, 2, and 3
[total dose/cycle = 300 mg/m^2]
Repeat cycle every 21 days for up to 10 cycles

Cisplatin-Fluorouracil (Bladder Cancer)

Use Bladder cancer

Regimen In combination with radiation therapy

Note: Begin infusion(s) 2 hours before radiation therapy on days 1, 3, 15, and 17:

Cisplatin: I.V.: 15 mg/m^2/day over 2 hours days 1, 2, 3, 15, 16, and 17
[total dose/cycle = 90 mg/m^2]

Fluorouracil: I.V.: 400 mg/m^2/day over 2 hours days 1, 2, 3, 15, 16, and 17
[total dose/cycle = 2400 mg/m^2]

Cisplatin-Fluorouracil (Cervical Cancer)

Use Cervical cancer

Regimen NOTE: Multiple variations are listed below.

Variation 1:

Cisplatin: I.V.: 75 mg/m^2 day 1
[total dose/cycle = 75 mg/m^2]

Fluorouracil: I.V.: 1000 mg/m^2/day continuous infusion days 1 to 4 (96 hours)
[total dose/cycle = 4000 mg/m^2]

Repeat cycle every 21 days

Variation 2:

Cisplatin: I.V.: 50 mg/m^2 day 1 starting 4 hours before radiotherapy
[total dose/cycle = 50 mg/m^2]

Fluorouracil: I.V.: 1000 mg/m^2/day continuous infusion days 2 to 5 (96 hours)
[total dose/cycle = 4000 mg/m^2]

Repeat cycle every 28 days

Variation 3:

Cisplatin: I.V.: 70 mg/m^2 day 1
[total dose/cycle = 70 mg/m^2]

Fluorouracil: I.V.: 1000 mg/m^2/day continuous infusion days 1 to 4 (96 hours)
[total dose/cycle = 4000 mg/m^2]

Repeat cycle every 21 days

Cisplatin-Fluorouracil (Esophageal Cancer)

Use Esophageal cancer

Regimen NOTE: Multiple variations are listed below.

Variation 1:

Cisplatin: I.V.: 100 mg/m^2/dose day 1
[total dose/cycle = 100 mg/m^2]

Fluorouracil: I.V.: 1000 mg/m^2/day continuous infusion days 1 to 5
[total dose/cycle = 5000 mg/m^2]

Repeat cycle every 28 days

Variation 2:

Cycles 1 to 3 (prior to surgery):

Cisplatin: I.V.: 100 mg/m^2/dose day 1
[total dose/cycle = 100 mg/m^2]

Fluorouracil: I.V.: 1000 mg/m^2/day continuous infusion days 1 to 5
[total dose/cycle = 5000 mg/m^2]

Treatment cycles 1-3 are 28 days each

Cycles 4 and 5 (postoperative):

Cisplatin: I.V.: 75 mg/m^2/dose day 1
[total dose/cycle = 75 mg/m^2]

Fluorouracil: I.V.: 1000 mg/m^2/day continuous infusion days 1 to 5
[total dose/cycle = 5000 mg/m^2]

Treatment cycles 4 and 5 are 28 days each

Variation 3 (in combination with radiation therapy):

Cycle 1:

Cisplatin: I.V.: 75 mg/m^2/dose day 1
[total dose/cycle = 75 mg/m^2]

Fluorouracil: I.V.: 1000 mg/m^2/day continuous infusion days 1 to 4
[total dose/cycle = 4000 mg/m^2]

Treatment cycle is 28 days

Cycles 2 to 4:
Cisplatin: I.V.: 75 mg/m^2/dose day 1
[total dose/cycle = 75 mg/m^2]
Fluorouracil: I.V.: 1000 mg/m^2/day continuous infusion days 1 to 4
[total dose/cycle = 4000 mg/m^2]
Repeat cycle every 21 days for 3 more cycles (total of 4 cycles)
Variation 4 (in combination with radiation therapy):
Cisplatin: I.V.: 100 mg/m^2/dose day 1
[total dose/cycle = 100 mg/m^2]
Fluorouracil: I.V.: 1000 mg/m^2/day continuous infusion days 1 to 4
[total dose/cycle = 4000 mg/m^2]
Repeat cycle every 28 days for total of 2 cycles
Variation 5 (in combination with radiation therapy):
Cisplatin: I.V.: 75 mg/m^2/dose day 1
[total dose/cycle = 75 mg/m^2]
Fluorouracil: I.V.: 1000 mg/m^2/day continuous infusion days 1 to 4
[total dose/cycle = 4000 mg/m^2]
Repeat cycle every 28 days for 4 cycles
Variation 6 (in combination with radiation therapy):
Cycles 1 and 2:
Cisplatin: I.V.: 75 mg/m^2/dose day 1
[total dose/cycle = 75 mg/m^2]
Fluorouracil: I.V.: 1000 mg/m^2/day continuous infusion days 1 to 4
[total dose/cycle = 4000 mg/m^2]
Treatment cycles 1 and 2 are 28 days each; cycle 2 is followed by a 2-week rest
Cycles 3 and 4 (begin cycle 3 at week 11):
Cisplatin: I.V.: 75 mg/m^2/dose day 1
[total dose/cycle = 75 mg/m^2]
Fluorouracil: I.V.: 1000 mg/m^2/day continuous infusion days 1 to 4
[total dose/cycle = 4000 mg/m^2]
Treatment cycles 3 and 4 are 28 days each
Variation 7 (in combination with radiation therapy):
Cycles 1 to 4:
Cisplatin: I.V.: 15 mg/m^2/day days 1 to 5
[total dose/cycle = 75 mg/m^2]
Fluorouracil: I.V.: 800 mg/m^2/day continuous infusion days 1 to 5
[total dose/cycle = 4000 mg/m^2]
Repeat cycles 1-4 every 21 days; cycle 4 is followed by a 1-week rest
Cycles 5 (begin cycle 5 at week 14):
Cisplatin: I.V.: 15 mg/m^2/day days 1 to 5
[total dose/cycle = 75 mg/m^2]
Fluorouracil: I.V.: 800 mg/m^2/day continuous infusion days 1 to 5
[total dose/cycle = 4000 mg/m^2]

Cisplatin-Fluorouracil (Head and Neck Cancer)

Use Head and neck cancer

Regimen NOTE: Multiple variations are listed below.
Variation 1:
Cisplatin: I.V.: 100 mg/m^2 day 1
[total dose/cycle = 100 mg/m^2]
Fluorouracil: I.V.: 1000 mg/m^2/day continuous infusion days 1 to 4
[total dose/cycle = 4000 mg/m^2]
Repeat cycle every 3 or 4 weeks
Variation 2:
Cisplatin: I.V.: 100 mg/m^2 day 1
[total dose/cycle = 100 mg/m^2]
Fluorouracil: I.V.: 1000 mg/m^2/day continuous infusion days 1 to 5
[total dose/cycle = 5000 mg/m^2]
Repeat cycle every 3 or 4 weeks

Variation 3:
Cisplatin: I.V.: 60 mg/m^2 day 1
[total dose/cycle = 60 mg/m^2]
Fluorouracil: I.V.: 800 mg/m^2/day continuous infusion days 1 to 5
[total dose/cycle = 4000 mg/m^2]
Repeat cycle every 14 days

Variation 4:
Cisplatin: I.V.: 20 mg/m^2/day days 1 to 5
[total dose/cycle = 100 mg/m^2]
Fluorouracil: I.V.: 200 mg/m^2/day days 1 to 5
[total dose/cycle = 1000 mg/m^2]
Repeat cycle every 3 weeks

Variation 5:
Cisplatin: I.V.: 80 mg/m^2 continuous infusion day 1
[total dose/cycle = 80 mg/m^2]
Fluorouracil: I.V.: 800 mg/m^2/day continuous infusion days 2 to 6
[total dose/cycle = 4000 mg/m^2]
Repeat cycle every 3 weeks

Variation 6:
Cisplatin: I.V.: 75 mg/m^2 day 1
[total dose/cycle = 75 mg/m^2]
Fluorouracil: I.V.: 1000 mg/m^2/day continuous infusion days 1 to 4
[total dose/cycle = 4000 mg/m^2]
Repeat cycle every 4 weeks

Variation 7:
Cisplatin: I.V.: 120 mg/m^2 day 1
[total dose/cycle = 120 mg/m^2]
Fluorouracil: I.V.: 1000 mg/m^2/day continuous infusion days 1 to 5
[total dose/cycle = 5000 mg/m^2]
Repeat cycle every 3 weeks

Variation 8:
Cisplatin: I.V.: 25 mg/m^2/day continuous infusion days 1 to 4
[total dose/cycle = 100 mg/m^2]
Fluorouracil: I.V.: 1000 mg/m^2/day days 1 to 4
[total dose/cycle = 4000 mg/m^2]
Repeat cycle every 3 weeks

Variation 9:
Fluorouracil: I.V.: 350 mg/m^2/day continuous infusion days 1 to 5
[total dose/cycle = 1750 mg/m^2]
Cisplatin: I.V.: 50 mg/m^2 day 6
[total dose/cycle = 50 mg/m^2]
Repeat cycle every 3 weeks

Variation 10:
Cisplatin: I.V.: 5 mg/m^2/day continuous infusion days 1 to 14
[total dose/cycle = 70 mg/m^2]
Fluorouracil: I.V.: 200 mg/m^2/day continuous infusion days 1 to 14
[total dose/cycle = 2800 mg/m^2]
With concurrent radiation therapy, cycle does not repeat

Cisplatin-Irinotecan (Small Cell Lung Cancer)

Use Lung cancer, small cell

Regimen

Cisplatin: I.V.: 60 mg/m^2 day 1
[total dose/cycle = 60 mg/m^2]
Irinotecan: I.V.: 60 mg/m^2/dose days 1, 8, and 15
[total dose/cycle = 180 mg/m^2]
Repeat cycle every 28 days for 4 cycles

Cisplatin-Paclitaxel (Intraperitoneal Regimen)

Use Ovarian cancer

Regimen Note: I.P. therapies administered in 2 liters warmed saline

Paclitaxel: I.V.: 135 mg/m^2 continuous infusion (over 24 hours) day 1
[total dose/cycle = 135 mg/m^2]
Cisplatin: I.P.: 100 mg/m^2 day 2
[total dose/cycle = 100 mg/m^2]
Paclitaxel: I.P.: 60 mg/m^2 day 8
[total dose/cycle = 60 mg/m^2]
Repeat cycle every 21 days for 6 cycles

Cisplatin-Paclitaxel (Ovarian Cancer)

Use Ovarian cancer

Regimen NOTE: Multiple variations are listed below.

Variation 1:
Paclitaxel: I.V.: 135 mg/m^2 continuous infusion over 24 hours day 1
[total dose/cycle = 135 mg/m^2]
Cisplatin: I.V.: 75 mg/m^2 day 2
[total dose/cycle = 75 mg/m^2]
Repeat cycle every 21 days for a total of 6 cycles

Variation 2:
Paclitaxel: I.V.: 175 mg/m^2 over 3 hours day 1
[total dose/cycle = 175 mg/m^2]
Cisplatin: I.V.: 75 mg/m^2 day 1
[total dose/cycle = 75 mg/m^2]
Repeat cycle every 21 days for a total of at least 6 cycles

Variation 3:
Paclitaxel: I.V.: 185 mg/m^2 over 3 hours day 1
[total dose/cycle = 185 mg/m^2; maximum: 400 mg/dose]
Cisplatin: I.V.: 75 mg/m^2 day 1
[total dose/cycle = 75 mg/m^2; maximum: 165 mg/dose]
Repeat cycle every 21 days

Cisplatin-Pemetrexed (Mesothelioma)

Use Malignant pleural mesothelioma

Regimen

Pemetrexed: I.V.: 500 mg/m^2 infused over 10 minutes day 1
[total dose/cycle = 500 mg/m^2]
Cisplatin: I.V.: 75 mg/m^2 infused over 2 hours day 1 (start 30 minutes after pemetrexed)
[total dose/cycle = 75 mg/m^2]
Repeat cycle every 21 days

Cisplatin-Vinblastine-Dacarbazine (Melanoma)

Use Melanoma

Regimen NOTE: Multiple variations are listed below.

Variation 1:
Cisplatin: I.V.: 20 mg/m^2/day days 2 to 5
[total dose/cycle = 80 mg/m^2]
Vinblastine: I.V.: 1.6 mg/m^2/day days 1 to 5
[total dose/cycle = 8 mg/m^2]
Dacarbazine: I.V.: 800 mg/m^2 day 1
[total dose/cycle = 800 mg/m^2]
Repeat cycle every 21 days

Variation 2:
Cisplatin: I.V.: 20 mg/m^2/day days 1 to 4
[total dose/cycle = 80 mg/m^2]
Vinblastine: I.V.: 2 mg/m^2/day days 1 to 4
[total dose/cycle = 8 mg/m^2]

Dacarbazine: I.V.: 800 mg/m^2 day 1
[total dose/cycle = 800 mg/m^2]
Repeat cycle every 21 days

Cisplatin-Vinblastine (NSCLC)

Use Lung cancer, nonsmall cell

Regimen NOTE: Multiple variations are listed below.

Variation 1:
Cisplatin: I.V.: 80 mg/m^2/day days 1, 22, 43, and 64
[total dose/treatment = 320 mg/m^2]
Vinblastine: I.V.: 4 mg/m^2/day days 1, 8, 15, 22, 29, 43, and 57
[total dose/treatment = 28 mg/m^2]

Variation 2:
Cisplatin: I.V.: 100 mg/m^2/day days 1, 29, and 57
[total dose/treatment = 300 mg/m^2]
Vinblastine: I.V.: 4 mg/m^2/day days 1, 8, 15, 22, 29, 43, and 57
[total dose/treatment = 28 mg/m^2]

Variation 3:
Cisplatin: I.V.: 100 mg/m^2/day days 1, 29, 57, and 85
[total dose/treatment = 400 mg/m^2]
Vinblastine: I.V.: 4 mg/m^2/day days 1, 8, 15, 22, 29, 43, 57, 71, and 85
[total dose/treatment = 36 mg/m^2]

Variation 4:
Cisplatin: I.V.: 120 mg/m^2/day days 1, 29, and 71
[total dose/treatment = 360 mg/m^2]
Vinblastine: I.V.: 4 mg/m^2/day days 1, 8, 15, 22, 29, 43, 57, and 71
[total dose/treatment = 32 mg/m^2]

Cisplatin-Vinorelbine

Use Cervical cancer

Regimen

Cisplatin: I.V.: 80 mg/m^2 day 1
[total dose/cycle = 80 mg/m^2]
Vinorelbine: I.V.: 25 mg/m^2/day days 1 and 8
[total dose/cycle = 50 mg/m^2]
Repeat cycle every 21 days

CMF

Use Breast cancer

Regimen NOTE: Multiple variations are listed below.

Variation 1:
Methotrexate: I.V.: 40 mg/m^2/day days 1 and 8
[total dose/cycle = 80 mg/m^2]
Fluorouracil: I.V.: 600 mg/m^2/day days 1 and 8
[total dose/cycle = 1200 mg/m^2]
Cyclophosphamide: Oral: 100 mg/m^2/day days 1 to 14
[total dose/cycle = 1400 mg/m^2]
Repeat cycle every 28 days

Variation 2 (>60 years of age):
Methotrexate: I.V.: 30 mg/m^2/day days 1 and 8
[total dose/cycle = 60 mg/m^2]
Fluorouracil: I.V.: 400 mg/m^2/day days 1 and 8
[total dose/cycle = 800 mg/m^2]
Cyclophosphamide: Oral: 100 mg/m^2/day days 1 to 14
[total dose/cycle = 1400 mg/m^2]
Repeat cycle every 28 days

CMF-IV

Use Breast cancer

Regimen

Cyclophosphamide: I.V.: 600 mg/m^2 day 1
[total dose/cycle = 600 mg/m^2]
Methotrexate: I.V.: 40 mg/m^2 day 1
[total dose/cycle = 40 mg/m^2]
Fluorouracil: I.V.: 600 mg/m^2 day 1
[total dose/cycle = 600 mg/m^2]
Repeat cycle every 21 or 28 days

CMFP

Use Breast cancer

Regimen

Cyclophosphamide: Oral: 100 mg/m^2/day days 1 to 14
[total dose = 1400 mg/m^2]
Methotrexate: I.V.: 30 or 40 mg/m^2/day days 1 and 8
[total dose = 60 or 80 mg/m^2]
Fluorouracil: I.V.: 400 or 600 mg/m^2/day days 1 and 8
[total dose = 800 or 1200 mg/m^2]
Prednisone: Oral: 40 mg/m^2/day days 1 to 14
[total dose = 560 mg/m^2]
Repeat cycle every 28 days

CMFVP (Cooper Regimen, VPCMF)

Use Breast cancer

Regimen

Cyclophosphamide: Oral: 2 mg/kg/day days 1 to 252
[total dose/cycle = 504 mg/kg]
Methotrexate: I.V.: 0.7 mg/kg day 1, weeks 1 to 8, 10, 12, 14, 16, 18, 20, 22, 24, 26, 28, 30, 32, 34, and 36
[total dose/cycle = 15.4 mg/kg]
Fluorouracil: I.V.: 12 mg/kg day 1, weeks 1 to 8, 10, 12, 14, 16, 18, 20, 22, 24, 26, 28, 30, 32, 34, and 36
[total dose/cycle = 264 mg/kg]
Vincristine: I.V.: 0.035 mg/kg (maximum: 2 mg) day 1, weeks 1 to 5, 8, 12, 16, 20, 24, 28, 32, and 36
[total dose/cycle = 0.455 mg/kg]
Prednisone: Oral: 0.75 mg/kg/day days 1 to 10, taper off over next 40 days
Administer one cycle only

CMV

Use Bladder cancer

Regimen

Cisplatin: I.V.: 100 mg/m^2 infused over 4 hours (start at least 12 hours after methotrexate) day 2
[total dose = 100 mg/m^2]
Methotrexate: I.V.: 30 mg/m^2/day days 1 and 8
[total dose = 60 mg/m^2]
Vinblastine: I.V.: 4 mg/m^2/day days 1 and 8
[total dose = 8 mg/m^2]
Repeat cycle every 21 days

CNF

Use Breast cancer

Regimen NOTE: Multiple variations are listed below.

Variation 1:
Cyclophosphamide: I.V.: 500 mg/m^2 day 1
[total dose/cycle = 500 mg/m^2]

Mitoxantrone: I.V.: 10 mg/m^2 day 1
[total dose/cycle = 10 mg/m^2]
Fluorouracil: I.V.: 500 mg/m^2 day 1
[total dose/cycle = 500 mg/m^2]
Repeat cycle every 21 days

Variation 2:
Cyclophosphamide: I.V.: 500-600 mg/m^2 day 1
[total dose/cycle = 500-600 mg/m^2]
Fluorouracil: I.V.: 500-600 mg/m^2 day 1
[total dose/cycle = 500-600 mg/m^2]
Mitoxantrone: I.V.: 10-12 mg/m^2 day 1
[total dose/cycle = 10-12 mg/m^2]
Repeat cycle every 21 days

CNOP

Use Lymphoma, non-Hodgkin

Regimen

Cyclophosphamide: I.V.: 750 mg/m^2 day 1
[total dose/cycle = 750 mg/m^2]
Mitoxantrone: I.V.: 10 mg/m^2 day 1
[total dose/cycle = 10 mg/m^2]
Vincristine: I.V.: 1.4 mg/m^2 day 1
[total dose/cycle = 1.4 mg/m^2]
Prednisone: Oral: 50 mg/m^2/day days 1 to 5
[total dose/cycle = 250 mg/m^2]
Repeat cycle every 21 days

CO

Use Retinoblastoma

Regimen

Cyclophosphamide: I.V.: 10 mg/kg/day days 1, 2, and 3
[total dose/cycle = 30 mg/kg]
Vincristine: I.V.: 1.5 mg/m^2 day 1
[total dose/cycle = 1.5 mg/m^2]
Repeat cycle every 21 days

CODOX-M

Use Lymphoma, non-Hodgkin

Regimen

Cytarabine: I.T.: 70 mg/day days 1 and 3
[total dose/cycle = 140 mg]
Cyclophosphamide: I.V.: 800 mg/m^2 day 1
followed by I.V.: 200 mg/m^2/day days 2 to 5
[total dose/cycle = 1600 mg/m^2]
Vincristine: I.V.: 1.5 mg/m^2/day days 1 and 8 (cycle 1); days 1, 8, and 15 (cycle 3)
[total dose/cycle = 3-4.5 mg/m^2]
Doxorubicin: I.V.: 40 mg/m^2 day 1
[total dose/cycle = 40 mg/m^2]
Methotrexate:
I.T.: 12 mg day 15
[total dose/cycle = 12 mg]
I.V.: 1200 mg/m^2 loading dose
followed by I.V.: 240 mg/m^2/hour for 23 hours day 10
[total dose/cycle = 6720 mg/m^2]
Leucovorin: I.V.: 192 mg/m^2 day 11
followed by I.V.: 12 mg/m^2 every 6 hours until methotrexate level <5 X 10^{-8}M
(begin 36 hours after the start of methotrexate infusion)
Sargramostim: SubQ: 7.5 mcg/kg/day day 13 until ANC >1000 cells/mm^3
Repeat cycle when ANC >1000 cells/mm^3

CODOX-M/IVAC

Use Lymphoma, non-Hodgkin (Burkitt)

Regimen

CODOX-M

Cyclophosphamide: I.V.: 800 mg/m^2/day days 1 and 2
[total dose/cycle = 1600 mg/m^2]
Vincristine: I.V.: 1.4 mg/m^2/day (maximum dose: 2 mg) days 1 and 10
[total dose/cycle = 2.8 mg/m^2; maximum dose: 4 mg/cycle]
Doxorubicin: I.V.: 50 mg/m^2 day 1
[total dose/cycle = 50 mg/m^2]
Methotrexate: I.V.: 3 g/m^2 day 10
[total dose/cycle = 3 g/m^2]
Leucovorin: I.V.: 200 mg/m^2 day 11
followed by Oral, I.V.: 15 mg/m^2 every 6 hours until methotrexate level <0.1 Mmol/L
Cytarabine: I.T.: 50 mg/day days 1 and 3
[total dose/cycle = 100 mg]
Methotrexate: I.T.: 12 mg day 1
[total dose/cycle = 12 mg]
Filgrastim: SubQ: Dose not specified, days 3 to 8 and day 12 until ANC >1000 cells/mm^3
Cycle alternates with IVAC (cycles begin when ANC >1000 cells/mm^3)

Note: Hydrocortisone 50 mg may be added to intrathecal therapy to reduce the incidence of side effects/chemical arachnoiditis.

IVAC

Ifosfamide: I.V.: 1500 mg/m^2/day days 1 to 5
[total dose/cycle = 7500 mg/m^2]
Mesna: I.V.: 1500 mg/m^2/day (in divided doses) days 1 to 5
[total dose/cycle = 7500 mg/m^2]
Etoposide: I.V.: 60 mg/m^2/day days 1 to 5
[total dose/cycle = 300 mg/m^2]
Cytarabine: I.V.: 2 g/m^2 every 12 hours, for 4 doses, days 1 and 2
[total dose/cycle = 8 g/m^2]
Methotrexate: I.T.: 12 mg day 5
[total dose/cycle = 12 mg]
Filgrastim: SubQ: Dose not specified, day 6 until ANC >1000 cells/mm^3
Cycle alternates with CODOX-M (cycles begin when ANC >1000 cells/mm^3)

Note: Hydrocortisone 50 mg may be added to intrathecal therapy to reduce the incidence of side effects/chemical arachnoiditis.

COMLA

Use Lymphoma, non-Hodgkin

Regimen

Cyclophosphamide: I.V.: 1500 mg/m^2 day 1
[total dose/cycle = 1500 mg/m^2]
Vincristine: I.V.: 1.4 mg/m^2/day (maximum dose: 2 mg) days 1, 8, and 15
[total dose/cycle = 4.2 mg/m^2]
Methotrexate: I.V.: 120 mg/m^2/day days 22, 29, 36, 43, 50, 57, 64, and 71
[total dose/cycle = 960 mg/m^2]
Leucovorin: Oral: 25 mg/m^2 every 6 hours for 4 doses (beginning 24 hours after each methotrexate dose)
[total dose/cycle = 800 mg/m^2]
Cytarabine: I.V.: 300 mg/m^2/day days 22, 29, 36, 43, 50, 57, 64, and 71
[total dose/cycle = 2400 mg/m^2]
Repeat cycle every 85 days

COMP

Use Lymphoma, Hodgkin disease; Lymphoma, non-Hodgkin disease

Regimen

Cyclophosphamide: I.V.: 1200 mg/m^2 day 1, cycle 1
[total dose/cycle = 1200 mg/m^2]
followed by I.V.: 1000 mg/m^2 day 1 on subsequent cycles
[total dose/cycle = 1000 mg/m^2]

Vincristine: I.V.: 2 mg/m^2/day (maximum dose: 2 mg) days 3, 10, 17, 24, cycle 1
[total dose/cycle = 8 mg/m^2]
followed by I.V.: 1.5 mg/m^2/day days 1 and 4, on subsequent cycles
[total dose/cycle = 3 mg/m^2]
Methotrexate: I.V.: 300 mg/m^2 day 12
[total dose/cycle = 300 mg/m^2]
Prednisone: Oral: 60 mg/m^2/day (maximum dose: 60 mg) days 3 to 30 then taper over next 7 days, cycle 1
[total dose/cycle = 1680 mg/m^2 then taper over next 7 days]
followed by Oral: 60 mg/m^2 (maximum dose: 60 mg) days 1 to 5, on subsequent cycles
[total dose/cycle = 300 mg/m^2]
Maintenance cycles repeat every 28 days

COP-BLAM

Use Lymphoma, non-Hodgkin

Regimen

Cyclophosphamide: I.V.: 400 mg/m^2 day 1
[total dose/cycle = 400 mg/m^2]
Vincristine: I.V.: 1 mg/m^2 day 1
[total dose/cycle = 1 mg/m^2]
Prednisone: Oral: 40 mg/m^2/day days 1 to 10
[total dose/cycle = 400 mg/m^2]
Bleomycin: I.V.: 15 mg day 14
[total dose/cycle = 15 mg]
Doxorubicin: I.V.: 40 mg/m^2 day 1
[total dose/cycle = 40 mg/m^2]
Procarbazine: Oral: 100 mg/m^2/day days 1 to 10
[total dose/cycle = 1000 mg/m^2]

COPE

Use Brain tumors

Regimen

Cycle A:
Vincristine: I.V.: 0.065 mg/kg/day (maximum: 1.5 mg) days 1 and 8
[total dose/cycle = 0.13 mg/kg]
Cyclophosphamide: I.V.: 65 mg/kg day 1
[total dose/cycle = 65 mg/kg]
Cycle B:
Cisplatin: I.V.: 4 mg/kg day 1
[total dose/cycle = 4 mg/kg]
Etoposide: I.V.: 6.5 mg/kg/day days 3 and 4
[total dose/cycle = 13 mg/kg]
Repeat cycle every 28 days in the following sequence: AABAAB

COPP

Use Lymphoma, non-Hodgkin

Regimen

Cyclophosphamide: I.V.: 450-650 mg/m^2/day days 1 and 8
[total dose/cycle = 900-1300 mg/m^2]
Vincristine: I.V.: 1.4-2 mg/m^2/day (maximum: 2 mg) days 1 and 8
[total dose/cycle = 2.8-4 mg/m^2]
Procarbazine: Oral: 100 mg/m^2/day days 1 to 14
[total dose/cycle = 1400 mg/m^2]
Prednisone: Oral: 40 mg/m^2/day days 1 to 14
[total dose/cycle = 560 mg/m^2]
Repeat cycle every 3-4 weeks

CP (Leukemia)

Use Leukemia, chronic lymphocytic

Regimen

Chlorambucil: Oral: 30 mg/m^2 day 1
[total dose/cycle = 30 mg/m^2]
Prednisone: Oral: 80 mg/day days 1 to 5
[total dose/cycle = 400 mg]
Repeat cycle every 14 days

CP (Ovarian Cancer)

Use Ovarian cancer

Regimen

Cyclophosphamide: I.V.: 750 mg/m^2 day 1
[total dose/cycle = 750 mg/m^2]
Cisplatin: I.V.: 75 mg/m^2 day 1
[total dose/cycle = 75 mg/m^2]
Repeat cycle every 21 days

CV

Use Retinoblastoma

Regimen

Cyclophosphamide: I.V.: 300 mg/m^2
[total dose/cycle = 300 mg/m^2]
Vincristine: I.V.: 1.5 mg/m^2
[total dose/cycle = 1.5 mg/m^2]
Repeat weekly for 6 weeks
followed by
Cyclophosphamide: I.V.: 200 mg/m^2
[total dose/cycle = 200 mg/m^2]
Vincristine: I.V.: 1.5 mg/m^2
[total dose/cycle = 1.5 mg/m^2]
Repeat weekly for 42 weeks

CVD-Interleukin-Interferon (Melanoma)

Use Melanoma

Regimen NOTE: Multiple variations are listed below.

Variation 1:
Cisplatin: I.V.: 20 mg/m^2/day days 1 to 4 and 22 to 25
[total dose/cycle = 160 mg/m^2]
Vinblastine: I.V.: 1.5 mg/m^2/day days 1 to 4 and 22 to 25
[total dose/cycle = 12 mg/m^2]
Dacarbazine: I.V.: 800 mg/m^2/day days 1 and 22
[total dose/cycle = 1600 mg/m^2]
Aldesleukin: I.V.: 9 million units/m^2/day continuous infusion days 5 to 8, 17 to 20, and 26 to 29
[total dose/cycle = 108 million units/m^2]
Interferon alfa-2b: SubQ: 5 million units/m^2/day days 5 to 9, 17 to 21, and 26 to 30
[total dose/cycle = 75 million units/m^2]
Repeat every 42 days (maximum of five 21-day cycles for cytokine [interleukin and interferon] component)

Variation 2:
Cisplatin: I.V.: 20 mg/m^2/day days 1 to 4
[total dose/cycle = 80 mg/m^2]
Vinblastine: I.V.: 1.6 mg/m^2/day days 1 to 4
[total dose/cycle = 6.4 mg/m^2]
Dacarbazine: I.V.: 800 mg/m^2 day 1
[total dose/cycle = 800 mg/m^2]
Aldesleukin: I.V.: 9 million units/m^2/day continuous infusion days 1 to 4
[total dose/cycle = 36 million units/m^2]

Interferon alfa-2a: SubQ: 5 million units/m^2/day days 1 to 5, 7, 9, 11, and 13
[total dose/cycle = 45 million units/m^2]
Repeat cycle every 21 days for a total of 6 cycles
Variation 3:
Cisplatin: I.V.: 20 mg/m^2/day days 1 to 4
[total dose/cycle = 80 mg/m^2]
Vinblastine: I.V.: 1.2 mg/m^2/day days 1 to 4
[total dose/cycle = 4.8 mg/m^2]
Dacarbazine: I.V.: 800 mg/m^2 day 1
[total dose/cycle = 800 mg/m^2]
Aldesleukin: I.V.: 9 million units/m^2/day continuous infusion days 1 to 4
[total dose/cycle = 36 million units/m^2]
Interferon alfa-2b: SubQ: 5 million units/m^2/day days 1 to 5, 8, 10, and 12
[total dose/cycle = 40 million units/m^2]
Repeat cycle every 21 days (maximum: 4 cycles)

CVP (Leukemia)

Use Leukemia, chronic lymphocytic

Regimen NOTE: Multiple variations are listed below.
Variation 1:
Cyclophosphamide: Oral: 300 or 400 mg/m^2/day days 1 to 5
[total dose/cycle = 1500 or 2000 mg/m^2]
Vincristine: I.V.: 1.4 mg/m^2 (maximum dose: 2 mg) day 1
[total dose/cycle = 1.4 mg/m^2]
Prednisone: Oral: 100 mg/m^2/day days 1 to 5
[total dose/cycle = 500 mg/m^2]
Repeat cycle every 21 days
Variation 2:
Cyclophosphamide: I.V.: 800 mg/m^2 day 1
[total dose/cycle = 800 mg/m^2]
Vincristine: I.V.: 1.4 mg/m^2 (maximum dose: 2 mg) day 1
[total dose/cycle = 1.4 mg/m^2]
Prednisone: Oral: 100 mg/m^2/day days 1 to 5
[total dose/cycle = 500 mg/m^2]
Repeat cycle every 21 days

CVP (Lymphoma, non-Hodgkin)

Use Lymphoma, non-Hodgkin

Regimen NOTE: Multiple variations are listed below.
Variation 1:
Cyclophosphamide: I.V.: 750 mg/m^2 day 1
[total dose/cycle = 750 mg/m^2]
Vincristine: I.V.: 1.2 mg/m^2 day 1
[total dose/cycle = 1.2 mg/m^2]
Prednisone: Oral: 40 mg/m^2/day days 1 to 5
[total dose/cycle = 200 mg/m^2]
Repeat cycle every 21 days for up to 10 cycles
Variation 2:
Cyclophosphamide: I.V.: 750 mg/m^2 day 1
[total dose/cycle = 750 mg/m^2]
Vincristine: I.V.: 1.2 mg/m^2 day 1 (maximum: 2 mg/dose)
[total dose/cycle = 1.2 mg/m^2 (maximum: 2 mg/dose)]
Prednisone: Oral: 40 mg/m^2/day days 1 to 5
[total dose/cycle = 200 mg/m^2]
Repeat cycle every 28 days for up to 8 cycles
Variation 3:
Cyclophosphamide: I.V.: 750 mg/m^2 day 1
[total dose/cycle = 750 mg/m^2]
Vincristine: I.V.: 1.4 mg/m^2 day 1 (maximum: 2 mg/dose)
[total dose/cycle = 1.4 mg/m^2 (maximum: 2 mg/dose)]
Prednisone: Oral: 40 mg/m^2/day days 1 to 5
[total dose/cycle = 200 mg/m^2]
Repeat cycle every 21 days for up to 8 cycles

Variation 4:
Cyclophosphamide: Oral: 400 mg/m^2/day days 1 to 5
[total dose/cycle = 2000 mg/m^2]
Vincristine: I.V.: 1.4 mg/m^2 day 1 (maximum: 2 mg/dose)
[total dose/cycle = 1.4 mg/m^2 (maximum: 2 mg/dose)]
Prednisone: Oral: 100 mg/m^2/day days 1 to 5
[total dose/cycle = 500 mg/m^2]
Repeat cycle every 21 days

Cyclophosphamide + Doxorubicin

Use Prostate cancer

Regimen
Doxorubicin: I.V.: 40 mg/m^2 day 1
[total dose/cycle = 40 mg/m^2]
Cyclophosphamide: I.V.: 800-2000 mg/m^2 day 1
[total dose/cycle = 800-2000 mg/m^2]
Filgrastim: SubQ: 5 mcg/kg/day days 2 to 10 (or until ANC >10,000 cells/μL)
[total dose/cycle = 45 mcg/kg or until ANC >10,000 cells/μL]
Repeat cycle every 21 days

Cyclophosphamide + Etoposide

Use Prostate cancer

Regimen
Cyclophosphamide: Oral: 100 mg/day days 1 to 14
[total dose/cycle = 1400 mg]
Etoposide: Oral: 50 mg/day days 1 to 14
[total dose/cycle = 700 mg]
Repeat cycle every 28 days

Cyclophosphamide + Vincristine + Dexamethasone

Use Prostate cancer

Regimen
Cyclophosphamide: Oral: 250 mg/day days 1 to 14
[total dose/cycle = 3500 mg]
Vincristine: I.V.: 1 mg/day days 1, 8, and 15
[total dose/cycle = 3 mg]
Dexamethasone: Oral: 0.75 mg twice daily days 1 to 14
[total dose/cycle = 21 mg]
Repeat cycle every 28 days

CYVADIC

Use Sarcoma

Regimen
Cyclophosphamide: I.V.: 500 mg/m^2 day 1
[total dose/cycle = 500 mg/m^2]
Vincristine: I.V.: 1.4 mg/m^2/day days 1 and 5
[total dose/cycle = 2.8 mg/m^2]
Doxorubicin: I.V.: 50 mg/m^2 day 1
[total dose/cycle = 50 mg/m^2]
Dacarbazine: I.V.: 250 mg/m^2/day days 1 to 5
[total dose/cycle = 1250 mg/m^2]
Repeat cycle every 21 days

DA

Use Leukemia, acute myeloid (induction)

Regimen Induction:
Daunorubicin: I.V.: 45 mg/m^2/day days 1, 2, and 3
[total dose/cycle = 135 mg/m^2]
Cytarabine: I.V.: 100 mg/m^2/day continuous infusion days 1 to 7
[total dose/cycle = 700 mg/m^2]

Dacarbazine-Carboplatin-Aldesleukin-Interferon

Use Melanoma

Regimen

Dacarbazine: I.V.: 750 mg/m^2/day days 1 and 22
[total dose/cycle = 1500 mg/m^2]
Carboplatin: I.V.: 400 mg/m^2/day days 1 and 22
[total dose/cycle = 800 mg/m^2]
Aldesleukin: SubQ: 4,800,000 units every 8 hours days 36 and 57
[total dose/cycle = 28,800,000 units]
then 4,800,000 units every 12 hours days 37 and 58
[total dose/cycle = 19,200,000 units]
then 4,800,000 units/day days 38 to 40, 43 to 47, 50 to 54, 59 to 61, 65 to 68, 71 to 75
[total dose/cycle = 120,000,000 units]
Interferon alpha-2a: SubQ: 6,000,000 units days 38, 40, 43, 45, 47, 50, 52, 54, 59, 61, 64, 66, 68, 71, 73, and 75
[total dose/cycle = 96,000,000 units]
Repeat cycle every 78 days for 3 cycles

Dartmouth Regimen

Use Melanoma

Regimen NOTE: Multiple variations are listed below.

Variation 1:
Cisplatin: I.V.: 25 mg/m^2/day days 1, 2, and 3
[total dose/cycle = 75 mg/m^2]
Dacarbazine: I.V.: 220 mg/m^2/day days 1, 2, and 3
[total dose/cycle = 660 mg/m^2]
Carmustine: I.V.: 150 mg/m^2 day 1 (every other cycle)
[total dose/cycle = 150 mg/m^2; every other cycle]
Tamoxifen: Oral: 10 mg twice daily (begin 1 week before chemotherapy)
[total dose/cycle = 420 mg]
Repeat cycle every 21 days

Variation 2:
Carmustine: I.V.: 150 mg/m^2 day 1
[total dose/cycle = 150 mg/m^2]
Cisplatin: I.V.: 25 mg/m^2/day days 1, 2, 3, 22, 23, and 24
[total dose/cycle = 150 mg/m^2]
Dacarbazine: I.V.: 220 mg/m^2/day days 1, 2, 3, 22, 23, and 24
[total dose/cycle = 1320 mg/m^2]
Tamoxifen: Oral: 10 mg twice daily days 1 to 42
[total dose/cycle = 840 mg]
Repeat cycle every 42 days

Variation 3:
Carmustine: I.V.: 150 mg/m^2 day 1
[total dose/cycle = 150 mg/m^2]
Cisplatin: I.V.: 25 mg/m^2/day days 1, 2, 3, 22, 23, and 24
[total dose/cycle = 150 mg/m^2]
Dacarbazine: I.V.: 220 mg/m^2/day days 1, 2, 3, 22, 23, and 24
[total dose/cycle = 1320 mg/m^2]
Tamoxifen: Oral: 160 mg/day days -6 to 0 (cycle 1 only)
[total dose/cycle = 1120 mg]
followed by Oral: 40 mg/day days 1 to 42
[total dose/cycle = 1680 mg]
Repeat cycle every 42 days

Variation 4:
Carmustine: I.V.: 150 mg/m^2 day 1
[total dose/cycle = 150 mg/m^2]
Cisplatin: I.V.: 25 mg/m^2/day days 1, 2, 3, 29, 30, and 31
[total dose/cycle = 150 mg/m^2]
Dacarbazine: I.V.: 220 mg/m^2/day days 1, 2, 3, 29, 30, and 31
[total dose/cycle = 1320 mg/m^2]

Tamoxifen: Oral: 10-20 mg twice daily days 1 to 56
[total dose/cycle = 1120-2240 mg]
Repeat cycle every 56 days
Variation 5:
Cisplatin: I.V.: 25 mg/m^2/day days 1, 2, and 3
[total dose/cycle = 75 mg/m^2]
Dacarbazine: I.V.: 220 mg/m^2/day days 1, 2, and 3
[total dose/cycle = 660 mg/m^2]
Carmustine: I.V.: 100 mg/m^2 day 1 (give in cycles 1, 3, and 6 **only**)
[total dose/cycles 1, 3, and 6 = 100 mg/m^2]
Tamoxifen: Oral: 160 mg loading dose immediately before cycle 1
[total dose/loading dose + cycle 1 = 580 mg]
followed by Oral: 20 mg daily days 1 to 21
[total dose/subsequent cycles = 420 mg]
Repeat cycle every 21 days
Note: Tamoxifen is continued until 3 weeks after last cycle.

DAT

Use Leukemia, acute myeloid (induction)

Regimen Induction:
Daunorubicin: I.V. bolus: 45 mg/m^2/day days 1, 2, and 3
[total dose/cycle = 135 mg/m^2]
Cytarabine: I.V. bolus: 200 mg/m^2
[total dose/cycle = 200 mg/m^2]
Thioguanine: Oral: 100 mg/m^2/day days 1 to 7
[total dose/cycle = 700 mg/m^2]

DAV

Use Leukemia, acute myeloid

Regimen
Daunorubicin: I.V.: 60 mg/m^2/day days 3, 4, and 5
[total dose/cycle = 180 mg/m^2]
Cytarabine I.V.: 100 mg/m^2/day continuous infusion days 1 and 2
[total dose/cycle = 200 mg/m^2]
followed by I.V.: 100 mg/m^2 over 30 minutes every 12 hours days 3 to 8 (12 doses)
[total dose/cycle = 1200 mg/m^2]
Etoposide: I.V.: 150 mg/m^2/day days 6, 7, and 8
[total dose/cycle = 450 mg/m^2]
Administer one cycle only

Decitabine (Low Dose Regimen)

Use Leukemia, chronic myelogenous; Myelodysplastic syndrome

Regimen
Decitabine: I.V.: 20 mg/m^2/day days 1 to 5
[total dose/cycle = 100 mg/m^2]
Repeat cycle every 28 days for at least 3 cycles

Docetaxel-Bevacizumab

Use Breast cancer

Regimen NOTE: Multiple variations are listed below.
Variation 1:
Docetaxel: I.V.: 100 mg/m^2 day 1
[total dose/cycle = 100 mg/m^2]
Bevacizumab: I.V.: 7.5 mg/kg day 1
[total dose/cycle = 7.5 mg/kg]
Repeat cycle every 21 days (administer docetaxel for up to 9 cycles, bevacizumab until disease progression or unacceptable toxicity)
Variation 2:
Docetaxel: I.V.: 100 mg/m^2 day 1
[total dose/cycle = 100 mg/m^2]

Bevacizumab: I.V.: 15 mg/kg day 1
[total dose/cycle = 15 mg/kg]
Repeat cycle every 21 days (administer docetaxel for up to 9 cycles, bevacizumab until disease progression or unacceptable toxicity)

Docetaxel-Carboplatin (Ovarian Cancer)

Use Ovarian cancer

Regimen NOTE: Multiple variations are listed below.

Variation 1:
Docetaxel: I.V.: 60 mg/m^2 day 1
[total dose/cycle = 60 mg/m^2]
Carboplatin: I.V.: Target AUC 6
[total dose/cycle = AUC = 6]
Repeat cycle every 21 days for 6 cycles

Variation 2:
Docetaxel: I.V.: 75 mg/m^2 day 1
[total dose/cycle = 75 mg/m^2]
Carboplatin: I.V.: AUC 5 day 1
[total dose/cycle = AUC = 5]
Repeat cycle every 21 days for 6 cycles

Docetaxel-Cisplatin

Use Lung cancer, nonsmall cell

Regimen

Docetaxel: I.V.: 75 mg/m^2 day 1
[total dose/cycle = 75 mg/m^2]
Cisplatin: I.V.: 75 mg/m^2 day 1
[total dose/cycle = 75 mg/m^2]
Repeat cycle every 21 days

Docetaxel-Cisplatin-Fluorouracil (Gastric/Esophageal Cancer)

Use Esophageal cancer; Gastric cancer

Regimen

Docetaxel: I.V.: 75 mg/m^2 day 1
[total dose/cycle = 75 mg/m^2]
Cisplatin: I.V.: 75 mg/m^2 day 1
[total dose/cycle = 75 mg/m^2]
Fluorouracil: I.V.: 750 mg/m^2/day continuous infusion days 1 to 5
[total dose/cycle = 3750 mg/m^2]
Repeat cycle every 21 days

Docetaxel-Cisplatin-Fluorouracil (Head and Neck Cancer)

Use Head and neck cancer

Regimen NOTE: Multiple variations are listed below.

Variation 1:
Docetaxel: I.V.: 75 mg/m^2 day 1
[total dose/cycle = 75 mg/m^2]
Cisplatin: I.V.: 75 mg/m^2 day 1
[total dose/cycle = 75 mg/m^2]
Fluorouracil: I.V.: 750 mg/m^2/day continuous infusion days 1 to 5
[total dose/cycle = 3750 mg/m^2]
Repeat cycle every 21 days for 4 cycles

Variation 2:
Docetaxel: I.V.: 75 mg/m^2 day 1
[total dose/cycle = 75 mg/m^2]
Cisplatin: I.V.: 75-100 mg/m^2 day 1
[total dose/cycle = 75-100 mg/m^2]
Fluorouracil: I.V.: 1000 mg/m^2/day continuous infusion days 1 to 4
[total dose/cycle = 4000 mg/m^2]
Repeat cycle every 21 days for total of 3 cycles

Docetaxel-Cyclophosphamide (TC)

Use Breast cancer

Regimen

Docetaxel: I.V.: 75 mg/m^2 day 1
[total dose/cycle = 75 mg/m^2]
Cyclophosphamide: I.V.: 600 mg/m^2 day 1
[total dose/cycle = 600 mg/m^2]
Repeat cycle every 21 days for 4 cycles

Docetaxel-FEC

Use Breast cancer

Regimen

Cycles 1, 2, and 3:
Docetaxel: I.V.: 80-100 mg/m^2 day 1
[total dose/cycle = 80-100 mg/m^2]
Repeat cycle every 21 days for 3 cycles
Cycles 4, 5, and 6 (FEC):
Fluorouracil: I.V.: 600 mg/m^2 day 1
[total dose/cycle = 600 mg/m^2]
Epirubicin: I.V.: 60 mg/m^2 day 1
[total dose/cycle = 60 mg/m^2]
Cyclophosphamide: I.V.: 600 mg/m^2 day 1
[total dose/cycle = 600 mg/m^2]
Repeat FEC cycle every 21 days for total of 3 cycles

Docetaxel-Oxaliplatin (Ovarian Cancer)

Use Ovarian cancer

Regimen

Docetaxel: I.V.: 75 mg/m^2/dose over 60 minutes day 1
[total dose/cycle = 75 mg/m^2]
Oxaliplatin: I.V.: 100 mg/m^2/dose over 2 hours day 1
[total dose/cycle = 100 mg/m^2]
Repeat cycle every 21 days

Docetaxel-Prednisone

Use Prostate cancer

Regimen

Docetaxel: I.V.: 75 mg/m^2 day 1
[total dose/cycle = 75 mg/m^2]
Prednisone: Oral: 5 mg twice daily
[total dose/cycle = 210 mg]
Repeat cycle every 21 days for up to 10 cycles

Docetaxel-Thalidomide

Use Prostate cancer

Regimen

Docetaxel: I.V.: 30 mg/m^2/day days 1, 8, and 15
[total dose/cycle = 90 mg/m^2]
Thalidomide: Oral: 200 mg daily (at bedtime)
[total dose/cycle = 5600 mg]
Repeat cycle every 28 days

Docetaxel-Trastuzumab

Use Breast cancer

Regimen

Cycle 1:
Docetaxel: I.V.: 100 mg/m^2 day 1
[total dose/cycle 1 = 100 mg/m^2]
Trastuzumab: I.V.: 4 mg/kg (loading dose) day 1 cycle 1
followed by I.V.: 2 mg/kg/day days 8 and 15 cycle 1
[total dose/cycle 1 = 8 mg/kg]

Treatment cycle is 21 days
Subsequent cycles:
Docetaxel: I.V.: 100 mg/m^2 day 1
[total dose/cycle = 100 mg/m^2]
Trastuzumab: I.V.: 2 mg/kg/day days 1, 8, and 15
[total dose/cycle = 6 mg/kg]
Repeat cycle every 21 days for a total of at least 6 cycles (continue weekly trastuzumab until disease progression)

Docetaxel-Trastuzumab-Carboplatin

Use Breast cancer

Regimen

Cycle 1:
Trastuzumab: I.V.: 4 mg/kg (loading dose) day 1 cycle 1
followed by I.V.: 2 mg/kg/day days 8 and 15 cycle 1
[total dose/cycle 1 = 8 mg/kg]
Docetaxel: I.V.: 75 mg/m^2 day 2
[total dose/cycle 1 = 75 mg/m^2]
Carboplatin: I.V.: AUC 6 day 2
[total dose/cycle 1 = AUC = 6]
Treatment cycle is 21 days
Subsequent cycles:
Trastuzumab: I.V.: 2 mg/kg/day days 1, 8, and 15
[total dose/cycle = 6 mg/kg]
Docetaxel: I.V.: 75 mg/m^2 day 1
[total dose/cycle = 75 mg/m^2]
Carboplatin: I.V.: AUC 6 day 1
[total dose/cycle = AUC = 6]
Repeat cycle every 21 days for a total of ~6 cycles (continue weekly trastuzumab for 1 year after chemotherapy, or until disease progression or unacceptable toxicity)

Docetaxel-Trastuzumab-Cisplatin

Use Breast cancer

Regimen

Cycle 1:
Trastuzumab: I.V.: 4 mg/kg (loading dose) day 1 cycle 1
followed by I.V.: 2 mg/kg/day days 8 and 15 cycle 1
[total dose/cycle 1 = 8 mg/kg]
Docetaxel: I.V.: 75 mg/m^2 day 2
[total dose/cycle 1 = 75 mg/m^2]
Cisplatin: I.V.: 75 mg/m^2 day 2
[total dose/cycle 1 = 75 mg/m^2]
Treatment cycle is 21 days
Subsequent cycles:
Trastuzumab: I.V.: 2 mg/kg/day days 1, 8, and 15
[total dose/cycle = 6 mg/kg]
Docetaxel: I.V.: 75 mg/m^2 day 1
[total dose/cycle = 75 mg/m^2]
Cisplatin: I.V.: 75 mg/m^2 day 1
[total dose/cycle = 75 mg/m^2]
Repeat cycle every 21 days for a total of ~6 cycles (continue weekly trastuzumab for 1 year after chemotherapy, or until disease progression or unacceptable toxicity)

Docetaxel-Trastuzumab-FEC

Use Breast cancer

Regimen

Cycle 1:
Trastuzumab: I.V.: 4 mg/kg (loading dose) day 1 cycle 1
followed by I.V.: 2 mg/kg/day days 8 and 15 cycle 1
[total dose/cycle 1 = 8 mg/kg]

Docetaxel: I.V.: 80-100 mg/m^2 day 1
[total dose/cycle 1 = 80-100 mg/m^2]
Treatment cycle is 21 days
Cycles 2 and 3:
Trastuzumab: I.V.: 2 mg/kg/day days 1, 8, and 15
[total dose/cycle = 6 mg/kg]
Docetaxel: I.V.: 80-100 mg/m^2 day 1
[total dose/cycle = 80-100 mg/m^2]
Treatment cycle is 21 days
Cycles 4, 5, and 6 (FEC):
Fluorouracil: I.V.: 600 mg/m^2 day 1
[total dose/cycle = 600 mg/m^2]
Epirubicin: I.V.: 60 mg/m^2 day 1
[total dose/cycle = 60 mg/m^2]
Cyclophosphamide: I.V.: 600 mg/m^2 day 1
[total dose/cycle = 600 mg/m^2]
Repeat FEC cycle every 21 days for total of 3 cycles

Docetaxel (Weekly Regimen)

Use Prostate cancer

Regimen

Docetaxel: I.V.: 40 mg/m^2 days 1, 8, and 15
[total dose/cycle = 120 mg/m^2]
Repeat cycle every 4 weeks

Docetaxel (Weekly)-Trastuzumab

Use Breast cancer

Regimen

Cycle 1:
Docetaxel: I.V.: 35 mg/m^2/day days 1, 8, and 15
[total dose/cycle 1 = 105 mg/m^2]
Trastuzumab: I.V.: 4 mg/kg (loading dose) day 0 cycle 1
followed by I.V.: 2 mg/kg/day days 8 and 15 cycle 1
[total dose/cycle 1 = 8 mg/kg]
Treatment cycle is 28 days
Subsequent cycles:
Docetaxel: I.V.: 35 mg/m^2/day days 1, 8, and 15
[total dose/cycle = 105 mg/m^2]
Trastuzumab: I.V.: 2 mg/kg/day days 1, 8, and 15
[total dose/cycle = 6 mg/kg]
Repeat cycle every 28 days

Dox-CMF (Sequential)

Use Breast cancer

Regimen

Doxorubicin: I.V.: 75 mg/m^2 day 1
[total dose/cycle = 75 mg/m^2]
Repeat cycle every 21 days for 4 cycles
followed by (after completing Cycle 4)
Cyclophosphamide: I.V.: 600 mg/m^2 day 1
[total dose/cycle = 600 mg/m^2]
Methotrexate: I.V.: 40 mg/m^2 day 1
[total dose/cycle = 40 mg/m^2]
Fluorouracil: I.V.: 600 mg/m^2 day 1
[total dose/cycle = 600 mg/m^2]
Repeat cycle every 21 days for 8 cycles

Doxorubicin + Ketoconazole

Use Prostate cancer

Regimen

Doxorubicin: I.V.: 20 mg/m^2 continuous infusion day 1
[total dose/cycle = 20 mg/m^2]
Ketoconazole: Oral: 400 mg 3 times/day days 1 to 7
[total dose/cycle = 8400 mg]
Repeat cycle every 7 days

Doxorubicin + Ketoconazole/Estramustine + Vinblastine

Use Prostate cancer

Regimen

Doxorubicin: I.V.: 20 mg/m^2/day days 1, 15, and 29
[total dose/cycle = 60 mg/m^2]
Ketoconazole: Oral: 400 mg 3 times/day days 1 to 7, 15 to 21, and 29 to 35
[total dose/cycle = 25,200 mg]
Estramustine: Oral: 140 mg 3 times/day days 8 to 14, 22 to 28, and 36 to 42
[total dose/cycle = 8820 mg]
Vinblastine: I.V.: 5 mg/m^2/day days 8, 22, and 36
[total dose/cycle = 15 mg/m^2]
Repeat cycle every 8 weeks

Doxorubicin (Liposomal)-Vincristine-Dexamethasone

Use Multiple myeloma

Regimen NOTE: Multiple variations are listed below.

Variation 1:
Doxorubicin, liposomal: I.V.: 40 mg/m^2 day 1
[total dose/cycle = 40 mg/m^2]
Vincristine: I.V.: 2 mg day 1
[total dose/cycle = 2 mg]
Dexamethasone: Oral or I.V.: 40 mg/day days 1 to 4
[total dose/cycle = 160 mg]
Repeat cycle every 4 weeks

Variation 2:
Doxorubicin, liposomal: I.V.: 40 mg/m^2 day 1
[total dose/cycle = 40 mg/m^2]
Vincristine: I.V.: 1.4 mg/m^2 (maximum: 2 mg) day 1
[total dose/cycle = 1.4 mg/m^2; maximum: 2 mg]
Dexamethasone: Oral: 40 mg/day days 1 to 4
[total dose/cycle = 160 mg]
Repeat cycle every 4 weeks

DTPACE

Use Multiple myeloma

Regimen

Dexamethasone: Oral: 40 mg/day days 1 to 4
[total dose/cycle = 160 mg]
Thalidomide: Oral: 400 mg/day
[total dose/cycle = 11,200 - 16,800 mg]
Cisplatin: I.V.: 10 mg/m^2/day continuous infusion days 1 to 4
[total dose/cycle = 40 mg/m^2]
Doxorubicin: I.V.: 10 mg/m^2/day continuous infusion days 1 to 4
[total dose/cycle = 40 mg/m^2]
Cyclophosphamide: I.V.: 400 mg/m^2 continuous infusion days 1 to 4
[total dose/cycle = 1600 mg/m^2]
Etoposide: I.V.: 40 mg/m^2 continuous infusion days 1 to 4
[total dose/cycle = 160 mg/m^2]
Repeat cycle every 4-6 weeks

DVP

Use Leukemia, acute lymphocytic

Regimen Induction:

Daunorubicin: I.V.: 25 mg/m^2/day days 1, 8, and 15
[total dose/cycle = 75 mg/m^2]
Vincristine: I.V.: 1.5 mg/m^2/day (maximum: 2 mg) days 1, 8, 15, and 22
[total dose/cycle = 6 mg/m^2]
Prednisone: Oral: 60 mg/m^2/day days 1 to 28 then taper over next 14 days
[total dose/cycle = 1680 mg/m^2 + taper over next 14 days]
Administer single cycle; used in conjunction with intrathecal chemotherapy

EAP

Use Gastric cancer

Regimen

Etoposide: I.V.: 120 mg/m^2/day days 4, 5, and 6
[total dose/cycle = 360 mg/m^2]
Doxorubicin: I.V.: 20 mg/m^2/day days 1 and 7
[total dose/cycle = 40 mg/m^2]
Cisplatin: I.V.: 40 mg/m^2/day days 2 and 8
[total dose/cycle = 80 mg/m^2]
Repeat cycle every 22-28 days

EC (NSCLC)

Use Lung cancer, nonsmall cell

Regimen

Etoposide: I.V.: 120 mg/m^2/day days 1, 2, and 3
[total dose/cycle = 360 mg/m^2]
Carboplatin: I.V.: AUC 6 day 1
[total dose/cycle = AUC = 6]
Repeat cycle every 21-28 days

EC (Small Cell Lung Cancer)

Use Lung cancer, small cell

Regimen NOTE: Multiple variations are listed below.

Variation 1:
Etoposide: I.V.: 100-120 mg/m^2/day days 1, 2, and 3
[total dose/cycle = 300-360 mg/m^2]
Carboplatin: I.V.: 325-400 mg/m^2 day 1
[total dose/cycle = 325-400 mg/m^2]
Repeat cycle every 28 days

Variation 2:
Etoposide: I.V.: 120 mg/m^2/day days 1, 2, and 3
[total dose/cycle = 360 mg/m^2]
Carboplatin: I.V.: AUC 6 day 1
[total dose/cycle = AUC = 6]
Repeat cycle every 21-28 days

EE

Use Wilms tumor

Regimen

Dactinomycin: I.V.: 15 mcg/kg/day days 1 to 5 of weeks 0, 5, 13, and 24
[total dose/cycle = 300 mcg/kg]
Vincristine: I.V.: 1.5 mg/m^2 day 1 of weeks 1-10, 13, 14, 24, and 25
[total dose/cycle = 21 mg/m^2]

EE-4A

Use Wilms tumor

Regimen

Dactinomycin: I.V.: 45 mcg/kg day 1 of weeks 0, 3, 6, 9, 12, 15, and 18
[total dose/cycle = 315 mcg/kg]
Vincristine: I.V.: 2 mg/m^2 day 1 of weeks 1-10, 12, 15, and 18
[total dose/cycle = 26 mg/m^2]

EFP

Use Gastric cancer

Regimen NOTE: Multiple variations are listed below.

Variation 1:
Etoposide: I.V.: 90 mg/m^2/day days 1, 3, and 5
[total dose/cycle = 270 mg/m^2]
Fluorouracil: I.V.: 900 mg/m^2/day (20-hour infusion) days 1 to 5
[total dose/cycle = 4500 mg/m^2]
Cisplatin: I.V.: 20 mg/m^2/day days 1 to 5
[total dose/cycle = 100 mg/m^2]
Repeat cycle every 24-28 days
Variation 2:
Etoposide: I.V.: 100 mg/m^2/day days 1, 3, and 5
[total dose/cycle = 300 mg/m^2]
Fluorouracil: I.V.: 800 mg/m^2/day (12-hour infusion) days 1 to 5
[total dose/cycle = 4000 mg/m^2]
Cisplatin: I.V.: 20 mg/m^2/day days 1 to 5
[total dose/cycle = 100 mg/m^2]
Repeat cycle every 3 weeks

ELF

Use Gastric cancer

Regimen

Leucovorin calcium: I.V.: 300 mg/m^2/day days 1, 2, and 3
[total dose/cycle = 900 mg/m^2]
followed by
Etoposide: I.V.: 120 mg/m^2/day days 1, 2, and 3
[total dose/cycle = 360 mg/m^2]
followed by
Fluorouracil: I.V.: 500 mg/m^2/day days 1, 2, and 3
[total dose/cycle = 1500 mg/m^2]
Repeat cycle every 21-28 days

EMA 86

Use Leukemia, acute myeloid

Regimen

Mitoxantrone: I.V.: 12 mg/m^2/day days 1, 2, and 3
[total dose/cycle = 36 mg/m^2]
Etoposide: I.V.: 200 mg/m^2/day continuous infusion days 8, 9, and 10
[total dose/cycle = 600 mg/m^2]
Cytarabine: I.V.: 500 mg/m^2/day continuous infusion days 1, 2, and 3 and days 8, 9, and 10
[total dose/cycle = 3000 mg/m^2]
Administer one cycle only

EMA/CO

Use Gestational trophoblastic tumor

Regimen NOTE: Multiple variations are listed below.

Variation 1:
Etoposide: I.V.: 100 mg/m^2/day days 1 and 2
[total dose/cycle = 200 mg/m^2]

Methotrexate: I.V.: 300 mg/m^2 continuous infusion over 12 hours day 1
[total dose/cycle = 300 mg/m^2]
Dactinomycin: I.V. push: 0.5 mg/day days 1 and 2
[total dose/cycle = 1 mg]
Leucovorin: Oral, I.M.: 15 mg twice daily for 2 days (start 24 hours after the start of methotrexate) days 2 and 3
[total dose/cycle = 60 mg]
Alternate weekly with:
Cyclophosphamide: I.V.: 600 mg/m^2 day 1
[total dose/cycle = 600 mg/m^2]
Vincristine: I.V. push: 0.8 mg/m^2 (maximum: 2 mg) day 1
[total dose/cycle = 0.8 mg/m^2]
Repeat cycle every 2 weeks

Variation 2:
Dactinomycin: I.V.: 0.5 mg/day days 1 and 2
[total dose/cycle = 1 mg]
Etoposide: I.V.: 100 mg/m^2/day days 1 and 2
[total dose/cycle = 200 mg/m^2]
Methotrexate: I.V. bolus: 100 mg/m^2 then 200 mg/m^2 continuous infusion over 12 hours day 1
[total dose/cycle = 300 mg/m^2]
Leucovorin: Oral, I.M.: 15 mg every 12 hours for 4 doses (start 24 hours after methotrexate) days 2 and 3
[total dose/cycle = 60 mg]
Vincristine: I.V.: 1 mg/m^2 day 8
[total dose/cycle = 1 mg/m^2]
Cyclophosphamide: I.V.: 600 mg/m^2 day 8
[total dose/cycle = 600 mg/m^2]
Repeat cycle every 2 weeks

Variation 3:
Dactinomycin: I.V.: 0.5 mg/day days 1 and 2
[total dose/cycle = 1 mg]
Etoposide: I.V.: 100 mg/m^2/day days 1 and 2
[total dose/cycle = 200 mg/m^2]
Methotrexate: I.V.: 300 mg/m^2 continuous infusion over 12 hours day 1
[total dose/cycle = 300 mg/m^2]
Leucovorin: Oral, I.M.: 15 mg every 12 hours for 4 doses (start 24 hours after start of methotrexate) days 2 and 3
[total dose/cycle = 60 mg]
Vincristine: I.V.: 1 mg/m^2 day 8
[total dose/cycle = 1 mg/m^2]
Cyclophosphamide: I.V.: 600 mg/m^2 day 8
[total dose/cycle = 600 mg/m^2]
Repeat cycle every 2 weeks

Variation 4:
Dactinomycin: I.V.: 0.35 mg/m^2/day days 1 and 2
[total dose/cycle = 0.7 mg/m^2]
Etoposide: I.V.: 100 mg/m^2/day days 1 and 2
[total dose/cycle = 200 mg/m^2]
Methotrexate: I.V. bolus: 100 mg/m^2 then 200 mg/m^2 continuous infusion over 12 hours day 1
[total dose/cycle = 300 mg/m^2]
Leucovorin: Oral, I.M.: 15 mg every 12 hours for 4 doses (start 24 hours after start of methotrexate) days 2 and 3
[total dose/cycle = 60 mg]
Vincristine: I.V.: 1 mg/m^2 day 8
[total dose/cycle = 1 mg/m^2]
Cyclophosphamide: I.V.: 600 mg/m^2 day 8
[total dose/cycle = 600 mg/m^2]
Repeat cycle every 2 weeks

Variation 5 (patients with brain metastases):
Dactinomycin: I.V.: 0.5 mg/day days 1 and 2
[total dose/cycle = 1 mg]
Etoposide:I.V.: 100 mg/m^2/day days 1 and 2
[total dose/cycle = 200 mg/m^2]
Methotrexate: I.V.: 1 g/m^2 continuous infusion over 12 hours day 1
[total dose/cycle = 1 g/m^2]
Leucovorin: I.M.: 20 mg/m^2 every 6 hours for 12 doses (start 24 hours after start of methotrexate) days 2, 3, and 4
[total dose/cycle = 240 mg/m^2]
Vincristine: I.V.: 1 mg/m^2 day 8
[total dose/cycle = 1 mg/m^2]
Cyclophosphamide: I.V.: 600 mg/m^2 day 8
[total dose/cycle = 600 mg/m^2]
Repeat cycle every 2 weeks

Variation 6 (patients with brain metastases):
Dactinomycin: I.V.: 0.5 mg/day days 1 and 2
[total dose/cycle = 1 mg]
Etoposide: I.V.: 100 mg/m^2/day days 1 and 2
[total dose/cycle = 200 mg/m^2]
Methotrexate: I.V.: 1 g/m^2 continuous infusion over 12 hours day 1
[total dose/cycle = 1 g/m^2]
Leucovorin: Oral, I.M.: 30 mg/m^2 every 12 hours for 6 doses (start 32 hours after start of methotrexate) days 2, 3, and 4
[total dose/cycle = 180 mg/m^2]
Vincristine: I.V.: 1 mg/m^2 day 8
[total dose/cycle = 1 mg/m^2]
Cyclophosphamide: I.V.: 600 mg/m^2 day 8
[total dose/cycle = 600 mg/m^2]
Repeat cycle every 2 weeks

Variation 7:
Dactinomycin: I.V.: 0.5 mg/day days 1 and 2
[total dose/cycle = 1 mg]
Etoposide: I.V.: 100 mg/m^2/day days 1 and 2
[total dose/cycle = 200 mg/m^2]
Methotrexate: I.V.: 1 g/m^2 continuous infusion over 24 hours day 1
[total dose/cycle = 1 g/m^2]
Leucovorin: Oral, I.M.: 15 mg every 8 hours for 9 doses (start 32 hours after start of methotrexate) days 2, 3, and 4
[total dose/cycle = 135 mg/m^2]
Vincristine: I.V.: 1 mg/m^2 day 8
[total dose/cycle = 1 mg/m^2]
Cyclophosphamide: I.V.: 600 mg/m^2 day 8
[total dose/cycle = 600 mg/m^2]
Repeat cycle every 2 weeks

Variation 8 (patients with lung metastases):
Dactinomycin: I.V.: 0.5 mg/day days 1 and 2
[total dose/cycle = 1 mg]
Etoposide: I.V.: 100 mg/m^2/day days 1 and 2
[total dose/cycle = 200 mg/m^2]
Methotrexate: I.V. bolus: 100 mg/m^2 then 200 mg/m^2 continuous infusion over 12 hours day 1
[total dose/cycle = 300 mg/m^2]
Leucovorin: Oral, I.M.: 15 mg every 12 hours for 4 doses (start 24 hours after start of methotrexate) days 2 and 3
[total dose/cycle = 60 mg]
Vincristine: I.V.: 1 mg/m^2 day 8
[total dose/cycle = 1 mg/m^2]
Cyclophosphamide: I.V.: 600 mg/m^2 day 8
[total dose/cycle = 600 mg/m^2]
Methotrexate: I.T.: 10 mg day 1 (every other cycle)
[total dose/cycle = 10 mg, every other cycle]
Repeat cycle every 2 weeks

Variation 9 (patients with lung metastases):
Dactinomycin: I.V.: 0.5 mg/day days 1 and 2
[total dose/cycle = 1 mg]
Etoposide: I.V.: 100 mg/m^2/day days 1 and 2
[total dose/cycle = 200 mg/m^2]
Methotrexate: I.V. bolus: 100 mg/m^2 then 200 mg/m^2 continuous infusion over 12 hours day 1
[total dose/cycle = 300 mg/m^2]
Leucovorin: Oral, I.M.: 15 mg every 12 hours for 4 doses (start 24 hours after start of methotrexate) days 2 and 3
[total dose/cycle = 60 mg]
Vincristine: I.V.: 1 mg/m^2 day 8
[total dose/cycle = 1 mg/m^2]
Cyclophosphamide: I.V.: 600 mg/m^2 day 8
[total dose/cycle = 600 mg/m^2]
Methotrexate: I.T.: 12.5 mg day 8
[total dose/cycle = 12.5 mg]
Repeat cycle every 2 weeks

EP (Adenocarcinoma)

Use Adenocarcinoma, unknown primary

Regimen
Cisplatin: I.V.: 60-100 mg/m^2 day 1
[total dose = 60-100 mg/m^2]
Etoposide: I.V.: 80-100 mg/m^2/day days 1, 2, and 3
[total dose = 240-300 mg/m^2]
Repeat cycle every 21 days

EP/EMA

Use Gestational trophoblastic tumor

Regimen NOTE: Multiple variations are listed below.
Variation 1:
Etoposide: I.V.: 150 mg/m^2 day 1
[total dose/cycle = 150 mg/m^2]
Cisplatin: I.V.: 25 mg/m^2 infused over 4 hours for 3 consecutive doses, day 1
[total dose/cycle = 75 mg/m^2]
Alternate weekly with:
Etoposide: I.V.: 100 mg/m^2 day 1
[total dose/cycle = 100 mg/m^2]
Methotrexate: I.V.: 300 mg/m^2 infused over 12 hours day 1
[total dose/cycle = 300 mg/m^2]
Dactinomycin: I.V. push: 0.5 mg day 1
[total dose/cycle = 0.5 mg]
Leucovorin: Oral, I.M.: 15 mg twice daily for 2 days (start 24 hours after the start of methotrexate) days 2 and 3
[total dose/cycle = 60 mg]
Variation 2:
Dactinomycin: I.V.: 0.5 mg/day days 1 and 2
[total dose/cycle = 1 mg]
Etoposide: I.V.: 100 mg/m^2/day days 1 and 2
[total dose/cycle = 200 mg/m^2]
Methotrexate: I.V.: 300 mg/m^2 continuous infusion over 12 hours day 1
[total dose/cycle = 300 mg/m^2]
Leucovorin: Oral, I.M.: 15 mg every 12 hours for 4 doses (start 24 hours after start of methotrexate) days 2 and 3
[total dose/cycle = 60 mg]
Etoposide: I.V.: 150 mg/m^2 day 8
[total dose/cycle = 150 mg/m^2]
Cisplatin: I.V.: 75 mg/m^2 day 8
[total dose/cycle = 75 mg/m^2]
Repeat cycle every 2 weeks

Epirubicin-Cisplatin-Capecitabine (Esophageal Cancer)

Use Esophageal cancer

Regimen

Epirubicin: I.V.: 50 mg/m^2 day 1
[total dose/cycle = 50 mg/m^2]
Cisplatin: I.V.: 60 mg/m^2 day 1
[total dose/cycle = 60 mg/m^2]
Capecitabine: Oral: 625 mg/m^2 twice daily days 1 to 21
[total dose/cycle = 26,250 mg/m^2]
Repeat cycle every 21 days for up to 8 cycles

Epirubicin-Cisplatin-Fluorouracil (Gastric/Esophageal Cancer)

Use Esophageal cancer; Gastric cancer

Regimen NOTE: Multiple variations are listed below.

Variation 1:
Epirubicin: I.V.: 50 mg/m^2 day 1
[total dose/cycle = 50 mg/m^2]
Cisplatin: I.V.: 60 mg/m^2 day 1
[total dose/cycle = 60 mg/m^2]
Fluorouracil: I.V.: 200 mg/m^2/day continuous infusion days 1 to 21
[total dose/cycle = 4200 mg/m^2]
Repeat cycle every 3 weeks for up to 8 cycles

Variation 2:
Epirubicin: I.V.: 50 mg/m^2 day 1
[total dose/cycle = 50 mg/m^2]
Cisplatin: I.V.: 60 mg/m^2 day 1
[total dose/cycle = 60 mg/m^2]
Fluorouracil: I.V.: 200 mg/m^2/day continuous infusion days 1 to 21
[total dose/cycle = 4200 mg/m^2]
Repeat cycle every 3 weeks for up to 6 cycles (3 cycles before surgery and 3 cycles postoperatively)

Epirubicin-Oxaliplatin-Capecitabine

Use Esophageal cancer; Gastric cancer

Regimen

Epirubicin: I.V.: 50 mg/m^2 day 1
[total dose/cycle = 50 mg/m^2]
Oxaliplatin: I.V.: 130 mg/m^2 day 1
[total dose/cycle = 130 mg/m^2]
Capecitabine: Oral: 625 mg/m^2 twice daily days 1 to 21
[total dose/cycle = 26,250 mg/m^2]
Repeat cycle every 21 days for up to 8 cycles

Epirubicin-Oxaliplatin-Fluorouracil (Esophageal Cancer)

Use Esophageal cancer

Regimen

Epirubicin: I.V.: 50 mg/m^2 day 1
[total dose/cycle = 50 mg/m^2]
Oxaliplatin: I.V.: 130 mg/m^2 day 1
[total dose/cycle = 130 mg/m^2]
Fluorouracil: I.V.: 200 mg/m^2/day continuous infusion days 1 to 21
[total dose/cycle = 4200 mg/m^2]
Repeat cycle every 21 days for up to 8 cycles

EP (NSCLC)

Use Lung cancer, nonsmall cell

Regimen

Etoposide: I.V.: 80-120 mg/m^2/day days 1, 2, and 3
[total dose/cycle = 240-360 mg/m^2]

Cisplatin: I.V.: 80-100 mg/m^2 day 1
[total dose/cycle = 80-100 mg/m^2]
Repeat cycle every 21-28 days

EPOCH

Use Lymphoma, non-Hodgkin

Regimen NOTE: Multiple variations are listed below.

Variation 1:
Etoposide: I.V.: 50 mg/m^2/day continuous infusion days 1 to 4
[total dose/cycle = 200 mg/m^2]
Vincristine: I.V.: 0.4 mg/m^2/day continuous infusion days 1 to 4
[total dose/cycle = 1.6 mg/m^2]
Doxorubicin: I.V.: 10 mg/m^2/day continuous infusion days 1 to 4
[total dose/cycle = 40 mg/m^2]
Cyclophosphamide: I.V.: 750 mg/m^2 day 5
[total dose/cycle = 750 mg/m^2]
Prednisone: Oral: 60 mg/m^2/day days 1 to 5
[total dose/cycle = 300 mg/m^2]
Repeat cycle (with cyclophosphamide dose adjustments if needed based on ANC) every 21 days (best response seen in a median of 4 cycles)

Variation 2:
Etoposide: I.V.: 50 mg/m^2/day continuous infusion days 1 to 4
[total dose/cycle = 200 mg/m^2]
Vincristine: I.V.: 0.4 mg/m^2/day continuous infusion days 1 to 4
[total dose/cycle = 1.6 mg/m^2]
Doxorubicin: I.V.: 10 mg/m^2/day continuous infusion days 1 to 4
[total dose/cycle = 40 mg/m^2]
Cyclophosphamide: I.V.: 750 mg/m^2 day 6
[total dose/cycle = 750 mg/m^2]
Prednisone: Oral: 60 mg/m^2/day days 1 to 6
[total dose/cycle = 360 mg/m^2]
Repeat cycle (with cyclophosphamide dose adjustments if needed based on ANC) every 21 days (best response seen in a median of 4 cycles)

EP/PE

Use Lung cancer, nonsmall cell

Regimen

Etoposide: I.V.: 120 mg/m^2/day days 1, 2, and 3
[total dose/cycle = 360 mg/m^2]
Cisplatin: I.V.: 60-120 mg/m^2 day 1
[total dose/cycle = 60-120 mg/m^2]
Repeat cycle every 21-28 days

EP (Small Cell Lung Cancer)

Use Lung cancer, small cell

Regimen NOTE: Multiple variations are listed below.

Variation 1:
Etoposide: I.V.: 100 mg/m^2/day days 1, 2, and 3
[total dose/cycle = 300 mg/m^2]
Cisplatin: I.V.: 100 mg/m^2 day 1
[total dose/cycle = 100 mg/m^2]
Repeat cycle every 21 days

Variation 2:
Etoposide: I.V.: 80 mg/m^2/day days 1, 2, and 3
[total dose/cycle = 240 mg/m^2]
Cisplatin: I.V.: 80 mg/m^2 day 1
[total dose/cycle = 80 mg/m^2]
Repeat cycle every 21-28 days

EP (Testicular Cancer)

Use Testicular cancer

Regimen NOTE: Multiple variations are listed below.

Variation 1:

Etoposide: I.V.: 100 mg/m^2/day days 1 to 5
[total dose/cycle = 500 mg/m^2]

Cisplatin: I.V.: 20 mg/m^2/day days 1 to 5
[total dose/cycle = 100 mg/m^2]

Repeat cycle every 21 days

Variation 2:

Etoposide: I.V.: 120 mg/m^2/day days 1, 2, and 3
[total dose/cycle = 360 mg/m^2]

Cisplatin: I.V.: 20 mg/m^2/day days 1 to 5
[total dose/cycle = 100 mg/m^2]

Repeat cycle every 3 or 4 weeks

Variation 3:

Etoposide: I.V.: 120 mg/m^2/day days 1, 3, and 5
[total dose/cycle = 360 mg/m^2]

Cisplatin: I.V.: 20 mg/m^2/day days 1 to 5
[total dose/cycle = 100 mg/m^2]

Repeat cycle every 3 weeks

Erlotinib-Paclitaxel-Carboplatin (NSCLC)

Use Lung cancer, nonsmall cell (in never smokers)

Regimen

Erlotinib: Oral: 150 mg once daily days 1 to 21
[total dose/cycle = 3150 mg]

Paclitaxel: I.V.: 200 mg/m^2/dose day 1
[total dose/cycle = 200 mg/m^2]

Carboplatin: I.V.: AUC 6 day 1
[total dose/cycle = AUC = 6]

Repeat cycle every 21 days (maximum: 6 cycles)

ESHAP

Use Lymphoma, non-Hodgkin

Regimen NOTE: Multiple variations are listed below.

Variation 1:

Etoposide: I.V.: 40 mg/m^2/day days 1 to 4
[total dose/cycle = 160 mg/m^2]

Methylprednisolone: I.V.: 250-500 mg/day days 1 to 5
[total dose/cycle = 1250-2500 mg]

Cytarabine: I.V.: 2000 mg/m^2 day 5
[total dose/cycle = 2000 mg/m^2]

Cisplatin: I.V.: 25 mg/m^2/day continuous infusion days 1 to 4
[total dose/cycle = 100 mg/m^2]

Repeat cycle every 21-28 days

Variation 2:

Etoposide: I.V.: 40 mg/m^2/day days 1 to 4
[total dose/cycle = 160 mg/m^2]

Methylprednisolone: I.V.: 500 mg/day days 1 to 5
[total dose/cycle = 2500 mg]

Cytarabine: I.V.: 2000 mg/m^2 day 5
[total dose/cycle = 2000 mg/m^2]

Cisplatin: I.V.: 25 mg/m^2/day continuous infusion days 1 to 4
[total dose/cycle = 100 mg/m^2]

Repeat cycle every 21-28 days

Variation 3:
Etoposide: I.V.: 60 mg/m^2/day days 1 to 4
[total dose/cycle = 240 mg/m^2]
Methylprednisolone: I.V.: 500 mg/day days 1 to 4
[total dose/cycle = 2000 mg]
Cytarabine: I.V.: 2000 mg/m^2 day 5
[total dose/cycle = 2000 mg/m^2]
Cisplatin: I.V.: 25 mg/m^2/day continuous infusion days 1 to 4
[total dose/cycle = 100 mg/m^2]
Repeat cycle every 21 days

Estramustine-Cyclophosphamide

Use Prostate cancer

Regimen

Cyclophosphamide: Oral: 2 mg/kg/day days 1 to 14
[total dose/cycle = 28 mg/kg]
Estramustine: Oral: 10 mg/kg/day days 1 to 14
[total dose/cycle = 140 mg/kg]
Repeat cycle every 28 days

Estramustine + Docetaxel

Use Prostate cancer

Regimen NOTE: Multiple variations are listed below.

Variation 1:
Docetaxel: I.V.: 20-80 mg/m^2 day 2
[total dose/cycle = 20-80 mg/m^2]
Estramustine: Oral: 280 mg 3 times/day days 1 to 5
[total dose/cycle = 4200 mg]
Repeat cycle every 21 days

Variation 2:
Docetaxel: I.V.: 20-80 mg/m^2 day 2
[total dose/cycle = 20-80 mg/m^2]
Estramustine: Oral: 14 mg/kg/day days 1 to 21
[total dose/cycle = 294 mg/kg]
Repeat cycle every 21 days

Variation 3:
Docetaxel: I.V.: 35 mg/m^2/day days 2 and 9
[total dose/cycle = 70 mg/m^2]
Estramustine: Oral: 420 mg 3 times/day for 4 doses, then 280 mg 3 times/day for 5 doses days 1, 2, 3, 8, 9, and 10
[total dose/cycle = 6160 mg]
Repeat cycle every 21 days

Variation 4:
Docetaxel: I.V.: 60 mg/m^2 day 2 cycle 1
[total dose/cycle = 60 mg/m^2]
followed by I.V.: 60-70 mg/m^2 day 2 (subsequent cycles)
[total dose/cycle = 60-70 mg/m^2]
Estramustine: Oral: 280 mg 3 times/day days 1 to 5
[total dose/cycle = 4200 mg]
Repeat cycle every 21 days for up to 12 cycles

Estramustine + Docetaxel + Calcitriol

Use Prostate cancer

Regimen

Cycle 1:
Calcitriol: Oral: 60 mcg (in divided doses) day 1
[total dose/cycle = 60 mcg]
Estramustine: Oral: 280 mg 3 times/day days 1 to 5
[total dose/cycle = 4200 mg]
Docetaxel: I.V.: 60 mg/m^2 day 2
[total dose/cycle = 60 mg/m^2]
Treatment cycle is 21 days

Subsequent cycles:
Calcitriol: Oral: 60 mcg (in divided doses) day 1
[total dose/cycle = 60 mcg]
Estramustine: Oral: 280 mg 3 times/day days 1 to 5
[total dose/cycle = 4200 mg]
Docetaxel: I.V.: 70 mg/m^2 day 2
[total dose/cycle = 70 mg/m^2]
Repeat cycle every 21 days for up to 12 cycles

Estramustine + Docetaxel + Carboplatin

Use Prostate cancer

Regimen

Docetaxel: I.V.: 70 mg/m^2 day 2
[total dose/cycle = 70 mg/m^2]
Estramustine: Oral: 280 mg 3 times/day days 1 to 5
[total dose/cycle = 4200 mg]
Carboplatin: I.V.: Target AUC 5 day 2
[total dose/cycle = AUC = 5]
Repeat cycle every 3 weeks

Estramustine + Docetaxel + Hydrocortisone

Use Prostate cancer

Regimen

Docetaxel: I.V.: 70 mg/m^2 day 2
[total dose/cycle = 70 mg/m^2]
Estramustine: Oral: 10 mg/kg/day days 1 to 5
[total dose/cycle = 50 mg/kg]
Hydrocortisone: Oral: 40 mg daily
[total dose/cycle = 840 mg]
Repeat cycle every 3 weeks

Estramustine + Docetaxel + Prednisone

Use Prostate cancer

Regimen

Estramustine: Oral: 280 mg 3 times/day days 1 to 5 and days 7 to 11
[total dose/cycle = 8400 mg]
Docetaxel: I.V.: 70 mg/m^2 day 2
[total dose/cycle = 70 mg/m^2]
Prednisone: Oral: 10 mg daily
[total dose/cycle = 210 mg]
Repeat cycle every 21 days for up to 6 cycles

Estramustine + Etoposide

Use Prostate cancer

Regimen NOTE: Multiple variations are listed below.

Variation 1:
Estramustine: Oral: 15 mg/kg/day days 1 to 21
[total dose/cycle = 315 mg/kg]
Etoposide: Oral: 50 mg/m^2/day days 1 to 21
[total dose/cycle = 1050 mg/m^2]
Repeat cycle every 4 weeks

Variation 2:
Estramustine: Oral: 10 mg/kg/day days 1 to 21
[total dose/cycle = 210 mg/kg]
Etoposide: Oral: 50 mg/m^2/day days 1 to 21
[total dose/cycle = 1050 mg/m^2]
Repeat cycle every 4 weeks

Variation 3:
Estramustine: Oral: 140 mg 3 times/day days 1 to 21
[total dose/cycle = 8820 mg]
Etoposide: Oral: 50 mg/m^2/day days 1 to 21
[total dose/cycle = 1050 mg/m^2]
Repeat cycle every 4 weeks

Estramustine-Paclitaxel

Use Prostate cancer

Regimen NOTE: Multiple variations are listed below.

Variation 1:
Paclitaxel: I.V.: 30-35 mg/m^2/day continuous infusion (given in 2-3 divided doses daily) either days 1 to 4 or days 2 to 5
[total dose/cycle = 120-140 mg/m^2]
Estramustine: Oral: 600 mg/m^2/day days 1 to 21
[total dose/cycle = 12,600 mg/m^2]
Repeat cycle every 21 days

Variation 2:
Paclitaxel: I.V. 60-107 mg/m^2 infused over 3 hours weekly for 6 weeks
[total dose/cycle = 360-642 mg/m^2]
Estramustine: Oral: 280 mg twice daily 3 days/week for 6 weeks
[total dose/cycle = 3360 mg]
Repeat cycle every 8 weeks

Variation 3:
Paclitaxel: I.V. 150 mg/m^2/day days 2, 9, and 16
[total dose/cycle = 450 mg/m^2]
Estramustine: Oral: 280 mg 3 times/day days 1, 2, 3, 8, 9, 10, 15, 16, and 17
[total dose/week = 7560 mg/m^2]
Repeat cycle every 4 weeks

Variation 4:
Paclitaxel: I.V.: 100 mg/m^2/day days 2, 9, and 16
[total dose/cycle = 300 mg/m^2]
Estramustine: Oral: 280 mg 3 times/day days 1, 2, 3, 8, 9, 10, 15, 16, and 17
[total dose/cycle = 7560 mg]
Repeat cycle every 4 weeks

Estramustine-Vinblastine

Use Prostate cancer

Regimen NOTE: Multiple variations are listed below.

Variation 1:
Estramustine: Oral: 10 mg/kg/day days 1 to 42
[total dose/cycle = 420 mg/kg]
Vinblastine: I.V.: 4 mg/m^2/day days 1, 8, 15, 22, 29, and 36
[total dose/cycle = 24 mg/m^2]
Repeat cycle every 8 weeks

Variation 2:
Estramustine: Oral: 600 mg/m^2/day days 1 to 42
[total dose/cycle = 25,200 mg/m^2]
Vinblastine: I.V.: 4 mg/m^2/day days 1, 8, 15, 22, 29, and 36
[total dose/cycle = 24 mg/m^2]
Repeat cycle every 8 weeks

Estramustine + Vinorelbine

Use Prostate cancer

Regimen NOTE: Multiple variations are listed below.

Variation 1:
Estramustine: Oral: 140 mg 3 times/day days 1 to 14
[total dose/cycle = 5880 mg]
Vinorelbine: I.V.: 25 mg/m^2/day days 1 and 8
[total dose/cycle = 50 mg/m^2]
Repeat cycle every 21 days

Variation 2:
Estramustine: Oral: 280 mg 3 times/day days 1, 2, and 3
[total dose/cycle = 2520 mg/m^2]
Vinorelbine: I.V.: 15 or 20 mg/m^2 day 2
[total dose/cycle = 15 or 20 mg/m^2]
Repeat cycle weekly for 8 weeks, then every other week

Etoposide-Carboplatin (Ovarian Cancer)

Use Ovarian cancer

Regimen

Etoposide: I.V.: 120 mg/m^2/day days 1, 2, and 3
[total dose/cycle = 360 mg/m^2]
Carboplatin: I.V.: 400 mg/m^2 day 1
[total dose/cycle = 400 mg/m^2]
Repeat cycle every 28 days for a total of 3 cycles

Etoposide-Vinblastine-Doxorubicin (Hodgkin)

Use Lymphoma, Hodgkin disease

Regimen

Etoposide: I.V.: 100 mg/m^2/day days 1, 2, and 3
[total dose/cycle = 300 mg/m^2]
Vinblastine: I.V.: 6 mg/m^2 day 1
[total dose/cycle = 6 mg/m^2]
Doxorubicin: I.V.: 50 mg/m^2 day 1
[total dose/cycle = 50 mg/m^2]
Repeat cycle every 28 days

FAC

Use Breast cancer

Regimen NOTE: Multiple variations are listed below.

Variation 1:
Fluorouracil: I.V.: 500 mg/m^2/day days 1 and 8
[total dose/cycle = 1000 mg/m^2]
or 500 mg/m^2 day 1
[total dose/cycle = 500 mg/m^2]
Doxorubicin: I.V.: 50 mg/m^2 day 1
[total dose/cycle = 50 mg/m^2]
Cyclophosphamide: I.V.: 500 mg/m^2 day 1
[total dose/cycle = 500 mg/m^2]
Repeat cycle every 21-28 days
Variation 2:
Fluorouracil: I.V.: 200 mg/m^2/day days 1, 2, and 3
[total dose/cycle = 600 mg/m^2]
Doxorubicin: I.V.: 40 mg/m^2 day 1
[total dose/cycle = 40 mg/m^2]
Cyclophosphamide: I.V.: 400 mg/m^2 day 1
[total dose/cycle = 400 mg/m^2]
Repeat cycle every 28 days
Variation 3:
Fluorouracil: I.V.: 400 mg/m^2/day days 1 and 8
[total dose/cycle = 800 mg/m^2]
Doxorubicin: I.V.: 40 mg/m^2 day 1
[total dose/cycle = 40 mg/m^2]
Cyclophosphamide: I.V.: 400 mg/m^2 day 1
[total dose/cycle = 400 mg/m^2]
Repeat cycle every 28 days
Variation 4:
Fluorouracil: I.V.: 600 mg/m^2/day days 1 and 8
[total dose/cycle = 1200 mg/m^2]
Doxorubicin: I.V.: 60 mg/m^2 day 1
[total dose/cycle = 60 mg/m^2]

Cyclophosphamide: I.V.: 600 mg/m^2 day 1
[total dose/cycle = 600 mg/m^2]
Repeat cycle every 28 days
Variation 5:
Fluorouracil: I.V.: 300 mg/m^2/day days 1 and 8
[total dose/cycle = 600 mg/m^2]
Doxorubicin: I.V.: 30 mg/m^2 day 1
[total dose/cycle = 30 mg/m^2]
Cyclophosphamide: I.V.: 300 mg/m^2 day 1
[total dose/cycle = 300 mg/m^2]
Repeat cycle every 28 days

FAM

Use Gastric cancer; Pancreatic cancer
Regimen NOTE: Multiple variations are listed below
Variation 1:
Fluorouracil: I.V.: 600 mg/m^2/day days 1, 8, 29, and 36
[total dose/cycle = 2400 mg/m^2]
Doxorubicin: I.V.: 30 mg/m^2/day days 1 and 29
[total dose/cycle = 60 mg/m^2]
Mitomycin: I.V.: 10 mg/m^2 day 1
[total dose/cycle = 10 mg/m^2]
Repeat cycle every 8 weeks
Variation 2:
Fluorouracil: I.V.: 600 mg/m^2/day days 29 to 32
[total dose/cycle = 2400 mg/m^2]
Doxorubicin: I.V.: 50 mg/m^2 day 1
[total dose/cycle = 50 mg/m^2]
Mitomycin: I.V.: 10 mg/m^2 day 3
[total dose/cycle = 10 mg/m^2]
Repeat cycle every 8 weeks
Variation 3:
Fluorouracil: I.V.: 500 mg/m^2/day days 1, 8, 21, and 28
[total dose/cycle = 2000 mg/m^2]
Doxorubicin: I.V.: 30 mg/m^2/day days 1 and 21
[total dose/cycle = 60 mg/m^2]
Mitomycin: I.V.: 10 mg/m^2 day 1
[total dose/cycle = 10 mg/m^2]
Repeat cycle every 6 weeks
Variation 4:
Fluorouracil: I.V.: 275 mg/m^2/day days 1 to 5 and 36 to 40
[total dose/cycle = 2750 mg/m^2]
Doxorubicin: I.V.: 30 mg/m^2/day days 1 and 36
[total dose/cycle = 60 mg/m^2]
Mitomycin: I.V.: 10 mg/m^2 day 1
[total dose/cycle = 10 mg/m^2]
Repeat cycle every 10 weeks
Variation 5:
Fluorouracil: I.V.: 600 mg/m^2/day days 1, 8, 22, and 29
[total dose/cycle = 2400 mg/m^2]
Doxorubicin: I.V.: 30 mg/m^2/day days 1 and 22
[total dose/cycle = 60 mg/m^2]
Mitomycin: I.V.: 10 mg/m^2 day 1
[total dose/cycle = 10 mg/m^2]
Repeat cycle every 6 weeks

FAMe

Use Gastric cancer
Regimen
Fluorouracil: I.V.: 325 mg/m^2/day days 1 to 5 and days 36 to 40
[total dose/cycle = 3250 mg/m^2]

Doxorubicin: I.V.: 40 mg/m^2 days 1 and 36
[total dose/cycle = 80 mg/m^2]
Lomustine: Oral: 110 mg/m^2 day 1
[total dose/cycle = 110 mg/m^2]
Repeat cycle every 10 weeks

FAMTX

Use Gastric cancer

Regimen NOTE: Multiple variations are listed below.

Variation 1:
Methotrexate: I.V.: 1500 mg/m^2 day 1
[total dose/cycle = 1500 mg/m^2]
Fluorouracil: I.V.: 1500 mg/m^2 (1 hour after methotrexate) day 1
[total dose/cycle = 1500 mg/m^2]
Leucovorin: Oral: 15 mg/m^2 every 6 hours for 48 hours (start 24 hours after methotrexate) day 2
[total dose/cycle = 120 mg/m^2]
Doxorubicin: I.V.: 30 mg/m^2 day 15
[total dose/cycle = 30 mg/m^2]
Repeat cycle every 28 days

Variation 2:
Methotrexate: I.V.: 1500 mg/m^2 day 1
[total dose/cycle = 1500 mg/m^2]
Fluorouracil: I.V.: 1500 mg/m^2 (1 hour after methotrexate) day 1
[total dose/cycle = 1500 mg/m^2]
Leucovorin: Oral: 30 mg/m^2 every 6 hours for 8 doses (start 24 hours after methotrexate)
[total dose/cycle = 240 mg/m^2]
followed by Oral: 30 mg/m^2 every 6 hours for 8 more doses if 24-hour methotrexate level ≥2.5 mol/L
[total cumulative dose/cycle = 480 mg/m^2]
Doxorubicin: I.V.: 30 mg/m^2 day 15
[total dose/cycle = 30 mg/m^2]
Repeat cycle every 28 days

Variation 3:
Methotrexate: I.V.: 1000 mg/m^2 day 1
[total dose/cycle = 1000 mg/m^2]
Fluorouracil: I.V.: 1500 mg/m^2 (1 hour after methotrexate) day 1
[total dose/cycle = 1500 mg/m^2]
Leucovorin: Oral: 15 mg every 6 hours for 8 doses (start 24 hours after methotrexate)
[total dose/cycle = 120 mg/m^2]
Doxorubicin: I.V.: 30 mg/m^2 day 15
[total dose/cycle = 30 mg/m^2]
Repeat cycle every 28 days

FAP

Use Gastric cancer

Regimen

Fluorouracil: I.V.: 300 mg/m^2/day days 1 to 5
[total dose/cycle = 1500 mg/m^2]
Doxorubicin: I.V.: 40 mg/m^2 day 1
[total dose/cycle = 40 mg/m^2]
Cisplatin: I.V.: 60 mg/m^2 day 1
[total dose/cycle = 60 mg/m^2]
Repeat cycle every 5 weeks

FEC

Use Breast cancer

Regimen

Fluorouracil: I.V.: 500 mg/m^2 day 1
[total dose/cycle = 500 mg/m^2]

Cyclophosphamide: I.V.: 500 mg/m^2 day 1
[total dose/cycle = 500 mg/m^2]
Epirubicin: I.V.: 100 mg/m^2 day 1
[total dose/cycle = 100 mg/m^2]
Repeat cycle every 21 days

FIS-HAM

Use Leukemia, acute lymphocytic; Leukemia, acute myeloid

Regimen

Fludarabine: I.V.: 15 mg/m^2/day every 12 hours days 1, 2, 8, and 9
[total dose/cycle = 120 mg/m^2]
Cytarabine: I.V.: 750 mg/m^2/day every 3 hours days 1, 2, 8, and 9
[total dose/cycle = 24,000 mg/m^2]
Mitoxantrone: I.V.: 10 mg/m^2/day days 3, 4, 10, and 11
[total dose/cycle = 40 mg/m^2]

FL

Use Prostate cancer

Regimen NOTE: Multiple variations are listed below.

Variation 1:
Flutamide: Oral: 250 mg every 8 hours
[total dose/cycle = 21,000 mg]
Leuprolide acetate: SubQ: 1 mg/day
[total dose/cycle = 28 mg]
Repeat cycle every 28 days

Variation 2:
Flutamide: Oral: 250 mg every 8 hours
[total dose/cycle = 67,500 mg]
Leuprolide acetate depot: I.M.: 22.5 mg day 1
[total dose/cycle = 22.5 mg]
Repeat cycle every 3 months

FLAG

Use Leukemia, acute myeloid

Regimen NOTE: Multiple variations are listed below

Variation 1:
Fludarabine: I.V.: 30 mg/m^2/day over 30 minutes days 1 to 5
[total dose/cycle = 150 mg/m^2]
Cytarabine: I.V.: 2 g/m^2/day over 4 hours days 1 to 5 (begin 4 hours after fludarabine infusion)
[total dose/cycle = 10 g/m^2]
Filgrastim: SubQ: 300 mcg 12 hours prior to start of fludarabine then 300 mcg/day days 2 through 5
[total dose/cycle = 1500 mcg]
followed by Filgrastim: SubQ: 300 mcg/day beginning one week after the end of treatment and continuing until complete neutrophil recovery

Variation 2:
Fludarabine: I.V.: 30 mg/m^2/day over 30 minutes days 1 to 5
[total dose/cycle = 150 mg/m^2]
Cytarabine: I.V.: 2 g/m^2/day over 4 hours days 1 to 5 (begin 3.5 hours after end of fludarabine infusion)
[total dose/cycle = 10 g/m^2]
Filgrastim: SubQ: 5 mcg/kg/day beginning 24 hours prior to start of fludarabine and continuing until ANC >500 cells/mm^3
May repeat cycle one time for partial remission

Variation 3:
Fludarabine: I.V.: 30 mg/m^2/day over 30 minutes days 1 to 5
[total dose/cycle = 150 mg/m^2]

Cytarabine: I.V.: 2 g/m^2/day over 2 hours days 1 to 5 (begin 4 hours after the start of fludarabine infusion)
[total dose/cycle = 10 g/m^2]
Filgrastim: SubQ or I.V.: 300 mcg/day beginning the day prior to start of chemotherapy and continuing during chemotherapy and until ANC >1000 cells/mm^3
May receive a second cycle
Variation 4:
Fludarabine: I.V.: 25 mg/m^2/day over 30 minutes days 1 to 5
[total dose/cycle = 125 mg/m^2]
Cytarabine: I.V.: 2 g/m^2/day over 4 hours days 1 to 5 (begin 4 hours after start of fludarabine infusion)
[total dose/cycle = 10 g/m^2]
Filgrastim: SubQ: 5 mcg/kg/day beginning 24 hours prior to start of cytarabine and continuing until ANC >500 cells/mm^3

FLAG-IDA

Use Leukemia, acute myeloid

Regimen

Fludarabine: I.V.: 30 mg/m^2/day days 1 to 5
[total dose/cycle = 150 mg/m^2]
Cytarabine: I.V.: 2 g/m^2/day days 1 to 5
[total dose/cycle = 10 g/m^2]
Idarubicin: I.V.: 10 mg/m^2/day days 1, 2, and 3
[total dose/cycle = 30 mg/m^2]
Filgrastim: 5 mcg/kg from day 6 until neutrophil recovery
Administer one cycle only

FLOX (Nordic FLOX)

Use Colorectal cancer

Regimen

Oxaliplatin: I.V.: 85 mg/m^2 day 1
[total dose/cycle = 85 mg/m^2]
Fluorouracil: I.V.: 500 mg/m^2/day days 1 and 2
[total dose/cycle = 1000 mg/m^2]
Leucovorin: I.V.: 60 mg/m^2/day days 1 and 2
[total dose/cycle = 120 mg/m^2]
Repeat cycle every 2 weeks

Fludarabine-Cyclophosphamide (CLL)

Use Leukemia, chronic lymphocytic

Regimen NOTE: Multiple variations are listed below.

Variation 1:
Fludarabine: I.V.: 25 mg/m^2/day days 1, 2, and 3
[total dose/cycle = 75 mg/m^2]
Cyclophosphamide: I.V.: 250 mg/m^2/day days 1, 2, and 3
[total dose/cycle = 750 mg/m^2]
Repeat cycle every 4 weeks for up to 6 cycles
Variation 2:
Fludarabine: I.V.: 30 mg/m^2/day days 1, 2, and 3
[total dose/cycle = 90 mg/m^2]
Cyclophosphamide: I.V.: 250 mg/m^2/day days 1, 2, and 3
[total dose/cycle = 750 mg/m^2]
Repeat cycle every 4 weeks for up to 6 cycles
Variation 3:
Cyclophosphamide: I.V.: 600 mg/m^2 day 1
[total dose/cycle = 600 mg/m^2]
Fludarabine: I.V.: 20 mg/m^2/day days 1 to 5
[total dose/cycle = 100 mg/m^2]
Repeat cycle every 4 weeks for up to 6 cycles

Variation 4:
Fludarabine: I.V.: 30 mg/m^2/day days 1, 2, and 3
[total dose/cycle = 90 mg/m^2]
Cyclophosphamide: I.V.: 300 mg/m^2/day days 1, 2, and 3
[total dose/cycle = 900 mg/m^2]
Repeat cycle every 4 weeks for up to 6 cycles
Variation 5:
Fludarabine: I.V.: 30 mg/m^2/day days 1, 2, and 3
[total dose/cycle = 90 mg/m^2]
Cyclophosphamide: I.V.: 300 mg/m^2/day days 1, 2, and 3
[total dose/cycle = 900 mg/m^2]
Repeat cycle every 4-6 weeks for up to 6 cycles

Fludarabine-Cyclophosphamide-Mitoxantrone-Rituximab

Use Lymphoma, non-Hodgkin

Regimen NOTE: Multiple variations are listed below.

Consider pretherapy cytoreduction with cyclophosphamide 200 mg/m^2/day for 3-5 days for patients with high tumor burden and/or lymphocytes >20,000/mm^3

Variation 1:
Rituximab: I.V.: 375 mg/m^2/dose day 1
[total dose/cycle = 375 mg/m^2]
Fludarabine: I.V.: 25 mg/m^2/day days 2, 3, and 4
[total dose/cycle = 75 mg/m^2]
Cyclophosphamide: I.V.: 200 mg/m^2/day days 2, 3, and 4
[total dose/cycle = 600 mg/m^2]
Mitoxantrone: I.V.: 8 mg/m^2/dose day 2
[total dose/cycle = 8 mg/m^2]
Repeat cycle every 28 days for total of 4 cycles
Variation 2 (with maintenance rituximab):
Rituximab: I.V.: 375 mg/m^2/dose day 1
[total dose/cycle = 375 mg/m^2]
Fludarabine: I.V.: 25 mg/m^2/day days 2, 3, and 4
[total dose/cycle = 75 mg/m^2]
Cyclophosphamide: I.V.: 200 mg/m^2/day days 2, 3, and 4
[total dose/cycle = 600 mg/m^2]
Mitoxantrone: I.V.: 8 mg/m^2/dose day 2
[total dose/cycle = 8 mg/m^2]
Repeat cycle every 28 days for total of 4 cycles
followed by:
Maintenance rituximab (begin 3 months after completion of cycle 4):
Rituximab: I.V.: 375 mg/m^2/dose day 1, 8, 15, and 22
[total dose/cycle = 1500 mg/m^2]
Repeat maintenance cycle (once) in 6 months

Fludarabine-Cyclophosphamide (NHL-Mantle Cell)

Use Lymphoma, non-Hodgkin (mantle cell lymphoma)

Regimen NOTE: Multiple variations are listed below.

Variation 1:
Fludarabine: I.V.: 20 mg/m^2/day days 1 to 5
[total dose/cycle = 100 mg/m^2]
Cyclophosphamide: I.V.: 800 mg/m^2/dose day 1
[total dose/cycle = 800 mg/m^2]
Repeat cycle every 3-4 weeks for up to a total of 5 cycles
Variation 2:
Fludarabine: I.V.: 20 mg/m^2/day days 1 to 5
[total dose/cycle = 100 mg/m^2]
Cyclophosphamide: I.V.: 1000 mg/m^2/dose day 1
[total dose/cycle = 1000 mg/m^2]
Repeat cycle every 3-4 weeks for up to a total of 5 cycles

Variation 3:
Fludarabine: I.V.: 25 mg/m^2/day days 1 to 4
[total dose/cycle = 100 mg/m^2]
Cyclophosphamide: I.V.: 1000 mg/m^2/dose day 1
[total dose/cycle = 1000 mg/m^2]
Repeat cycle every 3-4 weeks for up to a total of 5 cycles

Fludarabine-Cyclophosphamide-Rituximab (CLL)

Use Leukemia, chronic lymphocytic

Regimen

Cycle 1:
Rituximab: I.V.: 375 mg/m^2 day 1
[total dose/cycle = 375 mg/m^2]
Fludarabine: I.V.: 25 mg/m^2/day days 2, 3, and 4
[total dose/cycle = 75 mg/m^2]
Cyclophosphamide: I.V.: 250 mg/m^2/day days 2, 3, and 4
[total dose/cycle = 750 mg/m^2]
Treatment cycle is 4 weeks
Cycles 2-6:
Rituximab: I.V.: 500 mg/m^2 day 1
[total dose/cycle = 500 mg/m^2]
Fludarabine: I.V.: 25 mg/m^2/day days 1, 2, and 3
[total dose/cycle = 75 mg/m^2]
Cyclophosphamide: I.V.: 250 mg/m^2/day days 1, 2, and 3
[total dose/cycle = 750 mg/m^2]
Repeat cycle every 4 weeks

Fludarabine-Cyclophosphamide-Rituximab (NHL-Follicular)

Use Lymphoma, non-Hodgkin (Follicular lymphoma)

Regimen

Cycle 1:
Rituximab: I.V.: 375 mg/m^2 day 15
[total dose/cycle = 375 mg/m^2]
Fludarabine: I.V.: 25 mg/m^2/day days 1, 2, and 3
[total dose/cycle = 75 mg/m^2]
Cyclophosphamide: I.V.: 300 mg/m^2/day days 1, 2, and 3
[total dose/cycle = 900 mg/m^2]
Treatment cycle is 3 weeks
Cycles 2-4:
Rituximab: I.V.: 375 mg/m^2 day 1
[total dose/cycle = 375 mg/m^2]
Fludarabine: I.V.: 25 mg/m^2/day days 1, 2, and 3
[total dose/cycle = 75 mg/m^2]
Cyclophosphamide: I.V.: 300 mg/m^2/day days 1, 2, and 3
[total dose/cycle = 900 mg/m^2]
Each treatment cycle is 3 weeks

Fludarabine-Mitoxantrone

Use Lymphoma, non-Hodgkin

Regimen

Fludarabine: I.V.: 25 mg/m^2/day days 1, 2, and 3
[total dose/cycle = 75 mg/m^2]
Mitoxantrone: I.V.: 10 mg/m^2/dose day 1
[total dose/cycle = 10 mg/m^2]
Repeat cycle every 21 days for total of 6 cycles

Fludarabine-Mitoxantrone-Dexamethasone (NHL)

Use Lymphoma, non-Hodgkin

Regimen

Fludarabine: I.V.: 25 mg/m^2/day days 1, 2, and 3
[total dose/cycle = 75 mg/m^2]

Mitoxantrone: I.V.: 10 mg/m^2/dose day 1
[total dose/cycle = 10 mg/m^2]
Dexamethasone: I.V. or Oral: 20 mg/day days 1 to 5
[total dose/cycle = 100 mg]
Repeat cycle every 28 days for up to a total of 8 cycles

Fludarabine-Mitoxantrone-Dexamethasone-Rituximab

Use Lymphoma, non-Hodgkin

Regimen

Cycle 1:
Rituximab: I.V.: 375 mg/m^2/day days 1 and 8
[total dose/cycle = 750 mg/m^2]
Fludarabine: I.V.: 25 mg/m^2/day days 1, 2, and 3
[total dose/cycle = 75 mg/m^2]
Mitoxantrone: I.V.: 10 mg/m^2/dose day 1
[total dose/cycle = 10 mg/m^2]
Dexamethasone: I.V. or Oral: 20 mg/m^2/day days 1 to 5
[total dose/cycle = 100 mg/m^2]
Treatment cycle is 28 days

Cycles 2-5:
Rituximab: I.V.: 375 mg/m^2 day 1
[total dose/cycle = 375 mg/m^2]
Fludarabine: I.V.: 25 mg/m^2/day days 2, 3, and 4
[total dose/cycle = 75 mg/m^2]
Mitoxantrone: I.V.: 10 mg/m^2/dose day 2
[total dose/cycle = 10 mg/m^2]
Dexamethasone: I.V. or Oral: 20 mg/m^2/day days 1 to 5
[total dose/cycle = 100 mg/m^2]
Repeat cycle every 28 days

Cycles 6-8:
Fludarabine: I.V.: 25 mg/m^2/day days 1, 2, and 3
[total dose/cycle = 75 mg/m^2]
Mitoxantrone: I.V.: 10 mg/m^2/dose day 1
[total dose/cycle = 10 mg/m^2]
Dexamethasone: I.V. or Oral: 20 mg/m^2/day days 1 to 5
[total dose/cycle = 100 mg/m^2]
Repeat cycle every 28 days

followed by:

Interferon maintenance:
Interferon alfa-2b: SubQ: 3 million units/m^2 days 1 to 14
[total dose/cycle = 42 million units/m^2]
Dexamethasone: Oral: 8 mg/day days 1, 2, and 3
[total dose/cycle = 24 mg]
Repeat cycle every month for 1 year

Fludarabine-Mitoxantrone-Rituximab

Use Lymphoma, non-Hodgkin

Regimen

Fludarabine: I.V.: 25 mg/m^2/day days 1, 2, and 3
[total dose/cycle = 75 mg/m^2]
Mitoxantrone: I.V.: 10 mg/m^2/dose day 1
[total dose/cycle = 10 mg/m^2]
Repeat cycle every 21 days for total of 6 cycles

followed by:

Sequential rituximab (after completion of cycle 6):
Rituximab: I.V.: 375 mg/m^2/dose weekly for 4 doses
[total dose/4 weeks = 1500 mg/m^2]

Fludarabine-Rituximab (CLL)

Use Leukemia, chronic lymphocytic

Regimen

Rituximab: I.V.: 375 mg/m^2/day days 1 and 4 (cycle 1); day 1 (cycles 2 to 6)
Fludarabine: I.V.: 25 mg/m^2/day days 1 to 5
Repeat cycle every 4 weeks

Fluorouracil + Carboplatin

Use Head and neck cancer

Regimen NOTE: Multiple variations are listed below.

Variation 1:
Fluorouracil: I.V.: 600 mg/m^2/day continuous infusion days 1 to 4
[total dose/cycle = 2400 mg/m^2]
Carboplatin: I.V.: 70 mg/m^2/day days 1 to 4
[total dose/cycle = 280 mg/m^2]
Repeat cycle every 3 weeks for 3 cycles
Variation 2:
Carboplatin: I.V.: 400 mg/m^2 day 1
[total dose/cycle = 400 mg/m^2]
Fluorouracil: I.V.: 1000 mg/m^2/day continuous infusion days 1 to 4
[total dose/cycle = 4000 mg/m^2]
Repeat cycle every 28 days

Fluorouracil-Leucovorin

Use Colorectal cancer

Regimen NOTE: Multiple variations are listed below.

Variation 1 (Mayo Regimen):
Fluorouracil: I.V.: 425 mg/m^2/day days 1 to 5
[total dose/cycle = 2125 mg/m^2]
Leucovorin: I.V.: 20 mg/m^2/day days 1 to 5
[total dose/cycle = 100 mg/m^2]
Repeat cycle every 28 days
Variation 2:
Fluorouracil: I.V.: 400 mg/m^2/day days 1 to 5
[total dose/cycle = 2000 mg/m^2]
Leucovorin: I.V.: 20 mg/m^2/day days 1 to 5
[total dose/cycle = 100 mg/m^2]
Repeat cycle every 28 days
Variation 3:
Fluorouracil: I.V.: 500 mg/m^2 day 1
[total dose/cycle = 500 mg/m^2]
Leucovorin: I.V.: 20 mg/m^2 (2-hour infusion) day 1
[total dose/cycle = 20 mg/m^2]
or 500 mg/m^2 (2-hour infusion) day 1
[total dose/cycle = 500 mg/m^2]
Repeat cycle weekly
Variation 4:
Fluorouracil: I.V.: 600 mg/m^2 weekly for 6 weeks
[total dose/cycle = 3600 mg/m^2]
Leucovorin: I.V.: 500 mg/m^2 (3-hour infusion) weekly for 6 weeks
[total dose/cycle = 3000 mg/m^2]
Repeat cycle every 8 weeks
Variation 5:
Fluorouracil: I.V.: 600 mg/m^2 weekly for 6 weeks
[total dose/cycle = 3600 mg/m^2]
Leucovorin: I.V.: 500 mg/m^2 weekly for 6 weeks
[total dose/cycle = 3000 mg/m^2]
Repeat cycle every 8 weeks

Variation 6:
Fluorouracil: I.V.: 600 mg/m^2 weekly
[total dose/cycle = 600 mg/m^2]
Leucovorin: I.V.: 500 mg/m^2 (2-hour infusion) weekly
[total dose/cycle = 500 mg/m^2]
Repeat cycle weekly
Variation 7:
Fluorouracil: I.V.: 2600 mg/m^2 continuous infusion day 1
[total dose/cycle = 2600 mg/m^2]
Leucovorin: I.V.: 500 mg/m^2 continuous infusion day 1
[total dose/cycle = 500 mg/m^2]
Repeat cycle weekly
Variation 8:
Fluorouracil: I.V.: 2600 mg/m^2 continuous infusion day 1
[total dose/cycle = 2600 mg/m^2]
Leucovorin: I.V.: 300 mg/m^2 (maximum: 500 mg) continuous infusion day 1
[total dose/cycle = 300 mg/m^2; maximum: 500 mg]
Repeat cycle weekly
Variation 9:
Fluorouracil: I.V.: 2600 mg/m^2 continuous infusion once weekly for 6 weeks
[total dose/cycle = 15,600 mg/m^2]
Leucovorin: I.V.: 500 mg/m^2 weekly for 6 weeks
[total dose/cycle = 3000 mg/m^2]
Repeat cycle every 8 weeks
Variation 10:
Fluorouracil: I.V.: 2300 mg/m^2 continuous infusion day 1
[total dose/cycle = 2300 mg/m^2]
Leucovorin: I.V.: 50 mg/m^2 continuous infusion day 1
[total dose/cycle = 50 mg/m^2]
Repeat cycle weekly
Variation 11:
Fluorouracil: I.V.: 200 mg/m^2/day continuous infusion days 1 to 14
[total dose/cycle = 2800 mg/m^2]
Leucovorin: I.V.: 5 mg/m^2/day continuous infusion days 1 to 14
[total dose/cycle = 70 mg/m^2]
Repeat cycle every 28 days
Variation 12:
Cycle 1:
Fluorouracil: I.V.: 200 mg/m^2/day continuous infusion for 4 weeks
[total dose/cycle = 5600 mg/m^2]
Leucovorin: I.V.: 20 mg/m^2/day days 1, 8, 15, 22
[total dose/cycle = 80 mg/m^2]
Treatment cycle is 6 weeks
Subsequent cycles (starting week 7):
Fluorouracil: 200 mg/m^2 continuous infusion days 1 to 21
[total dose/cycle = 4200 mg/m^2]
Leucovorin: I.V.: 20 mg/m^2/day days 1, 8, and 15
[total dose/cycle = 60 mg/m^2]
Repeat cycle every 4 weeks

Fluorouracil-Leucovorin-Irinotecan (Saltz Regimen)

Use Colorectal cancer

Regimen

Fluorouracil: I.V.: 500 mg/m^2/day days 1, 8, 15, and 22
[total dose/cycle = 2000 mg/m^2]
Leucovorin: I.V.: 20 mg/m^2/day days 1, 8, 15, and 22
[total dose/cycle = 80 mg/m^2]
Irinotecan: I.V.: 125 mg/m^2/day days 1, 8, 15, and 22
[total dose/cycle = 500 mg/m^2]
Repeat cycle every 42 days

Fluorouracil-Leucovorin-Oxaliplatin (Gastric Cancer)

Use Gastric cancer

Regimen

Oxaliplatin: I.V.: 100 mg/m^2/dose over 2 hours day 1
[total dose/cycle = 100 mg/m^2]
Leucovorin: I.V.: 400 mg/m^2/dose over 2 hours day 1
[total dose/cycle = 400 mg/m^2]
Fluorouracil: I.V. bolus: 400 mg/m^2/dose over 10 minutes day 1
followed by I.V.: 3000 mg/m^2 continuous infusion over 46 hours day 1
[total dose/cycle = 3400 mg/m^2]
Note: Bolus fluorouracil and continuous infusion are both given on day 1.
Repeat cycle every 2 weeks for at least 6 cycles

Fluorouracil-Leucovorin-Oxaliplatin (Gastric/Esophageal Cancer)

Use Esophageal Cancer; Gastric Cancer

Regimen NOTE: Multiple variations are listed below.

Variation 1:
Oxaliplatin: I.V.: 85 mg/m^2/dose over 2 hours day 1
[total dose/cycle = 85 mg/m^2]
Leucovorin: I.V.: 200 mg/m^2/dose over 2 hours day 1
[total dose/cycle = 200 mg/m^2]
Fluorouracil: I.V.: 2600 mg/m^2/dose continuous infusion over 24 hours day 1
[total dose/cycle = 2600 mg/m^2]
Repeat cycle every 2 weeks

Variation 2:
Oxaliplatin: I.V.: 85 mg/m^2/dose over 2 hours day 1
[total dose/cycle = 85 mg/m^2]
Leucovorin: I.V.: 500 mg/m^2/day over 2 hours days 1 and 2
[total dose/cycle = 1000 mg/m^2]
Fluorouracil: I.V. bolus: 400 mg/m^2/day days 1 and 2
followed by I.V.: 600 mg/m^2/day continuous infusion over 22 hours days 1 and 2
[total dose/cycle = 2000 mg/m^2]
Note: Bolus fluorouracil and continuous infusion are both given on days 1 and 2.
Repeat cycle every 2 weeks

Fluorouracil-Mitomycin (Anal Cancer)

Use Anal cancer

Regimen NOTE: Multiple variations are listed below.

Variation 1 (in combination with radiotherapy):
Fluorouracil: I.V.: 1000 mg/m^2/day continuous infusion days 1 to 4 and days 29 to 32
[total dose/cycle = 8000 mg/m^2]
Mitomycin: I.V.: 10 mg/m^2/day (maximum: 20 mg/dose) days 1 and 29
[total dose/cycle = 20 mg/m^2; maximum: 40 mg]

Variation 2 (in combination with radiotherapy):
Fluorouracil: I.V.: 1000 mg/m^2/day continuous infusion days 1 to 4
[total dose/cycle = 4000 mg/m^2]
Mitomycin: I.V.: 10 mg/m^2/dose (maximum: 20 mg/dose) day 1
[total dose/cycle = 10 mg/m^2; maximum: 20 mg]
Repeat cycle in 28 days (total of 2 cycles)

FOIL (Colorectal Cancer)

Use Colorectal cancer

Regimen

Irinotecan: I.V.: 175 mg/m^2 day 1
[total dose/cycle = 175 mg/m^2]
Oxaliplatin: I.V.: 100 mg/m^2 day 1
[total dose/cycle = 100 mg/m^2]
Leucovorin: I.V.: 200 mg/m^2 day 1
[total dose/cycle = 200 mg/m^2]

Fluorouracil: I.V.: 3800 mg/m^2/day continuous infusion days 1 and 2
[total dose/cycle = 7600 mg/m^2]
Repeat cycle every 14 days

FOLFIRINOX (Pancreatic Cancer)

Use Pancreatic cancer

Regimen

Oxaliplatin: I.V.: 85 mg/m^2/dose over 2 hours day 1
[total dose/cycle = 85 mg/m^2]
Irinotecan: I.V.: 180 mg/m^2/dose over 90 minutes day 1
[total dose/cycle = 180 mg/m^2]
Leucovorin: I.V.: 400 mg/m^2/dose over 2 hours day 1
[total dose/cycle = 400 mg/m^2]
Fluorouracil: I.V. bolus: 400 mg/m^2/dose day 1
followed by I.V.: 2400 mg/m^2 continuous infusion over 46 hours beginning day 1
[total dose/cycle = 2800 mg/m^2]
Note: Bolus fluorouracil and continuous infusion are both given on day 1.
Repeat cycle every 14 days for 12 cycles or until disease progression or unacceptable toxicity

FOLFOX 1

Use Colorectal cancer

Regimen

Oxaliplatin: I.V.: 130 mg/m^2 day 1 (every other cycle)
[total dose/cycle = 130 mg/m^2]
Leucovorin: I.V.: 500 mg/m^2/day days 1 and 2
[total dose/cycle = 1000 mg/m^2]
Fluorouracil: I.V.: 1.5-2 g/m^2/day continuous infusion days 1 and 2
[total dose/cycle = 3-4 g/m^2]
Repeat cycle every 14 days

FOLFOX 2

Use Colorectal cancer

Regimen

Oxaliplatin: I.V.: 100 mg/m^2 day 1
[total dose/cycle = 100 mg/m^2]
Leucovorin: I.V.: 500 mg/m^2/day days 1 and 2
[total dose/cycle = 1000 mg/m^2]
Fluorouracil: I.V.: 1.5-2 g/m^2/day continuous infusion days 1 and 2
[total dose/cycle = 3-4 g/m^2]
Repeat cycle every 14 days

FOLFOX 3

Use Colorectal cancer

Regimen

Oxaliplatin: I.V.: 85 mg/m^2 day 1
[total dose/cycle = 85 mg/m^2]
Leucovorin: I.V.: 500 mg/m^2/day days 1 and 2
[total dose/cycle = 1000 mg/m^2]
Fluorouracil: I.V.: 1.5-2 g/m^2/day continuous infusion days 1 and 2
[total dose/cycle = 3-4 g/m^2]
Repeat cycle every 14 days

FOLFOX 4

Use Colorectal cancer

Regimen

Oxaliplatin: I.V.: 85 mg/m^2 day 1
[total dose/cycle = 85 mg/m^2]
Leucovorin: I.V.: 200 mg/m^2/day days 1 and 2
[total dose/cycle = 400 mg/m^2]

Fluorouracil: I.V. bolus: 400 mg/m^2/day days 1 and 2
[total dose/cycle = 800 mg/m^2]
followed by I.V.: 600 mg/m^2 continuous infusion (over 22 hours) days 1 and 2
[total dose/cycle = 1200 mg/m^2]
Note: Bolus fluorouracil and continuous infusion are both given on each day.
Repeat cycle every 14 days

FOLFOX 6

Use Colorectal cancer

Regimen

Oxaliplatin: I.V.: 100 mg/m^2 day 1
[total dose/cycle = 100 mg/m^2]
Leucovorin: I.V.: 400 mg/m^2 day 1
[total dose/cycle = 400 mg/m^2]
Fluorouracil: I.V. bolus: 400 mg/m^2 day 1
[total dose/cycle = 400 mg/m^2]
followed by I.V.: 2.4-3 g/m^2 continuous infusion (46 hours) extending over days 1 and 2
[total dose/cycle = 2.4-3 g/m^2]
Repeat cycle every 14 days

FOLFOX 7

Use Colorectal cancer

Regimen

Oxaliplatin: I.V.: 130 mg/m^2 day 1
[total dose/cycle = 130 mg/m^2]
Leucovorin: I.V.: 400 mg/m^2 day 1
[total dose/cycle = 400 mg/m^2]
Fluorouracil: I.V. bolus: 400 mg/m^2 day 1
[total dose/cycle = 400 mg/m^2]
followed by I.V.: 2.4 g/m^2 continuous infusion (46 hours) extending over days 1 and 2
[total dose/cycle = 2.4 g/m^2]
Repeat cycle every 14 days

FOLFOXIRI (Colorectal Cancer)

Use Colorectal cancer

Regimen

Irinotecan: I.V.: 165 mg/m^2 over 1 hour day 1
[total dose/cycle = 165 mg/m^2]
Oxaliplatin: I.V.: 85 mg/m^2 over 2 hours day 1
[total dose/cycle = 85 mg/m^2]
Leucovorin: I.V.: 200 mg/m^2 over 2 hours day 1
[total dose/cycle = 200 mg/m^2]
Fluorouracil: I.V.: 3200 mg/m^2/day continuous infusion over 48 hours beginning day 1
[total dose/cycle = 6400 mg/m^2]
Repeat cycle every 14 days (maximum: 12 cycles)

FU-LV-CPT-11

Use Colorectal cancer

Regimen NOTE: Multiple variations are listed below.

Variation 1:
Irinotecan: I.V.: 350 mg/m^2 day 1
[total dose/cycle = 350 mg/m^2]
Leucovorin: I.V.: 20 mg/m^2/day days 22 to 26
[total dose/cycle = 100 mg/m^2]
Fluorouracil: I.V.: 425 mg/m^2/day days 22 to 26
[total dose/cycle = 2125 mg/m^2]
Repeat cycle every 6 weeks

Variation 2:
Irinotecan: I.V.: 80 mg/m^2 day 1
[total dose/cycle = 80 mg/m^2]
Fluorouracil: I.V.: 2300 mg/m^2 continuous infusion day 1
[total dose/cycle = 2300 mg/m^2]
Leucovorin: I.V.: 500 mg/m^2 day 1
[total dose/cycle = 500 mg/m^2]
Repeat cycle weekly
or
Irinotecan: I.V.: 180 mg/m^2 day 1
[total dose/cycle = 180 mg/m^2]
Leucovorin: I.V.: 200 mg/m^2/day days 1 and 2
[total dose/cycle = 400 mg/m^2]
Fluorouracil: I.V.: 400 mg/m^2/day days 1 and 2
[total dose/cycle = 800 mg/m^2]
followed by I.V.: 600 mg/m^2/day continuous infusion days 1 and 2
[total dose/cycle = 1200 mg/m^2]
Repeat cycle every 2 weeks
Variation 3:
Irinotecan: I.V.: 175 mg/m^2 day 1
[total dose/cycle = 175 mg/m^2]
Leucovorin: I.V.: 250 mg/m^2 day 2
[total dose/cycle = 250 mg/m^2]
Fluorouracil: I.V.: 950 mg/m^2 day 2
[total dose/cycle = 950 mg/m^2]
or
Irinotecan: I.V.: 200 mg/m^2 day 1
[total dose/cycle = 200 mg/m^2]
Leucovorin: I.V.: 250 mg/m^2 day 2
[total dose/cycle = 250 mg/m^2]
Fluorouracil: I.V.: 850 mg/m^2 day 2
[total dose/cycle = 850 mg/m^2]
Repeat cycle every other week

FUP

Use Gastric cancer

Regimen

Fluorouracil: I.V.: 1000 mg/m^2/day continuous infusion days 1 to 5
[total dose/cycle = 5000 mg/m^2]
Cisplatin: I.V.: 100 mg/m^2 day 2
[total dose/cycle = 100 mg/m^2]
Repeat cycle every 28 days

FZ

Use Prostate cancer

Regimen NOTE: Multiple variations are listed below.

Variation 1:
Flutamide: Oral: 250 mg every 8 hours
[total dose/cycle = 21,000 mg]
Goserelin acetate: SubQ: 3.6 mg day 1
[total dose/cycle = 3.6 mg]
Repeat cycle every 28 days
Variation 2:
Flutamide: Oral: 250 mg every 8 hours
[total dose/cycle = 67,500 mg]
Goserelin acetate: SubQ: 10.8 mg day 1
[total dose/cycle = 10.8 mg]
Repeat cycle every 3 months

Gemcitabine-Capecitabine

Use Biliary adenocarcinoma; Pancreatic cancer

Regimen

Gemcitabine: I.V.: 1000 mg/m^2/day days 1 and 8
[total dose/cycle = 2000 mg/m^2]
Capecitabine: Oral: 650 mg/m^2 twice daily days 1 to 14
[total dose/cycle = 18,200 mg/m^2]
Repeat cycle every 21 days

Gemcitabine-Carboplatin (Bladder Cancer)

Use Bladder cancer

Regimen

Gemcitabine: I.V.: 1000 mg/m^2/day days 1 and 8
[total dose/cycle = 2000 mg/m^2]
Carboplatin: I.V.: AUC 5 day 1
[total dose/cycle = AUC = 5]
Repeat cycle every 21 days for up to 6 cycles

Gemcitabine-Carboplatin (NSCLC)

Use Lung cancer, nonsmall cell

Regimen NOTE: Multiple variations are listed below.

Variation 1:
Gemcitabine: I.V.: 1000 mg/m^2/dose days 1, 8, and 15
[total dose/cycle = 3000 mg/m^2]
Carboplatin: I.V.: AUC 5 day 1
[total dose/cycle = AUC = 5]
Repeat cycle every 28 days for up to 4 cycles

Variation 2:
Gemcitabine: I.V.: 1000 or 1100 mg/m^2/day days 1 and 8
[total dose/cycle = 2000 or 2200 mg/m^2]
Carboplatin: I.V.: AUC 5 day 8
[total dose/cycle = AUC = 5]
Repeat cycle every 28 days

Gemcitabine-Carboplatin (Ovarian Cancer)

Use Ovarian cancer

Regimen

Gemcitabine: I.V.: 1000 mg/m^2/day days 1 and 8
[total dose/cycle = 2000 mg/m^2]
Carboplatin: I.V.: AUC 4 day 1
[total dose/cycle = AUC = 4]
Repeat cycle every 21 days for 6-10 cycles

Gemcitabine-Cisplatin (Biliary Cancer)

Use Biliary adenocarcinoma

Regimen NOTE: Multiple variations are listed below.

Variation 1:
Gemcitabine: I.V.: 1250 mg/m^2/dose days 1 and 8
[total dose/cycle = 2500 mg/m^2]
Cisplatin: I.V.: 75 mg/m^2/dose day 1
[total dose/cycle = 75 mg/m^2]
Repeat cycle every 3 weeks

Variation 2:
Gemcitabine: I.V.: 1000 mg/m^2/dose days 1 and 8
[total dose/cycle = 2000 mg/m^2]
Cisplatin: I.V.: 70 mg/m^2/dose day 1
[total dose/cycle = 70 mg/m^2]
Repeat cycle every 3 weeks (maximum: 6 cycles)

Gemcitabine-Cisplatin (Bladder Cancer)

Use Bladder cancer

Regimen

Gemcitabine: I.V.: 1000 mg/m^2/day days 1, 8, and 15
[total dose/cycle = 3000 mg/m^2]
Cisplatin: I.V.: 70 mg/m^2 day 2
[total dose/cycle = 70 mg/m^2]
Repeat cycle every 28 days for 6 cycles

Gemcitabine-Cisplatin (Cervical Cancer)

Use Cervical cancer

Regimen

Gemcitabine: I.V.: 1250 mg/m^2/day days 1 and 8
[total dose/cycle = 2500 mg/m^2]
Cisplatin: I.V.: 50 mg/m^2 day 1
[total dose/cycle = 50 mg/m^2]
Repeat cycle every 21 days

Gemcitabine-Cisplatin (NSCLC)

Use Lung cancer, nonsmall cell

Regimen NOTE: Multiple variations are listed below.

Variation 1:
Gemcitabine: I.V.: 1000 mg/m^2/day days 1, 8, and 15
[total dose/cycle = 3000 mg/m^2]
Cisplatin: I.V.: 100 mg/m^2 day 1
[total dose/cycle = 100 mg/m^2]
Repeat cycle every 28 days

Variation 2:
Gemcitabine: I.V.: 1250 mg/m^2/day days 1 and 8
[total dose/cycle = 2500 mg/m^2]
Cisplatin: I.V.: 100 mg/m^2 day 1
[total dose/cycle = 100 mg/m^2]
Repeat cycle every 21 days

Variation 3:
Gemcitabine: I.V.: 1000 mg/m^2/day days 1 and 8
[total dose/cycle = 2000 mg/m^2]
Cisplatin: I.V.: 80 mg/m^2 day 1
[total dose/cycle = 80 mg/m^2]
Repeat cycle every 21 days

Variation 4:
Gemcitabine: I.V.: 1250 mg/m^2/day days 1 and 8
[total dose/cycle = 2500 mg/m^2]
Cisplatin: I.V.: 75 mg/m^2 day 1
[total dose/cycle = 75 mg/m^2]
Repeat cycle every 21 days for up to 6 cycles

Variation 5:
Gemcitabine: I.V.: 1000 mg/m^2/day days 1, 8, and 15
[total dose/cycle = 3000 mg/m^2]
Cisplatin: I.V.: 100 mg/m^2 day 15
[total dose/cycle = 100 mg/m^2]
Repeat cycle every 28 days

Variation 6:
Gemcitabine: I.V.: 1000 mg/m^2/day days 1, 8, and 15
[total dose/cycle = 3000 mg/m^2]
Cisplatin: I.V.: 100 mg/m^2 day 2
[total dose/cycle = 100 mg/m^2]
Repeat cycle every 28 days for 5 cycles

Variation 7:
Gemcitabine: I.V.: 1200 mg/m^2/day days 1, 8, and 15
[total dose/cycle = 3600 mg/m^2]

Cisplatin: I.V.: 100 mg/m^2 day 15
[total dose/cycle = 100 mg/m^2]
Repeat cycle every 28 days for up to 6 cycles
Variation 8 (patients ≥70 years of age):
Gemcitabine: I.V.: 1000 mg/m^2/day days 1 and 8
[total dose/cycle = 2000 mg/m^2]
Cisplatin: I.V.: 60 mg/m^2 day 1
[total dose/cycle = 60 mg/m^2]
Repeat cycle every 21 days for up to 6 cycles

Gemcitabine-Docetaxel (Bladder Cancer)

Use Bladder cancer

Regimen

Docetaxel: I.V.: 40 mg/m^2/day days 1 and 8
[total dose/cycle = 80 mg/m^2]
Gemcitabine: 800 mg/m^2/day days 1 and 8
[total dose/cycle = 1600 mg/m^2]
Repeat cycle every 21 days for up to 6 cycles

Gemcitabine-Docetaxel (Sarcoma)

Use Osteosarcoma; Soft tissue sarcoma

Regimen

Gemcitabine: I.V.: 675 mg/m^2/day days 1 and 8
[total dose/cycle = 1350 mg/m^2]
Docetaxel: I.V.: 100 mg/m^2 day 8
[total dose/cycle = 100 mg/m^2]
Repeat cycle every 21 days

Gemcitabine-Erlotinib

Use Pancreatic cancer

Regimen

Cycle 1:
Gemcitabine: I.V.: 1000 mg/m^2/day days 1, 8, 15, 22, 29, 36, and 43 (cycle 1 only)
[total dose/cycle 1 = 7000 mg/m^2]
Erlotinib: Oral: 100 mg once daily days 1 to 56
[total dose/cycle 1 = 5600 mg]
Treatment cycle is 56 days
Subsequent cycles:
Gemcitabine: I.V.: 1000 mg/m^2/day days 1, 8, and 15
[total dose/cycle = 3000 mg/m^2]
Erlotinib: Oral: 100 mg once daily days 1 to 28
[total dose/cycle = 2800 mg]
Repeat cycle every 28 days

Gemcitabine-Irinotecan

Use Pancreatic cancer

Regimen

Gemcitabine: I.V.: 1000 mg/m^2/day days 1 and 8
[total dose/cycle = 2000 mg/m^2]
Irinotecan: I.V.: 100 mg/m^2/day days 1 and 8
[total dose/cycle = 200 mg/m^2]
Repeat cycle 21 days

Gemcitabine-Oxaliplatin (Pancreatic Cancer)

Use Pancreatic cancer

Regimen

Gemcitabine: I.V.: 1000 mg/m^2/day (infused at 10 mg/m^2/minute) day 1
[total dose/cycle = 1000 mg/m^2]
Oxaliplatin: I.V.: 100 mg/m^2/day (over 2 hours) day 2
[total dose/cycle = 100 mg/m^2]
Repeat cycle every 14 days

Gemcitabine-Oxaliplatin-Rituximab (NHL)

Use Lymphoma, non-Hodgkin

Regimen

Oxaliplatin: I.V.: 100 mg/m^2/dose day 1
[total dose/cycle = 100 mg/m^2]
Gemcitabine: I.V.: 1000 mg/m^2/dose day 1
[total dose/cycle = 1000 mg/m^2]
Rituximab: I.V.: 375 mg/m^2/dose day 1
[total dose/cycle = 375 mg/m^2]
Repeat cycle every 3 weeks (for a total of 6-8 cycles)

Gemcitabine-Paclitaxel

Use Ovarian cancer

Regimen

Paclitaxel: I.V.: 80 mg/m^2 (infused over 60 minutes) days 1, 8, and 15
[total dose/cycle = 240 mg/m^2]
Gemcitabine: I.V.: 1000 mg/m^2/day (start at end of paclitaxel infusion) days 1, 8, and 15
[total dose/cycle = 3000 mg/m^2]
Repeat cycle every 4 weeks

Gemcitabine-Vinorelbine

Use Lung cancer, nonsmall cell

Regimen NOTE: Multiple variations are listed below.

Variation 1:
Gemcitabine: I.V.: 1200 mg/m^2/day days 1 and 8
[total dose/cycle = 2400 mg/m^2]
Vinorelbine: I.V.: 30 mg/m^2/day days 1 and 8
[total dose/cycle = 60 mg/m^2]
Repeat cycle every 21 days for 6 cycles

Variation 2:
Gemcitabine: I.V.: 1000 mg/m^2/day days 1, 8, and 15
[total dose/cycle = 3000 mg/m^2]
Vinorelbine: I.V.: 20 mg/m^2/day days 1, 8, and 15
[total dose/cycle = 60 mg/m^2]
Repeat cycle every 28 days for 6 cycles

Gemcitabine-Vinorelbine-Doxorubicin (Liposomal)

Use Lymphoma, Hodgkin disease

Regimen NOTE: Multiple variations are listed below.

Variation 1 (for transplant-naive patients):
Vinorelbine: I.V.: 20 mg/m^2/day days 1 and 8
[total dose/cycle = 40 mg/m^2]
Gemcitabine: I.V.: 1000 mg/m^2/day days 1 and 8
[total dose/cycle = 2000 mg/m^2]
Doxorubicin liposomal: I.V.: 15 mg/m^2/day days 1 and 8
[total dose/cycle = 30 mg/m^2]
Repeat cycle every 21 days for 2-6 cycles

Variation 2 (for patients with prior transplant):
Vinorelbine: I.V.: 15 mg/m^2/day days 1 and 8
[total dose/cycle = 30 mg/m^2]
Gemcitabine: I.V.: 800 mg/m^2/day days 1 and 8
[total dose/cycle = 1600 mg/m^2]
Doxorubicin liposomal: I.V.: 10 mg/m^2/day days 1 and 8
[total dose/cycle = 20 mg/m^2]
Repeat cycle every 21 days for 2-6 cycles

GEMOX (Biliary Cancer)

Use Biliary adenocarcinoma

Regimen

Gemcitabine: I.V.: 1000 mg/m^2 day 1
[total dose/cycle = 1000 mg/m^2]
Oxaliplatin: I.V.: 100 mg/m^2 day 2
[total dose/cycle = 100 mg/m^2]
Repeat cycle every 2 weeks

GEMOX (Testicular Cancer)

Use Testicular cancer

Regimen NOTE: Multiple variations are listed below.

Variation 1:
Gemcitabine: I.V.: 1000 mg/m^2/dose over 30 minutes days 1 and 8
[total dose/cycle = 2000 mg/m^2]
Oxaliplatin: I.V.: 130 mg/m^2/dose over 2 hours day 1
[total dose/cycle = 130 mg/m^2]
Repeat cycle every 21 days for a total of at least 2 cycles (maximum: 6 cycles)

Variation 2:
Gemcitabine: I.V.: 1250 mg/m^2/dose over 30 minutes days 1 and 8
[total dose/cycle = 2500 mg/m^2]
Oxaliplatin: I.V.: 130 mg/m^2/dose over 2 hours day 1
[total dose/cycle = 130 mg/m^2]
Repeat cycle every 21 days

HDMTX

Use Osteosarcoma

Regimen

Methotrexate: I.V.: 12 g/m^2/week for 2-12 weeks
[total dose/cycle = 24-144 g/m^2]
Leucovorin calcium rescue: Oral, I.V.: 15 mg/m^2 every 6 hours (beginning 30 hours after the beginning of the 4-hour methotrexate infusion) for 10 doses; **serum methotrexate levels must be monitored**
[total dose/cycle = 150 mg/m^2]

HIPE-IVAD

Use Neuroblastoma

Regimen

Cisplatin: I.V.: 40 mg/m^2/day days 1 to 5
[total dose/cycle = 200 mg/m^2]
Etoposide: I.V.: 100 mg/m^2/day days 1 to 5
[total dose/cycle = 500 mg/m^2]
Ifosfamide: I.V.: 3 g/m^2/day days 21 to 23
[total dose/cycle = 9 g/m^2]
Mesna: I.V.: 3 g/m^2/day continuous infusion days 21, 22, and 23
[total dose/cycle = 9 g/m^2]
Vincristine: I.V.: 1.5 mg/m^2 day 21
[total dose/cycle = 1.5 mg/m^2]
Doxorubicin: I.V.: 60 mg/m^2 day 23
[total dose/cycle = 60 mg/m^2]
Repeat cycle every 28 days

Hyper-CVAD + Imatinib

Use Leukemia, acute lymphocytic

Regimen

Cycle A: (Cycles 1, 3, 5, and 7)
Imatinib: Oral: 400 mg/day days 1 to 14
[total dose/cycle = 5600 mg]
Cyclophosphamide: I.V.: 300 mg/m^2 every 12 hours, for 6 doses, days 1, 2, and 3
[total dose/cycle = 1800 mg/m^2]

Mesna: I.V. 600 mg/m^2/day continuous infusion days 1, 2, and 3
[total dose/cycle = 1800 mg/m^2]
Vincristine: I.V.: 2 mg/day days 4 and 11
[total dose/cycle = 4 mg]
Doxorubicin: I.V.: 50 mg/m^2/day continuous infusion day 4
[total dose/cycle = 50 mg/m^2]
Dexamethasone: Oral, I.V.: 40 mg/day days 1 to 4 and 11 to 14
[total dose/cycle = 320 mg]

Cycle B: (Cycles 2, 4, 6, and 8)
Imatinib: Oral: 400 mg/day days 1 to 14
[total dose/cycle = 5600 mg]
Methotrexate: I.V.: 1 g/m^2/day continuous infusion day 1
[total dose/cycle = 1 g/m^2]
Leucovorin: I.V.: 50 mg then 15 mg every 6 hours, for 8 doses (start 12 hours after the end of the methotrexate infusion)
[total dose/cycle = 170 mg]
Cytarabine: I.V.: 3 g/m^2 every 12 hours for 4 doses, days 2 and 3
[total dose/cycle = 12 g/m^2]

Repeat every 6 weeks in the following sequence: ABABABAB

CNS Prophylaxis
Methotrexate: I.T.: 12 mg/day day 2
[total dose/cycle = 12 mg/day]
or 6 mg into Ommaya day 2
[total dose/cycle = 6 mg/day]
Cytarabine: I.T.: 100 mg/day day 7 or 8
[total dose/cycle = 100 mg/day]
Repeat cycle every 3 weeks for 3 or 4 cycles

Maintenance (POMP)
Imatinib: Oral: 600 mg/day
[total dose/cycle = 18,000 mg]
Vincristine: I.V.: 2 mg/day day 1
[total dose/cycle = 2 mg]
Prednisone: Oral: 200 mg/day days 1 to 5
[total dose/cycle = 1000 mg/m^2]
Repeat cycle every month (except months 6 and 13) for 13 months

Intensification
Imatinib: Oral: 400 mg/day days 1 to 14
[total dose/cycle = 5600 mg]
Cyclophosphamide: I.V.: 300 mg/m^2 every 12 hours, for 6 doses, days 1, 2, and 3
[total dose/cycle = 1800 mg/m^2]
Mesna: I.V.: 600 mg/m^2/day continuous infusion days 1, 2, and 3
[total dose/cycle = 1800 mg/m^2]
Vincristine: I.V.: 2 mg/day days 4 and 11
[total dose/cycle = 4 mg]
Doxorubicin: 50 mg/m^2/day continuous infusion day 4
[total dose/cycle = 50 mg/m^2]
Dexamethasone: I.V. or Oral: 40 mg/day days 1 to 4 and 11 to 14
[total dose/cycle = 320 mg]
Cycle is given in months 6 and 13 during maintenance

Hyper-CVAD (Leukemia, Acute Lymphocytic)

Use Leukemia, acute lymphocytic

Regimen NOTE: Multiple variations are listed below.

Variation 1:
Cycle A: (Cycles 1, 3, 5, and 7)
Cyclophosphamide: I.V.: 300 mg/m^2 every 12 hours, for 6 doses, days 1, 2, and 3
[total dose/cycle = 1800 mg/m^2]
Mesna: I.V.: 1200 mg/m^2/day continuous infusion days 1, 2, and 3
[total dose/cycle = 3600 mg/m^2]
Vincristine: I.V.: 2 mg/day days 4 and 11
[total dose/cycle = 4 mg]

Doxorubicin: I.V.: 50 mg/m^2 day 4
[total dose/cycle = 50 mg/m^2]
Dexamethasone: (route not specified): 40 mg/day days 1 to 4 and 11 to 14
[total dose/cycle = 320 mg]
Cycle B: (Cycles 2, 4, 6, and 8)
Methotrexate: I.V.: 1 g/m^2 continuous infusion day 1
[total dose/cycle = 1g/m^2]
Leucovorin: (route not specified): 15 mg every 6 hours, for 8 doses
(start 12 hours after end of methotrexate infusion)
[total dose/cycle = 120 mg]
Cytarabine: I.V.: 3 g/m^2 every 12 hours, for 4 doses, days 2 and 3
[total dose/cycle = 12 g/m^2]
Methylprednisolone: I.V.: 50 mg twice daily, for 6 doses, days 1, 2, and 3
[total dose/cycle = 300 mg/m^2]
Repeat every 6 weeks in the following sequence: ABABABAB

CNS Prophylaxis
Methotrexate: I.T.: 12 mg/day day 2
[total dose/cycle = 12 mg]
or 6 mg/day into Ommaya day 2
[total dose/cycle = 6 mg]
Cytarabine: I.T: 100 mg day 8
[total dose/cycle = 100 mg]
Repeat cycle every 3 weeks

Maintenance (POMP)
Mercaptopurine: Oral: 50 mg 3 times/day
[total dose/cycle = 4200-4650 mg]
Vincristine: I.V.: 2 mg day 1
[total dose/cycle = 2 mg]
Methotrexate: Oral: 20 mg/m^2/day days 1, 8, 15, and 22
[total dose/cycle = 80 mg/m^2]
Prednisone: Oral: 200 mg/day days 1 to 5
[total dose/cycle = 1000 mg/m^2]
or
Mercaptopurine: I.V.: 1 g/m^2/day days 1 to 5
[total dose/cycle = 5 g/m^2]
Vincristine: I.V.: 2 mg day 1
[total dose/cycle = 2 mg]
Methotrexate: I.V.: 10 mg/m^2/day days 1 to 5
[total dose/cycle = 50 mg/m^2]
Prednisone: Oral: 200 mg/day days 1 to 5
[total dose/cycle = 1000 mg/m^2]
Repeat cycles every month for 2 years

Variation 2:
Cycle A: (Cycles 1, 3, 5, and 7)
Cyclophosphamide: I.V.: 300 mg/m^2 every 12 hours, for 6 doses, days 1, 2, and 3
[total dose/cycle = 1800 mg/m^2]
Mesna: I.V.: 600 mg/m^2/day continuous infusion days 1, 2, and 3
[total dose/cycle = 1800 mg/m^2]
Vincristine: I.V.: 2 mg/day days 4 and 11
[total dose/cycle = 4 mg]
Doxorubicin: I.V.: 50 mg/m^2 day 4
[total dose/cycle = 50 mg/m^2]
Dexamethasone: Oral, I.V.: 40 mg/day days 1 to 4 and 11 to 14
[total dose/cycle = 320 mg]
Cycle B: (Cycles 2, 4, 6, and 8)
Methotrexate: I.V.: 1 g/m^2 continuous infusion day 1
[total dose/cycle = 1 g/m^2]
Leucovorin: I.V.: 50 mg (start 12 hours after end of methotrexate infusion)
followed by I.V.: 15 mg every 6 hours, for 8 doses
[total dose/cycle = 170 mg]
Cytarabine: I.V.: 3 g/m^2 every 12 hours, for 4 doses, days 2 and 3
[total dose/cycle = 12 g/m^2]
Repeat every 6 weeks in the following sequence: ABABABAB

CNS Prophylaxis
Methotrexate: I.T.: 12 mg day 2
[total dose/cycle = 12 mg]
or 6 mg into Ommaya day 2
[total dose/cycle = 6 mg]
Cytarabine: I.T.: 100 mg day 7
[total dose/cycle = 100 mg]
Repeat cycle every 3 weeks

Variation 3:
Cycle A: (Cycles 1, 3, 5, and 7)
Cyclophosphamide: I.V.: 300 mg/m^2 every 12 hours, for 6 doses, days 1, 2, and 3
[total dose/cycle = 1800 mg/m^2]
Mesna: I.V.: 600 mg/m^2/day continuous infusion days 1, 2, and 3
[total dose/cycle = 1800 mg/m^2]
Vincristine: I.V.: 2 mg/day days 4 and 11
[total dose/cycle = 4 mg]
Doxorubicin: I.V.: 50 mg/m^2 continuous infusion day 4
[total dose/cycle = 50 mg/m^2]
Dexamethasone: Oral, I.V.: 40 mg/day days 1 to 4 and 11 to 14
[total dose/cycle = 320 mg]
Cycle B: (Cycles 2, 4, 6, and 8)
Methotrexate: I.V.: 200 mg/m^2 day 1
followed by I.V.: 800 mg/m^2 continuous infusion day 1
[total dose/cycle = 1 g/m^2]
Leucovorin: I.V.: 50 mg (start 12 hours after end of methotrexate infusion)
followed by I.V.: 15 mg every 6 hours, for 8 doses
[total dose/cycle = 170 mg/m^2]
Cytarabine: I.V.: 3 g/m^2 every 12 hours, for 4 doses, days 2 and 3
[total dose/cycle = 12 g/m^2]
Repeat every 6 weeks in the following sequence: ABABABAB

CNS Prophylaxis
Methotrexate: I.T.: 12 mg day 2
[total dose/cycle = 12 mg]
or 6 mg into Ommaya day 2
[total dose/cycle = 6 mg]
Cytarabine: I.T.: 100 mg day 7 **or** 8
[total dose/cycle = 100 mg]
Repeat cycles every 3 weeks for 6 or 8 cycles

Maintenance (POMP)
Mercaptopurine: Oral: 50 mg 3 times/day
[total dose/cycle = 4200-4650 mg]
Vincristine: I.V.: 2 mg day 1
[total dose/cycle = 2 mg]
Methotrexate: Oral, I V: 20 mg/m^2/ day days 1, 8, 15, and 22
[total dose/cycle = 80 mg/m^2]
Prednisone: Oral: 200 mg/day days 1 to 5
[total dose/cycle = 1000 mg/m^2]
or
Mercaptopurine: I.V.: 1 g/m^2/day days 1 to 5
[total dose/cycle = 5 g/m^2]
Vincristine: I.V.: 2 mg day 1
[total dose/cycle = 2 mg]
Methotrexate: I.V.: 10 mg/m^2/day days 1 to 5
[total dose/cycle = 50 mg/m^2]
Prednisone: Oral: 200 mg/day days 1 to 5
[total dose/cycle = 1000 mg]
Repeat cycles every month (except months 7 and 11 or 9 and 12) for 2 years

Intensification
Etoposide: I.V.: 100 mg/m^2/day days 1 to 5
[total dose/cycle = 500 mg/m^2]

Pegaspargase: I.V.: 2500 units/m^2 day 1
[total dose/cycle = 2500 units/m^2]
Given during months 9 and 12 of maintenance
or
Methotrexate: I.V.: 100 mg/m^2/day days 1, 8, 15, and 22
[total dose/cycle = 400 mg/m^2]
Asparaginase: I.V.: 20,000 units/day days 2, 9, 16, and 23
[total dose/cycle = 80,000 units]
Given during months 7 and 11 of maintenance

Variation 4:

Cycle A: (Cycles 1, 3, 5, and 7)
Cyclophosphamide: I.V.: 300 mg/m^2 every 12 hours, for 6 doses, days 1, 2, and 3
[total dose/cycle = 1800 mg/m^2]
Mesna: I.V.: 600 mg/m^2/day continuous infusion days 1, 2, and 3
[total dose/cycle = 1800 mg/m^2]
Vincristine: I.V.: 2 mg/day days 4 and 11
[total dose/cycle = 4 mg]
Doxorubicin: I.V.: 50 mg/m^{2}day 4
[total dose/cycle = 50 mg/m^2]
Dexamethasone: (route not specified): 40 mg/day days 1 to 4 and 11 to 14
[total dose/cycle = 320 mg]

Cycle B: (Cycles 2, 4, 6, and 8)
Methotrexate: I.V.: 200 mg/m^2 day 1
followed by I.V.: 800 mg/m^2 continuous infusion day 1
[total dose/cycle = 1 g/m^2]
Leucovorin: (route not specified): 15 mg every 6 hours, for 8 doses (start 24 hours after end of methotrexate infusion)
[total dose/cycle = 120 mg]
Cytarabine: I.V.: 3 g/m^2 every 12 hours, for 4 doses, days 2 and 3
[total dose/cycle = 12 g/m^2]
Repeat every 6 weeks in the following sequence: ABABABAB

CNS Prophylaxis
Methotrexate: I.T.: 12 mg day 2
[total dose/cycle = 12 mg]
Cytarabine: I.T.: 100 mg day 8
[total dose/cycle = 100 mg]
Repeat cycle every 3 weeks for 4 or 8 cycles

Maintenance (POMP)
Mercaptopurine: Oral: 50 mg 3 times/day
[total dose/cycle = 4200-4650 mg]
Vincristine: I.V.: 2 mg day 1
[total dose/cycle = 2 mg]
Methotrexate: Oral: 20 mg/m^2/day days 1, 8, 15, and 22
[total dose/cycle = 80 mg/m^2]
Prednisone: Oral: 200 mg/day days 1 to 5
[total dose/cycle = 1000 mg/m^2]
or
Mercaptopurine: I.V.: 1 g/m^2/day days 1 to 5
[total dose/cycle = 5 g/m^2]
Vincristine: I.V.: 2 mg day 1
[total dose/cycle = 2 mg]
Methotrexate: I.V.: 10 mg/m^2/day days 1 to 5
[total dose/cycle = 50 mg/m^2]
Prednisone: Oral: 200 mg/day days 1 to 5
[total dose/cycle = 1000 mg/m^2]
or
Interferon alfa: SubQ: 5 million units/m^2 daily
[total dose/cycle = 140-155 million units/m^2]
Cytarabine: SubQ: 10 mg daily
[total dose/cycle = 280-310 mg]
Repeat cycles every month for 2 years

Variation 5:

Cycle A: (Cycles 1, 4, 6, and 8)

Cyclophosphamide: I.V.: 300 mg/m^2 every 12 hours, for 6 doses, days 1, 2, and 3 [total dose/cycle = 1800 mg/m^2]

Mesna: I.V.: 600 mg/m^2/day continuous infusion days 1, 2, and 3 [total dose/cycle = 1800 mg/m^2]

Vincristine: I.V.: 2 mg/day days 4 and 11 [total dose/cycle = 4 mg]

Doxorubicin: I.V.: 50 mg/m^2 continuous infusion day 4 [total dose/cycle = 50 mg/m^2]

Dexamethasone: Oral, I.V.: 40 mg/day days 1 to 4 and 11 to 14 [total dose/cycle = 320 mg]

Cycle B: (Cycles 3, 5, 7, and 9)

Methotrexate: I.V.: 200 mg/m^2 day 1

followed by I.V.: 800 mg/m^2 continuous infusion day 1 [total dose/cycle = 1 g/m^2]

Leucovorin: I.V.: 50 mg (start 12 hours after end of methotrexate infusion)

followed by I.V.: 15 mg every 6 hours, for 8 doses [total dose/cycle = 170 mg]

Cytarabine: I.V.: 3 g/m^2 every 12 hours, for 4 doses, days 2 and 3 [total dose/cycle = 12 g/m^2]

Cycle C: Liposomal Daunorubicin/Cytarabine (Cycle 2):

Daunorubicin, liposomal: I.V.: 150 mg/m^2/day days 1 and 2 [total dose/cycle = 300 mg/m^2]

Cytarabine: I.V.: 1.5 g/m^2/day continuous infusion days 1 and 2 [total dose/cycle = 3 g/m^2]

Prednisone: Oral: 200 mg/day days 1 to 5 [total dose/cycle = 1000 mg]

Administer in the following sequence: ACBABABA (Cycle C does not repeat)

CNS Prophylaxis

Methotrexate: I.T.: 12 mg day 2 [total dose/cycle = 12 mg]

or 6 mg into Ommaya day 2 [total dose/cycle = 6 mg]

Cytarabine: I.T.: 100 mg day 7 **or** 8 [total dose/cycle = 100 mg]

Repeat cycle every 3 weeks for 6 or 8 cycles

Maintenance (POMP)

Mercaptopurine: I.V.: 1 g/m^2/day days 1 to 5 [total dose/cycle = 5 g/m^2]

Vincristine: I.V.: 2 mg day 1 [total dose/cycle = 2 mg]

Methotrexate: I.V.: 10 mg/m^2/day days 1 to 5 [total dose/cycle = 50 mg/m^2]

Prednisone: Oral: 200 mg/day days 1 to 5 [total dose/cycle = 1000 mg]

Repeat cycles monthly, except months 6, 7, 18, and 19 for 3 years

Intensification

Methotrexate: I.V.: 100 mg/m^2/day days 1, 8, 15, and 22 [total dose/cycle = 400 mg/m^2]

Asparaginase: I.V.: 20,000 units/day days 2, 9, 16, and 23 [total dose/cycle = 80,000 units]

Given during months 6 and 18 of maintenance

Cyclophosphamide: I.V.: 300 mg/m^2 every 12 hours, for 6 doses, days 1, 2, and 3 [total dose/cycle = 1800 mg/m^2]

Mesna: I.V.: 600 mg/m^2/day continuous infusion days 1, 2, and 3 [total dose/cycle = 1800 mg/m^2]

Vincristine: I.V.: 2 mg/day days 4 and 11 [total dose/cycle = 4 mg]

Doxorubicin: I.V.: 50 mg/m^2/day continuous infusion day 4
[total dose/cycle = 50 mg/m^2]
Dexamethasone: Oral, I.V.: 40 mg/day days 1 to 4 and 11 to 14
[total dose/cycle = 320 mg]
Given during months 7 and 19 of maintenance

Hyper-CVAD (Lymphoma, non-Hodgkin)

Use Lymphoma, non-Hodgkin

Regimen

Cycle A: (Cycles 1, 3, 5, and 7)
Cyclophosphamide: I.V.: 300 mg/m^2 every 12 hours, for 6 doses, days 1, 2, and 3
[total dose/cycle = 1800 mg/m^2]
Vincristine: I.V.: 2 mg/day days 4 and 11
[total dose/cycle = 4 mg]
Doxorubicin: I.V.: 25 mg/m^2/day continuous infusion days 4 and 5
[total dose/cycle = 50 mg/m^2]
Dexamethasone: Oral, I.V.: 40 mg/day days 1 to 4 and 11 to 14
[total dose/cycle = 320 mg]
Cycle B: (Cycles 2, 4, 6, and 8)
Methotrexate: I.V.: 200 mg/m^2 day 1
followed by I.V.: 800 mg/m^2 continuous infusion day 1
[total dose/cycle = 1 g/m^2]
Leucovorin: Oral: 50 mg
followed by Oral: 15 mg every 6 hours, for 8 doses (start 24 hours after end of methotrexate infusion)
[total dose/cycle = 170 mg]
Cytarabine: I.V.: 3 g/m^2 every 12 hours, for 4 doses, days 2 and 3
[total dose/cycle = 12 g/m^2]
Repeat every 6 weeks in the following sequence: ABABABAB

Hyper-CVAD (Multiple Myeloma)

Use Multiple myeloma

Regimen

Cyclophosphamide: I.V.: 300 mg/m^2 every 12 hours, for 6 doses, days 1, 2, and 3
[total dose/cycle = 1800 mg/m^2]
Mesna: I.V.: 600 mg/m^2/day continuous infusion days 1, 2, and 3
[total dose/cycle = 1800 mg/m^2]
Doxorubicin: I.V.: 25 mg/m^2/day continuous infusion days 4 and 5
[total dose/cycle = 50 mg/m^2]
Vincristine: I.V.: 1 mg/day continuous infusion days 4 and 5
followed by I.V.: 2 mg day 11
[total dose/cycle = 4 mg]
Dexamethasone: Oral, I.V.: 20 mg/m^2/day days 1 to 5 and 11 to 14
[total dose/cycle = 180 mg/m^2]
Repeat cycle once if ≥50% reduction in myeloma protein

Maintenance

Cyclophosphamide: Oral: 125 mg/m^2 every 12 hours, for 10 doses, days 1 to 5
[total dose/cycle = 1250 mg/m^2]
Dexamethasone: Oral: 20 mg/m^2/day days 1 to 5
[total dose/cycle = 100 mg/m^2]
Repeat maintenance cycle every 5 weeks

Hyper-CVAD + Rituximab

Use Lymphona, non-Hodgkin (mantle cell)

Regimen

Cycle A: (Cycles 1, 3, 5 [and 7, if needed])
Rituximab: I.V.: 375 mg/m^2 day 1
[total dose/cycle = 375 mg/m^2]
Cyclophosphamide: I.V.: 300 mg/m^2 every 12 hours, for 6 doses, days 2, 3, and 4
[total dose/cycle = 1800 mg/m^2]

Mesna: I.V.: 600 mg/m^2 continuous infusion days 2, 3, and 4
[total dose/cycle = 1800 mg/m^2]
Vincristine: I.V.: 1.4 mg/m^2 (maximum: 2 mg) days 5 and 12
[total dose/cycle = 2.8 mg/m^2; maximum: 4 mg]
Doxorubicin: I.V.: 16.7 mg/m^2 continuous infusion days 5, 6, and 7
[total dose/cycle = 50.1 mg/m^2]
Dexamethasone: Oral, I.V.: 40 mg/day days 2 to 5 and 12 to 15
[total dose/cycle = 320 mg]
Cycle B: (Cycles 2, 4, 6 [and 8, if needed])
Rituximab: I.V.: 375 mg/m^2 day 1
[total dose/cycle = 375 mg/m^2]
Methotrexate: I.V.: 200 mg/m^2 day 2
followed by I.V.: 800 mg/m^2 continuous infusion day 2
[total dose/cycle = 1000 mg/m^2]
Leucovorin: Oral: 50 mg (start 12 hours after the end of the methotrexate infusion)
followed by Oral: 15 mg every 6 hours, for 8 doses
[total dose/cycle = 170 mg]
Cytarabine: I.V.: 3 g/m^2 every 12 hours, for 4 doses, day 3 and 4
[total dose/cycle = 12 g/m^2]
Repeat every 6 weeks in the following sequence: ABABABAB

ICE (Lymphoma, non-Hodgkin)

Use Lymphoma, non-Hodgkin

Regimen

Etoposide: I.V.: 100 mg/m^2/day days 1, 2, and 3
[total dose/cycle = 300 mg/m^2]
Carboplatin: I.V.: AUC 5 (maximum: 800 mg) day 2
[total dose/cycle = AUC = 5]
Ifosfamide: I.V.: 5000 mg/m^2 continuous infusion day 2
[total dose/cycle = 5000 mg/m^2]
Mesna: I.V.: 5000 mg/m^2 continuous infusion day 2
[total dose/cycle = 5000 mg/m^2]
Filgrastim: SubQ: 5 mcg/kg/day days 5-12 (cycles 1 and 2 only)
[total dose/cycle = 40 mcg/kg]
followed by SubQ: 10 mcg/kg/day day 5 through completion of leukaphoresis (cycle 3 only)
Repeat cycle every 2 weeks for 3 cycles

ICE (Sarcoma)

Use Osteosarcoma; Soft tissue sarcoma

Regimen

Ifosfamide: I.V.: 1500 mg/m^2/day days 1, 2, and 3
[total dose/cycle = 4500 mg/m^2]
Carboplatin: I.V.: 300-635 mg/m^2 day 3
[total dose/cycle = 300-635 mg/m^2]
Etoposide: I.V.: 100 mg/m^2/day days 1, 2, and 3
[total dose/cycle = 300 mg/m^2]
Mesna: I.V.: 500 mg/m^2 prior to each ifosfamide, and every 3 hours for 2 more doses/day days 1, 2, and 3
[total dose/cycle = 4500 mg/m^2]
Repeat cycle every 21-28 days

ICE-T

Use Breast cancer; Soft tissue sarcoma

Regimen

Ifosfamide: I.V.: 1250 mg/m^2/day days 1, 2, and 3
[total dose/cycle = 3750 mg/m^2]
Carboplatin: I.V.: 300 mg/m^2 day 1
[total dose/cycle = 300 mg/m^2]
Etoposide: I.V.: 80 mg/m^2/day days 1, 2, and 3
[total dose/cycle = 240 mg/m^2]

Paclitaxel: I.V.: 175 mg/m^2 day 4
[total dose/cycle = 175 mg/m^2]
Mesna: I.V.: 250 mg prior to ifosfamide days 1, 2, and 3
followed by: Oral: 500 mg at 4 and 8 hours after ifosfamide days 1, 2, and 3
[total dose/cycle = I.V. 750 mg; Oral: 3000 mg]
or
Mesna: I.V.: 1250 mg/m^2/day over 6 hours, days 1, 2, and 3
[total dose/cycle = 3750 mg/m^2]
Repeat cycle every 28 days

Idarubicin, Cytarabine, Etoposide (ICE Protocol)

Use Leukemia, acute myeloid

Regimen

Idarubicin: I.V.: 6 mg/m^2/day days 1 to 5
[total dose/cycle = 30 mg/m^2]
Cytarabine: I.V.: 600 mg/m^2/day days 1 to 5
[total dose/cycle = 3000 mg/m^2]
Etoposide: I.V.: 150 mg/m^2/day days 1, 2, and 3
[total dose/cycle = 450 mg/m^2]
Administer one cycle only

Idarubicin, Cytarabine, Etoposide (IDA-Based BF12)

Use Leukemia, acute myeloid

Regimen Induction:

Idarubicin: I.V.: 5 mg/m^2/day days 1 to 5
[total dose/cycle = 25 mg/m^2]
Cytarabine: I.V.: 2000 mg/m^2 every 12 hours days 1 to 5 (10 doses)
[total dose/cycle = 20,000 mg/m^2]
Etoposide: I.V.: 100 mg/m^2/day days 1 to 5
[total dose/cycle = 500 mg/m^2]
Second cycle may be given based on individual response; time between cycles not specified

IE

Use Soft tissue sarcoma

Regimen

Etoposide: I.V.: 100 mg/m^2/day days 1, 2, and 3
[total dose/cycle = 300 mg/m^2]
Ifosfamide: I.V.: 2500 mg/m^2/day days 1, 2, and 3
[total dose/cycle = 7500 mg/m^2]
Mesna: I.V.: 500 mg/m^2 prior to ifosfamide, after ifosfamide, and every 4 hours for 3 more doses (total of 5 doses/day) days 1, 2, and 3
[total dose/cycle = 7500 mg/m^2]
Repeat cycle every 28 days

IMVP-16

Use Lymphoma, non-Hodgkin

Regimen

Ifosfamide: I.V.: 4 g/m^2 continuous infusion over 24 hours day 1
[total dose/cycle = 4 g/m^2]
Mesna: I.V.: 800 mg/m^2 bolus prior to ifosfamide, then 4 g/m^2 continuous infusion over 12 hours concurrent with ifosfamide, then 2.4 g/m^2 continuous infusion over 12 hours after ifosfamide infusion day 1
[total dose/cycle = 7.2 g/m^2]
Methotrexate: I.V.: 30 mg/m^2/day days 3 and 10
[total dose/cycle = 60 mg/m^2]
Etoposide: I.V.: 100 mg/m^2/day days 1, 2, and 3
[total dose/cycle = 300 mg/m^2]
Repeat cycle every 21-28 days

Interleukin 2-Interferon Alfa-2

Use Renal cell cancer

Regimen

Weeks 1 and 4:

Aldesleukin: SubQ: 20 million units/m^2 3 times weekly
[total dose/cycle = 120 million units/m^2]

Interferon Alfa-2: SubQ: 6 million units/m^2 once weekly
[total dose/cycle = 12 million units/m^2]

Weeks 2, 3, 5, and 6:

Aldesleukin: SubQ: 5 million units/m^2 3 times weekly
[total dose/cycle = 60 million units/m^2]

Interferon Alfa-2: SubQ: 6 million units/m^2 3 times weekly
[total dose/cycle = 72 million units/m^2]

Repeat cycle every 56 days

Interleukin 2 (Low Dose)-Interferon Alfa 2b

Use Renal cell cancer

Regimen

Cycle 1:

Week 1:

Aldesleukin: SubQ: 5 million units/m^2 every 8 hours for 3 doses day 1
followed by SubQ: 5 million units/m^2/day days 2 to 5
[total dose/week 1 = 35 million units/m^2]

Interferon alfa-2b: SubQ: 5 million units/m^2 3 times/week
[total dose/week 1 = 15 million units/m^2]

Weeks 2-4:

Aldesleukin: SubQ: 5 million units/m^2/day days 1 to 5
[total dose/weeks 2-4 = 75 million units/m^2]

Interferon alfa-2b: SubQ: 5 million units/m^2 3 times/week
[total dose/weeks 2-4 = 45 million units/m^2]

Treatment cycle is 6 weeks

Cycles 2-6

Weeks 1-4:

Aldesleukin: SubQ: 5 million units/m^2/day days 1 to 5
[total dose/cycle = 100 million units/m^2]

Interferon alfa-2b: SubQ: 5 million units/m^2 3 times/week
[total dose/cycle = 60 million units/m^2]

Repeat cycle every 6 weeks for up to a total of 6 cycles

IPA

Use Hepatoblastoma

Regimen

Ifosfamide: I.V.: 500 mg/m^2 day 1
[total dose/cycle = 500 mg/m^2]
followed by I.V.: 1000 mg/m^2/day continuous infusion days 1 to 3
[total dose/cycle = 3000 mg/m^2]

Cisplatin: I.V.: 20 mg/m^2/day days 4 to 8
[total dose/cycle = 100 mg/m^2]

Doxorubicin: I.V.: 30 mg/m^2/day continuous infusion days 9 and 10
[total dose/cycle = 60 mg/m^2]

Repeat cycle every 21 days

Irinotecan-Cisplatin (Esophageal Cancer)

Use Esophageal cancer

Regimen

Cisplatin: I.V.: 30 mg/m^2/day days 1, 8, 15, and 22
[total dose/cycle = 120 mg/m^2]

Irinotecan: I.V.: 65 mg/m^2/day days 1, 8, 15, and 22
[total dose/cycle = 260 mg/m^2]

Repeat cycle every 6 weeks

IVAC

Use Lymphoma, non-Hodgkin

Regimen

Ifosfamide: I.V.: 1500 mg/m^2/day days 1 to 5
[total dose/cycle = 7500 mg/m^2]
Etoposide: I.V.: 60 mg/m^2/day days 1 to 5
[total dose/cycle = 300 mg/m^2]
Cytarabine: I.V.: 2 g/m^2 every 12 hours days 1 and 2
[total dose/cycle = 8 g/m^2]
Mesna: I.V.: 360 mg/m^2 every 3 hours days 1 to 5
[total dose/cycle = 14,400 mg/m^2]
Methotrexate: I.T.: 12 mg day 5
Sargramostim: SubQ: 7.5 mcg/kg day 7 until ANC >1000 cells/mm^3
Repeat when ANC >1000 cells/mm^3

Ixabepilone-Capecitabine

Use Breast cancer

Regimen

Capecitabine: Oral: 1000 mg/m^2 twice daily days 1 to 14
[total dose/cycle = 28,000 mg/m^2]
Ixabepilone: I.V.: 40 mg/m^2 day 1
[total dose/cycle = 40 mg/m^2]
Repeat cycle every 3 weeks

Larson Regimen

Use Leukemia, acute lymphocytic

Regimen

Cyclophosphamide: I.V.: 1200 mg/m^2 day 1
[total dose/cycle = 1200 mg/m^2]
Daunorubicin: I.V.: 45 mg/m^2/day days 1, 2, and 3
[total dose/cycle = 135 mg/m^2]
Vincristine: I.V.: 2 mg/day days 1, 8, 15, and 22
[total dose/cycle = 8 mg]
Prednisone: Oral or I.V.: 60 mg/m^2/day days 1 to 21
[total dose/cycle = 1260 mg/m^2]
Asparaginase: SubQ: 6000 units/m^2/day days 5, 8, 11, 15, 18, and 22
[total dose/cycle = 36,000 units/m^2]
Administer one cycle only

Lenalidomide-Dexamethasone

Use Multiple myeloma

Regimen

Lenalidomide: Oral: 25 mg/day days 1 to 21
[total dose/cycle = 525 mg]
Dexamethasone: Oral: 40 mg/day days 1 to 4, 9 to 12, and 17 to 20 (cycles 1 to 4)
[total dose/cycle = 480 mg]
Dexamethasone: Oral 40 mg/day days 1 to 4 (cycle 5 and beyond)
[total dose/cycle = 160 mg]
Repeat cycle every 28 days

Lenalidomide-Dexamethasone (Low Dose)

Use Multiple myeloma

Regimen

Lenalidomide: Oral: 25 mg/day days 1 to 21
[total dose/cycle = 525 mg]
Dexamethasone: Oral: 40 mg/day days 1, 8, 15, and 22
[total dose/cycle = 160 mg]
Repeat cycle every 28 days

Linker Protocol

Use Leukemia, acute lymphocytic

Regimen

Remission induction:

Daunorubicin: I.V.: 50 mg/m^2/day days 1, 2, and 3
[total dose/cycle = 150 mg/m^2]

Vincristine: I.V.: 2 mg/day days 1, 8, 15, and 22
[total dose/cycle = 8 mg]

Prednisone: Oral: 60 mg/m^2/day days 1 to 28
[total dose/cycle = 1680 mg/m^2]

Asparaginase: I.M.: 6000 units/m^2/day days 17 to 28
[total dose/cycle = 72,000 units/m^2]

If residual leukemia in bone marrow on day 14:

Daunorubicin: I.V.: 50 mg/m^2 day 15
[total dose/cycle = 50 mg/m^2]

If residual leukemia in bone marrow on day 28:

Daunorubicin: I.V.: 50 mg/m^2/day days 29 and 30
[total dose/cycle = 100 mg/m^2]

Vincristine: I.V.: 2 mg/day days 29 and 36
[total dose/cycle = 4 mg]

Prednisone: Oral: 60 mg/m^2/day days 29 to 42
[total dose/cycle = 840 mg/m^2]

Asparaginase: I.M.: 6000 units/m^2/day days 29 to 35
[total dose/cycle = 42,000 units/m^2]

Consolidation therapy:

Treatment A (cycles 1, 3, 5, and 7)

Daunorubicin: I.V.: 50 mg/m^2/day days 1 and 2
[total dose/cycle = 100 mg/m^2]

Vincristine: I.V.: 2 mg/day days 1 and 8
[total dose/cycle = 4 mg]

Prednisone: Oral: 60 mg/m^2/day days 1 to 14
[total dose/cycle = 840 mg/m^2]

Asparaginase: I.M.: 12,000 units/m^2/day days 2, 4, 7, 9, 11, and 14
[total dose/cycle = 72,000 units/m^2]

Treatment B (cycles 2, 4, 6, and 8)

Teniposide: I.V.: 165 mg/m^2/day days 1, 4, 8, and 11
[total dose/cycle = 660 mg/m^2]

Cytarabine: I.V.: 300 mg/m^2/day days 1, 4, 8, and 11
[total dose/cycle = 1200 mg/m^2]

Treatment C (cycle 9)

Methotrexate: I.V.: 690 mg/m^2 continuous infusion over 42 hours day 1
[total dose/cycle = 690 mg/m^2]

Leucovorin: I.V.: 15 mg/m^2 every 6 hours for 12 doses (start at end of methotrexate infusion)
[total dose/cycle = 180 mg/m^2]

Administer remission induction regimen for one cycle only. Repeat consolidation cycle every 28 days.

LOPP

Use Lymphoma, Hodgkin disease

Regimen

Chlorambucil: Oral: 10 mg/day days 1 to 10
[total dose/cycle = 100 mg/m^2]

Vincristine: I.V.: 1.4 mg/m^2/day (maximum dose: 2 mg) days 1 and 8
[total dose/cycle = 2.8 mg/m^2]

Procarbazine: Oral: 100 mg/m^2/day days 1 to 10
[total dose/cycle = 1000 mg/m^2]

Prednisone: Oral: 25 mg/m^2/day (maximum dose: 60 mg) days 1 to 14
[total dose/cycle = 350 mg/m^2]
or
Prednisolone: Oral: 25 mg/m^2/day (maximum dose: 60 mg) days 1 to 14
[total dose/cycle = 350 mg/m^2]
Repeat cycle every 28 days

M-2

Use Multiple myeloma

Regimen

Vincristine: I.V.: 0.03 mg/kg (maximum: 2 mg) day 1
[total dose/cycle = 0.03 mg/kg]
Carmustine: I.V.: 0.5-1 mg/kg day 1
[total dose/cycle = 0.5-1 mg/kg]
Cyclophosphamide: I.V.: 10 mg/kg day 1
[total dose/cycle = 10 mg/kg]
Melphalan: Oral: 0.25 mg/kg/day days 1 to 4
[total dose/cycle = 1 mg/kg]
or 0.1 mg/kg/day days 1 to 7 or 1 to 10
[total dose/cycle = 0.7 or 1 mg/kg]
Prednisone: Oral: 1 mg/kg/day days 1 to 7
[total dose/cycle = 7 mg/kg]
Repeat cycle every 35-42 days

MACOP-B

Use Lymphoma, non-Hodgkin

Regimen

Methotrexate: I.V. bolus: 100 mg/m^2 weeks 2, 6, 10
followed by I.V.: 300 mg/m^2 over 4 hours weeks 2, 6, and 10
[total dose/cycle = 1200 mg/m^2]
Doxorubicin: I.V.: 50 mg/m^2 weeks 1, 3, 5, 7, 9, and 11
[total dose/cycle = 300 mg/m^2]
Cyclophosphamide: I.V.: 350 mg/m^2 weeks 1, 3, 5, 7, 9, and 11
[total dose/cycle = 2100 mg/m^2]
Vincristine: I.V.: 1.4 mg/m^2 (maximum: 2 mg) weeks 2, 4, 6, 8, 10, and 12
[total dose/cycle = 8.4 mg/m^2; maximum: 12 mg]
Bleomycin: I.V.: 10 units/m^2 weeks 4, 8, and 12
[total dose/cycle = 30 units/m^2]
Prednisone: Oral: 75 mg/day for 12 weeks, then taper over 2 weeks
Leucovorin calcium: Oral: 15 mg/m^2 every 6 hours, for 6 doses (beginning 24 hours after methotrexate) weeks 2, 6, and 10
[total dose/cycle = 270 mg/m^2]
Administer one cycle

MAID

Use Soft tissue sarcoma

Regimen

Mesna: I.V.: 2500 mg/m^2/day continuous infusion days 1 to 4
[total dose/cycle = 10,000 mg/m^2]
Doxorubicin: I.V.: 20 mg/m^2/day continuous infusion days 1, 2, and 3
[total dose/cycle = 60 mg/m^2]
Ifosfamide: I.V.: 2500 mg/m^2/day continuous infusion days 1, 2, and 3
[total dose/cycle = 7500 mg/m^2]
Dacarbazine: I.V.: 300 mg/m^2/day continuous infusion days 1, 2, and 3
[total dose/cycle = 900 mg/m^2]
Repeat cycle every 21-28 days

m-BACOD

Use Lymphoma, non-Hodgkin

Regimen

Methotrexate: I.V.: 200 mg/m^2/day days 8 and 15
[total dose/cycle = 400 mg/m^2]
Leucovorin calcium: Oral: 10 mg/m^2 every 6 hours for 8 doses (beginning 24 hours after each methotrexate dose) days 9 and 16
[total dose/cycle = 160 mg/m^2]
Bleomycin: I.V.: 4 units/m^2 day 1
[total dose/cycle = 4 units/m^2]
Doxorubicin: I.V.: 45 mg/m^2 day 1
[total dose/cycle = 45 mg/m^2]
Cyclophosphamide: I.V.: 600 mg/m^2 day 1
[total dose/cycle = 600 mg/m^2]
Vincristine: I.V.: 1 mg/m^2 day 1
[total dose/cycle = 1 mg/m^2]
Dexamethasone: Oral: 6 mg/m^2/day days 1 to 5
[total dose/cycle = 30 mg/m^2]
Repeat cycle every 21 days

Melphalan-Prednisone-Thalidomide

Use Multiple myeloma

Regimen

Melphalan: Oral: 4 mg/m^2/day days 1 to 7
[total dose/cycle = 28 mg/m^2]
Prednisone: Oral: 40 mg/m^2/day days 1 to 7
[total dose/cycle = 280 mg/m^2]
Thalidomide: Oral: 100 mg/day days 1 to 28
[total dose/cycle = 2800 mg]
Repeat cycle every 28 days for 6 cycles
followed by
Thalidomide: Oral: 100 mg daily (as maintenance)

Methotrexate-Vinblastine (Desmoid Tumor)

Use Soft tissue sarcoma (Desmoid tumor)

Regimen

Methotrexate: I.V.: 30 mg/m^2 every 7-10 days
[total dose/treatment = 30 mg/m^2]
Vinblastine: I.V.: 6 mg/m^2 every 7-10 days
[total dose/treatment = 6 mg/m^2]
Continue treatment for 1 year (52 treatments)

MF

Use Breast cancer

Regimen

Methotrexate: I.V. 100 mg/m^2/day days 1 and 8
[total dose/cycle = 200 mg/m^2]
Fluorouracil: I.V.: 600 mg/m^2/day (start 1 hour after methotrexate) days 1 and 8
[total dose/cycle = 1200 mg/m^2]
Leucovorin: Oral, I.V.: 10 mg/m^2 every 6 hours for 6 doses (start 24 hours after methotrexate)
[total dose/cycle = 60 mg/m^2]
Repeat cycle every 28 days for 12 cycles

MINE

Use Lymphoma, non-Hodgkin

Regimen

Mesna: I.V.: 1.33 g/m^2/day concurrent with ifosfamide dose, then 500 mg orally (4 hours after each ifosfamide infusion) days 1, 2, and 3
[total dose/cycle = 3.99 g/m^2/1500 mg]

Ifosfamide: I.V.: 1.33 g/m^2/day days 1, 2, and 3
[total dose/cycle = 3.99 g/m^2]
Mitoxantrone: I.V.: 8 mg/m^2 day 1
[total dose/cycle = 8 mg/m^2]
Etoposide: I.V.: 65 mg/m^2/day days 1, 2, and 3
[total dose/cycle = 195 mg/m^2]
Repeat cycle every 28 days

MINE-ESHAP

Use Lymphoma, non-Hodgkin

Regimen

Mesna: I.V.: 1.33 g/m^2 concurrent with ifosfamide dose, then 500 mg orally (4 hours after ifosfamide) days 1, 2, and 3
[total dose/cycle = 4 g/m^2/1500 mg]
Ifosfamide: I.V.: 1.33 g/m^2/day days 1, 2, and 3
[total dose/cycle = 4 g/m^2]
Mitoxantrone: I.V.: 8 mg/m^2 day 1
[total dose/cycle = 8 mg/m^2]
Etoposide: I.V.: 65 mg/m^2/day days 1, 2, and 3
[total dose/cycle = 195 mg/m^2]
Repeat cycle every 21 days for 6 cycles, followed by 3-6 cycles of ESHAP

mini-BEAM

Use Lymphoma, Hodgkin disease

Regimen

Carmustine: I.V.: 60 mg/m^2 day 1
[total dose/cycle = 60 mg/m^2]
Etoposide: I.V.: 75 mg/m^2/day days 2 to 5
[total dose/cycle = 300 mg/m^2]
Cytarabine: I.V.: 100 mg/m^2 every 12 hours for 8 doses days 2 to 5
[total dose/cycle = 800 mg/m^2]
Melphalan: I.V.: 30 mg/m^2 day 6
[total dose/cycle = 30 mg/m^2]
Repeat cycle every 4-6 weeks

Mitomycin-Vinblastine

Use Breast cancer

Regimen

Mitomycin: I.V.: 20 mg/m^2 day 1
[total dose/cycle = 20 mg/m^2]
Vinblastine: I.V.: 0.15 mg/kg/day days 1 and 21
[total dose/cycle = 0.3 mg/kg]
Repeat cycle every 6-8 weeks

Mitoxantrone + Hydrocortisone

Use Prostate cancer

Regimen

Mitoxantrone: I.V.: 14 mg/m^2 day 1
[total dose/cycle = 14 mg/m^2]
Hydrocortisone: Oral: 40 mg daily
[total dose/cycle = 840 mg]
Repeat cycle every 3 weeks

Mitoxantrone-Prednisone (Prostate Cancer)

Use Prostate cancer

Regimen NOTE: Multiple variations are listed below.

Variation 1:
Mitoxantrone: I.V.: 12 mg/m^2 day 1
[total dose/cycle = 12 mg/m^2]

Prednisone: Oral: 5 mg twice daily
[total dose/cycle = 210 mg]
Repeat cycle every 21 days for up to a total of 10 cycles
Variation 2:
Cycle 1:
Mitoxantrone: I.V.: 12 mg/m^2 day 1
[total dose/cycle = 12 mg/m^2]
Prednisone: Oral: 5 mg twice daily
[total dose/cycle = 210 mg]
Treatment cycle is 21 days
Cycle 2 and beyond:
Mitoxantrone: I.V.: 12-14 mg/m^2 day 1 (increase to 14 mg/m^2 if no grade 3/4 adverse events)
[total dose/cycle = 12-14 mg/m^2]
Prednisone: Oral: 5 mg twice daily
[total dose/cycle = 210 mg]
Repeat cycle every 21 days for up to a maximum cumulative mitoxantrone dose of 144 mg/m^2
Variation 3:
Cycle 1:
Mitoxantrone: I.V.: 12 mg/m^2 day 1
[total dose/cycle = 12 mg/m^2]
Prednisone: Oral: 5 mg twice daily
[total dose/cycle = 210 mg]
Treatment cycle is 21 days
Cycles 2-8:
Mitoxantrone: I.V.: 12-14 mg/m^2 day 1 (increase to 14 mg/m^2 if granulocyte nadir is >1000/mm^3 and platelet nadir >50,000/ mm^3)
[total dose/cycle = 12-14 mg/m^2]
Prednisone: Oral: 5 mg twice daily
[total dose/cycle = 210 mg]
Treatment cycle is 21 days for up to a total of 8 cycles

MOP

Use Brain tumors

Regimen

Mechlorethamine: I.V.: 6 mg/m^2/day days 1 and 8
[total dose/cycle = 12 mg/m^2]
Vincristine: I.V.: 1.5 mg/m^2/day (maximum: 2 mg) days 1 and 8
[total dose/cycle = 3 mg/m^2]
Procarbazine: Oral: 100 mg/m^2/day days 1 to 14
[total dose/cycle = 1400 mg/m^2]
Repeat cycle every 28 days

MOPP/ABVD

Use Lymphoma, Hodgkin disease

Regimen NOTE: Multiple variations are listed below.

Variation 1:
Mechlorethamine: I.V.: 6 mg/m^2/day days 1 and 8
[total dose/cycle = 12 mg/m^2]
Vincristine: I.V.: 1.4 mg/m^2/day (maximum: 2 mg) days 1 and 8
[total dose/cycle = 2.8 mg/m^2]
Procarbazine: I.V.: 100 mg/m^2/day days 1 to 14
[total dose/cycle = 1400 mg/m^2]
Prednisone: Oral: 40 mg/m^2/day days 1 to 14 (during cycles 1, 4, 7, and 10 only)
[total dose/cycle = 560 mg/m^2]
Doxorubicin: I.V.: 25 mg/m^2/day days 29 and 43
[total dose/cycle = 50 mg/m^2]
Bleomycin: I.V.: 10 units/m^2/day days 29 and 43
[total dose/cycle = 20 units/m^2]
Vinblastine: I.V.: 6 mg/m^2/day days 29 and 43
[total dose/cycle = 12 mg/m^2]

Dacarbazine: I.V.: 375 mg/m^2/day days 29 and 43
[total dose/cycle = 750 mg/m^2]
Repeat cycle every 56 days

Variation 2:
Mechlorethamine: I.V.: 6 mg/m^2/day days 1 and 8
[total dose/cycle = 12 mg/m^2]
Vincristine: I.V.: 1.4 mg/m^2/day (maximum: 2 mg) days 1 and 8
[total dose/cycle = 2.8 mg/m^2]
Procarbazine: I.V.: 100 mg/m^2/day days 1 to 14
[total dose/cycle = 1400 mg/m^2]
Prednisone: Oral: 40 mg/m^2/day days 1 to 14 (during cycles 1 and 7 only)
[total dose/cycle = 560 mg/m^2]
Doxorubicin: I.V.: 25 mg/m^2/day days 29 and 43
[total dose/cycle = 50 mg/m^2]
Bleomycin: I.V.: 10 units/m^2/day days 29 and 43
[total dose/cycle = 20 units/m^2]
Vinblastine: I.V.: 6 mg/m^2/day days 29 and 43
[total dose/cycle = 12 mg/m^2]
Dacarbazine: I.V.: 375 mg/m^2/day days 29 and 43
[total dose/cycle = 750 mg/m^2]
Repeat cycle every 56 days

Variation 3:
Mechlorethamine: I.V.: 6 mg/m^2/day days 1 and 8
[total dose/cycle = 12 mg/m^2]
Vincristine: I.V.: 1.4 mg/m^2/day (maximum: 2 mg) days 1 and 8
[total dose/cycle = 2.8 mg/m^2]
Procarbazine: I.V.: 100 mg/m^2/day days 1 to 14
[total dose/cycle = 1400 mg/m^2]
Prednisone: Oral: 40 mg/m^2/day days 1 to 14 (every cycle)
[total dose/cycle = 560 mg/m^2]
Doxorubicin: I.V.: 25 mg/m^2/day days 29 and 43
[total dose/cycle = 50 mg/m^2]
Bleomycin: I.V.: 10 units/m^2/day days 29 and 43
[total dose/cycle = 20 units/m^2]
Vinblastine: I.V.: 6 mg/m^2/day days 29 and 43
[total dose/cycle = 12 mg/m^2]
Dacarbazine: I.V.: 375 mg/m^2/day days 29 and 43
[total dose/cycle = 750 mg/m^2]
Repeat cycle every 56 days

Variation 4:

MOPP Regimen:
Mechlorethamine: I.V.: 6 mg/m^2/day days 1 and 8
[total dose/cycle = 12 mg/m^2]
Vincristine: I.V.: 1.4 mg/m^2/day (maximum: 2 mg) days 1 and 8
[total dose/cycle = 2.8 mg/m^2]
Procarbazine: I.V.: 100 mg/m^2/day days 1 to 14
[total dose/cycle = 1400 mg/m^2]
Prednisone: Oral: 25 mg/m^2/day days 1 to 14
[total dose/cycle = 350 mg/m^2]

ABVD Regimen:
Doxorubicin: I.V.: 25 mg/m^2/day days 1 and 15
[total dose/cycle = 50 mg/m^2]
Bleomycin: I.V.: 6 units/m^2/day days 1 and 15
[total dose/cycle = 12 units/m^2]
Vinblastine: I.V.: 6 mg/m^2/day days 1 and 15
[total dose/cycle = 12 mg/m^2]
Dacarbazine: I.V.: 250 mg/m^2/day days 1 and 15
[total dose/cycle = 500 mg/m^2]
Each regimen cycle is 28 days. Administer regimens in alternating fashion as follows: 2 cycles of MOPP alternating with 2 cycles of ABVD for a total of 8 cycles

Variation 5 (pediatrics):
Mechlorethamine: I.V.: 6 mg/m^2/day days 1 and 8 [total dose/cycle = 12 mg/m^2]
Vincristine: I.V.: 1.4 mg/m^2/day days 1 and 8 [total dose/cycle = 2.8 mg/m^2]
Procarbazine: Oral: 100 mg/m^2/day days 1 to 14 [total dose/cycle = 1400 mg/m^2]
Prednisone: Oral: 40 mg/m^2/day days 1 to 14 [total dose/cycle = 560 mg/m^2]
Doxorubicin: I.V.: 25 mg/m^2/day days 29 and 42 [total dose/cycle = 50 mg/m^2]
Bleomycin: I.V.: 10 units/m^2/day days 29 and 42 [total dose/cycle = 20 units/m^2]
Vinblastine: I.V.: 6 mg/m^2/day days 29 and 42 [total dose/cycle = 12 mg/m^2]
Dacarbazine: I.V.: 150 mg/m^2/day days 29 to 33 [total dose/cycle = 750 mg/m^2]
Repeat cycle every 56 days for 4 cycles

Variation 6 (pediatrics):
Mechlorethamine: I.V.: 6 mg/m^2/day days 1 and 8 [total dose/cycle = 12 mg/m^2]
Vincristine: I.V.: 1.4 mg/m^2/day days 1 and 8 [total dose/cycle = 2.8 mg/m^2]
Procarbazine: Oral: 100 mg/m^2/day days 1 to 14 [total dose/cycle = 1400 mg/m^2]
Prednisone: Oral: 40 mg/m^2/day days 1 to 14 [total dose/cycle = 560 mg/m^2]
Doxorubicin: I.V.: 25 mg/m^2/day days 29 and 42 [total dose/cycle = 50 mg/m^2]
Bleomycin: I.V.: 10 units/m^2/day days 29 and 42 [total dose/cycle = 20 units/m^2]
Vinblastine: I.V.: 6 mg/m^2/day days 29 and 42 [total dose/cycle = 12 mg/m^2]
Dacarbazine: I.V.: 375 mg/m^2/day days 29 and 43 [total dose/cycle = 750 mg/m^2]
Repeat cycle every 56 days for 4 cycles

MOPP/ABV Hybrid

Use Lymphoma, Hodgkin disease

Regimen

Mechlorethamine: I.V.: 6 mg/m^2 day 1 [total dose/cycle = 6 mg/m^2]
Vincristine: I.V.: 1.4 mg/m^2 (maximum: 2 mg) day 1 [total dose/cycle = 1.4 mg/m^2]
Procarbazine: Oral: 100 mg/m^2/day days 1 to 7 [total dose/cycle = 700 mg/m^2]
Prednisone: Oral: 40 mg/m^2/day days 1 to 14 [total dose/cycle = 560 mg/m^2]
Doxorubicin: I.V.: 35 mg/m^2 day 8 [total dose/cycle = 35 mg/m^2]
Bleomycin: I.V.: 10 units/m^2 day 8 [total dose/cycle = 10 units/m^2]
Vinblastine: I.V.: 6 mg/m^2 day 8 [total dose/cycle = 6 mg/m^2]
Repeat cycle every 28 days

MOPP (Lymphoma, Hodgkin Disease)

Use Lymphoma, Hodgkin disease

Regimen NOTE: Multiple variations are listed below.

Variation 1:
Mechlorethamine: I.V.: 6 mg/m^2/day days 1 and 8 [total dose/cycle = 12 mg/m^2]

Vincristine: I.V.: 1.4 mg/m^2/day days 1 and 8
[total dose/cycle = 2.8 mg/m^2]
Procarbazine: Oral: 100 mg/m^2/day days 1 to 14
[total dose/cycle = 1400 mg/m^2]
Prednisone: Oral: 40 mg/m^2/day days 1 to 14 (cycles 1 and 4)
[total dose/cycle = 560 mg/m^2]
Repeat cycle every 28 days for 6-8 cycles

Variation 2:
Mechlorethamine: I.V.: 6 mg/m^2/day (maximum: 15 mg) days 1 and 8
[total dose/cycle = 12 mg/m^2]
Vincristine: I.V.: 1.4 mg/m^2/day (maximum: 2 mg) days 1 and 8
[total dose/cycle = 2.8 mg/m^2]
Procarbazine: Oral: 100 mg/m^2/day days 1 to 10
[total dose/cycle = 1000 mg/m^2]
Prednisone: Oral: 25 mg/m^2/day (maximum: 60 mg) days 1 to 14
[total dose/cycle = 350 mg/m^2]
or
Prednisolone: Oral: 25 mg/m^2/day (maximum: 60 mg) days 1 to 14
[total dose/cycle = 350 mg/m^2]
Repeat cycle every 28 days

Variation 3:
Mechlorethamine: I.V.: 6 mg/m^2/day days 1 and 8
[total dose/cycle = 12 mg/m^2]
Vincristine: I.V.: 1.4 mg/m^2/day days 1 and 8
[total dose/cycle = 2.8 mg/m^2]
Procarbazine: Oral: 50 mg day 1, 100 mg day 2, 100 mg/m^2/day days 3 to 14
[total dose/cycle = 150 mg / 1200 mg/m^2]
Prednisone: Oral: 40 mg/m^2/day days 1 to 14
[total dose/cycle = 560 mg/m^2]
Repeat cycle every 28 days

Variation 4:
Mechlorethamine: I.V.: 6 mg/m^2/day days 1 and 8
[total dose/cycle = 12 mg/m^2]
Vincristine: I.V.: 1.4 mg/m^2/day days 1 and 8
[total dose/cycle = 2.8 mg/m^2]
Procarbazine: Oral: 50 mg day 1, 100 mg day 2, 100 mg/m^2/day days 3 to 10
[total dose/cycle = 150 mg / 800 mg/m^2]
Prednisone: Oral: 40 mg/m^2/day days 1 to 14
[total dose/cycle = 560 mg/m^2]
Repeat cycle every 28 days

Variation 5:
Mechlorethamine: I.V.: 6 mg/m^2/day days 1 and 8
[total dose/cycle = 12 mg/m^2]
Vincristine: I.V.: 1.4 mg/m^2/day days 1 and 8
[total dose/cycle = 2.8 mg/m^2]
Procarbazine: Oral: 50 mg/m^2 day 1, then 100 mg/m^2/day days 2 to 14
[total dose/cycle = 1350 mg/m^2]
Prednisone: Oral: 40 mg/m^2/day days 1 to 14
[total dose/cycle = 560 mg/m^2]
Repeat cycle every 28 days

MOPP (Medulloblastoma)

Use Brain tumors

Regimen

Mechlorethamine: I.V.: 3 mg/m^2/day days 1 and 8
[total dose/cycle = 6 mg/m^2]
Vincristine: I.V.: 1.4 mg/m^2/day (maximum: 2 mg) days 1 and 8
[total dose/cycle = 2.8 mg/m^2]
Prednisone: Oral: 40 mg/m^2/day days 1 to 10
[total dose/cycle = 400 mg/m^2]

Procarbazine: Oral: 50 mg day 1
[total dose/cycle = 50 mg]
followed by Oral: 100 mg day 2
[total dose/cycle = 100 mg]
followed by Oral: 100 mg/m^2/day days 3 to 10
[total dose/cycle = 800 mg/m^2]
Repeat cycle every 28 days

MP (Multiple Myeloma)

Use Multiple myeloma

Regimen

Melphalan: Oral: 8-10 mg/m^2/day days 1 to 4
[total dose/cycle = 32-40 mg/m^2]
Prednisone: Oral: 40-60 mg/m^2/day days 1 to 4
[total dose/cycle = 160-240 mg/m^2]
Repeat cycle every 28-42 days

MTX/6-MP/VP (Maintenance)

Use Leukemia, acute lymphocytic

Regimen

Methotrexate: Oral: 20 mg/m^2 weekly
[total dose/cycle = 80 mg/m^2]
Mercaptopurine: Oral: 75 mg/m^2/day
[total dose/cycle = 2250 mg/m^2]
Vincristine: I.V.: 1.5 mg/m^2 day 1
[total dose/cycle = 1.5 mg/m^2]
Prednisone: Oral: 40 mg/m^2/day days 1 to 5
[total dose/cycle = 200 mg/m^2]
Repeat monthly for 2-3 years

MTX-CDDPAdr

Use Osteosarcoma

Regimen

Cisplatin: I.V.: 75 mg/m^2 day 1 of cycles 1-7, then 120 mg/m^2 for cycles 8, 9, and 10
Doxorubicin: I.V.: 25 mg/m^2/day days 1, 2, and 3 of cycles 1 to 7
Methotrexate: I.V.: 12 g/m^2/day days 21 and 28
Leucovorin calcium rescue: I.V.: 20 mg/m^2 every 3 hours (beginning 16 hours after completion of methotrexate) for 8 doses, then orally every 6 hours for 8 doses

MV

Use Leukemia, acute myeloid

Regimen Induction:

Mitoxantrone: I.V.: 10 mg/m^2/day days 1 to 5
[total dose/cycle = 50 mg/m^2]
Etoposide: I.V.: 100 mg/m^2/day days 1 to 5
[total dose/cycle = 500 mg/m^2]
Second cycle may be given based on individual response; time between cycles not specified

M-VAC (Bladder Cancer)

Use Bladder cancer

Regimen NOTE: Multiple variations are listed below.

Variation 1:
Methotrexate: I.V.: 30 mg/m^2/day days 1, 15, and 22
[total dose/cycle = 90 mg/m^2]
Vinblastine: I.V.: 3 mg/m^2/day days 2, 15, and 22
[total dose/cycle = 9 mg/m^2]
Doxorubicin: I.V.: 30 mg/m^2 day 2
[total dose/cycle = 30 mg/m^2]

Cisplatin: I.V.: 70 mg/m^2 day 2
[total dose/cycle = 70 mg/m^2]
Repeat cycle every 4 weeks

Variation 2:
Methotrexate: I.V.: 40 or 50 mg/m^2/day days 1, 15, and 22
[total dose/cycle = 120 or 150 mg/m^2]
Vinblastine: I.V.: 4 or 5 mg/m^2/day days 2, 15, and 22
[total dose/cycle = 12 or 15 mg/m^2]
Doxorubicin: I.V.: 40 or 50 mg/m^2 day 2
[total dose/cycle = 40 or 50 mg/m^2]
Cisplatin: I.V.: 100 mg/m^2 day 2
[total dose/cycle = 100 mg/m^2]
Repeat cycle every 4 weeks

Variation 3:
Methotrexate: I.V.: 30 mg/m^2/day days 1, 15, and 22
[total dose/cycle = 90 mg/m^2]
Vinblastine: I.V.: 3 mg/m^2 day 2
[total dose/cycle = 3 mg/m^2]
Doxorubicin: I.V.: 30 mg/m^2 day 2
[total dose/cycle = 30 mg/m^2]
Cisplatin: I.V.: 70 mg/m^2 day 2
[total dose/cycle = 70 mg/m^2]
Repeat cycle every 4 weeks

Variation 4:
Methotrexate: I.V.: 60 mg/m^2 day 1
[total dose/cycle = 60 mg/m^2]
followed by I.V.: 30 mg/m^2 day 16
[total dose/cycle = 30 mg/m^2]
Vinblastine: I.V.: 4 mg/m^2/day days 2 and 16
[total dose/cycle = 8 mg/m^2]
Doxorubicin: I.V.: 60 mg/m^2 day 2
[total dose/cycle = 60 mg/m^2]
Cisplatin: I.V.: 100 mg/m^2 day 2
[total dose/cycle = 100 mg/m^2]
Repeat cycle every 23 days

Variation 5:
Methotrexate: I.V.: 30 mg/m^2/day days 1, 16, and 23
[total dose/cycle = 90 mg/m^2]
Vinblastine: I.V.: 4 mg/m^2/day days 1, 16, and 23
[total dose/cycle = 12 mg/m^2]
Doxorubicin: I.V.: 60 mg/m^2 day 2
[total dose/cycle = 60 mg/m^2]
Cisplatin: I.V.: 100 mg/m^2 day 2
[total dose/cycle = 100 mg/m^2]
Repeat cycle every 23 days

Variation 6:
Methotrexate: I.V.: 30 or 35 mg/m^2 day 1
[total dose/cycle = 30 or 35 mg/m^2]
Vinblastine: I.V.: 3 or 3.5 mg/m^2 day 2
[total dose/cycle = 3 or 3.5 mg/m^2]
Doxorubicin: I.V.: 30 or 35 mg/m^2 day 2
[total dose/cycle = 30 or 35 mg/m^2]
Cisplatin: I.V.: 70 or 80 mg/m^2 day 2
[total dose/cycle = 70 or 80 mg/m^2]
Repeat cycle every 2 weeks

Variation 7:
Methotrexate: I.V.: 30 mg/m^2 day 1
[total dose/cycle = 30 mg/m^2]
Vinblastine: I.V.: 3 mg/m^2 day 2
[total dose/cycle = 3 mg/m^2]
Doxorubicin: I.V.: 30 mg/m^2 day 2
[total dose/cycle = 30 mg/m^2]

Cisplatin: I.V.: 70 mg/m^2 day 2
[total dose/cycle = 70 mg/m^2]
Repeat cycle every 14 days
Variation 8:
Methotrexate: I.V.: 30 mg/m^2/day days 1, 15, and 22
[total dose/cycle = 90 mg/m^2]
Vinblastine: I.V.: 3 mg/m^2/day days 1, 15, and 22
[total dose/cycle = 9 mg/m^2]
Doxorubicin: I.V.: 45 mg/m^2 day 2
[total dose/cycle = 45 mg/m^2]
Cisplatin: I.V.: 70 mg/m^2 day 2
[total dose/cycle = 70 mg/m^2]
Repeat cycle every 4 weeks
Variation 9:
Methotrexate: I.V.: 40 mg/m^2/day days 1 and 15
[total dose/cycle = 80 mg/m^2]
Vinblastine: I.V.: 4 mg/m^2/day days 1, 16, and 23
[total dose/cycle = 12 mg/m^2]
Doxorubicin: I.V.: 60 mg/m^2 day 2
[total dose/cycle = 60 mg/m^2]
Cisplatin: I.V.: 100 mg/m^2 day 2
[total dose/cycle = 100 mg/m^2]
Repeat cycle every 23 days
Variation 10:
Methotrexate: I.V.: 30 mg/m^2/day days 1, 15, and 22
[total dose/cycle = 90 mg/m^2]
Vinblastine: I.V.: 3 mg/m^2/day days 1, 16, and 22
[total dose/cycle = 9 mg/m^2]
Doxorubicin: I.V.: 30 mg/m^2 day 1
[total dose/cycle = 30 mg/m^2]
Cisplatin: I.V.: 70 mg/m^2 day 1
[total dose/cycle = 70 mg/m^2]
Repeat cycle every 4 weeks
Variation 11:
Methotrexate: I.V.: 30 mg/m^2/day days 1, 15, and 22
[total dose/cycle = 90 mg/m^2]
Vinblastine: I.V.: 3 mg/m^2/day days 2, 15, and 22
[total dose/cycle = 9 mg/m^2]
Doxorubicin: I.V.: 30 mg/m^2 day 2
[total dose/cycle = 30 mg/m^2]
Cisplatin: I.V.: 70 mg/m^2 day 2
[total dose/cycle = 70 mg/m^2]
Leucovorin: Oral: 15 mg every 6 hours for 4 doses days 2, 16, and 23
[total dose/cycle = 180 mg]
Repeat cycle every 4 weeks
Variation 12:
Methotrexate: I.V.: 30 mg/m^2/day days 1 and 15
[total dose/cycle = 60 mg/m^2]
Vinblastine: I.V.: 3 mg/m^2/day days 2 and 15
[total dose/cycle = 6 mg/m^2]
Doxorubicin: I.V.: 30 or 40 mg/m^2 day 3
[total dose/cycle = 30 or 40 mg/m^2]
Cisplatin: I.V.: 70 mg/m^2 day 2
[total dose/cycle = 70 mg/m^2]
Repeat cycle every 4 weeks
Variation 13:
Methotrexate: I.V.: 30 mg/m^2/day days 1 and 15
[total dose/cycle = 60 mg/m^2]
Vinblastine: I.V.: 3 mg/m^2/day days 2 and 15
[total dose/cycle = 6 mg/m^2]
Doxorubicin: I.V.: 30 or 40 mg/m^2 day 2
[total dose/cycle = 30 or 40 mg/m^2]

Cisplatin: I.V.: 70 mg/m^2 day 2
[total dose/cycle = 70 mg/m^2]
Repeat cycle every 4 weeks

M-VAC (Breast Cancer)

Use Breast cancer

Regimen

Methotrexate: I.V.: 30 mg/m^2/day days 1, 15, and 22
[total dose/cycle = 90 mg/m^2]
Vinblastine: I.V.: 3 mg/m^2/day days 2, 15, and 22
[total dose/cycle = 9 mg/m^2]
Doxorubicin: I.V.: 30 mg/m^2 day 2
[total dose/cycle = 30 mg/m^2]
Cisplatin: I.V.: 70 mg/m^2 day 2
[total dose/cycle = 70 mg/m^2]
Leucovorin: Oral: 10 mg every 6 hours for 6 doses days 2, 16, and 23
[total dose/cycle = 180 mg]
Repeat cycle every 4 weeks

M-VAC (Cervical Cancer)

Use Cervical cancer

Regimen

Methotrexate: I.V.: 30 mg/m^2/day days 1, 15, and 22
[total dose/cycle = 90 mg/m^2]
Vinblastine: I.V.: 3 mg/m^2/day days 2, 15, and 22
[total dose/cycle = 9 mg/m^2]
Doxorubicin: I.V.: 30 mg/m^2 day 2
[total dose/cycle = 30 mg/m^2]
Cisplatin: I.V.: 70 mg/m^2 day 2
[total dose/cycle = 70 mg/m^2]
Repeat cycle every 4 weeks

M-VAC (Endometrial Cancer)

Use Endometrial cancer

Regimen

Methotrexate: I.V.: 30 mg/m^2/day days 1, 15, and 22
[total dose/cycle = 90 mg/m^2]
Vinblastine: I.V.: 3 mg/m^2/day days 2, 15, and 22
[total dose/cycle = 9 mg/m^2]
Doxorubicin: I.V.: 30 mg/m^2/day day 2
[total dose/cycle = 30 mg/m^2]
Cisplatin: I.V.: 70 mg/m^2/day day 2
[total dose/cycle = 70 mg/m^2]
Repeat cycle every 4 weeks

M-VAC (Head and Neck Cancer)

Use Head and neck cancer

Regimen

Methotrexate: I.V.: 30 mg/m^2/day days 1, 15, and 22
[total dose/cycle = 90 mg/m^2]
Vinblastine: I.V.: 3 mg/m^2/day days 2, 15, and 22
[total dose/cycle = 9 mg/m^2]
Doxorubicin: I.V.: 30 mg/m^2 day 2
[total dose/cycle = 30 mg/m^2]
Cisplatin: I.V.: 70 mg/m^2 day 2
[total dose/cycle = 70 mg/m^2]
Repeat cycle every 4 weeks

MVPP

Use Lymphoma, Hodgkin disease

Regimen

Mechlorethamine: I.V.: 6 mg/m^2/day days 1 and 8
[total dose/cycle = 12 mg/m^2]
Vinblastine: I.V.: 4 mg/m^2/day days 1 and 8
[total dose/cycle = 8 mg/m^2]
Procarbazine: Oral: 100 mg/m^2/day days 1 to 14
[total dose/cycle = 1400 mg/m^2]
Prednisone: Oral: 40 mg/m^2/day days 1 to 14
[total dose/cycle = 560 mg/m^2]
Repeat cycle every 4-6 weeks

N4SE Protocol

Use Neuroblastoma

Regimen

Vincristine: I.V.: 0.05 mg/kg/day days 1 and 2
[total dose/cycle = 0.1 mg/kg]
Doxorubicin: I.V.: 15 mg/m^2/day days 1 and 2
[total dose/cycle = 30 mg/m^2]
Cyclophosphamide: I.V.: 30 mg/kg/day days 1 and 2
[total dose/cycle = 60 mg/kg]
Fluorouracil: I.V.: 1 mg/kg/day days 3, 8, and 9
[total dose/cycle = 3 mg/kg]
Cytarabine: I.V.: 3 mg/kg/day days 3, 8, and 9
[total dose/cycle = 9 mg/kg]
Hydroxyurea: Oral: 40 mg/kg/day days 3, 8, and 9
[total dose/cycle = 120 mg/kg]
Repeat cycle every 21-28 days

N6 Protocol

Use Neuroblastoma

Regimen

Course 1, 2, 4, and 6:
Cyclophosphamide: I.V.: 70 mg/kg/day days 1 and 2
[total dose/cycle = 140 mg/kg]
Doxorubicin: I.V.: 25 mg/m^2/day continuous infusion days 1, 2, and 3
[total dose/cycle = 75 mg/m^2]
Vincristine: I.V.: 0.033 mg/kg/day continuous infusion days 1, 2, and 3
[total dose/cycle = 0.099 mg/kg]
Vincristine: I.V.: 1.5 mg/m^2 day 9
[total dose/cycle = 1.5 mg/m^2]
Course 3, 5, and 7:
Etoposide: I.V.: 200 mg/m^2/day days 1, 2, and 3
[total dose/cycle = 600 mg/m^2]
Cisplatin: I.V.: 50 mg/m^2/day days 1 to 4
[total dose/cycle = 200 mg/m^2]

NFL

Use Breast cancer

Regimen NOTE: Multiple variations are listed below.

Variation 1:
Mitoxantrone: I.V.: 12 mg/m^2 day 1
[total dose/cycle = 12 mg/m^2]
Fluorouracil: I.V.: 350 mg/m^2/day days 1, 2, and 3
[total dose/cycle = 1050 mg/m^2]
Leucovorin: I.V.: 300 mg/m^2/day days 1, 2, and 3
[total dose/cycle = 900 mg/m^2]
Repeat cycle every 21 days

Variation 2:
Mitoxantrone: I.V.: 10 mg/m^2 day 1
[total dose/cycle = 10 mg/m^2]
Fluorouracil: I.V.: 1000 mg/m^2/day continuous infusion days 1, 2, and 3
[total dose/cycle = 3000 mg/m^2]
Leucovorin: I.V.: 100 mg/m^2/day days 1, 2, and 3
[total dose/cycle = 300 mg/m^2]
Repeat cycle every 21 days

OFAR (CLL)

Use Leukemia, chronic lymphocytic

Regimen

Cycle 1:
Oxaliplatin: I.V.: 25 mg/m^2/dose day 1 to 4
[total dose/cycle = 100 mg/m^2]
Fludarabine: I.V.: 30 mg/m^2/dose days 2 and 3
[total dose/cycle = 60 mg/m^2]
Cytarabine: I.V.: 1000 mg/m^2/dose over 2 hours days 2 and 3
[total dose/cycle = 2000 mg/m^2]
Rituximab: I.V.: 375 mg/m^2 day 3
[total dose/cycle = 375 mg/m^2]
Treatment cycle is 4 weeks

Cycles 2-6:
Oxaliplatin: I.V.: 25 mg/m^2/dose day 1 to 4
[total dose/cycle = 100 mg/m^2]
Fludarabine: I.V.: 30 mg/m^2/dose days 2 and 3
[total dose/cycle = 60 mg/m^2]
Cytarabine: I.V.: 1000 mg/m^2/dose over 2 hours days 2 and 3
[total dose/cycle = 2000 mg/m^2]
Rituximab: I.V.: 375 mg/m^2 day 1
[total dose/cycle = 375 mg/m^2]
Repeat cycle every 4 weeks (maximum: 6 cycles)

OPA

Use Lymphoma, Hodgkin disease

Regimen

Vincristine: I.V.: 1.5 mg/m^2/day (maximum dose: 2 mg) days 1, 8, and 15
[total dose/cycle = 4.5 mg/m^2]
Prednisone: Oral: 60 mg/m^2/day in 3 divided doses days 1 to 15
[total dose/cycle = 900 mg/m^2]
Doxorubicin: I.V.: 40 mg/m^2/day days 1 and 15
[total dose/cycle = 80 mg/m^2]
Second cycle may be given based on individual response; time between cycles not specified

OPEC

Use Neuroblastoma

Regimen

Vincristine: I.V.: 1.5 mg/m^2 day 1
[total dose/cycle = 1.5 mg/m^2]
Cyclophosphamide: I.V.: 600 mg/m^2 day 1
[total dose/cycle = 600 mg/m^2]
Cisplatin: I.V.: 100 mg/m^2 day 2
[total dose/cycle = 100 mg/m^2]
Teniposide: I.V.: 150 mg/m^2 day 4
[total dose/cycle = 150 mg/m^2]
Repeat cycle every 21 days

OPEC-D

Use Neuroblastoma

Regimen

Vincristine: I.V.: 1.5 mg/m^2 day 1
[total dose/cycle = 1.5 mg/m^2]
Cyclophosphamide: I.V.: 600 mg/m^2 day 1
[total dose/cycle = 600 mg/m^2]
Doxorubicin: I.V.: 40 mg/m^2 day 1
[total dose/cycle = 40 mg/m^2]
Cisplatin: I.V.: 100 mg/m^2 day 2
[total dose/cycle = 100 mg/m^2]
Teniposide: I.V.: 150 mg/m^2 day 4
[total dose/cycle = 150 mg/m^2]
Repeat cycle every 21 days

OPPA

Use Lymphoma, Hodgkin disease

Regimen

Vincristine: I.V.: 1.5 mg/m^2/day (maximum dose: 2 mg) days 1, 8, and 15
[total dose/cycle = 4.5 mg/m^2]
Prednisone: Oral: 60 mg/m^2/day in 3 divided doses days 1 to 15
[total dose/cycle = 900 mg/m^2]
Doxorubicin: I.V.: 40 mg/m^2/day days 1 and 15
[total dose/cycle = 80 mg/m^2]
Procarbazine: Oral: 100 mg/m^2/day in 2 or 3 divided doses days 1 to 15
[total dose/cycle = 1500 mg/m^2]
Second cycle may be given based on individual response; time between cycles not specified

Oxaliplatin-Cytarabine-Dexamethasone (NHL Regimen)

Use Lymphoma, non-Hodgkin

Regimen

Dexamethasone: I.V. or Oral: 40 mg/day days 1 to 4
[total dose/cycle = 160 mg]
Oxaliplatin: I.V.: 130 mg/m^2 over 2 hours day 1
[total dose/cycle = 130 mg/m^2]
Cytarabine: I.V.: 2000 mg/m^2 over 3 hours every 12 hours for 2 doses day 2
[total dose/cycle = 4000 mg/m^2]
Repeat cycle every 3 weeks

Oxaliplatin-Fluorouracil (Esophageal Cancer)

Use Esophageal cancer

Regimen In combination with radiation therapy:

Oxaliplatin: I.V.: 85 mg/m^2/day over 2 hours days 1, 15, and 29
[total dose/cycle = 255 mg/m^2]
Fluorouracil: I.V.: 180 mg/m^2/day continuous infusion days 8 to 42
[total dose/cycle = 6300 mg/m^2]

PAC (CAP)

Use Ovarian cancer

Regimen

Cisplatin: I.V.: 50 mg/m^2 day 1
[total dose/cycle = 50 mg/m^2]
Doxorubicin: I.V.: 50 mg/m^2 day 1
[total dose/cycle = 50 mg/m^2]
Cyclophosphamide: I.V.: 1000 mg/m^2 day 1
[total dose/cycle = 1000 mg/m^2]
Repeat cycle every 21 days for 8 cycles

PA-CI

Use Hepatoblastoma

Regimen NOTE: Multiple variations are listed below.

Variation 1:

Cisplatin: I.V.: 90 mg/m^2 day 1
[total dose/cycle = 90 mg/m^2]

Doxorubicin: I.V.: 20 mg/m^2/day continuous infusion days 2 to 5
[total dose/cycle = 80 mg/m^2]

Repeat cycle every 21 days

Variation 2:

Cisplatin: I.V.: 20 mg/m^2/day days 1 to 4
[total dose/cycle = 80 mg/m^2]

Doxorubicin: I.V.: 100 mg/m^2 continuous infusion day 1
[total dose/cycle = 100 mg/m^2]

Repeat cycle every 21-28 days

Paclitaxel-Bevacizumab

Use Breast cancer

Regimen

Paclitaxel: I.V.: 90 mg/m^2/day days 1, 8, and 15
[total dose/cycle = 270 mg/m^2]

Bevacizumab: I.V.: 10 mg/kg/day days 1 and 15
[total dose/cycle = 20 mg/kg]

Repeat cycle every 28 days

Paclitaxel-Carboplatin-Bevacizumab

Use Lung cancer, nonsquamous, nonsmall cell

Regimen

Paclitaxel: I.V.: 200 mg/m^2 infused over 3 hours day 1
[total dose/cycle = 200 mg/m^2]

followed by

Carboplatin: I.V.: Target AUC 6 day 1
[total dose/cycle = AUC = 6]

followed by

Bevacizumab: I.V.: 15 mg/kg day 1
[total dose/cycle = 15 mg/kg]

Repeat cycle every 21 days for 6 cycles

Paclitaxel-Carboplatin (Bladder Cancer)

Use Bladder cancer

Regimen

Paclitaxel: I.V.: 200 mg/m^2 or 225 mg/m^2 day 1
[total dose/cycle = 200 or 225 mg/m^2]

Carboplatin: I.V.: AUC 5-6 day 1
[total dose/cycle = AUC = 5-6]

Repeat cycle every 21 days

Paclitaxel-Carboplatin (Cervical Cancer)

Use Cervical cancer

Regimen NOTE: Multiple variations are listed below.

Variation 1:

Paclitaxel: I.V.: 175 mg/m^2 over 3 hours day 1
[total dose/cycle = 175 mg/m^2]

Carboplatin: I.V.: AUC 5 or 6 day 1
[total dose/cycle = AUC = 5 or 6]

Repeat cycle every 28 days for 6-9 cycles

Variation 2 (if patient has received prior pelvic radiation):

Paclitaxel: I.V.: 155 mg/m^2 over 3 hours day 1
[total dose/cycle = 155 mg/m^2]

...day 1
...5 or 6]
Carb...ys for 6-9 cycles
[tot...
Rep...

...atin-Etoposide

Use ...nknown primary
Regi...
Pa... ng/m^2 infused over 1 hour day 1
[t... 200 mg/m^2]
fo...
C... Target AUC 6
[... UC = 6]
E... l: 50 mg/day days 1, 3, 5, 7, and 9
...0 mg/day days 2, 4, 6, 8, and 10
...e/cycle = 750 mg]
R...cle every 21 days

Pa...el-Carboplatin-Gemcitabine

U... der cancer
Regim...
Pa...axel: I.V.: 200 mg/m^2 day 1
[total dose/cycle = 200 mg/m^2]
Gemcitabine: I.V.: 1000 mg/m^2/day days 1 and 8
[total dose/cycle = 2000 mg/m^2]
Carboplatin: I.V.: AUC 5 day 1
[total dose/cycle = AUC = 5]
Repeat cycle every 21 days

Paclitaxel-Cetuximab

Use Head and neck cancer

Regimen

Week 1:
Paclitaxel: I.V.: 80 mg/m^2 day 1
[total dose/week 1 = 80 mg/m^2]
Cetuximab: I.V.: 400 mg/m^2 (loading dose) day 1 (week 1 only)
[total loading dose (week 1) = 400 mg/m^2]
Subsequent weeks:
Paclitaxel: I.V.: 80 mg/m^2 day 1
[total dose/week = 80 mg/m^2]
Cetuximab: I.V.: 250 mg/m^2 day 1
[total dose/week = 250 mg/m^2]

Paclitaxel-Cisplatin (Cervical Cancer)

Use Cervical cancer

Regimen

Paclitaxel: I.V.: 135 mg/m^2 continuous infusion over 24 hours day 1
[total dose/cycle = 135 mg/m^2]
Cisplatin: I.V.: 50 mg/m^2 day 1
[total dose/cycle = 50 mg/m^2]
Repeat cycle every 21 days for 6 cycles

Paclitaxel-Cisplatin-Fluorouracil (Esophageal Cancer)

Use Esophageal cancer

Regimen

Paclitaxel: I.V.: 175 mg/m^2 over 3 hours day 1
[total dose/cycle = 175 mg/m^2]
Cisplatin: I.V.: 20 mg/m^2/day days 1 to 5 for cycles 1, 2, and 3
[total dose/cycle = 100 mg/m^2]
then 15 mg/m^2/day days 1 to 5
[total dose/cycle = 75 mg/m^2]

Fluorouracil: I.V.: 750 mg/m^2/day continuous infusion days 1 to 5
[total dose/cycle = 3750 mg/m^2]
Repeat cycle every 28 days

Paclitaxel + Estramustine + Carboplatin

Use Prostate cancer

Regimen

Paclitaxel: I.V.: 100 mg/m^2 day 3 each week
[total dose/cycle = 400 mg/m^2]
Estramustine: Oral: 10 mg/kg/day days 1 to 5 each week
[total dose/cycle = 200 mg/kg]
Carboplatin: I.V.: Target AUC 6 day 3
[total dose/cycle = AUC = 6]
Repeat cycle every 28 days

Paclitaxel + Estramustine + Etoposide

Use Prostate cancer

Regimen

Paclitaxel: I.V.: 135 mg/m^2 day 2
[total dose/cycle = 135 mg/m^2]
Estramustine: Oral: 280 mg 3 times/day days 1 to 14
[total dose/cycle = 11,760 mg]
Etoposide: Oral: 100 mg/day days 1 to 14
[total dose/cycle = 1400 mg]
Repeat cycle every 21 days

Paclitaxel-Gemcitabine

Use Bladder cancer

Regimen

Paclitaxel: I.V.: 200 mg/m^2 day 1
[total dose/cycle = 200 mg/m^2]
Gemcitabine: I.V.: 1000 mg/m^2/day days 1, 8, and 15
[total dose/cycle = 3000 mg/m^2]
Repeat cycle every 21 days for a maximum of 6 cycles

Paclitaxel-Ifosfamide-Cisplatin

Use Testicular cancer

Regimen

Paclitaxel: I.V.: 250 mg/m^2 continuous infusion day 1
[total dose/cycle = 250 mg/m^2]
Ifosfamide: I.V.: 1500 mg/m^2/day days 2 to 5
[total dose/cycle = 6000 mg/m^2]
Cisplatin: I.V.: 25 mg/m^2/day days 2 to 5
[total dose/cycle = 100 mg/m^2]
Mesna: I.V.: 500 mg/m^2 prior to ifosfamide and every 4 hours for 2 doses, days 2 to 5
[total dose/cycle = 6000 mg/m^2]
Repeat cycle every 21 days for 4 cycles

Paclitaxel-Vinorelbine

Use Breast cancer

Regimen NOTE: Multiple variations are listed below.

Variation 1:
Paclitaxel: I.V.: 135 mg/m^2 day 1
[total dose/cycle = 135 mg/m^2]
Vinorelbine: I.V.: 30 mg/m^2 day 1
[total dose/cycle = 30 mg/m^2]
Repeat cycle every 21 days

Variation 2:
Paclitaxel: I.V.: 150 mg/m^2 day 1
[total dose/cycle = 150 mg/m^2]

Vinorelbine: I.V.: 25 mg/m^2 day 1
[total dose/cycle = 25 mg/m^2]
Repeat cycle every 21 days
Variation 3:
Paclitaxel: I.V.: 135 mg/m^2 day 1
[total dose/cycle = 135 mg/m^2]
Vinorelbine: I.V.: 30 mg/m^2/day days 1 and 8
[total dose/cycle = 60 mg/m^2]
Repeat cycle every 28 days

PCE

Use Adenocarcinoma, unknown primary

Regimen

Paclitaxel: I.V.: 200 mg/m^2 day 1
[total dose/cycle = 200 mg/m^2]
Carboplatin: I.V.: AUC = 6 day 1
[total dose/cycle = AUC = 6]
Etoposide: Oral: 50 mg/day days 1, 3, 5, 7, and 9
and Oral: 100 mg/day days 2, 4, 6, 8, and 10
[total dose/cycle = 750 mg]
Repeat cycle every 3 weeks

PC (NSCLC)

Use Lung cancer, nonsmall cell

Regimen NOTE: Multiple variations are listed below.

Variation 1:
Paclitaxel: I.V.: 175-225 mg/m^2 day 1
[total dose/cycle = 175-225 mg/m^2]
Carboplatin: I.V.: Target AUC 5-7 day 1
[total dose/cycle = AUC = 5-7]
Repeat cycle every 21 days for 2-8 cycles
Variation 2:
Paclitaxel: I.V.: 175 mg/m^2 day 1
[total dose/cycle = 175 mg/m^2]
Cisplatin: I.V.: 80 mg/m^2 day 1
[total dose/cycle = 80 mg/m^2]
Repeat cycle every 21 days
Variation 3:
Paclitaxel: I.V.: 135 mg/m^2 continuous infusion day 1
[total dose/cycle = 135 mg/m^2]
Carboplatin: I.V.: AUC 7.5 day 2
[total dose/cycle = AUC = 7.5]
Repeat cycle every 21 days
Variation 4:
Paclitaxel: I.V.: 135 mg/m^2 continuous infusion day 1
[total dose/cycle = 135 mg/m^2]
Cisplatin: I.V.: 75 mg/m^2 day 2
[total dose/cycle = 75 mg/m^2]
Repeat cycle every 21 days

PCR

Use Leukemia, chronic lymphocytic

Regimen NOTE: Multiple variations are listed below.

Variation 1:
Cycle 1:
Cyclophosphamide: I.V.: 600 mg/m^2 day 1
[total dose/cycle = 600 mg/m^2]
Pentostatin: I.V.: 4 mg/m^2 day 1
[total dose/cycle = 4 mg/m^2]
Treatment cycle is 3 weeks

Cycles 2-6:
Cyclophosphamide: I.V.: 600 mg/m^2 day 1
[total dose/cycle = 600 mg/m^2]
Pentostatin: I.V.: 4 mg/m^2 day 1
[total dose/cycle = 4 mg/m^2]
Rituximab: I.V.: 375 mg/m^2 day 1
[total dose/cycle = 375 mg/m^2]
Repeat cycle every 3 weeks
Variation 2:
Cycle 1:
Pentostatin: I.V.: 2 mg/m^2 day 1
[total dose/cycle = 2 mg/m^2]
Cyclophosphamide: I.V.: 600 mg/m^2 day 1
[total dose/cycle = 600 mg/m^2]
Rituximab: I.V.: 100 mg/m^2 day 1 only
followed by I.V.: 375 mg/m^2/day days 3 and 5 only
[total dose/cycle 1 = 850 mg/m^2]
Treatment cycle is 3 weeks
Cycles 2-6:
Pentostatin: I.V.: 2 mg/m^2 day 1
[total dose/cycle = 2 mg/m^2]
Cyclophosphamide: I.V.: 600 mg/m^2 day 1
[total dose/cycle = 600 mg/m^2]
Rituximab: I.V.: 375 mg/m^2 day 1
[total dose/cycle = 375 mg/m^2]
Repeat cycle every 3 weeks

PCV (Brain Tumor Regimen)

Use Brain tumors

Regimen NOTE: Multiple variations are listed below.
Variation 1:
Lomustine: Oral: 110 mg/m^2 day 1
[total dose/cycle = 110 mg/m^2]
Procarbazine: Oral: 60 mg/m^2/day days 8 to 21
[total dose/cycle = 840 mg/m^2]
Vincristine: I.V.: 1.4 mg/m^2/day (maximum 2 mg) days 8 and 29
[total dose/cycle = 2.8 mg/m^2; maximum 4 mg]
Repeat cycle every 6 weeks for a total of 6 cycles
Variation 2:
Lomustine: Oral: 110 mg/m^2 day 1
[total dose/cycle = 110 mg/m^2]
Procarbazine: Oral: 60 mg/m^2/day days 8 to 21
[total dose/cycle = 840 mg/m^2]
Vincristine: I.V.: 1.4 mg/m^2/day (maximum: 2 mg) days 8 and 29
[total dose/cycle = 2.8 mg/m^2; maximum 4 mg]
Repeat cycle every 6 weeks for a total of 7 cycles
Variation 3:
Procarbazine: Oral: 75 mg/m^2/day days 8 to 21
[total dose/cycle = 1050 mg/m^2]
Lomustine: Oral: 130 mg/m^2 day 1
[total dose/cycle = 130 mg/m^2]
Vincristine: I.V.: 1.4 mg/m^2/day (no maximum) days 8 and 29
[total dose/cycle = 2.8 mg/m^2; no maximum]
Repeat cycle every 6 weeks for a total of 6 cycles
Variation 4:
Procarbazine: Oral: 75 mg/m^2/day days 8 to 21
[total dose/cycle = 1050 mg/m^2]
Lomustine: Oral: 130 mg/m^2 day 1
[total dose/cycle = 130 mg/m^2]
Vincristine: I.V.: 1.4 mg/m^2/day (no maximum) days 8 and 29
[total dose/cycle = 2.8 mg/m^2; no maximum]
Repeat cycle every 6 weeks for up to a total of 4 cycles

Variation 5:
Lomustine: Oral: 110 mg/m^2 day 1
[total dose/cycle = 110 mg/m^2]
Procarbazine: Oral: 60 mg/m^2/day days 8 to 21
[total dose/cycle = 840 mg/m^2]
Vincristine: I.V.: 1.4 mg/m^2/day days 8 and 29
[total dose/cycle = 2.8 mg/m^2]
Repeat cycle every 6-8 weeks for 1 year

PE-CAdO

Use Neuroblastoma

Regimen

Cisplatin: I.V.: 100 mg/m^2 day 1
[total dose/cycle = 100 mg/m^2]
Teniposide: I.V.: 160 mg/m^2 day 3
[total dose/cycle = 160 mg/m^2]
alternating with
Cyclophosphamide: I.V.: 300 mg/m^2/day days 1 to 5
[total dose/cycle = 1500 mg/m^2]
Doxorubicin: I.V.: 60 mg/m^2 day 5
[total dose/cycle = 60 mg/m^2]
Vincristine: I.V.: 1.5 mg/m^2/day days 1 and 5
[total dose/cycle = 3 mg/m^2]
Repeat cycle every 21 days

Pemetrexed (Bladder Cancer Regimen)

Use Bladder cancer

Regimen

Pemetrexed: I.V.: 500 mg/m^2 infused over 10 minutes day 1
[total dose/cycle = 500 mg/m^2]
Repeat cycle every 21 days

Pemetrexed-Carboplatin (Mesothelioma)

Use Malignant pleural mesothelioma

Regimen

Pemetrexed: I.V.: 500 mg/m^2 infused over 10 minutes day 1
[total dose/cycle = 500 mg/m^2]
Carboplatin: I.V.: AUC 5 infused over 30 minutes day 1 (start 30 minutes after pemetrexed)
[total dose/cycle = AUC = 5]
Repeat cycle every 21 days

Pemetrexed-Cisplatin (NSCLC)

Use Lung cancer, nonsmall cell

Regimen

Pemetrexed: I.V.: 500 mg/m^2/dose day 1
[total dose/cycle = 500 mg/m^2]
Cisplatin: I.V.: 75 mg/m^2/dose day 1
[total dose/cycle = 75 mg/m^2]
Repeat cycle every 21 days for up to 6 cycles

Pentostatin-Cyclophosphamide

Use Leukemia, chronic lymphocytic

Regimen

Cyclophosphamide: I.V.: 600 mg/m^2 day 1
[total dose/cycle = 600 mg/m^2]
Pentostatin: I.V.: 4 mg/m^2 day 1
[total dose/cycle = 4 mg/m^2]
Repeat cycle every 3 weeks for up to 6 cycles

PFL (Colorectal Cancer)

Use Colorectal cancer

Regimen

Cisplatin: I.V.: 25 mg/m^2/day continuous infusion days 1 to 5
[total dose/cycle = 125 mg/m^2]
Fluorouracil: I.V.: 800 mg/m^2/day continuous infusion days 2 to 5
[total dose/cycle = 3200 mg/m^2]
Leucovorin calcium: I.V.: 500 mg/m^2/day continuous infusion days 1 to 5
[total dose/cycle = 2500 mg/m^2]
Repeat cycle every 28 days

PFL (Head and Neck Cancer)

Use Head and neck cancer

Regimen NOTE: Multiple variations are listed below.

Variation 1:
Cisplatin: I.V.: 25 mg/m^2/day continuous infusion days 1 to 5
[total dose/cycle = 125 mg/m^2]
Fluorouracil: I.V.: 800 mg/m^2/day continuous infusion days 2 to 6
[total dose/cycle = 4000 mg/m^2]
Leucovorin: I.V.: 500 mg/m^2/day continuous infusion days 1 to 6
[total dose/cycle = 3000 mg/m^2]
Repeat cycle every 28 days

Variation 2:
Cisplatin: I.V.: 100 mg/m^2 day 1
[total dose/cycle = 100 mg/m^2]
Fluorouracil: I.V.: 600-1000 mg/m^2/day continuous infusion days 1 to 5
[total dose/cycle = 3000-5000 mg/m^2]
Leucovorin: Oral: 50 mg/m^2 every 4-6 hours days 1 to 6
[total dose/cycle = 1200-1800 mg/m^2]
Repeat cycle every 21 days

PFL + IFN

Use Head and neck cancer

Regimen

Cisplatin: I.V.: 100 mg/m^2 day 1
[total dose/cycle = 100 mg/m^2]
Fluorouracil: I.V.: 640 mg/m^2/day continuous infusion days 1 to 5
[total dose/cycle = 3200 mg/m^2]
Leucovorin calcium: Oral: 100 mg every 4 hours days 1 to 5
[total dose/cycle = 3000 mg/m^2]
Interferon alfa-2b: SubQ: 2 x 10^6 units/m^2 days 1 to 6
[total dose/cycle = 12 x 10^6 units/m^2]

POC

Use Brain tumors

Regimen

Prednisone: Oral: 40 mg/m^2/day days 1 to 14
[total dose/cycle = 560 mg/m^2]
Vincristine: I.V.: 1.5 mg/m^2/day (maximum dose: 2 mg) days 1, 8, and 15
[total dose/cycle = 4.5 mg/m^2]
Lomustine: Oral: 100 mg/m^2 day 1
[total dose/cycle = 100 mg/m^2]
Repeat cycle every 6 weeks

POG-8651

Use Osteosarcoma

Regimen

(Surgery at week 10)
Methotrexate: I.V.: 12 g/m^2 weeks 0, 1, 5, 6, 13, 14, 18, 19, 23, 24, 37, and 38
[total dose/cycle = 144 g/m^2]

Leucovorin: (route not specified): 15 mg every 6 hours for 10 doses, weeks 0, 1, 5, 6, 13, 14, 18, 19, 23, 24, 37, and 38
[total dose/cycle = 1800 mg]
Doxorubicin: I.V.: 37.5 mg/m^2/dose days 1 and 2 of weeks 2, 7, 25, and 28
followed by I.V.: 30 mg/m^2/dose days 1, 2, and 3 of week 20
[total dose/cycle = 390 mg/m^2]
Cisplatin: I.V.: 60 mg/m^2/day days 1 and 2, weeks 2, 7, 25, and 28
[total dose/cycle = 480 mg/m^2]
Cyclophosphamide: I.V.: 600 mg/m^2/day days 1, 2, and 3, weeks 15, 31, 34, 39, and 42
[total dose/cycle = 9000 mg/m^2]
Bleomycin: I.V.: 15 units/m^2/day days 1, 2, and 3, weeks 15, 31, 34, 39, and 42
[total dose/cycle = 225 units/m^2]
Dactinomycin: I.V.: 0.6 mg/m^2/day days 1, 2, and 3, weeks 15, 31, 34, 39, and 42
[total dose/cycle = 9 mg/m^2]
or
(Surgery at week 0)
Methotrexate: 12 g/m^2 weeks 3, 4, 8, 9, 13, 14, 18, 19, 23, 24, 37, and 38
[total dose/cycle = 144 g/m^2]
Leucovorin: (route not specified): 15 mg every 6 hours for 10 doses, weeks 3, 4, 8, 9, 13, 14, 18, 19, 23, 24, 37, and 38
[total dose/cycle = 1800 mg]
Doxorubicin: I.V.: 37.5 mg/m^2/day days 1 and 2, weeks 5, 10, 25, and 28 and 30 mg/m^2 days 1, 2, and 3, week 20
[total dose/cycle = 390 mg/m^2]
Cisplatin: I.V.: 60 mg/m^2/day days 1 and 2, weeks 5, 10, 25, and 28
[total dose/cycle = 480 mg/m^2]
Cyclophosphamide: I.V.: 600 mg/m^2/day days 1, 2, and 3, weeks 15, 31, 34, 39, and 42
[total dose/cycle = 9000 mg/m^2]
Bleomycin: I.V.: 15 units/m^2/day days 1, 2, and 3, weeks 15, 31, 34, 39, and 42
[total dose/cycle = 225 units/m^2]
Dactinomycin: I.V.: 0.6 mg/m^2/day days 1, 2, and 3, weeks 15, 31, 34, 39, and 42
[total dose/cycle = 9 mg/m^2]

POMP

Use Leukemia, acute lymphocytic
Regimen Maintenance:
Mercaptopurine: Oral: 50 mg 3 times/day
[total dose/cycle = 4200-4650 mg]
Methotrexate: Oral: 20 mg/m^2 once weekly
[total dose/cycle = 80 mg/m^2]
Vincristine: I.V.: 2 mg day 1
[total dose/cycle = 2 mg]
Prednisone: Oral: 200 mg/day days 1 to 5
[total dose/cycle = 1000 mg]
Repeat cycle monthly for 2 years

Pro-MACE-CytaBOM

Use Lymphoma, non-Hodgkin
Regimen
Prednisone: Oral: 60 mg/m^2/day days 1 to 14
[total dose/cycle = 840 mg/m^2]
Doxorubicin: I.V.: 25 mg/m^2 day 1
[total dose/cycle = 25 mg/m^2]
Cyclophosphamide: I.V.: 650 mg/m^2 day 1
[total dose/cycle = 650 mg/m^2]
Etoposide: I.V.: 120 mg/m^2 day 1
[total dose/cycle = 120 mg/m^2]
Cytarabine: I.V.: 300 mg/m^2 day 8
[total dose/cycle = 300 mg/m^2]
Bleomycin: I.V.: 5 units/m^2 day 8
[total dose/cycle = 5 units/m^2]

Vincristine: I.V.: 1.4 mg/m^2 (maximum dose:: 2 mg) day 8
[total dose/cycle = 1.4 mg/m^2]
Methotrexate: I.V.: 120 mg/m^2 day 8
[total dose/cycle = 120 mg/m^2]
Leucovorin: Oral: 25 mg/m^2 every 6 hours for 4 doses (start 24 hours after methotrexate dose) day 9
[total dose/cycle = 100 mg/m^2]
Repeat cycle every 21 days

PVA (POG 8602)

Use Leukemia, acute lymphocytic

Regimen

Induction:

Prednisone: Oral: 40 mg/m^2/day (maximum dose: 60 mg) given in 3 divided doses days 0 to 28
[total dose/cycle = 1160 mg/m^2]
Vincristine: I.V.: 1.5 mg/m^2/day (maximum dose: 2 mg) days 0, 7, 14, and 21
[total dose/cycle = 6 mg/m^2; maximum dose: 8 mg]
Asparaginase: I.M.: 6000 units/m^2 3 times per week for 2 weeks
[total dose/cycle = 36,000 units/m^2]
Intrathecal therapy (triple): Days 0 and 22
Leucovorin: Route and dose not specified: Single dose 24 hours after every intrathecal treatment days 1 and 23
Administer one cycle only

CNS consolidation:

Mercaptopurine: Oral: 75 mg/m^2/day days 29 to 43
[total dose/cycle = 1125 mg/m^2]
Intrathecal therapy (triple): Days 29 and 36
Leucovorin: Route and dose not specified: Single dose 24 hours after every intrathecal treatment days 30 and 37
Administer one cycle only

Intensification:

Regimen A:

Methotrexate: I.V.: 1000 mg/m^2 continuous infusion over 24 hours day 1
[total dose/cycle = 1000 mg/m^2]
Cytarabine: I.V.: 1000 mg/m^2 continuous infusion over 24 hours day 1 (start 12 hours after start of methotrexate)
[total dose/cycle = 1000 mg/m^2]
Leucovorin: I.M., I.V., or Oral: 30 mg/m^2 at 24 and 36 hours after the start of methotrexate
[total dose/cycle = 60 mg/m^2]
followed by I.M., I.V., or Oral: 3 mg/m^2 at 48, 60, and 72 hours after the start of methotrexate
[total dose/cycle = 9 mg/m^2]
Repeat cycle every 3 weeks for 6 cycles (administered weeks 7, 10, 13, 16, 19, and 22)
Intrathecal therapy (triple): Weeks 9, 12, 15, and 18
Leucovorin: Route and dose not specified: Single dose 24 hours after every intrathecal treatment weeks 9, 12, 15, and 18

or

Regimen B:

Methotrexate: I.V.: 1000 mg/m^2 continuous infusion over 24 hours day 1
[total dose/cycle = 1000 mg/m^2]
Cytarabine: I.V.: 1000 mg/m^2 continuous infusion over 24 hours day 1 (start 12 hours after methotrexate)
[total dose/cycle = 1000 mg/m^2]
Leucovorin: I.M., I.V., or Oral: 30 mg/m^2 at 24 and 36 hours after the start of methotrexate
[total dose/cycle = 60 mg/m^2]
followed by I.M., I.V., or Oral: 3 mg/m^2 at 48, 60, and 72 hours after the start of methotrexate
[total dose/cycle = 9 mg/m^2]

Repeat cycle every 12 weeks for 6 cycles (administer weeks 7, 19, 31, 43, 55, and 67)
Intrathecal therapy (triple): Weeks 9, 12, 15, and 18
Leucovorin: Route and dose not specified: Single dose 24 hours after every intrathecal treatment weeks 9, 12, 15, and 18

Maintenance:

Regimen A:

Methotrexate: I.M.: 20 mg/m^2 weekly, weeks 25 to 156
[total dose/cycle = 2640 mg/m^2]
Mercaptopurine: Oral: 75 mg/m^2 daily, weeks 25 to 156
[total dose/cycle = 69,300 mg/m^2]
Intrathecal therapy (triple): Every 8 weeks, weeks 26 through 105
Leucovorin: Route and dose not specified: Single dose 24 hours after every intrathecal treatment weeks 26 through 105
Prednisone: Oral: 40 mg/m^2/day (maximum dose: 60 mg) days 1 to 7 (given in 3 divided doses), weeks 8, 17, 25, 41, 57, 73, 89, and 105
[total dose/cycle = 2240 mg/m^2; maximum 3360 mg]
Vincristine: I.V.: 1.5 mg/m^2/day (maximum dose: 2 mg) day 1, weeks 8, 9, 17, 18, 25, 26, 41, 42, 57, 58, 73, 74, 89, 90, 105, and 106
[total dose/cycle = 24 mg/m^2; maximum dose: 32 mg]

or

Regimen B:

Methotrexate: I.M.: 20 mg/m^2 weekly, weeks 22-28, 34-40, 46-52, and 58-64
[total dose/cycle = 560 mg/m^2]
Mercaptopurine: Oral: 75 mg/m^2 daily for 7 weeks, weeks 22-28, 34-40, 46-52, and 58-64
[total dose/cycle = 14700 mg/m^2]

followed by

Methotrexate: I.M.: 20 mg/m^2 weekly, weeks 70 to 156
[total dose/cycle = 1720 mg/m^2]
Mercaptopurine: Oral: 75 mg/m^2 daily, weeks 70 to 156
[total dose/cycle = 45,150 mg/m^2]
Intrathecal therapy (triple): Every 8 weeks, weeks 26 through 105
Leucovorin: Route and dose not specified: Single dose 24 hours after every intrathecal treatment weeks 26 through 105
Prednisone: Oral: 40 mg/m^2/day (maximum dose: 60 mg) days 1 to 7 (given in 3 divided doses), weeks 8, 17, 25, 41, 57, 73, 89, and 105
[total dose/cycle = 2240 mg/m^2]
Vincristine: I.V.: 1.5 mg/m^2/day (maximum dose: 2 mg) day 1, weeks 8, 9, 17, 18, 25, 26, 41, 42, 57, 58, 73, 74, 89, 90, 105, and 106
[total dose/cycle = 24 mg/m^2; maximum dose: 32 mg]

PVB

Use Testicular cancer

Regimen NOTE: Multiple variations are listed below.

Variation 1:
Cisplatin: I.V.: 20 mg/m^2/day days 1 to 5
[total dose/cycle = 100 mg/m^2]
Vinblastine: I.V.: 0.2 mg/kg/day days 1 and 2
[total dose/cycle = 0.4 mg/kg]
Bleomycin: I.V.: 30 units/day days 2, 9, and 16
[total dose/cycle = 90 units]
Repeat cycle every 3 weeks

Variation 2:
Cisplatin: I.V.: 20 mg/m^2/day days 1 to 5
[total dose/cycle = 100 mg/m^2]
Vinblastine: I.V.: 0.15 mg/kg/day days 1 and 2
[total dose/cycle = 0.3 mg/kg]
Bleomycin: I.V.: 30 units/day days 2, 9, and 16
[total dose/cycle = 90 units]
Repeat cycle every 3 weeks

Variation 3:
Cisplatin: I.V.: 20 mg/m^2/day days 1 to 5
[total dose/cycle = 100 mg/m^2]
Vinblastine: I.V.: 6 mg/m^2/day days 1 and 2
[total dose/cycle = 12 mg/m^2]
Bleomycin: I.M.: 30 units/day days 2, 9, and 16
[total dose/cycle = 90 units]
Repeat cycle every 3 weeks

PVDA

Use Leukemia, acute lymphocytic

Regimen Induction:
Prednisone: Oral: 60 mg/m^2/day days 1 to 28
[total dose/cycle = 1680 mg/m^2]
Vincristine: I.V.: 1.5 mg/m^2/day days 1, 8, 15, and 22
[total dose/cycle = 6 mg/m^2]
Daunorubicin: I.V.: 25 mg/m^2/day days 1, 8, 15, and 22
[total dose/cycle = 100 mg/m^2]
Asparaginase: I.M., SubQ, or I.V.: 5000 units/m^2/day days 1 to 14
[total dose/cycle = 70,000 units/m^2]
Administer one cycle only; used in conjunction with intrathecal chemotherapy

R-CVP

Use Lymphoma, non-Hodgkin

Regimen
Rituximab: I.V.: 375 mg/m^2 day 1
[total dose/cycle = 375 mg/m^2]
Cyclophosphamide: I.V.: 750 mg/m^2 day 1
[total dose/cycle = 750 mg/m^2]
Vincristine: I.V.: 1.4 mg/m^2 day 1
[total dose/cycle = 1.4 mg/m^2]
Prednisone: Oral: 40 mg/m^2/day days 1 to 5
[total dose/cycle = 200 mg/m^2]
Repeat cycle every 21 days

Regimen A1

Use Neuroblastoma

Regimen
Cyclophosphamide: I.V.: 1.2 g/m^2 day 1
[total dose/cycle = 1.2 g/m^2]
Vincristine: I.V.: 1.5 mg/m^2 day 1
[total dose/cycle = 1.5 mg/m^2]
Doxorubicin: I.V.: 40 mg/m^2 day 3
[total dose/cycle = 40 mg/m^2]
Cisplatin: I.V.: 90 mg/m^2 day 5
[total dose/cycle = 90 mg/m^2]
Repeat cycle every 28 days

Regimen A2

Use Neuroblastoma

Regimen
Cyclophosphamide: I.V.: 1.2 g/m^2 day 1
[total dose/cycle = 1.2 g/m^2]
Etoposide: I.V.: 100 mg/m^2/day days 1 to 5
[total dose/cycle = 500 mg/m^2]
Doxorubicin: I.V.: 40 mg/m^2 day 3
[total dose/cycle = 40 mg/m^2]
Cisplatin: I.V.: 90 mg/m^2 day 5
[total dose/cycle = 90 mg/m^2]
Repeat cycle every 28 days

RICE

Use Lymphoma, non-Hodgkin

Regimen

Rituximab: I.V.: 375 mg/m^2/day days -2 and 1 (cycle 1)
[total dose/cycle = 750 mg/m^2]
Rituximab: I.V.: 375 mg/m^2 day 1 (cycles 2 and 3)
[total dose/cycle = 375 mg/m^2]
Etoposide: I.V.: 100 mg/m^2/day days 3, 4, and 5
[total dose/cycle = 300 mg/m^2]
Carboplatin: I.V.: AUC = 5 (maximum: 800 mg) day 4
[total dose/cycle = AUC = 5]
Ifosfamide: I.V.: 5000 mg/m^2 continuous infusion day 4
[total dose/cycle = 5000 mg/m^2]
Mesna: I.V.: 5000 mg/m^2 continuous infusion day 4
[total dose/cycle = 5000 mg/m^2]
Filgrastim: SubQ: 5 mcg/kg/day days 7 to 14 (cycles 1 and 2)
[total dose/cycle = 40 mcg/kg]
Filgrastim: SubQ: 10 mcg/kg/day days 7 to 14 (cycle 3)
[total dose/cycle = 80 mcg/kg]
Repeat cycle every 2 weeks

Rituximab-CHOP

Use Lymphoma, non-Hodgkin

Regimen

Rituximab: I.V.: 375 mg/m^2 day 1
[total dose/cycle = 375 mg/m^2]
Cyclophosphamide: I.V.: 750 mg/m^2 day 1
[total dose/cycle = 750 mg/m^2]
Doxorubicin: I.V.: 50 mg/m^2 day 1
[total dose/cycle = 50 mg/m^2]
Vincristine: I.V.: 1.4 mg/m^2 (maximum: 2 mg) day 1
[total dose/cycle = 1.4 mg/m^2; maximum: 2 mg]
Prednisone: Oral: 40 mg/m^2/day days 1 to 5
[total dose/cycle = 200 mg/m^2]
Repeat cycle every 21 days

Stanford V Regimen

Use Lymphoma, Hodgkin disease

Regimen NOTE: Multiple variations are listed below.

Variation 1:
Mechlorethamine: I.V.: 6 mg/m^2 day 1
[total dose/cycle = 6 mg/m^2]
Doxorubicin: I.V.: 25 mg/m^2/day days 1 and 15
[total dose/cycle = 50 mg/m^2]
Vinblastine: I.V.: 6 mg/m^2/day days 1 and 15
[total dose/cycle = 12 mg/m^2]
Vincristine: I.V.: 1.4 mg/m^2/day (maximum: 2 mg) days 8 and 22
[total dose/cycle = 2.8 mg/m^2; maximum: 4 mg]
Bleomycin: I.V.: 5 units/m^2/day days 8 and 22
[total dose/cycle = 10 units/m^2]
Etoposide: I.V.: 60 mg/m^2/day days 15 and 16
[total dose/cycle = 120 mg/m^2]
Prednisone: Oral: 40 mg/m^2 every other day for 9 weeks
followed by tapering of dose by 10 mg every other day, beginning at week 10
Repeat cycle every 28 days for 3 cycles; **Note:** In cycle 3, for patients ≥50 years of age, decrease vinblastine dose to 4 mg/m^2/dose and decrease vincristine dose to 1 mg/m^2/dose

Variation 2:
Mechlorethamine: I.V.: 6 mg/m^2/dose weeks 1, 5, and 9
[total dose/cycle = 18 mg/m^2]

Doxorubicin: I.V.: 25 mg/m^2/dose weeks 1, 3, 5, 7, 9, and 11
[total dose/cycle = 150 mg/m^2]
Vinblastine: I.V.: 6 mg/m^2/dose weeks 1, 3, 5, 7, 9, and 11
[total dose/cycle = 36 mg/m^2]
Vincristine: I.V.: 1.4 mg/m^2/dose (maximum: 2 mg) weeks 2, 4, 6, 8, 10, and 12
[total dose/cycle = 8.4 mg/m^2; maximum: 12 mg]
Bleomycin: I.V.: 5 units/m^2/dose weeks 2, 4, 6, 8, 10, and 12
[total dose/cycle = 30 units/m^2]
Etoposide: I.V.: 60 mg/m^2/day for 2 consecutive days, weeks 3, 7, and 11
[total dose/cycle = 360 mg/m^2]
Prednisone: Oral: 40 mg/m^2 every other day for 10 weeks
[total dose prior to taper = 1400 mg/m^2]
followed by tapering of prednisone dose during weeks 11 and 12
Treatment cycle is 12 weeks

TAC

Use Breast cancer

Regimen NOTE: Multiple variations are listed below.

Variation 1:
Docetaxel: I.V.: 75 mg/m^2 day 1
[total dose/cycle = 75 mg/m^2]
Doxorubicin: I.V.: 50 mg/m^2 day 1
[total dose/cycle = 50 mg/m^2]
Cyclophosphamide: I.V.: 500 mg/m^2 day 1
[total dose/cycle = 500 mg/m^2]
Repeat cycle every 3 weeks

Variation 2:
Docetaxel: I.V.: 60 mg/m^2 day 1
[total dose/cycle = 60 mg/m^2]
Doxorubicin: I.V.: 60 mg/m^2 day 1
[total dose/cycle = 60 mg/m^2]
Cyclophosphamide: I.V.: 600 mg/m^2 day 1
[total dose/cycle = 600 mg/m^2]
Repeat cycle every 3 weeks

TAD

Use Leukemia, acute myeloid

Regimen

Daunorubicin: I.V.: 60 mg/m^2/day days 3, 4, and 5
[total dose/cycle = 180 mg/m^2]
Cytarabine: I.V.: 100 mg/m^2/day continuous infusion days 1 and 2
[total dose/cycle = 200 mg/m^2]
followed by I.V.: 100 mg/m^2/day over 30 minutes every 12 hours days 3 to 8
[total dose/cycle = 1200 mg/m^2]
Thioguanine: Oral: 100 mg/m^2/day every 12 hours days 3 to 9
[total dose/cycle = 1400 mg/m^2]
Administer one cycle only

Tamoxifen-Epirubicin

Use Breast cancer

Regimen

Tamoxifen: Oral: 20 mg daily
[total dose/cycle = 560 mg]
Epirubicin: I.V.: 50 mg/m^2/day days 1 and 8
[total dose/cycle = 100 mg/m^2]
Repeat epirubicin cycle every 28 days for 6 cycles; continue tamoxifen for 4 years

TEX (Capecitabine + Docetaxel + Epirubicin)

Use Breast cancer

Regimen

Capecitabine: Oral: 1000 mg/m^2 twice daily days 1 to 14
[total dose/cycle = 28,000 mg/m^2]
Docetaxel: I.V.: 75 mg/m^2 day 1
[total dose/cycle = 75 mg/m^2]
Epirubicin: I.V.: 75 mg/m^2 day 1
[total dose/cycle = 75 mg/m^2]
Repeat cycle every 3 weeks

Thalidomide-Dexamethasone

Use Multiple myeloma

Regimen Note: Multiple variations are listed below.

Variation 1:
Thalidomide: Oral: 100 mg/day days 1 to 28
[total dose/cycle = 2800 mg]
Dexamethasone: Oral: 40 mg/day days 1 to 4
[total dose/cycle = 160 mg]
Repeat cycle every 28 days
Variation 2:
Thalidomide: Oral: 200 mg/day days 1 to 14 cycle 1
followed by Oral: 400 mg/day days 15 to 28 cycle 1
[total dose/cycle = 8400 mg]
Thalidomide: Oral: 400 mg/day days 1 to 28 (subsequent cycles)
[total dose/cycle = 11,200 mg]
Dexamethasone: Oral: 20 mg/m^2/day days 1 to 4, 9 to 12, and 17 to 20 cycle 1 (subsequent cycles)
[total dose/cycle = 240 mg/m^2]
followed by Oral: 20 mg/m^2/day days 1 to 4 (subsequent cycles)
[total dose/cycle = 80 mg/m^2]
Repeat cycle every 28 days
Variation 3:
Thalidomide: Oral: 100 mg/day days 1 to 7, 150 mg/day days 8 to 14, 200 mg/day days 15 to 21, 250 mg/day days 22 to 28, and 300 mg/day days 29 to 35 (cycle 1)
[total dose/cycle = 7000 mg]
Thalidomide: Oral: 300 mg/day days 1 to 35 (subsequent cycles)
[total dose/cycle = 10,500 mg]
Dexamethasone: Oral: 20 mg/m^2/day days 1 to 4, 9 to 12, and 17 to 20
[total dose/cycle = 240 mg/m^2]
Repeat cycle every 35 days
Variation 4:
Thalidomide: Oral: 200 mg/day days 1 to 28
[total dose/cycle = 5600 mg]
Dexamethasone: Oral: 40 mg/day days 1 to 4, 9 to 12, and 17 to 20 (odd cycles)
[total dose/cycle = 480 mg]
Dexamethasone: Oral: 40 mg/day days 1 to 4 (even cycles)
[total dose/cycle = 160 mg]
Repeat cycle every 28 days

TIP

Use Esophageal cancer; Head and neck cancer

Regimen

Paclitaxel: I.V.: 175 mg/m^2 day 1
[total dose/cycle = 175 mg/m^2]
Ifosfamide: I.V.: 1000 mg/m^2/day days 1, 2, and 3
[total dose/cycle = 3000 mg/m^2]

Mesna: I.V.: 400 mg/m^2/day before ifosfamide days 1, 2, and 3
plus I.V.: 200 mg/m^2 4 hours after ifosfamide days 1, 2, and 3
[total dose/cycle = 1800 mg/m^2]
Cisplatin: I.V.: 60 mg/m^2 day 1
[total dose/cycle = 60 mg/m^2]
Repeat cycle every 21-28 days

Topotecan-Cisplatin

Use Cervical cancer

Regimen Note: Body surface area capped at 2 m^2 maximum
Topotecan: I.V.: 0.75 mg/m^2/day days 1, 2, and 3
[total dose/cycle = 2.25 mg/m^2]
Cisplatin: I.V.: 50 mg/m^2 day 1 only
[total dose/cycle = 50 mg/m^2]
Repeat cycle every 21 days

Topotecan (Oral)-Cisplatin

Use Lung cancer, small cell

Regimen
Topotecan: Oral: 1.7 mg/m^2/day days 1 to 5
[total dose/cycle = 8.5 mg/m^2]
Cisplatin: I.V.: 60 mg/m^2 day 5 only
[total dose/cycle = 60 mg/m^2]
Repeat cycle every 21 days for 4 cycles (or for 2 cycles beyond best response)

Topotecan (Oral Regimen)

Use Lung cancer, nonsmall cell; Lung cancer, small cell; Ovarian cancer

Regimen
Topotecan: Oral: 2.3 mg/m^2/day days 1 to 5
[total dose/cycle = 11.5 mg/m^2]
Repeat cycle every 21 days

Topotecan (Weekly)

Use Lung cancer, small cell; Ovarian cancer

Regimen
Topotecan: I.V.: 4 mg/m^2/day days 1, 8, and 15
[total dose/cycle = 12 mg/m^2]
Repeat cycle every 28 days

Trastuzumab-Paclitaxel

Use Breast cancer

Regimen NOTE: Multiple variations are listed below.
Variation 1:
Cycle 1:
Paclitaxel: I.V.: 175 mg/m^2 day 1
[total dose/cycle = 175 mg/m^2]
Trastuzumab: I.V.: 4 mg/kg (loading dose) day 1
followed by I.V.: 2 mg/kg/day days 8 and 15
[total dose/cycle 1 = 8 mg/kg]
Treatment cycle is 21 days
Subsequent cycles:
Paclitaxel: I.V.: 175 mg/m^2 day 1
[total dose/cycle = 175 mg/m^2]
Trastuzumab: I.V.: 2 mg/kg/day days 1, 8, and 15
[total dose/cycle = 6 mg/kg]
Repeat cycle every 21 days for a total of at least 6 cycles
Variation 2:
Cycle 1:
Trastuzumab: I.V.: 4 mg/kg (loading dose) day 1
followed by I.V.: 2 mg/kg/day days 8 and 15
[total dose/cycle 1 = 8 mg/kg]

Paclitaxel: I.V.: 175 mg/m^2 day 2
[total dose/cycle = 175 mg/m^2]
Treatment cycle is 21 days
Subsequent cycles:
Trastuzumab: I.V.: 2 mg/kg/day days 1, 8, and 15
[total dose/cycle = 6 mg/kg]
Paclitaxel: I.V.: 175 mg/m^2 day 2
[total dose/cycle = 175 mg/m^2]
Repeat cycle every 21 days for a total of at least 6 cycles (continue weekly trastuzumab after chemotherapy until disease progression or unacceptable toxicity)

Trastuzumab-Paclitaxel-Carboplatin

Use Breast cancer

Regimen

Cycle 1:
Trastuzumab: I.V.: 4 mg/kg (loading dose) day 1
followed by I.V.: 2 mg/kg/day days 8 and 15
[total dose/cycle 1 = 8 mg/kg]
Paclitaxel: I.V.: 175 mg/m^2 day 2
[total dose/cycle = 175 mg/m^2]
Carboplatin: I.V.: AUC 6 day 2
[total dose/cycle = AUC = 6]
Treatment cycle is 21 days
Subsequent cycles:
Trastuzumab: I.V.: 2 mg/kg/day days 1, 8, and 15
[total dose/cycle = 6 mg/kg]
Paclitaxel: I.V.: 175 mg/m^2 day 2
[total dose/cycle = 175 mg/m^2]
Carboplatin: I.V.: AUC 6 day 2
[total dose/cycle = AUC = 6]
Repeat cycle every 21 days for a total of at least 6 cycles (continue weekly trastuzumab after chemotherapy until disease progression or unacceptable toxicity)

Trastuzumab-Paclitaxel (Weekly)

Use Breast cancer

Regimen NOTE: Multiple variations are listed below.

Variation 1:
Week 1:
Trastuzumab: I.V.: 4 mg/kg (loading dose) day 1
[total dose/week 1 = 4 mg/kg]
Paclitaxel: I.V.: 90 mg/m^2 day 2
[total dose/week 1 = 90 mg/m^2]
Subsequent weeks:
Paclitaxel: I.V.: 90 mg/m^2 day 1
[total dose/week = 90 mg/m^2]
Trastuzumab: I.V.: 2 mg/kg day 1
[total dose/week = 2 mg/kg]
Repeat weekly
Variation 2:
Week 1:
Trastuzumab: I.V.: 4 mg/kg (loading dose) day 1
[total dose/week 1 = 4 mg/kg]
Paclitaxel: I.V.: 80 mg/m^2 day 1
[total dose/week 1 = 80 mg/m^2]
Subsequent weeks:
Trastuzumab: I.V.: 2 mg/kg day 1
[total dose/week = 2 mg/kg]
Paclitaxel: I.V.: 80 mg/m^2 day 1
[total dose/week = 80 mg/m^2]
Repeat weekly

Tretinoin-Idarubicin

Use Leukemia, acute promyelocytic

Regimen NOTE: Multiple variations are listed below.

Variation 1:

Induction:

Tretinoin: Oral: 45 mg/m^2/day (in 2 divided doses) day 1 up to 90 days
[total dose/cycle = up to 4050 mg/m^2]
≤20 years: Oral: 25 mg/m^2/day (in 2 divided doses) day 1 up to 90 days
[total dose/cycle = up to 2250 mg/m^2]
Idarubicin: I.V.: 12 mg/m^2/day days 2, 4, 6, and 8 (omit day 8 for patients >70 years of age)
[total dose/cycle = 36-48 mg/m^2]

Consolidation (administer courses sequentially at 1-month intervals for 3 months):

Course 1:
Idarubicin: I.V.: 5 mg/m^2/day days 1 to 4
[total dose/cycle = 20 mg/m^2]
or
Idarubicin: I.V.: 7 mg/m^2/day days 1 to 4
[total dose/cycle = 28 mg/m^2]
Tretinoin: Oral: 45 mg/m^2/day (in 2 divided doses) days 1 to 15
[total dose/cycle = 675 mg/m^2]

Course 2:
Mitoxantrone: I.V.: 10 mg/m^2/day days 1 to 5
[total dose/cycle = 50 mg/m^2]
or
Mitoxantrone: I.V.: 10 mg/m^2/day days 1 to 5
[total dose/cycle = 50 mg/m^2]
Tretinoin: Oral: 45 mg/m^2/day (in 2 divided doses) days 1 to 15
[total dose/cycle = 675 mg/m^2]

Course 3:
Idarubicin: I.V.: 12 mg/m^2 day 1
[total dose/cycle = 12 mg/m^2]
or
Idarubicin: I.V.: 12 mg/m^2/day days 1 and 2
[total dose/cycle = 24 mg/m^2]
Tretinoin: Oral: 45 mg/m^2/day (in 2 divided doses) days 1 to 15
[total dose/cycle = 675 mg/m^2]

Maintenance:

Mercaptopurine: Oral: 50 mg/m^2 daily
[total dose/cycle = 4500 mg/m^2 (90 days)]
Methotrexate: I.M.: 15 mg/m^2 weekly
[total dose/cycle = 180 mg/m^2]
Tretinoin: Oral: 45 mg/m^2/day (in 2 divided doses) days 1 to 15
[total dose/cycle = 675 mg/m^2]
Repeat cycle every 3 months for 2 years

Variation 2:

Induction:

Tretinoin: Oral: 45 mg/m^2/day (in 2 divided doses) day 1 up to 90 days
[total dose/cycle = up to 4050 mg/m^2]
<15 years: Oral: 25 mg/m^2/day (in 2 divided doses) day 1 up to 90 days
[total dose/cycle = up to 2250 mg/m^2]
Idarubicin: I.V.: 12 mg/m^2/day days 2, 4, 6, and 8
[total dose/cycle = 48 mg/m^2]

Consolidation (administer courses sequentially at 1-month intervals for 3 months):

Course 1:
Idarubicin: I.V.: 5 mg/m^2/day days 1 to 4
[total dose/cycle = 20 mg/m^2]

Course 2:
Mitoxantrone: I.V.: 10 mg/m^2/day days 1 to 5
[total dose/cycle = 50 mg/m^2]

Course 3:
Idarubicin: I.V.: 12 mg/m^2 day 1
[total dose/cycle = 12 mg/m^2]
Maintenance:
Mercaptopurine: Oral: 90 mg/m^2 daily
[total dose/cycle = 8100 mg/m^2(90 days)]
Methotrexate: I.M.: 15 mg/m^2 weekly
[total dose/cycle = 180 mg/m^2]
Tretinoin: Oral: 45 mg/m^2/day (in 2 divided doses) days 1 to 15
[total dose/cycle = 675 mg/m^2]
Repeat cycle every 3 months for 2 years
Variation 3 (patients ≥60 years of age):
Induction:
Tretinoin: Oral: 45 mg/m^2/day (in 2 divided doses) day 1 up to 90 days
[total dose/cycle = up to 4050 mg/m^2]
Idarubicin: I.V.: 12 mg/m^2/day days 2, 4, 6, and 8 (omit day 8 for patients ≥70 years of age)
[total dose/cycle = 36-48 mg/m^2]
Consolidation (administer courses sequentially at 1-month intervals for 3 months):
Course 1:
Idarubicin: I.V.: 5 mg/m^2/day days 1 to 4
[total dose/cycle = 20 mg/m^2]
Tretinoin: Oral: 45 mg/m^2/day (in 2 divided doses) days 1 to 15 (if intermediate or high risk)
[total dose/cycle = 675 mg/m^2]
Course 2:
Mitoxantrone: I.V.: 10 mg/m^2/day days 1 to 5
[total dose/cycle = 50 mg/m^2]
Tretinoin: Oral: 45 mg/m^2/day (in 2 divided doses) days 1 to 15 (if intermediate or high risk)
[total dose/cycle = 675 mg/m^2]
Course 3:
Idarubicin: I.V.: 12 mg/m^2 day 1
[total dose/cycle = 12 mg/m^2]
Tretinoin: Oral: 45 mg/m^2/day (in 2 divided doses) days 1 to 15 (if intermediate or high risk)
[total dose/cycle = 675 mg/m^2]
Maintenance:
Mercaptopurine: Oral: 50 mg/m^2 daily
[total dose/cycle = 4500 mg/m^2 (90 days)]
Methotrexate: I.M.: 15 mg/m^2 weekly
[total dose/cycle = 180 mg/m^2]
Tretinoin: Oral: 45 mg/m^2/day (in 2 divided doses) days 1 to 15
[total dose/cycle = 675 mg/m^2]
Repeat cycle every 3 months for 2 years

TVTG

Use Leukemia, acute lymphocytic; Leukemia, acute myeloid

Regimen

Topotecan: I.V.: 1 mg/m^2/day continuous infusion days 1 to 5
[total dose/cycle = 5 mg/m^2]
Vinorelbine: I.V.: 20 mg/m^2/day days 0, 7, 14, and 21
[total dose/cycle = 80 mg/m^2]
Thiotepa: I.V.: 15 mg/m^2 day 2
Gemcitabine: I.V.: 3600 mg/m^2 day 7
Dexamethasone: Oral or I.V.: 45 mg/m^2/day days 7 to 14 (given in 3 divided doses)
[total dose/cycle = 315 mg/m^2]
Repeat cycle when ANC >500 cells/mm^3 and platelet count >75,000 cells/mm^3

VAC Alternating With IE (Ewing Sarcoma)

Use Ewing sarcoma

Regimen

Cycle A: (Odd numbered cycles)
Cyclophosphamide: I.V.: 1200 mg/m^2 day 1 (followed by mesna; dose not specified)
[total dose/cycle = 1200 mg/m^2]

Vincristine: I.V.: 2 mg/m^2 (maximum: 2 mg) day 1
[total dose/cycle = 2 mg/m^2; maximum 2 mg]
Doxorubicin: I.V.: 75 mg/m^2 day 1, for 5 cycles (maximum cumulative dose: 375 mg/m^2)
[total dose/cycle = 75 mg/m^2; maximum cumulative dose: 375 mg/m^2]
Dactinomycin: I.V.: 1.25 mg/m^2 day 1, begin cycle 11 (after reaching maximum cumulative doxorubicin dose)
[total dose/cycle = 1.25 mg/m^2]
Cycle B: (Even numbered cycles)
Ifosfamide: I.V.: 1800 mg/m^2/day days 1 to 5 (given with mesna)
[total dose/cycle = 9000 mg/m^2]
Etoposide: I.V.: 100 mg/m^2/day days 1 to 5
[total dose/cycle = 500 mg/m^2]
Alternate Cycles A and B, administering a cycle every 3 weeks (alternating in the following sequence: ABABAB) for 17 cycles

VAC Pulse

Use Rhabdomyosarcoma

Regimen

Vincristine: I.V.: 2 mg/m^2/dose (maximum dose: 2 mg/dose) every 7 days, for 12 weeks
Dactinomycin: I.V.: 0.015 mg/kg/day (maximum dose: 0.5 mg/day) days 1 to 5, every 3 months for 5 courses
Cyclophosphamide: Oral, I.V.: 10 mg/kg/day for 7 days, repeat every 6 weeks

VAC (Rhabdomyosarcoma)

Use Rhabdomyosarcoma

Regimen

Induction (weeks 1 to 17):
Vincristine: I.V. push: 1.5 mg/m^2 (maximum: 2 mg) day 1 of weeks 1 to 13, then one dose at week 17
Dactinomycin: I.V. push: 0.015 mg/kg/day (maximum: 0.5 mg) days 1 to 5 of weeks 1, 4, 7, and 17
Cyclophosphamide: I.V.: 2.2 g/m^2 day 1 of weeks 1, 4, 7, 10, 13, and 17
Continuation (weeks 21 to 44):
Vincristine: I.V. push: 1.5 mg/m^2 (maximum: 2 mg) day 1 of weeks 21 to 26, 30 to 35, and 39 to 44
Dactinomycin: I.V. push: 0.015 mg/kg/day (maximum: 0.5 mg) days 1 to 5 of weeks 21, 24, 30, 33, 39, and 42
Cyclophosphamide: I.V.: 2.2 g/m^2 day 1 of weeks 21, 24, 30, 33, 39, and 42

VAD

Use Multiple myeloma

Regimen

Vincristine: I.V.: 0.4 mg/day continuous infusion days 1 to 4
[total dose/cycle = 1.6 mg]
Doxorubicin: I.V.: 9 mg/m^2/day continuous infusion days 1 to 4
[total dose/cycle = 36 mg/m^2]
Dexamethasone: Oral: 40 mg/day days 1 to 4, 9 to 12, and 17 to 20
[total dose/cycle = 480 mg]
Repeat cycle every 28-35 days

VAD/CVAD

Use Leukemia, acute lymphocytic

Regimen Induction cycle:

Vincristine: I.V.: 0.4 mg/day continuous infusion days 1 to 4 and 24 to 27
[total dose/cycle = 3.2 mg]
Doxorubicin: I.V.: 12 mg/m^2/day continuous infusion days 1 to 4 and 24 to 27
[total dose/cycle = 96 mg/m^2]
Dexamethasone: Oral: 40 mg/day days 1 to 4, 9 to 12, 17 to 20, 24 to 27, 32 to 35, and 40 to 43
[total dose/cycle = 960 mg]

Cyclophosphamide: I.V.: 1 g/m^2 day 24
[total dose/cycle = 1 g/m^2]
Administer one cycle only

VATH

Use Breast cancer

Regimen

Vinblastine: I.V.: 4.5 mg/m^2 day 1
[total dose/cycle = 4.5 mg/m^2]
Doxorubicin: I.V.: 45 mg/m^2 day 1
[total dose/cycle = 45 mg/m^2]
Thiotepa: I.V.: 12 mg/m^2 day 1
[total dose/cycle = 12 mg/m^2]
Fluoxymesterone: Oral: 10 mg 3 times/day days 1 to 21
[total dose/cycle = 630 mg]
Repeat cycle every 21 days

VBAP

Use Multiple myeloma

Regimen

Vincristine: I.V.: 1 mg day 1
[total dose/cycle = 1 mg]
Carmustine: I.V.: 30 mg/m^2 day 1
[total dose/cycle = 30 mg/m^2]
Doxorubicin: I.V.: 30 mg/m^2 day 1
[total dose/cycle = 30 mg/m^2]
Prednisone: Oral: 100 mg/day days 1 to 4
[total dose/cycle = 400 mg]
Repeat cycle every 21 days

VBMCP

Use Multiple myeloma

Regimen

Vincristine: I.V.: 1.2 mg/m^2 (maximum: 2 mg) day 1
[total dose/cycle = 1.2 mg/m^2; maximum: 2 mg]
Carmustine: I.V.: 20 mg/m^2 day 1
[total dose/cycle = 20 mg/m^2]
Melphalan: Oral: 8 mg/m^2/day days 1 to 4
[total dose/cycle = 32 mg/m^2]
Cyclophosphamide: I.V.: 400 mg/m^2 day 1
[total dose/cycle = 400 mg/m^2]
Prednisone: Oral: 40 mg/m^2/day days 1 to 7 (all cycles)
[total dose/cycle = 280 mg/m^2]
followed by Oral: 20 mg/m^2/day days 8 to 14 (first 3 cycles only)
[total dose/cycle = 140 mg/m^2]
Repeat cycle every 35 days

VBP

Use Testicular cancer

Regimen

Vinblastine: I.V.: 0.15 mg/kg/day days 1 and 2
[total dose/cycle = 0.3 mg/kg]
Bleomycin: I.V.: 30 units/day days 2, 9, and 16
[total dose/cycle = 90 units]
Cisplatin: I.V.: 20 mg/m^2/day days 1 to 5
[total dose/cycle = 100 mg/m^2]
Repeat cycle every 21 days for 4 cycles

VCAP

Use Multiple myeloma

Regimen

Vincristine: I.V.: 1 mg/m^2 (maximum: 1.5 mg) day 1
[total dose/cycle = 1 mg/m^2]
Cyclophosphamide: Oral: 125 mg/m^2/day days 1 to 4
[total dose/cycle = 500 mg/m^2]
Doxorubicin: I.V.: 30 mg/m^2 day 1
[total dose/cycle = 30 mg/m^2]
Prednisone: Oral: 60 mg/m^2/day days 1 to 4
[total dose/cycle = 240 mg/m^2]
Repeat cycle every 21 days for 6-12 months

VD

Use Breast cancer

Regimen

Vinorelbine: I.V.: 25 mg/m^2/day days 1 and 8
[total dose/cycle = 50 mg/m^2]
Doxorubicin: I.V.: 50 mg/m^2 day 1
[total dose/cycle = 50 mg/m^2]
Repeat cycle every 3 weeks

VIM-D (Hodgkin Lymphoma)

Use Lymphoma, Hodgkin disease

Regimen

Cycle 1:
Etoposide: I.V.: 100 mg/m^2 day 1
[total dose/cycle = 100 mg/m^2]
Ifosfamide: I.V.: 4 g/m^2 continuous infusion over 24 hours day 1
[total dose/cycle = 4 g/m^2]
Mesna: I.V.: 1 g/m^2 bolus day 1, followed by 6 g/m^2 continuous infusion over 36 hours
[total dose/cycle = 7 g/m^2]
Mitoxantrone: I.V.: 10 mg/m^2 day 1
[total dose/cycle = 10 mg/m^2]
Dexamethasone: Oral: 40 mg/day days 1 to 5
[total dose/cycle = 200 mg]
Treatment cycle is 28 days
Cycle 2 and subsequent cycles (if mid-cycle neutrophil count >1500/mm^3; if not, continue with cycle 1 regimen):
Etoposide: I.V.: 100 mg/m^2/day days 1 and 2
[total dose/cycle = 200 mg/m^2]
Ifosfamide: I.V.: 4 g/m^2 continuous infusion over 24 hours day 1
[total dose/cycle = 4 g/m^2]
Mesna: I.V.: 1 g/m^2 bolus day 1, followed by 6 g/m^2 continuous infusion over 36 hours
[total dose/cycle = 7 g/m^2]
Mitoxantrone: I.V.: 10 mg/m^2 day 1
[total dose/cycle = 10 mg/m^2]
Dexamethasone: Oral: 40 mg/day days 1 to 5
[total dose/cycle = 200 mg]
Repeat cycle every 28 days for up to 6 cycles

Vincristine-Dactinomycin-Cyclophosphamide (Ovarian Cancer)

Use Ovarian cancer (germ cell tumor)

Regimen NOTE: Multiple variations are listed below.

Variation 1:
Vincristine: I.V.: 1.5 mg/m^2 (maximum: 2 mg) days 1, 8, 15, and 22 for 2-3 cycles
[total dose/cycle = 6 mg/m^2 (maximum: 8 mg)] for 2-3 cycles
Dactinomycin: I.V.: 300 mcg/m^2/day days 1 to 5
[total dose/cycle = 1500 mcg/m^2]

Cyclophosphamide: I.V.: 150 mg/m^2/day days 1 to 5
[total dose/cycle = 750 mg/m^2]
Repeat cycle every 4 weeks for at least 10 cycles; vincristine is only administered for 8-12 weeks
Variation 2:
Vincristine: I.V.: 1-1.5 mg/m^2 day 1
[total dose/cycle = 1-1.5 mg/m^2]
Dactinomycin: I.V.: 500 mcg/day days 1 to 5
[total dose/cycle = 2500 mcg]
Cyclophosphamide: I.V.: 5-7 mg/kg/day days 1 to 5
[total dose/cycle = 25-35 mg/kg]
Repeat cycle every 4 weeks for up to 12 cycles

Vinorelbine-Cisplatin

Use Lung cancer, nonsmall cell

Regimen NOTE: Multiple variations are listed below.
Variation 1:
Cisplatin: I.V.: 50 mg/m^2/day days 1 and 8
[total dose/cycle = 100 mg/m^2]
Vinorelbine: I.V.: 25 mg/m^2/day days 1, 8, 15, and 22
[total dose/cycle = 100 mg/m^2]
Repeat cycle every 28 days for total of 4 cycles
Variation 2:
Vinorelbine: I.V.: 25 mg/m^2/day days 1, 8, 15, and 22
[total dose/cycle = 100 mg/m^2]
Cisplatin: I.V.: 100 mg/m^2 day 1
[total dose/cycle = 100 mg/m^2]
Repeat cycle every 28 days
Variation 3:
Vinorelbine: I.V.: 30 mg/m^2 weekly
Cisplatin: I.V.: 120 mg/m^2/day days 1 and 29, then once every 6 weeks
Variation 4:
Vinorelbine: I.V.: 30 mg/m^2/day days 1, 8, and 15
[total dose/cycle = 90 mg/m^2]
Cisplatin: I.V.: 80 mg/m^2 day 1
[total dose/cycle = 80 mg/m^2]
Repeat cycle every 21 days for total of 4 cycles
Note: Vinorelbine treatment is discontinued after day 1 of cycle 4
Variation 5:
Vinorelbine: I.V.: 30 mg/m^2/day days 1, 8, 15, and 22
[total dose/cycle = 120 mg/m^2]
Cisplatin: I.V.: 100 mg/m^2 day 1
[total dose/cycle = 100 mg/m^2]
Repeat cycle every 28 days for total of 3 or 4 cycles
Note: Vinorelbine treatment is discontinued after day 1 of last treatment cycle

Vinorelbine-FEC

Use Breast cancer

Regimen
Cycles 1 and 2:
Vinorelbine: I.V.: 25 mg/m^2/day days 1, 8, and 15
[total dose/cycle = 75 mg/m^2]
Treatment cycle is 21 days
Cycle 3:
Vinorelbine: I.V.: 25 mg/m^2/day days 1 and 8
[total dose/cycle 3 = 50 mg/m^2]
Treatment cycle is 21 days
Cycles 4, 5, and 6 (FEC):
Fluorouracil: I.V.: 600 mg/m^2 day 1
[total dose/cycle = 600 mg/m^2]
Epirubicin: I.V.: 60 mg/m^2 day 1
[total dose/cycle = 60 mg/m^2]

Cyclophosphamide: I.V.: 600 mg/m^2 day 1
[total dose/cycle = 600 mg/m^2]
Repeat FEC cycle every 21 days for total of 3 cycles

Vinorelbine-Gemcitabine

Use Lung cancer, nonsmall cell

Regimen

Vinorelbine: I.V.: 20 mg/m^2/day days 1, 8, and 15
[total dose/cycle = 60 mg/m^2]
Gemcitabine: I.V.: 800 mg/m^2/day days 1, 8, and 15
[total dose/cycle = 2400 mg/m^2]
Repeat cycle every 28 days

Vinorelbine-Trastuzumab

Use Breast cancer

Regimen

Week 1:
Trastuzumab: I.V.: 4 mg/kg (loading dose) day 1 week 1
[total dose/week 1 = 4 mg/kg]
Vinorelbine: I.V.: 25 mg/m^2 day 1
[total dose/week 1 = 25 mg/m^2]
Subsequent weeks:
Trastuzumab: I.V.: 2 mg/kg (loading dose) day 1
[total dose/week = 2 mg/kg]
Vinorelbine: I.V.: 25 mg/m^2 day 1
[total dose/week = 25 mg/m^2]
Repeat weekly

Vinorelbine-Trastuzumab-FEC

Use Breast cancer

Regimen

Cycle 1:
Trastuzumab: I.V.: 4 mg/kg (loading dose) day 1 cycle 1
followed by I.V.: 2 mg/kg/day days 8 and 15 cycle 1
[total dose/cycle 1 = 8 mg/kg]
Vinorelbine: I.V.: 25 mg/m^2/day days 1, 8, and 15
[total dose/cycle 1 = 75 mg/m^2]
Treatment cycle is 21 days
Cycle 2:
Trastuzumab: I.V.: 2 mg/kg/day days 1, 8, and 15
[total dose/cycle = 6 mg/kg]
Vinorelbine: I.V.: 25 mg/m^2/day days 1, 8, and 15
[total dose/cycle 2 = 75 mg/m^2]
Treatment cycle is 21 days
Cycle 3:
Trastuzumab: I.V.: 2 mg/kg/day days 1, 8, and 15
[total dose/cycle = 6 mg/kg]
Vinorelbine: I.V.: 25 mg/m^2/day days 1 and 8
[total dose/cycle 3 = 50 mg/m^2]
Treatment cycle is 21 days
Cycles 4, 5, and 6 (FEC):
Fluorouracil: I.V.: 600 mg/m^2 day 1
[total dose/cycle = 600 mg/m^2]
Epirubicin: I.V.: 60 mg/m^2 day 1
[total dose/cycle = 60 mg/m^2]
Cyclophosphamide: I.V.: 600 mg/m^2 day 1
[total dose/cycle = 600 mg/m^2]
Repeat FEC cycle every 21 days for total of 3 cycles

VIP (Etoposide) (Testicular Cancer)

Use Testicular cancer

Regimen NOTE: Multiple variations are listed below.

Variation 1:

Etoposide: I.V.: 75 mg/m^2/day days 1 to 5
[total dose/cycle = 375 mg/m^2]
Ifosfamide: I.V.: 1200 mg/m^2/day days 1 to 5
[total dose/cycle = 6000 mg/m^2]
Cisplatin: I.V.: 20 mg/m^2/day days 1 to 5
[total dose/cycle = 100 mg/m^2]
Mesna: I.V.: 400 mg day 1 only
followed by I.V.: 1200 mg/day continuous infusion days 1 to 5
[total dose/cycle = 6400 mg]
Repeat cycle every 21 days for 4 cycles

Variation 2:

Etoposide: I.V.: 100 mg/m^2/day days 1 to 5
[total dose/cycle = 500 mg/m^2]
Ifosfamide: I.V.: 1200 mg/m^2/day days 1 to 5
[total dose/cycle = 6000 mg/m^2]
Cisplatin: I.V.: 20 mg/m^2/day days 1 to 5
[total dose/cycle = 100 mg/m^2]
Mesna: I.V.: 200 mg/m^2 every 4 hours, for 3 doses each day, days 1, 2, and 3
[total dose/cycle = 1800 mg/m^2]
Repeat cycle every 21 days

Variation 3:

Ifosfamide: I.V.: 2500 mg/m^2/day days 1 and 2
[total dose/cycle = 5000 mg/m^2]
Mesna: I.V.: 2400 mg/m^2/day days 1 and 2
[total dose/cycle = 4800 mg/m^2]
Etoposide: I.V.: 100 mg/m^2/day days 3, 4, and 5
[total dose/cycle = 300 mg/m^2]
Cisplatin: I.V.: 40 mg/m^2/day days 3, 4, and 5
[total dose/cycle = 120 mg/m^2]
Repeat cycle every 21 days

Variation 4:

Etoposide: I.V.: 75 mg/m^2/day days 1 to 5
[total dose/cycle = 375 mg/m^2]
Ifosfamide: I.V.: 1200 mg/m^2/day days 1 to 5
[total dose/cycle = 6000 mg/m^2]
Cisplatin: I.V.: 20 mg/m^2/day days 1 to 5
[total dose/cycle = 100 mg/m^2]
Mesna: I.V.: 120 mg/m^2 day 1 only
followed by I.V.: 1200 mg/m^2/day continuous infusion days 1 to 5
[total dose/cycle = 6120 mg/m^2]
Repeat cycle every 21 days for 4 cycles

VIP (Small Cell Lung Cancer)

Use Lung cancer, small cell

Regimen

Etoposide: I.V.: 75 mg/m^2/day days 1 to 4
[total dose/cycle = 300 mg/m^2]
Ifosfamide: I.V.: 1200 mg/m^2/day days 1 to 4
[total dose/cycle = 4800 mg/m^2]
Cisplatin: I.V.: 20 mg/m^2/day days 1 to 4
[total dose/cycle = 80 mg/m^2]
Mesna: I.V.: 300 mg/m^2 day 1 only
followed by I.V.: 1200 mg/m^2/day continuous infusion days 1 to 4
[total dose/cycle = 5100 mg/m^2]
Repeat cycle every 21 days

VIP (Vinblastine) (Testicular Cancer)

Use Testicular cancer

Regimen NOTE: Multiple variations are listed below.

Variation 1:

Vinblastine: I.V.: 0.11 mg/kg/day days 1 and 2
[total dose/cycle = 0.22 mg/kg]

Ifosfamide: I.V.: 1200 mg/m^2/day days 1 to 5
[total dose/cycle = 6000 mg/m^2]

Cisplatin: I.V.: 20 mg/m^2/day days 1 to 5
[total dose/cycle = 100 mg/m^2]

Mesna: I.V.: 400 mg day 1
followed by I.V.: 1200 mg/day continuous infusion days 1 to 5
[total dose/cycle = 6400 mg]

Repeat cycle every 21 days for 4 cycles

Variation 2:

Vinblastine: I.V.: 6 mg/m^2/day days 1 and 2
[total dose/cycle = 12 mg/m^2]

Ifosfamide: I.V.: 1500 mg/m^2/day days 1 to 5
[total dose/cycle = 7500 mg/m^2]

Cisplatin: I.V.: 20 mg/m^2/day days 1 to 5
[total dose/cycle = 100 mg/m^2]

Mesna: I.V.: 300 mg/m^2 3 times/day days 1 to 5
[total dose/cycle = 4500 mg/m^2]

Repeat cycle every 21 days for 4 cycles

VM

Use Breast cancer

Regimen

Variation 1:

Mitomycin: I.V.: 10 mg/m^2 days 1 and 28 for 2 cycles
[total dose/cycle = 20 mg/m^2]
followed by I.V.: 10 mg/m^2 day 1 only for subsequent cycles
[total dose/cycle = 10 mg/m^2]

Vinblastine: I.V.: 5 mg/m^2/day days 1, 14, 28, and 42 for 2 cycles
[total dose/cycle = 20 mg/m^2]
followed by I.V.: 5 mg/m^2/day days 1 and 21
[total dose/cycle = 10 mg/m^2]

Repeat cycle every 6-8 weeks

Variation 2:

Mitomycin: I.V.: 10 mg/m^2/day days 1 and 28 for 2 cycles
[total dose/cycle = 20 mg/m^2]
followed by I.V.: 10 mg/m^2 day 1 only for subsequent cycles
[total dose/cycle = 10 mg/m^2]

Vindesine: I.V.: 2 mg/m^2/day days 1, 14, 28, and 42 for 2 cycles
[total dose/cycle = 8 mg/m^2]
followed by I.V.: 2 mg/m^2/ day days 1 and 21 for subsequent cycles
[total dose/cycle = 4 mg/m^2]

Repeat cycle every 6-8 weeks

VP (Small Cell Lung Cancer)

Use Lung cancer, small cell

Regimen

Etoposide: I.V.: 100 mg/m^2/day days 1 to 4
[total dose/cycle = 400 mg/m^2]

Cisplatin: I.V.: 20 mg/m^2/day days 1 to 4
[total dose/cycle = 80 mg/m^2]

Repeat cycle every 21 days

V-TAD

Use Leukemia, acute myeloid

Regimen Induction:

Etoposide: I.V.: 50 mg/m^2/day days 1, 2, and 3
[total dose/cycle = 150 mg/m^2]

Thioguanine: Oral: 75 mg/m^2/day every 12 hours days 1 to 5
[total dose/cycle = 750 mg/m^2]

Daunorubicin: I.V.: 20 mg/m^2/day days 1 and 2
[total dose/cycle = 40 mg/m^2]

Cytarabine: I.V.: 75 mg/m^2/day continuous infusion days 1 to 5
[total dose/cycle = 375 mg/m^2]

Up to 3 cycles may be given based on individual response; time between cycles not specified

CHEMOTHERAPY REGIMEN INDEX

ADENOCARCINOMA, UNKNOWN PRIMARY

BRAIN TUMORS

Neuroblastoma

BREAST

HEAD AND NECK CANCER

HEMATOLOGIC/LEUKEMIA

Leukemia, Acute Lymphocytic

Leukemia, Acute Myeloid

Leukemia, Acute Promyelocytic

Leukemia, Chronic Lymphocytic

APPENDIX TABLE OF CONTENTS

Visit thePoint http://thepoint.lww.com/QL2010 for exclusive access to:

Apothecary/Metric Conversions

Pounds/Kilograms Conversion

Temperature Conversion

Pharmaceutical Manufacturers and Distributors

Multivitamin Products

Refer to the inside front cover of this book for your online access code.

ABBREVIATIONS & SYMBOLS COMMONLY USED IN MEDICAL ORDERS

Abbreviations Which May Be Used in This Reference

Abbreviation	Meaning
5-HT	5-hydroxytryptamine
AAP	American Academy of Pediatrics
ABG	arterial blood gases
ABW	adjusted body weight
AACT	American Academy of Clinical Toxicology
ACC	American College of Cardiology
ACE	angiotensin converting enzyme
ACLS	advanced cardiac life support
ACOG	American College of Obstetricians and Gynecologists
ACTH	adrenocorticotrophic hormone
ADH	alcohol dehydrogenase
ADHD	attention-deficit/hyperactivity disorder
ADLs	activities of daily living
AED	antiepileptic drug
AHA	American Heart Association
AIDS	acquired immune deficiency syndrome
AIMS	Abnormal Involuntary Movement Scale
ALS	amyotrophic lateral sclerosis
ALT	alanine aminotransferase
AMA	American Medical Association
ANC	absolute neutrophil count
aPTT	activated partial thromboplastin
ARB	angiotensin receptor blocker
ARDS	acute respiratory distress syndrome
AST	aspartate aminotransferase
AUC	area under the curve
BDI	Beck Depression Inventory
BEC	blood ethanol concentration
BLS	basic life support
BMI	body mass index
BMT	bone marrow transplant
BP	blood pressure
BPH	benign prostatic hyperplasia
BPRS	Brief Psychiatric Rating Scale
BSA	body surface area
BUN	blood urea nitrogen
CABG	coronary artery bypass graft
CAD	coronary artery disease
CAN	Canadian

Abbreviations Which May Be Used in This Reference *(continued)*

Abbreviation	Meaning
CAPD	continuous ambulatory peritoneal dialysis
CAS	chemical abstract service
CBC	complete blood count
CBT	cognitive behavioral therapy
Cl_{cr}	creatinine clearance
CDC	Centers for Disease Control and Prevention
CF	cystic fibrosis
CGI	Clinical Global Impression
CHD	coronary heart disease
CHF	congestive heart failure; chronic heart failure
CIE	chemotherapy-induced emesis
C-II	schedule two controlled substance
C-III	schedule three controlled substance
C-IV	schedule four controlled substance
C-V	schedule five controlled substance
CIV	continuous I.V. infusion
C_{max}	maximum plasma concentration
C_{min}	minimum plasma concentration
CMV	cytomegalovirus
CNS	central nervous system or coagulase negative staphylococcus
COLD	chronic obstructive lung disease
COPD	chronic obstructive pulmonary disease
COX	cyclooxygenase
CPK	creatine phosphokinase
CRF	chronic renal failure
CRP	C-reactive protein
CRRT	continuous renal replacement therapy
CSF	cerebrospinal fluid
CSII	continuous subcutaneous insulin infusion
CT	computed tomography
CVA	cerebrovascular accident
CVVH	continuous venovenous hemofiltration
CVVHD	continuous venovenous hemodialysis
CVVHDF	continuous venovenous hemodiafiltration
CYP	cytochrome
D_5W	dextrose 5% in water
DBP	diastolic blood pressure
DEHP	di(3-ethylhexyl)phthalate
DIC	disseminated intravascular coagulation
DM	diabetes mellitus
DMARD	disease modifying antirheumatic drug
DSC	discontinued
DSM-IV	Diagnostic and Statistical Manual
DVT	deep vein thrombosis

Abbreviations Which May Be Used in This Reference *(continued)*

Abbreviation	Meaning
EBV	Epstein-Barr virus
ECG	electrocardiogram
ECMO	extracorporeal membrane oxygenation
ECT	electroconvulsive therapy
ED	emergency department
EEG	electroencephalogram
EF	ejection fraction
EG	ethylene glycol
EGA	estimated gestational age
EIA	enzyme immunoassay
ELISA	enzyme-linked immunosorbent assay
EPS	extrapyramidal side effects
ESR	erythrocyte sedimentation rate
ESRD	end stage renal disease
EtOH	alcohol
FDA	Food and Drug Administration
FTT	failure to thrive
GABA	gamma-aminobutyric acid
GAD	generalized anxiety disorder
GERD	gastroesophageal reflux disease
GFR	glomerular filtration rate
GGT	gamma-glutamyltransferase
GI	gastrointestinal
GU	genitourinary
GVHD	graft versus host disease
HAM-A	Hamilton Anxiety Scale
HAM-D	Hamilton Depression Scale
HDL	high density lipoprotein
HF	heart failure
HFSA	Heart Failure Society of America
HIV	human immunodeficiency virus
HMG-CoA	3-hydroxy-3-methylglutaryl-coenzyme A
HOCM	hypertrophic obstructive cardiomyopathy
HPA	hypothalamic-pituitary-adrenal
HSV	herpes simplex virus
HTN	hypertension
HUS	hemolytic uremic syndrome
IBD	inflammatory bowel disease
IBS	irritable bowel syndrome
IBW	ideal body weight
ICD	implantable cardioverter defibrillator
ICH	intracranial hemorrhage
ICP	intracranial pressure
IDDM	insulin dependent diabetes mellitus

Abbreviations Which May Be Used in This Reference *(continued)*

Abbreviation	Meaning
IDSA	Infectious Diseases Society of America
IHSS	idiopathic hypertrophic subaortic stenosis
I.M.	intramuscular
INR	international normalized ration
Int. unit	international unit
IOP	intraocular pressure
IUGR	intrauterine growth retardation
I.V.	intravenous
JIA	juvenile idiopathic arthritis
JNC	Joint National Committee
KIU	kallikrein inhibitor unit
LAMM	L-α-acetyl methadol
LDH	lactate dehydrogenase
LDL	low density lipoprotein
LFT	liver function test
LGA	large for gestational age
LR	lactated ringers
LVEF	left ventricular ejection fraction
LVH	left ventricular hypertrophy
MADRS	Montgomery Asbery Depression Rating Scale
MAOIs	monamine oxidase inhibitors
MDD	major depressive disorder
MDRD	modification of diet in renal disease
mEq	milliequivalent
mg	milligram
MI	myocardial infarction
mL	milliliter
mm	millimeter
mM	millimolar
mm Hg	millimeters of mercury
MMSE	mini mental status examination
M/P	milk to plasma ratio
MPS I	mucopolysaccharidosis I
MRHD	maximum recommended human dose
MRI	magnetic resonance imaging
MUGA	multiple gated acquisition scan
NAS	neonatal abstinence syndrome
NF	National Formulary
NFD	Nephrogenic fibrosing dermopathy
ng	nanogram
NIDDM	Noninsulin dependent diabetes mellitus
NKA	no known allergies
NKDA	No known drug allergies
NMDA	n-methyl-d-aspartic acid

Abbreviations Which May Be Used in This Reference *(continued)*

Abbreviation	Meaning
NMS	neuroleptic malignant syndrome
NNRTI	non-nucleoside reverse transcriptase inhibitor
NRTI	nucleoside reverse transcriptase inhibitor
NS	normal saline
NSAID	nonsteroidal anti-inflammatory drug
NSF	nephrogenic systemic fibrosis
NSTEMI	Non-ST-elevation myocardial infarction
OA	osteoarthritis
OCD	obsessive-compulsive disorder
OHSS	ovarian hyperstimulation syndrome
OTC	over-the-counter
PAT	paroxysmal atrial tachycardia
PD	Parkinson disease; peritoneal dialysis
PDA	patent ductus arteriosus
PDE-5	phosphodiesterase-5
PE	pulmonary embolus
PEG tube	percutaneous endoscopic gastrostomy tube
PHN	post-herpetic neuralgia
PID	pelvic inflammatory disease
PMDD	premenstrual dysphoric disorder
PONV	postoperative nausea and vomiting
PPN	peripheral parenteral nutrition
PROM	premature rupture of membranes
PSVT	paroxysmal supraventricular tachycardia
PT	prothrombin time
PTSD	post-traumatic stress disorder
PTT	partial thromboplastin time
PUD	peptic ulcer disease
PVD	peripheral vascular disease
QT_c	corrected QT interval
QT_c-F	corrected QT interval by Fredricia formula
RA	rheumatoid arthritis
REM	rapid eye movement
RPLS	reversible posterior leukoencephalopathy syndrome
SA	sinoatrial
SAD	seasonal affective disorder
SAH	subarachnoid hemorrhage
SBE	subacute bacterial endocarditis
SBP	systolic blood pressure
S_{Cr}	serum creatinine
SERM	selective estrogen receptor modulator
SGA	small for gestational age
SGOT	serum glutamic oxaloacetic aminotransferase
SGPT	serum glutamic pyruvate transaminase

Abbreviations Which May Be Used in This Reference *(continued)*

Abbreviation	Meaning
SI	International System of Units or Systeme international d'Unites
SIADH	syndrome of inappropriate antidiuretic hormone secretion
SLE	systemic lupus erythematosus
SNRI	serotonin norepinephrine reuptake inhibitor
SSKI	saturated solution of potassium iodide
SSRIs	selective serotonin reuptake inhibitors
STD	sexually transmitted disease
STEM I	ST-elevation myocardial infarction
SubQ	subcutaneous
supp	suppository
SVT	supraventricular tachycardia
SWFI	sterile water for injection
syr	syrup
$T_{1/2}$	half-life
tab	tablet
TB	tuberculosis
TC	total cholesterol
TCA	tricyclic antidepressant
TD	tardive dyskinesia
TG	triglyceride
TIA	transient ischemic attack
TMA	thrombotic microangiopathy
T_{max}	time to maximum observed concentration, plasma
TNF	Tumor necrosis factor
TPN	total parenteral nutrition
tr, tinct	tincture
tsp	teaspoonful
UC	ulcerative colitis
ULN	upper limits of normal
URI	upper respiratory infection
USAN	United States Adopted Names
USP	United States Pharmacopeia
UTI	urinary tract infection
UV	ultraviolet
V_d	volume of distribution
VEGF	vascular endothelial growth factor
VF	ventricular fibrillation
VT	ventricular tachycardia
VTE	venous thromboembolism
vWD	von Willebrand disease
VZV	varicella zoster virus
YBOC	Yale Brown Obsessive-Compulsive Scale
YMRS	Young Mania Rating Scale

ABBREVIATIONS & SYMBOLS COMMONLY USED IN MEDICAL ORDERS

Common Weights, Measures, or Apothecary Abbreviations

Abbreviation	Meaning
<[1]	less than
>[1]	greater than
≤	less than or equal to
≥	greater than or equal to
ac	before meals or food
ad	to, up to
ad lib	at pleasure
AM	morning
AMA	against medical advice
amp	ampul
amt	amount
aq	water
aq. dest.	distilled water
ASAP	as soon as possible
a.u.[1]	each ear
bid	twice daily
bm	bowel movement
C	Celsius, centigrade
cal	calorie
cap	capsule
cc[1]	cubic centimeter
cm	centimeter
comp	compound
cont	continue
d	day
d/c[1]	discharge
dil	dilute
disp	dispense
div	divide
dtd	give of such a dose
Dx	diagnosis
elix, el	elixir
emp	as directed
et	and
ex aq	in water
F	Fahrenheit
f, ft	make, let be made
g	gram
gr	grain
gtt	a drop
h	hour
hs[1]	at bedtime
kcal	kilocalorie
kg	kilogram

Common Weights, Measures, or Apothecary Abbreviations *(continued)*

Abbreviation	Meaning
L	liter
liq	a liquor, solution
M	molar
mcg	microgram
m. dict	as directed
mEq	milliequivalent
mg	milligram
microL	microliter
mL	milliliter
mm	millimeter
mM	millimolar
mm Hg	millimeters of mercury
ng	nanogram
no.	number
noc	in the night
non rep	do not repeat, no refills
NPO	nothing by mouth
NV	nausea and vomiting
O, Oct	a pint
o.d.[1]	right eye
o.l.	left eye
o.s.[1]	left eye
o.u.[1]	each eye
pc, post cib	after meals
PM	afternoon or evening
P.O.	by mouth
P.R.	rectally
prn	as needed
pulv	a powder
q	every
qad	every other day
qd[1,2]	every day, daily
qh	every hour
qid	four times a day
qod[1,2]	every other day
qs	a sufficient quantity
qs ad	a sufficient quantity to make
Rx	take, a recipe
SL	sublingual
stat	at once, immediately
SubQ	subcutaneous
supp	suppository
syr	syrup
tab	tablet

Common Weights, Measures, or Apothecary Abbreviations *(continued)*

Abbreviation	Meaning
tal	such
tid	three times a day
tr, tinct	tincture
trit	triturate
tsp	teaspoon
u.d.	as directed
ung	ointment
v.o.	verbal order
w.a.	while awake
x3	3 times
x4	4 times

[1]ISMP error-prone abbreviation.

[2]JCAHO Do Not Use list.

Additional abbreviations used and defined within a specific monograph or text piece may only apply to that text.

References

The Institute for Safe Medication Practices (ISMP) list of Error-Prone Abbreviations, Symbols, and Dose Designations. Available at: http://www.ismp.org/Tools/errorproneabbreviations.pdf.

The Joint Commission Official "Do Not Use" list. Available at: http://www.jointcommission.org/PatientSafety/DoNotUseList/.

NORMAL LABORATORY VALUES FOR ADULTS

CHEMISTRY

Test	Values	Remarks
Serum / Plasma		
Acetone	Negative	
Albumin	3.2-5 g/dL	
Alcohol, ethyl	Negative	
Aldolase	1.2-7.6 IU/L	
Ammonia	20-70 mcg/dL	Specimen to be placed on ice as soon as collected.
Amylase	30-110 units/L	
Bilirubin, direct	0-0.3 mg/dL	
Bilirubin, total	0.1-1.2 mg/dL	
Calcium	8.6-10.3 mg/dL	
Calcium, ionized	2.24-2.46 mEq/L	
Chloride	95-108 mEq/L	
Cholesterol, total	≤200 mg/dL	Fasted blood required – normal value affected by dietary habits. This reference range is for a general adult population.
HDL cholesterol	40-60 mg/dL	Fasted blood required – normal value affected by dietary habits.
LDL cholesterol	<160 mg/dL	If triglyceride is >400 mg/dL, LDL cannot be calculated accurately (Friedewald equation). Target LDL-C depends on patient's risk factors.
CO_2	23-30 mEq/L	
Creatine kinase (CK) isoenzymes		
CK-BB	0%	
CK-MB (cardiac)	0%-3.9%	
CK-MM (muscle)	96%-100%	
CK-MB levels must be both ≥4% and 10 IU/L to meet diagnostic criteria for CK-MB positive result consistent with myocardial injury.		
Creatine phosphokinase (CPK)	8-150 IU/L	
Creatinine	0.5-1.4 mg/dL	
Ferritin	13-300 ng/mL	
Folate	3.6-20 ng/dL	
GGT (gamma-glutamyltranspeptidase)		
male	11-63 IU/L	
female	8-35 IU/L	
GLDH	To be determined	
Glucose (preprandial)	<115 mg/dL	Goals different for diabetics.
Glucose, fasting	60-110 mg/dL	Goals different for diabetics.
Glucose, nonfasting (2-h postprandial)	<120 mg/dL	Goals different for diabetics.
Hemoglobin A_{1c}	<8	
Hemoglobin, plasma free	<2.5 mg/100 mL	
Hemoglobin, total glycosolated (Hb A_1)	4%-8%	

CHEMISTRY *(continued)*

Test	Values	Remarks
Iron	65-150 mcg/dL	
Iron binding capacity, total (TIBC)	250-420 mcg/dL	
Lactic acid	0.7-2.1 mEq/L	Specimen to be kept on ice and sent to lab as soon as possible.
Lactate dehydrogenase (LDH)	56-194 IU/L	
Lactate dehydrogenase (LDH) isoenzymes		
LD_1	20%-34%	
LD_2	29%-41%	
LD_3	15%-25%	
LD_4	1%-12%	
LD_5	1%-15%	
Flipped LD_1/LD_2 ratios (>1 may be consistent with myocardial injury) particularly when considered in combination with a recent CK-MB positive result.		
Lipase	23-208 units/L	
Magnesium	1.6-2.5 mg/dL	Increased by slight hemolysis.
Osmolality	289-308 mOsm/kg	
Phosphatase, alkaline		
adults 25-60 y	33-131 IU/L	
adults ≥61 y	51-153 IU/L	
infancy-adolescence	Values range up to 3-5 times higher than adults	
Phosphate, inorganic	2.8-4.2 mg/dL	
Potassium	3.5-5.2 mEq/L	Increased by slight hemolysis.
Prealbumin	>15 mg/dL	
Protein, total	6.5-7.9 g/dL	
AST	<35 IU/L (20-48)	
ALT (10-35)	<35 IU/L	
Sodium	134-149 mEq/L	
Thyroid stimulating hormone (TSH)		
adults ≤20 y	0.7-6.4 mIU/L	
21-54 y	0.4-4.2 mIU/L	
55-87 y	0.5-8.9 mIU/L	
Transferrin	>200 mg/dL	
Triglycerides	45-155 mg/dL	Fasted blood required.
Troponin I	<1.5 ng/mL	
Urea nitrogen (BUN)	7-20 mg/dL	
Uric acid		
male	2-8 mg/dL	
female	2-7.5 mg/dL	
Cerebrospinal Fluid		
Glucose	50-70 mg/dL	
Protein	15-45 mg/dL	CSF obtained by lumbar puncture.

Note: Bloody specimen gives erroneously high value due to contamination with blood proteins

CHEMISTRY *(continued)*

Test	Values	Remarks
Urine **(24-hour specimen is required for all these tests unless specified)**		
Amylase	32-641 units/L	The value is in units/L and **not** calculated for total volume.
Amylase, fluid (random samples)		Interpretation of value left for physician, depends on the nature of fluid.
Calcium	Depends upon dietary intake	
Creatine		
male	150 mg/24 h	Higher value on children and during pregnancy.
female	250 mg/24 h	
Creatinine	1000-2000 mg/24 h	
Creatinine clearance (endogenous)		
male	85-125 mL/min	A blood sample must accompany urine specimen.
female	75-115 mL/min	
Glucose	1 g/24 h	
5-hydroxyindoleacetic acid	2-8 mg/24 h	
Iron	0.15 mg/24 h	Acid washed container required.
Magnesium	146-209 mg/24 h	
Osmolality	500-800 mOsm/kg	With normal fluid intake.
Oxalate	10-40 mg/24 h	
Phosphate	400-1300 mg/24 h	
Potassium	25-120 mEq/24 h	Varies with diet; the interpretation of urine electrolytes and osmolality should be left for the physician.
Sodium	40-220 mEq/24 h	
Porphobilinogen, qualitative	Negative	
Porphyrins, qualitative	Negative	
Proteins	0.05-0.1 g/24 h	
Salicylate	Negative	
Urea clearance	60-95 mL/min	A blood sample must accompany specimen.
Urea N	10-40 g/24 h	Dependent on protein intake.
Uric acid	250-750 mg/24 h	Dependent on diet and therapy.
Urobilinogen	0.5-3.5 mg/24 h	For qualitative determination on random urine, send sample to urinalysis section in Hematology Lab.
Xylose absorption test		
children	16%-33% of ingested xylose	
Feces		
Fat, 3-day collection	<5 g/d	Value depends on fat intake of 100 g/d for 3 days preceding and during collection.
Gastric Acidity		
Acidity, total, 12 h	10-60 mEq/L	Titrated at pH 7.

Blood Gases

	Arterial	Capillary	Venous
pH	7.35-7.45	7.35-7.45	7.32-7.42
pCO_2 (mm Hg)	35-45	35-45	38-52
pO_2 (mm Hg)	70-100	60-80	24-48
HCO_3 (mEq/L)	19-25	19-25	19-25
TCO_2 (mEq/L)	19-29	19-29	23-33
O_2 saturation (%)	90-95	90-95	40-70
Base excess (mEq/L)	-5 to +5	-5 to +5	-5 to +5

HEMATOLOGY

Complete Blood Count

Age	Hgb (g/dL)	Hct (%)	RBC (mill/mm^3)	RDW
0-3 d	15.0-20.0	45-61	4.0-5.9	<18
1-2 wk	12.5-18.5	39-57	3.6-5.5	<17
1-6 mo	10.0-13.0	29-42	3.1-4.3	<16.5
7 mo to 2 y	10.5-13.0	33-38	3.7-4.9	<16
2-5 y	11.5-13.0	34-39	3.9-5.0	<15
5-8 y	11.5-14.5	35-42	4.0-4.9	<15
13-18 y	12.0-15.2	36-47	4.5-5.1	<14.5
Adult male	13.5-16.5	41-50	4.5-5.5	<14.5
Adult female	12.0-15.0	36-44	4.0-4.9	<14.5

Age	MCV (fL)	MCH (pg)	MCHC (%)	Plts (x 10^3/mm^3)
0-3 d	95-115	31-37	29-37	250-450
1-2 wk	86-110	28-36	28-38	250-450
1-6 mo	74-96	25-35	30-36	300-700
7 mo to 2 y	70-84	23-30	31-37	250-600
2-5 y	75-87	24-30	31-37	250-550
5-8 y	77-95	25-33	31-37	250-550
13-18 y	78-96	25-35	31-37	150-450
Adult male	80-100	26-34	31-37	150-450
Adult female	80-100	26-34	31-37	150-450

WBC and Differential

Age	WBC (x $10^3/mm^3$)	Segs	Bands	Lymphs	Monos
0-3 d	9.0-35.0	32-62	10-18	19-29	5-7
1-2 wk	5.0-20.0	14-34	6-14	36-45	6-10
1-6 mo	6.0-17.5	13-33	4-12	41-71	4-7
7 mo to 2 y	6.0-17.0	15-35	5-11	45-76	3-6
2-5 y	5.5-15.5	23-45	5-11	35-65	3-6
5-8 y	5.0-14.5	32-54	5-11	28-48	3-6
13-18 y	4.5-13.0	34-64	5-11	25-45	3-6
Adults	4.5-11.0	35-66	5-11	24-44	3-6

Age	Eosinophils	Basophils	Atypical Lymphs	No. of NRBCs
0-3 d	0-2	0-1	0-8	0-2
1-2 wk	0-2	0-1	0-8	0
1-6 mo	0-3	0-1	0-8	0
7 mo to 2 y	0-3	0-1	0-8	0
2-5 y	0-3	0-1	0-8	0
5-8 y	0-3	0-1	0-8	0
13-18 y	0-3	0-1	0-8	0
Adults	0-3	0-1	0-8	0

Segs = segmented neutrophils.

Bands = band neutrophils.

Lymphs = lymphocytes.

Monos = monocytes.

Erythrocyte Sedimentation Rates and Reticulocyte Counts

Sedimentation rate, Westergren	Children	0-20 mm/h
	Adult male	0-15 mm/h
	Adult female	0-20 mm/h
Sedimentation rate, Wintrobe	Children	0-13 mm/h
	Adult male	0-10 mm/h
	Adult female	0-15 mm/h
Reticulocyte count	Newborns	2%-6%
	1-6 mo	0%-2.8%
	Adults	0.5%-1.5%

NORMAL LABORATORY VALUES FOR CHILDREN

	Normal Values	
CHEMISTRY		
Albumin	0-1 y	2-4 g/dL
	1 y to adult	3.5-5.5 g/dL
Ammonia	Newborns	90-150 mcg/dL
	Children	40-120 mcg/dL
	Adults	18-54 mcg/dL
Amylase	Newborns	0-60 units/L
	Adults	30-110 units/L
Bilirubin, conjugated, direct	Newborns	<1.5 mg/dL
	1 mo to adult	0-0.5 mg/dL
Bilirubin, total	0-3 d	2-10 mg/dL
	1 mo to adult	0-1.5 mg/dL
Bilirubin, unconjugated, indirect		0.6-10.5 mg/dL
Calcium	Newborns	7-12 mg/dL
	0-2 y	8.8-11.2 mg/dL
	2 y to adult	9-11 mg/dL
Calcium, ionized, whole blood		4.4-5.4 mg/dL
Carbon dioxide, total		23-33 mEq/L
Chloride		95-105 mEq/L
Cholesterol	Newborns	45-170 mg/dL
	0-1 y	65-175 mg/dL
	1-20 y	120-230 mg/dL
Creatinine	0-1 y	≤0.6 mg/dL
	1 y to adult	0.5-1.5 mg/dL
Glucose	Newborns	30-90 mg/dL
	0-2 y	60-105 mg/dL
	Children to Adults	70-110 mg/dL
Iron		
	Newborns	110-270 mcg/dL
	Infants	30-70 mcg/dL
	Children	55-120 mcg/dL
	Adults	70-180 mcg/dL
Iron binding	Newborns	59-175 mcg/dL
	Infants	100-400 mcg/dL
	Adults	250-400 mcg/dL
Lactic acid, lactate		2-20 mg/dL
Lead, whole blood		<10 mcg/dL
Lipase		
	Children	20-140 units/L
	Adults	0-190 units/L
Magnesium		1.5-2.5 mEq/L

		Normal Values
Osmolality, serum		275-296 mOsm/kg
Osmolality, urine		50-1400 mOsm/kg
Phosphorus	Newborns	4.2-9 mg/dL
	6 wk to 19 mo	3.8-6.7 mg/dL
	19 mo to 3 y	2.9-5.9 mg/dL
	3-15 y	3.6-5.6 mg/dL
	>15 y	2.5-5 mg/dL
Potassium, plasma	Newborns	4.5-7.2 mEq/L
	2 d to 3 mo	4-6.2 mEq/L
	3 mo to 1 y	3.7-5.6 mEq/L
	1-16 y	3.5-5 mEq/L
Protein, total	0-2 y	4.2-7.4 g/dL
	>2 y	6-8 g/dL
Sodium		136-145 mEq/L
Triglycerides	Infants	0-171 mg/dL
	Children	20-130 mg/dL
	Adults	30-200 mg/dL
Urea nitrogen, blood	0-2 y	4-15 mg/dL
	2 y to Adult	5-20 mg/dL
Uric acid	Male	3-7 mg/dL
	Female	2-6 mg/dL
ENZYMES		
Alanine aminotransferase (ALT)	0-2 mo	8-78 units/L
	>2 mo	8-36 units/L
Alkaline phosphatase (ALKP)	Newborns	60-130 units/L
	0-16 y	85-400 units/L
	>16 y	30-115 units/L
Aspartate aminotransferase (AST)	Infants	18-74 units/L
	Children	15-46 units/L
	Adults	5-35 units/L
Creatine kinase (CK)	Infants	20-200 units/L
	Children	10-90 units/L
	Adult male	0-206 units/L
	Adult female	0-175 units/L
Lactate dehydrogenase (LDH)	Newborns	290-501 units/L
	1 mo to 2 y	110-144 units/L
	>16 y	60-170 units/L

Blood Gases

	Arterial	Capillary	Venous
pH	7.35-7.45	7.35-7.45	7.32-7.42
pCO_2 (mm Hg)	35-45	35-45	38-52
pO_2 (mm Hg)	70-100	60-80	24-48
HCO_3 (mEq/L)	19-25	19-25	19-25
TCO_2 (mEq/L)	19-29	19-29	23-33
O_2 saturation (%)	90-95	90-95	40-70
Base excess (mEq/L)	-5 to +5	-5 to +5	-5 to +5

Thyroid Function Tests

T_4 (thyroxine)	1-7 d	10.1-20.9 mcg/dL
	8-14 d	9.8-16.6 mcg/dL
	1 mo to 1 y	5.5-16 mcg/dL
	>1 y	4-12 mcg/dL
FTI	1-3 d	9.3-26.6
	1-4 wk	7.6-20.8
	1-4 mo	7.4-17.9
	4-12 mo	5.1-14.5
	1-6 y	5.7-13.3
	>6 y	4.8-14
T_3 by RIA	Newborns	100-470 ng/dL
	1-5 y	100-260 ng/dL
	5-10 y	90-240 ng/dL
	10 y to Adult	70-210 ng/dL
T_3 uptake		35%-45%
TSH	Cord	3-22 μIU/mL
	1-3 d	<40 μIU/mL
	3-7 d	<25 μIU/mL
	>7 d	0-10 μIU/mL

ACQUIRED IMMUNODEFICIENCY SYNDROME (AIDS) - LAB TESTS AND APPROVED DRUGS FOR HIV INFECTION AND AIDS-RELATED CONDITIONS

This list of tests is not intended in any way to suggest patterns of physician's orders, nor is it complete. These tests may support possible clinical diagnoses or rule out other diagnostic possibilities. Each laboratory test relevant to AIDS is listed and weighted. Two symbols (**) indicate that the test is diagnostic, that is, documents the diagnosis if the expected is found. A single symbol (*) indicates a test frequently used in the diagnosis or management of the disease. The other listed tests are useful on a selective basis with consideration of clinical factors and specific aspects of the case.

Acid-Fast Stain
Acid-Fast Stain, Modified, *Nocardia* Species
Antimicrobial Susceptibility Testing, Fungi
Antimicrobial Susceptibility Testing, Mycobacteria
Arthropod Identification
Babesiosis Serological Test
Bacteremia Detection, Buffy Coat Micromethod
Bacterial Culture, Blood
Bacterial Culture, Bronchoscopy Specimen
Bacterial Culture, Sputum
Bacterial Culture, Stool
Bacterial Culture, Throat
Bacterial Culture, Urine, Clean Catch
$Beta_2$-Microglobulin
Blood and Fluid Precautions, Specimen Collection
Bronchial Washings Cytology
Bronchoalveolar Lavage Cytology
Brushings Cytology
Candida Antigen
Candidiasis Serologic Test
Cat Scratch Disease Serology
CD4/CD8 Enumeration
Cerebrospinal Fluid Cytology
Cryptococcal Antigen Titer
Cryptosporidium Diagnostic Procedures
Cytomegalic Inclusion Disease Cytology
Cytomegalovirus Antibody
Cytomegalovirus Antigen Detection
Cytomegalovirus Culture
Cytomegalovirus DNA Detection
Darkfield Examination, Syphilis
Electron Microscopy
Folic Acid, Serum
Fungal Culture, Biopsy or Body Fluid
Fungal Culture, Blood
Fungal Culture, Cerebrospinal Fluid
Fungal Culture, Sputum
Fungal Culture, Stool
Fungal Culture, Urine
Hemoglobin A_2
Hepatitis B Surface Antigen
Herpes Cytology
Herpes Simplex Virus Antigen Detection
Herpes Simplex Virus Culture
Histopathology
Histoplasmosis Antibody
Histoplasmosis Antigen
**HIV-1/HIV-2 Serology
HTLV-I/II Antibody
*Human Immunodeficiency Virus Culture
*Human Immunodeficiency Virus DNA Amplification

India Ink Preparation
Inhibitor, Lupus, Phospholipid Type
KOH Preparation
Leishmaniasis Serological Test
Leukocyte Immunophenotyping
Lymphocyte Enumeration Test
Lymphocyte Transformation Test
Microsporidia Diagnostic Procedures
Mycobacteria by DNA Probe
Mycobacterial Culture, Biopsy or Body Fluid
Mycobacterial Culture, Cerebrospinal Fluid
Mycobacterial Culture, Cutaneous and Subcutaneous Tissue
Mycobacterial Culture, Sputum
Mycobacterial Culture, Stool
Neisseria gonorrhoeae Culture and Smear
Nocardia Culture
Ova and Parasites, Stool
*p24 Antigen
Platelet Count
Pneumocystis carinii Preparation
Pneumocystis Immunofluorescence
Polymerase Chain Reaction
Red Blood Cell Indices
Risks of Transfusion
Skin Biopsy
Sputum Cytology
Toxoplasmosis Serology
VDRL, Serum
Viral Culture
Viral Culture, Blood
Viral Culture, Body Fluid
Viral Culture, Central Nervous System Symptoms
Viral Culture, Dermatological Symptoms
Viral Culture, Tissue
Virus, Direct Detection by Fluorescent Antibody
White Blood Count

PROVED AND INVESTIGATIONAL ANTIRETROVIRAL DRUGS

Antiretroviral Drugs

Generic Name	Also Known As	Brand Name	FDA Status
NUCLEOSIDE/NUCLEOTIDE ANALOG REVERSE TRANSCRIPTASE INHIBITORS (NRTIs)			
abacavir	ABC	Ziagen®	Approved
apricitabine	AVX754	—	Investigational
didanosine	ddI	Videx®; Videx® EC	Approved
elvucitabine	ACH-126,443; Beta-L-Fd4C	—	Investigational
emtricitabine	FTC	Emtriva®	Approved
lamivudine	3TC	Epivir®	Approved
stavudine	d4T	Zerit®	Approved
tenofovir	TDF	Viread®	Approved
zidovudine	ZDV	Retrovir®	Approved
—	RCV	Racivir	Investigational
NONNUCLEOSIDE REVERSE TRANSCRIPTASE INHIBITORS (NNRTIs)			
delavirdine	DLV	Rescriptor®	Approved
efavirenz	EFV	Sustiva®	Approved
etravirine	TMC 125	Intelence™	Approved
nevirapine	NVP	Viramune®	Approved
rilpivirine	TMC 278	—	Investigational
PROTEASE INHIBITORS (PIs)			
atazanavir	ATV	Reyataz®	Approved
darunavir	DRV	Prezista™	Approved
fosamprenavir	FPV	Lexiva®	Approved
indinavir	IDV	Crixivan®	Approved
lopinavir and ritonavir	LPV/RTV	Kaletra®	Approved
nelfinavir	NFV	Viracept®	Approved
ritonavir	RTV	Norvir®	Approved
saquinavir	SQV	Invirase®	Approved
tipranavir	TPV	Aptivus®	Approved
FIXED-DOSE COMBINATION PRODUCTS			
abacavir and lamivudine	ABC/3TC	Epzicom®, Kivexa™	Approved
abacavir, lamivudine, and zidovudine	ABC/3TC/ZDV	Trizivir®	Approved
efavirenz, emtricitabine and tenofovir	EFV/FTC/TDF	Atripla™	Approved
emtricitabine and tenofovir	FTC/TDF	Truvada®	Approved
zidovudine and lamivudine	ZDV/3TC	Combivir®	Approved
FUSION INHIBITORS			
enfuvirtide	ENF	Fuzeon®	Approved
—	TNX-355	—	Investigational
CHEMOKINE CORECEPTOR ANTAGONIST			
maraviroc	MVC	Selzentry™	Approved
vicriviroc	SCH-417690; SCH-D	—	Investigational

Antiretroviral Drugs *(continued)*

Generic Name	Also Known As	Brand Name	FDA Status
—	PRO 140	—	Investigational
—	INCB9741	—	Investigational
INTEGRASE INHIBITORS			
elvitegravir	GS-9137	—	Investigational
raltegravir	RAL	Isentress™	Approved
—	GSK364735	—	Investigational
MATURATION INHIBITORS			
bevirimat	PA-457	—	Investigational

DRUGS USED TO TREAT COMPLICATIONS OF HIV / AIDS

Brand Name	Generic Name (Synonym)	Use
Abelcet®, AmBisome®	amphotericin B, ABLC	Antifungal for aspergillosis
Bactrim™, Septra®	sulfamethoxazole and trimethoprim, SMZ/TMP	Antiprotozoal antibiotic used to treat and prevent *Pneumocystis carinii* pneumonia
Biaxin®	clarithromycin	Antibiotic used to treat and prevent *Mycobacterium avium*
Cytovene®	ganciclovir, DHPG	Antiviral used to treat CMV retinitis
DaunoXome®	daunorubicin citrate (liposomal)	Chemotherapy for Kaposi sarcoma
Diflucan®	fluconazole	Antifungal for candidiasis, cryptococcal meningitis
Doxil®	doxorubicin (liposomal)	Chemotherapy for Kaposi sarcoma
Eraxis™	anidulafungin	Antifungal (intravenous), used to treat *Candida* infections in the esophagus (candidiasis), blood stream (candidemia), and other forms of *Candida* infections, including abdominal abscesses and peritonitis (inflammation of the lining of the abdominal cavity)
Famvir®	famciclovir	Antiviral used to treat herpes
Foscavir®	foscarnet	Antiviral used to treat herpes and CMV retinitis
Gamimune® N	immune globulin, gamma globulin, IGIV	Immune booster used to prevent bacterial infections in children
Intron® A	interferon alfa-2b	Treat Kaposi sarcoma and hepatitis C
Marinol®	dronabinol	Treat loss of appetite
Megace®	megestrol acetate	Treat loss of appetite and weight
Mepron®	atovaquone	Antiprotozoal antibiotic used to treat and prevent *Pneumocystis carinii* pneumonia
Mycobutin®	rifabutin	Antimycobacterial used to prevent *Mycobacterium avium*
NebuPent®	pentamidine	Antiprotozoal antibiotic used to prevent *Pneumocystis carinii* pneumonia
Neutrexin®	trimetrexate glucuronate and leucovorin	Antiprotozoal antibiotic used to treat *Pneumocystis carinii* pneumonia
Panretin® Gel	alitretinoin gel 0.1%	AIDS-related Kaposi sarcoma
Procrit®, Epogen®	erythropoietin, EPO	Treat anemia related to AZT therapy
Roferon-A®	interferon alfa-2a	Treat Kaposi sarcoma and hepatitis C
Serostim®	somatropin rDNA	Treat weight loss
Sporanox®	itraconazole	Antifungal used to treat blastomycosis, histoplasmosis, aspergillosis, and candidiasis

DRUGS USED TO TREAT COMPLICATIONS OF HIV / AIDS *(continued)*

Brand Name	Generic Name (Synonym)	Use
Taxol®	paclitaxel	Kaposi sarcoma
Valcyte™	valganciclovir	Antiviral used to treat CMV retinitis
VFEND®	voriconazole	Antifungal for invasive aspergillosis and serious fungal infections due to *Fusarium sporotrichoides* and *Scedosporium apiospermum*, and Esophageal Candidiasis
Vistide®	cidofovir, HPMPC	Antiviral used to treat cytomegalovirus (CMV)
Vitrasert® Implant	ganciclovir insert	Antiviral used to treat CMV retinitis
Vitravene™ intravitreal injection	fomivirsen sodium injection	Antiviral used to treat CMV retinitis
Zithromax®	azithromycin	Antibiotic used to treat *Mycobacterium avium*

HERBS AND COMMON NATURAL AGENTS

The authors have chosen to include this list of natural products and their reported uses. Due to limited scientific evidence to support these uses, the information provided here is not intended as a cure for any disease, and should not be construed as curative or healing. In addition, the reader is strongly encouraged to seek other references that discuss this information in more detail, and that discuss important issues such as contraindications, warnings, precautions, adverse reactions, and interactions.

PROPOSED MEDICINAL CLAIMS

Herb	Reported Uses
Acetyl-L-carnitine (ALC)	AIDS; alcoholism; Alzheimer disease; angina; cerebral ischemia; congestive heart failure; coronary artery disease; depression; diabetes mellitus; diabetic peripheral neuropathy; erectile dysfunction; fatigue; fibromyalgia; fragile X syndrome; hyperlipoproteinemia; infertility; liver disease; mood disorder; myocardial infarction; neurologic function; neuropathy; nutritional deficiency; Parkinson disease; peripheral vascular disease; Peyronie disease; sickle cell disease; surgical uses; sperm motility; tuberculosis
Adrenal extract	Depression; fatigue, stress; fibromyalgia
Aloe (*Aloe* spp)	Aphthous stomatitis; cancer (prevention); constipation; diabetes; dry skin; genital herpes; gingivitis; healing agent for wounds, minor burns, and other minor skin irritations; irritable bowel syndrome; lichen planus; psoriasis vulgaris; seborrheic dermatitis; skin burns; ulcerative colitis
Alpha-Lipoic acid	Alcohol-induced liver damage; burning mouth syndrome; cardiovascular outcomes (in end-state renal disease); cataract prevention; chemotherapy and radiation (adjunct); circulation; coronary artery disease; diabetes, diabetic peripheral neuropathy; drug-induced cardiotoxicity; glaucoma; hypertension; insulin resistance; liver protective effects; multiple sclerosis; neuralgias; neurologic disorders, including stroke (preventive); skin aging
Andrographis (*Andrographis paniculata*)	Familial Mediterranean Fever (FMF); influenza; upper respiratory tract infection (treatment and prevention)
Aortic extract	Circulation structure, function, and integrity (arteries and veins); prevention of vascular disease including atherosclerosis, cerebral and peripheral arterial insufficiency, varicose veins, hemorrhoids, and vascular retinopathies such as macular degeneration
Arabinoxylan	Cancer; diabetes, type 2; HIV; immune support (antiviral and anticancer activity); leukopenia (chemotherapy-induced)
Arginine	Adrenoleukodystrophy (ALD); angina; burns; cancer; cardiovascular disease; chronic heart failure; circulation; critical illness; dental pain; erectile dysfunction; gastrointestinal cancer surgery; growth hormone reserve test/pituitary disorder diagnosis; heart protection during CABG; hypercholesterolemia; hypertension; immune support; inborn errors of urea synthesis; inflammatory bowel disease; increases lean body mass; male infertility; MELAS syndrome; migraine headache; myocardial infarction; neonatal outcomes; obesity (in type 2 diabetic patients); peripheral vascular disease/claudication; preeclampsia; pressure ulcers; recovery after surgery; sexual vitality and enhancement; transplants; wound healing
Arnica (*Arnica montana*)	Bruising; coagulation; diabetic retinopathy; osteoarthritis; pain; swelling (postoperative); trauma
Artichoke (*Cynara scolymus*)	Bile flow; dyspepsia (nonulcer); eczema and other dermatologic problems; hepatic protection/stimulation; hypercholesterolemia; indigestion; irritable bowel syndrome (IBS)
Ashwagandha (*Withania somnifera*)	Adaptogen/tonic (promote wellness); chemotherapy and radiation (adjunct); diabetes (type 2); diuresis; hypercholesterolemia; longevity/anti-aging; osteoarthritis; Parkinson disease; stress, fatigue, nervous exhaustion
Astragalus (*Astragalus membranaceus*) [Milk Vetch]	Adaptogen/tonic (promote wellness); antiviral activity; athletic performance (enhancement); burns; chemotherapy and radiation (adjunct); coronary artery disease; diabetes; heart failure; immune support; liver protection; mental performance; multiple sclerosis; otitis media; renal failure; smoking cessation; tissue oxygenation; tuberculosis
Bacopa (*Bacopa monniera*)	Alzheimer disease/senility; anxiety; epilepsy; irritable bowel syndrome (IBS); memory enhancement and improvement of cognitive function

PROPOSED MEDICINAL CLAIMS *(continued)*

Herb	Reported Uses
Barberry (*Berberis vulgaris*)	Bladder infection; bronchitis; sore throat; yeast infection
Beta-Carotene	Age-related maculopathy; AIDS; asthma; breast cancer; carotenoid deficiency; cataract prevention; cervical dysplasia; chromosome damage (reduction); chronic obstructive pulmonary disease (COPD); coronary heart disease (risk reduction; in combination); cystic fibrosis; diabetes; diabetes, type 2; esophageal cancer; gastric cancer; immune support; laryngeal cancer; LDL oxidation (decrease in males); lung cancer (preventive); lung function; macular degeneration; memory and cognition; night blindness; oral leukoplakia; osteoarthritis; photoprotection (erythropoietic protoporphyria); pregnancy-related complications
Betaine hydrochloride	Cardiovascular disease (in homocystinuric patients); cholesterol levels; digestive aid (hypochlorhydria and achlorhydria); hyperhomocysteinemia; hyperhomocysteinemia (in chronic renal failure patients); rosacea; steatohepatitis (nonalcoholic); weight loss
Bifidobacterium bifidum (*bifidus*)	Atopic dermatitis; constipation; Crohn disease; diarrhea; gastrointestinal microflora recolonization (anaerobic); *Helicobacter pylori* infection; immune function; irritable bowel syndrome (IBS); pouchitis; ulcerative colitis
Bilberry (*Vaccinium myrtillus*)	Circulation, peripheral; diabetes; diarrhea; dysmenorrhea; fibrocystic breast disease (FBD); hemorrhoids; ophthalmologic disorders (antioxidant) including myopia, diminished acuity, glaucoma; dark adaptation, macular degeneration, night blindness, diabetic retinopathy, cataracts; peptic ulcer disease; scleroderma; vascular disorders including varicose veins, capillary permeability/stability, phlebitis
Biotin (Vitamin H)	Cardiovascular disease (risk reduction; in combination); diabetes; diabetic peripheral neuropathy; hypertriglyceridemia; nails, brittle; pregnancy supplementation; seborrheic dermatitis; total parenteral nutrition (TPN); uncombable hair syndrome
Bismuth	Diarrhea; ulcers
Bitter melon (*Momordica charantia*)	Antiviral; cancer; diabetes, including impaired glucose tolerance (IGT)
Black cohosh (*Cimicifuga racemosa*)	Arthritis; depression (mild); menopause symptoms (including vasomotor); migraine; premenstrual syndrome (PMS)
Bladderwrack (*Fucus vesiculosus*)	Anticoagulant; antioxidant; bacterial and fungal infections; cancer; diabetes; fibrocystic breast disease (FBD); hypothyroidism; nutrient (rich source of iodine, potassium, magnesium, calcium, and iron)
Borage (*Borago officinalis*)	Acute respiratory distress syndrome; alcohol hangover; asthma; atopic dermatitis (treatment and prophylaxis); atopic eczema; cystic fibrosis; diabetic neuropathy; fatty acids (preterm infants); growth and development (infants); hyperlipidemia; infantile seborrheic dermatitis; malnutrition-inflammation complex syndrome; periodontitis; rheumatoid arthritis; stress; weight regain
Boron	Cognitive function improvement; osteoarthritis; osteoporosis; rheumatoid arthritis; vaginitis
Boswellia (*Boswellia serrata*)	Antiinflammatory; arthritis; asthma; brain tumors; Crohn disease; ulcerative colitis
Branched-chain amino acids (BCAAs)	Amyotrophic lateral sclerosis; anorexia; cardiac atrophy; cirrhosis; diabetes; energy metabolism improvement (in cirrhosis patients); exercise performance; hepatic encephalopathy; muscle development and lean body mass (increase); muscle fatigue and soreness; protein metabolism (in COPD patients); tardive dyskinesia
Bromelain (*Anas comosus*)	Arthritis (antiinflammatory; proteolytic); burn debridement; cancer; cervical dysplasia; chronic obstructive pulmonary disease (COPD); digestive enzyme; osteoarthritis of the knee; sinusitis; steatorrhea; urinary tract infection (UTI)
Bupleurum (*Bupleurum falcatum*)	Brain damage (minimal, children); chronic inflammatory disease; fatigue; hepatic protection; hepatitis; systemic lupus erythematosus (SLE); thrombocytopenic purpura

PROPOSED MEDICINAL CLAIMS *(continued)*

Herb	Reported Uses
Calcium	Antacid; black widow spider bite; blood pressure regulation; bone loss; bone stress injury prevention; cancer (prevention); colon cancer (distal); colorectal adenomas (recurrence); growth; hypercholesterolemia; hyperkalemia; hypermagnesemia; hyperparathyroidism; hyperphosphatemia; hypertension; kidney stones; lead toxicity; osteomalacia/rickets; osteoporosis (preventive); poison ivy (topical; lactate form); preeclampsia; pregnancy; premenstrual syndrome (PMS); weight loss in type 2 diabetic patients, fat metabolism, and weight gain prevention (in postmenopausal women); vaginal atrophy
Calendula (*Calendula officinalis*)	Antibacterial, antifungal, antiviral, antiprotozoal; otitis media; radiation dermatitis; skin inflammation; venous leg ulcers; wound healing
Caprylic acid	Antifungal/antiyeast; candidiasis; Crohn disease; dysbiosis; epilepsy (children)
Caprylidene	Alzheimer disease
Carnitine	Acute myocardial infarction (mortality); angina; arrhythmia; athletic performance (enhancement); attention-deficit hyperactivity disorder (ADHD); chronic obstructive pulmonary disease (COPD); congestive heart failure (CHF); diabetes; dialysis; diphtheria; erectile dysfunction; exercise performance; fatigue; hepatic encephalopathy; HIV/AIDS; Huntington disease; hypercholesterolemia; hyperlipoproteinemia; hyperthyroidism; male infertility; myocardial infarction; neonatal growth and breathing; obesity; peripheral vascular disease; postexercise metabolic stress and muscle damage; quality of life (maintenance hemodialysis patients); renal failure/dialysis; respiratory distress; sperm motility; weight loss
Cascara (*Rhamnus purshiana*)	Laxative
Cat's claw (*Uncaria tomentosa*)	Allergies; antiinflammatory; antimicrobial (antibacterial, antifungal, antiviral); antioxidant; arthritis; cancer; cervical dysplasia; Crohn disease; diverticulitis; endometriosis; fibromyalgia; immune support; multiple sclerosis; rosacea; systemic lupus erythematosus (SLE)
Cayenne (*Capsicum annuum, Capsicum frutescens*)	Antiinflammatory and analgesic (topical); cardiovascular circulatory support; cluster headache; digestive stimulant; fibromyalgia; postherpetic neuralgia; pruritus; rhinitis
Chamomile, German (*Matricaria chamomilla, Matricaria recutita*)	Anxiolytic; cardiovascular conditions; carminative, antispasmodic; colic; common cold; diaper rash; diarrhea (children); eczema; hemorrhagic cystitis; hemorrhoids; indigestion; insomnia (mild sedative); minor injury (topical antiinflammatory); mucositis (from chemotherapy); nausea/vomiting; oral health (as mouth rinse/gargle); stress/anxiety; teething; uterine tonic; vaginitis
Chasteberry (*Vitex agnus-castus*)	Acne vulgaris; cervical dysplasia; corpus luteum insufficiency; hyperprolactinemia and insufficient lactation; cyclic mastalgia; menopause; menorrhagia; menstrual disorders including amenorrhea, endometriosis, premenstrual syndrome (PMS); rosacea
Chitosan	Antibacterial; dental plaque; hyperlipidemia; periodontitis; renal failure; weight loss; wound healing
Chlorophyll	Antiinflammatory, antioxidant, and wound healing properties; bacteriostatic; cancer; chemoprevention; fibrocystic breast disease; herpes simplex, herpes zoster; leukopenia; odor absorbent/suppressant (breath freshener, toothpaste, mouthwash, and deodorant); pancreatitis; pneumonia; poisoning; protectant; rheumatoid arthritis; tuberculosis
Chondroitin sulfate	Coronary artery disease; interstitial cystitis; iron absorption enhancement; muscle soreness, delayed onset; ophthalmologic uses; osteoarthritis; overactive bladder; psoriasis
Chromium	Atherosclerosis; bone loss (postmenopausal women); cardiovascular disease (risk reduction; in combination); depression; diabetes, type 1; diabetes, type 2; glaucoma; hypercholesterolemia; hypertriglyceridemia; hypothyroidism; immunosuppression; insulin sensitivity (obese women with polycystic ovarian syndrome); premenstrual syndrome (PMS); weight loss
Clove (*Syzygium aromaticum*)	Anal fissures; analgesic (toothache and teething); anesthetic; antiseptic; fever; mosquito repellent; premature ejaculation (combination preparation)

PROPOSED MEDICINAL CLAIMS *(continued)*

Herb	Reported Uses
Coenzyme Q_{10}	Acute myocardial infarction; AIDS; Alzheimer disease; amyotrophic lateral sclerosis (ALS); angina; antioxidant; asthenozoospermia (idiopathic); cancer (preventive); cardiomyopathy; cardioprotection during surgery; chemotherapy (adjunct); chronic fatigue syndrome; congestive heart failure (CHF); Down syndrome; exercise performance; fibromyalgia; Friedreich ataxia; gingivitis; HMG-CoA reductase inhibitors (may cause depletion of this nutraceutical); hypercholesterolemia; hypertension; migraine; mitochondrial disease and Kearns-Sayre syndrome; multiple sclerosis; muscle pain (associated with HMG-CoA reductase inhibitors); muscular dystrophy; myelodysplastic syndromes; Parkinson disease; periodontal disease; renal failure; tinnitus; weight loss
Coleus (*Coleus forskohlii*)	Antiinflammatory action after cardiopulmonary bypass; asthma and allergies; eczema; glaucoma; hypertension and congestive heart failure (CHF); lactagogue; psoriasis
Collagen (Type II)	Arthritis (rheumatoid and osteo); burns (first- and second-degree); soft tissue correction; surgical and traumatic wounds; ulcers (pressure, venous stasis, diabetic); wound healing (topical)
Colostrum	Antiviral (mild); athletic performance (enhancement); body composition; colitis; cryptosporidiosis; diarrhea; flu prevention; HIV-associated diarrhea; *H. Pylori*; immune support; multiple sclerosis; prevention of NSAID-induced GI injury; shigellosis; sore throat; upper respiratory tract infection
Conjugated linoleic acid (CLA)	Cancer; muscle development and lean body mass (increase); obesity; oxidative stress and inflammatory disease in obese men; preeclampsia (in combination with calcium)
Copper	Age-related macular degeneration; anemia; atherosclerosis; copper deficiency; dental enamel demineralization (in combination with fluoride); growth promotion (children); marasmus; osteoporosis; plaque prevention; rheumatoid arthritis; systemic lupus erythematosus
Cordyceps (*Cordyceps sinensis*)	Adaptogen/tonic (promote wellness); antioxidant; asthma; chemotherapy and radiation (adjunct); endurance and stamina; fatigue; fibromyalgia; hepatitis B; hepatoprotection; hyperlipidemia; immunomodulator; lung, liver, and kidney function (general support); sexual vitality (males and females); tissue oxygenation
Cranberry (*Vaccinium macrocarpon*)	Achlorhydria and B_{12} absorption; antioxidant; bacterial and fungal infections; cancer (prevention); *H. pylori* infection; plaque; urinary tract infection, including prevention
Creatine	Athletic performance (enhancement) as energy production and protein synthesis for muscle building; chronic obstructive pulmonary disease; congestive heart failure (CHF); GAMT deficiency; Huntington disease; hyperlipidemia; ischemic heart disease; McArdle disease; muscle function and strength; mood; muscular dystrophy; Parkinson disease; resistance training in patients with Parkinson disease; schizophrenia; surgery (adjunct); traumatic brain injury, prevention of complications (children)
Cyclo-hispro	Diabetes, type 2; hypoglycemia
Damiana (*Turnera diffusa*)	Female sexual dysfunction; weight loss/obesity
Dandelion (*Taraxacum officinale*)	Leaf used as a diuretic; root used for disorders of bile secretion (choleretic), appetite stimulation, dyspepsia
Dehydroepiandrosterone (DHEA)	Adrenal insufficiency; AIDS/HIV; antiaging; cardiovascular disease; cervical cancer; chronic fatigue syndrome; cocaine withdrawal; cognitive function; Crohn disease; dementia; depression; diabetes, type 2; erectile dysfunction; extrapyramidal symptoms; fatigue; fibromyalgia; induction of labor; infertility; libido (premenopausal women); lupus; muscle mass and strength; obesity; perimenopausal symptoms; psoriasis; rheumatoid arthritis; schizophrenia; Sjögren syndrome
Devil's claw (*Harpagophytum procumbens*)	Antiinflammatory; back pain; osteoarthritis, gout, and other inflammatory conditions

PROPOSED MEDICINAL CLAIMS *(continued)*

Herb	Reported Uses
Docosahexaenoic acid (DHA)	Alzheimer disease; angina pectoris; appetite; arrhythmias; asthma; attention-deficit disorder and attention-deficit hyperactivity disorder (ADD/ADHD); bipolar disorder; cancer (prevention of colon cancer); cardiovascular disease; colon cancer; coronary heart disease (risk reduction); Crohn disease; cystic fibrosis; depression; diabetes; diabetes, type 2; dysmenorrhea; eczema; hypercholesterolemia; hypertension; hypertriglyceridemia; IgA nephropathy; immune support; infant eye/brain development; infection; lupus; nephrotic syndrome; preeclampsia; prevention of graft failure after heart bypass surgery; protection from cyclosporine toxicity in organ transplant patients; psoriasis; rheumatoid arthritis; schizophrenia; stroke (risk reduction); ulcerative colitis
Dong quai (*Angelica sinensis*)	Anemia; energy enhancement (particularly in females); hypertension; menopause, dysmenorrhea, premenstrual syndrome (PMS), and amenorrhea; menorrhagia; phytoestrogen; pulmonary hypertension
Echinacea (*Echinacea purpurea, Echinacea angustifolia*)	Antibacterial (topical; boils, abscesses, tonsillitis, poison ivy); antiviral; arthritis (*E. augustifolia*); genital herpes; immune support (cold and other upper respiratory infections); otitis media; radiation-associated leucopenia; upper respiratory infection; uveitis
Elder (*Sambucus nigra, Sambucus canadensis*)	Berry used as an antiviral, antioxidant, and for influenza; flower used as an antiinflammatory, for colds and influenza, diaphoretic, diuretic, fever, sinusitis, and sore throat
Ephedra (*Ephedra sinica*)	Allergies, sinusitis, hay fever; asthma; hypotension; sexual arousal; weight loss (monotherapy); weight loss (combination therapy)
Evening primrose (*Oenothera biennis*)	Amenorrhea; atopic dermatitis; attention-deficit disorder (ADD); bronchitis; depression; diabetes; diabetic peripheral neuropathy; eczema, dermatitis, and psoriasis; endometriosis; fatigue; fibrocystic breast disease (FBD); hypercholesterolemia; ichthyosis vulgaris; irritable bowel syndrome (IBS); mastalgia; menorrhagia; multiple sclerosis; obesity; omega-6 fatty acid supplementation; preeclampsia; premenstrual syndrome (PMS) and menopause; Raynaud phenomenon; rheumatoid arthritis; rosacea; scleroderma
Eyebright (*Euphrasia officinalis*)	Conjunctivitis; eye fatigue; catarrh of the eyes; hepatoprotection
Fennel (*Foeniculum vulgare* Mill.)	ACE inhibitor-associated cough; colic, infantile; dysmenorrhea; ultraviolet skin protection
Fenugreek (*Trigonella foenum-graecum*)	Diabetes; galactagogue; hypercholesterolemia
Feverfew (*Tanacetum parthenium*)	Antiinflammatory, rheumatoid arthritis; migraine headache (preventive); muscle soreness
Fish oils	Acne vulgaris; angina pectoris; arrhythmias; asthma; bipolar disorder; body weight improvement; cancer (prevention); cardiac death (sudden; preventive); cardiac support (general; proposed benefits); cardiovascular disease; circulation; cognitive performance; colon cancer; coronary heart disease (preventive); Crohn disease; cystic fibrosis; depression; diabetes, type 2; dysmenorrhea; eczema, psoriasis; fatigue; headache; heart disease and heart attack (risk reduction), including women and antiinflammatory effects in heart failure patients; herpes simplex 2; hypercholesterolemia; hypertension; hypertriglyceridemia; IgA nephropathy; immune support; infant eye/brain development; lupus; memory enhancement; multiple sclerosis; nephrotic syndrome; preeclampsia; premenstrual syndrome (PMS); prevention of graft failure after heart bypass surgery; protection from cyclosporine toxicity in organ transplant patients; psoriasis; Raynaud phenomenon; rheumatoid arthritis; rosacea; schizophrenia; scleroderma; stroke (risk reduction); ulcerative colitis
Flaxseed oil	Acne vulgaris; arthritis (rheumatoid); asthma; attention deficit hyperactivity disorder (ADHD); constipation; coronary heart disease (risk reduction); diabetes; hemorrhoids; dry eyes (Sjogren syndrome); hemorrhoids; hyperlipidemia; hypertension; menopausal symptoms; multiple sclerosis; omega-3 essential fatty acid source (cell wall and cellular membrane structure; cholesterol transport and oxidation); premenstrual syndrome (PMS); prostaglandins production; psoriasis; stroke (risk reduction); systemic lupus erythematosus (SLE)

PROPOSED MEDICINAL CLAIMS *(continued)*

Herb	Reported Uses
Folic acid	Alcoholism; Alzheimer disease; anemia; atherosclerosis; beta-thalassemia; cancer (preventive; colon and breast); cardiovascular morbidity or mortality in patients with chronic renal failure; cervical dysplasia; chronic fatigue syndrome; cognitive function; coronary heart disease (risk reduction); coronary restenosis (rate reduction by decreasing plasma homocysteine levels); Crohn disease; dementia and Alzheimer disease (risk reduction); depression; endothelial dysfunction (in type 2 diabetes); fragile X syndrome; gingivitis; hearing loss (slows progression); homocysteine; methotrexate toxicity; nitrate tolerance; osteoporosis; phenytoin-induced gingival hyperplasia; pregnancy (prevention of birth defects) and lactation; schizophrenia (risk reduction, by decreasing homocysteine levels); stroke; ulcer, aphthous; vitiligo
Gamma Linolenic Acid (GLA)	Acute respiratory distress syndrome; atopic dermatitis; attention-deficit hyperactivity disorder (ADHD); blood pressure control; cancer treatment (adjunct); diabetic neuropathy; immune enhancement; mastalgia; menopausal hot flashes; migraine; osteoporosis; preeclampsia; premenstrual syndrome (PMS); pruritus; rheumatoid arthritis; Sjögren syndrome; ulcerative colitis
Garcinia (*Garcinia cambogia*)	Exercise performance; halitosis; pancreatic function (supportive) and glucose regulation; weight loss
Garlic (*Allium sativum*)	Alopecia; antimicrobial (bacterial and fungal) including *Helicobacter pylori* infection and tinea pedis; antioxidant (practitioners should be aware that aged garlic extracts have been reported to improve this benefit); atherosclerosis; cancer (prevention); coagulation (mild inhibitor of platelet-activating factor); cryptococcal meningitis; cutaneous microcirculation; diabetes; hyperlipidemia; hypertension; immune support; peripheral vascular disease; tick repellant; upper respiratory tract infection
Ginger (*Zingiber officinale*)	Antiemetic, for nausea and vomiting in pregnancy, motion sickness; antiinflammatory (musculoskeletal); diverticulitis; indigestion/heartburn; motion sickness; osteoarthritis
Ginkgo (*Ginkgo biloba*)	Acute ischemic stroke; Alzheimer disease, dementia, age-related memory impairment; anxiety; asthma; chemotherapy (adjunct); chronic cochleovestibular disorders; cognitive function; depression; epilepsy; functional measures (in patients with multiple sclerosis); gastric cancer; glaucoma; headache; intermittent claudication; macular degeneration; memory enhancement; mountain sickness; multiple sclerosis; ocular blood flow; Parkinson disease; peripheral blood flow (cerebral vascular disease, peripheral vascular insufficiency, impotence, tinnitus, and depression); premenstrual syndrome (PMS); quality of life; Raynaud phenomenon; retinopathy; seasonal affective disorder (SAD); seizures; sexual dysfunction (antidepressant-induced); tinnitus; vertigo; vitiligo
Ginseng, Panax (*Panax ginseng*)	Adrenal tonic; bronchitis; cancer; congestive heart failure; COPD; dementia; diabetes; diabetic nephropathy; immune support; physical and mental performance including energy enhancement and chemotherapy and radiation (adjunct); radiation therapy side effects
Ginseng, Siberian (*Eleutherococcus senticosus*)	Adaptogen/tonic (promote wellness); athletic performance (enhancement); stress (decreased fatigue); immune support
Glucosamine	Chronic venous insufficiency; inflammatory bowel disease; knee injury recovery; osteoarthritis and joint structure support; rheumatoid arthritis and other inflammatory conditions; temporomandibular joint (TMJ)
Glutamine	Alcoholism; athletic performance (enhancement); cancer (adjunct); catabolic wasting; chemotherapy (prevention of adverse effects); critical illness; fibromyalgia; HIV (adjunct); HIV wasting; immune support; muscular dystrophy; peptic ulcer disease; postsurgical healing; ulcerative colitis and other inflammatory bowel diseases
Glutathione	Antioxidant, chemoprotection; hepatoprotection (alcohol-induced liver damage); immune support; male infertility; peptic ulcer disease; peripheral artery disease
Golden seal (*Hydrastis canadensis*)	Antimicrobial (antibacterial/antifungal); bronchitis, cystitis, and infectious diarrhea; fever; gallbladder; gastritis; heart failure; immune stimulation; infectious diarrhea; malaria (chloroquine resistant); mucous membrane tonifying (used in inflammation of mucosal membranes); narcotic concealment (urine analysis); sinusitis; sore throat; trachoma; urinary tract infection (UTI)

PROPOSED MEDICINAL CLAIMS *(continued)*

Herb	Reported Uses
Gotu kola (*Centella asiatica*)	Anxiety; cirrhosis; connective tissue (support); diabetic microangiopathy; hemorrhoids (topical); macular degeneration; memory enhancement; psoriasis; venous insufficiency; wound healing (topical)
Grapefruit seed (*Citrus paradisi*)	Antifungal, antibacterial, antiparasitic; diarrhea; diverticulitis; eczema; endometriosis; heart disease; irritable bowel syndrome (IBS); kidney stones; metabolic syndrome; rosacea; sinusitis; sore throat; ulcerative colitis; urinary tract infection (UTI)
Grapeseed (*Vitis vinifera*)	Agitation (aromatherapy); allergies, antiinflammatory, asthma; antioxidant; cardiovascular health; chloasma; circulation, platelet aggregation inhibitor, capillary fragility, arterial/venous insufficiency (intermittent claudification, varicose veins); diabetic retinopathy; edema; gingivitis; glaucoma; hyperlipidemia; macular degeneration; multiple sclerosis; Parkinson disease; scleroderma; sun protection
Green tea (*Camellia sinensis*)	Antioxidant, cancer and cardiovascular disease (preventive); chemotherapy and radiation (adjunct); common cold (prevention); diabetes; diarrhea; genital warts; gingivitis (prevention); human T-cell lymphocytic virus; hypercholesterolemia; hypertension; hypertriglyceridemia; macular degeneration; photoprotection; platelet-aggregation inhibitor; weight loss
Ground Ivy (*Glechoma hederacea*)	No reported therapeutic uses
Guggul (*Commiphora mukul*)	Acne vulgaris; hypercholesterolemia; hypothyroidism; obesity; osteoarthritis; rheumatoid arthritis; weight loss
Gymnema (*Gymnema sylvestre*)	Diabetes, blood sugar regulation; hyperlipidemia; weight loss
Hawthorn (*Crataegus oxyacantha*)	Angina; hypotension, hypertension, peripheral vascular disease, tachycardia; cardiotonic; congestive heart failure; heart failure
Hops (*Humulus lupulus*)	Menopausal symptoms; sedative/hypnotic (mild); rheumatic disease
Horse chestnut (*Aesculus hippocastanum*)	Scleroderma; venous insufficiency (varicose veins, hemorrhoids, deep venous thrombosis, lower extremity edema [oral and topical])
Horseradish (*Armoracia rusticana, Cochlearia armoracia*)	No reported therapeutic uses
Horsetail (*Equisetum arvense*)	Bone and connective tissue strengthening, including osteoporosis; diuretic; high mineral content (including silicic acid)
HuperzineA (*Huperzia serrata*)	Myasthenia gravis; senile dementia and Alzheimer disease
Hyaluronic acid	Aging; antioxidant; arthritis; immune system stimulant; osteoarthritis; skin conditions; urinary tract infections
Hydroxymethyl butyrate (HMB)	AIDS wasting; athletic performance (enhancement); muscle damage
5-Hydroxytryptophan (5-HTP)	Anxiety; cerebellar ataxia; depression; fibromyalgia; headache; migraine; schizophrenia; sleep disorders, insomnia (stimulates the production of melatonin); weight loss/obesity
Hyssop (*Hyssopus officinalis*)	Kidney inflammation
Inositol hexaphosphate (IP-6)	Cancer (preventive); intermittent claudication
Iodine	Bacterial conjunctivitis; bladder irrigation; bowel irrigation; cancer; cognitive function; corpus vitreous degeneration; fibrocystic breast disease (FBD); filarial lymphoedema; goiter (preventive); Graves disease; hypothyroidism; molluscum; mucolytic; ophthalmia neonatorum (preventive); oral intubation; periodontitis/gingivitis; pneumonia; postcesarean endometriosis; renal pelvic instillation sclerotherapy; skin disinfectant (wound cleansing); thyrotoxicosis; water purification
Ipriflavone	Menopausal symptoms; prevention of osteoporosis (men and women)
Iron	ACE inhibitor-associated cough; anemia; athletic performance; attention-deficit hyperactivity disorder (ADHD); blood transfusions (reduction); cognitive performance; hyposalivation; menorrhagia; nutritional status (infants/children); pregnancy; restless legs syndrome

PROPOSED MEDICINAL CLAIMS *(continued)*

Herb	Reported Uses
Isoflavones (soy)	Benign prostatic hyperplasia (BPH); bone mineral density (increase); cancer (preventive); cardiovascular effects; cervical dysplasia; chemotherapy (adjunct); cognitive function; diabetes; diarrhea; endometriosis; hypercholesterolemia; immune function; menopausal symptoms; menstrual migraine; osteoarthritis; osteoporosis; platelet function; premenstrual syndrome (PMS); prevention of bone loss; skin aging; weight loss
Kava kava (*Piper methysticum*)	Anxiety/stress, skeletal muscle relaxation, postischemic episodes; fibromyalgia; insomnia; muscle soreness
Kudzu (*Pueraria lobata*)	Alcoholism; cardiovascular disease/angina; deafness; diabetes; diabetic retinopathy; glaucoma; menopausal symptoms
Lactobacillus acidophilus	Allergies; bacterial vaginosis; colitis (collagenous); constipation; diarrhea (infantile, prevention, and chronic); eczema (preventive); gastrointestinal microflora recolonization; hepatic encephalopathy; hypercholesterolemia; immune support; irritable bowel syndrome (IBS); lactose intolerance; necrotizing enterocolitis; vaginal candidiasis
Lavender (*Lavendula officinalis*)	Anxiety; cancer; dementia (behavior disturbances); depression; hypnotic/sleep (aromatherapy); pain; perineal discomfort following childbirth; spasmolytic (oral); wound healing including minor burns (topical)
Lecithin	Acne vulgaris; dementia (ineffective); extrapyramidal disorders; hepatic steatosis; hypercholesterolemia
Lemon balm/Melissa (*Melissa officinalis*)	Agitation in dementia; antiviral (oral herpes virus); anxiety; attention-deficit hyperactivity disorder (ADHD); cognitive performance; colitis; dyspepsia; sedation (pediatrics); sleep quality; teething (topical)
Licorice (*Glycyrrhiza glabra*)	Adrenal insufficiency (licorice); aphthous ulcers/canker sores; atopic dermatitis; body fat mass reduction; Crohn disease; croup; expectorant and antitussive (licorice); familial Mediterranean fever (FMF); gastrointestinal ulceration (DGL chewable products); herpes simplex; hyperkalemia; viral hepatitis
Liver extract	Chronic fatigue syndrome; hepatitis; liver tonic; pernicious anemia
Lutein	Antioxidant; cataracts; colon cancer; macular degeneration; preeclampsia; visual acuity
Lycopene	Asthma (exercise induced); atherosclerosis; cancer (preventive; especially colon, lung, and prostate); immune enhancement; macular degeneration; oral submucous fibrosis
Lysine	Angina pectoris; growth and development (children); herpes simplex; osteoporosis; ulcer, aphthous
Magnesium	Acute tocolysis of preterm labor; arrhythmias/torsade de pointes; asthma; attention-deficit hyperactivity disorder (ADHD); cardiovascular disease; circulation; colic (magnesium salt); congestive heart failure (CHF); constipation; coronary artery disease; diabetes; dysmenorrhea; epilepsy; fatigue; fibromyalgia (magnesium salt); gallbladder (magnesium salt); hearing loss; heart disease; hypertension; hypoglycemia; insomnia; kidney stones; migraine headache; mitral valve prolapse (MVP); multiple sclerosis; muscle cramps; nervousness; neuropathic pain; osteoporosis; pain; preeclampsia/eclampsia; premenstrual syndrome (PMS); stress/anxiety; tension headache
Maitake (*Grifola frondosa*)	Cancer; diabetes; immune stimulation
Malic acid	Aluminum toxicity; fibromyalgia
Manganese	Diabetes; epilepsy; menstrual symptoms; osteoporosis
Marshmallow (*Althaea officinalis*)	Cough; croup; mucilaginous, demulcent; peptic ulcer disease; skin inflammatory conditions; sore throat
Mastic (*Pistacia lentiscus*)	Dental plaque; *H. pylori* inhibitor; peptic ulcer disease

PROPOSED MEDICINAL CLAIMS *(continued)*

Herb	Reported Uses
Melatonin	ADHD (sleep disorders); age-related macular degeneration; Alzheimer disease (sleep disorders); anxiety (preoperative); autism (sleep disorders); benzodiazepine tapering; bipolar disorder; cancer; cardioprotection; chemotherapy adverse effects; cognitive impairment; delayed sleep phase syndrome; depression (sleep disturbances); duodenal ulcer; dyspepsia; glaucoma; glycemic control; headache prevention; HIV/AIDS; hypertension; insomnia including elderly, children, and individuals with intellectual disabilities; irritable bowel syndrome; jet lag; menopause; nocturia; oxidative stress in dialysis patients (preventive); Parkinson disease; periodic limb movement disorder; preoperative sedation/ anxiolysis; Rett syndrome; sarcoidosis, chronic; schizophrenia (sleep disorders); seasonal affective disorder (SAD); sedation (children); seizure disorders; skin damage; sleep disturbances, in blind people; stroke; tardive dyskinesia; thrombocytopenia; tinnitus (sleep disorders); tuberous sclerosis; work-shift sleep disorder
Methionine	Acetaminophen toxicity; liver detoxification
Methyl sulfonyl methane (MSM)	Allergies; analgesic; arthritis (osteo and rheumatoid); interstitial cystitis; lupus; seasonal allergic rhinitis
Milk thistle (*Silybum marianum*)	*Amanita phalloides* mushroom toxicity; antidote for poisoning by Death Cup mushroom; antioxidant (specifically hepatic cells), acute/chronic hepatitis, jaundice, and stimulation of bile secretion/cholagogue; chemotherapy and radiation (adjunct); cirrhosis; constipation; diabetes; eczema; gallbladder; halitosis; hepatoprotective, including drug toxicities (ie, phenothiazines, butyrophenones, ethanol, and acetaminophen); hyperlipidemia; hyperthyroidism; psoriasis; rosacea
Modified citrus pectin (MCP)	Anticarcinogenic; detoxification (toxic elements); diarrhea; hypercholesterolemia; prostate cancer
Muira puama (*Ptychopetalum olacoides*)	Athletic performance (enhancement); erectile dysfunction; sexual vitality (males)
N-Acetyl cysteine (NAC)	Acetaminophen toxicity; acute respiratory distress syndrome (ARDS); acute respiratory infection; AIDS; angina; asthma (mucolytic, antioxidant); bronchitis; cancer; cardioprotection (during chemotherapy); cerebral adrenoleukodystrophy; chemotherapy adverse effects; chronic obstructive pulmonary disease (COPD); fatigue; glutathione production; heavy metal detoxification; HIV/AIDS; hyperthyroidism; hypothyroidism; influenza prevention; macular degeneration; multiple sclerosis; myocardial infarction; nephropathy (preventive); ovulation (induction in polycystic ovary syndrome); Parkinson disease; polycystic ovarian syndrome; renal impairment; scleroderma; sepsis; Sjögren syndrome; systemic lupus erythematosus (SLE)
Nicotinamide adenine dinucleotide (NADH)	Chronic fatigue syndrome; dementia; diabetes, type 1; hepatitis; Parkinson disease; stamina and energy
Octacosanol	Amyotrophic lateral sclerosis (ALS); hypercholesterolemia; Parkinson disease
Olive leaf (*Olea europaea*)	Acne vulgaris; antibacterial; antifungal, antiviral; Crohn disease; diabetes; diarrhea; diverticulitis; eczema; endometriosis; hypertension; multiple sclerosis; scleroderma; ulcerative colitis; urinary tract infection (UTI)
Pancreatic extract	Antiinflammatory; cancer (adjunct); celiac disease; digestive disturbances; food allergies; immune complex diseases; malabsorption
Para-Aminobenzoic acid (PABA)	Peyronie disease; scleroderma; vitiligo
Parsley (*Petroselinum crispum*)	Halitosis; antibacterial, antifungal
Passion flower (*Passiflora spp*)	Anxiety; congestive heart failure (CHF); hyperthyroidism; insomnia (sedative)
Peppermint (*Mentha piperita*)	Brain injury (aromatherapy); carminative, spasmolytic; colic; cough; cracked nipples (prevention); dyspepsia; gastrointestinal disorders, antispasmodic; indigestion; irritable bowel syndrome; motion sickness; nasal congestion; postherpetic neuralgia; postoperative nausea (inhalation); tension headache (topical)
Periwinkle (*Vinca minor*)	No reported therapeutic uses
Phenylalanine	Analgesic; depression; pain; Parkinson disease; reward deficiency syndrome in addiction; vitiligo

PROPOSED MEDICINAL CLAIMS *(continued)*

Herb	Reported Uses
Phosphatidyl choline (PC)	Alcohol-induced liver damage; Alzheimer disease; gallstones; hepatitis; hypercholesterolemia; tardive dyskinesia
Phosphatidyl serine (PS)	Alzheimer disease; depression; memory enhancement
Phosphorus	Bowel cleansing; burns; diabetic ketoacidosis; exercise performance; hypercalcemia; hypercalciuria; hyperparathyroidism; hypophosphatemia; kidney stones; refeeding syndrome prevention; total parenteral nutrition (TPN); vitamin D resistant rickets
Policosanol	Coronary heart disease; hypercholesterolemia; intermittent claudication; platelet aggregation inhibition; reactivity/brain activity
Potassium	Bone loss; cardiac arrhythmias; congestive heart failure (CHF); hypercalciuria; hypertension; kidney stones; molluscum contagiosum (topical); QT prolongation
Pregnenolone	Arthritis; hormone precursor (DHEA, cortisol, progesterone, estrogens, and testosterone); mental performance
Progesterone	Brain injury; breast cancer (preventive); dysmenorrhea; endometriosis; infertility; menopause; osteoporosis; premenstrual syndromes (PMS); preterm birth
Psyllium (*Plantago ovata, Plantago isphagula*)	Anal fissures; bulk-forming laxative (containing 10% to 30% mucilage); colon cancer; colonoscopy preparation; constipation; diarrhea; flatulence; halitosis; hemorrhoids; hypercholesterolemia; hyperglycemia; induction of labor; inflammatory bowel disease; irritable bowel syndrome (IBS); obesity
Pycnogenol (*Pinus pinaster*)	Asthma; attention-deficit hyperactivity disorder (ADHD); chronic venous insufficiency; climacteric syndrome; diabetes, type 2; diabetic microangiopathy; erectile dysfunction; gingival bleeding/plaque; hypertension; platelet aggregation (smokers); prevention of blood clots during long airplane flights; retinopathy; systemic lupus erythematosus (SLE); venous leg ulcers
Pygeum (*Pygeum africanum, Prunus africana*)	Benign prostatic hyperplasia (BPH)
Pyruvate	Athletic performance (enhancement); hyperlipidemia; photoaging; weight loss
Quercetin	Allergies; asthma; atherosclerosis; cardiovascular disease; cataracts; immune function; pancreatic cancer prevention; peptic ulcer disease; prostatitis; sinusitis
Red clover (*Trifolium pratense*)	Benign prostatic hyperplasia (BPH); endometriosis; hypercholesterolemia; liver and kidney detoxification (liquid extract); menopause; menorrhagia; osteoporosis; prostate cancer
Red yeast rice (*Monascus purpureus*)	Coronary heart disease; diabetes; hypercholesterolemia
Rehmannia (*Rehmannia glutinosa*)	Aplastic anemia (adjuvant); rheumatoid arthritis; Sheehan syndrome; systemic lupus erythematosus (SLE)
Reishi (*Ganoderma lucidum*)	Chemotherapy and radiation (adjunct); chronic hepatitis B; coronary heart disease; diabetes, type 2; fatigue; hypertension; immune support; poisoning (*Russula subnigricans*); postherpetic neuralgia; proteinuria; seizure disorder
Rose Hips (*Rosa canina*, *Various Rosa* spp)	Antioxidant; osteoarthritis
SAMe (S-adenosyl methionine)	Attention-deficit hyperactivity disorder (ADHD); cardiovascular disease; cholestasis; depression; fibromyalgia; headache; insomnia; liver disease; osteoarthritis; rheumatoid arthritis
Saw palmetto (*Serenoa repens*)	Androgenetic alopecia (topical); benign prostatic hyperplasia (BPH); prostatitis
Schisandra (*Schizandra chinensis*)	Adaptogen/tonic (to promote wellness); hepatic protection and detoxification; chemotherapy and radiation (adjunct); endurance, stamina, and work performance (enhancement); decreases fatigue

PROPOSED MEDICINAL CLAIMS *(continued)*

Herb	Reported Uses
Selenium	Acne vulgaris (with vitamin E); AIDS/HIV; asthma; atherosclerosis; bronchial asthma; burns; cancer (preventive); cardiomyopathy; cardiovascular disease; cataracts; chemotherapy and radiation (adjunct); chromosome damage (reduction); circulation; cystic fibrosis; dandruff; diabetes; dialysis; eczema; epilepsy; esophageal cancer; gastric cancer; hemorrhoids; herpes simplex 1 and 2; hypothyroidism; infection; infertility; intracranial pressure symptoms; low birth weight; lymphedema; macular degeneration; myotonic dystrophy; pancreatitis; preeclampsia; prostate cancer (preventive); psoriasis; rheumatoid arthritis; sepsis; thyroid conditions; tinea capitis; tinea versicolor; ulcerative colitis; uveitis
Senna (*Cassia senna*)	Bowel preparation for colonoscopy; laxative
Shark cartilage	Analgesia; cancer therapy; macular degeneration; osteoarthritis, rheumatoid arthritis; psoriasis
Skullcap (*Scutellaria lateriflora*)	Anxiety; cancer (*in vitro*); inflammation (*in vitro*)
Slippery Elm (*Ulmus fulva, Ulmus rubra*)	Cancer; diarrhea; gastrointestinal disorders; sore throat
Sodium	No reported therapeutic uses
Spirulina	Allergic rhinitis; arsenic poisoning; blepharospasm; chronic viral hepatitis; diabetes, type 2; fatigue; hypercholesterolemia; malnutrition; oral leukoplakia/cancer; skeletal muscle damage; weight loss
Spleen extract	Chemotherapy and radiation (adjunct); cold/influenza; fatigue; spleen function (supportive)
Stinging nettle (*Urtica dioica*)	Leaf used for allergic rhinitis, allergy, and hay fever symptoms, arthritis, joint pain, sinusitis, uric acid excretion; root used for benign prostatic hyperplasia (BPH)
St John's wort (*Hypericum perforatum*)	Antibacterial, antiinflammatory (topical: minor wounds, infections, bruises, muscle soreness, and sprains); antiviral; anxiety; atopic dermatitis; climacteric symptoms (combination therapy); mild to moderate depression, depression (children), seasonal affective disorder (SAD), melancholia, stress and anxiety, major depression; HIV; obsessive compulsive disorder (OCD); perimenopausal symptoms; premenstrual syndrome (PMS); smoking cessation; social phobia; somatoform disorders
Taurine	Congestive heart failure (CHF); cystic fibrosis; diabetes; energy; gallbladder; hypercholesterolemia; hypertension; iron deficiency anemia; liver disease; myotonic dystrophy; nutritional supplement (infant formula); nutritional support (TPN); obesity; seizure disorders; surgery; vaccine adjunct; vision problems
Tea tree (*Melaleuca alternifolia*)	**Not for ingestion**; acne vulgaris; antifungal, antibacterial; mouthwash for dental and oral health; burns, cuts, scrapes, insect bites, dandruff, lice, MRSA, onychomycosis, thrush
Thyme (*Thymus vulgaris*)	Alopecia areata; antifungal; bronchitis with cough; cough (upper respiratory origin); croup; dental plaque; inflammatory skin disorders
Thymus extract	Alopecia; arthritis; asthma; burns; cancer; chronic obstructive pulmonary disease; diabetes; fatigue; food allergies; glaucoma; human papilloma virus; HIV/AIDS; immune support; otitis media; respiratory tract infection; sinusitis; systemic lupus erythematosus (SLE)
Thyroid extract	Fatigue; immune support; fibromyalgia; hypothyroidism
Tocotrienols	Atherosclerosis; cancer (preventive); heart disease; hypercholesterolemia; skin (supportive, protective)
Tribulus (*Tribulus terrestris*)	Athletic performance (enhancement); coronary artery disease; infertility; muscle strength; sexual vitality
Turmeric (*Curcuma longa*)	Antioxidant; antiinflammatory; antirheumatic; cancer; cholelithiasis prevention, gallbladder disease; hypercholesterolemia; dysmenorrhea; dyspepsia; HIV; muscle soreness; osteoarthritis; peptic ulcer disease; rheumatoid arthritis; scabies; uveitis
Tylophora (*Tylophora asthmatica*)	Allergies; asthma
Tyrosine	Alzheimer disease; attention-deficit disorder and attention-deficit hyperactivity disorder (ADD/ADHD); cocaine cravings; depression; hypertension; hypothyroidism; narcolepsy; phenylketonuria (PKU); Rett syndrome; schizophrenia; stress; substance abuse

PROPOSED MEDICINAL CLAIMS *(continued)*

Herb	Reported Uses
Uva Ursi (*Arctostaphylos uva-ursi*)	Hyperpigmentation; urinary tract infections and kidney stone prevention
Valerian (*Valeriana officinalis*)	Anxiety; depression; hyperthyroidism; insomnia (sedative/hypnotic); premenstrual syndrome (PMS), menopause; restless motor syndromes and muscle spasms
Vanadium	Diabetes, type 1; diabetes, type 2; hypercholesterolemia; hypoglycemia; pneumonia
Vinpocetine	Acute ischemic stroke; Alzheimer disease and senility; cognitive function; hearing impairment; joint disorders; urinary incontinence
Vitamin A (Retinol)	Acne vulgaris; acute promyelocytic leukemia; AIDS; breast cancer; cancer (preventive); cataract preventive; cervical dysplasia; chemotherapy adverse effects; circulation; cold/influenza; Crohn disease; diarrhea; diverticulitis; eczema; esophageal cancer; fibrocystic breast disease (FBD); gastric cancer; glaucoma; goiter; hemorrhoids; HIV transmission; immune function; infant mortality; iron deficiency anemia; lung cancer; malaria; measles; menorrhagia; night blindness; norovirus; otitis media; pancreatic cancer; parasitic infections; photorefractive keratectomy; pneumonia; polyp prevention; pregnancy related complications; premenstrual syndrome (PMS); psoriasis; respiratory infection; retinitis pigmentosa; rosacea; skin aging, wrinkles; skin cancer preventive; sore throat; ulcerative colitis; urinary tract infection (UTI); weight loss; wound healing; xerophthalmia
Vitamin B_1 (Thiamine)	Alcoholism; Alzheimer disease; anemia (megaloblastic); cancer; cataract prevention; congestive heart failure (CHF); Crohn disease; diabetes; endothelial function; fibromyalgia; heart failure (cardiomyopathy); insomnia; metabolic disorders; neurological conditions (Bell palsy, trigeminal neuralgia, sciatica, sensory neuropathies); psychiatric illness; pyruvate dehydrogenase deficiency (PDH); total parenteral nutrition (TPN); Wernicke-Korsakoff syndrome (WKS); Wolfram syndrome (DIDMOAD)
Vitamin B_2	Anemia; anorexia/bulimia; cataracts; depression; esophageal cancer; ethylmalonic encephalopathy; malaria; migraine; neonatal jaundice; preeclampsia
Vitamin B_3	Acne vulgaris (4% niacinamide topical gel); age-related macular degeneration; atherosclerosis; cataracts; coronary disease (preventive); diabetes, type 1; diabetes, type 2; headache; hyperlipidemia (hypercholesterolemia, hypertriglyceridemia); impaired glucose tolerance; intermittent claudication; myocardial infarction (risk reduction); osteoarthritis; pellagra; phosphate control; Raynaud phenomenon; rheumatoid arthritis; schizophrenia; skin conditions
Vitamin B_5 (Pantothenic acid)	Adrenal support; allergies; arthritis; athletic performance (enhancement); attention-deficit hyperactivity disorder (ADHD); constipation; hyperlipidemia (pantethine, but not pantothenic acid, lowers cholesterol and triglycerides); osteoarthritis; radiation skin irritation; rheumatoid arthritis; wound healing
Vitamin B_6 (Pyridoxine)	Adverse effects of cycloserine (prevention); akathisia; Alzheimer disease; angioplasty; arthritis; asthma; attention-deficit hyperactivity disorder (ADHD); autism; birth outcomes; cardiovascular disease; carpal tunnel syndrome; coronary heart disease (risk reduction); coronary restenosis (rate reduction by lowering plasma homocysteine levels); dementia (risk reduction); depression (associated with oral contraceptives); diabetic peripheral neuropathy; epilepsy, B_6-dependant; headache; hereditary sideroblastic anemia; homocysteine (reduction); hyperkinetic syndrome; immune function; insomnia; kidney stones; lactation suppression; monosodium glutamate (MSG) sensitivity; nausea and vomiting (in pregnancy); peptic ulcer disease; premenstrual syndrome (PMS); pyridoxine dependent seizures in newborns; tardive dyskinesia
Vitamin B_{12} (Cobalamin)	AIDS; angioplasty; asthma; atherosclerosis (due to homocysteine elevation); breast cancer; coronary heart disease; coronary restenosis (rate reduction by lowering plasma homocysteine levels); Crohn disease; dementia and Alzheimer disease (risk reduction); depression; diabetic peripheral neuropathy; fatigue; homocysteine (reduction); Imerslund-Grasbeck disease; male infertility; megaloblastic anemia; memory loss; multiple sclerosis; pernicious anemia; radiation-induced mucosal injury; shaky leg syndrome; sickle cell disease; stroke; sulfite sensitivity
Vitamin B complex-25	See individual B vitamins

PROPOSED MEDICINAL CLAIMS *(continued)*

Herb	Reported Uses
Vitamin C	AIDS; alkaptonuria; allergies; Alzheimer disease; asthma; atherosclerosis; cancer; cardiovascular disease (negative report); cataracts; cervical dysplasia; chromosome damage (reduction); circulation; cold; constipation; coronary heart disease (preventive, in patients laking lipid-lowering agents, antioxidant); Crohn disease; diabetes; diabetes, type 2; diverticulitis; eczema; endometriosis; fatigue; fever; fibrocystic breast disease (FBD); fibromyalgia; gallbladder disease (risk reduction); gastroprotection; gingivitis; glaucoma; herpes simplex virus 1 and 2; *helicobacter pylori* (combination therapy); immune support; iron absorption enhancement; irritable bowel syndrome (IBS); ischemic heart disease; LDL oxidation (decrease in males); macular degeneration; multiple sclerosis; myocardial infarction (risk reduction); nitrate tolerance (preventive); osteoporosis; otitis media; pain (complex regional pain syndrome with wrist fracture); Parkinson disease; peptic ulcer disease; plaque; pregnancy; psoriasis; reflex sympathetic dystrophy (preventive); sinusitis; sore throat; stress/anxiety; stroke (preventive); sunburn; ulcerative colitis; urinary tract infection (UTI); vaginitis; wound healing
Vitamin D	Cancer, congestive heart failure; Crohn disease; diabetes; epilepsy (during anticonvulsant therapy); fall prevention; familial hypophosphatemia; Fanconi syndrome; hearing loss; hepatic osteodystrophy; hyperparathyroidism; hypertension; hypocalcemia; immune response (prevents reactivation of latent tuberculosis infection); immune response to hepatitis B vaccine; multiple sclerosis; muscle weakness; Myelodysplastic syndrome; nutritional status (breast-feeding women and infants); osteogenesis imperfecta; osteomalacia; osteoporosis including increase bone mineral density; physical performance; pigmented lesions; prostate cancer; proximal myopathy; psoriasis; renal osteodystrophy; rheumatoid arthritis; rickets; scleroderma; seasonal affective disorder (SAD); senile warts; tooth retention; weight loss (combination therapy)
Vitamin E	Acne vulgaris (with selenium); allergic rhinitis; Alzheimer disease; anemia; angina; arterial elasticity; asthma; atherosclerosis; Benign prostatic hyperplasia (BPH); bladder cancer; breast cancer; cancer (preventive); cardiovascular disease; cataracts; cervical dysplasia; chromosome damage (reduction); circulation; colon cancer (preventive); congestive heart failure; diabetes; diabetes, type 2; dyslipidemias; dysmenorrhea; eczema; endometriosis; epilepsy; esophageal caner; fibrocystic breast disease (FBD); G6PD deficiency; gallbladder; gastric cancer; glomerulosclerosis (kidney disease); hemorrhoids; hyperlipidemia; immune support; intermittent claudication; LDL oxidation (decrease in males); macular degeneration; mucositis (chemotherapy-induced); multiple sclerosis; myocardial infarction (risk reduction); neurotoxicity; osteoarthritis; Parkinson disease; peptic ulcer disease; peripheral circulation; photorefractive keratectomy; platelet aggregation; premenstrual syndrome (PMS); prostate cancer; psoriasis; respiratory infection (preventive); rheumatoid arthritis; scar prevention; scleroderma; steatohepatitis; sunburn; systemic lupus erythematosus (SLE); tardive dyskinesia; ulcerative colitis; uveitis; venous thromboembolism
Vitamin K	Hemorrhagic disease (in newborns); hepatitis C (preventive effects); hepatocellular carcinoma; osteoporosis, bone strength; synthesis of blood clotting factors; warfarin toxicity
White oak (*Quercus alba*)	Antiinflammatory (mild: throat and mouth as a soothing agent)
White willow (*Salix alba*)	Antipyretic; antiinflammatory; headache; low back pain; osteoarthritis; rheumatoid arthritis
Wild yam (*Dioscorea villosa*)	Female vitality (conversion to progesterone in the body is poor); hyperlipidemia; menopause

PROPOSED MEDICINAL CLAIMS *(continued)*

Herb	Reported Uses
Yohimbe (*Pausinystalia yohimbe*)	Autonomic failure; male erectile dysfunction; platelet aggregation inhibition; sexual side effects of SSRIs; sexual vitality (men and women); xerostomia (psychotropic drug induced)
Zinc	Acne vulgaris; alopecia areata; anorexia nervosa; aphthous ulcers; attention-deficit hyperactivity disorder (ADHD); benign prostatic hyperplasia (BPH); beta-thalassemia; boils; burns; cirrhosis; closed head injuries; cognitive deficits (children); common cold; Crohn disease; cystic fibrosis; dandruff; diabetes; diabetic neuropathy; diaper rash; diarrhea; diverticulitis; Down syndrome; exercise performance; fungal infections; gastric ulcer healing; Gilbert syndrome; halitosis; hepatic encephalopathy; hepatitis C; herpes simplex; HIV/AIDS; hyperlipidemia; immune support; infection; infertility; kwashiorkor; leg ulcers; leprosy; lower respiratory tract infection (children); macular degeneration; malaria; mucositis; muscle cramps; osteoporosis; otitis media; parasite infection; plaque/gingivitis; pneumonia; poisoning (arsenic); pregnancy; prostatitis (chronic); respiratory papillomatosis; rheumatoid arthritis; rosacea; sexual vitality (men); sickle cell anemia; skin conditions, eczema, psoriasis; sore throat; stomatitis; taste perception; tinnitus; trichomoniasis; ulcerative colitis; urecemic hypogeusia; viral warts; Wilson disease; wound healing

NEW DRUGS ADDED SINCE LAST EDITION

Brand Name	Generic Name	Use
AdreView™	iobenguane I 123	As an adjunct to other diagnostic tests, in the detection of primary or metastatic pheochromocytoma or neuroblastoma
Afinitor®	everolimus	Treatment of advanced renal cell cancer (RCC), after sunitinib or sorafenib failure
Banzel™	rufinamide	Adjunctive therapy in the treatment of generalized seizures of Lennox-Gastaut syndrome
Besivance™	besifloxacin	Treatment of bacterial conjunctivitis
Cerefolin® NAC	methylfolate, methylcobalamin, and acetylcysteine	Medicinal food for use in patients with neurovascular oxidative stress and/or hyperhomocysteinemia
Cinryze™	C1 inhibitor (human)	Routine prophylaxis against angioedema attacks in patients with hereditary angioedema (HAE) or inherited C1 inhibitor deficiency
Coartem®	artemether and lumefantrine	Treatment of acute, uncomplicated malaria infections due to *Plasmodium falciparum*
Durezol™	difluprednate	Treatment of inflammation and pain following ocular surgery
Dysport™	abobotulinumtoxinA	Treatment of cervical dystonia to reduce the severity of abnormal head position and neck pain in both toxin-naive and previously treated patients; temporary improvement in the appearance of moderate-to-severe glabellar lines associated with procerus and corrugator muscle activity in adults <65 years of age
Effient™	prasugrel	Reduces rate of thrombotic cardiovascular (eg, stent thrombosis) events in patients with unstable angina, non-ST-segment elevation MI, or ST-elevation MI (STEMI) managed with percutaneous coronary intervention (PCI)
Eovist®	gadoxetate	Contrast medium for magnetic resonance imaging (MRI) to detect and characterize lesions within focal liver disease
Epiduo™	adapalene and benzoyl peroxide	Topical treatment of acne vulgaris
Exforge HCT®	amlodipine, valsartan, and hydrochlorothiazide	Treatment of hypertension (not for initial therapy)
Fanapt™	iloperidone	Acute treatment of schizophrenia
Feraheme™	ferumoxytol	Treatment of iron-deficiency anemia in chronic kidney disease
Firmagon®	degarelix	Treatment of advanced prostate cancer
Ilaris®	canakinumab	Treatment of cryopyrin-associated periodic syndromes (CAPS), including familial cold autoinflammatory syndrome (FCAS) and Muckle-Wells syndrome (MWS)
Kapidex™	dexlansoprazole	Short-term (4 weeks) treatment of heartburn associated with nonerosive GERD; short-term (up to 8 weeks) treatment of all grades of erosive esophagitis; to maintain healing of erosive esophagitis for up to 6 months
Lusedra™	fospropofol	Monitored anesthesia care (MAC) sedation in patients undergoing diagnostic or therapeutic procedures

Brand Name	Generic Name	Use
Mozobil™	plerixafor	Mobilization of hematopoietic stem cells (HSC) for collection and subsequent autologous transplantation (in combination with filgrastim) in patients with non-Hodgkin lymphoma (NHL) and multiple myeloma (MM)
Multaq®	dronedarone	To reduce the risk of hospitalization related to paroxysmal or persistent atrial fibrillation (AF) or atrial flutter (AFl) in patients with a recent episode of AF/AFl and associated cardiovascular risk factors (eg, age >70 years, hypertension, diabetes, prior cerebrovascular accident, left atrial diameter ≥50 mm or left ventricular ejection fraction <40%), who are in normal sinus rhythm or will be cardioverted
Nucynta™	tapentadol	Relief of moderate-to-severe acute pain
Onglyza™	saxagliptin	Treatment of type 2 diabetes mellitus (noninsulin-dependent, NIDDM) as an adjunct to diet and exercise as monotherapy or in combination therapy with other antidiabetic agents to improve glycemic control
Phosphocol® P 32	chromic phosphate P 32	Treatment of peritoneal or pleural effusions caused by metastatic disease by intracavitary instillation; may be injected interstitially for the treatment of cancer
Promacta®	eltrombopag	Treatment of thrombocytopenia in patients with chronic immune (idiopathic) thrombocytopenic purpura (ITP) at risk for bleeding who have had insufficient response to corticosteroids, immune globulin, or splenectomy
Rapaflo™	silodosin	Treatment of signs and symptoms of benign prostatic hyperplasia (BPH)
RiaSTAP™	fibrinogen concentrate (human)	Treatment of acute bleeding episodes in patients with congenital fibrinogen deficiency (afibrinogenemia and hypofibrinogenemia)
Samsca™	tolvaptan	Treatment of clinically significant hypervolemic or euvolemic hyponatremia (associated with heart failure, cirrhosis or SIADH) with either a serum sodium <125 mEq/L or less marked hyponatremia that is symptomatic and resistant to fluid restriction
Saphris®	asenapine	Acute treatment of schizophrenia; treatment of acute mania or mixed episodes associated with bipolar I disorder
Savella™	milnacipran	Management of fibromyalgia
Simponi™	golimumab	Treatment of active rheumatoid arthritis (moderate-to-severe), active psoriatic arthritis, and active ankylosing spondylitis
Toviaz™	fesoterodine	Treatment of patients with an overactive bladder with symptoms of urinary frequency, urgency, or urge incontinence.
TriLipix™	fenofibric acid	Adjunct to dietary therapy for the treatment of severely elevated serum triglyceride levels; adjunct to dietary therapy for the reduction of low density lipoprotein cholesterol (LDL-C), total cholesterol (total-C), triglycerides, and apolipoprotein B (apo B) and to increase high density lipoprotein cholesterol (HDL-C) in patients with primary hypercholesterolemia or mixed dyslipidemia; adjunct to dietary therapy concomitantly with a statin to reduce triglyceride levels and increase HDL-C levels in patients with mixed dyslipidemia and coronary heart disease (CHD) or at risk for CHD

NEW DRUGS ADDED SINCE LAST EDITION

Brand Name	Generic Name	Use
Uloric®	febuxostat	Chronic management of hyperuricemia in patients with gout
Valstar®	valrubicin	Intravesical therapy of BCG-refractory bladder carcinoma in situ
Vimpat®	lacosamide	Adjunctive therapy in the treatment of partial-onset seizures

PENDING DRUGS OR DRUGS IN CLINICAL TRIALS

Proposed Brand Name or Synonym	Generic Name	Use
Acetavance™	acetaminophen (intravenous)	Pain, fever
Actemra®	tocilizumab	Rheumatoid arthritis
Acurox®	oxycodone and niacin	Pain
AP23573	deforolimus	Cancer
Arcoxia™	etoricoxib	Osteoarthritis
Arzerra™	ofatumumab	Monoclonal antibody
AVX754	apricitabine	HIV
Bepreve™	bepotastine	Allergic conjunctivitis
Bridion®	sugammadex	Reversal of nondepolarizing muscle relaxants
DAPD	amdoxovir	HIV
Daxas®	roflumilast	COPD
Fd4C	elvucitabine	HIV
Gemasense®	oblimersen	Chronic lymphocytic leukemia
Hexvix®	hexaminolevulinate	Diagnostic agent
Ilaris®	canakinaumab	Cryopyrin-associated periodic syndrome (CAPS)
Isovorin®	levofolinic acid	Colorectal cancer
Kiacta™	eprodisate	Amyloid A amyloidosis
Krystexxa®	pegloticase	Gout
Menveo®	menACWY-CRM	Meningitis
NBI-34060	indiplon	Insomnia
Nexavar®	sorafenib	Liver and kidney cancer
Orplanta®	satraplatin	Prostate cancer
prGCD	glucocerebrosidase	Gaucher disease
Provenge™	sipuleucel-T	Prostate cancer
Qlaira®	dienogest and estradiol valerate	Contraception
Reverset™	dexelvucitabine	HIV
Rezonic™	casopitant	Chemotherapy-induced nausea/vomiting
RSD1235	vernakalant	Atrial fibrillation
SCH417690	vicriviroc	HIV
SGN-35	brentuximab	Hodgkin
Spera™	satraplatin	Prostate cancer
Surfaxin®	lucinactant	Respiratory distress syndrome
SYR-322/Actos®	alogliptin and pioglitazone	Type 2 diabetes
TH9507	tesamorelin	HIV
TNX-355	ibalizumab	HIV
Vimovo®	naproxen and esomeprazole	Arthritis
Zimulti®	rimonabant	Weight loss agent

INDICATION / THERAPEUTIC CATEGORY INDEX

Antiseborrheic Agent, Topical

Estrogen and Androgen Combination

Keratolytic Agent

ACNE VULGARIS

ACQUIRED IMMUNODEFICIENCY SYNDROME (AIDS)

ANESTHESIA (GENERAL)

ANESTHESIA (LOCAL)

ANESTHESIA (OPHTHALMIC)

Local Anesthetic

ANGINA PECTORIS

Antiarrhythmic Agent, Class IV

Monoclonal Antibody

Nonsteroidal Antiinflammatory Drug (NSAID)

Corticosteroid, Topical

Vitamin

Vitamin, Fat Soluble

CEREBRAL PALSY

Skeletal Muscle Relaxant

CEREBROVASCULAR ACCIDENT (CVA)

Antiplatelet Agent

Fibrinolytic Agent

CERVICAL DYSTONIA

Neuromuscular Blocker Agent, Toxin

CHICKEN POX

Immune Globulin

CHOLELITHIASIS

Gallstone Dissolution Agent

CHOLERA

Vaccine

Antihistamine

CONJUNCTIVITIS (ALLERGIC)

DIABETES INSIPIDUS

Hormone, Posterior Pituitary

Vasopressin Analog, Synthetic

DIABETES MELLITUS, INSULIN-DEPENDENT (IDDM)

Antidiabetic Agent

DIABETES MELLITUS, NONINSULIN-DEPENDENT (NIDDM)

EPIDERMAL GROWTH FACTOR RECEPTOR (EGFR)

Antineoplastic Agent, Monoclonal Antibody

Epidermal Growth Factor Receptor (EGFR) Inhibitor

EPILEPSY

Anticonvulsant

Anticonvulsant, Sulfonamide

Antibiotic, Ophthalmic

EYE IRRITATION

Ophthalmic Agent, Miscellaneous

GAS PAINS

GASTRIC ULCER

GASTRITIS

HAY FEVER

Adrenergic Agonist Agent

Alpha/Beta Agonist

Antihistamine

Antihistamine/Decongestant/Analgesic

Antihistamine/Decongestant Combination

Histamine H_1 Antagonist

Histamine H_1 Antagonist, First Generation

HEADACHE (SINUS)

Analgesic, Nonnarcotic

Antihistamine/Analgesic

Antihistamine/Decongestant/Analgesic

Decongestant/Analgesic

HEADACHE (SINUS)

HEADACHE (TENSION)

Analgesic Combination (Opioid)

Analgesic, Miscellaneous

Analgesic, Narcotic

Analgesic, Nonnarcotic

Barbiturate

Barbiturate/Analgesic

Benzodiazepine

Skeletal Muscle Relaxant

HEADACHE (VASCULAR)

Analgesic, Nonnarcotic

HUMAN PAPILLOMAVIRUS (HPV) TYPES 6, 11, 16, 18

Vaccine

HUNTINGTON CHOREA

Monoamine Depleting Agent

HYDATIDIFORM MOLE (BENIGN)

Prostaglandin

HYPERACIDITY

Antacid

HYPERAMMONEMIA

Ammonium Detoxicant

HYPERCALCEMIA

Bisphosphonate Derivative

HYPERKALEMIA

HYPERKERATOSIS (FOLLICULARIS)

HYPERPARATHYROIDISM

Calcimimetic

Vitamin D Analog

HYPERPHOSPHATEMIA

Electrolyte Supplement, Oral

Phosphate Binder

HYPERPIGMENTATION

Topical Skin Product

HYPERPLASIA, VULVAR SQUAMOUS

Estrogen Derivative

Antihypertensive Agent

Antihypertensive Agent, Combination

Beta-Adrenergic Blocker

Beta-Adrenergic Blocker, Nonselective

Beta Blocker, Beta$_1$ Selective

Calcium Channel Blocker

Diuretic, Loop

Diuretic, Miscellaneous

Diuretic, Potassium Sparing

Diuretic, Thiazide

Diuretic, Thiazide-Related

Miscellaneous Product

Rauwolfia Alkaloid

Renin Inhibitor

Selective Aldosterone Blocker

Vasodilator

Vitamin, Fat Soluble

OBESITY

Nonsteroidal Antiinflammatory Drug (NSAID), COX-2 Selective

Prostaglandin

OSTEOPOROSIS

Analgesic, Nonnarcotic

Immunosuppressant Agent

Interleukin-12 Inhibitor

Interleukin-23 Inhibitor

Monoclonal Antibody

Psoralen

ROTAVIRUS GASTROENTERITIS

Vaccine

ROUNDWORMS

Anthelmintic

SALIVATION (EXCESSIVE)

Anticholinergic Agent

SARCOIDOSIS

Adrenal Corticosteroid

Corticosteroid, Topical

Antihistamine/Decongestant Combination

Cephalosporin (First Generation)

Cephalosporin (Second Generation)

Cephalosporin (Third Generation)

Cold Preparation

Decongestant/Analgesic

Decongestant/Anticholingeric Combination

Expectorant/Decongestant

Macrolide (Antibiotic)

SMALLPOX

Immune Globulin

Vaccine

SMOKING CESSATION

Antidepressant, Monoamine Oxidase Inhibitor

Partial Nicotine Agonist

Smoking Deterrent

SOFT TISSUE INFECTION

Aminoglycoside (Antibiotic)

Antibiotic, Carbapenem

Antibiotic, Miscellaneous

Antibiotic, Quinolone

Antifungal Agent, Systemic

Cephalosporin (First Generation)

Cephalosporin (Second Generation)

Cephalosporin (Third Generation)

SPASTICITY

TOXICITY, NONSPECIFIC (TREATMENT)

Antacid

Antidote

Diuretic, Osmotic

Electrolyte Supplement, Oral

Laxative

TOXOPLASMOSIS

Antibiotic, Miscellaneous

Folic Acid Antagonist (Antimalarial)

Sulfonamide

TRANSFUSION REACTION

Antihistamine

URINARY RETENTION

QUICK LOOK DRUG BOOK

Top 200 Prescribed Tablets and Capsules with Images

The Quick Look Drug Book 2010 Top 200 Prescribed Drugs insert displays actual color photographs of the most commonly prescribed tablets and capsules.

Drugs are listed alphabetically by generic name, and, where applicable, the trade name is listed. Dosages appear under each individual image.

Use the white scale at the bottom of each image to determine the actual size. The distance between each division on the scale is equivalent to 1/8 inch or 3.175 mm.

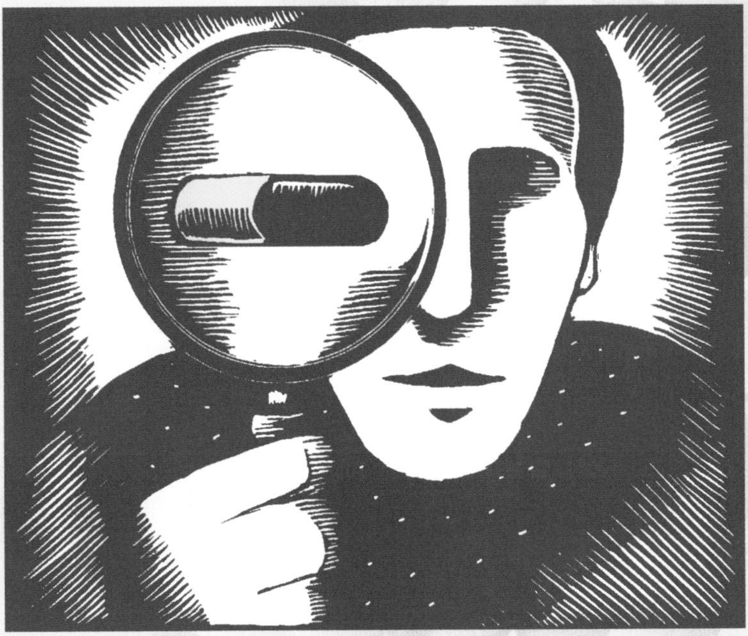

Acetaminophen and Codeine

(generic)

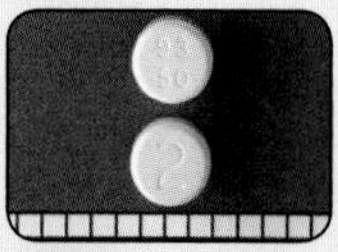

300/15 mg

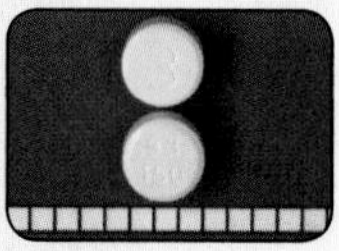

300/30 mg

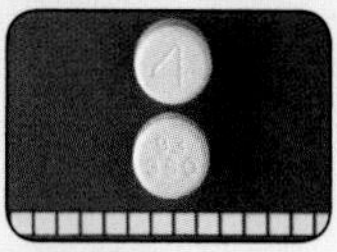

300/60 mg

Acyclovir

(generic)

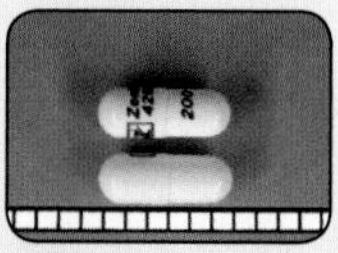

200 mg

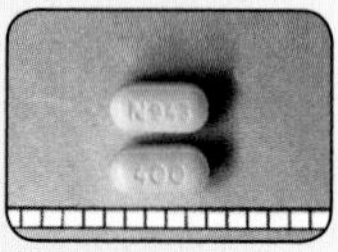

400 mg

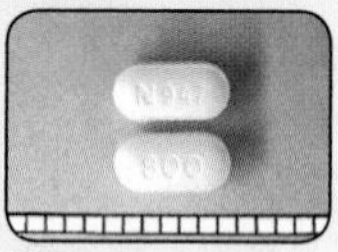

800 mg

Albuterol

(generic)

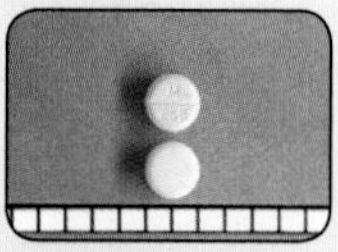

2 mg

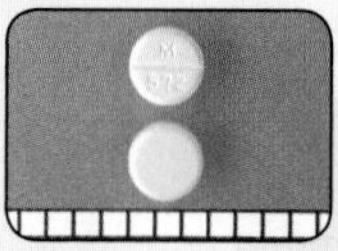

4 mg

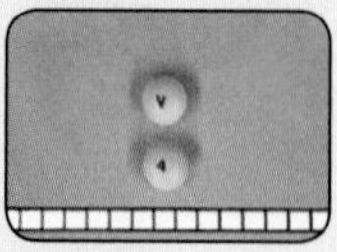

4 mg

Alendronate

(generic)

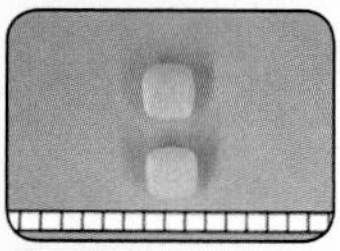

70 mg

Allopurinol

(generic)

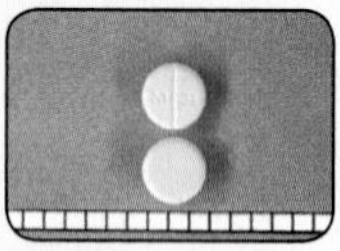

100 mg

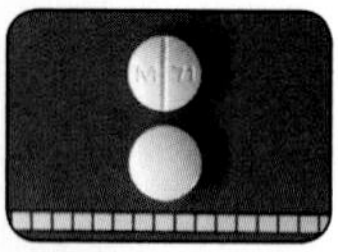

300 mg

Alprazolam

(generic)

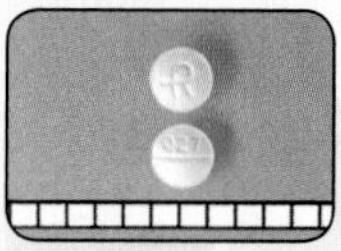

0.25 mg

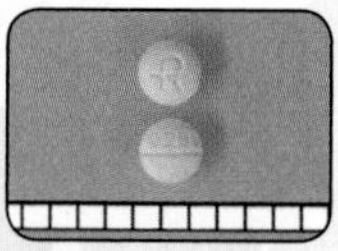

0.5 mg

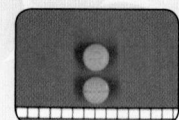

1 mg

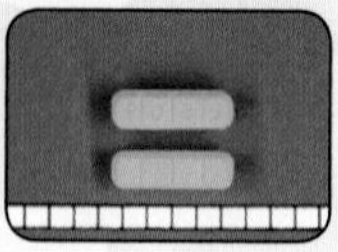

2 mg

Amitriptyline

(generic)

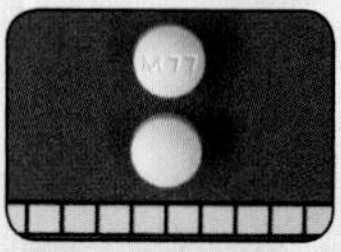

10 mg

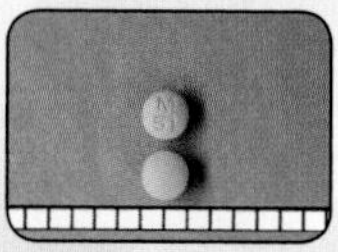

25 mg

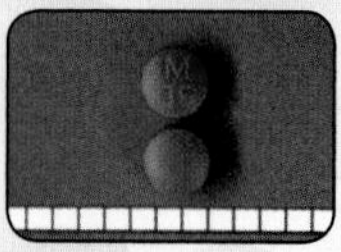

50 mg

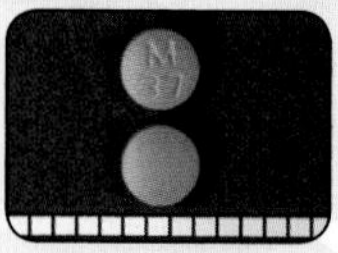

75 mg

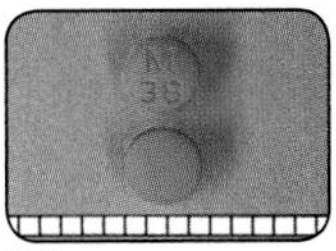
100 mg

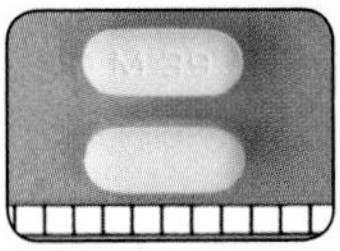
150 mg

Amoxicillin

(generic)

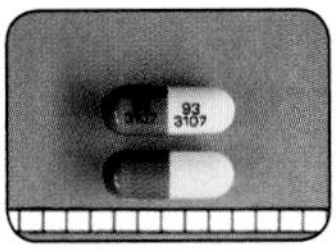
250 mg

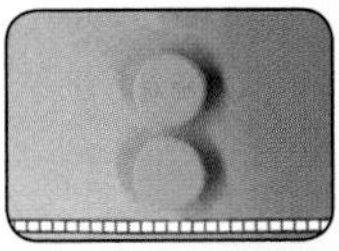
250 mg

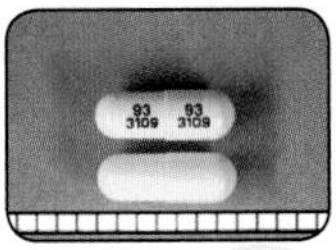
500 mg

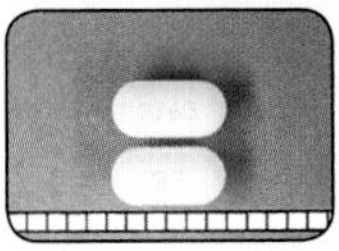
500 mg

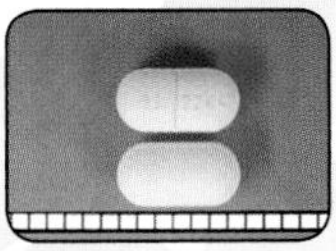
875 mg

Amoxicillin and Clavulanate Potassium

(generic)

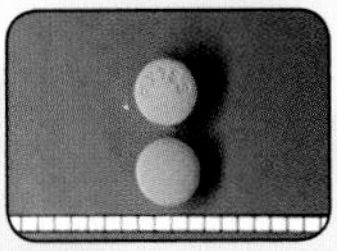
200/28.5 mg

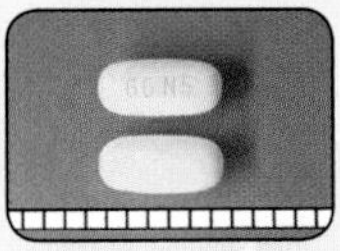
250/125 mg

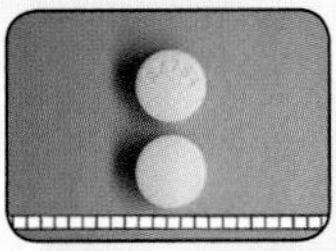
400/57 mg

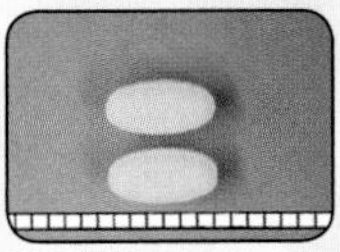
500/125 mg

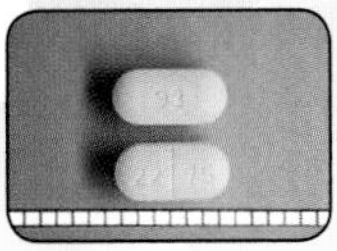
875/125 mg

Aripiprazole

Abilify®

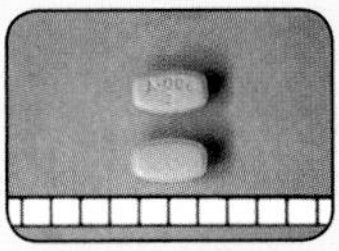
2 mg

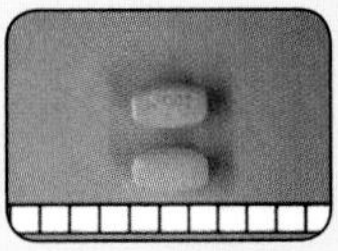
5 mg

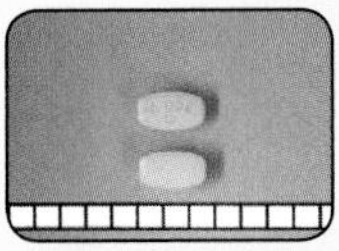
10 mg

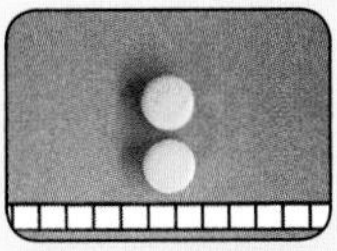
15 mg

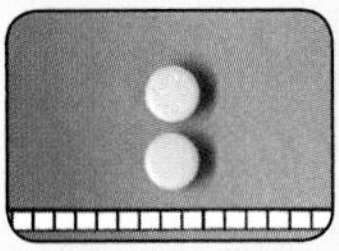
20 mg

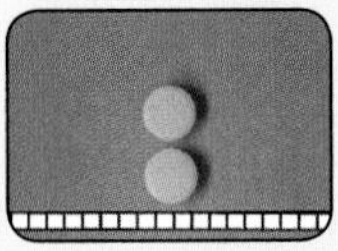
30 mg

Atenolol

(generic)

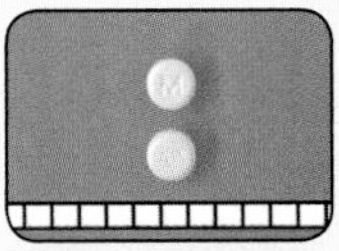
25 mg

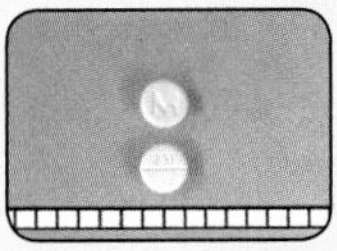
50 mg

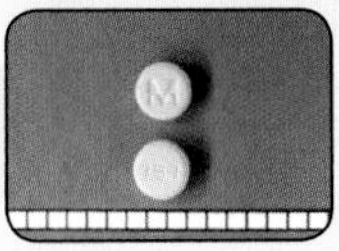
100 mg

Atorvastatin

Lipitor®

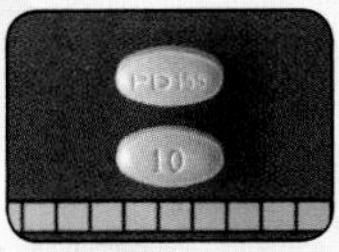
10 mg

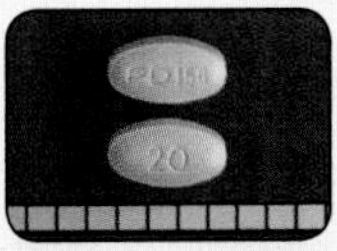
20 mg

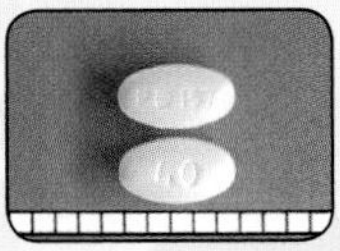
40 mg

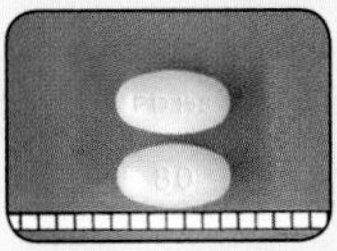
80 mg

Azithromycin
(generic)

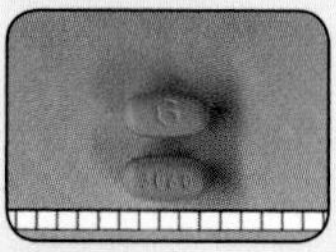
250 mg

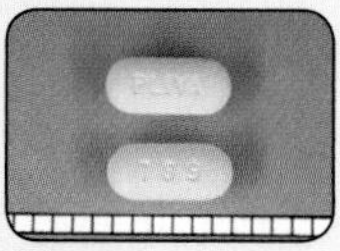
600 mg

Benazepril
(generic)

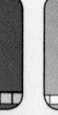

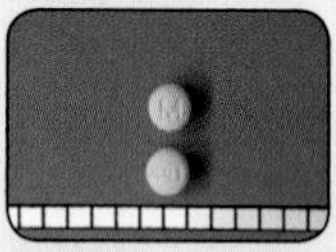
5 mg

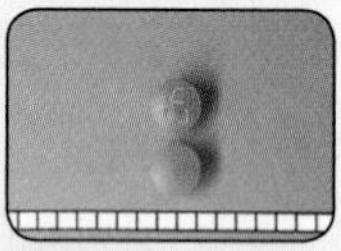
10 mg

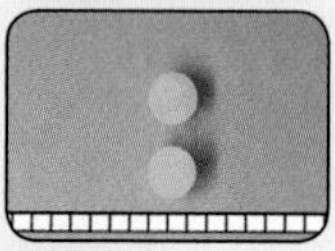
20 mg

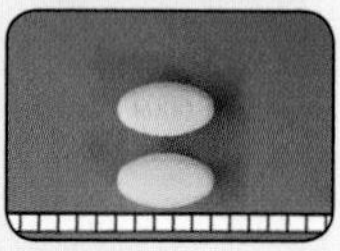
40 mg

Benzonatate
(generic)

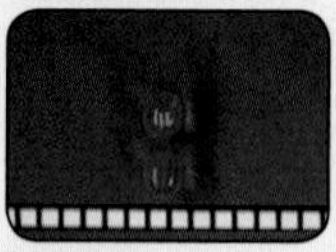
100 mg

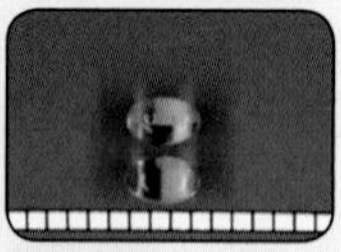
200 mg

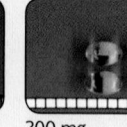

Bisoprolol and Hydrochlorothiazide
(generic)

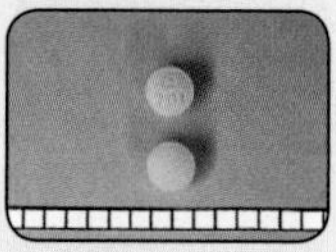
2.5/6.25 mg

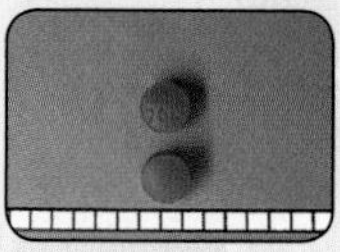
5/6.25 mg

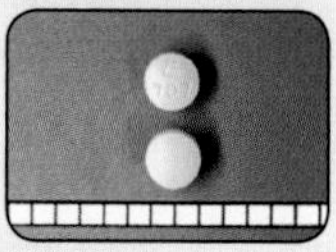
10/6.25 mg

Bupropion
(generic)

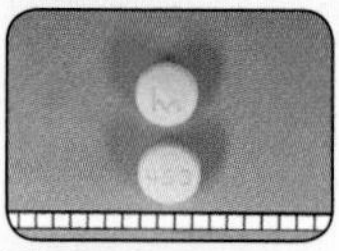
75 mg

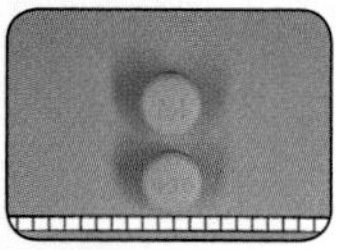
100 mg

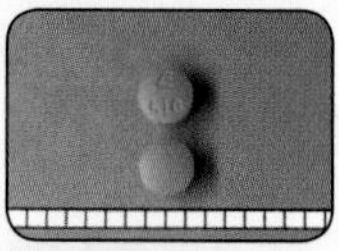
100 mg

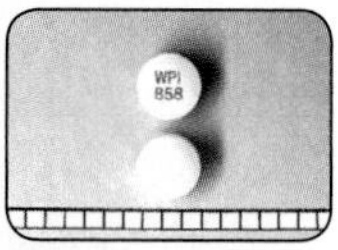

100 mg

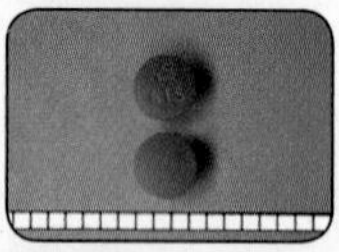
150 mg

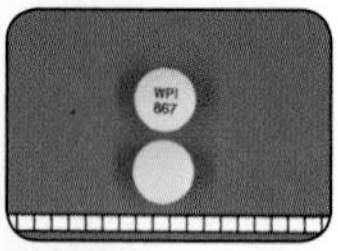

150 mg

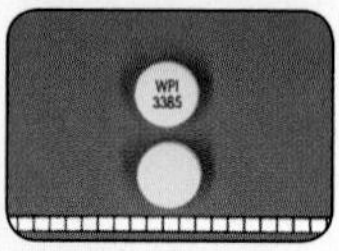

200 mg

Budeprion XL®

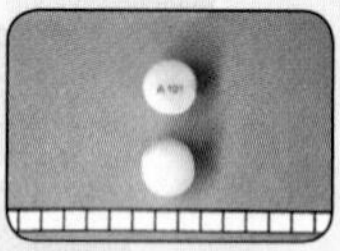

150 mg

Wellbutrin®

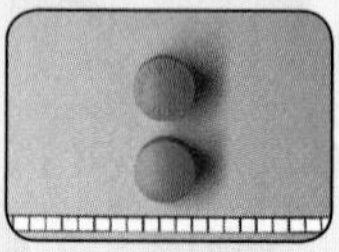
100 mg

Wellbutrin SR®

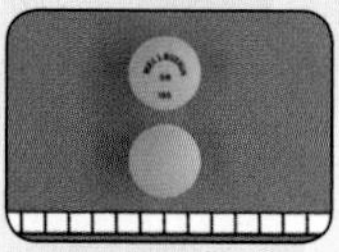
100 mg

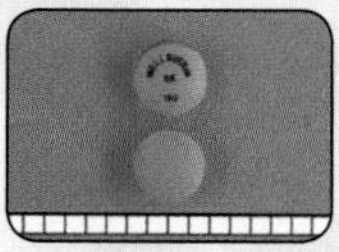
150 mg

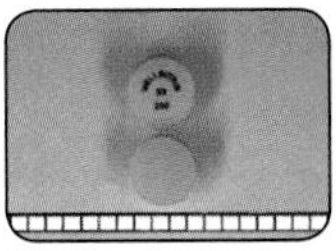
200 mg

Wellbutrin XL®

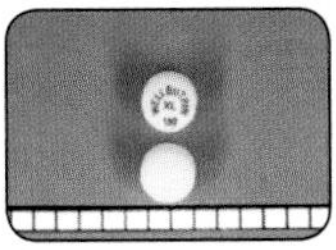
150 mg

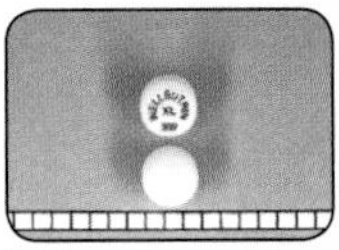
300 mg

Zyban®

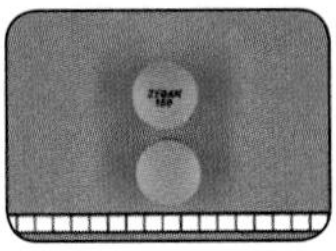
150 mg

Buspirone

(generic)

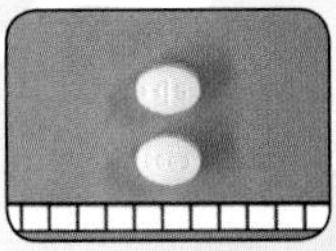
5 mg

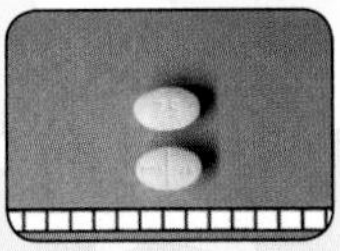
7.5 mg

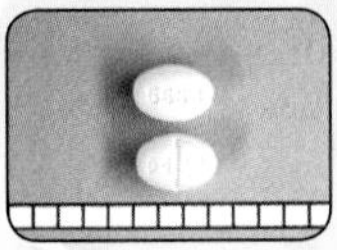
10 mg

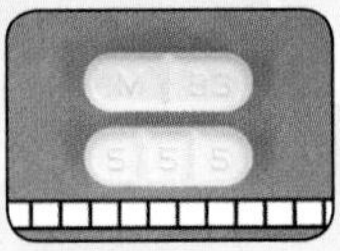
15 mg

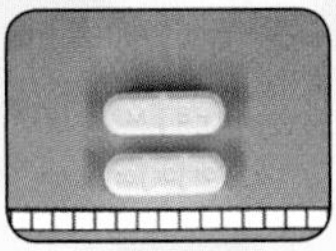
30 mg

Butalbital, Acetaminophen, and Caffeine

(generic)

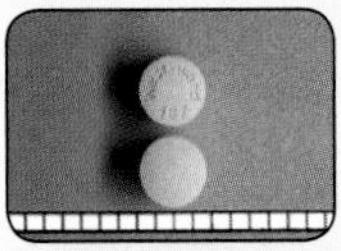
50/325/40 mg

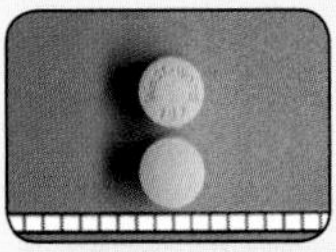
50/325/40 mg

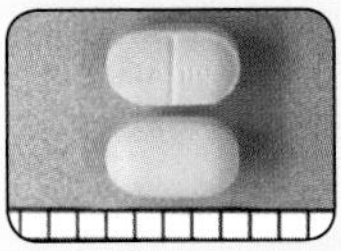
50/325/40 mg

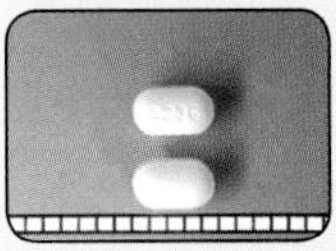
50/325/40 mg

Carisoprodol

(generic)

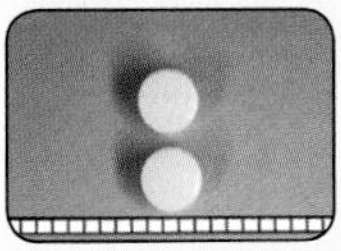
350 mg

Carvedilol

(generic)

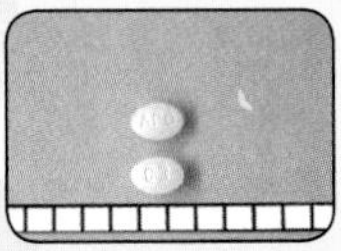
3.125 mg

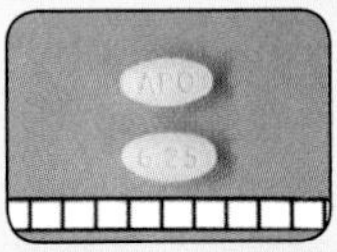
6.25 mg

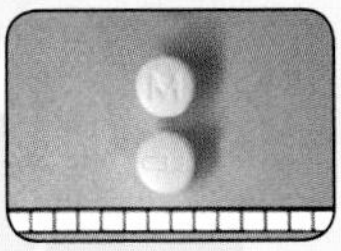
12.5 mg

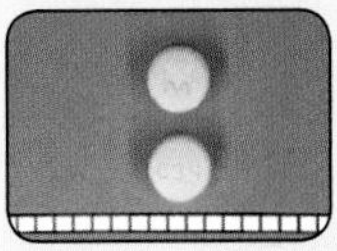
25 mg

Celecoxib

Celebrex®

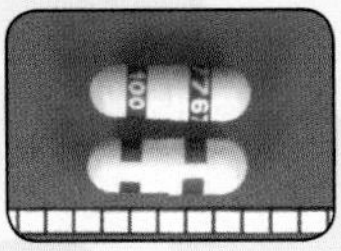
100 mg

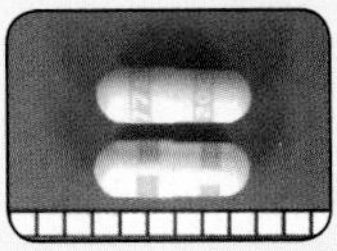
200 mg

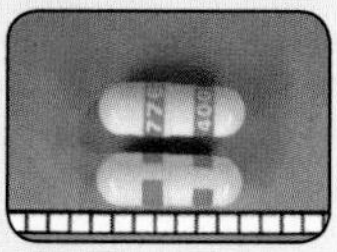

400 mg

Cephalexin

(generic)

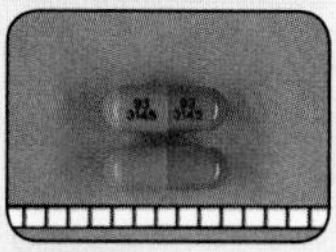

250 mg

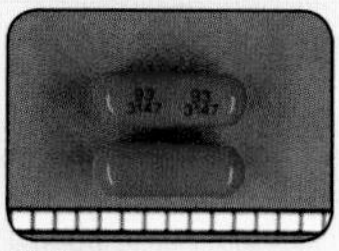

500 mg

Ciprofloxacin

(generic)

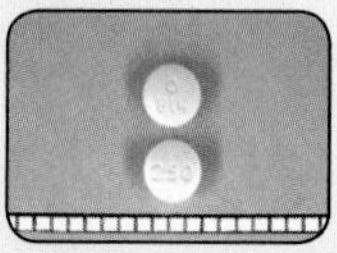

250 mg

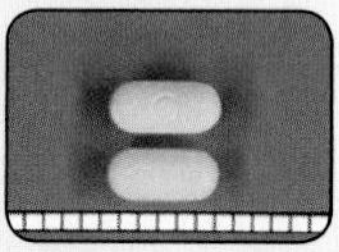

500 mg

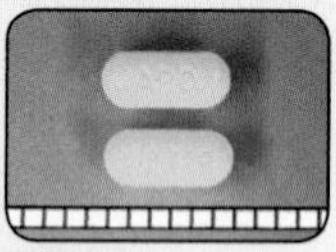

750 mg

Citalopram

(generic)

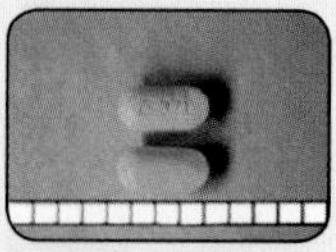

10 mg

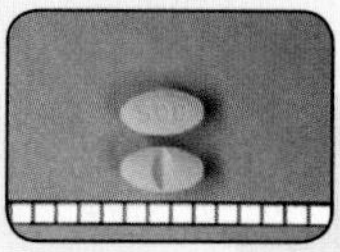

20 mg

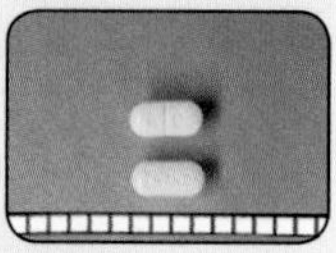

40 mg

Clindamycin

(generic)

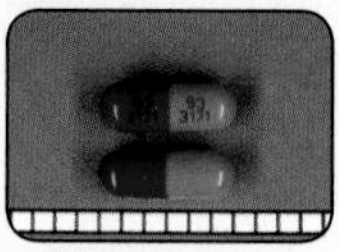

150 mg

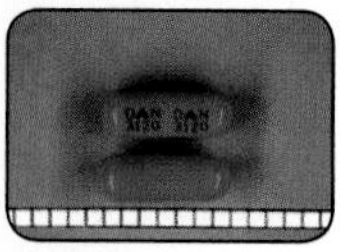

300 mg

Clonazepam

(generic)

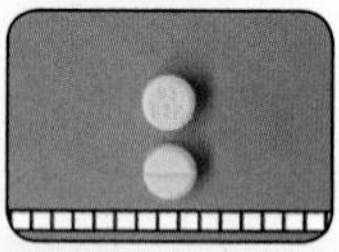

0.5 mg

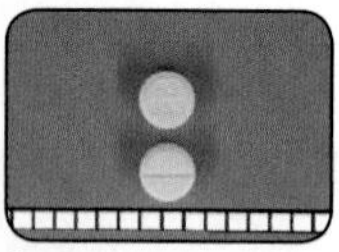

1 mg

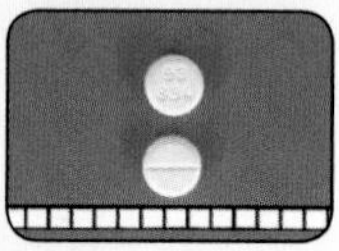

2 mg

Clonidine

(generic)

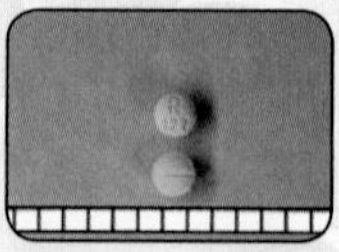

0.1 mg

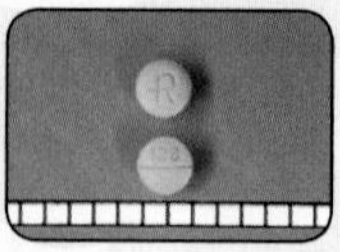

0.2 mg

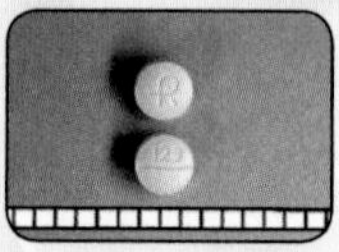

0.3 mg

Clopidogrel

Plavix®

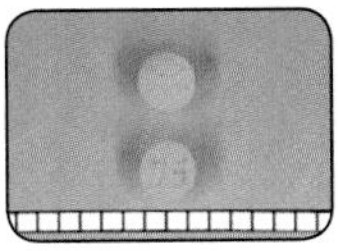
75 mg

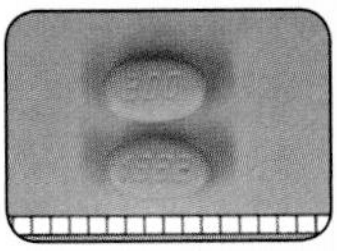
300 mg

Cyclobenzaprine

(generic)

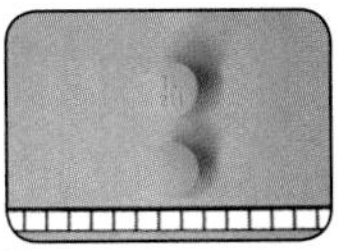
5 mg

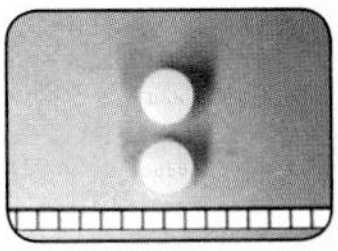
10 mg

Dextroamphetamine and Amphetamine

(generic)

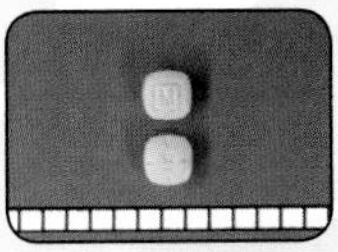
5 mg

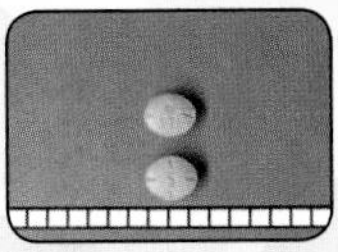
5 mg

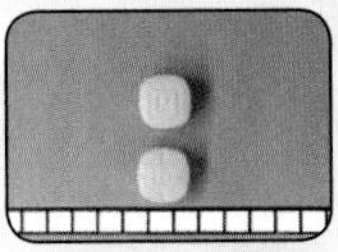
10 mg

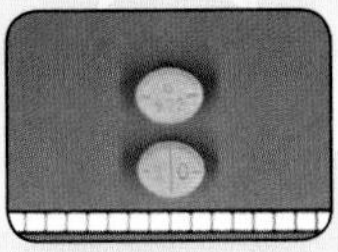
10 mg

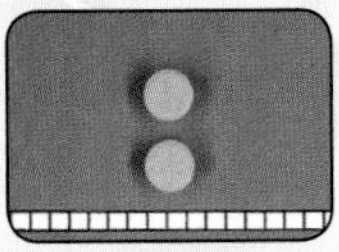
15 mg

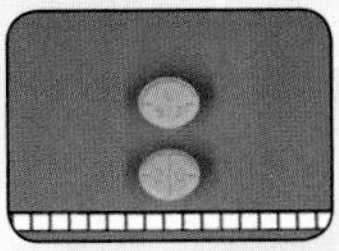
20 mg

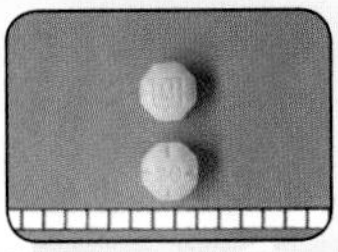
20 mg

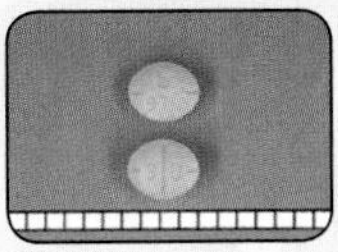
30 mg

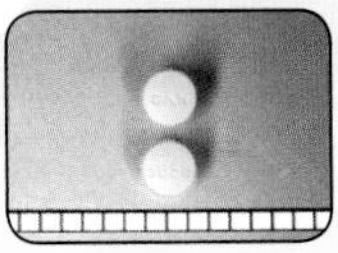
30 mg

Adderall®

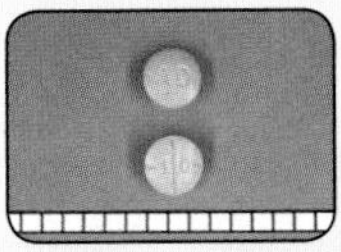
10 mg

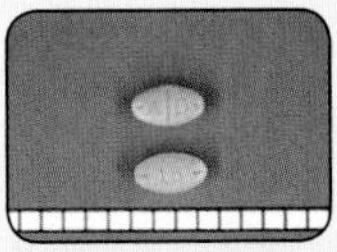
15 mg

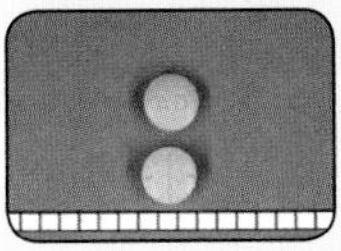
20 mg

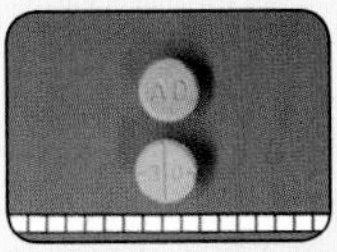
30 mg

Adderall XR®

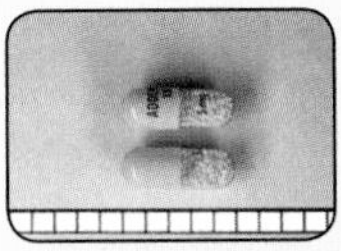
5 mg

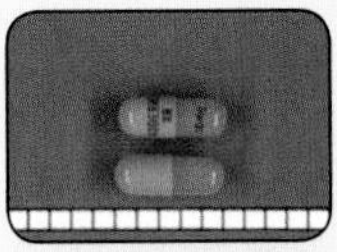
10 mg

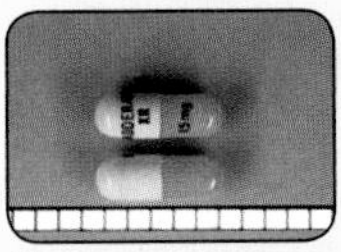
15 mg

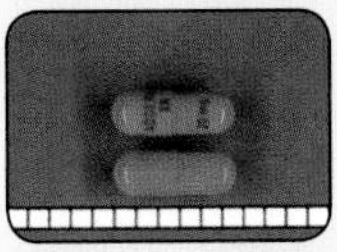
20 mg

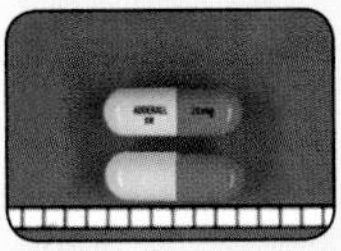
25 mg

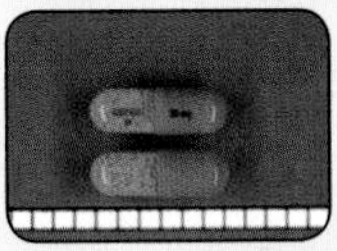
30 mg

Diazepam

(generic)

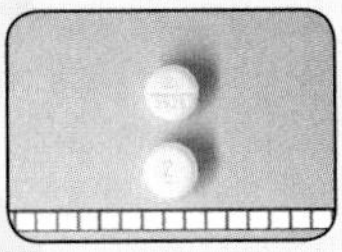
2 mg

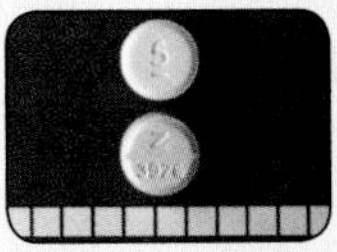
5 mg

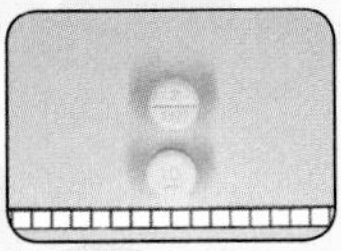
10 mg

Diclofenac
(generic)

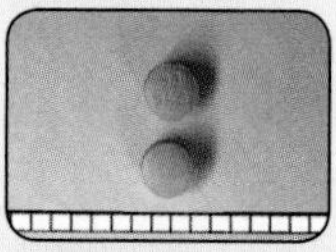
50 mg

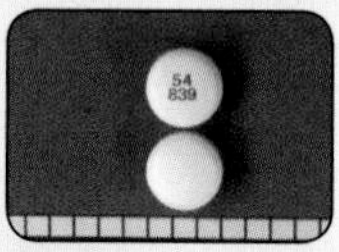

75 mg

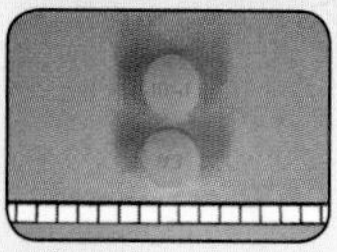
100 mg

Diltiazem
(generic)

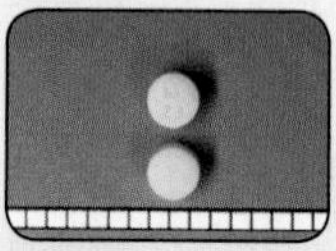
30 mg

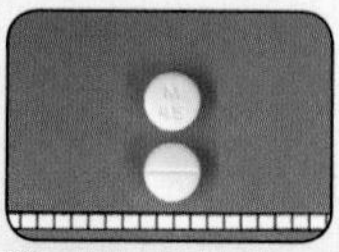
60 mg

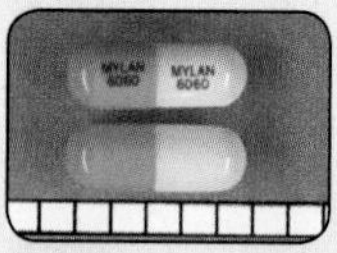

60 mg

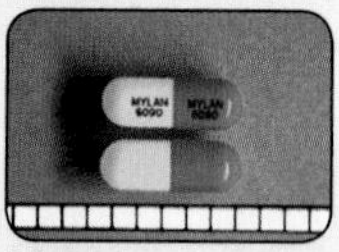

90 mg

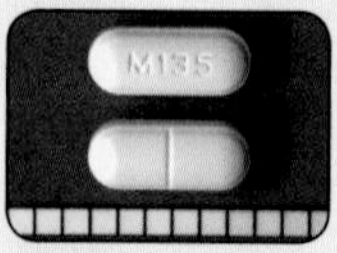

90 mg

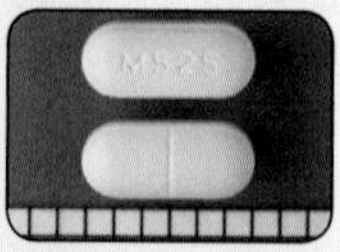

120 mg

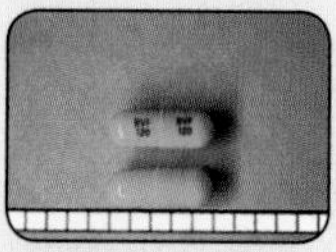
120 mg

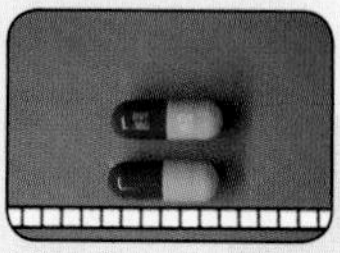
180 mg

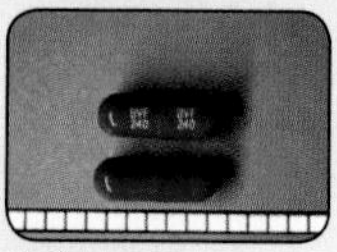
240 mg

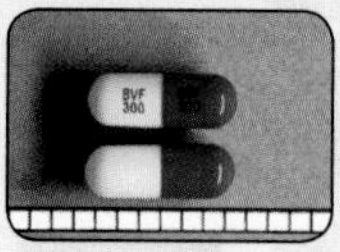

300 mg

Donepezil
Aricept®

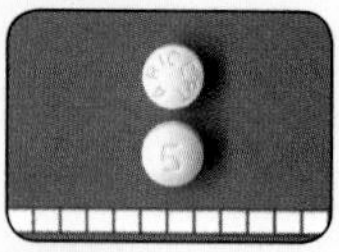

5 mg

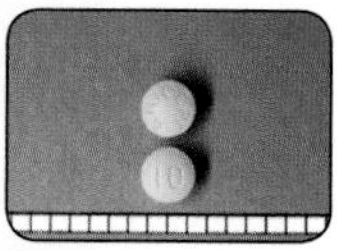

10 mg

Doxazosin
(generic)

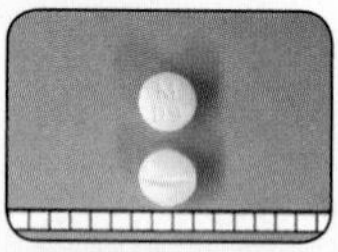
1 mg

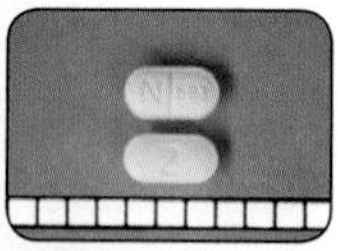

2 mg

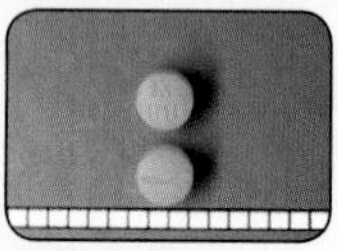
4 mg

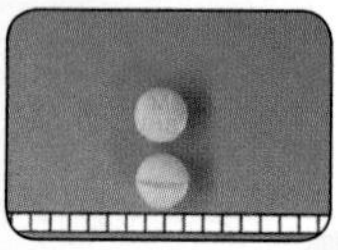
8 mg

Doxycycline
(generic)

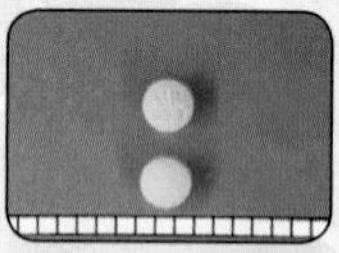
20 mg

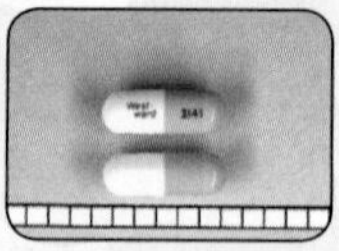
50 mg

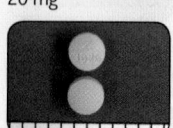
100 mg

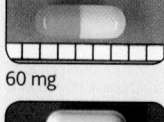

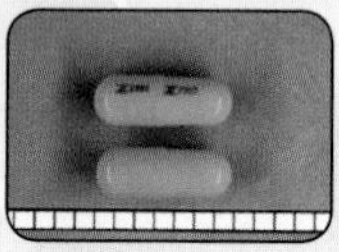
100 mg

Duloxetine
Cymbalta®

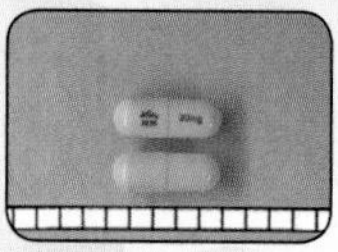
20 mg

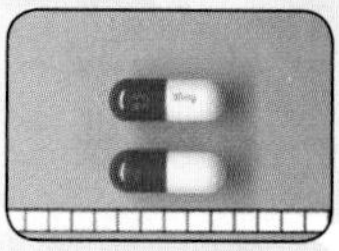
30 mg

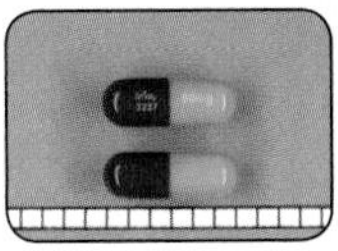
60 mg

Enalapril
(generic)

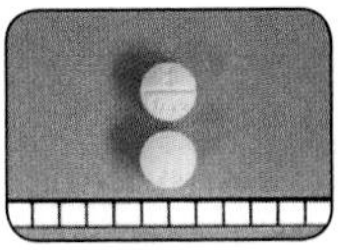
2.5 mg

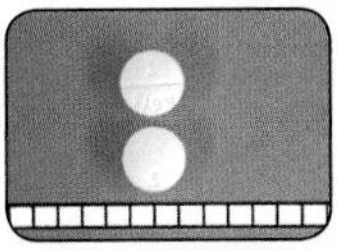
5 mg

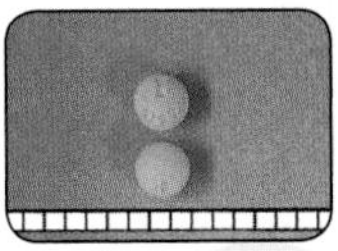
10 mg

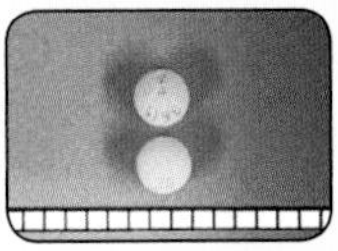
20 mg

Escitalopram
Lexapro®

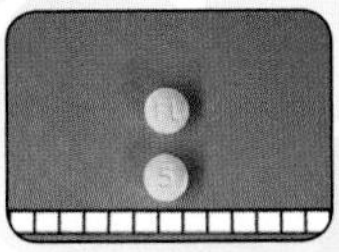
5 mg

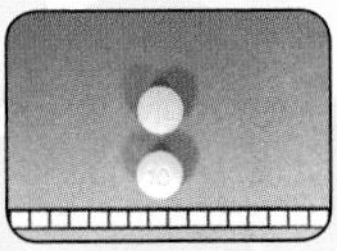
10 mg

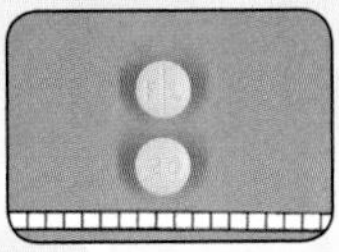
20 mg

Esomeprazole
Nexium®

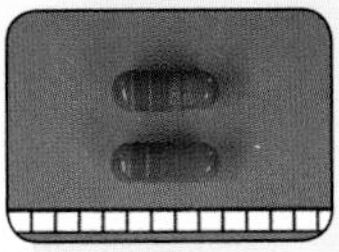
20 mg

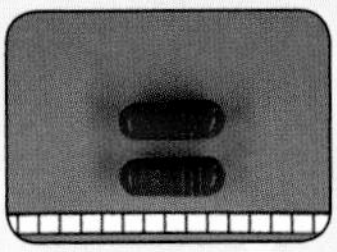
40 mg

Estradiol
(generic)

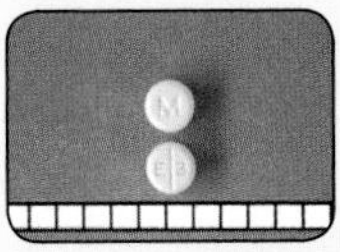
0.5 mg

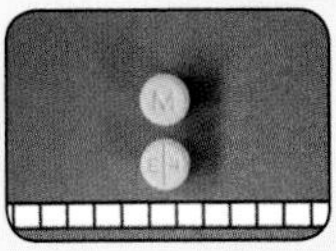
1 mg

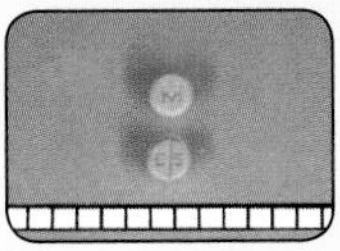
2 mg

Estrogens (Conjugated/Equine)
Premarin®

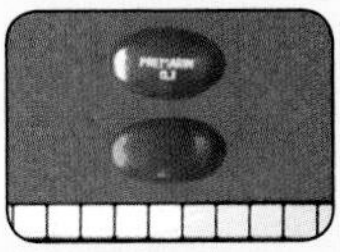
0.3 mg

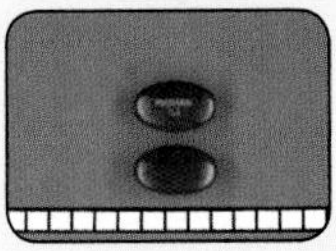
0.3 mg

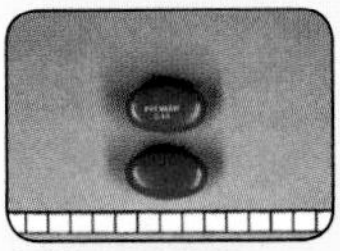
0.45 mg

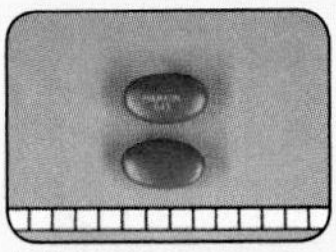
0.45 mg

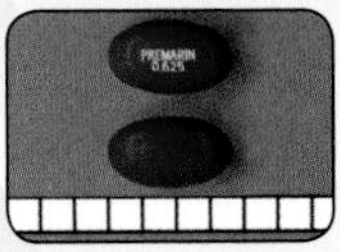
0.625 mg

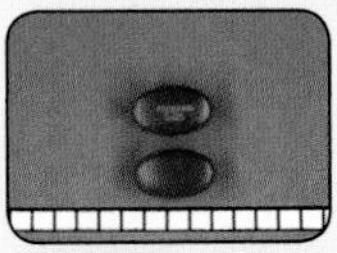
0.625 mg

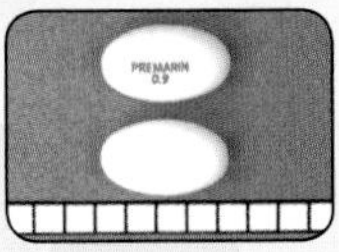
0.9 mg

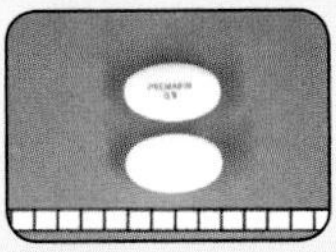
0.9 mg

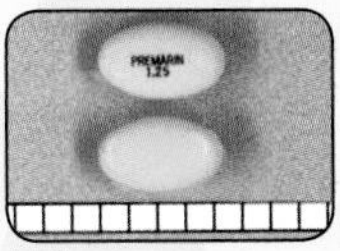
1.25 mg

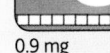

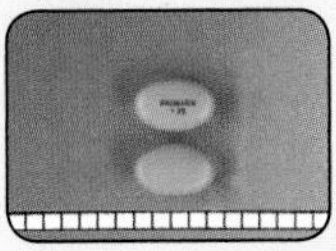
1.25 mg

Eszopiclone

Lunesta™

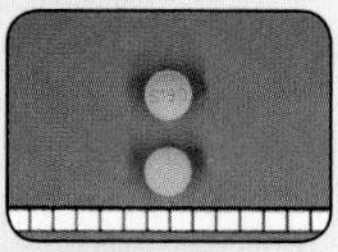

1 mg

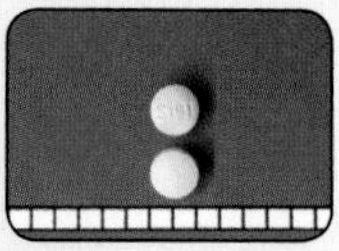

2 mg

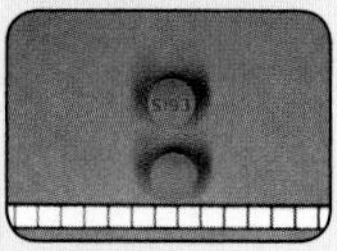

3 mg

Ethinyl Estradiol and Drospirenone

Yasmin®

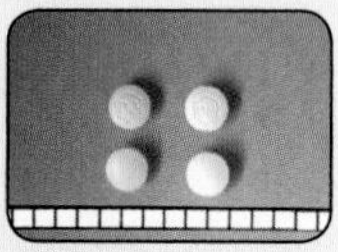

0.03/3 mg

Ethinyl Estradioll and Norgestimate

Tri-Sprintec® 28

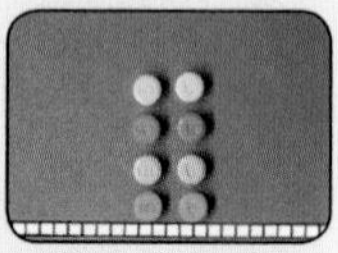

multiple # dosages

Ezetimibe

Zetia®

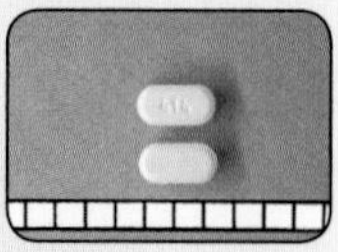

10 mg

Ezetimibe and Simvastatin

Vytorin®

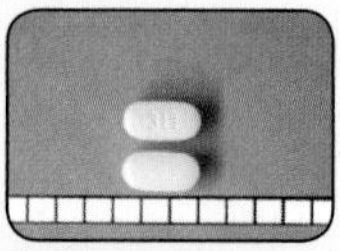

10/10 mg

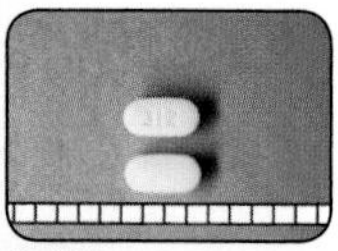

10/20 mg

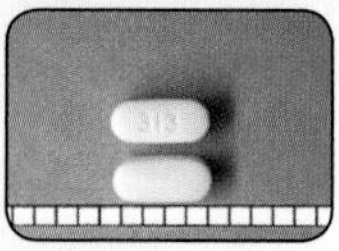

10/40 mg

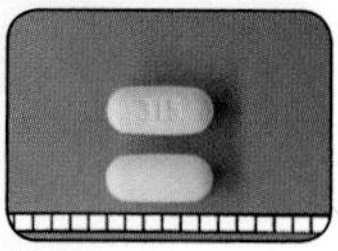

10/80 mg

Famotidine

(generic)

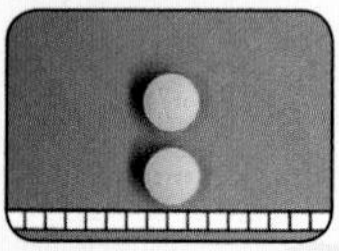

20 mg

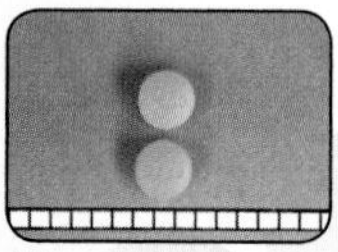

40 mg

Fenofibrate

TriCor®

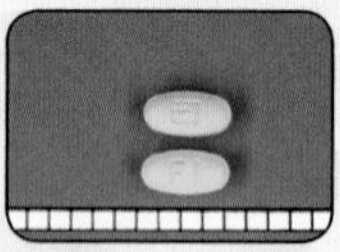

48 mg

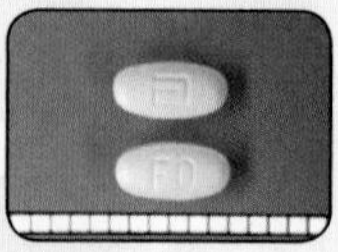

145 mg

(generic)

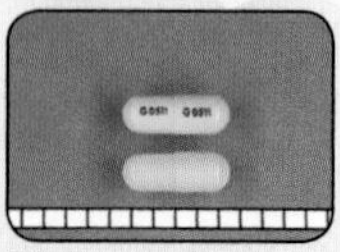

67 mg

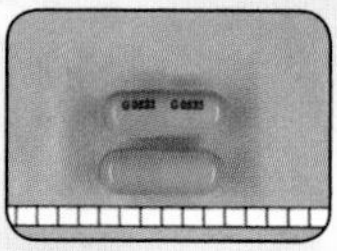

200 mg

Ferrous Sulfate
(generic)

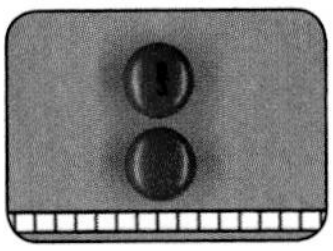
324 mg

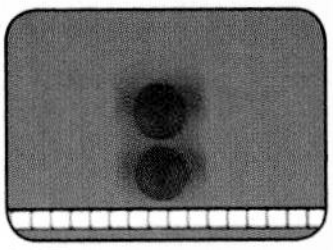
325 mg

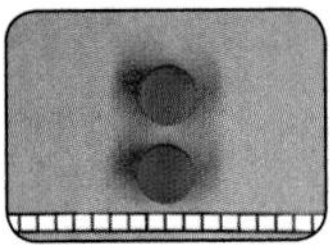
325 mg

Fexofenadine
(generic)

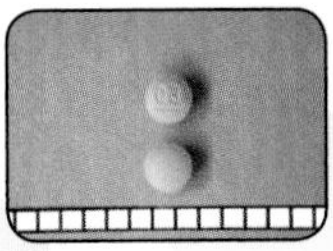
30 mg

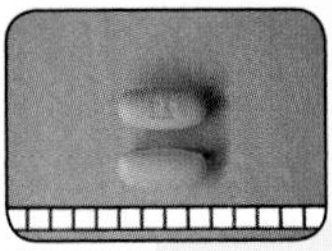
60 mg

Fluconazole
(generic)

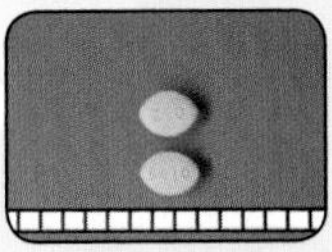
50 mg

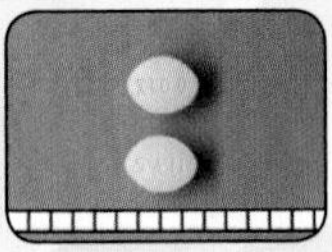
100 mg

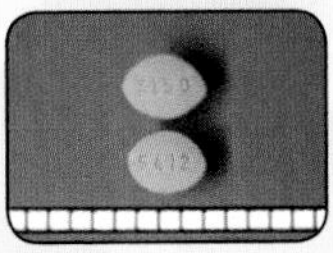
150 mg

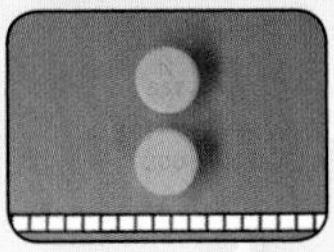
200 mg

Fluoxetine
(generic)

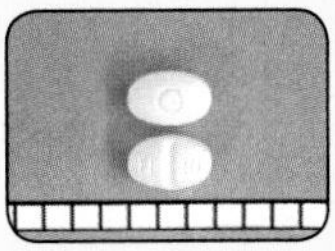
10 mg

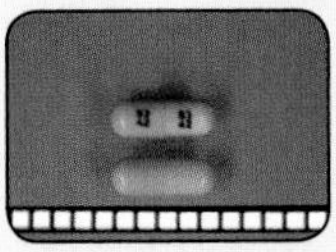
10 mg

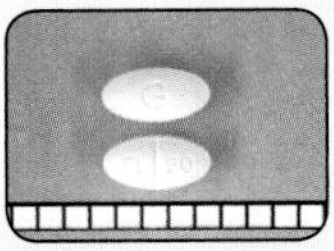
20 mg

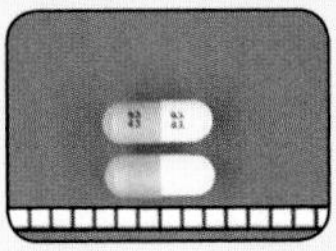
20 mg

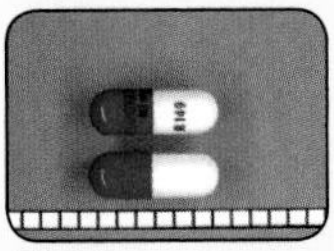
40 mg

Folic Acid
(generic)

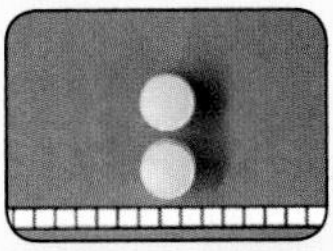
0.4 mg

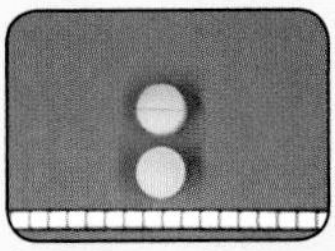
0.8 mg

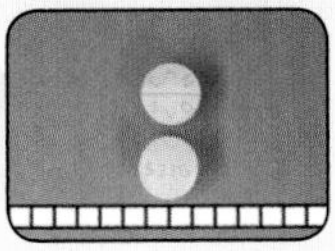
1 mg

Furosemide
(generic)

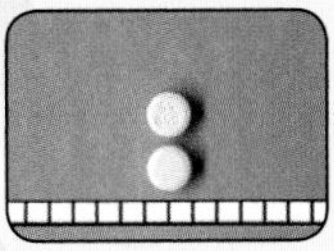
20 mg

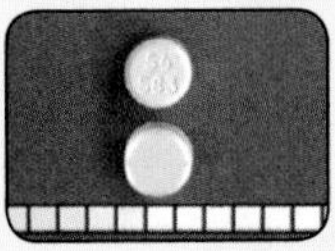
40 mg

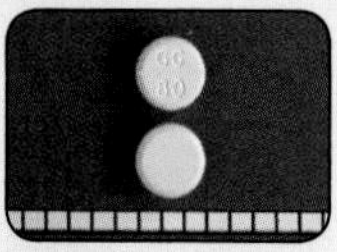

80 mg

Gabapentin

(generic)

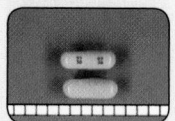

100 mg

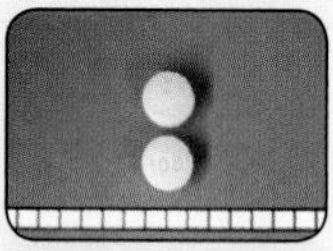

100 mg

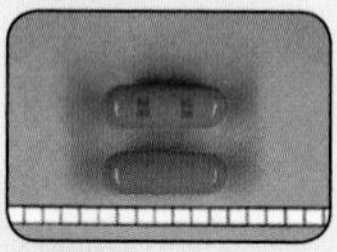

300 mg

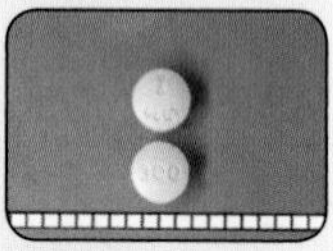

300 mg

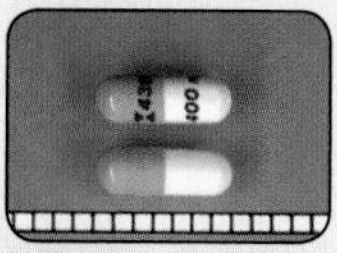

400 mg

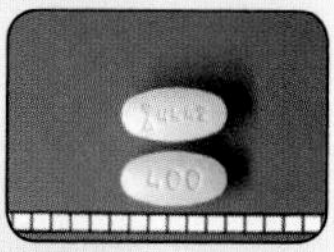

400 mg

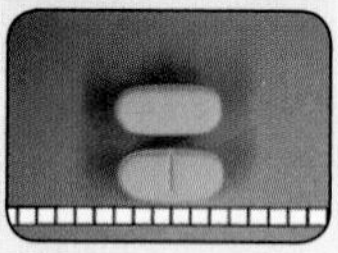

600 mg

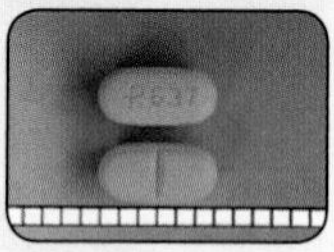

800 mg

Gemfibrozil

(generic)

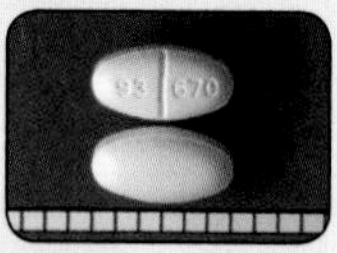

600 mg

Glimepiride

(generic)

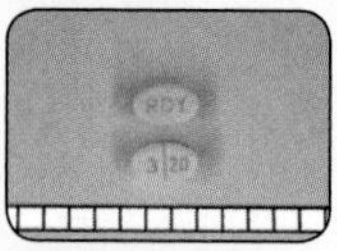

1 mg

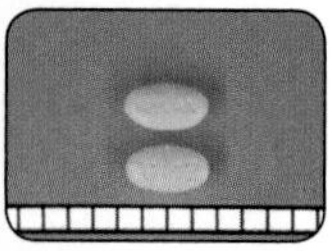

2 mg

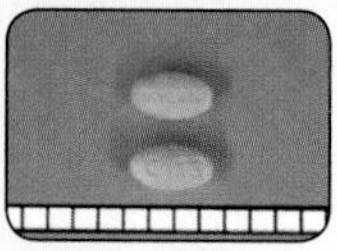

4 mg

Glipizide

(generic)

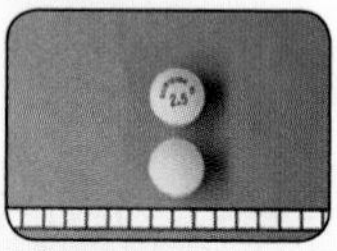

2.5 mg

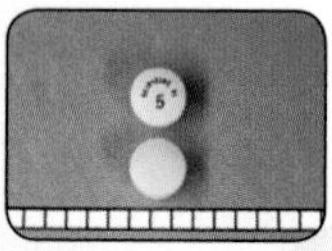

5 mg

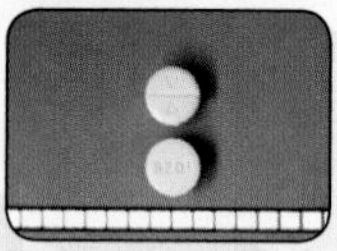

5 mg

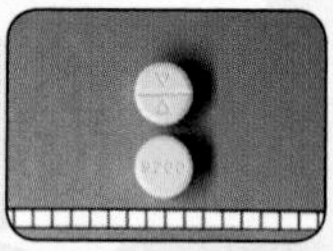

10 mg

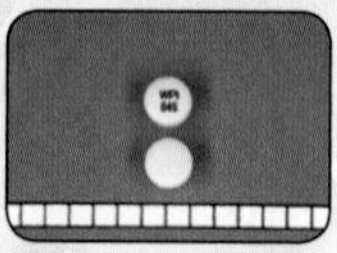

10 mg

Glyburide

(generic)

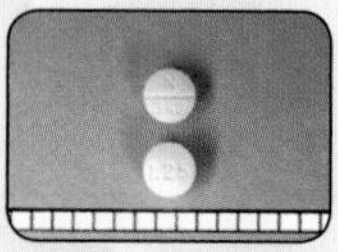

1.25 mg

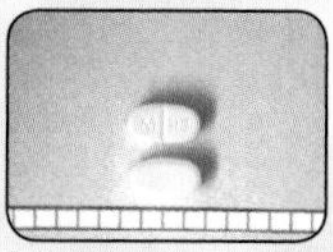

1.5 mg

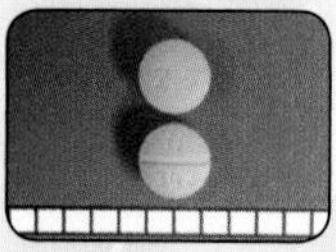

2.5 mg

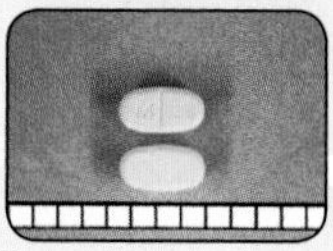

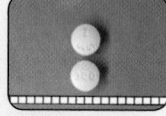

3 mg

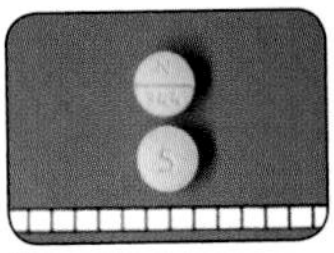
5 mg

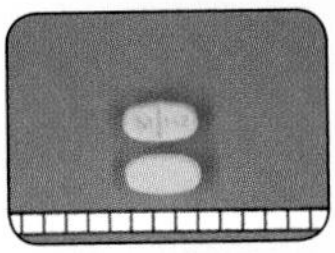
6 mg

Glyburide Metformin

(generic)

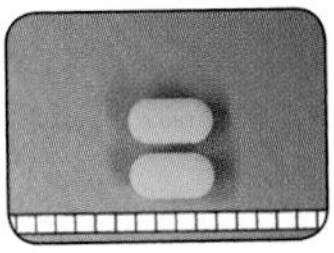
1.25/250 mg

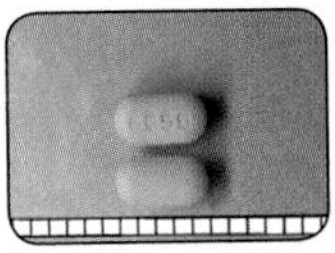
2.5/500 mg

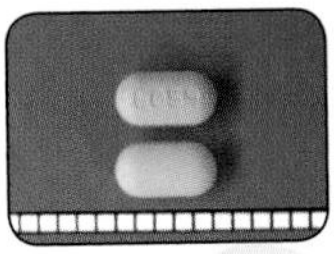
5/500 mg

Hydrochlorothiazide

(generic)

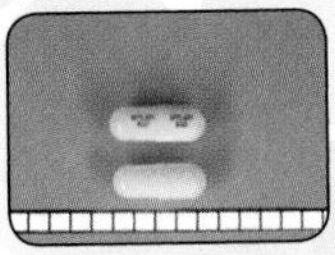
12.5 mg

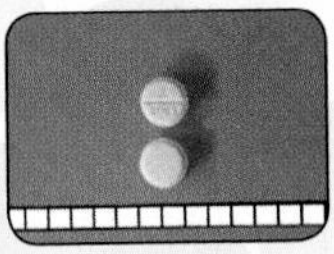
25 mg

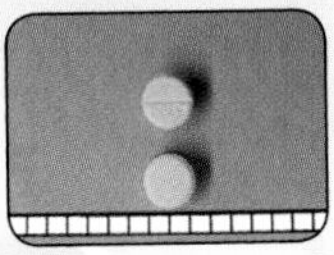
50 mg

Hydrocodone and Acetaminophen

(generic)

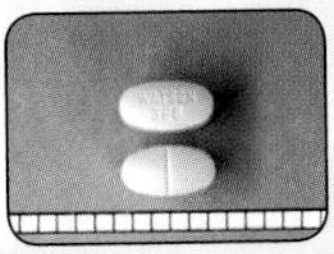
2.5/500 mg

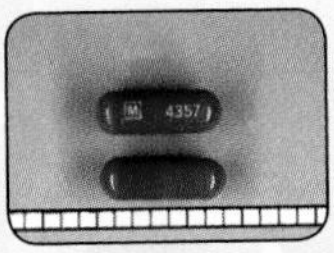

5/500 mg

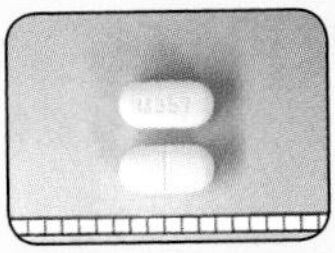
5/500 mg

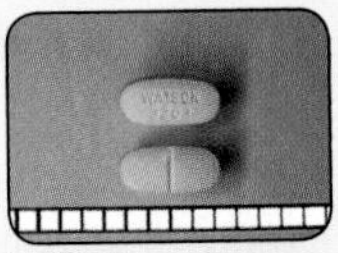
7.5/325 mg

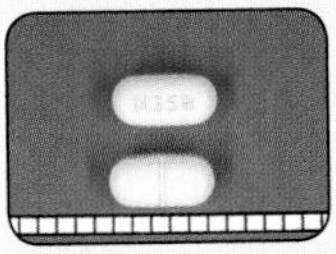
7.5/500 mg

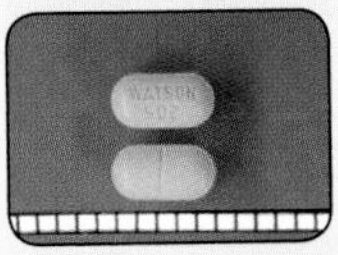
7.5/650 mg

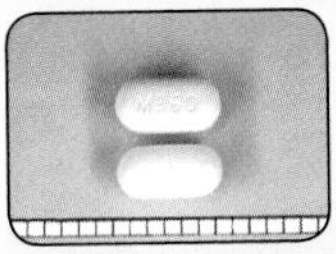
7.5/750 mg

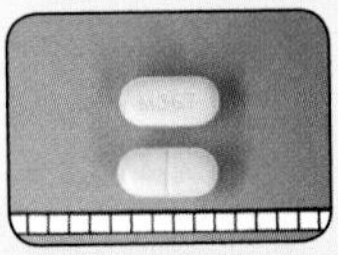
10/325 mg

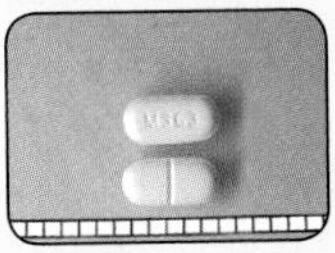
10/500 mg

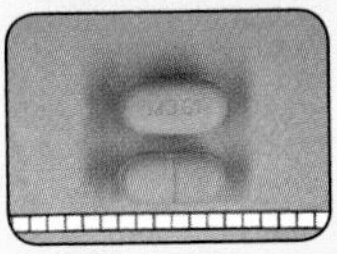
10/650 mg

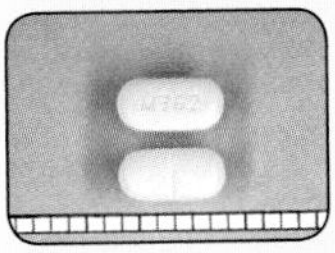
10/660 mg

Hydroxyzine

(generic)

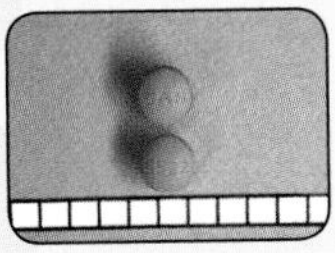
10 mg

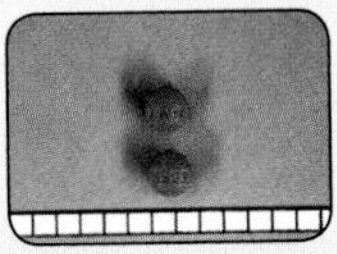
25 mg

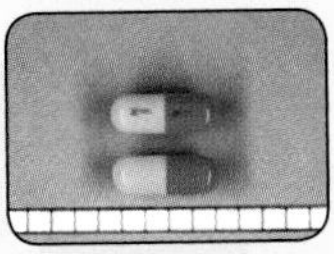
25 mg

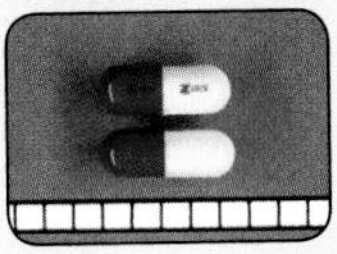
50 mg

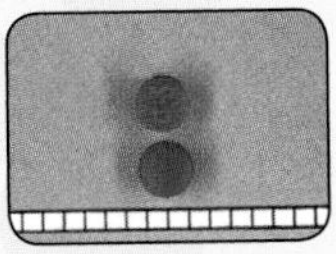
50 mg

Ibandronate

Boniva®

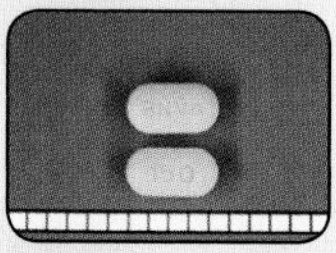

150 mg

Ibuprofen

(generic)

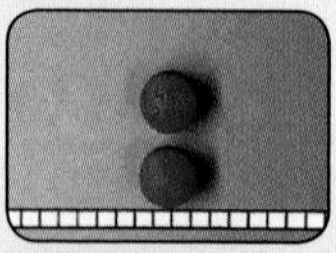

200 mg

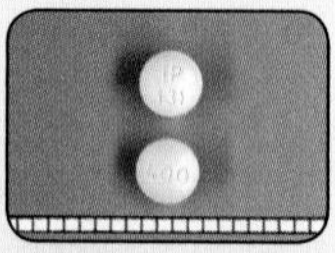

400 mg

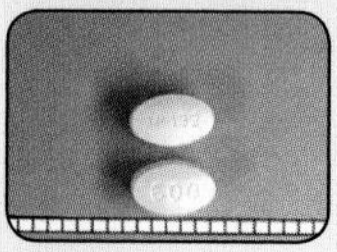

600 mg

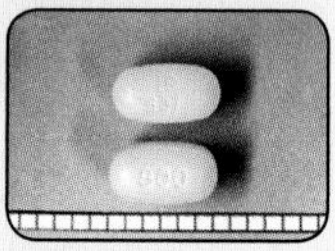

800 mg

Irbesartan

Avapro®

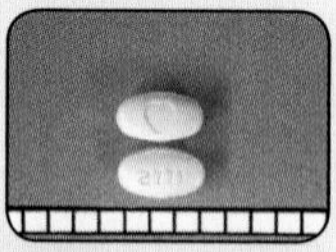

75 mg

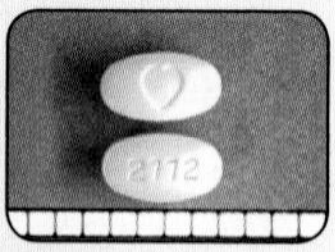

150 mg

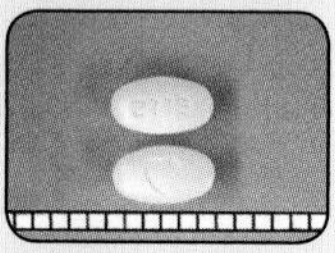

300 mg

Irbesartan and Hydrochlorothiazide

Avalide®

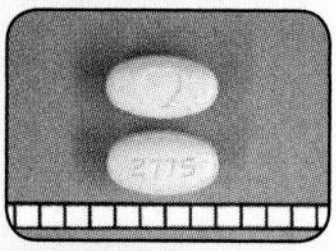

150/12.5 mg

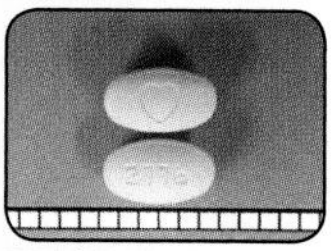

300/12.5 mg

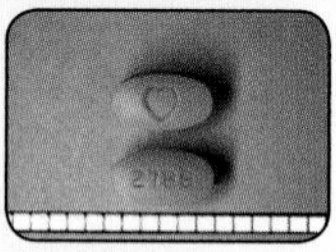

300/25 mg

Isosorbide Mononitrate

(generic)

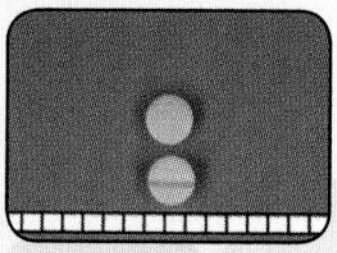

10 mg

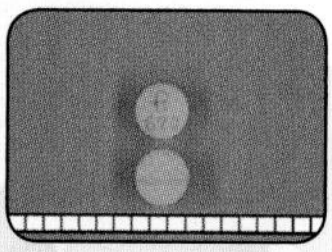

20 mg

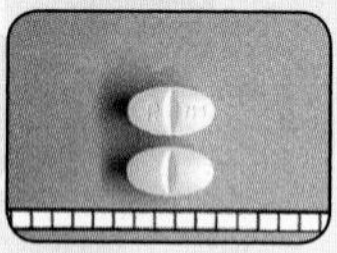

30 mg

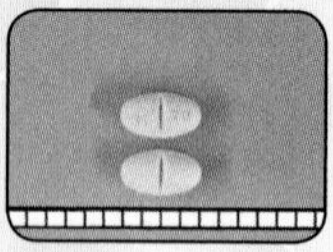

60 mg

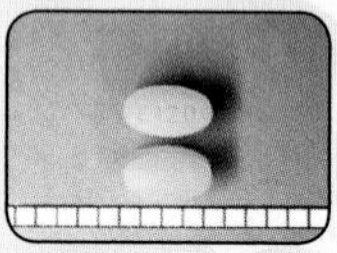

120 mg

Lamotrigine

(generic)

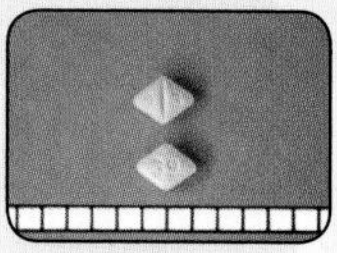

25 mg

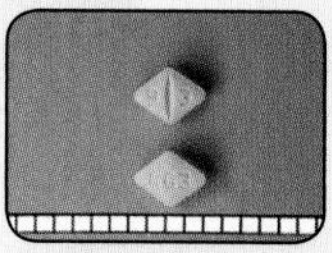

100 mg

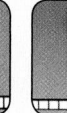

Lamictal®

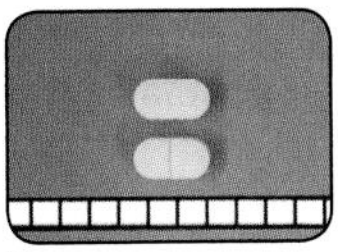
5 mg

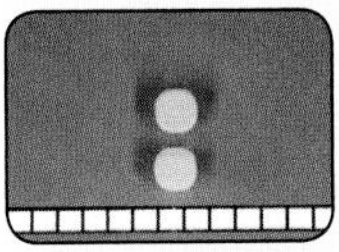
25 mg

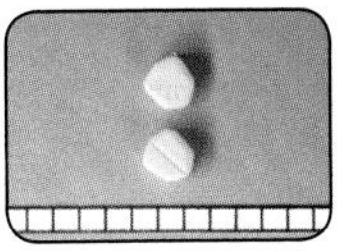
25 mg

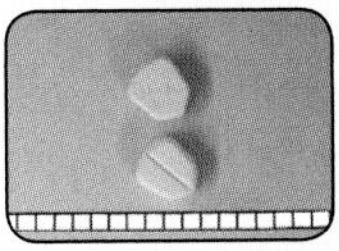
100 mg

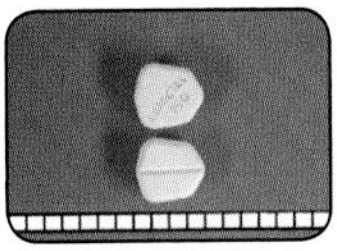
150 mg

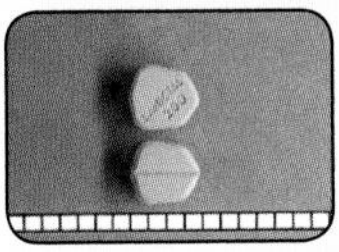
200 mg

Lansoprazole

Prevacid®

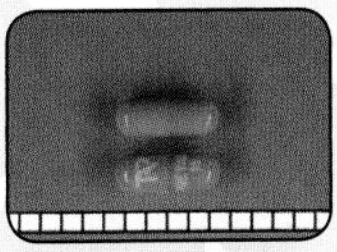
15 mg

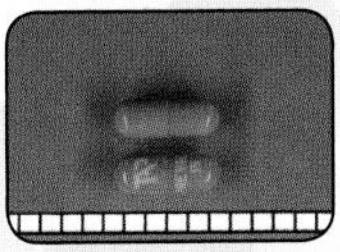
15 mg

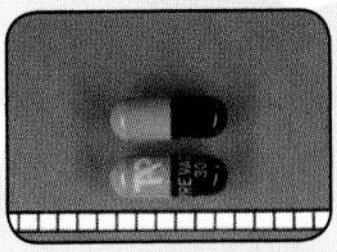
30 mg

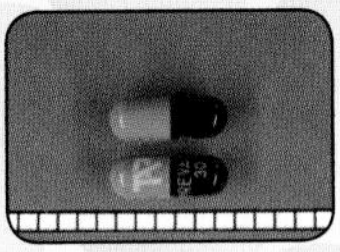
30 mg

Levofloxacin

Levaquin®

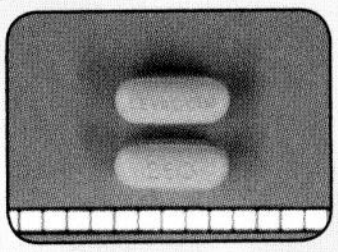
250 mg

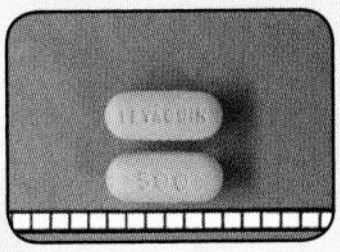
500 mg

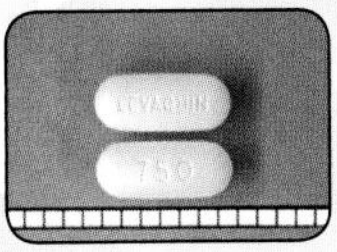
750 mg

Levothyroxine

(generic)

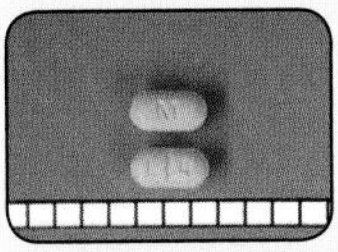
25 mcg

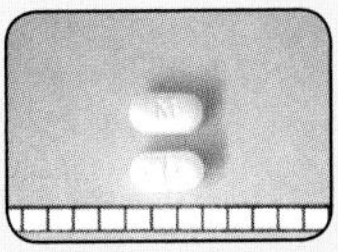
50 mcg

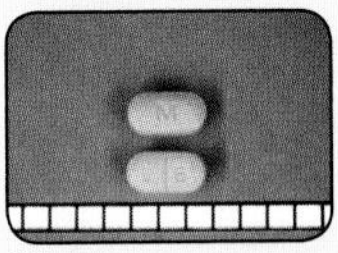
75 mcg

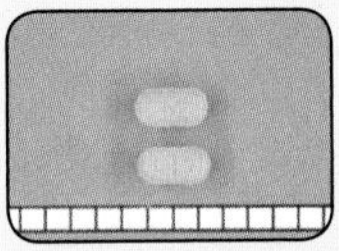
88 mcg

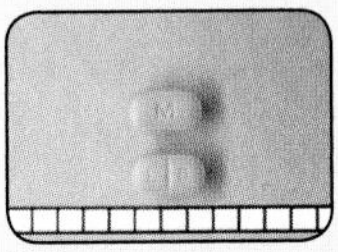
100 mcg

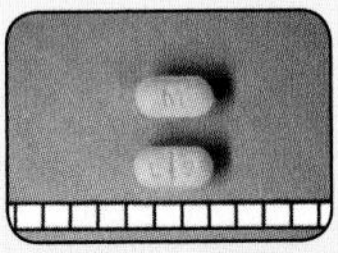
112 mcg

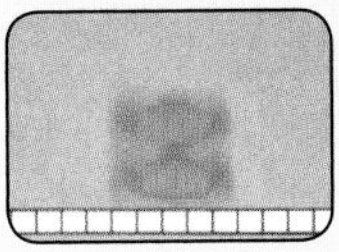
125 mcg

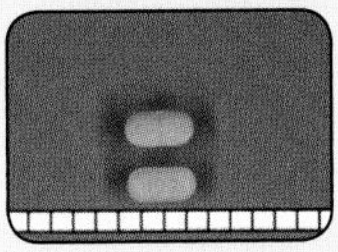
137 mcg

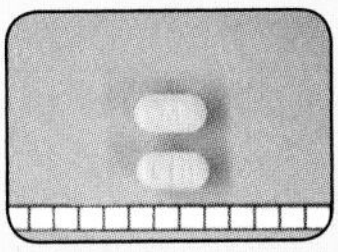
150 mcg

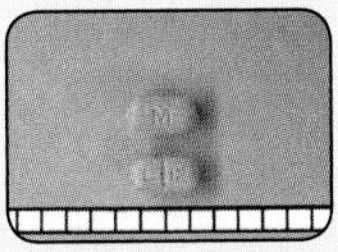
175 mcg

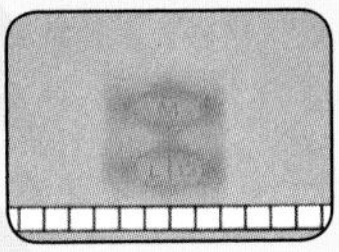
200 mcg

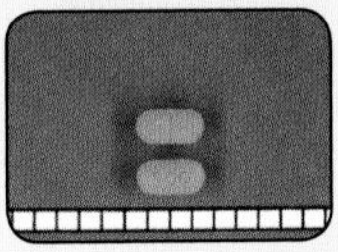
300 mcg

Levoxyl®

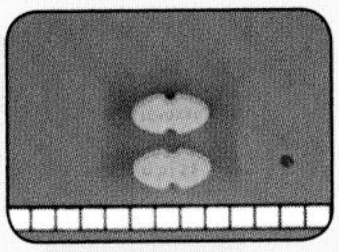
25 mcg

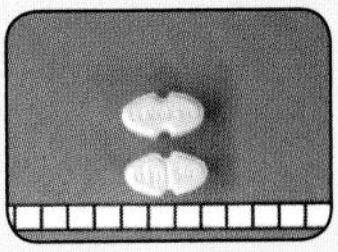
50 mcg

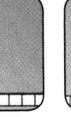

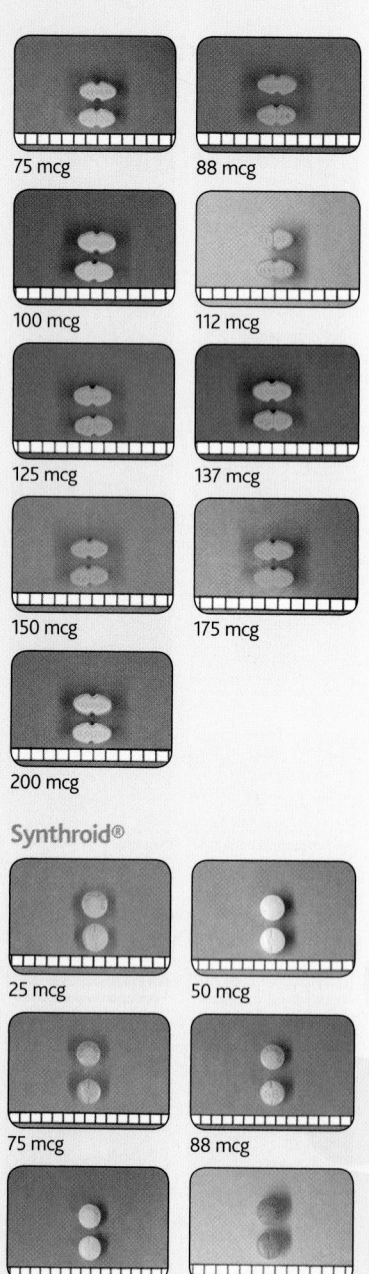

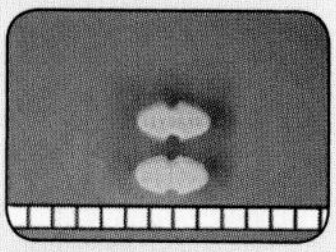
75 mcg

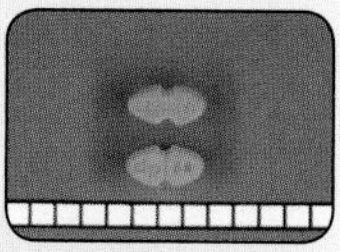
88 mcg

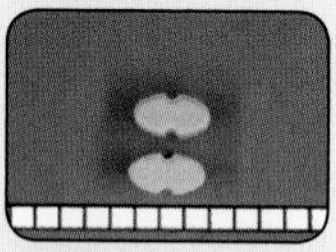
100 mcg

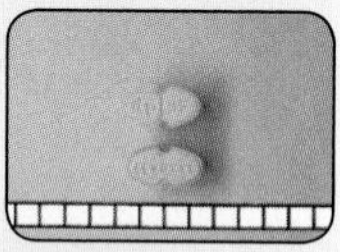
112 mcg

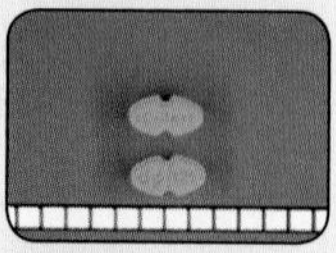
125 mcg

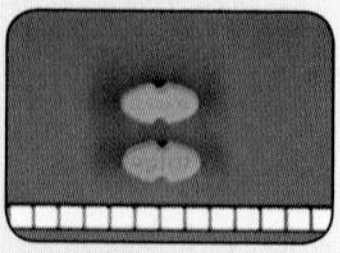
137 mcg

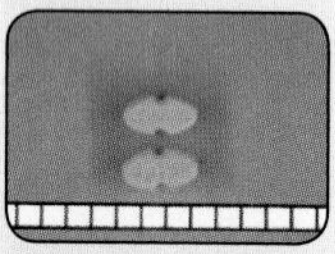
150 mcg

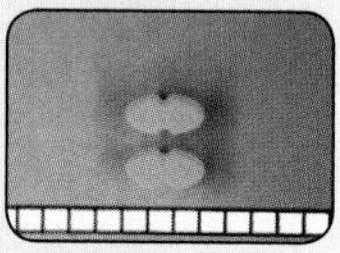
175 mcg

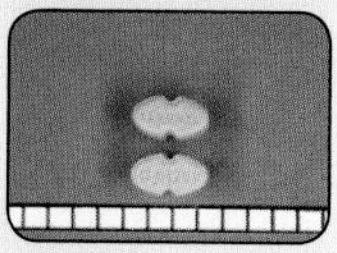
200 mcg

Synthroid®

25 mcg

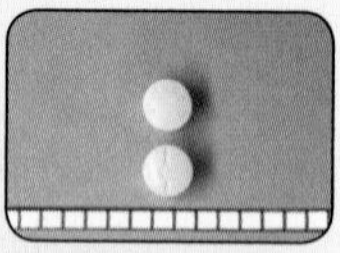
50 mcg

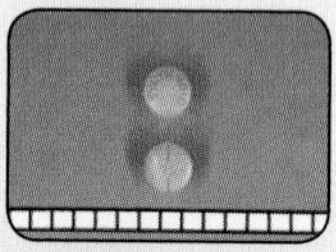
75 mcg

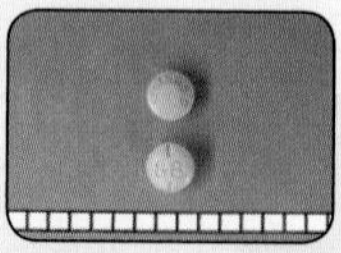
88 mcg

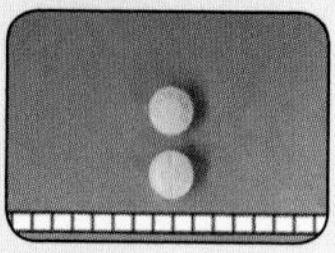
100 mcg

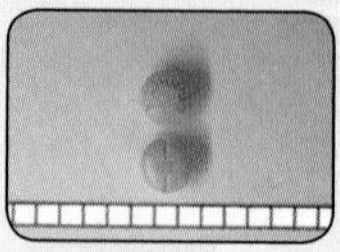
112 mcg

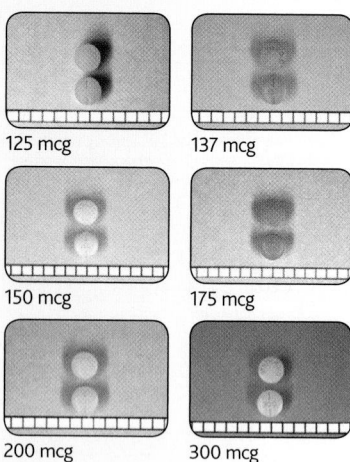

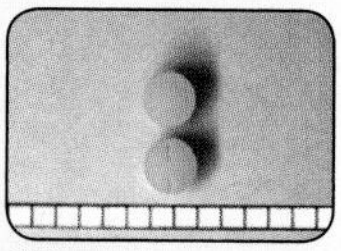
125 mcg

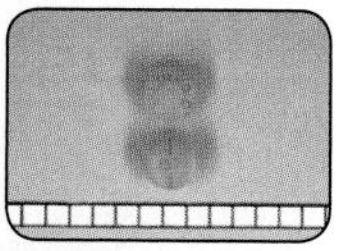
137 mcg

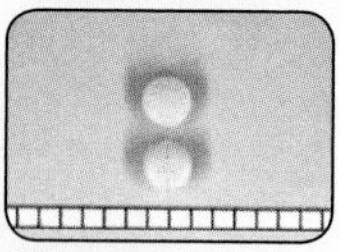
150 mcg

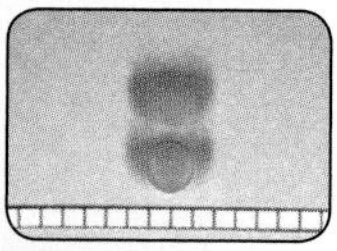
175 mcg

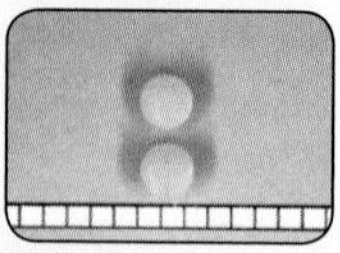
200 mcg

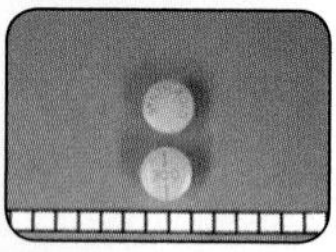
300 mcg

Lisinopril

(generic)

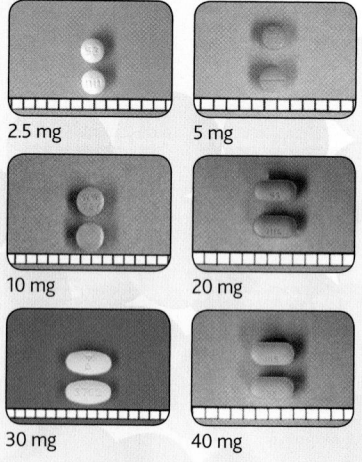

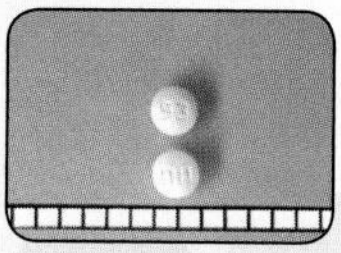
2.5 mg

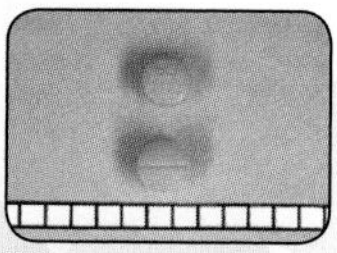
5 mg

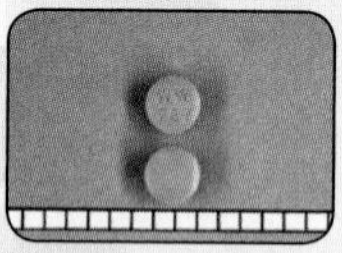
10 mg

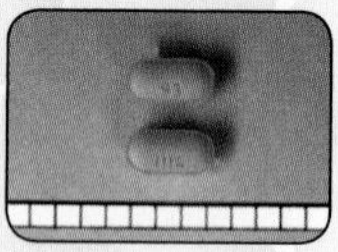
20 mg

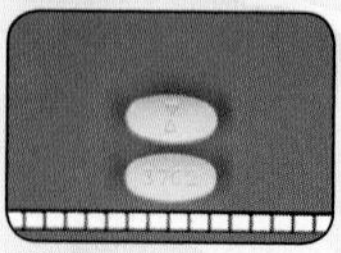
30 mg

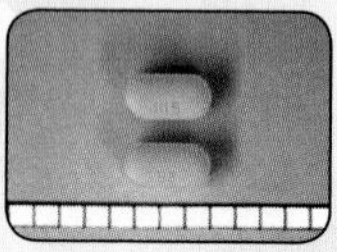
40 mg

Lisinopril and Hydrochlorothiazide

(generic)

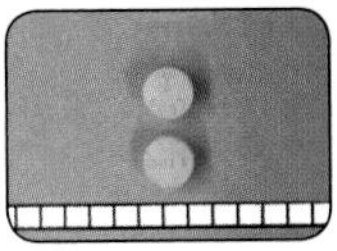
10/12.5 mg

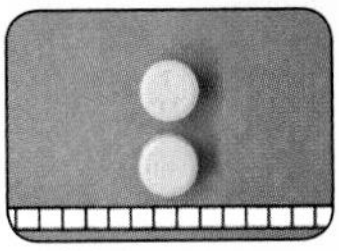
20/12.5 mg

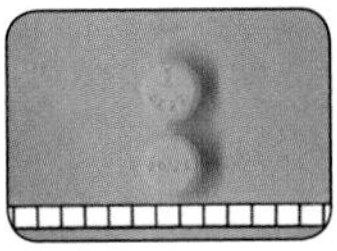
20/25 mg

Lorazepam

(generic)

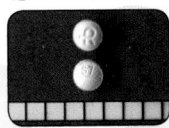
0.5 mg

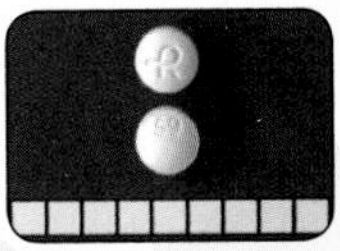
1 mg

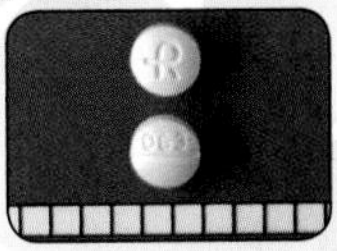
2 mg

Losartan

Cozaar®

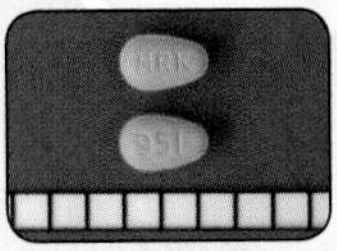
25 mg

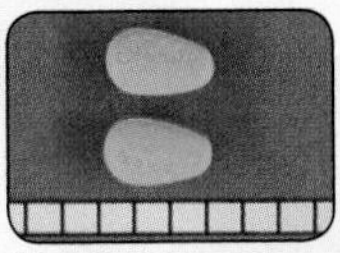
50 mg

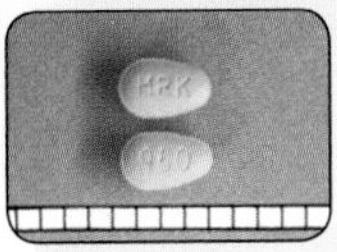
100 mg

Losartan and Hydrochlorothiazide

Hyzaar®

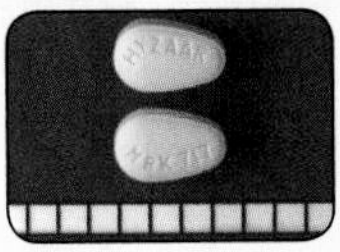
50/12.5 mg

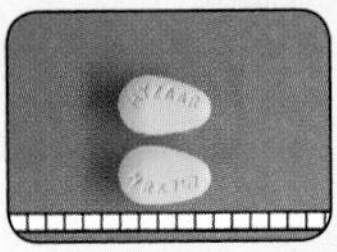
100/25 mg

Lovastatin

(generic)

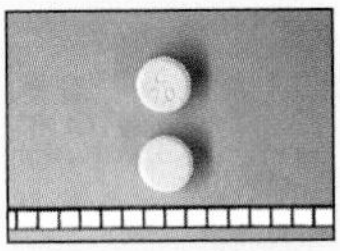
10 mg

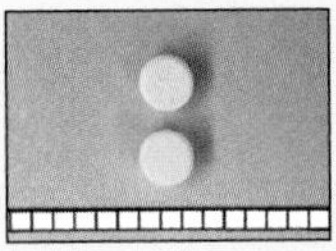
20 mg

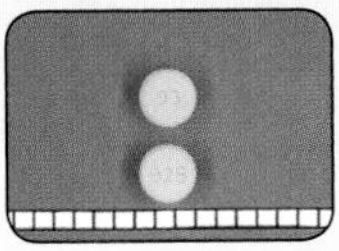
40 mg

Meclizine

(generic)

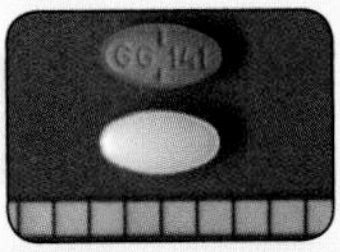
12.5 mg

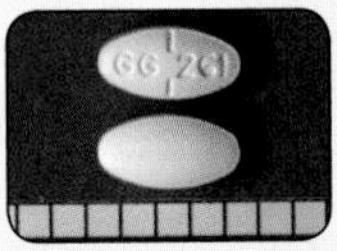
25 mg

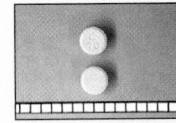

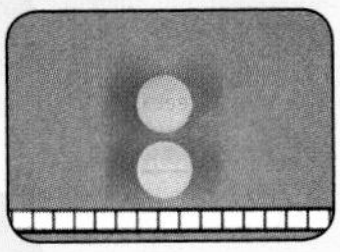
25 mg

Meloxicam

(generic)

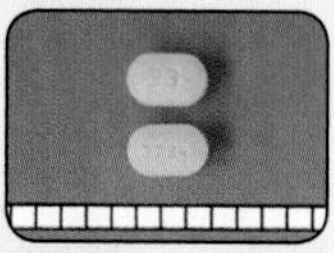

7.5 mg

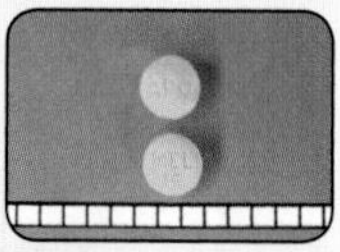

15 mg

Metformin

(generic)

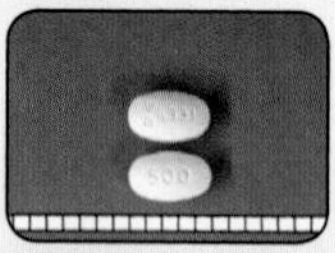

500 mg

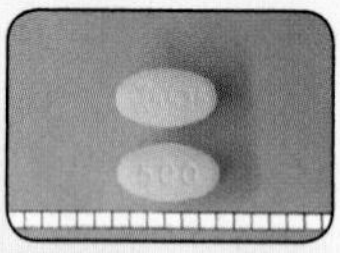

500 mg

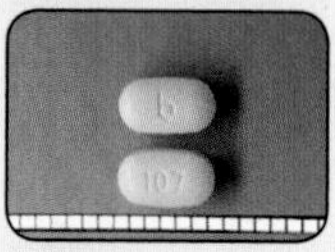

750 mg

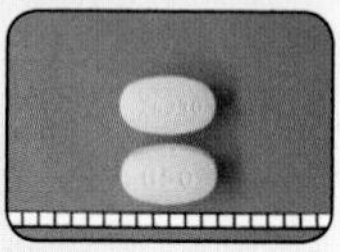

850 mg

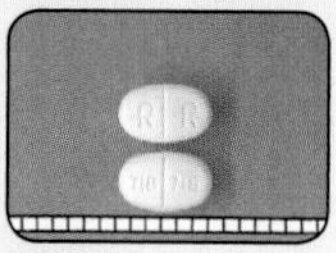

1000 mg

Methadone

(generic)

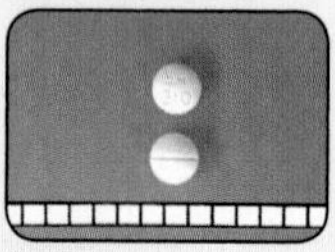

5 mg

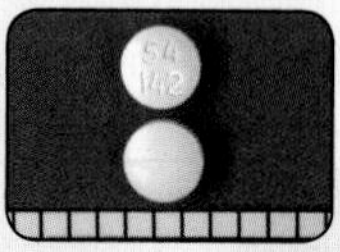

10 mg

Methocarbamol

(generic)

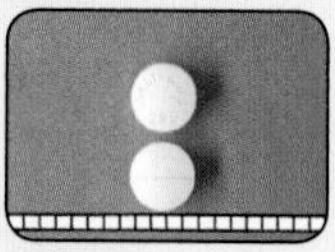

500 mg

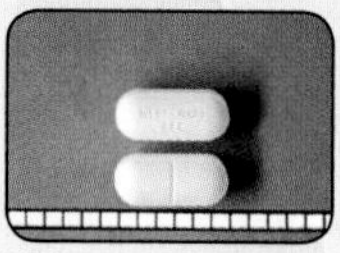

750 mg

Methocarbamol

(generic)

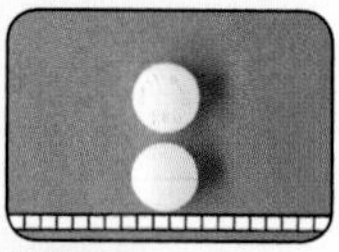

500 mg

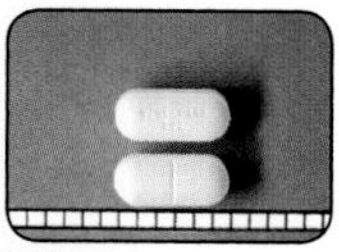

750 mg

Methotrexate

(generic)

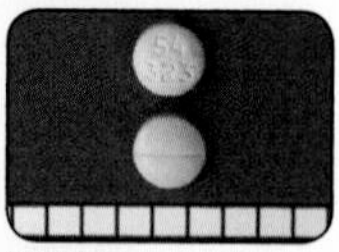

2.5 mg

Methylphenidate

(generic)

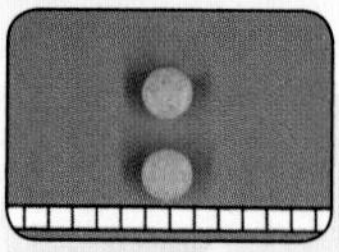

5 mg

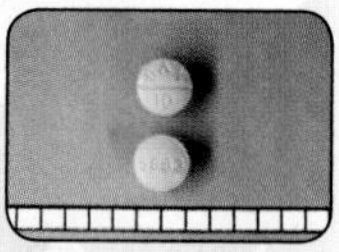

10 mg

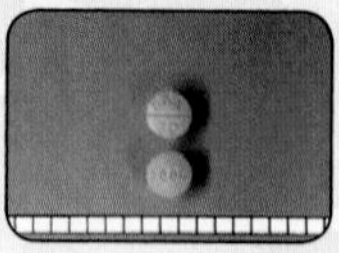

20 mg

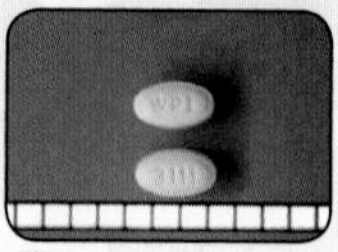

20 mg

Concerta®

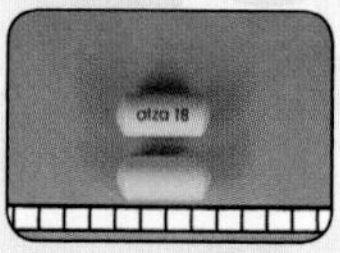

18 mg

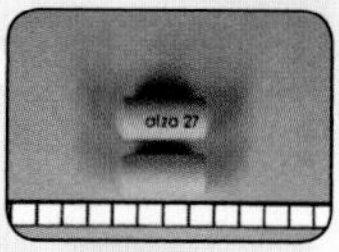

27 mg

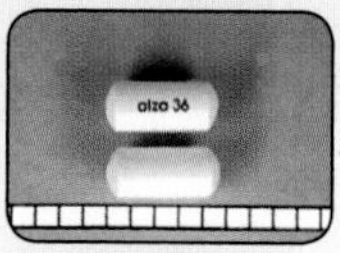

36 mg

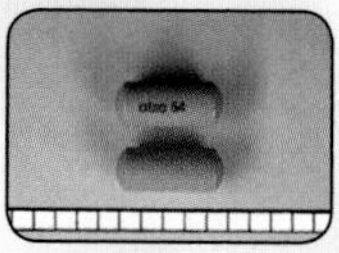

54 mg

Methylprednisolone
(generic)

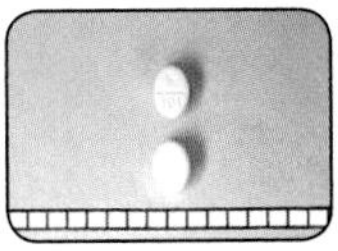
4 mg

Metoclopramide
(generic)

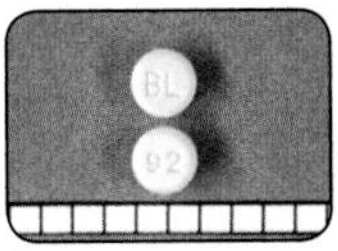
5 mg

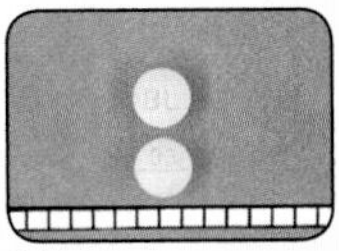
10 mg

Metoprolol
(generic)

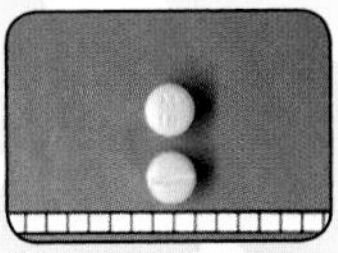
25 mg

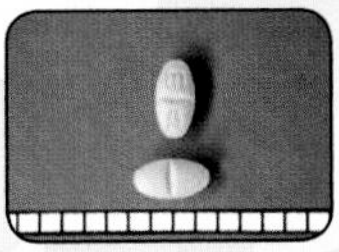
25 mg

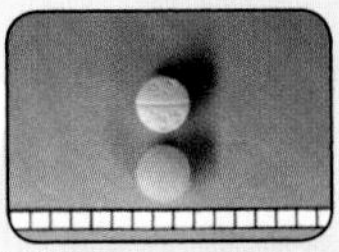
50 mg

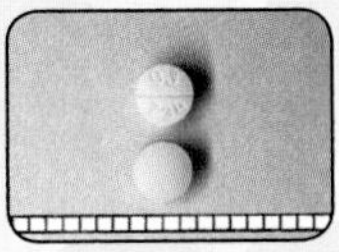
100 mg

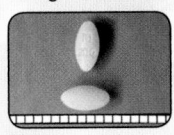
200 mg

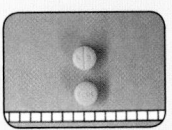

Metronidazole
(generic)

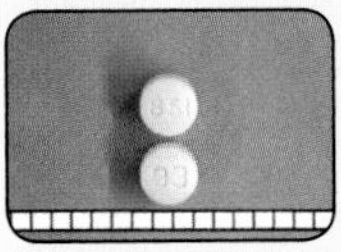
250 mg

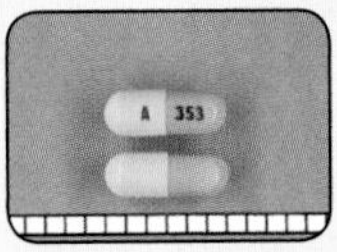
375 mg

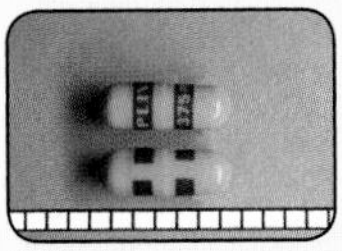
375 mg

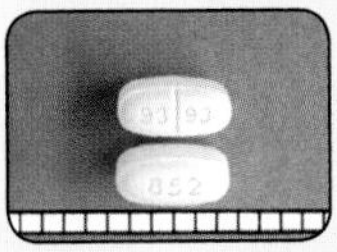
500 mg

Minocycline
(generic)

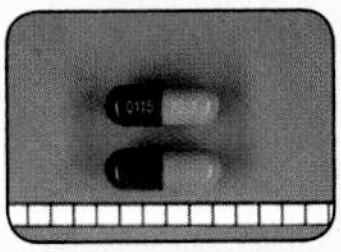
50 mg

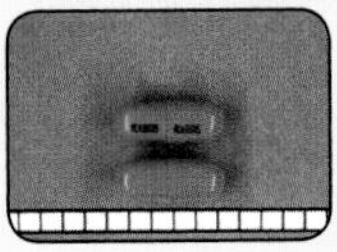
75 mg

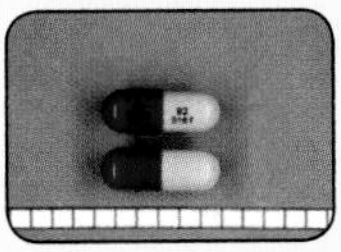
100 mg

Mirtazapine
(generic)

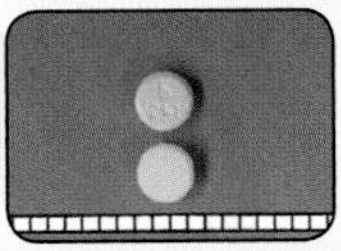
15 mg

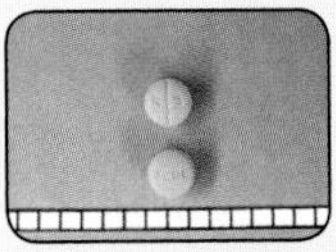
15 mg

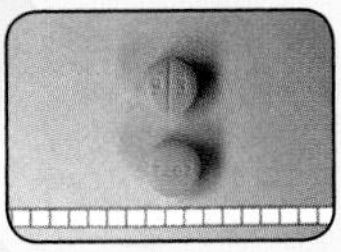
30 mg

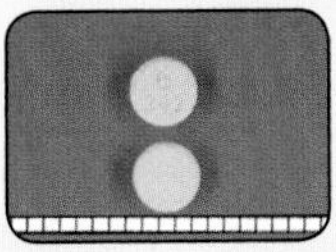
30 mg

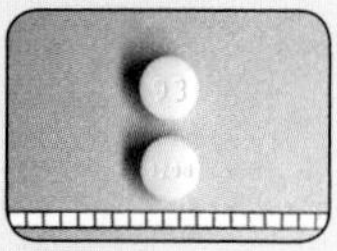

45 mg

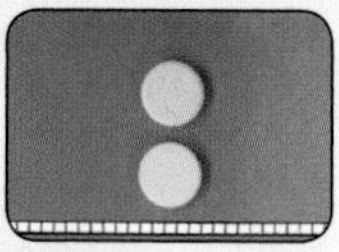

45 mg

Montelukast

Singulair®

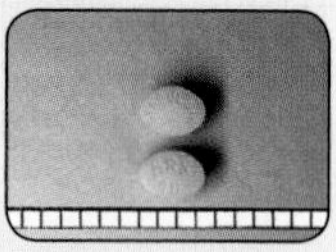

4 mg

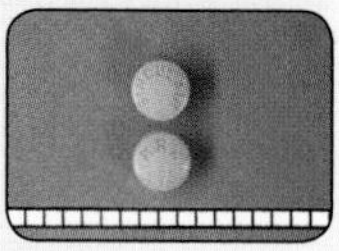

5 mg

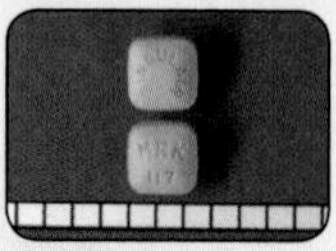

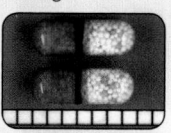

10 mg

Moxifloxacin

Avelox® ABC Pack

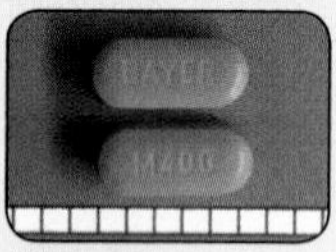

400 mg

Avelox®

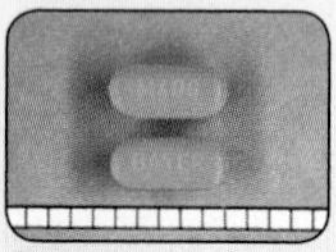

400 mg

Nabumetone

(generic)

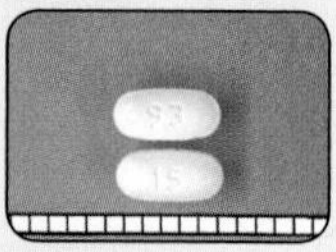

500 mg

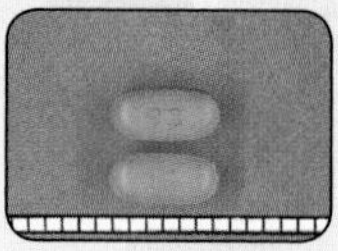

750 mg

Naproxen

(generic)

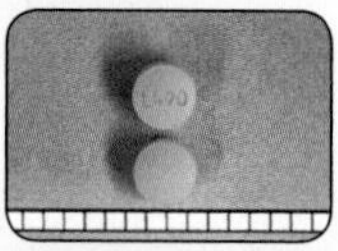

220 mg

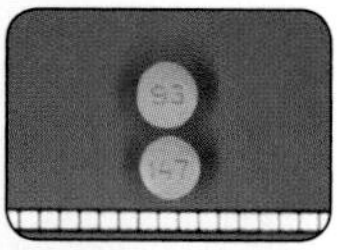

250 mg

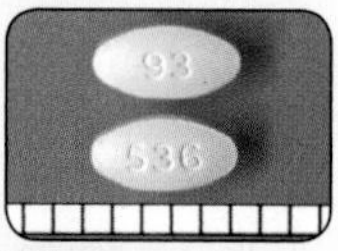

275 mg

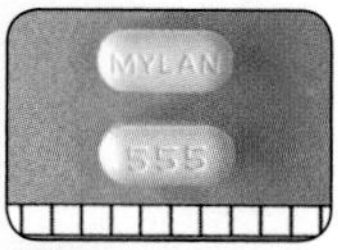

375 mg

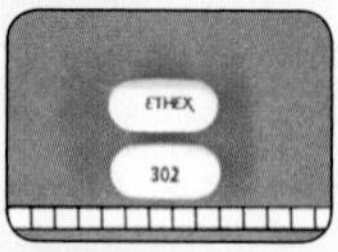

375 mg

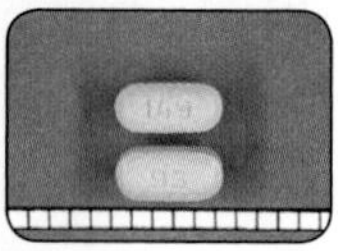

500 mg

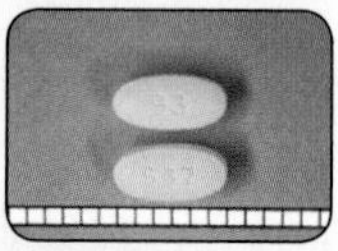

550 mg

Niacin

(generic)

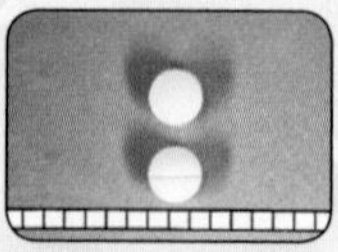

50 mg

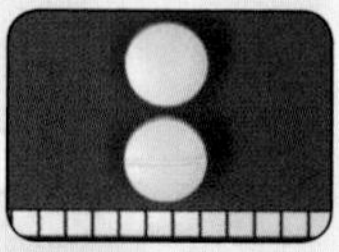

100 mg

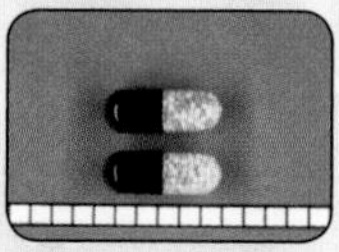

125 mg

250 mg

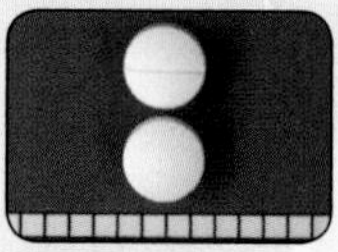

250 mg

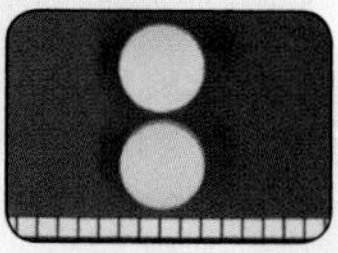

500 mg

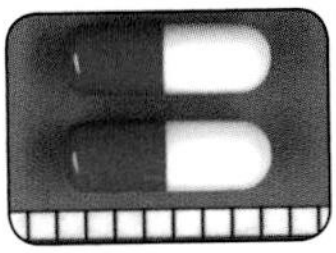

500 mg

Niaspan®

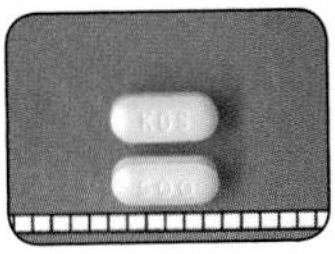

500 mg

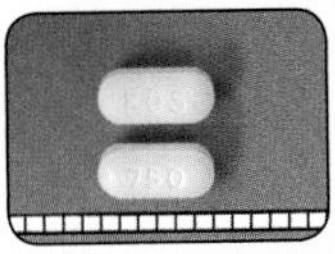

750 mg

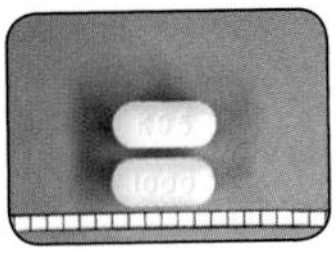

1000 mg

Nifedipine

(generic)

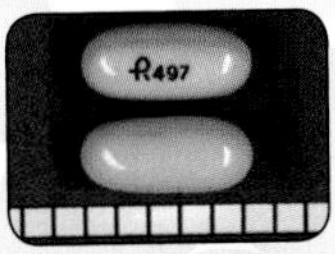

10 mg

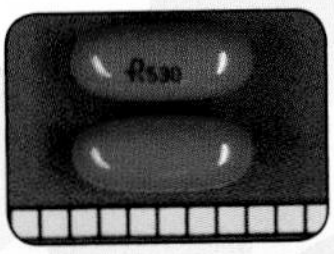

20 mg

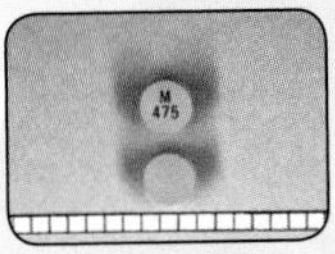

30 mg

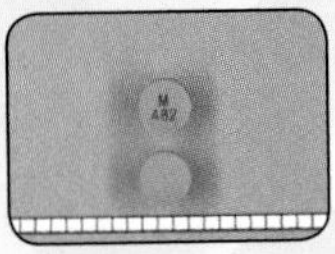

60 mg

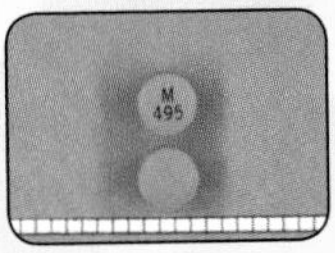

90 mg

Nitrofurantoin

(generic)

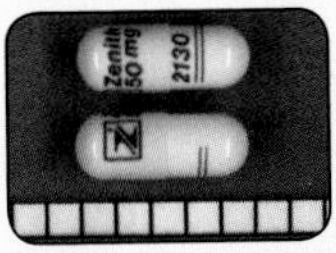

50 mg

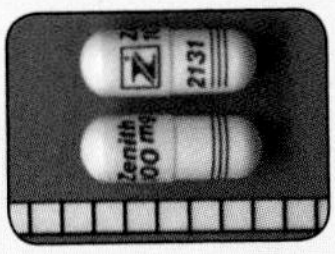

100 mg

Olanzapine

Zyprexa®

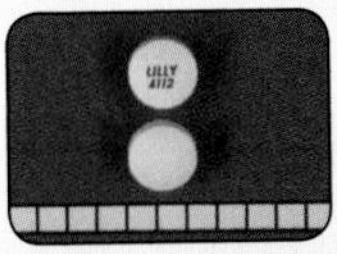

2.5 mg

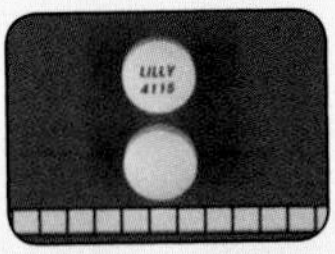

5 mg

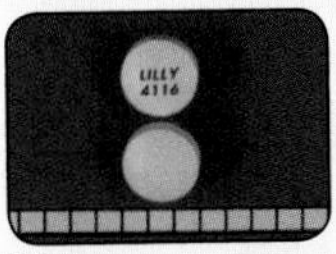

7.5 mg

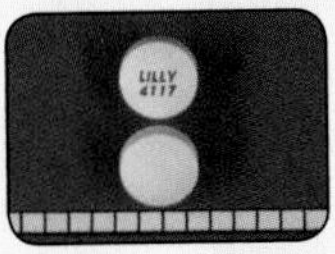

10 mg

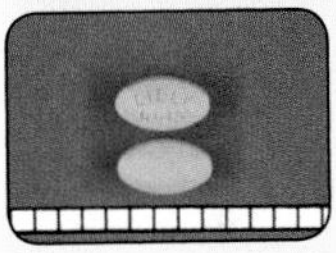

15 mg

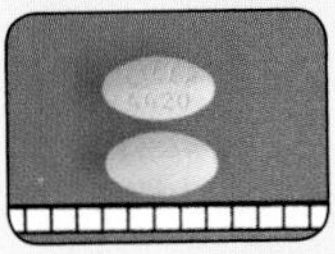

20 mg

Olmesartan

Benicar®

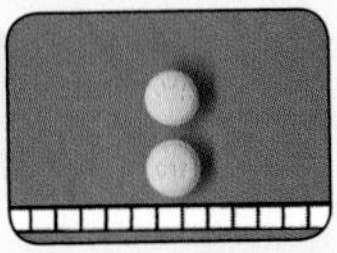

5 mg

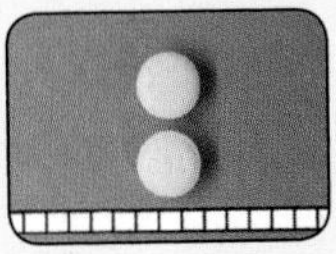

20 mg

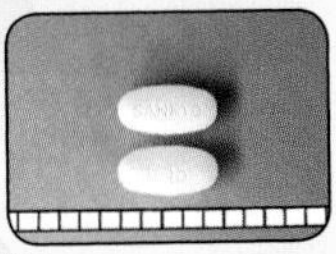

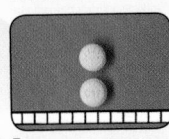

40 mg

Olmesartan and Hydrochlorothiazide

Benicar HCT®

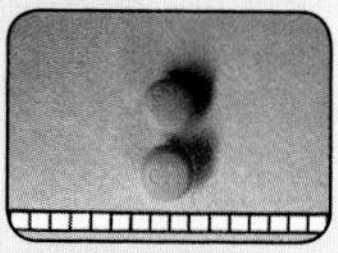

20/12.5 mg

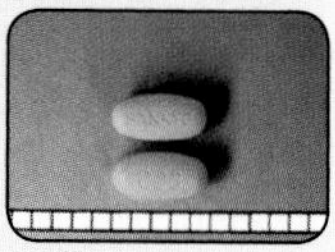

40/12.5 mg

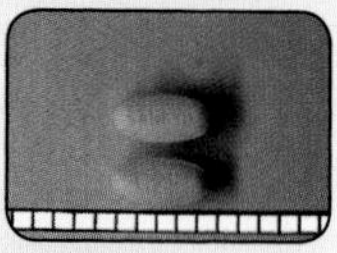

40/25 mg

Omeprazole

(generic)

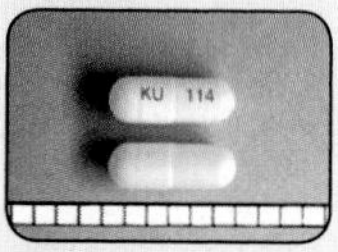

10 mg

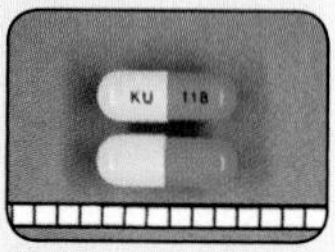

20 mg

Oxycodone

(generic)

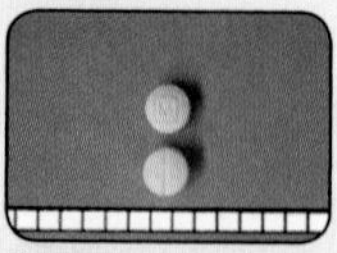

5 mg

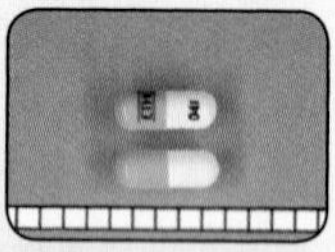

5 mg

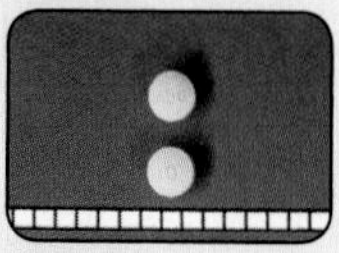

10 mg

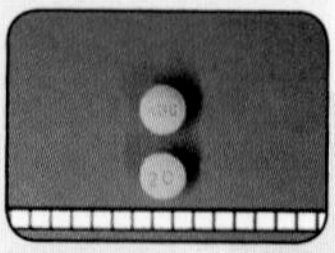

20 mg

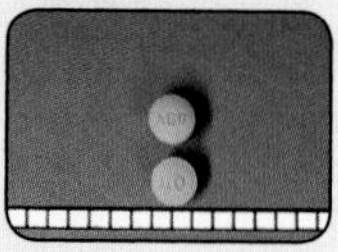

40 mg

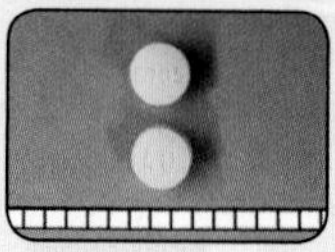

40 mg

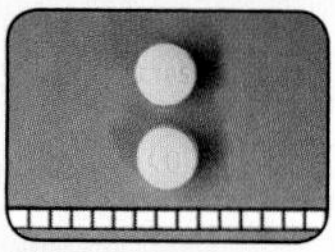

80 mg

OxyContin®

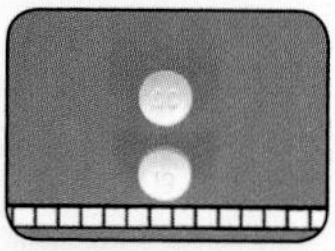

10 mg

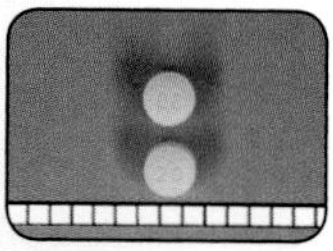

20 mg

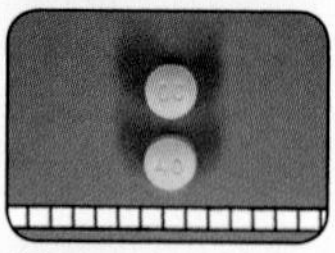

40 mg

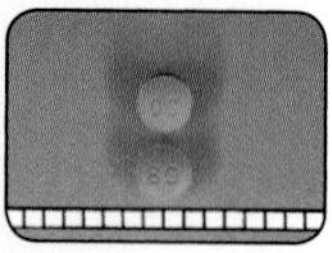

80 mg

Oxycodone and Acetaminophen

(generic)

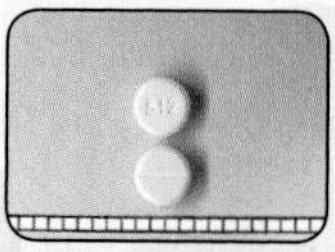

5/325 mg

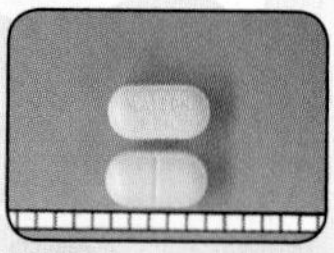

7.5/500 mg

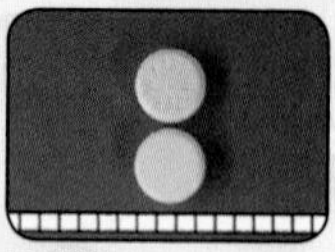

10/325 mg

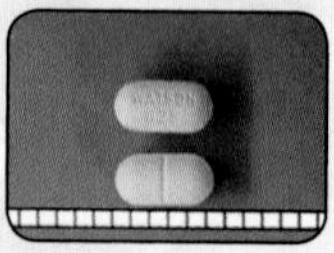

10/650 mg

Pantoprazole

(generic)

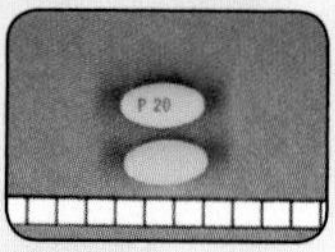

20 mg

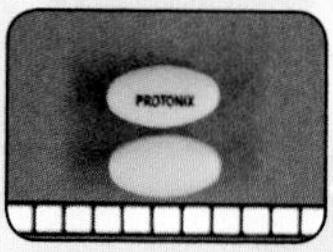

40 mg

Protonix®

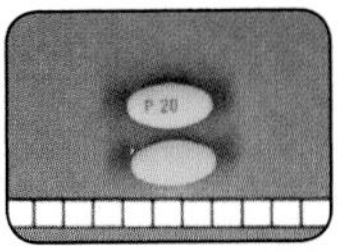

20 mg

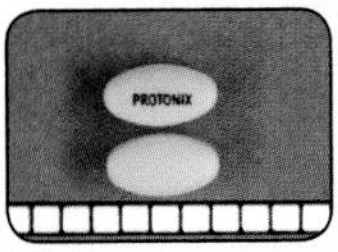

40 mg

Paroxetine

(generic)

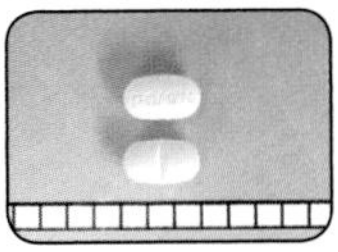
10 mg

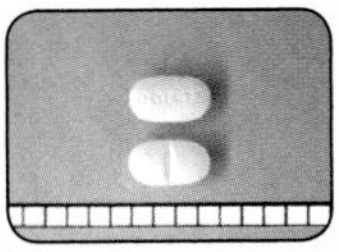
20 mg

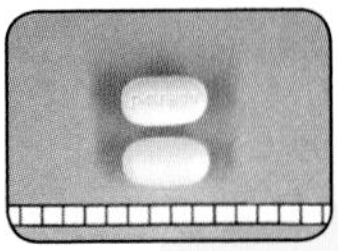
30 mg

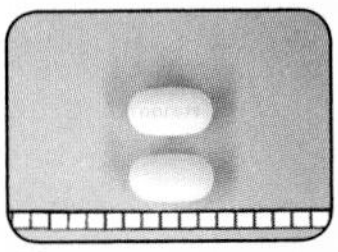
40 mg

Penicillin V Potassium

(generic)

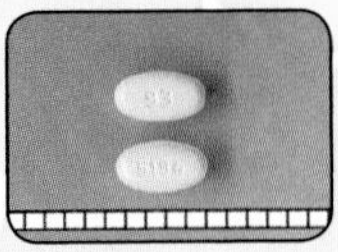
250 mg

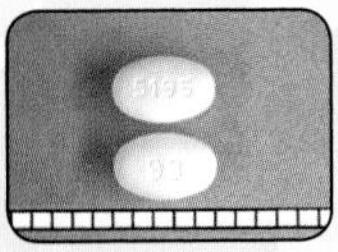
500 mg

Phentermin

(generic)

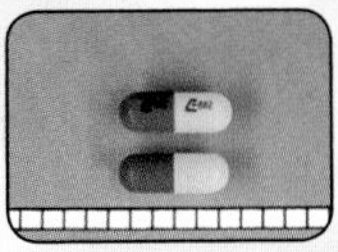
15 mg

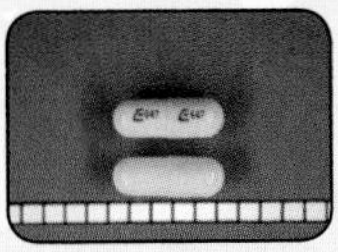
30 mg

Pioglitazone

Actos®

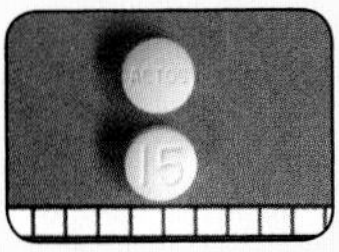
15 mg

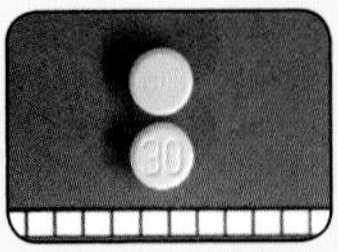

30 mg

Potassium Chloride

(generic)

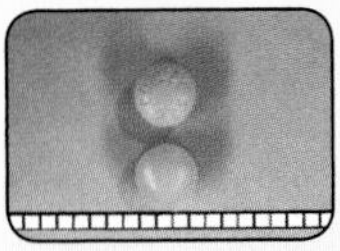
8 mEq

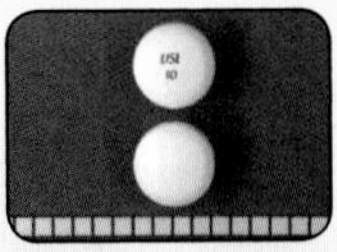
10 mEq

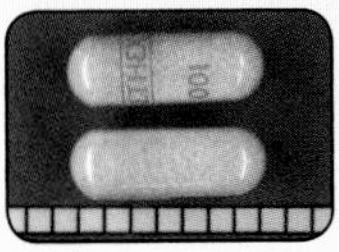
10 mEq

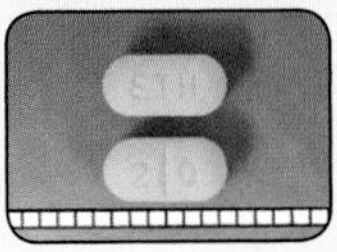
20 mEq

Klor-Con® 8

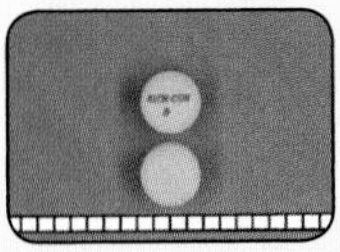
8 mEq

Klor-Con® 10

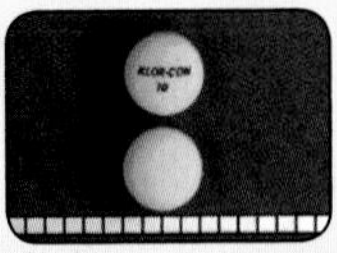
10 mEq

Pravastatin

(generic)

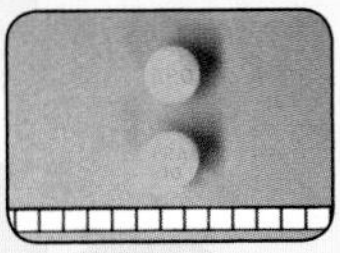
10 mg

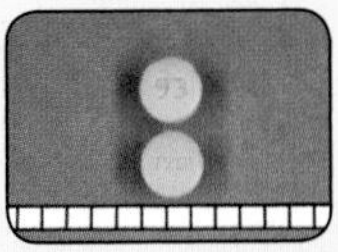
20 mg

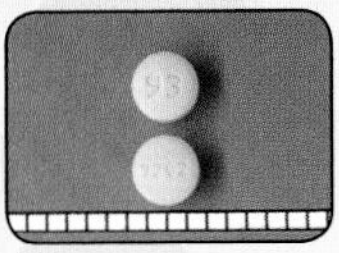
40 mg

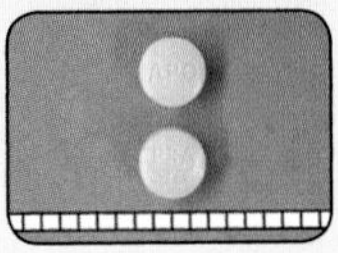
80 mg

Prednisone

(generic)

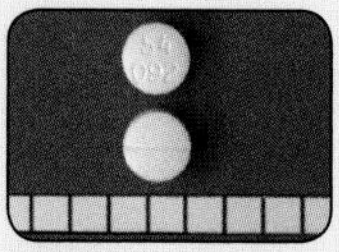

1 mg

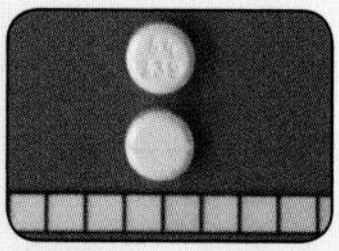

2.5 mg

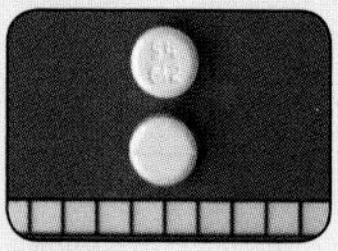

5 mg

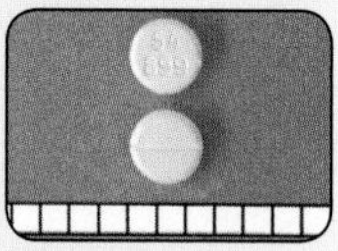

10 mg

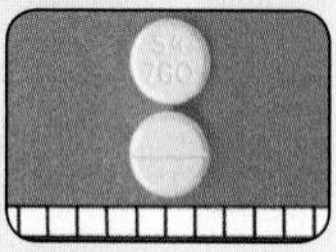

20 mg

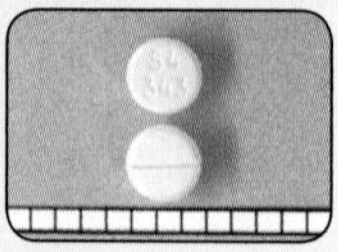

50 mg

Pregabalin

Lyrica®

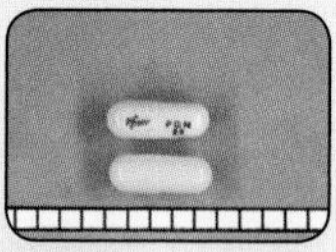

25 mg

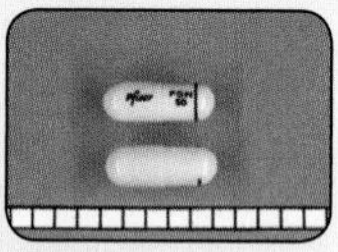

50 mg

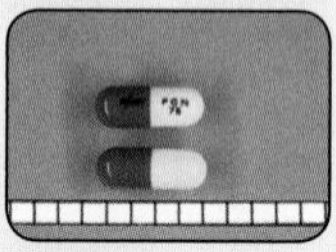

75 mg

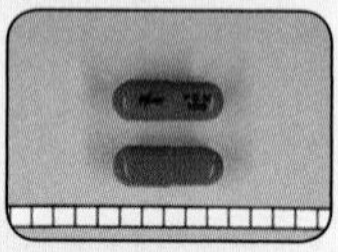

100 mg

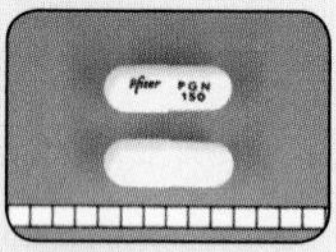

150 mg

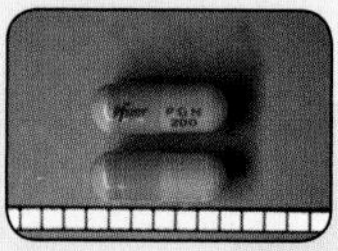

200 mg

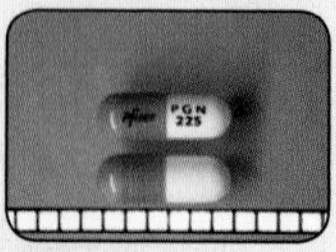

225 mg

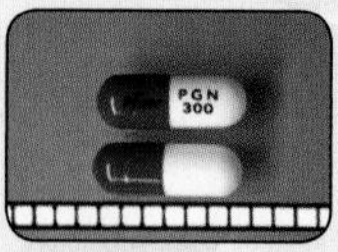

300 mg

Promethazine

(generic)

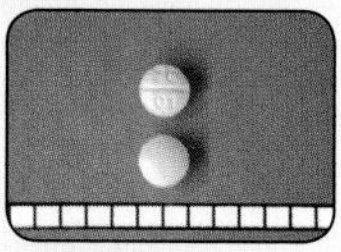

12.5 mg

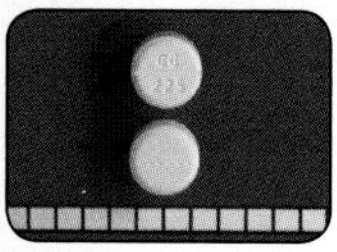

25 mg

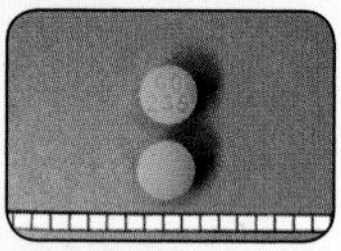

50 mg

Propoxyphene and Acetaminophen

(generic)

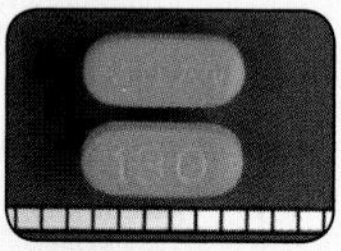

65/650 mg

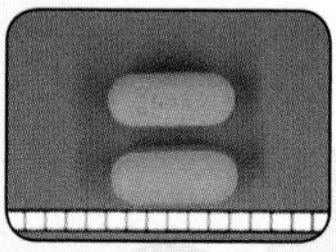

100/650 mg

Propranolol

(generic)

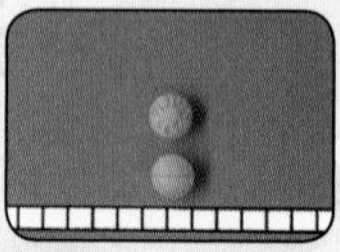

10 mg

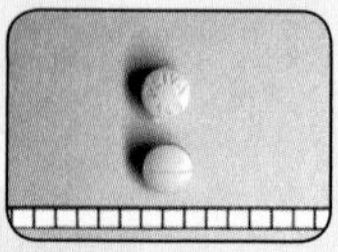

20 mg

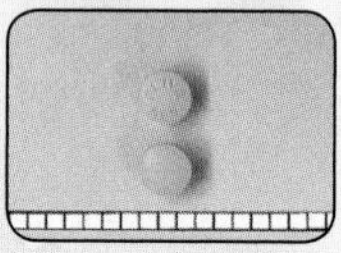

40 mg

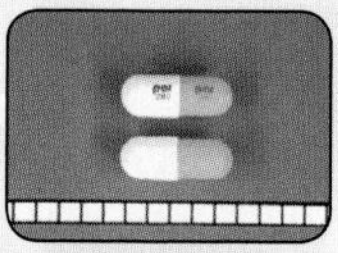

60 mg

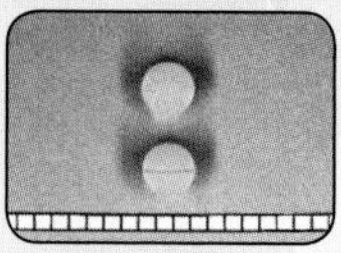

60 mg

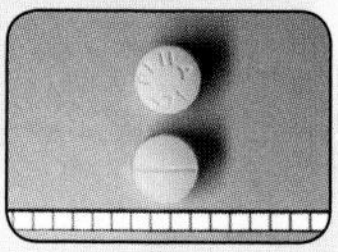

80 mg

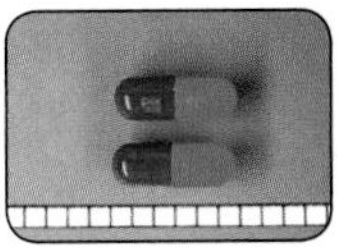
120 mg

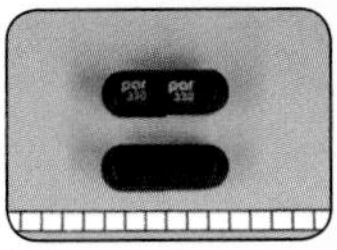
160 mg

Quetiapine

Seroquel®

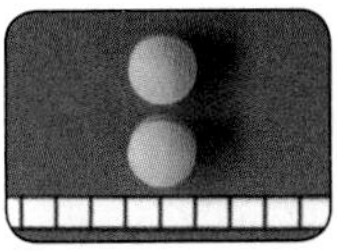
25 mg

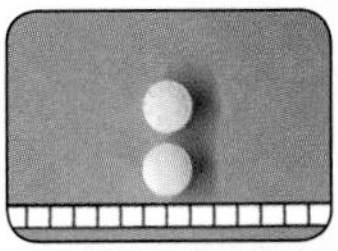
50 mg

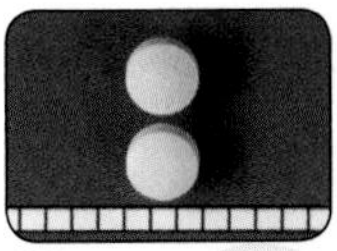
100 mg

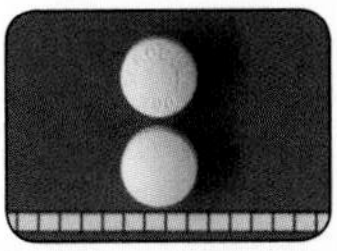
200 mg

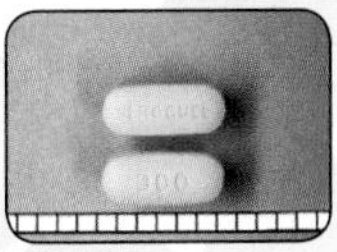
300 mg

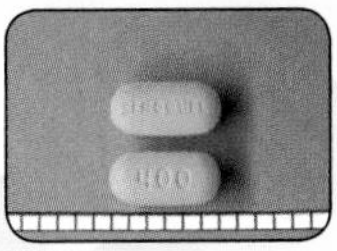
400 mg

Quinapril

(generic)

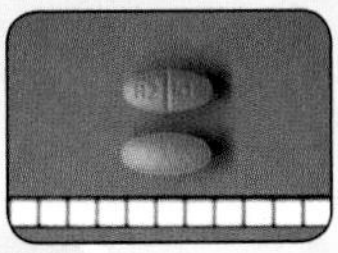
5 mg

Rabeprazole

Aciphex®

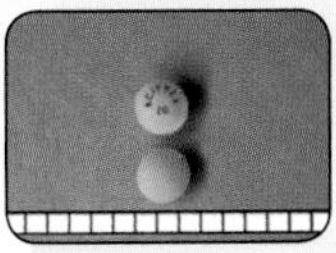
20 mg

Raloxifene

Evista®

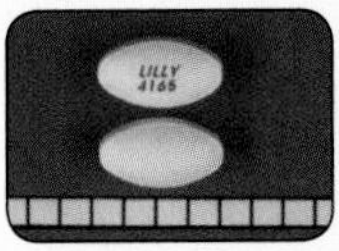
60 mg

Ramipril

(generic)

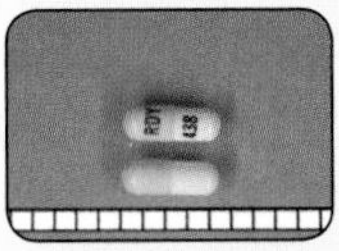
1.25 mg

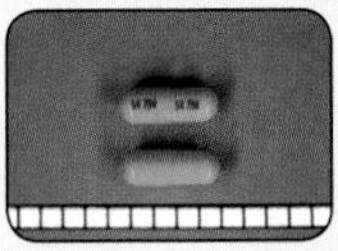
2.5 mg

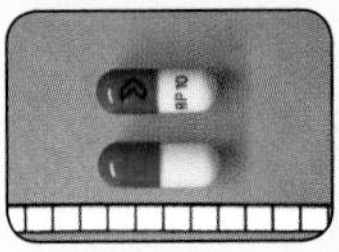
10 mg

Ranitidine

(generic)

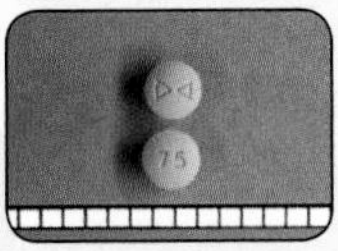
75 mg

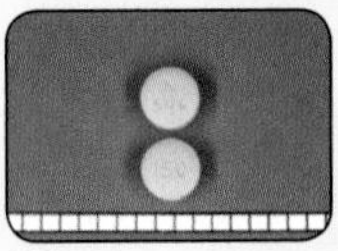
150 mg

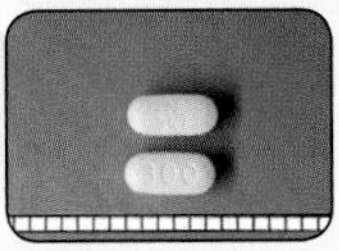
300 mg

Risedronate

Actonel®

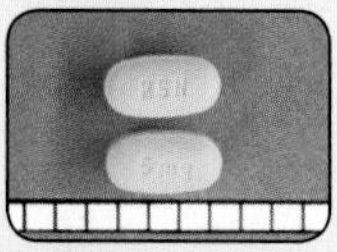

5 mg

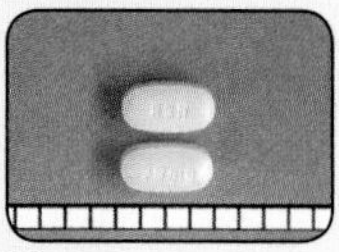

30 mg

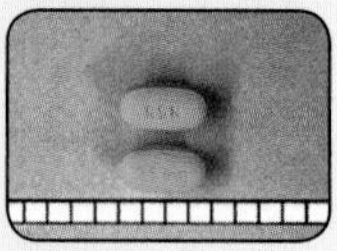

35 mg

Risperidone

(generic)

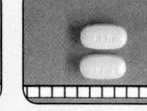

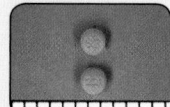

0.25 mg

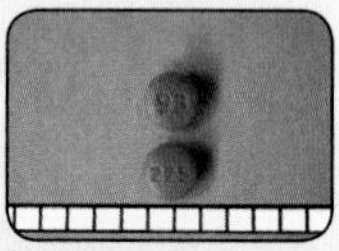

0.5 mg

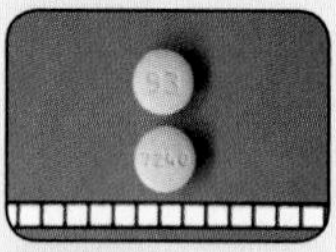

1 mg

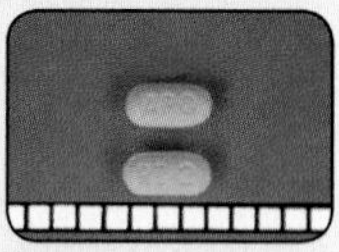

2 mg

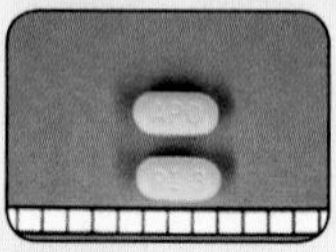

3 mg

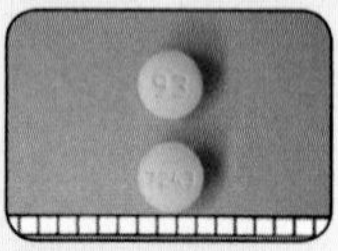

4 mg

Risperdal®

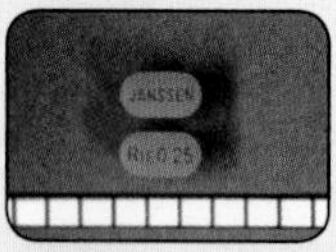

0.25 mg

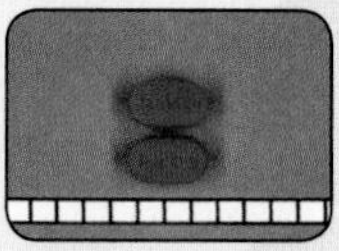

0.5 mg

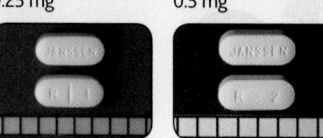

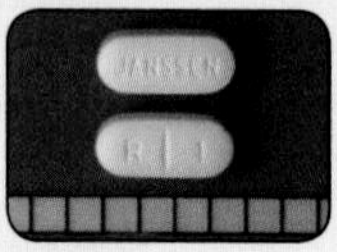

1 mg

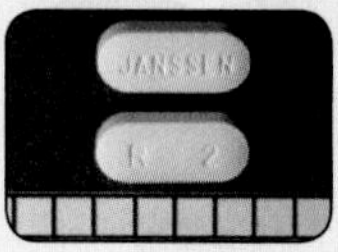

2 mg

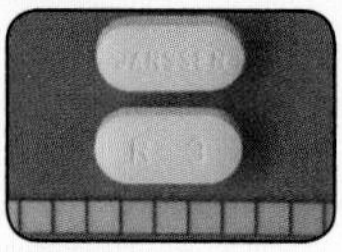

3 mg

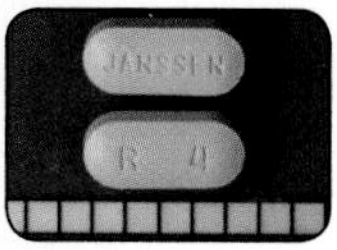

4 mg

Sertraline

(generic)

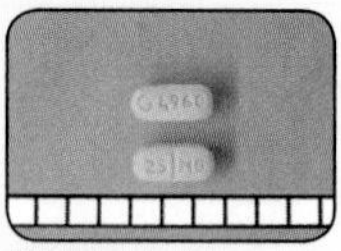

25 mg

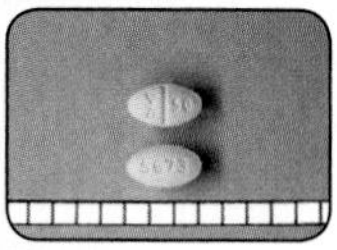

50 mg

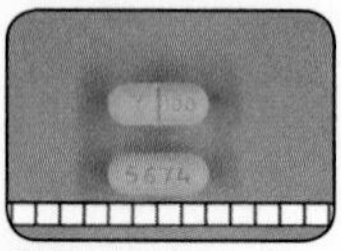

100 mg

Sildenafil

Viagra™

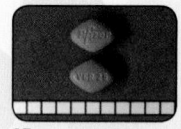

25 mg

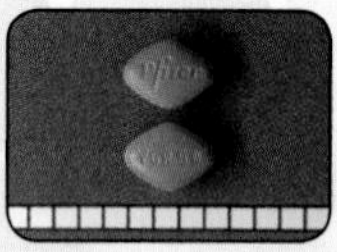

50 mg

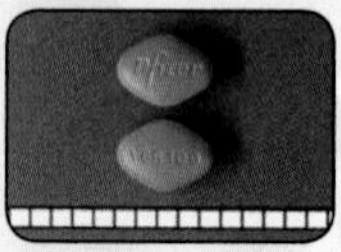

100 mg

Simvastin

(generic)

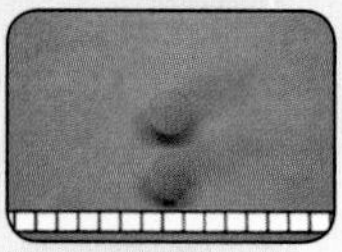

10 mg

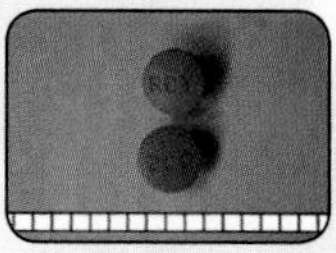

40 mg

Sitagliptin

Januvia™

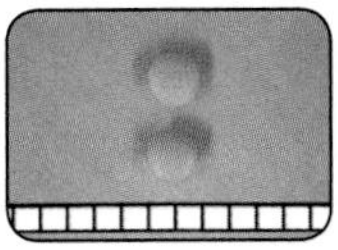
25 mg

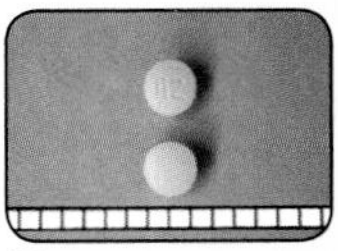
50 mg

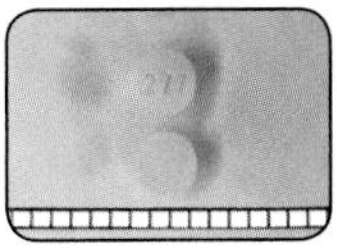
100 mg

Spironolactone

(generic)

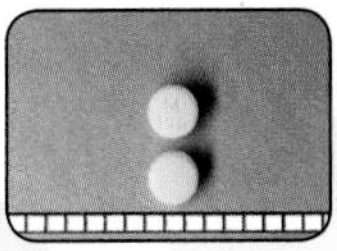
25 mg

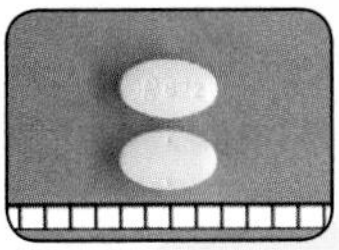
50 mg

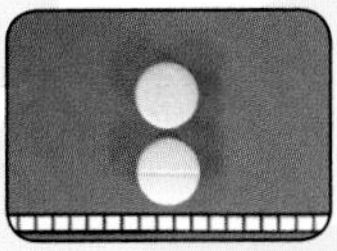
100 mg

Sulfamethoxazole and Trimethoprim

(generic)

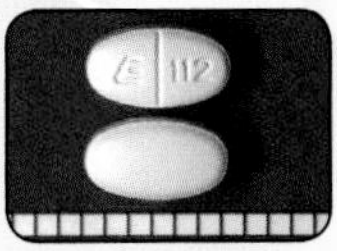
800/160 mg

Tadalafil

Cialis®

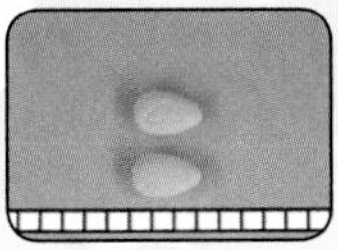
5 mg

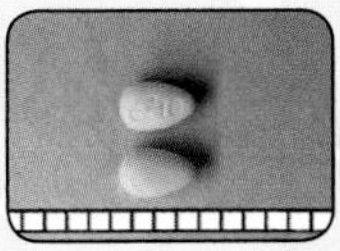
10 mg

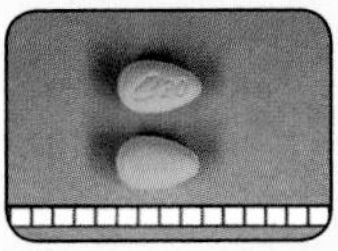
20 mg

Temazepam

(generic)

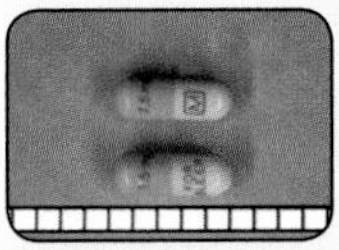
7.5 mg

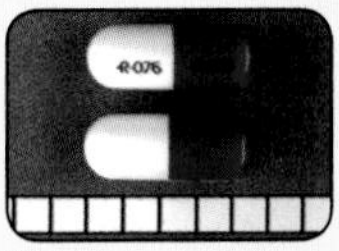
15 mg

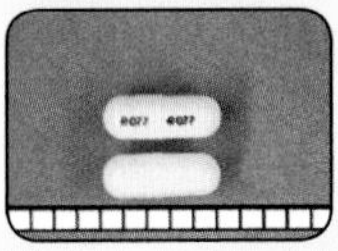
30 mg

Terazosin

(generic)

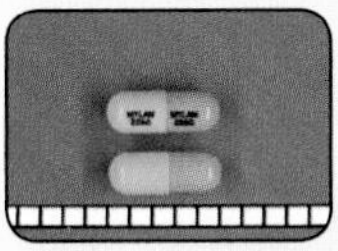
1 mg

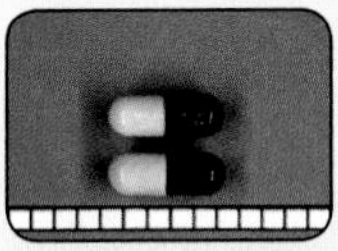
2 mg

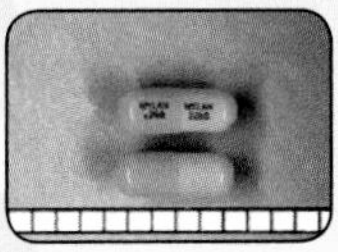
5 mg

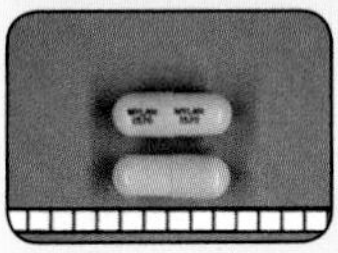
10 mg

Thyroid Desiccated

Armour® Thyroid

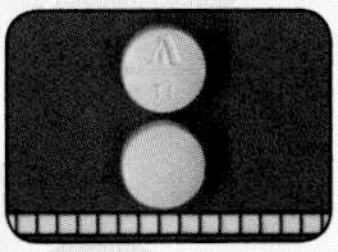
300 mg

Tizanidine
(generic)

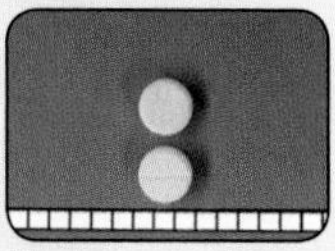
2 mg

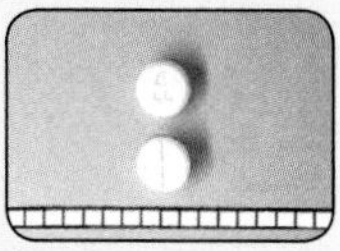
4 mg

Tolterodine
Detrol® LA

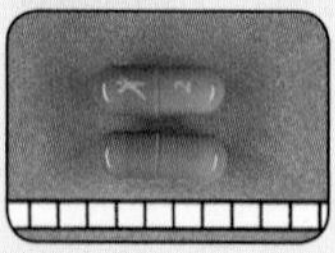
2 mg

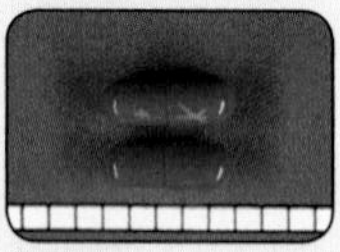
4 mg

Topiramate
Topamax®

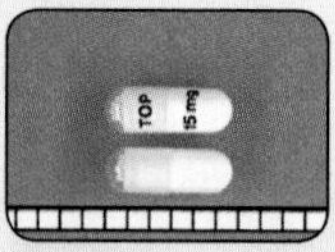

15 mg

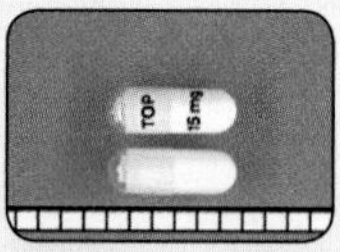

15 mg

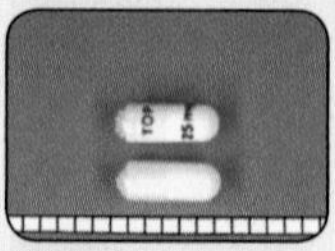
25 mg

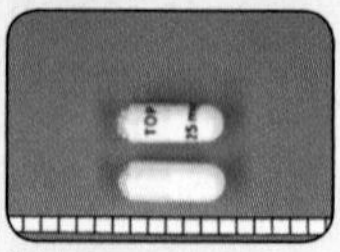
25 mg

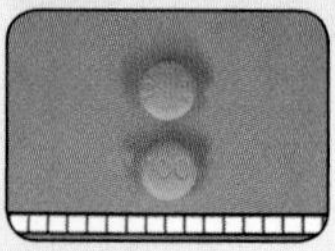
100 mg

Tramadol
(generic)

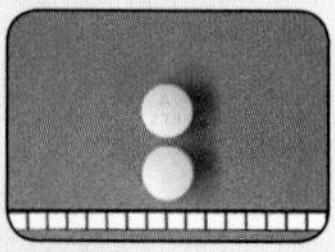
50 mg

Trazodone
(generic)

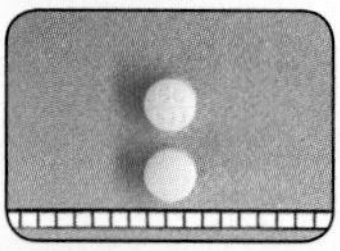
50 mg

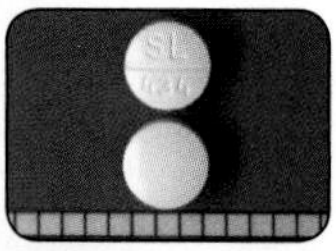
100 mg

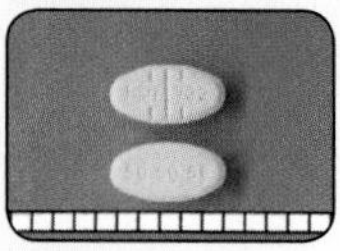
150 mg

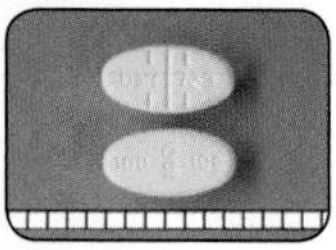
300 mg

Valacyclovir
Valtrex®

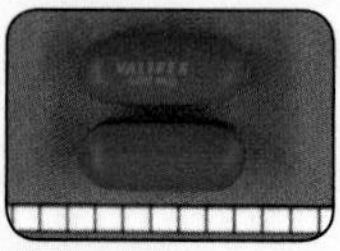
500 mg

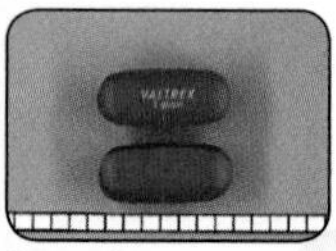
1 g

Valproic Acid and Derivatives
(generic)

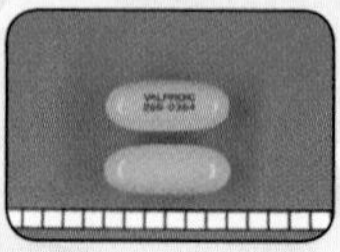
250 mg

Valsartan
Diovan®

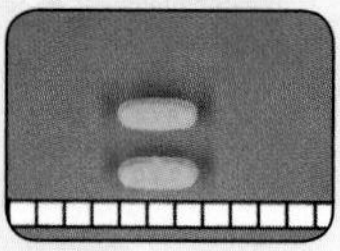
40 mg

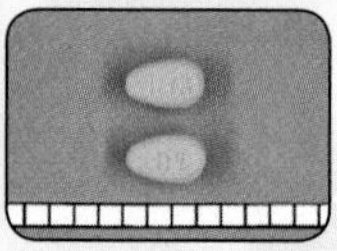
80 mg

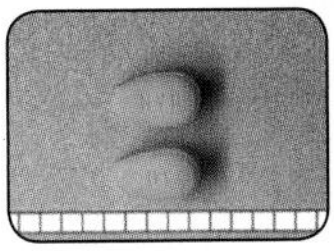
160 mg

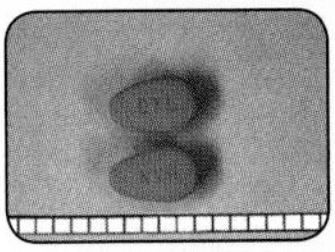
320 mg

Valsartan and Hydrochlorothiazide

Diovan HCT®

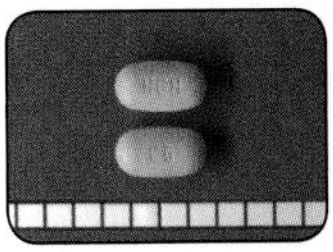
80/12.5 mg

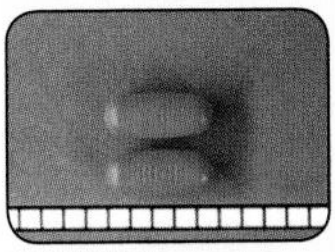
160/12.5 mg

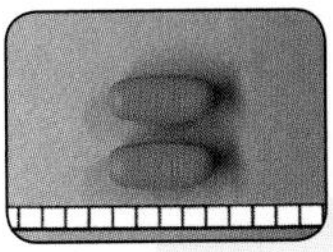
160/25 mg

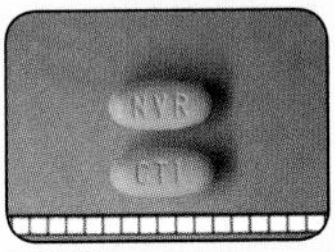
320/25 mg

Varenicline

Chantix®

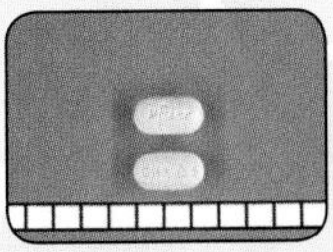
0.5 mg

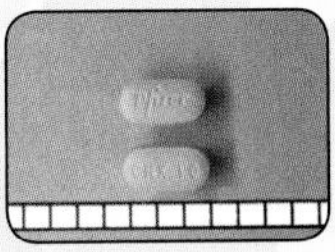
1 mg

Venlafaxine

(generic)

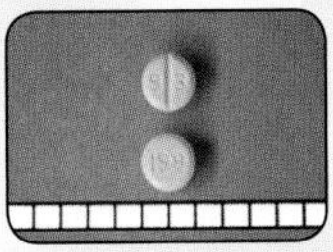
25 mg

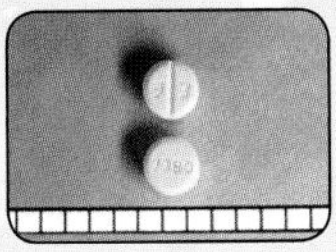
37.5 mg

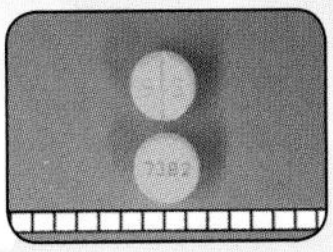
75 mg

Effexor XR®

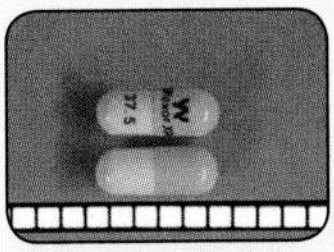
37.5 mg

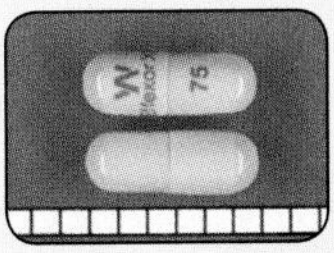
75 mg

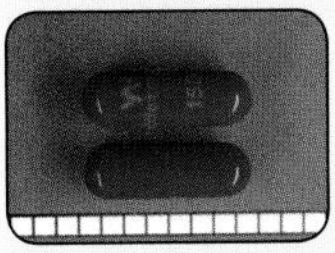
150 mg

Verapamil

(generic)

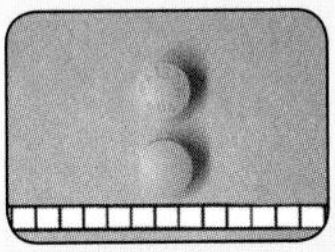
40 mg

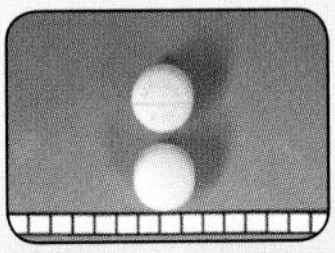
80 mg

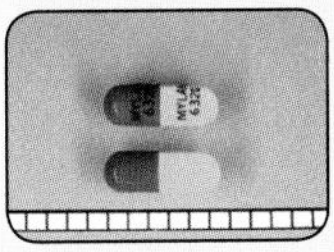
120 mg

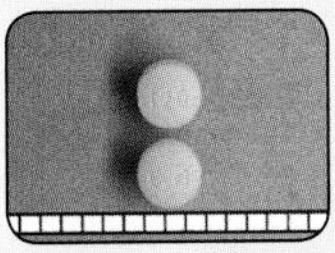
120 mg

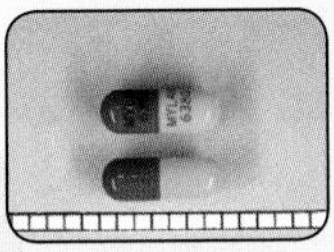
180 mg

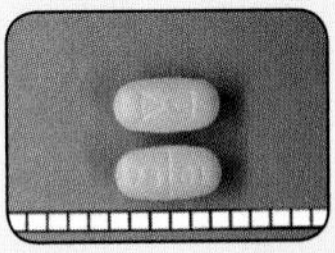
180 mg

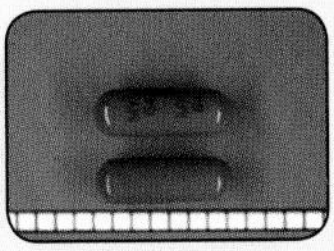
240 mg

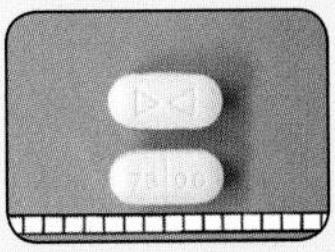
240 mg

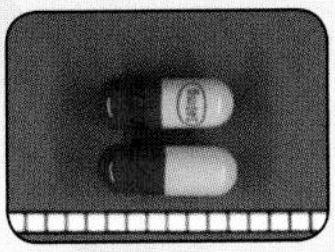
240 mg

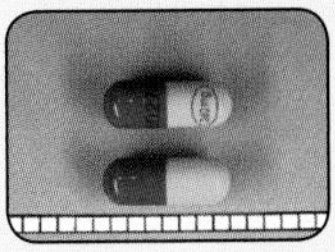
360 mg

Warfarin

(generic)

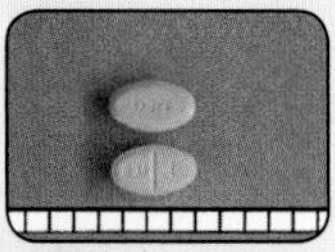

1 mg

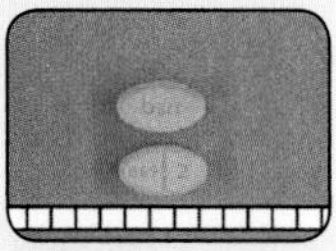

2 mg

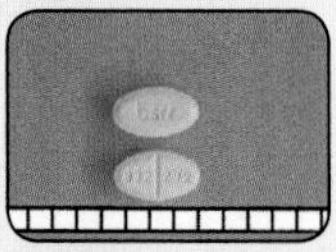

2.5 mg

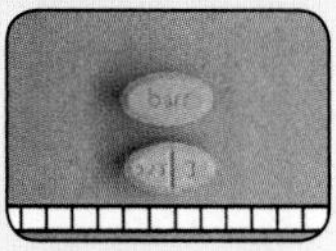

3 mg

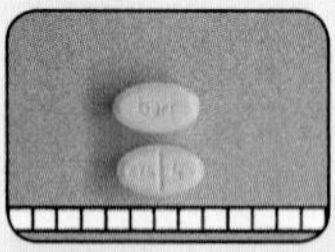

4 mg

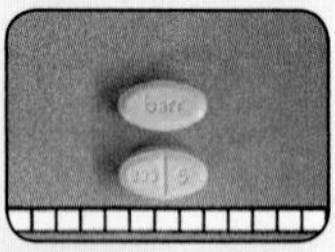

5 mg

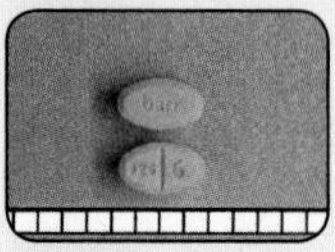

6 mg

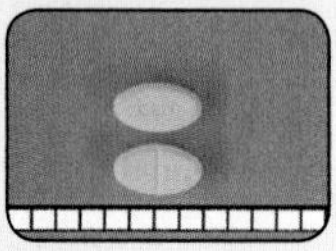

7.5 mg

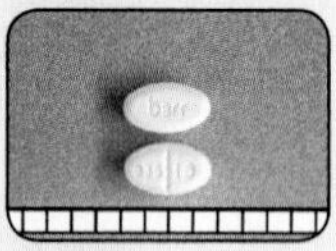

10 mg

Zolpidem

(generic)

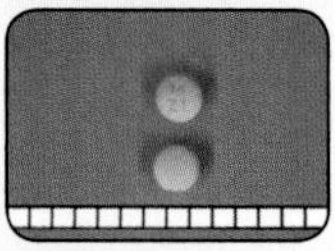

5 mg

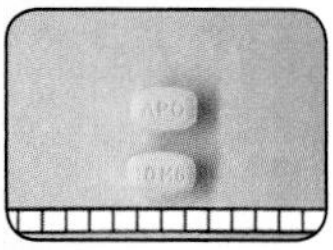

10 mg

Ambien®

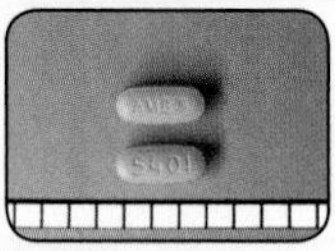

5 mg

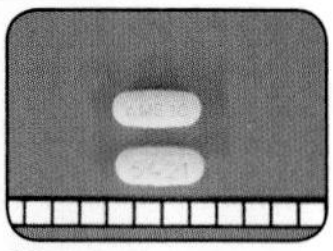

10 mg

Ambien CR

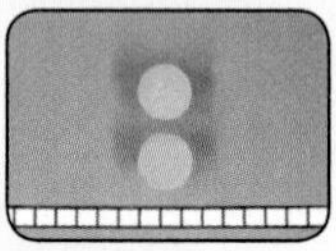

6.25 mg

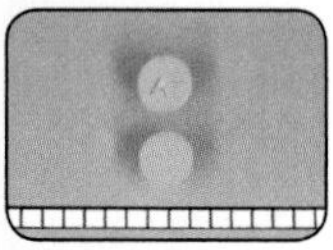

12.5 mg